THE HONOLULU INDEX
OF PLASTIC SURGERY
1971 A.D. to 1976 A.D.

THE McDOWELL INDEXES OF PLASTIC SURGICAL
LITERATURE
Edited By
FRANK McDOWELL, M.D., Sc.D.
Professor of Surgery, University of Hawaii
Professor of Clinical Surgery, Stanford University
Editor-in-Chief, *Plastic and Reconstructive Surgery*

VOLUME V

THE HONOLULU INDEX
OF PLASTIC SURGERY
1971 A.D. to 1976 A.D.

The Williams and Wilkins Co./Baltimore

Copyright ©, 1977
THE WILLIAMS & WILKINS COMPANY
428 E. Preston Street
Baltimore, Md. 21202, U.S.A.

Made in the United States of America

Library of Congress Cataloging in Publication Data

Main entry under title:
The Honolulu index of plastic surgery.

  (The McDowell indexes of plastic surgical literature; v. 5)
  1. Surgery, Plastic—Indexes. I. Series. [DNLM: 1. Surgery, Plastic—Bibliography.
2. Surgery, Plastic—Indexes. ZW0600 M138 v. 5]
Z6667.P5M33 vol. 5 [RD118] 016.617'95'08s
ISBN 0-683-06960-8   [016.617'95]   77-8303

Composed and printed at the
WAVERLY PRESS, INC.
Mt. Royal and Guilford Aves.
Baltimore, Md. 21202, U.S.A.

EDITOR'S FOREWORD

This is the fifth volume of five, which together comprise a nearly total index of the plastic surgical literature of the world from the beginning of time until now. The "McDowell Series" will occupy only 9 inches of space on a desktop, and it should prove an invaluable tool for the practicing surgeon, the surgical researcher, and the surgical teacher.

At first it was planned for the present volume, the Honolulu Index (1971 A.D. to 1976 A.D.), to contain only the items published in the main text of the journal *Plastic and Reconstructive Surgery* (PRS), or in its thousands of abstracts. Later, we decided to incorporate references to all of the other articles and books published on plastic surgical subjects throughout the world between July 1971 and July 1976. Thus, when you see a double reference in one entry, the first one marked "PRS" indicates the abstract while the second indicates the location of the full article.

Volume I of the "McDowell Series" was the Zeis Index, covering the period 900 B.C. to 1863 A.D. It was released in the spring of 1977. Volume II, the Patterson Index (1864 A.D. to 1920 A.D.), is being prepared now and is planned for publication in the fall of 1978. Volume III, the Leuz Index (1921 A.D. to 1946 A.D.), is in press and will be released in the fall of 1977. Volume IV, covering the original articles in PRS and those abstracted in PRS between 1946 and 1971, was released in 1971 as "The 25-Year Index of Plastic and Reconstructive Surgery." Copies are still available from the Williams & Wilkins Co.

This Volume V was compiled, edited, and checked in the Honolulu editorial office of *Plastic and Reconstructive Surgery,* and the staff deserves full credit for this large undertaking. Most of the work was done by Mary McDowell, Barbara Kramer, and Kitty Dabney—with strong assists from Freesia Kaneaiakala, Marie Hayashi, Mary Townsley, and Rena Shephard. For the references not derived from PRS, we relied heavily on the "Ongoing Current Bibliography of Plastic and Reconstructive Surgery," published every two months since 1973 by the National Library of Medicine. We have exercised considerable editorial license in combining subjects, splitting or deleting them, or adding others. In addition, much hand searching of the literature has been done by our staff, including your editor.

We wish to thank the Educational Foundation of ASPRS for sponsoring this series, and the Williams & Wilkins Co. (especially Mr. Dick Hoover and Mr. Robert Och) for help in so many ways during publication.

The plastic surgeon is, almost by definition, an innovator. Each deformity presented to him is different. Furthermore, each patient has a different set of contours, surrounding tissues, and healing tendencies—plus different ideas of how much surgery he wants and what the end result should be. Often, the plastic surgeon must individually design the operation (or series of operations) to meet the specific needs of the patient at hand. For this, in the past he has had to use his own imagination plus information from whatever relevant references he could slowly find by circuitous means. Now, with this index series, he can have instant access and easily obtain an instant focus on mankind's total experience with the problem facing him. That should make all the work that has gone into this series worthwhile!

Frank McDowell, M.D., Sc.D.

Honolulu, Hawaii
April 1977

NOTES ON THE USE OF THIS INDEX

In general, this index follows the format of *Index Medicus* and is easy to use. It is a subject index and author index, not a title index. The subject categories and the authors are interfiled throughout, in alphabetical order.

Within each subject category the individual entries are arranged chronologically. Within each year, the entries are listed alphabetically by journal title. (Articles are listed according to the time and place of their original publication, not according to the time of the abstract.)

In general, the author index carries only the names of the first authors, with the others listed as "*et al.*" In some cases, the second and third authors of articles which appeared originally in PRS have their own entries.

In searching subjects, it may be necessary to examine several categories. For example, to find an article entitled "Skin Grafting the Burned Foot" it may be necessary to look at the entries in the "Skin Grafting," "Burn," and "Foot" categories. The volume is compact enough that this will require but two or three minutes. Extensive cross references would have made it too large and too expensive.

After you have used the index a few times, we believe (and hope) you will become enthusiastic about this simple format. (Perhaps you will never want to fight with a computer again.)

A

AARNES, K.: Results of surgical correction of open bite using Kole's method. Fortschr. Kiefer. Gesichtschir., *18:*217, 1974(German)

AASS, A. S.: Complications to tracheostomy and long-term intubation, follow-up study. Acta Anaesthesiol. Scand., *19:*127, 1975

ABANDO, N. *et al*: Disseminated intravascular coagulation: an increasingly common phenomenon, PRS, *54:*239, 1974. Am. Surgeon, *40:*22, 1974

Abbe Flap: See *Cross-Lip Flap*

ABBES, M. *et al*: Difficult repair of 2 pharyngostomas with modified crosswise flaps. Ann. chir. plast., *16:*247, 1971 (French)

ABBES, M. *et al*: Role of surgery in treatment of lip tumors, 32 cases. J. Fr. Otorhinolaryngol., *21:*640, 1972 (French)

ABBES, M., DEMARD, F., AND AUBANEL, D.: Value of thermography in assessment of skin grafts and flaps, PRS, *55:*642, 1975. Ann chir. plast., *19:*325, 1974

ABBES, M. J. *et al:* Surgical science in France. Greater omentum in repair of complication following surgery and radiotherapy for certain cancers. Int. Surg., *59:*81, 1974

ABBOT, G. H. *et al*: Contoured laminated plastic seat for the treatment of recurrent ischial ulcerations resistant to other seat devices. Am. Correct. Ther. J., *26:*38, 1972

ABBOTT, W. M., AND AUSTEN, W. G.: Microcrystalline collagen as a topical hemostatic agent for vascular surgery, PRS, *54:*629, 1974. Surgery, *75:*925, 1974

ABBUD OCHOA, A. *et al*: Malignant melanoma. Clinico-pathological study of 92 patients in a 20-year period. Prensa Med. Mex., *36:*284, 1971 (German)

ABDEL-FATTAH, A. M. A.: Reappraisal of shaving and skin grafting for hypertrophic burn scars (with Moustafa), PRS, *57:*463, 1976

Abdominal Wall, Defects of

Flaps, repair of large incisional hernias with (Medgyesi), PRS, *51:*486, 1973. Scand. J. Plast. Reconstr. Surg., *6:*69, 1972

Abdominal wall, clostridial myonecrosis of (Eng, Casson, Berman), PRS, *52:*601, 1973. Am. J. Surg., *125:*367, 1973

Hernias, huge midline in scar tissue, repair (Chaimoff, Dintsman), PRS, *53:*110, 1974. Am. J. Surg., *125:*767, 1973

Abdominal wall defects, lyophilized corium grafts for repair (Prpic *et al*), PRS, *54:*700, 1974. Brit. J. Plast. Surg., *26:*35, 1973

Prune belly symdrome, subcellular muscle

Abdominal Wall, Defects of — Cont.

studies in (Mininberg *et al*), PRS, *52:*597, 1973. J. Urol., *109:*524, 1973

Abdominal wall defects, full-thickness, repair of (Mansberger, Kang), PRS, *54:*247, 1974. Am. Surgeon, *40:*117, 1974

Hernias, incisional, Teflon mesh used to repair (Kalsbeek), PRS, *54:*507, 1974. Arch. chir. neerl., *24:*71, 1974

Abdomen, postoperative eventrations, surgical plasty in septic conditions using nets of synthetic material (Hillskamp, Rainone), PRS, *55:*108, 1975. Bol. y trab. Acad. argent. cir., *58:*89, 1974

Abdominal wall defects reconstructed with xenograft corium (Prpic *et al*), PRS, *56:*678, 1975. Brit. J. Plast. Surg., *27:*125, 1974

Abdominal wall, full thickness defects in rats repaired avoiding visceral adhesions (Rayner), PRS, *56:*678, 1975. Brit. J. Plast. Surg., *27:*130, 1974

Abdominal wall, post-excisional defects, repair of (Wilson, Rayner), PRS, *56:*678, 1975. Brit. J. Plast. Surg., *27:*117, 1974

Abdominal wall, lower, neoplasms of, management of extensive, localized. Pubectomy and scrotal skin transfer technique (Skinner). Urology, *3:*34, 1974

Omphalocele and gastroschisis treated with biological dressings (Seashore, MacNaughton, Talbert), PRS, *56:*226, 1975. J. Pediat. Surg., *10:*9, 1975

Flap, groin, lined with dermal graft, to close abdominal hernia (Earle, Blackburn), PRS, *56:*447, 1975

Abdominal wall replacement with plastic mesh in ablative cancer surgery (Karakousis, Elias, Douglass), PRS, *57:*533, 1976. Surgery, *78:*4, 1975

Abdominoplasty

Abdominoplasty, in association with intracavitary surgeries (Franco), PRS, *50:*638, 1972. Rev. Bras. Cir., *61:*5, 1971

Abdominal dermolipectomy, geometrical planning for (Serson), PRS, *48:*605, 1971. Rev. espan. cir. plast., *4:*37, 1971

Panniculectomy, abdominal, after massive weight loss (Kamper, Galloway, Ashley), PRS, *50:*441, 1972

Plastic operations for pendulous abdomen in obese subjects (Szczawinski *et al*). Pol. Med. J., *11:*922, 1972

Abdomen, pendulous, plastic surgery in (Chachava *et al*). Vestn. Khir., *107:*89, 1972 (Russian)

Abdomen, upper, technic for surgical ap-

Abdominoplasty—Cont.

proach to, by use of esthetic incision (Del Soldato). Acta Gastroenterol. Latinoam., *5:*19, 1973. (Spanish)

Massive abdominal panniculectomy (Meyerowitz *et al).* J. A. M. A., *225:*408, 1973

Abdominoplasty, vertical (Fischl), PRS, *51:*139, 1973

Abdominoplasty (Grazer), PRS, *51:*617, 1973

Abdominoplasty: physiorespiratory, surgical, esthetic problems (Bellero *et al*), PRS, *56:*356, 1975. Riv. ital. chir. plast., *5:*417, 1973

Lipectomy, abdominal, added to laparocele treatment, advantages of (Guida, Picchi, Inzirillo), PRS, *56:*465, 1975. Riv. ital. chir. plast., *5:*445, 1973

Abdominal dermolipectomies, complications following (Francesconi *et al),* PRS, *56:*355, 1975. Riv. ital. chir. plast., *5:*455, 1973

Abdominoplasty (Cerveny), PRS, *55:*637, 1975. Acta chir. plast., *16:*178, 1974

Abdominal plastic surgery. "Horseshoe" technic (Elbaz). Ann. chir. plast., *19:*155, 1974 (French)

Abdominal fat, technique of excision of (Schwartz). Br. J. Plast. Surg., *27:*44, 1974

Panniculectomy following intestinal bypass (McCabe *et al*). Brit. J. Plast. Surg., *27:*346, 1974

Removal of panniculus adiposus (Drew). J. A. M. A., *229:*391, 1974

Abdomen, pendulous, surgical technic for treatment of, complicated by suprapubic eventration (Interlandi). Minerva Chir., *29:*208, 1974

Abdomen: surgical rehabilitation after massive weight reduction (McCraw), PRS, *53:*349, 1974

Abdominoplasty (Baroudi, Keppke, Netto), PRS, *54:*161, 1974

Dermolipectomy, anterolateral low, reconstruction of umbilicus in (Spadafora, Durand), PRS, *55:*509, 1975. Proc. 2nd Argent. Cong. Aesth. Surg., 66, 1974

Abdominal plastic surgery (Koechlin). Rev. Med. Suisse Romande., *94:*981, 1974 (French)

Adiposis, nosography of lipomatosis and lipodystrophy in light of present criticism (Lupo *et al),* PRS, *57:*683, 1976. Riv. ital. chir. plast., *6:*135, 1974

From massive weight loss to abdominal panniculectomy (Meyerowitz *et al).* R. N., *37:*1, 1974

Abdomen, massive, resection of (Hagerty *et al),* PRS, *55:*108, 1975. South. M. J., *67:*984, 1974

Abdominoplasty—Cont.

Difficulties of surgical treatment of abdominal dermodystrophies (Glicenstein). Ann. chir. plast., *20:*147, 1975 (French)

Note of surgical technic. The technic called "in a setting sun" in abdominal dermodystrophies (Vilain). Ann. chir. plast., *20:*239, 1975

Umbilicus, reconstruction of (Borges). Brit. J. Plast. Surg., *28:*75, 1975

Abdominal lipectomy (Pitanguy). Clin. Plast. Surg., *2:*401, 1975

Abdominal dermolipectomies (Regnault). Clin. Plast. Surg., *2:*411, 1975

Umbilicaplasty (Baroudi). Clin. Plast. Surg., *2:*431, 1975

Massive weight loss patient (Zook). Clin. Plast. Surg., *2:*457, 1975

Some considerations in surgical alteration of feminine silhouette (Vilain). Clin. Plast. Surg., *2:*467, 1975

Plastic surgery in treatment of obesity (Muhlbauer). Munch. Med. Wochenschr., *117:*747, 1975

Abdominoplasty by W technique (Regnault), PRS, *55:*265, 1975

Abdominal lipectomy: introduction of breast implants through abdominal route (Planas), PRS, *57:*434, 1976

ABE, S., AND NAGAI, Y.: Synovial collagenase – regulation and metabolism of enzyme activity and significance in pathogenesis of rheumatoid arthritis, PRS, *53:*114, 1974. Asian M. J., *16:*155, 1973

ABERDEEN, E. *et al*: Artificial airways in children. Surg. Clin. North Am., *54:*1155, 1974

ABLE, L. W.: Correction of hypospadias in infants. Tex. Med., *68:*97, 1972

ABLIN, R. J.: Autoallergy in burns (Letter to the Editor), PRS, *48:*170, 1971

ABOUCAYA, W. A.: The smile. Classification and criteria, applications in facial esthetics. Acad. Rev., *2:*2611, 1973

ABRAHAM, A. J.: Total reconstruction of upper and lower eyelids after loss of lids and globe, PRS, *48:*374, 1971

ABRAHAM, A. J.: Case of carbolic acid gangrene of the thumb. Br. J. Plast. Surg., *25:*282, 1972

ABRAHAM, E. A. *et al*: Whirlpool therapy in treating soft tissue wounds complicating fracture of extremities, PRS, *55:*720, 1975. Orthop. Rev., *4:*47, 1975

ABRAHAM, J. C., JABALEY, M. E., AND HOOPES, J. E.: Basal cell carcinoma of medial canthal region, PRS, *53:*688, 1974. Am. J. Surg., *126:*492, 1973

ABRAHAMS, J. I. *et al*: Treatment of urethral

stricture by free full-thickness skin graft (Devine) urethroplasty. Urology, *1:*93, 1973

ABRAHAMS, P. H.: Earlobe Z-plasty in Borneo, PRS, *53:*548, 1974

ABRAMCZYK, B.: Surgery for lop ears. Otolaryngol. Pol., *28:*307, 1974 (Polish)

ABRAMS, J. S., DEANE, R. S., AND DAVIS, J. H.: Adverse effects of salt and water retention on pulmonary function in patients with multiple trauma, PRS, *53:*500, 1974. J. Trauma, *13:*788, 1973

ABRAMSON, A. L.: Tracheotomy tube for management of enlarged neck. Trans. Am. Acad. Ophthalmol. Otolaryngol., *76:*1010, 1972

ABRAMSON, D. I. *et al:* Effect of repeated period of ischemia on sensory and motor latencies of median nerve in the hand at different temperatures. Arch. Phys. Med. Rehabil., *52:*455, 1971

ABRAMSON, M.: Treatment of parotid duct injuries. Laryngoscope, *83:*1764, 1973

ABREU, C. L.: Nasal deformities caused by inadequate posture during sleep, PRS, *51:*475, 1973. Rev. brasil. clin. terapeut., *1:*633, 1972

ABREU, C. DE L.: Wrinkles. Etiopathogenetic theory. Rev. Paul Med., *78:*93, 1971

ABROL, B. M., KAPUR, B. M., AND RAVEENDRAN, M.: Penetrating neck injury (unusual automobile accident). J. Laryng. & Otol., *86:*1253, 1972

ABSTON, S. *et al:* Gentamicin for septicemia in patients with burns. J. Infect. Dis., *124:*275, 1971, Suppl.

ABU-DALU, J. *et al:* Prophylactic regional lymph node excision in malignant melanoma. Harefuah, *80:*129, 1971 (Hebrew)

ACHACH, P. C.: Correction of swan-neck deformities and rosette deformities in the rheumatoid hand. Rev. Chir. Orthop., *58:*461, 1972 (French)

ACHARYYA, S. K.: Maxillofacial injuries in war, PRS, *56:*225, 1975. Indian J. Surg., *36:*392, 1974

ACHATZY, R.: Long-acting conduction anesthesia in surgery of the hand. Handchirurgie, *3:*119, 1971 (German)

ACHAUER, B. M.: Growth of homotransplanted ear cartilage in baby rabbits (with Allison, Furnas), PRS, *55:*479, 1975

ACHAUER, B. M. *et al:* Internal fixation in management of burned hand, PRS, *55:*112, 1975. Arch. Surg., *108:*814, 1974

ACKERMANNN, A. *et al:* Therapy of maxillofacial injuries, II. Magy. Traumatol. Orthop., *15:*69, 1972 (Hungarian)

ACLAND, R.: Signs of patency in small vessel anastomosis, PRS, *52:*325, 1973. Surgery, *72:*744, 1972

ACLAND, R.: Thrombus formation in microvascular surgery, experimental study of effects of surgical trauma, PRS, *52:*454, 1973. Surgery, *73:*766, 1973

ACLAND, R. D.: Does topical use of magnesium sulfate improve results in microvascular anastomoses? (Letter to the Editor), PRS, *56:*440, 1975

Acne Scars

Acne keloidalis (Cosman, Wolff), PRS, *50:*25, 1972

Acne conglobata of face, surgical treatment (Stellmach), PRS, *56:*471, 1975. J. Maxillofacial Surg., *3:*58, 1975

ACOSTA DE ALMEIDA, D. *et al:* Negroid nose. Int. Surg., *60:*554, 1975

Acrocephalosyndactylia: See *Craniofacial Surgery*

Actinomycosis

Disseminated actinomycosis with cutaneous and osseous foci (Godeau *et al*). Ann. Med. Interne (Paris), *122:*1129, 1971 (French)

Cervico-facial actinomycosis: a current disease? Apropos of 2 cases (Bonhomme *et al*). Ann. Otolaryngol. Chir. Cervicofac., *88:*350, 1972 (French)

Actinomycosis of the temporomandibular joint (Bradley). Brit. J. Oral Surg., *9:*54, 1971

Cervicofacial pseudo-actinomycoses caused by corynebacteriae (Junien-Lavillauroy *et al*). J. Fr. Otorhinolaryngol., *20:*1115, 1971 (French)

Actinomycosis of the parotid gland (Kowalska-Kulesza). Otolaryngol. Pol., *25:*455, 1971 (Polish)

Actinomycosis of the zygomaticotemporal region and the study of its infectious route (Funasaka *et al.*). Otolaryngology (Tokyo), *43:*923, 1971 (Japanese)

A case of combined lesions of the cervical lymph nodes from actinomycosis and tuberculosis (Pliner *et al*). Probl. Tuberk., *49:*78, 1971 (Russian)

Actinomycosis of the breast (Gogas *et al*). Int. Surg., *57:*664, 1972

Actinomycosis of the maxilla: review of literature and report of case (Goldstein *et al*). J. Oral Surg., *30:*362, 1972

Actinomycosis of the tongue (Uhler *et al*). Oral Surg., *34:*199, 1972

Facial actinomycosis (Stricker *et al*). Rev. Stomatol. Chir. Maxillofac., *73:*495, 1972 (French)

Actinomycosis—Cont.

Peculiarities in the clinical picture, diagnosis and treatment of actinomycosis of the jaws (Kuz'menko). Stomatologiia (Mosk.), *51:*77, 1972 (Russian)

Cervicofacial actinomycosis (Hartley, Schatten), PRS, *51:*44, 1973

Osteomyelitis of jaws, low grade, with actinomycosis (Stenhouse, MacDonald), PRS, *55:*508, 1975. Internat. J. Oral Surg., *3:*64, 1974

Actinomycosis of bone (Wilding *et al*). Aust. N. Z. J. Surg., *45:*61, 1975

Mandibular actinomycosis: report of case (Silbermann *et al*). J. Am. Dent. Assoc., *90:*162, 1975

Intraoral actinomycosis. Report of five cases (Stenhouse). Oral Surg., *39:*547, 1975

Acupuncture

China today, medicine and acupuncture anesthesia in (Capperauld), PRS, *51:*488, 1973. Surg. Gynec. & Obst., *135:*440, 1972

Acupuncture anesthesia, report of two cases (Ho *et al*). Am. J. Chin. Med., *1:*151, 1973

Acupuncture anesthesia, experience with, in cosmetic plastic surgery (Franklyn). Am. J. Chin. Med., *2:*345, 1974

Acupuncture in China (Wang), PRS, *54:*249, 1974. Anesth. & Analg., *53:*111, 1974

Acupuncture, western world's first detailed treatise: William Ten Rhijne's *De Acupunctura*. (Carrubba, Bowers), PRS, *55:*727, 1975. J. Hist. Med. & Allied Sc., *29:*371, 1974

Acupuncture and American doctor in China (Greentree), PRS, *56:*366, 1975. Surg. Gynec. & Obst., *139:*604, 1974

Acupuncture compared with 33 percent nitrous oxide for dental analgesia (Chapman, Gehrig, Wilson), PRS *56:*605, 1975. Anesthesiology, *42:*532, 1975

Acupuncture anesthesia (Shanghai Acupuncture Group), PRS, *56:*602, 1975. Chinese M. J., *1:*13, 1975

Syndrome, cervical, treatment by acupuncture (Laitinen), PRS, *57:*768, 1976. Scand. J. Rehab. Med., *7:*114, 1975

ADAMCZAK, T. *et al*: Evaluation of skin grafts subjected to bath hypotonic solutions. Pol. Przegl. Chir., *46:*509, 1974 (Polish)

ADAMS, A. P. *et al*: General anesthesia in adults. Int. Ophthalmol. Clin., *13:*83, 1973

ADAMSON, J. E.: Treatment of the stiff hand. Orthop. Clin. North Am., *1:*467, 1970

Adamson, J. E.: Comparative study of tendon

suture material in dogs (with Sruji), PRS, *50:*31, 1972

ADAMSON, J. E.: Studies on the action of dimethyl sulfoxide on the experimental pedicle flap (Follow-Up Clinic), PRS, *51:*88, 1972

ADAMSON, J. E.: Sensory rehabilitation of the injured thumb (Follow-Up Clinic), PRS, *52:*432, 1973

ADAMSON, J. E.: Acute submucous resection (Follow-Up Clinic), PRS, *52:*432, 1973

ADAMSON, J. E.: Five-year history of the American Society of Plastic and Reconstructive Surgeons, 1969–1973, PRS, *55:*445, 1975

ADAMUS, J.: Lymphographic observations following surgery of cervical lymphatic system. Otolaryngol. Pol., *27:*451, 1973 (Polish)

ADAMUS, J. *et al*: Cryosurgery in treatment of skin neoplasms. Pol. Tyg. Lek., *28:*440, 1973 (Polish)

ADAMUS, J. *et al*: Cryosurgery in treatment of oral neoplasms. Otolaryngol. Pol., *28:*41, 1974 (Polish)

ADAR, K. K. *et al*: Herpes simplex virus in idiopathic facial paralysis, PRS, *57:*400, 1976. J.A.M.A., *233:*527, 1975

ADDUCCI, J. F.: Amnion graft. Young helping aged. Minn. Med., *57:*626, 1974

ADELAAR, R. S., SOUCACOS, P. N., AND URBANIAK, J. R.: Autologous cortical bone grafts with microsurgical anastomosis of periosteal vessels, PRS, *57:*766, 1976. Surg. Forum, *25:*487, 1974

ADELL, R. *et al*: Intra-osseous anchorage of dental prostheses. II. Review of clinical approaches, PRS, *49:*102, 1972. Scand. J. Plast. Reconstr. Surg., *4:*19, 1970

ADELSON, H.: Prognathism—orthodontic and surgical management. N. Y. State Dent. J., *39:*477, 1973

ADERHOLD, M.: Lunate malacia, treatment by prosthesis, PRS, *53:*107, 1974. Chir. Praxis, *16:*81, 1972

ADHIA, G. D., AND ADHIA, R. G.: Photography of operative field—simple device, PRS, *54:*119, 1974. Indian J. Surg., *35:*593, 1973

ADKINS, K. F.: Lymphoid hyperplasia in oral mucosa. Aust. Dent. J., *18:*38, 1973

ADLER, C. I. *et al*: Metastatic bronchogenic carcinoma to maxilla: case report. J. Oral Surg., *31:*543, 1973

ADLER, H.: Tension strap osteosynthesis in unstable fractures of the metacarpal head. Monatsschr. Unfallheilkd., *72:*297, 1969 (German)

ADOUR, K. K.: Editorial: The bell tolls for decompression? N. Engl. J. Med., *292:*748, 1975

ADOUR, K. K., AND WINGERD, J.: Nonepidemic incidence of idiopathic facial paralysis, PRS,

*54:*239, 1974. J.A.M.A., *227:*653, 1974

ADUSS, H.: Craniofacial growth in complete unilateral cleft lip and palate. Angle. Orthod., *41:*202, 1971

AFANASSIEFF, A. *et al*: Results of 44 Cialit-preserved nerve homografts. Ann. chir. plast., *16:*284, 1971 (French)

AFRAPETIAN, M. KH.: Diagnosis and treatment of neurogenic tumors of the neck. Khirurgiia (Mosk.), *47:*53, 1971 (Russian)

AFSHIN, H., AND SHARMIN, R.; Hemangioma involving maxillary sinus, PRS, *56:*224, 1975. Oral Surg., *38:*204, 1974

AFTAB, M. *et al*: Basal cell carcinoma of conjunctiva. Brit. J. Ophthalmol., *57:*836, 1973

AGAZZI, C.: Treatment of lymphatic involvement in cancer of larynx and hypopharynx. Acta Otorhinolaryngol. Belg., *27:*1041, 1973 (French)

AGEEB, M. *et al*: Use of "Trasicor" in preventing rejection of allografts, PRS, *52:*463, 1973. Kasr el Fini J. Surg., *12:*10, 1971

AGERBERG, G. *et al*: Changes in the temporomandibular joint after surgical treatment. A radiologic follow-up study. Oral Surg., *32:*865, 1971

AGGARWAL, J. L.: Imperforate puncta with blocked nasolacrimal duct. Brit. J. Ophthalmol., *56:*788, 1972

AGGARWAL, S. B.: Off-midline forehead flap for the repair of small nasal defects (with Dhawan, Hariharan) PRS, *53:*537, 1974

AGOSTON, B.: Case of extensive globulomaxillary cyst. Fogorv. Sz., *65:*299, 1972 (Hungarian)

AGRIS, J., DINGMAN, R. O., AND WILENSKY, R. J.: Dissector for transaxillary approach in augmentation mammaplasty, PRS, *57:*10, 1976

AGUIRRE, J. A. O.: Skin grafts and rejection phenomenon, PRS, *52:*329, 1973. Rev. Latino Am. cir. plast., *14:*17, 1970

AGUIRRE, M. R., AND ENRIQUEZ DE SALAMANCA, F.: Method of probits in study of mortality from burns, PRS, *53:*493, 1974. Riv. ital. chir. plast., *4:*11, 1973

AHNEFELD, F. W.: General care of severe burns, PRS, *50:*204, 1972. Langenbecks Arch. Chir., *329:*900, 1971

AHSTROM, J. P., JR.: Treatment of established Volkmann's ischemic contracture of the forearm and hand. Curr. Pract. Orthop. Surg., *6:*213, 1975

AIACH, G.: Prevention of recurrence after Lefort I superior maxillary osteotomies for harelip. Rev. Stomatol. Chir. Maxillofac., *74:*327, 1973

AIACH, G.: Rhinoplasty and maxillary osteoto-

mies. Rev. Stomatol. Chir. Maxillofac., *75:*159, 1974 (French)

AIACHE, A.: Preservation of traumatically amputated fingertips (with Weiner, Silver), PRS, *49:*609, 1972

AIACHE, A. E.: Mammaplasty: technique for ptotic and moderately enlarged breast, PRS, *56:*677, 1975. Brit. J. Plast. Surg., *27:*318, 1974

AIACHE, A.E.: New soft, round, silicone gel breast implant (with Weiner, Silver), PRS, *53:*174, 1974

AIACHE, A. E., AND CHEN, M. T.: Reconstruction of a traumatic subtotal ear loss with two skin tubes. PRS, *49:*86, 1972. Letter to the Editor, PRS, *49:*332, 1972

AIACHE, A. E., AND DELAGI, E. F.: Pure sign of lumbrical function, PRS, *54:*312, 1974

AKERS, W. A., AND SULZBERGER, M. B.: Friction blister, PRS, *50:*98, 1972. Mil. Med., *137:*1, 1972

AKERSON, H. *et al*: Epidermoid cyst of tongue, case report. J. Oral Surg., *32:*117, 1974

AKHABADZE, A. F.: Cosmetology – one of the forms of specialized medical aid to the population. Sov. Med., *35:*122, 1972 (Russian)

AKIN, R. K. *et al*: Experience with intraoral vertical subcondylar osteotomy. J. Oral Surg., *33:*324, 1975

AKIN, R. K., KRELLER, A. J., III, AND WALTERS, P. J.: Sjögren's syndrome, PRS, *56:*462, 1975. Oral Surg., *33:*27, 1975

AKIN, R. K. *et al*: Paget's disease of bone. Report of a case. Oral Surg., *39:* 707, 1975

AKINOSI, J. O.: Multiple sublingual dermoid cysts. Brit. J. Oral Surg., *12:*235, 1974

AKINOSO, H. O. *et al*: Retrosternal parathyroid adenomas manifesting in the form of a giant-cell "tumor" of the mandible. Oral Surg., *39:*724, 1975

AKINYEMI, O. O.: Ankylosis of mandible from *cancrum oris* (with Oluwasanmi, Lagundoye), PRS, *57:*342, 1976

AKL, B. F. *et al*: Late assessment of results of cricopharyngeal myotomy for cervical dysphagia. Am. J. Surg., *128:*818, 1974

ALACH, G.: Use of extra-mucosal dissection in the treatment of certain vestibular stenoses. Ann. chir. plast., *19:*273, 1974 (French)

ALACH, G.: Modifications of the upper lip after rhinoplasty. Rev. Stomatol. Chir. Maxillofac., *75:*1119, 1974 (French)

ALAJMO, E.: Disease course and later results in malignant maxillary tumors. Monatsschr. Ohrenheilkd. Laryngorhinol., *106:*398, 1972 (German)

ALANI, H.: Reconstruction of mammary hypoplasia associated with chest wall deformities (with Hawtof, Ram), PRS, *57:*172, 1976

ALANIS, J., AND GUERRA, J.: Lymphosarcoma of maxillary antrum, PRS, *55:*117, 1975. Rev. Mex. Radiol., *28:*85, 1974

ALARCON-SEGOVIA, D., VELAZQUEZ-FORERO, F., AND GONZALEZ-JIMENEZ, Y.: Sjögren's syndrome in systemic *lupus erythematosus,* PRS, *56:*237, 1975. Ann. Int. Med., *81:*577, 1974

ALBANO, A. M. *et al*: New method for the fixation of the median palpebral ligament. Rev. Assoc. Med. Bras., *21:*291, 1975 (Portuguese)

ALBERS, S. W. *et al*: Eosinophilic granuloma of mandible. J. Oral Surg., *31:*841, 1973

ALBERT, P. S. *et al*: Fracture of Pearman penile implant. Urology, *3:*502, 1974

ALBERTENGO, A. G.: Burns in children: topical treatment. An. cir. (Rosario), *35:*42, 1970 (Spanish)

ALBERTENGO, A. G., AND ABRIATA, A. A.: Subcutaneous pedicled flaps in facial surgery, PRS, *51:*710, 1973. An. cir., *37:*20, 1972

ALBERTH, B.: Total upper lid substitute. Klin. Monatsbl. Augenheilkd., *165:*84, 1974 (German)

ALBERTSEN, J.: Aures alatae. A follow-up study of 104 patients operated on using Nordzell's method. Ugeskr. Laeger., *133:*2419, 1971 (Danish)

ALBIN, R. E.: Delayed volar advancement flap for thumb tip injuries (with Millender, Nalebuff), PRS, *52:*635, 1973

ALBOROVA, V. K. *et al*: Use of optic quantum generators (Lasers) for experimental removal of tattooing. Vestn. Dermatol. Venerol., *47:*35, 1973 (Russian)

ALBRECHT, K. F. *et al*: Surgical treatment of hypospadias and epispadias. Chirurg., *46:*503, 1975 (German)

ALBRECHTSEN, D.: Circulatory arrest following administration of succinylcholine in patients with extensive tissue damage. Tidsskr. nor. laegeforen., *93:*676, 1973 (Norwegian)

ALBRECHTSEN, R. *et al*: Extracardiac rhabdomyoma. Light and electron microscopic studies of two cases in the mandibular area, with a review of previous reports. Acta Otolaryngol. (Stockh.), *78:*458, 1974

ALBRIGHT, J. E. *et al*: Cementifying fibroma of mandible, case report. J. Oral Surg., *32:*294, 1974

ALCOCER ANDALON, A. *et al*: Transpositon of the greater epiplon in lymphedema caused by chronic venous insufficiency. Arch. Inst. Cardiol. Mex., *42:*444, 1972 (Spanish)

ALDASORO, G. E.: Surgical treatment of livedo reticularis. Int. Surg., *60:*44, 1975

ALDAY, E. S., AND GOLDSMITH, H. S.: Surgical

technique for omental lengthening based on arterial anatomy, PRS, *51:*354, 1973. Surg. Gynec. & Obst., *135:*103, 1972

ALEEM, A. A.: Diphallia: report of case, PRS, *51:*232, 1973. J. Urol., *108:*357, 1972

ALEKSANDROV, N. M. *et al*: Characteristics of anesthesiological care in certain operations of neck. Klin. Khir., *10:*23, 1974 (Russian)

ALEKSANDROV, N. M. *et al*: Anesthesia and resuscitation in operations for diseases and injuries of the tongue, and the floor of the mouth. Vestn. Khir., *112:*88, 1974 (Russian)

ALEKSANDROV, N. M. *et al*: Experience with anesthesia in the surgical treatment of maxillofacial and dental deformities. Stomatologiia (Mosk.), *54:*30, 1975 (Russian)

ALEKSANDROVA, D. I.: Treatment of patients having undergone surgery for venous lymphatic diseases of the limbs at the Sochi-Matsesta resort. Sov. Med., *35:*137, 1972 (Russian)

ALEXANDER, J. E.: Challenges in esthetic plastic surgery, PRS, *52:*337, 1973

ALEXANDER, J. M.: Alloplastic augmentation of middle-third facial deformities. J. Oral Surg., *34:*165, 1976

ALEXANDER, J. W.: Control of infection following burn injury, PRS, *49:*666, 1972. Arch. Surg., *103:*435, 1971

ALEXANDER, J. W., FISHER, M. W., AND MACMILLAN, B. G.: Immunological control of *Pseudomonas* infection in burn patients, PRS, *48:*90, 1971. Arch. Surg., *102:*31, 1971

ALEXANDER, J. W., SYKES, N. S., AND WHEELER, L. M.: Control of surface infection with antibiotic-impregnated Epigard, PRS, *52:*329, 1973. Surg. Forum, *23:*36, 1972

ALEXANDER, J. W. *et al*: Clinical evaluation of Epigard, new synthetic substitute for homograft and heterograft skin, PRS, *53:*500, 1974. J. Trauma, *13:*374, 1973

ALEXANDER, R. W. *et al*: Central mucoepidermoid tumor (carcinoma) of mandible. J. Oral Surg., *32:*541, 1974

ALEXANDER, R. W. *et al*: Postauricular approach for surgery of temporomandibular articulation. J. Oral Surg., *33:*346, 1975

ALFIERI, V.: Collins hand for arm amputees. Minerva Ortop., *21:*47, 1970 (Italian)

ALGVERE, P. *et al*: Pterional orbital decompression in progressive ophthalmopathy of Graves' disease 1. Short-term effects. Acta Ophthalmol. (Kbh.), *51:*461, 1973

ALGVERE, P. *et al*: Pterional orbital decompression in progressive ophthalmopathy of Graves' disease 2. Follow-up study. Acta Ophthalmol. (Kbh.), *51:*475, 1973

ALICHNEIWICZ, A. *et al*: Radical operation of

fibrous dysplasia of mandible with simultaneous reparative operation. Czas. Stomatol., 27:13, 1974 (Czechoslovakian)

ALIGA, A. *et al*: Proceedings: Giant proliferating epidermoid cyst. Ann. Dermatol. Syphilligr. (Paris), 102:409, 1975

ALLAN, J. C.: Micro-circulation of the skin of the normal leg, in varicose veins and in the post-thrombotic syndrome. S. Afr. J. Surg., 10:29, 1972

ALLAN, J. H. *et al*: Osteochondroma of mandible. Oral Surg., 37:556, 1974

ALLARDYCE, D. B.: Adverse effect of heparin in experimental fat embolism, PRS, 49:670, 1972. Surg. Forum, 22:203, 1971

ALLEN, A. M. *et al*: Skin infections in Vietnam, PRS, 52:103, 1973. Mil. Med., 137:295, 1972

ALLEN, H. E. *et al*: Skin dressings in treatment of contaminated wounds, PRS, 53:110, 1974. Am. J. Surg., 126:45, 1973

ALLEN, H. M. *et al*: Localization of deep abscesses with radioactive isotopes, PRS, 56:367, 1975. Henry Ford Hosp. M. J., 21:111, 1973

ALLEN, J. A. *et al*: Sweat responses of a hyperhidrotic subject. Brit. J. Dermatol., 90:277, 1974

ALLEN, M. S., JR. *et al*: Low-grade papillary adenocarcinoma of palate. Cancer, 33:153, 1974

ALLEN, S. D., JR., AND WILKERSON, J. L.: Importance of glucose-6-phosphate dehydrogenase screening in urologic practice, PRS, 50:539, 1972. J. Urol., 107:304, 1972

ALLEN, T. D., SPENCE, H. M., AND SALYER, K. E.: Reconstruction of external genitalia in exstrophy of bladder, PRS, 57:536, 1976. J. Urol., 111:830, 1974

ALLEN, T. H.: Subcutaneous mammectomy, new hope for benign breast disease. J. Arkansas Med. Soc., 69:153, 1972

ALLENDE, M. F.: Cryosurgery in basal cell carcinomas, PRS, 57:264, 1976. Med. Cut., 1:55, 1973

ALLGOWER, M.: Surgery and life-preservation. Praxis, 61:1255, 1972 (German)

ALLGOWER, M. *et al*: Burn toxin in mouse skin, PRS, 53:686, 1974. J. Trauma, 13:95, 1973

ALLIEU, Y.: Ulnar deviation. Arthroplasty of the matacarpophalangeal articulations. Rev. Chir. Orthop., 58:452, 1972 (French)

ALLIEU, Y.: Therapeutic deductions. Rev. Rhum. Mal. Osteoartic., 40:203, 1973 (French)

ALLIEU, Y.: Deformities of the fingers and thumb: surgical possibilities. Rev. Rhum. Mal. Osteoartic., 40:215, 1973 (French)

ALLIEU, Y. *et al*: Use of Jenning's barb wire in

tendon sutures. Absence of postoperative immobilization. Ann. Chir., 25:987, 1971 (French)

ALLIEU, Y. *et al:* Is there still a place for plastic and reconstructive surgery in treatment of open leg fractures? Ann. chir. plast., 17: 212, 1972 (French)

ALLIEU, Y. *et al*: Use of an external tutor in hand surgery. Acta Orthop. Belg., 39:988, 1973 (French)

ALLIEU, Y. *et al*: Valve of an external fixation device in the treatment of osteoarticular infections of the hand and fingers. Ann. Chir., 28:271, 1974 (French)

ALLIEU, Y. *et al*: Arthroplasties of metacarpophalangeal joints with Swanson implants in the rheumatic hand. Critical appraisal of results. Ann. Chir., 28:873, 1974 (French)

ALLING, C. C. *et al*: Synovial chondromatosis of temporomandibular joint. J. Oral Surg., 31:691, 1973

ALLING, C. C. *et al*: Compound, comminuted, complex maxillofacial fractures. J. Oral Surg., 32:415, 1974

ALLISON, G. R., ACHAUER, B. M., AND FURNAS, D. W.: Growth of homotransplanted ear cartilage in baby rabbits, PRS, 55:479, 1975

ALLISON, S. C. *et al*: Giant conjunctival cyst of orbit. Ann. Ophth., 5:199, 1973

ALMEIDA-GONZALVEZ, J. C., AND NORONHA, T.: Treatment of keratoses and cutaneous tumors with five percent 5-Fluorouracil, PRS, 52:599, 1973. Trab. Soc. Port. derm. ven., 18:83, 1970

ALMENDRAL LUCAS, J., AND MARTIN LABORDA, F.: Congenital shortness of urethra, PRS, 53:244, 1974. Rev. espań. cir., plast., 5:201, 1972

ALMEYDA, J., AND MANTELL, B.: Metastasizing basal cell carcinoma, PRS, 48:609, 1971. Proc. Roy. Soc. Med., 64:611, 1971

ALONSO, M. R. *et al*: Reconstruction of mandible. Otolaryngol. Clin. North Am., 5:501, 1972

ALONSO, M. R. *et al*: Minibikes, new factor in laryngotracheal trauma. Ann. Otol. Rhin. & Laryng., 82:800, 1973

Alopecia (See also *Hair, Free Flaps*)

Hair transplants in accidental baldness (Purita). Hospital (Rio de J.), 77:1303, 1970 (Portuguese)

Surgical possibilities in the treatment of baldness (Fevrier). Bord. Med., 4:3255, 1971 (French)

Alopecia, congenital universal (Podoswa, Laguna, Armendares), PRS, 57:267, 1976. Dermat. Ibero Lat. Am., 13:223, 1971

Alopecia—Cont.

Hair transplant (Smith). Arch. Otolaryng., *96:*227, 1972

Alopecia, cicatricial, narrow transposition flaps for reconstruction of (Hirata), PRS, *51:*602, 1973. Jap. J. Plast. Reconstr. Surg., *15:*292, 1972

Hair autografts (Editorial). Lancet, *2:*417, 1972

Hair transplantation (Orentreich). N. Y. State J. Med., *72:*578, 1972

Seborrheic alopecia. Surgical treatment by ligature of the scalp arteries (Marechal). Nouv. Presse Med., *1:*257, 1972 (French)

Hair transplants for male pattern baldness (Farber, Burks, Salinger), PRS, *51:*475, 1973. South. M. J., *65:*1380, 1972

Hairgrafting (Pirotta). Australas. J. Dermatol., *14:*121, 1973

Hair transplants in burn scars and other alopecias (Savin). Conn. Med., *37:*501, 1973

"Surgery of baldness." Therapeutic measure that cannot be patented (Muller). Hautarzt, *24:*130, 1973

Hair transplantation, treatment of baldness by (Auerbach, Pearlstein). J. M. Soc. New Jersey, *70:*119, 1973

Alopecia, transplantation of multiple skin flaps of haired part of head in (Kirpatovskii *et al*). Khirurgiia (Mosk.), *49:*112, 1973 (Russian)

Grafts, punch, combined with overlay sheet of split-skin graft for raw area in scalp (Hight, Anderton), PRS, *52:*663, 1973

Transplants, hair, for baldness (Cohen). South African M. J., *47:*3, 1973

Hair Transplant Surgery. By O'Tar T. Norwood. Charles C Thomas, Springfield, Ill., 1974. PRS, *54:*349, 1974

Alopecia, surgical correction of (Ditroi), PRS, *55:*632, 1975. Acta chir. plast., *16:*98, 1974

Frontal hairline in treatment of male pattern baldness (Mahe, Camblin), PRS, *54:*617, 1974. Ann. chir. plast., *19:*61, 1974

Secondary damage to hair follicles in full thickness skin autografts (Gloor). Arch. Dermat. Forsch., *249:*277, 1974

Hair transplantation, current trends in (Stough), PRS, *54:*104, 1974. Arch. Otolaryng., *98:*370, 1973

Hair transplantation with free scalp flap (Harii, Ohmori, Murakami), PRS, *55:*374, 1975. Jap. J. Plast. Reconstr. Surg., *17:*381, 1974

Clinical success of distant transfer of free skin flap in head and neck regions by microvascular anastomoses (Fujino *et al*). Keio J. Med., *23:*52, 1974

Hair transplantation with free scalp flaps

Alopecia—Cont.

(Harii, Ohmori, Ohmori), PRS, *53:*410, 1974

Adhesive, tissue, as an adjunct in hair transplantation (Wilkinson, Iglesias), PRS, *56:*103, 1975. South. M. J., *67:*1408, 1974

Parieto-occipital flaps in surgical treatment of baldness (Juri), *55:*456, 1975

Male pattern baldness: classification and incidence (Norwood), PRS, *57:*753, 1976. South. M. J., *68:*1359, 1975

Hair transplant (Monell), PRS, *57:*669, 1976. West. J. M., *123:*220, 1975

Baldness, reconstruction of sideburn for, after rhytidectomy (Juri, Juri, de Antueno), PRS, *57:*304, 1976

ALPERT, L. I. *et al*: Subungual basal cell epithelioma. Arch. Dermat., *106:*599, 1972

ALRICH, E. M., MANWARING, J. L., AND HORSLEY, J. S., III: Isolation perfusion: adjunct to surgical excision in primary treatment of melanoma of extremities, PRS, *49:*473, 1972. Am. J. Surg., *121:*583, 1971

ALSOP, D. G.: Bairnsdale ulcer. Aust. N. Z. J. Surg., *41:*317, 1972

ALTEMEIER, W. A. *et al*: Changing patterns in surgical infections, PRS, *52:*610, 1974. Ann. Surg., *178:*436, 1973

ALTER, M.: Variation in palmar creases. Am. J. Dis. Child., *120:*424, 1970

ALTON, H. R.: Posttraumatic orbits with lid deformities. Prosthetic correction. Int. Ophthalmol. Clin., *10:*869, 1971

ALTUNKOV, P. *et al*: Surgical treatment of case of Peutz-Jeghers disease. Khirurgiia (Sofiia), *26:*260, 1973 (Bulgarian)

ALTURA, B. M., AND ALTURA, B. T.: Effects of local anesthetics, antihistamines, and glucocorticoids on peripheral blood flow and vascular smooth muscle, PRS, *55:*644, 1975. Anesthesiology, *41:*197, 1974

ALVAREZ-Cordero, R. *et al*: New pharmacodynamic approach in treatment of shock—use of solution of glucose, insulin, and potassium in experimental shock, PRS, *56:*362, 1975. Cir. Cir., *42:*49, 1974

ALVES COSTA, E. *et al*: Use of silicone in temporomandibular ankylosis, PRS, *53:*365, 1974. Rev. brasil cir., *63:*73, 1973

AMA COMMITTEE ON CUTANEOUS HEALTH AND COSMETICS: Aging skin, PRS, *54:*383, 1974. Hospital Med., *10:*72, 1974

AMAR, R., AUBANIAC, J., AND BUREAU, H.: Our experience with muscle flaps applied to leg, PRS, *56:*230, 1975. Ann. chir. plast., *20:*61, 1975

AMAR INALSINGH, C. H.: Experience treating 501 patients with keloids, PRS, *57:*764, 1976.

Johns Hopkins Med. J., *134:*284, 1974

AMATO, G. A. *et al*: In situ squamous cell carcinoma of the skin. Clinical diagnosis, pathology and treatment. Rev. Bras. Pesqui. Mod. Biol., *7:*365, 1974

AMBROGGIO, G. *et al*: Use of mesh skin grafts in treatment of extensive burns. Minerva Chir., *26:*1406, 1971 (Italian)

AMBROGGIO, G., AND BORSETTI, G: Surgical treatment of burn scars, PRS, *56:*361, 1975. Riv. ital. chir. plast., *5:*261, 1973

AMBROGGIO, G., CAVALLERO, M., AND CATONE, A.: Trypsin and chymotrypsin toxicity in severely burned patients, PRS, *56:*361, 1975. Riv. ital. chir. plast., *5:*331, 1973

AMBROSE, J. *et al*: Anomalous extensor digiti minimi proprius causing tunnel syndrome in the dorsal compartment. Report of a case. J. Bone & Joint Surg. (Am.), *57:*706, 1975

AMBROSE, R. B.: Treatment of organic erectile impotence. Experience with the Scott procedure. J. Med. Soc. N.J., *72:*805, 1975

AMBROSE, S. S.: Repair of genital defects associated with persistent cloaca, PRS, *54:*504, 1974. J. Urol., *111:*256, 1974

AMBROSE, S. S. *et al*: Surgical embryology of the extrophy-epispadias complex. Surg. Clin. North Am., *54:*1379, 1974

AMERICAN ACADEMY OF ORTHOPAEDIC SURGEONS: *Symposium on Hand Tendon Surgery.* C. V. Mosby Co., St. Louis, 1975

American Association of Plastic Surgeons

American Association of Plastic Surgeons, PRS, *48:*409, 1971; *49:*113, 1972; *50:*642, 1972; *51:*495, 1973; *52:*604, 1973; *53:*507, 1974; *54:*634, 1974; *55:*262, 1975; *56:*608, 1975; *57:*411, 1976

American Association of Plastic Surgeons, presentation speech on occasion of Honorary Award to Jerome P. Webster (Edgerton), PRS, *50:*510, 1972

AMERICAN COLLEGE OF SURGEONS, COMMITTEE ON TRAUMA: *Early Care of the Injured Patient.* W. B. Saunders Co., Philadelphia, 1972. PRS, *55:*615, 1975

AMERICAN REPLANTATION MISSION: Replantation surgery in China, PRS, *52:*476, 1973

American Society for Aesthetic Plastic Surgery

American Society for Aesthetic Plastic Surgery, PRS, *48:*617, 1971; *50:*429, 643, 1972; *52:*333, 1973; *53:*119, 1974; *54:*253, 1974; *55:*262, 1975; *56:*482, 1975; *57:*271, 1976; Research Grants, *57:*685, 1976

American Society for Aesthetic Plastic Surgery, Honorary Award to Dr. Gustave Aufricht (Gurdin), PRS, *49:*70, 1972

American Society for Anesthetic Plastic Surgery — Cont.

History of American Society for Aesthetic Plastic Surgery (Crosby), PRS, *56:*506, 1975

American Society of Maxillofacial Surgeons

American Society of Maxillofacial Surgeons, PRS, *50:*104, 1972; *51:*240, 715, 1973; *53:*508, 695, 1974; *55:*392, 1975; *57:*550, 770, 1976

American Society of Plastic and Reconstructive Surgeons

The 39th Congress of the American Society of Plastic Surgery (Omori). Jap. J. Plast. Reconstr. Surg., *14:*189, 1971 (Japanese)

American Society of Plastic and Reconstructive Surgeons, PRS, *48:*204, 1971; *49:*242, 1972; *50:*104, 208, 1972; *51:*238, 715, 1973; *52:*110, 1973; *53:*377, 1974; *54:*122, 1974; *55:*390, 1975; *57:*549, 770, 1976

American Society of Plastic and Reconstructive Surgeons, 5-year history 1969–1973 (Adamson), PRS, *55:*445, 1975

ASPRS: Yesterday, today, and tomorrow (Gurdin) (Presidential Address), PRS, *53:*255, 1974

ASPRS, where are we going? (Hoopes), PRS, *56:*266, 1975

Educational Foundation of ASPRS, bibliography on, PRS, *48:*618, 1971

Educational Foundation of ASPRS, essay contest, PRS, *48:*412, 1971; *50:*207, 1972; *51:*242, 1973; *53:*121, 1974; *55:*264, 1975; *57:*274, 1976

Educational Foundation of ASPRS, winners of essay contest, PRS, *48:*411, 1971; *50:*207, 1972; *52:*333, 1973; *55:*128, 1975; *57:*130, 1976

Educational Foundation of ASPRS, meetings, annual, PRS, *49:*242, 1972; *50:*104, 1972; *51:*239, 1973; *53:*377, 1974; *54:*122, 1974; *55:*91, 1975; *57:*549, 1976

Educational Foundation of ASPRS, research grants, PRS, *54:*125, 1974; *55:*264, 1975; *57:*551, 1976

Educational Foundation of ASPRS, Symposia, PRS, *51:*113, 1973; *51:*715, 1973; *54:*123, 1974; *55:*393, 1975. Basic Science in Plastic Surgery, *55:*128, 1975; Breast, Female, *48:*520, 1971; Cancer of Head and Neck, *51:*614, 1973; Cleft Lip and Palate, *51:*241, 1973; *55:*527, 1975; Corrective Rhinoplasty, *54:*520, 1974; Craniofacial Anomalies, Diagnosis and Treatment, *57:*271, 1976; Esthetic Surgery, *48:*302, 1971; Esthetic Surgery of Breasts and Lipectomy, *53:*616,

American Society of Plastic and Reconstructive Surgeons—Cont.

1974; Hand Surgery, *49:*672, 1972; *52:*219, 1973; *50:*316, 1972; *51:*242, 1973; *56:*19, 1975; Hypospadias, Epispadias, Exstrophy of Bladder, *49:*483, 1972; Injured Human Face, *52:*336, 1973; Mammaplasty and Abdominoplasty, *55:*527, 1975; Mammaplasty and Lipectomy, *54:* 521, 1974; Microsurgery, *53:*616, 1974; *54:*384, 521, 1974; Neoplastic and Reconstructive Problems of Female Breast, *55:*128, 1975; Neurological Diseases of Upper Extremities, *57:*271, 1976; Office and Practice Management, *53:*616, 1974; *57:*271, 1976; Plastic Surgery of Orbital Region, *52:*692, 1973; Reconstruction of Auricle, *51:*495, 1973; Reconstruction of Jaw Deformity, *57:*411, 1976; Skin Tumors, *54:*384, 521, 1974; Treatment of Burns, *52:*607, 1973

AMERMAN, J. D. *et al*: Evaluation and rehabilitation of glossectomy speech behavior. J. Commun. Disord., 7:365, 1974

AMIES, D. R.: Orbital cellulitis. J. Laryng. & Otol., 88:559, 1974

AMINEV, A. M. *et al*: Experience in surgical treatment of congenital medial and lateral cysts and fistulae of neck. Stomatologiia (Mosk.), 52:83, 1973 (Russian)

AMIROV, A. G.: Instrument for suturing the mucosa of the nasal septum. Zh. Ushn. Nos. Gori. Bolezu., 0:113, 1974 (Russian)

AMMON, L. L.: Surviving enucleation. Am. J. Nurs., 72:1817, 1972

Amnion, Transplantation of (See also *Burns; Dressings*)

Amniotic membrane as living surgical dressing in human patients (Trelford *et al*). Oncology, 28:358, 1973

Amniotic membranes as temporary wound dressing (Robson *et al*), PRS, *52:*601, 1973. Surg. Gynec. & Obst., *136:*904, 1973

Wound dressing, physiologic, human amniotic membrane as (Colocho *et al*). Arch. Surg., *109:*370, 1974

Preliminary report on acceleration of wound healing by amnion membrane graft (Bapat *et al*). Indian J. Med. Res., 62:1342, 1974

Amnion graft. Young helping aged (Adducci). Minn. Med., 57:626, 1974

Burns and skin loss, lyophilized amnion in (Notea *et al*). Harefuah, 88:265, 1975 (Hebrew)

Amnion autografts, permanent structure (Trelford *et al*). J. Med. 6:243, 1975

AMPE, W. *et al*: Relative place of operation on

osseous planes and cartilaginous structures in treatment of protruding ears. Acta Otorhinolaryngol. Belg., 27:10, 1973 (French)

AMPHOUX, M.: Industry physician and accidents of the hand. Therapeutique, *44:* 567, 1968 (French)

ANAGNOSTOU, G. D., PAPADEMETRIOUS, D. G., AND TOUMAZANI, M. N.: Subcutaneous glomus tumors, PRS, *52:*599, 1973. Surg. Gynec. & Obst., *136:*945, 1973

ANASTASI, G. W., AND OLLSON, C. A.: Pedicle patch urethroplasty for cure of urethral stricture, PRS, *51:*1, 1973

ANASTASSOV, K. *et al*: Complete regeneration of the body of the ascending ramus and mandibular condyle in a child after disarticulation. Rev. Odontostomatol. (Paris), *4:*43, 1975 (French)

Anatomy (See also *Hands, Anatomy*)

Lubrication and Wear in Joints. Ed. by Verna Wright. J. B. Lippincott Co., Philadelphia, 1970. PRS, *48:*75, 1971

Sectional Anatomy and Tomography of the Head. By Guy D. Potter. Grune and Stratton, New York, 1971. PRS, *51:*84, 1973

Surgical Anatomy, Fifth Edition. Ed. by Barry J. Anson and Chester B. McVay. W. B. Saunders Co., Philadelphia, 1971. PRS, *48:*175, 1971

Innervation of superior pharyngeal constrictor muscle (Smith, Dedo), PRS, *48:*196, 1971. Ann. Otol. Rhin. & Laryng., *80:*92, 1971

Anatomical specimens, new method for permanent preservation of (Snow *et al*), PRS, *48:*387, 1971

Anatomy of the Head and Neck. By George H. Paff. W. B. Saunders Co., Philadelphia, 1973. PRS, *53:*468, 1974

Elbow, dynamic anatomy of the ulnar nerve at the (Apfelberg, Larson), PRS, *51:*76, 1973

Embryology: development of the cleft lip nose (Stark, Kaplan), PRS, *51:*413, 1973

Mastectomy, some anatomical considerations of subcutaneous (Goldman, Goldwyn), PRS, *51:*501, 1973

Nerve, facial, surgical anatomy as related to ancillary operations in rhytidoplasty (Correia, Zani), PRS, *52:*549, 1973

Human Engineering. The Body Re-Examined. By John Lenihan. George Brazillier Inc., New York, 1974. PRS, *56:*572, 1975

Anatomy, surgical, of orbital septum (Putterman, Urist), PRS, *54:*686, 1974. Ann. Ophth., *6:*290, 1974

Micro-anatomy, functional, of peripheral nerve trunks (Kuczynski), PRS, *54:*693,

Anatomy—Cont.
　　1974. Hand, *6:*1, 1974
　　Geniohyoid and genioglossus muscles (Moore, Russell), PRS, *55:*506, 1975. J. Oral Surg., *38:*2, 1974
　　Anatomy of a smile: its importance in the treatment of facial paralysis (Rubin), PRS, *53:*384, 1974
　　Surgical anatomy of the neck (Jurkiewicz *et al*). Surg. Clin. North Am., *54:*1269, 1974
　　Lips: study of development of *orbicularis oris* muscle (Fernandez Villoria), PRS, *55:*205, 1975
　　Deltopectoral flap, anatomical and hemodynamic approach (Daniel, Cunningham, Taylor), PRS, *55:*276, 1975
　　Vessels supplying several free flap donor sites (Taylor, Daniel), PRS, *56:*243, 1975
　　Nomenclature, anatomical, suggested, for nose (Schurter, Letterman), PRS, *57:*490, 1976

ANDERL, H.: Closing of extensive defects of face, PRS, *53:*104, 1974. Chir. Plast., *1:*53, 1971
ANDERL, H.: Simple method for correcting ectropion. Preliminary report, PRS, *49:*156, 1972
ANDERL, H.: Reconstruction of face through cross face nerve transplantation in facial paralysis, PRS, *53:*249, 1974. Chir. Plast., *2:*17, 1973
ANDERL, H.: Skin replacement on the penis. Langenbecks Arch. Chir., *339:*433, 1975 (German)
ANDERL, H.: Cross-face-nerve transplantation for repair of paralyzed facial musculature. In *Plastiche und Wiederherstellungs-Chirurgie* ed. Hohler; Schattauer, Stuttgart, 1975) pp. 137–42 (German)
ANDERL, H., AND WEISER, G.: Surgical treatment of pseudo-syndactyly in case of epidermolysis bullosa dystrophica, PRS, *53:*115, 1974. Chir. Plast., *1:*145, 1972
ANDERL, H., AND SEMENITZ, E.: Chronic recurrent tuberculous tenosynovitis of finger flexors, PRS, *52:*206, 1973. Handsurg., *4:*3, 1972
ANDERL, H. *et al*: Early skin coverage in extensive burns. Panminerva Med., *14:*220, 1972
ANDERL, H. *et al*: Septicaemia following early tangential excision of burns. Wien. Klin. Wochenschr., *86:*91, 1974 (German)
ANDERS, G. J. P. A. *et al*: Disturbed development of sexual organs in children, PRS, *57:*399, 1976. Stafleu's Wtnsch., Uitgevers. B.V., *93:* Monograph, 1975
ANDERSEN, E. B. *et al*: Letter: Axillary hyperhidrosis. J.A.M.A., *231:*1026, 1975
ANDERSEN, H. C. *et al*: Tracheal stenosis after intubation, tracheostomy and respirator therapy. Ugeskr. Laeger., *136:*2235, 1974 (Danish)
ANDERSEN, J. G.: Transverse metatarsal head resection—a radical approach to the problems of forefoot ulceration. Lepr. Rev., *46:*191, 1975
ANDERSON, C. B., MARR, J., AND JAFFE, B. M.: Anaerobic streptococcal infections simulating gas gangrene, PRS, *50:*422, 1972. Arch. Surg., *104:*196, 1972
ANDERSON, D. F.: Clinical characteristics of the genetic variety of cutaneous melanoma in man. Cancer, *28:*721, 1971
ANDERSON, D. K., AND PERRY, A. W.: Axillary hidradenitis, PRS, *55:*726, 1975. Arch. Surg., *110:*69, 1975
ANDERSON, J. R.: Straightening the crooked nose. Trans. Am. Acad. Ophthalmol. Otolaryngol., *76:*938, 1972
ANDERSON, J. R.: Philosophical considerations in revising cosmetic surgical operations. Otolaryngol. Clin. North Am., *7:*57, 1974
ANDERSON, J. R.: The tuck-up operation. A new technique of secondary rhytidectomy. Arch. Otolaryng., *101:*739, 1975
ANDERSON, L. G. *et al*: Familial osteodysplasia, PRS, *50:*633, 1972. J.A.M.A., *220:* 1687,1972
ANDERSON, ROBIN, AND HOOPES, JOHN: *Symposium on Malignancies of the Head and Neck.* Vol. XI. C. V. Mosby Co., St. Louis, 1975. PRS, *57:*373, 1973
ANDERSON, S., NIELSON, A., AND REYMANN, F.: Relationship between Bowen's disease and internal malignant tumors, PRS, *53:*370, 1974. Arch. Dermat., *108:*367, 1973
ANDERSON, V. S.: First branchial cleft cysts and sinuses (with Gaisford), PRS, *55:*299, 1975
ANDERTON, J. M. *et al*: Topical cocaine and general anesthesia: an investigation of the efficacy and side effects of cocaine on the nasal mucosae. Anesthesia, *30:*809, 1975
ANDINA, FRITZ: *Die Freien Hauttransplantationen.* Springer Verlag, Berlin, Heidelberg, New York, 1970. PRS, *48:*176, 1971
ANDRA, A.: Full thickness skin graft for primary repair of malignant facial tumors. Acta chir. plast. (Praha), *16:*85, 1974
ANDRA, A.: Full thickness skin grafts for closure of defects in radiation-damaged skin, PRS, *54:*625, 1974. J. Maxillo-facial Surg., *2:*9, 1974
ANDRA, A. *et al*: Oral surgical care in the Rostock district—a pilot study. Stomatol. D.D.R., *24:*582, 1974 (German)
ANDRADE, R.: Benign juvenile melanoma. A study of 51 lesions. Mod. Probl. Paediatr., *17:*212, 1975
ANDRADE, Z. A. *et al*: Nasal entomophthorosis.

Preliminary immunopathological study of new case. Am. J. Trop. Med. Hyg., *22:*361, 1972

ANDRADE MALABEHAR, R.: Benign juvenile melanoma: clinicopathological study of 51 lesions, PRS, *57:*677, 1976. Grac. Med. Mex., *110:*181, 1975

ANDRE, P.: Indications, technic and results of total subglossolaryngectomy. J. Fr. Otorhinolaryngol., *22:*881, 1973 (French)

ANDRE, P.: Treatment of cancerous adenopathies of the neck. J. Fr. Otorhinolaryngol., *24:*223, 1975 (French)

ANDRE, P. *et al*: Indications, methods and results of conservative surgery in the treatment of cancer of the sinus piriformis. Arch. Ital. Otol., *81:*247, 1970 (French)

ANDRE, P. *et al*: Major cervico-facial surgery and geriatrics. Ann. Otolaryngol. Chir. Cervicofac., *88:*295, 1971 (French)

ANDRE, P. *et al*: Indications, technics and results of conservative surgery in treatment of cancers in the piriform sinus. Probl. Actuels Otorhinolaryngol., *201:*24, 1972 (French)

ANDRE, P. *et al*: Laryngeal reconstruction after hemi-laryngo-pharyngectomy. Rev. Laryngol. Otol. Rhinol. (Bord.)., *93:*88, 1972 (French)

ANDRE, P. *et al*: Comparison of long-term carcinologic results between radical and conservative cervical surgery. Ann. Otolaryngol. Chir. Cervicofac., *92:*113, 1975 (French)

ANDRE, P. *et al*: Our procedure for pharyngoplasty in transmandibular pharyngectomies. Ann. Otolaryngol. Chir. Cervicofac., *92:*149, 1975 (French)

ANDREASEN, J. J. C. *et al*: Management of emotional reactions in seriously burned adults, PRS, *51:*107, 1973. New England J. Med., *286:*65, 1972

ANDREASEN, J. O. *et al*: Reversibility of surgically induced dental ankylosis in rats. Int. J. Oral Surg., *1:*98, 1972

ANDREASEN, N. J. *et al*: Long-term adjustment and adaptation mechanisms in severely burned adults. J. Nerv. Ment. Dis., *154:*352, 1972

ANDREASEN, N. J. C., NORRIS, A. S., AND HARTFORD, C. E.: Incidence of long term psychiatric complications in severely burned adults, PRS, *49:*666, 1972. Ann. Surg., *174:*785, 1971

ANDREEV, T. *et al*: Surgical treatment of hypospadias in childhood. Khirurgiia (Sofiia), *25:*304, 1972 (Bulgarian)

ANDREEVA, D. N. *et al*: Corrective surgery in scarring ectropion of the lower eyelid. Vestn. Khir., *107:*49, 1971 (Russian)

ANDREEVA, D. N. *et al*: Surgery for pendulous breast. Vestn. Khir., *111:*50, 1973 (Russian)

ANDREEVSKI, A.: Differential diagnosis and therapy of salivary gland tumor. God. Zb. Med. Fak. Skopje., *18:*207, 1972 (Croatian)

ANDREEVSKI, A. *et al*: Indications for surgical decompression in peripheral paralysis of facial nerve. God. Zb. Med. Fak. Skopje., *18:*215, 1972 (Serbian)

ADREN, L., AND EIKEN, O.: Arthrographic studies of wrist ganglions, PRS, *49:*663, 1972. J. Bone & Joint Surg., *53:*299, 1971

ANDREWS, M. J.: Incidence and pathogenesis of tracheal injury following tracheostomy with cuffed tube and assisted ventilation. Analysis of a 30 year prospective study. Brit. J. Surg., *58:*749, 1971

ANDREWS, M. J., AND PIERSON, E. G.: Incidence and pathogenesis of tracheal injury following cuffed tube tracheostomy with assisted ventilation – analysis of two-year prospective study, PRS, *49:*233, 1972. Ann. Surg., *173:*249, 1971

ANDREWS, P. E. *et al*: Carcinoma of the tonsil: a comparison of two treatment modalities. South. Med. J., *65:*982, 1972

ANDRIE, J. *et al*: Obwegeser's method of plastic surgery of edentulous mouth and vestibule of mouth. Cesk. Stomatol., *73:*122, 1973 (Czechoslovakian)

ANDRUSON, M. V.: Free skin grafting in surgical correction of cicatricial hand deformities. Ortop. Travmatol. Protez., *32:*1, 1971 (Russian)

ANDRUSON, M. V. *et al*: Our experience of fixing free skin grafts by overlap with cyacrin. Ortop. Travmatol. Protez., *33:*58, 1972 (Russian)

ANDRUSON, M. V. *et al*: Sutureless fixation of grafts in free skin plastic surgery (literature review). Ortop. Travmatol. Protez., *33:*78, 1972 (Russian)

Anesthesia (See also *Acupuncture; Anesthesia, Complications of; Anesthesia, Endotracheal; Anesthesia, Ketamine; and Anesthesia, Nerve Blocks*)

Analgesic, non-narcotic, pentazocine, evaluation of, in burned children. (Wilson, Priano, Traber), PRS, *48:*466, 1971

Anesthesia in an infant, hyperthermic reaction during. (Bergera, Friz), PRS, *48:*595, 1971

Tourniquet difficulty during intravenous regional anesthesia (Nizolek), PRS, *52:*323, 1973. South. M.J., *64:*1411, 1971

Thrombophlebitis, venous stasis on operating table. (Lewis, Mueller, Edwards), PRS, *52:*99, 1973. Am. J. Surg., *124:*780, 1972

Ventilation regulation during hemorrhage and its alterations in response to CO_2 (Baue, Nara), PRS, *51:* 710, 1973. Ann.

Anesthesia — Cont.

Surg., *176:* 80, 1972

Jugular vein, internal, puncture with margin of safety (Civetta, Gagel, Gemer), PRS, *51:*236, 1973. Anaesthesia, *36:*622, 1972

Diazepam treatment of local anesthetic induced seizures (Munson, Wagman), PRS, *51:*610, 1973. Anesthesiology, *27:*523, 1972

Hyperkalemia, succinylcholine-induced, and cardiac arrest (Baker *et al*). Arch. Otolaryng., *96:*464, 1972

Respiratory distress syndrome, fatal, after prolonged mechanical ventilation (Perna *et al*), PRS, *51:*353, 1973. J. Surg. Res., *11:*584, 1972

Hypotension, deliberate, for blepharoplasty and rhytidectomy (Stark) (Follow-Up Clinic), PRS, *49:*453, 1972

Epinephrine, adding a given concentration to a solution by needle drops (Bellinger), *50:*530, 1972

Epinephrine requirements for effective hemostasis in local anesthesia (Siegel, Vistnes), PRS, *51:*711, 1973. Surg. Forum, *23:*515, 1972

Hypnoanalgesia for major surgery. A psychodynamic process. (Scott). Am. J. Clin. Hypn., *16:*84, 1973

Diazepam, intravenous (Valium), adverse reactions to; report from Boston Collaborative Drug Surveillance Program (Greenblatt, Koch-Weser), PRS, *57:*541, 1976. Am. J. Med. Sci., *266:*261, 1973

Venous stasis on the operating table (Lewis, Mueller, Edwards), PRS, *52:*99, 1973. Am. J. Surg., *124:*780, 1972

Gases, tissue, PO_2 and PCO_2, measured by using silicone tube and capillary sampling technique (Kivisaari, Niinikoski), PRS, *52:*688, 1973. Am. J. Surg., *125:*623, 1973

Anesthesia, importance of changes in body temperature in pediatric surgery and (Dilworth), PRS, *53:*690, 1974. Anesth. & Intens. Care, *1:*480, 1973

Anesthesia, dental, in children (Bell), PRS, *53:*690, 1974. Anesth. & Intens. Care, *1:*540, 1973

Heat stroke, drug induced (Sarnquist, Larson), PRS, *53:*610, 1974. Anesthesiology, *39:*348, 1973

Anesthetized infants and children, effect of warming blanket on maintenance of body temperatures in (Goudsouzian, Morris, Ryan), PRS, *53:* 687, 1974. Anesthesiology, *39:*351, 1973

Anesthetic choice among anesthesiologists (Katz), PRS, *53:*376, 1974. Anesth. Analg., Cleve., *52:*373, 1973

Outpatients, general anesthesia in, renal hemodynamic effects (Everett *et al*), PRS,

Anesthesia — Cont.

*53:*373, 1974. Anesth. Analg., Cleve., *52:*470, 1973

Etidocaine — new long-acting local anesthetic agent (Lund, Cwik, Pagdanganan), PRS, *53:*372, 1974. Anesth. & Analg., Cleve., *52:*482, 1973

Anesthesia, outpatient, for pediatric ophthalmology (Nagel *et al*), PRS, *53:*373, 1974. Anesth. & Analg., Cleve., *52:*558, 1973

Anesthesia, outpatient, service for children (Steward), PRS, *53:*693, 1974. Anesth. & Analg., *52:*877, 1973

Outpatient anesthesia, experiences with (Thompson *et al*), PRS, *53:*693, 1974. Anesth. Analg., Cleve., *52:*881, 1973

Perphenazine side effects presenting in oral surgical practice (Smith). Brit. J. Oral Surg., *10:*349, 1973

Lung edema, gravitational, observed during assisted respiration (Leeming), PRS, *54:*502, 1974. Chest, *64:*719, 1973

Respiration, effects of ventral hernia on (Rives *et al*), PRS, *53:*605, 1974. Chir., Mem. Acad., *99:*547, 1973

Anesthesia, general, in adults (Adams *et al*). Int. Ophthalmol. Clin., *13:*83, 1973

Methoxyflurane nephrotoxicity (Cousins, Mazze), PRS, *53:*375, 1974. J.A.M.A., *225:*1611, 1973

Diazepam, intravenous, experience with use of, in outpatient procedures (Cheesman). J. Laryng. & Otol., *87:*1249, 1973

Circulation in profound hypothermia (Zarins, Skinner), PRS, *53:*115, 1974. J. Surg. Res., *14:*97, 1973

Pediatric otorhinolaryngological surgery, Fentanyl and droperidol in. Marginal notes on personal cases (Ciurea *et al*).Otorinolarngologie, *18:*419, 1973 (Rumanian)

Epinephrine, effective hemostasis with less, experimental and clinical study (Siegel, Vistnes, Iverson), PRS, *51:*129, 1973

Anesthesia (Penthrane) methoxyflurane, occasional occurrence of serious renal complications after (Olsen *et al*), PRS, *52:*160, 1973

Extremity, upper, tissue necrosis from vascular complications after arterial catheterization (Graham *et al*), PRS, *53:*487, 1974. Rev. Latino Am. cir. plast., *17:*37, 1973

Propanidide, maximum lethal dose (Landazuri, Flores, Lino), PRS, *53:*692, 1974. Rev. Latino Am. cir. plast., *17:*69, 1973

E. N. T. surgery, induced hypotension for (Loers *et al*). Z. Prakt. Anaesth., *8:*232, 1973 (German)

General anaesthesia for maxillo-facial surgery (Daubb). Z. Prakt. Anaesth., *8:*304,

Anesthesia — Cont.

1973 (German)

Pain, electrical inhibition of, PRS, *55:*261, 1975. Am. J. Med., *53:*208, 1974

Pain relief by subarachnoid hypothermic saline injection (Battista), PRS, *57:*767, 1976. Am. J. Surg., *128:*662, 1974

Lidocaine, effects on canine cerebral metabolism and circulation related to electroencephalogram (Sakabe *et al*), PRS, *54:*693, 1974. Anesthesiology, *40:*433, 1974

Insulin and anesthesia (Greene), PRS, *55:*259, 1975. Anesthesiology, *41:*75, 1974

Blood flow, cerebral, renal, and splanchnic, effects of anesthetics on (Larson *et al*), PRS, *55:*645, 1975. Anesthesiology, *41:*169, 1974

Temperatures, skin and rectal, during ether and halothane anesthesia in infants and children (Naito *et al*), PRS, *55:*644, 1975. Anesthesiology, *41:*237, 1974

Carbon dioxide, cardiovascular effects in man (Cullen, Eger), PRS, *55:*727, 1975. Anesthesiology, *41:*345, 1974

Isoflurane in surgical patients, cardiovascular effects (Graves, McDermott, Bidwai), PRS, *55:*727, 1975. Anesthesiology, *41:*486, 1974

Long-lasting anesthesia in plastic surgery and neurosurgery. Anesth. Analg. (Paris), *31:*181, 1974 (French)

Diazepam prophylaxis to avert convulsions induced by local anesthetic (De Jong, Heavner), PRS, *55:*120, 1975. Canad. Anaesth. Soc. J., *21:*153, 1974

Resuscitation, factors determining survival in cardiac arrest (Castagna, Weil, Shubin), PRS, *55:*250, 1975. Chest, *65:*527, 1974

Pain management, current techniques (Hardy), PRS, *56:*602, 1975. Cleveland Clin. Quart., *41:*177, 1974

Fetus, influence of anesthesia on (Smith), PRS, *55:*639, 1975. Clin. Obst. Gynec., *17:*145, 1974

Jaw and face, surgery of, effect of trimethaphan-camphor-sulfonate on blood pressure during neuroleptoanalgesia in (Schmelzle *et al*). Med. Welt., *25:*521, 1974 (German)

Premedication, effect on arterial blood gases (Carden, Hubbard, Petty), PRS, *54:*692, 1974. Mil. Med., *141:*476, 1974

Epinephrine, effect of local anesthesia with, on skin flap survival (Reinisch, Myers), PRS, *54:*324, 1974

Hematoma: prevention of bleeding following rhytidectomy (Barker), PRS, *54:*651, 1974

Anesthesia techniques and facial plastic surgery (Kean *et al*). Trans. Pa. Acad.

Anesthesia — Cont.

Ophthalmol. Otolaryngol., *27:*45, 1974

Head and neck surgery, anesthesiological problems in (Emanuelli *et al*). Tumori, *60:*491, 1974 (Italian)

Methoxyflurane anesthesia in pediatric patients (Stoelting, Peterson), PRS, *57:*681, 1976. Anesthesiology, *42:*16, 1975

Bronchomotor tone, regulation during anesthesia (Aviado), PRS, *57:*768, 1976. Anesthesiology, *42:*68, 1975

Pediatric surgery, specific therapy in water, electrolyte and blood-volume replacement during (Furman *et al*), PRS, *56:*237, 1975. Anesthesiology, *42:*187, 1975

Lidocaine and its metabolites in newborn (Blankenbaker, DeFazio), PRS, *57:*407, 1976. Anesthesiology, *42:*325, 1975

Morphine and hydromorphone, relative analgesic potencies in postoperative pain (Mahler, Forrest), PRS, *57:*267, 1976. Anesthesiology, *42:*602, 1975

Hyperkalemia induced by succinylcholine, pathophysiology of (Gronert, Theye), PRS, *57:*263, 1976. Anesthesiology, *43:*89, 1975

Innovar prededication, patient refusal of surgery following (Lee, Yeakel), PRS, *56:*604, 1975. Anesth. Analg., Cleve., *54:*224, 1975

Anesthesia orientation for medical students (Rosenberg), PRS, *57:*267, 1976. Anesth. Analg., Cleve., *54:*328, 1975

Aspirin-intolerant patients, anesthetic problems with (Barton), PRS, *57:*681, 1976. Anesth. Analg., Cleve., *54:*376, 1975

Anesthesia, regional, in children (Melman *et al*), PRS, *57:*405, 1976. Anesth. Analg., Cleve., *54:*387, 1975

Respiratory care in local anesthesia (Robertson, PRS, *56:*470, 1975. AORN, *21:*797, 1975

Anesthesia complication: idiopathic malignant hyperthermia (Bergman), PRS, *56:*235, 1975. Arch. Ophth., *93:*232, 1975

Hypnosis in anesthesia (Zaffiri). Minerva Med., *66:*3894, 1975 (Italian)

Anesthetic management and intraoperative care of patients undergoing major facial osteotomies (Davies, Munro), PRS, *55:*50, 1975

Thiopentone and methohexitone compared with intravenous steroid anesthetic Althesin (Carson), PRS, *56:*237, 1975. Proc. Roy. Soc. Med., *68:*108, 1975

Cocaine, use as topical anesthetic in nasal surgery (Feehan, Mancusi-Ungaro), PRS, *57:*62, 1976

Chlorpromazine to prevent postoperative hypertension, etiological factor in hematoma

Anesthesia — Cont.

after rhytidectomy (Berner, Morain, Noe), PRS, *57:*314, 1976

Anesthesia, Complications of (See also *Anesthesia*)

Anesthesia problems in patients with burns (Harrfeldt), PRS, *50:*203, 1972. Langenbeck's Arch. Chir., *329:*907, 1971

Hyperthermic reaction during anesthesia in infant (Bergera, Friz), PRS, *48:*595, 1971

Anesthesia, intravenous regional, tourniquet difficulty during (Nizolek), PRS, *52:*323, 1973. South. M. J., *64:*1411, 1971

Anesthetic induced seizures, local diazepam treatment of (Munson, Wagman), PRS, *51:*610, 1973. Anesthesiology, *27:*523, 1972

Cardiorespiratory resuscitation: emergency percutaneous transtracheal catheter and ventilator (Jacobs), PRS, *52:*106, 1973. J. Trauma, *12:*50, 1972

Pulmonary complications, postoperative, prevention of (Van de Water *et al*), PRS, *51:*355, 1973. Surg. Gynec. & Obst., *135:*229, 1972

Cardiorespiratory effects of Althesin and ketamine (Savage *et al*), PRS, *53:*373, 1974. Anesthesia, *28:*391, 1973

Anesthesia, general, in outpatients, renal hemodynamic effects (Everett *et al*), PRS, *53:*373, 1974. Anesth. & Analg., Cleve. *52:*470, 1973

Anesthesia, methoxyflurane, nephrotoxicity (Cousins, Mazze), PRS, *53:*375, 1974. J.A.M.A., *225:*1611, 1973

Hyperthermia, malignant, a catastrophic complication (Ryan, Kerr), PRS, *52:*602, 1973. J. Urol., *109:*879, 1973

Innovar premedication, patients' refusal of surgery after (Briggs, Ogg), PRS, *51:*158, 1973

Renal complications, serious, after methoxyflurane (Penthrane) anesthesia, occasional occurrence of (Olsen *et al*), PRS, *52:*160, 1973

Cardiovascular effects of isoflurane in surgical patients (Graves, McDermott, Bidwai), PRS, *55:*727, 1975. Anesthesiology, *41:*486, 1974

Blindness after ketamine anesthesia (Fine, Weissman, Finestone), PRS, *54:*248, 1974. Anesth. & Analg., *53:*72, 1974

Axillary approach to block brachial plexus, broken disposable needle during (Snow *et al*), PRS, *54:*249, 1974. Anesth. & Analg., *53:*89, 1974

Convulsions induced by local anesthetic: time course of diazepam prophylaxis (De

Anesthesia, Complications of — Cont.

Jong, Heavner), PRS, *55:*120, 1975. Canad. Anaesth. Soc. J., *21:*153, 1974

Anesthesia, teratology in (Smith), PRS, *55:*639, 1975. Clin. Obst. Gynec., *17:*145, 1974

Hypersensitivity to intravenous morphine sulfate (Cromwell, Zsigmond), PRS, *54:*224, 1974

Premedication, Innovar, patient refusal of surgery following (Lee, Yeakel), PRS, *56:*604, 1975. Anesth. Analg., Cleve., *54:*224, 1975

Anesthetic problems with aspirin-intolerant patients (Barton), PRS, *57:*681, 1976. Anesth. Analg., Cleve., *54:*376, 1975

Anesthesia, general, awareness, dreams, and hallucinations associated with (Wilson), PRS, *57:*682, 1976. Anesth. Analg., Cleve., *54:*609, 1975

Hyperthermia, idiopathic malignant: review and report of case (Bergman), PRS, *56:*235, 1975. Arch. Ophth., *93:*232, 1975

Anesthesia, Endotracheal

Endotracheal anesthesia in children during operations in the maxillofacial region (Vorob'eva *et al*). Stomatologiia (Mosk.), *50:*83, 1971 (Russian)

Intubation, prolonged, can we rehabilitate children exposed to? (Krivosic-Horber, Tempe, Gauthier-Lafaye). Anesth. Analg. (Paris), *29:*411, 1972 (French)

Resuscitation, cardiorespiratory, emergency percutaneous transtracheal catheter and ventilator (Jacobs), PRS, *52:*106, 1973. J. Trauma, *12:*50, 1972

Lacoorostomy with permanent intubation (Zakharov). Oftal. zhur., *27:*297, 1972 (Russian)

Intubation, emergency orotracheal, simple method for (Manchester, Mani, Masters), PRS, *49:*312, 1972

Rational tube for nasal tracheal intubation in buccal and oropharyngeal surgery (Le Mouel *et al*). Ann. Otolaryngol. Chir. Cervicofac., *90:*775, 1973 (French)

Epithelium, ciliated, lost in rapid tracheal injury by cuffed airways (Paegle, Ayres, Davis), PRS, *52:*462, 1973. Arch. Surg., *106:*31, 1973

Suction procedures, tracheo-bronchial damage with (Sacker *et al*), PRS, *53:*610, 1974. Chest, *64:*285, 1973

Intubation, nasotracheal, nasal necrosis complication (Zwillich, Pierson), PRS, *53:*681, 1974. Chest, *64:*376, 1973

Orotracheal intubation, emergency, simple

Anesthesia, Ketamine—Cont.

Ketamine and halothane, interaction in rats (White, Johnston), PRS, *57:*267, 1976. Anesthesiology, *42:*179, 1975

Anesthesia, Nerve Blocks

Nerve block, glossopharyngeal (Barton, Williams), PRS, *49:*105, 1972. Arch. Otolaryng., *93:*2, 1971

Nerve block, anterior ethmoid, for treatment of nasal fractures (Seitchick), PRS, *48:*187, 1971

Brachial plexus blockage, improved, with bupivacaine hydrochloride and carbonated lidocaine (Bromage, Gertel), PRS, *50:*631, 1972. Anesthesiology, *36:*479, 1972

Thigh, regional block of: uses in plastic surgery (Earle, Kiehn, DesPrez), PRS, *49:*134, 1972

Anesthesia, local, for hand surgery, under wrist block and upper arm tourniquet (Dupont *et al*), PRS, *50:*532, 1972

Axillary approach to brachial plexus anesthesia (Hopcroft), PRS, *52:*331, 1973. Anesth. & Intens. Care, *1:*3, 1973

Nerve blocks of head and neck, transient abducens paralysis following (Kepes, Foldes), PRS, *53:*246, 1974. Anesthesiology, *38:*893, 1973

Wrist block and local infiltration anesthesia, using upper arm tourniquet, hand surgery under (Dushoff, Dupont) (Letters to the Editor), PRS, *51:*685, 1973

Axillary blocks: rapid-onset, long-acting regional anesthetic technique (Cunningham, Kaplan), PRS, *56:*237, 1975. Anesthesiology, *41:*509, 1974

Needle, broken, during axillary approach to block brachial plexus (Snow *et al*), PRS, *54:*249, 1974. Anesth. & Analg., Cleve., *53:*89, 1974

Anesthetic agent, Etidocaine, with modified bilateral ulnar nerve block technique) Poppers *et al*), PRS, *54:*248, 1974. J. Anesth., *40:*13, 1974

Nerve blocks, selective peripheral, for reconstructive hand surgery (Connelly, Berry), PRS, *55:*109, 1975. M. J. Australia, *114:*94, 1974

Cervical plexus block, interscalene: single-injection technique (Winnie *et al*), PRS, *57:*543, 1976. Anesth. Analg., Cleve., *54:*370, 1975

Effects of peridural block (Stanton-Hicks *et al*), PRS, *57:*768, 1976. Anesthesiology, *42:*398, 1975

Ange, D. W. *et al:* Management of squamous cell carcinoma of tongue and floor of mouth after excisional biopsy. Radiology, *116:*143, 1975

Angela, G. G. *et al:* Histopathological and enzyme-cytological aspects in burn scars, PRS, *56:*360, 1975. Riv. ital. chir. plast., *5:*231, 1973

Angelats, J.: Surgical treatment of *hidradenitis suppurativa* of the axilla (with Tasche, Jayaram), PRS, *55:*559, 1975

Anita, N. H.: Review of surgery in leprosy. Int. J. Lepr., *39:*616, 1971

Anke, H. *et al:* Free full skin transplantation by the Corachan method. Zentralbl. Chir., *96:*799, 1971 (German)

Anneroth, G. *et al:* Primary melanoma in oral mucous membrane. Sven. Tandlak. Tidskr., *66:*27, 1973

Anneroth, G. *et al:* Calcifying odontogenic cyst. Oral Surg., *39:*794, 1975

Anneroth, G. *et al:* Benign cementoblastoma (true cementoma). Oral Surg., *40:*141, 1975.

Annis, D.: Sterile "use-once" clip applicator for skin closure. Brit. J. Surg., *60:*686, 1973

Announcements (See also American Association of Plastic Surgeons, American Society of Aesthetic Plastic Surgery American Society of Maxillofacial Surgeons, American Society of Plastic and Reconstructive Surgeons, and International Congress of Plastic Surgery, Courses, Societies, and Symposia)

Dow Corning award, first, given to Dr. Frank McDowell, PRS, *49:*363, 1972; second, given to Dr. H. Dean Hoskins, *51:*356, 1973; third, given to Dr. Charles E. Horton, *53:*377, 1974; fourth, given to Dr. Milton Edgerton, *55:*391, 1975

Basic Surgical Examination, PRS, *50:*106, 1972; *53:*507, 1975

New Film Review Section, PRS, *50:*316, 1972

Fellowship in Plastic Surgery in East Africa, PRS, *50:*429, 1972

Residency positions in plastic surgery in the United States, PRS, *50:*642, 1972

Plastic Surgery Chief Resident's Conference, PRS, *50:*644, 1972

National Archives of Plastic Surgery (Goldwyn) (Editorial), PRS, *51:*436, 1973

Postgraduate Fellowships Available at New York University, PRS, *52:*335, 1973

Survey of National Ambulatory Medical Care, PRS, *53:*252, 1974

Plastic and Reconstructive Surgery; Editorial Board meeting of, PRS, *52:*605, 1973; official organ of American Society for Aesthetic Plastic Surgery, PRS, *53:*120, 1974;

Announcements—Cont.
    of American Society of Maxillofacial Surgeons, PRS, *55:*263, 1975
    Establishment of Ralph Millard-Rudolph Light Chair of Plastic Surgery at University of Miami, PRS, *54:*123, 1974
    Congress of the French Chapter of the International College of Surgeons, organized by the Reims University Surgical Clinic, June 7, 8, and 9, 1974. Breast cancer, current problems. Conclusion (Romieu). Ann. Chir., *29:*877, 1975 (French)
    Cirugia Plastica Ibero-Latinoamericana, new plastic surgical journal, PRS, *55:*650, 1975
    American Cleft Palate Education Foundation, Essay Contest, PRS, *55:*733, 1975
    Graduate Fellowship in Plastic Surgery, PRS, *55:*733, 1975
    Subcutaneous Mastectomy Data Evaluation Center, PRS, *56:*241, 1975
    Care-Medico Seeks Doctors for Overseas Service, PRS, *56:*485, 1975
    Educational Assessment Examination— 1976, PRS, *57:*685, 1976
    Isambert Travel Fund, PRS, *57:*686, 1976

ANON, A. L.: Total osteotomy of face in treatment of Crouzon's syndrome. Rev. Clin. Esp., *137:*77, 1975 (Spanish)

ANSCOMBE, A. R.: Dexon absorbable suture material in general surgery, PRS, *53:*251, 1974. Internat. Surg., *57:*887, 1972

ANSELL, B., AND HARRISON, S.: Five-year follow-up of synovectomy of proximal interphalangeal joint in rheumatoid arthritis, PRS, *56:*596, 1975. Hand, *7:*34, 1975

ANSELL, B. M. *et al:* Farnham Park modular splint system. Rheumatol. Phys. Med., *11:*334, 1972

ANSELL, J. S.: Primary closure of exstrophy in the newborn: a preliminary report. Northwest Med., *70:*842, 1971

ANSON, BARRY J., AND MCVAY, CHESTER B.: *Surgical Anatomy,* Fifth Edition. W. B. Saunders Co., Philadelphia, 1971. PRS, *48:*175, 1971

ANTALIK, P. E. *et al:* Tumors of minor salivary gland origin. Trans. Pa. Acad. Ophthalmol. Otolaryngol., *28:*42, 1975

ANTHONY, J., AND CHANDRASEKHARA, M. K.: Penis agenesis, PRS, *54:*238, 1974. Internat. Surg., *58:*10, 1973

ANTIA, N.: Complications of free flap transfers to the mouth region (with Finseth, Kavarana), PRS, *56:*652, 1975

ANTIA, N. H.: The scope of plastic surgery in leprosy: a ten year progress report. Clin. Plast. Surg., *1:*69, 1974

ANTIA, N. H.: Significance of nerve involvement in leprosy, PRS, *54:*55, 1974

ANTIA, N. H. *et al:* Prefabricated silicone nasal implants, PRS, *52:*264, 1973

ANTIA, N. H., AND DAVER, B. M.: Endorsement of division of nasal lining to achieve pushback of palate, PRS, *55:*383, 1975. Indian J. Plast. Surg., *7:*3, 1974

Antibiotics

Bacitracin-neomycin surgical skin preparation, evaluation of (Saik, Walz, Rhoads), PRS, *51:*611, 1973. Am. J. Surg., *121:*557, 1971

Iatrogenic ototoxic hearing loss (Nilges, Northern), PRS, *49:*240, 1972. Ann. Surg., *173:*281, 1971

Hematomas, experimental bone, antibiotic penetration of (Wilson *et al*), PRS, *50:*310, 1972. J. Bone & Joint Surg., *53:*1622, 1971

Gentamycin-resistant *Pseudomonas,* evolution and spread of (Stone, Kolk), PRS, *49:*106, 1972. J. Trauma, *7:*586, 1971

Antibiotics and chemical adhesives, effect on infected wounds (Beasley *et al*), PRS, *49:*588, 1972. Mil. Med., *136:*566, 1971

Gentamycin therapy in renal failure (Chan, Benner, Hoeprick), PRS, *50:*634, 1972. Ann. Int. Med., *76:*773, 1972

Kanamycin, progressive neuro-ototoxicity of (Gonzalez, Miller, Wasilewski), PRS, *50:*312, 1972. Ann. Otol. Rhin. & Laryng., *81:*127, 1972

Antibiotics, preoperatively administered (Whitney, Anderson, Allansmith), PRS, *50:*93, 1972. Arch. Ophth., *87:*155, 1972

Penicillin preparations, long-acting, clinical-experimental evaluation of, in treatment of anaerobic infections (Grechukhin *et al*). Voen. Med. Zh., *4:*20, 1972 (Russian)

Antibiotics, resistance of surgical wound to antimicrobial prophylaxis and its mechanism of development (Edlich, Smith, Edgerton), PRS, *54:*114, 1974. Am. J. Surg., *126:*583, 1973

Infections, surgical, changing patterns in (Altemeier *et al*), PRS, *53:*610, 1974. Ann. Surg., *178:*436, 1973

Antibacterial agents, concentration in interstitial tissue fluid (Chisholm *et al*), PRS, *52:*462, 1973. Brit. M. J., *1:*569, 1973

Phagocytosis of the RES, attempts at interference with (Köhnlein, Lemperle, Scherer), PRS, *53:*376, 1974. Bruns' Beitr. klin. Chir., *220:*643, 1973

Hyperkalemia, cardiac arrest due to, following intravenous penicillin administration (Mercer, Logic), PRS, *53:*609, 1974. Chest, *64:*358, 1973

Antibiotics — Cont.

Intensive care, postoperative, candidiasis in cases of (Zierott, von Meissner), PRS, *53:*691, 1974. Chirurg, *44:*509, 1973

Congenital anomalies in rats and mice, produced by sulfonamides (Kato, Kitagawa), PRS, *53:*607, 1974. Congen. Anom., *13:*7, 1973

Antimicrobial therapy, complications of (Guckian), PRS, *53:*374, 1974. Fam. Phys., *8:*111, 1973

Antibiotics, topical, effect on healing of partial thickness skin wounds in rats (Burleson, Eiseman), PRS, *52:*461, 1973. Surg. Gynec. & Obst., *136:*958, 1973

Orthopedics and traumatology, evaluation of prophylactic antibiotics in (Kremmydas *et al*), PRS, *56:*471, 1975. Tr. 8th Panhellenic Cong. Surg. Soc. *A:* 308, 1973

Infections, *Candida:* pathogenesis and principles of treatment (Stone *et al*), PRS, *54:*702, 1974. Ann. Surg., *179:*697, 1974

Lidocaine, effect on antibacterial activity of 7 antibiotics (Barba *et al*), PRS, *55:*647, 1975. Arch. Ophth., *92:*514, 1974

Antibiotics to prevent wound infection, local use of (Bingham *et al*), PRS, *56:*362, 1975. Clin. Orthop., *99:*194, 1974

Infections, hospital, due to *Pseudomonas aeruginosa,* role of wounds in epidemiology of (Wysocki *et al*), PRS, *55:*258, 1975. Invest. Urol., *11:*370, 1974

Antibiotics, prophylactic, in clean orthopedic surgery (Pavel *et al*), PRS, *55:*388, 1975. J. Bone & Joint Surg., *56A:*777, 1974

Injections, intramuscular, contracture of deltoid muscle in adult after (Groves, Goldner), PRS, *55:*259, 1975. J. Bone & Joint Surg., *56A:*817, 1974

Antibiotics, systemic, efficacy in treatment of granulating wounds (Robson *et al*), PRS, *54:*695, 1974. J. Surg. Res., *16:*299, 1974

Antibiotic therapy, prophylactic, in surgery (MacLean), PRS, *57:*405, 1976. Canad. J. Surg., *18:*243, 1975

Prophylactic antibiotics in plastic and reconstructive surgery, current use of (Krizek, Koss, Robson), PRS, *55:*21, 1975

Preventive antibiotics in surgery (Burke), PRS, *57:*407, 1976. Postgrad. Med., *58:*65, 1975

Antimicrobial therapy of anaerobic infections (Finegold), PRS, *57:*406, 1976. Postgrad. Med., *58:*72, 1975

Infections in hospitals (Howells), PRS, *56:*237, 1975. Proc. Roy. Soc. Med., *68:*95, 1975

ANTOGNINI, F. *et al:* General anesthesia with association of gamma-OH (Sodium 4-hydroxy-butyrate) and neuroleptoanalgesic drugs in dental and maxillofacial surgery. Minerva Stomatol., *21:*255, 1972 (Italian)

ANTOGNINI, F. *et al:* Surgical treatment of oronasal fistula resulting from palatoplasty for cleft palate, using autogenous bone graft. Minerva Stomatol., *21:*276, 1972 (Italian)

ANTOGNINI, F. *et al:* Case of Mendelson's syndrome in patient with rigid intermaxillary block after Obwegeser-Dal Pont intervention for correction of prognathism. Mondo Odontostomatol., *14:*933, 1972 (Italian)

ANTOINE, T.: Plastic surgery for the correction of vaginal atresia. Wien. Klin. Wochenschr., *82:*559, 1970 (German)

ANTON'EV, A. A. *et al:* Preparation for plastic operations of skin and mucous membrane of external female genitalia in patients with urinary incontinence. Urol. Nefrol. (Mosk.), *38:*41, 1973

ANTONIADIS, A., PAPASOGLOU, O., AND MAKRIS, G.: Management of complicated hand fractures, PRS, *48:*393, 1971. Trans. 1st Panhellenic Cong. Orthop. Surg. & Traum., *1:*131, 1969

ANTOSZKIEWICZ, H. *et al:* Mandibulo-palpebral synkinesis following surgery for congenital ptosis. Klin. Oczna., *43:*823, 1973 (Polish)

Anus: See *Rectum*

ANZAI, T.: Effect of bromelain ointment on necrotic tissue, PRS, *52:*457, 1973. Jap. J. Plast. Reconstr. Surg., *15:*456, 1972

ANZE, M., SHIOYA, N., AND AKIYAMA, T.: Apparatus for correction of cryptotia, PRS, *49:*240, 1972. Jap. J. Plast. Reconstr. Surg., *14:*263, 1971

AOYAGI, F.: Reconstruction for aplasia of breast and pectoral region by microvascular transfer of free flap from buttock (with Fujino, Harashina), PRS, *56:*178, 1975. Discussion by Goldwyn, PRS, *56:*335, 1975

AOYAGI, F. *et al:* Operative method to correct saddle nose deformity, PRS, *56:*461, 1975. Jap. J. Plast. Reconstr. Surg., *17:*531, 1974

AOYAGI, F., FUJINO, T., AND OHSHIRO, T.: Detection of small vessels for microsurgery by Doppler flowmeter, PRS, *55:*372, 1975

APATENKO, A. K. *et al:* Glioma of nose. Arkh. Patol., *34:*72, 1972 (Russian)

Apert's Syndrome: See *Craniofacial Surgery*

APFELBERG, D. B. *et al:* Penetrating nasal trauma: report of unusual case and discussion of management. J. Trauma, *12:*821, 1972

APFELBERG, D. B., AND LARSON, S. J.: Dynamic anatomy of the ulnar nerve at the elbow, PRS, *51:*76, 1973

APFELBERG, D. B. *et al:* Funicular nerve grafting of the facial nerve. Surg. Forum., *24:*513, 1973

APFELBERG, D. B. *et al:* Treatment of chondritis in the burned ear by the local instillation of antibiotics, PRS, *53:*179, 1974

APFELBERG, D. B., AND GINGRASS, R. P.: Experimental funicular grafting of the facial nerve, PRS, *55:*195, 1975

APFELBERG, D. B. *et al:* Argon laser management of cutaneous vascular deformities. A preliminary report. West. J. Med., *124:*99, 1976

Apocrine Glands: See *Hyperhidrosis*

APPIANI SOTOMAYOR, E.: Esthetic approach for neck dissection, PRS, *49:*581, 1972. Prensa med. argent., *58:*1436, 1971

APPIANI SOTOMAYOR, E. *et al:* Reconstruction of the sternal wall for radionecrosis and cancer of said area. Prensa med. argent., *57:*789, 1971 (Spanish)

APPIANI SOTOMAYOR, E. *et al:* Diffusion factor for surgical edemas, PRS, *49:*585, 1972. Tribuna med. argent., *13:*B22, 1971

APTEKAR, R. G. *et al:* Metacarpophalangeal joint surgery in rheumatoid arthritis: long-term results. Clin. Orthop., *83:*123, 1972

APTEKAR, R. G. *et al:* Deforming non-erosive arthritis of the hand in systemic lupus erythematosus. Clin. Orthop., *100:*120, 1974

APTON, A. A.: Deformity due to heroin. Proc. Rudolph Virchow Med. Soc. City N.Y., *27:*19, 1968–69

APTON, A. A.: Surgical treatment of skin cancer. Proc. Rudolph Virchow Med. Soc. City N.Y., *111,* 1972–3

ARAI, K., AND FUKUDA, O.: Hand skin tube constructor, PRS, *49:*240, 1972. Jap. J. Plast. Reconstr. Surg., *14:*330, 1971

ARAI, K., FUKUDA, O., AND AKIYAMA, T.: Silicone mesh sheet as suspension material, PRS, *52:*463, 1973. Jap. J. Plast. Reconstr. Surg., *15:*447, 1972

ARAI, K. *et al:* Clinical application of collagen sheet as artificial skin (part one), PRS, *56:*365, 1975. Jap. J. Plast. Reconstr. Surg., *17:*405, 1974

ARAICO, J., VALDES, J. L., AND ORTIZ, J. M.: Internal wire splint for adduction contracture of the thumb, PRS, *48:*339, 1971

ARALBAEV, T. A.: Plastic surgery of skin in children. Sov. Zdravookhr. Kirg., *4:*58, 1973 (Russian)

ARANDES ADAN, R., AND PRATS ESTEVE, M.: Mammography, PRS, *48:*604, 1971. Barcelona Quirurgica, *15:*13, 1971

ARANHA, G. V.: Value of sinography in the management of decubitus ulcers (with Lopez), PRS, *53:*208, 1974

ARATA, J. *et al:* Dermatological evaluation of amikacin (BB-K8). Jpn. J. Antibiot., *27:*401, 1974 (Japanese)

ARBOUR, P.: Correction of post-traumatic saddle for middle third of nose. Can. J. Otolaryngol., *1:*304, 1972

ARBUZOV, S. N.: Recurrent keloid in the pedicle skin graft of the concha auriculae. Zdravookhr. Ross. Fed., *5:*111, 1974 (Russian)

ARCHER, W. HARRY: *Oral and Maxillofacial Surgery.* 5th edition. W. B. Saunders Co., Philadelphia, 1975

ARDEN, G. P., HARRISON, S. H., AND ANSELL, B. M.: Rheumatoid arthritis and surgical treatment, PRS, *48:*201, 1971. Brit. M.J., *4:* 604, 1970

ARDOUIN, M. *et al:* Injuries and pseudotumors of the orbit. Bull. Soc. Ophthalmol. Fr., *71:*744, 1971 (French)

ARENA, S.: Incisions. Laryngoscope, *85:*832, 1975

ARENS, J. F., LEJEUNE, F. E., AND WEBRE, D. R.: Maxillary sinusitis, complication of nasotracheal intubation, PRS, *54:*372, 1974. Anesthesiology, *40:*415, 1974

ARGAMASO, R. V.: Facial dimple: its formation by a simple technique, PRS, *48:*40, 1971

ARGAMASO, R. V.: Ear flaps. Eye Ear Nose Throat Mon., *51:*310, 1972

ARGAMASO, R. V.: Adjustable fascia lata sling for correction of blepharoptosis. Brit. J. Plast. Surg., *27:*274, 1974

ARGAMASO, R. V.: V-Y-S-plasty for closure of a round defect, PRS, *53:*99, 1974

ARGAMASO, R. V.: Rotation-transposition method for soft tissue replacement on distal segment of thumb, PRS, *54:*366, 1974

ARGAMASO, R. V.: An ideal donor site for the auricular composite graft. Brit. J. Plast. Surg., *28:*219, 1975

ARGAMASO, R. V. *et al:* Cross-leg flaps in children, PRS, *51:*662, 1973

ARIAGNO, R. P. *et al:* Chemexfoliation as an adjunct to facial rejuvenation. Trans. Am. Acad. Ophthalmol. Otolaryngol., *80:*536, 1975

ARIEL, I. M.: Extended radical groin dissection for melanomas of lower extremity, PRS, *48:*200, 1971. Surg. Gynec. & Obst., *132:*116, 1971

ARIEL, I. M.: Tridimensional resection of primary malignant melanoma. Surg. Gynec. Obst., *139:*601, 1974

ARIEL, I. M.: Results of treating malignant melanoma intralymphatically with radioactive isotopes. Surg. Gynec. & Obst., *139:*726, 1974

ARIEL, I. M.: Use of lymphangiography in melanoma, PRS, 56:113, 1975. Surgery, 76:654, 1974

ARIEL, I. M.: Tumors of connective tissue of skin. Rev. Surg., 32:153, 1975

ARIEL, I. M., AND CARON, A. S.: Diagnosis and treatment of malignant melanoma arising from skin of female breast, PRS, 51:347, 1973. Am. J. Surg., 124:384, 1972

ARIELY, E. et al: Maxillary resection prosthesis with magnetic connection to eye epithesis. Dtsch. Zahnaerztl. Z., 29:819, 1974 (German)

ARIENZA, B.: Mandibular prognathism. Rev. Asoc. Odontol. Argent., 59:12, 1971 (Spanish)

ARIENZA, B. et al: Upper maxillary protrusion. Surgical treatment. Ortodoncia, 37:143, 1973 (Spanish)

ARIFDZHANOV, A. K.: Method for the evaluation of the restoration of function of the soft palate following radical uranoplasty. Stomatologiia (Mosk.), 53:35, 1974 (Russian)

ARION, H. G.: Dynamic closure of lids in paralysis of *orbicularis* muscle, PRS, 50:629, 1972. Internat. Surg., 57:48, 1972

ARION, H. G.: On some mechanical properties of skin, PRS, 54:628, 1974. Ann. chir. plast., 19:37, 1974

ARIPOV, U. A. et al: Effect of autoantibodies on viability of autografts. Eksp. Khir. Anesteziol., 17:41, 1972 (Russian)

ARIT, N. et al: Cryo-sterilization of plastic implants. Zentralbl. Chir., 96:1131, 1971 (German)

ARIYAMITR, P. et al: Simple operation for correction of vaginal agenesis. J. Med. Assoc. Thai., 56:680, 1973

ARIYAN, S.: Severe acute radiation injuries of the hands (with Krizek), PRS, 51:14, 1973

ARIYAN, S. et al: Pseudohyperparathyroidism in head and neck tumors. Cancer, 33:159, 1974

ARIYAN, S., AND KRIZEK, T. J.: Tropical ulcers, PRS, 55:324, 1975

ARIYAN, S., AND GERSHON, R. K.: Role of BCG vaccination in producing tumor immunity, PRS, 56:430, 1975

ARLEN, M. et al: Chondrosarcoma of head and neck, PRS, 48:199, 1971. Am. J. Surg., 120:456, 1970

ARLEN, M. et al: Osseous metastasis: its relationship to primary carcinoma of head and neck. Am. J. Surg., 128:568, 1974

ARLON, H. G.: Covering of post-traumatic loss of cutaneous substance of the leg by cross legs, using a defatted flap, according to Colson's technic. Bull. Mem. Soc. Chir. Paris, 63:167, 1973 (French)

ARLOTTA, P. et al: Treatment of fracture of zygomatic arch by means of metallic osteo-synthesis. Rass. Int. Stomatol. Prat., 23:189, 1972 (Italian)

ARMA-SZLACHCIC, M. et al: Thiersch's graft used for shortening the healing process of leg ulcers. Dermatologica, 145:92, 1972 (German)

ARMSTRONG, D. et al: Torticollis: an analysis of 271 cases (Follow-Up Clinic), PRS, 49:565, 1972

ARMSTRONG, D. P., AND PETERS, A. S.: Cervical esophageal reconstruction after a laryngectomy and subtotal esophagectomy, PRS, 48:382, 1971

ARNAUD, A. et al: Extensive tracheal resection for post-tracheotomy stenosis or tumor. Postoperative radiological and functional study. Ann. Chir. Thorac. Cardiovasc., 13:73, 1974 (French)

ARNAUD, A. et al: Fractures of the orbital floor. Bull. Soc. Ophtalmol. Fr., 74:91, 1974 (French)

ARNERI, V.: Contraction of the hand in epidermolysis bullosa dystrophica and its surgical treatment. Med. Pregl., 28:451, 1975 (Serbian)

ARNERI, V.: Problem of surgical treatment of megaclitoris in cases of female hermaphroditism. Med. Pregl., 28:459, 1975 (Serbian)

ARNERI, V. et al: Our experiences in the treatment of skin hemangiomas. Vojnosanit. Pregl., 28:561, 1971 (Croatian)

ARNOLD, P. G., HARTRAMPF, C. R., AND JURKIEWICZ, M. J.: One-stage reconstruction of breast, using transposed greater omentum, PRS, 57:520, 1976

ARON, B. S. et al: Combination therapy in head and neck cancer. J.A.M.A., 233:177, 1975

ARONS, M. S.: Purposeful delay of the primary repair of cut flexor tendons in "some-man's-land" in children, PRS, 53:638, 1974. Discussion by Hartrampf, PRS, 54:95, 1974

ARONS, M. S., AND SAVIN, R. D.: Auricular cancer, some surgical and pathologic considerations, PRS, 51:607, 1973. Am. J. Surg., 122:770, 1971

ARONSOHN, R. B.: Complications of chemosurgery. Eye Ear Nose Throat Mon., 51:48, 1972

ARONSOHN, R. B.: Subcuticular closure in lower blepharoplasty. Eye Ear Nose Throat Mon., 51:143, 1972

AROUETE, M. J.: Correction of deep facial scars. Bull. Soc. Fr. Dermatol. Syphiligr., 78:498, 1971 (French)

ARRIGHI, E. et al: Lymphscrotum of filarial origin. Surgical treatment by lymphatico-venous fistula. Med. Trop. (Mars.), 32:305, 1972 (French)

ARRIGONI, G. et al: Reconstruction of the cheek in losses of substance caused by radionecrosis of the jaws. Rev. Stomatol. Chir. Maxillofac., *75:*224, 1974 (French)

ARSAC, M. *et al:* Successive bilateral cylindroma of parotid. Sem. Hop. Paris, *49:*2031, 1973 (French)

ARSENI, C. *et al:* Exophthalmic syndrome. Nosologic and neurosurgical considerations. Rev. Roum. Neurol., *7:*133, 1970

ARSENI, C. *et al:* Craniofacial mutilating injuries. Therapeutic problems. Rev. Chir. (Chir.), *23:*629, 1974 (Rumanian)

Arteries (See also *Carotid Arteries; Hands, Vascular Injuries; Maxillary Arteries*)

Balloon catheter tamponade of major vascular wounds (Smiley, Perry), PRS, *48:*515, 1971. Am. J. Surg., *121:*326, 1971

Femoral vessels, protection after groin dissection (Schweitzer), PRS, *49:*109, 1972. Am. J. Surg., *122:*223, 1971

Klippel-Trenaunay syndrome, congenital arteriovenous fistula and (Lindenauer), PRS, *50:*200, 1972. Ann. Surg., *174:*248, 1971

Femoral embolectomy, anterior tibial compartment syndrome complicating (Ransford, Provan), PRS, *48:*393, 1971. Canad. J. Surg., *14:*231, 1971

Coagulation, disseminated intravascular, and urologist (Seabaugh *et al),* PRS, *50:*540, 1972. J. Urol., *106:*267, 1971

Vascular graft, prosthetic, fibrosarcoma of thigh associated with (Herrmann *et al),* PRS, *48:*397, 1971. New England J. Med., *284:*91, 1971

Tourniquet, false aneurysm of ulnar artery after surgery employing a (Thio), PRS, *50:*540, 1972. Am. J. Surg., *123:*356, 1972

Aneurysms, arterial, of hand (Poirier, Stansel), PRS, *51:*230, 1973. Am. J. Surg., *124:*72, 1972

Allen's test, incorrect performance of ulnar artery flow erroneously presumed inadequate (Greenhow), PRS, *51:*603, 1973. Anesthesiology, *37:*356, 1972

Arterial repair failure, importance of venous occlusion in: an experimental study (Barcia, Nelson, Whelan), PRS, *50:*419, 1972. Ann. Surg., *175:*223, 1972

Muscle embolization, treatment of arteriovenous fistulas in cavernous hemangiomas of face (Bennett, Zook), PRS, *50:*84, 1972

Arteriovenous fistula, peripheral side to side (Hobson, Wright), PRS, *53:*606, 1974. Am. J. Surg., *126:*411, 1973

Arteriovenous fistulas, congenital, of head and neck (Coleman), PRS, *53:*489, 1974. Am. J. Surg., *126:*557, 1973

Aneurysm of radial artery, expanding, after

Arteries — Cont.

frequent puncture (Mathieu *et al*), PRS, *53:*245, 1974. Anesthesiology, *38:*401, 1973

Artery, facial, branches of (Mitz, Ricbourg, Lassau), PRS, *54:*500, 1974. Ann. chir. plast., *18:*339, 1973

Artery, prominent inferior labial (Howell, Freeman), PRS, *52:*678, 1973. Arch. Dermat. *107:*386, 1973

Head and neck, congenital arteriovenous fistulas of (Rappaport, Yim), PRS, *52:*454, 1973. Arch. Otolaryng., *97:*350, 1973

Fistulae, external carotid arteriovenous (Bruce, Walike, Goertzen), PRS, *54:*106, 1974. Arch. Otolaryng., *98:*332, 1973

Tibial compartment syndrome, anterior, following muscle hernia repair (Wolfort, Mogelvang, Fitzer), PRS, *52:*452, 1973. Arch. Surg., *106:*97, 1973

Femoral-axillary artery bypass for arm ischemia (Moseley, Porter), PRS, *52:*454, 1973. Arch. Surg., *106:*347, 1973

Aneurysms of hand (Kleinert, Burget, Morgan), PRS, *52:*595, 1973. Arch. Surg., *106:*554, 1973

Thigh injuries, massive, with vascular disruption: role of porcine skin grafting of exposed arterial vein grafts (Ledgerwood, Lucas), PRS, *53:*368, 1974. Arch. Surg., *107:*201, 1973

Thrombosis, arterial, possible link between smoking and; acute effect of cigarette smoking on platelet function (Levine), PRS, *53:*489, 1974. Circulation, *48:*619, 1973

Ergotamine, tongue necrosis attributed to, in temporal arteritis (Wolpaw, Brotten, Martin), PRS, *53:*241, 1974. J.A.M.A., *225:*514, 1973

Coagulation, disseminated intravascular (Barrocas), PRS, *52:*208, 1973. Mil. Med., *138:*9, 1973

Cancer, angiography in outlining solitary solid tumors of the head and neck (Mandel, Kiehn, Sykora), PRS, *52:*61, 1973

Carpal ganglion, radial artery occlusion by (Kelly), PRS, *52:*191, 1973

Thrombosis of ulnar arteries, bilateral, in hands (Eguro, Goldner), PRS, *52:*573, 1973

Vascular deficiency of upper extremity after arterial catheterization (Graham *et al*), PRS, *53:*487, 1974. Rev. Latino Am. cir. plast., *17:*37, 1973

Blood flow, limb, in congenital arteriovenous fistula (Yao *et al*), PRS, *52:*208, 1973. Surgery, *73:*80, 1973

Arterial occlusion following percutaneous femoral angiography, surgical management (Yellin, Shore), PRS, *52:*453, 1973.

Arteries — Cont.

Surgery, *73:*772, 1973

Doppler flowmeter to monitor traumatic arteriovenous fistula intraoperatively (Lichti, Erickson), PRS, *54:*505, 1974. Am. J. Surg., *127:*333, 1974

Coagulation, disseminated intravascular (Abando *et al*), PRS, *54:*239, 1974. Am. Surgeon, *40:*22, 1974

Vascular studies: thrombus formation in arterial and venous circulation in hypofibrinogenemic dogs (Olson), PRS, *55:*512, 1975. Europ. Surg., Res., *6:*176, 1974

Vessel repairs, evaluation of small-vessel flow (Wilgis *et al*), PRS, *55:*509, 1975. J. Bone & Joint Surg., *56A:*1199, 1974

Leg discrepancy, arteriovenous fistulae in management of (Kinmonth, Negus), PRS, *55:*249, 1975. J. Cardiovasc. Surg., *15:*447, 1974

Artery, subclavian, in head and neck surgery (Landa, Lesavoy), PRS, *55:*376, 1975. J. Maxillo-facial Surg., *2:*104, 1974

Vascular regeneration after different types of small bowel sutures (Juvara, Necula, Murgu), PRS, *54:*238, 1974. Lyon chir., *70:*52, 1974

Angiography, effect on arterial blood gases (Carden, Hubbard, Petty), PRS, *54:*692, 1974. Mil. Med., *141:*476, 1974

Zig-zag incision on a finger, importance of not damaging the volar digital arteries when using (Piggot, Black) (Letter to the Editor), PRS, *53:*80, 1974

Fistula, arteriovenous, spontaneous, arising from external carotid artery during pregnancy (Minami, Jafek, Cooper), PRS, *53:*230, 1974

Wrist, aneurysm of (Carneiro), PRS, *54:*483, 1974

Flowmeter, value in reconstructive arterial surgery (Cotton, Roberts), PRS, *55:*720, 1975. Proc. Roy Soc. Med., *67:*445, 1974

Claudication, rheological, importance of blood viscosity in (Dormandy, Hoare, Postelthwaite), PRS, *55:*720, 1975. Proc. Roy. Soc. Med., *67:*446, 1974

Artery, superficial temporal (Ricbourg, Mitz, Lassau), PRS, *57:*262, 1976. Ann. chir. plast., *20:*197, 1975

Juvenile temporal arteritis (Lie, Gordon, Titus), PRS, *57:*757, 1976. J.A.M.A., *234:*496, 1975

Femoral vessel protection with a de-epithelialized hypogastric flap (D'Hooghe, Hendrickx), PRS, *55:*87, 1975

Contracture, Dupuytren's, Doppler ultrasound detection of displaced neurovascular bundles in (Elsahy), PRS, *57:*104, 1976

ARTHUR, K., AND FARR, H. W.: Prognostic significance of histologic grade in epidermoid carcinoma of mouth and pharynx, PRS, *52:*102, 1972. Am. J. Surg., *124:*489, 1972

ARTSIMOVICH, N. G.: Immunological properties of preserved tissues, PRS, *55:*646, 1975. Acta chir. plast., *16:*96, 1974

ARTURSON, G.: Complete oxyhemoglobin dissociation curves in thermal trauma. Adv. Exp. Med. Biol., *33:*441, 1972

ARTURSON, G.: Maintenance of oxygen transport in severe thermal trauma, PRS, *53:*493, 1974. Riv. ital. chir. plast., *4:*32, 1973

ARTURSON, G., AND KHANNA, N. N.: Effects of hyperbaric oxygen, dimethyl sulfoxide, and Complamin on survival of experimental skin flaps, PRS, *49:*109, 1972. Scand. J. Plast. Reconstr. Surg., *4:*8, 1970

ARTURSON, G., AND PONTEN, B.: Effects of dimethyl sulfoxide (DMSO) on edema formation in experimental thermal trauma, PRS, *54:*696, 1974. Scand. J. Plast. Reconstr. Surg., *7:*74, 1973

ARTZ, C. P.: Changing concepts of electrical injury, PRS, *57:*538, 1976. Am. J. Surg., *128:*600, 1974

ARTZ, C. P.: What's new in burns? J. Med. Soc. N.J., *72:*1006, 1975

ARTZ, C. P., RITTENBURG, M. S., AND YARBROUGH, D. R.: Appraisal of allografts and xenografts as biological dressings for wounds and burns, PRS, *51:*236, 1973. Ann. Surg., *175:*934, 1972

ARTZ, C. P. *et al*: Topical burn wound therapy. Surg. Annu., *6:*349, 1974

ARTZ, T. D., AND POSCH, J. L.: Carpometacarpal boss, PRS, *53:*244, 1974. J. Bone & Joint Surg., *55A:*747, 1973

ARTZ, T. D., AND POSCH, J. L.: Use of cross-finger flap for treatment of congenital broad constricting bands of the fingers, PRS, *52:*645, 1973

ARZHANTSEV, P. Z.: Surgical interventions in the area of the temporomandibular joint. Voen. Med. Zh., *11:*23, 1971 (Russian)

ARZHANTSEV, P. Z.: Restoration of eyebrows with hairy flaps from chin using Filatov's flap. Voen. Med. Zh., *9:*38, 1974 (Russian)

ARZHANTSEV, P. Z.: New developments in plastic operations to close penetrating defects of face and neck using Filatov's tube flap. Voen. Med. Zh., *27:* July 1974 (Russian)

ARZHANTSEV, P. Z. *et al*: Surgical treatment of combined forms of bite anomalies in adults. Stomatologiia (Mosk.), *53:*38, 1974 (Russian)

ASAKURA, H. *et al*: Radiation therapy of keloids, PRS, *54:*118, 1974. Jap. J. Plast. Reconstr. Surg., *16:*496, 1973

ASCH, M., HUXTABLE, R., AND HAYS, D.: High

caloric parenteral therapy in infants and children, PRS, *50:*638, 1972. Arch. Surg., *104:*434, 1972

Asch, M. J. *et al*: Ocular complications associated with burns: review of five-year experience including 104 patients, PRS, *50:*205, 1972. J. Trauma, *11:*857, 1971

Asch, M. J. *et al*: Thermal injury involving bone: report of 32 cases. J. Trauma, *12:*135, 1972

Ascopa, H. S. *et al*: One stage correction of penile hypospadias using foreskin tube, PRS, *49:*104, 1972. Internat. Surg., *55:*435, 1971

Asensio, O: Variation of the rotation-advancement operation for repair of wide unilateral cleft lips, PRS, *53:*167, 1974. Discussions by Millard and Laub, PRS, *53:*340, 1974

Ashbell, T. S.: Storage of split-skin grafts on their donor sites (Letter to the Editor), PRS, *50:*178, 1972

Ashbell, T. S.: Exchange transfusion for flap surgery in sickle cell anemia, PRS, *51:*705, 1973. Surg. Forum, *23:*517, 1972

Ashbell, T. S. *et al*: Congenital malignant mesenchymoma of the face, PRS, *49:*348, 1972

Ashcraft, K. W. *et al*: Use of a one-way valve to aid in tracheostomy decannulation. J. Thorac. Cardiovasc. Surg., *64:*161, 1972

Ashken, M. H.: Personal experience with 37 Turner-Warwick scrotal inlay urethroplasties. Brit. J. Urol., *46:*313, 1974

Ashley, F.: Abdominal panniculectomy after massive weight loss (with Kamper, Galloway), PRS, *50:*441, 1972

Ashley, F. L.: Further studies on the natural-Y breast prosthesis, PRS, *49:*414, 1972

Ashley, F. L.: Silicone fluid injections for facial atrophy (with Rees, Delgado), PRS, *52:*118, 1973

Ashley, F. L.: Addendum to "Foreign body reactions to polyurethane covers of some breast prostheses," by Cocke *et al*, PRS, *56:*530, 1975

Ashley, F. L. Thompson, D. P., and Henderson, T.: Augmentation of surface contour by subcutaneous injections of silicone fluid, PRS, *51:*8, 1973

Ashley, F. L. *et al*: Preliminary investigation of peripheral nerve homograft storage technique, PRS, *52:*597, 1973. Rev. Latino Am. cir. plast., *14:*13, 1973

Ashworth, C., Williams, L. F., and Byrne, J. J.: Penetrating wounds of the neck. Reemphasis of the need for prompt exploration, PRS, *48:*612, 1971. Am. J. Surg., *121:*387, 1971

Askovitz, S. I.: Cancer of the tongue, results of treatment in 258 consecutive cases (with

Whitaker, Lehr), PRS, *50:*363, 1972

Aslamazova, V. I.: Contemporary viewpoints on tracheotomy. Vestn. Otorinolaringol., *33:*68, 1971 (Russian)

Associations: See *Societies*

Assor, D.: Bilateral carcinoma of parotid, one cancer arising in Warthin's tumor, PRS, *54:*234, 1974. Am. J. Clin. Path., *61:*270, 1974

Assor, D.: Epidermoid carcinoma with sebaceous differentiation in the vallecula. Report of a case. Am. J. Clin. Path., *63:*891, 1975

Astacio, J. N.: Papillary cystadenoma lymphomatosum associated with pleomorphic adenoma of parotid gland, PRS, *55:*507, 1975. Oral Surg., *38:*91, 1974

Astler, V. B.: Dr. Astler accepts the gavel, PRS, *56:*604, 1975. J. Florida M.A., *62:*32, 1975

Aston, S.: Effect of hematoma on thickness of pseudosheaths around silicone implants (with Williams, Rees), PRS, *56:*194, 1975

Aston, S. J., and Sparks, F. C.: Intraparotid neurilemmoma of facial nerve, PRS, *57:*116, 1976. Arch. Surg., *110:*757, 1975

Astrand, P.: Chewing efficiency before and after surgical correction of developmental deformities of jaws. Sven. Tandlak. Tidskr., *67:*135, 1974

Astrand, P. *et al*: Oblique sliding osteotomy of the mandibular rami in 55 patients with mandibular prognathism. Int. J. Oral Surg., *2:*89, 1973

Astrand, P., and Ericson, S.: Relation between fragments after oblique sliding osteotomy of mandibular rami and its influence on postoperative conditions, PRS, *55:*508, 1975. Int. J. Oral Surg., *3:*49, 1974

Astrup, P. *et al*: Moderate hypoxia exposure and fetal development, PRS, *56:*114, 1975. Arch. Environmental Health, *30:*15, 1975

Astvatsaturov, K. R. *et al*: Moscow therapeutic cosmetics clinic. The main stages of its practical and scientific and research activities. Vestn. Dermatol. Venerol., *46:*72, 1972 (Russian)

Ataisov, N. I. *et al*: General anesthesia in the active surgical management of the severely burned. Ortop. Travmatol. Protez., *0:*40, 1974 (Russian)

Atanasescu, I. *et al*: Results of exploratory fasciotomy of leg in predominantly venous edema. Chirurgia (Bucur.), *21:*429, 1972 (Rumanian)

Atanasov, A. K.: Indications for using direct blood transfusions in burns. Vrach. Delo., *7:*73, 1971 (Russian)

Atherton, J. D.: The natural history of the bilateral cleft. Angle. Orthod., *44:*269, 1974

ATHERTON, J. D. *et al*: Experimental surgical reduction of mandible of pig. Am. J. Orthod., *65:*158, 1974

ATHERTON, J. D., LOVIUS, B. B. J., AND MAISELS, D. O.: Growth of bony palate of pig consequent to transpositioning oral and nasal mucoperiosteum, PRS, *56:*110, 1975. Cleft Palate J., *11:*429, 1974

ATIASOV, N. I.: Use of venous bed of bones for multiple transfusion of blood and other fluids in patients with extensive burns. Probl. Gematol. Pereliv. Krovi., *16:*53, 1971 (Russian)

ATIASOV, N. I.: Experience with development and use of dermatomic dermatoplasty in burn patients. Ortop. Travmatol. Protez., *33:*64, 1972 (Russian)

ATIASOV, N. I. *et al*: Treatment of electric burns. Vestn. Khir., *111:*90, 1973 (Russian)

ATKINSON, K. B. *et al*: A note on volume determination in connexion with reconstructive surgery. In *Biostereometrics 74,* ed. Herron; Falls Church, Va.; Am. Soc. Photogrammetry, 1974, pp. 161-71

ATLAN, G. *et al*: Influence of tracheotomy or intubation cannulas on ventilatory work. Sem. Hop. Paris, *48:*2979, 1972 (French)

ATTENBOROUGH, N. R.: Recurrence of an odontogenic keratocyst in a bone graft: report of a case. Brit. J. Oral Surg., *12:*33, 1974

ATTIC, J. N., KHAFIF, R. A., AND STECKLER, R. M.: Elective neck dissection in papillary carcinoma of thyroid, PRS, *51:*702, 1973. Am. J. Surg., *122:*464, 1971

AUBRY, G. *et al*: Inclusion of windshield fragments in tegument and soft tissue of face. Rev. Stomatol. Chir. Maxillofac., *73:*575, 1972 (French)

AUDRETSCH, W.: Ultrasonic diagnosis of breast prosthesis implanted after operative treatment of tumors or augmentation (plastic) of the breast. Geburtshilfe Frauenheilkd., *35:*853, 1975 (German)

AUER, A. I. *et al*: Surgery for necrotic bites of brown spider. Arch. Surg., *108:*612, 1974

AUERBACH, R.: Letter: basal cell carcinoma. N.Y. State J. Med., *75:*2326, 1975

AUERBACH, R. AND PEARLSTEIN, H. H.: Treatment of baldness by hair transplantation. J.M. Soc. New Jersey, *70:*119, 1973

AUERBACH, R. *et al*: Ulcerative radiation dermatitis secondary to radon seeds. N.Y. State J. Med., *73:*2183, 1973

AUFRICHT, G.: Discussion of "A modified Aufricht reduction mammaplasty," by Meijer, PRS, *53:*132, 1974

AUGER, C. *et al*: Unusual histological appearance of a tumor of the palm of the hand (mixed tumor of the sweat glands?). Union. Med. Can., *102:*1973 (French)

AUGUST, G. P., CHANDRA, R., AND HUNG, W.: Prepubertal male gynecomastia, PRS, *52:*679, 1973. J. Pediat., *80:*259, 1972

AUGUST, P. J.: Cutaneous necrosis due to cetrimide application, PRS, *57:*127, 1976. Brit. M.J., *1:*70, 1975

AURIAT, J. *et al*: Surgical treatment of anterior tumors of floor of mouth. Ann. Otolaryngol. Chir. Cervicofac., *90:*648, 1973 (French)

Auricle: See *Ear*

AUSIN GARCIA, A., AND BERMUDEZ PIERNAGORDA, M.: Eyebrow reconstruction, buried graft method, PRS, *56:*590, 1975. Rev. españ. cir. plast., *6:*97, 1973

AUSTERMANN, K. H. *et al*: Influence of tongue asymmetries on the development of jaws and the position of teeth. Int. J. Oral Surg., *3:*261, 1974

AUSTIN, R. T.: Tracheostomy and prolonged intubation in the management of trauma. Injury, *2:*191, 1971

AUSTIN, T. A., AND TAMLYN, R. S. P.: Ketamine — revolutionary anesthetic agent for battle casualty, PRS, *53:*615, 1974. J. Roy. Army M. Corps, *18:*15, 1972

AUSTIN, W.: Eye complications with blepharoplasty or other eyelid surgery (with DeMere, Wood), PRS, *53:*634, 1974

AUVINEN, O. *et al*: Pharyngo-esophageal diverticula. Duodecim, *90:*1124, 1974 (Finnish)

AVAKOFF, J. C.: Dorsal nasal flap (Letter to the Editor), PRS, *53:*671, 1974

AVAKOFF, J. C. *et al*: Reconstruction of traumatic losses of external ear. South. Med. J., *65:*1471, 1972

AVELLAN, L.: The incidence of hypospadias in Sweden. Scand. J. Plast. Reconstr. Surg., *9:*129, 1975

AVIADO, D. M.: Regulation of bronchomotor tone during anesthesia, PRS, *57:*768, 1976. Anesthesiology, *42:*68, 1975

AVILA LOZADA, A. *et al*: Nasal surgery in childhood, clinical evaluation through 43 cases. Bol. Med. Hosp. Infant. Mex., *31:*799, 1974 (Spanish)

AVILES, E: Rhabdomyosarcoma of orbit, PRS, *55:*245, 1975. Internat. Surg., *59:*297, 1974

AVILES, E.: Management of pharyngoesophagostoma. Laryngoscope, *84:*317, 1974

AVILES, E., ARLEN, M., AND MILLER, T.: Plantar fibromatosis, PRS, *48:*295, 1971. Surgery, *69:*117, 1971

AWTY, M. D.: Removal of a large shell fragment from the nasopharynx. Oral Surg., *33:*513, 1972

AWTY, M. D. *et al*: Review of the treatment of facial injuries in the Nigerian Civil War. Trans. Int. Conf. Oral Surg., *4:*291, 1973

Axilla: See *Burn Contractures, Hidradenitis, Hyperhidrosis*

AYATS, J. P. *et al*: Facial deformity — surgical treatment. Trans. Int. Conf. Oral Surg., *4:*345, 1973

AYIM, F. N.: Tracheostomy dependence in children. Review of ten cases. East Afr. Med. J.: *49:*830, 1972

AYLIFFE, G. A. J. *et al*: *Pseudomonas aeruginosa* in hospital sinks, PRS, *55:*253, 1975. Lancet, *2:*578, 1974

AYTEMIZ, C. *et al*: Extramucous rhinoplasty, PRS, *57:*114, 1976. Bull. Milit. M. Acad., *16:*299, 1974

AZAZ, B. AND SHTEYER. A.: Dentigerous cysts associated with second mandibular bicuspids in children: report of 5 cases. J. Dent. Child., *40:*29, 1973

AZAZ, B., AND LUSTMAN, J.: Keratoacanthoma of lower lip, PRS, *56:*234, 1975. Oral Surg., *38:*918, 1974

AZEVEDO, N. *et al*.: Neuroleptoanalgesia in oncological surgery of the head and neck. Rev. Bras. Anestesiol., *22:*68, 1972 (Portugese)

AZIA, A. M., WEINBERG, B., AND CHALIAN, V. A.: Speech intelligibility following prosthetic obturation of surgically acquired maxillary defects, PRS, *55:*257, 1975. J. Prosth. Dent., *32:*87, 1974

AZNABAEV, M. T.: Forceps for the fixation of muscles elevating the upper eyelid in correction of blepharoptosis. Oftalmol. Zh., *28:*309, 1974 (Russian)

AZOLOV, V. V.: Certain problems of planning of surgical interventions on the hand and fingers in complications of burns and frostbite. Ortop. Travmatol. Protez., *34:*39, 1973 (Russian)

AZZOLINI, A., AND MANGIANTE, P.: On development of primary palate and nose in man, PRS, *49:*359, 1972. Rev. Ital. chir. plast., *3:*1, 1971

AZZOLINI, A., AND NOUVENNE, R.: Vascular hamartomata of masticatory muscles, PRS, *51:*107, 1973. Riv. ital. chir. plast., *3:*135, 1971

B

BA, J. *et al*: Esophagoplasty and labor. Orv. Hetil., *115:*2688, 1974 (Hungarian)

BAAB, G. H. *et al*: Malignant melanoma: the patient with an unknown site of primary origin. Arch. Surg., *110:*896, 1975

BABAEV, T. A.: Closure of perforations of the floor of the maxillary sinus. Stomatologiia (Mosk.), *51:*61, 1972 (Russian)

BABAIANTS, R. A.: Combined closure of open

defects of pharynx and cervical portion of esophagus by local tissues and Filatov's tube. Vestn. Otorinolaringol., *35:*96 1973 (Russian)

BABALANTS, R. S. *et al*: Clinical characteristics of skin cancer and comparative characteristics of different methods of its treatment at remote periods. Vestn. Dermatol. Venerol., *47:*3, 1973 (Russian)

BABENKO, Iu. S. *et al*: Comparative evaluation of the efficacy of antibiotics in the treatment of purulent infections of soft tissues of hands and fingers. Antibiotiki., *18:*844, 1973 (Russian)

BACHELOT, F. *et al*: Neoplasms of the floor of the mouth. Analysis of 70 cases. Sem. Hop. Paris, *48:*1413, 1972 (French)

BACHVAROFF, R., BROWNE, L. R., AND RAPAPORT, F. T.: Erythrocyte changes in severe thermal injury, PRS, *51:*706, 1973. Surg. Forum, *23:*502, 1972

BACIU, C. *et al*: Lumbrical plus syndrome. Rev. Chir. Orthop., *61:*153, 1975 (French)

BACK, S. *et al*: Plasma expansion in surgical patients with high central venous pressure (CVP); relationship of blood volume to hematocrit, CVP, pulmonary wedge pressure, and cardiorespiratory changes, PRS, *57:*407, 1976. Surgery, *78:*304, 1975

BACKHOUSE, K. M.: Extensor expansion of the rheumatoid hand. Ann. Rheum. Dis., *31:*112, 1972

BACKHOUSE, K. M. Surgery of some strictures and stenoses. Some tunnel syndromes. Compression problems in the hand. Ann. R. Coll. Surg. Engl., *50:*321, 1972

BACKHOUSE, K. M.: Innervation of hand, PRS, *57:*760, 1976. Hand, *7:*107, 1975

BACKHOUSE, K. M., AND CHURCHILL-DAVIDSON, D.: Anomalous *palmaris longus* muscle producing carpal tunnel-like compression, PRS, *56:*596, 1975. Hand, *7:*22, 1975

BACKSTROM, A. *et al*: Postoperative complications after combined treatment for carcinoma of tongue. Arch. Klin. Exp. Ohren Nasen Kehlkopfheilkd., *201:*273, 1972

BACKSTROM, A. *et al*: Prognosis of squamous cell carcinoma of gums with cytologically verified cervical lymph node metastases. J. Laryng. & Otol., *89:*391, 1975

BADACH-ROGOWSKI, W. *et al*: Skin grafting in the emergency management of a crushed hand with extensive skin defects. Chir. Narzadow. Ruchu Ortop. Pol., *37:*463, 1972 (Polish)

BADDELEY, H.: Kaposi's sarcoma, PRS, *55:*724, 1975. Proc. Roy. Soc. Med., *67:*866, 1974

BADEN, E. *et al*: Odontogenic gingival epithelial hamartoma: case report. J. Oral Surg., *31:*932, 1973

BADEN, M. *et al*: Upper airway obstruction in newborn, secondary to hemangiopericytoma. Can. Med. Assoc. J., *107*:1202, 1972

BADGER, G. A. *et al*: Desmoplastic fibroma of the mandible. Can. J. Otolaryngol., *3*:605, 1974

BADIM, J.: Guidelines for treatment of skin cancer, PRS, *57*:265, 1976. Rev. Col. bras. Cir., *1*:66, 1974

BADIM, J. *et al*: Gynecomastia, PRS, *51*:103, 1973. Rev. brasil. cir., *61*:141, 1971

BADIM, J. *et al*: Hypothenar region as donor area for lesions of fingertip volar surface, PRS, *53*:498, 1974. Rev. brasil. cir., *62*:163, 1973

BADIM, J., LESSA, S. F., AND CARREIRAO, S. E.: Marjolin's ulcer, PRS, *57*:125, 1976. Rev. Col. bras. Cir., *1*:261, 1974

BADOWSKI, A. *et al*: Case of sarcoma phylloides of the breast. Wiad. Lek., *28*:217, 1975 (Polish)

BAFNA, P. L., PANDE, S. K., AND BAID, J. C.: Replacement of soft tissue loss of distal phalanx of index finger, PRS, *55*:379, 1975. Indian J. Plast. Surg., *7*:23, 1974

BAGEANT, T. E., AND PETTY, W. C.: Ketamine and oxyhemoglobin dissociation curve, PRS, *53*:694, 1974. Anesth. & Analg., *52*:905, 1973)

BAGELY, D. H., JR. *et al*: Late Flavobacterium species meningitis after craniofacial exenteration. Arch. Intern. Med., *136*:229, 1976

BAGENYI, J. *et al*: Report on partial necrosis of tongue caused by endotracheal tube. Anaesthetist, *24*:136, 1975 (German)

BAGI, I.: Tooth reimplantation and transplantation problems in one of our own cases. Orv. Hetil., *115*:1110, 1974 (Hungarian)

BAGLEY, D. H., JR., *et al*: Effects of cryosurgery on facial nerve in monkeys. Surg. Forum, *24*:514, 1973

BAGSHAWE, K. D.: Chemotherapy; next decade, PRS, *55*:644, 1975. Proc. Roy. Soc. Med., *67*:745, 1974

BAHN, S. L.: Use of Scialom pins for fracture fixation. J. Oral Surg., *33*:268, 1975

BAHR, R. *et al*: Diagnosis and therapy of gas phlegmon. Med. Klin., *69*:859, 1974 (German)

BAIANBELEG, D.: Blood vessels of the human palmar aponeurosis. Arkh. Anat. Gistol. Embriol., *62*:82, 1972 (Russian)

BAILEY, B. H. *et al*: Rhabdomyosarcoma of maxillary sinus. Trans. Am. Acad. Ophthalmol. Otolaryngol., *76*:1375, 1972

BAILEY, B. J. *et al*: Olfactory neuroblastoma. Management and prognosis. Arch. Otolaryng., *101*:1, 1975

BAILEY, B. N.: Dermal arthroplasty. Hand, *3*:135, 1971

BAILEY, B. N.: Skin cover in hand injuries, PRS, *48*:606, 1971. Injury, *2*:294, 1971

BAILEY, B. N.: Surgical closure of sacral scores, PRS, *49*:475, 1972. Proc. Roy. Soc. Med., *64*:1148, 1971

BAILEY, B. N.: Composite reconstruction of the mandible and temporomandibular joint, following hemimandibulectomy (with Ho, Sykes), PRS, *53*:414, 1974

BAILEY, B. N. *et al*: Surgery of the hand in rheumatoid arthritis. Mod. Trends Rheumatol., *2*:240, 1971

BAILEY, B. N., AND DESAI, S. N.: Approach to treatment of hand burns, PRS, *53*:608, 1974. Injury, *4*:335, 1973

BAILLIE, E. E. *et al*: Glandular (seromucinous) hamartoma of the nasopharynx. Oral Surg., *38*:760, 1974

BAIROV, G. A.: Reconstructive plastic surgery in bladder exstrophy in newborn. Vestn. Khir., *97*:85, 1966 (Russian)

BAJARDI, A. *et al*: Tegumentary repair of lesions of the hand. Minerva Ortop., *20*:14, 1969 (Italian)

BAKAMJIAN, V. Y.: Technique for primary reconstruction of the palate after radical maxillectomy for cancer (Follow-Up Clinic), PRS, *49*:335, 1972

BAKAMJIAN, V. Y.: Surgical management of cancers of cheek J. Surg. Oncol., *6*:255, 1974

BAKAMJIAN, V. Y. *et al*: Concept of cure and palliation by surgery in advanced cancer of head and neck, PRS, *53*:688, 1974. Am. J. Surg., *126*:482, 1973

BAKAMJIAN, V. Y., AND HOLBROOK, L. A.: Prefabrication techniques in cervical pharyngoesophageal reconstruction, PRS, *55*:107, 1975. Brit. J. Plast. Surg., *26*:214, 1973

BAKAMJIAN, V. Y., AND SOUTHER, S. G.: Use of temporal muscle flap for reconstruction after orbito-maxillary resections for cancer, PRS, *56*:171, 1975

BAKER, B. B.: Nevus sebaceous of Jadassohn, PRS, *57*:403, 1976. Arch. Otolaryng., *101*:515, 1975

BAKER, B. B. *et al*: Succinylcholine-induced hyperkalemia and cardiac arrest. Arch. Otolaryng., *96*:464, 1972

BAKER, D. C., AND WEISMAN, B.: Post-irradiation carcinoma of larynx, PRS, *50*:310, 1972. Ann. Otol. Rhin. & Laryng., *80*:634, 1971

BAKER, D. C. JR. *et al*: Decannulation problems in infants. Ann. Otol. Rhin. & Laryng., *81*:555, 1972

BAKER, H. W.: Head and neck surgery: the pursuit of excellence. Am. J. Surg., *122*:433, 1971

BAKER, H. W.: Surgical management of oral cancer. Proc. Natl. Cancer Conf., 7:133, 1973

BAKER, J. L., JR., AND O'MALLEY, J. E.: Simplified splint for precise immobilization of mandible, PRS, 48:598, 1971

BAKER, J. L., JR., KOLIN, I. S., AND BARTLETT, E. S.: Psychosexual dynamics of patients undergoing mammary augmentation, PRS, 53:652, 1974

BAKER, J. L., JR., MARA, J. E., AND DOUGLAS, W. M.: Repair of concavity of thoracic wall with silicone elastomer implant. PRS, 56:212, 1975

BAKER, J. M.: Molten plastic injuries of hand (Follow-Up Clinic), PRS, 52:81, 1973

BAKER, S. P. et al: Recurrent problems in emergency room management of maxillofacial injuries. Clin. Plast. Surg., 2:65, 1975

BAKER, T. J., GORDON, H. L., AND WHITLOW, D. R.: Our present technique for rhytidectomy, PRS, 52:232, 1973

BAKER, T. J. et al: Long-term histological study of after chemical face peeling, PRS, 53:522, 1974

BAKIN, K. M.: Dacryocystorhinostomy using trephine-cutter and surgical brace. Oftalmol. Zh., 28:552, 1973 (Russian)

BAKIN, L. M.: Modification of dacryocystorhinostomy. Vestn. Oftalmol., 6:69, 1974 (Russian)

BAKIR, A. et al: Cylindromas of salivary glands. Bull. Cancer (Paris), 61:501, 1974 (French)

BAKSA, J. et al: Use of mesh dermatome in surgical treatment of thermal injuries in children. Orv. Hetil., 115:1347, 1974 (Hungarian)

BALABANOW, K. et al: Epidermolysis bullosa hereditaria dystrophica with severe mutilations in two girls. Hautarzt, 22:450, 1971 (German)

BALAN, E. H.: Pre- and postoperative documentation in orthopedic jaw surgery with special reference to prognathism. Fortschr. Kiefer. Gesichtschir., 18:124, 1974 (German)

BALAS, P.: Replantation of amputated extremities. Necessity for re-evaluation. Vasc. Surg., 7:1, 1973

BALAZS, G. et al: Surgical aspects of treatment of thyroid neoplasms following radiotherapy. Zentralbl. Chir., 98:1842, 1973 (German)

BALCHEV, G.: New procedure for the surgical treatment of pectus excavatus and pectus carinatus with a contribution of 26 case reports. Nauchni. Tr. Vssh. Med. Inst. Sofiia, 50:39, 1971

BALDAU, K. et al: On therapy planning in malignant melanoma. Radiobiol. Radiother. (Berl.), 16:51, 1975 (German)

Baldness: See Alopecia

BALDRIDGE, M.: Aberrant lacrimal gland in orbit, PRS, 48:293, 1971. Arch. Ophth., 84:758, 1970

BALES, C. R., RANDALL, P., AND LEHR, H. B.: Fractures of facial bones in children, PRS, 52:97, 1973. J. Trauma, 12:56, 1972

BALES, H. W.: Tissue transfers for functional reconstruction in thoracic surgery (with Cervino, Emerson), PRS, 54:437, 1974

BALKIN, S. W.: Treatment of corns by injectable silicone, PRS, 57:543, 1976. Arch. Dermat., 111:1143, 1975

BALLANTYNE, A. J.: Malignant melanoma of skin of head and neck, PRS, 48:200, 1971. Am. J. Surg., 120:425, 1970

BALLANTYNE, A. J.: Methods of repair after surgery for cancer of the pharyngeal wall, postcricoid area, and cervical esophagus. Am. J. Surg., 122:482, 1971

BALLANTYNE, A. J. et al: Surgical management of irradiation failures of nonfixed cancers of glottic region. Am. J. Roentgenol. Radium Ther. Nucl. Med. 120:164, 1974

BALLANTYNE, D. L., JR. et al: Circulating platelet levels in rat during rejection of xenogeneic skin. Thromb. Res., 4:177, 1974

BALLARD, R. et al: Synovial chondromatosis of temporomandibular joint. Cancer, 30:791, 1972

BALLEN, P. H. et al: Self-illuminating orbital retractor. Trans. Am. Acad. Ophthalmol. Otolaryngol., 76:519, 1972

BALLERSTAEDT, H.: Case demonstration: superficially spreading melanoma with nodous constituent. Z. Hautkr., 49:581, 1974 (German)

BALLIN, J. C.: In burns, another bug barricade, PRS, 57:401, 1976. Emerg. Med., 7:59, 1975

BALLINGER, WALTER F., AND DRAPANAS, THEODORE: Practice of Surgery. Current Review Volume II. C. V. Mosby Co., St. Louis, 1975. PRS, 57:374, 1976

BALNER, HANS, VAN BAKKUM, D. W., AND RAPAPORT, FELIX T.: Transplantation Today, Third Congress. Grune & Stratton, New York, 1971. PRS, 49:205, 1972

BALOGH, G.: Phlogosol therapy in inflammations of the oral mucosa. Ther. Hung., 22:83, 1974

BALOGH, G. et al: Recurrent mandibular myxoma. Fogorv. Sz., 65:116, 1972 (Hungarian)

BALON, L. R.: Use of free transplantation of previously cooled auricles of the external ear and local plastic surgery to replace defects in the nasal dorsum, apex, alae and septum. Vestn. Khir., 106:63, 1971 (Russian)

BALON, L. R.: Method of repairing defects and deformities of the nasal septum with free grafts of the concha auriculae. Vestn. Khir., *107*:80, 1971 (Russian)

BALON, L. R. *et al*: New principle of production of obturating apparatus in gaping defects of the esophagus and pharynx. Vestn. Khir., *115*:108, 1975 (Russian)

BALUYOT, S. T., JR., *et al*: Pre-irradiation tattooing. Arch. Otolaryng., *96*:151, 1972

BAMBER, D. B., RATCLIFFE, R., AND MCEWAN, T. E.: Clinical forum, ketamine for outpatient dental conservation in children, PRS, *53*:373, 1974. Anaesthesia, *28*:446, 1973

BANACH, J.: Usefulness of surgical diathermy for removal of abnormal attachment of labial frenum. Czas. Stomatol., *27*:405, 1974 (Polish)

BANDO, M.: Clinical review of patient with facial pachydermatocele in von Recklinghausen's disease, PRS, *52*:457, 1973. Jap. J. Plast. Reconstr. Surg., *15*:366, 1972

BANDO, M., FUKUDA, O., AND SOEDA, S.: Problems of free composite graft, PRS, *52*:461, 1973. Jap. J. Plast. Reconstr. Surg., *15*:420, 1972

BANDTLOW, O.: Diabetes mellitus causing facial palsy. Laryngol. Rhinol. Otol. (Stuttg.), *53*:661, 1974 (German)

BANGERTER, A.: Ophthalmological report to wound treatment of eyelids, PRS, *48*:194, 1971. Chir. Plast. et Reconstr., *6*:151, 1969

BANKS, P.: Incompetence of larynx: unusual postoperative complication. Brit. J. Oral Surg., *11*:94, 1973

BANKS, P.: Fixation of facial fractures. Current concepts. Brit. Dent. J., *138*:129, 1975

BANKS, P. *et al*: Method of localization and fixation for mid-facial osteotomies. Brit. J. Oral Surg., *12*:263, 1975

BANKS, P., AND MACKENZIE, I.: Condylotomy, clinical and experimental appraisal of surgical technique, PRS, *57*:531, 1976. J. Maxillofacial Surg., *3*:170, 1975

BANKS, P. *et al*: Criteria for condylotomy: a clinical appraisal of 211 cases. Proc. Roy. Soc. Med., *68*:601, 1975

BANOCZY, J. *et al*: Comparative study of the clinical picture and histopathologic structure of oral leukoplakia. Cancer, *29*:1230, 1972

BANOCZY, J. *et al*: Late results of periodontal surgical interventions. Fogorv. Sz., *67*:321, 1974 (Hungarian)

BANQUER DE BORELLO, E.: Treatment of peripheral facial paralysis and post-parotidectomy with ACTH-GEL. Report of 17 cases. Rev. Assoc. Odontol. Argent., *61*:5, 1973 (Spanish)

BANZET, P.: Digital gigantism. Ann. Chir., *25*:965, 1971 (French)

BANZET, P., DUFOURMENTEL, C., AND PAILHERET, J. P.: Clinical experience with chemo-

therapy in treatment of nevocarcinomas, PRS, *50*:636, 1972. Acta chir. belg., *70*:401, 1971

BANZET, P. *et al*: Present concepts of the treatment of malignant melanoma. Acta chir. belg., *74*:395, 1975 (French)

BANZET, P. *et al*: Melanotic tumours of the hand. Hand, *7*:183, 1975

BAPAT, C. V. *et al*: Preliminary report on acceleration of wound healing by amnion membrane graft. Indian. J. Med. Res., *62*:1342, 1974

BARABAN, M. R.: Student watches plastic surgery. New England J. Med., *288*:637, 1973

BARABAS, Z. *et al*: Mercury as foreign body in the hand. Magy. Traumatol. Orthop., *15*:299, 1972

BARACHINI, P.: Basal cell epithelioma on a burn cicatrix. G. Ital. Dermatol., *47*:26, 1972

BARADULINA, M. G. *et al*: Prophylactic removal of lymph nodes and cellular tissue of the neck in patients with laryngeal and laryngopharyngeal cancer. Vestn. Otorinolaringol., *33*:55, 1971 (Russian)

BARAKAT, N. J.: Leukoplakia of tongue treated by vermilionectomy. Rev. Dent. Liban., *21*:47, 1971

BARAKAT, N. J.: Extravasation cysts: case reports. Rev. Dent. Liban., *23*:59, 1973

BARAKAT, N. J.: Intermaxillary and internal wiring fixation. Review of techniques and report of cases. Rev. Dent. Liban., *24*:39, 1974

BARAN, N. K. *et al*: Growth potential of grafts, flaps, and tubes. Surg. Forum, *22*:481, 1971

BARAN, N. K., AND HORTON, C. E.: Growth of skin grafts, flaps, and scars in young mini-pigs, PRS, *50*:487, 1972

BARANCZAK, Z. *et al*: Results of surgical treatment of lateral occlusion by way of mandibular ramus osteotomy. Czas. Stomatol., *27*:1199, 1974 (Polish)

BARANCZAK, Z. *et al*: Analysis of morphological and functional conditions of the temporomandibular joints prior to and following treatment of prognathism. Czas. Stomatol., *28*:159, 1975 (Polish)

BARBA, M. *et al*: Effect of lidocaine on antibacterial activity of 7 antibiotics, PRS, *55*:647, 1975. Arch. Ophth., *92*:514, 1974

BARBARELLI, J. J. A.: Surgical treatment of gynecomastia, PRS, *53*:242, 1974. Prensa med. argent., *59*:1188, 1972

BARBOSA, JORGE FAIRBANKS: *Surgical Treatment of Head and Neck Tumors*. Grune & Stratton, New York, 1974. PRS, *57*:509, 1976

BARCAT, J. *et al*: Late results of Coffey's operation for bladder exstrophy in 10 cases. Ann. Chir. Infant., *12*:615, 1971 (French)

BARCIA, P. J., NELSON, T. G., AND WHELAN, T. J.: Importance of venous occlusion in arterial repair failure: experimental study, PRS, 50:419, 1972. Ann. Surg., 175:223, 1972

BARCLAY, S.: Letter: Cricopharyngeus. N. Z. Med. J., 80:314, 1974

BARDACH, J.: Use of pedunculated frontal flaps for rhinoplasty. Dtsch. Stomatol., 21:625, 1971 (German)

BARDACH, J. et al: Necrosis of scalp caused by perhydrol burns. Pol. Przegel. Chir., 46:559, 1974 (Polish)

BARDIN, J. et al: Tracheal healing following tracheostomy. Surg. Forum, 25:210, 1974

BARFOD, B.: Reconstruction of the nail fold. Hand, 4:85, 1972

BARFOD, B.: Reconstruction of nail fold, PRS, 52:594, 1973. Rev. Latino Am. cir. plast., 17:59, 1973

BARGA, J. L.: How to treat nosebleed, PRS, 53:602, 1974. Am. Fam. Phys., 8:66, 1973

BARINGER, J. R., AND SWOVELAND, P.: Recovery of herpes-simplex virus from human trigeminal ganglions, PRS, 52:321, 1973. New England J. Med., 288:648, 1973

BARINKA, L.: Management of case of true hermaphroditism with negative sex chromatin and an idiogram 46-XY. Brit. J. Plast. Surg., 25:427, 1972

BARINKA, L.: Present state of surgical treatment of lymphedemas of lower extremities. Acta Chir. Orthop. Traumatol. Cech., 41:557, 1974 (Czech)

BARINKA, L. et al: Artificial joints in experiments, PRS, 53:500, 1974. Acta chir. plast., 15:104, 1973

BARISONI, D.: Problem of infections and "open air" treatment of extensive burns. Fracastoro., 64:5, 1971

BARISONI, D. et al: Changes of immunoglobulin levels in burned patients, PRS, 56:360, 1975. Riv. ital. chir. plast., 5:319, 1973

BARKER, D. E.: Prevention of bleeding following a rhytidectomy, PRS, 54:651, 1974

BARKER, D. E.: Costs and charges for use of office operating room, PRS, 57:7, 1976

BARKER, D. J. et al: Buruli disease and patients' activities. East Afr. Med. J., 49:260, 1972

BARKER, HAROLD G.: The Continuing Education of the Surgeon. Charles C Thomas, Springfield, Ill., 1971. PRS, 48:590, 1971

BARKHASH, S. A. et al: Surgical treatment of ptosis complicated by synkinesis. Oftalmol. Zh., 27:567, 1973

BARKHAS, S. A. et al: Dacryocystorhinostomy in children by modification of Taumy's method. Oftalmol. Zh., 28:177, 1973 (Russian)

BARKLEY, H. T. et al: Management of cervical lymph node metastases in squamous cell carcinoma of tonsillar fossa, base of tongue, supraglottic larynx and hypopharynx, PRS, 52:103, 1973. Am. J. Surg., 124:462, 1972

BARLETTA, L. P. A.: Surgery of nasal pyramid and septum in one stage, combined rhinoplasty, PRS, 50:418, 1972. Prensa méd. argent., 59:112, 1972

BARLOVIC, M.: Problems of plastic surgery and prosthesis following surgical removal of maxillary malignoma. Med. Pregl., 28:467, 1975 (Serbian)

BARNAKO, D.: Flammable fabrics. J.A.M.A., 221;189, 1972

BARNEY, B. B.: Augmentation mammaplasty with two different kinds of prostheses in the same woman, PRS, 54:265, 1974

BARON, F. et al: Approaches used in E. N. T. oncological surgery. Rev. Laryngol. Otol. Rhinol. (Bord.). 94:521, 1973 (French)

BARON, S. H.: Rerouting the external auditory canal. A method of correcting congenital stenosis. Arch. Otolaryng., 101:238, 1975

BARON, S. H. et al: Mucoperiosteal flap in frontal sinus surgery (Sewall-Boyden-McNaught operation). Laryngoscope, 83:1266, 1973

BAROUDI, R.: Umbilicaplasty. Clin. Plast. Surg., 2:431, 1975

BAROUDI, R., KEPPKE, E. M., AND NETTO, F. T.: Abdomino-plasty, PRS, 54:161, 1974

BARR, N. R.: The Hand: Principles of Splint Making. Butterworth, London, 1974.

BARRAND, K. G. et al: Massive infiltrating cystic hygroma of neck in infancy. Arch. Dis. Child., 48:523, 1973

BARRERA, G., SERRANO-REBEIL, G., AND ORTIZ-MONASTERIO, F.: Nasal reconstruction of losses due to oncological surgery: 15 years' experience, PRS, 48:89, 1971. Mem. V Cong. Mexicano Dermat., 5:541, 1970

BARRETO, F.: Surgical management of the bilateral cleft lip (with Viale-Gonzalez, Ortiz-Monasterio), PRS, 51:530, 1973

BARROCAS, A.: Disseminated intravascular coagulation, PRS, 52:208, 1973. Mil. Med., 138:9, 1973

BARRON, J.: Education. Hand, 2:6, 1970

BARRON, J. N.: Structure and function of the skin of the hand. Hand, 2:93, 1970

BARRON, J. N.: Maribor method of burns treatment. A report on the work of Janzekovic at Maribor, Yugoslavia. Hand, 3:179, 1971

BARRON, J. N.: Instruments for hand surgery. Hand, 6:211, 1974

BARROW, M. V., AND SIMPSON, C. P.: Caution against use of lathyrogens, PRS, 50:101, 1972. Surgery, 71:309, 1972

BARSKII, A. V. et al: Skin auto- and homoplasty

in deep burns. Khirurgiia (Mosk.), *47:*20, 1971 (Russian)

BARSKY, A. J.: Burns of the dorsum of the hand, PRS, *48:*396, 1971. Hand, *3:*88, 1971

BARSKY, ARTHUR J: Recipient of the Special Honorary Citation of ASPRS, PRS, *53:*378, 1974. Barsky Society, PRS *57:*273, 1976

BARSKY, A. J.: Report on the CMRI hospital in Saigon (Letter to the Editor), PRS, *53:*464, 1974

BARTELS, R. J., AND HOWARD, R. C.: Congenital midline sinus of the upper lip, PRS, *52:*665, 1973

BARTELS, R. J., AND MARA, J. E.: Simple quick method for fixation of upper denture to maxilla, PRS, *56:* 221, 1975

BARTELS, R. J., AND MARA, J. E.: Simultaneous reduction of areola and augmentation mammaplasty, through periareolar incision, PRS, *56:*588, 1975

BARTELS, R. J., STRICKLAND, D. M., AND DOUGLAS, W. M.: New mastopexy operation for mild or moderate breast ptosis, PRS, *57:*687, 1976

BARTKOWSKI, S.: Principles of primary management of facial injuries. Pol. Przegl. Chir., *47:*529, 1975 (Polish)

BARTKOWSKI, S. *et al*: Critical evaluation of primary management of facial injuries according to records of Department of Stomatological Surgery of Medical Academy in Cracow. Pol. Przegl. Chir., *46:*15, 1974 (Polish)

BARTLETT, E. S.: Psychosexual dynamics of patients undergoing mammary augmentation (with Baker, Kolin), PRS, *53:*652, 1974

BARTLETT, R. H. *et al*: Hemodialysis in management of massive burns. Trans. Am. Soc. Artif. Intern. Organs, *19:*269, 1973

BARTON, M. D.: Anesthetic problems with aspirin-intolerant patients, PRS, *57:*681, 1976. Anesth. Analg., Cleve., *54:*376, 1975

BARTON, P. R.: Treatment of class II facial deformity. Segmental surgery. Brit. J. Oral Surg., *10:*265, 1973

BARTON, R. T.: The cuff: a mixed blessing. Surgery, *70:*800, 1971

BARTON, R. T.: Surgical treatment of carcinoma of the floor of the mouth. Surg. Gynec. Obst., *133:*971, 1971

BARTON, R. T.; Surgical treatment of carcinoma of pyriform sinus. Arch. Otolaryng., *97:*337, 1973

BARTON, R. T.: Mucosal melanomas of the head and neck. Laryngoscope, *85:*93, 1975

BARTON, R. T. *et al*: Technique for closure of the floor of the mouth in monobloc resection. Arch. Otolaryng., *101:*50, 1975

BARTON, R. W., REYNOLDS, D. G., AND SWAN, K. G.: Mesenteric circulatory responses to hemorrhagic shock in baboon, PRS, *50:*311, 1972. Ann. Surg., *175:*204, 1972

BARTON, S., AND WILLIAMS, J. D.: Glossopharyngeal nerve block, PRS, *49:*105, 1972. Arch. Otolaryng., *93:*2, 1971

BARTOSOVA, A.: Fibromatosis gingivae. Cesk. Stomatol., *72:*435, 1972 (Czechoslovakian)

BASCONES, *et al*: Extending Stensen's duct to eyeball. An. Esp. Odontoestomatol., *33:*9, 1974 (Spanish)

BASHIR, R. *et al*: Sex chromatin incidence and variation in group of Lebanese females, PRS, *52:*453, 1973. J. Med. Liban., *25:*5, 1972

BASILEVSKAIA, Z. V.: Early dermoplasty of decubitus ulcer in spine and spinal cord injuries. Khirurgiia (Mosk.), *11:*128, 1975 (Russian)

BASKETT, P. J.: Analgesia for the dressing of burns in children: a method using neuroleptanalgesia and Entonox. Postgrad. Med. J., *48:*138, 1972

BASORA, J. *et al*: Metastatic malignancy of the hand. Clin. Orthop., *108:*182, 1975

BASSET, A. *et al*: Diffuse recurring leukoplakia of the buccal cavity, with epitheliomatous degeneration. Bull. Soc. Fr. Dermatol. Syphiligr., *78:*160, 1971 (French)

BASSO RICCI, S. *et al*: Review of 445 recurrences of cutaneous epithelioma after surgery and radiotherapy. Tumori, *58:*361, 1972 (Italian)

BASTIAN, F. O.: Amyloidosis and carpal tunnel syndrome, PRS, *54:*620, 1974. Ab. J. Clin. Path., *61:*711, 1974

BASTOS, J. A. V., AND CARVALHO, J. R.: First care in treatment of burns, PRS, *55:*721, 1975. Ars Curandi, *7:*15, 1974

BATAILLE, R. *et al*: Mucoepidermoid tumors, two cases. Rev. Stomatol. Chir. Maxillofac., *74:*148, 1973 (French)

BATAILLE, R. *et al*: Several cases of primary or recurrent mandibular ameloblastomas treated by surgical curettage. Rev. Stomatol. Chir. Maxillofac., *75:*33, 1974 (French)

BATE, J. T.: Subcutaneous fasciotome. An instrument for relief of compression in anterior, lateral and posterior compartments of the leg from trauma and other causes. Clin. Orthop., *83:*235, 1972

BATESON, M. C.: Endocrine exophthalmos. Brit. Med. J., *4:*46, 1972

BATISSE, R. *et al*: Technique of anterior cartilaginous striation in correction of protruding ears. Ann. Otolaryngol. Chir. Cervicofac., *90:*389, 1973 (French)

BATRAK, S. P.: Use of embryonal tissue for therapeutic purposes. Vrach. Delo., *10:*127, 1971 (Russian)

BATSAKIS, J. G.: Neoplasms of minor and lesser major salivary glands, PRS, *51:*351, 1973.

Surg. Gynec. & Obst., *135:*289, 1972

BATSAKIS, JOHN G.: *Tumors of the Head and Neck.* Williams & Wilkins Co., Baltimore, 1974. PRS, *54:*479, 1974

BATSAKIS, J. G., AND McBURNEY, T. A.: Metastatic neoplasms to head and neck, PRS, *49:*360, 1972. Surg. Gynec. & Obst., *133:*783, 1971

BATSTONE, J. H. F.: Surgery of agenesis of external ear, PRS, *55:*715, 1975. Proc. Roy. Soc. Med., *67:*1199, 1974

Battered Child Syndrome (See also *Buttocks*)

Battered child syndrome, patterns of injury in (O'Neill *et al*), PRS, *53:*691, 1974. J. Trauma, *13:*332, 1973

Childhood accidents, common (Knowles), PRS, *54:*383, 1974. Hospital Med., *10:*48, 1974

Child abuse and neglect, priority problem for private physician (Green), PRS, *57:*680, 1976. Pediatr. Clin. N. Am., *22:*329, 1975

BATTERSBY, E. F. *et al*: Fenestrated tracheostomy tubes. Lancet, *2:*963, 1973

BATTEZZATI, M. *et al*: Phlebo-lymphatic surgery in treatment of post-phlebitic syndrome. Minerva Chir., *30:*410, 1975 (Italian)

BATTISTA, A. F.: Pain relief by subarachnoid hypothermic saline injection, PRS, *57:*767, 1976. Am. J. Surg., *128:*662, 1974

BATTLE, RICHARD: *Clinical Surgery: Plastic Surgery,* Vol. 4. J. B. Lippincott Co., Philadelphia, 1965

BATTLE, R. J. V.: Mechanics of nasal escape, PRS, *48:*515, 1971. Proc. Roy. Soc. Med., *64:*67, 1971

BAUDET, J.: Replantation of the mutilated external ear. New method. Nouv. Presse Med., *1:*344, 1972 (French)

BAUDET, J.: Successful replantation of a large severed ear fragment (Letter to the Editor), PRS, *51:*82, 1973

BAUDET, J. *et al*: New technic for the reimplantation of a completely severed auricle. Ann. chir. plast., *17:*67, 1972 (French)

BAUDET, J. *et al*: Reimplantation of pinna of mutilated ear. Rev. Laryngol. Otol. Rhinol. (Bord.), *93:*241, 1972 (French)

BAUDET, J. *et al*: Transfer by microanastomosis of a scalp flap in case of cicatricial baldness. Ann. chir. plast., *19:*313, 1974 (French)

BAUDET, J. *et al*: Prognostic value of thermography in operations of transplantation for saving a limb. J. Radiol. Electrol. Med. Nucl., *55:*239, 1974 (French)

BAUDET, J., AND LEMAIRE, J. M.: Abdominal flap in surgery of hand, PRS, *57:*265, 1976. Ann. chir. plast., *20:*215, 1975

BAUDET, J., LEMAIRE, J-M., AND GUIMBERTEAU, J-C.: Ten free groin flaps, PRS, *57:*577, 1976

BAUE, A. E., AND NARA, Y.: Regulation of ventilation during hemorrhage and its alterations in response to CO_2, PRS, *51:*710, 1973. Ann. Surg., *176:*80, 1972

BAUER, M. *et al*: Principles, methods and results of treatment of frontal bone defects. Chirurg., *45:*514, 1974 (German)

BAUER, M. *et al*: Reconstruction of frontal bone following frontobasal fractures. Z. Allgemeinmed., *50:*385, 1974 (German)

BAUER, U. *et al*: Aspergillus infection in skin transplantation and its therapy. Chirurg., *46:*279, 1975 (German)

BAUER, W. C. *et al*: Significance of positive margins in hemilaryngectomy specimens. Laryngoscope, *85:*1, 1975

BAUERMEISTER, A.: Surgery of the funnel chest. Bruns Beitr. Klin. Chir., *219:*241, 1972 (German)

BAUGHMAN, R. A.: Lingual thyroid and lingual thryoglossal tract remnants. Clinical and histopathologic study with review of literature. Oral Surg., *34:*781, 1972

BAUM, M: Should lymphadenectomy be discarded? I. Immunological considerations. J. R. Coll. Surg. Edinb., *18:*351, 1973

BAUM, M., EDWARDS, M. H., MAGAREY, C. J.: Organization of clinical trial on national scale: management of early cancer of breast. Brit. M. J., *4:*476, 1972

BAUM, S. M. *et al*: Central hemangioma of maxilla. J. Oral Surg., *30:*885, 1972

BAUMAL, A., HANSON, J., AND JEERAPAET, P.: Chromomycosis simulating basal cell carcinoma, PRS, *55:*640, 1975. Cutis, *14:*227, 1974

BAUMAN, L.: Melanoma in relatives. J.A.M.A., *218:*1300, 1971

BAUMANN, M.: Partial vestibuloplasty with secondary epithelization. Schweiz. Monatsschr. Zahnheilkd., *86:*17, 1976 (German)

BAUMANN, M., AND PAJAROLA, G.: Experiences on sequela of maxillary sinusitis following closure of curative oro-antral fistula, PRS, *57:*672, 1976. J. Maxillo-facial Surg., *3:*164, 1975

BAUMAN, M. L. *et al*: Intracranial metastatic malignant melanoma: long-term survival following subtotal resection. South. Med. J., *65:*344, 1972

BAUMANN, R. R.: Problems of jaw implants. H.N.O., *22:*191, 1974 (German)

BAUMBERGER, K. *et al*: Microsurgical treatment of cerebrospinal rhinorrhea. Schweiz. Med. Wochenschr., *104:*521, 1974 (German)

BAUMGARTEN, R. S., AND DESPREZ, J. D.: Morris bi-phasic external splint for mandibular fixation, PRS, *50:*66, 1972

BAUMGARTNER, R.: Proceedings: plastic hand splints. Hefte Unfallheilkd., *114:*297, 1973 (German)

BAUMGARTNER, R.: Hand splints made of plastics. Z. Unfallmed. Berufskr., *66:*188, 1973 (German)

BAUMRIND, S. *et al*: New system for integrated three dimensional craniofacial mapping. J. Dent. Res., *50:*1496, 1971

BAUTISTA, B. N., AND NERY, E. B.: Replacement of malformed fingernail with acrylic resin material, PRS, *55:*234, 1975

BAUX, S. *et al*: Technic and indications of net grafts. Outcome of the cicatrices. Ann. chir. plast., *16:*237, 1971 (French)

BAXTER, C. R.: Current status of burn research. J. Trauma, *14:*1, 1974

BAXTER, C. R. *et al*: Early management of thermal burns. Postgrad. Med., *55:*131, 1974

BAXTER, R. J. *et al*: Cosmetic nasal deformities complicating prolonged nasotracheal intubation in critically ill newborn infants, PRS, *57:*114, 1976. Pediatrics, *55:*884, 1975

BAYLIS, H. I. *et al*: Letter: Pyrex tubes in conjunctivodacryocystorhinostomy. Am. J. Ophth., *79:*887, 1975

BAYLIS, H. I. *et al*: Complications of Mohs' chemosurgical excision of eyelid and canthal tumors. Am. J. Ophth., *80:*116, 1975

BAYLOR, C. H. *et al*: Treatment of grease gun injuries. J. Occup. Med., *15:*799, 1973

BAZANT, B. *et al*: Covering of old and infected losses of the skin surface. Acta Chir. Orthop. Traumatol. Cech., *38:*230, 1971 (Czechoslovakian)

BAZHANOV, N. N. *et al*: Osteoplasty of defects of mandible with formalinized homotransplants. Stomatologiia (Mosk.), *51:*37, 1972 (Russian)

BAZHENOVA, A. P.: Surgical treatment of skin melanoma. Khirurgiia (Mosk.), *11:*26, 1975 (Russian)

BEAHRS, O. H.: Factors minimizing mortality and morbidity rates in head and neck surgery, PRS, *53:*692, 1974. Am. J. Surg., *126:*443, 1973

BEAHRS, O. H., AND CHONG, G. C.: Management of facial nerve in parotid gland surgery, PRS, *51:*349, 1973. Am. J. Surg., *124:*473, 1972

BEAL, D. D. *et al*: Surgery of the seventh cranial nerve. Alaska Med., *13:*137, 1971

BEAL, D. D. *et al*: Meatoplasty transposition flaps. Laryngoscope, *82:*404, 1972

BEAL, J. M.: Operation for lymphedema. Ill. Med. J., *142:*494, 1972

BEAL, J. M.: Surgical grand rounds. Carcinoma of lip. Ill. Med. J., *146:*462, 1974

BEAR, S. E.: Therapy for central non-odontogenic lesions of the jaws. Trans. Int. Conf. Oral Surg., *4:*33, 1973

BEAR, S. E. *et al*: Experimental use of stainless steel wire mesh in mandibular defects. J. Oral Surg., *31:*348, 1973

BEARD, C.: Ptosis: some newer concepts. Ann. Ophth., *3:*1047, 1971

BEARD, C.: Complications of ptosis surgery. Ann. Ophth., *4:*671, 1972

BEARD, C.: Observations on the treatment of basal cell carcinoma of the eyelids. The Wendell L. Huges Lecture. Trans. Am. Acad. Ophthalmol. Otolaryngol., *79:*664, 1975

BEARD, C. *et al*: *Transactions of the New Orleans Academy of Ophthalmology.* C. V. Mosby Co., St. Louis, 1974. PRS, *55:*355, 1975

BEARDMORE, G. L., AND DAVIS, N. C.: Multiple primary cutaneous melanomas, PRS, *57:*679, 1976. Arch. Dermat., *111:*603, 1975

BEARE, R.: Surgical repair of gross palatal defect, PRS, *48:*515, 1971. Proc. Roy. Soc. Med., *64:*71, 1971

BEARE, R. L. *et al*: Naso-labial full thickness graft. Brit. J. Plast. Surg., *25:*315, 1972

BEARS, R. L.: Basal cell carcinoma. Proc. Roy. Soc. Med., *66:*691, 1973

BEASLEY, H.: Fasanella-Servat operation. Tex. Med., *69:*83, 1973

BEASLEY, H.: Hyperthermia associated with ophthalmic surgery. Am. J. Ophth., *77:*76, 1974

BEASLEY, J. D., III *et al*: Effect of antibiotics and chemical adhesives on infected wounds, PRS, *49:*588, 1972. Mil. Med., *136:*566, 1971

BEASLEY, J. W. *et al*: Single stage repair of median cleft lip in an infant with premaxillary agenesis. S. D. J. Med., *24:*15, 1971

BEASLEY, R. W.: Local flaps for surgery of the hand. Orthop. Clin. North Am., *1:*219, 1970

BEASLEY, R. W.: Principles of tendon transfer. Orthop. Clin. North Am., *1:*433, 1970

BEASLEY, R. W.: Cosmetic considerations in surgery of the hand. Surg. Clin. North Am., *51:*471, 1971

BEAZLEY, J. M.: Letter: Congenital absence of vagina. Brit. Med. J., *3:*344, 1974

BEAZLEY, R. M., BAGLEY, D. H., AND KETCHAM, A. S.: Effect of cryosurgery on peripheral nerves, PRS, *54:*687, 1974. J. Surg. Res., *16:*231, 1974

BEAUCHEMIN, M.: Electric burns in the operating room (need for electronic technicians in today's hospital). Union. Med. Can., *100:*1806, 1971 (French)

BEAUVAIS, M. *et al*: Case of bilateral temporomandibular ankylosis. Rev. Stomatol. Chir. Maxillofac., *75:*851, 1974 (French)

BEBAIN, J. J. *et al*: Fronto-orbito-nasal fractures, PRS, *56:*353, 1975. Ann. Otolaryng., *10:*545, 1974

BECK, A. R., AND WESSER, D. R.: Constrictive digital injuries in infants, caused by human hair, PRS, *42:*420, 1972

BECK, F. *et al*: Late results of ulnar head resection. Monatsschr. Unfallheilkd., *72:*432, 1969 (German)

BECKER, R.: Treatment and its results in 38 ameloblastomas. Forschr. Kiefer. Gesichtschir., *15:*211, 1972 (German)

BECKER, R.: Stable compression plate fixation of mandibular fractures. Brit. J. Oral Surg., *12:*13, 1974

BECKER, R.: Surgical technic in combined treatment of cancer of the tongue and mouth floor. Acta Stomatol. Belg., *72:*247, 1975 (German)

BECKER, R. M.: Hypothalamic-pituitary derangements as a complication of severe facial injuries (with Daniel, Entin), PRS, *49:*548, 1972

BECKER, R. M., AND DANIEL, R. K.: Increased antidiuretic hormone production after trauma to craniofacial complex, PRS, *53:*690, 1974. J. Trauma, *13:*112, 1973

BECKER, S. N. *et al*: Pericardial effusion secondary to mucoepidermoid carcinoma of the parotid gland. A report of an unusual case. Cancer, *36:*1080, 1975

BECKER, W.: Medico-legal experiences in allegations of inadequate explanation and negligence. Laryngol. Rhinol. Otol. (Stuttg.), *53:*75, 1974 (German)

BECKETT, V. L. *et al*: Role of surgery in the rheumatoid hand. J. Ir. Med. Assoc., *66:*379, 1973

BECKMAN, J. S. *et al*: Lip cancer: surgical management. Am. J. Surg., *128:*732, 1974

BECKWITH, M. M.: Surgical rehabilitation after extensive losses in the lower face from war injuries (with Parsons, Thering), PRS, *49:*533, 1972

BECTON, J. L.: Repair of nerves in the hand—when? where? how? J. Med. Assoc. Ga., *65:*5, 1976

BECTON, J. L. *et al*: Nocardia infection of the hand. J. Bone & Joint Surg. (Am.), *52:*1443, 1970

BECTON, J. L. *et al*: Multiple-angled incision on the volar surface of the hand. Arch. Surg., *109:*582, 1974

BEDARD, C. H. *et al*: Osteitis fibrosa (brown tumor) of the maxilla. Laryngoscope, *84:*2093, 1974

BEDFORD, M. A.: *Color Atlas of Oro-Facial Diseases*. Year Book Medical Pub., Inc., Chicago, 1972

BEDNAREK, F. J., AND KUHNS, L. R.: Endotracheal tube placement in infants determined by suprasternal palpation, PRS, *57:*407, 1976. Pediatrics, *56:*224, 1975

BEDNARIK, J. *et al*: Peritendinous fibrosis of the dorsum of the hand. Acta Chir. Orthop. Traumatol. Cech., *38:*289, 1971 (Czechoslovakian)

BEEKHUIS, G. I.: Delayed skin grafting in head and neck surgery, PRS, *54:*625, 1974. J. Maxillo-facial Surg., *2:*3, 1974

BEEKHUIS, G. J.: Nasal tip projection. Eye, Ear, Nose, Throat Mon., *51:*92, 1972

BEEKHUIS, G. J.: "What's in a name?" Arch. Otolaryng., *100:*165, 1974

BEEKHUIS, G. J.: Saddle nose deformity, etiology, prevention, and treatment: augmentation rhinoplasty with polyamide. Laryngoscope, *84:*2, 1974

BEEKHUIS, G. J.: Surgical correction of saddle nose deformity. Trans. Am. Acad. Ophthalmol. Otolaryngol., *80:*596, 1975

BEESLEY, J. R. *et al*: Prophylactic antibiotics in minor hand injuries. Injury, *6:*366, 1975

BEETKE, E.: Salivary calculi (diagnosis and treatment). Zentralbl. Chir., *97:*1073, 1972 (German)

BEHERI, G. E., TALAAT, S. M., AND ZAKY, S.: Early liver changes in burns, role of A.T.P. and Trasylol in prevention, PRS, *56:*682, 1975. J. Kuwait M.A., *8:*77, 1974

BEHL, P. N.: Abrasion in treatment of nail disorders. Indian J. Dermatol., *18:*77, 1973

BEHL, P. N. *et al*: Treatment of vitiligo with autologous thin Thiersch's grafts. Int. J. Dermatol., *12:*329, 1973

BEHOUNKOVA, E.: Histologic examination of skin grafts stored at +4°C, PRS, *50:*543, 1972. Acta chir. plast., *13:*128, 1971

BEHRMAN, S. J.: Complications of sagittal osteotomy of the mandibular ramus. J. Oral Surg., *30:*554, 1972

BEKKE, J. P. H., AND SNOW, G. B.: Experience with cryosurgery in cases of new growth in oral cavity, PRS, *55:*376, 1975. Nederl. tijdschr. geneesk., *118:*1359, 1974

BELIK, I. E. *et al*: Burns in children. Ortop. Travmatol. Protez., *34:*8, 1973 (Russian)

BELINFANTE, L. S. *et al*: Teamwork approach to correct a severe prosthodontic problem. J. Am. Dent. Assoc., *91:*357, 1975

BELISARIO, J. C.: Local cytotoxic therapy of keratoacanthomas, PRS, *52:*599, 1973. Trans. Ibero-Latino Am. Cong. Dermat., *6:*349, 1970

BELISARIO, J. C.: Basal cell carcinoma, PRS, *51:*484, 1973. Med. Trib., *13:*21, 1972

BELL, F. A., III: Vestibuloplasty and floor of mouth revision with application of split-thickness skin graft. J. N.C. Dent. Soc., *57:*14, 1974

BELL, J. M.: Dental anesthesia in children,

PRS, *53:*690, 1974. Anesth. & Intens. Care, *1:*540, 1973

BELL, JOHN: *Observations on Italy.* Arno Press & The New York Times, New York, 1971. PRS, *57:*373, 1976

BELL, R. C.: *Monographs on Plastic Surgery.* Vol. 1. Oxford University Press, Inc., Fairlawn, N. J., 1973

BELL, R. C. *et al*: Advances in plastic surgery. Practitioner, *211:*441, 1973

BELL, W. H.: Correction of skeletal type of anterior open bite. J. Oral Surg., *29:*706, 1971

BELL, W. H.: Biologic basis for maxillary osteotomies. Am. J. Phys. Anthropol., *38:*279, 1973

BELL, W. H.: Immediate surgical repositioning of one-and two-tooth dento-osseous segments. Int. J. Oral Surg., *2:*265, 1973

BELL, W. H.: Le Fort I osteotomy for correction of maxillary deformities. J. Oral Surg., *33:*412, 1975

BELL, W. H. *et al*: Revascularization and bone healing after maxillary corticotomies. J. Oral Surg., *30:*640, 1972

BELL, W. H., AND CREEKMORE, T. D.: Surgical-orthodontic correction of mandibular prognathism. Am. J. Orthodontics, *63:*256, 1973

BELL, W. H. *et al*: Surgical correction of posterior crossbite. J. Oral Surg., *32:*811, 1974

BELL, W. H. *et al*: Bone healing and revascularization after total maxillary osteotomy, PRS, *57:*531, 1976. J. Oral Surg., *33:*253, 1975

BELLERO, V. *et al*: Abdominoplasty: physiorespiratory, surgical, esthetic problems, PRS, *56:*356, 1975. Riv. ital. chir. plast., *5:*417, 1973

BELLINGER, C. G.: Adding a given concentration of epinephrine to a solution by needle drops, PRS, *50:*530, 1972

BELLINGER, C. G., AND GOULIAN, D.: Secondary surgery in transsexuals, PRS, *51:*628, 1973

BELLMAN, H. *et al*: Influence of unusually high doses of vitamin C on healing of wounds and bones, and on prognosis of polytrauma, PRS, *52:*686, 1973. Zentralbl. Chir., *98:*510, 1973

BELOGLIADOVA, N. I.: Functional state and morphological changes in skin grafts following plastic surgery on the hand. Vestn. Khir., *106:*1971 (Russian)

BELOGLIADOVA, N. I.: Condition of reimplanted skin after operative treatment of chronic lympbedema. Klin. Khir., *3:*63, 1975 (Russian)

BELPOMME, C.: External osteosynthesis of distal fractures of phalanges by reposition-fixation of fingernail, PRS, *57:*118, 1976. J. Internat. Surg., *60:*219, 1975

BELTRAN-BROWN, F., AND NASRALLAH, R. E.:

Anorectal malformations, PRS, *51:*481, 1973. Cir. y cir. Mexico, *40:*57, 1972

BEM, J. C., AND GREAVES, M. W.: Prostaglandin E₁ effects in epidermal cell growth *in vitro,* PRS, *56:*474, 1975. Arch. Dermat. Forsch., *251:*35, 1974

BENAD, G.: Anesthesiologic aspects of general burn therapy in adults. Zentralbl. Chir., *97:*161, 1971 (German)

BENAGIANO, L.: On various methods of treatment of harelip and cleft palate. Minerva Stomatol., *19:*425, 1970

BENAIM, F.: Use of skin grafts in treatment of burns, PRS, *55:*111, 1975. Bol. y trab. Acad. argent. cir., *58:*102, 1974

BENAVENT, W. J.: Treatment of bilateral breast carcinomas in a patient with silicone-gel breast implants, PRS, *51:*588, 1973

BENCIVENGA, A.: New technic of pressure osteosynthesis in the hand. Chirurg., *45:*327, 1974 (German)

BENDER, LEONARD F.: *Prostheses and Rehabilitation After Arm Amputation.* Charles C Thomas, Springfield, Ill., 1974. PRS, *55:*487, 1975

BENDIK, A. L.: Etiopathogenesis and treatment of glossalgia. Stomatologiia (Mosk.), *52:*76, 1973 (Russian)

BENECSIK, R. *et al*: On the closure of the defect after tumor removal in the medial canthus. Klin. Monatsbl. Augenheilkd., *167:*685, 1975

BENEDICT, K. T., JR. *et al*: Hypothenar hammer syndrome. Radiology, *111:*57, 1974

BENEDITO, R.: Atomic explosion lesions, PRS, *48:*611, 1971. Rev. españ. cir. plast., *4:*47, 1971

BENENDO-KAPUSCINSKA, B. *et al*: Diagnostic possibilities of sialography in salivary gland tumors on basis of 100 cases confirmed surgically. Pol. Przegl. Radiol., *36:*721, 1972 (Polish)

BENFIELD, D. G.: On relief of respiratory obstruction in micrognathia by use of large nasogastric tube (Letter to the Editor), PRS, *56:*570, 1975

BEN-HUR, N.: Infestation and septicemia from *Candida albicans* in burns, caused by massive treatment with antibiotic and Sulfamylon, PRS, *53:*686, 1974. Riv. ital. chir. plast., *4:*45, 1973

BEN-HUR, N.: Discussion of "Vascularization of porcine skin heterografts," by Toranto, Salyer, Myers, PRS, *54:*352, 1974

BEN-HUR, N. *et al*: Phosphorus burns: the antidote: a new approach. Brit. J. Plast. Surg., *25:*245, 1972

BEN-HUR, N., AND NEUMAN, Z.: The fate of implanted living epithelial cells into the subcutis (Follow-Up Clinic), PRS, *49:*455, 1972

BENIRSCHKE, K. *et al*: True hemaphroditism and chimerism, case report. Trans. Pac. Coast Obstet. Gynecol. Soc., *39:*17, 1971

BENISCH, B. *et al*: Focal muscular hyperplasia of trachea, PRS, *54:*690, 1974. Arch. Otolaryng., *99:*226, 1974

BEN-MENACHEM, T. *et al*: Post-traumatic capillary hemangioma of the hand. A case report. J. Bone & Joint Surg. (Am.) *56A:*1741, 1974

BENNDORF, R.: Dystopia of lower molar in processus muscularis with genuine fusion with muscle. Dtsch. Zahn. Mund. Kieferheilkd., *62:*237, 1974 (German)

BENNETT, A. H.: Exstrophy of bladder treated by ureterosigmoidostomies. Long term evaluation. Urology, *2:*165, 1973

BENNETT, A. H., AND LAZARUS, J. M.: Bilateral nephrectomy performed on emergency basis for life-threatening malignant hypertension, PRS, *53:*501, 1974. Surg. Gynec. & Obst., *137:*451, 1973

BENNETT, J. F.: Evaluation of burn depth by the use of radioactive isotopes (Follow-Up Clinic), PRS, *48:*73, 1971

BENNETT, J. E.: Obituary on Harold M. Trusler, M.D., PRS, *51:*713, 1973

BENNETT, J. E.: Upper arm tourniquet tolerance in hand surgery (Letter to the Editor), PRS, *52:*660, 1973

BENNETT, J. E.: Skin and soft tissue injuries of hand in children, PRS, *57:*261, 1976. Pediatr. Clin. N. Am., *22:*443, 1975

BENNETT, J. E.: Discussion of "Arteriovenous malformations of the mandible, graduated surgical management," by Bryant, Maull, PRS, *56:*84, 1975

BENNETT, J. E.: Discussion of "Burned hands" by Huang, Larson, Lewis, PRS, *56:*442, 1975

BENNETT, J. E. *et al*: Mutilating injuries of the wrist. J. Trauma, *11:*1008, 1971

BENNETT, J. E., AND ZOOK, E. G.: Treatment of arteriovenous fistulas in cavernous hemangioma of face by muscle embolization, PRS, *50:*84, 1972

BENNETT, J. E., AND KAHN, R. A.: Surgical management of soft tissue defects of ankle-heel region, PRS, *53:*113, 1974. J. Trauma, *12:*696, 1973

BENNETT, J. P.: Sandwich pushback and lateral pharyngoplasty, PRS, *54:*694, 1974. Brit. J. Plast. Surg., *26:*16, 1973

BENNETT, J. P.: From noli-me-tangere to rodent ulcer: recognition of basal cell carcinoma, PRS, *57:*124, 1976. Brit. J. Plast. Surg., *27:*144, 1974

BENNETT, M.: The older cleft palate patient. (A clinical otologic-audiologic study.) Laryngoscope, *82:*1217, 1972

BENNETT, R. L.: Conservative management of

the wrist and hand in rheumatoid arthritis: the art of self-defense. South. Med. J., *66:*1267, 1973

BENOIST, M. *et al*: Dentofacial orthopedics and orthopedic surgery. Rev. Stomatol. Chir. Maxillofac., *76:*175, 1975 (French)

BENS, D. E., AND KREWER, S. E.: Hand gym: exercise apparatus for patient with rheumatoid arthritis, PRS, *55:*519, 1975. Arch. Phys. Med., *53:*477, 1974

BENSON, J. W.: Combined chemotherapy and cryosurgery for oral cancer. Am. J. Surg., *130:*596, 1975

BENTLEY, G. *et al*: Pre-operative assessment of the hand, hip, and knee in rheumatoid arthritis. Physiotherapy, *58:*83, 1972

BENTLEY-PHILLIPS, B. *et al*: Melanoma and trauma. A clinical study of Zulu feet under conditions of persistent and gross trauma. S. Afr. Med. J., *46:*535, 1972

BENTLEY-PHILLIPS, B., AND BAYLES, M. A. H.: Butylated hydroxytoluene as skin lightener, PRS, *54:*382, 1974. Arch. Dermat., *109:*216, 1974

BENVENISTE, R. J. *et al*: Nasal hemangiopericytoma. Arch. Otolaryng., *98:*358, 1973

BENVENISTE, R. J. *et al*: Teflon pharyngoplasty in incompetent velopharyngeal closure. Cleve. Clin. Q., *40:*93, 1973

BERADI, R. S. *et al*: Cancer of head and neck: 8-year experience. South. Med. J., *66:*1094, 1973

BERDAL, P.: Salivary gland tumors. Tidsskr. Nor. Laegeforen, *93:*1899, 1973 (Norwegian)

BERDIUK, I. V.: Determination of the optimal terms for surgical treatment of congenital clefts of the upper lip. Stomatologiia (Mosk.), *50:*63, 1971 (Russian)

BERECEK, K. H.: Treatment of decubitus ulcers. Nurs. Clin. North. Am., *10:*171, 1975

BERENS, J. J.: Thermal contact burns from streets and highways, PRS, *48:*296, 1971. J.A.M.A., *214:*2025, 1970

BERENYI, B.: Therapy of fractures of the zygomatic arch. Dtsch. Stomatol., *21:*599, 1971 (German)

BERENYI, B.: Open subcondylar osteotomy in treatment of mandibular deformities. Int. J. Oral Surg., *2:*81, 1973

BERENYI, B.: Oral surgical approach to the treatment of Sjögren's syndrome. Int. J. Oral Surg., *3:*309, 1974

BERENYI, B. *et al*: Surgical correction of jaw abnormalities causing severe facial deformities. Orv. Hetil., *116:*1767, 1975 (Hungarian)

BERES, K. *et al*: General anesthesia in surgical correction of prognathism. Fogorv. Sz., *68:*289, 1975 (Hungarian)

BERG, R. *et al*: Topographic and practical anatomy of articulatic temporomandibularis of various domestic animals with special reference to the possibility of discus articularis resection 1. Dog (anis familianis). Z. Exp. Chir., *5:*115, 1972 (German)

BERGAMASCHI, P. *et al*: On malignant melanoma and pregnancy and the puerperium. Minerva Ginecol., *25:*623, 1973 (Italian)

BERGAN, J. J., CONN, J., JR., AND TRIPPEL, O. H.: Severe ischemia of hand, PRS, *48:*94, 1971. Ann. Surg., *173:*301, 1971

BERGEN, R. P.: Protection against malpractice litigation. Arch. Otolaryng., *101:*182, 1975

BERGER, A.: Nerve-lesions due to electric current and thermal damage. Hefte Unfallheilkd., *0:*394, 1974 (German)

BERGER, A. *et al*: Avoidance of tracheotomy damage through a changed surgical technic. Langenbecks Arch. Chir., *327:*922, 1970 (German)

BERGER, A. *et al*: Clinical experiences with estriol succinate in surgery of the hand. Wien. Klin. Wochenschr., *82:*582, 1970 (German)

BERGER, A., MILLESI, H., AND SIMMA, W.: Treatment of large pilonidal sinus, PRS, *53:*249, 1974. Chir. Praxis, *17:*285, 1973

BERGER, C. J., DISQUE, F. C., AND TOPAZIAN, R. G.: Rhinocerebral mucormycosis, PRS, *57:*671, 1976. Oral Surg., *40:*27, 1975

BERGER, H. M. *et al*: Epidermoid carcinoma of the lip after renal transplantation. Report of two cases. Arch. Intern. Med., *128:*609, 1971

BERGER, J. C.: Suicide attempts related to congenital facial deformities, PRS, *51:*323, 1973

BERGER, R. A.: Use of silicone injections in facial defects, PRS, *57:*393, 1976. Arch. Otolaryng., *101:*525, 1975

BERGER, S. *et al:* Bacteremia after use of oral irrigation device, PRS, *55:* 260, 1975. Ann. Int. Med., *80:*570, 1974

BERGERA, J. J., AND FRIZ, R. F.: Hyperthermic reaction during anesthesia in an infant, PRS, *48:*595, 1971

BERGFELD, W. F. *et al*: Granuloma faciale – treatment by dermabrasion. Report of a case. Cleve. Clin. Q., *37:*215, 1970

BERGGREN, R. B.: Role of the plastic surgeon in undergraduate medical education (Editorial), PRS, *50:*75, 1972

BERGGREN, R. B.: Precise method for determination of the displacement in fractures of the midface (with Ferraro), PRS, *50:*447, 1972

BERGHAGEN, N. *et al*: Adenomatoid odontogenic tumor. Periodontal aspects on diagnosis and treatment. Sven. Tandlak. Tidskr., *66:*467, 1973

BERGLAND, O., AND BORCHGREVINK, H.: Role of nasal septum in midfacial growth in man elucidated by maxillary development in cer-

tain types of facial clefts, PRS, *56:*461, 1975. Scand. J. Plast. Reconstr. Surg., *8:*42, 1974

BERGLAND, O., AND SIDHU, S. S.: Occlusal changes from deciduous to early mixed dentition in unilateral complete clefts, PRS, *55:*514, 1975. Cleft Palate J., *11:*317, 1974

BERGMAN, J.: Idiopathic malignant hyperthermia: review and report of case, PRS, *56:*235, 1975. Arch. Ophth., *93:*232, 1975

BERGMAN, J. A.: Primary hemifacial hypertrophy, PRS, *52:* 593, 1973. Arch. Otolaryng., *97:* 490, 1973

BERGOEND, H. *et al*: Spindle cell epithelioma on an old keloid of the upper extremity after a burn. Functional restoration. Ann. chir. plast., *17:*142, 1972 (French)

BERGONZELLI, V.: Reconstruction and reparation in radical surgery of tumors. Cancro, *24:*369, 1971 (Italian)

BERGSMA, DANIEL: *Clinical Delineation of Birth Defects.* Williams & Wilkins Co., Baltimore, 1971. PRS, *50:*79, 1972

BERGSTROM, K. *et al*: Effect of superior labial frenectomy in cases with midline diastema. Am. J. Orthod., *63:*633, 1973

BERGSTROM, L. *et al*: Lightning-damaged ear, PRS, *55:*106, 1975. Arch. Otolaryng., *100:*117, 1974

BERGUER, A. S.: Fractures of middle third of face: technics of internal fixation. An. Esp. Odontoestomatol., *34:*103, 1975 (Spanish)

BERKE, R. N.: Surgical treatment of traumatic blepharoptosis, PRS, *51:*102, 1973. Am. J. Ophth., *72:*691, 1972

BERKOVITS, R. N. P. *et al*: Congenital laryngotracheoesophageal cleft, PRS, *55:*721, 1975. Arch. Otolaryng., *100:*442, 1974

BERKOWITZ, S., KRISCHER, J., AND PRUZANSKY, S.: Quantitative analysis of cleft palate casts, PRS, *55:*382, 1975. Cleft Palate J., *11:*134, 1974

BERKOWITZ, W. P. *et al*: Surgical management of severe lye burns of the esophagus by colon interposition. Ann. Otol. Rhin. & Laryng., *84:*576, 1975

BERKUTOV, A. N.: Hyperbaric oxygenation therapy of anaerobic wound infection (literature survey). Vestn. Khir., *113:*92, 1974 (Russian)

BERLIN, S. J. *et al*: Nerve tumors of the foot: diagnosis and treatment. J. Am. Podiatry Assoc., *65:*157, 1975

BERLINER, B. C. *et al*: Hypercalcemia associated with hypertension due to prolonged immobilization. An unusual complication of extensive burns. Pediatrics, *49:*92, 1972

BERLINGER, F. G., AND FLOWERS, H. H.: Some observations on treatment of snakebites in Vietnam, PRS, *52:*601, 1973. Mil. Med.,

*138:*139, 1973

BERMAN, D. N. Occlusion of the internal carotid artery associated with mandibular fracture. J. Oral Surg., *33:*134, 1975

BERMAN, W. E.: American Academy of Facial Plastic and Reconstructive Surgery, message from the president (Editorial). Arch. Otolaryng., *98:*365, 1973

BERMAN, W. E. *et al*: Complications in blepharoplasties and face lift operations. Otolaryngol. Clin. North Am., *7:*87, 1974

BERNADSKII, IuN. *et al*: Some functional indices of the external respiration in children with congenital cleft palate before and after operation. Stomatologiia (Mosk.), *49:*53, 1970 (Russian)

BERNARD, J. A.: Surgical treatment of lacrimal duct obstructions. Arch. Ophtalmol. (Paris), *32:*177, 1972 (French)

BERNARD, J. A. *et al*: Restoration of lacrimal canaliculi by means of a pigtail probe. Bull. Soc. Ophtalmol. Fr., *71:*419, 1971 (French)

BERNDORFER, A.: Facial clefts with concurrent cleft hands and cleft feet. Z. Orthop., *107:*344, 1970 (German)

BERNDORFER, A.: Clinical findings related to formal genesis of encephalocele, hydrocephaly and anencephaly, PRS, *51:*481, 1973. Rev. brasil. cir., *62:*137, 1972

BERNER, R. E.: Hypospadias. Calif. Med., *116:*56, 1972

BERNER, R. E., AND LAUB, D. R.: The spontaneous cure of massive fibrosarcoma (Follow-up Clinic), PRS, *50:*77, 1972

BERNER, R. E., MORAIN, W. D., AND NOE, J. M.: Postoperative hypertension as etiological factor in hematoma after rhytidectomy, prevention with chlorpromazine, PRS, *57:*314, 1976

BERNHARDT, H. W.: *Aeromonas hydrophila* wound infection (with Rosenthal, Phillips), PRS, *53:*77, 1974

BERNHOFT, C. H.: Ectoprosthesis after exenteration of the orbit. Nor. Tannlageforen Tid., *86:*57, 1976 (Norwegian)

BERNIMOULIN, J. P. *et al*: Free gingival grafts – clinical aspects and cytology of healing. Dtsch. Zahnaerztl. Z., *27:*357, 1972 (German)

BERNSTEIN, D.: Homologous nasal hump implant. Arch. Otolaryng., *98:*385, 1973

BERNSTEIN, L.: Dental occlusion and early repair of alveolar clefts. Arch. Otolaryng., *96:*395, 1972

BERNSTEIN, L.: Esthetic anatomy of nose. Laryngoscope, *82:*2000, 1972

BERNSTEIN, L.: Incisions and excisions in elective facial surgery. Arch. Otolaryng., *97:*238, 1973

BERNSTEIN, L.: Early submucous resection of nasal septal cartilage. Pilot study in canine pups. Arch. Otolaryng., *97:*273, 1973

BERNSTEIN, L.: Applied anatomy in corrective rhinoplasty. Arch. Otolaryng., *99:*67, 1974

BERNSTEIN, N. R.: Care of burned victims. New England J. Med., *286:*101, 1972

BERRY, E. P.: Planning and evaluating blepharoplasty, PRS, *54:*257, 1974

BERRY, F. A.: Craniofacial osteotomies and reconstructions in infants and young children (with Edgerton, Jane), PRS, *54:*13, 1974

BERSCHADSKY, M. *et al*: Atypical fibroxanthoma in the pharynx, PRS, *52:*443, 1973

BERTENYI, C.: Two cases of reconstruction of soft tissue defects of the face caused by human bite. Magy. Traumatol Orthop., *17:*126, 1974 (Hungarian)

BERTENYI, C. *et al*: Successful skin grafting in a case of pemphigus vulgaris. Brit. J. Plast. Surg., *26:*381, 1973

BERTENYI, C. *et al*: Rapid production of fresh granulation tissue suitable for transplantation following acquired chronic skin defects. Z. Haut. Geschlechtskr., *48:*153, 1973 (German)

BERTENYI, C. *et al*: Rehabilitation of severe case of acne conglobata through close dermatologic-surgical cooperation. Z. Hautkr., *49:*467, 1974 (German)

BERTHOLD, P. *et al*: Sulcus-extension surgery as pre-prosthetic treatment in front region of lower jaw. Clinical roentgenographic evaluation. Sven. Tandlak. Tidskr., *65:*255, 1972

BERTHOLD, V. H.: Experiences and therapeutic results with wire osteosynthesis in facial bone fractures. Zahn. Mund. Kieferheilkd., *62:*712, 1974 (German)

BERTOLINI, D., AND BARISONI, D.: Elastic compression in burn scar results, PRS, *56:*360, 1975. Riv. ital chir. plast., *5:*361, 1973

BERTOLINI, G. *et al*: Preliminary observations on use of ketamine in plastic and reconstructive surgery. Minerva Anestesiol., *39:*176, 1973) (Italian)

BERTOLINI, G. *et al*: Anesthesiological prospects in treatment of burns. Minerva Anestesiol., *39:*183, 1973 (Italian)

BERUCHASHVILI, L. Z. *et al*: Prevention of late complications of acrylate cranioplasty. Vopr. Neirokhir., *36:*41, 1972 (Russian)

BERUMEN-CERVANTES, U., CALDERON-LOPEZ, J., AND VILLARREAL-CANTU, R.: Clear cell sarcoma of tendons and aponeurosis, PRS, *55:*515, 1975. Sem. Med. Mexico, *81:*165, 1974

BES, J., AND DESCOTES, J.: Incidence of traumatic obstruction of superficial palmar arch in etiology of ischemia of the hand (30 out of 101 cases), PRS, *53:*107, 1974. J. Chir.,

*105:*261, 1973

BESHLEI, V. I. *et al*: Acquired lymphogenic edema of the extremities. Klin. Khir., *10:*52, 1972 (Russian)

BETHMANN, W. *et al*: Concomitant symptoms in cheilognathopalatoschisis in patients of the Thallwitz Clinic. Dtsch. Stomatol., *22:*907, 1972 (German)

BETHMANN, W. *et al*: Healing course and complications following surgery of cleft lip, maxilla and palate. Dtsch. Stomatol., *23:*633, 1973 (German)

BETHMANN, W. *et al*: Jaw development in cleft patients following primary and secondary velo-pharyngoplasty. Studies in the scope of the research project "the defect child." Dtsch. Zahn. Mund. Kieferheilkd., *60:*370, 1973 (German)

BETHMANN, W. *et al*: Differential diagnosis of maxillary antrum sinus and odontogenic cyst in dental X-ray film. Stomatol. D.D.R., *24:*126, 1974 (German)

BETKOWSKI, A.: Eosinophilic adenoma of parotid. Wiad. Lek., *27:*55, 1974 (Polish)

BETKOWSKI, A.: Branchiogenic carcinoma. Wiad. Lek., *27:*1671, 1974 (Polish)

BETKOWSKI, A. *et al*: Reticuloplasmacytoma of pharynx. Wiad. Lek., *27:* 751, 1974 (Polish)

BETSISHOV, V. K. *et al*: Classification and characteristics of operative treatment of deformities of the hand and fingers after burns. Ortop. Travmatol. Protez., *35:*5, 1974 (Russian)

BETTEX, M. *et al*: Long-term results of uretero-sigmoidostomies. Ann. Chir. Infant., *12:*423, 1971 (French)

BETTEX, M. *et al*: Letter: Gynecomastia in puberty. Anaesthesiol. Intensivmed. Prax., *9:*114, 1974 (German)

BETTMAN, OTTO: *Pictorial History of Medicine.* C C Thomas Co., Springfield, 1972.

BEVIN, A. G.: Hand trauma. N. C. Med. J., *31:*384, 1970)

BEVIN, A. G.: Aggressive combined management of the patient with hand injuries and hand surgery. Prog. Phys. Ther., *1:*191, 1970

BEVIN, A. G.: Metacarpal transfer. South. Med. J., *64:*1495, 1971

BEVIN, A. G.: Assessment of patients with injuries and surgical procedures of the hand. N. C. Med. J., *34:*197, 1973

BEYER, C. K.: Modified lacrimal probe. Arch. Ophth., *92:*157, 1974

BEYER, C. K. *et al*: Naso-orbital fractures, complications and treatment. Ophthalmologica, *163:*418, 1971

BEYER, C. K., AND CARROLL, J. M.: Moderately severe cicatricial entropion, PRS, *52:*450, 1973. Arch. Ophth., *89:*33, 1973

BEYER, C. K. *et al*: Anterior levator resection: problems and management. Trans. Am. Acad. Ophthalmol. Otolaryngol., *79:*687, 1975

BEZOUGLIS, C. P. *et al*: Use of skin strips in orthopedics. Ztschr. Orthop., *111:*617, 1973 (German)

BHANDARI, N. S., SHASTRI, K. D., AND SHARMA, M.: Double complete supernumerary breast on anterolateral aspect of right thigh: case report, PRS, *55:*247, 1975. Indian J. Surg., *36:*43, 1974

BHANGOO, K. S.: Histological changes following chemical face peeling (Letter to the Editor), PRS, *54:*599, 1974

BHANGOO, K. S., QUINLIVAN, J. K., AND CONNELLY, J.R.: Elastin fibers in scar tissue, PRS, *57:*308, 1976

BHANGOO, K. S., AND CHURCH, J. C. T.: Elastogenesis in healing wounds in bats, PRS, *57:*468, 1976

BHARGAVA, K. B. *et al*: Multiple neurilemmomas in ala nasi. J. Laryng. & Otol., *87:*823, 1973

BHARGAVA, K. S., AND ELHENCE, I. P.: Giant parotid tumors, PRS, *48:*604, 1971. Internat. Surg., *55:*448, 1971

BHASIN, D. *et al*: Radical metatarsectomy for intractable plantar ulceration in leprosy. Lepr. Rev., *43:*53, 1972

BHASKAR, S. N. *et al*: Pulsating water jet devices in debridement of combat wounds, PRS, *48:*612, 1971. Mil. Med., *136:*264, 1971

BHASKAR, S. N. *et al*: Tissue reaction to intrabony ceramic implants, PRS, *48:*299, 1971. Oral Surg., *31:*282, 1971

BHATIA, P. L. *et al*: Cranium bifidum occulta with juvenile fibromatosis of face. J. Laryng. & Otol., *87:*587, 1973

BIALOSTOZKY, L. Painless removal of sutures. Surgery, *76:*356, 1974

BIALOSTOZKY, L. *et al*: Fasciotomy in massive venous thrombosis. Arch. Inst. Cardiol. Mex., *41:*680, 1971 (Spanish)

BIALOSTOZKY, L. *et al*: Varicose ulcer, etiopathology and treatment. Prensa Med. Mex., *40:*92, 1975 (Spanish)

BIAS, H. I. *et al*: Implantable penile prostheses in impotent males. Urology, *5:*224, 1975

BICK, W.: Asymmetrical growth following repair of cleft lip, PRS, *56:*468, 1975. J. Maxillofacial Surg., *3:*7, 1975

BIGGAR, R. J. *et al*: Medical problems of ear piercing. N. Y. State J. Med., *75:*1460, 1975

BIEDERMANN, F. *et al*: Fibrous dysplasia of facial bones. Radiobiol. Radiother. (Berl.), *13:*189, 1972 (German)

BIENENGRABER, V. *et al*: Comparative histological studies on various methods for osteosynthesis in the mandible. Zahn. Mund. Kieferheilkd., *63:*668, 1975 (German)

BIERMANN, B. *et al*: Results of prognathism operations in the Westdeutsche Kieferklinik (West German Jaw Clinic). Differential analysis of the treatment in 98 cases. Fortschr. Kiefer. Gesichtschir., *18:*159, 1974 (German)

BILDER, J. *et al*: Discotemporal plastic treatment of hypermobile jaw joint. Cesk. Stomatol., *75:*190, 1975 (Czechoslovakian)

BILICH, G. L. *et al*: Anesthesia and treatment for burns in children. Khirurgiia (Mosk.), *47:* 32, 1971 (Russian)

BILLER, H. F.: Pedicled flaps: experimental and clinical study. Laryngoscope, *82:*1831, 1972

BILLER, H. F. *et al*: Delayed contralateral cervical metastases with laryngeal and laryngopharyngeal cancers. Laryngoscope, *81:*1499, 1971

BILLER, H. F. *et al*: Forehead flap. Technique and complications. Arch. Otolaryng., *97:*316, 1973

BILLER, H. F. *et al*: Angiofibroma: treatment approach. Laryngoscope, *84:*695, 1974

BILLINGHAM, RUPERT, AND SILVERS, WILLYS: *Immunobiology of Transplantation.* Prentice-Hall, Inc., Englewood Cliffs, N. J., 1971. PRS, *50:*399, 1972

BILLINGHAM, R. E. *et al*: Transplantation and cutaneous genetics. J. Invest. Dermatol., *60:*509, 1973

BILLINGS, B. L., AND LOWRY, L. D.: Tympanometry, impedence and aural reflex testing in cleft palate populations, PRS, *55:*380, 1975. Cleft Palate J., *11:*21, 1974

BILLROTH, T.: On uranoplasty (Classic Reprint), PRS, *50:*71, 1972

BILOW, H. *et al*: Interferences between the kind of injuries and wound healing in post-traumatic hand infections. Hefte Unfallheilkd., *107:*249, 1970 (German)

BINGHAM, H. G.: Discussion of "Simplified technique for free transfer of groin flaps, by use of Doppler probe," by Karkowski, Buncke, PRS, *56:*84, 1975

BINGHAM, H. G. *et al*: Should the pharyngeal flap be used primarily with palatoplasty? Cleft Palate J., *9:*319, 1972

BINGHAM, R. *et al*: Local use of antibiotics to prevent wound infection, PRS, *56:*362, 1975. Clin. Orthop., *99:*194, 1974

BINKERT, B.: Cholesteric liquid crystals: new visual aid to study of flap circulation (with Hoehn), PRS, *48:*209, 1971

BINNS, J. H.: Subcutaneous mastectomy and reconstruction in large breasts (with Kern), PRS, *54:*648, 1974

BINNS, P. M.: Experimental facial paralysis. Otolaryngol. Clin. North Am., 7:551, 1974

BINNS, P. M. *et al*: Facial nerve homografts. Arch. Otolaryng., *95:*342, 1972

BIRAN, S. *et al*: Malignant melanoma. Survey of 232 cases. Oncology, *28:*331, 1973

BIRCH, J. R.: Flammable fabrics and human burns, PRS, *48:*396, 1971. Canad. J. Surg., *14:*177, 1971

BIRCH, J. R., AND LINDSAY, W. K.: Evaluation of adults with repaired bilateral cleft lips and palates, PRS, *48:*457, 1971

BIRCHER, J. L.: Reflex algodystrophy and fractures of the hand. Acta Orthop. Belg., *39:*1024, 1973 (French)

BIRDSELL, D.: Surgical construction of male genitalia for the female-to-male transsexual (with Noe, Laub), PRS, *53:*511, 1974

BIRDSELL, D. C., AND BIRCH, J. R.: Anemia following thermal burns: survey of 109 children, PRS, *49:*236, 1972. Canad. J. Surg., *14:*345, 1971

BIRIUKOV, O. M.: Principles of restorative-reconstructive surgery in burns of the hands. Vestn. Khir., *105:*80, 1970 (Russian)

BIRKE, G. *et al*: Studies on burns. XV. Treatment with warm dry air, clinical results compared with those of earlier treatment series. Acta Chir. Scand. (Suppl.), *422:*1, 1971

BIRKE, W. P.: Difficulties in use of percutaneous osteosynthesis in the mandible. Dtsch. Gesundheitsw., *26:*1379, 1971 (German)

BIRKE, W. P.: Local complications in percutaneous osteosynthesis (Rostock model) of mandible. Beitr. Orthop. Traumatol., *19:*700, 1972 (German)

BIRKE, W. P.: Methods for improving fragment adaptation in percutaneous osteosynthesis using plastic bridges. Dtsch. Stomatol., *23:*721, 1973 (German)

BIRKE, W. P. *et al*: Late results following surgical correction of prominent ears. Dtsch. Gesundheitsw., *26:*2370, 1971 (German)

BIRKE, W. P. AND SONNENBURG, M.: Surgical treatment of facial fractures. Zahntechnik (Berl.), *13:*443, 1972 (German)

BIRKE, W. P. *et al*: Statistics of temporomandibular joint disorders from the viewpoint of maxillofacial surgery. Stomatol. D.D.R., *24:* 683, 1974 (German)

BIRKENSTOCK, W. E. *et al*: Combined Ehlers-Danlos and Marfan's syndromes, with case report. S. Afr. Med. J., *47:*2097, 1973

BIRNHOLZ, J. C. *et al*: Advanced laryngeal compression due to diffuse symmetric lipomatosis (Madelung's disease). Brit. J. Radiol., *46:*245, 1973

BIRNMEYER, G.: Parotid surgery with special care of facial nerve. Z. Laryngol. Rhinol. Otol., *52:*813, 1973 (German)

BIRO, V. *et al*: Flexor tendon injuries of the hand. Orv. Hetil., *114:*610, 1973 (Hungarian)

BIRO, V., HORVATH, A., AND HERBER, E.: Experimental tendon sheath formation out of vasal tissue, PRS, *55:*119, 1975. Bruns' Beitr. klin. Chir., *221:*319, 1974

BIRT, B. D. *et al*: Management of malignant tumors of the maxillary sinus. Otolaryngol. Clin. North Am., *9:*249, 1976

BISAGGIO, S.: Considerations about a case of silicoma, PRS, *50:*635, 1972. Folha med. Brazil, *63:*59, 1971

BISAGGIO, S.: Skin flaps in plastic surgery, PRS, *51:*109, 1973. Folha Med. Brazil, *63:*59, 1971

BISCHOFF, P.: Plastic and reconstructive procedures in cases of hypospadias, epispadias, and ectopic urinary bladder, PRS, *53:*244, 1974. Chir. Praxis, *16:*575, 1972; Part 2, *17:*73, 1973

BISHARA, S. E.: Cephalometric evaluation of facial growth in operated and non-operated individuals with isolated clefts of the palate. Cleft Palate J., *10:*239, 1973

BISHARA, S. E.: The influence of palatoplasty and cleft length on facial development. Cleft Palate J., *10:*390, 1973

BISHARA, S. E.: Treatment planning in maxillary prognathism. Am. J. Orthod., *64:*384, 1973; *65:*430, 1974

BISHARA, S. E.: Comparisons of effect of two palatal plasties on facial and dental relations, PRS, *55:*513, 1975. Cleft Palate J., *11:*261, 1974

BISHARA, S. E.: Effect of palatoplasty and cleft extent on facial and dental relations, PRS, *55:*513, 1975. Internat. J. Oral Surg., *3:*65, 1974

BISHARA, S. E.: Effects of the Wardill-Kilner (V/W-Y) palatoplasty on facial growth. Angle Orthod., *45:*55, 1975

BISHARA, S. E. *et al*: Surgical repositioning of the premaxilla in complete bilateral cleft lip and palate. Angle Orthod., *42:*139, 1972

BISHARA, S. E. *et al*: Cephalometric comparisons on the cranial base and face in individuals with isolated clefts of the palate. Cleft. Palate. J., *11:*162, 1974

BISHARA, S. E. *et al*: Relation between speech production and oro-facial structures in individuals with isolated clefts of the palate. Cleft Palate J., *12:*452, 1975

BISI, R. H.: Management of mandibular fractures in edentulous patients by intramedullary pinning. Laryngoscope, *83:*22, 1973

BISKCUPSKA-WIECKO, J.: Anthropometric studies of auricle from standpoint of reconstructive procedures in auricular hypoplasia. Oto-laryngol. Pol., *26:*537, 1972 (Polish)

BISKUPSKA-WIECKO, J. *et al*: Management of injuries of auricles and nose. Pol. Prezegl. Chir., *46:*619, 1974 (Polish)

Bites and Stings

Alligator bite (Doering *et al*). J.A.M.A., *218:*255, 1971

Facial reconstruction with tubed pedicle flaps in extensive soft tissue loss after a bear bite (Nara *et al*). Jap. J. Plast. Reconstr. Surg., *14:*502, 1971 (Japanese)

Survival after snake-bite with prolonged neurotoxic envenomation (Pearn). M. J. Australia, *2:*259, 1971

Corticosteroids and cryotherapy in treatment of rattlesnake bite (Clark), PRS, *48:*95, 1971. Mil. Med., *136:*42, 1971

Cat bites, Pasteurella multocida infections following animal injuries (Tindall, Harrison), PRS, *51:*485, 1973. Arch. Dermat., *105:*412, 1972

Arizona's lethal scorpion (Stahnke). Ariz. Med., *29:*490, 1972

Treatment of poisonous snake bites (Pogasian). Khirurgiia (Mosk.), *48:*129, 1972 (Russian)

Snakebitten hand (Snyder, Straight, Glenn), PRS, *49:*275, 1972

Dog bite avulsions of the lip, conservative concept (Musgrave, Garrett), PRS, *49:*294, 1972

Face, treatment of dog bite injuries, (Schultz, McMaster), PRS, *49:*494, 1972

Dog bite, loss of nasal ala from, immediate composite graft to (Wynn), PRS, *50:*188, 1972

Clinical development of three patients bitten by a viper (Laurencet *et al*). Schweiz. Med. Wochenschr., *102:*981, 1972 (French)

Treatment of injuries resulting from dog bites (Fritz). Wien. Klin. Wochenschr., *84:*12, 1972 (German)

Bites, 84 cases (Gournet). Ann. chir. plast., *18:*355, 1973 (French)

Snakebites in children (Henderson, Dujon), PRS, *54:*512, 1974. J. Pediat. Surg., *8:*729, 1973

Dog bites, role of primary closure (Thomson, Svitek), PRS, *52:*687, 1973. J. Trauma, *13:*20, 1973

Snakebites in Vietnam, treatment of (Berlinger, Flowers), PRS, *52:*601, 1973. Mil. Med., *138:*139, 1973

Early debridement in pit viper bite (Glass). Surg. Gynec. & Obst., *136:*774, 1973

Face bites, treatment of (Khaikin). Vestn. Khir., *109:*95, 1973 (Russian)

Bites and Stings—Cont.

Dog bite, replantation of composite graft of nasal ala (Elsahy), PRS, *55:*633, 1975. Acta chir. plast., *16:*124, 1974

Snakebite, excisional therapy in management of (Huang *et al*), PRS, *55:*121, 1975. Ann. Surg., *179:*598, 1974

Bites, necrotic, of brown spider, surgery for (Auer *et al*). Arch. Surg., *108:*612, 1974

Severe injury due to shark bite (Levy). Harefuah, *87:*258, 1974 (Hebrew)

Two cases of reconstruction of soft tissue defects of the face caused by human bite (Bertenyi). Magy. Traumatol Orthop., *17:*126, 1974 (Hungarian)

Bloodflow measured during the edema stage of snakebite by the Doppler flowmeter (Gurucharri, Henzel, Mitchell), PRS, *53:*551, 1974

Bites of the hand (Parks *et al*). Rocky Mt. Med. J., *71:*85, 1974

Rabies prevention in humans (Rubin, Corey), PRS, *56:*115, 1975. South. M.J., *67:*1472, 1974

Maxillofacial region, bite wounds in, treatment of (Rink). Stomatol. D.D.R., *24:*461, 1974 (German)

Bucloxic acid in plastic surgery (Deidier *et al*). Ann. chir. plast., *20:*343, 1975 (French)

Hand infections secondary to human bites (Shields *et al*). J. Trauma, *15:*235, 1975

Treatment of infected wounds and ulcers by coherent irradiation (Bogdanovich *et al*). Khirurgiia (Mosk.), *4:*56, 1975 (Russian)

Sepsis, selection of antibiotics for human bites of hand (Guba, Mulliken, Hoopes), PRS, *56:*538, 1975

Dogbite injuries in children (Chait, Spitz), PRS, *57:*126, 1976. South African M.J., *49:*718, 1975

Poisonous snakebite: a review. 2. Symptomatology and treatment (Van Mierop). J. Fla. Med. Assoc., *63:*201, 1976

BITSEFF, E. L.: Rapid transfer of thoracoacromial flaps to the face and neck (with Pollock, Ryan), PRS, *50:*433, 1972

BITTER, K.: Immunity suppression by bleomycinmethotrexate combined treatment in patients with epidermoid carcinoma of oral cavity, PRS, *54:*508, 1974. J. Maxillo-facial Surg., *2:*35, 1974

BIVENS, M. D., AND ZIMMERMANN, E. A.: Clear cell adenocarcinoma of vagina—reconstruction after radical surgery, PRS, *55:*511, 1975. Rocky Mountain M.J., *71:*512, 1974

BIVINS, B. A., MADAUSS, W. C., AND GRIFFIN, W. O.: Fat embolism syndrome: clinical study, PRS, *51:*486, 1973. South. M.J., *65:*937, 1972

BIXLER, D.: Heritability of clefts of lip and palate, PRS, *56:*108, 1975. Prosth. Dent., *33:*100, 1975

BIXLER, D., FOGH-ANDERSEN, P., AND CONNEALLY, P. M.: Incidence of cleft lip and palate in offspring of cleft parents, PRS, *51:*482, 1973. Clin. Genetics, *2:*155, 1971

BIZER, L. S.: Fibrosarcoma. Report of sixty-four cases, PRS, *49:*473, 1972. Am. J. Surg., *121:*586, 1971

BJARNASON, O.: Laryngectomy and radical neck dissection. Timarit. Hjukrunarfil. Isl., *48:*84, 1972 (Icelandic)

BJORDAL, R.: Treatment of ulcer venosum cruris. Tidsskr. Nor. Laegeforen, *95:*1809, 1975 (Norwegian)

BJORK, A., AND SKIELLER, V.: Growth in width of maxilla studied by implant method, PRS, *56:*354, 1975. Scand. J. Plast. Reconstr. Surg., *8:*25, 1974

BJORLIN, G. *et al*: Silicone implants for reconstruction of flabby alveolar ridges. Sven. Tandlak. Tidskr., *64:*789, 1971

BJORNSSON, A. *et al*: Paratuberculosis of the hand, PRS, *49:*584, 1972. Scand. J. Plast. Reconstr. Surg., *5:*156, 1971

BLACK, P. W.: Correction of a flat folded helix, PRS, *48:*86, 1971

BLACKFIELD, H. M. *et al*: Cinefluorographic analysis of the surgical treatment of cleft palate speech (Follow-Up Clinic), PRS, *49:*335, 1972

BLACKSTEIN, M. E. *et al*: Chemotherapy and palliative therapy in malignant disease of the maxillary sinus. Otolaryngol. Clin. North Am., *9:*291, 1976

Bladder Exstrophy

Bladder reconstruction. Method derived from that of Trendelenburg (Cendron). Ann. Chir. Infant., *12:*371, 1971 (French)

Disappointing results of reconstruction in the treatment of bladder exstrophy (Cukier *et al*). Ann. Chir. Infant., *12:*382, 1971 (French)

Treatment of bladder exstrophy. Bladder reconstruction. Dry repair (Mollard). Ann. Chir. Infant., *12:*385, 1971 (French)

Treatment of bladder exstrophy. 1. Bladder reconstruction. Extension plasties (Mollard). Ann. Chir. Infant., *12:*386, 1971 (French)

Treatment of bladder exstrophy. Bladder reconstruction. Osteotomy (Campo-Paysaa). Ann. Chir. Infant., *12:*387, 1971 (French)

Treatment of bladder exstrophy. Internal shunt. Vesicorectal implantations (Mollard). Ann. Chir. Infant., *12:*391, 1971 (French)

Bladder Exstrophy—Cont.

Ureterosigmoidostomy. Introduction (Mollard). Ann. Chir. Infant., *12:*393, 1971 (French)

Ureterocolonic transplantations. Palliative treatment of bladder exstrophy (Petit). Ann. Chir. Infant., *12:*394, 1971 (French)

Ureterocolonic implantation in the treatment of bladder exstrophy: 42 cases out of 68 bladder exstrophies from 1945 to 1969 (Pellerin *et al*). Ann. Chir. Infant., *12:*400, 1971 (French)

Long-term results of 16 ureterosigmoidostomies for bladder exstrophy (follow-up from 6 to 38 years) (Chatelain *et al*). Ann. Chir. Infant., *12:*408, 1971 (French)

Long-term results of ureterosigmoidostomies (Bettex *et al*). Ann. Chir. Infant., *12:*423, 1971 (French)

Intestinal bladders controlled by the anal sphincter. Technics and results (Duhamel). Ann. Chir. Infant., *12:*433, 1971 (French)

Ileal bladder controlled by the anal sphincter (Pous). Ann. Chir. Infant., *12:*443, 1971 (French)

Our experience with rectal bladders (Cendron). Ann. Chir. Infant., *12:*444, 1971 (French)

Treatment of bladder exstrophy. External shunt. Nephrostomy, ureterostomy, trigonostomy (Mollard). Ann. Chir. Infant., *12:*445, 1971 (French)

Transintestinal cutaneous ureterostomy for bladder exstrophy: 17 cases of which 13 use an ileal intraperitoneal loop and 4 a sigmoid loop (Pellerin *et al*). Ann. Chir. Infant., *12:*447, 1971 (French)

Transsigmoid cutaneous ureterostomies (Meli). Ann. Chir. Infant., *12:*450, 1971 (French)

Apropos of transsigmoid cutaneous ureterostomies (Brueziere). Ann. Chir. Infant., *12:*459, 1971 (French)

Apropos of the technic of ureterointestinal anastomosis (Lasserre). Ann. Chir. Infant., *12:*460, 1971 (French)

Apropos of Bricker's operation (Prevot). Ann. Chir. Infant., *12:*462, 1971 (French)

Treatment of bladder exstrophy. Practical problems of equipment (Cendron). Ann. Chir. Infant., *12:*464, 1971 (French)

Treatment of bladder exstrophy. Transformation of an external transintestinal shunt into an internal shunt (Cendron). Ann. Chir. Infant., *12:*465, 1971 (French)

Treatment of bladder exstrophy. Urinary results of the different methods (Mollard). Ann. Chir. Infant., *12:*467, 1971 (French)

Treatment of bladder exstrophy. Genital

Bladder Exstrophy—Cont.

problem (Cendron). Ann. Chir. Infant., *12:*473, 1971 (French)

Treatment of bladder exstrophy. Therapeutic indications (Cendron *et al*). Ann. Chir. Infant., *12:*481, 1971 (French)

Late results of Coffey's operation for bladder exstrophy in 10 cases (Barcat *et al*). Ann. Chir. Infant., *12:*615, 1971 (French)

Treatment of exstrophy of the bladder (Kimche *et al*). Harefuah, *80:*375, 1971 (Hebrew)

Bladder, incomplete exstrophy of (Ignatoff *et al*), PRS, *48:*514, 1971. J. Urol., *105:*579, 1971

Exstrophy of bladder, duplicate (Ellis), PRS, *50:*200, 1972. J. Urol., *106:*295, 1971

Primary closure of exstrophy in the newborn: a preliminary report (Ansell). Northwest Med., *70:*842, 1971

Exstrophy of the bladder (Johnston). Prog. Pediatr. Surg., *2:*147, 1971

New concept concerning treatment of exstrophy of the bladder: 20 years later (Boyce). Trans. Am. Assoc. Genitourin. Surg., *63:*121, 1971

Surgery of bladder exstrophy with ureterosigmoidostomy and cystectomy (Schmitt *et al*). Z. Urol. Nephrol., *64:*509, 1971 (German)

Genital function in males with vesical exstrophy and epispadias (Hanna *et al*). Brit. J. Urol., *44:*169, 1972

Indications for rectal bladder (Bracci). Bull. Soc. Internat. Chir., *31:*544, 1972 (Italian)

Bladder, ectopic urinary, plastic and reconstructive procedures (Bischoff), PRS, *53:*244, 1974. Chir. Praxis, *16:*575, 1972; Part 2, *17:*73, 1973

New concept concerning treatment of exstrophy of the bladder: 20 years later (Boyce). J. Urol., *107:*476, 1972

Exstrophied bladder, how well can it work? (Nisonson, Lattimer), PRS, *51:*604, 1973. J. Urol., *107:*664, 1972

Bladder, exstrophied, after anatomical closure, histologic analysis of (Rudin *et al*). J. Urol., *108:*802, 1972

Bladder exstrophy, surgery in (Romualdi). Minerva Pediatr., *24:*1168, 1972

Bladder exstrophy, possibilities of therapy (Wiltschke). Paediatr. Paedol., *7:*75, 1972 (German)

Female escutcheon in exstrophy of the bladder, reconstruction (Ship, Pelzer), PRS, *49:*643, 1972

Bladder, exstrophy of, one-stage reconstruction of the external genitalia in the female (Owsley, Hinman), PRS, *50:*227, 1972

Reply to the article by W. Schmitt and co-

Bladder Exstrophy — Cont.

workers: "Surgery of bladder exstrophy using ureterosigmoideostomy and cystectomy" in: Zschr. Urol., *64:*509, (Pompino). Z. Urol. Nephrol., *65:*289, 1972 (German)

Bladder exstrophy, rectal reservoir for (Strohmenger). Acta Urol. Belg., *41:*25, 1973

Bladder exstrophy, anomaly of external genitalia in female patients with (Jones). Am. J. Obstet. Gynecol., *117:*748, 1973

Successful treatment of severe hypokalaemic paralysis with respiratory insufficiency in patient with ureterosigmoidostomy (Chiari *et al*). Anaesthetist, *22:*280, 1973 (German)

Bladder exstrophy, reconstruction (Williams). Brit. J. Surg., *60:*203, 1973

Bladder exstrophy, notes on Boyce-Vest operation for (Marshall). J. Urol., *109:*111, 1973

Exstrophy of bladder, management of 140 cases (Megalli, Lattimer), PRS, *52:*597, 1973. J. Urol., *109:*246, 1973

Bladder exstrophy, management of infants with cloaca (Markland). J. Urol., *109:*740, 1973

Exstrophic human bladder, scanning and transmission electron microscopic studies of (Clark *et al*). J. Urol., *110:*481, 1973

Bladder exstrophy, ureterosigmoidostomy for, healthy pregnancy 24 years after, in spite of prolonged treatment with chloraminophen and corticosteroids for chronic rheumatoid arthritis (Suhler *et al*). J. Urol. Nephrol. (Paris), *79:*599, 1973 (French)

New urinary bladder made from rectum (Khadzhlev). Khirurgiia (Sofiia), *26:*168, 1973 (Bulgarian)

Urogenital system in children, certain abnormalities of, sex determination and its surgical correction in (Kushch). Klin. Khir., *8:*39, 1973

Bladder exstrophy, treated by cystosigmoidostomy, two cases. Fifteen year follow-up (Sesia). Minerva Urol., *25:*143, 1973 (Italian)

Urinary bladder exstrophy, treatment (Renkielski). Pol. Przegl. Chir., *45:*1201, 1973 (Polish)

Bladder exstrophy: vesicoplasty or urinary diversion? (Engle). Urology, *2:*20, 1973

Bladder exstrophy treated by ureterosigmoidostomies. Long term evaluation (Bennett). Urology, *2:*165, 1973

Urinary incontinence, preparation for plastic operations of skin and mucous membrane of external female genitalia in patients with (Anton'ev *et al*). Urol. Nefrol. (Mosk.), *38:*41, 1973

Bladder Exstrophy — Cont.

Bladder exstrophy, technic for repair of skin defect following Maydl-Ternovskii-Michelson operation for (Doleskii). Urol. Nefrol. (Mosk.), *38:*55, 1973 (Russian)

Ionic disorders in uro-ileal shunts (Mathieu *et al*). Arch. Fr. Pediatr., *31:*241, 1974 (French)

Bladder exstrophy, urinary, vesicosigmoanastomosis using Maydl method in (Murvanidze). Brantisl. Lek. Listy., *61:*396, 1974 (Slovakian)

Bladder, exstrophy of (Heras Perez), PRS, *56:*236, 1975. Cir. Españ., *28:*265, 1974

Exstrophic anomalies and their surgical reconstruction (Johnston *et al*). Curr. Probl. Surg., *1:*39, 1974

Urinary diversion, methods of (Kornitzer *et al*). Geriatrics, *29:*85, 1974

Anterior abdominal wall defects (Pathak *et al*). Indian. Pediatr., *11:*781, 1974

Urinary diversions, ureteroilial anastomosis in, comparison of Bricker and Wallace methods of (Esho *et al*). J. Urol., *111:*600, 1974

Urinary diversion, intestinal loop, in children (Richie). J. Urol., *111:*687, 1974

Bladder, exstrophy of, reconstruction of external genitalia in (Allen, Spence, Salyer), PRS, *57:*536, 1976. J. Urol., *111:*830, 1974

Bladder exstrophy, unilateral, and low male imperforate anus, duplication of hindgut (Emery *et al*). J. Urol., *112:*532, 1974

Urinary diversion in children by sigmoid conduit: its advantages and limitations (Kelalis). J. Urol., *112:*666, 1974

Cloacal exstrophy with the potential for urinary control: an unusual presentation (Koontz *et al*). J. Urol., *112:*828, 1974

Bladder exstrophy, children with, possibilities of operative treatment (Pompino). Munch. Med. Wochenschr., *116:*1187, 1974 (German)

Bladder exstrophy, vulvoplasty in cases of (Weed *et al*). Obstet. Gynecol., *43:*512, 1974

Bladder: external sphincterotomy (Schellhammer, Hackler, Bunts), PRS, *56:*106, 1975. Paraplegia, *12:*5, 1974

Surgical problems in various urologic diseases in childhood (Floretti *et al*). Pediatria (Napoli), *82:*398, 1974 (Italian)

Exstrophy, questions that worry children with (Feinberg *et al*). Pediatrics, *53:*242, 1974

Supracystic urinary drainage in children (Sztaba *et al*). Pol. Przegl. Chir., *46:*1453, 1974 (Polish)

Study of mucosa of ileocystoplasties and ileoureteroplasties. Preliminary note (Bocquet

Bladder Exstrophy — Cont.
et al). Sem. Hop. Paris, *50:*873, 1974
Surgical embryology of the exstrophy-epispa-
dias complex (Ambrose *et al*). Surg. Clin.
North Am., *54:*1379, 1974
Bladder exstrophy, urinary, complicated by
adenocarcinoma (Kandzari *et al*). Urology,
*3:*496, 1974
Surgical antireflux procedure for scarred or
exstrophic bladders, variation of technique
(Lattimer). Urology, *3:*508, 1974
Duplication of external genitalia in men (So-
tiropoulos *et al*). Urology, *4:*688, 1974
Modification of plastic repair of bladder ex-
strophy (Konstantinova). Urol. Nefrol.
(Mosk.), *32:*43, 1974 (Russian)
Derivation of the upper urinary ways in blad-
der exstrophy (Wagenknecht *et al*). Z.
Urol. Nephrol., *67:*589, 1974 (German)
Surgical correction of bladder exstrophy (de
Laval *et al*). Acta Urol. Belg., *43:*292, 1975
(French)
Accessory exstrophic bladder (Saadi). Brit. J.
Clin. Pract., *29:*275, 1975
Nonrefluxing colon conduit for temporary or
permanent urinary diversion in children
(Hendren). J. Pediatr. Surg., *10:*381, 1975
Exstrophy, genital aspects of (Johnston). J.
Urol., *113:*701, 1975
Exstrophy of the bladder. I. Long-term re-
sults in a series of 37 cases treated by ure-
terosigmoidostomy (Spence *et al*). J. Urol.,
*114:*133, 1975
Long-term results of ureterosigmoidostomy
in children with bladder exstrophy (Segura
et al). J. Urol., *114:*138, 1975
Bladder exstrophy operated by Lattimer's
technic. 10-year results (Cibert *et al*).
J. Urol. Nephrol. (Paris), 81:45, 1975
(French)
Neo-bladder made from the rectum in surgical care of uro-genital malformations (Nedelec *et al*). J. Urol. Nephrol. (Paris),
*81:*481, 1975 (French)
An assessment of the functional results of
various forms of surgery for epispadias and
exstrophy (Eckstein). Langenbecks Arch.
Chir., *339:*439, 1975 (German)
Round-table discussion on plastic and reconstructive surgery servicing function. Sexual function, urinary and fecal incontinence. Langenbecks Arch. Chir., *339:*459,
1975 (German)
Urinary diversion through isolated bowel
segments (Strohmenger *et al*). Langenbecks Arch. Chir., *340:*91, 1975 (German)
Incontinence, one-stage reconstruction for
exstrophy of bladder in girls (Furnas, Haq,
Somers), PRS, *56:*61, 1975. Discussion by

Bladder Exstrophy — Cont.
Devine, PRS, *56:*209, 1975
Exstrophy of the bladder. Fifty years' survival following cystosigmoidostomy. Case
report (Lindfors *et al*). Scand. J. Urol. Nephrol., *9:*282, 1975
Exstrophy of the bladder — an alternative
method of management (Hendren). J.
Urol., *115:*195, 1976
Considerations on malignant transformation
of congenital exstrophic bladder (Musierowicz *et al*). Wiad. Lek., *29:*153, 1976
(Polish)

BLAKE, G. B.: Back tube pedicle in head and
neck reconstruction. Brit. J. Plast. Surg.,
*28:*59, 1975
BLAKE, G. B. *et al*: Malignant tumors of ear and
their treatment. 1. Tumors of auricle. Brit. J.
Plast. Surg., *27:*67, 1974
BLAKE, J.: Immune studies in malignant mela-
noma. Brit. J. Surg., *58:*856, 1971
BLAKE, K. C. *et al*: Study of 99mTc-polyphos-
phate as a joint imaging agent. S. Afr. Med.
J., *48:*2292, 1974
BLAKEMORE, J. R. *et al*: Primary Ewing's sar-
coma of mandible: case report. J. Oral Surg.,
*33:*376, 1975
BLAKEMORE, J. R. *et al*: Maxillary exostoses.
Surgical management of an unusual case.
Oral Surg., *40:*200, 1975
BLANCHART, J. A.: Total rhinoplasties, PRS,
*48:*89, 1971. Rev. espan. cir. plast., *2:*21, 1969
BLANCK, C. *et al*: Poorly differentiated solid
parotid carcinoma. Acta Radiol. (Ther.)
(Stockh.), *13:*17, 1974
BLANCO, R., ARAMBURU, P. E., AND MALDON-
ADO, M.: Filling of first intermetacarpal
space in ulnar paralysis, PRS, *54:*620, 1974.
Bol. Sudamer. cir. Mano., *5:*38, 1973
BLANCO, R. H.: Digital transposition, PRS,
*49:*103, 1972. Bull. Soc. Plast. Surg. Cordoba
Argent., *1:*2, 1971
BLANCO LOPEZ, F. *et al*: Isolated lesions of penis
in children. An. Esp. Peadiatr., *7:*319, 1974
(Spanish)
BLANDY, J. P. *et al*: Technique and results of
one-stage island patch urethroplasty. Brit. J.
Urol., *47:*83, 1975
BLANKENBAKER, W. L., AND DeFAZIO, C. A.:
Lidocaine and its metabolites in newborn,
PRS, *57:*407, 1976. Anesthesiology, *42:*325,
1975

Blast Injuries

Multiple facial injuries (Hosxe *et al*). Maroc
Med., *52:*732, 1972 (French)
The Old Bailey bomb explosion (Caro *et al*).
Lancet, *1:*1433, 1973

Blast Injuries – Cont.

Thermonuclear weapon lesions of surgical interest (Dei Poli *et al*). Minerva Chir., *28:*558, 1973

Revised Fasanella-Servat ptosis operation (Bodian). Ann. Ophth., *7:*603, 1975

Military surgical team in Belfast (Boyd). Ann. R. Coll. Surg., Engl., *56:*15, 1975

Surgery of violence. 1. Civilian bomb injuries (Kennedy *et al*). Brit. Med. J., *1:*382, 1975

Tower of London bomb explosion (Tucker *et al*). Brit. Med. J., *3:*287, 1975

Surgical therapy of gunshot and explosion injuries (Hammer *et al*). Fortschr. Kiefer Gesichtschir., *19:*211, 1975 (German)

Current war injuries of extremities (Popovic *et al*). Vojnosanit. Pregl., *32:*546, 1975 (Serbian)

BLATT, I. M., AND FAILLA, A.: Acrylic implants for frontal bone defects, PRS, *50:*543, 1972. Mil. Med., *137:*22, 1972

BLAU, R. *et al*: Polyglycolic acid suture in strabismus surgery, PRS, *57:*394, 1976. Arch. Ophth., *93:*538, 1975

BLAUTH, W.: Surgical treatment of a case of dystrophic epidermolysis bullosa. Handchirurgie, *3:*129, 1971 (German)

BLAUTH, W. *et al*: Morphology and classification of symbrachydactylia. Handchirurgie, *3:*123, 1971 (German)

BLAUTH, W. *et al*: Art of incisions by syndactylyrecidives. Arch. Orthop. Unfallchir., *77:*97, 1973

BLAUTH, W. *et al*: Symbrachydactylias. Handchirurgie, *5:*121, 1973 (German)

BLEEKER, G. M.: *Proceedings, 2nd International Symposium on Orbital Disorders,* Amsterdam, 1973. Albert J. Phiebig, White Plains, N.Y., 1975

BLEEKER, G. M., AND LYLE, T. KEITH: *Fractures of the Orbit.* Williams & Wilkins Co., Baltimore, 1970. PRS, *48:*589, 1971

BLEIFELD, C. J., AND INGLIS, A. E.: Hand in systemic lupus erythematosus, PRS, *55:*570, 1975. J. Bone & Joint Surg., *56A:*1207, 1974

BLELOCK, J. A.: Intersex. Proc. Mine. Med. Off. Assoc., *50:*82, 1971

BLEMER, E. *et al*: Hand injury due to heat and simultaneous pressure "ironing machine injury." Munch. Med. Wochenschr., *116:*2185, 1974 (German)

BLEMER, E. *et al*: Localized neurofibromatosis of the right half of the face. In *Plastische und Wiederherstellungs-Chirurgie,* ed. Hohler; Schattauer, Stuttgart, 1975, pp. 357–61 (German)

Blepharoplasty

Palpebral fissure, lengthening and shortening the (Fox), PRS, *49:*356, 1972. Arch. Ophth., *86:*401, 1971

"Baggy eyelids," late report on an early operation for (Safian), PRS, *48:*347, 1971

Lid Surgery, Current Concepts. By Sidney A. Fox. Grune & Stratton, New York, 1972. PRS, *51:*580, 1973

Blepharoplasty, cosmetic, skin clamps in (Feldstein). Arch. Ophthalmol., *88:*659, 1972

Intradermal double eyelid operation and its follow-up results (Mutou *et al*). Brit. J. Plast. Surg., *25:*285, 1972

Malpractice and new legal decisions. II. Treatment of blepharoptosis following plastic surgery of eyelids (Terahata). Iryo, *26:*264, 1972 (Japanese)

Esthetic operations of the eyelids (Molenaar). Ned. tijdschr. geneeskd., *116:*68, 1972 (Dutch)

Blepharoplasty, upper, marginal incision for (Cronin), PRS, *49:*14, 1972

Blepharoplasty, causes and prevention of lower lid ectropion following (Edgerton), PRS, *49:*367, 1972

Blepharoplasty and rhytidectomy, deliberate hypotension for (Stark) (Follow-Up Clinic), PRS, *49:*453, 1972

Blepharoplasty, should incisions in the orbital septum be sutured in? (Tipton), PRS, *49:*613, 1972

Blepharoplasty, Trainor, for ptosis (Herceg, Harding), PRS, *49:*622, 1972

Blepharoplasty, correction of ectropion resulting from (Rees), PRS, *50:*1, 1972

Blepharoplasty, employment of carica papaya endopeptidase associated with benzidamine (Lopez), PRS, *52:*104, 1973. Tribuna Med. Argent., *15:*611, 1972

Blepharophimosis, surgical treatment of (Rougier). Ann. chir. plast., *18:*141, 1973 (French)

Blepharoplasty: baggy eyelids, true hernia (Putterman, Urist), PRS, *54:*686, 1974. Ann. Ophth., *5:*1029, 1973

Blepharoplasty, musculocutaneous flap in (Feldstein). Arch. Otolaryng., *97:*294, 1973

Blindness following blepharoplasty (Jafek, Kreiger, Morledge), PRS, *54:*105, 1974. Arch. Otolaryng., *98:*366, 1973

Blepharoplasty, sudden blindness following (Moser, DiPirro, McCoy), PRS, *51:*364, 1973

Retrobulbar hemorrhage, acute, during elective blepharoplasty (Hartley, Lester,

Blepharoplasty — Cont.

Schatten), PRS, *52:*8, 1973. Discussions by Lemoine, Rees, Newell, PRS, *52:*12, 1973

Blepharoplasty: brow lifting through a temporal scalp approach (Gleason), PRS, *52:*141, 1973

Eyelid, unesthetic (Hervouet). Rev. Prat., *23:*3149, 1973 (French)

Blepharophimosis syndromes, surgical correction of (Callahan). Trans. Am. Acad. Ophthalmol. Otolaryngol., *77:*687, 1973

Blepharoplasty, survey (Marlowe). Trans. Pa. Acad. Ophthalmol. Otolaryngol., *26:*114, 1973

Blepharochalasis (Stieglitz *et al*). Am. J. Ophth., *77:*100, 1974

Blepharoplasty complication — acute closed-angle glaucoma (Green, Kadri), PRS, *56:*676, 1975. Brit. J. Plast. Surg., *27:*25, 1974

Surgery of the Oriental eyelid (Sayoc). Clin. Plast. Surg., *1:*157, 1974

Blepharoplasties and face lift operations, complications in (Berman *et al*). Otolaryngol. Clin. North Am., *7:*87, 1974

Blepharoplasty, upper, use of double W-plasty (Courtiss, Webster, White), PRS, *53:*25, 1974

Intraorbital fat: anatomy for blepharoplasty (Hugo, Stone), PRS, *53:*381, 1974. Discussion by Castañares, PRS, *53:*587, 1974

Blepharoplasty, early relief of blindness occurring after (McDowell) (Editorial), PRS, *53:*581, 1974

Anatomy for a blepharoplasty (Hugo, Stone), PRS, *53:*381, 1974. Discussion by Castañares, PRS, *53:*587, 1974

Blepharoplasty, successful early relief of blindness occurring after (Hueston, Heinze), PRS, *53:*588, 1974. Discussion by Hepler, Sugimura, Straatsma, PRS, *57:*233, 1976

Blepharoplasty or other eyelid surgery, eye complications with (DeMere, Wood, Austin), PRS, *53:*634, 1974

Blepharoplasty, planning and evaluating (Berry), PRS, *54:*257, 1974

Supratarsal fixation in upper blepharoplasty (Sheen), PRS, *54:*424, 1974

Blepharoplasty, "dry eye" following (Swartz, Schultz, Seaton), PRS, *54:*644, 1974

Hemorrhage, orbital, from retrobulbar injection, central retinal artery closure during (Kraufhar, Seelenfreund, Froelich), PRS, *54:*382, 1974. Tr. Am. Acad. Ophth., *78:*65, 1974

Errors and complications of blepharoplasty (Muller). *In Plastische und Wiederherstel-*

Blepharoplasty — Cont.

lungs-Chirurgie, ed. Hohler; Schattauer, Stuttgart, 1975, pp. 81-3 (German)

Blepharoplasty, esthetic (Matton), PRS, *57:*529, 1976. Acta chir. belg., *74:*358, 1975

Anti-inflammatory agents, noncorticosteroidal, ocular compression and (Obstbaum, Podos), PRS, *57:*113, 1976. Am. J. Ophth., *79:*1008, 1975

Surgical revision of the upper eyelid fold (Cies *et al*). Am. J. Ophth., *80:*1019, 1975

Temporary blindness after cosmetic blepharoplasty (Putterman). Am. J. Ophth., *80:*1081, 1975

Keratoconjunctivitis sicca after lacrimal gland removal (Scherz, Dohlman), PRS, *56:*460, 1975. Arch. Ophth., *93:*281, 1975

Treatment of enophthalmic narrow palpebral fissure after blow-out fracture (Putterman *et al*). Ophthalmic Surg., *6:*45, 1975

Complications of blepharoplasty (Levine *et al*). Ophthalmic Surg., *6:*53, 1975

Blepharoplasty, temporary suspension of the lower lid after (Horton, Gursu), PRS, *55:*371, 1975

W-epicanthoplasty (Mulliken, Hoopes), PRS, *55:*435, 1975

Blepharoplasty, transconjunctival lower lid, for removal of fat (Tomlinson, Hovey), PRS, *56:*314, 1975

Blepharoplasty, "dry eye" complication after (Rees), PRS, *56:*375, 1975

Blepharocanthoplasty with eyebrow lift (Hinderer), PRS, *56:*402, 1975

Surgical repair of congenital colobomas (Gribor). Trans. Am. Acad. Ophthalmol. Otolaryngol., *79:*671, 1975

Anterior levator resection: problems and management (Beyer *et al*). Trans. Am. Acad. Ophthalmol. Otolaryngol., *79:*687, 1975

Surgical reconstruction of complications associated with fronto-ethmoid mucocele surgery (Guibor). Trans. Am. Acad. Ophthalmol. Otolaryngol., *80:*454, 1975

Blepharoplasty, keratoconjunctivitis sicca symptoms appearing after (Graham, Messner, Miller), PRS, *57:*57, 1976

Blepharoptosis

Blepharoptosis, congenital, analysis of the causes, types and factors important to the correction of (Spaeth), PRS, *48:*509, 1971. Am. J. Ophth., *71:*696, 1971

Blepharoptosis, is it correctable, and how? (Crawford). Ann. Ophth., *3:*452, 1971

Surgery for progressive familial myopathic ptosis (Fox). Ann. Ophth., *3:*1033, 1971

Blepharoptosis—Cont.

Blepharoptosis, some newer concepts (Beard). Ann. Ophth., *3:*1047, 1971

Prosthetic aids in blepharoptosis: shelf devices (Heyman). Int. Ophthalmol. Clin., *10:*803, 1971

Blepharoptosis (Reeh). Mil. Med., *136:*760, 1971

Ptosis complicated by blepharophimosis and epicanthus, surgical treatment of (Khrinenko). Oftalmol. Zh., *26:*433, 1971 (Russian)

Surgical methods and results in congenital ptosis (Wild). Z. Aerztl. Fortbild. (Jena), *65:*976, 1971 (German)

Blepharoptosis, traumatic, surgical treatment of (Berke), PRS, *51:*102, 1973. Am J. Ophth., *72:*691, 1972

Surgery for sectional blepharoptosis (Bodian *et al*). Am. J. Ophth., *73:*214, 1972

Correction of unilateral blepharoptosis with bilateral eyelid suspension (Callahan). Am. J. Ophth., *74:*321, 1972

Blepharoptosis in myasthenia gravis, surgical correction (Kapetansky). Am. J. Ophth., *74:*818, 1972

Orbital orbicularis sling operation for ptosis (Sarwar). Ann. Ophth., *4:*250, 1972

Complications of ptosis surgery (Beard). Ann. Ophth., *4:*671, 1972

Ptosis, congenital: new pedigree and classification (Cohen), PRS, *50:*93, 1972. Arch. Ophth., *87:*161, 1972

Clamp for strengthening Muller's muscle in the treatment of ptosis. Modification, theory, and clamp for the Fasanella-Servat ptosis operation (Putterman). Arch. Ophth., *87:*665, 1972

An external approach to ptosis repair (Bodian). Arch. Ophth., *88:*176, 1972

Ptosis: some anatomical and surgical considerations (El-D Barrada *et al*). Bull. Ophthalmol. Soc. Egypt, *65:*545, 1972

Subcuticular closure in lower blepharoplasty (Aronsohn). Eye, Ear, Nose, Throat Mon., *51:*143, 1972

Levator-Mueller's muscle resection through combined internal and external approach (Carbajal). Eye, Ear, Nose, Throat Mon., *51:*348, 1972

Ptosis, silicone mesh sheet as suspension material (Arai, Fukuda, Akiyama), PRS, *52:*463, 1973. Jap. J. Plast. Reconstr. Surg., *15:*447, 1972

Simple ptosis operation with modified tarsectomy (Walser). Klin. Monatsbl. Augenheilkd., *160:*589, 1972 (German)

Ptosis, Trainor blepharoplasty for (Herceg, Harding), PRS, *49:*622, 1972

Blepharoptosis—Cont.

Three-tailed fascial sling for blepharoptosis (Garcia) (Follow-Up Clinic), PRS, *50:*281, 1972

Caveat chirurgicus (Sullivan). Trans. Am. Ophthalmol. Soc., *70:*328, 1972

Blepharoptosis, jaw-winking, treated by Fasanella-Servat procedure. Am. J. Ophth., *75:*1016, 1973

Arion's sutures in blepharoptosis correction (Rama *et al*). Am. J. Ophth., *76:*276, 1973

Blepharoptosis clamp, modification of (Gershen). Am. J. Ophth., *76:*589, 1973

Blepharoptosis, jaw-winking (Lauring). Am. J. Ophth., *76:*604, 1973

Blepharoptosis repair with modification of Fasanella-Servat operation (Crawford). Can. J. Ophthalmol., *8:*19, 1973

Ptosis, upper eyelid, therapy of, at Ophthalmological Clinic on Olomouc (Hrivova). Cesk. Oftalmol., *29:*310, 1973 (Czeckoslovakian)

Ptosis, congenital, mandibulo-palpebral synkinesis following surgery for (Antoszkiewicz *et al*). Klin. Oczna., *43:*823, 1973 (Polish)

Diagnosis and surgical treatment of syndrome of unilateral paralysis of eyeball-elevating muscles (Kobiela-Krzystkowa *et al*). Klin. Oczna., *43:*1197, 1973 (Polish)

Blepharoptosis, treatment when complicated by synkinesis (Barkhash). Oftalmol. Zh., *27:*567, 1973

Eyelid ptosis, lower, surgical correction of. The anophthalmic orbit (Vistnes, Iverson, Laub), PRS, *52:*346, 1973

Ptosis: correction of complications after levator resections for blepharoptosis (Callahan), PRS, *52:*616, 1973

Simplified levator recession in treatment of overcorrected blepharoptosis (Putterman *et al*). Surg. Forum, *24:*504, 1973

Fasanella-Servat operation (Beasley). Tex. Med., *69:*83, 1973

Surgery for minimal ptosis: Fasanella-Servat operation, 1973 (Fasanella). Trans. Ophthalmol. Soc. U.K., *93:*425, 1973

Transconjunctival isolation and transcutaneous resection of levator palpebrae superioris muscle (Putterman *et al*). Am. J. Ophth., *77:*90, 1974

Blepharoptosis, overcorrected, simplified levator palpebrae superioris muscle recession to treat (Putterman *et al*). Am. J. Ophth., *77:*358, 1974

Oculopharyngeal muscular dystrophy (Johnson *et al*). Am. J. Ophth., *77:*872, 1974

Levator, surgical correction of ptosis by resection of (Castroviejo), PRS, *55:*245, 1975.

Blepharoptosis — Cont.

Ann. Ophth., *6:*163, 1974

Blepharoptosis, adjustable fascia lata sling for correction of (Argamaso). Brit. J. Plast. Surg., *27:*274, 1974

Ptosis as result of trauma (Crawford). Can. J. Ophthalmol., *9:*244, 1974

Blepharoptosis caused by previous tearing off of upper lid, surgical treatment of (Blochowa *et al*). Klin. Oczna., *44:*699, 1974 (Polish)

Progress in the field of eyelid and orbit surgery (Walser). Med. Klin., *69:*1720, 1974 (German)

Blepharoptosis, forceps for the fixation of muscles elevating the upper eyelid in correction of (Aznabaev). Oftalmol. Zh., *28:*309, 1974 (Russian)

Congenital ptosis in children, modification of operation of (Sergeeva *et al*). Oftalmol. Zh., *29:*146, 1974 (Russian)

Technics of tenorrhaphy of levator muscle in correction of ptosis of upper eyelid (Paklomova). Oftalmol. Zh., *29:*452, 1974 (Russian)

Fasanella-Servat operation for ptosis of upper eyelid (Souther, Corboy, Thompson), PRS, *53:*123, 1974

Blepharoptosis, use of temporal aponeurosis in correction of (Cardoso). Rev. Asoc. Med. Bras., *20:*229, 1974 (Portuguese)

Modified ptosis clamp (Bodian). Trans. Am. Acad. Ophthalmol. Otolaryngol., *78:*221, 1974

Common problems in ophthalmic plastic surgery (Carroll). Am. Fam. Physician, *12:*85, 1975

Progressive external ophthalmoplegia associated with retinal pigment epitheliopathy (Daniele, Cianchetti, Cao), PRS, *57:*755, 1976. Am. J. Ophth., *8:*585, 1975

Aniridia and congenital ptosis (Shields, Reed), PRS, *56:*223, 1975. Ann. Ophth., *7:*203, 1975

Ptosis of upper eyelid, simple levator resection operation (Fox), PRS, *56:*223, 1975. Ann. Ophth., *7:*315, 1975

Ptosis, revised Fasanella-Servat operation (Bodian), PRS, *56:*591, 1975. Ann. Ophth., *7:*603, 1975

Levator tuck, a simplified blepharoptosis procedure (Harris, Dortzbach), PRS, *57:*394, 1976. Ann. Ophth., *7:*873, 1975

Ptosis surgery, recent trends in (Crawford), PRS, *57:*529, 1976. Ann. Ophth., *7:*1263, 1975

Muller muscle-conjunctiva resection. Technique for treatment of blepharoptosis (Putterman *et al*). Arch. Ophth., *93:*619,

Blepharoptosis — Cont.

1975

Cure of ptosis by aponeurotic repair (Jones *et al*). Arch. Ophth., *93:*629, 1975

Modified Fasanella-Servat procedure for ptosis (Fox). Arch. Ophth., *93:*639, 1975

Arion's thread in ptosis surgery (Turut). Bull. Soc. Ophthalmol. Fr., *75:*347, 1975 (French)

Deformities of the midface resulting from malunited orbital and naso-orbital fractures (Converse *et al*). Clin. Plast. Surg., *2:*107, 1975

Correction of congenital ptosis by the method of levator shortening (Khrinenko). Oftalmol. Zh., *30:*304, 1975 (Russian)

Eyelids: problems and possibilities in ptosis surgery (Mustardé), PRS, *56:*381, 1975

Surgical judgment in ptosis repair (Tenzel). Trans. Am. Acad. Ophthalmol. Otolaryngol., *79:*679, 1975

External minimal ptosis procedure – external tarsoaponeurectomy (McCord). Trans. Am. Acad. Ophthalmol. Otolaryngol., *79:*683, 1975

Anatomic approach to corrective surgery for blepharoptosis (Hargiss). Trans. Am. Acad. Ophthalmol. Otolaryngol., *79:*696, 1975

Management of myogenic (myopathic) ptosis (Waller). Trans. Am. Acad. Ophthalmol. Otolaryngol., *79:*697, 1975

Functional dermatochalasia (Carroll). Minn. Med., *59:*15, 1976

Blepharospasm

Surgical treatment of essential blepharospasm (McCabe, Boles). Ann. Otol. Rhin. & Laryng., *81:*611, 1972

Complications in surgery for blepharospasm (Dortzbach). Am. J. Ophth., *75:*142, 1973

Blepharospasm. New approach to treatment (Castañares), PRS, *51:*248, 1973

Blepharospasm, essential (Reid *et al*). J. Ir. Med. Assoc., *67:*64, 1974

BLERACQUE, A. *et al*: Chondro-mucosal grafts. Bull. Soc. Ophtalmol. Fr., *72:*1125, 1972 (French)

BLESER, F., SZTUKA, J. C., AND MULLER, J. P.: Effect of hyperbaric oxygen, tham, and antibiotics on experimental burns in rats, PRS, *50:*95, 1972. Europ. Surg. Res., *3:*409, 1971

BLESSING, H. *et al*: Gracilis plastic surgery using Pickrell's technic. (Helv. Chir. Acta, *42:*231, 1975 (German)

BLEULER, K.: Radical neck dissection in recurrent laryngeal and hypopharyngeal carcinoma. O.R.L., *36:*7, 1974 (German)

BLICHERT-TOFT, M. *et al*: Clinical course of cystosarcoma phylloides related to histologic appearance. Surg. Gynec. & Obst., *140:*929, 1975

BLIZZARD, R. M.: Incomplete testicular feminization. Birth Defects, *7:*310, 1971

BLOCH, BERNARD, AND HASTINGS, GARTH W.: *Plastic Materials in Surgery,* Second Edition. Charles C Thomas, Springfield, Ill., 1972. PRS, *52:*83, 1973

BLOCHIN, V. N.: Hand injuries and rehabilitation. Beitr. Orthop. Traumatol., *17:*586, 1970 (German)

BLOCHOWA, B. *et al*: Surgical treatment of ptosis caused by previous tearing off of the upper lid. Klin. Oczna., *44:*699, 1974 (Polish)

BLOCK, M. A., HORN, R. C., JR., AND MILLER, J. M.: Hazards in diagnosis and management of certain thyroid nodules in children, PRS, *48:*198, 1971. Am. J. Surg., *120:*447, 1970

BLOCK, M. A., MILLER, J. M., AND HORN, R. C., JR.: Thyroid carcinoma with cervical lymph node metastasis. Effectiveness of total thyroidectomy and node dissection, PRS, *51:*702, 1973. Am. J. Surg., *122:*458, 1971

BLOCK, M. A. *et al*: Angiomatous lymphoid hamartomas: surgical implications. Ann. Surg., *176:*620, 1972

BLOCK, N., ROSEN, P., AND WHITMORE, W., JR.: Hemipelvectomy for advanced penile cancer, PRS, *54:*238, 1974. J. Urol., *110:*703, 1973

BLOCK, N. L., AND HOTCHKISS, R. S.: Malignant melanoma of the female urethra: report of case with 5-year survival and review of literature, PRS, *48:*518, 1971. J. Urol., *105:*251, 1971

BLOCKER, T. G., JR., AND MCCORMACK, R. M.: Obituary on Alexander Burns Wallace, F.R.C.S. (Ed.), Ph.D., PRS, *57:*269, 1976

BLOCKSMA, R.: Experience with dimethylsiloxane fluid in soft tissue augmentation, PRS, *48:*564, 1971

BLOCKSMAN, R. *et al*: Study of deformity following cleft palate repair in patients with normal lip and alveolus. Cleft Palate J., *12:*390, 1975

BLOCKSMA, R., LEUZ, C. A., AND MELLERSTIG, K. E.: Conservative program for managing cleft palates without use of mucoperiosteal flaps, PRS, *55:*160, 1975

BLOEM, J. J.: Distortion of hand and finger joints, PRS, *57:*118, 1976. Nederl. tijdschr. geneesk., *119:*472, 1975

BLOEM, J. J. A. M.: Treatment and prognosis of uncomplicated dislocated fractures of metacarpals and phalanges, PRS, *48:*392, 1971. Arch. chir. neerl., *23:*55, 1971

BLOEM, J. J. A. M.: Fracture of carpal scaphoid in child aged 4, PRS, *48:*392, 1971. Arch. chir. neerl., *23:*91, 1971

BLOEM, J. J. A. M., AND VAN DER WAAL, I.: Paraffinoma of face, PRS, *56:*473, 1975. Oral Surg., *38:*675, 1974

BLOKHIN, V. N.: Distraction-compression method in reconstructive surgery of the hand. Khirurgiia (Mosk.), *49:*10, 1973 (Russian)

BLOKHIN, V. N.: Trauma and restorative surgery of the hand. Ortop. Travmatol. Protez., *34:*1, 1973 (Russian)

BLOKHIN, V. N. *et al*: Rehabilitation measures in the treatment of hand injuries and deformities. Sov. Med., *36:*125, 1973 (Russian)

BLOKMANIS, A.: Esthesioneuroepithelioma: report of two cases and discussion of management. Can. J. Otolaryngol., *1:*43, 1972

BLOMFIELD, B.: Rhinoplasty. 2. Plea for discontinuance of submucous resection of septum operation. J. Otolaryngol. Soc. Aust., *3:*422, 1972

Blood, Abnormalities

Urologist, disseminated intravascular coagulation and (Seabaugh *et al*), PRS, *50:*540, 1972. J. Urol., *106:*267, 1971

Coumarin-congener therapy, cutaneous and subcutaneous necrosis as a complication of (Kahn, Stern, Rhodes), PRS, *48:*160, 1971

Platelet deaggregating agents, inhibition of experimental arterial thrombosis in dogs with (Danese, Haimov), PRS, *49:*586, 1972. Surgery, *70:*927, 1971

Hemodynamic consequences of moderate postoperative anemia in monkeys (Hoffbrand, Forsyth), PRS, *48:*400, 1971. Surg. Gynec. & Obst., *132:*61, 1971

Bleeding in central nervous system, severe complication of therapy with anticoagulants (Levy), PRS, *50:*95, 1972. Ther. Umsch., *28:*821, 1971

Heparin therapy, precise management (Boden *et al*), PRS, *52:*332, 1973. Am. J. Surg., *124:*777, 1972

Hemorrhagic necrosis of skin as complication of anticoagulant therapy (Von Empel, Smeenk), PRS, *52:*99, 1973. Arch. chir. neerl., *24:*353, 1972

Venous sampling sites for pulmonary shunt determination in injured patient (Horovitz, Carrico, Shires), PRS, *50:*205, 1972. J. Trauma, *11:*911, 1972

Coagulation mechanism in experimental pulmonary fat embolism (Soloway, Robinson), PRS, *52:*325, 1973. J. Trauma, *12:*630, 1972

Platelet dysfunction: important factor in massive bleeding from stress ulcer (Atik, Matini), PRS, *52:*324, 1973. J. Trauma, *12:*834, 1972

Heparin therapy, disseminated intravascular coagulation, diagnosis and treatment of

Blood, Abnormalities — Cont.
  a hemorrhagic diathesis after prostatectomy (Pickens, Lattimer), PRS, *52:*98, 1973. J. Urol., *108:*951, 1972
  Hemostyptic drugs, various, effects in rats (Koehnlein), PRS, *50:*462, 1972
  Oxygen delivery in man, effect of massive transfusion of stored blood on (Bowen, Fleming), PRS, *52:*330, 1973. Surg. Forum, *23:*17, 1972
  Transfusion, exchange, for flap surgery in sickle cell anemia (Ashbell), PRS, *51:*705, 1973. Surg. Forum, *23:*517, 1972
  Encephalocele, anterior, diagnosis and treatment (Poradowska *et al*), PRS, *54:*630, 1974. Acta chir. plast., *15:*137, 1973
  Fibrin degradation products in postoperative period (Smith, Ts'ao, Chung-Hsin), PRS, *53:*693, 1974. Am. J. Clin. Path., *60:*644, 1973
  Clotting time — an enigma (Sussman), PRS, *53:*694, 1974. Am. J. Clin. Path., *60:*651, 1973
  Tissue PO_2 and PCO_2, measured by using Silastic tube and capillary sampling technique (Kivisaari, Niinikoski), PRS, *52:*688, 1973. Am. J. Surg., *125:*623, 1973
  Heparinization of prosthetic heart valves (Schwartz *et al*), PRS, *53:*501, 1974. Circulation, suppl. #3, *47, 48:*85, 1973
  Platelet function, acute effect of cigarette smoking on (Levine), PRS, *53:*489, 1974. Circulation, *48:*619, 1973
  Platelet response and coagulation changes following massive blood replacement (Lim *et al*), PRS, *53:*690, 1974. J. Trauma, *13:*577, 1973
  Thrombosis, central venous: hazard of medical progress (Warden, Wilmore, Pruitt), PRS, *53:*489, 1974. J. Trauma, *13:*620, 1973
  Thrombosis, venous, small subcutaneous doses of heparin in prevention of (Gallus, Hirsh, Tuttle), PRS, *52:*331, 1973. New England J. Med., *288:*545, 1973
  Hemostatic agents, skin graft donor site as model for evaluation of (Wilkinson, Tenery, Zufi), PRS, *51:*541, 1973
  Blood loss in some major esthetic operations, autotransfusion for (Noone, Graham, Royster), PRS, *51:*559, 1973
  Hemolysis, fatal, from mafenide treatment of burns in patient with glucose-6-phosphate dehydrogenase deficiency (Marsicano, Hutton, Bryant), PRS, *52:*197, 1973
  Venous thrombosis, regimen to abolish (Rosengarten), PRS, *52:*687, 1973. Proc. Roy. Australasian Coll. Surg., *46:*737, 1973
  POR-8, use for hemostasis in plastic surgery (Manuel Lopez, Fernandez Jardon), PRS, *53:*614, 1974. Rev. espan. cir. plast., *5:*249,

Blood, Abnormalities — Cont.
  1973
  Encephaloceles, frontal (De Klerk *et al*). S. Afr. Med. J., *47:*1350, 1973
  Veins, thrombosis with cava catheters (Graudins, Duben, Popp), PRS, *52:*681, 1973. Zentralbl. Chir., *98:*274, 1973
  Hyperoxia, *in vivo,* age of red blood cells destroyed by (Carolla), PRS, *56:*107, 1975. Aerospace Med., *45:*1273, 1974
  Drug-induced bleeding (Soloway), PRS, *54:*622, 1974. Am. J. Clin. Path., *61:*622, 1974
  Heparin for disseminated intravascular coagulation (Abando *et al*), PRS, *54:*239, 1974. Am. Surgeon, *40:*22, 1974
  Intranasal meningoencephalocele (Schmidt *et al*), Arch. Otolaryng., *99:*402, 1974
  Bleeding time from incisions standardized by protruding skin fold method (Stavem). Brit. J. Haematol., *26:*153, 1974
  Frontoethmoidal encephalomeningocele with special reference to plastic reconstruction (Charoonsmith *et al*). Clin. Plast. Surg., *1:*27, 1974
  Thrombus formation in arterial and venous circulation in hypofibrinogenemic dogs (Olson), PRS, *55:*512, 1975. Europ. Surg. Res., *6:*176, 1974
  Hemostasis during hemorrhagic accidents in surgery with fibrinogen alteration (Boisseau), PRS, *56:*466, 1975. J. Chir., *108:*449, 1974
  Blood clotting properties, testing new materials *in vitro* (Vorlova), PRS, *56:*475, 1975. J. Polym. Med., *4:*119, 1974
  Hemoglobin II: immunogenic properties of stroma *vs.* stroma free hemoglobin solution (Cochin *et al*), PRS, *56:*473, 1975. J. Surg. Oncol., *6:*19, 1974
  Hemodialysis unit, immunity to hepatitis-B in (De la Concha *et al*), PRS, *55:*260, 1975. Lancet, *2:*461, 1974
  Blood coagulation in hemophilia — use of EACA (epsilon aminocarpoic acid) (Short, Ogle), PRS, *54:*247, 1974. Minnesota Med., *57:*77, 1974
  Blood viscosity: relationship of hematocrit levels to skin flap survival in the dog (Earle, Fratianne, Nunez), PRS, *54:*341, 1974
  Blood viscosity, importance in rheological claudication (Dormandy, Hoare, Postelthwaite), PRS, *55:*720, 1975. Proc. Roy. Soc. Med., *67:*446, 1974
  Skin necrosis following disseminated intravascular thrombotic syndrome (Franco, Callejo, Pedreno), PRS, *54:*693, 1974. Rev. españ. cir. plast., *7:*55, 1974
  Fronto-ethmoidal anterior encephalocele

Blood, Abnormalities — Cont.

(case report) (Kataye). Ann. Otolaryngol. Chir. Cervicofac., *92:*417, 1975 (French)

Hematoma, retropharyngeal, complication of therapy with anticoagulants (Owens *et al*), PRS, *57:*765, 1976. Arch. Otolaryng., *101:*565, 1975

Hemodialysis, maintenance, quality of life on (Levy, Wynbrandt), PRS, *57:*675, 1976. Lancet, *6:*1328, 1975

Blood coagulation alterations with trauma (Boehner), PRS, *57:*120, 1976. Pediat. Clin. N. Am., *22:*289, 1975

Blood clotting: iatrogenic platelet dysfunction, an emerging peril (Wolfe, Lian), PRS, *55:*602, 1975

Aspirin, influence on postoperative platelet kinetics and venous thrombosis (Clagett *et al*), PRS, *56:*115, 1975. Surgery, *77:*61, 1975

BLOOMENSTEIN, R. B.: Reconstruction of the external ear in children. J. Med. Soc. N.J., *69:*148, 1972

BLOOMENSTEIN, R. B.: Viability prediction in pedicle flaps by infrared thermography (Follow-Up Clinic), PRS, *52:*185, 1973

BLOOMENSTEIN, R. B.: Problems with thinner envelopes in some new breast implants (Letter to the Editor), PRS, *54:*213, 1974

BLUEMINK, E. *et al*: Sulphonamides and local treatment of burns. Lancet, *2:*1425, 1971

BLUESTONE, C. D.: Eustachian tube obstruction in the infant with cleft palate. Ann. Otol. Rhin. & Laryng., *80:*2, 1971

BLUESTONE, C. D. *et al*: Roentgenographic evaluation of eustachian tube function in infants with cleft and normal palates. Cleft Palate J., *9:*93, 1972

BLUESTONE, C. D. *et al*: Certain effects of cleft palate repair on eustachian tube function. Cleft Palate J., *9:*183, 1972

BLUESTONE, C. D. *et al*: Eustachian tube ventilatory function in relation to cleft palate. Ann. Otol. Rhin. & Laryng., *84:*333, 1975

BLUMLEIN, H. *et al*: Round-table discussion on "Therapy of facial injuries in general hospital." Langenbecks Arch. Chir., *334:*455, 1973 (German)

BOBEK, V.: Syndrome of arteriomesenterial duodenal compression in children with burns, PRS, *56:*469, 1975. Acta chir. plast., *16:*238, 1974

BOBIC, J.: Mixed tumor of parotid gland of enormous dimensions. Med. Arh., *25:*75, 1971 (Serbian)

BOCCHIOTTI, G., COLONNA, V., AND FUMAROLA, A.: Plastic reconstruction of lower lip following neoplastic exeresis. Cancro, *24:*197, 1971 (Italian)

BOCCHIOTTI, G. *et al*: Adipose tissue grafts and dermo-adipose grafts. Minerva Chir., *28:*1018, 1973 (Italian)

BOCHENEK, Z.: Diagnosis and surgical treatment of salivary gland diseases. Otolaryngol. Pol., *25:*597, 1971 (Polish)

BOCHNIK, H. J.: Psychiatry of aging. An outline for plastic surgery. In *Plastische und Wiederherstellungs-Chirurgie*, ed. by Hohler; pp. 3–12. Schattauer, Stuttgart, 1975 (German)

BOCK, O.: Significance of functional dentition analysis for surgical-orthopedic procedures. Fortschr. Kiefer. Gesichtschir., *18:*99, 1974 (German)

BOCQUET, L. *et al*: Study of mucosa of ileocystoplasties and ileo-ureteroplasties. Preliminary note. Sem. Hop. Paris, *50:*873, 1974

BOCZKOWSKI, K.: Results of treatment in cases of male hermaphroditism. Ginekol. Pol., *42:*1483, 1971 (Polish)

BOCZKOWSKI, K.: Therapy in male hermaphroditism. Ginekol. Pol., *44:*353, 1973 (Polish)

BODEA, I. *et al*: Fistulas of thyroglossal tract. Otorinolaringologie, *17:*425, 1972 (Rumanian)

BODEN, J. P. *et al*: Precise management of heparin therapy, PRS, *52:*332, 1973. Am. J. Surg., *124:*777, 1972

BODENHAM, D. C.: Complementary roles of otolaryngology and plastic surgery in major malignancies of middle ear, PRS, *50:*313, 1972. Proc. Roy. Soc. Med., *65:*248, 1972

BODIAN, M.: An external approach to ptosis repair. Arch. Ophth., *88:*176, 1972

BODIAN, M.: Modified ptosis clamp. Trans. Am. Acad. Ophthalmol. Otolaryngol., *78:*221, 1974

BODIAN, M.: Revised Fasanella-Servat ptosis operation, PRS, *56:*591, 1975. Ann. Ophth., *7:*603, 1975

BODIAN, M. *et al*: Surgery for sectional blepharoptosis. Am. J. Ophth., *73:*214, 1972

BODURTHA, A. J. *et al*: Clinical and immunological significance of human melanoma cytotoxic antibody, PRS, *55:*641, 1975. Cancer Res., *35:*189, 1975

BODY, J. *et al*: 343 injuries of fingers and hands treated in U. O. D. Ann. Chir., *27:*535, 1973 (French)

BOECKX, W. D., DE CONINCK, A., AND VANDERLINDEN, E.: Ten free flap transfers: use of intra-arterial dye injection to outline a flap exactly, PRS, *57:*716, 1976

BOEHNER, R. L.: Alterations in blood coagulation with trauma, PRS, *57:*120, 1976. Pediat. Clin. N. Am., *22:*289, 1975

BOENNINGHAUS, H. G.: Rhino-surgeon's responsibility at rhino-surgery of face skull adjoining base of skull. Arch. Otorhinolaryn-gol. (N.Y.), *207:*1, 1974 (German)

BOENNINGHAUS, H. G.: Rhinosurgical tasks in surgery of base of skull adjoining facial skull. Arch. Otorhinolaryngol. (N.Y.), *207:*397, 1974 (German)

BOENNINGHAUS, H. G. *et al:* Diagnosis and surgical indications of odontogenic and rhinogenic maxillary sinus diseases. Z. Laryngol. Rhinol. Otol., *52:*851, 1973 (German)

BOGATSKII, V. A.: Experience in surgical treatment of late radiation injuries. Stomatologiia (Mosk.), *51:*33, 1972 (Russian)

BOGDANOV, B.: Electric injuries. Med. Pregl., *28:*483, 1975 (Serbian)

BOGDANOV, B. *et al:* Some of our views on the surgical treatment of malignant melanoma. Med. Pregl., *28:*481, 1975 (Serbian)

BOGDANOV, E. A. *et al:* Surgery of fractures of the metacarpal bones and phalanges. Vestn. Khir., *102:*84, 1969 (Russian)

BOGDANOV, E. A. *et al:* Mental disorders in patients with severe hand injuries. Vestn. Khir., *113:*137, 1974 (Russian)

BOGDANOVA, S. V.: Treatment of hypospadias with a modification of the Duplay method. Vestn. Khir., *112:*74, 1974 (Russian)

BOGDANOVICH, U.Ia. *et al:* Treatment of infected wounds and ulcers by coherent irradiation. Khirurgiia (Mosk.), *4:*56, 1975 (Russian)

BOGGIO ROBUTTI, G.: Rare case of multiple craniofacial malformations, PRS, *57:*396, 1976. Riv. ital chir. plast., *6:*21, 1974

BOGGIO ROBUTTI, G., MUSIO, L., AND MAZZOLA, R.: Treatment of hemangioma by oral prednisone therapy, PRS, *53:*111, 1974. Chir. Plast., *1:*95, 1972

BOGI, I. *et al:* Correction of pseudoprognathism in adults. Fogorv. Sz., *68:*344, 1975 (Hungarian)

BOGORODZKI, B. *et al:* Juvenile melanoma of the bulbar conjunctiva. Klin. Oczna., *46:*67, 1976 (Polish)

BOGUMILL, G. P. *et al:* Tumors of the hand. Clin. Orthop., *108:*214, 1975

BOHLER, J.: Diagnosis and therapy of soft tissue infections in the hand. Hefte Unfallheilkd., *107:*221, 1970 (German)

BOHME, P. E. *et al:* Median cervical cysts and fistulae, their surgical correction with partial resection of the hyoid bone. Bruns Beitr. Klin. Chir., *218:*617, 1971 (German)

BOHMERT, H.: Fetal skin xenotransplants for temporary closure of extensive third degree burns. Fortschr. Med., *89:*836, 1971 (German)

BOHMERT, H.: Surgical treatment of lymph-edema of the arm after breast amputation. Fortschr. Med., *91:*228, 1973 (German)

BOHMERT, H.: Skin replacement in burns. Fortschr. Med., *91:*646, 1973

BOHMERT, H.: Skin replacement in burns using split skin net transplants and xenotransplants. Hefte Unfallheilkd., *116:*1, 1974 (German)

BOHMERT, H.: *Replacement of Skin in Burns with Split Thickness Skin Mesh Grafts and Xenotransplants.* Springer-Verlag, Berlin-Heidelberg-New York, 1974. PRS, *56:*82, 1975

BOHMERT, H. *et al:* Meshed autografts and xenografts to cover extensive burns, PRS, *50:*202, 1972. Langenbeck's Arch. Chir., *329:*918, 1971

BOHMERT, H. *et al:* Xenotransplantation as biologic dressing in severe burns, PRS, *48:*516, 1971. Med. & Hygiene, *955:*438, 1971

BOHMERT, H. *et al:* Therapy of severe burns. Med. Welt., *23:* 871, 1972 (German)

BOHMERT, H. *et al:* Management of lymph-edema with modified Thompson's method. Ther. Ggw., *113:*842, 1974 (German)

BOHN, A.: Cleft lip and cleft palate. Teamwork in treatment. 2. History. Present situation in Oslo. Tidsskr. Nor. Laegeforen, *93:*2463, 1973 (Norwegian)

BOHNDORF, W.: Clinical and therapeutical problems in metastases of the cervical lymph nodes. Fortschr. Geb. Roentgenstr. Nuklearmed., *116:*246, 1972 (German)

BOHRINGER, P. *et al:* Results after cystectomy connected with apicoectomy. Schweiz. Monatsschr. Zahnheilkd., *85:*186, 1975 (German)

BOHSALI, I.: Mattress suture otoplasty: histopathologic study. Eye, Ear, Nose & Throat Month., *52:*57, 1973

BOIARINOV, G. A. *et al:* Treatment of severely burned child with bilateral diffuse pneumonia. Ortop. Travmatol. Protez., *34:*58, 1973 (Russian)

BOIN, T. L.: Injuries of hamate bone, PRS, *54:*374, 1974. Hand, *5:*235, 1973

BOISHTIAN, V. E.: Technic of activation of lower lacrimal point. Oftalmol. Zh., *30:*309, 1975 (Russian)

BOISSEAU, M. R.: Practice of hemostasis during hemorrhagic accidents in surgery with fibrinogen alteration, PRS, *56:*466, 1975. J. Chir., *108:*449, 1974

BOJSEN-MOLLER, F. *et al:* Palmar aponeurosis and the central spaces of the hand. J. Anat., *117:*55, 1974

BOLCS, S.: Role of the disorder of the ethmoidal cells in the pathology of the tear ducts. Surv. Ophthalmol., *19:*57, 1974

BOLEO-TOME, J. DE P.: Facial tumors and medical collaboration. Rev. Port. Estomatol. Cir.

Maxillofac., *12:*95, 1971 (Portuguese)

BOLES, R. *et al*: Carcinoma in pleomorphic adenomas of salivary glands. Ann. Otol. Rhin. & Laryng., *82:*684, 1973

BOLINCHES BOLINCHES, R. *et al*: Anesthesia in epidermolysis bullosa. Rev. Esp. Anestesiol. Reanim., *21:*477, 1974 (Spanish)

BOLLINGER, T. E. *et al*: Basal cell adenoma of upper lip. Report of case. Oral Surg., *35:*600, 1973

BOLTON, H.: Primary tendon repair. Hand, *2:*56, 1970

BOLTON, P. M.: Effects of immune depression on chemical carcinogenesis in rat. I. Regional lymphadenectomy. Oncology, *27:*430, 1973

BOLUND, S. *et al*: Windshield lesions. Ugeskr. Laeger., *134:*2141, 1972 (Danish)

BOMBET, R.: On the lack of any effect of gravity on the survival of tubed flaps (with Myers, Cherry), PRS, *51:*428, 1973

BONAMICO, M. *et al*: Neurogenic tumor of the neck in the newborn, report of a case healed with only surgical treatment. Minerva Pediatr., *24:*266, 1972 (Italian)

BONANNO, P. C. *et al*: Primary bone grafting in management of facial fractures. N.Y. State J. Med., *75:*710, 1975

BONDAR, V. S.: Application of a combined flat pedicled graft for plastic surgery of trophic ulcers of the leg and foot. Vestn. Khir., *107:*116, 1971 (Russian)

BONDAR, V. S.: Surgical method of fixation of fractures of maxilla according to Adams. Stomatologiia (Mosk.), *52:*91, 1973 (Russian)

BONDAR, V. S. *et al*: Plastic surgery of cranial vault soft tissues. Vestn. Khir., *111:*94, 1973 (Russian)

BONDOC., C. C., AND BURKE, J. F.: Clinical experience with viable frozen human skin and frozen skin bank, PRS, *50:*99, 1972. Ann. Surg., *174:*371, 1971

Bone

Bone mineral metabolism, systemic effects of burns on (Kolar *et al*), PRS, *50:*541, 1972. Acta chir. plast., *13:*133, 1971. II. Influence of general anesthesia on, PRS, *57:*763, 1976. Acta chir. plast., *17:*56, 1975

Fracture healing, stimulation of, by direct current in rabbit fibula (Friedenberg *et al*), PRS, *50:*312, 1972. J. Bone & Joint Surg., *53:*1400, 1971

Bone hematomas, experimental, antibiotic penetration of (Wilson *et al*), PRS, *50:*310, 1972. J. Bone & Joint Surg., *53:*1622, 1971

Bones, long, combined lengthening and shortening of, Pierre-Robin syndrome in association with (Walden, Logosso, Bren-

Bone–Cont.

nan), PRS, *48:*80, 1971

Heat, effect on bone healing: disadvantage in use of power tools (Jacobs, Ray), PRS, *50:*638, 1972. Arch. Surg., *104:*687, 1972

Periostitis ossificans (Perriman, Uthman). Brit. J. Oral Surg., *10:*211, 1972

Bone defects, long, experimental, saline cartilage extract for healing (Herold, Hurvitz, Tadmor), PRS, *51:*487, 1973. Internat. Surg., *57:*246, 1972

Osteodysplasia, familial (Anderson *et al*), PRS, *50:*633, 1972. J.A.M.A., *220:*1687, 1972

Temperature measured in human cortical bone when drilling (Matthews, Hirsch), PRS, *50:*312, 1972. J. Bone & Joint Surg., *54:*297, 1972

Bone growth, fractures of facial bones in children (Bales, Randall, Lehr), PRS, *52:*97, 1973. J. Trauma, *12:*56, 1972

Bone hamate, injuries of (Boin), PRS, *54:*374, 1974. Hand, *5:*235, 1973

Bone, bonding porous metal to, effect of movement (Cameron, Pilliar, McNab), PRS, *53:*375, 1974. J. Biomed. Mater. Res., *7:*301, 1973

Bone, erosion by alloplastic implants (Jobe, Iverson, Vistnes), PRS, *51:*169, 1973. Discussions by Rees, Spira, PRS, *51:*174, 1973

Distraction, mandibular lengthening by gradual (Snyder *et al*), PRS, *51:*506, 1973

Bone changes in composite flaps after transfer to the head and neck region, investigation of (Conley *et al*), PRS, *51:*658, 1973. Discussion by Jurkiewicz, PRS, *52:*79, 1973

Cortical Bone Healing after Internal Fixation and Infection. By W. W. Rittman and S. M. Perren. Springer-Verlag, New York, 1974. PRS, *57:*91, 1976

Year Book of Orthopedics and Traumatic Surgery. Ed. by H. Herman Young. Year Book Medical Publishers, Chicago, 1974. PRS, *56:*81, 1975

Styloid bone, clinical and embryological study (Kootstra, Huffstadt, Kauer), PRS, *56:*228, 1975. Hand, *6:*185, 1974

Enchondromata of bones of hand–review of 40 cases (Noble, Lamb), PRS, *56:*227, 1975. Hand, *6:*275, 1974

Fracture healing accelerated distal to venous tourniquet (Kruse, Kelly), PRS, *55:*387, 1975. J. Bone & Joint Surg., *56A:*730, 1974

Bone plasty in the treatment of benign bone neoplasms and certain precancerous conditions (Stamatin *et al*), Ortop. Travmatol. Protez., *0:*25, 1974 (Russian)

Mandibular fractures, significance of persistent radiolucency of (Kappel *et al*), PRS, *53:*38, 1974

Bone—Cont.

Bone, membranous, fractures of, experimental study of healing (Craft *et al*), PRS, *53:*321, 1974

Bone, exposed, coverage by muscle transposition and skin grafting (Vasconez, Bostwick, McCraw), PRS, *53:*526, 1974

Bone growth, regeneration of tibial segment from periosteum (Cocke, Norton), PRS, *53:*675, 1974

Infants, craniofacial osteotomies and reconstructions in (Edgerton, Jane, Berry), PRS, *54:*13, 1974

Osteotomy: altering dimensions of canine face by induction of new bone formation (Calabrese, Winslow, Latham), PRS, *54:*467, 1974

Dacron felt, incorporation and tolerance in bones of rabbits (Crouse, Campo, Kodsi), PRS, *54:*471, 1974

Bone formation in palatal clefts subsequent to palatovomer plasty (Prydso *et al*), PRS, *56:*359, 1975. Scand. J. Plast. Reconstr. Surg., *8:*73, 1974

Bones, large segmental defects in, comparison of solid and split homotransplants in bridging (Lavrischeva, Grigoriev, Abakov), PRS, *57:*767, 1976. Acta chir. plast., *17:*27, 1975

Bones, long, congenital curving of (Eliachar *et al*), PRS, *57:*119, 1976. Ann. Pediat., *22:*61, 1975

Bone mineral and thenar muscle blood flow in forearms of lumberjacks (Karjalainen, Alhava, Valtola), PRS, *57:*761, 1976. Brit. J. Indust. Med., *32:*11, 1975

Fracture healing (Cruess, Dumont), PRS, *57:*764, 1976. Canad. J. Surg., *18:*403, 1975

Thermal properties of cancellous bone (Clattenburg *et al*), PRS, *57:*406, 1976. J. Biomed. Mater. Res., *9:*169, 1975

Bone cement, methylmethacrylate, contact dermatitis from (Fries *et al*), PRS, *57:*406, 1976. J. Bone & Joint Surg., *57A:*547, 1975

Bone, cryosurgical devitalization of, and its regeneration (Schargus *et al*), PRS, *57:*405, 1976. J. Maxillo-facial Surg., *3:*128, 1975

Osteotomy, maxillary, bone healing and revascularization after (Bell *et al*), PRS, *57:*531, 1976. J. Oral Surg., *33:*253, 1975

Bone, alveolar, healing of surgical defects produced with ultrasonic instrumentation, chisel, and rotary bur (Horton *et al*), PRS, *57:*257, 1976. J. Oral Surg., *39:*536, 1975

Fixation of bones, internal, design and applications of new device for (Crock), PRS, *56:*606, 1975. M. J. Australia, *1:*510, 1975

Bone absorption, mandibular, under silicone rubber chin implants, retrospective cepha-

Bone—Cont.

lometric analysis (Friedland, Coccaro, Converse), PRS, *57:*144, 1976

BONE, D. K. *et al*: Aspiration pneumonia. Prevention of aspiration in patients with tracheostomies. Ann. Thorac. Surg., *18:*30, 1974

BONE, R. C.: Management of solitary parotid mass. Postgrad. Med., *56:*119, 1974

Bone Derivatives, Grafting

Possibilities of use of Kiel bone chips in stomatologic practice. Dtsch. Zahnaerztl. Z., *28:*605, 1973 (German)

Bone graft, Kiel, use of, in restorative surgery in ENT fields (Renk). H.N.O., *21:*114, 1973 (German)

Implants, Kiel-bone, to chin and nose (Penn) (Follow-Up Clinic), PRS, *52;*432, 1973

Experimental bases for administration of the Kiel bone chip as bone substitute in jaw surgery (Wilfert *et al*). Dtsch. Zahnaerztl. Z., *27:*405, 1972 (German)

Bone matrix, decalcified, implantation in bone defects (Narang, Wells). Trans. Congr. Int. Assoc. Oral Surg., *4:*64, 1973

Bone defects, chemically modified osseous material for restoration of (Emmings). J. Periodontol., *45:*385, 1974

Bone matrix, decalcified allogenic, experimental osteogenesis in palatal defects (Narang, Wells), PRS, *55:*118, 1975. Oral Surg., *37:*153, 1974

*Bone Grafts, Free (*See also *Free Flaps)*

Epiphyseal transplants by flap and by free graft (Freeman) (Follow-Up Clinic), PRS, *48:*72, 1971

Bone grafts, massive osteo and osteo-articular, technic and results of 62 cases (Ottolenghi). Clin. Orthop., *87:*156, 1972

Bone grafts in dentistry, application of, clinicoroentgenographic studies on (Nam). J. Korean Dent. Assoc., *10:*351, 1972 (Korean)

Epiphyseal transplantation, experimental and clinical experiences in (Hoffman, Siffert, Simon), PRS, *50:*58, 1972

Ilium as source of bone grafts in children (Crockford, Converse), PRS *50:*270, 1972

Keratocyst in bone graft, remarkable recurrence (Persson). Int. J. Oral Surg., *2:*69, 1973

Iliac bone grafts, reason for taking from the left side in young patients (Smith) (Letter to the Editor), PRS, *52:*425, 1973

Osteogenesis after bone transplantation (Nade), PRS, *52:*686, 1973. Proc. Roy. Australasian Coll. Surg., *46:*261, 1973

Bone Grafts, Free—Cont.

Bone transplantation, problem of, in studies of Russian surgeons at beginning of 20th century (Mirskii). Vestn. Khir., *111:*141, 1973 (Russian)

Bone grafting and osteotomy to repair severe fronto-orbital lesion (Marchac *et al*), PRS, *55:*375, 1975. Ann. chir. plast., *19:*41, 1974

Autografts, bone membranous *vs* endochondral (Smith, Abramson), PRS, *54:*701, 1974. Arch. Otolaryng., *99:*203, 1974

Osteitis treatment by excision and graft at open operations by Papineau's method (Roy-Camille *et al*), PRS, *55:*253, 1975. Chirurgie, *100:*480, 1974

Bone grafts, use of (Kowalik *et al*). Czas. Stomatol., *27:*161, 1974 (Polish)

Trephine technique for obtaining small bone grafts (Braun), PRS, *54:*509, 1974. Hand, *6:*103, 1974

Bone graft survival, onlay, the influence of periosteum and calcitonin on (Knize), PRS, *53:*190, 1974

Skeletal reconstruction of extensive bilateral defect of anterior chest wall (Longacre, Maurer, Keirle), PRS, *53:*593, 1974

Tibial segment regeneration from periosteum (Cocke, Norton), PRS, *53:*675, 1974

Transfer, distant, of free, living bone graft by microvascular anastomoses (Ostrup, Fredrickson), PRS, *54:*274, 1974

Lip and palate, complete clefts of, primary early bone grafting of (Nylen *et al*), PRS, *56:*683, 1975. Scand. J. Plast. Reconstr. Surg., *8:*79, 1974

Bone grafting to treat cleft lip and palate, primary, orthodontic aspects (Friede, Johanson), PRS, *56:*680, 1975. Scand. J. Plast. Reconstr. Surg., *8:*88, 1974

Bone grafts, autologous cortical, with microsurgical anastomosis of periosteal vessels (Adelaar, Soucacos), PRS, *57:*766, 1976. Surg. Forum, *25:*487, 1974

Bone grafts, cancellous, from distal radius for use in hand surgery (MacCollum), PRS, *55:*477, 1975

Graft, bone, free vascularized; clinical extension of microvascular techniques (Taylor, Miller, Ham), PRS, *55:*533, 1975

Mandibular defects after radiation, reconstruction of, using a free, living bone graft transferred by microvascular anastomoses (Östrup, Fredrickson), PRS, *55:*563, 1975

Graft, bone, free, living (McDowell) (Editorial), PRS, *55:*612, 1975

Bone Grafts, Pedicled

Bone grafts, pedicled, in goats; vascular connections between soft tissues and bones

Bone Grafts, Pedicled—Cont.

(Medgyesi), PRS, *54:*509, 1974. Scand. J. Plast. Reconstr. Surg., *7:*110, 1973

Flap, composite island rib, for mandibular reconstruction (Ketchum, Masters, Robinson), PRS, *53:*471, 1974

Bone Grafts, Preserved (See also Bone Homografts)

Bone tissue conserved in plastic material and sterilized with gamma rays, biological properties of (Imamaliev, Gashimov), PRS, *55;*643, 1975. Acta chir. plast., *16:*129, 1974

Plastic closure of different skeletal segments with formalinized bone homotransplant (Kovanov *et al*). Eksp. Khir. Anesteziol., *2:*4, 1974 (Russian)

Bone preservation, use of self-hardening plastic material Protacryl for (Vodolatskii). Stomatologiia (Mosk.), *53:*38, 1974 (Russian)

Bone graft bank, clinical investigations as to value (Chakour), PRS, *54:*247, 1974. Ztschr. Orthop., *112:*207, 1974

Bone Grafts to Face (See also Craniofacial Surgery; Facial Bones; Jaw, Bone Graft to)

Lip, complete cleft, a study of the effects of early bone grafting (Jolleys, Robertson), PRS, *52:*208, 1973. Brit. J. Plast. Surg., *25:*229, 1972

Bone resorption, avoiding, under plastic chin implants (Parker), PRS, *53:*250, 1974. Arch. Otolaryng., *98:*100, 1973

Bone autografts, membranous *vs* endochondral (Smith, Abramson), PRS, *54:*701, 1974. Arch. Otolaryng., *99:*203, 1974

Osteoneogenesis: new method for facial reconstruction (Leake, Habal), PRS, *57:*125, 1976. Surg. Res., *18:*331, 1975

Bone Grafts to Mandible: See *Jaw, Bone Graft to*

Bone Grafts to Nose: See *Nose, Bone and Cartilage Autografts to*

Bone Grafts to Skull: See *Cranioplasty*

Bone Heterografts (See also Bone Grafts, Preserved)

Use of decalcified heterologous bone in plastic facial surgery (Sokolov). Vestn. Khir., *106:*100, 1971 (Russian)

Bone Homografts (See also Bone Grafts, Preserved)

Bone shavings, preserved homologous, regeneration of cranial bones after implanta-

Bone Homografts—Cont.

tion of (Kantorova, Timashkevich), PRS, *50:*206, 1972. Acta chir. plast., *13:*33, 1971

Bone transplants, brepho- and homo-, in maxillofacial surgery (Sevelyev, Sisolyatin), PRS, *53:*499, 1974. Acta chir. plast., *15:*65, 1973

Bone tissue transplants, homologous, reaction of hemapoietic system to (Bruskina), PRS, *55:*643, 1975. Acta chir. plast., *16:*141, 1974

Bone, allogenic, and autogenous marrow, use in extensive mandibular defects (Pike, Boyne), PRS, *55:*119, 1975. J. Oral Surg., *32:*177, 1974

Use of mandibular homografts in reconstructing jaw defects (Cantrell). Laryngoscope, *84:*1925, 1974

Oral surgery, homologous bone embryonic graft in (Sysoliatin *et al*). Stomatologiia (Mosk.), *53:*92, 1974 (Russian)

Comparison of solid and split homotransplants in bridging large segmental defects in long bones (Lavrischeva, Grigoriev, Abakov), PRS, *57:*767, 1976. Acta chir. plast., *17:*27, 1975

Bone Infections: See Osteomyelitis

BONGERT, H.: Treatment of complex, wound infected hand injuries following the principle of the "urgency with postponed surgical treatment" (Iselin). Hefte Unfallheilkd., *107:*243, 1970 (German)

BONHOMME, F. *et al*: Cervico-facial actinomycosis: a current disease? Apropos of 2 cases. Ann. Otolaryngol. Chir. Cervicofac., *88:*350, 1971 (French)

BONINI, P. A. *et al*: Urinary alpha glucosidase as measure of kidney damage in burns, PRS, *51:*107, 1973. Riv. ital. chir. plast., *2:*219, 1971

BONIUK, M.: Eyelids, lacrimal apparatus, and conjuctiva. Arch. Ophth., *90:*239, 1973

BONNABEAU, R. C. *et al*: Dermatofibrosarcoma protuberans. Report of case with multiple intrathoracic metastases and brief review of six others. W. Va. Med. J., *69:*107, 1973

BONNABEAU, R. C., JR. *et al*: Dermatofibrosarcoma protuberans. Report of case with pulmonary metastasis and multiple intrathoracic recurrences. Oncology, *29:*1, 1974

BONNEAU, R. A. *et al*: Stomal recurrence following laryngectomy. Arch. Otolaryng., *101:*408, 1975

BONNEFOUS, G.: Islet grafts for the loss of pulp substance in the fingers. Bull. Mem. Soc. Chir. Paris, *60:*411, 1970 (French)

BONNER, J. *et al*: Astrocytoma of the optic nerve and chiasm associated with mi-

crophthalmos and orbital cyst. Brit. J. Ophthalmol., *58:*828, 1974

BONOLA, A., AND MORELLI, E.: Congenital anomalies of hands and their treatment, PRS, *51:*103, 1973. Piccin, Padua, 1972

BONOLA, A., AND MORELLI, E.: *Le Deformita Congenite delle Mani ed il loro Trattamento.* Piccin Editore, Padua, Italy, 1972. PRS, *51:*443, 1973

BONVALLET, J. M.: Orthopedic treatment of fractures of phalanges. Immobilization on "plaster ball," PRS, *55:*249, 1975. Chirurgie, *100:*533, 1974

BOO-CHAI, K.: Three surgical instruments for cleft lip-palate repair. Brit. J. Plast. Surg., *24:*216, 1971

BOO-CHAI, K.: Unoperated adult bilateral cleft of the lip and palate. Brit. J. Plast. Surg., *24:*250, 1971

BOO-CHAI, K. *et al*: The origami cleft lip. Brit. J. Plast. Surg., *23:*248, 1970

Books (Alphabetically by Author)

American Academy of Orthopaedic Surgeons: *Symposium on Hand Tendon Surgery.* C. V. Mosby Co., St. Louis, 1975

American College of Surgeons, Committee on Trauma: *Early Care of the Injured Patient.* W. B. Saunders Co., Philadelphia, 1972. PRS, *55:*615, 1975

ANDERSON, ROBIN, AND HOOPES, JOHN: *Symposium on Malignancies of the Head and Neck.* Vol. XI. C. V. Mosby Co., St. Louis, 1975. PRS, *57:*373, 1976

ANSON, BARRY J., AND McVAY, CHESTER B.: *Surgical Anatomy,* Fifth Edition. W. B. Saunders Co., Philadelphia, 1971. PRS, *48:*175, 1971

ARCHER, W. H.: *Oral and Maxillofacial Surgery.* 5th Ed. W. B. Saunders Co., Philadelphia, 1975

BALLINGER, WALTER F., AND DRAPANAS, THEODORE: *Practice of Surgery.* Current Review, Volume II. C. V. Mosby Co., St. Louis, 1975. PRS, *57:*374, 1976

BALNER, HANS, VAN BEKKUM, D. W., AND RAPAPORT, FELIX T.: *Transplantation Today,* Third Congress. Grune & Stratton, New York, 1971. PRS, *49:*205, 1972

BARBOSA, JORGE FAIRBANKS: *Surgical Treatment of Head and Neck Tumors.* Grune & Stratton, New York, 1974. PRS, *57:*509, 1976

BARKER, HAROLD G.: *The Continuing Education of the Surgeon.* Charles C Thomas, Springfield, Ill., 1971. PRS, *48:*590, 1971

BARR, , N. R.: *The Hand: Principles of Splint Making.* Butterworth, London, 1974

BATSAKIS, JOHN G.: *Tumors of the Head and*

Books—Cont.

Neck. Williams & Wilkins Co., Baltimore, 1974. PRS, *54:*479, 1974

BATTLE, RICHARD: *Clinical Surgery: Plastic Surgery,* Vol. 4. J. B. Lippincott Co., Philadelphia, 1965

BEARD, C. *et al: Transactions of the New Orleans Academy of Ophthalmology.* C. V. Mosby Co., St. Louis, 1974. PRS, *55:*355, 1975

BEDFORD, M. A.: *Color Atlas of Oro-Facial Diseases.* Year Book Medical Pub., Inc., Chicago, 1972

BELL, JOHN: *Observations on Italy.* Arno Press & The New York Times, New York, 1971. PRS, *57:*373, 1976

BELL, R. C.: *Monographs on Plastic Surgery,* Vol. 1. Oxford University Press, Inc., Fair Lawn, N. J., 1973

BENDER, LEONARD F.: *Prostheses and Rehabilitation After Arm Amputation.* Charles C Thomas, Springfield, Ill., 1974. PRS, *55:*487, 1975

BERGSMA, DANIEL: *Clinical Delineation of Birth Defects.* Williams & Wilkins Co., Baltimore, 1971. PRS, *50:*79, 1972

BETTMAN, OTTO: *Pictorial History of Medicine.* Charles C Thomas Co., Springfield, 1972

BILLINGHAM, RUPERT, AND SILVERS, WILLYS: *Immunobiology of Transplantation.* Prentice-Hall, Inc., Englewood Cliffs, N. J., 1971. PRS, *50:*399, 1972

BLEEKER, G. M.: *Proceedings. 2nd International Symposium on Orbital Disorders,* Amsterdam, 1973. Albert J. Phiebig, White Plains, N. Y., 1975

BLEEKER, G. M., AND LYLE, T. KEITH: *Fractures of the Orbit.* Williams & Wilkins Co., Baltimore, 1970. PRS, *48:*589, 1971

BLOCH, BERNARD, AND HASTINGS, GARTH W.: *Plastic Materials in Surgery,* Second Edition. Charles C Thomas, Springfield, Ill., 1972. PRS, *52:*83, 1973

BOHMERT, H.: *Replacement of Skin in Burns with Split Thickness Skin Mesh Grafts and Xenotransplants.* Springer-Verlag, Berlin-Heidelberg-New York, 1974. PRS, *56:*82, 1975

BONOLA, A., AND MORELLI, E.: *Le Deformita Congenite delle Mani ed il loro Trattamento.* Piccin Editore, Padua, Italy, 1972. PRS, *51:*443, 1973

BORGES, ALBERT F.: *Elective Incisions and Scar Revision.* Little, Brown & Co., Boston, 1973. PRS, *54:*216, 1974

BRAVERMAN, IRWIN M.: *Skin Signs of Systemic Disease.* W. B. Saunders, Philadelphia, London, Toronto, 1975. PRS, *57:*657, 1976

BULBULIAN, ARTHUR H.: *Facial Prosthetics.* Charles C Thomas, Springfield, Ill., 1973. PRS, *52:*428, 1973

BZOCH, KENNETH R.: *Communicative Disorders Related to Cleft Lip and Palate.* Little, Brown & Co., Boston, 1972. PRS, *52:*572, 1973

CAILLIET, RENE: *Hand: Pain and Impairment.* F. A. Davis Co., Philadelphia, 1971. PRS, *49:*452, 1972

CAILLIET, RENE: *Hand Pain & Impairment.* 2nd edition. F. A. Davis Co., Philadelphia, 1975

CAILLIET, RENE: *Knee Pain and Disability.* F. A. Davis Co., Philadelphia, 1973. PRS, *55:*86, 1975

CAMERON, J. STEWART: *Proceedings of the European Dialysis and Transplant Association.* Vol. VIII. Williams & Wilkins Co., Baltimore, 1972. PRS, *51:*687, 1973

CHAMBERS, R. G. *et al: Cancer of the Head and Neck.* Excerpta Medica Co., Amsterdam, 1975

CHAPCHAL, G.: *Proceedings.* (Reconstruction Surgery and Traumatology Series, Vol. 15.) Albert J. Phiebig, White Plains, N. Y., 1975

CHAPCHAL, G.: *Reconstruction Surgery and Traumatology,* Volume 12. Albert J. Phiebig, White Plains, N. Y., 1971

CHAPCHAL, G.: *Reconstructive Surgery and Traumatology,* Vol. 14. Albert J. Phiebig, White Plains, N. Y., 1974

CHASE, ROBERT A.: *Atlas of Hand Surgery.* W. B. Saunders Co., Philadelphia, 1973. PRS, *53:*586, 1974

CONDON, ROBERT E., AND NYHUS, LLOYD M.: *Manual of Surgical Therapeutics,* Second Edition. Little, Brown & Co., Boston, 1972. PRS, *52:*82, 1973

CONLEY, JOHN J.: *Salivary Glands and the Facial Nerve.* Grune & Stratton, New York, 1975. PRS, *57:*658, 1976

CONLEY, JOHN, AND DICKINSON, JOHN T.: *Plastic and Reconstructive Surgery of the Face and Neck.* Grune & Stratton, New York: Georg Thieme Verlag, Stuttgart, 1972. PRS, *53:*86, 1974

CONVERSE, JOHN M.: *Surgical Treatment of Facial Injuries,* 3rd edition. Williams & Wilkins Co., Baltimore, 1974

COSTICH, EMMETT R., AND WHITE, RAYMOND P., JR.: *Fundamentals of Oral Surgery.* W. B. Saunders Co., Philadelphia, 1971

CRAMER, LESTER M., AND CHASE, ROBERT A.: *Symposium on the Hand,* Volume 3. C. V. Mosby Co., St. Louis, 1971. PRS, *50:*610,

Books — Cont.

1972

CRUESS, RICHARD L, AND MITCHELL, NELSON: *Surgery of Rheumatoid Arthritis.* J. B. Lippincott Co., Philadelphia, 1971

DANIELS, LUCILLE, AND WORTHINGHAM, CATHERINE: *Muscle Testing: Techniques of Manual Examination.* W. B. Saunders Co., Philadelphia, 1972. PRS, *53:*342, 1974

DAY, STACEY B. *et al: Curling's Ulcer: An Experiment of Nature.* Charles C Thomas, Springfield, Ill., 1972

DICKER, R. L., AND SYRACUSE, V. R.: *Consultation with a Plastic Surgeon.* Nelson-Hall Publishers, Chicago, 1975. PRS, *57:*741, 1976

Dorland's Illustrated Medical Dictionary, 25th Edition. W. B. Saunders Co., Philadelphia, 1974

DUKE-ELDER, SIR STEWART: *System of Ophthalmology.* Vol. XIV. *Injuries.* C. V. Mosby Co., St. Louis, 1972. PRS, *52:*571, 1973

DUNPHY, J. E.: *Wound Healing,* 2nd Ed. Med. Com., New York, 1974

EATON, RICHARD G.: *Joint Injuries of the Hand.* Charles C Thomas, Springfield, Ill., 1971. PRS, *49:*338, 1972

EDWARDS, CHARLES BEAVER: *Beyond Plastic Surgery.* Wayne State University Press, Detroit, 1972. PRS, *51:*329, 1973

ENGLISH, FRANK P., AND KEATS, WARREN A.: *Reconstructive and Plastic Surgery of the Eyelids.* Charles C Thomas, Springfield, Ill., 1975

ENLOW, E. H.: *Handbook of Facial Growth for Dental and Medical Students.* W. B. Saunders Co., Philadelphia, 1975

FABREGA, HORACIO, JR.: *Disease and Social Behavior — An Interdisciplinary Perspective.* M. I. T. Press, Cambridge, Mass., 1974. PRS, *55:*699, 1975

FALK, MERVYN L.: *A Cleft Palate Team Addresses the Speech Clinician.* Charles C Thomas, Springfield, Ill., 1971. PRS, *49:*568, 1972

FLATT, ADRIAN E.: *The Care of Minor Hand Injuries,* Third Edition. C. V. Mosby Co., St. Louis, 1972. PRS, *51:*210, 1973

FLATT, ADRIAN E.: *The Care of the Rheumatoid Hand,* 3rd Ed. C. V. Mosby Co., St. Louis, 1974. PRS, *56:*206, 1975

FLYNN, J. EDWARD: *Hand Surgery.* 2nd edition. Williams & Wilkins Co., Baltimore, 1975

FOX, DONNA RUSSELL, AND BLECHMAN, MARK: *Clinical Management of Voice Disorders.* Cliff Notes, Inc., Lincoln, Nebraska, 1975. PRS, *57:*657, 1976

Books — Cont.

FOX, SIDNEY A.: *Lid Surgery, Current Concepts.* Grune & Stratton, New York, 1972. PRS, *51:*580, 1973

FRAZIER, CLAUDE A.: *Is it Moral to Modify Man?* Charles C Thomas, Springfield, Ill., 1974. PRS, *55:*356, 1975

FRITSCHI, ERNEST P.: *Reconstructive Surgery in Leprosy.* Williams & Wilkins Co., Baltimore, 1971. PRS, *49:*567, 1972

GANS, BENJAMIN J.: *Atlas of Oral Surgery.* C. V. Mosby Co., St. Louis, 1972

GEORGIADE, NICHOLAS, AND HAGERTY, ROBERT: *Symposium on Management of Cleft Lip and Palate and Associated Deformities,* Vol. 8. C. V. Mosby Co., St. Louis, 1975. PRS, *56:*333, 1975

GIBSON, H. L.: *Medical Photography.* Eastman Kodak Co., Rochester, N. Y., 1973. PRS, *54:*602, 1974

GOHRBRANDT, E., GABKA, J., AND BERNDORFER, A.: *Handbuch der Plastischen Chirurgie,* Volume II, Chapters 21 and 22. Walter de Gruyter & Co., Berlin, 1973. PRS, *54:*93, 1974

GOLDWYN, ROBERT M.: *Physician Travelers.* Arno Press & The New York Times, New York, 1971. PRS, *50:*180, 1972

GOLDWYN, ROBERT M.: *The Unfavorable Result in Plastic Surgery: Avoidance and Treatment.* Little, Brown & Co., Boston, 1972. PRS, *52:*186, 1973

GOLDWYN, ROBERT M.: *Plastic and Reconstructive Surgery of the Breast.* Little, Brown & Co., Boston, 1976

GORLIN, ROBERT J.: *Syndromes of the Head and Neck.* 2nd Ed. McGraw-Hill Co., New York, 1976

GRABB, WILLIAM C., AND MYERS, M. BERT: *Skin Flaps.* Little, Brown & Co., Boston, 1976

GRABB, WILLIAM C., AND SMITH, JAMES W.: *Plastic Surgery. A Concise Guide to Clinical Practice.* Little, Brown & Co., Boston, 1973. PRS, *54:*602, 1974

GRABB, WILLIAM C., ROSENSTEIN, SHELDON W., AND BZOCH, KENNETH R.: *Cleft Lip and Palate. Surgical, Dental, and Speech Aspects.* Little, Brown & Co., Boston, 1971. PRS, *49:*337, 1972

GUIBOR, P., AND SMITH, B.: *Contemporary Oculoplastic Surgery.* Grune & Stratton Inc., New York, 1974

HALL, ROBERT M.: *Facial, Oral, and Reconstructive Surgery.* Vol. 3. Springer-Verlag, New York, 1973

HARDY, JAMES D.: *Human Organ Support and Replacement. Transplantation and Artificial Prostheses.* Charles C Thomas,

Books—Cont.

ing Co., Huntington, N. Y., 1971. PRS, *49:*568, 1972

MAIBACH, H. I., AND ROVEE, D. T.: *Epidermal Wound Healing.* Year Book Medical Publishers, Chicago, 1972. PRS, *52:*429, 1973

MAJNO, GUIDO: *The Healing Hand: Man and Wound in the Ancient World.* Harvard University Press, Cambridge, 1975. PRS, *57:*230, 1976

MASTERS, FRANK W., AND LEWIS, JOHN R., JR.: *Symposium on Aesthetic Surgery of the Face, Eyelid, and Breast,* Vol. IV. C. V. Mosby Co., St. Louis, 1972. PRS, *51:*687, 1973

MASTERS, FRANK W., AND LEWIS, JOHN R., JR.: *Symposium on Aesthetic Surgery of the Nose, Ears, and Chin.* C. V. Mosby Co., St. Louis, 1973. PRS, *54:*479, 1974

MATTER, P., BARCLAY, T. L., AND KONICKOVA, Z.: *Research in Burns.* Hans Huber Publishers, Bern, Stuttgart, Vienna, 1971. PRS, *50:*79, 1972

MAY, HANS: *Plastic and Reconstructive Surgery,* Third Edition, F. A. Davis Co., Philadelphia, 1971. PRS, *48:*589, 1971

McCOY, FREDERICK J. *et al: Year Book of Plastic and Reconstructive Surgery.* Year Book Medical Pub., Inc., Chicago, 1975

McDOWELL, FRANK, AND ENNA, CARL: *Surgical Rehabilitation in Leprosy.* Williams & Wilkins Co., Baltimore, 1974

McGREGOR, IAN A.: *Fundamental Techniques of Plastic Surgery and their Surgical Applications.* Williams & Wilkins Co., Baltimore, 1972. PRS, *53:*342, 1974

McGREGOR, IAN A.: *Fundamental Techniques of Plastic Surgery.* 6th edition. Longman, Inc., New York, 1975

MEYER, JON K.: *Clinical Management of Sexual Disorders.* Williams & Wilkins Co., Baltimore, 1976

MIEHLKE, ADOLF: *Surgery of the Facial Nerve.* W. B. Saunders Co., Philadelphia, 1973. PRS, *55:*85, 1975

MILFORD, LEE: *The Hand.* C. V. Mosby Co., St. Louis, 1971. PRS, *49:*338, 1972

MILLARD, D. RALPH, JR.: *Cleft Craft, the Evaluation of its Surgery,* Vol. 1: *The Unilateral Deformity.* Little, Brown & Co., Boston, 1976

MOLLER, GORAN: *Transplantation Reviews.* Vol. 7. *Immunological Surveillance Against Neoplasia.* Williams & Wilkins Co., Baltimore, 1971. PRS, *51:*86, 1973

MOLLOWITZ, D.: *The Accident Man.* Joh. Ambrosius Barth, Frankfurt, 1974. PRS, *56:*333, 1975

Books—Cont.

MONAFO, WILLIAM W. & PAPPALARDO, CARLOS: *The Treatment of Burns: Principles & Practice.* Warren H. Green, St. Louis, Mo., 1971

MONEY, JOHN, AND EHRHARDT, ANKE A.: *Man and Woman, Boy and Girl.* Johns Hopkins University Press, Baltimore, 1972. PRS, *52:*295, 1973

MONTGOMERY, WILLIAM WAYNE: *Surgery of the Upper Respiratory System.* Lea & Febiger, Philadelphia, 1971. PRS, *49:*205, 1972

MOORE, FRANCIS D.: *Transplant: The Give and Take of Tissue Transplantation.* Simon and Schuster, New York, 1972. PRS, *51:*84, 1973

MORLEY, MURIEL E.: *Cleft Palate & Speech.* 7th Ed. Longman, Inc., New York, 1971

MOTAMED, H. A.: *Color Anatomy and Kinesiology of the Hand.* Hosein A. Motamed, Chicago, 1973. PRS, *55:*699, 1975

MUSTARDÉ, JOHN CLARKE: *Plastic Surgery in Infancy and Childhood.* E. & S. Livingstone, Edinburgh, 1971. PRS, *49:*451, 1972

NORWOOD, O'TAR T.: *Hair Transplant Surgery.* Charles C Thomas, Springfield, Ill., 1974. PRS, *54:*349, 1974

ORTIZ-MONASTERIO, FERNANDO: Taliacotii's *De Curtorum Chirurgia per Insitionem.* Libreria Manuel Porrua, S. A., Mexico D. F., Mexico, 1973. PRS, *53:*466, 1974

PAFF, GEORGE H.: *Anatomy of the Head and Neck.* W. B. Saunders Co., Philadelphia, 1973. PRS, *53:*468, 1974

PAPARELLA, MICHAEL M., AND SHUMRICK, DONALD A.: *Otolaryngology, Volume III. Head and Neck.* W. B. Saunders Co., Philadelphia, 1973. PRS, *53:*218, 1974

PENN, JACK: *The Right to Look Human.* McGraw-Hill Book Co., Johannesburg, New York, 1974. PRS, *56:*664, 1975

PERRY, C. B. W.: *Rehabilitation of the Hand.* 3rd Ed. Butterworth, London, 1974.

PINDBORG, J. J.: *Atlas of Diseases of Oral Mucosa.* 2nd Ed. W. B. Saunders Co., Philadelphia, 1973.

PIPKIN, GARRETT, AND BUHLER, VICTOR: *The Illness of Trauma.* Charles C Thomas, Springfield, Ill., 1971. PRS, *50:*519, 1972

POLK, HIRAM C., JR., AND STONE, H. HARLAN: *Contemporary Burn Management.* Little, Brown & Co., Boston, 1971

POTTER, GUY D.: *Sectional Anatomy and Tomography of the Head.* Grune and Stratton, New York, 1971. PRS, *51:*84, 1973

POWERS, GENE R.: *Cleft Palate.* Bobbs-Merrill Co., Inc., Indianapolis, Ind., 1973.

POWLEY, PHILIP: *Trauma Surgery Excepting*

Books – Cont.

STEPHENSON, HUGH JR.: *Immediate Care of the Acutely Ill and Injured.* C. V. Mosby Co., St. Louis, 1974. PRS, *57:*509, 1976

STEPHENSON, KATHRYN LYLE: *The Year Book of Plastic and Reconstructive Surgery.* Year Book Medical Publishers, Inc., Chicago, 1974. PRS, *55:*355, 1975

SWANSON, ALFRED B.: *Flexible Implant Resection Arthroplasty in the Hand and Extremities.* C. V. Mosby Co., St. Louis, 1973. PRS, *54:*350, 1974

TANZER, RADFORD C., AND EDGERTON, MILTON T.: *Symposium on the Reconstruction of the Auricle.* C. V. Mosby Co., St. Louis, 1974. PRS, *56:*571, 1975

THOMPSON, R. V. S.: *Primary Repair of Soft Tissue Injuries.* Melbourne (Australia) University Press, 1969. PRS, *48:*276, 1971

TOULOUKIAN, ROBERT J., AND KRIZEK, THOMAS J.: *Diagnosis and Early Management of Trauma Emergencies: A Manual for the Emergency Service.* Charles C Thomas, Springfield, Ill., 1974. PRS, *56:*206, 1975

TUBIANA, R., HUESTON, J. T. *et al: Maladie de Dupuytren.* Second Edition. L'Expansion, Paris, 1972. PRS, *51:*210, 1973

VILAIN, RAYMOND *et al: Osteo-Articular Injuries of the Hand.* Expansion Scientifique Francaise, Paris, 1971. PRS, *49:*656, 1972

VILAIN, R., AND MICHON, J. *Infections de la Main Chez l'Enfant et l'Adulte.* Masson & Cie, Paris, 1972. PRS, *52:*661, 1973

VON PRINCE, K. M. P., AND YAEKEL, M.: *The Splinting of Burn Patients.* Charles C Thomas, Springfield, Ill., 1974. PRS, *56:*1975

VRABEC, R. *et al: Basic Problems in Burns: Proceedings.* Symposium, Prague, September 1973. Springer-Verlag, New York, 1975.

WACHSMUTH, W., AND WILHELM, A.: *Allgemeine und Spezielle Chirurgische Operationslehre: Die Operationen an der Hand.* Springer-Verlag, Berlin, 1972. PRS, *51:*580, 1973

WAITE, DANIEL E.: *Textbook of Practical Oral Surgery.* Lea & Febiger, Philadelphia, 1972.

WARKANY, JOSEPH: *Congenital Malformations: Notes and Comments.* Year Book Medical Publishers, Chicago, 1971. PRS, *52:*570, 1973

WECKESSER, ELDEN C.: *Treatment of Hand Injuries. Preservation and Restoration of Function.* Year Book Medical Publishers, Chicago, 1974. PRS, *55:*700, 1975

Books – Cont.

WEEKS, PAUL M. AND WRAY, R. CHRISTIE: *Management of Acute Hand Injuries. A Biological Approach.* C. V. Mosby Co., St. Louis, 1973. PRS, *54:*216, 1974

WHITEHEAD, E. D.: *Current Operative Urology.* Harper & Row, Hagerstown, Md., 1975. PRS, *57:*232, 1976

WILLIAMS, D. F. AND ROAF, ROBERT: *Implants in Surgery.* W. B. Saunders Co., London, Philadelphia, Toronto, 1973. PRS, *54:*480, 1974

WOLFF, DOROTHY, BELLUCCI, RICHARD J., AND EGGSTON, ANDREW A.: *Surgical and Microscopic Anatomy of the Temporal Bone.* Hafner Publishing Co. Inc., New York, 1971. PRS, *49:*656, 1972

YAWALKAR, S. J.: *Leprosy for Practitioners.* Popular Prakashan, Ltd., Bombay, India, 1974. PRS, *55:*616, 1975

YOEL, JOSE: *Pathology and Surgery of the Salivary Glands.* Charles C Thomas, Springfield, Ill., 1975. PRS, *57:*230, 1976

YOUNG, H. HERMAN: *Year Book of Orthopedics and Traumatic Surgery.* Year Book Medical Publishers, Chicago, 1974. PRS, *56:*81, 1975

YULES, RICHARD B.: *Atlas for Surgical Repair of Cleft Lip, Cleft Palate, and Noncleft Velopharyngeal Incompetence.* Charles C Thomas, Springfield, Ill., 1971. PRS, *50:*399, 1972

ZACARIAN, SETRAG A.: *Review of Cryosurgery of Tumors of the Skin and Oral Cavity.* Charles C Thomas, Springfield, Ill., 1973. PRS, *55:*486, 1975

BOOROM, J. A.: Heat loss in burn patients. A.O.R.N., J., *17:*80, 1973

BOOTH, D. F.: Use of direct bonding materials for fixation and stabilization in the correction of facial deformities. J. Oral Surg., *34:*142, 1976

BOOTH, D. F. *et al:* Massive osteolysis of mandible: attempt at reconstruction. J. Oral Surg., *32:*787, 1974

BORA, F. W., JR. *et al:* Radial meromelia. The deformity and its treatment. J. Bone & Joint Surg., (Am.), *52:*966, 1970

BORCBAKAN, C.: Early diagnosis of mouth cancer (analysis of 435 cases), PRS, *57:*123, 1976. J. Fac. M., Univ. Ankara, *22:*469, 1969

BORCBAKAN, C., AND UNER, O.: Evaluation of presurgical and postsurgical cephalometric examinations in prognathism, PRS, *57:*117, 1976. J. Fac. M., Univ. Ankara, *25:*1464, 1972

BORCBAKAN, C. *et al:* Salivary gland tumors (clinical research on 54 cases), PRS, *57:*116,

1976. Kanser, *3:*38, 1973

BORCHERT, K. *et al*: Problems of tracheotomy in the surgical routine. Zentralbl. Chir., *96:*1005, 1971 (German)

BORCHGREVINK, H. *et al*: Cleft lip and cleft palate. Primary cleft surgery. 3. Tidsskr. Nor. Laegeforen, *93:*2466, 1973 (Norwegian)

BORDIN, G. M. *et al.*: Distant cutaneous metastases in a patient with squamous-cell carcinoma of the lip. Oral Surg., *34:*445, 1972

BORDLEY, J. E. *et al*: Mucoceles of frontal sinus: causes and treatment. Ann. Otol. Rhin. & Laryng., *82:*696, 1973

BOREJKO, J.: X-ray treatment of postoperative recurrences of malignant salivary gland neoplasms. Pol. Przegl. Radiol., *36:*795, 1972 (Polish)

BORG, G. *et al*: Study of odontogenic cysts with special reference to comparisons between keratinizing and non-keratinizing cysts. Sven. Tandlak. Tidskr., *67:*311, 1974

BORGES, A. F.: Historical review of the Z- and W-plasty in revisions of linear scars, PRS, *49:*241, 1972. Internat. Surg., *56:*182, 1971

BORGES, ALBERT F.: *Elective Incisions and Scar Revision*. Little, Brown & Co., Boston, 1973. PRS, *54:*216, 1974

BORGES, A. F.: Five single Z-plasties, PRS, *55:*387, 1975. Virginia M. Month., *101:*618, 1974

BORGES, A. F.: Reconstruction of umbilicus. Brit. J. Plast. Surg., *28:*75, 1975

BORGES, A. F. *et al*: Original Z-plasty. Brit. J. Plast. Surg., *26:*237, 1973

BORGHGRAEF, C. *et al*: Immediate reconstruction of mandible by iliac bone graft in Africa. Acta Stomatol. Belg., *70:*301, 1973 (French)

BORGHOUTS, J. M. *et al*: Orbital corrections with the use of alloplastic material. Trans. Int. Conf. Oral Surg., *4:*321, 1973

BORGHOUTS, J. M. *et al*: Orbital correction by means of alloplastic materials. Ned. tijdschr. geneeskd., *118:*521, 1974 (Dutch)

BORGHOUTS, J. M. H. M.: Surgical treatment of chronic suppurative hidradenitis, PRS, *55:*121, 1975. Arch. chir. neerl., *26:*201, 1974

BORLAND, R. G. *et al*: Safety with lasers, PRS, *54:*383, 1974. Proc. Roy. Soc. Med., *66:*841, 1973

BORNSTEIN, L. A.: Treatment of burns in the recent Middle East conflict (with Levin), PRS, *54:*432, 1974

BORNSTEIN, L. A. *et al*: Use of water-soluble estrogens in plastic surgery. Harefuah, *83:*488, 1972 (Hebrew)

BORRAS, C., AZCOYTIA, M., AND DARGALLO, J.: Congenital camptodactyly of thumb, PRS, *56:*229, 1975. Barcelona Quirurgica, *18:*233, 1974

BORSETTI, G., AND AMBROGGIO, G.: Action of early surgical treatment in development of burn scars, PRS, *56:*361, 1975. Riv. ital. chir. plast., *5:*251, 1973

BORTHNE, A.: Intraorbital valve fracture. Acta Ophthalmol. (Kbh.), *51:*492, 1973

BORTNICK, E.: Evaluation of surgical techniques on nasal tip projection. Laryngoscope, *84:*1316, 1974

BORTOT, G. *et al*: Total parotidectomy with conservation of the facial nerve. Riv. Ital. Stomatol., *26:*446, 1971 (Italian)

BORTOT, G. *et al*: Unilateral mandibular resection-disarticulation by an intraoral method and immediate reconstruction by bone autograft. Riv. Ital. Stomatol., *26:*605, 1971 (Italian)

BOSCH, J.: Operative treatment of wry-neck. Follow-up study over period of 27 years. Wien. Klin. Wochenschr., *84:*688, 1972 (German)

BOSSLEY, C. J.: Industrial hand injuries in Pacific Island immigrants. N.Z. Med. J., *81:*191, 1975

BOSSUYT, M.: Experience with branchiogenic cysts. Acta Stomatol. Belg., *68:*425, 1971 (Dutch)

BOSTWICK, J., III: Coverage of exposed bone by muscle transposition and skin grafting (with Vasconez, McCraw), PRS, *53:*526, 1974

BOSTWICK, J., III, VASCONEZ, L. O., AND JURKIEWICZ, M. J.: Basal cell carcinoma of the medial canthal area, PRS, *55:*667, 1975

BOSTWICK, J., III, PENDERGRAST, W. J., JR., AND VASCONEZ, L. O.: Marjolin's ulcer: an immunologically privileged tumor? PRS, *57:*66, 1976

BOSWICK, J. A., JR.: Management of the burned hand. Orthop. Clin. North Am., *1:*311, 1970

BOSWICK, J. A., JR.: Burns of head and neck. Surg. Clin. North Am., *53:*97, 1973

BOSWICK, J. A., JR.: Rehabilitation of the burned hand. Clin. Orthop., *0:*162, 1974

BOSWICK, J. A.: Management of fresh burns of the hand and deformities resulting from burn injuries. Clin. Plast. Surg., *1:*621, 1974

BOSWICK, J. A. JR. *et al*: Emergency care of the burned patient. Surg. Clin. North Am., *52:*115, 1972

BOTHRA, R. *et al*: Cervical thymoma. Int. Surg., *60:*301, 1975

BOTTCHER, J.: Lymphography in case of combined toxoplasmosis of lymph nodes and stationary Hodgkin's disease. Roentgenblaetter, *27:*257, 1974 (German)

BOUCHE, J.: Minimum neurolysis in so-called frozen face paralysis. Ann. Otolaryngol. Chir. Cervicofac., *92:*203, 1975 (French)

BOUCHE, J. *et al*: Resection of tympanic plexus

in Frei's syndrome and recurrent parotiditis. Ann. Otolaryngol. Chir. Cervicofac., *88:*449, 1971 (French)

BOUCHER, A. H.: Ischiopedic bilateral congenital band, PRS, *55:*119, 1975. Bol. Soc. cir. Plast. Reconstr. Cordoba, *5:*21, 1974

BOUDREAU, R. G. *et al*: Maxillary "pocket inlay" vestibuloplasty. J. Oral Surg., *33:*601, 1975

BOUEZ, A. *et al*: Hemimandibulectomy for recurrence of ameloblastoma curetted and irradiated 16 years previously. Rev. Dent. Liban., *24:*1, 1974 (French)

BOUEZ, A. *et al*: Hemimandibulectomy after recurrent ameloblastoma curetted and irradiated 16 years before. Rev. Stomatol. Chir. Maxillofac., *75:*66, 1974 (French)

BOUMAN, F. G.: Reconstruction of breast after subcutaneous mastectomy, PRS, *55:*719, 1975. Arch. chir. neerl., *26:*343, 1974

BOUMAN, F. G.: Reconstructive surgery of the hand in contractures caused by epidermolysis bullosa. Ned. tijdschr. geneeskd., *118:*993, 1974 (Dutch)

BOURETZ, J. C.: Problems of tactics and approach. Unusual case of the hand. Rev. Chir. Orthop., *60 Suppl 2:*94, 1974 (French)

BOURGUET, J. *et al*: Fractures of malar bone (apropos of 149 cases). Ann. Otolaryngol. Chir. Cervicofac., *90:*55, 1973 (French)

BOURNE, I. H.: Vertical leg drainage of edema in treatment of leg ulcers, PRS, *57:*535, 1976. Brit. M. J., *2:*581, 1974

BOURREL, P.: Brand operation. Apropos of 12 personal cases. Ann. chir. plast., *13:*297, 1968 (French)

BOURREL, P.: Repeated exploration with interfascicular neurolysis after primary repair of lesions of the nerves of the hand. Value in tropical practice. Med. Trop. (Mars.), *30:*672, 1970 (French)

BOURREL, P.: Educational film: Zancolli's operation. Film commentary. Med. Trop. (Mars.), *32:*759, 1972 (French)

BOURREL, P.: Trauma-induced nerve sections without motor paralysis of the hand. Ann. Chir., *28:*831, 1974 (French)

BOURREL, P. *et al*: Functional restorations of hand mutilations caused by weapon explosions. Ann. chir. plast., *16:*215, 1971 (French)

BOURREL, P. *et al*: Treatment of keloid scars by subtotal excision and graft (14 cases). Ann. chir. plast., *17:*304, 1972 (French)

BOURREL, P. *et al*: Simplified method for thin skin graft. Value in tropical practice. Med. Trop. (Mars.), *32:*645, 1972 (French)

BOURREL, P. *et al*: Surgical treatment of claw-hand. Metacarpo-phalangeal capsular shortening and advancement of the trochleae

of the flexors (103 cases). Rev. Chir. Orthop., *60 Suppl 2:*243, 1974 (French)

BOURREL, P. *et al:* Aspects of cutaneous plastic surgery in the tropics. Ann. chir. plast., *20:*375, 1975 (French)

BOUTERIE, R. L., AND McLEAN, D. H.: Use of 0.5 per cent silver nitrate cream for burns, PRS, *49:*586, 1972. Am. J. Surg., *121:*576, 1971

BOUTIN, G. *et al*: Melanoma of nasal cavity. Union. Med. Can., *102:*1872, 1973 (French)

BOUVENG, R., SCHILDT, B., AND SORBO, B.: Studies on biosynthesis and transfer of labile methyl groups in experimental burn, PRS, *53:*109, 1974. Europ. Surg. Res., *5:*146, 1973

BOUWER, S.: Silicone implants in the hand. Acta Orthop. Belg., *58:*9, 1972

BOWE, J. J.: Primary excision in third degree burns (Follow-Up Clinic), PRS, *49:*565, 1972

BOWE, J. J.: Surgical approach to basal cell carcinoma. J. M. Soc. New Jersey, *70:*115, 1973

BOWE, J. J.: Congenital epulis tumor, PRS, *53:*227, 1974

BOWEN, D. A. *et al*: Traumatic air embolism. Med. Sci. Law, *16:*56, 1976

BOWEN, F. H.: Subfascial ligation (Linton operation) of the perforating leg veins to treat post-thrombophlebitic syndrome. Am. Surg., *41:*148, 1975

BOWEN, J.: Method for correction of prominent ears. Brit. J. Plast. Surg., *27:*92, 1974

BOWEN, J., AND MEARES, A.: Delayed local leg flaps, PRS, *56:*683, 1975. Brit. J. Plast. Surg., *27:*167, 1974

BOWEN, J. *et al*: Excision of deep burns with the carbon dioxide laser. Brit. J. Plast. Surg., *27:*322, 1974

BOWEN, J. C., AND FLEMING, W. H.: Effect of massive transfusion of stored blood on oxygen delivery in man, PRS, *52:*330, 1973. Surg. Forum, *23:*17, 1972

BOWEN, T. E., WHELAN, T. J., AND NELSON, T. G.: Sudden death after phosphorus burns: experimental observations of hypocalcemia, hyperphosphatemia, and electrocardiographic abnormalities following production of standard white phosphorus burn, PRS, *49:*667, 1972. Ann. Surg., *174:*779, 1971

BOWERMAN, J. E.: Review of reconstruction of mandible. Proc. Roy. Soc. Med., *67:*610, 1974

BOWERS, D. G.: Surgical repair of congenital lower lip sinuses, PRS, *49:*632, 1972

BOWERS, D. G.: Serious implications of multiple mucosal neuromata, PRS, *56:*554, 1975

BOWERS, D. G., AND GRUBER, H.: Use of acrylic obturators to protect suture lines in the hard palate, PRS, *51:*98, 1973

BOWERS, M. P.: Management of traumatic facial nerve injuries. J. Natl. Med. Assoc., 67:103, 1975

BOXER, R. J.: Reconstruction of the male external genitalia. Surg. Gynec. & Obst., 141:939, 1975

BOYCE, W. H.: New concept concerning treatment of exstrophy of the bladder: 20 years later. Trans. Am. Assoc. Genitourin. Surg., 63:121, 1971

BOYCE, W. H.: New concept concerning treatment of exstrophy of the bladder: 20 years later. J. Urol., 107:476, 1972

BOYD, N. A.: Military surgical team in Belfast. Ann. R. Coll. Surg. Engl., 56:15, 1975

BOYES, J. H.: Regional surgeon – new kind of specialist (Editorial), PRS, 56:199, 1975

BOYES, J. H., AND STARK, H. H.: Flexor tendon grafts in fingers and thumb, study of factors influencing results in 1000 cases, PRS, 50:630, 1972. J. Bone & Joint Surg., 53:1332, 1971

BOYKO, A. et al: Osteopetrosis: report of case. J. Oral Surg., 32:859, 1974

BOYLE, R. W. et al: Revascularization of the hand in a patient with complete interruption of the radial and ulnar arteries. Arch. Phys. Med. Rehabil., 54:229, 1973

BOYNE, P. J.: Methods of osseous reconstruction of mandible following surgical resection, PRS, 53:365, 1974. J. Biomed. Mater. Res., 7:195, 1973.

BOYNE, P. J.: Use of marrow-cancellous grafts in regeneration of mandibular bone. Trans. Congr. Int. Assoc. Oral Surg., 4:58, 1973

BOYNE, P. J.: Restoration of deficient edentulous ridges by bone grafting and use of subperiosteal metal implants. Int. J. Oral Surg., 3:278, 1974

BOYNE, P. J.: Use of marrow-cancellous bone grafts in maxillary alveolar and palatal clefts. J. Dent. Res., 53:821, 1974

BOYNE, P. J. et al: Secondary bone grafting of residual alveolar and palatal clefts. J. Oral Surg., 30:87, 1972

BOYNE, P. J. et al: Evaluation of a compression intraosseous fixation device in mandibular fractures. Oral Surg., 33:696, 1972

BOYNE, P. J. et al: Treatment of long standing bilateral fracture non- and mal-union in atrophic edentulous mandibles. Int. J. Oral Surg., 3:213, 1974

BOYSEN, G. et al: Cerebral blood flow and internal carotid artery flow during carotid surgery. Stroke, 1:253, 1970

BOZDUGANOV, A. et al: Histological and histochemical examinations of skin after irradiation by ruby laser. Radiobiol. Radiother. (Berl.), 14:703, 1973 (German)

BOZEK, J. et al: Late results of surgical treatment of benign lingual tumors in children. Pediatr. Pol., 45:1193, 1973 (Polish)

BOZZAY, L.: Salivary calculus of sublingual gland. Forgorv. Sz., 67:134, 1974 (Hungarian)

BRAATZ, J. H., McALISTAR, B. R., AND BROADDUS, M. D.: Ultrasound and plantar warts: a double blind study, PRS, 54:699, 1974. Mil. Med., 139:199, 1974

BRACCI, U.: Indications for rectal bladder. Bull. Soc. Internat. Chir., 31:544, 1972 (Italian)

BRACKEN, R. B., AND DIOKNO, A. C.: Melanoma of penis and urethra, PRS, 54:621, 1974. J. Urol., 111:198, 1974

BRACKMANN, D. E. et al: Glomus jugulare tumors: effect of irradiation. Trans. Am. Acad. Ophthalmol. Otolaryngol., 76:1423, 1972

BRADHAM, G.: Direct measurement of total metabolism of burned patient, PRS, 51:234, 1973. Arch. Surg., 105:410, 1972

BRADLEY, E. L.: Management of penetrating injuries carotid artery. J. Trauma, 13:248, 1973

BRADLEY, P.: Actinomycosis of the temporomandibular joint. Brit. J. Oral Surg., 9:54, 1971

BRADLEY, P. F. et al: Cryosurgery of bone. An experimental and clinical assessment. Oral Surg., 13:111, 1975

BRADY, M. P., AND O'SULLIVAN, D. J.: Bull man's hand: unusual occupational lesion, PRS, 57:262, 1976. J. Cardiovasc. Surg., 16:157, 1975

BRAIN, D. J.: Cryosurgery in benign conditions of nose and throat. Proc. Roy. Soc. Med., 67:72, 1974

BRALEY, S. A.: Use of silicones in plastic surgery, retrospective view, PRS, 51:280, 1973

BRAMI, S.: Case of post-traumatic ischemic necrosis of the tongue. Rev. Stomatol. Chir. Maxillofac., 76:455, 1975 (French)

BRAMI, S. et al: Treatment of facial asymmetries by one-stage maxillary and mandibular bilateral osteotomies. Int. J. Oral Surg., 3:239, 1974

BRAMLEY, P.: Odontogenic keratocyst – an approach to treatment. Int. J. Oral Surg., 3:337, 1974

BRAMLEY, P. A. et al: Secondary enlargement of the mandibular coronoid process. Brit. J. Surg., 59:426, 1972

Branchial Cysts (See also *Lateral Cervical Fistula*)

Experience with branchiogenic cysts (Bossuyt). Acta Stomatol. Belg., 68:425, 1971 (Dutch)

Accessory tragi (Brownstein *et al*). Arch Der-

Branchial Cysts—Cont.

mat., *104:*625, 1971

On a case of total branchial fistula (Obreja *et al*). Otorinolaringologie, *16:*345, 1971 (Rumanian)

Branchio-skeleto-genital syndrome, new hereditary syndrome (Elsahy, Waters). PRS, *48:*542, 1971

Embryonal remnant with parotid symptomatology (Pelerin). Rev. Laryngol. Otol. Rhinol. (Bord.), *92:*851, 1971 (French)

Unilateral transverse facial cleft—a method of surgical closure (Mansfield *et al*). Brit. J. Plast. Surg., *25:*29, 1972

Pre-auricular sinus: clinical features and the problems of recurrence (Sykes). Brit. J. Plast. Surg., *25:*175, 1972

Cervicoaural fistula (Novak). Cesk. Otolaryngol., *21:*86, 1972 (Czechoslovakian)

Malformative aspects involving the 1st branchial arch. Report of 3 cases (Caramia *et al*). Minerva Med., *63:*490, 1972 (Italian)

Anomalies of the first branchial cleft (Trail *et al*). South. Med. J., *65:*716, 1972

Branchial cyst, midline cervical cleft of neck with associated (French, Bale). Am. J. Surg., *125:*376, 1973

Problems raised by fistula of low parotid region (originating from first branchial pocket) (Peri *et al*). Ann. chir. plast., *18:*83, 1973

Cysts, branchial, and fistulas (Sancho Rodriguez-Fornos, Narbona Arnau), PRS, *54:*111, 1974. Cir. Españ., *27:*339, 1973

Sinus and pouch, first branchial cleft (Pap). PRS, *52:*583, 1973

Branchial cleft, first, anomalies of (Dougall), PRS, *55:*252, 1975. J. Pediat. Surg., *9:*203, 1974

Branchial cleft cysts and sinuses in children (Buckingham, Lynn), PRS, *54:*378, 1974. Mayo Clin. Proc., *49:*172, 1974

Surgical treatment of congenital neck fistulae in childhood (Epel'baum). Stomatologiia (Mosk.), *53:*89, 1974 (Russian)

Anomalies, first branchial cleft cysts and sinuses (Gaisford, Anderson). PRS, *55:*299, 1975

BRAND, K. G. *et al*: Etiological factors, stages and role of foreign body in foreign body tumorigenesis, PRS, *56:*111, 1975. Cancer Res., *35:*279, 1975

BRAND, P. W.: Tendon transfers for median and ulnar nerve paralysis. Orthop. Clin. North Am., *1:*447, 1970

BRAND, P. W.: Evaluation of the hand and its function. Orthop. Clin. North Am., *4:*1127, 1973

BRAND, P. W.: Rehabilitation of the hand with motor and sensory impairment. Orthop. Clin. North Am., *4:*1135, 1973

BRAND, P. W.: Biomechanics of tendon transfer. Orthop. Clin. North Am., *5:*205, 1974

BRAND, P. W.: Discussion of "Skin, dartos, and nerve biopsies as aids to diagnosis in leprosy," by Pandya. PRS, *54:*218, 1974

BRAND, P. W.: Discussion of "Preventing recurrent tissue breakdowns after pressure 'sore' closures," by Rogers, Wilson. PRS, *56:*573, 1975

BRANDAO, C., TORRES, P., AND ALVES, J.: Carcinoma of male breast, report on 12 cases, PRS, *50:*630, 1972. Folia med. Brazil, *64:*23, 1972

BRANDAO, G. S. *et al*: Bilateral nasolabial cyst. Oral Surg., *37:*480, 1974

BRANDESKY, G.: Experimental studies of function of pedicled muscle flaps in diaphragmatic defects, PRS, *54:*620, 1974. Ztschr. Kinderchir., *14:*260, 1974

BRANDIS, H. J. VON: Breast surgery—a marginal field? A report. Chirurg., *42:* Suppl 9, 65, 1971 (German)

BRANDT, H. P.: Contributions to the therapy of epiphora. Klin. Monatsbl. Augenheilkd., *167:*105, 1975 (German)

BRANDT, K. A.: Bandage-free method for the covering of hand-burns. Handchirurgie, *2:*203, 1970 (German)

BRANEMARK, P. I. *et al*: Intra-osseous anchorage of dental prostheses. I. Experimental studies, PRS, *48:*97, 1971. Scand. J. Plast. Reconstr. Surg., *3:*81, 1969

BRANEMARK, P. I. *et al*: Repair of defects in mandible, PRS, *49:*470, 1972. Scand. J. Plast. Reconstr. Surg., *4:*100, 1970

BRANEMARK, P. I. *et al*: Reconstruction of the defective mandible. Scand. J. Plast. Reconstr. Surg., *9:*116, 1975

BRANLEY, P. A.: Treatment of cysts of jaws, PRS, *49:*232, 1972. Proc. Roy Soc. Med., *64:*547, 1971

BRANNON, W., OCHSNER, M. D., AND FUSELIER, H. A., JR.: Anterior urethral strictures: experience with free graft urethroplasty, PRS, *52:*680, 1973. J. Urol., *109:*265, 1973

BRANTIGAN, C. O.: Delayed major vessel hemorrhage following tracheostomy, PRS, *53:*604, 1974. J. Trauma, *13:*235, 1973

BRANTIGAN, C. O. *et al*: Cricothyroidotomy: elective use in respiratory problems requiring tracheotomy. J. Thorac. Cardiovasc. Surg., *71:*72, 1976

BRANZOVSKY, T.: Desmoid of the abdominal wall. Rozhl. Chir., *51:*87, 1972 (Czechoslovakian)

BRARA, N. S., KATHPALIA, P. M. L., AND CHAR,

R. D.: War injuries of upper extremity, PRS, *56:*228, 1975. Indian J. Surg., *36:*379, 1974

BRASFIELD, R. D., AND GUPTA, T. K. S.: Von Recklinghausen's disease: clinicopathological study, PRS, *50:*309, 1972. Ann. Surg., *175:*86, 1972

BRASHER, W. J. *et al*: Complications of free grafts of oral mucosa. J. Periodontol., *46:*133, 1975

BRAUER, R. O.: Treatment of the double cleft of the primary and secondary palate with a protruding premaxilla. Jap. J. Plast. Reconstr. Surg., *14:*41, 1971

BRAUER, R. O.: Observations and measurements of nonoperative setback of premaxilla in double cleft patients (Follow-Up Clinic), PRS, *50:*280, 1972

BRAUER, R. O.: Retropharyngeal implantation of silicone gel pillows for velopharyngeal incompetence, PRS, *51:*254, 1973

BRAUN, R. M.: Nail-gun injury of the hand. J. Bone & Joint Surg. (Am.), *53:*383, 1971

BRAUN, R.M.: Trephine technique for obtaining small bone grafts, PRS, *54:*509, 1974. Hand, *6:*103, 1974

BRAUN, R. M. *et al*: Quantitative results following implant arthroplasty of the proximal finger joints in the arthritic hand. Clin. Orthop., *83:*135, 1972

BRAUN, R. M. *et al*: Preliminary experience with superficialis-to-profundus tendon transfer in the hemiplegic upper extremity. J. Bone & Joint Surg. (Am.), *56:*466, 1974

BRAUN-FALCO, O.: Malignant melanomas of the skin from the dermatologic viewpoint. Chirurg., *45:*345, 1974 (German)

BRAVERMAN, IRWIN M.: *Skin Signs of Systemic Disease*. W. B. Saunders, Philadelphia, London, Toronto, 1975. PRS, *57:*657, 1976

BRAY, A. E.: Use of serum-blocking factor as an indicator of residual tumor following primary excision. J. Surg. Res., *19:*341, 1975

Breasts (See also *Gynecomastia; Mammaplasty; Mastectomy, Subcutaneous; Mammaplasty, Mastopexy*)

Breast surgery – a marginal field? A report (Brandis). Chirurg., *42:* Suppl 9, 65, 1971 (German)

Necrosis, cutaneous and subcutaneous, as complication of coumarin-congener therapy (Kahn, Stern, Rhodes), PRS, *48:*160, 1971

Breast operations, noncosmetic, aesthetic considerations in (Bryant). Am. Surgeon, *38:*524, 1972

Estrogen therapy, benign breast disease in women on (Fechner), PRS, *50:*96, 1972.

Breasts – Cont.

Cancer, *29:*273, 1972

Adenomammectomy: technique and advantages (Rice). Northwest. Med., *71:*375, 1972

Mondor's disease, observations on 14 patients and survey of literature (Sivula, Somer), PRS, *54:*117, 1974. Ann. chir. et gynaec. Fenniae, *62:*361, 1973

Suction drainage in breast surgery. Brit. Med. J., *3:*554, 1973

Granuloma, lipophagic, of female breast (Moguilevsky, Barbarelli, Zanniello), PRS, *57:*397, 1976. Bol. y trab. Soc. argent. cir., *35:*581, 1974

Modifications to breasts. Brit. Med. J., *3:*135, 1974

Progesterone: treatment of macromastia in actively enlarging breast (Mayl, Vasconez, Jurkiewicz), PRS, *54:*6, 1974

Breast, subareolar abscess of, chronic, areolar reconstruction for (Golden *et al*). Surg. Gynec. & Obst., *138:*609, 1974

New instrument for mammary surgery (Zenteno). Brit. J. Plast. Surg., *28:*164, 1975

Axillary breasts. An aesthetic deformity of the trunk (Kaye). Clin. Plast. Surg., *2:*397, 1975

Ectopic mammary gland on the back (Eckert *et al*). Dtsch. Med. Wochenschr., *100:*1395, 1975 (German)

Letter: Terminology (Notes). J.A.M.A., *234:*1321, 1975

Breasts, Augmentation: See *Mammaplasty, Augmentation*

Breasts, Cancer

Carcinoma of male breast (Cortese, Cornell), PRS, *49:*238, 1972. Ann. Surg., *173:*275, 1971

Mammography, accuracy, clinical value and limitations (Marx *et al*), PRS, *51:*103, 1973. Arch. chir. neerl., *23:*315, 1971

Mammography (Arandes Adan, Prats Esteve), PRS, *48:*604, 1971. Barcelona Quirurgica, *15:*13, 1971

Breast, foreign body granuloma of, incident to malignant tumor (Yamazaki *et al*), PRS, *50:*305, 1972. Geka Surg. Ther. Osaka, *33:*1283, 1971

Limb, upper, bi-hinged chest-arm flap for lymphedema of (Hirshowitz, Goldan), PRS, *48:*52, 1971

Breast, female, diagnosis and treatment of malignant melanoma arising from skin of (Ariel, Caron), PRS, *51:*347, 1973. Am. J. Surg., *124:*384, 1972

Breast carcinoma, "inoperable," successful result using zinc chloride fixative (Sonne-

Breasts, Cancer—Cont.

land), PRS, *51:*347, 1973. Am. J. Surg., *124:*391, 1972

Mammary gland cancer in University Hospital of Caracas (Heredia *et al*), PRS, *52:*600, 1973. Biol. Soc. Venezuelana Cir., *26:*295, 1972

Breast cancer, early, management of, organization of clinical trial on national scale (Baum, Edwards, Magarey). Brit. M. J., *4:*476, 1972

Breast carcinoma involving thoracic wall, treatment of local recurrences (Bruck), PRS, *53:*113, 1974. Chir. Plast., *1:*265, 1972

Carcinoma of male breast, report on 12 cases (Brandao, Torres, Alves), PRS, *50:*630, 1972. Folia med. Brazil, *64:*23, 1972

Breast cancer, modern trends in the surgical treatment (Schwaiger), PRS, *53:*365, 1974. Langenbecks Arch. Chir., *332:*619, 1972

Carcinoma of female breast, recurrent, treatment of (Grady), PRS, *55:*719, 1975. Rocky Mountain M. J., *72:*24, 1972

Male breast carcinoma (Donegan, Perez-Mesa), PRS, *52:*460, 1973. Arch. Surg., *106:*273, 1973

Carcinoma, mammary, resection of thoracic wall and local flap repair for recurrences of (Korlof *et al*). Brit. J. Plast. Surg., *26:*322, 1973

Lymphangiosarcoma, brawny arm complication after mastectomy (Mosiman). Helv. Chir. Acta, *40:*651, 1973 (French)

Xeroradiography of breast (Phillips, Lutterbeck, Wilkolm), PRS, *55:*379, 1975. Internat. Surg., *58:*607, 1973

Breast cancer treated without recurrence, chronic lymphedema after (Mayer *et al*), PRS, *54:*111, 1974. Lyon chir., *69:*401, 1973

Cancer, breast, silicone granulomatous disease simulating (Kuiper), PRS, *52:*452, 1973. Mich. Med., *72:*215, 1973

Breast carcinomas, treatment of bilateral, in a patient with silicone-gel breast implants (Benavent), PRS, *51:*588, 1973

Carcinoma: value of mammography in cosmetic surgery of the breasts (Perras, Papillon), PRS, *52:*132, 1973

Cystic disease of the breast, chronic, treatment by subcutaneous mastectomy (Pennisi, Capozzi), PRS, *52:*520, 1973

Cancer, breast, early, detection and management of (McDivitt). Proc. Natl. Cancer Conf., *7:*269, 1973

Cancer, breast, surgery from Halsted to 1972 (Lewison). Proc. Natl. Cancer Conf., *7:*272, 1973

Aesthetic excisional biopsy of a nipple lesion

Breasts, Cancer—Cont.

(Golden *et al*). Am. J. Surg., *128:*445, 1974

Breast esthetics and carcinology (Vilain), PRS, *54:*620, 1974. Ann. chir. plast., *19:*1, 1974

Mammary gland, male, malignant tumors of, report of 16 cases (Krakovic). Bruns Beitr. Klin. Chir., *221:*35, 1974 (German)

Cancer, breast, minimal, treatment of (Wanebo *et al*). Cancer, *33:*349, 1974

Breast disease, appraisal of mammography for (Peck, Lowman), PRS, *54:*373, 1974. Conn. Med., *38:*103, 1974

Breast disease, mammography in 50 cases (Pandya *et al*), PRS, *55:*247, 1975. Indian J. Surg., *36:*102, 1974

Breast cancer patients, epidemiologic comparison (Craig, Comstock, Geiser), PRS, *55:*724, 1975. J. Nat. Cancer Inst., *53:*1577, 1974

Mammography at Mayo Clinic—a year's experience (Karsell), PRS, *56:*106, 1975. Mayo Clin. Proc., *49:*954, 1974

Value of plate thermography in the diagnosis of the breast (Muhlberger *et al*). Munch. Med. Wochenschr., *116:*2047, 1974 (German)

Breast cancer, simple mastectomy with immediate reconstruction (Horton *et al*), PRS, *53:*42, 1974

Breast cancer, recurrent, a transverse abdominal flap for reconstruction after radical operations (Tai, Hasegawa), PRS, *53:*52, 1974

Breast cancer, bilateral, 10 years after an augmentation mammaplasty (Johnson, Lloyd), PRS, *53:*88, 1974

Mammaplasty, augmentation, effect on mammography and thermography (Rintala, Svinhufvud), PRS, *54:*390, 1974

Breast carcinoma, conservative surgical treatment (Mason), PRS, *55:*719, 1975. Proc. Roy. Soc. Med., *67:*473, 1974

Prophylaxis of breast cancer (Eder). Wien. Klin. Wochenschr., *86:*153, 1974 (German)

Paget's disease, mammary and extramammary (Bussolati, Pich), PRS, *57:*260, 1976. Am. J. Clin. Path., *80:*117, 1975

Breast cancer, a surgical dilemma (Leis). Ann. Chir., *29:*852, 1975 (French)

Cancer: biological basis for management of benign disease of the breast; case against subcutaneous mastectomy (Peacock), PRS, *55:*14, 1975. Discussion by Watson, PRS, *55:*225, 1975

Carcinoma, obscure, incidence of, in subcutaneous mastectomy (Pennisi, Capozzi), PRS, *56:*9, 1975. Discussion by Snyder-

Breasts, Cancer — Cont.

man, PRS, *56:*208, 1975

Breast cancer, prognosis in young women (Gogas, Skalkeas), PRS, *57:*533, 1976. Surgery, *78:*339, 1975

Cancer, breast reconstruction after radical mastectomy (Guthrie), PRS, *57:*14, 1976

Cancer, breast, reconstruction after mastectomy (Hartwell *et al*), PRS, *57:*152, 1976

Cancer, breast, reconstruction after mastectomy (Snyderman) (Editorial), PRS, *57:*224, 1976

Mastectomy: one-stage reconstruction of breast, using transposed greater omentum (Arnold, Hartrampf, Jurkiewicz), PRS, *57:*520, 1976

Breast, Cystosarcoma Phylloides

Cystosarcoma phylloides of the mammary gland (Kucharski *et al*). Pol. Przegl. Chir., *43:*1791, 1971 (Polish)

Cystosarcoma phylloides. Treatment by subcutaneous mastectomy with immediate prosthetic implantation (Mandel *et al*), PRS, *50:*630, 1972. Am. J. Surg., *123:*718, 1972

Giant fibroadenoma of breast (Burghard *et al*). Fortschr. Geb. Roentgenstr. Nuklearmed., *117:*607, 1972 (German)

Cystosarcoma phylloides (Lawrence). Indian J. Cancer, *9:*231, 1972

Breast, cystosarcoma phylloides of — conservative procedures or amputation? (Klein *et al*). Pol. Tyg. Lek., *27:*1401, 1972 (Polish)

Breast, giant fibroadenoma of, in young (Lengyel *et al*). Orv. Hetil., *114:*2545, 1973 (Hungarian)

Cystosarcoma phylloides, giant, case (Falardeau *et al*). Union Med. Can., *102:*1528, 1973 (French)

Cystosarcoma phylloides of breast (Halverson *et al*). Am. Surg., *40:*295, 1974

Cystosarcoma phylloides, recurrent, radical treatment (Faraci *et al*). Ann. Surg., *180:*796, 1974

Cystosarcoma phylloides (giant fibro-adenoma) in adolescent females: clinicopathological study (Nambiar *et al*). Brit. J. Surg., *61:*113, 1974

Subcutaneous mastectomy (Molenar). Clin. Plast. Surg., *1:*427, 1974

Cystosarcoma phylloides (Turnbull *et al*). J. R. Coll. Surg. Edinb., *19:*104, 1974

Cystosarcoma phylloides in twelve-year-old girl (Kelsh). N. C. Med. J., *35:*295, 1974

Mixed tumor of female breast of unusual duration and size (Williams *et al*). South Med. J., *68:*97, 1975

Breasts, Cystosarcoma Phylloides — Cont.

Clinical course of cystosarcoma phylloides related to histologic appearance (Blichert-Toft *et al*). Surg. Gynec. & Obst., *140:*929, 1975

Case of sarcoma phylloides of the breast (Badowski *et al*). Wiad. Lek., *28:*217, 1975 (Polish)

Hypertrophic breast (Gaudenz). Praxis, *65:*164, 1976 (German)

Breasts, Deformity (See also *Mammaplasty*)

Breast and mammarian region, plastic surgery of (Lupo, Boggio-Robutti), PRS, *49:*357, 1972. Minerva med., Italy, Monograph, 1971

Treatment of asymmetry of the breasts (Grant). South Med. J., *64:*1097, 1971

Breasts, excessively large, neurologic changes with (Kaye), PRS, *50:*305, 1972. South. M. J., *65:*177, 1972

Breast plasty in scar deformation and defects after deep burns (Mukhin), PRS, *54:*501, 1974. Acta chir. plast., *15:*176, 1973

Breast plasties with omentum magnum in prethoracic transposition (Kiricuta, Popescu), PRS, *53:*242, 1974. Chir. plast., *2:*47, 1973

Breasts, virginal hypertrophy of, use of an antiestrogen after a reduction mammaplasty to prevent recurrence of (Sperling, Gold), PRS, *52:*439, 1973

Breast deformities in young women, surgical correction (Henrik *et al*). Tidsskr. Nor. Laegeforen, *93:*1044, 1973 (Norwegian)

Breast, grossly hypertrophied in puberty, surgical and hormonal management (Lejour, Loriaux, Hardy), PRS, *55:*636, 1975. Ann. chir. plast., *19:*347, 1974

Breast deformities and their surgical repair (Schurter *et al*). J. Invest. Dermatol., *63:*138, 1974

Breast enlargement, significance of (Wehby, Salti), PRS, *56:*677, 1975. Lebanese M. J., *27:*719, 1974

Hypertrophy of breast: reduction mammaplasty by "B" technique (Regnault), PRS, *53:*19, 1974

Breast surgery, cosmetic, evaluation of mammaplasty techniques in a municipal teaching hospital (Bromberg, Song, Norwitz), PRS, *53:*33, 1974

Hypertrophy, mammary: Will Durston's "mammaplasty" (Letterman, Schurter), PRS, *53:*48, 1974

Breasts, axillary (Kaye), PRS, *53:*61, 1974

Breast, modified Aufricht reduction mammaplasty (Meijer), PRS, *53:*129, 1974. Discus-

Breasts, Deformity — Cont.

sion by Aufricht, PRS, *53:*132, 1974

Breast: simplified design for reduction mammaplasty (Gerow, Spira, Hardy), PRS, *53:*271, 1974

Mammary hypertrophy: reduction mammaplasty for extremely large breasts (Gsell), PRS, *53:*643, 1974

Breast, macromastia in the actively enlarging, treatment of (Mayl, Vasconez, Jurkiewicz), PRS, *54:*6, 1974

Breasts, unequal, volume measurements of (Kirianoff), PRS, *54:*616, 1974

Breast hypertrophy, functional alterations in (Pitanguy *et al*), PRS, *57:*673, 1976. Rev. brasil. cir., *64:*209, 1974

Breast masses, pediatric, surgical management (Turbey, Dudgeon), PRS, *57:*674, 1976. Pediatrics, *56:*736, 1975

Breast, hypertrophic: reduction mammaplasty with an L-shaped suture line (Meyer, Kesselring), PRS, *55:*139, 1975

Breasts, hypertrophied, new technique for reduction (Ribeiro), PRS, *55:*330, 1975

Biesenberger technique of reduction mammaplasty, variation of (Carlsen, Tershakowec), PRS, *55:*653, 1975

Anomaly, congenital unilateral hypoplasia or absence of breast (Pierre, Jouglard), PRS, *56:*146, 1975

Mammaplasty, correction of asymmetrical breasts (Elliott, Hoehn, Greminger), PRS, *56:*260, 1975

Breast, new technique for reduction mammaplasty (Johnson) (Letter to the Editor), PRS, *57:*372, 1976

Asymmetry of breasts, correction of (Elsahy), PRS, *57:*700, 1976

Breast implant, giant, for unilateral aplasia (Marchac, Alkhatib), PRS, *57:*749, 1976

Breasts, Hypoplasia (See also *Mammaplasty, Augmentation*)

Breast, infant, radiation to, mammary hypoplasia following (Skalkeas, Gogas, Pavlatos), PRS, *52:*679, 1973. Acta chir. plast., *14:*240, 1972

Hypoplasia of the breast, a psychosocial disease (van de Lande *et al*). Ned. tijdschr. geneeskd., *116:*428, 1972 (Dutch)

Breast, unilateral hypoplastic, plastic surgery for; report of 8 cases (Corso), PRS, *50:*134, 1972

Breast, hypoplastic and aplastic, plasty using adipodermal grafts (Bruckner, Lenz), PRS, *56:*355, 1975. Acta chir. plast., *16:*216, 1974

Breast, absence of, or unilateral congenital hypoplasia, treatment of (Pierre, Joug-

Breasts, Hypoplasia — Cont.

lard), PRS, *56:*146, 1975

Hypoplasia, mammary, associated with chest wall deformities, reconstruction of (Hawtof, Ram, Alani), PRS, *57:*172, 1976

Hypoplasia, correction of asymmetries of breasts (Elsahy), PRS *57:*700, 1976

Breasts, Nipple Operations

Nipple reduction (Pitanguy, Cansancao), PRS, *49:*582, 1972. Rev. brasil. cir., *61:*73, 1971

Nipple and areola reconstruction by split-skin graft from normal side (Millard), PRS, *50:*350, 1972

Nipple, congenital inversion, in identical twins (Lamont). Brit. J. Plast. Surg., *26:*178, 1973

Nipple transposition, single dermal pedicle for, in subcutaneous mastectomy, reduction mammaplasty, or mastopexy (Weiner *et al*), PRS, *51:*115, 1973

Areolar sharing to reconstruct the absent nipple (Wexler, Oneal), PRS, *51:* 176, 1973

Nipple lesion, aesthetic excisional biopsy of (Golden *et al*). Am. J. Surg., *128:*445, 1974

Nipple, cosmetic reduction, with functional preservation (Sperli). Brit. J. Plast. Surg., *27:*42, 1974

Nipple sensation following breast reduction and free nipple transplantation (Townsend), PRS, *56:*678, 1975. Brit. J. Plast. Surg., *27:*308, 1974

Areolae, large, planning an augmentation mammaplasty (Snyder), PRS, *54:*132, 1974

Areola and nipple reconstruction in the burned breast, "double bubble" technique (Bunchman *et al*), PRS, *54:*531, 1974

Breast: inversion of human female nipple with simple method of treatment (Schwager *et al*), PRS, *54:*564, 1974

Nipple, inverted (Pitanguy *et al*), PRS, *57:*673, 1976. Rev. brasil. cir., *64:*199, 1974

Breast feeding aided by correcting inverted nipples (Otte), PRS, *56:*605, 1975. Am. J. Nursing, *75:*454, 1975

Nipple hypertrophy. Physiologic reduction by circumcision (Regnault). Clin. Plast. Surg., *2:*391, 1975

Areola, breast, reconstruction of, by intradermal tattooing and transfer (Rees), PRS, *55:*620, 1975

Nipple and areola reconstruction (Guida, Picchi, Inzirillo), PRS, *56:*454, 1975

Areola reduction and simultaneous augmentation mammaplasty, through periareolar incision (Bartels, Mara), PRS, *56:*588, 1975

Areola method for recontouring domed nipple

Breasts, Nipple Operations—Cont.

(Vecchione), PRS, *57:*30, 1976

Breast, alternative operation for inverted nipple (Elsahy), PRS, *57:*438, 1976

Nipple reconstruction (Silsby), PRS, *57:*667, 1976

Breasts, Ptosis of (See also *Mammaplasty, Reduction; Mastectomy,. Subcutaneous; Mammaplasty, Mastopexy*)

Ptosis, mammary gland, indications of the Aries-Pitanguy technique in (Lejour), PRS, *50:*199, 1972. Acta chir. belg., *70:*5, 1971

Dermal mastopexy technique, subcutaneous mastectomy with immediate reconstruction of the breasts, using the (Goulian, McDivitt), PRS, *50:*211, 1972

Neurologic changes with excessively large breasts (Kaye), PRS, *50:*305, 1972. South. M. J., *65:*177, 1972

Breast, ptotic and moderately enlarged, mammaplasty for (Aiache), PRS, *56:*677, 1975. Brit. J. Plast. Surg., *27:*38, 1974

Breast hypertrophy and ptosis, new data on surgery of (Mitz), PRS, *55:*248, 1975. J. chir., *107:*595, 1974

Ptosis of breasts, reduction mammaplasty by "B" technique (Regnault), PRS, *53:*19, 1974

Mammary hyperinvolution and ptosis (North). Brit. J. Plast. Surg., *28:*310, 1975

Breast, ptotic: reduction mammaplasty with an L-shaped suture line (Meyer, Kesselring), PRS, *55:*139, 1975

Breasts, pendulous: inframammary-based dermofat flaps in mammary reconstruction following a subcutaneous mastectomy (Letterman, Schurter), PRS, *55:*156, 1975

Ptosis of breasts, new technique for reduction mammaplasty (Ribeiro), PRS, *55:*330, 1975

Ptosis, subcutaneous mastectomy, excess skin problem in (Hartley, Schatten, Griffin), PRS, *56:*5, 1975

Mammaplasty, technique for subcutaneous mastectomy and immediate reconstruction in ptotic breast (Georgiade, Hyland), PRS, *56:*121, 1975

Breast ptosis, mild or moderate, new mastopexy operation for (Bartels, Strickland, Douglas), PRS, *57:*687, 1976

Breasts, Reconstruction of

Breast reconstruction: a plea for saving the uninvolved nipple (Millard *et al*). Am. J. Surg., *122:*763, 1971

Is it permissible to reconstruct a breast with prosthesis after mastectomy for cancer? When and how? (Picaud *et al*). Ann. chir.

Breasts, Reconstruction of—Cont.

plast., *17:*278, 1972 (French)

Mammary reconstruction, further experience with our technique (Fernandez), PRS, *51:*347, 1973. Bol. y trab. Acad. argent. cir., *56:*129, 1972

Breast reconstruction after breast amputation (Millesi). Dtsch. Med. Wochenschr., *97:*785, 1972 (German)

Breast reconstruction (Georgiade). N. C. Med. J., *33:*524, 1972

Split-skin graft from normal side for nipple and areola reconstruction (Millard), PRS, *50:*350, 1972

Total reconstruction of the breast after the removal of a bilateral giant fibroadenoma (Carvalho). Rev. Asoc. Med. Bras., *18:*95, 1972 (Portuguese)

Symposium on Neoplastic & Reconstructive Problems of the Female Breast. Vol. 7. Ed. by Reuven K. Snyderman. C. V. Mosby Co., St. Louis, 1973

Breast, use of buttock to reconstruct (Orticochea). Brit. J. Plast. Surg., *26:*304, 1973

Breast, missing, single stage reconstruction of (Pontes). Brit. J. Plast. Surg., *26:*377, 1973

Breast reconstruction: areolar sharing to reconstruct the absent nipple (Wexler, Oneal), PRS, *51:*176, 1973

Mas⁺ ᵗomy, reconstruction of breast following (De Cholnoky) (Follow-Up Clinic), PRS, *52:*435, 1973

A note on volume determination in connexion with reconstructive surgery (Atkinson *et al*). In *Biostereometrics 74*, ed. by Herron; pp. 161–71. Falls Church, Va.; Am. Soc. Photogrammetry, 1974

Breast and thoracic wall, radionecrosis of, reconstructive surgery (Matton, D'Hooghe), PRS, *56:*226, 1975. Acta chir. belg., *73:*301, 1974

Breast reconstruction after subcutaneous mastectomy (Bouman), PRS, *55:*719, 1975. Arch. chir. neerl., *26:*343, 1974

Surgical reconstruction of the breast (Kohnlein). Med. Klin., *69:*1647, 1974 (German)

Cancer of breast, simple mastectomy with immediate reconstruction (Horton *et al*), PRS, *53:*42, 1974

Breast reconstruction after radical mastectomy (Miller *et al*). Am. Fam. Physician, *11:*97, 1975

Letter: Breast reconstruction (Paulshock). Am. Fam. Physician, *12:*30, 1975

Reconstruction surgery of the breast (Strombeck). Arch. Gynaekol., *219:*121, 1975 (German)

Subcutaneous mastectomy with immediate

Breasts, Reconstruction of—Cont.

reconstruction of the breast (Poate). Aust. N. Z. J. Surg., *45:*383, 1975

Breast restoration after mastectomy for cancer (Chong *et al*). Mayo Clin. Proc., *50:*453, 1975

Breast reconstruction after mastectomy, indications for (Van Dongen, Lichtveld), PRS, *57:*397, 1976. Nederl. tijdschr. geneesk., *119:*997, 1975

Mammary reconstruction following subcutaneous mastectomy, inframammary-based dermofat flaps in (Letterman, Schurter), PRS, *55:*156, 1975

Breast areola, reconstruction by intradermal tattooing and transfer (Rees), PRS, *55:*620, 1975

Breast reconstruction for aplasia by microvascular transfer of free flap from buttock (Fujino, Harashina, Aoyagi), PRS, *56:*178, 1975. Discussion by Goldwyn, PRS, *56:*335, 1975

Breast, areola and nipple reconstruction (Guida, Picchi, Inzirillo), PRS, *56:*454, 1975

Breast reconstruction after radical mastectomy (Guthrie), PRS, *57:*14, 1976

Breast reconstruction after mastectomy for cancer (Hartwell *et al*), PRS, *57:*152, 1976

Breast reconstruction after mastectomy for cancer (Snyderman) (Editorial), PRS, *57:*224, 1976

Breast, one-stage reconstruction, using transposed greater omentum (Arnold, Hartrampf, Jurkiewicz), PRS, *57:*520, 1976

Breast, nipple reconstruction (Silsby), PRS, *57:*667, 1976

Breasts, Reduction: See Mammaplasty, Reduction

Breasts, Subcutaneous Excision: See Mastectomy, Subcutaneous

Breasts, Supernumerary

Breast cystic lesions of dorsal supernumerary in male (Brightmore), PRS, *48:*605, 1971. Proc. Roy. Soc. Med., *64:*662, 1971

Supernumerary breast, double complete, on anterolateral aspect of right thigh: case report (Bhandari, Shastri, Sharma), PRS, *55:*247, 1975. Indian J. Surg., *36:*43, 1974

Polymastia — axillary breast (Carreirao, Lessa), PRS, *57:*533, 1976. Rev. brasil. cir., *53:*77, 1975

Breasts, Suspension of: See Mammaplasty, Mastopexy

BREDIN, H. C. *et al*: Surgical correction of male epispadias with total incontinence. J. Urol., *109:*904, 1973

BREISTEIN, L.: Regeneration of the cartilaginous nasal septum in the rat, after resection. Its influence on facial growth (with Kvinnsland), PRS, *51:*190, 1973

BREJCHA, M., AND FARA, M.: Osseous changes in middle clefts of nose, PRS, *50:*633, 1972. Acta chir. plast., *13:*141, 1971

BRENNAN, D. G., AND CULLINAN, W. L.: Object identification and naming in cleft palate children, PRS, *55:*382, 1975. Cleft Palate J., *11:*188, 1974

BRENNAN, H. G. *et al*: Submentoplasty. Classification and theoretical outline of management. Arch. Otolaryng., *95:*24, 1972

BRENNAN, H. G., AND PARKES, M. L.: Septal surgery: high septal transfixion, PRS, *54:*234, 1974. Internat. Surg., *58:*732, 1973

BRENNAN, M. *et al*: Growth of *Candida albicans* in nutritive solutions given parenterally, PRS, *50:*312, 1972. Arch. Surg., *103:*705, 1971

BRENNER, R. L.: Dacryocystorhinostomy in children. Tex. Med., *70:*71, 1974

BRENT, B.: Effective safety devices for the Padgett dermatome, PRS, *51:*467, 1973

BRENT, B.: Magnetic surgical instrument stand, PRS, *52:*318, 1973

BRENT, B.: Ear reconstruction with an expansile framework of autogenous rib cartilage, PRS, *53:*619, 1974

BRENT, B: Reconstruction of ear, eyebrow, and sideburn in the burned patient, PRS, *55:*312, 1975

BRENT, B.: Earlobe construction with an auriculo-mastoid flap, PRS, *57:*389, 1976

BRESLOW, A.: Tumor thickness, level of invasion and node dissection in stage I cutaneous melanoma. Ann. Surg., *182:*572, 1975

BRETTEVILLE-JENSEN, G.: Radical sweat gland ablation for axillary hyperhidrosis, PRS, *55:*114, 1975. Brit. J. Plast. Surg., *26:*158, 1973

BRETTEVILLE-JENSEN, G.: Reconstruction of lower lip after central excisions. Brit. J. Plast. Surg., *26:*247, 1973

BRETTEVILLE-JENSEN, G.: Mammaplasty with reduced blood loss: effect of noradrenalin, PRS, *56:*677, 1975. Brit. J. Plast. Surg., *27:*31, 1974

BRETTEVILLE-JENSEN, G.: Surgical treatment of gynecomastia. Brit. J. Plast. Surg., *28:*177, 1975

BRETTEVILLE-JENSEN, G. *et al*: Surgical treatment of axillary hyperhidrosis in 123 patients. Acta Derm. Venereol. (Stockh.), *55:*73, 1975

BREUNSBACH, J. *et al*: Interpretation of the 99mTcO-4-salivary gland scans. Fortschr.

Geb. Roentgenstr. Nuklearmed., *121:*500, 1974 (German)

BREWERTON, D. A.: Tenography in the rheumatoid hand. Hand, *2:*46, 1970

BREWITT, H. *et al*: Basalioma of the eyelids. Klin. Monatsbl. Augenheilkd., *166:*503, 1975 (German)

BREWITT, H. *et al*: Lid basaliomas with malignant courses. Klin. Monatsbl. Augenheilkd., *166:*770, 1975 (German)

BREYTENBACH, H. S. *et al*: Clinical characteristics and genetic identity of basal cell nevus syndrome (Gorlin-Goltz syndrome). S. Afr. Med. J., *49:*544, 1975. (Afrikaans)

BRIANT, T. D.: Switch flaps from anterior chest and nape of neck. Can. J. Otolaryngol., *1:*299, 1972

BRIANT, T. D.: Complementary specialties. Can. J. Otolaryngol., *2:*205, 1973 (French)

BRIANT, T. D.: Spontaneous pharyngeal fistula and wound infection following laryngectomy. Laryngoscope, *85:*829, 1975

BRIANT, T. D. *et al*: Carcinoma of nasal premaxillary complex. Can. J. Otolaryngol., *1:*30, 1972

BRIANT, T. D. *et al*: Carcinoma of hypopharynx. Can. J. Otolaryngol., *2:*4, 1973

BRIANT, T. D. *et al*: Inverted papilloma of nose and paranasal sinuses. Can. J. Otolaryngol., *3:*180, 1974

BRIANT, T. D. R., FITZPATRICK, P. J., AND BOOK, H.: Radiological treatment of juvenile nasopharyngeal angiofibromas, PRS, *48:*198, 1971. Ann. Otol. Rhin. & Laryng., *79:*1108, 1970

BRIANTSEVA, L. N.: Several operations for restoring thumb opposition. Vestn. Khir., *106:*68, 1971 (Russian)

BRIANTSEVA, L. N. *et al*: Reconstructive surgery of the hand in patients with leprosy. Vestn. Khir., *111:*67, 1973 (Russian)

BRICHE, G. *et al*: Oral surgery in orthodontic practice. Stomatologia (Athenai), *28:*259, 1971

BRIDGER, A. J.: Cosmetic rhinoplasty – the prerogative of plastic surgeon or rhinologist. J. Otolaryngol. Soc. Aust., *3:*428, 1972

BRIDGER, M. W.: Hemangioma of the nasal bones. J. Laryng. & Otol., *90:*191, 1976

BRIEDIS, J.: Dupuytren's contracture, lack of complications with open palm technique, PRS, *56:*680, 1975. Brit. J. Plast. Surg., *27:*218, 1974

BRIGGS, R. M., AND OGG, M. J.: Patients' refusal of surgery after Innovar premedication, PRS, *51:*158, 1973

BRIGHTMORE, T. G. T.: Cystic lesion of dorsal supernumerary breast in male, PRS, *48:*605,

1971. Proc. Roy. Soc. Med., *64:*662, 1971

BRIHAYE, J. *et al*: Local gigantism of the hand associated with a plexiform neurofibroma of the ulnar nerve. Report of a case. J. Neurosurg. Sci., *18:*271, 1974

BRIHAYE, J. *et al*: Injuries of the fronto-orbitomalar region. Rev. Stomatol. Chir. Maxillofac., *75:*246, 1974 (French)

BRIX, M. *et al*: Oroileoanastomosis in total oesophagoplasty. Bratisl. Lek. Listy., *63:*395, 1975 (Slovakian)

BROADBENT, T. R.: Four-flap Z-plasty (with Woolf), PRS, *49:*48, 1972

BROADBENT, T. R.: Continuing education and plastic surgery (Editorial), PRS, *57:*88, 1976

BROADBENT, T. R., AND WOOLF, R. M.: Hypospadias, two-stage repair, PRS, *50:*539, 1972. Rocky Mountain M. J., *68:*37, 1971

BROADBENT, T. R., AND WOOLF, R. M.: Gunshot wounds of face: initial care, PRS, *52:*107, 1973. J. Trauma, *12:*229, 1972

BROADBENT, T. R., AND WOOLF, R. M.: Bilateral cleft lip repairs. Review of 160 cases and description of present management, PRS, *50:*36, 1972

BROCHERIOU, C. *et al*: Giant calculi of submandibular gland. Case. Rev. Stomatol. Chir. Maxillofac., *73:*517, 1972 (French)

BROCHERIOU, C. *et al*: Muco-epidermoid tumors of the salivary glands. Description of 30 cases. Rev. Stomatol. Chir. Maxillofac., *75:*1039, 1974 (French)

BROCKMULLER, K. D. *et al*: Controlled hypotension in orthopedic jaw operations. Fortschr. Kiefer. Gesichtschir., *18:*117, 1974 (German)

BRODEUR, A. *et al*: Surgical treatment of bedsores. Union Med. Can., *102:*1921, 1973 (French)

BRODKIN, R. H. *et al*: Basal cell carcinoma. J.A.M.A., *228:*463, 1974

BRODRIBB, A. J. M., AND RICKETTS, C. R.: Effect of zinc in healing of burns, PRS, *49:*359, 1972. Injury, *3:*25, 1971

BRODY, G. S.: Immobilization of tiny hands. Hand, *3:*97, 1971

BRODY, G. S.: Facial reanimation. Calif. Med., *116:*55, 1972

BRODY, G. S., AND McCORRISTON, J. R.: Experimental transplantation of small bowel mucosa to the rectum (Follow-Up Clinic), PRS, *50:*183, 1972

BROEDERS, G. H. B. *et al*: True hermaphroditism with XX/XY/XXY chromosome pattern, PRS, *55:*387, 1975. Nederl. tijdschr. geneesk., *118:*726, 1974

BROGAN, W. F. *et al*: Decline in the incidence of cleft lip and palate in Western Australia, 1963 to 1972. M. J. Australia, *2:*8, 1974

BROMAGE, P. R., AND GERTEL, M.: Improved brachial plexus blockage with bupivacaine hydrochloride and carbonated lidocaine, PRS, *50*:631, 1972. Anesthesiology, *36*:479, 1972

BROMBERG, B. E.: Mandibular bone grafts (Follow-Up Clinic), PRS, *48*:172, 1971

BROMBERG, B. E.: Recovery in Pseudomonas septicemia (Follow-Up Clinic), PRS, *51*:88, 1973

BROMBERG, B. E.: Primary vaginal reconstruction after pelvic exenteration (with Song, Cramer), PRS, *51*:509, 1973

BROMBERG, B. E., SONG, I. C., AND WALDEN, R. H.: Hydrotherapy of chemical burns (Follow-Up Clinic), PRS, *49*:453, 1972

BROMBERG, B. E., SONG, I. C., AND CRAIG, G. T.: Split rib mandibular reconstruction, PRS, *50*:357, 1972

BROMBERG, B. E., SONG, I. C., AND NORWITZ, S.: Evaluation of mammaplasty techniques in a municipal teaching hospital, PRS, *53*:33, 1974

BROMIGE, M. R.: Severe compound comminuted fracture of the mandible. Brit. J. Oral Surg., *9*:29, 1971

BRONNER, A. *et al*: Technic and results of treatment of traumatic canalicular sections using Worst's "pig tail" sound. Bull. Soc. Ophtalmol. Fr., *73*:939, 1973 (French)

BRONNER, A. *et al*: Tumor of the lacrimal apparatus. Investigations and therapeutic management. Bull. Soc. Ophthalmol. Fr., *74*:643, 1974 (French)

BRONNER, A. *et al*: Course of conjunctival melanocancer, therapeutic management. Apropos of 2 cases. Bull. Soc. Ophtalmol. Fr., *74*:647, 1974 (French)

BROOKS, J. E.: Cystic hygroma of neck. Laryngoscope, *83*:117, 1973

BROTMAN, R.: Letter: hand injuries caused by opening safety containers. Am. J. Hosp. Pharm., *32*:455, 1975

BROTSOS, A.: Surgical treatment of mandibular prognathism. Hell. Stomatol. Chron., *16*:171, 1972 (Greek)

BROUCHERIOU, C. *et al*: Ewing's sarcoma localized to the mandible. 2 cases. Rev. Stomatol. Chir. Maxillofac., *75*:877, 1974 (French)

BROVKINA, A. F.: Reasons for complications stemming from orbital surgery and measures to prevent them. Vestn. Oftalmol., *1*:31, 1972 (Russian)

BROVKINA, A. F. *et al*: Orbital spatula – light guide. Vestn. Oftalmol., *1*:79, 1973 (Russian)

BROVKINA, A. F. *et al*: Orbitotomy performed with use of ultrasonic instruments. Vestn. Oftalmol., *2*:46, 1975

BROWAND, B. C. *et al*: Central mucoepidermoid tumors of the jaws. Report of nine cases and review of the literature. Oral Surg., *40*:631, 1975

Browlift

Eyebrow, ptosis of, surgical correction (English *et al*). Br. J. Ophthalmol., *57*:761, 1973

Forehead lift: brow lifting through temporal scalp approach (Gleason), PRS, *52*:141, 1973

Repair of drooping brow and upper eyelid, secondary to facial nerve palsy (Luxenberg). Trans. Am. Acad. Ophthalmol. Otolaryng., *77*:721, 1973

Brow-lift operation (Rafaty *et al*). Arch. Otolaryng., *101*:467, 1975

Brow lift with blepharocanthoplasty (Hinderer), PRS, *56*:402, 1975

Brow lift, forehead rhytidoplasty and (Viñas, Caviglia, Cortinas), PRS, *57*:445, 1976

BROWN, BARRETT: Prize in Plastic Surgery, PRS, *52*:605, 1973; *52*:659, 1973; *54*:705, 1974; *56*:687, 1975

BROWN, C. B.: Case report: vestibuloplasty – skin and palatal mucosal grafts. J. Mich. State Dent. Assoc., *55*:70, 1973

BROWN, F. C., AND LEUY, J.: Keratoacanthoma, unusual case report, PRS, *52*:327, 1973. Cutis, *8*:585, 1972

BROWN, F. C., AND TAN, E. M.: Immunological reaction in keratoacanthoma, spontaneously resolving skin tumor, PRS, *53*:496, 1974. Cancer Res., *33*:2030, 1973

BROWN, G. E. *et al*: Flap repair of cervical esophageal stricture, PRS, *55*:379, 1975. Australian & New Zealand J. Surg., *44*:133, 1974

BROWN, H.: Closed crush injuries of the hand and forearm. Orthop. Clin. North Am., *1*:253, 1970

BROWN, H., AND FLYNN, J. E.: Abdominal flap for hand neuromas and entrapped nerves, PRS, *52*:595, 1973. J. Bone & Joint Surg., *55A*:575, 1973

BROWN, H. C.: Current concepts of burn pathology and mechanisms of deformity in the burned hand. Orthop. Clin. North Am., *4*:987, 1973

BROWN, H. G.: Functional anatomy of the hand. Orthop. Clin. North Am., *1*:199, 1970

BROWN, H. G.: Electrical and cold injuries of the hand. Orthop. Clin. North Am., *1*:321, 1970

BROWN, J. B.: Closure of surface defects with free skin grafts and with pedicle flaps. Woman Physician, *26*:75, 1971

BROWN, J. B., AND FRYER, M. P.: Hemangiomas: role of plastic surgery in early treatment for prevention of deformities and in the repair of late lesions and defects (Follow-Up Clinic), PRS, 50:77, 1972

BROWN, L.: Nice adventure for a woman. Infirm. Can., 15:24, 1973 (French)

BROWN, L. H.: Treatment of burns of the hands. J. Okla. State Med. Assoc., 63:141, 1970

BROWN, P. W.: Zancolli capsulorrhaphy for ulnar claw hand—appraisal of 44 cases, PRS, 48:512, 1971. J. Bone & Joint Surg., 52A:868, 1970

BROWN, R. F.: Compound fractures of tibia: soft tissue defect. Proc. Roy. Soc. Med., 65:625, 1972

BROWN, R. G., VASCONEZ, L. O., AND JURKIEWICZ, M. J.: Transverse abdominal flaps and the deep epigastric arcade, PRS, 55:416, 1975

BROWN, S. H., JR., NEERHOUT, R. C., AND FONKALSRUD, E. W.: Prednisone therapy in management of large hemangiomas in infants and children, PRS, 50:96, 1972. Surgery, 71:168, 1972

BROWN, V. K. H.: Decontamination procedures for skin exposed to phenolic substances, PRS, 56:114, 1975. Arch. Environmental Health, 30:1, 1975

BROWNE, E. Z.: Successful replantation of a totally severed thumb (with Snyder, Stevenson), PRS, 50:553, 1972

BROWNE, E. Z., JR., AND SNYDER, C. C.: Carpal tunnel syndrome caused by hand injuries, PRS, 56:41, 1975

BROWNE, R. M.: Metaplasia and degeneration in odontogenic cysts in man. J. Oral Pathol., 1:145, 1972

BROWNE, S. G.: Summary of recent abstracts. 8. Leprosy Trop. Dis. Bull., 69:863, 1972

BROWNSTEIN, M., AND SHAPIRO, L.: Trichlelemoma, PRS, 57:264, 1976. Arch. Dermat., 107:866, 1973

BROWNSTEIN, M. H. et al: Accessory tragi. Arch. Dermat., 104:625, 1971

BROWNSTEIN, M. H., AND HELWIG, E. B.: Spread of tumors to skin, PRS, 52:460, 1973. Arch. Dermat., 107:80, 1973

BROWNSTEIN, M. H., AND HELWIG, E. B.: Subcutaneous dermoid cysts, PRS, 52:457, 1973. Arch. Dermat., 107:237, 1973

BROWNSTEIN, M. H., SHAPIRO, L., AND SLEVIN, R.: Fistula of dorsum of nose, PRS, 54:377, 1974. Arch. Dermat., 109:227, 1974

BROZMAN, M.: Revascularization of free skin grafts in dependence on recipient bed, PRS, 55:643, 1975. Acta chir. plast., 16:136, 1974

BROZMAN, M.: Carcinoma of lower lip. Rozhl. Chir., 54:430, 1975 (Slovakian)

BROZMAN, M. et al: Suture of palate and secondary repair of pharyngeal flap. Acta chir. plast. (Praha), 14:218, 1972

BRUCE, M., WALIKE, J., AND GOERTZEN, E.: External carotid arteriovenous fistulae, PRS, 54:106, 1974. Arch. Otolaryng., 98:332, 1973

BRUCE, R. A.: Trichinosis associated with oral squamous cell carcinoma, PRS, 57:265, 1976. Oral Surg., 33:136, 1975

BRUCHET, P. et al: Tolerance of the cortical bone to silicone materials. Ann. chir. plast., 20:227, 1975 (French)

BRUCHIE, H.: Examining the blood supply of the hand following injuries. Handchirurgie, 2:147, 1970 (German)

BRUCHIE, H. et al: Results following surgical treatment of Dupuytren's contracture. Handchirurgie, 2:27, 1970 (German)

BRUCHLE, H.: First aid in fresh complex hand injuries. Hefte Unfallheilkd., 107:241, 1970 (German)

BRUCHLE, H.: Extensor tendon injuries of the back of the hand and wrist. Monatsschr. Unfallheilkd., 73:503, 1970 (German)

BRUCK, H. G.: Experiences with dermatovaginal plastic surgery. Wien. Klin. Wochenschr., 82:562, 1970 (German)

BRUCK, H. G.: Use of free transplanted dermis flaps in modern plastic surgery. Bruns Beitr. Klin. Chir., 218:664, 1971 (German)

BRUCK, H. G.: Possibilities and indications of dermis grafts, PRS, 48:519, 1971. Med. & Hygiene, 955:443, 1971

BRUCK, H. G.: Clinical use of POR 8 in plastic and reconstructive surgery. Wien. Med. Wochenschr., 121:691, 1971 (German)

BRUCK, H. G.: Treatment of local recurrences in breast carcinoma involving thoracic wall, PRS, 53:113, 1974. Chir. Plast., 1:265, 1972

BRUCK, H. G.: Corrective rhinoplasty. Study of 5,000 personal cases. Arch. Otolaryng., 97:441, 1973

BRUCK, H. G.: Management of skin defects. Closure of skin defect by free transplants. Basic principles of application and technique. Langenbecks Arch. Chir., 334:567, 1973 (German)

BRUCK, H. M. et al: Opportunistic fungal infection of burn wound with Phycomycetes and Aspergillus, PRS, 49:107, 1972. Arch. Surg., 102:476, 1971

BRUCK, H. M. et al: Studies on occurrence and significance of yeasts and fungi in burn wound, PRS, 51:350, 1973. Ann. Surg., 176:108, 1972

BRUCK, H. M., AND PRUITT, B. A., JR.: Curling's ulcer in children, 12-year review of 63 cases, PRS, 52:101, 1973. J. Trauma, 12:490, 1972

BRUCKE, P. *et al*: Comments on paper by P. Wilflingseder: Reconstruction of trachea using segment transplant from nasal septum. Wien. Klin. Wschr., *84:*226, 1972. Wien. Klin. Wchr., *84:*797, 1972 (German)

BRUCKE, P. *et al*: Resection of benign tracheal stenoses following tracheostomy and longtime intubation. Bruns Beitr. Klin. Chir., 220, 387, 1973 (German)

BRUCKNER, H.: Standardization of corrective surgery in macromastias and breast ptoses. Zentralbl. Chir., *98:*817, 1973 (German)

BRUCKNER, H.: Reconstruction of hand in epidermolysis bullosa. Zentralbl. Chir., *99:*328, 1974 (German)

BRUCKNER, H.: Errors and dangers of mammaplasty. Zentralbl. Chir., *100:*1266, 1975

BRUCKNER, H., AND LENZ, P.: Plasty of hypoplastic and aplastic breast using adipodermal grafts, PRS, *56:*355, 1975. Acta chir. plast., *16:*216, 1974

BRUCKNER, W. L. *et al*: Influence of pure virus infection on wound healing, PRS, *52:*329, 1973. Surg. Forum, *23:*41, 1972

BRUDVIK, J. S.: Custom cast splints for oral surgical procedures, PRS, *55:*506, 1975. Oral Surg., *38:*15, 1974

BRUDZYNSKA-CHAREWICZ, S. *et al*: Bacteriological and clinical studies of the use of sulfamylon in the treatment of burns. Pol. Przegl. Chir., *44:*783, 1972 (Polish)

BRUEZIERE, J.: Apropos of transsigmoid cutaneous ureterostomies. Ann. Chir. Infant., *12:*459, 1971 (French)

BRUG, E. *et al*: Auxiliary chemotherapy in bacterial infections of the hand. Arzneim. Forsch., *21:*586, 1971 (German)

BRUG, E. *et al*: Bacteriological analysis and chemotherapeutic sequelae of purulent hand infections. Handchirurgie, *3:*93, 1971 (German)

BRUNER, J. M.: Presents McIndoe Lecture, PRS, *51:*717, 1973

BRUNER, J. M.: Contributions of Sir Archibald McIndoe to surgery of the hand. Ann. R. Coll. Surg. Engl., *53:*1, 1973

BRUNER, J. M.: Surgical exposure of flexor tendons in the hand. Ann. R. Coll. Surg. Engl., *53:*84, 1973

BRUNER, J. M.: Moto perpetuo – (Paganini). A theme for surgery of the hand. Hand, *6:*115, 1974

BRUNER, J. M.: Surgical exposure of the flexor pollicis longus tendon. Hand, *7:*241, 1975

BRUNIAUX, J. *et al*: Long-lasting anesthesia in plastic surgery and neurosurgery. Anesth. Analg. (Paris), *31:*181, 1974 (French)

BRUNNER, U. *et al*: Use of cutaneous homografts in surgical treatment of large varicose ulcers. Phlebologie, *26:*249, 1973 (French)

BRUSATI, R.: Correction of prognathism associated with maxillary retrusion (with Rusconi), PRS, *48:*558, 1971

BRUSATI, R. *et al*: Dermal-epidermal free grafts in preprosthetic surgery. Riv. Ital. Stomatol., *26:*731, 1971 (Italian)

BRUSATI, R. *et al*: Large calculus of submandibular gland, case report. J. Oral Surg., *31:*710, 1973

BRUSATI, R. *et al*: Maxillary anterior segmentary osteotomy: experimental research on vascular supply of osteotomised segment. Fortschr. Kiefer. Gesichtschir., *18:*90, 1974

BRUSIS, T.: New marking instrument for otoplasty. Ztschr. Laryng. Rhin. Otol., *52:*51, 1973 (German)

BRUSKINA, V. Y.: Reaction of hemapoietic system to transplantation of homologous bone tissue, PRS, *55:*643, 1975. Acta chir. plast., *16:*141, 1974

BRYAN, R. S. *et al*: Metastatic lesions of the hand and forearm, PRS, *56:*235, 1975. Clin. Orthop., *101:*167, 1974

BRYAN, R. S. *et al*: Primary epithelioid sarcoma of the hand and forearm. A review of thirteen cases. J. Bone & Joint Surg. (Am.), *56:*458, 1974

BRYANT, F. L.: Early nonsurgical decompression of facial nerve. J. Louisiana M. Soc., *125:*85, 1973

BRYANT, L. R., TRINKLE, J. K., AND DUBILIER, L.: Reappraisal of tracheal injury from cuffed tracheostomy tubes, PRS, *48:*392, 1971. J.A.M.A., *215:*625, 1971

BRYANT, W. M.: Aesthetic considerations in noncosmetic breast operations. Am. Surgeon, *38:*542, 1972

BRYANT, W. M.: Internal stent for securing large skin grafts on small animals, PRS, *52:*106, 1973. J. Surg. Res., *13:*241, 1972

BRYANT, W. M.: Ketamine anesthesia and intranasal or intraoral operations, PRS, *51:*562, 1973

BRYANT, W. M.: When patients inquire about breast augmentation, PRS, *55:*508, 1975. Human Sexuality, *8:*127, 1974

BRYANT, W. M., AND MAULL, K. I.: Arteriovenous malformations of mandible, graduated surgical management, *55:*690, 1975. Discussion by Bennett, PRS, *56:*84, 1975

BRYCE, D.: Conventional surgical management of carcinoma of the hypopharynx. J. Laryng. & Otol., *85:*1221, 1971

BRYCE, D. P.: Conventional pharyngolaryngectomy in surgical management of hypopharyngeal cancer. Can. J. Otolaryngol., *1:*231, 1972

BRYGMAN, A.: Traumatic scalping of penile and

scrotal skin. Pol. Przegl. Chir., Suppl *44:*1157, 1972 (Polish)

BUCH, V. I.: Clinical and functional assessment of the hand after metacarpophalangeal capsulotomy, PRS, *53:*452, 1974

BUCHAN, A. C.: Deep burns—burn contractures. Hand, *3:*90, 1971

BUCHAN, N. G.: Cleft ear lobe: a method of repair with preservation of the earring canal. Brit. J. Plast. Surg., *28:*296, 1975

BUCHAN, N. G.: Experience with thermoplastic splints in the post-burn hand. Brit. J. Plast. Surg., *28:*8193, 1975

BUCHAN, N. G. *et al*: Successful surgical treatment of lipoid proteinosis. Brit. J. Dermatol., *90:*561, 1974

BUCKFIELD, P.: Major congenital faults in newborn infants—a pilot study in New Zealand, PRS, *54:*118, 1974. New Zealand M. J., *78:*196, 1973

BUCK-GRAMCKO, D.: Management of flexor tendon injuries of the hand. The causes of primary suture failure. Monatsschr. Unfallheilkd., *72:*55, 1969 (German)

BUCK-GRAMCKO, D.: Primary care for injured hands. Handchirurgie, *2:*47, 1970 (German)

BUCK-GRAMCKO, D.: Unusual therapeutic method in extensor tendon rupture with bone involvement. Handchirurgie, *2:*210, 1970 (German)

BUCK-GRAMCKO, D.: Pollicization of the index finger. Method and results in aplasia and hypoplasia of the thumb, PRS, *50:*306, 1972. J. Bone & Joint Surg., *53:*1605, 1971

BUCK-GRAMCKO, D.: Operative treatment of congenital malformations of the hand. Hand, *4:*33, 1972

BUCK-GRAMCKO, D.: Crush and wringer injuries of hand, PRS, *51:*476, 1973. Langenbecks Arch. Chir., *332:*465, 1972

BUCK-GRAMCKO, D.: Treatment of motor disturbances of hand and fingers, PRS, *53:*367, 1974. Bruns' Beitr. Klin. Chir., *220:*522, 1973

BUCK-GRAMCKO, D.: Proceedings: Complications of superficial infections of the hand. Langenbecks Arch. Chir., *334:*505, 1973 (German)

BUCK-GRAMCKO, D.: Surgical treatment of congenital malformations of the hand. Handchirurgie, *7:*53, 1975 (German)

BUCK-GRAMCKO, D. *et al*: Expert opinion of hand injuries. Monatsschr. Unfallheilkd., *73:*474, 1970 (German)

BUCKINGHAM, J. M., AND LYNN, H. B.: Branchial cleft cysts and sinuses in children, PRS, *54:*378, 1974. Mayo Clin. Proc., *49:*172, 1974

BUCKO, C. D., AND STEINMULLER, D.: Reinnervation after orthotopic grafting of peripheral

nerve segments in inbred rats, PRS, *53:*326, 1974

BUCKWALTER, J. A. *et al*: Is childhood thyroid cancer a lethal disease? Ann. Surg., *18:*632, 1975

BUDER, G., AND PAPE, K.: Clinical studies on lip carcinoma. Deutsche Stomatol., *22:*746, 1972 (German)

BUDHRAJA, S. N. *et al*: Cryosurgery. Indian J. Med. Sci., *27:*343, 1973

BUDHRAJA, S. N., PASUPATHY, N. K., AND PERIANAYAGAM, W. J.: Salivary gland tumors in Pondicherry, PRS, *55:*634, 1975. Indian J. Surg., *36:*235, 1974

BUEHRIE, R. *et al*: Mixed salivary gland tumor of palate in child. Arch. Otolaryng., *96:*163, 1972

BUENO, R. A. *et al*: Surgical treatment of axillary hyperhidrosis. J. Tenn. Med. Assoc., *68:*544, 1975

BUFALINI, C. *et al*: Reconstructive tegumentary surgery of lower limb. Arch. Putti. Chir. Organi. Mev., *26:*126, 1971 (Italian)

BUGAJ, J.: Case of Peutz-Jeghers syndrome. Pol. Przegl. Chir., *46:*1153, 1974 (Polish)

BUGLAEV, A. I.: Disability and work capacity in the sequelae of deep burns of the legs. Ortop. Travmatol. Protez., *32:*69, 1971 (Russian)

BUKER, R. H. *et al*: Causalgia and transthoracic sympathectomy, PRS, *52:*322, 1973. Am. J. Surg., *124:*724, 1972

BULACIO NUÑEZ, A. W.: New theory regarding the lines of skin tension, PRS, *53:*663, 1974

BULAENKO, I. P. *et al*: Hand and finger injuries. Voen. Med. Zh., *3:*37, 1972 (Russian)

BULBULIAN, ARTHUR H.: *Facial Prosthetics.* Charles C Thomas, Springfield, Ill., 1973. PRS, *52:*428, 1973

BULL, J. C., JR.: Soft silicone bag for antral inflation, PRS, *51:*223, 1973

BULL, J. P.: Revised analysis of mortaliy due to burns. Lancet, *2:*1133, 1971

BULL, J. P.: Revised analysis of mortality due to burns, PRS, *50:*420, 1972. Lancet, *2:*7734, 1972

BULL, J. P.: Current trends in research on burns. Proc. Roy. Soc. Med. *65:*27, 1972

BULLENS, R.: Present day assessment of osteosynthesis using a metal wire in the treatment of mandibular fractures. Rev. Stomatol. Chir. Maxillofac., *73:*156, 1972 (French)

BULLENS, R.: Immediate reconstruction of lower lip and chin following total resection for extensive cancer. Acta Stomatol. belg., *71:*63, 1974 (Dutch)

BULLENS, R. *et al*: Considerations in van Myrhaug's operation for habitual dislocation of temporomandibular joint. Acta Stomatol.

belg., *70:*199, 1973 (Dutch)

BULLOUGH, V. L.: Transsexualism in history. Arch. Sex Beh., *4:*561, 1975

BUNCHMAN, H. H., II AND LEWIS, S. R.: Treatment of lymphedema. PRS, *54:*64, 1974

BUNCHMAN, H. H., II *et al:* Prevention and reconstruction in the burned breast. The "double bubble" technique. PRS, *54:*531, 1974

BUNCHMAN, H. H. 2ND *et al:* Prevention and management of contractures in patients with burns of the neck. Am. J. Surg., *130:*700, 1975

BUNCKE, H. J., JR.: Autotransplant of omentum to large scalp defect, with microsurgical vascularization (with McLean). PRS, *49:*268, 1972

BUNCKE, H. J., JR.: Use of the Saran Wrap cuff in microsurgical arterial repairs (with McLean). PRS, *51:*624, 1973

BUNCKE, H. J., JR.: First successful distant transfer of an island flap in man (Editorial). PRS, *52:*178, 1973

BUNCKE, H. J., JR.: Commentary on "Replantation of a completely amputated distal thumb without venous anastomosis," by Serafin, Kutz, and Kleinert. PRS, *52:*581, 1973

BUNCKE, H. J.: Improved patency rates in microvascular surgery when using magnesium sulfate and a silicone rubber vascular cuff (with Nomoto, Chater). PRS, *54:*157, 1974

BUNCKE, H. J.: Simplified technique for free transfer of groin flaps, by use of Doppler probe, (with Karkowski). PRS, *55:*682, 1975. Discussion by Bingham, PRS, *56:*84, 1975

BUNCKE, H. J.: Study of washout solutions for microvascular replantation and transplantation (with Harashina). PRS, *56:*542, 1975

BUNCKE, H. J. *et al:* Thumb replacement: great toe transplantation by microvascular anastomosis, PRS, *55:*109, 1975. Brit. J. Plast. Surg., *26:*194, 1973

BUNDIN, V. N.: Microtrauma of the hand and fingers in vegetable growers and ways of prevention of suppurative complications. Ortop. Travmatol. Protez., *35:*58, 1974 (Russian)

BÜNTE, H., AND HUSEMANN, B.: Acute metabolic disorders after intestinal short circuit operations because of massive obesity, PRS, *53:*365, 1974. Bull. Soc. Internat. Chir., *32:*415, 1973

BUNTE, M.: Surgical treatment of dysgnathia in Mobius' syndrome. Fortschr. Kiefer. Gesichtschir., *18:*256, 1974 (German)

BURATTI, G. *et al:* Surgical treatment of the "boutonniere" deformity. Experience with the I. Matev method. Minerva Ortop., *23:*22, 1972 (Italian)

BURCH, M.: Surgery of lacrimal drainage system. Klin. Monatsbl. Augenheilkd., *163:*717, 1973 (German)

BURCH, M. S. *et al:* Regional odontodysplasia with associated midline mandibular cyst, case report. J. Oral Surg., *31:*44, 1973

BURCHELL, G., AND STACK, G.: Exsanguination of arm and hand. PRS, *54:*236, 1974. Hand, *5:*124, 1973

BUREN, E. A., AND RYAN, R. F.: Standardization of measurements in medicine by conversion to the metric system, PRS, *54:*459, 1974

BURG, G. *et al:* Chemosurgery. Surgical removal of chemically fixed tumor tissue with microscopic control. Hautarzt, *23:*16, 1972 (German)

BURG, G. *et al:* Chemosurgery of basaliomas. Z. Hautkr., *49:*713, 1974 (German)

BURGE, H. A. S.: Significance and management of metastatic lymph nodes in neck, PRS, *56:*464, 1975. Proc. Roy. Soc. Med., *68:*77, 1975

BURGHARD, A. *et al:* Giant fibroadenoma of breast. Fortschr. Geb. Roentgenstr. Nuklearmed., *117:*607, 1972 (German)

BURI, P.: Experiences with Goldsmith's omental transposition. Vasa, *1:*45, 1972 (German)

BURIAN, F.: *Plastic Surgery Atlas.* Macmillan Publishing Co., Inc., Riverside, N. J., 1968.

BURKE, J. F.: Preventive antibiotics in surgery, PRS, *57:*407, 1976. Postgrad. Med., *58:*65, 1975

BURKE, J. F. *et al:* Primary burn excision and immediate grafting: method shortening illness. J. Trauma, *14:*386, 1974

BURKE, J. F. *et al:* Temporary skin transplantation and immunosuppression for extensive burns. New England J. Med., *290:*269, 1974

BURKHALTER, W., CHRISTENSEN, R. C., AND BROWN, P.: Extensor indicis proprius opponensplasty, PRS, *53:*243, 1974. J. Bone & Joint Surg., *55A:*725, 1973

BURKHALTER, W. E.: Open injuries of the lower extremity. Surg. Clin. North Am., *53:*1439, 1973

BURKHALTER, W. E. *et al:* Metacarpophalangeal flexor replacement for intrinsic-muscle paralysis. J. Bone & Joint Surg. (Am.), *55:*1667, 1973

BURKHARDT, B. R.: Alternative to the total-thigh flap for coverage of massive decubitus ulcers, PRS, *49:*433, 1972

BURKHARDT, B. R.: Immediate or early excision and skin grafting of full-thickness burns of the palm. Report of two cases, PRS, *49:*572, 1972

BURKHARDT, E.: Chronic diseases of the synovial sheath (from hand surgery consulting hour). Beitr. Orthop. Traumatol., *19:*377,

1972 (German)

BURKHARDT, K.: Prognosis and therapy of burns in infants, PRS, *53:*608, 1974. Riv. ital. chir. plast., *4:*27, 1973

BURKLE, H.: Case of forced straightening. Quintessenz, *24:*91, 1973 (German)

BURKLE, H.: Case of forced positional change (redressement force). Quintessence Int., *5:*39, 1974

BURLESON, R., AND EISEMAN, B.: Nature of bond between partial-thickness skin and wound granulation, PRS, *51:*353, 1973. Surgery, *72:*315, 1972

BURLESON, R., AND EISEMAN, B.: Effect of skin dressing and topical antibiotics on healing of partial thickness skin wounds in rats, PRS, *52:*461, 1973. Surg. Gynec. & Obst., *136:*958, 1973

BURLIBASA, C. *et al:* Auto-transplantation of motor nerves after surgery of parotid neoplasms with involvement of the facial nerve. Stomatologia (Bucur.), *19:*81, 1972 (Rumanian)

BURLIBASA, C. *et al:* Decalcified bone homotransplant used for repair of an extensive mandibular defect remaining after removal of recurrent ameloblastoma. Rev. Chir. (Stomatol.), *21:*359, 1974 (Rumanian)

BURMAN, M.: Pigmented villonodular synovitis. Localized tumor on dorsum of hand. N.Y. State J. Med., *73:*2174, 1973

BURMEISTER, L. F. *et al:* Prediction of hand strength in elementary school children. Hand, *7:*123, 1975

BURMISTROV, V. M. *et al:* Use of Filatov's pedicled flap in treatment of burns and their sequelae. Vestn. Khir., *111:*75, 1973 (Russian)

BURN, J. I.: Multiple tumors of arm. Proc. Roy. Soc. Med., *65:*750, 1972

Burn Scars (See also *Burns, Contractures; Burns, Skin Grafting*)

Burned patient, techniques for decreasing scar formation and contractures in (Larson *et al*), PRS, *49:*586, 1972. J. Trauma, *11:*807, 1971

Burn scar as immunologically privileged site (Futrell, Myers), PRS, *52:*326, 1973. Surg. Forum, *23:*129, 1972

Burns, deep, of breast, plasty for scar deformation (Mukhin), PRS, *54:*501, 1974. Acta chir. plast., *15:*176, 1973

Burn scar on face, extensive, tension releasing graft for (Matsumoto *et al*), PRS, *53:*607, 1974. J. Jap. Accident Med. Assoc., *21:*329, 1973

Burns, treatment and prevention of scars following (Schmidt-Tintemann). Munch.

Burn Scars—Cont.

Med. Wochenschr., *115:*718, 1973 (German)

Scars, marginal, of skin grafted burns in rats, effect of 1-tri-iodothyronine on (Zamick, Mehregan), PRS, *51:*71, 1973

Burn scars, histopathological and enzymecytological aspects in (Angela *et al*), PRS, *56:*360, 1975. Riv. ital. chir. plast., *5:*231, 1973

Hydroxyproline activity in formation of burn scars (Cavallero, Magliacani, Rinaudo), PRS, *56:*361, 1975. Riv. ital. chir. plast., *5:*241, 1973

Burn scars, action of early surgical treatment in development of (Borsetti, Ambroggio), PRS, *56:*361, 1975. Riv. ital. chir. plast., *5:*251, 1973

Burn scars, surgical treatment of (Ambroggio, Borsetti), PRS, *56:*361, 1975. Riv. ital. chir. plast., *5:*261, 1973

Burn scars and burns, initial treatment of (Zdravic), PRS, *56:*361, 1975. Riv. ital. chir. plast., *5:*305, 1973

Burn scar treatment, morphological and functional results (Petrolati, Gnucci, Dell'Antonio), PRS, *56:*361, 1975. Riv. ital. chir. plast., *5:*345, 1973

Burn scar results, elastic compression in (Bertolini, Barisoni), PRS, *56:*360, 1975. Riv. ital. chir. plast., *5:*361, 1973

Burns, treatment and hypertrophic scars (Raff). Wien Med. Wochenschr., *115:*395, 1973

Breast, burn scars, nipple and areola reconstruction with the "double bubble" technique (Bunchman *et al*), PRS, *54:*531, 1974

Effect of different local treatment upon cicatrization in burns of children (Dietrich *et al*). In *Plastische und Wiederherstellungs-Chirurgie*, ed. Hohler; Stuttgart; Schattauer, 1975. pp. 267–77 (German)

Scar hypertrophy in burned hands (Huang, Larson, Lewis), PRS, *56:*21, 1975. Discussion by Bennett, PRS, *56:*442, 1975

Correction of the postburn deformity of the left breast (Mirov). Vestn. Khir., *114:*85, 1975 (Russian)

Burn scars, hypertrophic, reappraisal of shaving and skin grafting for (Moustafa, Abdel-Fattah), PRS, *57:*463, 1976

Burn Shock (See also *Burns*)

Urgency of fluid administration in resuscitation of burn shock (Leape). J. Surg. Res., *11:*513, 1971

Clinical use of a 10 percent solution of placental albumin (Mel'nik *et al*). Probl. Gematol. Pereliv. Krovi., *16:*7, 1971 (Russian)

Burn Shock — Cont.

Shortcomings in the treatment of burns in the shock period (Konigova *et al*). Rozhl. Chir., *50:*600, 1971 (Czechoslovakian)

Resuscitation, hypertonic lactate saline, in thermal injury (Moylan, Reckler, Mason), PRS, *49:*665, 1972. Surg. Forum, *22:*49, 1971

Coagulation defects in burned patients (Gehrke *et al*), PRS, *49:*359, 1972. Surg. Gynec. & Obst., *133:*613, 1971

Bacteriologic nature and prevention of contamination to intravenous catheters (Crenshaw *et al*), PRS, *50:*424, 1972. Am. J. Surg., *123:*264, 1972

Thermal injury involving bone: report of 32 cases (Asch *et al*). J. Trauma, *12:*135, 1972

Thrombocytes, blood levels in burned patients (Hergt), PRS, *52:*326, 1973. J. Trauma, *12:*599, 1972

Transfusion of whole blood in burn shock (Murazian). Khirurgiia (Mosk.), *48:*23, 1972 (Russian)

Burns, use of new vasoconstrictor in management of (Clarke *et al*). M. J. Australia, *2:*361, 1972

Burn shock treated with hypertonic sodium solutions (Monafo, Chuntrasakul, Ayvozian), PRS, *54:*241, 1974. Am. J. Surg., *126:*778, 1973

Modern concepts of surgical shock (Stortenbeek). Arch. chir. neerl., *25:*215, 1973

Shock, burn, pathophysiology, sequential hemodynamic alterations (Shoemaker *et al*), PRS, *53:*493, 1974. J. Surg. Res., *14:*64, 1973

Coagulation, disseminated intravascular, in burned patients (McManus, Eurenius, Pruitt), PRS, *53:*492, 1974. J. Trauma, *13:*416, 1973

Thrombocyte behavior during scalding shock in rabbit (Loew, Langer, Bochum), PRS, *53:*607, 1974. Langenbecks Arch. Chir., *333:*71, 1973

Burn shock, efficacy of hypertonic lactated saline solution (Monafo), PRS, *54:*240, 1974. Rev. Latino Am. cir. plast., *17:*65, 1973

Burn shock treatment by colloid infusion and electrolyte infusion (Hall, Sorensen), PRS, *53:*491, 1974. Scand. J. Plast. Reconstr. Surg., *7:*67, 1973

Electrical burn of scalp and skull (Luce, Hoopes). PRS, *54:*359, 1974

Denudation of frontal and parietal · bones after burn (Munchhoff). In *Plastische und Wiederherstellungs Chirurgie*, ed. by Hohler; pp. 317–20. Schattauer, Stuttgart, 1975 (German)

Burn Shock — Cont.

Burn shock, hypertonic balanced sodium solution in (Fox), PRS, *57:*401, 1976. Internat. Surg., *60:*348, 1975

Resuscitation, shock, choice of intravenous fluid in (Rowe, Arango), PRS, *57:*122, 1976. Pediat. Clin. N. Am., *22:*269, 1975

Cardiac assistance devices in gravely burned patient, plea for improved monitoring and use of (Fox) (Editorial), PRS, *56:*328, 1975

BURNAM, J. A.: Nasolabial flap in reconstruction of the nose. J. Fla. Med. Assoc., *59:*32, 1972

BURNS, H. *et al:* Surgery in rheumatoid arthritis of hand. N.Y. State J. Med., *71:*340, 1971

BURNS, K. H., AND HARRISON, H. N.: Effect of cleansing agents used on burn wound (Betadine, Joy), hydrotherapy, and presence of residual cream on absorption of Sulfamylon into burn wound, PRS, *52:*326, 1973. J. Trauma, *12:*903, 1972

BURNS, P. E.: Letter: Breast prosthesis. Lancet, *2:*1259, 1975

Burns (See also *Hands, Burns*)

Burned adults, severely, incidence of long-term psychiatric complications in (Andreasen *et al*), PRS, *49:*666, 1972. Ann. Surg., *174:*785, 1971

Catheter embolism, paradoxical (Nash, Moylan), PRS, *48:*198, 1971. Arch. Surg., *102:*213, 1971

Universal challenge (Dressler). Arch. Surg., *103:*434, 1971

Weight loss and energy balance in burned patients (Gump, Kinney), PRS, *49:*666, 1972. Arch. Surg., *103:*442, 1971

Burns, current problems in: perspective (Haynes), PRS, *49:*665, 1972. Arch. Surg., *103:*454, 1971

Emergency aid and transport of seriously burnt patients (Lareng *et al*). Cah. Anesthesiol., *19:*1049, 1971 (French)

Children with thermal burns, survey of 109 cases of anemia following (Birdsell, Birch), PRS, *49:*236, 1972. Canad. J. Surg., *14:*345, 1971

Pediatric disaster — bathtub burn (Thomson, Shore), PRS, *49:*472, 1972. Canad. J. Surg., *14:*399, 1971

On the depth of burns and healing time in grade II thermal burns (Goris). Chirurgia (Bucur.), *20:*735, 1971 (Rumanian)

Zinc, effect in healing of burns (Brodribb, Ricketts), PRS, *49:*359, 1972. Injury, *3:*25, 1971

Burn problems illustrated by a case (Stadaas *et al*). J. Oslo City Hosp., *21:*97, 1971

Burns–Cont.

Circulatory changes following circumferential extremity burns evaluated by the ultrasonic flowmeter: an analysis of 60 thermally injured limbs (Moylan *et al*). J. Trauma, *11:*763, 1971

Burned children, bereaved, editorial on talking to (Morse), PRS, *49:*586, 1972. J. Trauma, *11:*894, 1971

Thrombolysis, positive effects on superficial extent of standardized burns in animals (Hettich, Otten, Henne), PRS, *50:*204, 1972. Langenbecks Arch. Chir., *329:*899, 1971

Plastic surgery in a developing country (Nylen). Nord. Med., *86:*1220, 1971 (Swedish)

Burn, severe, respiratory insufficiency in patients with (Tahara *et al*), PRS, *49:*237, 1972. Operation, *25:*765, 1971

Disability and work capacity in the sequelae of deep burns of the legs (Buglaev). Ortop. Travmatol. Protez., *32:*69, 1971 (Russian)

Burn depth, evaluation by use of radioactive isotopes (Bennett) (Follow-Up Clinic), PRS, *48:*73, 1971

How children live after disfiguring burns (Quinby *et al*). Psychiatry Med., *2:*146, 1971

Nutrition, the red cell and burns (Wilmore). Rev. Surg., *28:*451, 1971

Urinary alpha glucosidase as measure of kidney damage in burns (Bonini *et al*), PRS, *51:*107, 1973. Riv. ital. chir. plast., *2:*219, 1971

Effects of threshold burns on distant microcirculation (Jelenko *et al*). Surg. Forum, *22:*53, 1971

Urinary output, simple method for continuous evaluation in severely burned children (Goris), PRS, *49:*107, 1972. Surg. Gynec. & Obst., *132:*695, 1971

Problems with burns illustrated by a case (Stadaas *et al*). Tidsskr. Nor. Laegeforen, *91:*2007, 1971 (Norwegian)

Research in Burns. Ed. by P. Matter, T. L. Barclay, and Z. Konickova. Hans Huber Publishers, Bern, Stuttgart, Vienna, 1971. PRS, *50:*79, 1972

Burned persons, occurrence and development of psychopathologic phenomena and relation to severity of burns, age, and premorbid personality (Pavlovsky), PRS, *52:*327, 1973. Acta chir. plast., *4:*112, 1972

Temperature measurements, subcutaneous, in non-contact burn (Prouza, Moserova, Janecek), PRS, *52:*684, 1973. Acta chir. plast., *14:*168, 1972

Hormone levels, growth in burned subjects

Burns–Cont.

(Dolecek *et al*), PRS, *52:*684, 1973. Acta chir. plast., *14:*179, 1972

Predisposing causes of burns (Escott), PRS, *52:*684, 1973. Acta chir. plast., *14:*236, 1972

Complete oxyhemoglobin dissociation curves in thermal trauma (Arturson). Adv. Exp. Med. Biol., *33:*441, 1972

Burned children, superior mesenteric artery syndrome in (Ogbuokiri, Low, MacMillan), PRS, *51:*234, 1973. Am. J. Surg., *124:*75, 1972

Tracheostomy in thermally injured patients: a review of five years' experience (Moylan *et al*). Am. Surg., *38:*119, 1972

Will it happen again? (Swartz). Arch. Surg., *104:*19, 1972

Adrenal cortical function in severe burns (Wise, Margraf, Ballinger), PRS, *51:*606, 1973. Arch. Surg., *105:*213, 1972

Burned patient, severely, fibrin split products in (Meyers), PRS, *51:*606, 1973. Arch. Surg., *105:*404, 1972

Burned patient, direct measurement of total metabolism of (Bradham), PRS, *51:*234, 1973. Arch. Surg., *105:*410, 1972

Tissue oxygen tension changes in acute burn edema, topography of (Remensnyder), PRS, *51:*606, 1973. Arch. Surg., *105:*477, 1972

Colorimetric estimation of blood loss during surgery of burns (Mahler *et al*). Brit. J. Plast. Surg., *25:*130, 1972

Blood gases altered in acute burns (Robinson *et al*), PRS, *52:*209, 1973. Brit. J. Plast. Surg., *25:*250, 1972

Intensive care of patients with burns–investment, costs and clinical aspects (Ganzoni). Helvet. chir. acta, *39:*607, 1972 (German)

Long-term adjustment and adaptation mechanisms in severely burned adults (Andreasen *et al*). J. Nerv. Ment. Dis., *154:*352, 1972

Postburn effects of antitoxicants of long-term utility of ethyl linoleate as water-holding lipid for topical use (Jelenko, Wheeler), PRS, *51:*350, 1973. J. Surg. Res., *12:*161, 1972

Burned patients, blood levels of thrombocytes in (Hergt), PRS, *52:*326, 1973. J. Trauma, *12:*599, 1972

Restrictive effects of thoracic burns in children (Quinby). J. Trauma, *12:*646, 1972

Hyperplasia, thymic, in children recovering from thermal burns (Gelfand *et al*), PRS, *52:*327, 1973. J. Trauma, *12:*813, 1972

Burns, stress ulcer: preventable disease

Burns–Cont.

(Chernov *et al*), PRS, *52:*326, 1973. J. Trauma, *12:*831, 1972

Ethyl linoleate: waterholding lipid of skin. A. The evidence (Jelenko, Wheeler, Scott), PRS, *52:*210, 1973. B. Effects on *in vivo* burn eschar, PRS, *52:*211, 1973. J. Trauma, *12:*968, 974, 1972

Heterotopic calcification following burns (Munster *et al*), PRS, *52:*210, 1973. J. Trauma, *12:*968, 1972

Classification of burns of the lower limbs (Volkov *et al*). Khirurgiia (Mosk.), *48:*28, 1972 (Russian)

Medical disability evaluation of patients with thermal burns (Pechatnikova *et al*). Khirurgiia (Mosk.), *48:*46, 1972 (Russian)

Burned adults, seriously, management of emotional reactions in (Andreasen *et al*), PRS, *51:*107, 1973. New England J. Med., *286:*65, 1972

Accidental burns and poisoning of children in the home (Holdaway). N. Z. Med. J., *75:*280, 1972

Maintenance of function of the burn patient (Jaeger). Phys. Ther., *52:*627, 1972

Current trends in research on burns (Bull). Proc. Roy. Soc. Med., *65:*27, 1972

Pulmonary microembolization in severe thermal injury (Rapaport *et al*). Proc. Soc. Exp. Biol. Med., *139:*1013, 1972

Burning and the healing of children (Galdston). Psychiatry, *35:*57, 1972

Burn patient, record card for (Ortiz-Monasterio, Araico, Trigos), PRS, *52:*325, 1973. Rev. Latino Am. cir. plast., *16:*25, 1972

Emergency care of the burned patient (Boswick *et al*). Surg. Clin. North Am., *52:*115, 1972

Thermal injury, essential fatty acid deficiency in red cell membrane following; correction with parenteral fat emulsion (Wilmore, Helmkamp, Pruitt), PRS, *51:*705, 1973. Surg. Forum, *23:*499, 1972

Erythrocyte changes in severe thermal injury (Bachvaroff, Browne, Rapaport), PRS, *51:*706, 1973. Surg. Forum, *23:*502, 1972

Plasma renin-like activity (RLA) and angiotensin II levels after major burns (Dolecek *et al*), PRS, *54:*506, 1974. Acta chir. plast., *15:*166, 1973

Feet, burned, in children (Heimburger *et al*), PRS, *52:*684, 1973. Am. J. Surg., *125:*575, 1973

Burned children, gastrointestinal series in evaluation of (Law *et al*), PRS, *53:*491, 1974. Am. J. Surg., *126:*366, 1973

Burns, thermal. Retrospective study on 240

Burns – Cont.

patients. I. Distribution of material and admission factors (Sundell). Ann. Chir. Gynaecol. Fenn., *62:*339, 1973

Burns, thermal. Retrospective study on 192 fresh burns. II. Care of burn wound and mortality (Sundell), Ann. Chir. Gynaecol. Fenn., *62:*344, 1973

Burns, mechanisms of erythrocyte destruction after (Loebl, Baxter, Curreri), PRS, *54:*112, 1974. Ann. Surg., *178:*681, 1973

Microcirculation, distant, threshold burning effects on (Jelenko *et al*), PRS, *52:*456, 1973; *55:*113, 1975. Arch. Surg., *106:*317, 1973. Am. Surgeon, *40:*388, 1974

Fire victims, human, carbon monoxide toxicity in (Zarem, Rattenborg, Harmel), PRS, *54:*112, 1974. Arch. Surg., *107:*1, 1973

Burns, extensive, prevention of early histopathological changes in liver in (Talaat *et al*), PRS, *55:*112, 1975. Brit. J. Plast. Surg., *26:*132, 1973

Lyell's syndrome treated in specialized burn unit (Tubiana *et al*), PRS, *52:*456, 1973. Chirurgie, *99:*40, 1973

Vitamin E and its relation to heart disease (Olson), PRS, *54:*119, 1974. Circulation, *48:*179, 1973

Medical education, epidemiology and surgery (Sorensen). Int. J. Epidemiol., *2:*387, 1973

Burn pathophysiology in man, sequential hemodynamic alterations (Shoemaker *et al*), PRS, *53:*493, 1974. J. Surg. Res., *14:*64, 1973

Oxygen transport and acid base alterations in burns (Vladeck *et al*), PRS, *53:*609, 1974. J. Surg. Res., *14:*74, 1973

Artery, superior mesenteric, syndrome as consequence of burn injury (Reckler *et al*), PRS, *53:*493, 1974. J. Trauma, *12:*979, 1973

Burned patient, gastric secretion in (Harrison, Gaisford, Wechsler), PRS, *52:*211, 1973. J. Trauma, *12:*1041, 1973

Burned patients, disseminated intravascular coagulation in (McManus, Eurenius, Pruitt), PRS, *53:*492, 1974. J. Trauma, *13:*416, 1973

Cardiac output following circumferential burn (Turbow), PRS, *53:*608, 1974. J. Trauma, *13:*535, 1973

Pulmonary burns, new approach (Noe, Constable), PRS, *53:*686, 1974. J. Trauma, *13:*1015, 1973

Burn patients treated with multiple blood transfusions, matching of compatible blood in (Minev *et al*). Khirurgiia (Sofiia), *26:*113, 1973 (Bulgarian)

Burns, changes of hexosamines and sialic

Burns—Cont.

acids in blood serum in (Zaidenberg et al). Klin. Med. Mosk., 51:86, 1973 (Russian)

Burns (Moncrief). New England J. Med., 288:444, 1973

Pregnancy, severe burns in (Stage), PRS, 54:240, 1974. Obst. & Gynec., 42:259, 1973

Burns in children (Belik et al). Ortop. Travmatol. Protez., 34:8, 1973 (Russian)

Burned child, severely, with bilateral diffuse pneumonia treatment of (Boiarinov et al). Ortop. Travmatol. Protez., 34:58, 1973 (Russian)

Burns, work of specialized children's care centers for, and their needs (Vozdvizhenskii et al). Ortop. Travmatol. Protez., 34:69, 1973

Burns program, Shriners, role of the orthopedic hospital in (Sullivan), PRS, 51:293, 1973

Maintenance of oxygen transport in severe thermal trauma (Arturson), PRS, 53:493, 1974. Riv. ital. chir. plast., 4:32, 1973

Burns of head and neck (Boswick). Surg. Clin. North Am., 53:97, 1973

Hydroxyproline of urine after thermal injury in burns (Spanos et al), PRS, 56:469, 1975. Tr. 8th Panhellenic Cong. Surg. Soc., A: 314, 1973

Burns, deep circular, of inferior extremities (Ivanova), PRS, 52:598, 1973. Zentralbl. Chir., 98:331, 1973

Burns, fatal, in old people (Hajek, Vrabec, Topinka), PRS, 55:639, 1975. Acta chir. plast., 16:164, 1974

Syndrome, arteriomesenterial duodenal compression in children with burns (Bobek), PRS, 56:469, 1975. Acta chir. plast., 16:238, 1974

Burned children, psychiatric classification system for (Seligman). Am. J. Psychiatry, 131: 41, 1974

Burn injury, massive, tracheostomy complicating. Plea for conservatism (Eckhauser et al). Am. J. Surg., 127:418, 1974

Electrosurgery, burns from miniature ECG electrodes (Finlay et al), PRS, 55:639, 1975. Anesthesiology, 41:263, 1974

Burns in tropical countries (Sinha). Clin. Plast. Surg., 1:121, 1974

Burns in children (MacMillan). Clin. Plast. Surg., 1:633, 1974

Outpatient burns (Haynes). Clin. Plast. Surg., 1:645, 1974

Accidents, common childhood (Knowles). PRS, 54:383, 1974. Hospital Med., 10:48, 1974

K. U. M. C. Burn Center. First six months

Burns—Cont.

(Robinson). J. Kans. Med. Soc., 75:233, 1974

Burns, liver changes in, role of A.T.P. and Trasylol in prevention (Beheri, Talaat, Zaky), PRS, 56:682, 1975. J. Kuwait M. A., 8:77, 1974

Erythrocyte survival following thermal injury (Loebl et al), PRS, 55:252, 1975. J. Surg. Res., 16:96, 1974

Burn research, current status (Baxter). J. Trauma, 14:1, 1974

Venous occlusion, importance in dermal ischemia after thermal injury (Massiha, Monafo), PRS, 57:538, 1976. J. Trauma, 14:705, 1974

Burns in light of A. V. Vishnevskii's school of thought (Sologub et al). Khirurgiia (Mosk.), 9:21, 1974 (Russian)

Skin viability, enzyme analysis as test (Georgiade, King, O'Fallon), PRS, 53:67, 1974

Burn experience, initial, in recent Middle East conflict (Levin, Bornstein), PRS, 54:432, 1974

Pediatric burn unit, chickenpox epidemic in (Weintraub et al). Surgery, 76:490, 1974

Hormone, human growth, and high caloric feedings, anabolic effects following thermal injury (Wilmore et al), PRS, 55:112, 1975. Surg. Gynec. & Obst., 138:875, 1974

Active sodium transport inhibition in erythrocytes from burned patients (Curreri et al), PRS, 56:469, 1975. Surg. Gynec. & Obst., 139:538, 1974

Treatment of burn trauma under the conditions of a garrison hospital (Shvarts). Voen. Med. Zh., 1:40, 1974 (Russian)

Basic Problems in Burns: Proceedings. Symposium, Prague, September, 1973. Ed. by R. Vrabec et al. Springer-Verlag, New York, 1975

Reactions to Injury and Burns and their Clinical Importance. By S. Sevitt. J. B. Lippincott Co., Philadelphia, 1975. PRS, 56:444, 1975

Burns, systemic effects on bone mineral metabolism (Kolar et al), PRS, 50:541, 1972. Acta chir. plast., 13:133, 1971. II. Influence of general anesthesia, PRS, 57:763, 1976. Acta chir. plast., 17:56, 1975

Catheters, indwelling (Degroot, Kunin), PRS, 56:596, 1975. Am. J. Nursing, 75:448, 1975

What is clinical smoke poisoning (Zikria et al), PRS, 56:598, 1975. Ann. Surg., 181:151, 1975

Serum levels of fibrin split products after thermal injury (Curreri, Wilterdink, Bax-

Burns—Cont.

ter), PRS, *56:*233, 1975. Ann. Surg., *181:*157, 1975

Heparin and protamine sulfate, effect on coagulation dynamics following thermal injury (Curreri, Wilterdink, Baxter), PRS, *56:*232, 1975. Ann. Surg., *181:*161, 1975

Leukocyte chemotaxis suppressed *in vitro* by chemotherapeutic agents in thermal injuries (Warden *et al*), PRS, *57:*263, 1976. Ann. Surg., *181:*363, 1975

Tower of London bomb explosion (Tucker *et al*). Brit. Med. J., *3:*287, 1975

What's new in burns? (Artz). J. Med. Soc. N. J., *72:*1006, 1975

Burn, minor, tetanus following (Larkin *et al*). J. Trauma *15:*546, 1975

Breast, burned female (Rubin). N. Y. State J. Med., *75:*865, 1975

Psychological reactions to facial and hand burns in young men. Can I see myself through your eyes? (Solnit *et al*). Psychoanal. Study Child., *30:*549, 1975

Diadermic micro-thermometry (Dioguardi, Musajo Somma), PRS, *57:*762, 1976 (Italian). Riv. ital. chir. plast., *7:*505, 1975

The past and present of the Soviet military-field surgery (Vishnevskii *et al*). Sov. Med., *5:*3, 1975 (Russian)

Burns, inhalation injury in, fiberoptic bronchoscopy after (Moylan, Adib, Birnbaum), PRS, *56:*598, 1975. Surg. Gynec. & Obst., *140:*541, 1975

Health and disease in rural Ethiopia (Finseth *et al*). Yale J. Biol. Med., *48:*105, 1975

Burns of the Upper Extremity. By Roger E. Salisbury. W. B. Saunders Co., Philadelphia, 1976

Burns, Anesthesia for

Anesthesia and treatment for burns in children (Bilich *et al*). Khirurgiia (Mosk.), *47:*32, 1971

Burns, problems of anesthesia in patients with (Harrfeldt), PRS, *50:*203, 1972. Langenbecks Arch. Chir., *329:*907, 1971

Anesthesiologic aspects of general burn therapy in adults (Benad). Zentralbl. Chir., *97:*161, 1971 (German)

Analgesia for burns dressing using methoxyflurane (Marshall *et al*). Brit. J. Anaesth, *44:*80, 1972

Methoxyflurane analgesia for burns dressings and other painful ward procedures in children (Firn). Brit. J. Anaesth., *44:*517, 1972

Repeated methoxyflurane analgesia for

Burns, Anesthesia for—Cont.

burns dressings (Calverley). Brit. J. Anaesth., *44:*628, 1972

Anesthesiologic risk in extensively burned patient (Castello *et al*). Minerva Anestesiol., *38:*553, 1972 (Italian)

General therapy and anesthesia of patients with burns (Harrfeldt). Monatsschr. Unfallheilkd., *75:*103, 1972 (German)

History of analgesia in burns (Murray). Postgrad. Med. J., *48:*124, 1972

Methoxyflurane analgesia for burns dressings (Packer). Postgrad. Med. J., *48:*128, 1972

Effect of methoxyflurane analgesia on renal function in burned patients: an investigation (Laird *et al*). Postgrad. Med. J., *48:*133, 1972

Analgesia for the dressing of burns in children: a method using neuroleptanalgesia and Entonox (Baskett). Postgrad. Med. J., *48:*138, 1972

Problems of anaesthesia in the burnt child (Bush). Postgrad. Med. J., *48:*148, 1972

General anaesthesia in the adult burned patient (Howie). Postgrad. Med. J., *48:*152, 1972

Ketamine anaesthesia for burns surgery (Sage *et al*). Postgrad. Med. J., *48:*156, 1972

Use of ketamine chloride in anesthesia of the burn patient (Martinez Trens *et al*). Rev. Esp. Anestesiol. Reanim., *19:*144, 1972 (Spanish)

Ketalar in burns (Pocta *et al*). Rozhl. Chir., *51:*7, 1972 (Czechoslovakian)

Burn patients, single-drug anesthesia using ketamine in, clinical studies on (Klose *et al*). Anaesthesist, *22:*121, 1973 (German)

Burns, ketamine in subjects with, use of (Marynen). Anesth. Analg. (Paris), *30:*1043, 1973

Burned children, anesthesia in under-5-year-olds (Ensel *et al*). Anesth. Analg. (Paris), *30:*1093, 1973 (French)

Burns, anesthesiological prospects in treatment of (Bertolini *et al*). Minerva Anestesiol., *39:*183, 1973 (Italian)

Halothane anesthesia in burn patient: nine consecutive anesthetics in one having 30 percent second- and third-degree burns (Seebert). South. Med. J., *66:*1057, 1973

Circulatory arrest following administration of succinylcholine in patients with extensive tissue damage (Albrechtsen). Tidsskr. Nor. Laegeforen, *93:*676, 1973 (Norwegian)

Topical refrigeration analgesia for skin transplantation in patients with burns

Burns, Anesthesia for—Cont.

(Magierski). Anaesth. Resusc. Intensive Ther., 2:77, 1974

General anesthesia in the active surgical management of the severely burned (Atiasov et al). Ortop. Travmatol. Protez., 0:40, 1974 (Russian)

Technics of anesthesia and resuscitation in severely burned patients (Giralt Prat et al). Rev. Esp. Anestesiol. Reanim., 21:539, 1974 (Spanish)

Repeated general anesthesia (Chernokozhev). Vestn. Khir., 113:83, 1974 (Russian)

Anesthesia in burns (Zhillis et al). Khirurgiia (Mosk.), 4:33, 1975 (Russian)

Hypnosis in anesthesia (Zaffiri). Minerva Med., 66:3894, 1975 (Italian)

Burns, Cancer in

Marjolin's ulcer (Editorial). Ill. Med. J., 140:500, 1971

Burn scar carcinoma, avoidable sequelae of burns? (Reichmann). Z. Aerztl. Fortbild. (Jena.), 65:1197, 1971 (German)

Spindle cell epithelioma on an old keloid of the upper extremity after a burn. Functional restoration (Bergoend et al). Ann. chir. plast., 17:142, 1972 (French)

Carcinoma arising in a post-burn scar (Rintala et al). Duodecim, 88:639, 1972 (Finnish)

Basal cell epithelioma on a burn cicatrix (Barachini). G. Ital. Dermatol., 47:26, 1972 (Italian)

Fibrosarcoma in the burn scar (Niimura), PRS, 52:457, 1973. Saigai Igaku, Disaster Med., 15:366, 1972

Carcinoma, scar tissue—experience in 24 cases (Namba, Yanase, Horiuchi), PRS, 54:115, 1974. Jap. J. Plast. Reconstr. Surg., 16:549, 1973

Burn scar carcinoma and hypercalcemia (Gerner, Moore), PRS, 55:113, 1975. Erratum, PRS, 56:241, 1975. Ann. Surg., 7:95, 1974

Marjolin's ulcer (Badim, Lessa, Carreirao), PRS, 57:125, 1976. Rev. Col. bras. Cir., 1:261, 1974

Marjolin's ulcer: immunologically privileged tumor? (Bostwick, Pendergrast, Vasconez), PRS, 57:66, 1976

Burns, Chemical

Burns, phosphorus, experimental observations on (Bowen, Whelan, Nelson), PRS, 49:667, 1972. Ann. Surg., 174:779, 1971

Some characteristics of chemical burns in

Burns, Chemical—Cont.

metallurgists (Demchenko). Klin. Khir., 10:69, 1971 (Russian)

Results of conservative and surgical treatment of chemical and thermal eye burns based on clinical research between 1957 and 1966 (Szymankiewicz). Klin. Oczna., 41:559, 1971 (Polish)

Decompression incision in finger burns—chemical burn of the finger (Oara et al). Orthop. Surg. (Tokyo), 22:881, 1971 (Japanese)

Hydrofluoric acid burns (Iverson, Laub, Madison), PRS, 48:107, 1971

Early surgical treatment of deep chemical burns (Orlov et al). Voen. Med. Zh., 8:33, 1971 (Russian)

Incidence, therapy and prognosis of chemical eye burns (Pietruschka et al). Z. Aerztl. Fortbild. (Jena.), 65:835, 1971 (German)

Phosphorus burns: the antidote: a new approach (Ben-Hur et al). Brit. J. Plast. Surg., 25:245, 1972

Case of carbolic acid gangrene of the thumb (Abraham). Brit. J. Plast. Surg., 25:282, 1972

Use of inorganic reducing agents to neutralize the toxic effect of "chronic alkalis" in thermochemical burns (Pamurzin et al). Farmakol. Toksikol., 35:498, 1972 (Russian)

Hydrotherapy for chemical burns (Bromberg). Follow-Up Clinic, PRS, 49:453, 1972

Mafenide acetate in treatment of caustic chemical burns (Jepsen). Vet. Med. Small Anim. Clin., 67:52, 1972

Chemical burns (Folesky). Z. Aerztl. Fortbild. (Jena), 66:365, 1972 (German)

Surgical therapy of esophageal erosions and their consequences (Zuhlke et al). Bruns Beitr. Klin. Chir., 220:792, 1973 (German)

Necrosis of scalp caused by perhydrol burns (Bardach et al). Pol. Przegl. Chir., 46:559, 1974 (Polish)

Reconstruction of a subcutaneous artificial esophagus into a retrosternal one (Masiukova et al). Vestn. Khir., 112:113, 1974 (Russian)

Surgical management of severe lye burns of the esophagus by colon interposition (Berkowitz et al). Ann. Otol. Rhin. & Laryng., 84:576, 1975

Oroileoanastomosis in total oesophagoplasty (Brix et al). Bratisl. Lek. Listy., 63:395, 1975 (Slovakian)

Surgical mesh technic for covering large skin defects (Konz). Hautarzt, 26:277, 1975 (German)

Hydrotherapy, effect on clinical course and

Burns, Chemical—Cont.

pH of experimental cutaneous chemical burns (Gruber, Laub, Vistnes), PRS, *55:*200, 1975

Surgical injuries and methemoglobinemia due to explosion of an oxidizing mixture (Jonecko *et al*). Wiad. Lek., *29:*158, 1976 (Polish)

Burns, Complications of (See also *Burns, Infections; Curling's Ulcer*)

Acalculous cholecystitis in burned patients (Munster, Goodwin, Pruitt), PRS, *50:*541, 1972. Am. J. Surg., *122:*591, 1971

Energy balance and weight loss in burned patients (Gump, Kinney), PRS, *49:*666, 1972. Arch. Surg., *103:*442, 1971

Anemia following thermal burns: survey of 109 children (Birdsell, Burch), PRS, *49:*236, 1972. Canad. J. Surg., *14:*345, 1971

Respiratory insufficiency in patients with severe burn (Tahara *et al*), PRS, *49:*237, 1972. Operation, *25:*765, 1971

Kidney damage in burns, urinary alpha glucosidase as measure of (Bonini *et al*), PRS, *51:*107, 1973. Riv. ital. chir. plast., *2:*219, 1971

Burned patients, coagulation defects in (Gehrke *et al*), PRS, *9:*359, 1972. Surg. Gynec. & Obst., *133:*613, 1971

Periurethral abscess in patients with major burns (Stone *et al*). Am. Surg., *38:*318, 1972

Renal failure, gentamicin therapy in (Chan, Benner, Hoeprick), PRS, *50:*634, 1972. Ann. Int. Med., *76:*773, 1972

Burn edema formation in primates, kinetics of (Leape), PRS, *51:*706, 1973. Ann. Surg., *176:*223, 1972

Burns, severe, adrenal cortical function in (Wise, Margraf, Ballinger), PRS, *51:*606, 1973. Arch. Surg., *105:*213, 1972

Fibrin split products in severely burned patient (Meyers), PRS, *51:*606, 1973. Arch. Surg., *105:*404, 1972

Pulmonary ventilation altered in acute burns (Robinson *et al*), PRS, *52:*209, 1973. Brit. J. Plast. Surg., *25:*250, 1972

Fatal tetanus complicating a small partial-thickness burn (Marshall *et al*). J. Trauma, *12:*91, 1972

Joint limitation in burns: analysis of results of physical therapy in 681 patients (Dobbs, Curreri), PRS, *52:*101, 1973. J. Trauma, *12:*242, 1972

Burned children, thymic hyperplasia in (Gelfand *et al*), PRS, *52:*327, 1973. J. Trauma, *12:*813, 1972

Calcification, heterotopic, following burns

Burns, Complications of—Cont.

(Munster *et al*), PRS, *52:*210, 1973. J. Trauma, *12:*968, 1972

Hypercalcemia associated with hypertension due to prolonged immobilization. An unusual complication of extensive burns (Berliner *et al*). Pediatrics, *49:*92, 1972

Thermal injury, severe, erythrocyte changes in (Bachvaroff, Browne, Rapaport), PRS, *51:*706, 1973. Surg. Forum, *23:*502, 1972

Liver impairment in burns, clinical manifestations of (Chlumsky *et al*), PRS, *54:*624, 1974. Acta chir. plast., *15:*238, 1973

Anemia of thermal injury, role of erythropoietin in (Robinson *et al*), PRS, *53:*608, 1974. Ann. Surg., *178:*565, 1973

Erythrocyte destruction after burns (Loebl, Baxter, Curreri), PRS, *54:*112, 1974. Ann. Surg., *178:*681, 1973

Pulmonary artery pressure monitoring in acute burn management (German, Allyn, Bartlett), PRS, *53:*370, 1974. Arch. Surg., *106:*788, 1973

Carbon monoxide toxicity in human fire victims (Zarem, Rattenborg, Harmel), PRS, *54:*112, 1974. Arch. Surg., *107:*1, 1973

Liver, prevention of early histopathological changes in extensive burns (Talaat *et al*), PRS, *55:*112, 1975. Brit. J. Plast. Surg., *26:*132, 1973

Burned patients, fatally, sequential oxygen transport and acid base alterations (Vladeck *et al*), PRS, *53:*609, 1974. J. Surg. Res., *14:*74, 1973

Burn injury, superior mesenteric artery syndrome as consequence of (Reckler *et al*), PRS, *53:*493, 1974. J. Trauma, *12:*979, 1973

Burn, circumferential, abdominal compression following, cardiovascular responses (Turbow), PRS, *53:*608, 1974. J. Trauma, *13:*535, 1973

Burns in patient with glucose-6-phosphate dehydrogenase deficiency, fatal hemolysis from mafenide treatment of (Marsicano, Hutton, Bryant), PRS, *52:*197, 1973

Burns, chondritis of ear in (Stadaas). Tidsskr. Nor. Laegeforen, *93:*678, 1973 (Norwegian)

Burns, hydroxyproline of urine after (Spanos *et al*), PRS, *56:*469, 1975. Tr. 8th Panhellenic Cong. Surg. Soc., *A:* 314, 1973

Burns, suppurative arthritis in (Schreiber, Dolgina, Schljapzew), PRS, *52:*683, 1973. Zentralbl. chir., *98:*328, 1973

Burns, children with, syndrome of arteriomesenterial duodenal compression in (Bobek), PRS, *56:*469, 1975. Acta chir. plast., *16:*238, 1974

Pneumonia, postburn, eschar major factor in

Burns, Complications of—Cont.

(Dressler, Skornik), PRS, *54:*379, 1974. Am. J. Surg., *127:*413, 1974

Burns, full-thickness, threshold effects on distant microcirculation (Jelenko *et al*), PRS, *52:*456, 1973. Arch. Surg., *106:*317, 1973; PRS, *55:*113, 1975. Am. Surgeon, *40:*388, 1974

Complications of thermal injury (Pruitt). Clin. Plast. Surg., *1:*667, 1974

Liver changes, early, in burns, role of A.T.P. and Trasylol in prevention (Beheri, Talaat, Zaky), PRS, *56:*682, 1975. J. Kuwait M. A., *8:*77, 1974

Burn injury, dermal ischemia in: importance of venous occlusion (Massiha, Monafo), PRS, *57:*538, 1976. J. Trauma, *14:*705, 1974

Burned ear, chondritis treated by local instillation of antibiotics (Apfelberg *et al*), PRS, *53:*179, 1974

Burned patients, inhibition of active sodium transport in erythrocytes from (Curreri *et al*), PRS, *56:*469, 1975. Surg. Gynec. & Obst., *139:*538, 1974

Keratoplasty, penetrating, in patient with 75% third degree burns (Older, Allansmith), PRS, *56:*223, 1975. Ann. Ophth., *7:*309, 1975

Fibrin split products elevated following thermal injury (Curreri, Wilterdink, Baxter), PRS, *56:*233, 1975. Ann. Surg., *181:*157, 1975

Respiratory problems complicating burn injury (Jelenko, Garrison, McKinley), PRS, *57:*538, 1976. Postgrad. Med., *58:*97, 1975

Bronchoscopy, fiberoptic, after thermal injury (Moylan, Adib, Birnbaum), PRS, *56:*598, 1975. Surg. Gynec. & Obst., *140:*541, 1975

Burns, Contractures

Deep burns—burn contractures (Buchan). Hand, *3:*90, 1971

Treatment of scar contracture of the perineal region (Nanba). Jap. J. Plast. Reconstr. Surg., *14:*382, 1971 (Japanese)

Burn contracture of neck, use of local flap for (Jabaley, Nguyen, Nguyen), PRS, *48:*288, 1971

Cicatricial deformation of the perioral region following burns and their treatment (Mukhin *et al*). Vestn. Khir., *107:*3, 1971 (Russian)

Local skin flaps in treatment of cutaneous contractures, sequelae of burns of the anterior and lateral sides of the neck (Janvier *et al*). Ann. chir. plast., *17:*26, 1972 (French)

Burns, Contractures—Cont.

Burns, contractures of extremities following, Z-plasty in treatment of (Kobus *et al*). Chir. Narzadow. Ruchu Ortop. Pol., *37:*529, 1972 (Polish)

Burn injuries, management of neck contractures resulting from (Pap), PRS, *51:*351, 1973. Internat. Surg., *57:*413, 1972

Axillary burns in children, clinical experience with (Law, Hoefer, MacMillan), PRS, *52:*101, 1973. J. Trauma, *12:*34, 1972

Surgery of cicatricial contracture of the upper extremities after deep burns (Dmitriev). Khirurgiia (Mosk.), *48:*31, 1972 (Russian)

Burn contractures in child (Dey). M. J. Australia, *2:*604, 1972

Skin plastic surgery in scar contractures of the neck following burns (Dmitriev *et al*). Ortop. Travmatol. Protez., *33:*7, 1972 (Russian)

On the problem of reconstruction after burns (Schrudde). Panminerva Med., *14:*241, 1972

Surgical repair and reconstruction of the burned surface (Damiani *et al*). Panminerva Med., *14:*245, 1972

Cicatrical contracture of fingers treated by temporary surgical syndactyly (Fittipaldi, Lanatta), PRS, *53:*243, 1974. Rev. españ. cir. plast., *5:*221, 1972

Contractures after secondary repair of burned neck, devices for preventing (Colin, Janvier), PRS, *54:*113, 1974. Ann. chir. plast., *18:*15, 1973

Labiomandibular areas in burn patients, problems posed by restoration of (Janvier *et al*). Ann. chir. plast., *18:*255, 1973 (French)

Burn patients, keloid and finger contractures in (Robitaille *et al*), PRS, *54:*113, 1974. Arch. Phys. Med., *54:*515, 1973

Burns of face, extensive, reconstruction of large perioral defects and correction of stenosis and distortion due to (Levignac). J. Maxillo-facial Surg., *1:*129, 1973

Burns, deep, contractures, deformities and cicatricial-trophic ulcers of lower extremities after, surgical treatment of (Dmitriev). Ortop. Travmatol. Protez., *34:*33, 1973 (Russian)

Burns, treatment of severe deformities and contractures of lower extremities resulting from (Ivanova *et al*). Ortop. Travmatol. Protez., *34:*38, 1973 (Russian)

Contractures, cicatricial, and its morphological foundation, plastic surgery of skin in treatment of (Gusarev). Ortop. Travmatol. Protez., *34:*61, 1973 (Russian)

Burns, Contractures — Cont.

Contractures: role of the orthopedic hospital in the Shriners burns program (Sullivan), PRS, *51:*293, 1973

Burns, effect of, on development of jaws and teeth (Kufner). Cesk. Stomatol., *74:*172, 1974 (Czechoslovakian)

Control and prevention of hypertrophic scarring and contracture (Noordhoff). Clin. Plast. Surg., *1:*49, 1974

Neck contractures, management of (Sawhney), PRS, *55:*384, 1975. Indian J. Plast. Surg., *7:*6, 1974

Burn, untreated, microstomia secondary to, cheiloplasty for correction (Friedlander *et al*). J. Oral Surg., *32:*525, 1974

Burns, use of ultrasonics for prevention of contractures after (Razvozova). Ortop. Travmatol. Protez., *34:*13, 1974 (Russian)

Burn contractures of the neck: natural history and surgical treatment (Remensnyder). In *Plastische und Wiederherstellungs-Chirurgie*, ed. by Hohler; pp. 259-66. Stuttgart; Schattauer, 1975

Contractures of neck, scar, treatment with Filatov pedicled flap in children (Shchipacheva), PRS, *57:*766, 1976. Acta chir. plast., *17:*49, 1975

Prevention and management of contractures in patients with burns of the neck (Bunchman *et al*). Am. J. Surg., *130:*700, 1975

Epithelialization and wound contracture in rabbits, effects of cortisone acetate, methylprednisolone and medroxyprogesterone on (Lenco, McKnight, MacDonald), PRS, *56:*470, 1975. Ann. Surg., *181:*67, 1975

Advantages of double releases in axillary, antecubital and popliteal contractures (Noe *et al*). J. Trauma, *15:*762, 1975

Separation of short stumps of shoulders from cicatricial adhesion to skin of chest (Keier). Ortop. Travmatol. Protez., *4:*67, 1975 (Russian)

Evaluation of biochemical changes in blood of patients with severe burns during reconstructive operation on the skin (Korolev *et al*). Sov. Med., *8:*149, 1975 (Russian)

Flap, lateral-volar finger, in treatment of burn syndactyly (MacDougal, Wray, Weeks), PRS, *57:*167, 1976

Burns, use of Filatov's pedicled flap in treatment of, and their sequelae (Burmistrov *et al*). Vestn. Khir., *111:*75, 1976

Burns, Debridement of

Burns, tangential excision: experimental study using animal model (Groves, Law-

Burns, Debridement of — Cont.

rence), PRS, *49:*359, 1972. Injury, *3:*30, 1971

Scalp avulsion and reconstruction (Jeremiah), PRS, *48:*604, 1971. Internat. Surg., *55:*265, 1971

Fluid debridement of the burn wound (Gerow *et al*). J. Trauma, *11:*1021, 1971

Burn eschar, histopathological study (Vistnes, Hogg), PRS, *48:*56, 1971

Burns, enzymatic debridement of (Levine, Seifter, Levenson), PRS, *49:*665, 1972. Surg. Forum, *22:*57, 1971

Eschars of major burns, early tangential excision of (Monafo, Aulenbacher, Pappalardo), PRS, *50:*634, 1972. Arch. Surg., *104:*503, 1972

Plasma jet — plasma scalpel surgery (Hishimoto, Goldman), PRS, *53:*110, 1974. Asian M. J., *15:*264, 1972

Burns, tangential excision and grafting (Jackson, Stone), PRS, *52:*210, 1973. Brit. J. Plast. Surg., *25:*416, 1972

Debriding, effect of bromelain ointment on necrotic tissue (Anzai), PRS, *52:*457, 1973. Jap. J. Plast. Reconstr. Surg., *15:*456, 1972

Device for dissection of necrotic skin (necrotome) (Plakhotniuk *et al*). Ortop. Travmatol. Protez., *33:*71, 1972 (Russian)

Burns, series of skin, with necrectomy immediately after electrolytic stabilization (Griswold) (Follow-Up Clinic), PRS, *49:*83, 1972

Effect of collagenase on the necrolysis of burn wounds delayed by antibiotic therapy (Zimmermann *et al*). Res. Exp. Med. (Berl.), *157:*244, 1972 (German)

Sutilains as enzymatic debriders for burn wounds (Silverstein *et al*), PRS, *52:*212, 1973. Surg. Forum, *23:*31, 1972

Histological examination of tangentially excised and grafted burns (Stone, Lawrence), PRS, *54:*696, 1974. Brit. J. Plast. Surg., *26:*20, 1973

Burns, tangential excision; studies of metabolic activity of recipient areas for skin grafts (Lawrence, Carney), PRS, *54:*695, 1974. Brit. J. Plast. Surg., *26:*93, 1973

Burns, staged excision of eschars in (Fang). Chinese Med. J., *4:*200, 1973

Burns, treatment by shaving eschars off. Chinese Med. J., *4:*208, 1973

Sutilains ointment as topical debriding agent in burns (Grossman). Internat. Surg., *58:*93, 1973

Plasma scalpel, wound healing of mouse skin incised with (Link *et al*), PRS, *54:*113, 1974. J. Surg. Res., *14:*505, 1973

Burns, Debridement of–Cont.

Burns, acute third degree, laser excision followed by immediate autograft replacement (Stellar *et al*), PRS, *53:*685, 1974. J. Trauma, *13:*45, 1973

Burns, laser excision of, letter to editor (Mendelson). J. Trauma, *13:*575, 1973

Burn debridement, Travase, an effective enzyme for (Pennisi, Capozzi, Friedman), PRS, *51:*371, 1973

Debridement of burn eschar and necrotic tissue, use of water-insoluble papain (WIP) for (Shapira, Giladi, Neuman), PRS, *52:*279, 1973

Debridement of experimental skin burns of pigs with bromelain, a pineapple stem enzyme (Levine *et al*), PRS, *52:*413, 1973

Burns, facial, enzymatic debridement (Yacomotti), PRS, *53:*491, 1974. Prensa med. argent., *60:*1055, 1973

Burns, enzymatic debridement (Levine, Seifter, Levenson). Rev. Surg., *30:*72, 1973

Trypsin and chymotrypsin toxicity in severely burned patients (Ambroggio, Cavallero, Catone), PRS, *56:*361, 1975. Riv. ital. chir. plast., *5:*331, 1973

Burns, debriding by grid escharotomy (Richards, Feller), PRS, *53:*685, 1974. Surg. Gynec. & Obst., *137:*843, 1973

Eschar: major factor in postburn pneumonia (Dressler, Skornik), PRS, *54:*379, 1974. Am. J. Surg., *127:*413, 1974

Child, burned, controlled hypotension for surgical excision (Szyfelbein, Ryan), PRS, *55:*515, 1975. Anesthesiology, *41:*501, 1974

Burned patients, subanesthetic ketamine for debridement or dressing change (Slogoff *et al*), PRS, *54:*628, 1974. Anesth. & Analg., *53:*354, 1974

Burns, third degree, use of carbon dioxide laser for debridement (Levine *et al*), *54:*240, 1974. Ann. Surg., *179:*246, 1974

Burns, chemical debridement of (Levenson *et al*), PRS, *55:*514, 1975. Ann. Surg., *180:*670, 1974

Burns, deep, treatment of necrotic scab in (Melega), PRS, *55:*721, 1975. Ars Curandi, *7:*42, 1974

Tangential excision (Monafo). Clin. Plast. Surg., *1:*591, 1974

The excision of burns (Ganzoni *et al*). Helv. Chir. Acta., *41:*221, 1974 (German)

Experimental use of collagenase in the debridement of thermally damaged skin (Moserova *et al*). J. Hyg. Epidemiol. Microbiol. Immunol. (Praha.), *18:*494, 1974

Clinical experience with enzymatic debridement of burned skin with the use of collagenase (Vrabec *et al*). J. Hyg. Epidemiol.

Burns, Debridement of–Cont.

Microbiol. Immunol. (Praha.), *18:*496, 1974

Burns, acute, carbon dioxide laser excision of, with immediate autografting (Fidler *et al*), PRS, *55:*253, 1975. J. Surg. Res., *17:*1, 1974

Burn wound sepsis, enzymatic debridement, experimental (Krizek, Robson, Groskin), PRS, *55:*515, 1975. J. Surg. Res., *17:*219, 1974

Burns, sepsis following enzymatic debridement, continuing problem of (Hummel *et al*). J. Trauma, *14:*572, 1974

Burns scab, period of detachment in children and indications for autoplastic operations (Ivanova *et al*). Ortop. Travmatol. Protez., *35:*28, 1974 (Russian)

Burn care, pediatric, primary excision, innovation in (Sheehy). R. N., *37:*21, 1974

Nursing care after primary excision (Kunsman). R. N., *37:*25, 1974

Septicaemia following early tangential excision of burns (Anderl *et al*). Wien. Klin. Wochenschr., *86:*91, 1974 (German)

Selective early excision of burns and its significance for the prophylaxis of burn complications (Olivari). In *Plastische und Wiederherstellungs-Chirurgie*, ed. by Hohler; pp. 227–36. Schattauer, Stuttgart, 1975 (German)

Burn, full-thickness, electrosurgical excision of (Lewis, Quinby), PRS, *56:*233, 1975. Arch. Surg., *2:*191, 1975

Scalpel, plasma, to excise burns (Link, Zook, Glover), PRS, *55:*657, 1975

Tangential excisions, laser, scalpel, electrosurgical, of third degree burns (Levine *et al*), PRS, *56:*286, 1975

Burns, Electrical

Severe electrical burns with impeding renal failure (Reckling *et al*). J. Kans. Med. Soc., *72:*410, 1971

Treatment of electrical injuries (Sturim). J. Trauma, *11:*959, 1971

Functional reconstruction of electric burn of the hand (Ishinada *et al*). Orthop. Surg. (Tokyo), *22:*882, 1971 (Japanese)

Successful resuscitation in injuries caused by electric current (Malatskii *et al*). Ortop. Travmatol. Protez., *32:*72, 1971 (Russian)

Low voltage skin burns (Jarvis *et al*). Pediatrics, *48:*831, 1971

Burn, deep electrical, regeneration of skull following (Worthen), PRS, *48:*1, 1971

Burn, electrical, reconstruction of lips and buccal commissure after (Gonzalez, Ojeda), PRS, *49:*237, 1972. Semana med. Mexico, *68:*101, 1971

Burns, Electrical—Cont.

Electromyographic findings in high voltage electrical burns: two cases (Hoover *et al*). South. Med. J., *64:*1392, 1971

Electric burns in the operating room (need for electronic technicians in today's hospital) (Beauchemin). Union Med. Can., *100:*1806, 1971 (French)

Electric burns and neurologic manifestations (Laurencon *et al*). Ann. chir. plast., *17:*54, 1972 (French)

Electrical burns of the mouth in children (Mladick). Arch. Dermat., *105:*296, 1972

Visceral injuries, unusual complication of electrical burn (Newsome, Curreri, Eurenius), PRS, *51:*606, 1973. Arch. Surg., *105:*494, 1972

Thermal trauma: a review of 22 electrical burns of the lip (Gormley *et al*). J. Oral Surg., *30:*531, 1972

Treatment of an electric burn of the face (Lebedeva). Stomatologiia (Mosk.), *51:*77, 1972 (Russian)

Plastic surgery of a large defect of skull soft tissue following burn wound due to electric current (Opolski *et al*). Wiad. Lek., *25:*383, 1972 (Polish)

Electrocardiographic changes in a patient struck by lightning (Karobath *et al*). Wien. Klin. Wochenschr., *84:*428, 1972 (German)

Burns caused by electric arc (Stieglitz *et al*). Z. Aerztl. Fortbild. (Jena), *66:*364, 1972 (German)

Abdomen, electrical burn, case report (Kaushik). Aust. N. Z. J. Surg., *43:*186, 1973

Treatment of 246 electrical burns. Chinese Med. J., *4:*213, 1973

Burns, hand, caused by electric fires (Stone), PRS, *53:*370, 1974. Injury, *4:*240, 1973

Burns, electrical, of upper extremity, management of (Salisbury *et al*), PRS, *51:*648, 1973

Electrical injuries, clinical experience in 100 cases (Kuo), PRS, *53:*490, 1974. Riv. ital. chir. plast., *4:*51, 1973

Management of electrical injuries of extremities (Kay *et al*). Surg. Clin. North Am., *53:*1459, 1973

Burns, electric, treatment of (Atiasov *et al*). Vestn. Khir., *111:*90, 1973 (Russian)

Electrical injury, changing concepts of (Artz), PRS, *57:*538, 1976. Am. J. Surg., *128:*600, 1974

Burns, electrosurgical, from miniature ECG electrodes (Finlay *et al*), PRS, *55:*639, 1975. Anesthesiology, *41:*263, 1974

Nerve-lesions due to electric current and thermal damage (Berger). Hefte Unfallheilkd., *0:*394, 1974 (German)

Burns, Electrical—Cont.

Burn, electrical, severe, with injury to sacrum and rectum, surgical tactics in (Matiashin *et al*). Klin. Khir., *10:*68, 1974 (Russian)

Electrical burns of lip, tongue flap for reconstruction (Zarem, Greer), PRS, *53:*310, 1974

Burn, electrical, of scalp and skull (Luce, Hoopes), PRS, *54:*359, 1974

Amputation and prosthesis after electric trauma of the upper limbs (Sarkisov *et al*). Vestn. Khir., *113:*103, 1974 (Russian)

Electrical burns of mouth (Wagner, Schwartz), PRS, *56:*232, 1975. Emergency Med., *7:*275, 1975

Problems of plastic and reconstructive surgery in the face (Buschmann). Fortschr. Med., *93:*1691, 1975 (German)

Burns, electrical, of mouth in children: method for assessing results (Orgel *et al*). J. Trauma, *15:*285, 1975

Spinal cord injury following electrical accidents: case reports (Levine *et al*). J. Trauma, *15:*459, 1975

Skin substitution in neck and facial burns (Zellner). Magy. Traumatol. Orthop., *18:*265, 1975 (Hungarian)

Electric injuries (Bogdanov). Med. Pregl., *28:*483, 1975 (Serbian)

Amputation of the extremities in burns (Iudenich *et al*). Voen. Med. Zh., *10:*15, 1975 (Russian)

Burns, Experimental

Serum and chorionic gonadotrophins, experimental thermal injury (Zalis, Rosales, Prince), PRS, *48:*516, 1971. Bol. Soc. argent. Cir., *31:*161, 1970

Burned rat, topical antisepsis studies in (Skornik, Dressler), PRS, *49:*666, 1972. Arch. Surg., *103:*469, 1971

Burns, experimental, in rats, effect of hyperbaric oxygen, tham, and antibiotics on (Bleser, Sztuka, Muller), PRS, *50:*95, 1972. Europ. Surg. Res., *3:*409, 1971

Enhanced survival in burned mice treated with antiserum prepared against normal and burned skin (Holder *et al*). J. Trauma, *11:*1041, 1971

Burns, standardized, in animals, positive effects of thrombolysis on superficial extent of (Hettich, Otten, Henne), PRS, *50:*204, 1972. Langenbecks Arch. Chir., *329:*899, 1971

Experimental principles of local therapy for burns. I. (Kohnlein). Monatsschr. Unfallheilkd., *14:*464, 1971 (German)

Burns, Electrical – Cont.

Effect of silver lactate and silver sulfadiazine on experimental burn wound sepsis (Cossman *et al*). Surg. Forum, *22:*495, 1971

Study of the cicatrization of experimental burns in rats (Flandre *et al*). Therapie, *26:*517, 1971 (French)

Burn, non-contact, subcutaneous temperature measurements in (Prouza, Moserova, Janecek), PRS, *52:*684, 1973. Acta chir. plast., *14:*168, 1972

Critical factors in resuscitation of the severely burned rat: the relative merit of volume, tonicity, sodium load, and concentration of the solution used (Casali *et al*). Ann. Surg., *175:*138, 1972

Burned rat, effect of antimicrobic therapy on lung bacterial clearance in (Dressler, Skornik), PRS, *50:*421, 1972. Ann. Surg., *175:*241, 1972

Kinetics of burn edema formation in primates (Leape), PRS *51:*706, 1973. Ann. Surg., *176:*223, 1972

Coagulation, intravascular, in experimental dog burns (Encke, Grozinger), PRS, *52:*211, 1973. Bull. Soc. Internat. Chir., *5:*445, 1972

"Burn toxin," specific, formation in mouse skin by thermal injuries (Stadtler *et al*), PRS, *51:*482, 1973. Europ. Surg. Res., *4:*198, 1972

Burns, experimental, effect of elemental diet on mortality rates and gastrointestinal lesions in (Langlois, Williams, Gurd), PRS, *52:*211, 1973. J. Trauma, *12:*771, 1972

Burns, studies in. X. Ethyl linoleate: water-holding lipid of skin. A. The evidence (Jelenko, Wheeler, Scott), PRS, *52:*210, 1973; B. Effects on *in vivo* burn eschar, PRS, *52:*211, 1973. J. Trauma, *12:*968, and 974, 1972

Wound healing with ordinary adhesive tape. A clinical and experimental study (Stenstrom *et al*). Scand. J. Plast. Reconstr. Surg., *6:*40, 1972

Burns, lymphocytotherapy in experimental *Pseudomonas sepsis* (Munster), PRS, *52:*329, 1973. Surg. Forum, *23:*42, 1972

Burns, major, plasma renin like activity (RLA) and angiotensin II levels after (Dolecek *et al*), PRS, *54:*506, 1974. Acta chir. plast., *15:*166, 1973

Burn, standard non-contact, subcutaneous temperature dynamics during thermal injury (Moserova, Prouzas), PRS, *54:*506, 1974. Acta chir. plast., *15:*247, 1973

Burning effects, threshold, on distant microcirculation (Jelenko *et al*), PRS, *52:*456,

Burns, Experimental – Cont.

1973. Arch. Surg., *106:*317, 1973; PRS, *55:*113, 1975. Am. Surgeon, *40:*388, 1974

Protection of damaged tissue by skin cover (Lawrence, Stone), PRS, *54:*696, 1974. Brit. J. Plast. Surg., *26:*101, 1973.

Burn, experimental studies on biosynthesis and transfer of labile methyl groups (Bouveng, Schildt, Sorbo), PRS, *53:*109, 1974. Europ. Surg. Res., *5:*146, 1973

Burn toxin in mouse skin (Allgower *et al*), PRS, *53:*686, 1974. J. Trauma, *13:*95, 1973

Burns, behavior of thrombocytes during scalding shock in rabbit (Loew, Langer, Bochum), PRS, *53:*607, 1974. Langenbecks Arch. Chir., *333:*71, 1973

Skin grafted burns in rats, effect of 1-triiodothyronine on marginal scars of (Zamick, Mehregan), PRS, *51:*71, 1973

Burns, experimental skin, of pigs, debridement of, with bromelain, a pineapple stem enzyme (Levine *et al*), PRS, *52:*413, 1973

Burns, experimental, effects of dimethyl sulfoxide (DMSO) on edema formation in (Arturson, Ponten), PRS, *54:*696, 1974. Scand. J. Plast. Reconstr. Surg., 7:74, 1973

Burns, new method for covering large surface area wounds with autografts. I. *In vitro* multiplication of rabbit-skin epithelial cells (Freeman *et al*), PRS, *55:*114, 1975. Arch. Surg., *108:*721, 1974

Burns, new method for covering large surface wounds with autografts. II. Surgical application of tissue culture expanded rabbit-skin autografts (Igel *et al*), PRS, *55:*114, 1975. Arch. Surg., *108:*724, 1974

Biosynthesis and transfer of labile methyl groups in experimental burn (Bouveng, Schildt, Sorbo), PRS, *53:*109, 1974. Europ. Surg. Res., *5:*146, 1973

Burn wound sepsis, experimental, topical povidone-iodine ointment in (Robson, Schaerf, Krizek), PRS, *54:*328, 1974

Burns, survival time of rats in severe heat (O'Hara *et al*), PRS, *57:*127, 1976. J. Appl. Physiol., *38:*724, 1975

Burns, chemical experimental cutaneous, effect of hydrotherapy on clinical course and pH of (Gruber, Laub, Vistnes), PRS, *55:*200, 1975

Burns, effect of early surgical excision and homografting on survival of burned rats and of intraperitoneally-infected burned rats (Levine, Salisbury, Mason), PRS, *56:*423, 1975

Blister and second degree burn in guinea pigs: effect of exposure (Wheeler, Miller), PRS, *57:*74, 1976

Burns, Eyes and Eyelids: See *Eye, Burns of*

Burns, Face

Management of facial burns (Sekiguchi *et al*). Shujutsu, *25:*1127, 1971 (Japanese)

Facial burns (Pennisi *et al*). Med. Trial Tech. Q., *18:*361, 1972

Treatment of an electric burn of the face (Lebedeva). Stomatologiia (Mosk.), *51:*77, 1972 (Russian)

Burns, deep facial, correction of cicatricial deformations and defects of nose after (Kabakov *et al*). Vestn. Khir., *111:*91, 1973

Burns, facial, reconstruction of ear, eyebrow, and sideburn (Brent), PRS, *55:*312, 1975

Burns, Fluid Therapy

Burned patient, what constitutes proper solution for resuscitation of severely (Caldwell *et al*), PRS, *50:*541, 1972. Am. J. Surg., *122:*655, 1971

Evaluation of fluid resuscitation in the burned patient (Sundell). Ann. Chir. Gynaecol. Fenn., *60:*192, 1971

Fluid administration and vasodilator (Hydralazine), influence on hemodynamic changes in early postburn patient (Pruitt, Mason, Moncrief), PRS, *49:*587, 1972. J. Trauma, *11:*36, 1971

Simplified formula for calculating fluid requirements in severely burned patients (Nasilowski). Pol. Tyg. Lek., *26:*1950, 1971 (Polish)

Evaporative water loss from burns under different environmental conditions (Lamke). Scand. J. Plast. Reconstr. Surg., *5:*77, 1971

Burnt skin, evaporative water loss from normal and (Lamke), PRS, *49:*665, 1972. Thesis, Dept. of Surg., Linkoping Univ., Sweden, 1971

Intravenous therapy, prevention of infection of scalp vein sites of needle insertion during (Crenshaw *et al*), PRS, *51:*354, 1973. Am. J. Surg., *124:*43, 1972

Burned patients, Evans formula revisited (Hutcher, Haynes), PRS, *52:*101, 1973. J. Trauma, *12:*453, 1972

Burns, severe, tris buffer in (Cramer). Follow-Up Clinic, PRS, *50:*401, 1972

Resuscitation with hypertonic lactate saline in thermal injury (Moylan, Reckler, Mason), PRS, *52:*598, 1973. Am. J. Surg., *125:*580, 1973

Hypernatremic state in hypermetabolic burn patients (Warden *et al*), PRS, *52:*598, 1973. Arch. Surg., *106:*420, 1973

Sodium concentration, tissue, after thermal burns (Day, Leape), PRS, *52:*212, 1973. J. Trauma, *12:*1063, 1973

Burns, Fluid Therapy—Cont.

Hydration of burned patients in first 48 hours (Souza), PRS, *55:*722, 1975. Ars Curandi, *7:*34, 1974

Hospital burn units (Marcondes, Rufatto), PRS, *55:*721, 1975. Ars Curandi, *7:*64, 1974

Cannulation, venous, trouble with I-V in the long run (Munster), PRS, *56:*597, 1975. Emergency Med., *7:*230, 1975

Fluid administration, intermittent intravenous, chronic cannulation for (Mostardi *et al*), PRS, *57:*127, 1976. J. Appl. Physiol., *38:*750, 1975

Acidosis of burns, early, relationship to extent of burn and management (Eggleston, Feierabend), PRS, *57:*762, 1976. Surgery, *77:*641, 1975

Burns, Heat Regulation and

Heat production failure in the postburn period (Caldwell *et al*), PRS, *50:*205, 1972. J. Trauma, *11:*936, 1971

Burn patients, heat loss in (Boorom). A.O.R.N., *17:*80, 1973

Temperature dynamics, subcutaneous, during thermal injury (Moserova, Prouzas), PRS, *54:*506, 1974. Acta chir. plast., *15:*247, 1973

Thermal regulation in patients after healing of large deep burns (McGibbon *et al*). PRS, *52:*164, 1973

Heat production and heat loss in burn patients, effect of ambient temperature on (Wilmore *et al*), PRS, *57:*121, 1976. J. Appl. Physiol., *38:*593, 1975

Burns, Homografts and Heterografts for (See also *Amnion; Burns, Topical Therapy*)

Use of cutaneous homografts in severely burned patients (Faguer *et al*). Ann. Chir., *25:*919, 1971 (French)

Supplement to the cutaneous homograft case report presented in 1950 (Caby). Chirurgie, *97:*722, 1971 (French)

Fetal skin xenotransplants for temporary closure of extensive third degree burns (Bohmert). Fortschr. Med., *89:*836, 1971

Skin auto- and homoplasty in deep burns (Barskii *et al*). Khirurgiia (Mosk.), *47:*20, 1971 (Russian)

Evaluation of homotransplantation of skin preserved by lyophilization and freezing (Donetskii *et al*). Khirurgiia (Mosk.), *47:*22, 1971 (Russian)

Autografts and xenografts, meshed, to cover extensive burns (Bohmert *et al*), PRS, *50:*202, 1972. Langenbeck's Arch. Chir., *329:*918, 1971

Burns, severe, xenotransplantation as bio-

Burns, Homografts for, etc.—Cont.

logic dressing in (Bohnert *et al*), PRS, *48:*516, 1971. Med. & Hygiene, *955:*438, 1971

Primary homotransplantation (biological dressing) without excision in the treatment of burns (Novak *et al*). Orv. Hetil., *112:*3078, 1971 (Hungarian)

Burns, thermal, use of pigskin in treatment (Wood *et al*). Am. J. Surg., *124:*720, 1972

Burns, comparative characteristics of human and porcine staphylococci and their differentiation in xenografting procedures (Smith, Bettge). Appl. Microbiol., *24:*929, 1972

Combined autograft and homograft cover in extensive deep burns (Sawhney). Brit. J. Plast. Surg., *25:*141, 1972

Porcine skin grafts (Capozzi). Calif. Med., *116:*56, 1972

Burns, use of preserved skin for resurfacing of (Mahler *et al*). Harefuah, *82:*122, 1972 (Hebrew)

Resurfacing of burns with preserved skin (Mahler *et al*). Isr. J. Med. Sci., *8:*141, 1972

Heterografting of partial thickness burns, early (Lee). J. Trauma, *12:*818, 1972

Burns, heterotopic calcification following (Munster *et al*), PRS, *52:*210, 1973. J. Trauma, *12:*968, 1972

Burns, deep thermal, in children, surgical treatment of, by means of free autologous and homologous skin transplantations (Shindarski *et al*). Khirurgiia (Sofiia), *25:*267, 1972 (Bulgarian)

Mowlem-Jackson auto-homologous grafts in large surface burns (Kopp). Monatsschr. Unfallheilkd., *75:*268, 1972 (German)

Burns, healing of second degree. Comparison of effects of early application of homografts and coverage with tape (Miller, White). PRS, *49:*552, 1972

Autograft rejection induced by homografting (Cramer) (Follow-Up Clinic), PRS. *50:*401, 1972

Allogenic skin grafting in treatment of burns (Nasilowski). Pol. Tyg. Lek., *27:*509, 1972 (Polish)

Burns, use of heterografts as first surgical dressing (Sturla *et al*), PRS, *52:*598, 1973. Rev. argent. cir., *23:*49, 1972

Quantitative comparison of biological dressings (Robson *et al*). Surg. Forum, *23:*503, 1972

Burned patients, value of excision-homograft in (Lagrot *et al*). Ann. Chir., *27:*191, 1973 (French)

Burns, successful treatment of extensive deep. Chinese Med. J., *4:*205, 1973

Burns, Homografts for, etc.—Cont.

Burns, extensive third degree, review on management (Editorial). Chinese Med. J., *11:*673, 1973 (Chinese)

Homografts of skin, Epigard, a substitute for (Alexander). J. Trauma, *13:*374, 1973

Cable from Cathay (Malt, McDowell). New England J. Med., *228:*1353, 1973

Immune response, cellular, of humans to pigskin (McCabe *et al*), PRS, *51:*181, 1973

Burns, massive, use of tissue-matched meshed homografts in treatment of (Rhoads *et al*). Rev. Surg., *30:*451, 1973

Burns, deep dermal, use of homografts in (Zdrawic), PRS, *53:*686, 1974. Riv. ital. chir. plast., *4:*19, 1973

Burns, skin transplantation in, use of immunological enhancement in (Munster *et al*). Surg. Forum, *24:*48, 1973

Burns, colonization of by Streptococcus faecalis related to contaminated porcine xenografts (Smith *et al*). Tex. Rep. Biol. Med., *31:*47, 1973

Burns, porcine skin dressings for (Stinson). Am. J. Nurs., *74:*111, 1974

Burned child, skin transplants with immunosuppressive therapy (Diethelm *et al*), PRS, *55:*639, 1975. Ann. Surg., *180:*814, 1974

Preliminary report on comparative use of lyophilized homograft and zenograft in closure of raw areas (Hackett *et al*). Brit. J. Surg., *61:*427, 1974

Burns, skin replacement in, using split skin net transplants and xenotransplants (Bohmert). Hefte Unfallheilkd., *116:*1, 1974 (German)

Burns in children, immediate heterografting of (Lilly, Peck), PRS, *55:*252, 1975. J. Pediat. Surg., *9:*335, 1974

Burned patients, heterografted, anti-porcine antibodies in (Harris, Abston), PRS, *55:*113, 1975. J. Surg. Res., *16:*599, 1974

Burned patients, technique for obtaining porcine heterografts for use on (Shircliffe *et al*). J. Trauma, *14:*168, 1974

Burns, allo- and xeno-grafts of fresh and cryopreserved skin, comparison of clinical activity of (Donati *et al*). Minerva Med., *65:*3654, 1974

Burns, extensive, temporary skin transplantation and immunosuppression for (Burke *et al*). New England J. Med., *290:*269, 1974

Comparative evaluation of certain methods of skin preservation (Margolin). Ortop. Travmatol. Protez., *35:*26, 1974 (Russian)

Burns, absence of vascularization in porcine skin grafts on mice (Pandya, Zarem). PRS, *53:*211, 1974

Burn, second degree: deleterious effect of

Burns, Homografts for, etc.—Cont.

split-skin homograft coverage on split-skin graft donor sites (Miller). PRS, *53:*316, 1974

Vascularization of porcine skin heterografts (Toranto, Salyer, Myers), PRS, *54:*195, 1974. Discussion by Ben-Hur, PRS, *54:*352, 1974

Bacteriological control of dermo-epidermal transplants from pig's carcasses (Moserova *et al*). Rozhl. Chir., *53:*631, 1974 (Czechoslovakian)

Preserved cadaver skin for the coverage of large-scale third-degree burns (Zellner). Zentralbl. Chir., *99:*1105, 1974 (German)

Burns, thermal, treated by amniotic membranes (Visuthikosol, Buri), PRS, *56:*232, 1975. Asian J. Mod. Med., *11:*17, 1975

Prolonged retention of glutaraldehyde-treated skin homografts in humans (Schechter *et al*). Brit. J. Plast. Surg., *28:*198, 1975

Transplantation and preservation of tissue-typized skin in burns (Zellner *et al*). Chirurg., *46:*319, 1975 (German)

Treatment of burn wounds with the skin of the convalescents (Sokolov). Khirurgiia (Mosk), *4:*21, 1975 (Russian)

Xenograft in the treatment of burns (Istvan). Magy. Traumatol. Orthop., *18:*314, 1975 (Hungarian)

Surgery in China: part 1 (Critchley). M. J. Australia, *1:*693, 1975

Panniculectomy specimens as a convenient and inexpensive source of homograft skin (Swartz, Rueckert, Brown). PRS, *55:*628, 1975

Homografting, early surgical excision and, effect on survival of burned rats and of intraperitoneally-infected burned rats (Levine, Salisbury, Mason). PRS, *56:*423, 1975

Pigskin, on the cutaneous porcine heterograft (Habal) (Editorial). PRS, *57:*367, 1976

Burns, Immunology of

Lymphocytic reactivity studies, evaluation in patients with thermal burns (Daniels *et al*), PRS, *49:*107, 1972. J. Trauma, *11:*595, 1971

Autoallergy in burns (Ablin) (Letter to the Editor). PRS, *48:*170, 1971

Immunotherapy for severe burns in children (Craig) (Follow-Up Clinic). PRS, *48:*368, 1971

Reticuloendothelial system function in severe thermal injury (Converse *et al*), PRS, *50:*202, 1972. Surg. Forum, *22:*493, 1971

Burned subjects, plasma immunoreactive in-

Burns, Immunology of—Cont.

sulin and growth hormone levels in (Dolecek *et al*), PRS, *52:*684, 1973. Acta chir. plast., *14:*179, 1972

Burns, host defence mechanisms in. New horizons in surgical immunobiology (Munster). Ann. R. Coll. Surg. Engl., *51:*69, 1972

Effect of autoantibodies on viability of autografts (Aripov *et al*). Eksp. Khir. Anesteziol., *17:*41, 1972 (Russian)

Immunologic reactivity in burned patients and autoplasty (Matusis *et al*). Khirurgiia (Mosk.), *48:*36, 1972 (Russian)

Lymphocytotherapy in experimental *Pseudomonas* sepsis (Munster), PRS, *52:*329, 1973. Surg. Forum, *23:*42, 1972

Burned patients, anemia of, role of erythropoietin in (Robinson *et al*), PRS, *53:*608, 1974. Ann. Surg., *178:*565, 1973

Leukocytic response as a monitor of immunodepression in burn patients (McCabe, Rebuck, Kelly), PRS, *52:*456, 1973. Arch. Surg., *106:*155, 1973

Burned patients, changes of immunoglobulin levels in (Barisoni *et al*), PRS, *56:*360, 1975. Riv. ital. chir. plast., *5:*319, 1973

Lymphocyte depletion and serum complement perturbations following acute burn trauma (Farrell *et al*), PRS, *52:*456, 1973. Surgery, *73:*697, 1973

Use of immunological enhancement in skin transplantation in burns (Munster *et al*). Surg. Forum, *24:*48, 1973

Burned patients, impaired function of polymorphonuclear leukocytes in (Grogan, Miller), PRS, *53:*608, 1974. Surg. Gynec. & Obst., *137:*784, 1973

Immunosuppressive therapy with skin transplants for severely burned child (Diethelm *et al*), PRS, *55:*639, 1975. Ann. Surg., *180:*814, 1974

Burn neutrophil function, immunologic and nutritional evaluation of (Lennard *et al*). J. Surg. Res., *16:*286, 1974

Burns, thermal, gunshot wounds and skin grafts, pemphigus-like antibodies in sera of patients with (Dahl *et al*). Mil. Med., *139:*196, 1974

Survey of the current status of the clinical uses of antilymphocyte serum (Monaco *et al*). Surg. Gynec. & Obstet., *142:*417, 1976

Burns, Infections

Burned patients, vaccination against *Pseudomonas* infection in: aspects and problems (Taidelli, Savani, Grisotti), PRS, *50:*308, 1972. Acta chir plast., *13:*94, 1971

Infection and superinfection of burn patients. Is the burn center a septic ghetto? (Vilain).

Burns, Infections — Cont.

Anesth. Analg. (Paris), *28:*761, 1971 (French)

Pseudomonas infection in burn patients, immunological control (Alexander, Fisher, MacMillan), PRS, *48:*90, 1971. Arch. Surg., *102:*31, 1971

Burn wound, opportunistic fungal infection with Phycomycetes and Aspergillus (Bruck *et al*), PRS, *49:*107, 1972. Arch. Surg., *102:*476, 1971

Candida septicemia (Williams, Chandler, Orloff), PRS, *49:*239, 1972. Arch. Surg., *103:*8, 1971

Candida albicans, growth of, in nutritive solutions given parenterally (Brennan *et al*), PRS, *50:*312, 1972. Arch. Surg., *103:*705, 1971

Colonization with gentamicin-resistant Pseudomonas aeruginosa, pyocine type 5, in a burn unit (Shulman *et al*). J. Infect. Dis., *124:*18, 1971, Suppl

Gentamicin for septicemia in patients with burns (Abston *et al*). J. Infect. Dis., *124:*275, 1971, Suppl

Pseudomonas, gentamicin-resistant, evolution and spread of (Stone, Kolk), PRS, *49:*106, 1972. J. Trauma, *7:*586, 1971

Myocardial contractility in sepsis, effect of digitalis on (Cann *et al*), PRS, *49:*475, 1972. Surg. Forum, *22:*1, 1971

Burn wound studies on occurrence and significance of yeasts and fungi (Bruck *et al*), PRS, *51:*350, 1973. Ann. Surg., *176:*108, 1972

Lung bacterial clearance in burned rat, effect of antimicrobial therapy on (Dressler, Skornik), PRS, *50:*421, 1972. Ann. Surg., *175:*241, 1972

Mode of transmission of Pseudomonas aeruginosa in a burn unit and an intensive care unit in a general hospital (Kominos *et al*). Appl. Microbiol., *23:*309, 1972

Burn patients, experience with Candida infections in (MacMillan, Law, Holder), PRS, *50:*634, 1972. Arch. Surg., *104:*509, 1972

Burn patients, study of surgical infections among (Ramires), PRS, *51:*706, 1973. Asian J. Med., *8:*512, 1972

Pseudomonas, experiments in local burn treatment (Köhnlein, Dietrich), PRS, *52:*212, 1973. Chir. Plast., *1:*207, 1972

Pseudomonas pyocyaneus infections, treatment with combined carbenicillin and gentamycin (Michaeli, Medini), PRS, *50:*637, 1972. Harefuah, *72:*312, 1972

Burned patients, successful treatment of can-

Burns, Infections — Cont.

dida septicemia with new antimycotic, Clotrimazole (Bay b 5097) (Liljedahl, Fris, Wickman), PRS, *52:*101, 1973. Injury, *4:*157, 1972

Control by ventilation of airborne bacterial transfer between hospital patients, and its assessment by means of a particle tracer. 3. Studies with an airborne-particle tracer in an isolation ward for burned patients (Hambraeus *et al*). J. Hyg. (Camb.), *70:*299, 1972

Prevention of bacterial growth and local infection in burn wounds (Linkner *et al*). J. Pediatr. Surg., *7:*310, 1972

Heparin treatment of live *Escherichia coli* bacteremia in rats (Horwitz *et al*), PRS, *52:*106, 1973. J. Surg. Res., *13:*120, 1972

Amphotericin B in systemic candidiasis in burned patient (Law *et al*), PRS, *52:*326, 1973. J. Trauma, *12:*543, 1972

Pathogenesis and clinical picture of burn sepsis (Vishnevskii *et al*). Klin. Med. (Mosk.), *50:*7, 1972 (Russian)

Bacteremia in burned patients (Kolker *et al*). Khirurgiia (Mosk.), *48:*31, 1972 (Russian)

Pyocyanens infection in burned patients. Immunitary protection (Moyen *et al*). Nouv. Presse Med., *1:*947, 1972 (French)

Infection associated with burns (Lowbury). Postgrad. Med. J., *48:*338, 1972

Sepsis in burns, prevention and treatment of (Lowbury), PRS, *50:*202, 1972. Proc. Roy. Soc. Med., *65:*23, 1972

Immunological control of *pseudomonas* infection in burns. R. I. Med. J., *55:*88, 1972

Carbenicillin, clinical use in extensive burns (Franco Diaz, Alonso Rosa), PRS, *53:*247, 1974. Rev. españ. cir. plast., *5:*209, 1972

Pseudomonas aeruginosa, control of surface infection with antibiotic-impregnated Epigard (Alexander, Sykes, Wheeler), PRS, *52:*329, 1973. Surg. Forum, *23:*36, 1972

Pseudomonas sepsis, lymphocytotherapy in (Munster), PRS, *52:*329, 1973. Surg. Forum, *23:*42, 1972

Anaerobic infections, clinical-experimental evaluation of long-acting penicillin preparations in treatment (Grechukhin *et al*). Voen. Med. Zh., *4:*20, 1972 (Russian)

Burn illness, septic shock in (Matejicek *et al*), PRS, *54:*507, 1974. Acta chir. plast., *15:*263, 1973

Candidiasis in cases of postoperative intensive care (Zierott, von Meissner), PRS, *53:*691, 1974. Chirurg, *44:*509, 1973

Pseudomonas aeruginosa identified and serologically typed by fluorescent antibody

Burns, Infections — Cont.
technique (Nashimura, Tagagi, Kotani), PRS, *52:*687, 1973. Japan J. Exp. Med., *43:*43, 1973
Bacteremia in burned patient (Mamattah *et al*). J. Clin. Pathol., *26:*388, 1973
Candida serology: an aid in diagnosis of deep-organ candidiasis (Jones, Brennan, Kundsin), PRS, *54:*119, 1974. J. Surg. Res., *14:*235, 1973
Escherichia coli in vitro and in the germfree mouse to inhibit *Candida albicans* (Hummel *et al*), PRS, *54:*118, 1974. J. Surg. Res., *15:*53, 1973
Pseudomonas epidemiology in a burn intensive care unit (MacMillan *et al*), PRS, *54:*378, 1974. J. Trauma, *13:*627, 1973
Pseudomonas septicemia, recovery in (Bromberg) (Follow-Up Clinic), PRS, *51:*88, 1973
Burned patient, severely, disseminated candidiasis in (Rayner), PRS, *51:*461, 1973
Burns, infestation and septicemia from *Candida albicans* caused by massive treatment with antibiotic and Sulfamylon (Ben-Hur), PRS, *53:*686, 1974. Riv. ital. chir. plast., *4:*45, 1973
Biopsies, use in burn patient care (Pruitt, Foley), PRS, *52:*683, 1973. Surgery, *73:*887, 1973
Neutrophil bactericidal function assessed by stimulated nitroblue tetrazolium test to predict wound sepsis in burned patients (Curreri *et al*), PRS, *52:*683, 1973. Surgery, *74:*6, 1973
Granulocyte and platelet production suppressed by *Pseudomonas* burn wound infection (Newsome, Euremius), PRS, *52:*209, 1973. Surg. Gynec & Obst., *136:*373, 1973
Leukocytes, polymorphonuclear, impaired function in patients with burns and other trauma (Grogan, Miller), PRS, *53:*608, 1974. Surg. Gynec. & Obst., *137:*784, 1973
Arthritis, suppurative, in burns (Schreiber, Dolgina, Schljapzew), PRS, *52:*683, 1973. Zentralbl. chir., *98:*328, 1973
Candida sepsis: pathogenesis and principles of treatment (Stone *et al*), PRS, *54:*702, 1974. Ann. Surg., *179:*697, 1974
Fungal septicemia in surgical patients (Rodrigues, Wolff), PRS, *55:*645, 1975. Ann. Surg., *180:*741, 1974
Pseudomonas aeruginosa, role of wounds in epidemiology of nosocomial infections due to (Wysocki *et al*), PRS, *55:*258, 1975. Invest. Urol., *11:*370, 1974
Burn patients, use of quantitative biopsy cultures in bacteriologic monitoring of (Loebl

Burns, Infections — Cont.
et al), PRS, *55:*114, 1975. J. Surg. Res., *16:*1, 1974
Macronumbers of microorganisms (Mason, Lindberg), PRS, *55:*113, 1975. Lancet, *2:*292, 1974
Pseudomonas aeruginosa in hospital sinks (Ayliffe *et al*), PRS, *55:*253, 1975. Lancet, *2:*578, 1974
Burns, large, upper extremity fungal invasions secondary to (Salisbury, Silverstein, Goodwin), PRS, *54:*654, 1974
Infection in patients with burns (Pavkova *et al*), PRS, *54:*623, 1974. Rozhl. chir., *53:*195, 1974
Hyperalimentation in patients with potential sepsis (Copeland *et al*), PRS, *54:*379, 1974. Surg. Gynec & Obst., *138:*377, 1974
Bacteremia and postmortem microbiology in burned children (Smith *et al*), PRS, *56:*469, 1975. Am. J. Clin. Path., *63:*502, 1975
Pseudomonas septicemia, metastatic gangrene of lid in (Treister *et al*), PRS, *57:*113, 1976. Ann. Ophth., *7:*639, 1975
Bacterial invasion in burns (Ballin), PRS, *57:*401, 1976. Emerg. Med., *7:*59, 1975
Antibiotics, prophylactic, current use in plastic and reconstructive surgery (Krizek, Koss, Robson), PRS, *55:*21, 1975
Excision, early surgical, and homografting, effect of, on survival of burned rats and of intraperitoneally-infected burned rats (Levine, Salisbury, Mason), PRS, *56:*423, 1975

Burns, Mortality in

Burns, death causes after (Hajek *et al*), PRS, *50:*201, 1972. Acta chir. plast., *12:*78, 1971
Revised analysis of mortality due to burns (Bull). Lancet, *2:*1133, 1971
Burns, changing patterns in mortality of (Lynch *et al*), PRS, *48:*329, 1971
Cocoanut Grove Disaster (Maxwell Finland) (Davidson). J. Infect. Dis., *125:*Suppl 58, 1972
Burns, revised analysis of mortality due to (Bull), PRS, *50:*420, 1972. Lancet, *2:*7734, 1972
Mortality in burns, values of lethal area 50 in patients of various ages (Hajek), PRS, *54:*506, 1974. Acta chir. plast., *15:*162, 1973
Burn injury mortality over a period of 10 years (Vladovic-Relja, Montani, Zecevic), PRS, *54:*623, 1974. Acta chir. plast., *15:*231, 1973
Burned patients treated by the exposure method, mortality and causes of death in (Sørensen, Hall), PRS, *51:*59, 1973

Burns, Skin Grafting—Cont.

Burns, skin replacement (Bohmert). Fortschr. Med., *91:*646, 1973

Burns, full thickness, in children, simple technique of primary excision (Murray *et al*). J. R. Coll. Surg. Edinb.,*18:*176, 1973

Burns, donor sites, Gelfoam dressings for (Patkin *et al*). M. J. Australia, *2:*750, 1973

Burns, deep, patients with, osteonecrectomy and skin plasty in (Iukhin). Ortop. Travmatol. Protez., *34:*18, 1973 (Russian)

Burned patients, severely, restoration of integument in (Matchin). Ortop. Travmatol. Protez., *34:*53, 1973 (Russian)

Burned patients, auto-dermoplasty in, results of outcome of (Rusakov *et al*). Ortop. Travmatol. Protez., *34:*56, 1973 (Russian)

Aerophoresis of penicillin in early postoperative period after skin autoplasty in patients with thermal trauma (Kamrash *et al*). Ortop. Travmatol. Protez., *34:*60, 1973 (Russian)

Burned hand, delayed primary excision and skin grafting of (Krizek *et al*), PRS, *51:*524, 1973

Burns: effect of Silastic sheet dressings on the healing of split-skin graft donor sites (Harris, Filarski, Hector), PRS, *52:*189, 1973

Burns, children, plastic surgery of skin in (Aralbaev). Sov. Zdravookhr. Kirg., *4:*58, 1973 (Russian)

Autografting large burns from limited donor sites (Zawacki, Asch), PRS, *53:*498, 1974. Surgery, *74:*774, 1973

Burn disease, functional state of restored skin cover in persons who have suffered (Starchenko). Vestn. Khir., *110:*82, 1973 (Russian)

Burns, skin grafting of (Zani), PRS, *55:*725, 1975. Ars Curandi, *7:*49, 1974

Burns, use of skin grafts in treatment of (Benaim), PRS, *55:*111, 1975. Bol. y trab. Acad. argent. cir., *58:*102, 1974

Rosette inhibition test in skin grafted patients (Chapel *et al*). Brit. Med. J., *2:*236, 1974

Preparing and closing the burn wound (Shuck). Clin. Plast. Surg., *1:*577, 1974

Burn excision, primary, and immediate grafting: method shortening illness (Burke *et al*). J. Trauma, *14:*386, 1974

Burns, split skin transplantation (Hohle *et al*). Monatsschr. Unfallheilkd., *77:*189, 1974 (German)

Treatment of burns by split skin grafting (Clery). Nurs. Times, *70:*1893, 1974

Use of mesh dermatome in surgical treatment of thermal injuries in children

Burns, Skin Grafting—Cont.

(Baksa *et al*). Orv. Hetil., *115:*1347, 1974 (Hungarian)

Skin grafting burned patient who has *epidermolysis bullosa,* new method for (Skivolocki, Harris, Boles), PRS, *53:*355, 1974

Burned breast, nipple and areola reconstruction—"double bubble" technique (Bunchman *et al*), PRS, *54:*531, 1974

Skin grafts subjected to bath hypotonic solutions, evaluation of (Adamczak *et al*). Pol. Przegl. Chir., *46:*509, 1974 (Polish)

Plastic surgery and burns (Weeks). Surg. Gynec. & Obstet., *138:*212, 1974

Closure of large burn wounds in children (Frittsshe *et al*). Vestn. Khir., *112:*103, 1974 (Russian)

Replacement of Skin in Burns with Split Thickness Skin Mesh Grafts and Xenotransplants. By H. Bohmert. Springer-Verlag, Berlin-Heidelberg-New York, 1974. PRS, *56:*82, 1975

Clinical and histological results after extensive split skin transplantation (Kunert *et al*). In *Plastische und Wiederherstellungs-Chirurgie,* ed. by Hohler; pp. 251–7. Stuttgart; Schattauer, 1975 (German)

Split skin transplantation after grinding off hypertrophic burn scars (Zeitz *et al*). In *Plastische und Wiederherstellungs-Chirurgie,* ed. by Hohler; Stuttgart; Schattauer, 1975 pp. 327–9 (German)

Burned patients, appraisal of prognostic significance of various factors in results of autotransplantation of skin in (Shalimov *et al*), PRS, *57:*762, 1976. Acta chir. plast., *17:*42, 1975

Burn wound from the surgical point of view (Janzekovic). J. Trauma, *15:*42, 1975

Editorial: Transplantation and burns. Lancet, *1:*1017, 1975

Burns and transplantation (Koumans). Lancet, *1:*1190, 1975

Skin substitution in neck and facial burns (Zellner). Magy. Traumatol. Orthop., *18:*265, 1975 (Hungarian)

Free skin transplantation (Huffstadt). Ned. tijdschr. geneeskd., *119:*589, 1975 (Dutch)

Burned female breast (Rubin). N.Y. State J. Med., *75:*865, 1975

Prognostic value of cytological characteristics of the burn wound prior to autodermoplasty (Rusakov *et al*). Ortop. Travmatol. Protez., *2:*62, 1975 (Russian)

Evaluation of biochemical changes in blood of patients with severe burns during reconstructive operation on the skin (Korolev *et al*). Sov. Med., *8:*149, 1975 (Russian)

Burns, Topical Therapy—Cont.

Burns, effect of bromelain ointment on necrotic tissue (Anzai), PRS, *52:*457, 1973. Jap. J. Plast. Reconstr. Surg., *15:*456, 1972

Silver nitrate cream treatment in burns, some interesting and unanticipated findings (Foerster). J. Okla. State Med. Assoc., *65:*262, 1972

Treatment of burns in children using 0.5 per cent silver nitrate spray locally. A preliminary report (Shah *et al*). J. Postgrad. Med., *18:*74, 1972

Pseudomonas aeruginosa, experimental burn wound sepsis: variations in response to topical agents (Krizek, Cossman), PRS, *52:*325, 1973. J. Trauma, *12:*553, 1972

Use of 0.5 percent silver nitrate in burns: results in 220 patients (Hartford *et al*). J. Trauma, *12:*682, 1972

Burn wound epsis, experimental, laboratory evaluation of topical silver nitrate in (Dressler, Skornik), PRS, *52:*211, 1973. J. Trauma, *12:*791, 1972

Burn wound, effect of cleansing agents used on (Burns, Harrison), PRS, *52:*326, 1973. J. Trauma, *12:*903, 1972

Burned skin, absorption of C^{14}-labeled Sulfamylon acetate through (Harrison *et al*), PRS, *53:*492, 1974. J. Trauma, *12:*986, 1972

Sulfamylon solution dressings in the management of burn wounds (Shuck, Einfeldt, Trainor), PRS, *53:*492, 1974. J. Trauma, *12:*999, 1972

Effects of topical chemoprophylaxis on transferable antibiotic resistance in burns (Roe *et al*). Lancet, *2:*109, 1972

Burns, alternate forms of local treatment of (Lowbury *et al*), PRS, *50:*420, 1972. Lancet, *2:*7734, 1972

Adult burns. A three-year survey with assessment of sulfamylon (Pegg). M. J. Australia, *1:*350, 1972

Use of silver sulphadiazine in the treatment of burns at Royal Perth Hospital (McDougall). M. J. Australia, *1:*979, 1972

Burns, third degree, primary excision in (Bowe) (Follow-Up Clinic), PRS, *49:*565, 1972

Bacteriological and clinical studies of the use of sulfamylon in the treatment of burns (Brudzynska-Charewicz *et al*). Pol. Przegl. Chir., *44:*783, 1972 (Polish)

Effect of the pH of solutions used topically on the bacterial flora of burn wounds (Zietkiewicz *et al*). Pol. Tyg. Lek., *27:*949, 1972 (Polish)

Burns, topical therapy of (Ryan). Postgrad. Med., *52:*105, 1972

Burns, Topical Therapy—Cont.

Burn wound care with neosporin (Bush, Stone), PRS, *51:*482, 1973. South M. J., *65:*1083, 1972

Infection, surface, control with antibiotic-impregnated Epigard (Alexander, Sykes, Wheeler), PRS, *52:*329, 1973. Surg. Forum, *23:*36, 1972

Problems of sulfamylon treatment for burns (Shimazaki *et al*). Surg. Ther. (Osaka), *26:*589, 1972 (Japanese)

Ultra thin silicone polymer membrane: a new synthetic skin substitute. (Kornberg *et al*). Trans. Am. Soc. Artif. Intern. Organs, *18:*39, 1972

Burn wound therapy (Still, Georgiade). Am Surgeon, *39:*82, 1973

Burns, stimulation of granulation tissue in (Viljanto). Ann. Chir. Gynaec. Fenn., *62:*18, 1973

Burn wound management (Hunt *et al*). Heart, Lung, *2:*690, 1973

Burns, Sutilains ointment as topical debriding agent in (Grossman). Internat. Surg., *58:*93, 1973

Burn wound cover, prosthetic, compared with porcine heterograft (O'Neill), PRS, *54:*506, 1974. J. Pediat. Surg., *5:*705, 1973

Burned skin, absorption of Sulfamylon acetate from 5% aqueous solution (Harrison, Bales, Jacoby), PRS, *53:*685, 1974. J. Trauma, *12:*994, 1973

Epigard, clinical evaluation of (Alexander *et al*), PRS, *53:*500, 1974. J. Trauma, *13:*374, 1973

Exposure method, mortality and causes of death in burned patients treated by the (Sørensen, Hall), PRS, *51:*59, 1973

Travase, effective enzyme for burn debridement (Pennisi, Capozzi, Friedman), PRS, *51:*371, 1973

Mafenide treatment of burns in patient with glucose-6-phosphate dehydrogenase deficiency, fatal hemolysis from (Marsicano, Hutton, Bryant), PRS, *52:*197, 1973

Burn eschar and necrotic tissue, use of water-insoluble papain (WIP) for debridement of (Shapira, Giladi, Neuman), PRS, *52:*279, 1973

Dressings, use of commercial porcine skin for (Elliott, Hoehn), PRS, *52:*401, 1973

Burns, open and closed treatment with povidone-iodine (Georgiade, Harris), PRS, *52:*640, 1973. Discussion by Pruitt, PRS, *53:*82, 1973

Burn treatment with Sulfamylon cream and Sulfamylon solution (Shuck), PRS, *54:*112, 1974. Rev. Latino Am. cir. plast., *17:*75,

Burns, Topical Therapy—Cont.
1973

Burns, open air treatment (Teich-Alasia), PRS, *53:*491, 1974. Riv. ital. chir. plast., *4:*1, 1973

Sulfamylon, massive treatment in burns causing infestation and septicemia from *Candida albicans* (Ben-Hur), PRS, *53:*686, 1974. Riv. ital. chir. plast., *4:*45, 1973

Burned patients, severely, trypsin and chymotrypsin toxicity in (Ambroggio, Cavallero, Catone), PRS, *56:*361, 1975. Riv. ital. chir. plast., *5:*331, 1973

Burn wound eschar, in vitro evaluation of enzymatic debridement of (Silverstein *et al*). Surgery, *73:*15, 1973

Burn wound sepsis, experimental, evaluation of 5% Sulfamylon cream in control of (Skornik, Dressler), PRS, *53:*492, 1974. Surgery, *74:*540, 1973

Burn wounds, preparation of, for autodermatoplasty (Makarevich *et al*). Voen. Med. Zh., *1:*31, 1973 (Russian)

Burn wound in rats, effect of synthetic dressing formed on: comparison of allografts, collagen sheets, and polyhydroxyethylmethacrylate in control of wound infection (Nathan *et al*). Appl. Microbiol., *28:*465, 1974

Burns, what's new in treatment of (Melega), PRS, *55:*721, 1975. Ars Curandi, *7:*68, 1974

Burn wound, preparing and closing (Shuck). Clin. Plast. Surg., *1:*577, 1974

Burn wounds, local antibacterial therapy during preparation of, for autodermoplasty (Pakhomov *et al*). Khirurgiia (Mosk.), *9:*37, 1974 (Russian)

Antibiotics instilled locally to treat chondritis in the burned ear (Apfelberg *et al*), PRS, *53:*179, 1974

Sepsis, burn wound, experimental, topical providone-iodine ointment in (Robson, Schaerf, Krizek), PRS, *54:*328, 1974

Burned subjects and their wounds, topical lipid protection of (Jelenko *et al*), PRS, *54:*623, 1974. Surgery, *75:*892, 1974

Topical burn wound therapy (Artz *et al*). Surg. Annu., *6:*349, 1974

Development of a synthetic burn covering (Schwope *et al*). Trans. Am. Soc. Artif. Inter. Organs, *20A:*103, 1974

Synthetic products used in surgery, late effects of (Gevorkian). Zh. Eksp. Klin. Med., *14:*35, 1974

Hydrotherapy in cauterization wounds (Rothmann, Vakilzadeh, Rupec), PRS, *56:*599, 1975. Arch. Dermat. Forsch., *251:*281, 1975

Dressing, biological: treatment of thermal

Burns, Topical Therapy—Cont.

burns by amniotic membranes (Visuthikosol, Buri), PRS, *56:*232, 1975. Asian J. Mod. Med., *11:*17, 1975

Mafenide acetate solution dressings: an adjunct in burn wound care (Shuck *et al*). J. Trauma, *15:*595, 1975

Use of plastubol for the treatment of burns (Vinogradova *et al*). Khirurgiia (Mosk.), *4:*30, 1975 (Russian)

Cold water treatment as first aid in burned patients (Klasen), PRS, *57:*122, 1976. Nederl. tijdschr. geneesk., *119:*601, 1975

Laser, scalpel, electrosurgical, tangential excisions of third degree burns (Levine *et al*), PRS, *56:*256, 1975

Travase, effect on heat-injured skin (Zawacki), PRS, *56:*111, 1975. Surgery, *77:*132, 1975

Exposure, effect of: blister and second degree burn in guinea pigs (Wheeler, Miller), PRS, *57:*74, 1976

Burns, Toxins in

Burn toxins, research on (Stadtler *et al*), PRS, *50:*308, 1972. Ther. Umsch., *28:*847, 1971

Toxic substance, isolation and characterization of, produced in mouse skin by thermal energy (Cueni, Allgower, Schoenenberger), PRS, *50:*95, 1972. Zurich J. Exp. Med., *156:*110, 1971

Thermal injuries, formation of specific "burn toxin" in mouse skin by (Stadtler *et al*), PRS, *51:*482, 1973. Europ. Surg. Res., *4:*198, 1972

Burn toxic factor, purified, and its competitin (Rosenthal, Hawley, Hakim), PRS, *50:*421, 1972. Surgery, *71:*527, 1972

Endotoxin in serum, determination of (Konickova, Matejicek, Vrabec), PRS, *54:*506, 1974. Acta chir. plast., *15:*170, 1973

Toxin, burn, in mouse skin (Allgower *et al*), PRS, *53:*686, 1974. J. Trauma, *13:*95, 1973

Burns, Treatment

Contemporary Burn Management. By Hiram C. Polk, Jr. and H. Harlan Stone. Little, Brown & Co., Boston, 1971

The Management & Nursing of Burns, 2nd Ed. By J. E. Laing and J. Harvey. Medical Examination Pub. Co., Inc., Flushing, N. Y., 1971.

The Treatment of Burns: Principles & Practice. By William W. Monafo and Carlos Pappalardo. Warren H. Green, St. Louis, Mo., 1971.

Studies on burns. XV. Treatment with warm

Burns, Treatment—Cont.

dry air, clinical results compared with those of earlier treatment series (Birke *et al*). Acta Chir. Scand. (Suppl.), *422:*1, 1971

Wound, burn, and its care (Pruitt, Curreri), PRS, *49:*667, 1972. Arch. Surg., *103:*461, 1971

Treatment of severe burns (Muir). Drugs, *1:*429, 1971

Use of hyperbaric oxygen in experimental burns (Rudakov). Eksp. Khir. Anesteziol., *16:*82, 1971 (Russian)

Maribor method of burns treatment. A report on the work of Janzekovic at Maribor, Yugoslavia (Barron). Hand, *3:*179, 1971

Treatments of the granulation wounds— therapeutic experience in extensive thermal burns (Kurata *et al*). Jap. J. Plast. Reconstr. Surg., *14:*150, 1971 (Japanese)

Protective isolation in a burns unit: the use of plastic isolators and air curtains (Lowbury *et al*). J. Hyg. (Camb.), *69:*529, 1971

Treatment of thermal burns (Hirayama). J. Jap. Med. Assoc., *66:*490, 1971 (Japanese)

Comments on current burn therapy (Shea). J. Med. Assoc. Ga., *60:*373, 1971

Burns, severe, general care of (Ahnefeld), PRS, *50:*204, 1972. Langenbecks Arch. Chir., *329:*900, 1971

Hyperbaric oxygen therapy in a caisson using pure oxygen (Hanquet *et al*). Laval. Med., *42:*647, 1971 (French)

Effects of cooling on the microvasculature after thermal injury (Wiedeman *et al*). Microvasc. Res., *3:*154, 1971

Experimental basis of typical treatment of burns. II (Kohnlein). Monatsschr. Unfallheilkd., *74:*507, 1971 (German)

Therapeutic experience in heat-press injury (Ishida *et al*). Orthop. Surg. (Tokyo), *22:*878, 1971 (Japanese)

Restoration of the function of the upper extremities in deformities following burns (Grigor'ev *et al*). Ortop. Travmatol. Protez., *32:*15, 1971 (Russian)

Burned children, evaluation of a non-narcotic analgesic, pentazocine, in (Wilson, Priano, Traber), PRS, *48:*466, 1971

Neovascularization, stimulation of, comparative efficacy of fresh and preserved skin grafts (O'Donoghue, Zarem), PRS, *48:*474, 1971

Use of venous bed of bones for multiple transfusion of blood and other fluids in patients with extensive burns (Atiasov). Probl. Gematol. Pereliv. Krovi., *16:*53, 1971 (Russian)

Burns, treatment of today (Evans), PRS,

Burns, Treatment—Cont.

*50:*203, 1972. Proc. Roy. Soc. Med., *64:*1295, 1971

Surgical treatment of burns (Kracmer *et al*). Rozhl. Chir., *50:*595, 1971 (Czechoslovakian)

Therapy of burns in Egypt (Vrabec). Rozhl. Chir., *50:*652, 1971 (Czechoslovakian)

Oral zinc therapy in thermal burns (Lawhorn *et al*). South. Med. J., *64:*1538, 1971

First aid in mass treatment of burns (Tasic). Srp. Arh. Celok. Lek., *99:*51, 1971 (Serbian)

Burn therapy—current appraisal (Haynes). Surg. Annu., *3:*125, 1971

Deep dermal burns treated by excision, skin grafts, and tri-iodothyronine (Zamick *et al*). Surg. Forum, *22:*491, 1971

Burned children, severely, simple method for the continuous evaluation of the urinary output in (Goris), PRS, *49:*107, 1972. Surg. Gynec. & Obst., *132:*695, 1971

Treatment of serious burns (Malm). Tidsskr. Nor. Laegeforen, *91:*2033, 1971 (Norwegian)

Principles of regional treatment of burns (Mindikoglu). Turk. Tip. Cemiy. Mecm., *37:*107, 1971 (Turkish)

Modified apparatus for intraosseous infusions and irrigation of burns (Varavva). Vestn. Khir., *106:*107, 1971 (Russian)

Errors in the treatment of burns (Schraiber). Voen. Med. Zh., *8:*24, 1971 (Russian)

Comparative evaluation of the detoxification properties of different transfusion media during the treatment of burns (Fomina). Voen. Med. Zh., *8:*35, 1971 (Russian)

Indications for using direct blood transfusions in burns (Atanasov). Vrach. Delo., *7:*73, 1971 (Russian)

Antibiotics and corticosteroids in the corticosteroids treatment of burns (Wittels). Wien. Klin. Wochenschr., *83:*936, 1971 (German)

First aid in skin burns (Hochleitner). Z. Allgemeinmed. *47:*1438, 1971 (German)

Burns and their treatment (Wittels). Z. Haut. Geschlechtskr., *46:*761, 1971 (German)

Results in the treatment of burns (Reding). Zentralbl. Chir., *96:*1032, 1971 (German)

Nursing Care of the Patient with Burns. By Florence G. Jacoby. C. V. Mosby Co., St. Louis, 1972.

Burns, thermal, current management (Pruitt, Moylan). Adv. Surg., *6:*237, 1972

Use of an air-fluidized bed in the care of patients with extensive burns (Newsome *et al*). Am. J. Surg., *124:*52, 1972

Burns, Treatment—Cont.

Value of "tissue circulation" treatment in plastic and reconstructive surgery. Results with Hydrosarpan 711. Comparison with placebo (Laurencon *et al*). Ann. chir. plast., *17:*221, 1972 (French)

Muscle transposition in deep localized burns (Ger *et al*). Arch. Surg., *104:*710, 1972

Analgesia for burnt patients: a symposium. Brit. Med. J., *2:*418, 1972

Indications for and technic of suspension therapy of injured extremities (Zollinger *et al*). Helv. Chir. Acta, *39:*367, 1972 (German)

Burns, treatment of, at Karolinska Hospital (Liljedahl). Int. J. Vitam. Nutr. Res., *12:*184, 1972 (German)

Decompression dermotomy (Gaspard, Cohen, Gaspar), PRS, *50:*538, 1972. J.A.M.A., *220:*831, 1972

Disordered blood coagulation in burned children receiving high molecular weight dextran (Thomas *et al*). J. Clin. Pathol., *25:*473, 1972

Nutrition in the burned patient (Love). J. Miss. State Med. Assoc., *13:*391, 1972

Aggressive outpatient care of burns (Nance *et al*). J. Trauma, *12:*144, 1972

Burns: analysis of results of physical therapy in 681 patients (Dobbs, Curreri), PRS, *52:*101, 1973. J. Trauma, *12:*242, 1972

Burn formulae, Evans formula revisited (Hutcher, Haynes), PRS, *52:*101, 1973. J. Trauma, *12:*453, 1972

Burn formulae (Moncrief). J. Trauma, *12:*538, 1972

Burns, plastic surgery for in the middle-aged and elderly (Lomakin). Khirurgiia, *49:*17, 1972

Burn injuries, current treatment methods in (Zellner). Krankenpflege, *26:*47, 1972 (German)

Blood-volume changes and transfusion requirements of burned patients after the shock phase of injury (Hinton *et al*). Lancet, *1:*913, 1972

Burns and hyperbaric oxygenation (Sosath). Med. Klin., *67:*1638, 1972 (German)

Therapy of burn injuries (Zellner). Med. Klin., *67:*657, 1972 (German)

Therapy of severe burns (Bohmert *et al*). Med. Welt., *23:*871, 1972 (German)

Care of burned victims (Bernstein). New England J. Med., *286:*101, 1972

Treatment of burns in a non-urban community hospital (Smith *et al*). Northwest. Med., *71:*103, 1972

Terms of dermoplasty of burn wounds in children (based on cytology of wound exudate)

Burns, Treatment—Cont.

(Edinak). Ortop. Travmatol. Protez., *33:*11, 1972 (Russian)

Tris buffer in severe burns (Cramer) (Follow-Up Clinic), PRS, *50:*401, 1972

Burned surface, early surgical treatment (Janzekovic). Panminerva Med., *14:*228, 1972

Considerations on the surgical treatment of deep burns (4th degree) (Ionesco *et al*). Panminerva Med., *14:*237, 1972

Burned surface, surgical repair and reconstruction (Damiani *et al*). Panminerva Med., *14:*245, 1972

Surgery and life-preservation (Allgower). Praxis, *61:*1255, 1972 (German)

Wound excision and closure as applied to burns (Jackson), PRS, *50:*204, 1972. Proc. Roy. Soc. Med., *65:*23, 1972

Effect of exercise therapy on rheographic values in patients with burns (Zubenko). Vrach. Delo., *4:*131, 1972 (Russian)

Symposium on the Treatment of Burns, Volume 5. Ed. by John B. Lynch and Stephen R. Lewis. C. V. Mosby Co., St. Louis, 1973. PRS, *53:*585, 1974

Burned feet in children, acute and reconstructive care (Heimburger *et al*), PRS, *52:*684, 1973. Am. J. Surg., *125:*575, 1973

Burns, bactericidal effect of air-fluidized bed (Sharbaugh, Gargest, Wright), PRS, *52:*602, 1973. Am. Surgeon, *39:*253, 1973

Burned child, aspects of management of (Overton *et al*). Anaesth. Intensive Care, *1:*535, 1973

Burns, extensive, in children, medical aspect of treatment of, 8 cases (Cloup *et al*). Ann. chir. plast., *18:*325, 1973 (French)

Burn patients, 10% intravenous fat emulsion for parenteral nutrition (Wilmore *et al*), PRS, *53:*686, 1974. Ann. Surg., *178:*503, 1973

Burn management, acute, pulmonary artery pressure monitoring (German, Allyn, Bartlett), PRS, *53:*370, 1974. Arch. Surg., *106:*788, 1973

Burns, severe, experiences in treatment of (Koehnlein, Härtwig, Hartung), PRS, *53:*370, 1974. Bull. Soc. Internat. Chir., *32:*509, 1973

Treatment of extensive 3rd degree burns. Chinese Med. J., *4:*195, 1973

Successful treatment in a case of extensive deep burns. Chinese Med. J., *4:*205, 1973

Treatment of deep burns by shaving off eschars. Chinese Med. J., *4:*208, 1973

Burn therapy in foreign countries. Chinese Med. J., *4:*241, 1973

Burns, extensive third degree, review of

Burns, Treatment—Cont.

management for 14 years (Chinese PLA Burns Unit), PRS, *54:*241, 1974. Chinese M. J., *11:*148, 1973

Review on management of extensive third degree burns. Chinese Med. J., *11:*673, 1973 (Chinese)

Burn unit, specialized, to treat Lyell's syndrome (Tubiana *et al*), PRS, *52:*456, 1973. Chirurgie, *99:*40, 1973

Burn patient, care of, modern trends in (Polk). D. M., *1:*39, 1973

Burns in childhood, surgical treatment (Helbig). Fortschr. Med., *91:*982, 1973 (German)

Heparin to treat large burns in humans (Saliba, Dempsey, Kruggel), PRS, *53:*246, 1974 J.A.M.A., *225:*261, 1973

Heparinization for disseminated intravascular coagulation (Barrocas), PRS, *52:*208, 1973. Mil. Med., *138:*9, 1973

Burns, treatment of extensive deep by surgery (Deutschmann). Munch. Med. Wochenschr., *115:*395, 1973

Burns, thermal, modern principles of therapy of patients with (Grigor'ev). Ortop. Travmatol. Protez., *34:*1, 1973 (Russian)

Burns, deep, extensive, active surgical treatment in (Pakhomov). Ortop. Travmatol. Protez., *34:*13, 1973 (Russian)

Burns, patients with, experience with active surgical treatment of (Galustov). Ortop. Travmatol. Protez., *34:*49, 1973 (Russian)

Burns, active surgical treatment (Iakushev). Ortop. Travmatol. Protez., *34:*51, 1973 (Russian)

Burns, experience with work of children's units for treatment of, and norms for their demand (Vozdvizhenskii *et al*). Ortop. Travmatol. Protez., *34:*69, 1973 (Russian)

Burns, dorsal, of hand, dynamic splinting for (Salisbury, Palm), PRS, *51:*226, 1973

Burned patients: thermal regulation in patients after the healing of large deep burns (McGibbon *et al*), PRS, *52:*164, 1973

Burns, late periods of, personal experiences in treatment (Kobus *et al*). Pol. Tyg. Lek., *28:*1811, 1973 (Polish)

Burns in infants, prognosis and therapy (Burkhardt), PRS, *53:*608, 1974. Riv. ital. chir. plast., *4:*27, 1973

Edema formation in experimental burns, effect of dimethyl sulfoxide (DMSO) on (Arturson, Ponten), PRS, *54:*696, 1974. Scand. J. Plast. Reconstr. Surg., *7:*74, 1973

Burn patient care, use of biopsies (Pruitt, Foley), PRS, *52:*683, 1973. Surgery, *73:*887, 1973

Treatment of thermal injuries (Castillo).

Burns, Treatment—Cont.

Surg. Clin. North Am., *53:*627, 1973

Burns, massive, hemodialysis in management of (Bartlett *et al*). Trans. Am. Soc. Artif. Intern. Organs, *19:*269, 1973

Burns, skeletal suspension in treatment of (Matchin). Vestn. Khir., *111:*79, 1973 (Russian)

The Splinting of Burn Patients. By K. M. P. Von Prince and M. Yaekel. Charles C Thomas, Springfield, Ill., 1974. PRS, *56:*664, 1975

Burn management, current practices in (Shuck). Am. Surg., *40:*145, 1974

Burned child, extensively, use of controlled hypotension for primary surgical excision (Szyfelbein, Ryan), PRS, *55:*515, 1975. Anesthesiology, *41:*501, 1974

Burned child, parenteral nutrition of (Popp, Law, MacMillan), PRS, *54:*378, 1974. Ann. Surg., *179:*219, 1974

Burns, prevention of necrosis and reversal of capillary stasis (Zawacki), PRS, *55:*113, 1975. Ann. Surg., *180:*98, 1974

Burn patient, overall treatment of (Melega *et al*), PRS, *55:*722, 1975. Ars Curandi, *7:*10, 1974

Burns, first care in treatment (Bastos, Carvalho), PRS, *55:*721, 1975. Ars Curandi, *7:*15, 1974

Burn units, hospital (Marcondes, Rufatto), PRS, *55:*721, 1975. Ars Curandi, *7:*64, 1974

Preparing and closing the burn wound (Shuck). Clin. Plast. Surg., *1:*577, 1974

Burn therapy and trauma at Dallas, PRS, *55:*384, 1975. Contemp. Surg., *4:*31, 1974

Burns in childhood, treatment (Heikkinen). Duodecim, *90:*262, 1974 (Finnish)

Burn treatment methods compared by probit analysis (Waisbren, Stein, Collentine), PRS, *56:*232, 1975. J.A.M.A., *231:*255, 1974

Burns, extensive, treatment (Zawacki). New England J. Med., *290:*862, 1974

Burns, enormous deep, success in healing and saving lives in patients with (McDowell) (Editorial), PRS, *54:*209, 1974

Burns and treatment of thermal injuries, present and future trends in research on (Rudowski). Pol. Przegl. Chir., *46:*73, 1974 (Polish)

Burns, thermal, early management (Baxter *et al*). Postgrad. Med., *55:*131, 1974

Burn therapy, recent progress in (Donati), PRS, *57:*401, 1976. Riv. ital. chir. plast., *6:*41, 1974

Burns, surgical treatment of, modern orientations (Teich-Alasia), PRS, *57:*676, 1976. Riv. ital. chir. plast., *6:*279, 1974

Lower extremities, poorly healing wounds of,

Burns, Treatment — Cont.

complex treatment of (Jezek *et al*). Rozhl. Chir., *53:*635, 1974 (Czechoslovakian)

Burns, treatment of (Munchhoff). Schwest. Rev., *12:*26, 1974

Burns, plastic surgery and (Weeks). Surg. Gynec. & Obstet., *138:*212, 1974

Burns, patients with, use of multiple systemic antibiotics in treatment of (Hartford *et al*). Surg. Gynec. & Obstet., *138:*837, 1974

Burns, anabolic effects of human growth hormone and high caloric feedings following (Wilmore *et al*), PRS, *55:*112, 1975. Surg. Gynec. & Obst., *138:*875, 1974

Treatment of burns with hyperbaric oxygen (Hart *et al*). Surg. Gynec. & Obstet., *139:*693, 1974

Burns (Thomsen). Zentralbl. Chir., *99:*1098, 1974 (German)

Burns, thermal, in children, characteristics of treatment of (Klimenko *et al*). Klin. Khir., *3:*38, 1975 (Russian)

Past and present management burns (Janzekovic). Magy. Traumatol. Orthop., *18:*260, 1975 (Hungarian)

Burned patients, treatment of (Huffstadt, Klasen, Eisma), PRS, *57:*263, 1976. Nederl. tijdschr. geneesk., *119:*595, 1975

Outcome of the treatment of the wounded of the G. K. Zhukov Partisan Unit in Ukraine (Ermakov). Ortop. Travmatol. Protez., *4:*81, 1975 (Russian)

Bath-bed for burn management (McComb, Annear), PRS, *55:*102, 1975

Burns, plasma scalpel excision of (Link, Zook, Glover), PRS, *55:*657, 1975

Burns, mud bed in treatment of (Caffee, Zawacki), PRS, *56:*456, 1975

Burned child, evaluation and treatment of (O'Neill), PRS, *57:*121, 1976. Pediat. Clin. N. Am., *22:*407, 1975

Present-time problems of the treatment of burns (Orlov *et al*). Vestn. Khir., *114:*69, 1975 (Russian)

Results of treatment of patients with deep burns (Iukhin *et al*). Vestn. Khir., *114:*78, 1975 (Russian)

Child, burned, misery of (McDowell) (Editorial), PRS, *57:*369, 1976

Behavior modification therapy in recalcitrant burned child, use of (Zide, Pardoe), PRS, *57:*378, 1976

BURPEE, J. F., AND EDWARDS, P.: Fournier's gangrene, PRS, *50:*633, 1972. J. Urol., *107:*812, 1972

BURRIE, C., HENKEMEYER, H., AND RUEDI, T.:

Surgical treatment of infected bone defects, PRS, *49:*588, 1972. Langenbeck's Arch. Chir., *330:*54, 1971

BURSTON, W. R.: Presurgical facial orthopaedics in relationship to the overall management of cleft lip and palate conditions. Ann. R. Coll. Surg. Engl., *48:*31, 1971

BURT, G. B.: Role of steroids in prevention of circumferential capsular scarring in augmentation mammaplasty (with Peterson), PRS, *54:*28, 1974

BURTON, D. S. *et al:* Surgical treatment of malignant soft-tissue tumors of the extremities in the adult. Clin. Orthop., *84:*144, 1972

BURTON, F. C.: Versatile mammaplasty pattern of Wise (with Parsons, Shaw), PRS, *55:*1, 1975

BURTON, R. I.: Implant arthroplasty in the hand. An introduction. Orthop. Clin. North Am., *4:*313, 1973

BURTON, R. I. *et al:* Common hand injuries in the athlete. Orthop. Clin. North Am., *4:*809, 1973

BURTON, R. I., AND LITTLER, J. W.: Nontraumatic soft tissue afflictions of hand, PRS, *57:*534, 1976. Curr. Probl. Surg., *5:*56, 1975

BURZYNSKI, N. J. *et al:* Craniocarpotarsal dysplasia syndrome, PRS, *57:*528, 1976. Oral Surg., *39:*893, 1975

BUSCHMANN, A: Incurable case in the area of facial surgery. Fortschr. Med., *92:*1063, 1974 (German)

BUSCHMANN, A.: Problems of plastic and reconstructive surgery in the face. Fortschr. Med., *93:*1691, 1975 (German)

BUSCHMANN, A.: Surgery of hypospadias, Langenbecks Arch. Chir., *339:*417, 1975 (German)

BUSH, C. A., AND STONE, H. H.: Care of burn wound with neosporin, PRS, *51:*482, 1973. South. M. J., *65:*1083, 1972

BUSH, G. H.: Problems of anaesthesia in the burnt child. Postgrad. Med. J., *48:*148, 1972

BUSSCHOP, J. *et al:* Technic of free autologous mucosal grafts. Rev. Belge. Med. Dent., *30:*215, 1975 (Dutch)

BUSSOLATI, G., AND PICH, A.: Mammary and extramammary Paget's disease, PRS, *57:*260, 1976. Am. J. Clin. Path., *80:*117, 1975

BUTIUKOVA, V. A.: Blunt injuries to the soft tissues of the orbit. Oftalmol. Zh., *26:*609, 1971 (Russian)

BUTLER, B. JR.: Initial management of hand wounds. Mil. Med., *134:*1, 1969

BUTLER, C.: Salivary gland tumours. J. Laryng. & Otol., *86:*775, 1972

BUTLER, N. R., PECKHAM, C., AND SHERIDAN,

M.: Speech defects in children, aged 7: national study, PRS, *52:*455, 1973. Brit. M. J., *1:*253, 1973

BUTSON, A. R. C.: Effects and prevention of frostbite in wound healing, PRS, *56:*599, 1975. Canad. J. Surg., *18:*145, 1975

BUTTERS, A. G. *et al:* Free skin grafts on the parietal pleura; report of a case. Brit. J. Plast. Surg., *24:*412, 1971

BUTTERWORTH, R. F. *et al:* Device for treating pressure sores around the ankle. M. J. Australia, *2:*1135, 1971

Buttock (See also *Battered Child Syndrome; Lipodystrophy; Pilonidal Cysts*)

Sacroiliac region, topography of fat in (Georgiadis, Katsas), PRS, *49:*110, 1972. Acta Chir. Hellenica, *18:*289, 1971

Technics and hazards of intragluteal injections (Schierhorn). Dtsch. Gesundheitsw. *26:*2360, 1971 (German)

Dermolipectomies crurales (Pitanguy). Ann. chir. plast., *17:*40, 1972 (French)

Battered buttock syndrome – fat fractures. A report on a group of traumatic lipomata (Meggitt *et al*). Brit. J. Surg., *59:*165, 1972

Traumatic displacement of fat. Brit. Med. J., *2:*309, 1972

Battered buttock syndrome. Can. Med. Assoc. J., *106:*1280, 1972

Ischemic necrosis of muscles of the buttock. A case report (Kaufman *et al*). J. Bone & Joint Surg. (Am.), *54:*1079, 1972

Surgical correction of the Duchenne-Trendelenburg phenomenon (Fishkin *et al*). Ortop. Travmatol. Protez., *33:*6, 1972 (Russian)

Total-thigh flap, alternative to, for coverage of massive decubitus ulcers (Burkhardt), PRS, *49:*433, 1972

Fibrinolysis in lymphangioma (Kornfalt *et al*). Acta Paediatr. Scand., *62:*538, 1973

Cruro-femoro-gluteal or circumgluteal plasty (Delerm, Cirotteau). Ann. chir. plast., *18:*31, 1973 (French)

Sarcoma of buttock, reappraisal of surgical management (Wanebo *et al*), PRS, *52:*460, 1973. Cancer, *31:*97, 1973

Gluteal augmentation (Cocke, Ricketson), PRS, *52:*93, 1973

Granuloma, aluminum hydroxide (Savage), PRS, *54:*118, 1974. Proc. Roy. Soc. Med., *66:*984, 1973

Weber-Christian disease, soft tissue defects in (McCabe *et al*). Brit. J. Plast. Surg., *27:*107, 1974

Sacral area in young paraplegics, use of long

Buttock – Cont.

island flap to bring sensation to (Dibbell), PRS, *54:*220, 1974

Treatment of steatomery in the female: theory and practice (Vilain). Ann. chir. plast., *20:*135, 1975 (French)

Surgical correction of steatomeries (Vilain). Clin. Plast. Surg., *2:*449, 1975

Plastic surgery in treatment of obesity (Muhlbauer). Munch. Med. Wochenschr., *117:*747, 1975

Thigh and hip deformity, experience with Pitanguy method of correction of trochanteric lipodystrophy (Hoffman, Simon), PRS, *55:*551, 1975

Buttock, unusual congenital dermal sinus of (Rigg, Martyn), PRS, *56:*581, 1975

Plastic surgical treatment of obesity (Sanders). Proc. R. Soc. Med., *68:*664, 1975

Body sculpturing (Tearston *et al*). Surg. Clin. North Am., *55:*151, 1975

BUZELIN, J. M. *et al:* Management of penoscrotal skin avulsions. Ann. Urol. (Paris), *5:*263, 1971 (French)

BYERLY, W. G., AND PENDSE, P. D.: War surgery in forward surgical hospital in Vietnam: continuing report, PRS *48:*612, 1971. Mil. Med., *136:*221, 1971

BYERS, R. M. *et al:* Malignant tumors of submaxillary gland, PRS, *53:*682, 1974. Am. J. Surg., *126:*458, 1973

BYRD, D. L., KINDRICK, R. D., AND DUNSWORTH A. R.: Myxoma of maxilla: report of case. J. Oral Surg., *31:*123, 1973

BYRD, D. L., ALLEN, J. W., AND DUNSWORTH, A. R.: Ameloblastoma originating in wall of primordial cyst: report of case. J. Oral Surg., *31:*301, 1973

BYRHE, R. P. *et al:* Transpositional genioplasty. J. Oral Surg., *32:*145, 1974

BYRNE, J. E. *et al:* Corrosion of metal fracture fixation appliances. J. Oral Surg., *31:*639, 1973

BYRNE, M. P., KOSMALA, R. L., AND CUNNINGHAM, M. P.: Ameloblastoma with regional and distant metastases, PRS, *57:*540, 1976. Am. J. Surg., *128:*91, 1974

BYRNE, R. P. *et al:* Ramus "C" osteotomy with body sagittal split. J. Oral Surg., *32:*259, 1974

BYSTRENIN, V. A. *et al:* Use of a correcting negative mask in cosmetic operations on the external nose. Vestn. Otorinolaringol., *1:*43, 1975 (Russian)

BYSTROM, E. B., SANGER, R. G., AND STEWART, R.: Syndrome of ectrodactyly, ectodermal dysplasia, and clefting, PRS, 57:543, 1976. J. Oral Surg., 33:192, 1975

BYSTROM, J. et al: Induratio penis plastica (Peyronie's disease). Results after excision and dermofat grafting, PRS, 54:691, 1974. Scand. J. Plast. Reconstr. Surg., 7:137, 1973

BZOCH, KENNETH R.: Communicative Disorders Related to Cleft Lip and Palate. Little, Brown & Co., Boston, 1972. PRS, 52:572, 1973

C

CABREAR TRIGO, J. S.: Reconstructive hemilaryngectomy, PRS, 48:294, 1971. Prensa méd. argent., 57:1946, 1970

CABY, F.: Supplement to the cutaneous homograft case report presented in 1950. Chirurgie, 97:722, 1971 (French)

CACHIN, Y. et al: Results of surgical treatment of cancers of hypopharynx. Experience at Institut Gustave-Roussy, Villejuif, 1960–1970. Acta Otorhinolaryngol. Belg., 27:1010, 1973 (French)

CACHIN, Y. et al: Giant mixed parotid tumor. Ann. Otolaryngol. Chir. Cervicofac., 90:363, 1973 (French)

CACHIN, Y. et al: Combination of radiotherapy and surgery in the treatment of head and neck cancers. Cancer Treat. Rev., 2:177, 1975

CADARIU, E. et al: Free nerve graft in case of facial paralysis after petro-mastoid evidement (functional recovery). Otorinolaringologie, 18:121, 1973 (Rumanian)

CADENAT, H. et al: Laterognathism due to condylar agenesis treated with functional equipment. Orthod. Fr., 41:289, 1970 (French)

CADENAT, H. et al: Use of Muller's plates (A-O technic) in mandibular fractures. Rev. Stomatol. Chir. Maxillofac., 72:483, 1971 (French)

CADENAT, H. et al: Case of labio-mental hemangiopericytoma. Rev. Stomatol. Chir. Maxillofac., 73:49, 1972 (French)

CADENAT, H. et al: Tongue flaps, vascularization, morphology and use. Ann. chir. plast., 18:223, 1973 (French)

CADENAT H. et al: Results of the use of Muller plates in mandibular osteosynthesis. Rev. Stomatol. Chir. Maxillofac., 74:230, 1973 (French)

CADENAT, H. et al: Preoperative prosthesis in hemi resections of the maxillary bone. Rev. Stomatol. Chir. Maxillofac., 74:682, 1973 (French)

CADENAT, H. et al: Tongue flaps in plastic surgery. Rev. Stomatol. Chir. Maxillofac., 74:690, 1973 (French)

CADENAT, H. et al: Use of Kirschner wires in facial fractures. Rev. Stomatol. Chir. Maxillofac., 74:698, 1973 (French)

CADENAT, H. et al: Orthopedic treatment of cleft lip and palate in the newborn. Rev. Stomatol. Chir. Maxillofac., 74:706, 1973 (French)

CADENAT, H. et al: Management of a mandibular ameloblastoma recurrence. Rev. Stomatol. Chir. Maxillofac., 75:65, 1974 (French)

CADENAT, H. et al: Technic of closures of orostomes in irradiated skin. Rev. Stomatol. Chir. Maxillofac., 75:222, 1974 (French)

CADENAT, H. et al: Access to the pharyngeal extension of the parotid. Rev. Stomatol. Chir. Maxillofac. 75:893, 1974 (French)

CADY, B. et al: Contemporary treatment of malignant melanoma. Am. J. Surg., 129:472, 1975

CAFFEE, H. H., AND ZAWACKI, B. E.: Use of mud bed in treatment of burns, PRS, 56:456, 1975

CAGIE, J. D. et al: Radionuclide, radiographic and histologic evaluation of mandibular bone grafts, PRS, 55:716, 1975. J. Maxillo-facial Surg., 2:179, 1974

CAHAN, W. G.: Surgical management of melanoma metastatic to the lung: problems in diagnosis and management. Prog. Clin. Cancer, 6:205, 1975

CAHOON, J. R. et al: Concept of protection potential applied to corrosion of metallic orthopedic implants, PRS, 57:266, 1976. J. Biomed. Mater. Res., 9:259, 1975

CAHUZAC, M. et al: Our experience in treatment of hypospadias. Surgical technic. Apropos of 195 cases. Chirurgie, 98:148, 1972 (French)

CAHUZAC, M. et al: Hand surgery in infantile hemiplegia; technics – results. Chirurgie, 99:859, 1973 (French)

CAHUZAC, M. et al: Hemiplegic hand in children with cerebral palsy. Place of surgical treatment. Rev. Chir. Orthop., 59:321, 1973 (French)

CAILLIET, RENE: Hand: Pain and Impairment. F. A. Davis Co., Philadelphia, 1971. PRS, 49:452, 1972. 2nd edition, 1975

CAILLIET, RENE: Knee Pain and Disability. F. A. Davis Co., Philadelphia, 1973. PRS, 55:86, 1975

CAIRNS, A. B. JR.: Dermal grafts – a viable alternative. Trans. Am. Acad. Ophthalmol. Otolaryngol., 80:510, 1975

CAJGFINGER, H. et al: Septoplasty or reposition of the nasal septum, basic element of rhinoplasty (its functional and esthetic value). J. Med. Lyon, 52:1513, 1971 (French)

CAJGFINGER, H. *et al:* Dislocation of cartilaginous nasal septum in newborn infants. J. Fr. Otorhinolaryngol., *22:*62, 1973 (French)

CAJGFINGER, H. *et al:* Further case of fibrous dysplasia of face with misleading symptomatology. J. Fr. Otorhinolaryngol., *22:*67, 1973 (French)

CAJKOVA, E.: Problems of facial paralysis in children. Cesk. Pediatr., *29:*488, 1974 (Slovakian)

CALABRESE, C. T., WINSLOW, R. B., AND LATHAM, R. A.: Altering the dimensions of the canine face by the induction of new bone formation, PRS, *54:*467, 1974

CALABRETTA, A. M. *et al:* Treatment of facial fractures. Pa. Med., *77:*62, 1974

CALAMEL, P. M.: Median transit tongue flap, PRS, *51:*315, 1973

CALAS, E.: Tissue repair in atonic ulcerations of the lower limbs. Angieologie, *23:*143, 1971 (French)

CALATRAVA, L.: Curative treatment of malignant midline granuloma of face, PRS, *57:*539, 1976. J. Maxillo-facial Surg., *3:*160, 1975

CALBERG, G.: Surgical anatomy, kinesiology and propedeutics of the hand. Brux. Med., *51:*329, 1971 (French)

CALBERG, G.: Burned hand. Current ideas on burns of the hand. Brux. Med., *54:*265, 1974 (French)

CALCATERRA, T. C.: Antral-ethmoid decompression of endocrine exophthalmos. Ann. Ophth., *3:*1004, 1971

CALCATERRA, T. C., CHERNEY, E. F., AND SAFFOURI, M.: Cutaneous vascular anatomy of pectoral skin flaps, PRS, *53:*613, 1974. Ann. Otol. Rhin. & Laryng., *82:*691, 1973

CALCATERRA. T. C. *et al:* Forehead reconstruction with silicone elastomer sponge. Arch. Otolaryng., *98:*389, 1973

CALCATERRA, T. C. *et al:* Neurilemmoma of the sphenoid sinus. Arch. Otolaryng., *100:*383, 1974

CALCATERRA, T. *et al:* Dysphagia secondary to cricopharyngeal muscle dysfunction, surgical management. Arch. Otolaryng., *101:*726, 1975

CALCATERRA, T. C. *et al:* Antral-ethmoidal decompression in Graves' disease. Five-year experience. West. J. Med., *124:*87, 1976

CALDANI, P. *et al:* Technic for rapid grafting of large surfaces. Minerva Chir., *26:*1390, 1971 (Italian)

CALDARELLI, D. D. *et al:* Hemangiopericytoma of the maxilla. Arch. Otolaryng., *102:*49, 1976

CALDAROLA, L. *et al:* Radical neck dissection in advanced tumors of the head and neck. Considerations on 52 cases. Cancro, *27:*187, 1974 (Italian)

CALDWELL, F. T. *et al:* What constitutes proper solution for resuscitation of severely burned patient? PRS, *50:*541, 1972. Am. J. Surg., *122:*655, 1971

CALDWELL, F. T. *et al:* On failure of heat production in immediate postburn period, PRS, *50:*205, 1972. J. Trauma, *11:*936, 1971

CALDWELL, R. D. *et al:* Clinical Pathological Conference. Case 6. Carcinoma of maxillary antrum in 8-year-old child. J. Oral Surg., *32:*367, 1974

CALENOFF, L.: Angiography of the hand: guidelines for interpretation. Radiology, *102:*331, 1972

CALLAHAN, A.: Correction of unilateral blepharoptosis with bilateral eyelid suspension. Am. J. Ophth., *74:*321, 1972

CALLAHAN, A.: Correction of complications after levator resections for blepharoptosis, PRS, *52:*616, 1973

CALLAHAN, A.: Surgical correction of blepharophimosis syndromes. Trans. Am. Acad. Ophthalmol. Otolaryngol., *77:*687, 1973

CALLI, L. J. JR.: Cleft lip/palate with tetralogy of Fallot. Birth Defects, *7:*261, 1971

Calluses (See also *Plantar Warts*)

    Callus, painful metatarsal, treatment of the chronic by a tendon transfer (Kiehn, Earle, Des Prez), PRS, *51:*154, 1973

    Calluses, plantar, plantar warts, and such (McDowell) (Editorial), PRS, *51:*196, 1973

CALVERLEY, R. K.: Repeated methoxyflurane analgesia for burns dressings. Brit. J. Anaesth., *44:*628, 1972

CAMERON, H. U., PILLIAR, R. M., AND MCNAB, I.: Effect of movement on bonding of porous metal to bone, PRS, *53:*375, 1974. J. Biomed. Mater. Res., *7:*301, 1973

CAMERON, J. D.: Treatment of glass injuries to the hand at work. Hand, *2:*52, 1970

CAMERON, J. D.: Cases of severe vascular injury to the hand. Hand, *2:*74, 1970

CAMERON, J. L., REYNOLDS, J., AND ZUIDEMA, G. D.: Aspiration in patients with tracheostomies, PRS, *52:*206, 1973. Surg. Gynec. & Obst., *136:*68, 1973

CAMERON, J. STEWART: *Proceedings of the European Dialysis and Transplant Association.* Vol. VIII. Williams & Wilkins Co., Baltimore, 1972, PRS, *51:*687, 1973

CAMERON, P.: Mood as indicant of happiness: age, sex, social class, and situational differences, PRS, *57:*267, 1976. J. Gerontol., *30:*216, 1975

CAMERON, R. R.: Restoring the overhang of the upper lip in repairs of the oral commissure (with Wall, Latham), PRS, 49:626, 1972

CAMERON, R. R., CONRAD, R. N., AND LATHAM, W. D.: Preserved composite tendon allografts: development of circulation, PRS, 48:94, 1971. Woman Physician, 25:788, 1970

CAMERON, R. R., LITTON, C., CONRAD, R. N., AND LATHAM, W. D.: Use of dermal flaps for attachment of rhytidoplasty flaps, PRS, 51:596, 1973

CAMERON, R. R., LATHAM, W. D., AND DOWLING, J. A.: Reconstructions of the nose and upper lip with nasolabial flaps, PRS, 52:145, 1973

CAMILLO, A. A.: Radionecrosis of jaws: its prophylaxis, PRS, 48:603, 1971. Rev. port. Oral. Surg., 2:207, 1970

CAMINITI, G.: Peridural anesthesia in arterial diseases of lower limbs. Minerva Anestesiol., 40:313, 1974

CAMMACK, K. V. et al: Advanced neoplasms of head and neck. Treatment with combined radiation and chemotherapy. Rocky Mt. Med. J., 69:54, 1972

CAMPAILLA, E. et al: Note on skeletal lesions in scleroderma with three case reports. Bull. Hosp. Joint Dis., 32:100, 1971

CAMPBELL, P. M. et al: Orthodontically corrected midline diastemas. A histologic study and surgical procedure. Am. J. Orthod., 67:139, 1975

CAMPBELL, R. L. et al: Primary reticulum-cell sarcoma of mandible. Review of literature and report of case. Oral Surg., 39:918, 1975

CAMPBELL, R. M.: Dermatome grafting of the totally denuded testes (Follow-Up Clinic), PRS, 50:280, 1972

CAMPO, R. D.: Incorporation and tolerance of Dacron felt in bones of rabbits (with Crouse, Kodsi), PRS, 54:471, 1974

CAMPO-PAYSAA, A.: Treatment of bladder exstrophy. Bladder reconstruction. Osteotomy. Ann Chir. Infant., 12:387, 1971 (French)

CANALE, T. J., AND COX, R. H.: Decompression of the facial nerve in Melkersson's syndrome, PRS, 55:715, 1975. Arch. Otolaryng., 100:373, 1974

Cancer (See also Anatomical Areas; Neoplasms)

Nevocarcinomas, clinical experience with chemotherapy in treatment of (Banzet, Dufourmentel, Pailheret), PRS, 50:636, 1972. Acta chir. belg., 70:401, 1971

Metastasis of V2 carcinoma in rabbits, effect of Dextran on (Schatten) (Follow-Up Clinic), PRS, 50:78, 1972

Cancer – Cont.

Tumors, solid malignant, localized leukocyte mobilization in patients with (Steiner et al), PRS, 51:484, 1973. Schweiz. med. Wchnschr., 102:1165, 1972

Mitomycin-C in treatment of advanced malignant tumors (Tepmongkol), PRS, 52:213, 1973. Siriraj Hosp. Gaz., 24:1265, 1972

Tumors, malignant, arising de novo in immunosuppressed organ transplant recipients (Penn, Starzl), PRS, 51:483, 1973. Transplantation, 14:407, 1972

Rhabdomyosarcoma in children, improved outlook with multidisciplinary approach (Jaffe et al), PRS, 52:600, 1973. Am. J. Surg., 125:482, 1973

Scapula, elastofibroma dorsi – unusual soft tissue tumor simulating sarcoma (Harry, Kruger, McLaughlin), PRS, 53:111, 1974. Am. J. Surg., 125:773, 1973

Rhabdomyosarcoma, reasonable surgery for (Kilman et al), PRS, 53:612, 1974. Ann. Surg., 178:346, 1973

Schwannoma, malignant, clinicopathological study (Ghosh et al), PRS, 51:708, 1973. Cancer, 31:184, 1973

Verrucous carcinoma, perineural invasion and anaplastic transformation (Damian, Buskin, Echevarria), PRS, 54:245, 1974. Cancer, 32:395, 1973

Tumors, malignant, replantation of limbs after resection – report of 8 cases (Shanghai Sixth Peoples Hospital), PRS, 55:255, 1975. Chinese M. J., 6:72, 1973

Liposarcoma, subcutaneous (Weitzner). Int. J. Dermatol. 12:283, 1973

Tumor, melanoameloblastoma, in 3-month-old girl (Nagathan, Krishnamurthy), PRS, 54:381, 1974. J. Pediat. Surg., 6:977, 1973

Children, soft part sarcomas in (Exelby). Proc. Natl. Cancer Conf., 7:619, 1973

Cancer, mechanisms of spread (Cole). Surg. Gynec. & Obstet., 137:853, 1973

Pseudosarcoma (atypical fibroxanthoma) (Paterson). Brit. J. Dermatol., 90:359, 1974

Malignant disease, repair of large full-thickness post-excisional defects of abdominal wall in (Wilson, Rayner), PRS, 56:678, 1975. Brit. J. Plast. Surg., 27:117, 1974

Metastasis facilitated by antithymocyte globulin (James, Salisbury), PRS, 54:244, 1974. Cancer Res., 34:367, 1974

Methotrexate, intermittent high-dose, for children with malignant tumors (Pratt et al), PRS, 55:516, 1975. Cancer Res., 34:3326, 1974

Tumors, malignant, effect of route of admin-

Cancer—Cont.

istration and effusion on methotrexate pharmacokinetics (Wan *et al*), PRS, *55:*516, 1975. Cancer Res., *34:*3487, 1974

Tumors, chemotherapy of next decade (Bagshawe), PRS, *55:*644, 1975. Proc. Roy. Soc. Med., *67:*745, 1974

Metastasis of tumors, factors in (Williams), PRS, *55:*723, 1975. Proc. Roy. Soc. Med., *67:*847, 1974

Cancerous disease, patient with—towards independence and subsequently (Downie). Queens Nurs. J., *16:*254, 1974.

Children with malignant neoplasms, school phobia in (Lansky *et al*), PRS, *57:*766, 1976. Am. J. Dis. Child., *129:*42, 1975

Malignant cells *in vivo*, human, macrophage-mediated destruction of (Mansell *et al*), PRS, *56:*472, 1975. J. Nat. Cancer Inst., *54:*471, 1975

Myoblastoma, congenital granular-cell (Cussen, Mahon), PRS, *56:*472, 1975. J. Pediat. Surg., *10:*249, 1975

Malignant tumors formed against the background of ulcers, osteomyelitic fistulas and scars (Dryzhak). Klin. Khir., *10:*78, 1975 (Russian)

Leukemia, acute monomyelocytic, presenting as felon (Chang, Whitaker, LaRossa), PRS, *55:*623, 1975

Cancer, Antral: See Maxillary Neoplasms; Maxillary Resection; Paranasal Sinus Neoplasms

Cancer, Basal Cell

Significance of a single injury in the causation of basal-cell carcinoma of the skin (Ewing). Aust. N. Z. J. Surg., *41:*140, 1971

Turban tumors (cylindromatosis) (Harper). Birth Defects, *7:*338, 1971

Curettage and electrodesiccation as a method of treatment of epitheliomas of the skin (Crissey). J. Surg. Oncol., *3:*287, 1971

Rodent ulcer (Hofmann). Klin. Monatsbl. Augenheilkd., *159:*460, 1971 (German)

Basal cell carcinoma of the face. Problems of treatment and rehabilitation (Drepper). Minerva Stomatol., *20:*249, 1971 (German)

Basal cell carcinomas of the face, malignant degeneration of; basal-squamous carcinoma (Stellmach, Rehrmann, Koch), PRS, *48:*471, 1971

Metastasizing basal cell carcinoma (Almeyda, Mantell), PRS, *48:*609, 1971. Proc. Roy. Soc. Med., *64:*611, 1971

Surgical therapy of basal cell carcinoma. Correlation of the macroscopic and micro-

Cancer, Basal Cell—Cont.

scopic control of excision with recurrence (Rintala). Scand. J. Plast. Reconstr. Surg., *5:*87, 1971

Metastatic basal cell epithelioma discovered by chemosurgery (Mikhail *et al*). Arch. Dermat., *105:*103, 1972

Subungual basal cell epithelioma (Alpert *et al*). Arch. Dermat., *106:*599, 1972

Chemosurgery for facial neoplasms (Mohs). Arch. Otolaryng., *95:*62, 1972

Carcinoma, basal cell metastasis in bone (Cornelius), PRS, *50:*635, 1972. Arch. Surg., *104:*848, 1972

Combined cytostatic and surgical treatment of extensive basal cell epitheliomata (Weber *et al*). Brit. J. Dermatol., *86:*408, 1972

Five-Fluorouracil and Bucky rays in the treatment of superficial basaliomas (Trnka). Cesk. Dermatol., *47:*80, 1972 (Czechoslovakian)

Carcinoma, basal cell, follow-up study of treatment with 5-fluorouracil ointment (Reymann). Dermatologica, *144:*205, 1972

Basalioma therapy from dermatologist's viewpoint (Kleine-Natrop *et al*). Dermatol. Monatsschr., *158:*884, 1972 (German)

Chemosurgery. Surgical removal of chemically fixed tumor tissue with microscopic control (Burg *et al*). Hautarzt, *23:*16, 1972 (German)

Nasal cancers. Individuality of treatment (Converse). J.A.M.A., *219:*348, 1972

"Bell's palsy" caused by basal cell carcinomas (May, Lucente), PRS, *50:*635, 1972. J.A.M.A., *220:*159, 1972

Basal cell carcinoma as seen by plastic surgeon (Ryan *et al*). J. La. State Med. Soc., *124:*361, 1972

Cancer of the lip (Yonkers *et al*). Laryngoscope, *82:*625, 1972

En bloc ethmoidectomy for cancer. (A progress report.) (Ross *et al*). Laryngoscope, *82:*682, 1972

Basal cell carcinoma: treatment by the Mohs technique (Robins *et al*). Laryngoscope, *82:*965, 1972

Chemosurgery (Mohs' technique) in the treatment of epitheliomas (Tolman). Med. Clin. North Am., *56:*739, 1972

Carcinoma, basal cell (Belisario), PRS, *51:*484, 1973. Med. Trib., *13:*21, 1972

Ear skin-cartilage plastic surgery for eyelid margin tumors (Hanselmayer *et al*). Ophthalmologica, *165:*464, 1972 (German)

Radiation injury, local, and its surgical treatment. Report of 170 cases (Homlström, Johanson). Scand. J. Plast. Reconstr. Surg., *6:*156, 1972

Cancer, Basal Cell – Cont.

Skin cancer (Jensen *et al*). Ugeskr. Laeger., *134:*107, 1972 (Danish)

Basal and squamous carcinoma (Clabaugh). Am. Fam. Phys., *7:*78, 1973

Carcinoma, basal cell, of medial canthal region (Abraham, Jabaley, Hoopes), PRS, *53:*688, 1974. Am. J. Surg., *126:*492, 1973

Carcinoma, basal cell, adequacy of surgical excision (Rakofsky). Ann. Ophth., *5:*596, 1973

Bowen's disease, relationship to internal malignant tumors (Anderson, Nielson, Reymann), PRS, *53:*370, 1974. Arch. Dermat., *108:*367, 1973

Effects of new laser systems on skin (Goldman). Arch. Dermat., *108:*385, 1973

Carcinoma, basal cell, in children (Milstone, Helwig), PRS, *53:*688, 1974. Arch. Dermat., *108:*523, 1973

Carcinoma, basal cell, of skin, treatment with curettage (Reymann), PRS, *53:*612, 1974. Arch. Dermat., *108:*528, 1973

Follow-up after treatment of basal cell carcinoma, value of (Epstein), PRS, *54:*381, 1974. Arch. Dermat., *108:*798, 1973

Carcinoma, basal cell, of nail bed (Hoffman), PRS, *54:*380, 1974. Arch. Dermat., *108:*828, 1973

Carcinoma, basal cell, margins, how accurate is visual assessment? (Epstein), PRS, *54:*381, 1974. Brit. J. Dermat., *89:*37, 1973

Carcinoma, basal cell, of conjunctiva (Aftab *et al*). Brit. J. Ophthalmol., *57:*836, 1973

Carcinoma, basal cell, surgical treatment, ten years' experience in. Study of factors associated with recurrence (Taylor *et al*). Brit. J. Surg., *60:*522, 1973

Rodent ulcer, surgical treatment (Moustafa, Ghazaly), PRS, *53:*494, 1974. Bull. Alexandria Fac. Med., *8:*24, 1973

Basaliomas, recurrent, analysis of therapy of (Sebastian *et al*). Dermatol. Monatsschr., *159:*216, 1973 (German)

Carcinoma, basal cell – formation of metastases of basal cell epithelioma (Go *et al*). Hautarzt, *24:*449, 1973 (German)

Scalp and skull, combined resection for basal cell cancer (Pratt, Trembly, Goodof). J. Maine M. A., *64:*29, 1973

Carcinoma, basal cell, surgical approach to (Bowe). J. M. Soc. New Jersey, *70:*115, 1973

Carcinoma, basal cell, horrifying: study of 33 cases and comparison with 435 non-horror cases and report on four metastatic cases (Jackson *et al*). J. Surg. Oncol., *5:*431, 1973

Carcinoma, basal cell, cryosurgery in (Al-

Cancer, Basal Cell – Cont.

lende), PRS, *57:*264, 1976. Med. Cut., *1:*55, 1973

Basal cell carcinoma of the skin, an appraisal of the treatment of (Griffith, McKinney), PRS, *51:*565, 1973

Fluorouracil-5 in treatment of skin lesions (Snyderman) (Follow-Up Clinic), PRS, *52:*298, 1973

Carcinoma, basal cell (Bears). Proc. Roy. Soc. Med., *66:*691, 1973

Therapeutic possibilities in multiple epitheliomas of trunk skin (Schnellen *et al*). Z. Haut. Geschlechtskr., *48:*287, 1973 (German)

Basalioma, recurrent, treatment of (Kleine-Natrop). Arch. Geschwulstforsch., *43:*75, 1974 (German)

History of basal cell carcinoma (Bennett), PRS, *57:*124, 1976. Brit. J. Plast. Surg., *27:*144, 1974

Scalp, basal cell carcinoma of, harmless osteoporosis of skull underlying (Herbert *et al*). Brit. J. Plast. Surg., *27:*248, 1974

Immunotherapy, topical, of basal cell carcinomas with dinitrochlorobenzene (Levis *et al*), PRS, *54:*245, 1974. Cancer Res., *33:*3036, 1974

Basal cell carcinoma, chromomycosis simulating (Baumal, Hanson, Jeerapaet), PRS, *55:*640, 1975. Cutis, *14:*227, 1974

Carcinoma, basal cell, cosmetic results after treatment (Epstein), PRS, *56:*104, 1975. Cutis, *14:*825, 1974

Surgical therapy of extended skin tumors of the torso (Petres *et al*). Hautarzt, *5:*566, 1974 (German)

Carcinoma, basal cell (Brodkin *et al*). J.A.M.A., *228:*463, 1974

Carcinoma, basal cell, treatment (Letter). J.A.M.A., *229:*1581, 1974

Carcinomas, basal cell, why do they recur (or not recur) following treatment? (Jackson). J. Surg. Oncol., *6:*245, 1974

Excision or radiation of basaliomas of the lids (Wilke). Klin. Monatsbl. Augenheilkd., *165:*676, 1974 (German)

Cryosurgical treatment of recurrent head and neck malignancies – a comparative study (Goode *et al*). Laryngoscope, *84:*1950, 1974

Cancer, skin, basal cell, plastic surgical treatment of (Greeley). Mil. Med., *141:*443, 1974

Cryosurgery and basal cell epitheliomas. Clinical and histological study (Leigheb *et al*). Minerva Med., *65:*3676, 1974

Carcinoma, basal cell, and peripheral amelo-

Cancer, Basal Cell — Cont.
blastoma (Simpson). Oral Surg., *38:*233, 1974

Carcinoma, morphoic basal cell, with invasion of orbit (Gilkes, Borrie), PRS, *55:*385, 1975. Proc. Roy. Soc. Med., *67:*437, 1974

Carcinoma sebaceum (adenoma sebaceum malignum) (Wojnerowicz). Przegl. Dermatol., *61:*865, 1974 (Polish)

Carcinoma, basal cell, multiple, treated with curettage (Reymann). Ugeskr. Laeger, *136:*2523, 1974 (Danish)

Chemosurgery of basaliomas (Burg *et al*). Z. Hautkr., *49:*713, 1974 (German)

X-ray injury of the skin and its treatment (Olivari *et al*). In *Plastische und Wiederherstellungs-Chirurgie,* ed. by Holhler; pp. 341–51. Stuttgart; Schattauer, 1975 (German)

Laser therapy of human benign and malignant neoplasms of the skin (Wagner *et al*). Acta Radiol. (Ther.) (Stockh.), *14:*417, 1975

Complications of Mohs' chemosurgical excision of eyelid and canthal tumors (Baylis *et al*). Am. J. Ophth., *80:*116, 1975

Carcinoma, multiple basal cell, and internal malignant tumors (Moller, Nielsen, Reymann), PRS, *57:*679, 1976. Arch. Dermat., *111:*585, 1975

Carcinoma, basal cell, and basal cell carcinoma-like changes overlying dermatofibromas (Goette, Helwig), PRS, *57:*540, 1976. Arch. Dermat., *111:*589, 1975

Carcinoma of skin, multiple basal cell (Reymann), PRS, *57:*679, 1976. Arch. Dermat., *111:*877, 1975

Punch excision technique for removing basal cell epithelioma (Montes *et al*). Geriatrics, *30:*65, 1975

Dermatome excision of multiple basaliomas of the trunk skin (Konz). Hautarzt, *26:*647, 1975 (German)

Epithelioma, basal cell: treat on sight (Epstein). Int. J. Dermatol., *14:*263, 1975

The "turban" nevoid basal cell syndrome. Current management with surgery, chemotherapy and immunotherapy (Habal *et al*). Int. Surg., *60:*493, 1975

Basaliomas, biological behavior of (Koch, Pfeifle, Kreidler), PRS, *56:*472, 1975. J. Maxillo-facial Surg., *3:*35, 1975

Treatment of skin cancer by cryosurgery (Woolridge *et al*). Mo. Med., *72:*28, 1975

Letter: Basal cell carcinoma (Auerbach). N. Y. State J. Med., *75:*2326, 1975

Complications following use of cheek flap rotation to reconstruct lower lid (Weiss). Ophthalmic Surg., *6:*42, 1975

Cancer, Basal Cell — Cont.
Basal-cell carcinoma of the vermilion mucosa and skin of the lip (Weitzner). Oral Surg., *39:*634, 1975

Carcinoma, unusual basal cell, lip reconstruction following resection (Kelly, Klein), PRS, *57:*539, 1976. Oral Surg., *40:*19, 1975

Carcinoma, basal cell, cryosurgery for (Vistnes, Harris, Fajardo), PRS, *55:*71, 1975

Carcinoma, basal cell, of medial canthal area (Bostwick, Vasconez, Jurkiewicz), PRS, *55:*667, 1975

Clinical characteristics and genetic identity of the basal cell nevus syndrome (Gorlin-Goltz syndrome) (Breytenbach *et al*). S. Afr. Med. J., *49:*544, 1975 (Afrikaans)

Metastasizing basal cell carcinoma (Lildholdt, Sogaard), PRS, *57:*678, 1976. Scand. J. Plast. Reconstr. Surg., *9:*170, 1975

Treatment of basal cell epitheliomas and actinic keratoses (Jansen). J.A.M.A., *235:*1152, 1976

Cancer incidence (Cosman, Heddle, Crikelair), PRS, *57:*50, 1976

Cancer, Burn Scars: See *Burns, Cancer in*

Cancer, Cheek: See *Mouth Neoplasms*

Cancer, Ear: See *Ear, Neoplasms of*

Cancer, Epidermoid: See *Cancer, Squamous Cell*

Cancer, Eyelid: See *Eyelids, Neoplasms of*

Cancer, Face: See *Facial Neoplasms, Skin Neoplasms, etc.*

Cancer, Hand: See *Hands, Neoplasms of*

Cancer, Head and Neck (See also *Neck Dissections and specific anatomical area*)

Head and neck, cryosurgery of (Von Leden). Acta Otorinolaryngol. Iber. Am., *22:*275, 1971 (Spanish)

Lymphoma of head and neck masquerading as carcinoma (Elias, Mittelman), PRS, *49:*360, 1972. Am. J. Surg., *122:*424, 1971

Cancer of scalp and skull, major resection for, with immediate complete reconstruction in 14 cases (Gaisford) (Follow-Up Clinic), PRS, *48:*369, 1971

Cancer surgery, replantation of the mandible in (Harding) (Follow-Up Clinic), PRS, *48:*586, 1971

Cancer, Head and Neck – Cont.

Head and neck tumors, surgery and chemotherapy in (Hurley *et al*) (Follow-Up Clinic), PRS, *48:*587, 1971

Head and neck surgery, reconstruction in (Matthews), PRS, *49:*240, 1972. Proc. Roy. Soc. Med., *64:*731, 1971

Chemotherapy-surgery combination for treatment of carcinomas of mouth and jaw (Routledge), PRS, *49:*238, 1972. Proc. Roy. Soc. Med., *64:*737, 1971

Drooling in patients with cancer of head and neck, parotid duct transplantation for correction of (Cohen, Holmes, Edgerton), PRS *49:*361, 1972. Surg. Gynec. & Obst., *133:*633, 1971

Metastatic neoplasms to head and neck (Batsakis, McBurney), PRS, *49:*360, 1972. Surg. Gynec. & Obst., *133:*783, 1971

Stell, P. M., and Maran A. G. D.: *Head and Neck Surgery.* J. B. Lippincott Co., Philadelphia, 1972. PRS, *52:*295, 1973

Reticulum cell sarcoma in head and neck surgery (Larsen, Hill, Rotzer), PRS, *50:*421, 1972. Am. J. Surg., *123:*338, 1972

Arterial infusion chemotherapy for cancer of head and neck, factors influencing success of (Donegan, Harris), PRS, *51:*608, 1973. Am. J. Surg., *123:*549, 1972

Cancer, head and neck, treated by intra-arterial infusion therapy (Freckman), PRS *52:*214, 1973. Am. J. Surg., *124:*501, 1972

Cancer, head and neck, methotrexate plus bacillus Calmette-Guerin (BCG) and isoniazid in treatment (Donaldson), PRS, *52:*216, 1973. Am. J. Surg., *124:*527, 1972

Cancer, head and neck, preoperative irradiation in (Moore, Mullins, Scott), PRS, *52:*213, 1973. Am. J. Surg., *124:*555, 1972

Cancer, head and neck, deltopectoral flap in surgery of (Pradier *et al*), PRS, *51:*485, 1973. Bol y Trab. Acad. argent. cir., *56:*204, 1972

Head and neck neoplasia, cryosurgery in treatment of (Holden). Brit. J. Surg., *59:*709, 1972

Head and neck, use of regional flaps in reconstructive surgery of (Ogura *et al*). Can. J. Otolaryngol., *1:*290, 1972

Practical course of regional, plastic and constructive surgery. I. Free, primary skin transplantation in head and neck surgery. Basic considerations, technique and indication (Nagel). H.N.O., *20:*319, 1972 (German)

Head and neck, method of treatment of vascular tumor (Ono *et al*). J. Otolaryngol. Japan, *75:*1091, 1972 (Japanese)

Head and neck surgery, major, use of re-

Cancer, Head and Neck – Cont.

gional flaps in (Conley). J. Otolaryngol. Soc. Aust., *3:*303, 1972

Head and neck tumors, cryosurgery for. Experimental and clinical considerations (Neel). Minn. Med., *55:*886, 1972

Pneumonia, chronic aspiration, life-endangering, surgical treatment; use of epiglottic flap to arytenoids (Habal, Murray), PRS, *49:*305, 1972

Oropharyngeal cancer surgery, massive, catastrophic postoperative breakdown after, management of; survival in a perilous situation (Mladick *et al*), PRS, *49:*316, 1972

Maxillectomy, radical, for cancer, primary reconstruction of palate after (Bakamjian) (Follow-Up Clinic), PRS, *49:*335, 1972

Lymphatic cannulation of head and neck (Smith) (Follow-Up Clinic), PRS, *49:*454, 1972

Flap, deltopectoral, complications with (Gingrass *et al*), PRS, *49:*501, 1972

Head and neck, use of composite flaps containing bone for major repairs (Conley), PRS, *49:*522, 1972

Metastatic head and neck neoplastic cell, radiophosphorus uptake by (Kiehn) (Follow-Up Clinic), PRS, *50:*183, 1972

Neuroleptoanalgesia in oncological surgery of the head and neck (Azevedo *et al*). Rev. Bras. Anestesiol., *22:*68, 1972 (Portuguese)

Cryogenic surgery of the head and neck (Hoki). Saishin Igaku, *27:*691, 1972 (Japanese)

Cancer, head and neck, newer concepts of reconstructive surgery in patients with (Salyer, Nickell), PRS, *51:*485, 1973. South. M. J., *65:*1364, 1972

Flap, deltopectoral, for reconstruction of radiated cancer of the head and neck (Krizek, Robson), PRS, *52:*105, 1973. Surg. Gynec. & Obst., *135:*787, 1972

Head and neck region, radical cancer surgery, use of deltopectoral flap in (Siemssen *et al*). Ugeskr. Laeger., *134:*2137, 1972 (Danish)

An Atlas of Head and Neck Surgery, Second Edition. By John M. Lore, Jr. W. B. Saunders Co., Philadelphia, 1973. PRS, *54:*94, 1974

Otolaryngology, Volume III. Head and Neck. By Michael M. Paparella and Donald A. Shumrick. W. B. Saunders Co., Philadelphia, 1973. PRS, *53:*218, 1974

Cancers, head and neck, Applications of electron beam in management of lymphatics of neck in (Tapley *et al*). Am. J. Roentgenol. Radium Ther. Nucl. Med., *117:*575, 1973

Cancer, head and neck, advanced, concept of

Cancer, Head and Neck — Cont.

cure and palliation by surgery in (Bakamjian *et al)*, PRS, *53:*688, 1974. Am. J. Surg., *126:*482, 1973

Head and neck reconstruction, split flap in (Krizek, Robson), PRS, *53:*613, 1974. Am. J. Surg., *126:*488, 1973

Chemoimmunotherapy for cancer of head and neck (Donaldson), PRS, *53:*688, 1974. Am. J. Surg., *126:*507, 1973

Hydroxyurea in treatment of neoplasms of head and neck (Richards, Chambers), PRS, *53:*688, 1974. Am. J. Surg., *126:*513, 1973

Cancer, head and neck, far advanced, six year survival under combined therapy program (Lipshutz, Lerner), PRS, *53:*497, 1974. Am. J. Surg., *126:*519, 1973

Cancer, head and neck, intra-arterial infusion chemotherapy in (Snow, Sindram), PRS, *54:*246, 1974. Arch. chir. neerl., *25:*363, 1973

Head and neck, skin flaps to reconstruct (Lichtfeld, Snow), PRS, *54:*117, 1974. Arch. chir. neerl., *25:*379, 1973

Head and neck tumors, cryogenic surgery in (Von Leden). Arch. Klin. Exp. Ohren Nasen Kehlkopfheilkd., *250:*84, 1973 (German)

Head and neck surgery, risks of, in previously irradiated patients (Joseph *et al)*. Arch. Otolaryng., *97:*381, 1973

Head and neck, synovial sarcoma of (Krugman *et al)*. Arch. Otolaryng., *98:*53, 1973

Head and neck, adenoid cystic carcinoma of, report of 30 cases (Ramsden *et al)*. Aust. N. Z. J. Surg., *43:*102, 1973

Tumors, head and neck, which involve bone, some aspects of surgical treatment of (Wilson, Westbury). Brit. J. Radiol., *46:*151, 1973

Rhabdomyosarcoma of head and neck in children (Donaldson *et al)*, PRS, *52:*214, 1973. Cancer, *31:*26, 1973

Tumors, epidermoid, of head, neck, and esophagus, hypercalcemia in (Stephens, Hansen, Muggia), PRS, *54:*108, 1974. Cancer, *31:*1487, 1973

Chemotherapy, regional arterial, for advanced carcinoma of head and neck (Oberfield, Cady, Booth), PRS, *54:*235, 1974. Cancer, *32:*82, 1973

Alcoholics, head and neck cancer in (Kissin *et al)*, PRS, *52:*685, 1973. J.A.M.A., *224:*1174, 1973

Head and neck region, malignant tumor of, treatment through team work with radiology department (Sato). J. Otolaryngol. Jap., *76:*1301, 1973 (Japanese)

Cancer, Head and Neck — Cont.

Head and neck cancer. Should lymphadenectomy be discarded? (Harrison). J. R. Coll. Surg. Edin. *18:*357, 1973

Head and neck, malignancy of, massive surgery for palliation in (Tucker *et al)*. Laryngoscope, *83:*1635, 1973

Head and neck cancer; comprehensive team approach (Mladick *et al)*. Med. Trial Tech. Q., *177:*82, 1973

Head and neck operations after radiation therapy (Goode). Oral Surg., *36:*170, 1973

Head and neck, reconstructive plastic surgery, symposium on. Rehabilitative responsibilities and philosophies (Lederer). Otolaryngol. Clin. North Am., *5:*405, 1973

Visor flap reconstruction for massive oropharyngeal defect (Griffin *et al)*, PRS, *51:*457, 1973. Discussion by Edgerton, PRS, *51:*582, 1973

Head and neck region, investigation of bone changes in composite flaps after transfer to (Conley *et al)*. PRS *51:*658, 1973. Discussion by Jurkiewicz, PRS, *52:*79, 1973

Cranio-orbital resection and neck dissection for recurrent mixed tumor of the lacrimal gland (Habal, Murray), PRS, *51:*689, 1973

Angiography, use of, in outlining solitary solid tumors of the head and neck (Mandel, Kiehn, Sykora), PRS, *52:*61, 1973

Head and neck, malignant neoplasms of, role of plastic surgery in complex treatment of (Pasnikowski). Pol. Tyg. Lek., *28:*1743, 1973 (Polish)

Head and neck surgery, nutritional care after (Noone *et al)*. Postgrad. Med., *53:*80, 1973

Adenoid cystic carcinoma of head and neck (Newton *et al)*, PRS, *52:*600, 1973. Proc. Roy. Australasian Coll. Surgeons, *46:*720, 1973

Cutaneous gliomas of hand (Saavedra Gonzales *et al)*. Rozhl. Chir., *52:*822, 1973 (Czechoslovakian)

Head and neck cancer, 8-year experience (Beradi *et al)*. South Med. J., *66:*1094, 1973

Head and neck surgery, management of complications in (Zarem). Surg. Clin. North Am., *53:*191, 1973

Head and neck, complications in cryosurgery in (Strome). Trans. Am. Acad. Ophthalmol. Otolaryngol., *77:*1372, 1973

Cancer, head and neck, advanced, surgical management (Vrachnos, Paraskevas, Stylogiannis), PRS, *56:*473, 1975. Tr. 8th Panhellenic Cong. Surg. Soc., *A:*190, 1973

Cancer, metastatic, in elderly patients, surgical treatment of (Merlo). Vopr. Onkol., *19:*57, 1973 (Russian)

Cancer, Head and Neck — Cont.

Surgical Treatment of Head and Neck Tumors. Ed. Jorge Fairbanks Barbosa. Grune & Stratton, New York, 1974. PRS, *57:*509, 1976

Tumors of the Head and Neck. By John G. Batsakis. Williams & Wilkins Co., Baltimore, 1974. PRS *54:*479, 1974

Head and neck, certain cancerous diseases, combination therapy in (Raven). Am. J. Roentgenol. Ther. Nucl. Med., *120:*178, 1974

Head and neck tumors, advanced, aggressive management (Rafla *et al*). Am. J. Roentgenol. Radium Ther. Nucl. Med., *120:*608, 1974

Cancer, head and neck, in Utah (Smart), PRS, *57:*540, 1976. Am. J. Surg., *128:*463, 1974

Cancer, head and neck, cryosurgery for (Weaver, Smith), PRS, *57:*540, 1976. Am. J. Surg., *128:*466, 1974

Synovial sarcoma of the head and neck (Jacobs *et al*). Am. J. Surg., *128:*527, 1974

Head and neck cancer, immunologic abnormalities in (Eilber *et al*). Am. J. Surg., *128:*534, 1974

Osseous metastasis: its relationship to primary carcinoma of head and neck (Arlen *et al*). Am. J. Surg., *128:*568, 1974

Head and neck cancer, triple drug intra-arterial infusion combined with X-ray therapy and surgery for (Cruz *et al*). Am. J. Surg., *128:*573, 1974

Results of high dose radiation and surgery in the treatment of advanced cancer of the head and neck (Carifi *et al*). Am. J. Surg., *128:*580, 1974

Head and neck, fibrosarcoma of: clinical analysis of 40 cases (Swain *et al*). Ann. Otol. Rhin. & Laryngol., *83:*439, 1974

Chemotherapy of malignant melanoma with dimethyl triazeno imidazole carboxamide (DITC) and nitrosourea derivatives (BCNU, CCNU) (Hill *et al*), PRS, *55:*117, 1975. Ann. Surg., *180:*167, 1974

Vascular complications of head and neck surgery (Miller, Bergstrom), PRS, *55:*107, 1975. Arch. Otolaryng., *100:*136, 1974

Head and neck, diagnosis of malignant neoplasms. Scintiscanning with gallium citrate 67. (Kornblut *et al*). Arch. Otolaryng., *100:*201, 1974

Deltopectoral flaps (Zirkle, Thompson), PRS, *54:*690, 1974. Arch. Surg., *108:*770, 1974

Cancer, head and neck, recurrent (Williams), PRS, *57:*124, 1976. Brit. J. Surg., *61:*691, 1974

Head and neck tumors, pseudohyperparathy-

Cancer, Head and Neck — Cont.

roidism in (Ariyan *et al*). Cancer, *33:*159, 1974

Head and neck cancer, preoperative irradiation for: prospective study (Lawrence *et al*). Cancer, *33:*318, 1974

Chemotherapy, bleomycin, and concurrent methotrexate. Phase II study of (Lokich, Frei), PRS, *55:*256, 1975. Cancer Res., *34:*2240, 1974

Otorhinolaryngology, chemodectomas in (Ritter). H.N.O., *22:*6, 1974

Head and neck, dermatofibrosarcoma protuberans of (Hempel). H.N.O., *22:*176, 1974 (German)

Management of fistulae of the head and neck after radical surgery (Stell *et al*). J. Laryng. & Otol., *88:*819, 1974

Head and neck tumor surgery, elective tracheostomy in (Shaw *et al*). J. Leg. Med., *88:*599, 1974

Tumors of head and neck in infancy and childhood, statistical evaluation of (Koch), PRS, *54:*628, 1974. J. Maxillo-facial Surg., *2:*26, 1974

Head and neck operations, mortality in (Kogge, Koch), PRS, *54:*625, 1974. J. Maxillo-facial Surg., *2:*32, 1974

Philosophy of head and neck cancer surgery (Steckler *et al*). J. Prosthet. Dent., *32:*307, 1974

Head and neck cancer patient, prosthetic rehabilitation of (Schaaf *et al*). J. Surg. Oncol., *6:*311, 1974

Clinical success of distant transfer of free skin flap in head and neck regions by microvascular anastomoses (Fujino *et al*). Keio J. Med., *23:*47, 1974

Tumors, head and neck, radiation induced (Modan *et al*), PRS, *54:*498, 1974. Lancet, *1:*227, 1974

Cryosurgical treatment of recurrent head and neck malignancies — a comparative study (Goode *et al*). Laryngoscope, *84:*1950, 1974

Chemotherapy to treat advanced squamous carcinoma of head and neck (Stephens), PRS, *55:*386, 1975. M. J. Australia, *2:*587, 1974

Chemotherapy of thyroid cancer with Adriamycin (Gottlieb, Hill), PRS, *54:*373, 1974. New England J. Med., *290:*193, 1974

Head and neck, ablative surgery of, physiologic problems following (Summers). Otolaryngol. Clin. North Am., *7:*217, 1974

Cutaneous reactivity, delayed, in head and neck cancer patients, prognostic significance of (Mandel, Kiehn), PRS, *53:*72, 1974

Cancer: core resection, composite regional

Cancer, Head and Neck — Cont.

ear resection (Mladick *et al*), PRS, *53:*281, 1974

Hemimandibulectomy, composite reconstruction of mandible and temporomandibular joint following (Ho, Bailey, Sykes), PRS, *53:*414, 1974

Head and neck tumors, cryosurgery as therapeutic modality in treatment of (Miller). Proc. Roy. Soc. Med., *67:*69, 1974

Head and neck neoplasia, indications and limitations of cryosurgery in (Holden). Proc. Roy. Soc. Med., *67:*76, 1974

Chemotherapy of next decade (Bagshawe), PRS, *55:*644, 1975. Proc. Roy. Soc. Med., *67:*745, 1974

Flap, deltopectoral, for reconstruction in head and neck cancer (Pradier *et al*), PRS, *54:*626, 1974. Rev. argent. cir., *26:*32, 1974

Melanoblastoma of head and neck, advanced metastasizing, is radical neck dissection of value? (Kluzak), PRS, *54:*619, 1974. Rozhl. chir., *53:*204, 1974

Flap, deltopectoral, variations in use (Nickell, Salyer, Vargas), PRS, *54:*700, 1974. South. M. J., *67:*697, 1974

Myoblastoma, granular cell, of head and neck (Thawley, Ogura), PRS, *55:*515, 1975. South. M.J., *67:*1020, 1974

Head and neck surgery, regional flaps in (Komorn). Tex. Med., *70:*70, 1974

Effect of premedication with droperidol, atropine and promedol on basic indices of blood circulation in patients with tumors of the head and neck (Guliaev *et al*). Vestn. Akad. Med. Nauk., 7:65, 1974 (Russian)

Cancer of the Head and Neck. By R. G. Chambers, *et al.* Excerpta Medica Co., Amsterdam, 1975

Symposium on Malignancies of the Head and Neck. Vol. XI. Ed. by Robin Anderson and John Hoopes. C. V. Mosby Co., St. Louis, 1975. PRS, *57:*373, 1976

Significance of local malignant lesions of the neck diagnosed accidentally during parathyroid exploration (Lenquist *et al*). Acta Chir. Scand., *141:*721, 1975

Olfactory neuroblastoma. Management and prognosis (Bailey *et al*). Arch. Otolaryng., *101:*1, 1975

Role of surgery in head and neck cancer with fixed nodes (Santos *et al*). Arch. Otolaryng., *101:*645, 1975

Head and neck reconstruction, back tube pedicle in (Blake). Brit. J. Plast. Surg., *28:*59, 1975

Cancer, recurrent, head and neck, management of (Editorial). Brit. Med. J., *2:*54, 1975

Cancer, Head and Neck — Cont.

Head and neck tumors, randomized clinical trial of fast neutrons compared with X or gamma rays in treatment (Catterall, Sutherland, Bewley), PRS, *57:*402, 1976. Brit. M.J., *2:*653, 1975

Intravenous hyperalimentation in patients with head and neck cancer (Copeland *et al*). Cancer, *35:*606, 1975

Limitations of surgery in the treatment of head and neck cancer (Stell). Can. J. Otolaryngol., *4:*508, 1975

Chemosurgery in treatment of cancer (Mikhail). Int. J. Dermatol., *14:*33, 1975

Cancer, head and neck, combination therapy in (Aron *et al*). J.A.M.A., *233:*177, 1975

Temporal or frontotemporal flap in cervicofacial oncology (Desaulty *et al*). J. Fr. Otorhinolaryngol., *24:*521, 1975 (French)

Temporo-frontal flap. Its value in post-irradiation buccal-pharyngeal surgery (Junien-Lavillauroy *et al*). J. Fr. Otorhinolaryngol., *24:*763, 1975 (French)

Rehabilitation for patients following head and neck surgery (Downie). J. Laryng. & Otol., *89:*1281, 1975

Head and neck, diagnostic and therapeutic regime for reducing mortality after resection of tumors in (Reil *et al*). J. Maxillofacial Surg., *3:*54, 1975

Clinical-pathological conference: case 10, part 2. Neurofibrosarcoma (Carpenter *et al*). J. Oral Surg., *33:*38, 1975

On mucoepidermoid tumors with rare locations in laryngological areas (Schmid *et al*). Laryngol. Rhinol. Otol. (Stuttg.), *54:*290, 1975 (German)

Histological examinations on the hemostatic effect of freezing during surgical procedures in the head and neck (Ganz *et al*). Laryngol. Rhinol. Otol. (Stuttg.), *54:*328, 1975 (German)

Regional neck lymph nodes and primary tumors. 1. Neck lymph node metastases (Simon). Laryngol. Rhinol. Otol. (Stuttg.), *54:*997, 1975 (German)

Pneumonia, chronic aspiration, further experiences with arytenoid-epiglottic flap for (Vecchione, Habal, Murray), PRS, *55:*318, 1975

Stress fracture of clavicle after radical neck dissection (Cummings, First), PRS, *55:*366, 1975

Dermal-fat flap, free deltopectoral, microvascular, transfer of (Fujino, Tanino, Sugimoto), PRS, *55:*428, 1975

Head and neck region, fiberoptic endoscopy in (Dellon, Hall, Chretien), PRS, *55:*466, 1975

Cancer, Head and Neck — Cont.

Rhabdomyosarcoma: deltoscapular flap (Doldan, Shatkin), PRS, *55:*708, 1975

Head and neck cancer, influence of immunologic responsiveness on; therapeutic implications (Woods) (Editorial), PRS, *56:*77, 1975

Cancer, head and neck, use of temporal muscle flap for reconstruction after orbito-maxillary resections for (Bakamjian, Souther), PRS, *56:*171, 1975

Cancer, head and neck, use of folded forehead flap for reconstruction after large excision of full thickness of cheek (Kavarana), PRS, *56:*629, 1975

Cancer, head and neck, complications of free flap transfer to mouth region (Finseth, Kavarana, Antia), PRS, *56:*652, 1975

Plastic closure of extensive defects of the maxillofacial area following extensive surgical operations for cancer (Shental *et al*). Stomatologiia (Mosk.), *54:*36, 1975 (Russian)

Head and neck surgery, silicone rubber drain in (Fleming *et al*). Trans. Am. Acad. Ophthalmol. Otolaryngol., *80:*254, 1975

Neurilemmoma of the head and neck (Conley *et al*). Trans. Am. Acad. Ophthalmol. Otolaryngol., *80:*459, 1975

Neurilemmomas of the face and oral cavity (Partyka *et al*). Czas. Stomatol., *29:*147, 1976 (Polish)

Rehabilitation problems of head and neck cancer patients (Shedd). J. Surg. Oncol., *8:*11, 1976

Resection of rhabdomyosarcoma of the neck. An office procedure (Farley). Minn. Med., *59:*24, 1976

Cancer patients, skin testing for prognosis or therapy formulation in: *caveat emptor* (Mandel), PRS, *57:*621, 1976. Discussion by Humphrey, PRS, *57:*743, 1976

Chemotherapy, synergistic effect of salicylates on methotrexate toxicity (Mandel), PRS, *57:*733, 1976

Resection and immediate reconstruction for patients with "inoperable" recurrent head and neck cancer (Robson). Surg. Clin. North Am., *56:*111, 1976

Cancer, Immunology of

Immunosuppressive and oncogenic effects of heterologous antilymphocyte serum, analysis of (Zipp, Kountz), PRS, *49:*109, 1972. Am. J. Surg., *122:*204, 1971

Tumors, human evidence for antigenicity with reference both to melanoma and acute leukemia (Fairley), PRS, *49:*473, 1972. Proc. Roy. Soc. Med., *64:*1044, 1971

Cancer, Immunology of — Cont.

Immunological Aspects of Neoplasia I, and *Immunological Aspects of Neoplasia II, Series Haematologica,* Vols. 4 & 5. Munksgaard, Copenhagen, Denmark, 1972. PRS, *54:*349, 1974

Methotrexate plus bacillus Calmette-guerin (CG) and isoniazid in treatment of cancer of the head and neck (Donaldson), PRS, *52:*216, 1973. Am. J. Surg., *124:*527, 1972

Tumor immunity and the mechanism of polyinosinic-polycytidylic acid inhibition of tumor growth (Kreider, Benjamin). J. Natl. Cancer Inst., *49:*1303, 1972

Leukocyte mobilization, localized, in patients with solid malignant tumors (Steiner *et al*), PRS, *51:*484, 1973. Schweiz. med. Wchnschr., *102:*1165, 1972

Immunotherapy, non-specific and specific, in patients with melanoma (Siegler *et al*), PRS, *50:*636, 1972. Surgery, *72:*162, 1972

Immunoglobulin levels in cancer patients (Mandel, Dvorak, DeCosse), PRS, *51:*708 1973. Surg. Forum, *23:*513, 1972

Cancer, head and neck, chemoimmunotherapy for (Donaldson), PRS, *53:*688, 1974. Am. J. Surg., *126:*507, 1973

Mumps virus and BCG vaccine in metastatic melanoma (Minton), PRS, *52:*600, 1973. Arch. Surg., *106:*503, 1973

Immunosuppressed patients, skin tumors in (Marshall), PRS, *54:*115, 1974. Australian & New Zealand J. Surg., *43:*214, 1973

Immunoglobulins, salivary, in patients with oropharyngeal and bronchopulmonary carcinoma (Mandel, Dvorak, DeCosse), PRS, *54:*108, 1974. Cancer, *31:*1408, 1973

Immunotherapy of malignant melanoma (McCarthy *et al*), PRS, *54:*245, 1974. Cancer, *32:*97, 1973

Immunological reaction in keratoacanthoma, spontaneously resolving skin tumor (Brown, Tan), PRS, *53:*496, 1974. Cancer Res., *33:*2030, 1973

Globulin, rabbit anti-rat lymphocyte, effects in rats of intravenous injection on diuresis and blood pressure (Dalton, Davison), PRS, *53:*614, 1974. Europ. Surg. Res., *5:*116, 1973

Immunologic effects of BCG in patients with malignant melanoma (Chess *et al*), PRS, *53:*497, 1974. J. Nat. Cancer Inst., *51:*57, 1973

Mycobacterium bovis, tumor regression after intralesional injection of (Hanna *et al*), PRS, *54:*509, 1974. J. Nat. Cancer Inst., *51:*1897, 1973

Immune factors in host resistance, fate of methylcholanthrene tumor cells in bone

Cancer, Neck: See Neck Dissections; Neck Neoplasms

Cancer, Nose: See Nose, Neoplasms

Cancer, Parotid: See Parotid Neoplasms; Salivary Gland Neoplasms

Cancer, Pharynx: See Pharyngeal Neoplasms

Cancer, Salivary Gland: See Parotid Neoplasms; Salivary Gland Neoplasms

Cancer, Skin: See Cancer, Basal Cell; Cancer, Squamous Cell; Skin, Neoplasms

Cancer, Squamous Cell

Modified blepharoplasty for malignant lid tumours (Mortada et al). Bull. Ophalmol. Soc. Egypt, 63:421, 1970

Spindle-cell variant of squamous carcinoma (Lichtiger, Mackay, Tessemer), PRS, 48:199, 1971. Cancer, 26:1311, 1970

Surgical treatment of stomal recurrences in cancer of the larynx (Kuehn et al). Am. J. Surg., 122:445, 1971

Carcinoma of the posterior pharyngeal wall (Wilkins). Am. J. Surg., 122:477, 1971

Ultraconservative management of superficially invasive epidermoid carcinoma of the true vocal cord (Stutsman et al). Ann. Otol. Rhin. & Laryngol., 80:507, 1971

Multiple self-healing squamous epithelioma (Ferguson-Smith et al). Birth Defects, 7:157, 1971

Curettage and electrodesiccation as a method of treatment for epitheliomas of the skin (Crissey). J. Surg. Oncol., 3:287, 1971

Squamous cell carcinoma of tonsillar fossa, base of tongue, supraglottic larynx and hypopharynx, cervical lymph node metastases (Barkley et al), PRS, 52:103, 1973. Am. J. Surg., 124:462, 1972

Squamous cell cancer of supraglottic larynx, surgery and radiation in treatment (Flynn, Jesse, Lindberg), PRS, 52:102, 1973. Am. J. Surg., 124:477, 1972

Squamous cell carcinoma of oral cavity, treatment (Fayos, Lampe), PRS, 52:102, 1973. Am. J. Surg., 124:493, 1972

Role of radiation therapy and of surgery in the management of localized epidermoid carcinoma of the maxillary sinus (Kurohara et al). Am. J. Roentgenol. Radium Ther. Nucl. Med., 114:35, 1972

Planned preoperative irradiation and surgery for advanced cancer of the oral cavity, pharynx and larynx (Roswit et al). Am. J. Roentgenol. Radium Ther. Nucl. Med., 114:59, 1972

Cancer, Squamous Cell—Cont.

Experiences with plastic surgery in therapy (Petres). Arch. Derm. Forsch., 244:156, 1972 (German)

Use of scalp flaps following resection of oral cancer (Dhawan et al). Aust. N. Z. J. Surg., 41:363, 1972

Nasal cancers. Individuality of treatment (Converse). J.A.M.A., 219:348, 1972

Segmental sagittal splitting of the mandible in the surgical treatment of carcinoma of the floor of the mouth (Perl). J. Oral Surg., 30:656, 1972

Carcinoma, squamous cell, of penis, surgical management of (Skinner, Leadbetter, Kelley), PRS, 50:542, 1972. J. Urol., 107:273, 1972

Cancer of the lip (Yonkers et al). Laryngoscope, 82:625, 1972

En bloc ethmoidectomy for cancer. (A progress report.) (Ross et al). Laryngoscope, 82:682, 1972

Surgery in cancer of head and neck. Use of posterior surgical flap (Lenczyk et al). N. Y. State J. Med., 72:239, 1972

Carcinoma, squamous cell, in epidermolysis bullosa dystrophica, autografting in the treatment of (Eastwood), PRS, 49:93, 1972

Management of major nasal defects (Remark et al) South. Med. J., 65:623, 1972

Carcinoma of the tonsil: a comparison of two treatment modalities (Andrews et al). South. Med. J., 65:982, 1972

Skin cancer (Jensen et al). Ugeskr. Laeger., 134:107, 1972 (Danish)

Carcinoma, squamous, of floor of the mouth (Flynn, Mullins, Moore), PRS, 53:497, 1974. Am. J. Surg., 126:477, 1973

Verrucose squamous carcinoma (Elliot, MacDougall, Elliott), PRS, 52:215, 1973. Ann. Surg., 177:21, 1973

Carcinoma, squamous cell, of skin (Honeycutt, Jansen), PRS, 54:380, 1974. Arch. Dermat., 108:670, 1973

Carcinoma, squamous, of ear (Lewis), PRS, 52:600, 1973. Arch. Otolaryng., 97:41, 1973

Carcinoma, postoperative recurrent squamous cell in head and neck, radiotherapy for (Deutsch et al), PRS, 54:108, 1974. Arch. Otolaryng., 98:316, 1973

Pemphigus and malignancy (Saikia). Brit. J. Dermatol., 88:407, 1973

Squamous cell carcinoma of hypopharynx, treatment (Inoue, Shigematsu, Sato), PRS, 52:460, 1973. Cancer, 31:649, 1973

Collagenolytic activities of squamous cell carcinoma of skin (Hashimoto et al), PRS, 54:116, 1974. Cancer Res., 33:2790, 1973

Cancer, Squamous Cell – Cont.

Carcinoma, squamous cell, late development of, in a split-skin graft lining a vagina (Steffanoff), PRS, *51:*454, 1973

Carcinoma, squamous, in a split-skin graft lining the vagina (Crow) (Letter to the Editor), PRS, *52:*293, 1973

Spinalioma, metastasizing, treated with bleomycin, clinical picture and histology of (Post). Z. Hautkr., *48:*1019, 1973 (German)

Cancer, squamous, of floor of mouth, marginal resection of mandible in (Flynn, Moore), PRS, *57:*540, 1976. Am. J. Surg., *128:*490, 1974

Carcinoma, squamous cell, and Bowen's disease of nail bed (Mikhail), PRS, *55:*256, 1975. Arch. Dermat., *110:*267, 1974

Epidermoid carcinoma, inadequately excised, management of (Glass, Perez-Mesa), PRS, *54:*246, 1974. Arch. Surg., *108:*50, 1974

Tumors, epidermoid, concurrent methotrexate and bleomycin chemotherapy (Lokich, Frei), PRS, *55:*256, 1975. Cancer Res., *34:*2240, 1974

Carcinoma, squamous cell, diagnosed as keratoacanthoma (Mikhail), PRS, *54:*381, 1974. Cutis, *13:*378, 1974

The philosophy of head and neck cancer surgery (Steckler *et al*). J. Prosthet. Dent., *32:*307, 1974

Carcinoma, squamous cell, of oral cavity, pharynx, and larynx, recurrence patterns in (Gilbert, Kagan), PRS, *56:*363, 1975. J. Surg. Oncol., *6:*257, 1974

Carcinoma, head and neck, advanced squamous, treated by chemotherapy (Stephens), PRS, *55:*386, 1975. M. J. Australia, *2:*587, 1974

Carcinoma, squamous, arising in an artificial vagina (Dellon) (Letter to the Editor), PRS, *53:*584, 1974

Malignant transformation of leg ulcers. Apropos of three cases (Nguyen *et al*). Phlebologie, *27:*215, 1974 (French)

In situ squamous cell carcinoma of the skin. Clinical diagnosis, pathology and treatment. (Amato *et al*). Rev. Bras. Pesqui. Mod. Biol., *7:*365, 1974

Advances in the surgical treatment of skin tumors (Wilflingseder). Wien. Med. Wochenschr., *124:*593, 1974 (German)

Cervical metastasis from an unknown primary (Fried *et al*). Ann. Otol. Rhin. & Laryngol., *84:*152, 1975

Carcinoma, squamous cell, invasive, of conjunctiva (Iliff, Marback, Green), PRS, *56:*235, 1975. Arch. Ophth., *93:*119, 1975

Cancer, Squamous Cell – Cont.

Carcinoma, squamous cell, of skin of pinna (Shiffman), PRS, *57:*403, 1976. Canad. J. Surg., *18:*279, 1975

Carcinoma, bowenoid squamous cell, of digits (Gottlieb, Newman), PRS, *57:*679, 1976. Cutis, *16:*108, 1975

Carcinoma, squamous cell, in epidermolysis bullosa dystrophica (Gipson), PRS, *57:*760, 1976. Hand, *7:*179, 1975

Daily practice: appreciation of the oncologic risk of oral lichen planus (Castermans-Elias *et al*). Rev. Belge. Med. Dent., *30:*33, 1975 (French)

Carcinoma, epidermoid: Marjolin's ulcer, immunologically privileged tumor? (Bostwick, Pendergrast, Vasconez), PRS, *57:*66, 1976

Carcinoma, squamous cell, arising in mandibular cyst (Herceg, Harding), PRS, *57:*383, 1976

Cancer, Tongue: See *Tongue, Neoplasms*

CANCURA, W.: Therapy of parotid gland tumors. Wien. Med. Wochenschr., Suppl *31:*3, 1975 (German)

CANIZARO, P. C., PRAGER, M. D., AND SHIRES, T. G.: Infusion of Ringer's lactate solution during shock, PRS, *51:*710, 1973. Am. J. Surg., *122:*494, 1971

CANJI, V. *et al:* Lateral cysts of the neck. Med. Pregl., *28:*537, 1975 (Serbian)

CANN, M. S. *et al:* Effect of digitalis on myocardial contractility in sepsis, PRS, *49:*475, 1972. Surg. Forum, *22:*1, 1971

CANNELL, H.: Cell-mediated and humoral immune responses to primary oral cancers, PRS, *55:*385, 1975. J. Maxillo-facial Surg., *2:*108, 1974

CANNIFF, J. P.: Longstanding bilateral intracapsular fracture dislocation on the condyles treated by closed condylotomy. Trans. Congr. Int. Assoc. Oral Surg., *4:*336, 1973

CANNON, B.: Discussion of "Cross-foot flap," by Taylor, Hopson, PRS, *56:*83, 1975

CANNON, B.: Interfascicular nerve grafting: early experiences at Massachusetts General Hospital (with Finseth, Constable), PRS, *56:*492, 1975

CANNON, B.: Discussion of "Free musculocutaneous flap," by Harii *et al*, PRS, *57:*511, 1976

CANTEGREL, C.: Study of 1,000 ulcers treated in a non-hospitalized clientele. Phlebologie, *27:*141, 1974 (French)

Canthoplasty: See *Eyelids, Canthoplasty*

CANTRELL, R. W.: Use of mandibular homografts in reconstructing jaw defects. Laryngoscope, *84:*1925, 1974

CAPETANAKIS, J.: Juvenile melanoma disseminatum. Brit. J. Dermatol., *92:*207, 1975

CAPINPIN, A.: Survey of chemical peeling of the face (with Litton, Fournier), PRS, *51:*645, 1973

CAPITAINE, P. *et al:* Ameloblastic odontoma in a very young child. Rev. Stomatol. Chir. Maxillofac., *76:*447, 1975 (French)

CAPLAN, H.: Craft of rhinoplasty. Can. J. Otolaryngol., *1:*102, 1972

CAPLAN, H.: Profileoplasty. Can. J. Otolaryngol., *2:*347, 1973

CAPOZZI, A.: Porcine skin grafts. Calif. Med., *116:*56, 1972

CAPOZZI, A.: Transposition of fat in cervicofacial rhytidectomy (with Pennisi), PRS, *49:*423, 1972

CAPOZZI, A.: Travase, effective enzyme for burn debridement (with Pennisi, Friedman), PRS, *51:*371, 1973

CAPOZZI, A.: Treatment of chronic cystic disease of the breast by subcutaneous mastectomy (with Pennisi), PRS, *52:*520, 1973

CAPOZZI, A.: Incidence of carcinoma in subcutaneous mastectomy (with Pennisi), PRS, *56:*9, 1975. Discussion by Snyderman, PRS, *56:*208, 1975

CAPPERAULD, I.: Acupuncture anesthesia and medicine in China today, PRS, *51:*488, 1973. Surg. Gynec. & Obst., *135:*440, 1972

CAPRARO, V. J. *et al:* Creation of a neovagina. A simplified technic. Obstet. Gynecol., *39:*545, 1972

CAPRARO, V. J. *et al:* Vaginal agenesis. Am. J. Obstet. Gynecol., *124:*98, 1976

CAPUTO, R., AND PRANDI, G.: Inverse ungual pterygium, PRS, *57:*267, 1976. Arch. Dermat., *108:*817, 1973

CARACCIOLO, P. R.: Review of surgical treatment of 90 cases of cancer of thyroid. Int. Surg., *58:*402, 1973

CARACCIOLO, P. R.: Surgical treatment of 150 cases of squamous cell carcinoma of the mouth. Int. Surg., *60:*546, 1975

CARACINO, A. M.: Topical treatment of secondary pyogenic cutaneous infections with gentamycin sulfate. G. Ital. Dermatol., *46:*530, 1971 (Italian)

CARAMIA, G. *et al:* Malformative aspects involving the 1st branchial arch. Report of 3 cases. Minerva Med., *63:*490, 1972 (Italian)

CARAPETO, F. J. *et al:* Adenoacanthoma: review of 20 cases, compared with literature. Dermatologica, *145:*269, 1972

CARAVEL, J. B.: Traumatic section of lacrimal canaliculi, therapeutical attitudes and results. Ann. chir. plast., *18:*371, 1973 (French)

CARAVEL, J. B. *et al:* Osteosynthesis of middle face by screwed plates. Rev. Stomatol. Chir. Maxillofac., *75:*256, 1974 (French)

CARAYON, A. *et al:* Peripheral nerve surgery in leprous neuritis (technics, value and respective indications of procedures). Med. Trop. (Mars.), *32:*23, 1972 (French)

CARAYON, A. *et al:* Selection of cases and results of direct surgery of 535 mixed nerves in leprosy. Med. Trop. (Mars.), *32:*157, 1972 (French)

CARAYON, A., VAN DROOGENBROECK, J. B., GIRANDEAU, P.: Evaluation of palliative surgery in leprotic paralysis of foot. Med. Trop., *32:*695, 1972 (French)

CARBAJAL, U. M.: Levator-Mueller's muscle resection through combined internal and external approach. Eye, Ear, Nose, Throat Mon., *51:*348, 1972

CARBAJAL, U. M.: Sliding bridge graft in exenteration of the orbit. Trans. Ophthalmol. Soc., N.Z., *25:*136, 1973

Carbon Dioxide Freezing: See *Cryotherapy*

Carcinoma: See *Cancer*

CARDEN, E. T.: Plastic surgery monopoly? New England J. Med., *288:*164, 1973

CARDEN, W. D., HUBBARD, R. B., AND PETTY, C.: Effect of premedication and angiography on arterial blood gases, PRS, *54:*692, 1974. Mil. Med., *141:*476, 1974

Cardiac Arrest (See also *Anesthesia; Shock*)

Cardiac arrest in operating room (McClure, Skardasis, Brown), PRS, *50:*540, 1972. Am. Surgeon, *38:*241, 1972

Penicillin administration, intravenous, cardiac arrest due to hyperkalemia following (Mercer, Logic), PRS *53:*609, 1974. Chest, *64:*358, 1973

Cardiac arrest, factors determining survival in patients with (Castagna, Weil, Shubin), PRS, *55:*250, 1975. Chest, *65:*527, 1974

CARDINAL, E. D.: Vulvar elephantiasis, PRS, *54:*377, 1974. Rev.Medico, *24:*43, 1974

CARDO, V. A. JR., *et al:* Surgical removal of nasopalatine cyst, case report. N. Y. State Dent. J., *39:*484, 1973

CARDOSO, A. D.: Use of temporal aponeurosis in correction of blepharoptosis. Rev. Assoc. Med. Bras., *20:*229, 1974 (Portuguese)

CARDOSO, A. D. *et al:* Planning reduction rhinoplasties. Rev. Assoc. Med. Bras., *18:*401, 1972 (Portuguese)

CARDOSO DE CASTRO, C.: Mammaplasty with curved incisions, PRS, *57:*596, 1976

CARIATI, E. *et al:* Recent evaluations on treatment of lymphedema, PRS, *57:*399, 1976. J. Cardiovasc. Surg., *16:*192, 1975

CARIFI, V. G. *et al:* Results of high dose radiation and surgery in the treatment of advanced cancer of the head and neck. Am. J. Surg., *128:*580, 1974

CARL, P. *et al:* Operative treatment of male pseudohermaphroditism. Urologe(A)., *14:*178, 1975 (German)

CARL, W. *et al:* Oral surgery and patient who has had radiation therapy for head and neck cancer. Oral Surg., *36:*651, 1973

CARL, W., SAKO, K., AND SCHAFF, N.: Dental complications in treatment of rhabdomyosarcoma of oral cavity in children, PRS, *56:*223, 1975. Oral Surg., *38:*367, 1974

CARLIER, F. *et al:* Section of facial nerves and periocular muscles in photosensitive Papio papio. Electroencephalogr. Clin. Neurophysiol., *35:*13, 1973 (French)

CARLIER, G. *et al:* Palatal neoplasms of salivary origin, 10 cases. Acta Stomatol. Belg., *69:*257, 1972 (French)

CARLIER, G. *et al:* Numerical data on the recurrence of ameloblastomas. Rev. Stomatol. Chir. Maxillofac., *75:*37, 1974 (French)

CARLIER, G. *et al:* Depressed fractures of the upper part of the face. Rev. Stomatol. Chir. Maxillofac., *75:*238, 1974 (French)

CARLIER, G. *et al:* Three hundred thirty eight tumors of the parotid region. Acta Stomatol. Belg. 72:*465, 1975 (French)

CARLIN, G. A.: Personally fabricated chin implants, PRS, *51:*121, 1973

CARLIN, G. A.: Knee-to-knee syndrome, PRS, *53:*353, 1974

CARLIN, R. *et al:* Malignant lymphoma of nasolacrimal sac. Am. J. Ophth., *78:*511, 1974

CARLSEN, L., AND TERSHAKOWEC, M. G.: Variation of Biesenberger technique of reduction mammaplasty, PRS, *55:*653, 1975

CARLSON, L. E.: Below-elbow control of an externally powered hand. Bull. Prosthet. Res., *10:*43, 1970

CARNEIRO, R. S.: Aneurysm of wrist, PRS, *54:*483, 1974

CARNEY, P. J. *et al:* Structural correlates of nasality. Cleft Palate J., *8:*307, 1971

CARO, D. *et al:* The Old Bailey bomb explosion. Lancet, *1:*1433, 1973

CAROLLA, R. L.: Age of red blood cells destroyed by *in vivo* hyperoxia, PRS, *56:*107, 1975. Aerospace Med., *45:*1273, 1974

CARON, A. S. *et al:* Osteogenic sarcoma of the facial and cranial bones. A review of forty-three cases. Am. J. Surg., *122:*719, 1971

CARONNI, ERNESTO P.: *Congenital Anomalies of the Eyelids.* Minerva Medical Press, Turin, Italy, 1967. PRS, *50:*518, 1972

CARONNI, E. P.: New method to correct nasolabial angle in rhinoplasty, PRS, *50:*338, 1972

Carotid Arteries

Cerebral blood flow and internal carotid artery flow during carotid surgery. (Boysen *et al*). Stroke, *1:*253, 1970

Circulation patterns during clamping of the carotid arteries as determined by cutaneous carotid photoplethysmography (Fuster *et al*). Acta Neurol. Lat. Am., *17:*273, 1971

Carotid body tumors, surgical treatment of (Krause-Senties), PRS, *49:*237, 1972. Arch. Inv. Med. Mex., *2:*25, 1971

Case of acute nasal bleeding requiring unilateral ligation of the external carotid artery (Kekelidze). Vestn. Otorinolaringol., *33:*108, 1971 (Russian)

Carotid neurifibroma in a child (Slim *et al*). Am. J. Surg., *123:*343, 1972

Effect of peripheral resistance on carotid blood flow after carotid-subclavian bypass (Cook *et al*). Arch. Surg., *105:*9, 1972

Carotid arteries, intraoperative injuries of, and their surgical correction (Flora *et al*). Bruns Beitr. Klin. Chir., *219:*716, 1972 (German)

Carotid artery surgery and intermittent monocular blindness (amaurosis fugax) (Houck *et al*). J. S. C. Med. Assoc., *68:*57, 1972

Experimental evaluation of some methods of plastic operations on the common carotid artery (Paszenko *et al*). Neurol. Neurochir. Pol., *6:*447, 1972 (Polish)

Carotid artery, forehead flap rotation to protect (Smalley, Cunningham), PRS, *49:*96, 1972

Carotid artery, protection by fascia lata in head and neck surgery (Foote, Chandler), PRS, *51:*351, 1973. South. M.J., *65:*1225, 1972

Rapid microvascular repair using plastic adhesive (Shintani *et al*). Stroke, *3:*34, 1972

Aneurysm of a saphenous vein graft to the common carotid artery (Carrasquilla *et al*). Vasc. Surg., *6:*66, 1972

External carotid artery ligation in epistaxis (Viktorov *et al*). Vestn. Otorinolaringol., *34:*115, 1972 (Russian)

Carotid artery, open severance (Grohmann). Z. Aerztl. Fortbild., Jena, *66:*1031, 1972 (German)

Carotid artery, resected, clinicopathologic study of (Huvos, Leaming, Moore), PRS,

Carotid Arteries — Cont.

53:488, 1974. Am. J. Surg., *126:*570, 1973

Carotid arteriovenous fistulae, external (Bruce, Walike, Goertzen), PRS, *54:*106, 1974. Arch. Otolaryng., 98:332, 1973

Carotid arteries, intraoperative injuries of (Flora). Deutsch. Med. Wochenschr., 98:716, 1973

Cerebral insufficiency with common carotid kinking (Kia-Noury), PRS, *54:*239, 1974. Internat. Surg., 58:9, 1973

Carotid arteries, penetrating injuries of (Bradley). J. Trauma, 13:248, 1973

Carotid artery rupture (Shumrick). Laryngoscope, 83:1051, 1973

Carotid body tumors: 16-year follow-up of 7 malignant cases (Martin, Rosenfeld, McSwain), PRS, *53:*612, 1974. South. M.J., 66:1236, 1973

Carotid artery protection, dermis grafts for (Smithdeal, Corso, Strong), PRS, *57:*536, 1976. Am. J. Surg., *128:*484, 1974

Carotid artery, traumatic injuries in civilian practice (DiVincenti *et al*). Am. Surg., *40:*277, 1974

Carotid artery, operation for aneurysm of, high in neck; new and an old technique (Hershey). Angiology, 25:24, 1974

Carotid artery rupture, experimental analysis of causative factors and protective methods in (Swain *et al*), PRS, *55:*110, 1975. Arch. Otolaryng., 99:235, 1974

Carotid artery and dermal graft (Yim *et al*), PRS, *54:*692, 1974. Arch. Otolaryng., 99:242, 1974

Carotid artery replacement with saphenous vein graft for other than arteriosclerotic obstructive disease (Stueber *et al*). Med. Ann. D.C., *43:*237, 1974

Experiments on cryosurgery of tumors of great blood vessels in neck (Ganz). Minerva Med., 65:3645, 1974

Carotid artery, external, spontaneous arteriovenous fistula arising from, during pregnancy (Minami, Jafek, Cooper), PRS, 53:230, 1974

Transparotid approach in mandibular ameloblastoma recurrences (Gouiric *et al*). Rev. Stomatol. Chir. Maxillofac., 75:58, 1974 (French)

Carotid intimal tear following blunt craniocervical trauma, delayed presentation of (Crissey *et al*). Surgery, 75:543, 1974

Carotid arteries, external and internal, complete traumatic transection of (Merguet). Thorax-chirurgie, 22:68, 1974 (German)

Carotid artery protection, blood supply to levator scapulae muscle relative to (Smith *et*

Carotid Arteries — Cont.

al). Trans. Am. Acad. Ophthalmol. Otolaryngol., 78:1128, 1974

Injury of the left common carotid artery (Iupatov *et al*). Vestn. Khir., *112:*105, 1974 (Russian)

Carotid, common, closed injury of (Piscevic *et al*). Vojnosanit. Pregl., *31:*119, 1974 (Serbian)

Carotid arteries, external and internal, post-traumatic nasal hemorrhage requiring unilateral ligation of (Pavlovskii). Zh. Ushn. Nos. Gorl. Bolezn., 105, Mar–Apr., 1974 (Russian)

Transsternal radical neck dissection. Postoperative complications and management (Sisson *et al*). Arch. Otolaryng., *101:*46, 1975

Complications of dermal graft protection of carotid artery (Dedo *et al*). Arch. Otolaryng., *101:*649, 1975

Elective carotid artery resection (Martinez *et al*). Arch. Otolaryng., *101:*744, 1975

Emergency care of severe facial injuries (Eade). Clin. Plast. Surg., 2:73, 1975

Arterial epistaxis (Shaheen). J. Laryng. & Otol., 89:17, 1975

Muscle and facial grafts in carotid artery protection (Sadoyama). Laryngoscope, 85:841, 1975

Fistula, carotid-cavernous sinus, occurring after a rhinoplasty (Song, Bromberg), PRS, 55:92, 1975

Carotid artery, trigone, rhabdomyoma in (Gawronski *et al*). Patol. Pol., 26:287, 1975 (Polish)

Dermal grafts — a viable alternative (Cairns). Trans. Am. Acad. Ophthalmol. Otolaryngol., 80:510, 1975

Injury of the right common carotid artery (Dekster *et al*). Vestn. Khir., *115:*105, 1975 (Russian)

Carpal Tunnel Syndrome

Carpal tunnel syndrome in pregnancy (Nicholas, Noone, Graham), PRS, *48:*513, 1971. Hand, 3:80, 1971

Anomalous muscle belly of the flexor digitorum superficialis causing carpal-tunnel syndrome. Report of a case (Smith). J. Bone & Joint Surg. (Am.), 53:1215, 1971

Essential acroparesthesia and the carpal tunnel syndrome (Chatin *et al*). Lyon Med., 18:Suppl. 85, 1971 (French)

Gilliat and Wilson's test in carpal tunnel syndrome (Fernandez Sabata, Yaya Huaman), PRS, *51:*232, 1973. Med. Clin., 46:349, 1971

Carpal Tunnel Syndrome — Cont.

Case of carpal tunnel syndrome due to lumbricalis anomaly (Kojima *et al*). Orthop. Surg. (Tokyo), *22:*746, 1971 (Japanese)

Surgery of some strictures and stenoses. Some tunnel syndromes. Compression problems in the hand (Backhouse). Ann. R. Coll. Surg. Engl., *50:*321, 1972

Case of carpal tunnel syndrome on the basis of an abnormally long lumbrical muscle (Eriksen). Acta Orthop. Scand., *44:*275, 1973

Vascularization of flexor tendons within the carpal tunnel and the hand (Zbrodowski). Chir. Narzadow. Ruchu. Ortop. Pol., *38:*589, 1973 (Polish)

Carpal tunnel syndrome (Stack), PRS, *53:*367, 1974. Fam. Phys., *8:*88, 1973

Kienbock's disease treated by neurolysis of median nerve in carpal tunnel (Codega, Codega, Kus), PRS, *53:*246, 1974. Internat. Surg., *58:*378, 1973

Palmar cutaneous branch of median nerve and approach to carpal tunnel (Taleisnik), PRS, *53:*684, 1974. J. Bone & Joint Surg., *55:*1212, 1973

Carpal tunnel syndrome in patients with myxedematous arthropathy (Frymoyer, Bland), PRS, *52:*207, 1973. J. Bone & Joint Surg., *55A:*78, 1973

Carpal tunnel syndrome, internal neurolysis as adjunct to treatment of (Curtis, Eversmann), PRS, *53:*246, 1974. J. Bone & Joint Surg., *55A:*733, 1973

Thrombosis of persistent median artery, acute carpal tunnel syndrome secondary to (Maxwell, Kepes, Ketchum), PRS, *53:*368, 1974. J. Neurosurg., *38:*774, 1973

Carpal tunnel: variations of motor branch of median nerve at wrist (Graham), PRS, *51:*90, 1973

Entrapment, nerve, in the wrist and hand, anomalous muscles and (Still, Kleinert), PRS, *52:*394, 1973

Amyloidosis and carpal tunnel syndrome (Bastian), PRS, *54:*620, 1974. Am. J. Clin. Path., *61:*711, 1974

Carpal tunnel syndrome, proximal pain in (Cherington), PRS, *54:*237, 1974. Arch. Surg., *108:*69, 1974

An unusual cause of carpal tunnel syndrome (Engeron *et al*). Cah. Med., *15:*25, 1974

Anatomical model of the mesotenon of the flexor tendons in the carpal tunnel (Zbrodowski). Chir. Narzadow. Ruchu. Ortop. Pol., *39:*57, 1974 (Polish)

Palmar incision for release of the carpal tunnel (Rowland). Clin. Orthop., *0:*89, 1974

Carpal Tunnel Syndrome — Cont.

Carpal tunnel syndrome, *flexor digitorum superficialis indicis* and (Neviaser), PRS, *56:*230, 1975. Hand, *6:*155, 1974

Carpal tunnel syndrome, incipient, anomalous *flexor sublimis* muscle with (Hayes), PRS, *53:*479, 1974

Muscle, anomalous *palmaris longus*, producing carpal tunnel-like compression (Backhouse, Churchill-Davidson), PRS, *56:*596, 1975. Hand, *7:*22, 1975

Carpal tunnel syndrome: importance of sensory nerve conduction studies in diagnosis (Hoffman), PRS, *57:*400, 1976. J.A.M.A., *233:*983, 1975

An unusual cause of carpal tunnel syndrome (Engeron *et al*). J. Iowa Med. Soc., *65:*25, 1975

Syndrome, carpal tunnel, caused by hand injuries (Browne, Snyder), PRS, *56:*41, 1975

Nerve, median and ulnar, entrapment in hand, place of resection of hood of hamate in treatment of (Wissinger), PRS, *56:*501, 1975

Median carpal tunnel syndrome following a vascular shunt procedure in the forearm (Mancusi-Ungaro, Corres, Di Spaltro), PRS, *57:*96, 1976

CARPENDALE, M.: Comparison of four beds in prevention of tissue ischemia in paraplegic patients, PRS, *56:*115, 1975. Paraplegia, *12:*21, 1974

CARPENTER, P. A. *et al:* Clinical-pathological conference: Case 10, part 2. Neurofibrosarcoma. J. Oral Surg., *33:*38, 1975

CARRARO, J. J. *et al:* Enlargement of coronoid process of jaw, PRS, *54:*687, 1974. Bol. y trab. Acad. argent. cir., *57:*469, 1973

CARRARO, J. J., CAFFESSE, R. G., AND ALBANO, E.: Temporomandibular joint syndrome: influence of first symptom on initial therapeutic response, PRS, *53:*682, 1974. J. Prosth. Dent., *30:*87, 1973

CARRASQUILLA, C. *et al:* Aneurysm of a saphenous vein graft to the common carotid artery. Vasc. Surg., *6:*66, 1972

CARREIRAO, S. E., AND LESSA, S.: Polymastia — axillary breast, PRS, *57:*533, 1976. Rev. brasil. cir., *53:*77, 1975

CARROLL, J. M., AND BEYER, C. K.: Conjunctivodacryocystorhinostomy using silicone rubber lacrimal tubes. Arch. Ophth., *89:*113, 1973

CARROLL, R. E., AND DICK, H. M.: Arthrodesis of the wrist for rheumatoid arthritis, PRS, *50:*307, 1972. J. Bone & Joint Surg., *53:*1365, 1971

CARROLL, R. E., AND BERMAN, A. T.: Glomus tumors of hand, PRS, *51:*104, 1973. J. Bone & Joint Surg., *54A:*691, 1972

CARROLL, R. G.: Evaluation of tracheal tube cuff designs. Crit. Care Med., *1:*45, 1973

CARROLL, R. G. *et al:* Proper use of large diameter, large residual volume cuffs. Crit. Care Med., *1:*153, 1973

CARROLL, R. G. *et al:* Recommended performance specifications for cuffed endotracheal and tracheostomy tubes: joint statement of investigators, inventors and manufacturers. Crit. Care Med., *1:*155, 1973

CARROLL, R. P.: Common problems in ophthalmic plastic surgery. Am. Fam. Physician, *12:*85, 1975

CARROLL, R. P.: Functional dermatochalasia. Minn. Med., *59:*15, 1976

CARROLL, R. P. *et al:* Mustarde suturing forceps. Am. J. Ophth., *78:*860, 1974

CARRUBBA, R. W., AND BOWERS, J. Z.: Western world's first detailed treatise on acupuncture: William Ten Rhijne's *De Acupunctura,* PRS, *55:*727, 1975. J. Hist. Med. & Allied Sc., *29:*371, 1974

CARSON, I. W.: Review of methods for evaluation of recovery from anesthesia and comparative study of intravenous steroid anesthetic Althesin with methohexitone and thiopentone, PRS, *56:*237, 1975. Proc. Roy. Soc. Med., *68:*108, 1975

CARSTAM, N.: What is happening in hand surgery? Lakartidningen, *71:*2840, 1974 (Swedish)

CARSTAM, N., AND EIKEN, O.: Kirner's deformity of little finger, PRS, *49:*234, 1972. J. Bone & Joint Surg., *52A:*1663, 1970

CARSTENS, P. H. B., AND SCHRODT, G. R.: Ultrastructure of sclerosing hemangioma, PRS, *57:*678, 1976. Am. J. Path., *77:*377, 1974

CARTER, S. J. *et al:* Infections of the hand. Orthop. Clin. North Am., *1:*455, 1970

Cartilage Grafts

Autograft, ground cartilage (Gallo), PRS, *50:*99, 1972. Med. Colombiana, *42:*17, 1971

Rib growth cartilage, transplantation; experimental study and possible use in primary cleft lip repairs (Kluzak), PRS, *49:*61, 1972

Mucochondrial graft, autogenous, tracheal reconstruction with (Krizek, Kirchner), PRS, *50:*123, 1972

Cartilage, rib growth, autotransplantation of (Kluzak), PRS, *53:*499, 1974. Acta Chir. orthop. Trauma cech., *40:*89, 1973

Cartilage graft, retrocondylar, for treatment of mandibular retrognathism (Lachard, Vitton). Ann. chir. plast., *18:*50, 1973 (French)

Cartilage Grafts – Cont.

Cartilage, articular, value of preserving in transarticular joint amputations (Graham *et al*), PRS, *53:*495, 1974. J. Surg. Res., *14:*524, 1973

Antigenicity of cartilage grafts (Heyner), PRS, *53:*613, 1974. Surg. Gynec. & Obst., *136:*298, 1973

Growth hormone, response of transplanted articular cartilage to (Yablon, Frazblau, Leach), PRS, *54:*510, 1974. J. Bone & Joint Surg., *56A:*322, 1974

Cartilage, articular, synovectomy and (Schulitz), PRS, *54:*247, 1974. Ztschr. Orthop., *112:*118, 1974

Arthritis formation of articular cartilage from free perichondrial grafts (Skoog, Johansson), PRS, *57:*1, 1976

Cartilage Grafts, Ear

Ear cartilage grafts, young rabbit, transplanted in young rabbits, does growth occur in? (Peer) (Follow-Up Clinic), PRS, *49:*208, 1972

Ear cartilage grafts, use for nasal tip reconstructions (Falces, Gorney), PRS, *50:*147, 1972

Cartilage, auricular, for auricle reconstruction (Kruchinski), PRS, *53:*601, 1974. Acta chir. plast., *15:*72, 1973

Cartilage, autogenous rib in expansile framework for ear reconstruction (Brent), PRS, *53:*619, 1974

Cartilage Grafts, Experimental

Growth potential of autografts of cartilage from nasal septum in rat (Kvinnsland), PRS, *52:*557, 1973

Perichondrial graft, free, placed across defect in a rabbit's trachea, growth of cartilage from (Sohn, Ohlsén), PRS, *53:*55, 1974

Homotransplanted ear cartilage, growth in baby rabbits (Allison, Achauer, Furnas), PRS, *55:*479, 1975

Cartilage, mandibular condylar, in rat, effects of hydrocortisone (Priest), PRS, *56:*225, 1975. Proc. Roy. Soc. Med., *68:*128, 1975

Cartilage Grafts, Homografts and Heterografts

Cartilage, heterologous, evaluation of transplantation stored frozen and in 70° alcohol (Pankin, Chirkova), PRS, *54:*510, 1974. Acta chir. plast., *15:*155, 1973

Grafts, cartilage, antigenicity of (Heyner), PRS, *53:*613, 1974. Surg. Gynec. & Obst., *136:*298, 1973

Concha auriculae, allo-, homo- and autografts of supporting skeleton of (compara-

Cartilage Grafts, Homografts and Heterografts — Cont.

tive results) (Lapchenko *et al*). Zh. Ushn. Nos. Gori. Bolezn., *33:*48, 1973 (Russian)

Immunogenicity of homograft articular cartilage (Langer, Gross), PRS, *54:*507, 1974. J. Bone & Joint Surg., *56A:*297, 1974

Homograft cartilage and skin reconstruction (Mathias), PRS, *57:*125, 1976. Arch. Otol., *101:*301, 1975

Growth of homotransplanted ear cartilage in baby rabbits (Allison, Achauer, Furnas), PRS, *55:*479, 1975

Cartilage Grafts, Preserved (See also *Cartilage Grafts, Homografts)*

Cartilage, preserved human, fate of (Rasi) (Follow-Up Clinic), PRS, *49:*83, 1972

Cartilage, heterologous, stored frozen in 70 degrees alcohol, comparative evaluation of transplantation of. Experimental-clinical investigation (Pankin *et al*). PRS, *54:*510, 1974. Acta chir. plast. *15:*155, 1973

CARUSO, A. C.: Treatment of arthrosis of the hands. Prensa Med. Argent., *58:*629, 1971 (Spanish)

CARVALHAL FRANCA, J. G.: Treatment of comminuted fractures of malar bone and floor of orbital cavity using hydropneumatic method of immobilization, PRS, *48:*510, 1971. Rev. Latino Am. cir. plast., *13:*106, 1969

CARVALHAL FRANCA, J. G.: Lip reconstruction employing lingual flap, PRS, *49:*102, 1972. Assoc. med. Brasil, *17:*123, 1971

CARVALHO, F. DOS S.: Total reconstruction of the breast after the removal of a bilateral giant fibroadenoma. Rev. Assoc. Med. Bras., *18:*95, 1972 (Portuguese)

CARVALHO, R. R. *et al:* Hemifacial spasm: results of surgical treatment in 14 cases. Arq. Neuropsiquiatr., *31:*91, 1973 (Portuguese)

CASALI, R. E. *et al:* Critical factors in resuscitation of the severely burned rat: the relative merit of volume, tonicity, sodium load, and concentration of the solution used. Ann. Surg., *175:*138, 1972

CASE, T. D., AND LAPIANA, F. G.: Benign fibrous tumor of orbit, PRS, *57:*256, 1976. Ann. Ophth., *7:*813, 1975

CASESA, P. R.: Disabilities of hand under social security. N.Y. State J. Med., *73:*2569, 1973

CASSON, P. R., BONANNO, P. C., AND CONVERSE, J. M.: Midface degloving procedure, PRS, *53:*102, 1974

CASTAGNA, J., WEIL, W., AND SHUBIN, H.: Factors determining survival in patients with cardiac arrest, PRS, *55:*250, 1975. Chest, *65:*527, 1974

CASTAÑARES, S.: Blepharospasm, new approach to treatment, PRS, *51:*248, 1973

CASTAÑARES, S.: Discussion of "Anatomy for a blepharoplasty," by Hugo, Stone, PRS, *53:*587, 1974

CASTAÑARES, S.: Plastic construction of an artificial vagina (Follow-Up Clinic), PRS, *54:*605, 1974

CASTAÑARES, S.: Facial nerve paralyses coincident with, or subsequent to, rhytidectomy, PRS, *54:*637, 1974

CASTELAIN, P. Y.: Successive nevocarcinomas complicating Dubreuilh's melanosis evolving over period of 38 years. Bull. Soc. Fr. Dermatol. Syphiligr., *79:*276, 1972 (French)

CASTELLANI, A.: A note on infantile and juvenile leucodermata and their palliative cosmetic treatment. Arch. Ital. Sci. Med. Trop. Parassitol., *51:*49, 1970

CASTELLO, C. *et al:* Anesthesiologic risk in extensively burned patient. Minerva Anestesiol., *38:*553, 1972 (Italian)

CASTERMANS, A.: Policy of treatment of cleft lip and palate. Rev. Med. Liege, *27:*Suppl 137, 1972 (French)

CASTERMANS, A.: Surgical treatment of exophthalmos (Letter to the Editor), PRS, *57:*90, 1976

CASTERMANS-ELIAS, S. *et al:* Daily practice: appreciation of the oncologic risk of oral lichen planus. Rev. Belge. Med. Dent., *30:*33, 1975 (French)

CASTILLO, J.: Treatment of thermal injuries. Surg. Clin. North Am., *53:*627, 1973

CASTILLO, L. A. *et al:* Clinical and electrobiological basis for surgery in primary peripheral facial paralysis. Indications for emergency surgery. Rev. Laryngol. Otol. Rhinol. (Bord.), *96:*65, 1975

CASTRO, E. B. *et al:* Tumors of the major salivary glands in children, PRS, *50:*97, 1972. Cancer, *29:*312, 1972

CASTRO, E. B., HAJDU, S. I., AND FORTNER, J. G.: Surgical therapy of fibrosarcoma of extremities: reappraisal, PRS, *53:*371, 1974. Arch. Surg., *107:*284, 1973

CASTRO FARINA, I.: Employment of skin homografts in epidermolysis bullosa, PRS, *48:*611, 1971. Rev. españ. cir. plast., *4:*109, 1971

CASTRO FERREIRA, M., PSILLAKIS, M. J., AND SPINA, V.: *Cutis laxa:* its physiopathology and surgical treatment, PRS, *52:*682, 1973. Rev. Assoc. Med. Brasil, *19:*9, 1973

CASTROVIEJO, R.: Modified Wheeler's operation for senile spastic entropion. Harefuah, *85:*462, 1973 (Hebrew)

CASTROVIEJO, R.: Surgical correction of ptosis by resection of levator, PRS, *55:*245, 1975. Ann. Ophth., *6:*163, 1974

CASTROVIEJO, R.: Modification of Wheeler's operation for senile spastic entropion, PRS, 55:245, 1975. Ann. Ophth., 6:171, 1974

CASTRUP, W. et al: So-called eosinophilic soft-tissue granuloma. Strahlentherapie, 148:139, 1974 (German)

CATALANOTTO, F. A.: Eosinophilic granuloma of bone in childhood: report of case. J. Dent. Child., 41:33, 1974

CATALOGLU, C.: Surgical and prosthetic treatment of maxillary prognathism and case. Dentoral. (Istanbul), 4:180, 1972 (Turkish)

CATANIA, C. V. et al: End results of surgical treatment of 622 cases of tumors of the salivary glands. Tumori, 60:307, 1974 (Italian)

CATANIA, V. C.: Instant prosthetic substitution after resection and disarticulation of mandible. Minerva Chir., 26:1418, 1971 (Italian)

CATANIA, V. C.: Experiences in treatment of parotid gland neoplasms. Minerva Chir., 26:1422, 1971 (Italian)

CATANIA, V. C. et al: Prosthetic reconstruction of mandible. Minerva Med., 64:3641, 1973 (Italian)

CATANIA, V. C. et al: New perspectives in prosthetic replacement of mandible after resection or disarticulation. Tumori, 59:137, 1973 (Italian)

CATE, H. W. et al: External shunt in the treatment of idiopathic priapism. J. Urol., 114:726, 1975

CATON, R. B. et al: Complex odontoma in maxillary sinus. Oral Surg., 36:658, 1973

CATTERALL, M., SUTHERLAND, I., AND BEWLEY, D. K.: Randomized clinical trial of fast neutrons compared with X or gamma rays in treatment of advanced tumors of head and neck, PRS, 57:402, 1976. Brit. M. J., 2:653, 1975

CATTONI, M.: Vestibular extension in periodontal surgery. Edjan and Mejchar technic. Rev. Dent. (St. Domingo), 18:5, 1972 (Spanish)

CAUCCI, M.: Plastic repair of hypospadias. Minerva Pediatr., 26:1525, 1974 (Italian)

CAVALLERO, M., MAGLIACANI, G., AND RINAUDO, M. T.: Activity of hydroxyproline in formation of burn scars, PRS, 56:361, 1975. Riv. ital. chir. plast., 5:241, 1973

CAVALLO, C. A. et al: Chylothorax complicating radical neck dissection. Am. Surg., 41:266, 1975

CAVANAGH, H. D. et al: Multicentric sebaceous adenocarcinoma of meibomian gland. Am. J. Ophth., 77:326, 1974

CAVIGLIA, C.: Forehead rhytidoplasty and brow lifting (with Viñas, Cortinas), PRS, 57:445, 1976

CAVINA, C.: Surgical correction of case of mi-

crognathism. Minerva Stomatol., 21:211, 1972 (Italian)

CAVO, J. W. et al: Flow resistance in tracheotomy tubes. Surg. Forum, 23:490, 1972

CAWSON, R. A.: Myxoma of mandible with 35-year follow-up. Brit. J. Oral Surg., 10:59, 1972

CECILIANI, L., AND TOLU, P.: Surgical treatment of rheumatoid hand, PRS, 51:104, 1973. Minerva ortop., 22:175, 1971

CELESNIK, F.: Classification of cheilognathopalatoschisis. Chir. Maxillofac. Plast., 7:59, 1970 (German)

CELESNIK, F.: Treatment of hare lip and cleft palate. Rev. Stomatol. Chir. Maxillofac., 71:559, 1970 (French)

CELESNIK, F.: Surgical anatomy of intraglandular portion of facial nerve, PRS, 53:603, 1974. J. Maxillo-facial Surg., 1:65, 1973

CELESNIK, F.: General problems of the cleft lip and palate. Minerva Stomatol., 23:171, 1974 (Italian)

CELIS-BLAUBACH, A. et al: Idiopathic hemifacial spasm. New method of surgical treatment. Acta Otolaryngol. (Stockh.), 77:221, 1974

CELLERINO, N. A.: Brief notes on malignant melanomas. Prensa med. argent., 58:1601, 1971 (Spanish)

CELLI, L., AND CAROLI, A.: Revival of sensation in transplantations and cutaneous grafts of hand, PRS, 51:104, 1973. Riv. Chir. della Mano, 8:23, 1972

CENDELIN, E.: Diagnosis and therapy of mixed salivary gland tumors. Dtsch. Stomatol., 22:509, 1972 (German)

CENDRON, J.: Bladder reconstruction. Method derived from that of Trendelenbourg. Ann. Chir. Infant., 12:371, 1971 (French)

CENDRON, J.: Our experience with rectal bladders. Ann. Chir. Infant., 12:444, 1971 (French)

CENDRON, J.: Treatment of bladder exstrophy. Practical problems of equipment. Ann. Chir. Infant., 12:464, 1971 (French)

CENDRON, J.: Treatment of bladder exstrophy. Transformation of an external transintestinal shunt into an internal shunt. Ann. Chir. Infant., 12:465, 1971 (French)

CENDRON, J.: Treatment of bladder exstrophy. Genital problems. Ann. Chir. Infant., 12:473, 1971 (French)

CENDRON, J.: Treatment of hypospadias, PRS, 48:607, 1971. Proc. Roy. Soc. Med., 64:125, 1971

CENDRON, J.: Epispadias. Seventy cases. Urol. Int., 27:291, 1972 (French)

CENDRON, J. et al: Ureterosigmoidostomies in

bladder exstrophy. J. Urol. Nephrol. (Paris), 76:380, 1970 (French)

CENDRON, J. et al: Treatment of bladder exstrophy. Therapeutic indications. Ann. Chir. Infant., 12:481, 1971 (French)

CENTARO, A. et al: Re-establishment of vaginal function through the creation of neo-vagina. Description of simple and reasonable method. Ann. Ostet. Ginecol. Med. Perinat., 94:79, 1974 (Italian)

CERNEA, P. et al: Malignant parotid cystadenolymphoma. Histological and ultrastructural study. Rev. Stomatol. Chir. Maxillofac., 74:141, 1973 (French)

CERNEA, P. et al: Recurrences of ameloblastomas of the jaws. Statistical study; therapeutic indications. Rev. Stomatol. Chir. Maxillofac., 75:18, 1974 (French)

CERNEA, P. et al: Malignant mandibular schwannoma. Rev. Stomatol. Chir. Maxillofac., 75:1103, 1974 (French)

CERNEA, P. et al: Electrocoagulation of epitheliomas of the mouth floor. Study of 254 cases. Acta Stomatol. Belg., 72:221, 1975 (French)

CERNY, E. et al: Plastic correction of postoperative depressions on forehead using alloplastic substances. Cesk. Otolaryngol., 22:277, 1973 (Czechoslovakian)

CERNY, L.: Resection of maxillary nerve in pterigopalatine fossa. Cesk. Otolaryngol., 22:298, 1973 (Czechoslovakian)

CERNY, L. et al: Surgical treatment of facial paralysis in Melkersson-Rosenthal syndrome. Z. Laryngol. Rhinol. Otol., 51:525, 1972 (German)

CERNY, L. J. et al: Reinnervation after resection of facial nerve. Acta Otolaryngol. (Stockh.), 77:102, 1974

CERVENKA, J.: Cleft lip of Ayagutak, the Eskimo. Cleft Palate J., 11:235, 1974

CERVENY, J.: Oldest presentation of cleft lip in Czechoslovakia, PRS, 54:505, 1974. Acta chir. plast., 15:195, 1973

CERVENY, J.: Reconstruction of abdominal wall of venter pendulus, PRS, 55:637, 1975. Acta chir. plast., 16:178, 1974

CERVINO, A. L., BALES, H. W., AND EMERSON, G. L.: Tissue transfers for functional reconstruction in thoracic surgery, PRS, 54:437, 1974

CESARI, M.: In a cultural mission of the People's Republic of China: reimplantation of limbs. Chir. Organi. Mov., 61:655, 1974 (Italian)

CESARINI, J. P. et al: Dubreuilh's melanosis in cervicofacial carcinology: precancerous state or in-situ cancer? J. Fr. Otorhinolaryngol., 20:1037, 1971 (French)

CEVESE, P. G. et al: Postoperative chylothorax. Six cases in 2,500 operations, with survey of world literature. J. Thorac. Cardiovasc. Surg., 69:966, 1975

CHABORA, A. J., AND HOROWITZ, S. L.: Cleft lip and cleft palate: one genetic system, PRS, 56:231, 1975. Oral Surg., 38:181, 1974

CHABRIER, R.: Corrective rhinoplasty. Inf. Dent., 55:45, 1973 (French)

CHACHAVA, M. K. et al: Plastic surgery in pendulous abdomen. Vestn. Khir., 107:89, 1972 (Russian)

CHACO, J.: Electromyography as a diagnostic tool in soft palate insufficiency. Harefuah, 78:116, 1970 (Hebrew)

CHADFIELD, H. W.: Severe rhinophyma. Brit. J. Dermatol., 88:517, 1973

CHAIMOFF, C., AND DINTSMAN, M.: Repair of huge midline hernias in scar tissue, PRS, 53:110, 1974. Am. J. Surg., 125:767, 1973

CHAIT, D. et al: Management of cystic hygromas. Surg. Gynec. & Obstet., 139:55, 1974

CHAIT, L.: Use of extensor pollicis longus tendon as distal extension for opponens transfer (with Kaplan, Dinner), PRS, 57:186, 1976

CHAIT, L. A.: Treatment of contact burns of the palm in children. S. Afr. Med. J., 49:1839, 1975

CHAIT, L. A., AND SPITZ, L.: Dogbite injuries in children, PRS, 57:126, 1976. S. Afr. Med. J., 49:718, 1975

CHAKOUR, K.: Clinical investigations as to value of bank bone graft, PRS, 54:249, 1974. Ztschr. Orthop., 112:207, 1974

CHAKOUR, K. et al: Improvement of function as a result of substitutive radialis operation because of radialis-paresis. Ztschr. Orthop., 112:341, 1974 (German)

CHAKRAVORTY, R. C., AND SCHATZKI, P. F.: Lateral sublingual dermoid, PRS, 57:756, 1976. Oral Surg., 39:862, 1975

CHALAZONITES, I. et al: Treatment of unusually large mandibular cysts. Stomatologia (Athenai), 28:249, 1971 (Multi-language)

CHALIAN, V. A. et al: Custom designing and fabricating silicone implants for mandibular defects. J. Am. Dent. Assoc., 89:1128, 1974

CHALMERS, J.: Abnormalities of the hand associated with generalised developmental disorders of the skeleton. Hand, 4:11, 1972

CHAMBERS, R. G. et al: Cancer of the Head and Neck. Excerpta Medica Co., Amsterdam, 1975

CHAMBERS, R. G. et al: Palatal reconstruction utilizing retrieved forehead flap. J. Surg. Oncol., 7:191, 1975

CHAMPY, M.: Anomalous flexibility of nasal septum following subperichondral resection,

PRS, 56:104, 1975. Ann. chir. plast., 19:339, 1974

CHAMPY, M. et al: Nasal atresia with breathing impairment in an infant. Ann. chir. plast., 19:189, 1974 (French)

CHAMPY, M. et al: Use of Dal Pont's hooks in facial injuries. Rev. Stomatol. Chir. Maxillofac., 75:783, 1974 (French)

CHAN, E. et al: Boutonniere deformity. Ill. Med. J., 146:532, 1974

CHAN, R. A., BENNER, E. J., AND HOEPRICK, P. D.: Gentamicin therapy in renal failure, PRS, 50:634, 1972. Ann. Int. Med., 76:773, 1972

CHANDER, J.: Epignathus, PRS, 55:636, 1975. Indian J. Surg., 36:242, 1974

CHANDLER, A.: Modifications of conjunctivodacryocystostomy procedure, PRS, 57:754, 1976. Am. J. Ophth., 80:522, 1975

CHANDLER, A. C. JR. et al: Conjunctivodacryocystostomy. Am. J. Ophth., 77:830, 1974

CHANDLER, J. R.: Cryosurgery of malignant neoplasms of the head and neck. J.A.M.A., 221:387, 1972

CHANDLER, J. R.: Cryosurgery for recurrent carcinoma of oral cavity. Arch. Otolaryng., 97:319, 1973

CHANDLER, J. R.: Cryosurgery for recurrent cancer of head and neck. Otolaryngol. Clin. North. Am., 7:193, 1974

CHANDLER, J. R. et al: Cryosurgery in the management of tumors of the head and neck. South. Med. J., 64:1440, 1971

CHANDLER, S. A.: Functional stimulation of disabled limbs. Hand, 3:15, 1971

CHANDRA, R. et al: Permanent records of cleft lip, nose and palate abnormalities. Brit. J. Plast. Surg., 27:139, 1974

CHANDRA, R., SHARMA, R. N., AND YADWA, V. N. S.: Otomandibular dysostosis, PRS, 55:377, 1975. Indian J. Plast. Surg., 7:16, 1974

CHANDRA, R., YADAVA, V. N. S., AND SHARMA, R. N.: Persistent buccopharyngeal membrane, PRS, 54:678, 1974

CHANDRAN, S.: Causes of enucleation in West Malaysia. Singapore Med. J., 14: 497, 1973

CHANEY, R. et al: Management of tracheal stenosis secondary to prolonged ventilation utilizing a cuffed tracheostomy tube – a case report. J. Indiana State Med. Assoc., 64:1196, 1971

CHANG, J. C.: Canalicular blockage. Aust. J. Ophthalmol., 1:58, 1973

CHANG, W. H. J., THOMS, O. J., AND WHITE, W. L.: Avulsion injury of the long flexor tendons, PRS, 50:260, 1972

CHANG, W. H. J., GOMEZ, N. H., AND EDEL-

STEIN, L. M.: Use of lyophilized pig skin for donor site cover, PRS, 55:118, 1975. Brit. J. Plast. Surg., 26:147, 1973

CHANG, Y., WHITAKER, L. A., AND LaROSSA, D.: Acute monomyelocytic leukemia presenting as a felon, PRS, 55:623, 1975

CHANTERELLE, A. et al: Approach and treatment of injuries of orbital floor via conjunctiva. Ann. chir. plast., 19:159, 1974 (French)

CHANTRAINE, A. et al: Decubitus ulcer and its incidence in rehabilitation of neurological patients. J. Belge. Rhumatol. Med. Phys., 28:386, 1973 (French)

CHAPCHAL, G.: Reconstruction Surgery and Traumatology, Volume 12. Albert J. Phiebig, White Plains, N.Y., 1971

CHAPCHAL, G.: Reconstructive Surgery and Traumatology, Vol. 14. Albert J. Phiebig, White Plains, N. Y., 1974

CHAPCHAL, G.: Proceedings. (Reconstruction Surgery and Traumatology Series, Vol. 15.) Albert J. Phiebig, White Plains, N. Y., 1975

CHAPEL, H. M. et al: Rosette inhibition test in skin grafted patients. Brit. Med. J., 2:236, 1974

CHAPMAN, C. R., GEHRIG, J. D., AND WILSON, M. E.: Acupuncture compared with 33 percent nitrous oxide for dental analgesia, PRS, 56:605, 1975. Anesthesiology, 42:532, 1975

CHAPNICH, P.: Review of hyperparathyroidism and an interesting case presenting with a giant cell lesion. Trans. Int. Conf. Oral Surg., 4:44, 1973

CHAR, F.: Cleft lip/palate in the Waardenburg syndrome. Birth Defects, 7:258, 1971

CHARACHON, R. et al: Surgical treatment of traumatic facial paralysis. Ann. Otolaryngol. Chir. Cervicofac., 92:213, 1975 (French)

CHAROONSMITH, T. et al: Frontoethmoidal encephalomeningocele with special reference to plastic reconstruction. Clin. Plast. Surg., 1:27, 1974

CHASE, ROBERT A.: Atlas of Hand Surgery. W. B. Saunders Co., Philadelphia, 1973. PRS, 53:586, 1974

CHASE, R. A.: Reconstructive procedures after irreversible nerve damage in the upper extremity. Clin. Neurosurg., 17:142, 1969

CHASE, R. A.: Early salvage in acute hand injuries with a primary island flap, PRS, 48:521, 1971

CHASE, R. A.: Surgery of hand (in two parts), PRS, 51:477, 1973. New England J. Med., 287:1174, and 1227, 1972

CHASE, R. A.: Treatment of acute hand injuries. Proc. Mine. Med. Off. Assoc., 51:9, 1972

CHASE, R. A.: Tendon injuries. Proc. Mine. Med. Off. Assoc., 51:14, 1972

CHASE, R. A.: Oxygen tension and wound healing, PRS, *50:*98, 1972. Surgery, *71:*150, 1972

CHASE, R. A.: Surgical work loads, PRS, *50:*206, 1972. Surgery *71:*475, 1972

CHASE, R. A. *et al:* Surgical manpower. Symposium. Arch. Surg., *108:*637, 1974

CHATELAIN, C. *et al:* Long-term results of ureterosigmoidostomies for bladder exstrophy. J. Urol. Nephrol. (Paris), *76:*385, 1970 (French)

CHATELAIN, C. *et al:* Long-term results of 16 ureterosigmoidostomies for bladder exstrophy (follow-up from 6 to 38 years). Ann. Chir. Infant., *12:*408, 1971 (French)

CHATER, N. L.: Improved patency rates in microvascular surgery when using magnesium sulfate and a silicone rubber vascular cuff (with Nomoto, Buncke), PRS, *54:*157, 1974

CHATIN, B. *et al:* Essential acroparesthesia and the carpal tunnel syndrome. Lyon Med., *18:*Suppl.:85, 1971 (French)

CHATTERJEE, S. K. *et al:* Restoration of finger flexion by biceps brachil. J. Indian Med. Assoc., *55:*333, 1970

CHATTERJI, P.: Nasal syringadenomas. J. Laryng. & Otol., *88:*89, 1974

CHAUDHURI, P.: Ameloblastoma of upper jaw. J. Laryngol. Otol., *89:*457, 1975

CHAUSSE, J. M.: Results of surgical treatment of ankylosis of temporomandibular joint. Schweiz. Monatsschr. Zahnheilkd., *83:*23, 1973 (German)

CHAUSSE, J. M.: Standard method for the correction of symmetrical "bird-face." Fortschr. Kiefer. Gesichtschir., *18:*182, 1974 (German)

CHAUSSE, J. M.: Facial malformations and their surgical treatment. Rev. Otoneurooph-talmol., *46:*437, 1974 (French)

CHAVATZAS, D., AND JAMIESON, C.: Simple method for approximate measurement of skin blood pressure, PRS, *55:*119, 1975. Lancet, *1:*711, 1974

CHAVES, E. *et al:* Leiomyosarcoma in skin. Case report. Acta Derm. Venereol (Stockh.), *52:*288, 1972

CHAVES, E., AND OLIVEIRA, A. M.: Congenital hemangioma of parotid gland in six-month-old child, PRS, *53:*111, 1974. Folha Med. Brazil, *65:*385, 1972

CHAVEZ-PEON, P., ALBERU-GOMEZ, J., AND WOLPERT-BARRAZA, E.: Transplant of small intestine in dog: new approach to immunological problem, PRS, *56:*474, 1975. Cir. Cir., *42:*35, 1974

CHAYEN, J., AND BITENSKY, L.: Lysosomal enzymes and inflammation with particular reference to rheumatoid diseases, PRS, *49:*361, 1972. Ann. Rheumat. Dis., *30:*522, 1971

CHEAH, J. S. *et al:* Unusual cause of hypothyroidism (following excision of lingual thyroid) in Chinese boy. Med. J. Malaysia, *27:*217, 1973

Cheek (See also *Face; Mouth; Zygoma*)

Cheek reconstruction with bipolar scalp flap, new variation of (Narayanan) (Letter to the Editor), PRS, *48:*274, 1971

Cheek bones, flat (platyzygion) (Spadafora, De Los Rios, Toledo Rios), PRS, *49:*581, 1972. Prensa med. argent., *58:*1946, 1971

Cheek skin, tuberous hemangioma of (Spadafora, De Los Rios), PRS, *49:*475, 1972. Prensa Univ. Arg., *5:*6825, 1971

Cheek defects, cervico-temporo-frontal S-plasty for repair of (Greco *et al*). Ann. chir. plast., *18:*319, 1973 (French)

Cheek, case of juvenile angiofibroma (Parker), PRS, *50:*248, 1974. Arch. Otolaryng., *98:*129, 1973

Cheek, unusual penetrating injury of (Sykes). Injury, *4:*347, 1973

Malar bone fracture: case report with serious delayed sequelae (Rogers, Nardi), PRS, *52:*205, 1973. M.J. Australia, *1:*175, 1973

Cheek augmentation, transoral Silastic (Jabaley, Hoopes, Cochran), PRS, *56:*676, 1975. Brit. J. Plast. Surg., *27:*98, 1974

Cheek loss, full-thickness, use of unlined skin flaps in repair of (Gabriel). Ceylon Med. J., *19:*28, 1974

Repair of facial defect using free skin island flap with vascular anastomoses, case report. Chinese Med. J., *3:*163, 1974 (Chinese)

Cheek reconstruction using cylindrical flap of abdominal skin (Preferansow *et al*). Czas. Stomatol., *27:*265, 1974 (Polish)

Healing of lined and unlined parasitic and nonparasitic flaps (Whitaker *et al*). J. Surg. Oncol., *6:*511, 1974

Clinical success of distant transfer of free skin flap in head and neck regions by microvascular anastomoses (Fujino *et al*). Keio J. Med., *23:*47, 1974

Repair of defects in the cheeks and lips (Haas). Laryngol. Rhinol. Otol. (Stuttg.), *53:*695, 1974 (German)

Soft tissue glass impaction. Oral Surg., *32:*161, 1974

Cheek, skin defects of, reconstructed with large island flap (Lejour), PRS, *56:*473, 1975. Acta chir. belg., *74:*183, 1975

Cheek reconstruction with a doubly folded forehead flap (D'Hooghe *et al*). Acta Stomatol. Belg., *72:*111, 1975

Cheek — Cont.

Analysis of mortality and morbidity in 100 composite resections for oral carcinoma (Robins *et al*). Am. J. Surg., *130:*178, 1975

Malar implants for improvement of facial appearance (Hinderer), PRS, *56:*157, 1975

Cheeks, flaccidity of, cutaneous resection with quadrangular preauricular incision (Spadafora, Durand, de los Rios), PRS, *57:*670, 1976. Prensa Univ. Arg., *6:*8361, 1975

CHESSMAN, A. D.: Experience with use of intravenous diazepam in outpatient procedures. J. Laryng. & Otol., *87:*1249, 1973

CHESSMAN, A. D.: Antral packing, PRS, *55:*634, 1975. Proc. Roy. Soc. Med., *67:*716, 1974

Cheiloplasty: See *Lip*

Chemical Peeling

Face, chemical peeling of (Serson Neto, Martins), PRS, *49:*477, 1972. Ars Curandi, *2:*52, 1971

Phenol skin tightening for better dermabrasion (Dupont *et al*), PRS, *50:*588, 1972

Chemosurgery: survey of chemical peeling of face (Litton, Fournier, Capinpin), PRS, *51:*645, 1973

Chemical peel for facial wrinkles (Stough *et al*). Am. Fam. Physician, *10:*106, 1974

Face, chemical peeling (Ludin *et al*). Conn. Med., *38:*353, 1974

Chemical face peeling, long-term histological study of skin after (Baker *et al*), PRS, *53:*522, 1974

Chemical face peeling, complications of (Spira, Gerow, Hardy), PRS, *54:*397, 1974

Chemical face peeling, histological changes following (Bhangoo) (Letter to the Editor), PRS, *54:*599, 1974

Decontamination procedures for skin exposed to phenolic substances (Brown), PRS, *56:*114, 1975. Arch. Environmental Health, *30:*1, 1975

Chemical peels, skin pigmentation, current concepts and relevance to plastic surgery (Morgan, Gilchrest, Goldwyn), PRS, *56:*617, 1975

Chemexfoliation as an adjunct to facial rejuvenation (Ariagno *et al*). Trans. Am. Acad. Ophthalmol. Otolaryngol., *80:*536, 1975

CHEN, F. H.: Male urinary incontinence. Correction with ischiocavernous muscles collaring method. Urology, *4:*348, 1974

CHEN, S. Y. *et al:* Ultrastructure of the keratinizing and calcifying odontogenic cyst. Oral Surg., *39:*769, 1975

CHEN, Y. M., AND CHAVIN, W.: Melanogenesis in human melanomas, PRS, *56:*112, 1975. Cancer Res., *35:*606, 1975

CHENG, S. F.: Seborrheic keratosis of penis. Urology, *3:*595, 1974

CHEREVATENKO, D. L.: Treatment of mandibular fractures in the aged. Stomatologiia (Mosk), *53:*46, 1974 (Russian)

CHERGESHTAV, I. *et al:* Photoplethysmography of Filatov's skin flap. Stomatologiia, *52:*50, 1973

CHERINGTON, M.: Proximal pain in carpal tunnel syndrome, PRS, *54:*237, 1974. Arch. Surg., *108:*69, 1974

CHERINGTON, M., AND GINSBURG, S.: Wound botulism, PRS, *56:*596, 1975. Arch. Surg., *110:*436, 1975

CHERNAVSKII, V. A. *et al:* Transosseous osteosynthesis in fractures of the metacarpal bones. Ortop. Travmatol. Protez., *1:*10, 1975 (Russian)

CHERNOKOZHEV, KH.: Repeated general anesthesia. Vestn. Khir., *113:*83, 1974 (Russian)

CHERNOV, M. S. *et al:* Stress ulcer: a preventable disease, PRS, *52:*326, 1973. J. Trauma, *12:*831, 1972

CHERNYKH, V. G.: Modification of drainage tube for formation of anastomosis between frontal sinus and nasal cavity. Zh. Ushn. Nos. Gorl. Bolezn., *33:*82, 1973 (Russian)

CHERRICK, H. M. *et al:* Leiomyomas of oral cavity. Review of literature and clinicopathologic study of 7 new cases. Oral Surg., *35:*54, 1973

CHERRY, G.: On the lack of any effect of gravity on the survival of tubed flaps (with Myers, Bombet), PRS, *51:*428, 1973

CHERUBINO, M. *et al:* Surgical, radiological and combined treatment of latero-cervical metastases. Arch. Ital. Otol., *80:*297, 1969 (Italian)

CHESNEY, J.: Peyronie's disease, PRS, *57:*262, 1976. Brit. J. Urol., *47:*209, 1975

CHESS, L. *et al:* Immunologic effects of BCG in patients with malignant melanoma: specific evidence for stimulation of "secondary" immune response, PRS, *53:*497, 1974. J. Nat. Cancer Inst., *51:*57, 1973

Chest (See also *Breast, Deformity; Funnel Chest*)

Thoracic wall, breast carcinoma involving, treatment of local recurrences (Bruck), PRS, *53:*113, 1974. Chir. Plast., *1:*265, 1972

Thoracic wall reconstruction after removal of large tumor mass (Saubier *et al*), PRS, *51:*103, 1973. Lyon chir., *68:*256, 1972

Omentum, greater, transposition for reconstruction of chest wall (Dupont, Menard), PRS, *49:*263, 1972

Chest—Cont.

Pacemaker, covering exposed (Coburn, Blank, Campbell), PRS, *50:*622, 1972

Disease, Mondor's observations on 14 patients and survey of literature (Sivula, Somer), PRS, *54:*117, 1974. Ann. chir. et gynaec. Fenniae, *62:*361, 1973

Chest, cutaneous vascular anatomy of pectoral skin flaps (Calcaterra, Cherney, Saffouri), PRS, *53:*613, 1974. Ann. Otol. Rhin. & Laryng., *82:*691, 1973

Thoracic radiodermatitis treated with pediculated autoplasty of large mesentery followed by skin graft (Texier *et al*), PRS, *53:*243, 1974. Chirurg., *99:*262, 1973

Chest wall, anterior, immediate reconstruction of an extensive bilateral defect of (Longacre, Maurer, Keirle), PRS, *53:*593, 1974

Tissue transfers for functional reconstruction in thoracic surgery (Cervino, Bales, Emerson), PRS, *54:*437, 1974

Thoracic wall defect, extensive, arm flap repair of (Farina), PRS, *54:*680, 1974

Chest wall, repair of concavity of, with silicone elastomer implant (Baker, Mara, Douglas), *56:*212, 1975

Chest wall defects, one-stage coverage with giant bipedicled flap (LeWinn, Guthrie, Kovachev), PRS, *56:*336, 1975

Chest wall deformities associated with mammary hypoplasia, reconstruction of (Hawtof, Ram, Alani), PRS, *57:*172, 1976

Chi, S. *et al:* Cleft lip and cleft palate in New South Wales. M. J. Australia, *2:*1172, 1970

Chiadek, V.: Problem of laryngopharyngeal and pharyngeal carcinomas. Cesk. Otolaryngol., *21:*102, 1972 (Czechoslovakian)

Chiang, C. S.: Case of ossifying fibroma of the maxillary sinus. Otolaryngology (Tokyo), *43:*367, 1971 (Japanese)

Chiari, R. *et al:* Successful treatment of severe hypokalaemic paralysis with respiratory insufficiency in patient with ureterosigmoidostomy. Anaesthesist, *22:*280, 1973 (German)

Chien, K. Y. *et al:* Esophagoplasty for corrosive stricture of esophagus, analysis of 60 cases. Ann. Surg., *179:*510, 1974

Chierici, G. *et al:* Morphogenetic experiments in cleft palate: mandibular response. Cleft Palate J., *10:*51, 1973

Chierici, G. J.: Re-do pharyngeal flap (with Owsley, Lawson), PRS, *57:*180, 1976

Chignell, R.: Iatrogenic disorders of nose and throat. Proc. Roy. Soc. Med., *65:*679, 1972

Chilvers, A. S., and Kinmonth, J. B.: Operations for lymphedema of lower limbs, PRS, *57:*262, 1976. J. Cardiovasc. Surg., *16:*115, 1975

Chin

Hypermentonism (Pitanguy, Cansancao), PRS, *50:*94, 1972. Rev. brasil. cir., *61:*119, 1971

Chin, alloplastic reconstruction of, in bird face, by intraosseous anchorage of plastic implants (Spreter von Kreudenstein). Zanaerztl. Prax., *22:*37, 1971 (German)

Submentoplasty. Classification and theoretical outline of management (Brennan *et al*). Arch. Otolaryng., *95:*24, 1972

Bone resorption under plastic chin implants. Follow-up of a preliminary report (Robinson). Arch. Otolaryng., *95:*30, 1972

Mentoplasty, augmentation, reflections (Tresley *et al*). Laryngoscope, *82:*2092, 1972

Chin, ptosis of—the witches' chin (Gonzalez-Ulloa), PRS, *50:*54, 1972

Chin, making permanent dimple (Guerrero-Santos, Ramirez, Rivera), PRS, *50:*88, 1972

Chin, making cleft in (Cinelli), PRS, *50:*91, 1972

Chin, double, surgical treatment (Viñas *et al*), PRS, *50:*119, 1972

Prognathic profile (Quetglas, Perez, Escribano), PRS, *54:*104, 1974. Rev. españ. cir. plast., *5:*235, 1972

Chin implants, plastic, avoiding bone resorption under (Parker), PRS, *53:*250, 1974. Arch. Otolaryng., *98:*100, 1973

Mentoplasty (Newton). Can. J. Otolaryngol., *2:*235, 1973

Profileoplasty (Caplan). Can. J. Otolaryngol., *2:*347, 1973

Chin, consideration of, in surgical-orthodontic procedures (Norton *et al*). Isr. J. Dent. Med., *22:*124, 1973

Chin (Lund *et al*). Mayo Clin. Proc., *48:*417, 1973

Chin implants, personally fabricated (Carlin), PRS, *51:*121, 1973

Alloplastic implants, bone deformation beneath (Jobe, Iverson, Vistnes), PRS, *51:*169, 1973. Discussions by Rees and Spira, PRS, *51:*174, 1973

Senile hypoplastic chin associated with submandibular adiposity (Pitanguy *et al*), PRS, *54:*233, 1974. Rev. brasil. cir., *63:*217, 1973

Case report (Poulton). Angle Orthod., *44:*167, 1974

Face, middle and lower, bony deformities of, assessment and management of (Henderson). Brit. J. Plast. Surg., *27:*287, 1974

Notes on esthetic surgery in the Indonesian

Chin — Cont.

(Wiratmadja). Clin. Plast. Surg., *1:*173, 1974

Esthetic aspects in the planning of chin operations (Schule). Fortschr. Kiefer. Gesichtchir., *18:*114, 1974 (German)

Facial profile, surgical and esthetic aspects of (D'ottaviano *et al*). Int. J. Oral Surg., *3:*243, 1974

Genioplasty with reference to resorption and hinge sliding osteotomy (Fitzpatrick). Int. J. Oral Surg., 3:247, 1974

Transpositional genioplasty (Byrhe *et al*). J. Oral Surg., *32:*145, 1974

Soft tissue procedures adjunctive to orthognathic surgery for improvement of facial balance (Turvey *et al*). J. Oral Surg., *32:*572, 1974

Mandibular symphysis, particulate marrow graft for restoration of (Mitchell *et al*). Oral Surg., *37:*196, 1974

Cervico-mentoplasty with rhytidectomy (Snyder), PRS, *54:*404, 1974

Chin implants, silicone, for chin augmentation (Wray, Moore, Weeks), PRS, *54:*510, 1974. South. M.J., *67:*456, 1974

Tolerance of the cortical bone to silicone materials (Bruchet *et al*). Ann. chir. plast., *20:*227, 1975 (French)

Chin reduction in profileplasty (Simons, Lawson), PRS, *57:*528, 1976. Arch. Otolaryng., *101:*207, 1975

Orthosurgical teamwork (Olsen *et al*). J. Am. Dent. Assoc., *90:*998, 1975

Chin reconstruction in cosmetic surgery (Fitzpatrick), PRS, *57:*112, 1976. J. Oral Surg., *39:*522, 1975

Depression, submental, occurring after rhytidectomy, repair of (Wilkinson), PRS, *57:*33, 1976

Cephalometric analysis, retrospective, of mandibular bone absorption under silicone rubber chin implants (Friedland, Coccaro, Converse), PRS, *57:*144, 1976

CHINA BURNS UNIT: Review of management of extensive third degree burns in 14 successive years, PRS, *54:*241, 1974. Chinese M. J., *11:*148, 1973

CHINA COORDINATING GROUP FOR RESEARCH ON ETIOLOGY OF ESOPHAGEAL CANCER: Epidemiology and etiology of esophageal cancer in North China — preliminary report, PRS, *57:*759, 1976. Chinese M. J., *1:*167, 1975

CHINA, KWANGCHOW CHUNG SHAN MEDICAL COLLEGE: Experience in replantation of severed fingers, PRS, *55:*248, 1975. Chinese M. J., *6:*71, 1973

CHINA, KWANGCHOW CHUNG SHAN MEDICAL

COLLEGE: Experimental study of effect of ilex pubescens on vessels of isolated organs, with report on clinical use in limb replantation, PRS, *55:*250, 1975. Chinese M. J., *2:*28, 1974

CHINA, LANCHOW GENERAL HOSPITAL: Reconstruction of missing thumbs with improved "cocked hat" operation, PRS, *55:*637, 1975. Chinese M. J., *10:*177, 1974

CHINA, PEKING ANESTHESIA COORDINATING GROUP: Clinical application of ketamine anesthesia, PRS, *55:*646, 1975. Chinese M. J., *7:*121, 1974

CHINA, PEKING CHISCHUEITAN HOSPITAL: Replantation of severed limbs — analysis of 40 cases, PRS, *55:*254, 1975. Chinese M. J., *6:*67, 1973

CHINA, SHANGHAI ACUPUNCTURE ANESTHESIA COORDINATING GROUP: Acupuncture anesthesia, PRS, *56:*602, 1975. Chinese M. J., *1:*13, 1975

CHINA, SHANGHAI FIRST MEDICAL COLLEGE: Orbital hemangioma, clinical analysis of 79 cases, PRS, *55:*633, 1975. Chinese M. J., *9:*162, 1974

CHINA, SHANGHAI SIXTH PEOPLE'S HOSPITAL: Replantation of severed limbs and fingers, PRS, *51:*703, 1973. Chinese M. J., *1:*1, 1973

CHINA, SHANGHAI SIXTH PEOPLE'S HOSPITAL: Replantation of limbs after resection of neoplastic segment, PRS, *55:*255, 1975. Chinese M. J., *6:*72, 1973

CHINESE PLA BURNS UNIT: Review of management of extensive third degree burns in 14 successive years, PRS, *54:*241, 1974. Chinese M. J., *11:*148, 1973

CHING, N. *et al:* Letter: Cuff pressure measurements. Chest, *66:*604, 1974

CHING, N. P. *et al:* The contribution of cuff volume and pressure in tracheostomy tube damage. J. Thorac. Cardiovasc. Surg., *62:*402, 1971

CHING, N. P. *et al:* Clinical experience with new low-pressure high-volume tracheostomy cuffs. Importance of limiting intracuff pressure. N. Y. State J. Med., *74:*2379, 1974

CHIOSSONE LARES, E.: Surgery of the facial nerve with anatomic and functional preservation of the ear. Acta Otorinolaryngol. Iber. Am., *22:*599, 1971 (Spanish)

CHIR, M.: *Plastic Surgery*. J. B. Lippincott Co., Philadelphia, 1969.

CHISHOLM, G. D. *et al:* Concentration of antibacterial agents in interstitial tissue fluid, PRS, *52:*462, 1973. Brit. M. J., *1:*569, 1973

CHISTIKHIN, V. S.: Bilateral stress pneumothorax during tracheostomy. Khirugiia (Mosk.), *0:*138, 1974 (Russian)

CHIZHIKOV, V. M. *et al:* Case of resection of a full congenital lateral fistula of the neck with simultaneous tonsillectomy. Zh. Ushn. Nos. Gorl. Bolezn., *32*:101, 1972 (Russian)

CHIU, G. W. *et al:* Ideal penile dressing. Urology, *5*:670, 1975

CHLUMSKY, J. *et al:* Clinical manifestation of impairment of liver in course of burn disease, PRS, *54*:624, 1974. Acta chir. plast., *15*:238, 1973

Choanal Atresia: See *Nose, Choanal Atresia*

CHODOSH, P. L.: Cricopharyngeal myotomy in the treatment of dysphagia. Laryngoscope, *85*:1862, 1975

CHOHAN, B. S. *et al:* Orbital meningoencephalocele communicating with lacrimal sac, case report. Clin. Pediatr. (Phila.), *13*:330, 1974

CHONG, G. C., BEAHRS, O. H., AND WOOLNER, L. B.: Surgical management of acinic cell carcinoma of parotid gland, PRS, *54*:246, 1974. Surg. Gynec. & Obst., *138*:65, 1974

CHONG, G. C. *et al:* Management of parotid gland tumors in infants and children. Mayo Clin. Proc., *50*:279, 1975

CHONG, G. C. *et al:* Breast restoration after mastectomy for cancer. Mayo Clin. Proc., *50*:453, 1975

CHONG, J. K.: Pedicled tendon transfer (Letter to the Editor), PRS, *50*:398, 1972

CHONG, J. K., AND WINSLOW, R. B.: Simple technique for correction of "whistling" deformity in repaired cleft lips, PRS, *48*:84, 1971

CHONG, J. K. *et al:* Combined two-stage tenoplasty with silicone rods for multiple flexor tendon injuries in "no-man's-land." J. Trauma., *12*:104, 1972

CHOU, C. C. *et al:* Evaluation of temporomandibular arthrography in temporomandibular joint dysfunction; analysis of 67 cases. Chinese Med. J., *10*:601, 1973 (Chinese)

CHOUARD, CH. H.: Results and indications of chordal neurolysis in facial paralysis. Ann. Otolaryngol. Chir. Cervicofac., *89*:507, 1972 (French)

CHOUARD, C. H.: Electrical examination and surgical indications in facial paralysis. Ann. Otolaryngol. Chir. Cervicofac., *92*:195, 1975 (French)

CHOUBRAC, P. *et al:* Ambulatory enteral nutrition. A new method. Nouv. Presse Med., *3*:1959, 1974 (French)

CHOUDHURY, A. R.: Non-endocrine unilateral proptosis. Trans. Ophthalmol. Soc. U. K., *93*:673, 1973

CHOUKAS, N. C.: Modified palatal flap technique for closure of oroantral fistulas. J. Oral Surg., *32*:112, 1974

CHOUKAS, N. C. *et al:* Histological study of

regeneration of inferior alveolar nerve. J. Oral Surg., *32*:347, 1974

CHOWDHURY, J.: Oxyphenbutazone in plastic surgery, PRS, *55*:388, 1975. Indian J. Plast. Surg., *7*:26, 1974

CHRETIEN, P. B.: Fiberoptic endoscopy in the head and neck region (with Dellon, Hall), PRS, *55*:466, 1975

CHRETIEN, P. B.: Defining malignant potential of giant pigmented nevus (with Dellon, Edelson), PRS, *57*:611, 1976

CHRETIEN, P. B. *et al:* Quantitative dinitrochlorobenzene contact sensitivity in preoperative and cured cancer patients. Natl. Cancer Inst. Monogr., *39*:263, 1973

CHRIST, T. F. *et al:* Papilliferous ameloblastic fibroma. Oral Surg., *34*:806, 1972

CHRISTENSEN, D. R., MASHBERG, A., TURK, M. H.: Correction of extreme dilation of Stensen's duct resulting from chronic partial obstruction. J. Oral Surg., *31*:136, 1973

CHRISTENSEN, D. R. *et al:* Soft tissue closure of unilateral congenital maxillary alveolar cleft. J. Oral Surg., *33*:872, 1975

CHRISTIANSEN, R. L. *et al:* Habilitation of severe craniofacial anomalies – the challenge of new surgical procedures: an NIDR workshop. Cleft Palate J., *12*:167, 1975

CHRISTIANSEN, T. A. *et al:* Juvenile nasopharyngeal angiofibroma. Trans. Am. Acad. Ophthalmol. Otolaryngol., *78*:1140, 1974

CHUDAKOV, O. P.: Elimination of penetrating palatal defects by using a flat epithelialized skin flap. Vestn. Khir., *110*:86, 1973 (Russian)

CHUDAKOV, O. P.: Epithelized skin flap in plastic surgery for gaping defects of pharyngeal walls and jugular portion of esophagus. Vestn. Khir., *111*:83, 1973 (Russian)

CHUDAKOVA, T. N.: Double skin flap using A. K. Tych Tychinkina's method in plastic surgery. Khirurgiia (Mosk.), *48*:49, 1972 (Russian)

CHUDAKOVA, T. N.: Experience in the use of double skin flap (A. K. Tychinkina's method). Khirurgiia (Sofiia), *25*:49, 1972 (Russian)

CHUDEN, H.: Decompression of the retrobular space and the optic nerve. H.N.O., *22*:320, 1974 (German)

CHUNG, C. K., AND HEFFERNAN, A. H.: Clear cell hidradenoma with metastasis, PRS, *48*:177, 1971

CHUNG SHAN HOSPITAL, SHANGHAI: Subclavian venipuncture and catheterization by supraclavicular approach, PRS, *54*:692, 1974. Chinese M. J., *5*:81, 1974

CHUNG SHAN MEDICAL COLLEGE, KWANGHOW: Experience in replantation of severed fingers, PRS, *55:*248, 1975. Chinese M. J., *6:*71, 1973

CHUNG SHAN MEDICAL COLLEGE, KWANGCHOW: Experimental study of effect of ilex pubescens on vessels of isolated organs, with report on clinical use in limb replantation, PRS, *55:*250, 1975. Chinese M. J., *2:*28, 1974

CHUNPRAPAPH, B.: Replantation of portions of 4 fingers in one hand, PRS, *55:*248, 1975. New England J. Med., *291:*460, 1974

CHURCH, J. C. T.: Elastogenesis in healing wounds in bats, PRS, *57:*468, 1976

CHURCH, R. E.: Relapsing polychondritis. Proc. Roy. Soc. Med., *64:*1194, 1971

CHUTKOW, J. G., SHARBROUGH, F. W., AND RILEY, F. C., JR.: Simultaneous blindness following bilateral neck dissection, PRS, *53:*374, 1974. Mayo Clin. Proc., *48:*713, 1973

CHVAPIL, M.: Discussion of "Disruption of healed scars in scurvy—result of disequilibrium in collagen metabolism," by Cohen, Keiser, PRS, *57:*376, 1976

CHWIROT, R.: Isolated neurofibroma of the orbit. Klin. Oczna., *42:*781, 1972 (Polish)

CHWIROT, R.: Capody's orbitoplasty by means of Meller's epithelial graft. Klin. Oczna., *43:*49, 1973 (Polish)

CHWIROT, R.: Meller's free epithelial graft in reconstructive eyelid surgery. Klin. Oczna., *44:*381, 1974 (Polish)

CHWIROT, R.: Total upper lid reconstruction following excision of extensive carcinoma. Klin. Oczna., *44:*597, 1974 (Polish)

CHWIROT, R.: Advances in orbital surgery. Klin. Oczna., *45:*575, 1975 (Polish)

CHYTILOVA, M. *et al:* Should a plastic surgeon take part in treatment of patients with multiple injuries? Cas. Lek. Cesk., *110:*673, 1971 (Czechoslovakian)

CIABURRO, H.: Simplifying the Le Fort I type of maxillary osteotomy (with Dupont, Prévost), PRS, *54:*142, 1974

CIABURRO, H. *et al:* Forward traction in correction of retrodisplaced maxilla, PRS, *52:*687, 1973. Canad. M. A. J., *108:*1511, 1973

CIANI, A.: Intraoral approach in mandibular osteosynthesis. Rass. Int. Stomatol. Prat., *23:*163, 1972 (Italian)

CIBERT, J. *et al:* Bladder exstrophy operated by Lattimer's technic. 10-year results. J. Urol. Nephrol. (Paris), *81:*45, 1975 (French)

CIES, W. A., AND BARTLETT, R. E.: Modification of Mustardé and Hughes methods of reconstructing lower lid, PRS, *57:*755, 1976. Ann. Ophth., *7:*1497, 1975

CIES, W. A. *et al:* Surgical revision of the upper eyelid fold. Am. J. Ophth., *80:*1019, 1975

CIMORRA, G. A., FERREIRA, V., AND MARTINEZ-TELLO, F. J.: Spontaneous facial nerve paral-

ysis associated with an ipsilateral benign parotid tumor, PRS, *50:*523, 1972

CINCA, D. *et al:* Remarks on case of laterocervical Schwannoma. Ann. Otolaryngol. Chir. Cervicofac., *90:*307, 1973 (French)

CINELLI, J. A.: Making a cleft in the chin, PRS, *50:*91, 1972

CINOTTI, V.: Retrospective study of 102 cases of epistaxis. V. Med. Pregl., *27:*343, 1974 (Serbian)

CISLAGHI, E.: Reconstructive prosthesis in extensive resections of mandible for neoplasms. Minerva Chir., *26:*1411, 1971 (Italian)

CISLAGHI, E.: Titanium blades for supporting prostheses after maxillary resection. Tumori, *58:*13, 1972 (Italian)

CIUREA, M. *et al:* Aspects of controversy concerning tracheostomy and prolonged tracheal intubation in young children. Current status of the problem. Otorinolaringologie, *18:*107, 1973 (Rumanian)

CIUREA, M. *et al:* Fentanyl and droperidol in pediatric otorhinolaryngological surgery. Marginal notes on personal cases. Otorinolaringologie, *18:*419, 1973 (Rumanian)

CIVATTE, J.: Mucoid cysts and trauma. Arch. Belg. Dermatol. Syphiligr., *29:*217, 1973 (French)

CIVETTA, M., GAGEL, J. C., AND GEMER, M.: Internal jugular vein puncture with margin of safety, PRS, *51:*236, 1973. Anaesthesia, *36:*622, 1972

CLABAUGH, W. *et al:* Frey's syndrome. Arch. Dermat., *106:*597, 1972

CLABAUGH, W. A.: Basal cell and squamous cell carcinoma of skin. Am. Fam. Physician, *7:*78, 1973

CLABAUGH, W. A.: Tattoo removal by superficial dermabrasion, PRS, *55:*401, 1975

CLAGETT, G. P. *et al:* Influence of aspirin on postoperative platelet kinetics and venous thrombosis, PRS, *56:*115, 1975. Surgery, *77:*61, 1975

CLAIMONT, A. A. *et al:* Papillomas of the nasal and paranasal cavities. South. Med. J., *68:*41, 1975

CLARK, A. W. *et al:* Active enhancement of mouse skin allografts: effect of Bordetella pertussis and regional lymphadenectomy. Brit. J. Surg., *61:*325, 1974

CLARK, C., WEAVER, A. W., AND SMITH, D. B.: Post maxillectomy rhinorrhea, PRS, *57:*395, 1976. Arch. Otolaryng., *101:*492, 1975

CLARK, D. D., RICKER, J. H., AND MACCOLLUM, M. S.: Efficacy of local steroid injection in the treatment of stenosing tenovaginitis, PRS, *51:*179, 1973

CLARK, G. L. *et al:* Surgical prevention and correction of deformities in the rheumatoid hand. Md. State Med. J., *22:*47, 1973

CLARK, G. M.: Photoelastic analysis of nasal support, PRS, *49:*101, 1972. Arch. Otolaryng., *93:*3, 1971

CLARK, HENRY B. JR.: *Practical Oral Surgery.* 3rd ed. Lea & Febiger, Philadelphia, 1965

CLARK, M. *et al:* Scanning and transmission electron microscopic studies of exstrophic human bladder. J. Urol., *110:*481, 1973

CLARK, R. W.: Cryotherapy and corticosteroids in treatment of rattlesnake bite, PRS, *48:*95, 1971. Mil. Med., *136:*42, 1971

CLARKE, A. M. *et al:* Chlorhexidine with silversulphadiazine in the treatment of burns. M. J. Australia, *2:*446, 1971

CLARKE, A. M. *et al:* Use of new vasoconstrictor in management of burns. M. J. Australia, *2:*361, 1972

CLARKE, P. R.: Proceedings: Endocrine exophthalmos treated by orbital decompression. J. Neurol. Neurosurg. Psychiatry, *38:*822, 1975

Classic Reprints (See also *History of Plastic Surgery)*

Stevens, A. H.: Staphyloraphe, or palate suture, successfully performed, PRS, *48:*61, 1971

Smith, N.: Suture of the palate, PRS, *48:*61, 1971

Liston, R.: Closure of cleft palate, PRS, *48:*167, 1971

Warren, J. M.: Operations for fissure of soft and hard palate, PRS, *48:*271, 1971

Mettauer, J. P.: On staphyloraphy, PRS, *48:*364, 1971

Fergusson, W.: Observations on cleft palate and on staphyloraphy, PRS, *48:*365, 1971

Liston, R.: Cleft palate – velosynthesis, PRS, *48:*366, 1971

Monks, G. H.: Correction, by operation, of some nasal deformities and disfigurements, PRS, *48:*485, 1971

Langenbeck, B.: New method for operation on complete congenital cleft of the hard palate, PRS, *49:*323, 1972

Langenbeck, B.: Uranoplasty by means of raising mucoperiosteal flaps, PRS, *49:*326, 1972

Schoenborn, K.: On a new method of staphylorrhaphy, PRS, *49:*558, 1972

Schoenborn, K.: Presentation of a patient after staphyloplasty, PRS, *49:*560, 1972

Billroth, T.: On uranoplasty, PRS, *50:*71, 1972

Dorrance, G. M.: Lengthening the soft palate in cleft palate operations, PRS, *50:*275, 1972

Lanz, O.: Die transplantation betreffend

Classic Reprints – Cont.

(Concerning transplantation), PRS, *50:*395, 1972

Le Fort, R.: Experimental study of fractures of the upper jaw, PRS, *50:*497, 1972

Le Fort, R.: Experimental study of upper jaw fractures, PRS, *50:*600, 1972

Stein, S. A. V.: Lip repair (cheiloplasty) performed by a new method, PRS, *53:*332, 1974

Franco, P.: The cure of cleft lips in 1561, PRS, *57:*84, 1976

De la Faye, G.: Observations on cleft lip, PRS, *57:*216, 1976

Malgaigne, J. F.: Cleft lip, du bec-de-lièvre, PRS, *57:*359, 1976

Mirault, G.: Cleft lip, letter on operation of, PRS, *57:*502, 1976

CLATTENBURG, R. *et al:* Thermal properties of cancellous bone, PRS, *57:*406, 1976. J. Biomed. Mater. Res., *9:*169, 1975

Clawhand (See also *Hands, Deformities, Acquired; Hands, Reconstructive Surgery)*

Contraction, flexion of fingers or toes, combined method of rotation flap and free skin graft to (Morotomi *et al),* PRS, *50:*311, 1972. Jap. J. Plast. Reconstr. Surg., *14:*377, 1971

Contractures, non-ischemic, of intrinsic muscles of hand (Smith), PRS, *49:*665, 1972. J. Bone & Joint Surg., *53A:*1313, 1971

Claw finger deformity, capsulodesis and pulley advancement for correction of (Leddy *et al),* PRS, *51:*477, 1973. J. Bone & Joint Surg., *54A:*1465, 1972

Fingers, cicatricial contracture, treated by temporary surgical syndactyly (Fittipaldi, Lanatta), PRS, *53:*243, 1974. Rev. Españ. cir. plast., *5:*221, 1972

Fowler procedure for correction of the paralytic claw hand (Enna, Riordan), PRS, *52:*352, 1973

Fibroblasts, presence in ischemic contracture of intrinsic musculature of hand (Madden, Carlson, Hines), PRS, *56:*595, 1975. Surg. Gynec. & Obst., *140:*509, 1975

CLAWSON, D. K. *et al:* Functional assessment of the rheumatoid hand. Clin. Orthop. 77:203, 1971

CLAYPOOLE, W. H., WARREN, D. W., AND BRADLEY, D. P.: Effect of cleft palate on oral port constriction during fricative productions, PRS, *55:*382, 1975. Cleft Palate J., *11:*95, 1974

CLAYTON, M. L., AND FERLIC, D. C.: Tendon transfer for radial rotation of wrist in rheumatoid arthritis, PRS, *55:*637, 1975. Clin. Orthop., *100:*176, 1974

Cleft Hand: See *Hands, Deformities, Acquired*

Cleft Lip

Atlas for Surgical Repair of Cleft Lip, Cleft Palate, and Noncleft Velopharyngeal Incompetence. By Richard B. Yules. Charles C Thomas, Springfield, Ill., 1971. PRS, *51:*399, 1972

Cleft Lip and Palate. Surgical, Dental, and Speech Aspects. Ed. by William C. Grabb, Sheldon W. Rosenstein, and Kenneth R. Bzoch. Little, Brown & Co., Boston, 1971. PRS, *49:*337, 1972

Clefts of lip, unilateral, importance of folding down muscle stumps in the operation of (Fara), PRS, *50:*541, 1972. Acta chir. plast., *13:*162, 1971

Congenital labio-palatine fissures (Tresserra Llaurado). An. Esp. Odontoestomatol., *30:*407, 1971 (Spanish)

Congenital labio-palatine fissures (Tresserra Llaurado). An. Esp. Odontoestomatol., *30:*483, 1971 (Spanish)

Management of cleft lip and palate. Introduction (Tulley). Ann. R. Coll. Surg. Engl., *48:*30, 1971

Cleft lip and palate, sinusitis in children with (Jaffe, DeBlanc), PRS, *49:*105, 1972. Arch. Otolaryng., *93:*5, 1971

Three surgical instruments for cleft lip-palate repair (Boo-Chai). Brit. J. Plast. Surg., *24:*216, 1971

Fresh look at Le Mesurier: the problem of the drifting ala (Mustarde). Brit. J. Plast. Surg., *24:*258, 1971

Field guide to cleft lip repair (Heycock). Brit. J. Surg., *58:*567, 1971

The importance of physiological reconstruction of the orbicularis oris muscle for esthetic and functional result in operations of unilateral cleft lip (Fara). Cesk Stomatol., *71:*358, 1971 (Czech)

Role of the lip adhesion procedure in cleft lip repair (Hamilton *et al*). Cleft Palate J., *8:*1, 1971

Recent trends in early treatment of cleft lip and palate (Robertson). Dent. Pract. Dent. Rec., *21:*326, 1971

Two stage surgery for cleft lip, jaw, palate and velum (Koch). Dtsch. Stomatol., *21:*635, 1971 (German)

Electromyographic studies on palatal, pharyngeal and lip muscles during phonation and deglutition in patients with cleft palate (Pruszewicz *et al*). H.N.O., *19:*77, 1971 (German)

Cleft Lip — Cont.

Reconstruction of cleft lip and palate (Neuman). Harefuah, *81:*563, 1971 (Hebrew)

Selection of procedure in unilateral cleft lip repair (Theogaraj). Indian Pediatr., *8:*774, 1971

Congenital prolabial-maxillary scar: a possible minor expression of cleft lip (Pomerance). J. Pediatr., *78:*868, 1971

Primary treatment of cleft lip and cleft palate (Perko *et al*). Minerva Stomatol., *20:*193, 1971 (Italian)

Surgical treatment of cheilognathopalatoschisis (Stea). Mondo Odontostomatol., *14:*101, 1971 (Italian)

3 years experience in the early orthodontic management and subsequent surgery of cleft lip and palate in children (Kontor *et al*). Orv. Hetil., *112:*1957, 1971 (Hungarian)

Harelips (Jost). Probl. Actuels Otorhinolaryngol., *223:*1971 (French)

Cleft lip, crossed denuded flap as a complement to the Millard technique in correction of (Guerrero-Santos *et al*), PRS, *48:*506, 1971

Determination of the optimal terms for surgical treatment of congenital clefts of the upper lip (Berdiuk). Stomatologiia (Mosk), *50:*63, 1971 (Russian)

Surgical treatment of congenital cleft lip in newborn infants (Znamenskii). Vestn. Khir., *106:*66, 1971 (Russian)

Cleft Lip and Palate. By R. B. Ross and M. C. Johnston. Williams & Wilkins Co., Baltimore, 1972. PRS, *51:*444, 1973

Communicative Disorders Related to Cleft Lip and Palate. Ed. by Kenneth R. Bzoch. Little, Brown & Co., Boston, 1972. PRS, *52:*572, 1973

Cleft lip and palate treatment in Prague (Fara), PRS, *52:*682, 1973. Acta chir. plast., *14:*201, 1972

Current trends in primary osteoplasty in cleft lip (Clooster). Acta Stomatol. Belg., *69:*309, 1972 (Dutch)

Preliminary observations on 105 cases of hare lip operated on with Skoog's periosteal flap (Rosselli *et al*). Ann. chir. plast., *17:*106, 1972 (French)

Ten-year survey of cleft lip and cleft palate in the Southwest Region (Wilson). Brit. J. Plast. Surg., *25:*224, 1972

Repair of unilateral cleft lip nasal deformities (Hugo *et al*). Cleft Palate J., *8:*257, 1971

Studies on the status of cleft surgery (Hochstein). Dtsch. Gesundheitsw., *27:*993, 1972 (German)

Cleft Lip — Cont.

Concomitant symptoms in cheilognathopala-toschisis in patients of the Thallwitz Clinic (Bethmann *et al*). Dtsch. Stomatol., *22:*907, 1972 (German)

Cleft lip repair, primary (Tange), PRS, *52:*455, 1973. Jap. J. Plast. Reconstr. Surg., *15:*412, 1972

Cleft lips, complete, primary nostril recon-struction in round nostril technique (Wynn), PRS, *49:*56, 1972

Cleft lip repairs, primary, experimental study of transplantation of rib growth cartilage and possible use in (Kluzak), PRS, *49:*61, 1972

Cleft lip-palate patients, study of 100, oper-ated upon 22–27 years ago by one surgeon (Pickrell *et al*), PRS, *49:*149, 1972

Cleft lips in Malaysians (Sivaloganathan), PRS, *49:*176, 1972

Cleft lip repair, single, geometry of (Sawhney), PRS, *49:*518, 1972

Lip adhesion operation in cleft lip surgery (Randall) (Follow-Up Clinic), PRS, *50:*182, 1972

Methods of treatment of cleft lip and cleft palate (Clooster). Rev. Belge. Med. Dent., *27:*334, 1972 (Dutch)

Policy of treatment of cleft lip and palate (Castermans). Rev. Med. Liege, *27:* Suppl 137, 1972 (French)

Evolution of techniques in cheiloplasty for cleft-lip (and study of a few complementary measures) (Delaire *et al*). Rev. Stomatol. Chir. Maxillofac., *73:*337, 1972 (French)

Reduction of bleeding by vasoconstrictive drugs infiltration in the surgery cleft lip and cleft palate (Popescu *et al*). Stomatolo-gia (Bucur.), *19:*51, 1972 (Rumanian)

Foundations of planning of plastic operation of the upper lip in children with congenital complete bilateral cleft lip, alveolar process and palate (Kasparova). Stomatolo-giia (Mosk.), *51:*52, 1972 (Russian)

Effect of surgical treatment of psychic read-aptation of patients with congenital and acquired defects of the face (Matveev *et al*). Stomatologiia (Mosk.), *51:*54, 1972 (Rus-sian)

Cleft lip and palate treatment and organiza-tion of the patient care in Finland (Solvio *et al*). Suom. Hammaslaak. Toim., *68:*32, 1972 (Finnish)

Surgical treatment of cleft lip and palate (Rintala). Suom. Hammaslaak. Toim., *68:*35, 1972 (Finnish)

Cleft lip and palate management (Stark, Ka-plan), PRS, *50:*540, 1972. Tribuna Med. Mexico, *21:*11, 1972

Cleft Lip — Cont.

Clefts, unilateral, shape of nose before opera-tional repair (Hajnis, Figalova), PRS, *53:*681, 1974. Acta chir. plast., *15:*11, 1973

Cleft lip, oldest presentation in Czechoslo-vakia (Cerveny), PRS, *54:*505, 1974. Acta chir. plast., *15:*195, 1973

Theory and empiricism in surgical treatment of orofacial clefts (Fara). Acta Univ. Carol. (Med. Monogr.) (Praha.), *56:*31, 1973

An important contribution of the Millard flap to cleft lip surgery (Dey). Aust. N. Z. J. Surg., *42:*271, 1973

Some unusual aspects of clefts of the lip (Dey). Aust. N. Z. J. Surg., *43:*171, 1973

Planning the repair of cleft lip deformities (Onizuka). Brit. J. Plast. Surg., *26:*181, 1973

Clinical research in cleft lip and cleft palate: the state of the art (Spriestersbach *et al*). Cleft Palate J., *10:*113, 1973

Lip and palate, cleft (Hagerty, Mylin), PRS, *53:*490, 1974. Contemp. Surg., *3:*44, 1973

Modern views on treatment of clefts of upper lip, alveolar process and palate (Perczyn-ska-Partyka). Czas. Stomatol., *26:*547, 1973 (Polish)

Healing course and complications following surgery of cleft lip, maxilla and palate (Bethmann *et al*). Dtsch. Stomatol., *23:*633, 1973 (German)

Cleft lip repair, philtrum reconstruction in (Fukuda, Arai), PRS, *53:*369, 1974. Jap. J. Plast. Reconstr. Surg., *16:*355, 1973

Wave-line procedure in the repair of cleft lip (Holtje *et al*). J. Maxillo-facial Surg., *1:*198, 1973

Cleft lip and palate children, asymmetric for-mation in permanent dentition (Ranta), PRS, *54:*694, 1974. Scand. J. Plast. Re-constr. Surg., *7:*59, 1973

Team work and clinical research in the treat-ment of cleft lip and palate (Heilquist). Sven. Tandlak. Tidskr., *66:*145, 1973

Cleft lip and palate, differentiation of (Eman-uel *et al*), PRS, *54:*111, 1974. Teratology, *7:*271, 1973

Is our treatment of children with cleft palate-cleft lip rational? (Eskeland). Tidsskr. Nor. Laegeforen, *93:*2459, 1973 (Norwe-gian)

Cleft lip and cleft palate. Teamwork in treat-ment. 2. History. Present situation in Oslo (Bohn). Tidsskr. Nor. Laegeforen, *93:*2463, 1973 (Norwegian)

Cleft lip and cleft palate. Primary cleft sur-gery. 3 (Borchgrevink *et al*). Tidsskr. Nor. Laegeforen, *93:*2466, 1973 (Norwegian)

Cleft lip and cleft palate. Prosthetic treat-

Cleft Lip, Bilateral — Cont.

illa in bilateral cleft lip, jaw and palate (Ivankievicz *et al*). Fogorv. Sz., *67*:161, 1974 (Hungarian)

Proceedings: Early closure of the prolabium in piercing cleft lip, jaw and palate (Hollmann). Munch. Med. Wochenschr., *116*:1064, 1974 (German)

Cleft lip deformities, bilateral, secondary correction with Millard's midline muscular closure (Oneal, Greer, Nobel), PRS, *54*:45, 1974

Premaxilla, recession of, in bilateral cleft lip and palate (Monroe) (Follow-Up Clinic), PRS, *54*:482, 1974

Repositioning and surgical retention of the median tubercle in the sequelae of bilateral labio-maxillary cleft (Michelet *et al*). Rev. Stomatol. Chir. Maxillofac., *75*:83, 1974 (French)

Cleft lip and palate, bilateral, early management (Hotz, Perko), PRS, *56*:467, 1975. Scand. J. Plast. Reconstr. Surg., *8*:104, 1974

Longitudinal study of postoperative changes in the soft-tissue profile in bilateral cleft lip and palate from birth to 6 years (Hanada *et al*). Am. J. Orthod., *67*:363, 1975

Two sisters with unoperated bilateral cleft lip and palate, age 6 and 4 years (Pruzansky *et al*). Brit. J. Plast. Surg., *28*:251, 1975

Primary repair of the bilateral cleft lip nose (McComb). Brit. J. Plast. Surg., *28*:262, 1975

Electromyographic verification of viable muscle tissue following a double-pendulum flap procedure for surgical repair of bilateral cleft lip (Moceri *et al*). Cleft Palate J., *12*:405, 1975

Clefts, bilateral, construction of upper lip, columella, and *orbicularis* muscle (Rehrmann), PRS, *56*:468, 1975

Cleft lip and palate, bilateral, maxillary arch alignment using pinned coaxial screw appliance (Georgiade, Latham), PRS, *56*:52, 1975

Cleft Lip, Facial Growth: See Cleft Palate, Growth

Cleft Lip, Median

Median cleft of the lower lip and mandible: a case report (Millard *et al*). Brit. J. Plast. Surg., *24*:391, 1971

Single stage repair of median cleft lip in an infant with premaxillary agenesis (Beasley *et al*). S. D. J. Med., *24*:15, 1971

Cleft, median, of upper lip and jaw (Pen-

Cleft Lip, Median — Cont.

kava), PRS, *56*:358, 1975. Acta chir. plast., *16*:201, 1974

Cleft, middle, of upper lip and jaw (Pekava), PRS, *54*:506, 1974. Cesk. stomatol., *2*:142, 1974

Cleft, median lip, a true hare lip (Lehman, Cuddapah), PRS, *56*:109, 1975. Cleft Palate J., *11*:497, 1974

Cleft, median, microforms of, with bilateral supernumerary canine teeth (Novak), PRS, *54*:630, 1974. Czas. Stomatol., *2*:148, 1974

Lip, upper, median cleft of (Sharma), PRS, *53*:155, 1974

Cleft, midline, of lower lip and mandible (Ojeda *et al*), PRS, *57*:263, 1976. Cir. Plast. Ibero-Latino Am., *1*:51, 1975

Cleft Lip, Presurgical Orthopedics: See Cleft Palate Orthodontia

Cleft Lip, Secondary Deformity (See also *Nose; Cleft Lip Deformities*)

Pyriform aperture margin, chondroplasty of, in residual deformities of unilateral cleft lip (Kozin), PRS, *50*:95, 1972. Acta chir. plast., *13*:7, 1971

Treatment of nose stenoses (Masing). Arch. Klin. Exp. Ohren Nasen Kehlkopfheilkd., *199*:352, 1971 (German)

Nostril asymmetry not a microform of cleft lip (Pashayan *et al*). Cleft Palate J., *8*:185, 1971

Columella reconstruction, new method of, using a cross lip flap (Onizuka, Tai, Kondo), PRS, *50*:305, 1972. Jap. J. Plast. Reconstr. Surg., *14*:373, 1971

New technic for repairing the nostril deformity in cleft lip (Uchida). Jap. J. Plast. Reconstr. Surg., *14*:405, 1971 (Japanese)

"Whistling" deformity in repaired cleft lips, simple technique for correction of (Chong, Winslow), PRS, *48*:84, 1971

One stage correction of the sequelae of unilateral harelip (Lassus). Rev. Stomatol. Chir. Maxillofac., *72*:323, 1971 (French)

Repair of columella base deformity in unilateral cleft lip (Onizuka). Brit. J. Plast. Surg., *25*:33, 1972

Simple method for the repair of minor postoperative cleft lip "whistling" deformity (Johnson). Brit. J. Plast. Surg., *25*:152, 1972

Reconstruction of the prominence of the columellar sill of the nose (Onizuka *et al*). Jap. J. Plast. Reconstr. Surg., *15*:175, 1972 (Japanese)

Cleft Lip, Secondary Deformity—Cont.

Cleft lip nose, use of anthropometry in assessing (Lindsay, Farkas), PRS, *49:*286, 1972

Bone grafting in secondary cleft lip and palate (Stenström) (Follow-Up Clinic), PRS, *49:*333, 1972

Lip defects, use of tongue flaps to resurface, and close palatal fistulae in children (Jackson), PRS, *49:*537, 1972

Results after midface-osteotomies (Freihofer) J. Maxillo-facial Surg., *1:*30, 1973

Combined correction of the upper jaw and nose in patients with schisis (Steolinga *et al*). Ned. tijdschr. geneeskd., *117:*1604, 1973 (Dutch)

Rhinoplasty: crossed alar wing procedure for correction of late deformity in the unilateral cleft lip nose (Whitlow, Constable), PRS, *52:*38, 1973

Midfacial retrusion, mild, advancement of soft tissues to correct (O'Connor *et al*), PRS, *52:*42 1973

Prevention of recurrence after Lefort I superior maxillary osteotomies for harelip (Aiach). Rev. Stomatol. Chir. Maxillofac., *74:*327, 1973 (French)

Use of tongue flaps in the treatment of sequelae of cleft lip and palate (Gola *et al*). Rev. Stomatol. Chir. Maxillofac., *74:*626, 1973 (French)

Cleft lip and cleft palate. Secondary surgery. 6 (Eskeland *et al*). Tidsskr. Nor. Laegeforen, *93:*2481, 1973 (Norwegian)

Results of the complex treatment of facial deformities, bite disorders after congenital unilateral cleft lip and palate, and surgery (Limberg *et al*). Tsitologiia, *15:*105, 1973 (Russian)

Results of the complex treatment of facial deformities, bite disorders after congenital unilateral cleft lip and palate, and surgery (Limberg *et al*). Vestn. Khir., *111:*105, 1973 (Russian)

Lip, complicated reconstruction after mutilating operation of, and bilateral cleft of primary and secondary palate (Penkava), PRS, *54:*623, 1974. Acta chir. plast., *16:*8, 1974

Correction of a nostril deformity secondary to cleft lip and palate (Vinageras Guarneros *et al*). Bol. Med. Hosp. Infant. Mex., *31:*771, 1974 (Spanish)

Cleft lip nasal deformities, new method for correcting (Elsahy), PRS, *55:*383, 1975. Cleft Palate J., *11:*214, 1974

Maxillofacial osteotomy following unsatisfactory results of surgical correction of cleft

Cleft Lip, Secondary Deformity—Cont.

palate and lip (Curioni *et al*). Minerva Stomatol., *23:*59, 1974 (Italian)

Reconstruction of nose deformities associated with unilateral cleft lip (Kallay). Orv. Hetil., *115:*1946, 1974 (Hungarian)

Lip adhesion, preliminary, secondary correction of bilateral clefts with Millard's midline muscular closure (Oneal, Greer, Nobel), PRS, *54:*45, 1974

Cleft lip repair, primary and secondary, muscle reconstruction in (Randall, Whitaker, LaRossa), PRS, *54:*316, 1974

Cleft lip and palate, bilateral, recession of premaxilla in (Monroe) (Follow-Up Clinic), PRS, *54:*482, 1974

Cleft lip, elongation of (Zenteno), PRS, *54:*240, 1974. Rev. españ. cir. plast., *7:*13, 1974

Delayed corrections of labio-maxillary clefts: soft palate (Neuner *et al*). Rev. Stomatol. Chir. Maxillofac., *75:*68, 1974 (French)

Internasal vestibular flap in cheilorhinoplasty for sequelae of cleft (Stricker *et al*). Rev. Stomatol. Chir. Maxillofac., *75:*71, 1974 (French)

Delayed corrections of labio-maxillary clefts: nose and upper lip (Meyer). Rev. Stomatol. Chir. Maxillofac., *75:*74, 1974 (French)

Surgical treatment of maxillary sequelae of labio-palatine clefts. Pterygo-maxillary disjunction (Lachard *et al*). Rev. Stomatol. Chir. Maxillofac., *75:*77, 1974 (French)

Repositioning and surgical retention of the median tubercle in the sequelae of bilateral labio-maxillary cleft (Michelet *et al*). Rev. Stomatol. Chir. Maxillofac., *75:*83, 1974 (French)

Corrective osteotomies in the sequelae of operations for congenital labio-maxillo-palatine malformations (Popescu *et al*). Rev. Stomatol. Chir. Maxillofac., *75:*86, 1974 (French)

Maxillofacial osteotomy in sequelae of labio-maxillary and palatine clefts (Curioni). Rev. Stomatol. Chir. Maxillofac., *75:*96, 1974 (French)

Follow-up study of cleft lip and palate patients treated with orthodontics, secondary bone grafting, and prosthetic rehabilitation (Johanson *et al*). Scand. J. Plast. Reconstr. Surg., *8:*121, 1974

Cleft lip patients, nasal deformities and their treatment in secondary repair (Malek), PRS, *56:*461, 1975. Scand. J. Plast. Reconstr. Surg., *8:*136, 1974

Indications for and results of Abbe flap (Momma, Koberg, Mai), PRS, *56:*352,

Cleft Lip and Palate Etiology—Cont.

Cleft lip and palate incidence in offspring of cleft patients (Bixler, Fogh-Andersen, Conneally), PRS, *51:*482, 1973. Clin. Genetics, *2:*155, 1971

Morphogenesis of cleft palate induced by exogenous factors. I. The sensitivity period after the administration of cortisone (Dostal *et al*). Folia Morphol. (Praha), *19:*88, 1971

Epidemiological aspects of cleft lip and cleft palate (Schade). Ned. Tijdschr. Trandheelkd., *78:*300, 1971 (Dutch)

Vascular patterns in normal and cleft primary and secondary palate in human embryos (Frederiks), PRS, *52:*209, 1973. Brit. J. Plast. Surg., *25:*207, 1972

Chemically induced abnormalities of the masticatory skull in experimental animals. I. Effect of cyclophosphamide and 6-mercaptopurine on embryonic and fetal development of the rat (Schmitz *et al*). Dtsch. Zahn. Mund. Kieferheilkd., *59:*385, 1972 (German)

Sex ratio and cleft lip with or without cleft palate (Niswander *et al*). Lancet, *2:*858, 1972

Dilantin and hare-lip (Dunstone). M. J. Australia, *2:*54, 1972

New data on the embryology of congenital labiopalatine defects (Talmant *et al*). Rev. Stomatol. Chir. Maxillofac., *73:*257, 1972 (French)

Etiology of cleft lip and cleft palate in humans and in animal experiments (Pfeifer *et al*). Experientia, *29:*225, 1973 (German)

Updating the genetics of cleft lip and palate (Fraser). Birth Defects, *10:*107, 1974

Vitamin A, effect on potentiality of rat palatal processes to fuse *in vivo* and *in vitro* (Nanda), PRS, *55:*383, 1975. Cleft Palate J., *11:*123, 1974

Frequency of cleft lip and palate in northern Israel (Tal *et al*). Isr. J. Med. Sci., *10:*515, 1974

Decline in the incidence of cleft lip and palate in Western Australia, 1963 to 1972 (Brogan *et al*). M. J. Australia, *2:*8, 1974

Induction of cleft palate by amniotic sac puncture (Schade). Acta Morphol. Neerl. Scand., *13:*104, 1975

Embryology of cleft lip and cleft palate (Johnston *et al*). Clin. Plast. Surg., *2:*195, 1975

Diazepam, prenatal exposure, association between cleft lip with or without cleft palate and (Safra, Oakley), PRS, *57:*676, 1976. Lancet, *9:*478, 1975

Letter: cleft lip and palate and pregnancy

Cleft Lip and Palate Etiology—Cont.

tests (Brogan). M. J. Australia, *1:*44, 1975

Lip and palate clefts, heritability of (Bixler), PRS, *56:*108, 1975. Prosth. Dent., *33:*100, 1975

Is it possible to prevent the occurrence of cleft lip and cleft palate (Gabka). Zahnaerztl. Mitt., *65:*762, 1975 (German)

Cleft Lip and Palate, Nursing Care

Feeding cleft palate babies—today's babies, today's methods (Kelly). Cleft Palate J., *8:*61, 1971

Cleft palate care, nursing device for use in (Shirley, Cocke). PRS, *48:*83, 1971

Cleft lip and palate. 2. Nursing care (Pressland). Nurs. Times, *69:*1406, 1973

Nursing of children with congenital cleft lip and palate during the first year of life (Kovalenko *et al*). Stomatologiia (Mosk.), *53:*41, 1974 (Russian)

Cleft Palate (See also Cleft Palate, Velopharyngeal Incompetence)

A Cleft Palate Team Addresses the Speech Clinician. Ed. by Mervyn L. Falk. Charles C Thomas, Springfield, Ill., 1971. PRS, *49:*568, 1972

Atlas for Surgical Repair of Cleft Lip, Cleft Palate, and Noncleft Velopharyngeal Incompetence. By Richard B. Yules. Charles C Thomas, Springfield, Ill., 1971. PRS, *50:*399, 1972

Cleft Lip and Palate. Surgical, Dental, and Speech Aspects. Ed. by William C. Grabb, Sheldon W. Rosenstein, and Kenneth R. Bzoch. Little, Brown & Co., Boston, 1971. PRS, *49:*337, 1972

Cleft Palate & Speech. 7th Ed. By Muriel E. Morley. Longman, Inc., New York, 1971.

Congenital labio-palatine fissures (Tresserra Llaurado). An. Esp. Odontoestomatol., *30:*407, 1971 (Spanish)

Restoration of maxillary cleft using periosteum flaps in case of complete labio-palatine cleft (Santoni-Rugiu *et al*). Ann. chir. plast., *16:*326, 1971 (French)

Timing and choice of operation for primary repairs of clefts of the lip and palate (Maisels). Ann. R. Coll. Surg. Engl., *48:*32, 1971

Children with cleft lip and palate, sinusitis in (Jaffe, DeBlanc), PRS, *49:*105, 1972. Arch. Otolaryng., *93:*5, 1971

Oral and respiratory flora of individuals with normal and repaired palatal clefts (Crawford *et al*). Cleft Palate J., *8:*166, 1971

Recent trends in the early treatment of cleft

Cleft Palate — Cont.

constr. Surg., *8:*1, 1972

Cleft Palate. By Gene R. Powers. Bobbs-Merrill Co., Inc., Indianapolis, Ind., 1973.

Palate closure, course in embryos of different mouse strains (Dostal, Jelinek), PRS, *53:*490, 1974. Acta chir. plast., *15:*23, 1973

Theory and empiricism in surgical treatment of orofacial clefts (Fara). Acta Univ. Carol. (Med. Monogr.) (Praha.), *56:*31, 1973

Problem of tissue deficiency in cleft palate: an experiment in mobilising the palatine bones of cleft dogs (Latham *et al*). Brit. J. Plast. Surg., *26:*252, 1973

Histology of the premaxillary-vomerine suture in a bilateral cleft case (Friede). Cleft Palate J., *10:*14, 1973

Clinical research in cleft lip and cleft palate: the state of the art (Spriestersbach *et al*). Cleft Palate J., *10:*113, 1973

Oral-pharyngeal movements during swallowing and speech (Flowers *et al*). Cleft Palate J., *10:*181, 1973

Palate and lip, cleft (Hagerty, Mylin), PRS, *53:*490, 1974. Contemp. Surg., *3:*44, 1973

Healing course and complications following surgery of cleft lip, maxilla and palate (Bethmann *et al*). Dtsch. Stomatol., *23:*633, 1973 (German)

Intra- and postoperative complications in surgical repair of clefts in infancy (Schettler). J. Maxillo-facial Surg., *1:*40, 1973

Present view on bone grafting in cleft palate (a review of the literature) (Koberg). J. Maxillo-facial Surg., *1:*185, 1973

Technic of isolated veloplasty (Kontor). Magy. Traumatol. Orthop., *16:*215, 1973 (Hungarian)

Evaluation of the surgical treatment of 175 children with cleft of secondary palate (Kawiak). Probl. Med. Wieku. Rozwoj., *3:*193, 1973 (Polish)

Team work and clinical research in the treatment of cleft lip and palate (Hellquist). Sven. Tandlak. Tidskr. *66:*145, 1973

Cleft lip and cleft palate. Primary cleft surgery. 3 (Borchgrevink *et al*). Tidsskr. Nor. Laegeforen, *93:*2466, 1973 (Norwegian)

Muscle closure in cleft palate repair (Hayward). Trans. Int. Conf. Oral Surg., *4:*74, 1973

Results of the complex treatment of facial deformities, bit disorders after congenital unilateral cleft lip and palate, and surgery (Limberg *et al*). Vestn. Khir., *111:*105, 1973 (Russian)

Contribution to the assessment of the preoperative condition of the nose in patients

Cleft Palate — Cont.

with palatoschisis (Hajnis *et al*). Acta chir. plast. (Praha), *16:*1, 1974

Embryonic tissue studies, rapid technique for contrast in secondary palate development (Dostal, Behounkova), PRS, *56:*367, 1975. Acta chir. plast., *16:*243, 1974

Early bone grafting in clefts of the lip, maxilla and palate (Nakajima). Acta Med. (Fukuoka), *44:*17, 1974 (Japanese)

Aspects of plastic surgery. Cleft lip and palate — management (Muir). Brit. Med. J., *3:*162, 1974

Palate and lip, cleft, educational level of patients with (Lahti, Rintala, Soivio), PRS, *55:*252, 1975. Cleft Palate J., *11:*36, 1974

Electrical stimulation of soft palate (Peterson), PRS, *55:*382, 1975. Cleft Palate J., *11:*72, 1974

Casts, cleft palate, quantitative analysis of (Berkowitz, Krischer, Pruzansky), PRS, *55:*382, 1975. Cleft Palate J., *11:*134, 1974

Cleft palate children, object identification and naming (Brennan, Cullinan), PRS, *55:*382, 1975. Cleft Palate J., *11:*188, 1974

Airway, nasopharyngeal, in cleft palate, effect of restorative procedures on (Warren, Trier, Bevin), PRS, *56:*108, 1975. Cleft Palate J., *11:*367, 1974

Cleft palate preschoolers, clinical use of Peabody picture vocabulary test with (McWilliams), PRS, *56:*110, 1975. Cleft Palate J., *11:*439, 1974

Status of research in cleft palate anatomy and physiology, July 1973, part 1 (Dickson *et al*). Cleft Palate J., *11:*471, 1974

Treatment of cleft hard palate using lyophilized cartilage plate. Preliminary communication (Krajnik *et al*). Czas. Stomatol., *27:*711, 1974 (Polish)

Use of mucosal-periosteal flaps from the vomer in the treatment of asymmetrical palatal clefts (Puk). Czas. Stomatol., *27:*1037, 1974 (Polish)

Cleft palate, primary closure using palatal mucosal flap to prevent growth impairment (Peiko), PRS, *54:*622, 1974. J. Maxillo-facial Surg., *2:*40, 1974

A surgeon's view of the congenitally cleft maxilla (Dey). M. J. Australia, *1:*708, 1974

General problems of the cleft lip and palate (Celesnik). Minerva Stomatol., *23:*171, 1974 (Italian)

Proceedings: early closure of the prolabium in piercing cleft lip, jaw and palate (Hollmann). Munch. Med. Wochenschr., *116:*1064, 1974 (German)

Current status of the treatment of cheilognathopalatoschisis (Coerdt). Munch. Med.

Cleft Palate – Cont.

Wochenschr., *116*:1207, 1974 (German)

Palatine shelves, spatial changes during horizontalization of (Dostal, Jelinek), PRS, *54*:629, 1974. Rozhl. chir., *53*:171, 1974

Timing of hard palate repair (Robertson, Jolleys), PRS, *56*:468, 1975. Scand. J. Plast. Reconstr. Surg., *8*:49, 1974

Flap, periosteal, in surgery for cleft lip and palate, bone forming capacity (Rintala *et al*), PRS, *56*:681, 1975. Scand. J. Plast. Reconstr. Surg., *8*:58, 1974

Flap, periosteal, effect on cleft width and formation of alveolar ridge in relation to bite level (Ranta *et al*), PRS, *56*:682, 1975. Scand. J. Plast. Reconstr. Surg., *8*:62, 1974

Cleft palate managed by modified Dunn procedure with skin graft to vomer flaps (Stenström, Thilander), PRS, *56*:682, 1975. Scand. J. Plast. Reconstr. Surg., *8*:67, 1974

Clefts, palatal, bone formation subsequent to palato-vomer plasty (Prydso *et al*), PRS, *56*:359, 1975. Scand. J. Plast. Reconstr. Surg., *8*:73, 1974

Lip and palate, cleft, final results from delayed treatment (Ortiz-Monasterio *et al*), PRS, *56*:468, 1975. Scand. J. Plast. Reconstr. Surg., *8*:109, 1974

Cleft palate timing of primary repair (Evans, Renfrew), PRS, *56*:360, 1975. Scand. J. Plast. Reconstr. Surg., *8*:153, 1974

Method for the evaluation of the restoration of function of the soft palate following radical uranoplasty (Arifdzhanov). Stomatologiia (Mosk.), *53*:35, 1974 (Russian)

Symposium on Management of Cleft Lip and Palate and Associated Deformities. Vol. 8. Ed. by Nicholas Georgiade and Robert Hagerty. C. V. Mosby Co., St. Louis, 1975. PRS, *56*:333, 1975

Status of research in cleft lip and palate: anatomy and physiology, part 2 (Dickson *et al*). Cleft Palate J., *12*:131, 1975

Review of the results of two different surgical procedures for the repair of clefts of the soft palate only (Musgrave *et al*). Cleft Palate J., *12*:281, 1975

Surgical repair of cleft palate (Lindsay). Clin. Plast. Surg., *2*:309, 1975

Evaluation of therapeutic results in the surgical treatment of cleft palate using lyophilized plates of xenogenous cartilage (Krajnik *et al*). Czas. Stomatol., *28*:497, 1975 (Polish)

New guiding principles in the treatment of clefts (Oblak). J. Maxillo-facial Surg., *3*:231, 1975

Cleft palate rehabilitation, total maxillary osteotomy for (Pederson, Blatto), PRS,

Cleft Palate – Cont.

57:121, 1976. J. Oral Surg., *39*:669, 1975

Cleft palate, soft palate repair by levator muscle reconstruction and buccal mucosal flap (Kaplan). PRS, *56*:129, 1975

Palate, cleft, conservative program for managing without use of mucoperiosteal flaps (Blocksma, Leuz, Mellerstig). PRS, *55*:160, 1975

Clefts, rapid expansion in (Matthews). PRS, *56*:396, 1975

Naso-alveolar openings, plea for primary closure of, during cleft palate repairs (Tucker) (Letter to the Editor). PRS, *55*:614, 1975

Surgical treatment of unilateral upper cleft palate in children using our own method (Debowska-Wojcik). Pol. Przegl. Chir., *47*:45, 1975 (Polish)

Palatoplasty: a comparative study (Krause *et al*). Trans. Am. Acad. Ophthalmol. Otolaryngol., *80*:551, 1975

Time plan for the treatment of cheilognathouranoschisis (Schilli *et al*). Z. Allgemeinmed., *51*:1312, 1975 (German)

Cleft Palate, Complications

Sinusitis in children with cleft lip and palate (Jaffe, DeBlanc), PRS, *49*:105, 1972. Arch. Otolaryng., *93*:5, 1971

Nasal floor, closure of secondary palatal fistulae with intraoral tissue and bone grafting (Jackson), PRS, *52*:100, 1973. Brit. J. Plast. Surg., *25*:93, 1972

Palatal fistulae, use of tongue flaps to resurface lip defects and close, in children (Jackson). PRS, *49*:537, 1972

Clefts, middle ear complications in (Fara, Hrivnakova, Horak), PRS, *53*:607, 1974. Acta chir. plast., *15*:7, 1973

Osteoplasty of alveolus and hard palate followed by development of cleft upper jaw (Schmid *et al*), PRS, *55*:381, 1975. J. Maxillo-facial Surg., *2*:92, 1974

Osteotomy, total maxillary, for cleft palate rehabilitation (Pederson, Blatto), PRS, *57*:121, 1976. J. Oral Surg., *39*:669, 1975

Maxillary arch alignment in bilateral cleft lip and palate infant using pinned coaxial screw appliance (Georgiade, Latham). PRS, *56*:52, 1975

Cleft Palate, Ear Problems

Eustachian tube obstruction in the infant with cleft palate (Bluestone). Ann. Otol. Rhin. & Laryngol., *80*:2, 1971

Middle ear exudates as regular findings in cleft lip, jaw and palate (Quante *et al*). Arch. Klin. Exp. Ohren Nasen Kehlkopfheilkd., *199*:483, 1971 (German)

Cleft Palate, Ear Problems — Cont.

Observations on hearing levels of preschool cleft palate children (Harrison *et al*). J. Speech Hear. Disord., *36:*252, 1971

Middle ear problems associated with cleft palate (Shimo). Can. J. Otolaryngol., *1:*9, 1972

Roentgenographic evaluation of eustachian tube function in infants with cleft and normal palates (Bluestone *et al*). Cleft Palate J., *9:*93, 1972

Certain effects of cleft palate repair on eustachian tube function (Bluestone *et al*). Cleft Palate J., *9:*183, 1972

Hearing problems in velar insufficiency (Morgon *et al*). J. Fr. Otorhinolaryngol., *21:*891, 1972 (French)

Otolaryngological evaluation of the cleft palate patient (King). Laryngoscope, *82:*276, 1972

The older cleft palate patient. A clinical otologic-audiologic study (Bennett). Laryngoscope, *82:*1217, 1972

Longitudinal study of the efficacy of adenoidectomy in children with cleft palate and secretory otitis media (Severeid). Trans. Am. Acad. Opthalmol. Otolaryngol., *76:*1319, '1972

Tonsillectomy in patients with cleft palate (Muhler). Z. Laryngol. Rhinol. Otol., *51:*806, 1972 (German)

Effect on middle ear disease of fracture of the pterygoid hamulus during palatoplasty (Noone *et al*). Cleft Palate J., *10:*23, 1973

Prevention of hearing damage in cleft palate patients (Koch *et al*). Dtsch. Stomatol., *23:*816, 1973 (German)

Eustachian tube function in cleft lip and palate patients (Cole, Cole, Intaraprasong), PRS, *54:*695, 1974. Arch. Otolaryng., *99:*337, 1974

Cleft palate population, tympanometry, impedence and aural reflex testing in (Billings, Lowry), PRS, *55:*380, 1975. Cleft Palate J., *11:*21, 1974

Cleft palate population otolaryngic findings in (Lowry, Billings, Leonard), PRS, *55:*251, 1975. Cleft Palate J., *11:*62, 1974

Palate, cleft aural form discrimination of children with (Pressel, Hochberg), PRS, *55:*251, 1975. Cleft Palate J., *11:*66, 1974

Cleft palate males 7 and 8 years old, speech sound discrimination (Finnegan), PRS, *55:*382, 1975. Cleft Palate J., *11:*111, 1974

Sucking exercise for adenoidal atrophy (Massengill, Quinn), PRS, *55:*376, 1975. Cleft Palate J., *11:*196, 1974

Follow-up study of cleft children treated with primary-bone grafting. II. Audiological as-

Cleft Palate, Ear Problems — Cont.

pects (Korsan-Bengsten *et al*). Scand. J. Plast. Reconstr. Surg., *8:*161, 1974

Ear pathology and hearing loss in cleft palate. Treatment of cleft palate in Bergen (Moller). Tidsskr. Nor. Laegeforen, *94:*2078, 1974 (Norwegian)

Palatal clefts and hearing (Fombeur *et al*). Ann. chir. plast., *20:*295, 1975 (French)

Hearing disorders in children operated on for cleft palate (Fombeur *et al*). Ann. Otolaryngol. Chir. Cervicofac., *92:*436, 1975 (French)

Eustachian tube ventilatory function in relation to cleft palate (Bluestone *et al*). Ann. Otol. Rhin. & Laryngol., *84:*333, 1975

Middle ear problems-associated with cleft palate. An internationally-oriented review (Paradise). Cleft Palate J., *12:*17, 1975.

Cleft palates middle ear effusions in babies (Soudijn *et al*). Cleft Palate J., *12:*229, 1975

Current concepts of treatment of ear disease in cleft palate children and adults (Yules). Cleft Palate J., *12:*315, 1975

Hearing acuity before and after pharyngeal flap procedure (LeWorthy, Schliesser), PRS, *56:*49, 1975

Hearing acuity before and after pharyngeal flap procedure (Kaplan) (Letter to the Editor). PRS, *56:*205, 1975

Cleft Palate, Elongation of

Cleft palate operations, lengthening soft palate in (Dorrance) (Classic Reprint). PRS, *50:*275, 1972

Palate, cleft, sandwich pushback and lateral pharyngoplasty (Bennett), PRS, *54:*694, 1974. Brit. J. Plast. Surg., *26:*16, 1973

Palatal pushback and pharyngeal flap operation, combined (Kaplan) (Follow-Up Clinic). PRS, *51:*206, 1973

Vomerine flaps, use of, to cover raw area on nasal surface in cleft palate pushbacks (Horton *et al*). PRS, *51:*421, 1973

Pushback operations, results of, in treatment of submucous cleft palate (Massengill, Pickrell, Robinson). PRS, *51:*432, 1973

Palate pushback, division of nasal lining to achieve (Antia, Daver). PRS, *55:*383, 1975. Indian J. Plast. Surg., *7:*3, 1974

Pushback operation for complete unilateral cleft palate (Honjow, Isshiki, Morimoto). PRS, *53:*306, 1974

Palate, soft, repaired by levator muscle reconstruction and buccal mucosal flap (Kaplan). PRS, *56:*129, 1975

Nasopharyngeal pushback in treatment of velopharyngeal insufficiency (Smith *et al*). Arch. Otolaryng., *102:*83, 1976

Cleft Palate, Elongation of—Cont.

Comparative-study of results of the von Langenbeck and the V-Y pushback palatoplasties (Krause *et al*). Cleft Palate J., *13:*11, 1976

Pushback and pharyngeal flap operations, combined, cephalometric study of facial growth in children after (Pearl, Kaplan). PRS, *57:*480, 1976

Cleft Palate, Extra-Oral Flaps for

Cleft palate repair, the tube flap (Evans). PRS, *48:*395, 1971. Proc. Roy. Soc. Med., *64:*73, 1971

Elimination of penetrating palatal defects by using a flat epithelialized skin flap (Chudakov). Vestn. Khir., *110:*86, 1973 (Russian)

Cleft Palate, Genetics of (See also *Cleft lip and Palate, Etiology*

Cleft palate, incidence in offspring of cleft parents (Bixler, Fogh-Andersen, Conneally), PRS, *51:*482, 1973. Clin. Genetics, *2:*155, 1971

Congenital malformations, cleft lip and palate in particular, in children of epileptic women (Elshove, Van Eck), PRS, *49:*359, 1972. Nederl. tijdschr. geneesk., *115:*1371, 1971

Clefts, genetic counseling, empirical recurrence risk figures for (Tolarova), PRS, *52:*683, 1973. Acta chir. plast., *14:*234, 1972

Cleft palate formation, possible genesis for (Smiley). PRS, *50:*390, 1972

Embryos of different mouse strains, course of palate closure in (Dostal, Jelinek), PRS, *53:*490, 1974. Acta chir. plast., *15:*23, 1973

Lip and palate, cleft, in Bohemia, epidemiological study (Klásková-Buriánová), PRS, *54:*505, 1974. Acta chir. plast., *15:*258, 1973

Clefts, families with, cephalometric study of (Figalova, Smahel), PRS, *56:*358, 1975. Acta chir. plast., *16:*247, 1974

Cleft lip and palate: one genetic system (Chabora, Horowitz), PRS, *56:*231, 1975. Oral Surg., *38:*181, 1974

Pathogenesis of submucous cleft palate (Poswillo), PRS, *56:*359, 1975. Scand. J. Plast. Reconstr. Surg., *8:*34, 1974

Clinical epidemiological studies on harelip and cleft palate (Otsuka). J. Otolaryngol. Jpn., *78:*345, 1975 (Japanese)

Clefts of lip and palate, heritability of (Bixler), PRS, *56:*108, 1975. Prosth. Dent., *33:*100, 1975

Cleft Palate Growth (See also *Cleft Palate; Cleft Palate, X-ray Studies*)

Influence of selecting the time for staphylorraphia upon maxillary and facial growth (Longacre *et al*). Ann. chir. plast., *13:*241, 1968 (French)

Cleft lip and palate patients in Uppsala, jaw orthopedic and orthodontic treatment for (Hellquist), PRS, *49:*236, 1972. Scand. J. Plast. Reconstr. Surg., *4:*11, 1970

Craniofacial growth in complete unilateral cleft lip and palate (Aduss). Angle Orthod., *41:*202, 1971

Growth mechanism of the human face with special reference to cleft lip and palate conditions (Latham). Ann. R. Coll. Surg. Engl., *48:*30, 1971

Timing and choice of operation for primary repairs of clefts of the lip and palate (Maisels). Ann. R. Coll. Surg. Engl., *48:*32, 1971

Influence of primary osteoplasty on the treatment of patients with clefts of the lip, palate and jaw (Schrudde). Brit. J. Plast. Surg., *24:*189, 1971

Age factors in operative treatment of children with congenital clefts of the upper lip and palate (Mukhin *et al*). Bull. Eksp. Biol. Med., *71:*60, 1971 (Russian)

Effect of early bone grafting on the growth of upper jaw in cleft lip and palate children. A computer evaluation (Rehrmann). Minerva Chir., *26:*874, 1971

Age factors in operative treatment of children with congenital clefts of the upper lip and palate (Mukhin *et al*). Stomatologiia Mosk., *50:*60, 1971 (Russian)

Discussion of the right age for the surgical treatment of children with congenital cleft lip and palate (Kats). Stomatologiia Mosk., *50:*75, 1971 (Russian)

Morphology of the orbital region in adults following the cleft lip-palate repair in childhood (Farkas *et al*). Am. J. Phys. Anthropol., *37:*65, 1972

A series of cleft lip and palate children five years after undergoing orthopedic and bone grafting procedures (Rosenstein *et al*). Angle Orthod., *42:*1, 1972

Cleft lip and palate, complete, a study of the effects of early bone grafting (Jolleys, Robertson), PRS, *52:*208, 1973. Brit. J. Plast. Surg., *25:*229, 1972

Hourglass maxillary collapse in repaired postalveolar clefts of the palate (Crikelair *et al*). Cleft Palate J., *9:*13, 1972

Facial growth of children with cleft lip and/or

Cleft Palate Growth – Cont.

to unilateral cleft lip and palate surgery: a comparison of the effects of different surgical approaches (Onizuka *et al*). Cleft Palate J., *12:*444, 1975

Clefts in lip, alveolus, and palate, morphogenesis of (Oblak), PRS, *57:*675, 1976. J. Maxillo-facial Surg., *3:*182, 1975

Cleft lip and palate cases, midface anthropometry on cephalometric radiograph in (Wepner, Hollman), PRS, *57:*537, 1976. J. Maxillo-facial Surg., *3:*188, 1975

Cleft, oral, conservative program for managing without use of mucoperiosteal flaps (Blocksma, Leuz, Mellerstig). PRS, *55:*160, 1975

Cleft: mobile unit for detection and care of craniofacial anomalies (Ortiz-Monasterio). PRS, *55:*186, 1975

Lip and palate, bilateral cleft, maxillary arch alignment using pinned coaxial screw appliance (Georgiade, Latham). PRS, *56:*52, 1975

Maxilla, collapsed – rapid expansion in clefts (Matthews). PRS, *56:*396, 1975

Cranial base, growth of cartilages of, preliminary studies on *Rattus norvegicus* (Roberts), PRS, *56:*225, 1975. Proc. Roy. Soc. Med., *68:*130, 1975

Time plan for the treatment of cheilognathouranoschisis (Schilli *et al*). Z. Allgemelomed., *51:*1312, 1975 (German)

Flap, pharyngeal, and pushback operations, combined cephalometric study of facial growth in children after (Pearl, Kaplan). PRS, *57:*480, 1976

Cleft Palate Obturators

Prosthetic or surgical therapy in congenital palatal defects in the adult (Hochstein). Dtsch. Stomatol., *21:*663, 1971 (German)

Speech, poor, following pharyngeal flap operation (Owsley, Creech, Dedo), PRS, *52:*325, 1973. Cleft Palate J., *9:*312, 1972

Significance of Passavant's pad in post-obturator patients (Weiss). Folia Phoniatr. (Basel), *24:*51, 1972

Speech intelligibility analysis, presurgical maxillary prosthesis (Kipfmueller, Lang), PRS, *52:*204, 1973. J. Prosth. Dent., *28:*620, 1972

Obturators, acrylic, to protect suture lines in hard palate (Bowers, Gruber). PRS, *51:*98, 1973

Speech intelligibility following prosthetic obturation of surgically acquired maxillary defects (Azia, Weinberg, Chalian), PRS, *55:*257, 1975. J. Prosth. Dent., *32:*87, 1974

Cleft Palate Obturators – Cont.

Speech pathologist's role in dealing with obturator-wearing school children (Weiss), PRS, *56:*110, 1975. J. Speech & Hearing Disorders, *39:*153, 1974

Obturator, superiorly based (Tautin, Schaaf), PRS, *56:*105, 1975. Prosth. Dent., *33:*96, 1975

Cleft Palate Operations, Anesthesia for

Naso-tracheal fluorothane nitrous oxide anesthesia in uranoplasty (Golovatenko). Stomatologiia (Mosk.), *51:*80, 1972 (Russian)

Difficulties and modifications of intubation technique in infants with labial, alveolar and palatal clefts (Zawistowska *et al*). Anaesth. Resusc. Intensive Ther., *1:*211, 1973

Cleft Palate Orthodontia

Presurgical facial orthopaedics in relationship to the overall management of cleft lip and palate conditions (Burston). Ann. R. Coll. Surg. Engl., *48:*31, 1971

Early maxillary orthopedics in relation to maxillary cleft repair by periosteoplasty (Hellquist). Cleft Palate J., *8:*36, 1971

Dental occlusion and early repair of alveolar clefts (Bernstein). Arch. Otolaryng., *96:*395, 1972

Some observations on rapid expansion followed by bone grafting in cleft lip and palate (Robertson *et al*). Cleft Palate J., *9:*236, 1972

Post-orthodontic retention and post-prosthodontic occlusion in adult complete unilateral and bilateral cleft subjects (Ramstad). Cleft Palate J., *10:*34, 1973

Orthopedic treatment of cleft lip and palate in the newborn (Cadenat *et al*). Rev. Stomatol. Chir. Maxillofac., *74:*706, 1973. (French)

Results of the complex treatment of facial deformities, bite disorders after congenital unilateral cleft lip and palate, and surgery (Limberg *et al*). Tsitologiia, *15:*105, 1973. (Russian)

Cleft palate casts, quantitative analysis of (Berkowitz, Krischer, Pruzansky), PRS, *55:*382, 1975. Cleft Palate J., *11:*134, 1974

Cleft lip and palate, pre-surgical orthopedic treatment (Graf-Pinthus, Bettex), PRS, *55:*513, 1975. Cleft Palate J., *11:*253, 1974

Occlusion, changes from deciduous to early mixed dentition in unilateral complete clefts (Bergland, Sidhu), PRS, *55:*514, 1975. Cleft Palate J., *11:*317, 1974

Orthopedics, presurgical, in treatment of unilateral cleft lip and palate (O'Donnell,

Cleft Palate Orthodontia—Cont.

Krischer, Shiere), PRS, *56:*108, 1975. Cleft Palate J., *11:*374, 1974

Cleft lip and palate patients, longitudinal analysis of maxillary growth in (Mapes *et al*), PRS, *56:*109, 1975. Cleft Palate J., *11:*450, 1974

Experience with orthodontic treatment before surgical correction of unilateral and bilateral cleft lip and palate in infants (Rehak *et al*). Orv. Hetil., *115:*2672, 1974 (Hungarian)

Cleft lip, jaw, and palate patients, incidence of pseudoprognathism and other serious orthodontic anomalies in (Mullerova, Brousilova, Pasek), PRS, *54:*623, 1974. Rozhl. chir., *53:*164, 1974

Orthodontic aspects of treating cleft lip and palate by primary bone grafting (Friede, Johanson), PRS, *56:*680, 1975. Scand. J. Plast. Reconstr. Surg., *8:*88, 1974

Coordinated orthodontic and surgical treatment of cleft lip, jaw and palate. A contribution on the prevention of delayed adverse effects (Hotz-Jenny *et al*). Schweiz. Med. Wochenschr., *104:*718, 1974 (German)

Orthodontic and bone grafting procedures in a cleft lip and palate series: an interim cephalometric evaluation (Rosenstein). Angle Orthod., *45:*227, 1975

Management of dental arch deformity in cleft lip and palate (Ross). Clin. Plast. Surg., *2:*325, 1975

Orthodontic treatment of children with unilateral cleft palate before uranoplasty (Isaeva). Stomatologiia (Mosk.), *54:*54, 1975 (Russian)

Cleft Palate, Pharyngeal Flap for (See also *Cleft Palate, Velopharyngeal Incompetence*)

Pedicle tubing, increase of biological value of pharyngeal flap by (Fara). PRS, *50:*201, 1972. Acta chir. plast., *12:*57, 1971

Indication and the results of pharyngeal flap operation (Isshiki *et al*). Arch. Klin. Exp. Ohren Nasen Kehlkopfheilkd., *200:*158, 1971

Pharyngeal flap, conversion of inferiorly-based, to superiorly-based position (McEvitt). PRS, *48:*36, 1971

Pharyngeal flap, indications for, in primary repair of cleft palate (Weisman). PRS, *48:*568, 1971

Suture of palate and secondary repair of pharyngeal flap (Brozman *et al*). Acta chir. plast. (Praha.), *14:*218, 1972

Velopharyngeal competence and incompetence following pharyngeal flap surgery:

Cleft Palate, Pharyngeal Flap for—Cont.

videofluoroscopic study in multiple projections (Skolnick *et al*). Cleft Palate J., *9:*1, 1972

Histology and electromyography of primary pharyngeal flaps (Fara *et al*). Cleft Palate J., *9:*64, 1972

Palate, cleft, pharyngeal surgery: meningitis following accidental rupture of meningocele (Cronin, Penoff), PRS, *52:*100, 1973. Cleft Palate J., *9:*215, 1972

Pharyngeal flaps, comparison of superior and inferior based posterior (Whitaker *et al*), PRS, *52:*100, 1973. Cleft Palate J., *9:*304, 1972

Pharyngeal flap operation, poor speech following (Owsley, Creech, Dedo), PRS, *52:*325, 1973. Cleft Palate J., *9:*312, 1972

Pharyngeal flap, operation of, postoperative progress (Isshiki, Honjo, Shiba). J. Otolaryngol. Jap., *75:*1063, 1972 (Japanese)

Pharyngeal flap, elusive dynamic, new approach, preliminary report (McCoy, Zahorsky). PRS, *49:*160, 1972

Pharyngeal flaps, nasality in patients with, radiographic technique for demonstrating causes (Skolnic, McCall), PRS, *54:*689, 1974. Brit. J. Plast. Surg., *26:*12, 1973

Combined pharyngeal flap and palate pushback procedure: improvements in technique (Jobe). Brit. J. Plast. Surg., *226:*384, 1973

Pharyngeal flap as a primary and secondary procedure (Curtin *et al*). Cleft Palate J., *10:*1, 1973

Pharyngeal flap surgery and voice quality—factors related to success and failure (Schulz *et al*). Cleft Palate J., *10:*166, 1973

Complications following poster or pharyngeal flap surgery (Graham *et al*). Cleft Palate J., *10:*176, 1973

Cleft palate speech, surgical goals in, and introduction of lateral port control (LPC) pharyngeal flap (Hogan), PRS, *54:*505, 1974. Cleft Palate J., 10:331, 1973

Normal speech recovery after pharyngeal flap operation, case (Imazato *et al*). Jap. J. Oral Surg., *19:*166, 1973 (Japanese)

Pharyngeal flap and palatal pushback operation, combined (Kaplan) (Follow-Up Clinic), PRS, *51:*206, 1973

Pharyngeal flaps, bilateral transverse, for repair of cleft palate (Kapetansky), PRS, *52:*52, 1973

Flap, bilateral island sandwich, combined with superiorly based pharyngeal flap for velopharyngeal incompetency (Winslow *et al*), PRS, *55:*513, 1975. Cleft Palate J., *11:*272, 1974

Cleft Palate, Pharyngeal Flap for—Cont.

Flap, pharyngeal, bleeding following Teflon pharyngoplasty (Sturim), PRS, *55:*514, 1975. Cleft Palate J., *11:*292, 1974

Cleft palate, new anteriorly superiorly based pharyngeal flap (Massengill, Georgiade), PRS, *55:*512, 1975. Cleft Palate J., *11:*333, 1974

Osteomyelitis and disc space involvement, following pharyngeal flap operation (Tucker, Hubbard), PRS, *53:*477, 1974

Velopharyngeal flap operation, superiorly based, age factor and reduction of open nasality (Leanderson *et al*), PRS, *56:*681, 1975. Scand. J. Plast. Reconstr. Surg., *8:*156, 1974

Further experience with pharyngeal flap in the cleft palate patient (Jones). Trans. Pac. Coast Otoophthalmol. Soc., *55:*85, 1974

Clinical investigation of the efficacy of primary nasopalatal pharyngoplasty (Dalston *et al*). Cleft Palate J., *12:*177, 1975

Delayed pharyngeal flap success: report of a case (Neiman *et al*). Cleft Palate J., *12:*244, 1975

Combined use of levator retrodisplacement and pharyngeal flap for congenital palate insufficiency (Fisher *et al*). Cleft Palate J., *12:*270, 1975

Flaps, cross palatopharyngeal, pharyngoplasty through (Heller), PRS, *57:*117, 1976. J. Maxillo-facial Surg., *3:*94, 1975

Pharyngeal flap augmentation (Cosman, Falk), PRS, *55:*149, 1975

Flap, new folded pharyngeal (Isshiki, Morimoto), PRS, *55:*461, 1975

Pharyngeal flap, is late severance feasible? (Fujino) (Letter to the Editor), PRS, *55:*483, 1975

Pharyngeal flap procedure, hearing acuity before and after (LeWorthy, Schliesser), PRS, *56:*49, 1975

Pharyngeal flap procedure, hearing acuity before and after (Kaplan) (Letter to the Editor), PRS, *56:*205, 1975

Repeated superiorly based pharyngeal flap operation for persistent velopharyngeal incompetence (Hirshowitz *et al*). Cleft Palate J., *13:*45, 1976

Pharyngeal flap, redone (Owsley, Lawson, Chierici), PRS, *57:*150, 1976

Pharyngeal flap, posterior, preservation of, during maxillary advancement (Ruberg, Randall, Whitaker), PRS, *57:*335, 1976

Pharyngeal flap and pushback operations, combined, cephalometric study of facial growth in children after (Pearl, Kaplan), PRS, *57:*480, 1976

Cleft Palate Pushback: See *Cleft Palate, Elongation of*

Cleft Palate, Secondary Operations (See also *Cleft Lip, Secondary Deformity*

Secondary cleft palate (Clooster). Acta Stomatol. Belg., *67:*467, 1970 (Dutch)

Surgical therapy of jaw deformities caused by cleft lip and cleft palate. Indications and late results (Perko). Osterr. Z. Stomatol., *67:*287, 1970 (German)

Maxillofacial surgery of harelip and cleft palate (Dirlewanger). Rev. Med. Suisse Romande, *90:* 337, 1970 (French)

Treatment of mandibular prognathism in cleft palate patients (Quinn *et al*). Am. J. Orthod., *59:*76, 1971

Our experience with secondary osteoplasty in the treatment of cleft palate (Petrovic). Dtsch. Zahn. Mund. Kieferheilkd., *57:* 230 1971 (German)

Palate, soft, temporal muscle transfers to incompetent, progress report (Kiehn *et al*), PRS, *48:*335, 1971

Pharyngoplasty, bilateral, as aid to velopharyngeal closure (Sullivan) (Follow-Up Clinic), PRS, *48:*587, 1971

Fistulae, secondary palatal, closure with intraoral tissue and bone grafting (Jackson), PRS, *52:*100, 1973. Brit. J. Plast. Surg., *25:* 93, 1972

Secondary bone grafting in cleft palate: a follow-up of 145 patients (Hogeman *et al*). Cleft Palate J., *9:*39, 1972

Secondary bone grafting of residual alveolar and palatal clefts (Boyne *et al*). J. Oral Surg., *30:* 87, 1972

Surgical treatment of oronasal fistula resulting from palatoplasty for cleft palate, using autogenous bone graft (Antognini *et al*). Minerva Stomatol., *21:*276, 1972 (Italian)

Teflon pharyngoplasty (Sturim, Jacob), PRS, *49:*180, 1972

Objective analysis of persistent deformities of the palate following surgical interventions and assessment of the results of uranostaphyloplasty (Zausaev). Stomatologiia (Mosk.), *51:*51, 1972 (Russian)

Maxillary osteotomies in cleft palate repairs (Grocott). Brit. J. Plast. Surg., *26:*261, 1973

Further experience with tongue flap in cleft palate repair (Guerrero-Santos *et al*). Cleft Palate J., *10:*192, 1973

Primary, early secondary or late secondary osteoplasty in cleft surgery? Clinical and animal experimental study (Harle). Dtsch. Zahnaerztl. Z., *28:*612, 1973 (German)

Cleft Palate Secondary Operations – Cont.

Correction of jaw position in an adult cleft patient (Obwegeser). Dtsch. Zahnaerztl. Z., *28:* 688, 1973 (German)

Use of tongue flaps in the treatment of sequelae of cleft lip and palate (Gola *et al*). Rev. Stomatol. Chir. Maxillofac., *74:*626, 1973 (French)

Tongue flaps in plastic surgery (Cadenat *et al*). Rev. Stomatol. Chir. Maxillofac., *74:*690, 1973 (French)

Cleft lip and cleft palate. Secondary surgery. 6 (Eskeland *et al*). Tidsskr. Nor. Laegeforen, *93:*2481, 1973 (Norwegian)

Palate, cleft, effect of restorative procedures on nasopharyngeal airway in (Warren, Trier, Bevin), PRS, *56:*108, 1975. Cleft Palate J., *11:*367, 1974

Results after mobilization of the mid-facial bone structure (Freihofer). Fortschr. Kiefer. Gesichtschir., *18:*219, 1974 (German)

Use of marrow-cancellous bone grafts in maxillary alveolary and palatal clefts (Boyne). J. Dent. Res., *53:*821, 1974

Delayed corrections of labio-maxillary clefts: soft palate (Neuner *et al*). Rev. Stomatol. Chir. Maxillofac., *75:*68, 1974 (French)

Comparative study of late postoperative results following plastic surgery of the palate (Shchegoleva). Stomatologiia (Mosk.), *53:*39, 1974 (Russian)

Reconstruction of the defect of alveolar process of the maxilla using bone graft as a pre-prosthetic arrangement in adult patients with cleft palate (Petrovic). Cesk. Stomatol., *75:*131, 1975 (Slovakian)

Observations of patients with late surgery for cleft palate (Herwerth *et al*). Fogorv. Sz., *68:*164, 1975 (Hungarian)

Bone brephroplasty in cleft palate (Ruzin *et al*). Stomatologiia (Mosk.), *54:*38, 1975 (Russian)

Cleft Palate, Social Problems

Insights into the total cleft palate child (Walton). J. Arkansas Med. Soc., *67:*131, 1970

Congenital malformations in community, detection of incidence (Weatherall), PRS, *48:*91, 1971. Proc. Roy. Soc. Med., *63:*1251, 1970

Cleft palate and the person: psychologic studies of its impact (Clifford). South. Med. J., *64:*1516, 1971

Public health in Pennsylvania, reminiscences, cleft palate program (Ivy), PRS, *48:*400, 1971. Tr. Coll Physicians Phila., *38:*174, 1971

Psychological findings in adulthood of 98 cleft

Cleft Palate, Social Problems – Cont.

lip-palate children (Clifford, Crocker, Pope), PRS, *50:*234, 1972

Effect of surgical treatment on psychic readaptation of patients with congenital and acquired defects of the face (Mateev *et al*). Stomatologiia (Mosk.), *51:*54, 1972 (Russian)

Educational, occupational, and marital status of cleft palate adults (McWilliams *et al*). Cleft Palate J., *10:*223, 1973

Exposure of medical and dental students to the disorder of cleft palate (Lass *et al*). Cleft Palate J., *10:*306, 1973

Parents working with parents: the cleft palate program (Irwin *et al*). Cleft Palate J., *10:*360, 1973

The intellectual function of cleft palate children compared on the basis of cleft type and sex (Lamb *et al*). Cleft Palate J., *10:*367, 1973

Rehabilitation of persons with congenital cleft palate (Mulfay *et al*). Otorinolaringologie, *18:*359, 1973 (Rumanian)

Cleft palate and normal children, comparison of written language ability (Ebert, McWilliams, Wolf), PRS, *55:*381, 1975. Cleft Palate J., *11:*17, 1974

Cleft lip and palate, educational level of patients with (Lahti, Rintala, Soivio), PRS, *55:*252, 1975. Cleft Palate J., *11:*36, 1974

Cleft palate adults, sociological aspects. I. Marriage (Peter, Chinsky), PRS, *55:*514, 1975. II. Education, PRS, *56:*109, 1975. Cleft Palate J., *11:*295, 443, 1974

Vocabulary test, Peabody picture, clinical use with cleft palate preschoolers (McWilliams), PRS, *56:*110, 1975. Cleft Palate J., *11:*439, 1974

Cleft lip and palate, surgical and social pediatric viewpoints in treatment of (Schmid), PRS, *55:*111, 1975. Ztschr. Kinderchir., *15:*9, 1974

Behavior and achievement of cleft palate children (Richman). Cleft Palate J., *13:*4, 1976

Survey of publications for parents of cleft palate children: a preliminary report (Pannbacker). Cleft Palate J., *13:*57, 1976

Letter: For parents of new-born babies with cleft lip/palate – pamphlet (Pruzansky *et al*). Cleft Palate J., *13:* 76, 1976

Cleft Palate Speech (See also *Cleft Palate, Velopharyngeal Incompetence*)

Palatal stimulant to decrease velopharyngeal gap (Massengill, Quinn, Pickrell), PRS, *48:*296, 1971. Ann. Otol. Rhin. & Lar-

Cleft Palate Speech — Cont.

Nasality, open, method for correction — lateral velopharyngoplasty (Reichert), PRS, *55:*381, 1975. J. Maxillo-facial Surg., *2:*95, 1974

Learning rate and retrieval from memory of speech-like stimuli, effects of low-pass filtering on (Novak, Davis), PRS, *57:*683, 1976. J. Speech & Hearing Res., *17:*279, 1974

Obturator-wearing school children, speech pathologist's role in dealing with (Weiss), PRS, *56:*110, 1975. J. Speech & Hearing Disorders, *39:*153, 1974

Cleft palate, complete unilateral, pushback operation for, (Honjow, Isshiki, Morimoto), PRS, *53:*306, 1974

Cleft palate surgery, submucous, evaluation of (Dellon, Hoopes) (Letter to the Editor), PRS, *53:*338, 1974. Reply from Dr. Pickrell, PRS, *53:*339, 1974

Cleft lip and palate, age factor and reduction of open nasality following superiorly based velopharyngeal flap operation in 124 cases (Leanderson *et al*), PRS, *56:*681, 1975. Scand. J. Plast. Reconstr. Surg., *8:*156, 1974

Role of Passavant's ridge in cleft palate speech (Honjo *et al*). Arch. Otorhinolaryngol. (N.Y.), *211:*203, 1975

Speech results after Millard island flap repair in cleft palate and other velopharyngeal insufficiencies (Lewin *et al*). Cleft Palate J., *12:*263, 1975

Patterns of velopharyngeal closure in subjects with repaired cleft palate and normal speech: a multi-view videofluoroscopic analysis (Skolnick *et al*). Cleft Palate J., *12:*369, 1975

Relation between speech production and orofacial structures in individuals with isolated clefts of the palate (Bishara *et al*). Cleft Palate J., *12:*452, 1975

Changes of cheek pressure during swallowing following expansion of the maxillary dental arch in repaired cleft palates (Sakuda *et al*). J. Oral Rehabil., *2:*145, 1975

Surgical procedures in cleft-palate patients with reference to phonetic function: primary and secondary methods (Scheunemann). Langenbecks Arch. Chir., *339:*355, 1975 (German)

Cleft palate speech: pharyngeal flap augmentation (Cosman, Falk), PRS, *55:*149, 1975

Speech, hypernasal: velopharyngeal incompetence without overt cleft palate (Minami *et al*), PRS, *55:*573, 1975

Phonetic results of velopharyngoplasties. Apropos of 67 cases (Souyris *et al*). Rev. Sto-

Cleft Palate Speech — Cont.

matol. Chir. Maxillofac., *76:*423, 1975 (French)

Speech, hypernasal; the re-do pharyngeal flap (Owsley, Lawson, Chierici), PRS, *57:*180, 1976

Cleft Palate, Submucous

Cleft palates, submucous (Fara, Hrivnakova, Sedlackova), PRS, *51:*481, 1973. Acta chir. plast., *13:*221, 1971

Perforation in a case of submucous cleft palate due to an aphthous ulcer (Weijerman *et al*). Brit. J. Oral Surg., *10:*217, 1972

Submucous cleft palate; its incidence, natural history, and indications for treatment (Weatherley-White *et al*), PRS, *49:*297, 1972

Cleft palate, submucous, and the general practitioner (Lowry, Courtemanche, MacDonald), PRS, *53:*489, 1974. Canad. M.A.J., *109:*995, 1973

Submucous cleft palate, results of pushback operations in treatment of (Massengill, Pickrell, Robinson), PRS, *51:*432, 1973

Submucous cleft palate surgery, evaluation of (Dellon, Hoopes) (Letter to the Editor), PRS, *53:*338, 1974. Reply from Dr. Pickrell, PRS, *53:*339, 1974

Palate, submucous cleft, pathogenesis of (Poswillo), PRS, *56:*359, 1975. Scand. J. Plast. Reconstr. Surg., *8:*34, 1974

Palatopharyngeal disproportion, velopharyngeal incompetence without overt cleft palate (Minami *et al*), PRS, *55:*573, 1975

Cleft Palate, Velopharyngeal Incompetence
(See also *Cleft Palate, Speech; Cleft Palate, X-ray studies)*

Velopharyngeal gap, use of a palatal stimulant to reduce (Massengill, Quinn, Pickrell), PRS, *48:*296, 1971. Ann. Otol. Rhin. & Laryng., *80:*135, 1971

Radiological evaluation of velopharyngeal closure (Skolnick *et al*). (J.A.M.A., *218:*96, 1971

Temporal muscle transfers to incompetent soft palate, progress report (Kiehn *et al*), PRS, *48:*335, 1971

Velopharyngeal closure, bilateral pharyngoplasty as aid to (Sullivan) (Follow-Up Clinic), PRS, *48:*587, 1971

Nasal escape, mechanics of (Battle), PRS, *48:*515, 1971. Proc. Roy. Soc. Med., *64:*67, 1971

X-ray image intensifier, use in management of nasal escape (Heycock), PRS, *48:*394, 1971. Proc. Roy. Soc. Med., *64:*70, 1971

Palatopharyngeal closure, means of indirect

Cleft Palate, Velopharyngeal
Incompetence — Cont.
evaluation of (Tytar *et al)*. Zh. Ushn. Nos.
Gorl. Bolezn., *31:*85, 1971 (Russian)
Velopharyngeal incompetence, comparison of
superior and inferior based posterior pharyngeal flaps (Whitaker *et al)*, PRS,
*52:*100, 1973. Cleft Palate J., *9:*304, 1972
Electorhinopneumography as an objective
method of assessment of velopharyngeal
insufficiency in cleft-palate patients (Tronczynska). Folia Phoniatr. (Basel), *24:*371,
1972
An approach to palatopharyngeal incompetence (Ghosh *et al)*. J. Laryng. & Otol.,
*86:*709, 1972
Pharyngoplasty, Teflon (Sturim, Jacob),
PRS, *49:*180, 1972
Nasal escape, simple test for (Furlow), PRS,
*49:*355, 1972
Rhinolalia aperta (Gorman). Va. Med. Mon.,
*99:*1077, 1972
Pharyngoplasty, lateral, and sandwich pushback (Bennett), PRS, *54:*694, 1974. Brit. J.
Plast. Surg., *26:*16, 1973
Velopharyngeal competence and primary
cleft palate surgery, 1960-1971: a critical
review (Morris). Cleft Palate J., *10:*62,
1973
Teflon pharyngoplasty in incompetent velopharyngeal closure (Benveniste *et al)*.
Cleve. Clin. Q., *40:*93, 1973
Velopharyngeal incompetence, contribution
to the problem of (Perko), PRS, *53:*246,
1974. J. Maxillo-facial Surg., *1:*96, 1973
Velopharyngeal incompetence, retropharyngeal implantations of silicone gel pillows
for (Brauer), PRS, *51:*254, 1973
Cleft palate pushbacks, use of vomerine flaps
to cover raw area on the nasal surface in
(Horton *et al)*, PRS, *51:*421, 1973
Palate, cleft, bilateral transverse pharyngeal
flaps for repair of (Kapetansky), PRS,
*52:*52, 1973
Pharynx, dynamic muscle sphincter of, indications and convenient surgical moment
(Orticochea), PRS, *54:*619, 1974. Ann. chir.
plast., *19:*5, 1974
Pharyngo-palatoplasty with free transplantation of *palmaris longus* (Song, Bromberg), PRS, *56:*677, 1975. Brit. J. Plast.
Surg., *27:*337, 1974
Nasality and velopharyngeal gap, effect of
muscle exercise on (Powers, Starr), PRS,
*55:*251, 1975. Cleft Palate J., *11:*28, 1974
Velopharyngeal insufficiency: effect of cleft
palate on oral port constriction during fricative productions (Claypoole, Warren,
Bardley), PRS, *55:*382, 1975. Cleft Palate
J., *11:*95, 1974

Cleft Palate, Velopharyngeal
Incompetence — Cont.
Adenoid atrophy, velopharyngeal incompetence and sucking exercises (Massengill,
Quinn), PRS, *55:*376, 1975. Cleft Palate J.,
*11:*196, 1974
Rhinophonia, noninvasive electrometric de-
tection of nasal escape in patients with
(Habal, Mardam-Rey), PRS, *55:*386, 1975.
Cleft Palate J., *11:*209, 1974
Velopharyngeal incompetency treated by bi-
lateral island sandwich flap combined with
superiorly based pharyngeal flap (Winslow
et al), PRS, *55:*513, 1975. Cleft Palate J.,
*11:*272, 1974
Velopharyngeal closure in normal individuals, fibrescopic examination of (Matsuya,
Miyazaki, Yamaoka), PRS, *55:*514, 1975.
Cleft Palate J., *11:*286, 1974
Pharyngoplasty, Teflon; bleeding complica-
tions with pharyngeal flap construction in
humans following (Sturim), PRS, *55:*514,
1975. Cleft Palate J., *11:*292, 1974
Velopharyngeal competency assessment for
children with cleft palates (Van Demark),
PRS, *55:*514, 1975. Cleft Palate J., *11:*310,
1974
Velopharyngeal closure during speech and
non-speech activities in normals, 3-dimen-
sional cinefluoroscopic analysis of
(Shprintzen *et al)*, PRS, *56:*114, 1975. Cleft
Palate J., *11:*412, 1974
Velopharyngeal competence, comparison of
Danish and Iowa children with cleft palates (Van Demark), PRS, *56:*109, 1975.
Cleft Palate J., *11:*463, 1974
Open nasal speech following adenoidectomy
and tonsillectomy (van Gelder). J. Com-
mun. Disord., *7:*263, 1974
Velopharyngoplasty, lateral: new method for
correction of open nasality (Reichert),
PRS, *55:*381, 1975. J. Maxillo-facial Surg.,
*2:*95, 1974
Nasopharyngoscopic assessment of pharyn-
goplasty (Pigott), PRS, *56:*354, 1975.
Scand. J. Plast. Reconstr. Surg., *8:*148,
1974
Cleft velum, functional findings in, correc-
tion by intravelar plastic operation
(Kriens), PRS, *55:*111, 1975. Ztschr. Kin-
derchir., *15:*21, 1974
Prediction of velopharyngeal competency
(Demark *et al)*. Cleft Palate J., *12:*5, 1975
Velopharyngeal function in cleft palate
(Skolnick). Clin. Plast. Surg., *2:*285, 1975
The determination of velopharyngeal incom-
petence by aerodynamic and acoustical
techniques (Warren). Clin. Plast. Surg.,
*2:*299, 1975
Developing a direct, objective measure of ve-

Cleft Palate, Velopharyngeal
  Incompetence — Cont.
lopharyngeal inadequacy (Schwartz). Clin. Plast. Surg., 2:305, 1975

A biased approach to the treatment of velopharyngeal incompetence (Hogan). Clin. Plast. Surg., 2:319, 1975

Palate: pharyngeal flap augmentation (Cosman, Falk), PRS, 55:149, 1975

Velopharyngeal inadequacy, new folded pharyngeal flap for (Isshiki, Morimoto), PRS, 55:461, 1975

Velopharyngeal incompetence without overt cleft palate (Minami et al), PRS, 55:573, 1975

Flap, pharyngeal, redone (Owsley, Lawson, Chierici), PRS, 57:180, 1976

Velopharyngeal incompetence, cephalometric study of facial growth in children after combined pushback and pharyngeal flap operations (Pearl, Kaplan), PRS, 57:480, 1976

Cleft Palate, X-Ray Studies

A cephalometric radiographic evaluation of pharyngeal flap surgery for correction of palatopharyngeal incompetence (Musgrave). Cleft Palate J., 8:118, 1971

Radiological evaluation of velopharyngeal closure (Skolnick et al). J.A.M.A., 218:96, 1971

Cleft palate speech, cinefluorographic analysis of surgical treatment of (Owsley) (Follow-Up Clinic). PRS, 49:335, 1972

Palatography. "A study of velo-pharyngeal closure" (Kamdar et al). Australas. Radiol., 17:26, 1973

Cephalometric evaluation of facial growth in operated and non-operated individuals with isolated clefts of the palate (Bishara). Cleft Palate J., 10:239, 1973

Videofluoroscopy as an aid in the management of velopharyngeal insufficiency. J. Maine Med. Assoc., 64:89, 1973

Cephalometric study of families with clefts (Figalova, Smahel), PRS, 56:358, 1975. Acta chir. plast., 16:247, 1974

Permanent records of cleft lip, nose and palate abnormalities (Chandra et al). Brit. J. Plast. Surg., 27:139, 1974

Cephalometric comparisons on the cranial base and face in individuals with isolated clefts of the palate (Bishara et al). Cleft Palate J., 11:162, 1974

Cephalometric radiograph, midface anthropometry on, in cleft lip and palate cases (Wepner, Hollmann), PRS, 57:537, 1976. J. Maxillo-facial Surg., 3:188, 1975

CLEMENTSCHITSCH, F.: Motility disorders of the eye in injuries of the osseous orbit (oral surgery report). Wien. Med. Wochenschr., 122 Suppl 5:3, 1972 (German)

CLEMIS, J. D. et al: Intramuscular hemangioma in head and neck. Can. J. Otolaryngol., 4:339, 1975

CLEMONS, J. E. et al: Reattachment of totally amputated auricle. Arch. Otolaryng., 97:269, 1973

CLERICI, E. et al: Poly-DL-alanyl skin isograft rejection by purified anti-poly-DL-alanyl antibodies. Tissue Antigens, 4:21, 1974

CLERMONT, H. G., AND WILLIAMS, J. S.: Lymph lysosomal enzyme acid phosphatase in hemorrhagic shock, PRS, 51:710, 1973. Ann. Surg., 176:90, 1972

CLERY, A. B.: Treatment of burns by split skin grafting. Nurs. Times, 70:1893, 1974

CLIFFORD, E.: Cleft palate and the person: psychologic studies of its impact. South. Med. J., 64:1516, 1971

CLIFFORD, E., CROCKER, E. C., AND POPE, B. A.: Psychological findings in the adulthood of cleft lip-palate children, PRS, 50:234, 1972

CLIFFORD, P.: Nasal septum in repairing surgical defects of palate. J. Laryng. & Otol., 87:655, 1973

CLIMO, M. S.: Keratosis palmaris et plantaris — some prospective thoughts (Letter to the Editor); Reply (Kisner), PRS, 52:568, 1973

CLIMO, M. S., BLOCK, L. I., AND ALEXANDER, J. E.: Extra-osseous Kirschner wire fixation for an unstable depressed fracture of the frontal bone, PRS, 52:200, 1973

CLODIUS, L.: The surgical management of postmastectomy lymphedema of the arm, PRS, 49:585, 1972. Chir. Praxis, 15:273, 1971

CLODIUS, L.: Life of Theodor Billroth, PRS, 50:72, 1972

CLODIUS, L.: Biographical sketch of Lanz by Dr. Leo Clodius (Classic Reprint), PRS, 50:396, 1972

CLODIUS, L.: Reconstruction of the nasolabial fold. PRS, 50:467, 1972

CLODIUS, L.: Facial scars and lymph outflow. Praxis, 62:336, 1973 (German)

CLODIUS, L.: Peripheral facial paralysis as asymmetry problem. Helv. Chir. Acta, 42:157, 1975 (German)

CLODIUS, L.: Xeroradiography examination in orbitonasal surgery (with Maillard, Otto), PRS, 55:664, 1975

CLODIUS, L., AND SMAHEL, J.: Thin and thick pedicle flaps. PRS, 51:485, 1973. Acta chir. plast., 14:30, 1972

CLODIUS, L. et al: Dependence of skinflap survival on their thickness and on the quality of the flap bed, as monitored by vital staining, pH measurements and clinical observation.

Helv. chir. acta, *39:*419, 1972 (German)

CLODIUS, L., UHLSCHMID, G., AND MADRITSCH, W.: Secondary lymphedema of arm, PRS, *53:*605, 1974. Helv. chir. acta, *40:*659, 1973

CLODIUS, L., AND SMAHEL, J.: Reverse dermal-fat flap: an alternative cross-leg flap. PRS, *52:*85, 1973

CLOOSTER, R. VAN: Secondary cleft palate. Acta Stomatol. Belg., *67:*467, 1970 (Dutch)

CLOOSTER, R. VAN: Current trends in primary osteoplasty in cleft lip. Acta Stomatol. Belg., *69:*309, 1972 (Dutch)

CLOOSTER, R. VAN: Methods of treatment of cleft lip and cleft palate. Rev. Belge. Med. Dent., *27:*334, 1972 (Dutch)

CLOUP, M. *et al*: Medical aspect of treatment of extensive burns in children, 8 cases. Ann. chir. plast., *18:*325, 1973 (French)

COATES, H. L. *et al*: Glandular tumors of palate, PRS, *56:*462, 1975. Surg. Gynec. & Obst., *140:*589, 1975

COBBETT, J. R.: Free graft. Hand, *2:*112, 1970

COBURN, R. J.: Expanding hematoma after rhytidectomy, retrospective study (with Rees, Lee). PRS, *51:*149, 1973

COBURN, R. J.: Use of inflatable breast implants (with Rees, Guy). PRS, *52:*609, 1973

COBURN, R. J. *et al*: Platelet activity in allograft rejection. Surg. Forum, *22:*476, 1971

COBURN, R. J., BLANK, H. L., AND CAMPBELL, R. M.: Covering an exposed pacemaker. PRS, *50:*622, 1972

COCCARO, P. J.: Cephalometric analysis in diagnosis and treatment planning of craniofacial dysostoses (with Firmin, Converse). PRS, *54:*300, 1974

COCCARO, P. J.: Retrospective cephalometric analysis of mandibular bone absorption under silicone rubber chin implants (with Friedland, Converse). PRS, *57:*144, 1976

COCERO, E. *et al*: Electroneurophysiology in control of reparative surgery of cancer of lip. Arch. Neurobiol. (Madr.), *37:*31, 1974 (Spanish)

COCHET, B.: The diabetic hand. Praxis, *62:*1055, 1973 (French)

COCHIN, A. *et al*: Hemoglobin II: immunogenic properties of stroma *vs.* stroma free hemoglobin solution, PRS, *56:*473, 1975. J. Surg. Oncol. *6:*19, 1974

COCHRAN, A. J. *et al*: Postoperative depression of tumor-directed cell-mediated immunity in patients with malignant disease. Brit. Med. J., *4:*67, 1972

COCHRAN, A. J. *et al*: Cell-mediated immunity in malignant melanoma. Lancet, *1:*1340, 1972

COCHRAN, A. J. *et al*: Tumor-directed cellular immunity in malignant melanoma and its modification by surgical treatment. Yale J. Biol. Med., *46:*650, 1973

COCKE, W. M.: Principles of surgery for pressure sores. J. Tenn. Med. Assoc., *64:*949, 1971

COCKE, W. M.: Dexon – a new suture material: its use in plastic surgery. South. Med. J., *65:*629, 1972

COCKE, W. M.: Reconstructive surgery of lower extremity injuries. J. Tenn. Med. Assoc., *66:*1039, 1973

COCKE, W. M., AND DAVIS, W. G.: Reconstruction in Landouzy-Dejerine progressive muscular dystrophy, PRS, *48:*77, 1971

COCKE, W. M., AND RICKETSON, G.: Gluteal augmentation, PRS, *52:*93, 1973

COCKE, W. M., AND NORTON, C.: Regeneration of tibial segment from periosteum, PRS, *53:*675, 1974

COCKE, W. M., LEATHERS, H. K., AND LYNCH, J. B.: Foreign body reactions to polyurethane covers of some breast prostheses, PRS, *56:*527, 1975

CODD, R. D. *et al*: An adaptive multi-functional hand prosthesis. J. Physiol. (Lond.), *232:*55P, 1973

CODEGA, G., CODEGA, O., AND KUS, H.: Neurolysis of median nerve in carpal tunnel as surgical treatment of Kienbock's disease, PRS, *53:*246, 1974. Internat. Surg., *58:*378, 1973

CODEGA, G. *et al*: Complication after alloplastic thigh augmentation. Polim. Med., *4:*153, 1974

CODEGA, G. *et al*: Elastic redressing-training devices in flexure contractures of the fingers. Polim. Med., *4:*189, 1974 (Polish)

CODINA, J. *et al*: Epidermolysis bullosae, PRS, *53:*615, 1974. Rev. españ. cir. plast., *4:*145, 1971

CODLING, B. W. *et al*: Histiocytosis presenting as swelling of orbit and eyelid. Brit. J. Ophthalmol., *56:*517, 1972

COERDT, I.: Errors in indications for plastic operations. Langenbecks Arch. Chir., *327:*652, 1970 (German)

COERDT, I.: Current status of the treatment of cheilognathopalatoschisis. Munch. Med. Wochenschr., *116:*1207, 1974 (German)

COEVORDEN, J. J., AND HORREE, W. A.: Benign tumors of parotid gland, PRS, *54:*106, 1974. Arch. chir. neerl., *25:*435, 1973

COFFIN, F.: Twelve years of free skin vestibuloplasty. Trans. Int. Conf. Oral Surg., *4:*195, 1973

COGAN, M. I.: Related maxillary sinus problem: diagnosis and treatment of second division trigeminal neuralgia. Trans. Int. Conf. Oral Surg., *4:*179, 1973

COHEN, B. E., AND ELIN, R. J.: Enhanced resistance to certain infections in vitamin A-treated mice, PRS, *54:*192, 1974

COHEN, C. *et al*: Effect of RL-A locus and NLC

locus on graft survival in rabbit. Transplantation, *18:*150, 1974

COHEN, G.: Harry's angels. Brit. Med. J., *4:*288, 1972

COHEN, H. B.: Congenital ptosis: a new pedigree and classification, PRS, *50:*93, 1972. Arch. Ophth., *87:*161, 1972

COHEN, I. K.: Hypertrophic scars and keloids (with Ketchum, Masters), PRS, *53:*140, 1974

COHEN, I. K.: Secondary reconstruction of cervical esophagus (with Petty, Theogaraj), PRS, *56:*70, 1975

COHEN, I. K., AND EDGERTON, M. T.: Transbuccal flaps for reconstruction of the floor of the mouth, PRS, *48:*8, 1971

COHEN, I. K., KEISER, H. R., AND SJOERDSMA, A.: Collagen synthesis in human keloid and hypertrophic scar, PRS, *50:*205, 1972. Surg. Forum, *22:*488, 1971

COHEN, I. K., HOLMES, E. C., AND EDGERTON, M. T.: Parotid duct transplantation for correction of drooling in patients with cancer of head and neck, PRS, *49:*361, 1972. Surg. Gynec. & Obst., *133:*663, 1971

COHEN, I. K. *et al*: Histamine and collagen synthesis in keloid and hypertrophic scar, PRS, *51:*709, 1973. Surg. Forum, *23:*509, 1972

COHEN, I. K., AND CHRETIEN, P. B.: Control of hemorrhage from internal jugular vein by balloon catheter, PRS, *52:*462, 1973. Surg. Gynec. & Obst., *136:*791, 1973

COHEN, I. K., AND KEISER, H. R.: Disruption of healed scars in scurvy — result of disequilibrium in collagen metabolism, PRS, *57:*213, 1976. Discussion by Chvapil, PRS, *57:*376, 1976

COHEN, M. H. *et al*: Staging laparotomy in the treatment of metastatic melanoma of the lower extremities. Ann. Surg., *182:*710, 1975

COHEN, N.: Surgical treatment of pressure sores. Harefuah, *80:*86, 1971 (Hebrew)

COHEN, N. *et al*: Review of 57 cases of keratoacanthoma, PRS, *49:*138, 1972

COHEN, S.: Transplants for baldness. South African M. J., *47:*3, 1973

COHEN, S. R., DAVIS, D. M., AND KRAMKOWSKI, R. S.: Clinical manifestations of chromic acid toxicity: nasal lesions in electroplate workers, PRS, *54:*371, 1974. Cutis, *13:*558, 1974

COIFFMAN, F.: New aspects in free scalp transplants, PRS, *51:*485, 1973. Rev. Latino Am. cir. plast., *16:*21, 1972

COIFFMAN, F.: How to improve circulation in pedicled skin flaps, PRS, *55:*518, 1975. Rev. Latino Am. cir. plast., *17:*21, 1973

COIN, C. G.: Tomography of temporomandibular joint, PRS, *55:*377, 1975. Dent. Radiogr. Photogr., *47:*23, 1974

COKER, S. B. *et al*: Safe alternative to tracheos-

tomy in acute epiglottis. Am. J. Dis. Child., *129:*136, 1975

COLBURN, J. F. *et al*: Myxoma of mandibular condyle — surgical excision with immediate reconstruction. J. Oral Surg., *33:*351, 1975

COLE, J., AND COLE, S.: Ortega hypothesis, PRS, *51:*487, 1973. Science, *178:*368, 1972

COLE, P.: Nasal turbinate function. Can. J. Otolaryngol., *2:*259, 1973

COLE, R.: Neurovascular flap repair of fingertip amputations, PRS, *52:*595, 1973. Proc. Roy. Australasian Coll. Surgeons, *46:*399, 1973

COLE, R., COLE, J., AND INTARAPRASONG, S.: Eustachian tube function in cleft lip and palate patients, PRS, *54:*695, 1974. Arch. Otolaryng., *99:*337, 1974

COLE, W. G.: Fat embolism: a current concept, PRS, *54:*627, 1974. M. J. Australia, *1:*535, 1974

COLE, W. H.: Mechanisms of spread of cancer. Surg. Gynec. & Obstet., *137:*853, 1973

COLEMAN, B. H.: Congenital atresia of the ear: the otological problem. Proc. Roy. Soc. Med., *67:*1203, 1974

COLEMAN, C. C.: Diagnosis and treatment of congenital arteriovenous fistulas of the head and neck, PRS, *53:*489, 1974. Am. J. Surg., *126:*557, 1973

COLEMAN, W. P., III: Use of student-written programmed texts for the teaching of "core" knowledge in surgery (with Ryan), PRS, *53:*429, 1974

COLETTI, G. D.: A simple treatment for localized alveolar osteitis. Ann. Dent., *33:*46, 1974

COLIN, B., AND JANVIER, H.: Devices for preventing retractions after secondary repair of burned neck, PRS, *54:*113, 1974. Ann. chir. plast., *18:*15, 1973

Collagen (See also *Keloid; Scars, Hypertrophic; Wound Healing*)

Collagen, studies on biology during wound healing. III. Dynamic metabolism of scar collagen and remodeling of dermal wounds (Madden, Peacock), PRS, *51:*235, 1973. Ann. Surg., *174:*511, 1971

Enzymes, lysosomal, and inflammation with particular reference to rheumatoid diseases (Chayen, Bitensky), PRS, *49:*361, 1972. Ann. Rheumat. Dis., *30:*522, 1971

Lathyrogens, effect on development of midfacial structures in rat (Stivers, Steffek, Yarington), PRS, *49:*586, 1972. J. Surg. Res., *11:*415, 1971

Collagen synthesis, defective, in inguinal herniation (Wagh, Read), PRS, *52:*103, 1973. Am. J. Surg., *124:*819, 1972

Collagen synthesis and wound repair, inhibitory effects of vitamin E on (Ehrlich, Tarver, Hunt), PRS, *50:*421, 1972. Ann.

Collagen — Cont.

Surg., *175:*235, 1972

Biology and pathology at molecular level of connective tissue fibrous proteins (Lapiere), PRS, *51:*609, 1973. Arch. belges dermat. et syph., *28:*15, 1972

Enzymes, proteolytic, oral, double-blind study on effect, in postsurgical hand inflammation (Garcia-Velazco, Araico), PRS, *50:*632, 1972. Arch. Int. Med. Mex., *3:*7, 1972

Isografts and homografts of tendons, collagen metabolism in (Tobias, Seiffert), PRS, *52:*105, 1973. Brit. J. Plast. Surg., *25:*83, 1972

Enzymes, proteolytic, clinical effect after reconstructive hand surgery (McCue, Webster, Gieck), PRS, *51:*231, 1973. Internat. Surg., *57:*479, 1972

Elbow, tennis, radial tunnel syndrome (Roles, Maudsley), PRS, *52:*679, 1973. J. Bone & Joint Surg., *54B:*499, 1972

Glucose-6-phosphate dehydrogenase screening, importance in urologic practice (Allen, Wilkerson), PRS, *50:*539, 1972. J. Urol., *107:*304, 1972

Collagen maturation in healing wounds in young and old rats (Holm-Pedersen, Viidik), PRS, *51:*108, 1973. Scand. J. Plast. Reconstr. Surg., *6:*24, 1972

Lathyrogens, caution against use of (Barrow, Simpson), PRS, *50:*101, 1972. Surgery, *71:*309, 1972

Collagen-glycosaminoglycan in healing wounds, byssal thread formation (Keiter, Bakowski, Weeks), PRS, *52:*328, 1973. Surg. Forum, *23:*27, 1972

Histamine and collagen synthesis in keloid and hypertrophic scar (Cohen *et al*), PRS, *51:*709, 1973. Surg. Forum, *23:*509, 1972

³H-collagen turnover in skin grafts (Klein, Rudolph), PRS, *51:*352, 1973. Surg. Gynec. & Obst., *135:*49, 1972

Benzidamine associated with carica papaya endopeptidase, employment in plastic surgery (Lopez), PRS, *52:*104, 1973. Tribuna Med. Argent., *15:*611, 1972

Collagenase, synovial — regulation and metabolism of enzyme activity and significance in pathogenesis of rheumatoid arthritis (Abe, Nagai), PRS, *53:*114, 1974. Asian M. J., *16:*155, 1973

Chondroitin-sulfates used as prophylaxis for adhesions in peritonitis caused by enterococci (Sailer, Stauch), PRS, *53:*366, 1974. Bruns' Beitr. klin. chir., *220:*637, 1973

Tissue, biological, stochastic model for elasticity in simple elongation (Soong, Huang), PRS, *53:*375, 1974. J. Bio-Mechanics, *6:*451, 1973

Collagen — Cont.

Collagen destruction by triamcinolone, inhibition of (Rudolph, Klein), PRS, *53:*692, 1974. J. Surg. Res., *14:*435 1973

Steroid, local injection, efficacy of, in treatment of stenosing tenovaginitis (Clark, Ricker, MacCollum), PRS, *51:*179, 1973

Pseudosheath pocket around silicone implants, fate of (Thomson), PRS, *51:*667, 1973

Granulation tissue: contractile fibroblast. Its relevance in plastic surgery (Montandon *et al*), PRS, *52:*286, 1973

Curvature of penis: Peyronie's disease (Horton, Devine), PRS, *52:*503, 1973

Collagen in thrombus formation in microvascular surgery (Acland), PRS, *52:*454, 1973. Surgery, *73:*766, 1973

Biopolymers and Biomechanics of Connective Tissue. Ed. by F. Hartmann, C. Hartung, and H. Zeidler. Springer-Verlag, New York, 1974. PRS, *57:*231, 1976

Letter: Collagenases: human and bacterial (Kirman). New England J. Med., *291:*1363, 1974

Triamcinolone for hypertrophic scars and keloids (Ketchum, Cohen, Masters), PRS, *53:*140, 1974

India, South, study of 1,000 patients with keloids (Ramakrishnan, Thomas, Sundarajan), PRS, *53:*276, 1974

Steroids, role in prevention of circumferential capsular scarring in augmentation mammaplasty (Peterson, Burt), PRS, *54:*28, 1974

Collagen, microcrystalline, as topical hemostatic agent for vascular surgery (Abbott, Austen), PRS, *54:*629, 1974. Surgery, *75:*925, 1974

Skin grafts, pathways of radioactive collagen loss from (Rudolph, Klein), PRS, *55:*114, 1975. Surg. Gynec. & Obst., *138:*55, 1974

Skin grafts, pathways of radioactive collagen loss from (Rudolph, Klein), PRS, *55:*114, 1975. Surg. Gynec. & Obst., *138:*55, 1974

Enzymes, oral proteolytic, in treatment of sprained ankles (Craig), PRS, *57:*262, 1976. Injury, *6:*313, 1975

Pseudosheaths around silicone implants, effect of hematoma on thickness (Williams, Aston, Rees). PRS, *56:*194, 1975

Estrogens, pregnancy, presumptive evidence of effect on keloid growth (Moustafa, Abdel-Fattah). PRS, *56:*450, 1975

Prostheses, inflatable breast, use of soluble steroids within (Perrin). PRS, *57:*163, 1976

Cell size and growth characteristics of cultured fibroblasts isolated from normal and keloid tissue (Russell, Witt). PRS, *57:*207, 1976

Collagen — Cont.

Collagen metabolism disequilibrium, disruption of healed scars in scurvy, result of (Cohen, Keiser), PRS, *57:*213, 1976. Discussion by Chvapil, PRS, *57:*376, 1976

Steroid instillation, failure of, to prevent capsular contracture after augmentation mammaplasty (Price) (Letter to the Editor). PRS, *57:*371, 1976

Elastogenesis in healing wounds in bats (Bhangoo, Church). PRS, *57:*468, 1976

COLLIER, M.: Progressive facial hemiatrophy with megalocornea, micropupil and central nebular dystrophy of the cornea. Acta Ophthalmol. (Kbh.), *49:*946, 1971 (French)

COLLINS, D. W.: Some new thoughts on hand prostheses. Hand, *3:*9, 1971

COLLINS, W. F., JR.: Discussion of "Single fascicular recordings: intraoperative diagnostic tool for management of peripheral nerve lesions," by Williams, Terzis. PRS, *57:*744, 1976

COLOCHO, G. *et al*: Human amniotic membrane as physiologic wound dressing. Arch. Surg., *109:*370, 1974

COLSON, P. *et al*: Clinical and ultrastructural study of fragmented skin grafts. Ann. chir. plast., *16:*299, 1971 (French)

COLSON, P. *et al*: Case of dorsal burns of the hand. Tissue contracture. Grafts and flaps. Ann. chir. plast., *17:*34, 1972 (French)

COLUCCIO, A.: Postponed tracheostomy. Minerva chir., *28:*148, 1973 (Italian)

Columella: See *Nose and Rhinoplasty*

COLVILLE, J.: Tendon graft function, PRS, *54:*375, 1974. Hand, *5:*152, 1973

COMAN, C. *et al*: Surgical treatment of congenital deformities of thoracic wall in children. Pediatria (Bucur.), *22:*543, 1973 (Rumanian)

COMER, T. T. *et al*: Delayed massive hemorrhage from tracheostomy, PRS, *55:*508, 1975. J. Cardiovasc. Surg., *15:*389, 1974

COMIS, R. L. *et al*: Integration of chemotherapy into combined modality therapy of solid tumors. IV. Malignant melanoma. Cancer Treat. Rev., *1:*285, 1974

COMMITTEE ON CUTANEOUS HEALTH AND COSMETICS OF AMA: The aging skin, PRS, *54:*383, 1974. Hospital Med., *10:*72, 1974

COMMITTEE ON MEDICINE IN SOCIETY: Measures employed to prolong life in terminal illness, PRS, *53:*114, 1974. N. Y. Acad. M., *49:*349, 1973

Composite Flap (See also *Free Flaps*)

Musculocutaneous flap, immediate and heroic substitute for the method of delay (Orticochea), PRS, *52:*105, 1973. Brit. J. Plast.

Composite Flap — Cont.

Surg., *25:*106, 1972

Composite flaps containing bone for major repairs in the head and neck (Conley), PRS, *49:*522, 1972

Pedicle flaps, bone-muscle-skin, in surgery of head and neck (Conley). Trans. Am. Acad. Ophthalmol. Otolaryngol., *76:*936, 1972

Flaps, composite, investigation of bone changes in after transfer to the head and neck region (Conley *et al)*, PRS, *51:*658, 1973. Discussion by Jurkiewicz, PRS, *52:*79, 1973

Island rib flap, composite, mandibular reconstruction (Ketchum, Masters, Robinson), PRS, *53:*471, 1974

Flaps, fascio-muscle, to repair defects in leg (Robbins), PRS, *57:*460, 1976

Composite Graft

Theory and practice of free composite graft (Soeda). Jap. J. Plast. Reconstr. Surg., *14:*97, 1971 (Japanese)

Composite grafts, eye socket reconstruction with (Orticochea), PRS, *48:*343, 1971

Use of free transplantation of previously cooled auricles of the external ear and local plastic surgery to replace defects in the nasal dorsum, apex, alae and septum (Balon). Vestn. Khir., *106:*63, 1971 (Russian)

Labial composite graft, problems of (Bando, Fukuda, Soeda), PRS, *52:*461, 1973. Jap. J. Plast. Reconstr. Surg., *15:*420, 1972

Ear skin-cartilage plastic surgery for eyelid margin tumors (Hanselmayer *et al).* Ophthalmologica, *165:*464, 1972 (German)

Head and neck region, survey of use of composite grafts in (Walter). Otolaryngol. Clin. North Am., *5:*571, 1972

Composite grafts of skin and fat (Rees) (Follow-Up Clinic), PRS, *49:*84, 1972

Composite grafts, ear reconstruction by (Rubin) (Follow-Up Clinic), PRS, *49:*454, 1972

Composite lip grafts, free (Walker, Sawhney), PRS, *50:*142, 1972

Composite graft, immediate, to loss of nasal ala from dog bite (Wynn), PRS, *50:*188, 1972

Grafts, auricular, to reconstruct lower portion of nasal pyramid (Dufourmentel, Le Pesteur), PRS, *54:*499, 1974. Ann. chir. plast., *18:*199, 1973

Composite grafts of skin and fat (Sweeney), PRS, *54:*700, 1974. Brit. J. Plast. Surg., *26:*72, 1973

Ideal donor site for the auricular composite graft (Argamaso). Brit. J. Plast. Surg., *28:*219, 1975

COMPTE, J., AND LISBONNE, M.: Submucosal septal resection followed by immediate reconstruction by bone grafting, PRS, *54*:618, 1974. Ann. chir. plast., *19*:55, 1974

COMTE, J. *et al*: Submucous resection of nasal septum and immediate reconstruction by bone graft. Ann. chir. plast., *19*:55, 1974 (French)

COMTET, J. J. *et al*: Short palmar muscle with a double insertion, including a fasciculus on the 5th metacarpal acting as an adductor. Lyon Med., *225*:1161, 1971 (French)

COMTET, J. J. *et al*: Value of an enzyme inhibitor in cicatrization (animal experimentation; application to hand surgery). Ann. chir. plast., *17*:145, 1972 (French)

COMTET, J. J. *et al*: Comparative study of two series of preserved nerve grafts in dogs, PRS, *52*:98, 1973. Lyon chir., *68*:352, 1972

CONDON, ROBERT E., AND NYHUS, LLOYD M.: *Manual of Surgical Therapeutics*, Second Edition. Little, Brown & Co., Boston, 1972. PRS, *52*:82, 1973

CONE, J., AND HUESTON, J. T.: Psychological aspects of hand injury, PRS, *54*:236, 1974. M.J. Australia, *1*:104, 1974

Congenital Defects and Deformities (See also *Anatomical Area*)

Defects, extensive, of face, closing of (Anderl), PRS, *53*:104, 1974. Chir. Plast., *1*:53, 1971

Nasopharynx, anterior, congenital absence of nose and; report of two cases (Gifford, Swanson, MacCollum), PRS, *50*:5, 1972

Tail, human (Fara, Smahel), PRS, *54*:512, 1974. Acta chir. plast., *15*:184, 1973

Pectoralis muscle, congenital absence of (Ramirez, Marti), PRS, *53*:604, 1974. An. med. cir., *53*:293, 1973

Congenital anomaly, baby with tail (White, Wexler), PRS, *54*:382, 1974. J. Pediat. Surg., *8*:833, 1973

Congenital defects, major, in newborn infants—pilot study in New Zealand (Buckfield), PRS, *54*:118, 1974. New Zealand M.J., *78*:196, 1973

Moebius syndrome associated with mother taking thalidomide during gestation (Elsahy), PRS, *51*:93, 1973

Hemifacial microsomia, corrective treatment of skeletal asymmetry in (Converse *et al*), PRS, *52*:221, 1973

Congenital constriction band of thigh (Owen-Smith), PRS, *54*:503, 1974. Australian & New Zealand J. Surg., *44*:57, 1974

Congenital band, ischiopedic bilateral (Boucher), PRS, *55*:119, 1975. Bol. Soc. cir. Plast. Reconstr. Cordoba, *5*:21, 1974

Congenital Defects and Deformities—Cont.

Constriction, ring, of extremities (Vrebos), PRS, *56*:602, 1975. Brux. Med., *54*:693, 1974

Teratology in anesthesia (Smith), PRS, *55*:639, 1975. Clin. Obst. Gynec., *17*:145, 1974

Limb amputee, congenital lower, conservative management of (Varma *et al*), PRS, *55*:249, 1975. Indian J. Surg., *36*:193, 1974

Congenital annular bands (pseudoainhum) associated with other congenital abnormalities (Izumi, Arnold), PRS, *55*:519, 1975. J.A.M.A., *229*:1208, 1974

Otomandibular deformity: pathogenesis as guide to reconstruction (Poswillo), PRS, *55*:378, 1975. J. Maxillo-facial Surg., *2*:64, 1974

Hanhart's syndrome (Wexler, Novark), PRS, *54*:99, 1974

Defects, inborn and developmental, genetic counseling in (Tolarova), PRS, *54*:629, 1974. Rozhl. chir., *53*:151, 1974

Congenital anomalies (Sousa-Lennox), PRS, *54*:629, 1974. Semana med. Mexico, *79*:243, 1974

Congenital malformations (Ho, Kaufman, McAlister), PRS, *57*:762, 1976. Am. J. Dis. Child., *129*:714, 1975

Congenital curving of long bones (Eliacher *et al*), PRS, *57*:119, 1976. Ann. Pediat., *22*:61, 1975

Teratogenic exposure, syndrome of multiple congenital anomalies associated with (Nora, Nora), PRS, *56*:110, 1975. Arch. Environmental Health, *30*:17, 1975

Polydactyly, surgical management of (Franciosi, Barney, Kramer), PRS, *57*:760, 1976. Foot Surg., *14*:103, 1975

Congenital malformation, adaptation of parents to birth of infant with (Drotar *et al*), PRS, *57*:682, 1976. Pediatrics, *56*:710, 1975

Moebius syndrome, surgical treatment of by platysma and *temporalis* muscle transfers (Edgerton, Tuerk, Fisher), PRS, *55*:305, 1975

Congenital anomalies, correlation with hypospadias (Wehnert), PRS, *56*:466, 1975. Ztschr. Urol., *67*:857, 1975

Syndrome, aglossia-adactylia (Stallard, Saad), PRS, *57*:92, 1976

CONKLIN, W. W.: Transplantation of third molar into edentulous site. Oral Surg., *38*:193, 1974

CONLEY, JOHN: *Face-Lift Operation*. Charles C Thomas, Springfield, Ill., 1968.

CONLEY, J.: Evolution of skin flap technique. J. Laryng. & Otol., *85*:1242, 1971

CONLEY, J.: Use of regional flaps in major head and neck surgery. J. Otolaryngol. Soc. Aust., 3:303, 1972

CONLEY, J.: Use of composite flaps containing bone for major repairs in the head and neck, PRS, 49:522, 1972

CONLEY, J.: Regional composite-swivel flap in surgery. Arch. Klin. Exp. Ohren Nasen Kehlkopfheilkd., 205:78, 1973 (German)

CONLEY, J.: Regional plastic surgery. Arch. Otolaryng., 101:205, 1975

CONLEY, J.: Regional skin flaps in partial laryngectomy. Laryngoscope, 85:942, 1975

CONLEY, J.: Rare, inexorable, lethal benign mixed tumor of parotid (Letter to the Editor), PRS, 56:205, 1975

CONLEY, J., LATTES, R., AND ORR, W.: Desmoplastic malignant melonoma (rare variant of spindle cell melanoma), PRS, 49:587, 1972. Cancer, 28:914, 1971

CONLEY, J. et al: Squamous cell cancer of buccal mucosa. Review of 90 cases. Arch. Otolaryng., 97:330, 1973

CONLEY, J. et al: Investigation of bone changes in composite flaps after transfer to the head and neck region, 51:658, 1973. Discussion by Jurkiewicz, PRS, 52:79, 1973

CONLEY, J., AND JANECKA, I.: Neurilemmoma of the facial nerve, PRS, 52:55, 1973

CONLEY, J., AND PACK, G.: Melanoma of mucous membranes of head and neck, PRS, 54:699, 1974. Arch. Otolaryng., 99:315, 1974

CONLEY, J., AND DINGMAN, D.: Adenoid cystic carcinoma in the head and neck (cylindroma), PRS, 55:106, 1975. Arch. Otolaryng., 100:81, 1974

CONLEY, J. et al: Schwann cell tumors of facial nerve. Laryngoscope, 84:958, 1974

CONLEY, J. et al: Long-standing facial paralysis rehabilitation. Laryngoscope, 84:2155, 1974

CONLEY, J. et al: Prognosis of malignant tumors of the parotid gland with facial paralysis. Arch. Otolaryng., 101:39, 1975

CONLEY, J. et al: Neurilemmoma of the head and neck. Trans. Am. Acad. Ophthalmol. Otolaryngol., 80:459, 1975

CONLEY, J. J.: Regional bone-muscle-skin pedicle flaps in surgery of head and neck. Trans. Am. Acad. Ophthalmol. Otolaryngol., 76:963, 1972

CONLEY, J. J.: Some reflections on our specialty. Ann. Otol. Rhin. & Laryngol., 84:729, 1975

CONLEY, JOHN, AND DICKINSON, JOHN T.: Plastic and Reconstructive Surgery of the Face and Neck. Grune & Stratton, New York; Georg Thieme Verlag, Stuttgart, 1972. PRS, 53:86, 1974

CONLEY, JOHN J.: Salivary Glands and the Facial Nerve. Grune & Stratton, New York, 1975. PRS, 57:658, 1976

CONN, J. JR. et al: Hand ischemia: hypothenar hammer syndrome. Proc. Inst. Med. Chic., 28:83, 1970

CONN, J. JR. et al: Hypothenar hammer syndrome: posttraumatic digital ischemia. Surgery, 68:1122, 1970

CONNELL, H. C., AND EVANS, J. C.: Mucoepidermoid carcinoma of the salivary gland, PRS, 52:213, 1973. Am. J. Surg., 124:519, 1972

CONNELLY, F. J.: Superior sulcus deformity. Prosthetic correction. Int. Ophthalmol. Clin., 10:799, 1971

CONNELLY, J. R.: Elastin fibers in scar tissue (with Bhangoo, Quinlivan), PRS, 57:308, 1976

CONNOLE, P. W.: Mandibular cancellous bone grafts: discussion of 25 cases. J. Oral Surg., 32:745, 1974

CONOLLY, W. B.: Complications following the early treatment of hand injuries: an analysis of 100 cases. Aust. N. Z. J. Surg., 42:145, 1972

CONOLLY, W. B., AND GOULSTON, E.: Surgical amputation through digit, PRS, 52:595, 1973. Proc. Roy. Australasian Coll. Surgeons, 46:241, 1973

CONOLLY, W. B.: Spontaneous healing and wound contraction of soft tissue wounds of hand, PRS, 54:690, 1974. Hand, 6:26, 1974

CONOLLY, W. B.: Spontaneous healing of hand wounds. Aust. N. Z. J. Surg., 44:393, 1975

CONOLLY, W. B., AND BERRY, F. R.: Selective peripheral nerve blocks for reconstructive hand surgery, PRS, 55:109, 1975. M.J. Australia, 2:94, 1974

CONNOR, J. N.: Prosthodontist and continuing treatment for maxillofacial patients, case report. Aust. Dent. J., 18:281, 1973

CONRAD, F. G.: Treatment of malignant melanoma: wide excision alone versus lymphadenectomy, PRS, 50:636, 1972. Arch. Surg., 104:587, 1972

CONRAD, F. G.: Cures achieved in patients with metastatic malignant melanoma of the skin. Cancer, 30:144, 1972

CONRAD, F. G.: Surgical treatment of Stage I melanoma. Arch. Surg., 106:740, 1973

CONROY, W. C.: Salvage of an amputated ear (Letter to the Editor), PRS, 49:564, 1972

CONROY, W. C.: Septoplasty with pin fixation, PRS, 54:683, 1974

CONSIGLIO, V.: Reminiscence of a pioneer of plastic surgery: Gustavo Sanvenero-Rosselli. Minerva Med., 65:4380, 1974 (Italian)

CONSTABLE, J. D.: Crossed alar wing procedure for correction of late deformity in the unilateral cleft lip nose (with Whitlow), PRS,

*52:*38, 1973

CONSTABLE, J. D.: Interfascicular nerve grafting: early experiences at Massachusetts General Hospital (with Finseth, Cannon), PRS, *56:*492, 1975

CONSTABLE, J. D., SCAPICCHIO, A. P., AND OPITZ, B.: Studies of the effects of diapulse treatment of various aspects of wound healing in experimental animals, PRS, *48:*610, 1971. J. Surg. Res., *11:*254, 1971

CONSTANT, E., GREEN, R. L., AND WAGNER, D. K.: Salmonella osteomyelitis of both hands and hand-foot syndrome, PRS, *48:*300, 1971. Arch. Surg., *102:*148, 1971

CONSTANT, E., AND DAVIS, D. G.: The premalignant nature of the sebaceous nevus of Jadassohn, PRS, *50:*257, 1972

CONSTANT, E., DAVIS, D. G., AND MALDONADO, W. E.: Disseminated cytomegalovirus infection associated with death in a patient with severe facial injuries, PRS, *51:*336, 1973

CONSTANT, E., DAVIS, D. G., AND EDMINSTER, R.: Bronchogenic cyst of suprasternal area, PRS, *52:*88, 1973

CONSTANT, E., HAREBOTTLE, N. H., AND DAVIS, D. G.: Synovial chondromatosis of the hand, PRS, *54:*353, 1974

CONSTANTINIDES, G. *et al*: Primary orbital nevocarcinoma. Bull. Soc. Ophthalmol. Fr., *74:*517, 1974 (French)

Contractures: See *Burns, Contractures*

Contractures, Dupuytren's

New approach to the excision of Dupuytren contractures in the hand (Verstreken). Acta Orthop. Belg., *37:*290, 1971

Three cases of fibromatosis (Lampe). Nord. Med., *85:*291, 1971 (Danish)

Dupuytren's contracture, etiological role of trauma (Zachariae), PRS, *49:*583, 1972. Scand. J. Plast. Reconstr. Surg., *5:*116, 1971

Fibromatosis, plantar (Aviles, Arlen, Miller), PRS, *48:*295, 1971. Surgery, *69:*117, 1971

Dupuytren's contracture (Nigst), PRS, *50:*306, 1972. Ther. Umsch., *28:*818, 1971

Dupuytren's contracture (Fragiadakis), PRS, *50:*94, 1972. Trans. 7th Panhellenic Cong. Surg. Soc., *1:*241, 1971

Maladie de Dupuytren. Ed. by R. Tubiana, J. T. Hueston, *et al.* Second Edition. L'Expansion, Paris, 1972. PRS, *51:*210, 1973

Dupuytren's disease (Quetglas), PRS, *52:*679, 1973. Acta chir. plast., *14:*244, 1972

Dupuytren's contracture, surgical correction by limited fasciectomy (Sakellarides),

Contractures, Dupuytren's—Cont.

PRS, *54:*109, 1974. Acta orthop. belg., *38:*190, 1972

Tumors, soft tissues, differential diagnosis of fibromatosis (Krieg, Puls), PRS, *51:*107, 1973. Bruns' Beitr. klin. Chir., *219:*450, 1972

Dupuytren's contracture, operative treatment of (Rukavina), PRS, *51:*478, 1973. Bruns' Beitr. klin, Chir., *219:*551, 1972

Dupuytren's contracture (Ketchum, Robinson, Masters), PRS, *51:*348, 1973. J. Kansas M. Soc., *73:*108, 1972

Fibromatosis, isolated plantar (Warthan, Rudolph, Gross), PRS, *54:*379, 1974. Arch. Dermat., *108:*823, 1973

Dupuytren's contracture, experience with McCash's "open palm" technique (Salvi), PRS, *54:*376, 1974. Hand, *5:*161, 1973

Dupuytren's disease: contractile fibroblast, its relevance in plastic surgery (Montandon *et al*), PRS, *52:*286, 1973

Dupuytren's Disease. Ed. by J. T. Hueston and R. Tubiana. Grune & Stratton, New York, 1974. PRS, *57:* 740, 1976

Palmar Fascia. By H. B. Stack. Longman, London, 1974

Dupuytren's contracture (Orlando, Smith, Goulian), PRS, *56:*680, 1975. Brit. J. Plast. Surg., *27:*211, 1974

Dupuytren's contracture, lack of complications with open palm technique (Briedis), PRS, *56:*680, 1975. Brit. J. Plast. Surg., *27:*218, 1974

Tumors and tumor-like lesions of the hand (Warda *et al*). Chir. Narzadow. Ruchu Ortop. Pol., *39:*773, 1974 (Polish)

Dupuytren's contracture, patterns of the diseased fascia in fingers. Displacement of the neurovascular bundle (McFarlane), PRS, *54:*31, 1974

Dupuytren's disease, pattern of (Rettig, Oest), PRS, *54:*247, 1974. Ztschr. Orthop., *112:*187, 1974

Multifocal form of fibromatosis palmaris (Tysziewicz *et al*). Chir. Narzadow. Ruchu Ortop. Pol., *40:*89, 1975 (Polish)

Dupuytren's contracture, Doppler ultrasound detection of displaced neurovascular bundles in (Elsahy), PRS, *57:*104, 1976

Contractures, Volkmann's

Volkmann's contracture associated with prolonged external pressure on forearm (Osborne, Dorey, Harvey), PRS, *51:*348, 1973. Arch. Surg., *104:*794, 1972

Volkmann's ischemia, iatrogenic—result of pressure due to transfusion (Maer *et al*), PRS, *51:*231, 1973. Internat. Surg., *57:*415,

Contractures, Volkmann's — Cont.
1972
Ischemic contracture of hand, inpending; early diagnosis and management (Spinner et al), PRS, *50:*341, 1972
Ischemic tissue, cell swelling factor in (Leth), PRS, *53:*501, 1974. Circulation, *48:*455, 1973
Volkmann's ischemia treated by transfibular fasciotomy (Feagin, White), PRS, *53:*110, 1974. Mil. Med., *138:*497, 1973
Treatment of established Volkmann's ischemic contracture of the forearm and hand (Ahstrom). Curr. Pract. Orthop. Surg., *6:*213, 1975
Treatment of established Volkmann's contracture (Tsuge). J. Bone & Joint Surg. (Am.), *57:*925, 1975

Conu, A. *et al*: Malignant melanoma developing in intrauterine life. Rom. Med. Rev., *15:*41, 1971
Converse, John M. (with V. H. Kazanjian): *Surgical Treatment of Facial Injuries.* 3rd Ed. Williams & Wilkins Co., Baltimore, 1974
Converse, J. M.: Nasal cancers. Individuality of treatment. J.A.M.A., *219:*348, 1972
Converse, J. M.: *Orbicularis* advancement flap for the restoration of the angle of the mouth, PRS, *49:*99, 1972
Converse, J. M.: Ilium as a source of bone grafts in children (with Crockford), PRS, *50:*279, 1972
Converse, J. M.: Robert H. Ivy, M.D., D.D.S. A tribute, PRS, *51:*411, 1973
Converse, J. M.: Turnover island flap of *gluteus maximus* muscle for repair of sacral decubitus ulcer (with Stallings, Delgado), PRS, *54:*52, 1974
Converse, J. M.: On "medicalese." A plea for proper English usage (Editorial), PRS, *54:*206, 1974
Converse, J. M.: Cephalometric analysis in diagnosis and treatment planning of craniofacial dysostoses (with Firmin, Coccaro), PRS, *54:*300, 1974
Converse, J. M.: Correction of drooping lateral portion of cleft lip following LeMesurier repair, PRS, *55:*501, 1975
Converse, J. M.: Obituary on Varaztad H. Kazanjian, M.D., PRS, *55:*524, 1975
Converse, J. M.: "Over and out" flap for restoration of corner of mouth, PRS, *56:*575, 1975
Converse, J. M.: Retrospective cephalometric analysis of mandibular bone absorption under silicone rubber chin implants (with Friedland, Coccaro), PRS, *57:*144, 1976
Converse, J. M.: Bridge flap for reconstruction of full-thickness defect of upper lip, PRS,

*57:*442, 1976
Converse, J. M. *et al*: Tripartite osteotomy of the mid-face for orbital expansion and correction of the deformity in craniostenosis. Brit. J. Plast. Surg., *24:*365, 1971
Converse, J. M., and Betson, R. J., Jr.: A 20-year follow-up of a patient with a hemifacial atrophy treated by a buried de-epithelized flap, PRS, *48:*278, 1971
Converse, J. M. *et al*: Reticuloendothelial system function in severe thermal injury, PRS, *50:* 202, 1972. Surg. Forum, *22:* 493, 1971
Converse, J. M., and Fleury, A. F.: Note on frontal encephalocele: case report with a 20-year follow-up, PRS, *49:*343, 1972
Converse, J. M., and Stallings, J. O.: Eradication of large auricular keloids by excision, skin grafting, and intradermal injection of triamcinolone acetonide solution, PRS, *49:*461, 1972
Converse, J. M. *et al:* Infections in plastic surgery. Surg. Clin. North Am., *52:*1459, 1972
Converse, J. M. *et al:* Simianism: surgical orthodontic correction of bimaxillary protrusion. J. Maxillo-facial Surg., *1:*8, 1973
Converse, J. M. *et al:* On hemifacial microsomia, first and second branchial arch syndrome, PRS, *51:*268, 1973
Converse, J. M. *et al:* Corrective treatment of the skeletal asymmetry in hemifacial microsomia, PRS, *52:*221, 1973
Converse, J. M. *et al:* Conjunctival approach in orbital fractures, PRS, *52:*656, 1973
Converse, J. M. *et al:* Craniofacial surgery for ocular hypertelorism and craniofacial stenosis. Trans. Am. Acad. Ophthalmol. Otolaryngol., *77:*1352, 1973
Converse, J. M. *et al:* Craniofacial surgery. Clin. Plast. Surg., *1:*499, 1974
Converse, J. M. *et al:* Hemifacial microsomia (dysostosis otomandibularis). Fortschr. Keifer. Gesichtschir., *18:*53, 1974
Converse, J. M. *et al:* Bilateral facial microsomia. Diagnosis, classification, treatment, PRS, *54:*413, 1974
Converse, J. M. *et al:* Diagnosis and treatment of maxillomandibular dysplasias. Am. J. Orthod., *68:*625, 1975
Converse, J. M. *et al:* Deformities of the midface resulting from malunited orbital and naso-orbital fractures. Clin. Plast. Surg., *2:*107, 1975
Converse, J. M., Wood-Smith, D., and McCarthy, J. G.: Report on a series of 50 craniofacial operations, PRS, *55:* 283, 1975
Converse, J. M., McCarthy, J. G., and Wood-Smith, D.: Orbital hypotelorism. Pathogenesis, associated facio-cerebral

anomalies, surgical correction, PRS, *56:*389, 1975

CONWAY, J. *et al:* Videotaped and real-time color television in rhinoplasty training. Can. J. Otolaryngol., *2:*282, 193.

COOK, C. H. *et al:* Effect of peripheral resistance on carotid blood flow after carotid-subclavian bypass. Arch. Surg., *105:*9, 1972

COOK, H. P.: Teflon implantation in temporomandibular arthroplasty. Oral Surg., *33:*706, 1972

COOK, R. M. *et al:* Mandibular sagittal split osteotomy — a clinical and cephalometric review. Trans. Int. Conf. Oral Surg., *4:*232, 1973

COOKE, B. E. D.: Leukoplakia buccalis, an enigma, PRS, *57:*258, 1976. Proc. Roy. Soc. Med., *68:*337, 1975

COOKE, J. P., AND OLSON, R. M.: Blood flow during 2-Torr exposures at different decompression rates, PRS, *57:*120, 1976. J. Applied Physiol., *38:* 643, 1975.

COOL, J. C. *et al:* Hand prosthesis with adaptive internally powered fingers. Med. Biol. Eng., *9:*33, 1971

COOPER, C. T.: Hansen's disease: a podiatrist's experience. J. Am. Podiatry Assoc., *65:*300, 1975

COOPER,E. H.: Partial myotomy in temporomandibular pain dysfunction: preliminary communication. Brit. J. Oral Surg., *10:*154, 1972

COOPER, J. C. *et al:* Coronoid ostochondroma presenting as a corono-zygomatic ankylosis. A case report. Brit. Dent. J., *137:*99, 1974

COOPER, T. P. *et al:* Hemangioma of the scrotum: a case report review and comparison with varicocele. J. Urol., *112:*623, 1974

COPELAND, E. M. *et al:* Axillary metastases from unknown primary sites. Ann. Surg., *178:*25, 1973

COPELAND, E. M., III *et al:* Use of hyperalimentation in patients with potential sepsis, PRS, *54:*379, 1974. Surg. Gynec. & Obst., *138:* 377, 1974

COPELAND, E. M. *et al:* Intravenous hyperalimentation in patients with head and neck cancer. Cancer, *35:*606, 1975.

COPEMAN, P. W. *et al:* Immunological associations of halo nevus with cutaneous malignant melanoma. Brit. J. Dermatol., *88:* 127, 1973

COPHIGNON, J. *et al:* Extended subfrontal approach to tumors of the orbit. Neurochirurgie, *20:*161, 1974 (French)

COPLEY, J. *et al:* Long-standing facial paralysis rehabilitation. Laryngoscope, *84:*2155, 1974

COPPILINO, S. *et al:* Replantation of an almost totally amputated limb. Minerva Med., *62:*4732, 1971 (Italian)

CORAN, A. G.: Long-term total intravenous feeding of infants using peripheral veins, PRS, *54:*697, 1974. J. Pediat. Surg., *8:*801, 1973

CORBOY, J. M.: Fasanella-Servat operation for ptosis of the upper eyelid (with Souther, Thompson), PRS, *53:*123, 1974

CORDEIRO, A. K. *et al:* Surgical treatment of postmastectomy lymphedema of the upper limb. J. Cardiovasc. Surg. (Torino), Spec. No.: 125, 1973

CORKILL, G., AND HASELDEN, F. G.: Experience in treatment of burns in an underdeveloped country, PRS, *48:*296, 1971. Internat. Surg., *54:*445, 1970

CORNELIUS, C. E.: Bone: site of metastatic basal cell carcinoma, PRS, *50:*635, 1972. Arch. Surg., *104:*848, 1972

CORNET, L. *et al:* Soft tissue of the hand and fingers. J. Chir. (Paris), *108:*143, 1974 (French)

CORONEL, S. *et al:* Hemangiopericytoma of gum. Rev. Stomatol. Chir. Maxillofac., *73:*295, 1972 (German)

CORRAO, F., BEVERAGGI, E. A., AND PIETRAVELLO, A. F.: Clinicosurgical treatment of synergistic necrotizing cellulitis, PRS, *57:*764, 1976. Bol. y trab. soc. argent. cir., *36:*271, 1975

CORREA ITURRASPE, M., AND PANIGATTI, L. P.: Practical substitute for throw-away blades of skin graft knives and dermatomes, PRS, *49:*476, 1972. Bol. y trab. Soc. argent. cir., *32:*238, 1971

CORREIA, P., AND ZANI, R.: Masseter muscle rotation in the treatment of inferior facial paralysis, PRS, *52:*370, 1973

CORREIA, P., AND ZANI R.: Surgical anatomy of the facial nerve as related to ancillary operations in rhytidoplasty, PRS, *52:*549, 1973

CORREIA, P. C., MELEGA, J. M., AND CARVALHO, R. J.: Plastic surgery of protruding ear, PRS, *53:*680, 1974. Ars Curandi, *5:*148, 1972

CORRY, R. J., AND RUSSELL, P. S.: Replantation of severed fingers, PRS, *54:*502, 1974. Ann. Surg., *179:*225, 1974

CORSO, P. F.: Plastic surgery for the unilateral hypoplastic breast. A report of 8 cases, PRS, *50:*134, 1972

CORSO, P. F., AND SCHACHTER, A.: Making a folded denture or intraoral prosthesis for insertion into a small mouth, PRS, *52:*94, 1973

CORSO, P. F., AND ZUNIRI, J. S.: Breast-halving incision for subcutaneous mastectomy, PRS, *56:*1, 1975

CORT, D. F.: Nasal tip replantation, PRS, *52:*194, 1973

CORTES. E. P. *et al:* Amputation and adriamycin in primary osteosarcoma. New England J. Med., *29:*998, 1974

CORTESE, A. F., AND CORNELL, G. N.: Carcinoma of male breast, PRS, *49:*238, 1972. Ann. Surg., *173:*275, 1971

CORTEZ, L. M., AND PANPEY, G. A.: *Mycobacterium marinum* infection of hand, PRS, *52:*322, 1973. J. Bone & Joint Surg., *55A:*363, 1973

CORTINAS, J. L.: Forehead rhytidoplasty and brow lifting (with Viñas, Caviglia), PRS, *57:*445, 1976

CORVERA, J., SOMONTE, R., AND GONZALEZ-ROMERO, A.: Facial pain and some forms of epistaxis, treatment by surgery in pterygomaxillary fossa, PRS, *52:*98, 1973. Tribuna Med. Mexico, *23:*3, 1972

CORWIN, T. R., AND GREER, D. M., JR.: Prognathism in a patient with Hand-Schuller-Christian's disease, PRS, *57:*513, 1976

CORY, C. C. *et al:* Unilateral proptosis in newborn. Brit. J. Ophthalmol., *58:*110, 1974

COSKEY, R. J., AND MEHREGAN, A.: Spindle cell nevi in adults and children, PRS, *53:*611, 1974. Arch. Dermat., *108:*535, 1973

COSMA, D., AND POPESCU, L.: Conservative treatment of cervico-facial suppuration, PRS, *57:*670, 1976. J. Maxillo-facial Surg., *3:*198, 1975

COSMAN, B., AND CRIKELAIR, G. F.: Tissue additions in forked flap columella lengthening, PRS, *48:*395, 1971. Acta chir. plast., *12:*197, 1970

COSMAN, B., AND WOLFF, M.: Acne keloidalis, PRS, *50:*25, 1972

COSMAN, B., AND WOLFF, M.: Correlation of keloid recurrence with completeness of local excision: negative report, PRS, *50:*163, 1972

COSMAN, B., AND CRIKELAIR, G. F.: Mandibular hypoplasia and the late development of glossopharyngeal airway obstruction, PRS, *50:*573, 1972

COSMAN, B., AND KEYSER, J. J.: Eye abnormalities and skeletal deformities in Pierre Robin syndrome, PRS, *56:*109, 1975. Cleft Palate J., *11:*404, 1974

COSMAN, B., AND WOLFF, M.: Bilateral earlobe keloids, PRS, *53:*540, 1974

COSMAN, B., AND FALK, A. S.: Pharyngeal flap augmentation, PRS, *55:*149, 1975

COSMAN, B., HEDDLE, S. B., AND CRIKELAIR, G. F.: Increasing incidence of melanoma, PRS, *57:*50, 1976

Cosmetics

Cosmetics, allergy to, what goes on under make-up (Taub), PRS, *57:*681, 1976. Eye, Ear, Nose & Throat Month., *54:*278, 1975

COSSMAN, D. V. *et al:* Effect of silver lactate and silver sulfadiazine on experimental burn wound sepsis. Surg. Forum, *22:*495, 1971

COSSU, G. *et al:* Treatment of severe lymphedema of the extremities by venous-lymphatic anastomosis. Atti. Accad. Med. Lomb., *27:*55, 1972 (Italian)

COSTA, E. A. *et al:* Contribution to technique of maxilla osteotomy in maxillary protrusions, PRS, *54:*688, 1974. Rev. brasil cir., *63:*307, 1973

COSTANZA, M. E. *et al:* Therapy of malignant melanoma with imidazole carboxamide and bis-chloroethyl nitrosourea. Cancer, *30:*1457, 1972

COSTELLO, L. C., BALKISSOON, B., AND STACEY, R.: Hypocitricemic effect of surgical stress, PRS, *54:*119, 1974. J. Surg. Res., *15:*182, 1973

COSTER, C. W.: Connective tissue activation, PRS, *48:*398, 1971. Arth. & Rheum., *14:*41, 1971

COSTICH, EMMETT R., AND WHITE, RAYMOND P., JR.: *Fundamentals of Oral Surgery.* W. B. Saunders Co., Philadelphia, 1971

COTE, A. C. *et al:* Synthetic implants in otorhinolaryngology. Can. J. Otolaryngol., *2:*263, 1973 (French)

COTTON, L. T., AND ROBERTS, V. C.: Value of blood flow measurement in reconstructive arterial surgery, PRS, *55:*720, 1975. Proc. Roy. Soc. Med., *67:*445, 1974

COTTON, R. T.: Use of rhomboid flap in facial surgery. Can. J. Otolaryngol., *3:*51, 1974

COUDERC, J. L. *et al:* Early skin graft in the treatment of palpebral burns. Bull. Soc. Ophtalmol. Fr., *74:*1159, 1974 (French)

COUDRY, H. *et al:* Surgical treatment of tongue cancers. J. Fr. Otorhinolaryngol., *22:*869, 1973 (French)

COURAGE, G. R. *et al:* Healing of mylohyoid musculature after vestibuloplasty involving lingual side of mandible ("lowering floor of mouth"). Oral Surg., *34:*581, 1972

Courses, Study (See also *Symposia*)

Course on Rhinoplasty in Buenos Aires, PRS, *48:*204, 1971

Cleft Lip and Palate Course in Mexico, PRS, *48:*412, 1971; *50:*431, 1972; *52:*219, 1973; *55:*129, 1975

Courses in Hand Surgery, PRS, *49:*114, 1972; *51:*114, 1973; *54:*126, 521, 1974; *56:*486, 1975; *57:*273, 1976

International Course on Esthetic Plastic Surgery in Argentina, PRS, *50:*105, 1972; *51:*357, 718, 1973; *54:*124, 125, 1974; *55:*733, 1975

Course on How to Start a Solo Plastic Surgi-

Courses, Study—Cont.

cal Practice, PRS, *50:*545, 1972; *53:*380, 1974

Plastic Surgical Course in Scotland, PRS, *50:*545, 1972; *52:*692, 1973; *55:*128, 1975

Course on Implant Surgery for Joints and Tendons in the Hand, PRS, *54:*384, 1974

Course on Facial Traumatology in Spain, PRS, *54:*385, 1974

Post-Graduate Course in Plastic Surgery, PRS, *54:*385, 1974

Plastic Surgical Course at UCLA, PRS, *55:*395, 1975

Esthetic Surgery Course in Barcelona, PRS, *55:*733, 1975

Course in Surgical Techniques for Cleft Lip and Palate, PRS, *56:*241, 1975

International Workshop on Facial Prosthetics, PRS, *56:*485, 1975

Course on Management of Severe Facial Injuries, PRS, *56:*608, 1975

COURAUD, L. *et al*: Late cataclysmic tracheal hemorrhage following tracheotomy: new surgical success and over-all results of 10 operations. Ann. Chir. Thorac. Cardiovasc., *11:*401, 1972 (French)

COURSEY, D. L.: Staphylococcal endocarditis following septorhinoplasty. Arch. Otolaryng., *99:*454, 1974

COURTISS, E. H.: On the use of razor blade fragments as scalpels (Letter to the Editor), PRS, *50:*608, 1972

COURTISS, E. H.: Nasal tip correction in rhinoplasty (with Webster, White), PRS, *51:*384, 1973

COURTISS, E. H., WEBSTER, R. C., AND WHITE, M. F.: Use of double W-plasty in upper blepharoplasty, PRS, *53:*25, 1974

COURTISS, E. H., WEBSTER, R. C., AND WHITE, M. F.: Selection of alternatives in augmentation mammaplasty, PRS, *54:*552, 1974

COUSINS, M., AND MAZZE, R.: Methoxyflurane nephrotoxicity, PRS, *53:*375, 1974. J.A.M.A., *225:*1611, 1973

COVE, P.: Unusual presentation of rhabdomyosarcoma: a case report. Brit. J. Oral Surg., *12:*240, 1974

COWAN, D. L.: Laryngeal and tracheal stenosis: an adapted speaking aid tracheostomy tube. J. Laryng. & Otol., *89:*531, 1975

COWAN, R. J., AND CONLEY, M. M.: Surface area of hand and digits, PRS, *52:*679, 1973. Canad. J. Surg., *16:*187, 1973

Cox, C. W. JR.: Technique for conjunctivo-dacryocystorhinostomy. Am. J. Ophth., *72:*931, 1971

Cox, K. R.: Survival with melanoma, PRS, *52:*685, 1973. Proc. Roy. Australasian Coll.

Surg., *46:*630, 1973

Cox, K. R.: Regional cutaneous metastases in melanoma of limb, PRS, *55:*257, 1975. Surg. Gynec. & Obst., *139:*385, 1974

Cox, K. R.: Survival after amputation for recurrent melanoma. Surg. Gynec. & Obst., *139:*720, 1974

Cox, K. R.: Survival after regional perfusion for limb melanoma. Aust. N. Z. J. Surg., *45:*32, 1975

Cox, P. M., JR. *et al*: Respiratory therapy. Pressure measurements in endotracheal cuffs: common error. Chest, *65:*84, 1974

CRABTREE, J. A.: Herpes zoster oticus and facial paralysis. Otolaryngol. Clin. North Am., *7:*369, 1974

CRAFT, P. D. *et al*: Experimental study of healing of fractures of membranous bone, PRS, *53:*321, 1974

CRAIG, G. T.: Split-rib mandibular reconstruction (with Bromberg, Song), PRS, *50:*357, 1972

CRAIG, R. D.: Management of deformities following electric fire burns. Hand, *4:*247, 1972

CRAIG, R. D. *et al*: Correction of facial contour defects by precision-made silastic implants. Brit. J. Plast. Surg., *28:*67, 1975

CRAIG, R. D. P.: Immunotherapy for severe burns in children (Follow-Up Clinic), PRS, *48:*368, 1971

CRAIG, R. P.: Quantitative evaluation of use of oral proteolytic enzymes in treatment of sprained ankles, PRS, *57:*262, 1976. Injury, *6:*313, 1975

CRAIG, T. V., COMSTOCK, G. W., AND GEISER, P. B.: Epidemiologic comparison of breast cancer patients with early and late onset of malignancy and general population controls, PRS, *55:*724, 1975. J. Nat. Cancer Inst., *53:*1577, 1974

CRAMER, L. M.: Treatment of facial paralysis produced by combat wounds (with Morgan), PRS, *53:*647, 1974

CRAMER, LESTER, M., AND CHASE, ROBERT A.: *Symposium on the Hand,* Volume III. C. V. Mosby Co., St. Louis, 1971. PRS, *50:*610, 1972

CRAMER, L. M., AND HINSHAW, J. R.: Autograft rejection induced by homografting (Follow-Up Clinic), PRS, *50:*401, 1972

CRAMER, L. M., AND HINSHAW, J. R.: Further use of tris buffer in treatment of severely burned patients (Follow-Up Clinic), PRS, *50:*401, 1972

CRAMER, M. S.: Primary vaginal reconstruction after pelvic exenteration (with Song, Bromberg), PRS, *51:*509, 1973

CRANIN, A. M. *et al*: Anchor oral endosteal implant. J. Biomed. Mater. Res., *7:*235, 1973

CRANIN, A. N. AND DENNISON, T. A.: Simplified method of fixation after segmental orthodontic surgery. J. Oral Surg., *31:*109, 1973

Craniofacial Injuries (See also *Facial Injuries*)

First aid in jaw and cranio-facial injuries (Mehnert *et al*). Z. Allgemeinmed., *47:*1436, 1971 (German)

Craniofacial injuries due to impalement on an auto gearshift lever (Steckler *et al*). J. Trauma, *12:*161, 1972

Dura mater defects, biological material for bridging (Meskhia *et al*), PRS, *53:*692, 1974. Acta chir. plast., *15:*33, 1973

Brain abscess complicating use of halo traction (Victor, Bresnan, Keller), PRS, *52:*602, 1973. J. Bone & Joint Surg., *55A:*635, 1973

Craniofacial complex, increased antidiuretic hormone production after trauma to (Becker, Daniel), PRS, *53:*690, 1974. J. Trauma, *13:*112, 1973

Temporal bone, giant cell reparative granuloma in (Katz, Hirschi), PRS, *55:*723, 1975. Arch. Otolaryng., *100:*380, 1974

Craniofacial trauma and acute alcoholism: problem of differential diagnosis (Small), PRS, *54:*372, 1974. J. Oral Surg., *32:*275, 1974

Craniofacial mutilating injuries. Therapeutic problems (Arseni *et al*). Rev. Chir. (Chir.), *23:*629, 1974 (Rumanian)

Head injuries, primary surgical management (Fromm, Schaefer), PRS, *57:*396, 1976. Aktuel Chir., *10:*219, 1975

Craniofacial border area, heavy injuries of (Stricker *et al*), PRS, *57:*758, 1976 (French). Ann. chir. plast., *20:*285, 1975

Naso-orbital fracture, xeroradiography examinations in (Maillard, Otto, Clodius), PRS, *55:*664, 1975

Facio-orbito-cranio missile wounds (Dillon *et al*). Surg. Neurol. *4:*515, 1975

Craniofacial Surgery (See also *Acrocephalosyndactylia; Crouzon's Syndrome: Hypertelorism: Hypotelorism*)

Tripartite osteotomy of the mid-face for orbital expansion and correction of the deformity in craniostenosis (Converse *et al*). Brit. J. Plast. Surg., *24:*365, 1971

Challenge and opportunity in craniofacial anomalies (Pruzansky). Cleft Palate J., *8:*239, 1971

One stage surgical and dental-orthopaedic correction of bimaxillary and cranio-facial dysostoses (Hogeman *et al*). Dtsch. Zahn. Mund. Kieferheilkd., *57:*277, 1971

Treatment of facial dysmorphias in craniofacial dysostosis, Crouzon's and Apert's dis-

Craniofacial Surgery—Cont.

eases. Total osteotomy and sagittal displacement of the facial massive. Faciostenosis, sequelae of Le Fort 3 fracture (Tessier). Dtsch. Zahn. Mund. Kieferheilkd., *57:*302, 1971 (French)

Cranio-orbito-facial osteotomies in severe malformations (Stricker *et al*). Minerva Stomatol., *20:*161, 1971

Treatment of facial dysmorphisms in craniofacial dysostosis (DCF). Crouzon and Apert diseases. Total osteotomy of the facial massif. Sagittal displacement of the facial massif (Tessier). Neurochirurgie, *17:*295, 1971 (French)

Craniofacial dysostoses, relationship of craniostenoses to, and to faciostenoses. Study with therapeutic implications (Tessier), PRS, *48:*224, 1971

Apert's and Crouzon's diseases. Definitive plastic surgical treatment of the severe facial deformities of craniofacial dysostosis (Tessier), PRS, *48:*419, 1971

Midface, sliding forward under cranium (Editorial) (McDowell), PRS, *48:*495, 1971

Face, total osteotomy of middle third of, for faciostenosis or for sequelae of Le Fort III fractures (Tessier), PRS, *48:*533, 1971

Surgical advances in the treatment of rare craniofacial anomalies (Edgerton). South. Med. J., *64:*1348, 1971

Craniofacial osteotomy (Kaplan *et al*). Calif. Med., *116:*53, 1972

Changing concepts in the treatment of craniofacial anomalies (Curtin). Cleft Palate J., *9:*269, 1972

Crouzon's disease (craniofacial dysostosis). Modern diagnosis and treatment (Kushner *et al*). J. Neurosurg., *37:*434, 1972

Apertognathia—an interdisciplinary approach: report of case (Hershman *et al*). J. Oral Surg., *30:*743, 1972

Orbitary, orbito-facial, orbito-craniofacial osteotomies (Stricker *et al*). Rev. Otoneuroophtalmol., *44:*441, 1972 (French)

Midface osteotomies for correction of facial deformities (Lewin *et al*). Trans. Am. Acad. Ophthalmol. Otolaryngol., *76:*946, 1972

Craniofacial dysostosis (Romodanov, Liashchenko). Zh. Nevropatol. Psikhiatr., *72:*1487, 1972 (Russian)

Orbital walls, combined craniofacial resection for tumor involving (Wilson, Westbury), PRS, *54:*685, 1974. Brit. J. Plast. Surg., *26:*44, 1973

Le Fort III osteotomy, craniofacial, permitting advancement of the middle third of face (Dufourmentel, Marchac), PRS, *54:*107, 1974. Chirurgie, *99:*755, 1973

Craniofacial Surgery—Cont.

Structural goals in craniofacial surgery (Whitaker *et al*). Cleft Palate J., *12:*23, 1975

Habilitation of severe craniofacial anomalies—the challenge of new surgical procedures: an NIDR workshop (Christiansen *et al*). Cleft Palate J.. *12:*167. 1975

Craniofacial deformities, surgery of (Jane). J. Neurol. Neurosurg. Psychiatry, *38:*409, 1975

Radical one-stage correction of craniofacial anomalies (Epstein *et al*). J. Neurosurg., *42:*522, 1975

Treatment of exophthalmia and retrognathia (van der Meulen *et al*). Ned. tijdschr. geneeskd., *119:*1757, 1975 (Dutch)

Recent progress in plastic surgery, especially on craniofacial surgery (Ohmori). Neurol. Surg. (Tokyo), *3:*277, 1975 (Japanese)

Dysplasia, craniocarpotarsal, syndrome (Burzynski *et al*), PRS, *57:*528, 1976. Oral Surg., *39:*893, 1975

Craniofacial surgery: anesthetic management and intraoperative care of patients undergoing major facial osteotomies (Davies, Munro), PRS, *55:*50, 1975

Cranio-orbito-facial surgery: team approach (Munro), PRS, *55:*170, 1975

Craniofacial anomalies, mobile unit for detection and care of (Ortiz-Monasterio), PRS, *55:*186, 1975

Apert's disease: 50 cranio-facial operations (Converse, Wood-Smith, McCarthy), PRS, *55:*283, 1975

Faciostenosis, xeroradiography examinations in (Maillard, Otto, Clodius), PRS, *55:*664, 1975

Facio-cerebral anomalies, orbital hypotelorism (Converse, McCarthy, Wood-Smith), PRS, *56:*389, 1975

Le Fort III osteotomy to correct dish-face deformity resulting from facial trauma (Lewis *et al*). S. Afr. Med. J., *49:*1915, 1975

Problems of face and neck surgery near the orbital base of the skull (Mennig). Z. Aerztl. Fortbild. (Jena.), *69:*949, 1975 (German)

Late Flavobacterium species meningitis after craniofacial exenteration (Bagely *et al*). Arch. Intern. Med., *136:*229, 1976

Freeman-Sheldon "whistling face" syndrome (Rinsky *et al*). J. Bone & Joint Surg., (Am.), *58:*148, 1976

Flap, posterior pharyngeal, preservation of, during maxillary advancement (Ruberg, Randall, Whitaker). PRS, *57:*335, 1976

Craniofacial reconstruction: ocular management of orbital hypertelorism (Lloyd). Trans. Am. Ophthamol. Soc., *73:*123, 1976

Cranioplasty

Cranial bones, regeneration of, after implantation of preserved homologous bone shavings (Kantorova, Timashkevich), PRS, *50:*206, 1972. Acta chir. plast., *13:*33, 1971

Skull regeneration following deep electrical burn (Worthen). PRS, *48:*1, 1971

Osteotomy of skull and face (Stricker *et al*). Ann. chir. plast., *17:*233, 1972 (French)

Skull defects, repair with autogenous bone (Nickell, Jurkiewicz, Salyer), PRS, *51:*353, 1973. Arch. Surg., *105:*431, 1972

Craniostenosis and cranio-facial dysmorphism. Principles of new method of treatment and its results (Rougerie *et al*). Neurochirurgie, *18:*429, 1972 (French)

Tumors, recurrent, regional cranio-orbital resection with delayed reconstruction (Murray *et al*), PRS, *50:*97, 1972. Surg. Gynec. & Obst., *134:*437, 1972

Cranioplasty, acrylate, prevention of late complications of (Beruchashvili *et al*). Vopr. Neirokhir., *36:*41, 1972 (Russian)

Facial, Oral, and Reconstructive Surgery. By Robert M. Hall. Vol. 3. Springer-Verlag, New York, 1973

Cranioplasties of skull dome (Pastoriza *et al*). Ann. chir. plast., *18:*261, 1973 (French)

Halo traction complicated by brain abscess (Victor, Bresnan, Keller), PRS, *52:*602, 1973. J. Bone & Joint Surg., *55A:*635, 1973

Cranioplasty, silastic (Lehman). Ohio State Med. J., *69:*441, 1973

Skull, and scalp, congenital defect of, due to arteriovenous malformation (Vasconez). PRS, *51:*692, 1973

Bone grafting of skull defects (Korlof, Nylen, Rietz). PRS, *52:*378, 1973

Facial anomaly, hypertelorism, analysis of 20 cases (Psillakis, Pereira, Ishida), PRS, *52:*451, 1973. Rev. bras. clin. terap., *2:*55, 1973

Cranioplasty with roentgenocontrast acrylic plates (Vologodskala *et al*). Vestn. Khir., *110:*118, 1973 (Russian)

Cranial vault soft tissues, plastic surgery of (Bondar *et al*). Vestn. Khir., *111:*94, 1973 (Russian)

Tumors of ethmoid and sphenoid sinuses, problems in (Lapayowker, Ronis), PRS, *56:*677, 1975. Adv. Oto-rhino-laryngol., *21:*19, 1974

Maxillofacial and craniofacial surgery, osteosynthesis using screws and plates in (Souyris *et al*). Ann. chir. plast., *19:*131, 1974 (French)

Cranioplasty, value of: repair of vault of skull (Stricker *et al*), PRS, *56:*103, 1975. Ann. chir. plast., *19:*289, 1974

Cranioplasty—Cont.

Skull defects, titanium cranioplasty for (Gordon, Blair), PRS, *54:*688, 1974. Brit. M. J., *2:*478, 1974

Skull growth, influence of unilateral operations on, with reference to soft tissue only (Duker, Harle), PRS, *54:*618, 1974. J. Maxillo-facial Surg., *2:*44, 1974

Tantalum plate cranioplasty, delayed infection following (Mirabile, Pawl, Hart), PRS, *54:*702, 1974. Mil. Med., *140:*398, 1974

Craniostenosis, results of surgical treatment of 26 cases (Skaropoulos *et al*). Rev. Otoneuroophtalmol., *46:*453, 1974 (French)

Cranioplasty: method of prefabricating alloplastic plates (Maniscalco *et al*). Surg. Neurol., *2:*339, 1974

Skull, exposed, surgical closure of (Widmaier), PRS, *57:*527, 1976. J. Maxillo-facial Surg., *3:*149, 1975

Skull, cloverleaf syndrome, case report (Muller *et al*). J. Neurosurg., *43:*86, 1975

Some elective procedures for cranioplasty (Fontana *et al*). Minerva Chir., *30:*665, 1975 (Italian)

Grafts, split-rib, technique for embedding in cranioplasty (Marchac, Cophignon), PRS, *55:*237, 1975

Cranioplasty, reduction, stabilized by temporary use of a breast prosthesis intracranially (Thomson, Hoffman), PRS, *55:*704, 1975

Gardner's syndrome, extra-abdominal manifestations of (Neale, Pickrell, Quinn), PRS, *56:*92, 1975

Osteo-cranioplasty, method with Silastic (Fontana), PRS, *57:*767, 1976 (Italian). Riv. ital. chir. plast., *7:*539, 1975

CRANLEY, J. J.: Letter: Venous stasis. Surgery, *77:*730, 1975

CRASSELT, C. *et al*: Functional palliative operations in the carpal region. Beitr. Orthop. Traumatol., *20:*399, 1974 (German)

CRAWFORD, B. S., AND VIVAKANANTHAN, C.: Treatment of giant cystic hygroma of neck, PRS, *54:*697, 1974. Brit. J. Plast. Surg., *26:*69, 1973

CRAWFORD, C. L.: Letter: Nerve grafting in leprosy. Lancet, *2:*326, 1975

CRAWFORD, H. H.: Dura replacement, experimental study of derma autografts and preserved dura homografts (Follow-Up Clinic), PRS, *48:*73, 1971

CRAWFORD, J. J. *et al*: Oral and respiratory flora of individuals with normal and repaired palatal clefts. Cleft Palate J., *8:*166, 1971

CRAWFORD, J. S.: Ptosis: is it correctable, and how? Ann. Ophth., *3:*452, 1971

CRAWFORD, J. S.: Repair of blepharoptosis with modification of Fasanella-Servat operation. Can. J. Ophthalmol., *8:*19, 1973

CRAWFORD, J. S.: Ptosis as result of trauma. Can. J. Ophthalmol., *9:*244, 1974

CRAWFORD, J. S.: Recent trends in ptosis surgery, PRS, *57:*529, 1976. Ann. Ophth., *7:*1263, 1975

CREECH, B. J., AND THORNE, F. L.: Pocket photoplethysmograph, an aid in determining the viability of pedicle flaps, PRS, *49:*380, 1972

CREECH, B. J., DeVITO, R. V., AND EADE, G. G.: Viability of split-skin grafts from pigs following incubation on autologous blood or serum for various periods, PRS, *51:*572, 1973

CREELY, J. J., JR., AND PETERSON, H. D.: Carcinoma of the lip, PRS, *55:*106, 1975. South. M. J., *67:*779, 1974

CRENSHAW, C. A. *et al*: Bacteriologic nature and prevention of contamination to intravenous catheters, PRS, *50:*424, 1972. Am. J. Surg., *123:*264, 1972

CRENSHAW, C. A. *et al*: Prevention of infection of scalp vein sites of needle insertion during intravenous therapy, PRS, *51:*354, 1973. Am. J. Surg., *124:*43, 1972

CREPY, C.: Our experience with chemotherapy in the treatment of orofacial cancers. Rev. Stomatol. Chir. Maxillofac., *75:*166, 1974 (French)

CREPY, C. *et al*: Case of parotid angioma. Rev. Stomatol. Chir. Maxillofac., *73:*213, 1972 (French)

CREPY, C. *et al*: Muco-epidermoid cancer of minor vestibular salivary gland. Rev. Stomatol. Chir. Maxillofac., *73:*223, 1972 (French)

CREPY, C. *et al*: Wisdom teeth and inferior alveolar nerve. Tomographic localization. Rev. Stomatol. Chir. Maxillofac., *74:*548, 1973 (French)

CRIKELAIR, G. F.: Problem of somatic delusions in patients seeking cosmetic surgery (with Druss, Symonds), PRS, *48:*246, 1971

CRIKELAIR, G. F.: Excerpts from chairman's address to American Board of Plastic Surgery (Editorial), PRS, *48:*492, 1971

CRIKELAIR, G. F.: Influence of surgical pathology on plastic surgical procedures. Brit. J. Plast. Surg., *25:*329, 1972

CRIKELAIR, G. F.: Burn prevention. J. Trauma, *12:*363, 1972

CRIKELAIR, G. F.: Rhinophyma skin grafts, PRS, *49:*98, 1972

CRIKELAIR, G. F.: Mandibular hypoplasia and the late development of glossopharyngeal airway obstruction (with Cosman), PRS, *50:*573, 1972

CRIKELAIR, G. F.: An accounting to the American Society of Plastic and Reconstructive

Surgeons. Presidential address, PRS, *51:*243, 1973

CRIKELAIR, G. F.: Obituary on Joseph A. Tamerin, M.D., PRS, *56:*480, 1975

CRIKELAIR, G. F.: Increasing incidence of melanoma (with Cosman, Heddle), PRS, *57:*50, 1976

CRIKELAIR, G. F. *et al*: Hourglass maxillary collapse in repaired postalveolar clefts of the palate. Cleft Palate J., *9:*13, 1972

CRIKELAIR, G. F. *et al*: Critical look at the "blowout" fracture, PRS, 49:374, 1972

CRIKELAIR, G. F., AND WOLF, C. E.: Preoperative work-ups and near catastrophes (Letter to the Editor), PRS, *53:*216, 1974

CRILE, G., JR.: Discussion of "Subcutaneous mastectomy for central tumors of the breast with immediate reconstruction" by Freeman, PRS, *51:*445, 1973

Crissey, J. T.: Curettage and electrodesiccation as a method of treatment for epitheliomas of the skin. J. Surg. Oncol., *3:*287, 1971

CRISSEY, M. M. *et al*: Delayed presentation of carotid intimal tear following blunt craniocervical trauma. Surgery, *75:*543, 1974

CRISTIAN, V.: Methods of surgical treatment of post-thrombophlebitic syndrome. Chirurgia (Bucur.), *23:*31, 1974 (Rumanian)

CRISTIAN, V.: Surgical treatment of post-thrombophlebitic syndrome in ulceration stage. Chirurgia (Bucur.), *23:*223, 1974 (Rumanian)

CRITCHLEY, J.: Surgery in China, part I. M. J. Australia, *1:*693, 1975

CROCE, E. J., PUROHIT, R. C., AND JANOVSKI, N. A.: Congenital absence of skin (aplasia cutis congenita), PRS, *53:*376, 1974. Arch. Surg., *106:*732, 1973

CROCENZI, F.: Successful filling of atrophic calf of leg with a dermal-fat graft, PRS, *49:*351, 1972

CROCK, H. V.: Design and applications of a new device for internal fixation of bones, PRS, *56:*606, 1975. M. J. Australia, *1:*510, 1975

CROCKER, M. C.: Psychological findings in the adulthood of 98 cleft lip-palate children (with Clifford, Pope), PRS, *50:*234, 1972

CROCKETT, D. J.: Millard "crane flap" for acute hand injuries. Hand, *2:*156, 1970

CROCKETT, D. J.: Aspects of plastic surgery. Scars. Brit. Med. J., *2:*648, 1974

CROCKETT, D. J.: Rigid fixation of bones of the hand using K wires bonded with acrylic resin. Hand, *6:*106, 1974

CROCKETT, D. J.: Diagnostic coding in a plastic surgery unit. Brit. J. Plast. Surg., *28:*286, 1975

CROCKFORD, D., AND CONVERSE, J. M.: Ilium as a source of bone grafts in children, PRS,

*50:*270, 1972

CROMWELL, T. A., AND ZSIGMOND, E. K.: Hypersensitivity to intravenous morphine sulfate, PRS, *54:*224, 1974

CRONIN, J.: Fibrosarcoma of paranasal air sinuses. J. Laryng. & Otol., *87:*667, 1973

CRONIN, T., AND PENOFF, J.: Pharyngeal surgery: meningitis following accidental rupture of a meningocele, PRS, *52:*100, 1973. Cleft Palate J., *9:*215, 1972

CRONIN, T. D.: Marginal incision for upper blepharoplasty, PRS, *49:*14, 1972

CRONIN, T. D. *et al*: Bilateral clefts of the primary palate. Cleft Palate J., *8:*349, 1971

CROOKS, L. C.: Correcting mandibular prognathism A.O.R.N., *17:*66, 1973

CROS, P. *et al*: Discussion of indications for alveolar segmental osteotomy of the jaws. Rev. Stomatol. Chir. Maxillofac., *75:*107, 1974 (French)

CROSBY, J. F., JR.: History of the American Society for Aesthetic Plastic Surgery, PRS, *56:*506, 1975

CROSS, D. E.: Recent developments in tracheal cuffs. Resuscitation, *2:*77, 1973

CROSS, J.P. *et al*: Should adenotonsillectomy be done in cleft palate patient? Va. Med. Mon., *98:*338, 1971

Cross-Arm Flap

Cross arm flap, value in reconstructive surgery of the hand (Teich-Alasia, Barberis), PRS, *53:*113, 1974. Chir. Plast., *1:*134, 1972

Cross-Finger Flap

Cross finger flaps in hand (Johnson, Iverson), PRS, *49:*663, 1972. J. Bone & Joint Surg., *53:*913, 1971

Graft, radial innervated cross-finger pedicled, for thumb reconstruction (Miura), PRS, *52:*595, 1973. J. Bone & Joint Surg., *55A:*563, 1973

Flap, cross-finger, use for treatment of congenital broad constricting bands of fingers (Artz, Posch), PRS, *52:*645, 1973

Cross-Leg Flap

Thrombophlebitis, cross-leg flaps in patients over fifty years of age (Stark, Kaplan), PRS, *52:*207, 1973. Brit. J. Plast. Surg., *25:*20, 1972

Cross-leg flaps, new fixation device for (Stern), PRS, *50:*194, 1972

Complications of cross-leg flap operation (Dawson). Proc. Roy. Soc. Med., *65:*626, 1972

Covering of post-traumatic loss of cutaneous substance of the leg by cross legs, using a

Cross-Leg Flap — Cont.

defatted flap, according to Colson's technic (Arlon). Bull. Mem. Soc. Chir. Paris, *63*:167, 1973 (French)

Cross-leg flaps in children (Argamaso *et al*), PRS, *51*:662, 1973

Cross-leg flap, alternative: reverse dermal-fat flap (Clodius, Smahel), PRS, *52*:85, 1973

Cross-leg flaps. A review of eleven personal cases (Jamra). Med. Liban., *27*:591, 1974

Cross-leg (arm-leg), new fixation method for open fractures (Nylén) (Follow-Up Clinic), PRS, *54*:604, 1974

Cross-foot flap (Taylor, Hopson), PRS, *55*:677, 1975. Discussion by Cannon, PRS, *56*:83, 1975

Cross-Lip Flap (See also *Cleft Lip, Secondary Deformity*)

Cross lip flap, new method of columella reconstruction using (Onizuka, Tai, Kondo), PRS, *50*:305, 1972. Jap. J. Plast. Reconstr. Surg., *14*:373, 1971

Electromyography in full thickness flaps rotated between upper and lower lips (Hardy) (Follow-Up Clinic), PRS, *48*:72, 1971

Airway, oral, for use around edematous lip adhesions (Rubin, Marshall), PRS, *49*:354, 1972

Estlander flaps, bilateral, total reconstruction of a lower lip with (Murray), PRS, *49*:658, 1972

Flap, cross-lip, unusual, for hemifacial atrophy (Fischl). New York J. Med., *73*:313, 1973

Flap, lip, procedures by Stein (Petersen), PRS, *54*:499, 1974. Scand. J. Plast. Reconstr. Surg., *7*:82, 1973

Abbe flap, indications for and results of (Momma, Koberg, Mai), PRS, *56*:352, 1975. Scand. J. Plast. Reconstr. Surg., *8*:142, 1974

Cross-Thigh Flap

Cross thigh flap, bilateral (Kojima, Ichinose, Onitsuka), PRS, *51*:609, 1973. Operation, Japan, *26*:1065, 1972

CROUSE, G. S., CAMPO, R. D., AND KODSI, M. S.: Incorporation and tolerance of Dacron felt in the bones of rabbits, PRS, *54*:471, 1974

Crouzon's Syndrome (See also *Craniofacial Surgery*)

Craniostenoses, relationship of, to craniofacial dysostoses and to faciostenoses. Study with therapeutic implications (Tessier),

Crouzon's Syndrome — Cont.

PRS, *48*:224, 1971

Crouzon's and Apert's diseases, definitive plastic surgical treatment of the severe facial deformities of craniofacial dysostosis (Tessier), PRS, *48*:419, 1971

Syndromes, Apert's and Crouzon's, palatal anomalies in (Peterson, Pruzansky), PRS, *56*:109, 1975. Cleft Palate J., *11*:394, 1974

Syndrome, Crouzon, craniofacial hereditary (Pilger). Int. J. Orthod., *12*:25, 1974

Crouzon's disease, advancement of middle third of face without bone grafting (Popescu), PRS, *55*:716, 1975. J. Maxillo-facial Surg., *2*:219, 1974

Crouzon's disease: cephalometric analysis in diagnosis and treatment planning of craniofacial dysostoses (Firmin, Coccaro, Converse), PRS, *54*:300, 1974

Osteotomies, craniofacial, feasibility in infants and young children (Edgerton *et al*), PRS, *56*:464, 1975. Scand. J. Plast. Reconstr. Surg., *8*:164,1974

Syndromes, Crouzon's and Apert's, craniofacial surgery (Ortiz-Monasterio *et al*), PRS, *57*:116, 1976. Bol. Med. Hosp. Infant., *32*:587, 1975

Osteotomies, major facial, anesthetic management and intraoperative care of patients undergoing (Davies, Munro), PRS, *55*:50, 1975

Orbito-cranio-facial surgery: team approach (Munro), PRS, *55*:170, 1975

Mobile unit for detection and care of craniofacial anomalies (Ortiz-Monasterio), PRS, *55*:186, 1975

Crouzon's disease: 50 craniofacial operations (Converse, Wood-Smith, McCarthy), PRS, *55*:283, 1975

Syndrome, Crouzon's total osteotomy of face in treatment of (Anon). Rev. Clin. Esp., *137*:77, 1975 (Spanish)

CROW, M. L.: Squamous carcinoma in a split-skin graft lining the vagina (Letter to the Editor), PRS, *52*:293, 1973

CROWELL, N. T. *et al*: Pseudo mandibular prognathism corrected by total maxillary osteotomy. J. Oral Surg., *31*:18, 1973

CROWSON, W. N.: Fatal necrotizing fasciitis developing after tooth extraction, PRS, *53*:602, 1974. Am. Surgeon, *39*:525, 1973

CRUESS, RICHARD L., AND MITCHELL, NELSON: *Surgery of Rheumatoid Arthritis.* J. B. Lippincott Co., Philadelphia, 1971

CRUESS, R. L., AND DUMONT, J.: Fracture healing, PRS, *57*:764, 1976. Canad. J. Surg., *18*:403, 1975

CRUICKSHANK, G. W. *et al*: Total maxillary

osteotomy and retropositioning of the maxilla: report of case. J. Oral Surg., *30:*586, 1972

CRUTCHER, W. A., AND MOSCHELLA, S. L.: Surgical management of axillary hyperhidrosis, PRS, *55:*248, 1975. Cutis, *14:*367, 1974

CRUZ, A. B., JR., *et al*: Triple drug intra-arterial infusion combined with X-ray therapy and surgery for head and neck cancer. Am. J. Surg., *128:*573, 1974

CRUZ, A. D., AND CHANDLER, J. R.: Management of penetrating wound of neck, PRS, *54:*107, 1974. Surg. Gynec. & Obst., *137:*458, 1973

Cryotherapy

Cancer, requisites for successful cryogenic surgery of (Neel, Ketcham, Hammond), PRS, *48:*398, 1971. Arch. Surg., *102:*45, 1971

Cryo-bistoury and electric bistoury in plastic surgery (Dogo). Cancro, *24:*337, 1971 (Italian)

Cryosurgery, critical look at (Gill, Long), PRS, *50:*100, 1972. Internat. Surg., *56:*344, 1971

Cryosurgical therapy of benign lesions of the skin and mucous membranes (Hansen), PRS, *50:*424, 1972. Internat. Surg., *56:*403, 1971

Cryotherapy and corticosteroids in the treatment of rattlesnake bite (Clark), PRS, *48:*95, 1971. Mil. Med., *136:*42, 1971

Cryosurgery. 2. Advantages and disadvantages of various forms of cryosurgery (Dieterich *et al*). Z. Aerztl. Fortbuild. (Jena), *65:*948, 1971 (German)

Cryotherapy of intraoral leukoplakia (Sako, Marchetta, Hayes), PRS, *52:*102, 1973. Am. J. Surg., *124:*482, 1972

Cryosurgery, head and neck, curative, palliative, and adjunctive uses (DeSanto). Laryngoscope, *82:*1282, 1972

Cryosurgery in treatment of hemangiomas (Jarzab). Polski tygodnik lek., *27:*2025, 1972 (Polish)

Cryogenic surgery of the head and neck (Hoki). Saishin Igaku, *27:*691, 1972 (Japanese)

Cryotherapy, use in management of intraoral hemangiomas (Huang *et al*), PRS, *51:*707, 1973. South. M. J., *65:*1123, 1972

Cryosurgery in dermatologic office practice, with special reference to basal cell carcinoma (Spiller). Tex. Med., *68:*84, 1972

Review of Cryosurgery of Tumors of the Skin and Oral Cavity. By Setrag A. Zacarian. Charles C Thomas, Springfield, Ill., 1973. PRS, *55:*486, 1975

Cryosurgery of inoperable malignant tumors

Cryotherapy—Cont.

(Largiader), PRS, *53:*371, 1974. Bull. Soc. Internat. Chir., *32:*466, 1973

Cryosurgery (Budhraja *et al*). Indian J. Med. Sci., *27:*343, 1973

Cryosurgery in basal cell carcinomas (Allende), PRS, *57:*264, 1976. Med. Cut., *1:*55, 1973

Cryosurgical device with adjustable cooling capacity (Zubashich *et al*). Med. Tekh., *3:*44, 1973 (Russian)

Freezing, autografts, canine small intestinal, preservation of structure and function in, after (LaRossa *et al*), PRS, *52:*174, 1973

Cryosurgical treatment of rhinophyma (Nolan), PRS, *52:*437, 1973

Cryosurgery in treatment of skin neoplasms (Adamus). Pol. Tyg. Lek., *28:*440, 1973

Cryosurgery in treatment of intraoral hemangiomas (Kayhan *et al*). Rev. Laryngol. Otol. Rhinol. (Bord.), *94:*245, 1973

Cryosurgery: complications in head and neck (Strome). Trans. Am. Acad. Ophthalmol. Otolaryngol., *77:*1327, 1973

Cryotherapy, local, in treatment of benign and malignant tumors of otorhinolaryngeal organs (Potapov *et al*). Vestn. Otorinolaringol., *35:*8, 1973 (Russian)

Otorhinolaryngology, cryotherapy in (D'Hont). Acta Otorhinolaryngol. Belg., *28:*274, 1974 (French)

Cryosurgery for head and neck cancer (Weaver, Smith), PRS, *57:*540, 1976. Am. J. Surg., *128:*466, 1974

Oral cavity, cryosurgery of, in rhesus monkeys, tissue response to (Natiella *et al*). Arch. Pathol., *98:*183, 1974

Cryosurgical device with adjustable cold output (Zubashich *et al*). Biomed. Eng. (N.Y.), *7:*175, 1974

Management of keratosis and carcinoma in situ with cryosurgery (Miller). Can. Otolaryngol., *3:*557, 1974

Heat and cold, therapeutic (Lehmann *et al*), PRS, *56:*475, 1975. Clin. Orthop., *99:*207, 1974

Cryosurgery, clinical application (Ohtsuka *et al*), PRS, *55:*384, 1975. Jap. J. Plast. Reconstr. Surg., *17:*371, 1974

Cryosurgery, effect on peripheral nerves (Beazley, Bagley, Ketcham), PRS, *54:*687, 1974. J. Surg. Res., *16:*231, 1974

Cryosurgical treatment of recurrent head and neck malignacies—a comparative study (Goode *et al*). Laryngoscope, *84:*1950, 1974

Cryosurgery and basal cell epitheliomas. Clinical and histological study (Leigheb *et al*). Minerva Med., *65:*3676, 1974

Cryotherapy — Cont.

Cryotherapy in plastic surgery (Fontana *et al*). Minerva Med., *65:*3677, 1974 (Italian)

Cryosurgery for new growth in oral cavity (Bekke, Snow), PRS, *55:*376, 1975. Nederl. tijdschr. geneesk., *118:*1359, 1974

Oral tumors, cryosurgery in treatment of (Adamus *et al*). Otolaryngol. Pol., *28:*41, 1974 (Polish)

Nose and throat, cryosurgery in benign conditions of (Brain). Proc. Roy. Soc. Med., *67:*72, 1974

Otorhinolaryngology, assessment of cryotherapy in (McKelvie). Proc. Roy. Soc. Med., *67:*78, 1974

Oral mucosa, controlled cryosurgical treatment of, results of comparative animal experimental studies on (Hausamen *et al*.) Z. W. R., *83:*262 1974 (German)

Cryosurgery in tumors of oral cavity and face, basis, technique and indication for (Hausamen), PRS, *56:*470, 1975. J. Maxillo-facial Surg., *3:*41, 1975

Cryosurgical devitalization of bone and its regeneration (Schargus *et al*), PRS, *57:*405, 1976. J. Maxillo-facial Surg., *3:*128, 1975

Cryosurgery of hemangioma, clinical experience (Jarzab), PRS, *57:*539, 1976. J. Maxillo-facial Surg., *3:*146, 1975

Cryosurgery, postoperative sequelae of (Marciani *et al*). J. Oral Surg., *33:*485, 1975

Cryosurgery of bone. An experimental and clinical assessment (Bradley *et al*). Oral Surg., *13:*111, 1975

Cryosurgery for basal cell carcinoma, evaluation of (Vistnes, Harris, Fajardo), PRS, *55:*71, 1975

Cryosurgery for facial skin lesions (Leopard). Proc. Roy. Soc. Med., *68:*606, 1975

Cryosurgery of the oral mucous membranes (Poswillo). Proc. R. Soc. Med., *68:*608, 1975

Cryosurgical augmentation of tumor immunity, *in vitro* demonstration of (Faraci *et al*), PRS, *56:*599, 1975. Surgery, *77:*433, 1975

Practical Cryosurgery. By H. B. Holden. Year Book Co., Chicago, 1976

Cryptotia: See Ear Deformities, Congenital

CRYSDALE, W. S.: Septorhinoplasty surgery in children. Can. J. Otolaryngol., *2:*211, 1973

CRYSDALE, W. S.: Delayed decannulation — investigation and management. Can. J. Otolaryngol., *3:*156, 1974

CSIBA, A. *et al*: Ultrastructure of fibromatous ameloblastoma. Morphol. Igazsagugyi. Orv. Sz., *13:*183, 1973 (Hungarian)

CSICSKO, J. F. *et al*: Cervicomediastinal hygroma with pulmonary hypoplasia in new-

born. Am. J. Dis. Child., *128:*557, 1974

CUBEY, R. B.: Consideration of aetiology of lip plug carcinoma with special reference to local geographical tumor incidence. Brit. J. Cancer, *30:*95, 1974

CUBEY, R. B.: Lip-plug carcinoma and its management by modified Abbe flap. Brit. J. Plast. Surg., *28:*80, 1975

CUCCIA, C. A. Treatment of cancer of skin. Del. Med. J., *45:*323, 1973

CUCIN, R. L.: Predicting the extent of viability in flaps by measurement of gas tensions, using a gas spectrometer (with Guthrie, Goulian), PRS, *50:*385, 1972

CUENI, L. B., ALLGOWER, M., AND SCHOENENBERGER, G. A.: Isolation and characterization of a toxic substance produced in mouse skin by thermal energy, PRS, *50:*95, 1972. Zurich J. Exp. Med., *156:*110, 1971

CUEVAS-SOSA, A. *et al*: Brachydactyly with absence of middle phalanges and hypoplastic nails. A new hereditary syndrome. J. Bone & Joint Surg. (Br.), *53:*101, 1971

CUKIER, J. *et al*: Disappointing results of reconstruction in the treatment of bladder exstrophy. Ann. Chir. Infant., *12:*382, 1971 (French)

CULLEN, D. J., AND EGER, E. I., II: Cardiovascular effects of carbon dioxide in man, PRS, *55:*727, 1975. Anesthesiology, *41:*345, 1974

CULLEN, S. I.: Topical methenamine therapy for hyperhidrosis, PRS, *57:*543, 1976. Arch. Dermat., *111:*1158, 1975

CULLITON, B. J.: Medical devices: should they be cleared before marketing? PRS, *53:*691, 1974. Science, *182:*565, 1973

CULP, D. A.: Traumatisms of scrotum, PRS, *56:*106, 1975. Tribuna Med., *28:*15, 1975

CULP, O. S.: Treatment of epispadias with and without urinary incontinence. Experience with 46 patients. J. Urol., *109:*120, 1973

CULP, O. S.: Anomalies of male genitalia, PRS, *55:*250, 1975. Hum. Sexuality, *8:*126, 1974

CULVER, J. E. JR. *et al*: Chondrosarcoma of the hand arising from a pre-existent benign solitary enchondroma. Clin. Orthop., *113:*128, 1975

CUMMINGS, C. W.: Incidence of nodal metastases in T_2 supraglottic carcinoma. Arch. Otolaryng., *99:*268, 1974

CUMMINGS, C. W.: Preservation of mandibular arch in floor of mouth carcinoma employing temporary pharyngostome. J. Laryng. & Otol., *88:*329, 1974

CUMMINGS, C. W., AND FIRST, R.: Stress fracture of clavicle after radical neck dissection, PRS, *55:*366, 1975

CUNAT, J. J. *et al*: Changes in mandibular morphology after surgical correction of prognathism: case report. J. Oral Surg., *31*:694, 1973

CUNLIFFE, W. J.: Acne vulgaris. Brit. Med. J., *4*:667, 1973

CUNNINGHAM, C. D. *et al*: Desmoplastic fibroma of the mandible. A case report. Ann. Otol. Rhin. & Laryng., *84*:125, 1975

CUNNINGHAM, D. M.: Deltopectoral flap: anatomical and hemodynamic approach (with Daniel, Taylor), PRS, *55*:276, 1975

CUNNINGHAM, D. M., AND SCHWARZ, G.: Dorsal dislocation of the index metacarpophalangeal joint, PRS, *56*:654, 1975

CUPERMAN, A.: Nerve repair in the hand, PRS, *49*:471, 1972. Rev. Latino Am. cir. plast., *15*:17, 1971

CUPERMAN, D. A.: Flag flap, PRS, *49*:103, 1972. Rev. Latino Am. cir. plast., *14*:17, 1970

CURIONI, C.: Maxillofacial osteotomy in sequelae of labio-maxillary and palatine clefts. Rev. Stomatol. Chir. Maxillofac., *75*:96, 1974 (French)

CURIONI, C.: Multiple osteotomies in a single surgical stage. Rev. Stomatol. Chir. Maxillofac., *75*:116, 1974 (French)

CURIONI, C. *et al*: Maxillofacial osteotomy following unsatisfactory results of surgical correction of cleft palate and lip. Minerva Stomatol., *23*:59, 1974 (Italian)

CURIONI, C. *et al*: Multiple osteotomy at a single stage. Minerva Stomatol., *23*:106, 1974. (Italian)

CURIONI, C. *et al*: New dynamic functional method in surgical treatment of skeletal open-bite. Minerva Stomatol., *23*:175, 1974

Curling's Ulcer

Curling's ulcer, statistical research of (Grisotti, Savoia, Taidelli), PRS, *50*:308, 1972. Acta chir. plast., *13*:83, 1971

Curling's ulcer (Vrabec, Kolar, Drugova), PRS, *50*:541, 1972. Acta chir. plast., *13*:176, 1971

Gastrointestinal complications in burns (Kolar *et al*). Med. Klin., *66*:1617, 1971 (German)

Curling's Ulcer: An Experiment of Nature. By Stacey B. Day *et al*. Charles C Thomas, Springfield, Ill., 1972

Stress ulcers in patients with major burns (Stone). Am. Surg., *38*:107, 1972

Stress ulcers, therapy (Raithel, Mühe, Decker), PRS, *51*:110, 1973. Chirurg., *43*:328, 1972

Children, Curling's ulcer in, 12-year review of 63 cases (Bruck, Pruitt), PRS, *52*:101, 1973. J. Trauma, *12*:490, 1972

Gastrointestinal lesions in experimental burns, effect of elemental diet (Langlois,

Curling's Ulcer—Cont.

Williams, Gurd), PRS, *52*:211, 1973. J. Trauma, *12*:771, 1972

Stress ulcer: preventable disease (Chernov *et al*), PRS, *52*:326, 1973. J. Trauma, *12*:831, 1972

Stress ulcer following burns (Druner *et al*). Med. Welt., *23*:707, 1972 (German)

Stress ulcers produced by bile salts during experimental shock (Hamza, Den Besten), PRS, *50*:100, 1972. Surgery, *71*:161, 1972

Gastric secretion in burned patient (Harrison, Gaisford, Wechsler), PRS, *52*:211, 1973. J. Trauma, *12*:1041, 1973

Digestive complications in patients with severe burns (Ley), PRS, *57*:263, 1976. Acta chir. belg., *74*:277, 1975

Duodenitis and duodenal ulceration after burns, acute (Czaja *et al*), PRS, *57*:122, 1976. J.A.M.A., *232*:621, 1975

CURRAN, J. B. *et al*: Traumatic (hemorrhagic) bone cyst of mandible, report of unusual case. J. Can. Dent. Assoc., *39*:853, 1973

CURRAN, J. B. *et al*: Benign (true) cementoblastoma of mandible. Oral Surg., *35*:168, 1973

CURRERI, P. W. *et al*: Intracellular cation alterations following major trauma: effect of supranormal caloric intake, PRS, *49*:476, 1972. J. Trauma, *11*:390, 1971

CURRERI, P. W. *et al*: Stimulated nitroblue tetrazolium test to assess neutrophil antibacterial function: prediction of wound sepsis in burned patients, PRS, *52*:683, 1973. Surgery, *74*:6, 1973

CURRERI, P. W. *et al*: Inhibition of active sodium transport in erythrocytes from burned patients, PRS, *56*:469, 1975. Surg. Gynec. & Obst., *139*:538, 1974

CURRERI, P. W., WILTERDINK, M. E., AND BAXTER, C. R.: Characterization of elevated fibrin split products following thermal injury, PRS, *56*:233, 1975. Ann. Surg., *181*:157, 1975

CURRERI, P. W., WILTERDINK, M. E., AND BAXTER, C. R.: Coagulation dynamics following thermal injury: effect of heparin and protamine sulfate, PRS, *56*:232, 1975. Ann. Surg., *181*:161, 1975

CURRERI, R. C. *et al*: Complex odontoma of the maxillary sinus: report of case. J. Oral Surg., *33*:45, 1975

CURRIE, G.: Role of circulating antigen as an inhibitor of tumour immunity in man. Brit. J. Cancer., *28*:suppl. 1, 153, 1973

CURRIE, G.: Role of circulating antigen as inhibitor of tumor immunity in man. Brit. J. Cancer, *153*:61, 1973

CURRIE, G. A.: Effect of active immunization with irradiated tumor cells on specific serum inhibitors of cell-mediated immunity in patients with disseminated cancer. Brit. J. Cancer, 28:25, 1973

CURRY, J. T., III et al: Use of malleable metal mesh in open mandibular reductions. Report of 9 cases. Oral Surg., 38:335, 1974

CURTIN, J. W.: Changing concepts in the treatment of craniofacial anomalies. Cleft Palate J., 9:269, 1972

CURTIN, J. W.: Supplementary procedure for improvement of nerve paralysis (Follow-Up Clinic), PRS, 49:84, 1972

CURTIN, J. W.: Basic plastic surgical techniques in repair of facial lacerations. Surg. Clin. North Am., 53:33, 1973

CURTIN, J. W.: Reconstructive surgical procedures in myelodysplasia, PRS, 54:505, 1974. South. M. J., 67:406, 1974

CURTIN, J. W. et al: Pharyngeal flap as a primary and secondary procedure. Cleft Palate J., 10:1, 1973

CURTIS, M. L. et al: Osteosarcoma of jaws: report of case and review of literature. J. Oral Surg., 32:125, 1974

CURTIS, R., AND EVERSMANN, W.: Internal neurolysis as adjunct to treatment of carpal tunnel syndrome, PRS, 53:246, 1974. J. Bone & Joint Surg., 55A:733, 1973

CURTIS, R. M.: Fundamental principles of tendon transfer. Orthop. Clin. North Am., 5:231, 1974

CURTIS, R. M.: Tendon transfers in the patient with spinal cord injury. Orthop. Clin. North Am., 5:415, 1974

CURTIS, R. M.: Reeducation of sensation in hand after nerve injury and repair (with Dellon, Edgerton), PRS, 53:297, 1974

CURTIS, T. A. et al: Forgotton patient in maxillofacial prosthetics. J. Prosthet. Dent., 31:662, 1974

CURUTCHET, H. P. et al: Value of the autogenous dermal graft for carotid artery protection. Surgery, 71:876, 1972

CUSSEN, L. J., AND MAHON, R. A.: Congenital granular-cell myoblastoma, PRS, 56:472, 1975. J. Pediat. Surg., 10:249, 1975

CUSTER, J. et al: Studies in management of contaminated wound. V. Assessment of effectiveness of pHisoHex and Betadine surgical scrub solutions, PRS, 49:587, 1972. Am. J. Surg., 121:572, 1971

CUTRIGHT, D. E. et al: Effect of vancomycin, streptomycin and tetracycline pulsating jet lavage on contaminated wounds, PRS 50:98, 1972. Mil. Med., 136:810, 1971

CUTRIGHT, D. E. et al: Repair of fractures of the orbital floor using biodegradable polylactic

acid. Oral Surg., 33:28, 1972

CUTRIGHT, D. E. et al: Biodegradable tendon gliding device. Hand, 7:228, 1975

CUTTINO, C. L. et al: Immediate management of facial gunshot wounds: report of case. J. Oral Surg., 30:674, 1972

CVEJIC, D.: Surgery of alae nasi. Med. Glas., 25:75, 1971 (Croatian)

CVETNIC, V. et al: Nasal injuries in newborn infants. Lijec. Vjesn., 95:693, 1973 (Croatian)

CWIORO, F.: Surgical treatment of prognathism by means of splitting the mandibular ramus. Czas. Stomatol., 25:833, 1972 (Polish)

Cystic Hygroma (See also *Lymphangioma*)

Cystic lymphangioma in children: report of 32 cases including lesions at rare sites (Singh, Baboo, Pathak), PRS, 48:517, 1971. Surgery, 69:947, 1971

Lymphangioma, cystic, of neck, case (Gignoux et al). J. Fr. Otorhinolaryngol., 21:519, 1972

Cystic hygroma, massive infiltrating, of neck in infancy (Barrand et al). Arch. Dis. Child., 48:523, 1973

Hygroma, giant cystic, of neck, treatment of (Crawford, Vivakananthan), PRS, 54:697, 1974. Brit. J. Plast. Surg., 26:69, 1973

Cystic hygroma, cervicomediastinal, in infancy, one-stage operation for (Mills et al). J. Thorac. Cardiovasc. Surg., 65:608, 1973

Cystic hygroma of neck (Brooks). Laryngoscope, 83:117, 1973

Lymphangioma, cavernous, of neck, limited (Kruk-Zagajewska et al). Otolaryngol. Pol., 27:233, 1973

Cervicomediastinal hygroma with pulmonary hypoplasia in newborn (Csicsko et al). Am. J. Dis. Child., 128:557, 1974

Cystic hygroma colli in adult (Miller et al) (Johns Hopkins Med. J., 134:233, 1974

Lymphangioma, cystic, of neck, case (Martin et al). J. Fr. Otorhinolaryngol., 23:255, 1974 (French)

Hygroma, cystic, in children – report of 126 cases (Ninh, Ninh), PRS, 55:252, 1975. J. Pediat. Surg., 9:191, 1974

Lymphangioma, cervical, case (Kamieniec et al). Otolaryngol. Pol., 28:99, 1974 (Polish)

Cystic hygromas, management of (Chait et al). Surg. Gynec. & Obst., 139:55, 1974

Lymphangioma of tongue associated with cervical cystic hygroma and anterior open bite (Mendex et al), PRS, 57:757, 1976. O Medico, 79:199, 1975

Hygroma, "piecemeal principle" (Weisman), PRS, 57:570, 1976

Cysts and Fistulas (See also *Branchial Cysts, Dermoid Cysts, Jaw Cysts, Lateral Cervical Fistula, Pilonidal Cysts, Sebaceous Cysts, Thyroglossal Cysts and Fistulas)*

Fistulas, post-surgical, new technique for (Medina), PRS, *50:*424, 1972. Rev. Latino Am. cir. plast., *15:*25, 1972

Fistula of low parotid region, problems raised by (originating from first branchial pocket) (Peri *et al*). Ann. chir. plast., *18:*83, 1973 (French)

Cysts and fistulas, medial, surgery of, from cosmetic point of view (Pihrt). Cesk. Otolaryngol., *22:*246, 1973 (Czechoslovakian)

Cyst, bronchogenic, of suprasternal area (Constant, Davis, Edminster), PRS, *52:*88, 1973

Pouch, and sinus, first branchial cleft (Pap), PRS, *52:*583, 1973

Cysts, extravasation, case reports (Barakat). Rev. Dent. Liban., *23:*59, 1973

Cysts, mucinous, and mucinous pseudocysts (Dubin), PRS, *53:*611, 1974. Univ. Mich. M. J., *39:*78, 1973

Sinus, dermal, unusual congenital, of buttock (Rigg, Martyn), PRS, *56:*581, 1975

Cyst, nasolabial (Renard, Morgan), PRS, *57:*240, 1976

Cervical mass, migrating (Futrell, Izant), PRS, *57:*660, 1976

Cysts and Fistulas, Branchial: See *Branchial Cysts*

Cysts and Fistulas, Thyroglossal: See *Thyroglossal Cysts and Fistulas*

Cysts, Dermoid: See *Dermoid Cysts*

Cysts, Implantation: See *Implantation Cysts*

Cysts, Sebaceous: See *Sebaceous Cysts*

CZAJA, A. J. *et al*: Acute duodenitis and duodenal ulceration after burns, PRS, *57:*122, 1976. J.A.M.A., *232:*621, 1975

CZARNECKI, H. *et al*: Usefulness of cyanoacrylic glues in otorhinolaryngology. Otolaryngol. Pol., *28:*141, 1974 (Polish)

CZERWINSKI, F. *et al*: Healing of mandibular defects in guinea pigs treated with preparation Vasculat in light of radiological and biochemical studies. Czas. Stomatol., *27:*287, 1974 (Polish)

CZETI, I: Surgical correction of labium duplex by W-plasty. Forgorv. Sz., *66:*186, 1973 (Hungarian)

D

DABROWSKI, W.: Regional intravenous administration of hydrocortisone in the treatment of the rheumatoid hand. I. Methods. Reumatologia, *13:*301, 1975 (Polish)

DABSKA, M. *et al*: Sarcoma aponeuroticum (sarcoma of the aponeurosis). Pol. Tyg. Lek., *28:*99, 1973 (Polish)

Dacryocystorhinostomy (See also *Lacrimal Apparatus*

Modified technique of external dacryocystorhinostomy (Pico). Am. J. Ophth., *72:*679, 1971

Technique for conjunctivo-dacryocystorhinostomy (Cox). Am. J. Ophth., *72:*931, 1971

Conjunctivorhinostomy, office (Raine). Ann. Ophth., *3:*1097, 1971

Three cases of dacryocystorhinostomy (Takayama *et al*). Otolaryngology (Tokyo), *43:*673, 1971 (Japanese)

Dacryocystorhinostomy, endoscopic observations on internal surface of lacrimal sac following (Tajima, Maruyama, Ikegami). Acta Soc. Ophthalmol. Japan, *76:*1242, 1972 (Japanese)

Dacryocystitis, chronic, polyethylene intubation of nasolacrimal duct in, review of 40 cases with one-year follow-up (Singh, Garg). Brit. J. Ophth., *56:*914, 1972

Canthal region, dacryocystography in midfacial fractures (Stranc, Bunce), PRS, *52:*96, 1973. Brit. J. Plast. Surg., *25:*269, 1972

Dacryocystorhinostomy, modified (Sood *et al*). Indian J. Ophthalmol., *20:*127, 1972

Dacryocystorhinostomy in lacrimal fistula, few observations on (Saxena). Indian J. Ophthalmol., *20:*133, 1972

Dacryocystorhinostomy, severe epistaxis after (Saxena *et al*). Indian J. Ophthalmol., *20:*136, 1972

Dacryocystorhinostomy, external, cosmetic aspect (Sultanov). Oftal. zhur., *27:*302, 1972 (Russian)

Conjunctivodacryocystorhinostomy using silicone rubber lacrimal tubes (Carroll, Beyer). Arch. Ophth., *89:*113, 1973

Dacryocystorhinostomy – our experience with 100 cases (Hosni *et al*). Eye, Ear, Nose, Throat Mon., *52:*251, 1973

Dacryocystorhinostomy, endoscopic observation of lacrimal sac following (Tajima, Ikegami), PRS, *54:*118, 1974. Jap. J. Ophth., *17:*175, 1973

Dacryocystorhinostomy in children by modification of Taumy's method (Barkhash *et*

Dacryocystorhinostomy—Cont.
al). Oftalmol. Zh., *28:*177, 1973 (Russian)

Dacryocystorhinostomy using trephine-cutter and surgical brace (Bakin). Oftalmol. Zh., *28:*552, 1973 (Russian)

Dacryocystorhinostomy, Bonnacolto, modified (Spira, Gerow, Hardy), PRS, *52:*511, 1973

Dacryocystorhinostomy, results of, analysis of causes for failure (Welham *et al*). Trans. Ophth. Soc. U.K., *93:*601, 1973

Conjunctivodacryocystostomy (Chandler *et al*). Am. J. Ophth., *77:*830, 1974

Dacryocystorhinostomy: Kasper operation (Taiara, Sargent, Smith), PRS, *56:*104, 1975. Ann. Ophth., *6:*1333, 1974

Dacryocystorhinostomy, endonasal (Jokinen *et al*). Arch. Otolaryng., *100:*41, 1974

Dacryocystorhinostomy: microsurgical approach (Kursar). J. Am. Osteopath. Assoc., *73:*387, 1974

Dacryocystorhinostomy, Toti's, diaphanoscopy in (Stepanik). Klin. Monatsbl. Augenheilkd., *164:*270, 1974

Dacryocystorhinostomy in children (Brenner). Tex. Med., *70:*71, 1974

Dacrocystorhinostomy (Verdich). Ugeskr. Laeger., *136:*1196, 1974 (Danish)

Conjunctivodacryocystostomy procedure, modifications of (Chandler), PRS, *57:*754, 1975. Am. J. Ophth., *80:*522, 1975

Dacryocystorhinostomy with nasolacrimal duct prosthesis (Thorton *et al*). Ophthalmic Surg., *6:*50, 1975

Dacryocystorhinostomy, external, comparative evaluation of effectiveness of three modifications of (Sultanov). Vestn. Oftalmol., *3:*77, 1975 (Russian)

DADD, M., KOSSOFF, G., AND HUGHES, H.: Ultrasonic display of orbital contents, PRS, *54:*618, 1974. M. J. Australia, *1:*580, 1974

DA FONSECA, G. D.: Experimental study on fractures of mandibular condylar process, PRS, *55:*508, 1975. Internat. J. Oral Surg., *3:*89, 1974

DAFTARY, D. K. *et al*: Presence of Candida in 723 oral leukoplakias among Indian villagers. Scand. J. Dent. Res., *80:*75, 1972

DAGHER, R., SELZER, M. L., AND LAPIDES, J.: Carcinoma of penis and anti-circumcision crusade, PRS, *53:*245, 1974. J. Urol., *110:*79, 1973

DAHL, C. H., BACCARI, M. E., AND ARFAI, P.: A silicone gel inflatable mammary prosthesis, PRS, *53:*234, 1974

DAHL, D. S. *et al*: Comparison between cavernosaphenous and cavernospongiosum shunting in the treatment of idiopathic priapism: a report of 5 operations. J. Urol., *112:*614, 1974

DAHL, ERIK: *Craniofacial Morphology in Congenital Clefts of the Lip and Palate: An X-Ray Cephalometric Study of Young Adult Males.* Institute of Orthodontics, Copenhagen, 1967. PRS, *48:*372, 1971

DAHL, I. *et al*: Fibrosarcoma in early infancy. Pathol. Eur., *8:*193, 1973

DAHL, I. *et al*: Cutaneous and subcutaneous leiomyosarcoma. A clinicopathologic study of 47 patients. Pathol. Eur., *9:*307, 1974

DAHL, M. V. *et al*: Pemphigus-like antibodies in sera of patients with thermal burns, gunshot wounds and skin grafts. Mil. Med., *139:*196, 1974

DAHLIN, D. C., AND SALVADOR, A. H.: Cartilaginous tumors of soft tissues of hand and feet, PRS, *55:*385, 1975. Mayo Clin. Proc., *49:*721, 1974

DAIEFF, C. Y.: Need of mini-cast for nose. Ann. chir. plast., *18:*189, 1973 (French)

DAIEFF, C. Y. *et al*: Eight cases of sagittal osteotomies of the mandibular rami. Rev. Stomatol. Chir. Maxillofac., *75:*145, 1974 (French)

DAIEFF, C. Y. *et al*: Oral resection-reconstruction of the mandible because of fibroma. Rev. Stomatol. Chir. Maxillofac., *75:*859, 1974 (French)

DAIL, W. G., JR., AND EVAN, A. P., JR.: Neural and vascular development in human phallus, PRS, *55:*250, 1975. Invest. Urol., *11:*427, 1974

DALE, W. A.: The swollen leg. Curr. Probl. Surg., *1:*66, 1973

DALSTON, R. M. *et al*: Clinical investigation of the efficacy of primary nasopalatal pharyngoplasty. Cleft Palate J., *12:*177, 1975

DALTON, R. G., AND DAVISON, A. M.: Effects in rats of intravenous injection of rabbit anti-rat lymphocyte globulin on diuresis and blood pressure, PRS, *53:*614, 1974. Europ. Surg. Res., *5:*116, 1973

DALTON, W. E.: Muscle transposition in treatment of severe wounds, PRS, *55:*640, 1975. South. M. J., *67:*1203, 1974

DALY, J. M. *et al*: Postoperative oral and intravenous nutrition, PRS, *55:*645, 1975. Ann. Surg., *180:*709, 1974

DALY, K. M.: "Don't wave good-bye." Am. J. Nurs., *74:*1641, 1974

DALY, T. E., DRANE, J. B., AND MacCOMB, W. S.: Management of problems of teeth and jaw in patients undergoing irradiation, PRS, *52:*213, 1973. Am. J. Surg., *124:*539, 1972

DALY, T. E. *et al*: Management of teeth related to treatment of oral cancer. Proc. Natl. Cancer Conf., *7:*147, 1973

DAME, H., SCHUH, F. D., AND HULL, D. C.: Verrucous carcinoma of buccal mucosa, PRS,

55:517, 1975. South. M. J., 67:1070, 1974

DAMIANI, R. et al: Reconstructive surgical therapy in cicatricial sequelae of burns. Ann. Ital. Chir., 46:352, 1970 (Italian)

DAMIANI, R. et al: Surgical reparative therapy of burns. Ann. Ital. Chir., 46:367, 1970.

DAMIANI, R. et al: Destructive lesions of nose. Minerva Chir., 26:1429, 1971 (Italian)

DAMIANI, R. et al: Surgical repair of ulcer due to venous stasis in lower limbs. Minerva Chir., 26:1471, 1971 (Italian)

DAMIANI, R. et al: Surgical repair and reconstruction of burned surface. Panminerva Med., 14:245, 1972

DANCZAK, S.: Results of treatment of cancer of floor of mouth in Warsaw Oncological Institute. J. Radiol. Electrol. Med. Nucl., 53:470, 1972 (French)

DANCZAK, Z.: Topical treatment of carcinoma of the mouth floor. Nowotwory, 22:139, 1972 (Polish)

DANE, T. E. B. et al: Prospective study of complications after tracheostomy for assisted ventilation. Chest, 67:398, 1975

DANESE, C., CREE, I. C., AND SINGER, A.: Vascular problems in replantation of limbs, PRS, 53:606, 1974. Arch. Surg., 107:715, 1973

DANESE, C. A., AND HAIMOV, M.: Inhibition of experimental arterial thrombosis in dogs with platelet-deaggregating agents, PRS, 49:586, 1972. Surgery, 70:927, 1971

D'ANGELO, M.: Clinical experimentation of DA 2370 (Zepelin) in oral surgery. Minerva Stomatol., 21:270, 1972 (Italian)

D'ANGELO, M. et al: Mucoepidermoid tumors of minor salivary glands. Clinical note. Minerva Stomatol., 23:116, 1974 (Italian)

DANIEL, D. M.: Acutely swollen hand in drug user, PRS, 53:683, 1974. Arch. Surg., 107:548, 1973

DANIEL, G., ENTIN, M. A., AND KAHN, D. S.: Autogenous transplantation in dog of metacarpophalangeal joint with preserved neurovascular bundle, PRS, 49:104, 1972. Canad. J. Surg., 14:253, 1971

DANIEL, H. T.: Maxillary osteotomy—surgical orthodontics. J. Ky. Dent. Assoc., 24:13, 1972

DANIEL, R. K.: Personal communications (Letter to the Editor), PRS, 49:203, 1972

DANIEL, R. K.: Anatomy of several free flap donor sites (with Taylor), PRS, 56:243, 1975

DANIEL, R. K.: Toward an anatomical and hemodynamic classification of skin flaps (Letter to the Editor), PRS, 56:330, 1975

DANIEL, R. K., AND MIDGLEY, R. D.: Facial fractures in snowmobile injuries, PRS, 49:38, 1972

DANIEL, R. K., BECKER, R. M., AND ENTIN, M. A.: Hypothalamic-pituitary derangements as a complication of facial injuries, PRS, 49:548, 1972

DANIEL, R. K. et al: Experimental arterial flaps. Surg. Forum, 23:507, 1972

DANIEL, R. K., AND WILLIAMS, H. B.: Free transfer of skin flaps by microvascular anastomoses, PRS, 52:16, 1973

DANIEL, R. K., AND TAYLOR, G. I.: Distant transfer of an island flap by microvascular anastomoses, PRS, 52:111, 1973

DANIEL, R. K., CUNNINGHAM, D. M., AND TAYLOR, G. I.: Deltopectoral flap: anatomical and hemodynamic approach, PRS, 55:276, 1975

DANIEL, R. K., TERZIS, J., AND SCHWARZ, G.: Neurovascular free flaps: preliminary report, PRS, 56:13, 1975

DANIEL, R. K., TERZIS, J., AND MIDGLEY, R. D.: Restoration of sensation to anesthetic hand by free neurovascular flap from foot, PRS, 57:275, 1976

DANIEL, W. W., AND COOGLER, C. E.: Statistical applications in physical medicine, PRS, 56:604, 1975. Part I: Am. J. Phys. Med., 53:271, 1974; Part II: 54:25, 1975

DANIELE, S., CIANCHETTI, C., AND CAO, A.: Progressive external ophthalmoplegia associated with retinal pigment epitheliopathy, PRS, 57:755, 1976. Am. J. Ophth., 8:585, 1975

DANILEVICIUS, Z.: The beauty, the beast, and the breast. J.A.M.A., 223:683, 1973

DANIELS, J. C. et al: Evaluation of lymphocyte reactivity studies in patients with thermal burns, PRS, 49:107, 1972. J. Trauma, 11:595, 1971

DANIELS, LUCILLE, AND WORTHINGHAM, CATHERINE: Muscle Testing: Techniques of Manual Examination. W. B. Saunders Co., Philadelphia, 1972. PRS, 53:342, 1974

DANIELSON, D. A.: Human skin as elastic membrane, PRS, 53:375, 1974. J. Bio-Mechanics, 6:539, 1973

DANILEWICZ, B.: Remote results of nerve suture performed following traumatic lesions of the peripheral nerves of the lower limbs. Pol. Przegl. Chir., 43:1369, 1971 (Polish)

DANIS, R. K.: Alternative in management of lingual thyroid: excision with implantation, PRS, 54:371, 1974. J. Pediat. Surg., 8:869, 1973

DANN. J. J. III et al: Soft tissue changes associated with total maxillary advancement: a preliminary study. J. Oral Surg., 34:19, 1976

DANON, J. et al: Attempt at objective assessment of cosmetic damage. Application to several cases of facial scars. Ann. chir. plast., 17:155, 1972 (French)

DANOPOULOS, E. D., AND DANOPOULOU, I. E.: Urea treatment of skin malignancies, PRS, 54:508, 1974. Lancet, 1:115, 1974

DANTZIG, P. I.: Immunosuppressive and cyto- toxic drugs in dermatology, PRS, *57:*768, 1976. Arch. Dermat., *110:*393, 1975

DAPUNT, O. *et al*: Operative reduction of the enlarged clitoris. Geburtshilfe Frauen- heilkd., *30:*433, 1970 (German)

DARBY, C. W. *et al*: Letter: Testosterone cream; use or abuse? Lancet, *2:*598, 1974

DARDIK, H., DARDIK, I., AND LAUFMAN, H.: Clinical use of polyglycolic acid polymer as new absorbable synthetic suture, PRS, *49:*477, 1972. Am. J. Surg., *121:*656, 1971

DARDOUR, J. C.: Thermography and hand inju- ries. Ann. chir. plast., *20:*45, 1975 (French)

DARDOUR, J. C. *et al*: A plea for rehabilitation in sensitivity alterations of the hand. Ann. Chir., *29:*999, 1975 (French)

DA REIS, P. D. *et al*: Surgical closure of oroan- tral fistulas. Rev. Bras. Odontol., *30:*134, 1973 (Portuguese)

DARGENT, M. *et al*: Lymph node problem in treatment of cancers of lower lip. Ann. Oto- laryngol. Chir. Cervicofac., *90:*609, 1973 (French)

DAS, S. *et al*: Oncocytoma of tongue in a child. J. Pediat. Surg., *11:*113, 1976

DAS, S. K. *et al*: An anomalous flexor digitorum sublimis to index finger with absent lumbri- cal. Brit. J. Plast. Surg., *28:*299, 1975

DAS GUPTA, T. K.: Current concepts on malig- nant melanoma. Surg. Annu., *2:*183, 1970

DAS GUPTA, T. K.: Management of soft tissue sarcomas. Surg. Gynec. & Obst., *137:*1012, 1973

DA SILVA, N.: Treatment of facial fractures. Rev. Port. Estomatol. Cir. Maxillofac., *14:*99, 1973 (Portuguese)

D'ASSUMPÇÃO, E. A.: Gigantic cleft palate ther- apeutically occluded with a pharyngeal flap, PRS, *48:*395, 1971. J. Brit. M., *19:*43, 1970

D'ASSUMPÇÃO, E. A.: Hypospadias retractor. Brit. J. Plast. Surg., *24:*417, 1971

D'ASSUMPÇÃO, E. A.: *Proboscis lateralis*, PRS, *55:*494, 1975

DASTOOR, H. D.: Severe oculo-orbital injuries, PRS, *56:*460, 1975. Internat. Surg., *60:*217, 1975

DATTA, N. S., AND RHEINSCHILD, G. W.: Doughnut scrotum, PRS, *48:*608, 1971. J. Urol., *105:*692, 1971

DATTA, N. S. *et al*: Transposition of penis and scrotum in two brothers, PRS, *48:*607, 1971. J. Urol., *105:*739, 1971

DATTA, N. S., AND KERN, F. B.: Silicone granu- loma of penis, PRS, *52:*596, 1973. J. Urol., *109:*840, 1973

DAUBB, I.: General anaesthesia for maxillo-fa- cial surgery. Z. Prakt. Anaesth., *8:*304, 1973 (German)

DAUDERIS, I. P.: Remote results of the surgical treatment of the post-thrombophlebitic syn- drome. Khirugiia (Mosk.), *47:*55, 1971 (Rus- sian)

DAUSS, I. *et al*: Problems and experiences of anesthesia in surgery of infants with cleft lips. Dtsch. Zahn. Mund. Kieferheilkd., *62:*252, 1974 (German)

DAUTREY, J. *et al*: Surgical treatment of upper prognathism. Acta Stomatol. Belg., *68:*335, 1971 (French)

DAVER, B. M., AND ANTIA, N. H.: Large Indian forehead rhinoplasty, PRS, *55:*360, 1975

DAVEY, W. W.: Surgery of jaw tumors, PRS, *50:*536, 1972. Trop. Doctor, *1:*170, 1972

DAVID, D. J.: Skin trauma in patients receiving systemic corticosteroid therapy, PRS, *50:*637, 1972. Brit. M. J., *2:*614, 1972

DAVID, D. J.: Exploration of orbital floor through conjunctival approach, PRS, *54:*500, 1974. Australian & New Zealand J. Surg., *44:*25, 1974

DAVID, M. *et al*: Treatment of lymphedema. Thompson's operation. Nouv. Presse Med., *1:*2327, 1972 (French)

DAVID, T. J.: Differential diagnosis of the cleft hand and cleft foot malformations. Hand, *6:*58, 1974

DAVIDOFF, S. M.: Davidoff's craniofacial osteo- synthesis and its indications. Dtsch. Stoma- tol., *21:*589, 1971 (German)

DAVIDSON, C. S.: Cocoanut Grove Disaster (Maxwell Finland). J. Infect. Dis., *125:*Suppl 58, 1972

DAVIDSON, T. J. *et al*: Emotional aspects of new prostheses for previously treated maxillofa- cial patients. J. Prosthet. Dent., *34:*55, 1975

DAVIES, A. S.: Traumatic defects of orbital floor. Brit. J. Oral Surg., *10:*133, 1972

DAVIES, D. *et al*: Preliminary assessment of radical surgery in cleft palate deformities. J. S. Afr. Speech Hear. Assoc., *19:*3, 1972

DAVIES, D., MORRISON, G., AND MILLER, B. H.: Reduplication of mouth and mandible. Brit. J. Plast. Surg., *26:*84, 1973

DAVIES, D. W., AND MUNRO, I. R.: Anesthetic management and intraoperative care of pa- tients undergoing major facial osteotomies, PRS, *55:*50, 1975

DAVIES, P.: Proximal obstruction of inferior canaliculus treated by superior canaliculot- omy. Proc. Roy. Soc. Med., *67:*815, 1974

DAVIES, P. A.: Management of Pierre Robin syndrome. Dev. Med. Child. Neurol., *15:*359, 1973

DAVIES, R. M.: Burn dressing, PRS, *50:*95, 1972. Proc. Roy. Soc. Med., *64:*1289, 1971

DAVIES, W. H. *et al*: Long-term ridge augmen- tation with rib graft, PRS, *57:*259, 1976. J.

Maxillo-facial Surg., *3*:103, 1975

DAVIS, D. G.: Premalignant nature of the sebaceous nevus of Jadassohn (with Constant), PRS, *50*:257, 1972

DAVIS, D. G., AND CONSTANT, E.: Transverse palatal wire for treatment of vertical maxillary fractures, PRS, *48*:191, 1971

DAVIS, E. *et al*: Hemangioma of bone. Arch. Otolaryng., *99*:443, 1974

DAVIS, G. N.: Office surgery and pursuit of excellence (Editorial), PRS, *54*:345, 1974

DAVIS, JOHN STAIGE: Society of Plastic Surgeons of Maryland, PRS, *48*:301, 1971

DAVIS, J. W.: Treatment of hypospadias by the Byars technique (with Nosti), PRS, *52*:128, 1973

DAVIS, L.: Why the declining census in university hospitals? PRS, *52*:689, 1973. Surg. Gynec. & Obst., *136*:785, 1973

DAVIS, N.: Letter: Treatment of primary melanoma by intralesional vaccina before excision. Lancet, *2*:922, 1975

DAVIS, N. C.: Regional lymph nodes in malignant melanoma: is routine excision indicated? Prog. Clin. Cancer, *6*:183, 1975

DAVIS, N. C. *et al*: Elective lymph-node dissection for melanoma. Brit. J. Surg., *58*:820, 1971

DAVIS, N. C. *et al*: Surgery of primary melanoma: problems and practice. M. J. Australia, *2*:778, 1972

DAVIS, N. C., COHEN, J., AND RAO, A.: Incidence of surgical wound infection: prospective study of 20,822 operations, PRS, *53*:371, 1974. Australian & New Zealand J. Surg., *43*:75, 1973

DAVIS, N. C., AND LITTLE, J. H.: Role of frozen section in diagnosis and management of malignant melanoma, PRS, *54*:700, 1974. Brit. J. Surg., *61*:505, 1974

DAVIS, P. K. *et al*: Complications of silastic implants. Experience with 137 consecutive cases. Brit. J. Plast. Surg., *24*:405, 1971

DAVIS, W. B.: Obituary on Edward A. Kitlowski, M.D., PRS, *48*:615, 1971

DAVIS, W. E. *et al*: Use of the Doppler ultrasonic flowmeter for pedicle flaps. Ann. Otol. Rhin. & Laryng., *84*:213, 1975

DAVIS, W. E. *et al*: Unusual case of temporomandibular joint ankylosis, PRS, *57*:758, 1976. Oral Surg., *40*:194, 1975

DAVIS, W. H. *et al*: Transoral rib grafting for mandibular alveolar atrophy – a progress report. Trans. Int. Conf. Oral Surg., *4:* 206, 1973

DAVIS, W. H. *et al*: Long-term ridge augmentation with rib graft. J. Maxillo-facial Surg., *3*:103, 1975

DAVYDOV, S. N., AND ZHVITIASHVLI, O. D.: For-

mation of vagina from peritoneum of Douglas' pouch, PRS, *54*:622, 1974. Acta chir. plast., *16*:35, 1974

DAWSON, R. L.: Interpretation of skin loss and the preliminary treatment. Hand, *2*:134, 1970

DAWSON, R. L.: Complications of cross-leg flap operation. Proc. Roy. Soc. Med., *65*:626, 1972

DAY, C., AND LEAPE, L. L.: Tissue sodium concentration after thermal burns, PRS, *52*:212, 1973. J. Trauma, *12*:1063, 1973

DAY, STACEY B. *et al*: *Curling's Ulcer: An Experiment of Nature.* Charles C Thomas, Springfield, Ill., 1972

DAYAL, V. S. *et al*: Cricopharyngeal myotomy for dysphagia in oculopharyngeal muscular dystrophy. Report of a case. Arch. Otolaryng., *102*:115, 1976

DAYKHES, A. I.: Reconstructive operations for leprous disfigurement of face, PRS, *52*:321, 1973. Acta chir. plast., *14*:101, 1972

DAYTON, G. O., JR.: Surgery of the orbit. Radiol. Clin. North Am., *10*:11, 1972

DE ALBENTIIS. D. *et al*: An original technic for reconstruction of the extensor apparatus. Minerva Chir., *25*:852, 1970 (Italian)

DEAN, R. H., PINKERTON, J. A., AND FOSTER, J. H.: Use of monofilament suture in vascular surgery, PRS, *57*:407, 1976. Surgery, *78*:165, 1975

DE ANTUENO, J.: Modification of Kapetansky technique for repair of whistling deformities of upper lip (with Juri, Juri), PRS, *57*:70, 1976

DE ANTUENO, J.: Reconstruction of sideburn for alopecia after rhytidectomy (with Juri, Juri), PRS, *57*:304, 1976

DEBOWSKA-WOJCIK, D.: Surgical treatment of unilateral upper cleft palate in children using our own method. Pol. Przegl. Chir., *47*:45, 1975 (Polish)

Debridement (See also *Burns, Debridement of*)

Enzymic fasciotomy (Hueston), PRS, *48*:512, 1971. Hand, *3*:38, 1971

Fluid debridement of the burn wound (Gerow *et al*). J. Trauma, *11*:1021, 1971

Enzyme therapy as a method of preparing trophic ulcers and protractedly nonhealing wounds for dermato-autoplasty (Grigorian *et al*). Klin. Khir., *9*:1, 1971 (Russian)

Water jet devices, pulsating, in debridement of combat wounds (Bhaskar *et al*), PRS, *48*:612, 1971. Mil. Med., *136*:264, 1971

Jet lavage, pulsating, effect of vancomycin, streptomycin, and tetracycline on contaminated wounds (Cutright *et al*), PRS, *50*:98, 1972. Mil. Med., *136*:810, 1971

Enzymatic debridement of burns (Levine, Seifter, Levenson), PRS, *49*:665, 1972.

Debridement — Cont.

Surg. Forum, *22:*57, 1971

Water jet lavage, pulsating, effectiveness in treatment of contaminated crush wounds (Gross, Cutright, Bhaskar), PRS, *51:*352, 1973. Am. J. Surg., *124:*373, 1972

Enzymatic debridement of burn eschar, experiments in local burn treatment (Köhnlein, Dietrich), PRS, *52:*212, 1973. Chir. Plast., *1:*207, 1972

Bromelain ointment, effect on necrotic tissue (Anzai), PRS, *52:*457, 1973. Jap. J. Plast. Reconstr. Surg., *15:*456, 1972

Jet lavage, pulsating and antiseptic agents, effect on contaminated wounds (Gross *et al*), PRS, *50:*542, 1972. Mil. Med., *137:*145, 1972

Effect of water lavage on removal of tissue fragments from crush wounds. (Grower *et al*). Oral Surg., *33:*1031, 1972

Enzymatic burn wound debridement *in vitro* and *in vivo*, laboratory evaluation (Silverstein *et al*), PRS, *52:*212, 1973. Surg. Forum, *23:*31, 1972

Water jet in surgical preparation of hands (Gross *et al*), PRS, *53:*114, 1974. Am. J. Surg., *126:*49, 1973

Debriding agent, Sutilains ointment as topical, in burns (Grossman). Internat. Surg., *58:*93, 1973

Enzymatic debridement of facial burns (Yacomotti), PRS, *53:*491, 1974. Prensa med. argent., *60:*1055, 1973

Debridement, enzymatic, of burns (Levine, Seifter, Levenson). Rev. Surg., *30:*72, 1973

Preparing and closing the burn wound (Shuck). Clin. Plast. Surg., *1:*577, 1974

Burns in children (MacMillan). Clin. Plast. Surg., *1:*633, 1974

Outpatient burns (Haynes). Clin. Plast. Surg., *1:*645, 1974

Enzymatic debridement of burn wound sepsis, evaluation (Krizek, Robson, Groskin), PRS, *55:*515, 1975. J. Surg. Res., *17:*219, 1974

Primary wound care in the casualty department (Hugh). M. J. Australia, *2:*631, 1974

Letter: Collagenases: human and bacterial (Kirman). New England J. Med., *29:*1363, 1974

Topical burn wound therapy (Artz *et al*). Surg. Annu., *6:*349, 1974

Electrosurgical excision of full-thickness burn (Lewis, Quinby), PRS, *56:*233, 1975. Arch. Surg., *2:*191, 1975

Wound cleansing by high pressure irrigation (Rodeheaver *et al*), PRS, *57:*402, 1976. Surg. Gynec. & Obst., *141:*357, 1975

DE CAMPORA, E. *et al*: Congenital lateral fistulae of the neck. Clinical and therapeutic aspects. Valsalva, *43:*97, 1967 (Italian)

DE CESARE, W. F. *et al*: High pressure injection injuries to the hand. J. Iowa Med. Soc., *65:*461, 1975

DECHAMPLAIN, R. W.: Mandibular reconstruction. J. Oral Surg., *31:*448, 1973

DECHERD, J. W., LEYDEN, J. J., AND HOLTZAPPLE, P. G.: Facial pyoderma gangrenosum preceding ulcerative colitis, PRS, *55:*645, 1975. Cutis, *14:*208, 1974

DE CHOLNOKY, T.: Reconstruction of the breast following mastectomy (Follow-Up Clinic), PRS, *52:*435, 1973

DE CONINCK, A.: Ten free flap transfers: use of intra-arterial dye injection to outline a flap exactly (with Boeckx, Vanderlinden), PRS, *57:*716, 1976

DE CONINCK, A. *et al*: Therapeutic aspects of mandibular osteoradionecrosis. Acta Stomatol. Belg., *70:*387, 1973 (French)

DE CONINCK, A. *et al*: Nasal keratoacanthoma. Reconstruction by island flap. Acta Otorhinolaryngol. Belg., *28:*193, 1974 (French)

DE CONINCK, A. *et al*: Autologous transplants with vascular microsutures, PRS, *57:*266, 1976. Ann. chir. plast., *20:*163, 1975

DECROIX, G. *et al*: Nerve decompression in traumatic facial paralysis. Lille Med., *17:*1237, 1972

Decubitus Ulcer: See *Pressure Sores*

DEDO, D. D. *et al*: Complications of dermal graft protection of carotid artery. Arch. Otolaryng., *101:*649, 1975

DE DULANTO, F.: Dermatologic plastic surgery. Medico-social aspects. Actas Dermosifiliogr., *63:*369, 1972 (Spanish)

DE DULANTO, F. *et al*: Perialar semilunar excision and malignant tumors of upper lip. Actas Dermosfiliogr., *62:*371, 1971 (Spanish)

DEFFEZ, J. P.: Origin and development of large jaw cysts linked to the dental system. Rev. Stomatol. Chir. Maxillofac., *75:*885, 1974 (French)

DEFFEZ, J. P. *et al*: Surgical treatment of upper incisive protrusions in adolescents. Rev. Stomatol. Chir. Maxillofac., *75:*111, 1974 (French)

DEFFEZ, J. P. *et al*: Complementary orthopedic treatments after surgical treatment of upper incisor protrusion in adolescents. Rev. Stomatol. Chir. Maxillofac., *75:*134, 1974 (French)

DEFINE, D.: Treatment of congenital radial club hand. Clin. Orthop., *73:*153, 1970

DEFRIES, H. O.: Management of maxillofacial

injuries; medical viewpoint, PRS, *49:*580, 1972. Mil. Med., *136:*558, 1971

DeFRIES, H. O.: Reconstruction of tongue. Ann. Otol. Rhin. & Laryng., *83:*471, 1974

DeFRIES, H. O., MARBLE, H. B., AND SELL, K. W.: Reconstruction of mandible, PRS, *49:*102, 1972. Arch. Otolaryng., *93:*4, 1971

DE GANDT, J. B. *et al:* Ameloblastoma of the maxillary sinus. Acta Otorhinolaryngol. Belg., *28:*365, 1974 (French)

DEGEN, I. L.: Modeling and transfer of composite bone autografts in tubed flaps, PRS, *48:*518, 1971. Acta chir. plast., *12:*133, 1970

DE GEUS, J. J.: Burned hand. Nurs. times, *70:*988, 1974

DEGNI, M.: New technique of drainage of subcutaneous tissue of limbs with nylon net for treatment of lymphedema. Vasa, *3:*329, 1974

DEGROOT, J., AND KUNIN, C. M.: Indwelling catheters, PRS, *56:*596, 1975. Am. J. Nursing, *75:*448, 1975

DEGTIAREVA, S. I. *et al:* Mistakes in the treatment of injuries of nerves of the palm and fingers. Ortop. Travmatol. Protez., *34:*24, 1973 (Russian)

DEGTIAREVA, S. I. *et al:* Surgical treatment of deformities of the hand and fingers with the aid of Volkov-Oganesian apparatus. Ortop. Travmatol. Protez, *35:*24, 1974 (Russian)

DeHAAN, B. B., ELLIS, H., AND WILKS, M.: Role of infection in wound healing, PRS, *54:*698, 1974. Surg. Gynec. & Obst., *138:*693, 1974

DEIDIER, C. M.: Vascular pathogenesis of eschars and its surgical treatment. Angeiologie, *23:*135, 1971 (French)

DEIDIER, C. M. *et al:* Bucloxic acid in plastic surgery. Ann. chir. plast., *20:*343, 1975 (French)

DEIGERT, F. A.: Lymphatics, lymphedema and lymphangiosarcoma. Rocky Mt. Med. J., *72:*210, 1975

DEI POLI, G. *et al:* Thermonuclear weapon lesions of surgical interest. Minerva Chir., *28:*558, 1973 (Italian)

DE JACOBY, L. F. *et al:* Clinical results with Edlan and Mejchar's vestibuloplasty. Dtsch. Zahnaerztl. Z., *30:*581, 1975 (German)

DE JONG, R. H., AND HEAVNER, J. E.: Convulsions induced by local anesthetic: time course of diazepam prophylaxis, PRS, *55:*120, 1975. Canad. Anaesth. Soc. J., *21:*153, 1974

DEKKER, J. G. *et al:* Histologic study of free mucosal graft from cheek used in preprosthetic surgery. Int. J. Oral Surg., *2:*284, 1973

DE KLERK, D. J. *et al:* Laboratory training in microsurgical techniques for neurosurgery. S. Afr. Med. J., *46:*1740, 1972

DE KLERK, D. J. *et al:* Frontal encephaloceles. S. Afr. Med. J., *47:*1350, 1973

DEKSTER, B. G. *et al:* Injury of the right common carotid artery. Vestn. Khir., *115:*105, 1975 (Russian)

DE LA CAFFINIERE, J. Y.: Theoretical basis for surgery of proximal pulley in injuries of *flexor longus* tendon of fingers, PRS, *55:*511, 1975. Ann. chir. plast., *19:*201, 1974

DE LA CAFFINIERE, J. Y., MOZAS, F., AND ACHACH, P. C.: Joint destruction in rheumatoid arthritis of hand, PRS, *56:*465, 1975. Rev. chir. orthop., *61:*61, 1975

DE LA CONCHA, E. *et al:* Immunity of hepatitis-B in hemodialysis unit, PRS, *55:*260, 1975. Lancet, *2:*461, 1974

DELACROIX, R. *et al:* Repair of extensive radionecrosis of the thoracic wall using soft tissues from the paralyzed upper limb. Ann. Chir. Thorac. Cardiovasc., *14:*185, 1975 (French)

DeLaCRUZ, A., AND CHANDLER, J. R.: Management of penetrating wounds of neck, PRS, *53:*603, 1974. Surg. Gynec. & Obst., *137:*458, 1973

DE LA FAYE, G.: Observations on cleft lip (Classic Reprint), PRS, *57:*216, 1976

DELAGE, C., SHANE, J. J., AND JOHNSON, F. B.: Mammary silicone granuloma, PRS, *54:*373, 1974. Arch. Dermat., *108:*105, 1973

DELAGI, E. F.: Pure sign of lumbrical function (with Aiache), PRS, *54:*312, 1974

DELAIRE, J.: Surgical treatment of mandibular laterognathies. Orthod. Fr., *41:*269, 1970 (French)

DELAIRE, J.: Reconstruction of the uvula and posterior parts of congenital cleft palates. Ann. chir. plast., *17:*99, 1972 (French)

DELAIRE, J.: New surgical treatment method for temporomandibular ankyloses. Conservation of the meniscus of attempt at reconstruction of an equivalent structure and mobilization in propulsion. Actual Odontostomatol. (Paris), *110:*173, 1975 (French)

DELAIRE, J.: Primary cheilorhinoplasty for congenital unilateral labiomaxillary fissure. Trial schematization of a technique. Rev. Stomatol. Chir. Maxillofac., *76:*193, 1975 (French)

DELAIRE, J. *et al:* Contention in fractures of the zygomatic bone. Rev. Stomatol. Chir. Maxillofac., *72:*623, 1971 (French)

DELAIRE, J. *et al:* Surgical treatment of osteoradionecrosis of jaw. J. Fr. Otorhinolaryngol., *21:*635, 1972 (French)

DELAIRE, J. *et al:* Evolution of techniques in cheiloplasty for cleft-lip (and study of a few complementary measures). Rev. Stomatol.

Chir. Maxillofac., *73:*337, 1972 (French)

DELAIRE, J. *et al*: Two cases of coronoid process osteitis. Exceptional localization of mandibular osteitis. Rev. Stomatol. Chir. Maxillofac., *74:*29, 1973 (French)

DELAIRE, J. *et al*: Intramaxillary position of tooth germs and dental apices in relation to Francfort's plane. Incidences in maxillary osteotomies. Rev. Stomatol. Chir. Maxillofac., *74:*281, 1973 (French)

DELAIRE, J. *et al*: Case of pseudotumoral osteitis of mandibular angle in children. Rev. Stomatol. Chir. Maxillofac., *74:*321, 1973 (French)

DELAIRE, J. *et al*: Functional treatment of fractures of mandibular condyle and its neck. Rev. Stomatol. Chir. Maxillofac., *76:*331, 1975 (French)

DE LA MATA PAGES, R.: Surgical treatment of odontogenic cysts. Rev. Esp. Estomatol., *21:*413, 1973 (Spanish)

DE LA PLAZA, R.: Reconstruction of extensive full-thickness defects of oral walls, following cancer excision, PRS, *57:*530, 1976. Cir. Plast. Ibero-Latino Am., *1:*35, 1975

DE LATHOUWER, C. *et al*: Simple technic for immediate reconstruction of mandibular arch after surgery for cancer exeresis: importance of stainless steel pins. Acta Stomatol. Belg., *70:*315, 1973 (French)

DE LATHOUWER, L. *et al*: Two cases of osteogenic sarcoma of the mandible; indications for immediate reconstruction. Acta Chir. Belg., *73:*49, 1974 (French)

DE LAVAL, J. *et al*: Surgical correction of bladder exstrophy. Acta Urol. Belg., *43:*292, 1975 (French)

DE LEO, A. A. *et al*: Incidence of bacteremia following oral prophylaxis on pediatric patients, PRS, *55:*120, 1975. Oral Surg., *37:*37, 1974

DELERM, A. AND CIROTTEAU, Y.: Cruro-femoro-gluteal or circumgluteal plasty. Ann. chir. plast., *18:*31, 1973 (French)

DELERM, A. *et al*: Cheiloplasty of thin lips: Proposal of a technic. Ann. chir. plast., *20:*243, 1975 (French)

DELGADO, J. P.: Silicone fluid injections for facial atrophy (with Rees, Ashley), PRS, *52:*118, 1973

DELGADO, J. P.: Turnover island flap of *gluteus maximus* muscle for repair of sacral decubitus ulcer (with Stallings, Converse), PRS, *54:*52, 1974

DELGERT, F. A.: Lymphatics, lymphedema and lymphangiosarcoma. Rocky Mt. Med. J., *72:*210, 1975

DEL HOYO, J. A. *et al*: Partial corticotomies and osteotomies. Rev. Stomatol. Chir. Maxillofac., *75:*131, 1974 (French)

DELILKAN, A. E. *et al*: Elective postoperative I.P.P.V. for extensive head and neck skin grafting. Anaesth. Intensive Care, *3:*68, 1975

DELINER, L. P.: Tumors of mandible and maxilla in children, PRS, *54:*235, 1974. Cancer, *32:*112, 1973

DELISLE, M. J. *et al*: Isotopic examination of melanoma with labelled iodoquine. Bull. Soc. Fr. Dermatol. Syphiligr., *79:*163, 1972 (French)

DELIYANNAKIS, E.: Peripheral nerve and root disturbances following active immunization against smallpox and tetanus, PRS, *48:*608, 1971. Mil. Med., *136:*458, 1971

DELLON, A. L.: Squamous carcinoma arising in an artificial vagina (Letter to the Editor), PRS, *53:*584, 1974

DELLON, A. L. *et al*: Evaluating recovery of sensation in the hand following nerve injury. Johns Hopkins Med. J., *130:*235, 1972

DELLON, A. L., AND KETCHAM, A. S.: Surgical treatment of Stage I melanoma, PRS, *53:*370, 1974. Arch. Surg., *106:*738, 1973

DELLON, A. L., CURTIS, R. M., AND EDGERTON, M. T.: Reeducation of sensation in the hand after nerve injury and repair, PRS, *53:*297, 1974

DELLON, A. L., AND HOOPES, J. E.: Evaluation of submucous cleft palate surgery (Letter to the Editor), PRS, *53:*338, 1974. Reply from Dr. Pickrell, PRS, *53:*339, 1974

DELLON, A. L. *et al*: Immunobiology of skin cancer, PRS, *55:*341, 1975

DELLON, A. L., HALL, C. A., AND CHRETIEN, P. B.: Fiberoptic endoscopy in the head and neck region, PRS, *55:*466, 1975

DELLON, A. L., WITEBSKY, F. G., AND TERRILL, R. E.: Denervated Meissner corpuscle, sequential histological study after nerve division in Rhesus monkey, PRS, *56:*182, 1975

DELLON, A. L., EDELSON, R. L., AND CHRETIEN, P. B.: Defining malignant potential of giant pigmented nevus, PRS, *57:*611, 1976

DELMAN, M.: New use of the Bowman probe in dacrycystorhinostomy. Ann. Ophth., *4:*505, 1972

DEL SOLDATO, G.: Technic for surgical approach to upper abdomen by use of esthetic incision. Acta Gastroenterol. Latinoam., *5:*19, 1973 (Spanish)

DELUCA, F. N. *et al*: Median nerve compression complicating tendon graft prosthesis, PRS, *57:*398, 1976. J. Bone & Joint Surg., *57A:*553, 1975

DE MACEDO, N. F., BAROUDI, R., AND TOZZI NETTO, F.: Reconstruction of thumb using amputated phalanges, PRS, *57:*534, 1976. Cir. Plast. Ibero-Latino Am., *1:*97, 1975

DE MACEDO, N., BAROUDI, R., AND TOZZI-NETTO, F.: Reconstruction of thumb, PRS,

*57:*674, 1976. Rev. Iber. Latinoamericana Cir. Plast., *1:*293, 1975

DEMARK, R. V. *et al*: Prediction of velopharyngeal competency. Cleft Palate J., *12:*5, 1975

DEMCHENKO, P. S.: Some characteristics of chemical burns in metallurgists. Klin. Khir., *10:*69, 1971 (Russian)

DEMELLO, F. J. *et al*: Comparative study of experimental Clostridium perfringens infection in dogs treated with antibiotics, surgery, and hyperbaric oxygen. Surgery, *73:*936, 1973

DEMERE, M.: Case against primary repair of seventh nerve (Follow-Up Clinic), PRS, *48:*172, 1971

DeMere, McCarthy: Plastic Surgeon Chairman of New Committee of American Bar Association, PRS, *52:*219, 1973

DeMERE, M.: Views of several prominent attorneys on the preoperative showing of photographs of results in other patients (Letter to the Editor), PRS, *54:*91, 1974

DeMERE, M., WOOD, T., AND AUSTIN, W.: Eye complications with blepharoplasty or other eyelid surgery, PRS, *53:*634, 1974

DEMETRIADES, A. G. *et al*: Management of facial and dental anomalies. Basic principles of orthodontic and plastic reconstruction. Odontostomatol. Proodos., *26:*151, 1972 (Greek)

DEMETRIADES, A. G. *et al*: Surgical and orthodontic management of Class 3 malocclusion. Odontostomatol. Proodos., *26:*183, 1972 (Greek)

DEMIAN, S. D. E., BUSKIN, F. L., and ECHEVARRIA, R. A. : Perineural invasion and anaplastic transformation of verrucous carcinoma, PRS, *54:*245, 1974. Cancer, *32:*395, 1973

DEMIANIUK, D. G.: Treatment of suppurative diseases of the fingers and hand. Klin. Khir., *8:*56, 1972 (Russian)

DEM'IANIUK, D. G.: Microtrauma of the hand and fingers and its complications in the rural economy. Ortop. Travmatol. Protez., *34:*58, 1973 (Russian)

DEMICHEV, N. P. *et al*: Characteristics of treatment of hand and finger tendon injuries in patients of middle and old age. Ortop. Travmatol. Protez., *32:*10, 1971 (Russian)

DEMICHEV, N. P. *et al*: Our position with respect to anesthesia in reconstructive surgery of the wrist. Ortop. Travmatol. Protez., *32:*19, 1971 (Russian)

DEMIDOV, P. A. *et al*: Treatment of resistant forms of vasomotor-allergic rhinitis as preliminary stage to rhinoplasty. Vestn. Otorinolaringol., *34:*56, 1972 (Russian)

DEMJEN, S.: Operative methods of palatoplastics in consideration of the posterior neurovascular bundle. Acta chir. plast. (Praha.), *14:*149, 1972

DE MOULIN, D.: Treatment of facial fractures in Hippocrates' time, PRS, *55:*718, 1975. Arch. chir. neerl., *26:*283, 1974

DEMPSEY, W. C.: Subpectoral implants in augmentation mammaplasty (Follow-Up Clinic), PRS, *52:*300, 1973

DE MURPHY, C. A., AND TOVAR ZAMORA, E.: Utility of techniques with radionuclides in renal transplant, PRS, *56:*357, 1975. Prensa Med. Mex., *39:*247, 1974

DeMUTH, W. E., JR.: Mechanism of shotgun wounds, PRS, *49:*475, 1972. J. Trauma, *11:*219, 1971

DENDY, R. A.: Facial nerve paralysis following sagittal split mandibular osteotomy, case report. Brit. J. Oral. Surg., *11:*101, 1973

DENECKE, H. J.: Infratemporal approach to the orbit and pterygopalatine fossa. Monatsschr. Ohrenheilkd. Laryngorhinol., *105:*150, 1971 (German)

DENECKE, H. J.: Experiences with Italian plastic surgery of nose and face. Laryngol. Rhinol. Otol. (Stuttg.), *53:*248, 1974 (German)

DeNIORD, R. N. *et al*: Pectus excavatum — surgical management. Va. Med. Mon., *99:*614, 1972

Dentigerous Cysts: See *Jaw Cysts*

DE PADUA BERTELLI, A. *et al*: Tumors of parapharyngeal region. II. Neural tumors, chemodectomas, chordomas, branchial cysts. Surgical treatment. Conclusions. Rev. Paul. Med., *82:*103, 1973 (Portuguese)

DePALMA, A. F., AHMAD, I., AND FLANNERY, G.: Treatment of giant cell tumors in bone, PRS, *55:*640, 1975. Clin. Orthop., *100:*76, 1974

DE PALMA, R. G.: Surgical therapy for venous stasis. Surgery, *76:*910, 1974

DePALMA, R. G. *et al*: Structure and function of hepatic mitochondria in hemorrhage and endotoxemia, PRS, *48:*201, 1971. Surg. Forum, *21:*3, 1970

DE PENA PEREZ, R. *et al*: Digitopalmar steal syndrome with peripheral arteriovenous fistula. Med. Welt., *15:*601, 1971 (German)

DEREUME-DE CORTE, M. T.: Use of the pigtail catheter in reconstruction of the lacrimal ducts. Bull. Soc. Belge. Ophtalmol., *159:*590, 1971 (French)

DE REZENDE, J. R.: Universal internal immediate mandibular prosthesis. Rev. Fac. Odontol. Sao Paulo, *10:*57, 1972 (Portuguese)

Dermabrasion

Dermabrasion for nodular cutaneous elastosis with cysts and comedones. Favre-Racouchot syndrome (English *et al*). Arch. Dermat., *104:*92, 1971

Dermal Grafts—Cont.

ulcers (Thompson, Ell), PRS, *54:*290, 1974

Dermis fat graft for correction of eyelid deformity of enophthalmos (Hawtof). Mich. Med., *74:*331, 1975

Graft, dermal, to line groin flap for closure of abdominal hernia (Earle, Blackburn), PRS, *56:*447, 1975

Razor dermatome, adjustable (Huang), PRS, *57:*264, 1976. Surgery, 77:703, 1975

Dermoid Cysts

Marsupialization of inoperable orbital dermoids (Kennedy). Trans. Am. Ophthalmol. Soc., *68:*146, 1970

Dermoid cysts of the nose (Skolnik *et al)*. Laryngoscope, *81:*1632, 1971

Cysts, intraosseous dermoid and epidermoid, in jaw region (Heidsieck). Fortschr. Kiefer. Gesichtschir., *15:*220, 1972 (German)

Subcutaneous dermoid cysts (Brownstein, Helwig), PRS, *52:*457, 1973. Arch. Dermat., *107:*237, 1973

Dermal sinus, lateral, associated with an intradiploic cyst (Green). Brit. J. Plast. Surg., *26:*202, 1973

Epidermoid cyst, proliferating (Vulcan, Georgescu), PRS, *57:*255, 1976. Dermat. Vener., *18:*47, 1973

Dermoid cyst of head, face, and neck (Gupta *et al)*, PRS, *54:*377, 1974. Indian M. Gaz., *12:*557, 1973

Cyst, dermoid, large sublingual (Stewart *et al)*. J. Oral Surg., *31:*620, 1973

Multiple sublingual dermoid cysts (Akinosi). Brit. J. Oral Surg., *12:*235, 1974

Cysts, dermoid, epidermoid and teratomatous, of tongue and floor of mouth (Gold *et al)*. J. Oral Surg., *32:*107, 1974

Dermoid cyst with lingual sinus tract, case report (Korchin). Oral Surg., *37:*175, 1974

Cysts, epidermoid, and polyposis coli (Leppard), PRS, *55:*640, 1975. Proc. Roy. Soc. Med., *67:*1036, 1974

Proceedings: Giant proliferating epidermoid cyst (Aliga *et al)*. Ann. Dermatol. Syphilligr. (Paris), *102:*409, 1975

Congenital double columella (Rawat *et al)*. Brit. J. Plast. Surg., *28:*153, 1975

Cyst, dermoid, of floor of mouth (Oatis *et al)*, PRS, *56:*597, 1975. J. Oral Surg., *39:*192, 1975

Cyst, lateral sublingual dermoid (Chakravorty, Schatzki), PRS, *57:*756, 1976. Oral Surg., *39:*862, 1975

Dermoid tumors, frontonasal, diagnosis and management (Griffith), PRS, *57:*692, 1976

DE ROO, T.: Lymphangiographic studies in series of 55 patients with malignant melanoma.

Lymphology, *6:*6, 1973

DERZHAVIN, V. M. *et al*: Peculiarities of preoperative preparation and postoperative management of patients with defects of genitourinary system development. (Vestn. Khir., *97:*89, 1966 (Russian)

DE SALAMANCA, E. F.: Capsulodesis *versus* proximal activation? Ann. Chir., *29:*987, 1975 (French)

DESANTO, L. W.: Curative, palliative, and adjunctive uses of cryosurgery in head and neck. Laryngoscope, *82:*1282, 1972

DESANTO, L. W.: Selection of treatment for *in situ* and early invasive carcinoma of the glottis. Can. J. Otolaryngol., *3:*552, 1974

DESANTO, L. W.: Lingual flap reconstruction after resection for cancer. Trans. Am. Acad. Ophthalmol. Otolaryngol., *78:*1135, 1974

DESANTO, L. W. *et al*: Selection of patients and choice of operation for orbital decompression in Graves ophthalmopathy. Laryngoscope, *83:*945, 1973

DESANTO, L. W. *et al*: Mandibular osteotomy and lingual flaps. Use in patients with cancer of the tonsil area in tongue base. Arch. Otolaryng., *101:*652, 1975

DESAULTY, A. *et al*: Temporal or frontotemporal flap in cervicofacial oncology. J. Fr. Otorhinolaryngol., *24:*521, 1975 (French)

DESAULTY, A. *et al*: Significance of myotomy of cricopharyngeal muscle and the surface fibers of the esophagus in pharyngo-esophageal dyskinesia. Apropos of 7 cases. J. Fr. Otorhinolaryngol., *24:*527, 1975 (French)

DE SAXE, B. M.: Breast augmentation. Results in series of 150 cases. S. Afr. Med. J., *48:*737, 1974

DE SEBASTIAN, G.: Frigore facial paralysis. Surgical problems. Acta Otorinolaryngol. Iber. Am., *23:*565, 1972 (Spanish)

DESJARDINS, R. P. *et al*: Etiology and management of hypermobile mucosa overlying the residual alveolar ridge. J. Prosthet. Dent., *32:*619, 1974

DESMOND, J. W., AND LAWS, A. K.: Blood volume and capacitance vessel compliance in the quadriplegic patient, PRS, *55:*110, 1975. Canad. Anaesth. Soc. J., *21:*421, 1974

DESMONS, F. *et al*: Value of early detection by phlebography of venous abnormalities with voluminous angiomas in newborns and very young infants. Bull. Soc. Fr. Dermatol. Syphiligr., *79:*523, 1972 (French)

DE SOUZA, F. M. *et al*: Planned pharyngostome. Laryngoscope, *85:*848, 1975

DE SOUZA, L. J. *et al*: Swallowing and speech after radical total glossectomy with tongue prosthesis. Oral Surg., *39:*356, 1975

DESPREZ, J. D.: Regional block of the thigh: uses in plastic surgery (with Earle, Kiehn),

PRS, *49:*134, 1972

DESPREZ, J. D.: Morris bi-phasic external splint for mandibular fixation (with Baumgarten), PRS, *50:*66, 1972

DESPREZ, J. D.: Treatment of chronic, painful metatarsal callus by a tendon transfer (with Kiehn, Earle), PRS, *51:*154, 1973

DESPREZ, J. D. *et al*: Response of oral carcinoma to preoperative methotrexate infusion therapy, PRS, *48:*199, 1971. Am. J. Surg., *102:*461, 1970

DESPREZ, J. D., AND KIEHN, C. L.: Valvular obstruction of nasal airway, PRS, *56:*307, 1975

DESSAPT, B. *et al*: Muscle grafts. Anatomical study and technic for the removal of *extensor digitorum brevis* and *palmaris longus* muscles. Ann. chir. plast., *19:*235, 1974 (French)

DETTMAR, H.: One-stage surgical correction of hypospadias. Urologe, *9:*131, 1970 (German)

DEUTSCH, A. R.: Distichiasis and epicanthus. Study of one family. Ann. Ophth., *3:*168, 1971

DEUTSCH, M. *et al*: Radiotherapy for postoperative recurrent squamous cell carcinoma in head and neck, PRS, *54:*108, 1974. Arch. Otolaryng., *98:*316, 1973

DEUTSCH, M. *et al*: Primary malignant melanoma of the vagina. Oncology, *30:*509, 1974

DEUTSCHMANN, R. *et al*: Dysontogenetic tumors of maxilla in infancy. Paediatr. Grenzgeb., *11:*141, 1972 (German)

DEUTSCHMANN, W.: Primary surgical treatment of extensive deep burns. Munch. Med. Wochenschr., *115:*395, 1973

DEUTSCHMANN, W.: Early treatment of injuries of the soft facial tissues. Zentralbl. Chir., *11:*641, 1975

DE VAAL, O. M.: Transsexualism, form of gender dysphoria, PRS, *55:*726, 1975. Geneesk. gids., *6:*20, 1975

DEVAN, S. K. *et al*: Surgical management of ankylosis of temporomandibular joint. J. Indian Dent. Assoc., *45:*355, 1973

DEVERIDGE, R. J. *et al*: Gas gangrene. M. J. Australia, *1:*1106, 1973

Devices, Medical

Zimfoam pad: comfortable mattress for outpatient surgery (McKinney, Monn), PRS, *52:*446, 1973

Devices, medical, should they be cleared before marketing? (Culliton), PRS, *53:*691, 1974. Science, *182:*565, 1973

Microfiche reader-printer, PRS, *54:*631, 1974. Am. J. Phys. Med., *53:*47, 1974

Appliance to prevent self-inflicted trauma in semicomatose patients (Piercell, Waite, Nelson), PRS, *56:*353, 1975. J. Oral Surg., *32:*903, 1974

Devices, Medical – Cont.

Products, current, PRS, *55:*260, 1975. Med. Electronics & Data, *5:*68, 1974

Perineal urethrostomy, modification of Foley catheter for use in (Tolhurst), PRS, *55:*503, 1975

DEVINE, C. J., JR.: Studies of urethral bleeding in dogs (with Everingham, Horton), PRS, *51:*312, 1973

DEVINE, C. J., JR.: Plication of the *tunica albuginea* to straighten the curved penis (with Horton), PRS, *52:*32, 1973

DEVINE, C. J., JR.: Peyronie's disease (with Horton), PRS, *52:*503, 1973

DEVINE, C. J., JR.: Discussion of "One-stage reconstruction for exstrophy of the bladder in girls" by Furnas, Haq, Somers, PRS, *56:*209, 1975

DEVINE, C. J., JR., AND HORTON, C. E.: Chordee without hypospadias, PRS, *53:*245, 1974. J. Urol., *110:*264, 1973

DEVINE, C. J., JR., AND HORTON, C. E.: Surgical treatment of Peyronie's disease with dermal graft, PRS, *54:*504, 1974. J. Urol., *111:*44, 1974

DEVINE, C. J., JR., AND HORTON, C. E.: Use of dermal graft to correct chordee, PRS, *57:*675, 1976. J. Urol., *113:*56, 1975

DEVINE, K. D.: Patient has lump in neck, PRS, *57:*118, 1976. Postgrad. Med., *57:*131, 1975

DEVITO, R. V.: Viability of split-skin grafts from pigs following incubation on autologous blood or serum for various periods (with Creech, Eade), PRS, *51:*572, 1973

DE VIVIE, E. R. *et al*: Early and late results of funnel chest operation after method of Jensen, Schmidt, and Garamella, PRS, *53:*105, 1974. Bruns' Beitr. klin. Chir., *220:*284, 1973

DE VLEESCHOUWER, L. *et al*: Lipoma of the tongue. Arch. Belg. Dermatol. Syphiligr., *27:*123, 1971 (Dutch)

DEVLIN, D. H.: Participation on Hospital Committees. J. Oral Surg., *32:*487, 1974

DE WET, H. C.: Use of a drum dermatome in reduction mammaplasty, PRS, *52:*448, 1973

DEWHURST, C. J.: Aetiology and management of intersexuality. Clin. Endocrinol. (Oxf.), *4:*625, 1975

DEY, D. L.: Total care of children with cleft lip and cleft palate. M. J. Australia, *2:*738, 1970

DEY, D. L.: Treatment of hypospadias. M. J. Australia, *1:*110, 1972

DEY, D. L.: Burn contractures in child. M. J. Australia, *2:*604, 1972

DEY, D. L.: An important contribution of the Millard flap to cleft lip surgery. Aust. N.Z. J. Surg., *42:*271, 1973

DEY, D. L.: Some unusual aspects of clefts of

the lip. Aust. N.Z. J. Surg., *43:*171, 1973

DEY, D. L.: Oblique facial clefts, PRS, *52:*258, 1973

DEY, D. L.: Hemifacial atrophy: repair with buried flap, PRS, *56:*590, 1975. Australian & New Zealand J. Surg., *44:*379, 1974

DEY, D. L.: A surgeon's view of the congenitally cleft maxilla. M. J. Australia, *1:*708, 1974

DEY, D. L., AND COHEN, D.: Surgery of female epispadias, PRS, *48:*295, 1971. Surgery, *69:*542, 1971

DHAWAN, I. K. *et al*: Use of scalp flaps following resection of oral cancer. Aust. N.Z. J. Surg., *41:*363, 1972

DHAWAN, I. K., AGGARWAL, S. B., AND HARIHARAN, S.: Off-midline forehead flap for repair of small nasal defects, PRS, *53:*537, 1974

D'HONT, G.: Cryotherapy in otorhinolaryngology. Acta Otorhinolaryngol. Belg., *28:*274, 1974 (French)

D'HOOGHE, P.: Simple apparatus for expanding split-skin grafts, PRS, *57:*387, 1976

D'HOOGHE, P., AND HENDRICKX, E.: Simplified technique of skin transplantation, PRS, *57:*766, 1976. Acta chir. belg., *5:*500, 1975

D'HOOGHE, P. *et al*: Cheek reconstruction with doubly folded forehead flap. Acta Stomatol. Belg., *72:*111, 1975

D'HOOGHE, P., AND HENDRICKX, E. E. M.: Protection of femoral vessels with a de-epithelialized hypogastric flap, PRS, *55:*87, 1975

DIAMOND, L. S., AND GOULD, V. E.: Macrodactyly of foot, surgical syndactyly after wedge resection, PRS, *54:*691, 1974. South. M.J., *67:*645, 1974

DIAMOND, M.: Transsexualism. M. J. Australia, *1:*51, 1974

DIAZ, J. E. *et al*: Perforation of the deep palmar arch produced by surgical wire after tenorrhaphy. A case report and review of the literature. J. Bone & Joint Surg. (Am.), *57:*1150, 1975

DIAZ, R. R. *et al*: Maxillary prognathism. Surgical and prosthetic therapy. Rev. Esc. Odontol. Tucuman., *38:*43, 1972 (Spanish)

DIAZ-BALLESTEROS, F., PARAMO-DIAZ, M., AND LOPEZ-SILVA, J.: Osteolytic hemangiomatosis of the extremities, PRS, *52:*454, 1973. Cir. Cir., *40:*215, 1972

DIBBELL, D. G.: Use of a long island flap to bring sensation to the sacral area in young paraplegics, PRS, *54:*220, 1974

DIBBELL, D. G. *et al*: Hydrofluoric acid burns of hand, PRS, *48:*516, 1971. J. Bone & Joint Surg., *52A:*931, 1970

DICKER, R. L., AND SYRACUSE, V. R.: *Consultation with a Plastic Surgeon*. Nelson-Hall Publishers, Chicago, 1975. PRS, *57:*741, 1976

DICKIE, W. R. *et al*: Crypto-hypospadias − re

view of 38 cases. Brit. J. Plast. Surg., *26:*227, 1973

DICKIE, W. R., AND WILLIAMS, C. W.: Hypospadias, critical assessment of management, PRS, *54:*579, 1974

DICKINSON, J. T.: Otolaryngologic and ophthalmologic reconstructive plastic surgery. Trans. Pa. Acad. Ophthalmol. Otolaryngol., *26:*98, 1973

DICKINSON, J. T. *et al*: Alloplastic implants. Otolaryngol. Clin. North Am., *5:*481, 1972

DICKINSON, J. T. *et al*: Chemoexfoliation and dermabrasion. Trans. Pa. Acad. Ophthalmol. Otolaryngol., *26:*9, 1973

DICKINSON, J. T. *et al*: Minor surgery for benign and malignant facial lesions. Am. Fam. Physician, *10:*102, 1974

DICKSON, D. R.: Normal and cleft palate anatomy. Cleft Palate J., *9:*280, 1972

DICKSON, D. R. *et al*: Status of research in cleft palate anatomy and physiology, July 1973, part 1. Cleft Palate J., *11:*471, 1974

DICKSON, D. R. *et al*: Status of research in cleft lip and palate: anatomy and physiology, part 2. Cleft Palate J., *12:*131, 1975

DICKSON, R. A. *et al*: Hand function − a practical method of assessment. Brit. J. Surg., *59:*316, 1972

DICKSON, R. A. *et al*: Assessment of hand function. 1. Measurement of individual digits. Hand, *4:*207, 1972

DICKSON, R. C.: Maxillary cyst. Proc. Mine. Med. Off. Assoc., *50:*81, 1971

DIECKMANN, J.: Malignant synovioma of temporomandibular joint. Dtsch. Zahnaerztl. Z., *27:*854, 1972 (German)

DIECKMANN, J. *et al*: Surgical treatment of multiple mandibular fractures by means of wire osteosynthesis. Fortschr. Kiefer. Gesichtschir., *19:*97, 1975 (German)

DIEDRICH, P. *et al*: Studies on the width of the gingiva proper after vestibuloplasty with and without periosteal fenestration. Dtsch. Zahnaerztl. Z., *27:*346, 1972 (German)

DIETERICH, F. *et al*: Cryosurgery. 2. Advantages and disadvantages of various forms of cryosurgery. Z. Aerztl. Fortbild. (Jena), *65:*948, 1971 (German)

DIETERT, S. E.: Papillary cystadenoma lymphomatosum (Warthin's tumor) in patients in general hospital over a 24-year period. Am. J. Clin. Pathol., *63:*866, 1975

DIETHELM, A. G. *et al*: Treatment of severely burned child with skin transplantation modified by immunosuppressive therapy, PRS, *55:*639, 1975. Ann. Surg., *180:*814, 1974

DIETRICH, F. E. *et al*: Effect of different local treatment upon cicatrization in burns of children. In *Plastische und Wiederherstellungs-*

Chirurgie, ed. by Hohler; pp. 267–77. Stuttgart; Schattauer, 1975 (German)

DIETZEL, F. *et al*: Tumor therapy with high frequency hyperthermia (Decimeter-waves). Animal experiments. Biomed. Tech. (Stuttg.), *16:*213, 1971 (German)

DIJKSTRA, R.: Electric stimulation in a case of median-nerve reconstruction. Arch. chir. neerl., *24:*337, 1972

DIJKSTRA, R., AND SILLEVIS SMITH, W. G.: Treatment of X-ray ulcers by omental transposition, PRS, *57:*123, 1976. Arch. chir. neerl., *27:*35, 1975

DILLON, J. D., JR. *et al*: Facio-orbito-cranio missile wounds. Surg. Neurol. *4:*515, 1975

DILWORTH, N. M.: Importance of changes in body temperature in pediatric surgery and anesthesia, PRS, *53:*690, 1974. Anesth. & Intens. Care, *1:*480, 1973

DIMICK, A. R.: Management of patients with thermal injuries. Am. Surg., *37:*637, 1971

DIMITRIU, A. V. *et al*: Left cervicotomy for esophageal foreign body. Rev. Chir. (Otorinolaringol.), *19:*369, 1974 (Rumanian)

DIMMICK, J. E. *et al*: Complications of intravenous alimentation in seriously ill infants, PRS, *55:*120, 1975. Canad. J. Surg., *17:*186, 1974

DIMOUPOULOS, J. *et al*: Diagnosis, surgical and radiotherapeutic treatment of malignant tumors of the upper jaw. Strahlentherapie, *147:*416, 1974

DINER, J.: Facial restoration. J. Arkansas Med. Soc., *71:*304, 1975

DINGMAN, D.: On the collectivization of American medicine (Letter to the Editor), PRS, *50:*508, 1972

DINGMAN, D. L.: Resection of base of skull for sarcoma of midface. Trans. Am. Acad. Ophthalmol. Otolaryngol., *76:*1371, 1972

DINGMAN, D. L.: Surgical correction of lesions of the temporomandibular joints (with Dingman, Lawrence), PRS, *55:*335, 1975. Discussion by Kiehn, PRS, *55:*484, 1975

DINGMAN, D. L., AND PICKENS, J. E.: Plastic surgery operatory unit, PRS, *56:*673, 1975

DINGMAN, R. O.: Fate of amputated tissues of the head and neck following replacement (with Grabb), PRS, *49:*28, 1972

DINGMAN, R. O.: Restoration of the oral commissure (with Fairbanks), PRS, *49:*411, 1972

DINGMAN, R. O.: Severe bleeding during and after face-lifting operations under general anesthesia (Letter to the Editor), PRS, *50:*608, 1972

DINGMAN, R. O., AND GRABB, W. C.: Costal cartilage homografts preserved by radiation (Follow-Up Clinic), PRS, *50:*516, 1972

DINGMAN, R. O., DINGMAN, D. L., AND LAW-

RENCE, R. A.: Surgical correction of lesions of the temporomandibular joints, PRS, *55:*335, 1975. Discussion by Kiehn, PRS, *55:*484, 1975

DINNER, M.: Use of *extensor pollicis longus* tendon as distal extension for *opponens* transfer (with Kaplan, Chait), PRS, *57:*186, 1976

DINNER, M. I. *et al*: Immediate reconstruction in ablative head and neck surgery. S. Afr. Med. J., *49:*1863, 1975

DIOGUARDI, D., AND MUSAJO SOMMA, A.: Diadermic micro-thermometry, PRS, *57:*762, 1976 (Italian). Riv. ital. chir. plast., *7:*505, 1975

DION, M.: Mammaplasty. Infirm, Can., *15:*21, 1973 (French)

DIOP, L. *et al*: Pseudomalignant, craniofacial fibrous osteodysplasia (a case). Bull. Soc. Med. Afr. Noire Lang. Fr., *15:*260, 1970 (French)

DIOP, L. *et al*: Lagrot's operation and Rizzali-Esmach operation in the treatment of temporomaxillary ankylosis, sequellae of noma. Bull. Soc. Med. Afr. Noire Lang. Fr., *15:*263, 1970 (French)

DIOP, L. *et al*: An exceptional form of noma. Bull. Soc. Med. Afr. Noire Lang. Fr., *16:*599, 1971 (French)

DIABAL, K. *et al*: Mesh graft plastic in the therapy of leg ulcers. Cesk. Dermatol., *46:*267, 1971 (Czechoslovakian)

D'IAKONOV, M. F.: Immediate and remote results of treatment of trophic leg ulcers at the Vangou health resort. Sov. Med., *35:*140, 1972 (Russian)

DIPIRRO, E.: Sudden blindness following blepharoplasty (with Moser, McCoy), PRS, *51:*364, 1973

DIRLEWANGER, A.: Maxillofacial surgery of harelip and cleft palate. Rev. Med. Suisse Romande, *90:*337, 1970 (French)

DISLEIEV, B. *et al*: Two unusual cases of neck tumors. Khirurgiia (Sofiia), *23:*408, 1970 (Bulgarian)

DITMARS, D. M., JR.: Soft tissue changes in the hands of drug addicts (with McCabe), PRS, *52:*538, 1973

DITROI, S.: Surgical correction of alopecia, PRS, *55:*632, 1975. Acta chir. plast., *16:*98, 1974

DITROI, S.: Reconstruction of dorsum nasi by osteoperiosteal grafts, PRS, *55:*634, 1975. Acta chir. plast., *16:*171, 1974

DIUKOV, IU. I.: Industrial injuries of the hand sustained in metallurgy plants. Ortop. Travmatol. Protez., *33:*58, 1972 (Russian)

DIVINCENTI, F. C. *et al*: Traumatic carotid artery injuries in civilian practice. Am. Surg., *40:*277, 1974

DJALILIAN, M. *et al*: Significance of jugular

vein invasion by metastatic carcinoma in radical neck dissection, PRS, *53*:604, 1974. Am. J. Surg., *126*:566, 1973

DJINDJIAN, R.: Embolization, new technique, PRS, *54*:630, 1974. Nouvelle Presse Med., *3*:1475, 1974

DLABAL, K. *et al*: Mesh graft plastic in the therapy of leg ulcers. Cesk Dermatol., *46*:267, 1971 (Czech)

DMITRIEV, G. I.: Reconstructive surgery in severe deformation of the hand after deep burns. Ortop. Travmatol. Protez., *31*:26, 1970 (Russian)

DMITRIEV, G. I.: Surgery of cicatricial contracture of the upper extremities after deep burns. Khirurgiia (Mosk.), *47*:30, 1971 (Russian)

DMITRIEV, G. I.: Surgery of cicatricial contracture of the upper extremities after deep burns. Khirurgiia (Mosk.), *48*:31, 1972 (Russian)

DMITRIEV, G. I.: Surgical treatment of contractures, deformities and cicatricial trophic ulcers of lower extremities after deep burns. Ortop. Travmatol. Protez., *34*:33, 1973 (Russian)

DMITRIEV, G. I. *et al*: Skin plastic surgery in scar contractures of the neck following burns. Ortop. Travmatol. Protez., *33*:7, 1972 (Russian)

DMITRIEVA, Z. E. *et al*: Indications for skin transplantation on a wide nourishing pedicle in injuries to the hand. Ortop. Travmatol. Protez., *31*:45, 1970 (Russian)

DOBACZEWSKI, Z.: Radiological appearance of maxillary sinuses prior to treatment of oroantral fistula and during late control examinations. Czas. Stomatol., *27*:1043, 1974 (Polish)

DOBACZEWSKI, Z.: Long-term study after treatment of oroantral fistulae. Czas. Stomatol., *28*:707, 1975 (Polish)

DOBBELAERE, F. *et al*: Spitz's nevus. Arch. Belg. Dermatol., *29*:339, 1973 (French)

DOBBS, E. R., AND CURRERI, P. W.: Burns: analysis of results of physical therapy in 681 patients, PRS, *52*:101, 1973. J. Trauma, *12*:242, 1972

DOBERNECK, R. C.: Evaluation of wound complications after neck dissection and composite resection utilizing transverse cervical incisions, PRS, *52*:322, 1973. Surgery, *73*:261, 1973

DOBERNECK, R. C.: Diagnosis and treatment of solitary mass in neck. Am. Surg., *40*:181, 1974

DOBERNECK, R. C. *et al*: Deglutition after resection of oral, laryngeal and pharyngeal cancers. Surgery, *75*:87, 1974

DOBREV, IA. *et al*: Case of successfully operated thyroid cancer infiltrating great vessels on the left side of the neck. Khirurgiia (Sofiia), *24*:214, 1971 (Bulgarian)

DOBROSSY, L., RONAY, P., MOINAR, L.: Malignant papillary cystadenoma lymphomatosum. Oncology, *26*:457, 1972

DOBYNS, J. H. *et al*: Rheumatoid hand repairs. Orthop. Clin. North Am., *2*:629, 1971

DOBYNS, J. H. *et al*: Bowler's thumb: diagnosis and treatment, PRS, *51*:347, 1973. J. Bone & Joint Surg., *54A*:751, 1972

DOCIU, I. *et al*: Camptodactyly. Apropos of 25 cases. Sem. Hop. Paris, *51*:1175, 1975 (French)

DODICK, J. M., GALLIN, M. A., AND KWITKO, M. L.: Concomitant blowout fracture of orbit and rupture of globe, PRS, *48*:293, 1971. Arch. Ophth., *84*:707, 1970

DOERING, E. J. III *et al*: Alligator bite. J.A.M.A., *218*:255, 1971

DOFFING, K., NELSON, G. D., AND KENDALL, T. E.: Skin carrier for the Padgett mesh dermatome, PRS, *50*:299, 1972

DOGO, G.: Cryo-bistoury and electric bistoury in plastic surgery. Cancro, *24*:337, 1971 (Italian)

DOKA, V. *et al*: Psychosomatic development of women with artificial vagina. Cesk. Gynekol., *39*:187, 1974 (Slovakian)

DOKISH, IU. M. *et al*: Late results of treating injuries to the flexor tendons of the fingers and hand. Vestn. Khir., *108*:93, 1972 (Russian)

DOLDAN, F. G., AND SHATKIN, S.: Deltoscapular flap, PRS, *55*:708, 1975

DOLECEK, R., AND MAHAFFEY, W.: Uncoupling phenomenon and metabolic block after burns, PRS, *48*:396, 1971. Acta chir. plast., *12*:217, 1970

DOLECEK, R. *et al*: Plasma immunoreactive insulin and growth hormone levels in burned subjects, PRS, *52*:684, 1973. Acta chir. plast., *14*:179, 1972

DOLECEK, R. *et al*: Plasma renin like activity (RLA) and angiotensin levels after major burns, PRS, *54*:506, 1974. Acta chir. plast., *15*:166, 1973

DOLESKII, S. I.: Technic for repair of skin defect following Maydl-Ternovskii-Michelson operation for bladder exstrophy. Urol. Nefrol. (Mosk.), *38*:55, 1973 (Russian)

DOLEZALOWA, M. *et al*: Aspergillosis as a postoperative complication of a jaw cyst. Pol. Tyg. Lek., *30*:437, 1975 (Polish)

DOLLING, D., AND FRANKE, D.: Scaphoid fractures in child and their "specialties," PRS, *51*:478, 1973. Bruns' Beitr. klin. Chir., *219*:462, 1972

DOL'NITSKII, O. V. *et al*: So-called bilateral muscular torticollis. Ortop. Travmatol. Protez., *35:*69, 1974

DOMARUS, H. *et al*: Experimental results of mandibular nearthrosis. Zahnaerztl. Prax., *24:*147, 1973 (German)

DOMARUS, H. V.: Technique for reconstruction of blowout fractures of medial orbital wall, PRS, *54:*619, 1974. J. Maxillo-facial Surg., *2:*55, 1974

DOMARUS, H. V.: Residual nasal deformity after Wegener's granuloma, PRS, *56:*216, 1975

DOMASCHK, W.: Possibilities of use of Kiel bone chips in stomatologic practice. Dtsch. Zahnaerztl. Z., *28:*605, 1973 (German)

DOMENECI LLAVALLOL, O.: Surgical treatment of rosacea. Acta Otorinolaryngol. Iber. Am., *24:*94, 1973 (Spanish)

DOMKE, H.: Surgical care of naso-lacrimal duct stenosis following middle face fractures. Dtsch. Gesundheitsw., *27:*2141, 1972 (German)

DOMOTOR, E.: Gerdox treatment in hand-surgery. Ther. Hung., *23:*27, 1975

DONALD, P. J.: Leading with nose, PRS, *57:*755, 1976. Emerg. Med., *7:*27, 1975

DONALD, P. J.: Mandibular and maxillary osteotomy, PRS, *57:*673, 1976. West. J. Med., *123:*219, 1975

DONALDSON, R. C.: Methotrexate plus bacillus Calmette-Guerin (BCG) and isoniazid in treatment of cancer of head and neck, PRS, *52:*216, 1973. Am. J. Surg., *124:*527, 1972

DONALDSON, R. C.: Chemoimmunotherapy for cancer of head and neck, PRS, *53:*688, 1974. Am. J. Surg., *126:*507, 1973

DONALDSON, R. C. *et al*: Uveitis and vitiligo associated with BCG treatment for malignant melanoma, PRS, *56:*113, 1975. Surgery, *76:*771, 1974

DONALDSON, S. S. *et al*: Rhabdomyosarcoma of the head and neck in children, PRS, *52:*214, 1973. Cancer, *31:*26, 1973

DONATI, L.: Recent progress in burn therapy, PRS, *57:*401, 1976. Riv. ital. chir. plast., *6:*41, 1974

DONATI, L. *et al*: Comparison of clinical activity of allo- and xeno-grafts of fresh and cryopreserved skin. Minerva Med., *65:*3654, 1974

DONATI, R. M. *et al*: Effect of germ-free state on wound healing, PRS, *48:*610, 1971. J. Surg. Res., *11:*163, 1971

DONEGAN, W. L., AND HARRIS, H. S.: Factors influencing success of arterial infusion chemotherapy for cancer of head and neck, PRS, *51:*608, 1973. Am. J. Surg., *123:*549, 1972

DONEGAN, W. L., AND PEREZ-MESA, C. M.: Carcinoma of male breast, PRS, *52:*460, 1973.

Arch. Surg., *106:*273, 1973

DONETSKII, D. A. *et al*: Evaluation of homo-transplantation of skin preserved by lyophilization and freezing. Khirurgiia (Mosk.), *47:*22, 1971 (Russian)

DONNELLAN, M. J. *et al*: Clinicopathologic study of cutaneous melanoma of head and neck, PRS, *52:*103, 1973. Am. J. Surg., *124:*450, 1972

DONOFF, R. B. *et al*: Keratocysts of jaws. J. Oral Surg., *30:*880, 1972

DONOHUE, W. B.: Immediate mandibular reconstruction following resection. J. Can. Dent. Assoc., *39:*720, 1973

DONOVAN, W.: Lack of effect of skin cycle on survival of experimental skin flaps in rats (with Myers, Falterman), PRS, *57:*650, 1976

DOR, P. *et al*: Prophylactic antibiotics in oral, pharyngeal and laryngeal surgery for cancer (double blind study). Laryngoscope, *83:*1992, 1973

DOREMIEUX, J., REZIEINER, S., AND KOHLER, J. J.: Fournier's disease. Apropos of 3 cases. J. Urol. Nephrol. (Paris), *78:*696, 1972 (French)

DORMANDY, J. A., HOARE, E., AND POSTEL-THWAITE, J.: Importance of blood viscosity in rheological claudication, PRS, *55:*720, 1975. Proc. Roy. Soc. Med., *67:*446, 1974

DORNER, K. R.: Malpractice: positive steps for plastic surgeons. Mich. Med., *74:*298, 1975

DORNETTE, W. H. L.: Medical injury insurance – possible remedy for malpractice problem, PRS, *53:*115, 1974. J. Legal Med., *1:*29, 1973

DOROFEEV, V. I. *et al*: Osteosynthesis of maxillary fractures with metal nails. Voen. Med. Zh., *6:*66, 1975 (Russian)

DOROGI, J. *et al*: Pediatric aspects of treatment of hemangioma of skin. Orv. Hetil., *113:*2522, 1972 (Hungarian)

DORPH, S., OIGAARD, A., AND JENSEN, J.: Tomography in diagnosis of tumors in paranasal region, PRS, *55:*257, 1975. Adv. Otorhinolaryng., *21:*41, 1974

DORRANCE, G. M.: Lengthening the soft palate in cleft palate operations (Classic Reprint), PRS, *50:*275, 1972

DORSEY, J. W.: Urinary diversion by anterior transposition of urethra, PRS, *48:*607, 1971. J. Urol., *105:*725, 1971

DORTZBACH, R. K.: Complications in surgery for blepharospasm. Am. J. Ophth., *75:*142, 1973

DORTZBACH, R. K., AND CALLAHAN, A.: Repair of cicatricial entropion of upper eyelids, PRS, *48:*89, 1971. Arch. Ophth., *85:*82, 1971

DOS REIS, S. M.: Oroantral fistulas following dental extraction. Rev. Port. Estomatol. Cir. Maxilofac., *14:*79, 1973 (Portuguese)

Dos Reis, S. M.: Lithiasis of aberrant lingual salivary gland. Rev. Port. Estomatol. Cir. Maxilofac., *14*:191, 1973 (Portuguese)

Dos Reis, S. M. *et al*: Malignant tumors in maxillofacial surgery. Rev. Port. Estomatol. Cir. Maxilofac., *15*:71, 1974

Dossantos, G. M. *et al*: Fracture of mandible. Treatment by osteosynthesis by extraoral approach, case report. Rev. Fac. Odontol. Sao Jose dos Campos, *1*:15, 1972 (Spanish)

Dostal, M., and Jelinek, R.: Morphogenesis of cleft palate induced by exogenous factors, PRS, *48*:395, 1971. Acta chir. plast., *12*:206, 1970

Dostal, M. *et al*: Morphogenesis of cleft palate induced by exogenous factors. I. The sensitivity period after the administration of cortisone. Folia Morphol. (Praha), *19*:88, 1971

Dostal, M., and Jelinek, R.: Course of palate closure in embryos of different mouse strains, PRS, *53*:490, 1974. Acta chir. plast., *15*:23, 1973

Dostal, M., and Behounkova, E.: Rapid technique for contrasting embryonic tissues in secondary palate development studies, PRS, *56*:367, 1975. Acta chir. plast., *16*:243, 1974

Dostal, M., and Jelinek, R.: Spatial changes during horizontalization of palatine shelves, PRS, *54*:629, 1974. Rozhl. chir., *53*:171, 1974

D'Ottaviano, N. *et al*: Surgical and esthetic aspects of the facial profile. Int. J. Oral Surg., *3*:243, 1974

Douek, E. *et al*: Recent advances in pathology of olfaction, PRS, *57*:682, 1976. Proc. Roy. Soc. Med., *68*:467, 1975

Dougall, A. J.: Anomalies of first branchial cleft, PRS, *55*:252, 1975. J. Pediat. Surg., *9*:203, 1974

Douglas, J. S., Jr., and Eby, C. S.: Silicone for immersion foot prophylaxis, where and how much to use, PRS, *52*:97, 1973. Mil. Med., *137*:386, 1972

Douglas, W. M.: New mastopexy operation for mild or moderate breast ptosis (with Bartels, Strickland), PRS, *57*:687, 1976

Dowie, D. A.: Amputation stump management—preliminary report on use of shrink plastic film as surgical dressing in amputation surgery, PRS, *57*:122, 1976. M.J. Australia, *2*:127, 1975

Dowling, J. A.: Reconstructions of the nose and upper lip with nasolabial flaps (with Cameron, Latham), PRS, *52*:145, 1973

Downie, P. A.: Rehabilitation of cancer patient. 2. Paraplegia, amputations and head and neck surgery. Nurs. Mirror, *135*:36, 1972

Downie, P. A.: Patient with cancerous disease—towards independence and subsequently. Queens Nurs. J., *16*:254, 1974

Downie, P. A.: Rehabilitation for patients following head and neck surgery. J. Laryng. & Otol., *89*:1281, 1975

Doyle, D. E., and Passey, V.: Keloid management and present status, PRS, *57*:123, 1976. Eye, Ear, Nose & Throat Month., *54*:239, 1975

Doyle, J. C. *et al*: Spontaneous regression of malignant melanoma. M. J. Australia, *2*:551, 1973

Draf, W.: One stage reconstruction of hypopharynx following total laryngopharyngectomy. Laryngol. Rhinol. Otol. (Stuttg.), *54*:572, 1975 (German)

Drastichova, V., Samohyl, J., and Slavetinska, A.: Strengthening sutured skin wound with ultrasound in experiments of animals, PRS, *53*:611, 1974. Acta chir. plast., *15*:114, 1973

Drepper, H.: Basal cell carcinoma of the face. Problems of treatment and rehabilitation. Minerva Stomatol., *20*:249, 1971 (German)

Dressings and Drains

Wide-mesh net for immobilization of skin grafts (Freeman) (Follow-Up Clinic), PRS, *49*:207, 1972

Barton bandage, use of modified head halter for (Green), PRS, *49*:466, 1972

Skin grafting, use of foam rubber sponge in tie-over dressings for (Wexler, Neuman), PRS, *50*:301, 1972

Quantitative comparison of biological dressings (Robson, Samburg, Krizek), PRS, *51*:706, 1973. Surg. Forum, *23*:504, 1972; PRS, *53*:689, 1974. J. Surg. Res., *14*:431, 1973

Ultra thin silicone polymer membrane: a new synthetic skin substitute. A preliminary study (Kornberg *et al*). Trans. Am. Soc. Artif. Intern. Organs, *18*:39, 1972

Biological material for bridging *dura mater* defects (Meskhia *et al*), PRS, *53*:692, 1974. Acta chir. plast., *15*:33, 1973

Skin dressings in treatment of contaminated wounds (Allen *et al*), PRS, *53*:110, 1974. Am. J. Surg., *126*:45, 1973

Suction drainage, new principle for postoperative. Suction flow drainage in head and neck surgery (Hallen *et al*). Ann. Otol. Rhin. & Laryng., *82*:370, 1973

Biological dressings for skin graft donor sites (Salisbury *et al*), PRS, *52*:456, 1973. Arch. Surg., *106*:705, 1973

Skin defects, chronic and acute, treatment with autologous skin homogenizate (Klein, Kohler), PRS, *52*:461, 1973. Bruns' Beitr. klin. Chir., *220*:214, 1973

Elastic membrane, human skin as (Daniel-

Dressings and Drains – Cont.

son), PRS, *53:*375, 1974. J. Bio-Mechanics, *6:*539, 1973

Surgical tape wound closure: disenchantment (Ellenberg) (Follow-Up Clinic), PRS, *52:*80, 1973

Porcine skin grafts, commercial, use for wound dressings (Elliott, Hoehn), PRS, *52:*401, 1973

Suction drain for small areas, "home-made" (Kaye), PRS, *52:*447, 1973

Pressure dressing, use of acrylic fiber in (Herndon, Morgan), PRS, *52:*591, 1973

Polyurethane foam in tie-over dressing (Minami, Holderness, Vistnes), PRS, *52:*672, 1973

Wound dressing, temporary, amniotic membranes as (Robson *et al)*, PRS, *52:*601, 1973. Surg. Gynec. & Obst., *136:*904, 1973

Dressing, skin, effect on healing of partial thickness skin wounds in rats (Burleson, Eiseman), PRS, *52:*461, 1973. Surg. Gynec. & Obst., *136:*958, 1973

Human dura as skin substitute (Schnellen). Z. Hautkr., *48:*999, 1973 (German)

Collagen sheet, clinical application as artificial skin (Arai *et al)*, PRS, *56:*365, 1975. Jap. J. Plast. Reconstr. Surg., *17:*405, 1974

Heterografts: absence of vascularization in porcine skin grafts on mice (Pandya, Zarem), PRS, *53:*211, 1974

Dressing, Plastubol spray, in management of extensive surgical wounds (Kabza, Pasz), PRS, *56:*471, 1975. Wiad. Lek., *27:*1275, 1974

Dressings, biological, to treat gastroschisis and omphalocele (Seashore, MacNaughton, Talbert), PRS, *56:*226, 1975. J. Pediat. Surg., *10:*9, 1975

Dressing, surgical, shrink plastic film for amputation surgery (Dowie), PRS, *57:*122, 1976. M.J. Australia, *2:*127, 1975

Bolus dressing, simple method for changing (Levin, Masters), PRS, *55:*500, 1975

Dressings, biological, panniculectomy specimens as a convenient and inexpensive source of homograft skin (Swartz, Rueckett, Brown), PRS, *55:*628, 1975

Dressings, method to keep moist prior to delayed skin grafting (Jackson), PRS, *56:*347, 1975

Polyurethane foam dressing (Lyofoam), new, epidermal wound healing under (Winter), PRS, *56:*531, 1975

DRESSLER, D. P.: Universal challenge. Arch. Surg., *103:*434, 1971

DRESSLER, D. P., AND SKORNIK, W. A.: Effect of antimicrobial therapy on lung bacterial

clearance in burned rat, PRS, *50:*421, 1972. Ann. Surg., *175:*241, 1972

DRESSLER, D. P., AND SKORNIK, W. A.: Laboratory evaluation of topical silver nitrate in experimental burn wound sepsis, PRS, *52:*211, 1973. J. Trauma, *12:*791, 1972

DRESSLER, D. P., AND SKORNIK, W. A.: Eschar: a major factor in postburn pneumonia, PRS, *54:*379, 1974. Am. J. Surg., *127:*413, 1974

DREVER, J. M.: Simple method for obtaining fascia lata grafts, PRS, *50:*196, 1972

DREW, E. J.: Removal of panniculus adiposus. J.A.M.A. *229:*391, 1974

DREWS, R.: Primary malignant melanoma of orbit in Negro, PRS, *56:*591, 1975. Arch. Ophth., *93:*335, 1975

DREYER, C. J., AND PRESTON, C. B.: Classification of cleft lip and palate in animals, PRS, *55:*514, 1975. Cleft Palate J., *11:*327, 1974

DRINKER, H., KNORR, N. J., AND EDGERTON, M. T.: Factitious wounds, psychiatric and surgical dilemma, PRS, *50:*458, 1972

DRONAMRAJU, K. R.: Epilepsy and cleft lip and palate. Lancet, *2:*867, 1970

DROTAR, D. *et al*: Adaptation of parents to birth of infant with congenital malformation, PRS, *57:*682, 1976. Pediatrics, *56:*710, 1975

DROUILLAT, J. P.: Treatment of granulomas and cysts (discussion of their surgical treatment). Rev. Odontostomatol. (Paris), *4:*123, 1975 (French)

Drugs

Pentazocine, non-narcotic analgesic, evaluation of, in burned children (Wilson, Priano, Traber), PRS, *48:*466, 1971

Drugs in children, side effects (Kosenow), PRS, *53:*115, 1974. Chir. Praxis, *16:*143, 1972

Chemotherapeutic agents for cancer, used in non-neoplastic diseases (Hall), PRS, *54:*114, 1974. Cancer, *31:*1256, 1973

Medication, preoperative work-ups and near catastrophes (Crikelair, Wolf) (Letter to the Editor), PRS, *53:*216, 1974

Morphine sulfate, intravenous, hypersensitivity to (Cromwell, Zsigmond), PRS, *54:*224, 1974

Use of sodium nitroprusside as a hypotensive agent in plastic surgery (Hester). Postgrad. Med. J., *50:*582, 1974

Nose surgery, use of cocaine as topical anesthetic in (Feehan, Mancusi-Ungaro), PRS, *57:*62, 1975

DRUNER, H. U. *et al*: Stress ulcer following burns. Med. Welt., *23:*707, 1972 (German)

DRUSS, R. G., SYMONDS, F. C., AND CRIKELAIR, G. F.: Problems of somatic delusions in patients seeking cosmetic surgery, PRS, *48:*246, 1971

DRYZHAK, V. I.: Results of treating skin cancer relapses. Vopr. Onkol., *18:*73, 1972 (Russian)

DRYZHAK, V. I.: Malignant tumors formed against the background of ulcers, osteomyelitic fistulas and scars. Klin. Khir., *10:*78, 1975 (Russian)

DUBE, V. E., AND PAULSON, J. F.: Metastatic hemangiopericytoma cured by radiotherapy, case report, PRS, *55:*388, 1975. J. Bone & Joint Surg. *56A:*833, 1974

DUBEN, W.: Etiology and treatment of ischemic contractures of the forearm and hand. Handchirurgie, *1:*63, 1969 (German)

DUBIN, H. V.: Mucinous cysts and mucinous pseudocysts, PRS, *53:*611, 1974. Univ. Mich. M. J., *39:*78, 1973.

DUBROV, IA. G.: Injury of the tendons of the hand. Ortop. Travmatol. Protez., *5:*75, 1975 (Russian)

DUBS-BUCHSER, R. *et al*: Basal cell carcinoma of the nasal dorsum 22 years after implantation of a bony strut for saddle nose. Laryngol. Rhinol. Otol. (Stuttg.), *53:*392, 1974 (German)

DUCHATEAU, C., AND CARTEAU, G.: Calculation of degrees of mandibular prognathism. Orthod. Fr., *42:*566, 1971 (French)

DUCKER, T. B. *et al:* Surgical aspects of peripheral nerve trauma. Curr. Probl. Surg., 1, Sept., 1974

DUCKLER, L.: Squamous cell carcinoma developing in an artificial vagina. Obstet. Gynecol., *40:*35, 1972

DUCOURTIOUX, J. L.: Problems of cutaneous closing. Bull. Mem. Soc. Chir. Paris, *61:*310, 1971 (French)

DUCOURTIOUX, J. L.: Technic and indications for crural dermolipectomies. Ann. chir. plast., *17:*204, 1975 (French)

DUCREY, N. *et al*: Fractures of the orbital floor. Ophthalmologica, *163:*254, 1971 (French)

DUDGEON, D. L. *et al*: Multiple teratomas of head and neck. J. Pediat., *85:*139, 1974

DUERKSEN, R. L.: Orbital decompression of malignant exophthalmos. Trans. Pa. Acad. Ophthalmol. Otolaryngol., *25:*113, 1972

DUFFY, M.: Concerning the absence of muscle in the prolabium (Letter to the Editor), PRS, *49:*450, 1972

DUFFY, M. M.: Restoration of orbicularis oris muscle continuity in the repair of bilateral cleft lip. Brit. J. Plast. Surg., *24:*48, 1971

DUFOURMENTEL, C., AND MARCHAC, D.: Rise of plastic surgery. Current advances, future prospects. Rev. Prat., *22:*19, 1972 (French)

DUFOURMENTEL, C., AND LePESTEUR, J.: Composite auricular grafts in reconstruction of

lower portion of nasal pyramid, PRS, *54:*499, 1974. Ann. chir. plast., *18:*199, 1973

DUFOURMENTEL, C., AND MARCHAC, D.: Craniofacial LeFort III osteotomy permitting advancement of middle third of face, PRS, *54:*107, 1974. Chirurgie, *99:*755, 1973

DUHAMEL, B.: Intestinal bladders controlled by the anal sphincter. Technics and results. Ann. Chir. Infant., *12:*433, 1971 (French)

DUJOVNY, M. *et al*: Orbitocranial foreign body, case report. Ophthalmologica, *168:*261, 1974

DUJOVNY, M., VAS, R., AND OSGOOD, C. P.: Bipolar jeweler's forceps with automatic irrigation, for coagulation in microsurgery, PRS, *56:*585, 1975

DUKART, R. C. *et al*: Cherubism: case report. J. Oral Surg., *32:*782, 1974

DUKE-ELDER, SIR STEWART: *System of Ophthalmology*. Vol. XIV. *Injuries*. C. V. Mosby Co., St. Louis, 1972. PRS, *52:*571, 1973

DUKER, J.: Experimental animal research into segmental alveolar movement after corticotomy, PRS, *57:*395, 1976. J. Maxillo-facial Surg., *3:*81, 1975

DUKER, J., AND HARLE, F.: Influence of unilateral operations with reference to soft tissue only, on growth of skull, PRS, *54:*618, 1974. J. Maxillo-facial Surg., *2:*44, 1974

DULAC, G. L.: Respective indications for radiation and surgery in treatment of primary localization of epitheliomas of floor of mouth. J. Radiol. Electrol. Med. Nucl., *53:*467, 1972 (French)

DULONG DE ROSNAY, C. *et al*: Bacteriological research on the use of Sterlane in the treatment of burns. Bord. Med., *4:*2587, 1971 (French)

DUMAS, P., AND FREIDEL, M.: Sagittal osteotomy of the ascending branch of the mandible by the endobuccal approach to correct prognathism, PRS, *50:*418, 1972. J. Fr. Otorhinolaryng., *21:*317, 1972

DUMAS, P., AND FREIDEL, M.: Surgical treatment of prognathism by sagittal osteotomy of ascending rami, PRS, *53:*105, 1974. Lyon Chir., *69:*258, 1973

DUMAS, P. *et al*: Delayed correction of the primary palate in the treatment of unilateral labio-alveolar clefts. Rev. Stomatol. Chir. Maxillofac., *75:*90, 1974 (French)

DUNAEVSKII, V. A. *et al*: Tracheostomy in system of resuscitation and anesthesiological measures in maxillofacial surgery. Tsitologiia, *15:*74, 1973 (Russian)

DUNAEVSKII, V. A. *et al*: Postoperative bronchopulmonary complications in malignant neoplasms of maxillofacial localization. Vestn. Khir., *113:*69, 1974 (Russian)

DUNCAN, D. J.: Bell's palsy: review of current

treatment. J. Am. Osteopath. Assoc., *73*:150, 1973

DUNCAN, J. *et al*: Low-velocity gunshot wounds of the hand. Arch. Surg., *109*:395, 1974

DUNCKER, H. R.: Anatomy and surgical treatment of syndactylism (with Lösch), PRS, *50*:167, 1972

DUNN, A. W.: Trapezius paralysis after minor surgical procedures in posterior cervical triangle. South Med. J., *67*:312, 1974

DUNN, C., DUNN, D. L., AND MOSER, K. M.: Determinants of tracheal injury by cuffed tracheostomy tubes, PRS, *54*:501, 1974. Chest, *65*:128, 1974

DUNNE, J. H., AND JOHNSON, W. C.: Necrotizing skin lesions in heroin addicts, PRS, *50*:538, 1972. Arch. Dermat., *105*:544, 1972

DUNPHY, J. E.: *Wound Healing*. 2nd Ed. Med. Com., New York, 1974

DUNPHY, J. E.: Surgery in the 21st century, PRS, *54*:511, 1974. Surgery, *75*:332, 1974

DUNSTONE, M.: Dilantin and hare-lip. M. J. Australia, *2*:54, 1972

DUNSWORTH, A. R.: Zygomatic complex fracture with an avulsed tooth causing malocclusion: case report. J. Oral Surg., *32*:131, 1974

DUPAL, H. D.: Diplopia as sequel of fractures of orbital wall. Case studies on rhinological diagnosis and therapy. Wien. Med. Wochenschr., *124*:716, 1974 (German)

DUPARC, J. *et al*: Sub-clavicular tube flaps in reconstructive surgery of the hand. Ann. Chir., *25*:1023, 1971 (French)

DUPARC, J. *et al*: Plasties of opposition by tendinous transplantation through the interosseous membrane. Rev. Chir. Orthop., *57*:29, 1971 (French)

DUPARC, J. *et al*: Recent lesions of flexor tendons at finger level, PRS, *53*:243, 1974. Ann. Chir., *27*:467, 1973

DUPARC, J., AND ROUX, F.: Sensitivity of hand restored by transfer of heterodigital skin transplant including its fascicular and nervous pedicle, PRS, *53*:112, 1974. Ann. Chir., *27*:497, 1973

DUPERRAT, B. *et al*: Monstrous keloid. Bull. Soc. Fr. Dermatol. Syphiligr., *79*:210, 1972 (French)

DUPONT, C.: Hand surgery under wrist block and local infiltration anesthesia, using an upper arm tourniquet (Letter to the Editor), PRS, *51*:685, 1973

DUPONT, C., AND MENARD, Y.: Transposition of the greater omentum for reconstruction of chest wall, PRS, *49*:263, 1972

DUPONT, C. *et al*: Hand surgery under wrist block and local infiltration anesthesia, using an upper arm tourniquet, PRS, *50*:532, 1972

DUPONT, C. *et al*: Phenol skin tightening for better dermabrasion, PRS, *50*:588, 1972

DUPONT, C., CIABURRO, H., AND PREVOST, Y.: Simplifying the Le Fort I type of maxillary osteotomy, PRS, *54*:142, 1974

DUPUIS, A.: Tumors of parotid region. Rev. Stomatol. Chir. Maxillofac., *74*:493, 1973 (French)

DUPUIS, A.: Surgical treatment for permanent facial paralysis. Rev. Stomatol. Chir. Maxillofac., *74*:499, 1973 (French)

DUPUIS, A. *et al*: Treatment of osteoradionecrosis by bone removal and grafting. Rev. Stomatol. Chir. Maxillofac., *73*:410, 1972

DUPUIS, A. *et al*: Diplopia due to fracture of the roof of the orbit. Rev. Stomatol. Chir. Maxillofac., *74*:620, 1973 (French)

DUPUIS, A. *et al*: Techniques and indications for superior maxillary osteotomies. Rev. Stomatol. Chir. Maxillofac., *75*:1055, 1974 (French)

DUPUIS, J. F.: Use of flag flap for coverage of small area on palm (with Vilain), PRS, *51*:397, 1973

DUPUIS, J. F., DEBRAY, G., AND VILAIN, R.: Treatment of ischiatic bedsores by ischiectomy associated with muscular plasty. Ann. chir. plast., *18*:27, 1973 (French)

DUPUIS, M. A.: Muscular interventions in orthopedic surgery of the maxillo-facial skeleton. Orthod. Fr., *41*:335, 1970 (French)

DUPUIS, R. H. *et al*: Letter: who treats facial fractures? J. Trauma, *14*:990, 1974

Dupuytren's Contracture: See Contracture, Dupuytren's

DURAND, J. C. *et al*: Role of surgery in treatment of cancers of floor of mouth. J Radiol. Electrol. Med. Nucl., *53*:473, 1972 (French)

DURAND, J. C. *et al*: Role of surgery in cancers of gingiva in Fondation Curie. J. Radiol. Electrol. Med. Nucl., *53*:481, 1972 (French)

DURILIN, I. A. *et al*: Filatov's flap in otorhinolaryngology (on the centenary of the birth of Academician V. P. Filatov). Zh. Ushn. Nos. Gorl. Bolezn., *2*:4, 1975 (Russian)

DURKOVSKY, J. *et al*: Problem of lip cancer metastases. Neoplasma, *19*:653, 1972

DURRANI, K. M.: Surgical repair of defects from noma (cancrum oris), PRS, *52*:629, 1973

DURRANI, K. M., SHAH, P. I., AND KAKALIA, G. R.: Interurethral fenestration for a case of double urethra with hypospadias, PRS, *52*:98, 1973. J. Urol., *108*:586, 1972

DUSHOFF, I. M.: Hand surgery under wrist block and local infiltration anesthesia, using an upper arm tourniquet (Letter to the Editor), PRS, *51*:685, 1973

DUSHOFF, I. M.: About face, PRS, *55*:505, 1975. Emerg. Med., *6*:25, 1974

DUTESCU, N. *et al*: Experiences in the treatment of complex mid-facial fractures. Dtsch. Stomatol., *21:*585, 1971 (German)

DUTESCU, N. *et al*: Management of metastatic adenopathies in cancer of the mouth. Stomatologia (Bucur.), *18:*425, 1971 (Rumanian)

DUTESCU, N. *et al*: Lipoma of submandibular space with osseous metaplasia. Oral Surg., *35:*611, 1973

DUTHIE, A. M.: Harare staff clinical conference. Tracheostomy versus naso-tracheal intubation. Cent. Afr. J. Med., *17:*222, 1971

DUTTA, A.: Rhinolith. J. Oral Surg., *31:*876, 1973

DUTTA, T. *et al*: Rare combination of duplication of genito-urinary tract, hindgut, vertebral column and other associated anomalies. Brit. J. Urol., *46:*577, 1974

DUVALL, A. J., III, *et al*: Juvenile nasopharyngeal angiofibroma. Minn. Med., *56:*283, 1973

DUVERNE, M. J.: Role of plastic surgery in treatment of benign and malignant tumors of face and scalp. J. Med. Lyon, *53:*1063, 1972 (French)

DVORAKOVA, M. *et al*: Absence of *musculus palmaris longus* in the Prague population. Cas. Lek. Cesk., *114:*1365, 1975

DWORECKA, F. *et al*: New device for the restoration of partially amputated hands. Mt. Sinai J. Med. N. Y., *38:*462, 1971

DYBKOWSKA-KLOS, H.: Oral lipofibromas. Czas. Stomatol., *28:*987, 1975 (Polish)

DYRAS, M. *et al*: Late results of separation of raphe palati in malocclusion. Czas. Stomatol., *27:*635, 1974 (Polish)

DZIUK, E. *et al*: Accidental irradiation of skin on hands with a proton beam of 4 MeV. energy. Strahlentherapie, *148:*685, 1973

E

EADE, G. G.: Viability of split-skin grafts from pigs following incubation on autologous blood or serum for various periods (with Creech, DeVito), PRS, *51:*572, 1973

EADE, G. G.: Radial incision for gynecomastia excisions, PRS, *54:*495, 1974

EADE, G. G.: Emergency care of severe facial injuries. Clin. Plast. Surg., *2:*73, 1975

Ear (See also *Otoplasty; Replantation*)

Ear, middle, complication in clefts (Fara, Hrivnakova, Horak), PRS, *53:*607, 1974. Acta chir. plast., *15:*7, 1973

Earring, preservation of perforation for repair of torn earlobe with (Pardue), PRS, *51:*472, 1973

Ear, chondritis of, in burns (Stadaas) Tidsskr. Nor. Laegeforen, *93:*678, 1973

Ear—Cont.
(Norwegian)

Bilateral pseudocysts of auricle in female (Santos *et al*). Ann. Otol. Rhin. & Laryng., *83:*9, 1974

Technic and application of retroauricular insular flap (Tolsdorff *et al*). Laryngol. Rhinol. Otol. (Stuttg.), *53:*887, 1974 (German)

Ear piercing, medical problems of (Biggar *et al*) N. Y. State J. Med., *75:*1460, 1975

Epidermal cyst of the external acoustic canal (Marusiak). Vestn. Otorinolaringol., *3:*102, 1975 (Russian)

Ear Deformities, Acquired

Relapsing polychondritis (Church). Proc. Roy. Soc. Med., *64:*1194, 1971

Acquired atresia of external auditory canal (Marlow). Arch. Otolaryng., *96:*380, 1972

Keloids, large auricular, eradication by excision, skin grafting, and intradermal injection of triamcinolone acetonide solution (Converse, Stallings), PRS, *49:*461, 1972

Ear deformities: relapsing polychondritis (Jones), PRS, *51:*331, 1973

Ear, "cauliflower," experimental production of, in rabbits (Pandya), PRS, *52:*534, 1973

Ear, external, absence or major loss of part of (Fine, Robinson, Barnhart), PRS, *54:*371, 1974. J. Prosth. Dent., *31:*313, 1974

Earlobe keloids, bilateral (Cosman, Wolff), PRS, *53:*540, 1974

Earlobe Z-plasty in Borneo (Abrahams), PRS, *53:*548, 1974

Cleft ear lobe: a method of repair with preservation of the earring canal (Buchan). Brit. J. Plast. Surg., *28:*296, 1975

Earlobes, cleft, method for repair of (Hamilton, LaRossa), PRS, *55:*99, 1975

Ear Deformities, Congenital (See also *Ear, Reconstruction of; Otoplasty*)

Microtia, congenital (Stallings *et al*), PRS, *49:*233, 1972. Arch. Otolaryng., *94:*176, 1971

Helix, correction of flat folded (Black), PRS, *48:*86, 1971

Cupped ear, surgical correction of (Kislov), PRS, *48:*121, 1971

Ear, total reconstruction of, in congenital microtia (Spina, Kamakura, Psillakis), PRS, *48:*349, 1971

Mandible, case of laterognathism supported by residue of Meckel's cartilage (Mangiante), PRS, *51:*102, 1973. Riv. ital. chir. plast., *3:*233, 1971

Aures alatae. A follow-up study of 104 patients operated on using Nordzell's method

Ear Deformities, Congenital — Cont.

(Albertsen). Ugeskr. Laeger., *133:*2419, 1971 (Danish)

Shell ear deformity, method of repairing (Maris), PRS, *51:*475, 1973. Acta chir. plast., *14:*47, 1972

Ears, classification of auricular anomalies and significance for their surgical treatment (Kruchinski), PRS, *52:*677, 1973. Acta chir. plast., *14:*225, 1972

Cryptotia, treatment using Teflon string (Ohmori, Matsumoto), PRS, *49:*33, 1972

Microtia, condition of auditory ossicles in; findings in 57 middle ear operations (Harada, Ishii), PRS, *50:*48, 1972

Trefoil flap, repair of cryptotic ear with (Wesser), PRS, *50:*192, 1972

Ear morphology in cleft lip and palate anomaly (Farkas *et al*). Arch. Otorhinolaryngol. (N.Y.), *206:*57, 1973

Conchal hypertrophy and correction of protruding ears (Schneider, Clodius), PRS, *55:*105, 1975. Brit. J. Plast. Surg., *26:*115, 1973

Ear, prominent, a simplified method for correcting the (Kaye) (Follow-Up Clinic), PRS, *52:*184, 1973

Concha-mastoid sutures, correction of prominent ears by (Furnas) (Follow-Up Clinic), PRS, *52:*434, 1973

Cryptotia: pathology and repair (Washio), PRS, *52:*648, 1973

Restoration of pinna in congenital microtia (Iarchuk). Zh. Ushn. Nos. Gorl. Belezn., *33:*46, 1973 (Russian)

Ear anomalies, temporal bone findings in trisomy D (Saito *et al*). PRS, *55:*717, 1975. Arch. Otolaryng., *100:*386, 1974

Ears of cleft palate patients, tympanometry, impedence and aural reflex testing (Billings, Lowry). PRS, *55:*380, 1975. Cleft Palate J., *11:*21, 1974

Congenital deformities of the auricle (Omori) Clin. Plast. Surg., *1:*3, 1974

Microtic ear reconstructed with silicone rubber frame (Ohmori, Matsumoto, Nakai). PRS, *56:*352, 1975. Jap. J. Plast. Reconstr. Surg., *17:*484, 1974

Pinna, surgery of anomalies of position and shape (Haas). Laryngol. Rhinol. Otol. (Stuttg.), *53:*93, 1974 (German)

Earlobe crease, diagonal: prevalence and implications as coronary risk factor (Lichstein *et al*). PRS, *54:*371, 1974. New England J. Med., *290:*615, 1974

Microtia: survey of 180 cases in 10 years (Fukuda). PRS, *53:*458, 1974

Microtia, reconstruction using silicone framework, follow-up study (Ohmori, Mat-

Ear Deformities, Congenital — Cont.

sumoto, Nakai). PRS, *53:*555, 1974

Ear, small defects of helix, rotation flap repair for (Elsahy). PRS, *53:*598, 1974

Ears, prominent, correcting (Pandeya, Furnas) (Letter to the Editor). PRS, *53:*670, 1974

Congenital lop ear, simplified technique for correction (Kaye, Lotuaco). PRS, *54:*667, 1974

Ear, middle and inner, dysplasias in different types of malformation (Mundnich). PRS, *56:*352, 1975. Proc. Roy. Soc. Med., *67:*1197, 1974

Agenesis of external ear, surgery of (Batstone). PRS, *55:*715, 1975. Proc. Roy. Soc. Med., *67:*1199, 1974

Ear abnormalities excluding agenesis, surgery of (Maisels). PRS, *55:*714, 1975. Proc. Roy. Soc. Med., *67:*1201, 1974

Congenital atresia of the ear: the otological problem (Coleman). Proc. Roy. Soc. Med., *67:*1203, 1974

Rerouting the external auditory canal. A method of correcting congenital stenosis (Baron). Arch. Otolaryng., *101:*238, 1975

Ear, constricted (cup and lop) (Tanzer). PRS, *55:*406, 1975

Ear, Injuries of, (See also *Ear, Reconstruction; Replantation*)

Ear part, severed, pocket principle for reattachment (Mladick *et al*). PRS, *48:*219, 1971

Successful replantation of a severed half ear (McDowell), PRS *48:*281, 1971

Accidental injuries of the ears (Fischer). Hippokrates, *43:*251, 1972 (German)

Earlobe, torn, repair of, with preservation of perforation for earring (Pardue). PRS, *51:*472, 1973

Ear reattachment by the modified pocket principle (Mladick, Carraway). PRS, *51:*584, 1973

"Cauliflower ear" in rabbits, experimental production of (Pandya). PRS, *2:*534, 1973

Lightning damaged ear (Bergstrom *et al*). PRS, *55:*106, 1975. Arch. Otolaryng., *100:*117, 1974

Reconstruction of severed ears by implanting cartilage (Lo). Chinese Med. J., *54:*714, 1974 (Chinese)

Frostbite of ears treated with flurandrenolide ointment (Kobak). PRS, *57:*529, 1976. Eye, Ear, Nose & Throat Month., *54:*31, 1974

Chondritis in burned ear treated by local instillation of antibiotics (Apfelberg *et al*). PRS, *53:*179, 1974

Management of injuries of auricles and nose

Ear, Injuries of—Cont.
(Biskupska-Wiedo *et al*). Pol. Przegl. Chir., *46:*619, 1974 (Polish)
Cleft earlobes, method for repair of (Hamilton, LaRossa). PRS, *55:*99, 1975

Ear, Neoplasms of

Cancer, auricular, some surgical and pathologic considerations (Arons, Savin). PRS, *51:*607, 1973. Am. J. Surg.,*122:*770, 1971
Ear, middle, and mastoid neoplasm (Goodman). PRS, *49:*238, 1972. Ann. Otol. Rhin. & Laryng., *80:*419, 1971
Two cases of unusual tumors of the ear (Mitrovic *et al*). Med. Glas., *25:*86, 1971 (Croatian)
Ear defect, "button" skin repair of (Gordon). PRS, *48:*190, 1971
Otolaryngology and plastic surgery, complementary roles in major malignancies of the middle ear (Bodenham). PRS, *50:*313, 1972. Proc. Roy. Soc. Med., *65:*248, 1972
Glomus jugulare tumors: effect of irradiation (Brackmann *et al*). Trans. Am. Acad. Ophtalmol. Otolaryngol. 76:1423, 1972
Ear, external, epitheliomas of (Kokoschka *et al*). Z. Haut. Geschiechtskr., *47:*779, 1972 (German)
Ear and mandible, unusual tumors of (Horowitz) Arch. Klin. Exp. Ohren Nasen Kehlkopfheilkd., *205:*203, 1973 (German)
Ear, squamous carcinoma of (Lewis). PRS, *52:*600, 1973. Arch. Otolaryng., *97:*41, 1973
Hamartomas of ear and nose (Kacker *et al*). J. Laryng. & Otol., *87:*801, 1973
Cancer, external ear, *en bloc* subtotal temporal bone resection for (Yamada *et al*). J. Neurosurg., *39:*370, 1973
Carcinoma, ear, external (Jeppson *et al*). O. R. L., *35:*336, 1973
Ear, cylindroma of (Riabina *et al*). Vestn. Otorinolaringol., *35:*93, 1973 (Russian)
Diagnosis and treatment of cylindromas of otorhinolaryngologic organs (Opanashchenko *et al*). Zh. Ushn. Nos. Gorl. Bolezn., *33:*104, 1973 (Russian)
Surgical treatment (Matton *et al*). Acta chir. Belg., *73:*189, 1974 (French)
Ear, malignant tumors of auricle (Blake, Wilson). PRS, *57:*125, 1976. Brit. J. Plast. Surg., *27:*67, 1974
Ear, malignant tumors of external auditory meatus, middle ear cleft, and temporal bone (Wilson *et al*). PRS, *57:*124, 1976. Brit. J. Plast. Surg., *27:*77, 1974
Carcinoma of middle ear and temporal bone, total resection of temporal bone (Wu *et al*). PRS, *55:*635, 1975. Chinese M. J., *2:*23, 1974

Ear, Neoplasms of—Cont.
Ganglioneuroma of the auricle. Case report (Szmeja *et al*). Otolaryngol. Pol., *28:*687, 1974 (Polish)
Core resection, composite regional ear resection (Mladick *et al*). PRS, *53:*281, 1974
Helix of ear, small defects of, rotation flap repair for (Elsahy). PRS, *53:*598, 1974
Ear, squamous cell carcinomas of skin of pinna (Shiffman). PRS, *57:*403, 1976. Canad. J. Surg., *18:*279, 1975
Carcinoma, external auditory canal. Extended exeresis of canal before irradiation (Gaillard *et al*). J. Fr. Otorhinolaryngol., *24:*137, 1975 (French)
Carcinoma of the external ear (Skonieczny *et al*). Otolaryngol. Pol., *29:*61, 1975 (Polish)

Ear, Reconstruction of

Simple precedure for reconstruction of the lower part of the auricle (Preaux). Ann. chir. plast., *16:*60, 1971 (French)
"Button" skin repair of an ear defect (Gordon). PRS, *48:*190, 1971
Mastoid shell. Uses in ear aplasia and external ear amputations (Muler *et al*). Ann. Otolaryngol. Chir. Cervicofac., *89:*547, 1972
Simple island flap for reconstruction of concha-helix defects (Masson). Brit. J. Plast. Surg., *25:*399, 1972
Ear flaps (Argamaso). Eye Ear Nose & Throat Mon., *51:*310, 1972
Reconstruction of the external ear in children (Bloomenstein). J. Med. Soc. N. J., *69:*148, 1972
Meatoplasty transposition flaps (Beal *et al*). Laryngoscope, *82:*404, 1972
Ear, burned, reconstruction of (Lawrence *et al*). Otolaryngol. Clin. North Am., *5:*667, 1972
Anthropometric studies of auricle from standpoint of reconstructive procedures in auricular hypoplasia (Biskcupska-Wiecko). Otolaryngol. Pol., *26:*537, 1972 (Polish)
Ear loss, subtotal, reconstruction with two skin tubes (Aiache, Chen). PRS, *49:*86, 1972 (Discussion by Wynn, PRS, *49:*332, 1972)
Ear implants, Silastic, our experiences with (Lynch *et al*). PRS, *49:*283, 1972
Auricular loss, partial, reconstruction of (Nagel). PRS, *49:*340, 1972
Ear framework, silicone, our experiences with, a report of 17 ears in 15 patients (Monroe). PRS, *49:*428, 1972
Ear reconstruction by composite grafts (Rubin) (Follow-Up Clinic). PRS, *49:*454,

Ear, Reconstruction of—Cont.
1972
Auricle, reconstruction of (Walter). PRS, *50:*418, 1972
Earlobe reconstruction by use of preauricular flap (Pitanguy *et al*). PRS, *51:*602, 1973. Rev. brasil. cir., *62:*51, 1972
Ear, external, reconstruction of traumatic losses of (Avakoff *et al*). South. Med. J., *65:*1471, 1972
Reparative surgery of the nose and ear (Omori). Surg. Ther. (Osaka), *26:*548, 1972 (Japanese)
External ear reconstruction using skin from the retroauricular area and preserved cartilage (Kovlenko *et al*). Vestn. Khir., *103:*114, 1972 (Russian)
Auricle reconstruction using reinforced auricular cartilage (Kruchinski). PRS, *53:*601, 1974. Acta chir. plast., *15:*72, 1973
Ear, human external, reconstruction of, in animal experiments (Nagel). Arch. Klin. Exp. Ohren Nasen Kehlkopfheilkd., *205:*166, 1973 (German)
Silastic frameworks in total reconstruction of auricle (Wray *et al*). Brit. J. Plast. Surg., *26:*296, 1973
Synthetic implants, plastic surgery application of (Gerow *et al*). Med. Instrum., *7:*96, 1973
Auricle reconstruction, symposium on, PRS, *51:*495, 1973
Symposium on the Reconstruction of the Auricle. Ed. by Radford C. Tanzer and Milton T. Edgerton. C. V. Mosby Co., St. Louis, 1974. PRS, *56:*571, 1975
Restoration of the external ear in aplasias using skin grafts in the canal (Poncet *et al*). Ann. Otolaryngol. Chir. Cervicofac., *91:*526, 1974 (French)
Ear, external, surgery of (McLaren). J. Laryng. & Otol., *88:*23, 1974
Two cases of reconstruction of soft tissue defects of the face caused by human bite (Bertenyl). Magy. Traumatol. Orthop., *17:*126, 1974 (Hungarian)
Ear reconstruction, protective guard for use during (Tanzer, Chaisson). PRS, *53:*236, 1974
Otoplasty in microtic ear: survey of 180 cases in 10 years (Fukuda). PRS, *53:*458, 1974
Ear reconstruction with expansile framework of autogenous rib cartilage (Brent). PRS, *53:*619, 1974
Helix, sommersault flap for reconstruction of (Tofield). Brit. J. Plast. Surg., *28:*71, 1975
Auricular defects, partial, laminate-plasty reconstruction of (Pless). PRS, *57:*394, 1976. Scand. J. Plast. Reconstr. Surg.,

Ear, Reconstruction of—Cont.
*9:*40, 1975
Correction of partial defects of the pinna (Kruchinskil *et al*). Vestn. Otorinolaringol., *4:*10, 1975 (Russian)
Earlobe construction with auriculo-mastoid flap (Brent). PRS, *57:*389, 1976

EARLE, A. S.: Treatment of the chronic, painful metatarsal callus by a tendon transfer (with Kiehn, DesPrez). PRS, *51:*154, 1973
EARLE, A. S., KIEHN, C. L., AND DESPREZ, J. D.: Regional block of the thigh: uses in plastic surgery. PRS, *49:*134, 1972
EARLE, A. S., FRATIANNE, R. B., AND NUNEZ, F. D.: Relationship of hematocrit levels to skin flap survival in the dog. PRS, *54:*341, 1974
EARLE, A. S., AND BLACKBURN, W. W.: Closure of abdominal hernia with groin flap lined with dermal graft. PRS, *56:*447, 1975
EASTRIDGE, C. E.: Pharyngo-esophageal diverticulum. South. Med. J., *65:*745, 1972
EASTWOOD, D. S.: Autografting in the treatment of squamous cell carcinoma in epidermolysis bullosa dystrophica. PRS, *49:*93, 1972
EATON, RICHARD G.: *Joint Injuries of the Hand.* Charles C Thomas, Springfield, Ill. 1971. PRS, *49:*338, 1972
EBBEHOJ, J.: New operation for priapism, PRS, *56:*357, 1975. Scand. J. Plast. Reconstr. Surg., *8:*241, 1974
EBERLE, R. C.: Facial reanimation in facial paralysis. Otolaryngol. Clin. North Am., *5:*631, 1972
EBERT, P. R., MCWILLIAMS, B. J., AND WOOLF, G.: Comparison of written language ability of cleft palate and normal children, PRS, *55:*381, 1975. Cleft Palate J., *11:*17, 1974
EBNER, H. *et al*: Skin carcinomas in the region of the lower extremities. Wien. Klin. Wochenschr., *83:*459, 1971 (German)
EBNER, H. *et al*: Treatment of keratoacanthoma. Wien. Med. Wochenschr., *125:*91, 1975 (German)
EBSKOV, B.: Kinesiological recording of motion with particular emphasis on electrogoniometers, PRS, *49:*583, 1972. Scand J. Plast. Reconstr. Surg., *5:*96, 1971
ECHTERNACH, J. L.: Electrophysiological testing in facial nerve dysfunction. Phys. Ther., *54:*843, 1974
ECKE, M.: Current problems in children's urology. Z. Urol. Nephrol., *67:*623, 1974 (German)
ECKERT, M. *et al*: Ectopic mammary gland on the back. Dtsch. Med. Wochenschr., *100:*1395, 1975 (German)
ECKHARDT, D. *et al*: Diagnostic significance of

tomography of the hand in rheumatoid arthritis. Radiol. Diagn. (Berl.), *14:*215, 1973 (German)

ECKHAUSER, F. E. *et al*: Tracheostomy complicating massive burn injury. Plea for conservatism. Am. J. Surg., *127:*418, 1974

ECKSTEIN, H. B.: Problems of primary closure of myelomeningoceles, PRS, *49:*471, 1972. Proc. Roy. Soc. Med., *64:*1143, 1971

ECKSTEIN, H. B.: An assessment of the functional results of various forms of surgery for epispadias and exstrophy. Langenbecks Arch. Chir., *339:*439, 1975 (German)

Ectropion

Cicatricial ectropion in epidermolysis bullosa and in congenital ichthyosis: its plastic repair (Hill *et al*). Can. J. Ophthalmol., *6:*89, 1971

Corrective surgery in scarring ectropion of the lower eyelid (Andreeva *et al*). Vestn. Khir., *107:*49, 1971 (Russian)

Sutureless fixation of free skin transplants during removal of cicatricial deformities of the eyelids (Poliakova *et al*). Vestn. Oftalmol., *3:*56, 1971 (Russian)

Surgery of senile ectropion and entropion (Fox). Ann. Ophth., *4:*217, 1972

Eyelid, upper, retraction, surgical treatment of (Putterman, Urist). PRS, *50:*417, 1972. Arch. Ophth., *87:*401, 1972

Ectropion, spastic, surgery for (Vodovozov). Oftalmol. Zh., *27:*390, 1972

Ectropion, simple method for correcting, preliminary report (Anderl). PRS, *49:*156, 1972

Ectropion, lower lid, causes and prevention of, following blepharoplasty (Edgerton). PRS, *49:*367, 1972

Ectropion resulting from blepharoplasty, correction of (Rees). PRS, *50:*1, 1972

Congenital upper eyelid eversion and Down's syndrome (Gilbert *et al*). Am. J Ophth., *75:*469, 1973

Ectropion, cicatricial, associated with lamellar ichthyosis (Shindle, Leone). Arch. Ophth., *89:*62, 1973

Original Z-plasty (Borges *et al*). Brit. J. Plast. Surg., *26:*237, 1973

Ectropion, cicatricial, of lower lid (Singha *et al*). Indian J. Ophthalmol., *21:*82, 1973

Ectropion from burns of eyelids: treatment of eyelid deformities due to burns (Silverstein, Peterson). PRS, *51:*38, 1973

Ectropion: correction of complications after levator resections for blepharoptosis (Callahan). PRS, *52:*616, 1973

Classification of post-burn cicatricial deformations of the eyelids (Ter-Andriasov).

Ectropion—Cont.

Voen. Med. Zh., *8:*20, 1973 (Russian)

Ultrastructural changes in senile atrophy of *orbicularis oculi* muscle (Radnot *et al*). Am. J. Ophth., *78:*689, 1974

Total eversion of upper lids (Roussos). Ann. Ophth., *6:*633, 1974

Ichthyosis congenita (Katowitz *et al*). Arch. Ophth., *91:*208, 1974

Ectropion, severe cicatricial, surgical correction (Guibor, Smith). PRS, *55:*633, 1975. Arch. Ophth., *92:*304, 1974

Surgical management of paralyzed *orbicularis oculi* (Rich). Trans. Am. Acad. Ophthalmol. Otolaryngol., *78:*622, 1974

Ectropion after lower lid strain due to scar adherence (Hartel). In *Plastische und Wiederherstellungs-Chirurgie*, ed. by Hohler; pp. 323-4. Stuttgart; Schattauer, 1975 (German)

Common problems in ophthalmic plastic surgery (Carroll). Am. Fam. Physician, *12:*85, 1975

Repair of cicatricial ectropion by horizontal shortening and pedicle flap (Leone). Ophthalmic Surg., *6:*47, 1975

EDEL, A.: Use of a free connective tissue graft to increase the width of attached gingiva. Oral Surg., *39:*341, 1975

EDELSON, R. L.: Defining malignant potential of giant pigmented nevus (With Dellon, Chretien). PRS, *57:*611, 1976

EDER, H.: Prophylaxis of breast cancer. Wien. Klin. Wochenschr., *86:*153, 1974 (German)

EDER, M.: After care in Hodgkin's disease (pathology). Fortschr. Geb. Roentgenstr. Nuklearmed. Suppl: 116-7 1973 (German)

EDGELL, P. G.: Psychiatrist joins surgery of appearance symposium—personal point of view. Can. J. Otolaryngol., *2:*72, 1973

EDGERTON, M. T., JR.: Transbuccal flaps for reconstruction of the floor of the mouth (with Cohen). PRS, *48:*8, 1971

EDGERTON, M. T., JR.: Surgical advances in the treatment of rare craniofacial anomalies. South. Med. J., *64:*1348, 1971

EDGERTON, M. T., JR.: Reconstruction. J.A.M.A., *221:*1258, 1972

EDGERTON, M. T., JR.: Causes and prevention of lower lid ectropion following blepharoplasty. PRS, *49:*367, 1972

EDGERTON, M. T., JR.: Factitious wounds; a psychiatric and surgical dilemma (with Drinker, Knorr). PRS, *50:*458, 1972

EDGERTON, M. T., JR.: Honorary award of American Association of Plastic Surgeons to Dr. Jerome P. Webster. Presentation speech. PRS, *50:*510, 1972

EDGERTON, M. T., JR.: Discussion of "Visor flap reconstruction of massive oropharyngeal defect," by Griffin *et al.* PRS, *51:*582, 1973

EDGERTON, M. T., JR.: Transsexualism – a surgical problem? (Editorial). PRS, *52:*74, 1973

EDGERTON, M. T., JR.: Rehabilitation of oral cavity by plastic surgery after cancer resections. Proc. Natl. Cancer Conf., *7:*199, 1973

EDGERTON, M. T., JR.: The surgical treatment of male transsexuals. Clin. Plast. Surg., *1:*285, 1974

EDGERTON, M. T., JR.: Reeducation of sensation in hand after nerve injury and repair (with Dellon, Curtis). PRS, *53:*297, 1974

EDGERTON, M. T., JR.: Role of plastic surgery in academic medicine. Presidential address. PRS, *54:*523, 1974

EDGERTON, M. T., JR.: New hope for the child with major craniofacial deformity. Birth Defects, *11:*297, 1975

EDGERTON, M. T., JR.: Plastic surgeon's obligations to the emotionally disturbed patient (Editorial). PRS, *55:*81, 1975

Edgerton, Milton T., Jr.: 1974 Dow Corning Award Given to. PRS, *55:*391, 1975

EDGERTON, M. T., JR.: Cross-hand finger transfer. PRS, *57:*281, 1976

EDGERTON, M. T., JR.: Surgical correction of absent nasal alae of Johanson-Blizzard syndrome (with Fox, Golden). PRS, *57:*484, 1976

EDGERTON, M. T., JR.: Frontonasal dysplasia with alar clefts in two sisters; genetic considerations and surgical correction (with Fox, Golden). PRS, *57:*553, 1976

EDGERTON, M. T., JR., AND KNORR, N. J.: Motivational patterns of patients seeking cosmetic (esthetic) surgery, PRS, *48:*551, 1971

EDGERTON, M. T., JANE, J. A., AND BERRY, F. A.: Craniofacial osteotomies and reconstructions in infants and young children, PRS, *54:*13, 1974

EDGERTON, M. T. *et al*: Feasibility of craniofacial osteotomies in infants and young children, PRS, *56:*464, 1975. Scand. J. Plast. Reconstr. Surg., *8:*164, 1974

EDGERTON, M. T., TUERK, D. B., AND FISHER, J. C.: Surgical treatment of Moebius syndrome by platysma and *temporalis* muscle transfers. PRS, *55:*305, 1975

EDINAK, B. I.: Terms of dermoplasty of burn wounds in children (based on cytology of wound exudate). Ortop. Travmatol. Protez., *33:*11, 1972 (Russian)

EDISON, B. D.: Frey's syndrome: diagnosis and treatment, Eye, Ear, Nose & Throat Mon., *53:*50, 1974

Editorials

Filed under this heading are also articles and books of a general or philosophical nature, even though they were not written as editorials.

The Continuing Education of the Surgeon. Ed. by Harold G. Barker. Charles C Thomas, Springfield, Ill., 1971. PRS, *48:*590, 1971

Marjolin's ulcer. Ill. Med. J., *140:*500, 1971

Ill-fated JCAH, or who is going to inspect hospitals? (McDowell). PRS, *48:*65, 1971

Fifth International Congress of Plastic Surgery, President's Address (Rank). PRS, *48:*207, 1971

Excerpts from chairman's address to American Board of Plastic Surgery (Crikelair). PRS, *48:*492, 1971

Sliding the midface forward under the cranium (McDowell). PRS, *48:*495, 1971

Ameloblastomas in young people. Subperiosteal resections. Rev. Stomatol. Chir. Maxillofac., *72:*667, 1971 (French)

The Case for American Medicine: A Realistic Look at our Health Care System. By Harry Schwartz. David McKay Co., New York, 1972. PRS, *53:*85, 1974

Laryngology, new horizons in (Von Leden). Acta Otolaryngol. (Stockh.), *74:*332, 1972

Mortality, comparative, for various surgical operations in older versus younger age groups (Ziffren *et al*). J. Am. Geriatr. Soc., *20:*485, 1972

Hair autografts. Lancet. *2:*417, 1972

Cosmetic surgery and the university hospital (Goldwyn). PRS, *49:*76, 1972

Case of the elusive Mr. Lucas, the mysterious Major Heitland, *et al.* (McDowell). PRS, *49:*77, 1972

Promotion of verbal and written communication of ideas to professional colleagues (Ivy). PRS, *49:*200, 1972

"Personal" communications (Daniel) (Letter to the Editor). PRS, *49:*203, 1972

What's new in esthetic surgery (Gurdin). PRS, *49:*448, 1972

Experimental method (Grabb). PRS, *49:*563, 1972

Whither subcutaneous mastectomy? (Freeman). PRS, *49:*654, 1972

On subcutaneous mastectomy (Weiner). PRS, *49:*654, 1972

Role of the plastic surgeon in undergraduate medical education (Berggren). PRS, *50:*75, 1972

Preoperative selection and counseling of patients for rhinoplasty (Thomson). PRS, *50:*174, 1972

Department of negative results (McDowell). PRS, *50:*507, 1972

Voice of Polite Dissent (McDowell). PRS, *50:*507, 1972

Medicine, American, on collectivization of

EDLAN, A.: Pre-prosthetic surgery – a new technique in edentulous lower jaw. Trans. Congr. Int. Assoc. Oral Surg., *4:*191, 1973

EDLICH, R., SMITH, Q., AND EDGERTON, M.: Resistance of surgical wound to antimicrobial prophylaxis and its mechanism of development, PRS, *54:*114, 1974. Am. J. Surg., *126:*583, 1973

EDLICH, R. F. *et al*: Studies in management of contaminated wound. VI. Therapeutic value of gentle scrubbing in prolonging limited period of effectiveness of antibiotics in contaminated wounds, PRS, *49:*668, 1972. Am. J. Surg., *121:*668, 1971. VIII. Assessment of tissue adhesives for repair of contaminated tissue, PRS, *49:*361, 1972. Am. J. Surg., *122:*394, 1971

EDSMYR, F. *et al*: Radiotherapy in treatment of keloids in East Africa. East Afr. Med. J., *50:*457, 1973

EDSON-SPERLI, A.: Considerations on aesthetic plastic surgery of face, PRS, *53:*239, 1974. Rev. Latino Am. cir. plast., *17:*15, 1973

EDWARDS, B. F.: Bilateral temporal neurotomy for frontalis hypermotility (Follow-Up Clinic), PRS, *48:*370, 1971

EDWARDS, CHARLES BEAVER: *Beyond Plastic Surgery.* Wayne State University Press, Detroit, 1972. PRS, *51:*329, 1973

EDWARDS, D. H.: Spectrum of hand injuries. Hand, *7:*46, 1975

EDWARDS, J. M.: Malignant melanoma: surgical aspects of treatment. Proc. Roy. Soc. Med., *65:*140, 1972

EDWARDS, J. M. *et al*: Lymphangiography and surgery in lymphangioma of the skin. Brit. J. Surg., *59:*36, 1972

EDWARDS, M.: Letter: cleft lip and palate. Brit. Med. J., *3:*578, 1974

EFIMOV, I. S. *et al*: Free skin plasty in traumatic lesions of foot. Klin. Khir., *10:*49, 1973 (Russian)

EGGLESTON, F. C., AND FEIERABEND, T. C.: Early acidosis of burns: relationship to extent of burn and management, PRS, *57:*762, 1976. Surgery, *77:*641, 1975

EGOROV, E. A. *et al*: Indications for endonasal dacryocystorhinostomy. Vestn. Oftalmol., *5:*75, 1974 (Russian)

EGURO, H., AND GOLDNER, J. L.: Bilateral thrombosis of the ulnar arteries, in the hands, PRS, *52:*573, 1973

EGYEDI, P.: An experimental investigation into the relapse problem in vestibuloplasties with secondary epithelialization. Aust. Dent. J., *17:*67, 1972

EGYEDI, P.: Degloving nose, PRS, *55:*375, 1975. J. Maxillo-facial Surg., *2:*101, 1974

EGYEDI, P., AND BEYAZIT, E.: Marsupialization of large cysts of maxillas into the maxillary sinus and/or nose. Follow-up investigation. Trans. Congr. Int. Assoc. Oral Surg., *4:*81, 1973

EHLER, E. *et al*: Lever effects on mandible. 4. Lever lengths of mandible in dogs following experimental exclusion of masticatory muscles. Anat. Anz., *134:*425, 1973 (German)

EHLERS, G., AND STEPHAN, T.: Quantitative histochemical investigations on DNA content of facultatives and obligatory precanceroses of skin, PRS, *51:*107, 1973. Arch. Derm. Forsch., *243:*114, 1972

Ehlers-Danlos Syndrome

Cutis laxa with abnormal copper metabolism, case (Ferreira *et al*). Brit. J. Plast. Surg., *26:*283, 1973

Ehlers-Danlos syndrome, coexisting with a Martin-Gruber anastomosis. A case report (Posner). Ohio State Med. J., *69:*453, 1973

Cutis laxa, its physiopathology and surgical treatment (Castro Ferreira, Psillakis), PRS, *52:*682, 1973. Rev. Assoc. Med. Brasil, *19:*9, 1973

Syndromes, Ehlers-Danlos and Marfan's, combined with case report (Birkenstock *et al*). S. Afr. Med. J., *47:*2097, 1973

Hip dislocation in Ehlers-Danlos syndrome (Milkovska-Dimitrova, Ilief), PRS, *54:*511, 1974. Lyon chir., *70:*38, 1974

Cutis laxa (Hashimoto, Kanzaki), PRS, *57:*539, 1976. Arch. Dermat., *111:*861, 1975

Syndrome, Ehlers-Danlos, contribution to (Fuxa *et al*). Klin. Monatsbl. Augenheilkd., *166:*247, 1975

EHRICHT, R.: Contribution to the construction of resection prostheses in cases of limited oral aperture. Dtsch. Zahnaerztl. Z., *29:*948, 1974 (German)

EHRIG, U. *et al*: Fibrous dysplasia of bone and primary hyperparathyroidism. Ann. Intern. Med., *77:*234, 1972

EHRING, F. *et al*: Rehabilitation even for disfigured persons. Oeff. Gesundheitswes., *34:*529, 1972 (German)

EHRLICH, H. P., TARVER, H., AND HUNT, T. K.: Inhibitory effects of vitamin E on collagen synthesis and wound repair, PRS, *50:*421, 1972. Ann. Surg., *175:*235, 1972

EHRLICH, H. P., GRISLIS, G., AND HUNT, T. J.: Metabolic and circulatory contributions to oxygen gradients in wounds, PRS, *51:*352, 1973. Surgery, *72:*578, 1972

EICHER, E. *et al*: Alternatives to amputation in extreme Dupuytren's contracture. Handchirurgie, 2:56, 1970 (German)

EICHER, W. et al: Psychological aspects in plastic surgery of the breast. Fortschr. Med., 92:1407, 1974 (German)

EICHER, W. et al: Proceedings: psychological aspects in augmentation and reduction plasties. Arch. Gynaekol., 219:157, 1975 (German)

EIGENTHALER, L.: Motility disorders of the eye in injuries of the osseous orbit (accident surgery report). Wien. Med. Wochenschr., 122: Suppl 5:2, 1972 (German)

EILBER, F. R. et al: Immunologic abnormalities in head and neck cancer. Am. J. Surg., 128:534, 1974

EILBER, F. R. et al: Adjuvant immunotherapy with BCG in treatment of regional-lymph-node metastases from malignant melanoma. New England J. Med., 294:237, 1976

EINHORN, I. H. et al: Prognostic correlations and response to treatment in advanced metastatic malignant melanoma, PRS, 55:115, 1975. Cancer Res., 34:1995, 1974

EISEMAN, G.: Augmentation mammaplasty by the trans-axillary approach, PRS, 54:229, 1974

EJIDE, A. O.: Present and future role of plastic surgery in Africa. A viewpoint. East Afr. Med. J., 52:599, 1975

ELBAZ, C.: Surgical treatment of lymphedema of the lower limb (current orientations). Phlebologie, 24:253, 1971 (French)

ELBAZ, J. S.: Abdominal plastic surgery. "Horse shoe" technic. Ann. chir. plast., 19:155, 1974 (French)

ELBAZ, J. S.: Technique of mammaplasty with J-shaped scar, PRS, 57:260, 1976. Ann. chir. plast., 20:101, 1975

ELBAZ, J. S. et al: L-form cicatrix in breast plastic surgery. Ann. chir. plast., 17:283, 1972 (French)

ELBER, F. R. et al: Immunologic abnormalities in head and neck cancer. Am. J. Surg., 128:534, 1974

ELBROND, O. et al: Combined irradiation and surgical treatment of cancer of the nasal cavity and the nasal sinuses. Ugeskr. Laeger, 134:1149, 1972 (Danish)

ELBROND, O. et al: Carcinoma of tongue. Incidence and management of regional lymph node metastasis. Acta Otolaryngol. (Stockh.), 75:310, 1973

ELBROND, O. et al: Carcinoma linguae. Series of 96 patients. Acta Radiol. (Ther.) (Stockh.), 12:465, 1973

EL-D BARRADA, A. et al: Ptosis: some anatomical and surgical considerations. Bull. Ophthalmol. Soc. Egypt, 65:545, 1972

EL-DEIRY, A.: Maxillary sinus carcinoma. Can.

J. Otolaryngol., 2:101, 1973

EL-DOMEIRI, A. A. et al: Sweat gland carcinoma: clinico-pathological study of 83 patients, PRS, 48:93, 1971. Ann. Surg., 173:270, 1971

EL-DOMEIRI, A. A., AND PAGLIA, M. A.: Carcinoma of scrotum, radical excision and repair using ox fascia: case report, PRS, 50:94, 1972. J. Urol., 106:575, 1971

EL-DOMEIRI, A. A. et al: Management of oral and pharyngeal cancer: a multidisciplinary approach. Surg. Clin. North Am., 55:107, 1975

Elephantiasis: See Lymphedema

EL-FALAKY, M. H.: Use of bipedicled flaps in the management of pretibial skin defects. Aust. N.Z. J. Surg., 41:253, 1972

ELIACHAR, E. et al: Congenital curving of long bones, PRS, 57:119, 1976. Ann. Pediat., 22:61, 1975

ELIAS, A. C. et al: Orthodontic surgery: important part of treatment of skeletal malocclusions. Case presentation. Int. J. Orthod., 11:75, 1973

ELIAS, A. C. et al: Orthodontic treatment during intermaxillary immobilization period following surgical correction of prognathism. Oral Surg., 37:526, 1974

ELIAS, E. G., AND MITTELMAN, A.: Lymphoma of head and neck masquerading as carcinoma, PRS, 49:360, 1972. Am. J. Surg., 122:424, 1971

ELIAS, S., AND CHVAPIL, M.: Zinc and wound healing in normal and chronically ill rats, PRS, 53:495, 1974. J. Surg. Res., 15:59, 1973

ELIN, R. J.: Enhanced resistance to certain infections in vitamin A-treated mice (with Cohen), PRS, 54:192, 1974

ELINEK, R.: Treatment of cancer of the vestibule of the larynx and of the root of the tongue. Vestn. Otorinolaringol., 34:89, 1972 (Russian)

ELIOPOULOS, C. et al: Hemipelvectomy—indications, technic and results on 4 cases, PRS, 56:473, 1975. Tr. 8th Panhellenic Cong. Surg. Soc., A: 263, 1973

ELKEN, O.: Aspects of rheumatoid hand surgery. Acta Orthop. Belg., 58:9, 1972

ELL, P. J.: Dermal overgrafting in treatment of venous stasis ulcers, a substitute for skin flap repairs in some injuries of the extremities (with Thompson), PRS, 54:290, 1974

ELLEGAST, H.: Motility disorders of the eye in injuries of the osseous orbit (x-ray report). Wien. Med. Wochenschr., 122: Suppl 5:7, 1972 (German)

ELLENBERG, A. H.: Surgical tape wound closure: disenchantment (Follow-Up Clinic),

PRS, *52:*80, 1973

ELLIOT, G. B., MacDOUGALL, J. A., AND EL-LIOTT, J. D. A.: Problems of verrucose squamous carcinoma, PRS, *52:*215, 1973. Ann. Surg., *177:*21, 1973

ELLIOTT, R. A., JR.: Injuries to the extensor mechanism of the hand. Orthop. Clin. North Am., *1:*335, 1970

ELLIOTT, R. A., JR.: Splints for mallet and boutonniere deformities, PRS, *52:*282, 1973

ELLIOTT, R. A., JR., AND HOEHN, H. G.: Use of commercial porcine skin for wound dressings, PRS, *52:*401, 1973

ELLIOTT, R. A., JR., HOEHN, J. G., AND GREMINGER, R. F.: Correction of asymmetrical breasts, PRS, *56:*260, 1975

ELLIS, B. P., AND TAUBE, E.: Clofazimine ointment in treatment of trophic ulcers. South African M.J., *47:*378, 1973

ELLIS, D. A.: Development of aging face. Can. J. Otolaryngol., *2:*231, 1973

ELLIS, D. G.: Duplicate exstrophy of bladder, PRS, *50:*200, 1972. J. Urol., *106:*295, 1971

ELLIS, D. J. *et al*: Aneurysmal bone cyst of the maxilla. Oral Surg., *34:*26, 1972

ELLIS, D. J. *et al*: Osteomyelitis, iatrogenic osteolysis, pathologic fracture and bone graft. Oral Surg., *37:*364, 1974

ELLIS, H.: Hyperhidrosis and its surgical management, PRS, *57:*538, 1976. Postgrad. Med., *58:*191, 1975

ELLIS, J. S.: Peripheral nerve injuries, PRS, *56:*230, 1975. Hand, *6:*142, 1974

ELLISON, M. R., KELLY, K. J., AND FLATT, A. E.: Results of surgical synovectomy of digital joints in rheumatoid disease, PRS, *50:*631, 1972. J. Bone & Joint Surg., *53:*1041, 1971

ELLISON, M. R. *et al*: Ulnar drift of the fingers in rheumatoid disease. Treatment by crossed intrinsic tendon transfer. J. Bone & Joint Surg. (Am.), *53:*1061, 1971

EL-MOFTY, S.: Surgical treatment of ankylosis of temporomandibular joint, PRS, *55:*106, 1975. J. Oral Surg., *32:*202, 1974

EL-NAGGAR, A. M.: Globus fixus as rare complication to orbitotomy, irradiation of lid tumors or plastic reconstruction of lids. Bull. Ophthalmol. Soc. Egypt, *64:*535, 1971

ELNER, A. *et al*: Combined radiological and surgical therapy of cancer of the ethmoid. Acta Otolaryngol., *78:*270, 1974

ELOMAA, M. *et al*: Melanotic neuroectodermal tumor of infancy. Case report and review. Proc. Finn. Dent. Soc., *69:*227, 1973

ELSAHY, N. I.: Scrotal and penile lymphedema as complication of testicular prosthesis, PRS, *52:*207, 1973. J. Urol., *108:*595, 1972

ELSAHY, N. I.: New method for correction of traumatic footdrop, PRS, *50:*614, 1972

ELSAHY, N. I.: Use of Foley catheter in perineal urethrostomy, PRS, *53:*488, 1974. Acta chir. plast., *15:*131, 1973

ELSAHY, N. I.: Modified striped Y – a systematic classification for cleft lip and palate. Cleft Palate J., *10:*247, 1973

ELSAHY, N. I.: Moebius syndrome associated with the mother taking thalidomide during gestation, PRS, *51:*93, 1973

ELSAHY, N. I.: Replantation of composite graft of nasal ala, PRS, *55:*633, 1975. Acta chir. plast., *16:*124, 1974

ELSAHY, N. I.: New method for correcting cleft lip nasal deformities, PRS, *55:*383, 1975. Cleft Palate J., *11:*214, 1974

ELSAHY, N. I.: Reverse pollicization for thumb reconstruction, PRS, *56:*357, 1975. Hand, *6:*233, 1974

ELSAHY, N. I.: Rotation flap repair for small defects of helix of ear, PRS, *53:*598, 1974

ELSAHY, N. I.: Use of dermal flaps in treatment of protruding ears, PRS, *57:*755, 1976. Acta chir. plast., *17:*71, 1975

ELSAHY, N. I.: Doppler ultrasound detection of displaced neurovascular bundles in Dupuytren's contracture, PRS, *57:*104, 1976

ELSAHY, N. I.: Alternative operation for inverted nipple, PRS, *57:*438, 1976

ELSAHY, N. I.: Syphilitic elephantiasis of the penis and scrotum, PRS, *57:*601, 1976

ELSAHY, N. I.: Correction of asymmetries of the breasts, PRS, *57:*700, 1976

ELSAHY, N. I., AND WATERS, W. R.: Branchioskeleto-genital syndrome, new hereditary syndrome, PRS, *48:*542, 1971

ELSAHY, N. I., AND VISTNES, L. M.: Alternate method in treatment of zygomatic fractures, PRS, *53:*603, 1974. Acta chir. plast., *15:*51, 1973

ELSAS, F. J. *et al:* Benign pigmented tumors, arising in acquired conjunctival melanosis. Am. J. Ophth., *78:*229, 1974

ELSHOVE, J., AND VAN ECK, J. H. M.: Congenital malformations, cleft lip and palate in particular, in children of epileptic women, PRS, *49:*359, 1972. Nederl. tijdschr. geneesk., *115:*1371, 1971

ELWOOD, J. M., AND LEE, J. A. H.: Trends in mortality from primary tumors of skin in Canada, PRS, *54:*509, 1974 Canad. M. A. J., *110:*913, 1974

EMANUEL, I. *et al*: Epidemiological differentiation of cleft lip and palate: a population study of clefts in King County, Washington, 1956–1965, PRS, *54:*111, 1974. Teratology, *7:*271, 1973

EMANUELLI, H. *et al*: Anesthesiological problems in head and neck surgery. Tumori, 60:491, 1974 (Italian)

Embolism

Fat emoblism, post-traumatic, pathogenesis of (Kerstell), PRS, *49:*671, 1972. Am. J. Surg., *121:*712, 1971

Embolectomy, femoral, anterior tibial compartment syndrome complicating (Ransford, Provan), PRS *48:*393, 1971. Canad. J. Surg., *14:*231, 1971

Fat embolism, experimental, adverse effect of heparin in (Allardyce), PRS *49:*670, 1972. Surg. Forum, *22:*203, 1971

Embolism, pulmonary, venous stasis on operating table (Lewis, Mueller, Edwards), PRS, *52:*99, 1973. Am. J. Surg. *124:*780, 1972

Embolism, pulmonary fat, coagulation mechanism in (Soloway, Robinson), PRS, *52:*325, 1973. J. Trauma, *12:*630, 1972

Fat embolism syndrome, clinical study (Bivins, Madauss, Griffin), PRS, *51:*486, 1973. South. M. J., *65:*937, 1972

Children, posttraumatic fat embolism in (Weisz, Rang, Salter), PRS, *53:*500, 1974. J. Trauma, *13:*529, 1973

Embolism, pulmonary, small subcutaneous doses of heparin in prevention of venous thrombosis (Gallus, Hirsh, Tuttle), PRS, *52:*331, 1973. New England J. Med., *288:*545, 1973

Fat embolization prophylaxis, use of hypertonic glucose (Horne, Horne), PRS, *54:*624, 1974. Arch. Int. Med., *133:*288, 1974

Fat embolism, current concept (Cole), PRS, *54:*627, 1974. M. J. Australia, *1:*535, 1974

EMERSON, E. B., JR.: Improved tracheotomy tube obdurator. Am. Fam. Physician, *10:*155, 1974

EMERSON, G. L.: Tissue transfers for functional reconstruction in thoracic surgery (with Cervino, Bales), PRS, *54:*437, 1974

EMERY, F. M.: Speaking valve for attachment to tracheostomy tube. Brit. Med. J., *2:*466, 1972

EMERY, J. A. *et al*: Duplication of hindgut: low male imperforate anus and unilateral exstrophy of bladder. J. Urol., *112:*532, 1974

EMERY, J. M. *et al*: Management of orbital floor fractures. Am. J. Ophth., *74:*299, 1972

EMERY, J. M., AND VON NOORDEN, G. K.: "Pseudo" blowout fractures called diagnostic pitfalls, PRS, *57:*754, 1976. Clin. Trends Ophth., *13:*7, 1975

EMERYK, B. *et al:* Evaluation of surgical treatment of facial nerve lesions based on clinical and electromyographic findings. Neurol. Neurochir. Pol., *7:*467, 1973 (Polish)

EMISTEIN, R. A., AND KATZ, A.D.: Parotid area

swelling caused by a prominent transverse process of atlas, PRS, *57:*395, 1976. Arch. Otolaryng., *101:*558, 1975

EMERSON, R. W.: Multicentric pigmented Bowen's disease of perineum, PRS, *57:*399, 1976. Proc. Roy. Soc. Med., *68:*345, 1975

EMMETT, A. J. J.: Finger resurfacing by multiple subcutaneous pedicle or louvre flaps, PRS, *56:*683, 1975. Brit. J. Plast. Surg., *27:*370, 1974

EMMETT, A. J. J.: Four V-flap repair of preputial stenosis, alternative to circumcision, PRS, *55:*687, 1975

EMMINGS, F. G.: Chemically modified osseous material for the restoration of bone defects. J. Peridontol., *45:*385, 1974

EMRL, J.: Hand injuries caused by blank cartridges. Acta Chir. Orthop. Traumatol. Cech., *40:*556, 1973 (Czechoslovakian)

Encephaloceles and Meningoceles

Myelomeningoceles, problems of primary closure of (Eckstein), PRS, *49:*471, 1972. Proc. Roy. Soc. Med., *64:*1143, 1971

Meningocele, accidental rupture, meningitis following (Cronin, Penoff), PRS, *52:*100, 1973. Cleft Palate J., *9:*215, 1972

Bone changes in meningomyelocele (Tosovsky, Strykal, Kolikova), PRS, *51:*234, 1973. Kinderchir., *11:*254, 1972

Encephalocele, frontal, note on (Converse, Fleury), PRS, *49:*343, 1972

Encephalocele, hydrocephaly, and anencephaly, clinical findings related to formal genesis of (Berndorfer), PRS, *51:*481, 1973. Rev. brasil. cir., *62:*137, 1972

Meningoencephalocele, diagnosis and treatment (Poradowska *et al*), PRS, *54:*630, 1974. Acta chir. plast., *15:*137, 1973

Myelomeningocele, large, closure of (Salasin, Briggs), PRS, *51:*464, 1973

Frontoethmoidal encephalomeningocele, large (Mulliken), PRS, *51:*592, 1973

Meningoencephalocele, intranasal (Schmidt *et al*). Arch. Otolaryng., *99:*402, 1974

Meningoencephalocele, intransal (Rao *et al*). Int. Surg., *59:*421, 1974

Cooperation of a neurosurgeon and plastic surgeon during the surgical treatment of encephalocele sincipitalis (Mircevski *et al*). Med. Pregl., *28:*529, 1975 (Serbian)

Encephaloceles, frontonasal tumors, diagnosis and management (Griffith), PRS, *57:*692, 1976

ENCKE, A., AND GROZINGER, K. H.: Studies of intravascular coagulation in experimental dog burns, PRS, *52:*211, 1973. Bull. Soc. Internat. Chir., *5:*445, 1972

ENDO, N. *et al:* Study on recovery of masticatory function with surgical mandibular reconstruction. Jap. J. Oral Surg., *19:*441, 1973 (Japanese)

ENEROTH, C. M.: Salivary gland tumors in parotid gland, submandibular gland and palate region, PRS, *49:*237, 1972. Cancer, *27:*1415, 1971

ENEROTH C. M., HENRIKSON, C. O., AND JAKOBSSON, P. A.: Effect of fractionated radiotherapy on salivary gland function, PRS, *51:*476, 1973. Cancer, *30:*1147, 1972

ENEROTH, C. M. *et al:* Malignancy of melanocytoblastoma. Analysis of malignant skin melanomas of head and neck region. H.N.O., *21:*208, 1973 (German)

ENEROTH, C. M. *et al:* Malignancy in pleomorphic adenoma. Clinical and microspectrophotometric study. Acta Otolaryngol. (Stockh.), 77:426, 1974

ENFORES, B., AND HERNGREN, L.: Nasal glomus, PRS, *57:*670, 1976. J. Laryng. & Otol., *89:*863, 1975

ENG, K. *et al:* Clostridial myonecrosis of abdominal wall, PRS, *52:*601, 1973. Am. J. Surg., *125:*367, 1973

ENGDAHL, E.: Significance of periosteum in bone regeneration in the maxilla-premaxilla after bone resection (surgical experimental and histological study in growing rabbits). 2. Nord. Med., *86:*1221, 1971 (Swedish)

ENGDAHL, E.: Bone regeneration in maxillary defects. An experimental investigation on the significance of the periosteum and various media (blood, surgicel, bone marrow and bone grafts) on bone formation and maxillary growth. Scand. J. Plast. Reconstr. Surg., *8:*1, 1972

ENGEL, M. F.: Dimethyl sulfoxide in treatment of scleroderma, PRS, *52:*332, 1973. South. M. J., *65:*71, 1972

ENGEL, R. M.: Bladder exstrophy: vesicoplasty or urinary diversion? Urology, *2:*20, 1973

ENGEL, R. M.: Surgical construction of the male external genitalia. Clin. Plast. Surg., *1:*299, 1974

ENGEL, R. M. *et al:* Hypospadias: experience with new one-stage repair (Hodgson urethroplasty). Md. State Med. J., *20:*45, 1971

ENGEL, R. M. E., AND SCOTT, W. W.: Hypospadias: results with the Hodgson urethroplasty, PRS, *52:*208, 1973. J. Urol., *109:*115, 1973

ENGELHARDT, A. *et al:* Experimental results with the power-feedback system of an electrical hand prosthesis. Biomed. Tech. (Stuttg.), *17:*238, 1972 (German)

ENGELMAN, E. R. *et al:* Traumatic amputation of the penis. J. Urol., *112:*774, 1974

ENGELMAN, E. R. *et al:* Lipogranulomatosis of external genitalia. Urology, *3:*358, 1974

ENGERON, O. *et al:* An unusual cause of carpal tunnel syndrome. Cah. Med., *15:*25, 1974

ENGERON, O. *et al:* An unusual cause of carpal tunnel syndrome. J. Iowa Med. Soc., *65:*25, 1975

ENGLISH, D. T. *et al:* Dermabrasion for nodular cutaneous elastosis with cysts and comedones. Favre-Racouchot syndrome. Arch. Dermat., *104:*92, 1971

ENGLISH, FRANK P., AND KEATS, WARREN A.: *Reconstructive and Plastic Surgery of the Eyelids.* Charles C Thomas, Springfield, Ill., 1975

ENGLISH, F. P. *et al:* Reconstruction of lower eyelid utilizing upper eyelid. Aust. N.Z. J. Surg., *42:*33, 1972

ENGLISH, F. P. *et al:* Palpebral spring in facial palsy. M. J. Australia, *1:*223, 1972

ENGLISH, F. P. *et al:* Surgical correction of ptosis of eyebrow. Brit. J. Ophthalmol., *57:*761, 1973

ENGLISH, F. P. *et al:* Cilia graft. Brit. J. Ophthalmol., *57:*763, 1973

ENGLISH, G. M. *et al:* Surgical treatment of invasive angiofibroma. Arch. Otolaryng., *96:*312, 1972

ENGRAV, L. H. *et al:* Experimental effects of heparin or magnesium sulfate on patency of microvascular anastomoses, PRS, *55:*618, 1975

ENKER, W. E. *et al:* Experience in operative management of penetrating injuries of neck. Surg. Clin. North Am., *53:*87, 1973

ENLOW, E. H.: *Handbook of Facial Growth for Dental and Medical Students.* W. B. Saunders Co., Philadelphia, 1975

ENNA, C. D.: Neurolysis and transposition of ulnar nerve in leprosy. J. Neurosurg., *40:*734, 1974

ENNA, C. D. *et al:* Redundant and wrinkled facial skin in lepromatous leprosy. Correlation of clinical and histopathological findings. Int. J. Lepr., *42:*297, 1974

ENNA, C. D. *et al:* Temperature studies of the hand and its claw deformities due to peripheral nerve paralysis in leprosy. Hand, *5:*10, 1973

ENNA, C. D., AND RIORDAN, D. C.: Fowler procedure for correction of the paralytic claw hand, PRS, *52:*352, 1973

ENNA, C. D. (with Frank McDowell): *Surgical Rehabilitation in Leprosy.* Williams & Wilkins Co., Baltimore, 1974

ENNA, C. D. *et al:* A clinical assessment of

neurolysis for leprous involvement of the ulnar nerve. Int. J. Lepr., *42*:162, 1974

Enophthalmos

Correction of enophthalmos and deep supratarsal sulcus by posterior subperiosteal glass bead implantation (Taiara *et al*). Brit. J. Ophthalmol., *57*:741, 1973

Eye trauma, late treatment of enophthalmos (Stallings, Pakiam, Cory), PRS, *54*:686, 1974. Brit. J. Plast. Surg., *26*:57, 1973

Anophthalmic orbit, correction of enophthalmos in (Iverson, Vistnes, Siegel), PRS, *51*:545, 1973

Enophthalmos, posttraumatic, correction of (Spira, Gerow, Hardy), PRS, *55*:632, 1975. Acta chir. plast., *16*:107, 1974

Dermis fat graft for correction of the eyelid deformity of enophthalmos (Hawtof). Mich. Med., *74*:331, 1975

ENSEL, J. *et al*: Anesthesia in under-5-year-old burned children. Anesth. Analg. (Paris), *30*:1093, 1973 (French)

ENTERLINE, P. E. *et al*: Effects of "free" medical care on medical practice—Quebec experience, PRS, *53*:251, 1974. New England J. Med., *288*:1152, 1973)

ENTIN, M. *et al*: Classification of congnital malformations of the hand and upper extremity. Hand, *4*:215, 1972

ENTIN, M. A.: Hypothalamic-pituitary derangements as a complication of severe facial injuries (with Daniel, Becker), PRS, *49*:548, 1972

ENTIN, M. A.: Philosophy of tendon repair. Orthop. Clin. North Am., *4*:859, 1973

ENTIN, M. A.: Self-fulfilling prophecies: reflections on the future of A.S.S.H. J. Bone & Joint Surg. (Am.), *56*:1088, 1974

ENTIN, M. A. *et al:* Scleroderma hand: a reappraisal. Orthop. Clin. North Am., *4*:1031, 1973

Entropion

Distichiasis and epicanthus. Study of one family (Deutsch). Ann. Ophth. *3*:168, 1971

Entropion, cicatricial, of upper eyelids, repair of (Dortzbach, Callahan), PRS, *48*:89, 1971. Arch. Ophth., *85*:82, 1971

Senile entropion. A new concept for correction (Jones *et al*). Am. J. Ophth., *74*:327, 1972

Surgery of senile ectropion and entropion (Fox). Ann. Ophth., *4*:217, 1972

Entropion, cicatricial, moderately severe (Beyer, Carroll), PRS, *52*:450, 1973. Arch. Ophth., *89*:33, 1973

Entropion—Cont.

Inferior aponeurosis vs orbital septum tucking for senile entropion (Hargiss). Arch. Ophth., *89*:210, 1973

Entropion, bilateral, congenital, of upper eyelids (Firat *et al*). Brit. J. Ophthalmol., *57*:753, 1973

Entropion, senile spastic, modified Wheeler's operation for (Castroviejo). Harefuah, *85*:462, 1973

Entropion: correction of complications after levator resections for blepharoptosis (Callahan), PRS, *52*:616, 1973

Entropion, senile spastic, modification of Wheeler's operation for (Castroviejo), PRS, *55*:245, 1975. Ann. Ophth., *6*:171, 1974

Entropion, cicatricial, tarsotomy for correction of (Halasa *et al*). Ann. Ophth., *6*:837, 1974

Mucous membrane grafting (Welsh). Arch. Ophth., *92*:362, 1974

Mucous membrane grafting for cicatricial entropion (Leone). Ophthalmic Surg., *5*:24, 1974

Entropion of lower lid: repair by double triangle tarsectomy (Yassin *et al*). Ophthalmic Surg., *5*:65, 1974

Common problems in ophthalmic plastic surgery (Carroll). Am. Fam. Physician, *12*:85, 1975

Orbicularis resection, internal tarsus, for senile spastic entropion (Leone), PRS, *57*:257, 1976. Ann. Ophth., *7*:1004, 1975

Simple office procedure for the repair of senile entropion (Magnuson). Ophthalmic Surg., *6*:83, 1975

Senile (atonic) entropion (Fox). Ann. Ophth., *8*:167, 1976

ENZINGER, F. M.: Epitheloid sarcoma. A sarcoma simulating a granuloma or a carcinoma. Cancer *26*:1029, 1970

EPEL'BAUM, L. M.: Surgical treatment of congenital neck fistulae in childhood. Stomatologiia (Mosk.), *53*:89, 1974 (Russian)

Epicanthus

Epicanthus: W-epicanthoplasty (Mulliken, Hoopes), PRS, *55*:435, 1975

Epidermolysis Bullosa

Epidermolysis bullosa, involvement of hand in (Horner, Wiedel, Bralliar), PRS, *49*:663, 1972. J. Bone & Joint Surg., *53*:1347, 1971

Epidermolysis bullosa, employment of skin homografts in (Castro Fariña), PRS, *48*:611, 1971. Rev. españ. cir. plast., *4*:109, 1971

Epidermolysis Bullosa—Cont.

Epidermolysis bullosae (Codina *et al*), PRS, *53:*615, 1974. Rev. españ. cir. plast., *4:*145, 1971

Epidermolysis bullosa dystrophica, surgical treatment of pseudo-syndactyly in a case of (Anderl, Weiser), PRS, *53:*115, 1974. Chir. Plast., *1:*145, 1972

Epidermolysis bullosa dystrophica, squamous cell carcinoma in, autografting in treatment (Eastwood), PRS, *49:*93, 1972

Epidermolysis bullosa, new method for skin grafting burned patient who has (Skivolocki, Harris, Boles), PRS, *53:*355, 1974

Epidermolysis bullosa, anesthesia in (Bolinches Bolinches *et al*). Rev. Esp. Anestesiol. Reanim., *21:*477, 1974 (Spanish)

Epidermolysis bullosa dystrophica, squamous cell carcinoma in (Gipson), PRS, *57:*760, 1976 Hand, *7:*179, 1975

Epiglottis

Subtotal reconstructive surgery in the treatment of laryngeal cancers (Piquet *et al*). Ann. Otolaryngol. Chir. Cervicofac., *91:*311, 1974 (French)

View from within (Flannagan). J. Pract. Nurs., *24:*32, 1974

Epiglottis, benign mesenchymoma of, in infant (Timar *et al*). Orv. Hetil., *115:*873, 1974 (Hungarian)

Letter: Procedures to prevent chronic aspiration (Murray). New England J. Med., *293:*561, 1975

EPINETTE, W. W., AND HURWITZ, R. M.: Acquired *cheilitis glandularis simplex,* PRS, *51:*334, 1973

Epispadias (See also *Bladder Exstrophy)*

Epispadias, female, the surgery of (Dey, Cohen), PRS, *48:*295, 1971. Surgery, *69:*542, 1971

Epispadias of the double urethra (Solov'ev). Vestn. Khir., *107:*90, 1971 (Russian)

Genital function in males with vesical exstrophy and epispadias (Hanna *et al*). Brit. J. Urol., *44:*169, 1972

Epispadias, female, functional urethral reconstruction in (Harrold, Champion, Ford), PRS, *50:*539, 1972. J. Urol., *107:*144, 1972

Epispadias. Seventy cases (Cendron) Urol. int., *27:*291, 1972 (French)

Epispadias procedures, plastic and reconstructive (Bischoff), PRS, *53:*244, 1974. Chir. Praxis, *16:*575, 1972; Part 2, *17:*73, 1973

Epispadias—Cont.

Epispadias, male, surgical correction of (with total incontinence) (Bredin *et al*). J. Urol., *109:*904, 1973

Epispadias with and without urinary incontinence, treatment of. Experience with 46 patients (Culp). J. Urol., *109:*120, 1973

Epispadias, incomplete subsymphyseal (Kondo *et al*). Jap. J. Urol., *64:*421, 1973 (Japanese)

Penis: technique for epispadias repair (Khanna), PRS, *52:*365, 1973

Epispadias and bladder exstrophy, gynecologic complications (Stanton). Am J. Obstet. Gynecol., *119:*749, 1974

Epispadias with incontinence (Klauber, Williams), PRS, *54:*504, 1974. J. Urol., *111:*110, 1974

Epispadias repair, urodynamic measurements following (Festge *et al*). Zentralbl. Chir., *99:*337, 1974

Epistaxis

Epistaxis, management in Osler-Weber-Rendu disease; recurrence of telangiectases within a nasal skin graft (McCabe, Kelly), PRS, *50:*114, 1972

Epistaxis, facial pain treated by surgery in pterygomaxillary fossa (Corvera, Somonte, Gonzalez-Romero), PRS, *52:*98, 1973. Tribuna Med. Mexico, *23:*3, 1972

Nosebleed, how to treat (Barga), PRS, *53:*602, 1974. Am. Fam. Phys., *8:*66, 1973

Septal dermoplasty for von Willebrand's disease in children (Letson *et al*). Laryngoscope, *83:*1078, 1973

Epistaxis, cyclic, severe, medical and surgical aspects of (Tainmont). Acta Otorhinolaryngol. Belg., *28:*187, 1974 (French)

Epistaxis, recurrent, after multiple arterial ligation, use of angiography in case of (Taylor *et al*). Brit. J. Surg., *61:*721, 1974

Epistaxis, intractable, on management of (Shapiro). Eye, Ear, Nose, Throat Mon., *53:*153, 1974

Epistaxis, managing (Smith). Postgrad. Med., *55:*143, 1974

Retrospective study of 102 cases of epistaxis (Cinotti). V. Med. Pregl., *27:*343, 1974 (Serbian)

Detachment of mucosa and perichondrium of nasal septum with subsequent ligation of terminal branch of anterior ethmoid artery for stopping nasal hemorrhaging (Ulasovets). Zh. Ushn. Nos. Gorl. Bolezn., 104, Mar–Apr., 1974

Severe emergency epistaxis (Poncet *et al*). Ann. Otolaryngol. Chir. Cervicofac.,

Epistaxis – Cont.

92:145, 1975 (French)

Arterial epistaxis (Shaheen). J. Laryng. & Otol., 89:17, 1975

Epistaxis (Pearson), PRS, 57:257, 1976. Postgrad. Med., 57:116, 1975

Internal maxillary artery ligation for posterior epistaxis (Geroulis *et al*). Surg. Forum, 26:531, 1975

Air-fluid levels in the sphenoid sinus in epistaxis and nasal packing (Ogawa *et al*). Radiology, 118:351, 1976

EPKER, B. N.: Open surgical management of nasoorbital-ethmoid facial fractures. Trans. Congr. Int. Assoc. Oral. Surg., 4:323, 1973

EPKER, B. N.: Middle-third facial osteotomies: their use in correction of acquired and developmental dentofacial and craniofacial deformities. J. Oral Surg., 33:491, 1975

EPKER, B. N., AND HENNY, F. A.: Intraoral sebaceous gland adenoma, PRS, 48:609, 1971. Cancer, 27:987, 1971

EPSTEEN, C. M. *et al:* Maxillofacial injuries and craniocerebral trauma. Int. Surg., 57:315, 1972

EPSTEIN, E.: Effect of biopsy on the prognosis of melanoma. J. Surg. Oncol., 3:251, 1971

EPSTEIN, E.: Value of follow-up after treatment of basal cell carcinoma, PRS, 54:381, 1974. Arch. Dermat., 108:798, 1973

EPSTEIN, E.: How accurate is visual assessment of basal carcinoma margins? PRS, 54:381, 1974. Brit. J. Dermat., 89:37, 1973

EPSTEIN, E.: Cosmetic results after treatment of basal cell carcinoma, PRS, 56:104, 1975. Cutis, 14:825, 1974

EPSTEIN, E.: Basal cell epithelioma: treat on sight. Int. J. Dermatol., 14:263, 1975

EPSTEIN, F. *et al:* Correction of ocular hypertelorism. Childs Brain, 1:288, 1975

EPSTEIN, F. J. *et al:* Radical one-stage correction of craniofacial anomalies. J. Neurosurg., 42:522, 1975

EPSTEIN, M. J.: Malignant schwannomas of the hand: a review. Bull. Hosp. Joint Dis., 32:136, 1971

EPSTEIN, W. L. *et al:* Halo nevi and melanoma, PRS, 53:248, 1974. J. A. M. A., 225:373, 1973

ERICKSON, G. E. *et al:* Mandibular asymmetry. J. Am. Dent. Assoc., 89:1369, 1974

ERICSON, S. *et al:* Results of apicoectomy of maxillary canines, premolars and molars with special reference to oroantral communication as prognostic factor. Int. J. Oral Surg., 3:386, 1974

ERIKSEN, J.: Case of carpal tunnel syndrome on the basis of an abnormally long lumbrical muscle. Acta Orthop. Scand., 44:275, 1973

ERIKSON, U. *et al*: Congenital vascular malformations of the hand. Acta Radiol. (Diagn.) (Stockh.), 14:753, 1973

ERIKSSON, E. *et al*: Varicose ulcers. Scand. J. Soc. Med., 3:13, 1975

ERIKSSON, G.: Keratinization of human split skin autografts. Light and electron microscopic study. Scand. J. Plast. Reconstr. Surg., 7:15, 1973

ERMAKOV, M. A.: Outcome of the treatment of the wounded of the G. K. Zhukov Partisan Unit in Ukraine. Ortop. Travmatol. Protez., 4:81, 1975 (Russian)

ERWIG, R. *et al*: Single-step higher repositioning of the alveolar process in the treatment of open bite due to rickets. Fortschr. Kiefer. Gesichtschir., 18:207, 1974 (German)

ESCH, W.: Autologous free grafting of ureter with dogs, PRS, 57:120, 1976. Acta chir. Austria, 7:43, 1975

ESCH, W.: Penis erection in hypospadias. Z. Urol. Nephrol., 68:575, 1975 (German)

ESCHWEGE, F. *et al*: Treatment of adenocarcinomas of the larynx. Can. J. Otolaryngol., 4:290, 1975

ESCOBAR ALDASORO, G. *et al*: Results of the treatment of arteriovenous malformations of the extremities by means of muscle embolization. Preliminary report. Arch. Inst. Cardiol. Mex., 42:247, 1972 (Spanish)

ESCOTT, J. E.: Predisposing causes of burns, two unusual case reports, PRS, 52:684, 1973. Acta chir. plast., 14:236, 1972

ESHO, J. O. *et al*: Comparison of Bricker and Wallace methods of ureteroilial anastomosis in urinary diversions. J. Urol., 111:600, 1974

ESKELAND, G.: Scars and scar revision. Tidsskr. Nor. Laegeforen, 93:1067, 1973 (Norwegian)

ESKELAND, G.: Is our treatment of children with cleft palate-cleft lip rational? Tidsskr. Nor. Laegeforen, 93:2459, 1973 (Norwegian)

ESKELAND, G. *et al:* Cleft lip and cleft palate. Secondary surgery. 6. Tidsskr. Nor. Laegeforen, 93:2481, 1973 (Norwegian)

ESKICI, A.: Surgery of cysts from the nasal cavity: methods and results. Dtsch. Zahnaerztl. Z., 29:742, 1974 (Eng. Abstr.)

Esophageal Diverticula

Esophageal diverticula, cervical, surgical technic of (Rossetti). Helv. Chir. Acta, 38:237, 1971 (German)

Safeguards in the repair of pharyngoesophageal diverticulum (Van De Water). Surg. Gynec. & Obst., 133:851, 1971

Pharyngo-esophageal diverticulum (Eastridge). South. Med. J., 65:745, 1972

Esophageal diverticula, treatment of (Hoff-

Esophageal Diverticula—Cont.

man *et al*). Zentralbl. Chir., *98:*1501, 1973 (German)

Pharyngo-esophageal diverticula (Auvinen *et al*). Duodecim, *90:*1124, 1974 (Finnish)

Late results of one-step excision of an esophageal diverticulum (Misterka). Wiad. Lek., *27:*15, 1974 (Polish)

Value of the myotomy for the management of a cervical esophageal diverticulum (Gignoux *et al*). Ann. Chir., *29:*847, 1975 (French)

Esophagoplasty

Esophagoplasty, subtotal, by combined cervico-abdominal route: its possible use in megaesophagus (Ferreira). Rev. Paul. Med., *82:*133, 1973 (Portuguese)

Esophagus, corrosive stricture of, esophagoplasty for, analysis of 60 cases (Chien *et al*). Ann. Surg., *179:*510, 1974

Stricture, cervical esophageal, flap repair (Brown *et al*), PRS, *55:*379, 1975. Australian & New Zealand J. Surg., *44:*133, 1974

Pharyngotomy for colonic anastomosis during total esophagoplasty (Laccourreye *et al*). J. Chir., *107:*83, 1974 (French)

Esophageal surgery, free autodermoplasty in (Sardak *et al*). Klin. Khir., *3:*16, 1974 (Russian)

Esophagoplasty and labor (Ba *et al*). Orv. Hetil., *115:*2688, 1974 (Hungarian)

Reconstruction of pharynx and cervical part of esophagus following pharyngolaryngectomy (Witwicka *et al*). Otolaryngol. Pol., *28:*657, 1974 (Polish)

Importance of preservation of vascular pedicles in esophagoplasties. Results observed in 60 patients with caustic stenosis of esophagus operated on consecutively (Silva *et al*). Rev. Assoc. Med. Bras., *20:*219, 1974 (Portuguese)

Reconstruction of a subcutaneous artificial esophagus into a retrosternal one (Masiukova *et al*). Vestn. Khir., *112:*113, 1974 (Russian)

Technic of joining an artificial esophagus and the pharynx (Khitrov *et al*). Vestn. Khir., *113:*105, 1974 (Russian)

Surgical management of severe lye burns of the esophagus by colon interposition (Berkowitz *et al*). Ann. Otol. Rhin. & Laryng., *84:*576, 1975

Orolleoanastomosis in total oesophagoplasty (Brix *et al*). Bratisl. Lek. Listy., *63:*395, 1975 (Slovakian)

New principle of production of obturating apparatus in gaping defects of the esophagus

Esophagoplasty—Cont.

and pharynx (Balon *et al*). Vestn. Khir., *115:*108, 1975 (Russian)

Esophagus

Cervical esophageal reconstruction after a laryngectomy and subtotal esophagectomy (Armstrong, Peters), PRS, *48:*382, 1971

Esophagus, everted anastomoses, in piglet (Kormfalt, Okmian, Jonsson), PRS, *53:*683, 1974. Ztschr. Kinderchir., *13:*306, 1973

Esopharyngostomas, huge, appearing after total laryngectomy for irradiated laryngeal cancer, treatment for (Kiricuta, Popescu, Suceava), PRS, *56:*464, 1975. Ann. oto-laryng., *91:*585, 1974

Congenital laryngotracheoesophageal cleft (Berkovits *et al*), PRS, *55:*721, 1975. Arch. Otolaryng., *100:*442, 1974

Esophagus, cervical, stricture of, flap repair (Brown *et al*), PRS, *55:*379, 1975. Australian & New Zealand J. Surg., *44:*133, 1974

Esophageal speech proficiency, relation to auditory function (Martian, Hoops), PRS, *56:*594, 1975. J. Speech & Hearing Res., *17:*80, 1974

Osteochondromatous choristoma of esophagus (Minami, Tsang, Haber), PRS, *53:*94, 1974

Swallowing, some aspects of dysphagia (Thomas), PRS, *55:*718, 1975. Proc. Roy. Soc. Med., *67:*477, 1974

Esophageal replacement with lyophilic dura in dogs (Herefrath *et al*), PRS, *54:*619, 1974. Ztschr. Kinderchir., *14:*146, 1974

Esophageal speech aid, modified Tokyo larynx (Nelson, Parkin, Potter), PRS, *57:*396, 1976. Arch. Otolaryng., *101:*107, 1975

Esophageal cancer in North China, epidemiology and etiology of (Coordinating Group for Research on Etiology of Esophageal Cancer in North China), PRS, *57:*759, 1976. Chinese M. J., *1:*167, 1975

Cervical esophagus, secondary reconstruction of (Petty, Theogaraj, Cohen), PRS, *56:*70, 1975

Esophagus, cervical, repair of fistula by microvascular transfer of free skin flap (Fujino, Saito), PRS, *56:*549, 1975

ESPAILLAT, L.: Treatment of facial paralysis by static suspension with dermal flaps (with Guerrero-Santos, Ramirez), PRS, *48:*325, 1971

ESPAILLAT, L.: Muscular lift in cervical rhytidoplasty (with Guerrero-Santos, Morales), PRS, *54:*127, 1974

ESSER, E. *et al*: Clinical picture and therapy of

intraoral leukoplakia. Dtsch. Zahn. Mund. Keiferheilkd., *60:*378, 1973 (German)

ESTABROOKS, L. N. *et al*: Role of condylotomy with interpositional silicone rubber in temporomandibular joint ankylosis. Oral Surg., *34:*2, 1972

Esthetic Surgery (See also *Abdominoplasty, Blepharoplasty, Mammaplasty, Otoplasty, Rhinoplasty, Rhytidectomy*)

Exophthalmos, endocrine, antral-ethmoid decompression of (Calcaterra). Ann. Ophth., *3:*1004, 1971

Obstetric remissness, syndrome of (Gonzalez-Ulloa, Flores), PRS, *48:*95, 1971. Internat. Surg., *55:*63, 1971

Facial dimple: its formation by a simple technique (Argamaso), PRS, *48:*40, 1971

Esthetic surgery, the first woman to do. Dr. Suzanne Noel (Regnault, Stephenson), PRS, *48:*133, 1971

Delusions, somatic, in patients seeking cosmetic surgery (Druss, Symonds, Crikelair), PRS, *48:*246, 1971

Cosmetic surgery, performance by residents in plastic surgery in city hospitals (Gorney) (Letter to the Editor), PRS, *48:*362, 1971

Frontalis hypermotility, bilateral temporal neurotomy for (Edwards) (Follow-Up Clinic), PRS, *48:*370, 1971

Lipectomy, submental, simplified technique in (Weisman), PRS, *48:*443, 1971

Cosmetic (esthetic) surgery, motivational patterns of patients seeking (Edgerton, Knorr), PRS, *48:*551, 1971

Wrinkles and etiopathogenic theory (Lacerda Abreu), PRS, *50:*417, 1972. Rev. paulista med. Brazil, *78:*93, 1971

Cosmetic surgery (Petersen) (Ugeskr. Laeger, *133:*2441, 1971 (Danish)

Age changes in the forehead area and a surgical method of treating them (Mirov). Vestn. Dermatol. Venerol., *45:*74, 1971 (Russian)

Symposium on Aesthetic Surgery of the Face, Eyelid, and Breast, Vol. IV. Ed. by Frank W. Masters and John R. Lewis, Jr. C. V. Mosby Co., St. Louis, 1972. PRS, *51:*687, 1973

Exophthalmos, endocrine (Bateson). Brit. Med. J., *4:*46, 1972

Face, wrinkles in (Malbec, Quaife, Arce-Gonzalez), PRS, *50:*198, 1972. El Dia Medico Argentina, *44:*15, 1972

Cosmetic surgery, breast (Holder). J.A.M.A., *222:*1101, 1972

Esthetic plastic surgery, development and place in medical practice (Reich), PRS,

Esthetic Surgery—Cont.

*51:*712, 1973. M. J. Australia, *1:*1152, 1972

Graves' disease, surgical management of ophthalmopathy in. Transfrontal orbital decompression (Riley). Mayo Clin. Proc., *47:*986, 1972

Cosmetic surgery and the university hospital (Goldwyn) (Editorial), PRS, *49:*76, 1972

"Crow's-feet," complete face and forehead lifting with double traction (Regnault), PRS, *49:*123, 1972

Facial rhytidoplasties, earlobe tailoring during (Loeb), PRS, *49:*485, 1972

Exophthalmos, unilateral (Hartley, Schatten), PRS, *49:*576, 1972

Exophthalmos, surgical correction; history technique and long-term follow-up (Moran, Letterman, Schurter), PRS, *49:*595, 1972

Witches' chin, ptosis of the chin (Gonzalez-Ulloa), PRS, *50:*54, 1972

Dimple, permanent, in the chin, making (Guerrero-Santos, Ramirez, Rivera), PRS, *50:*88, 1972

Cleft in chin, making (Cinelli), PRS, *50:*91, 1972

Double chin, surgical treatment of (Viñas *et al*), PRS, *50:*119, 1972

Glabellar rhytidoplasty, new approach (Rosenthal), PRS, *50:*361, 1972

Skin tightening with phenol, for better dermabrasion (Dupont *et al*), PRS, *50:*588, 1972

Cosmetology—one of the forms of specialized medical aid to the population (Akhabadze). Sov. Med., *35:*122, 1972 (Russian)

Exophthalmos, endocrine, medial decompression of orbit for (Smith). Trans. Ophthalmol. Soc. U.K., *92:*485, 1972

Orbital decompression of malignant exophthalmus (Duerksen). Trans. Pac. Acad. Ophthalmol. Otolaryngol., *25:*113, 1972

Moscow therapeutic cosmetics clinic. The main stages of its practical and scientific and research activities. (Astvatsaturov *et al*). Vestn. Dermatol. Venerol., *46:*72, 1972 (Russian)

Atlas of Aesthetic Plastic Surgery. By John R. Lewis, Jr. Little, Brown & Co., Boston, 1973. PRS, *53:*673, 1974

Cosmetic Facial Surgery. By Thomas D. Rees and Donald Wood-Smith. W. B. Saunders Co., Philadelphia, 1973. PRS, *52:*427, 1973

"Doctor, Make Me Beautiful!" By James W. Smith and Samm Sinclair Baker. David McKay Co., New York, 1973. PRS, *53:*219, 1974

Symposium on Aesthetic Surgery of the Nose, Ears, and Chin. Ed. by Frank W.

Esthetic Surgery—Cont.

Masters and John R. Lewis, Jr. C. V. Mosby Co., St. Louis, 1973. PRS, *54:*479, 1974

Exophthalmos, unilateral, diagnosis and therapy of (Profeta). Acta Neurol. (Napoli), *28:*85, 1973 (Italian)

Orbital decompression, pterional, in progressive ophthalmopathy of Graves' disease. 1. Short-term effects (Algvere *et al*). Acta Ophthalmol. (Kbh.), *51:*475, 1973

Orbital decompression, pterional, in progressive ophthalmopathy of Graves' disease. 2. Follow-up study (Algvere *et al*). Acta Ophthalmol. (Kbh.), *51:*475, 1973

Exophthalmos, edematous, Ogura's technic in (Freyss *et al*). Bull. Soc. Ophtalmol. Fr., *73:*253, 1973 (French)

Exophthalmos, unilateral, role of sarcoidosis in etiology of (Urvoy *et al*). Bull. Soc. Ophtalmol. Fr., *73:*581, 1973 (French)

Exophthalmos, neurosurgeon's interest in. 1. Diagnosis of exophthalmos (Naito *et al*). Keio J. Med., *22:*85, 1973

Exophthalmos, neurosurgeon's interest in. 2. Surgical approach (Naito *et al*). Keio J. Med., *22:*93, 1973

Exophthalmos, malignant, of both eyes (Krawczykowa *et al*). Klin. Oczna, *43:*835, 1973 (Polish)

Cosmetic surgery (Editorial). Lancet, *2:*1136, 1973

Selection of patients and choice of operation for orbital decompression in Graves' ophthalmopathy (DeSanto *et al*). Laryngoscope, *83:*945, 1973

Hemostasis, effective, with less epinephrine. Experimental and clinical study (Siegel, Vistnes, Iverson), PRS, *51:*129, 1973

Hematoma, expanding, after rhytidectomy (Rees, Lee, Coburn), PRS, *51:*149, 1973

Autotransfusion for blood loss in some major esthetic operations (Noone, Graham, Royster), PRS, *51:*559, 1973

Flaps, dermal, use for attachment of rhytidoplasty flaps (Cameron *et al*), PRS, *51:*596, 1973

Earlobe, preventing pulled-down or deformed, in rhytidectomies (Lindgren, Carlin), PRS, *51:*598, 1973

Lipectomy: abdominoplasty (Grazer), PRS, *51:*617, 1973

Face, survey of chemical peeling of (Litton, Fournier, Capinpin), PRS, *51:*645, 1973

Rhytidectomy, pattern for postauricular incision in (Letterman, Schurter), PRS, *51:*697, 1973

Intraocular pressure: acute retrobulbar hemorrhage during elective blepharoplasty

Esthetic Surgery—Cont.

(Hartley, Lester, Schatten), PRS, *52:*8, 1973. Discussions by Lemoine, Rees, Newell, PRS, *52:*12, 1973

Eyelid surgery: brow lifting through a temporal scalp approach (Gleason), PRS, *52:*141, 1973

Esthetic plastic surgery, challenges in (Alexander), PRS, *52:*337, 1973

Cosmetic surgery: plea for balance. Presidential address (Monroe), PRS, *52:*471, 1973

Esthetic plastic surgery of face, psychological aspects (Edson-Sperli), PRS, *53:*239, 1974. Rev. Latino Am. cir. plast., *17:*15, 1973

Exophthalmos, atypical intermittent, due to hyperplasia of lacrimal gland associated with dacryolithiasis (Nalto *et al*). Surg. Neurol., *1:*84, 1973

Orbitotomy, lateral, evolution of (Stallard) (Presidential Address). Trans. Ophthalmol. Soc. U.K., *93:*3, 1973

Exophthalmos, non-endocrine with unilateral proptosis (Choudhury). Trans. Ophthalmol. Soc. U.K., *93:*673, 1973

Proptosis, unilateral, in newborn (Cory *et al*). Brit. J. Ophthalmol., *58:*110, 1974

Forehead wrinkles, total permanent removal (LeRoux, Jones), PRS, *56:*675, 1975. Brit. J. Plast. Surg., *27:*359, 1974

Cosmetic surgery (Horton *et al*). Brit. Med. J., *3:*566, 1974

Case of von Recklinghausen's disease with unilateral pulsating exophthalmos (Shibata *et al*). Clin. Neurol., *14:*512, 1974 (Japanese)

Notes on esthetic surgery in the Indonesian (Wiratmadja). Clin. Plast. Surg., *1:*173, 1974

Fee entitlement in failed cosmetic surgery (Rieger). Dtsch. Med. Wochenschr., *99:*2068, 1974 (German)

Retro-orbital fibrosis in Ormond's disease (Lenhard *et al*). Dtsch. Med. Wochenschr., *99:*2286, 1974 (German)

Exophthalmos, methods of correcting (Naumann). Laryngol. Rhinol. Otol. (Stuttg.), *53:*469, 1974 (German)

Exophthalmos, malignant, surgical results of orbital decompression for (Ogura *et al*). Laryngoscope, *84:*637, 1974

Cosmetic surgery, physiologic and, facial analysis in patient evaluation for (Patterson *et al*). Laryngoscope, *84:*1004, 1974

Aesthetic surgery to improve appearance of female body (Reich), PRS, *56:*236, 1975. M. J. Australia, *2:*767, 1974

Cosmetic surgical operations, revising, philosophical considerations in (Anderson). Otolaryngol. Clin. North Am., *7:*57, 1974

Esthetic Surgery—Cont.

Augmentation, alloplastic thigh, complication after (Fornaroli), PRS, *56:*357, 1975. Polymers in Med., *4:*153, 1974

Malar prominences, building out as addition to rhytidectomy (Gonzalez-Ulloa), PRS, *53:*293, 1974. Discussion by Stark, PRS, *53:*469, 1974

Thighs: surgical rehabilitation after massive weight reduction (McGraw), PRS, *53:*349, 1974

Skin, long-term histological study of, after chemical face peeling (Baker *et al*), PRS, *53:*522, 1974

Eyelids, anatomy for blepharoplasty (Hugo, Stone), PRS, *53:*381, 1974. Discussion by Castañares, PRS, *53:*587, 1974

Eyelid, lower: successful early relief of blindness occurring after blepharoplasty (Hueston, Heinze), PRS, *53:*588, 1974. Discussion by Hepler, Sugimura, Straatsma, PRS, *57:*233, 1976

Male, rhytidectomy in (Hamilton), PRS, *53:*629, 1974

Cervicofacial rhytidoplasty: should the subcutaneous tissues be plicated in a face lift? (Tipton), PRS, *54:*1, 1974

Esthetic surgery result, a plea for showing the average (Goldwyn) (Editorial), PRS, *54:*88, 1974

Rhytidoplasty, cervical, muscular lift in (Guerrero-Santos, Espaillat, Morales), PRS, *54:*127, 1974

Lipectomy, abdominal (Baroudi, Keppke, Netto), PRS, *54:*161, 1974

Asymmetry, natural facial, as a preoperative and postoperative consideration (Gorney, Harries), PRS, *54:*187, 1974

Intravenous morphine sulfate, hypersensitivity to (Cromwell, Zsigmond), PRS, *54:*224, 1974

Orbital fat: planning and evaluating blepharoplasty (Berry), PRS, *54:*257, 1974

Face lift incision at front of ear, variation (Stark), PRS, *54:*369, 1974

Aesthetic surgery, whither? (Fredricks), PRS, *54:*387, 1974

Face peeling, chemical, complications of (Spira, Gerow, Hardy), PRS, *54:*397, 1974

Face lift: cervico-mentoplasty with rhytidectomy (Snyder), PRS, *54:*404, 1974

Fixation, supratarsal, in upper blepharoplasty (Sheen), PRS, *54:*424, 1974

Moustache, hair transplantation to upper lip to create (Villis), PRS, *54:*606, 1974

Paralysis, facial, coincident with, or subsequent to, rhytidectomy (Castañares), PRS, *54:*637, 1974

Esthetic Surgery—Cont.

"Dry eye" following blepharoplasty (Swartz, Schultz, Seaton), PRS, *54:*644, 1974

Rhytidectomy, prevention of bleeding following (Barker), PRS, *54:*651, 1974

Forehead wrinkles, surgical treatment of (Spina *et al*), PRS, *55:*244, 1975. Rev. Hosp. clin., *29:*76, 1974

On Le Fort III osteotomy for Crouzon's disease in children. Report of a four-year follow-up in one patient (Hogeman *et al*). Scand. J. Plast. Reconstr. Surg., *8:*169, 1974

Transantral orbital decompression in dysthyroid eye disease (Taylor). Trans. Ophthalmol. Soc. N. Z., *26:*51, 1974

Medicine and surgery of the profile (Vilain). Ann. chir. plast., *20:*113, 1975 (French)

Lift, brow (Rafaty), PRS, *57:*393, 1976. Arch. Otolaryng., *101:*467, 1975

Westmore Bros. launch paramedical makeup service (Editorial). Eye Ear Nose Throat Mon., *54:*34, 1975

Transcranial orbital decompression in severe cases of unilateral exophthalmos (Palva *et al*). J. Laryng. & Otol., *89:*1123, 1975

Proceedings: endocrine exophthalmos treated by orbital decompression (Clarke). J. Neurol. Neurosurg. Psychiatry, *38:*822, 1975

Exophthalmos. More commonly encountered neurosurgical lesions (Smigiel *et al*). Mayo Clin. Proc., *50:*345, 1975

Treatment of exophthalmia and retrognathia (van der Meulen *et al*). Ned. tijdschr. geneeskd., *119:*1757, 1975 (Dutch)

Psychological factors influencing patient satisfaction with the results of esthetic plastic surgery (Reich), PRS, *55:*5, 1975

Exophthalmos, surgical treatment of (Lanier), PRS, *55:*56, 1975

Face lift, should the subcutaneous tissue be plicated in? (Gurdin) (Letter to the Editor), PRS, *55:*84, 1975

Lipectomy, abdominal, by W technique (Regnault), PRS, *55:*265, 1975

Incision, face-lift, modification, to facilitate suturing around earlobe (Hirshowitz), PRS, *55:*368, 1975

Lid, lower, temporary suspension after blepharoplasty (Horton, Gursu), PRS, *55:*371, 1975

Lipodystrophy, trochanteric, experience with Pitanguy method of correction (Hoffman, Simon), PRS, *55:*551, 1975

Cheeks, hypoplasia of malar bone: implants for improvement of facial appearance (Hinderer), PRS, *56:*157, 1975

Face lift, segmental approach (Lewis), PRS,

Esthetic Surgery—Cont.
56:297, 1975
Transconjunctival lower lid blepharoplasty for removal of fat (Tomlinson, Hovey), PRS, 56:314, 1975
Adam's apple, laryngeal chondroplasty for appearance (Wolfort, Parry), PRS, 56:371, 1975
Eyelids: "dry eye" complication after blepharoplasty (Rees), PRS, 56:375, 1975
Esthetic plastic surgery, parable of 3 doyens (Stark), PRS, 56:487, 1975
Profiloplasty, rhinoplasty and additional techniques of (Hinderer), PRS, 57:756, 1976. Rev. Iber. Latinoamericana Cir. Plast., 1:245, 1975
Esthetic surgery, causes of failure in mammaplasty (Piotti), PRS, 57:759, 1976 (Italian). Riv. ital. chir. plast., 7:447, 1975
Surgical reduction of adipose tissue hypercellularity in man (Kral). Scand. J. Plast. Reconstr. Surg., 9:140, 1975
Peer review of cosmetic surgeons (Smith). Eye Ear Nose Throat Mon., 55:17, 1976
Considerations in cosmetic plastic surgery (Goldberg *et al*). J. S. C. Med. Assoc., 72:7, 1976
Face-lift, repair of submental depression occurring after (Wilkinson), PRS, 57:33, 1976
Dry eye, keratoconjunctivitis sicca symptoms appearing after blepharoplasty (Graham, Messner, Miller), PRS, 57:57, 1976
Face-lift, male, sideburn relationship (Sturman), PRS, 57:248, 1976
Hair, sideburn reconstruction for alopecia after rhytidectomy (Juri, Juri, de Antueno), PRS, 57:304, 1976
Rhytidectomy, hematoma after, postoperative hypertension as etiological factor, prevention with chlorpromazine (Berner, Morain, Noe), PRS, 57:314, 1976
Forehead rhytidoplasty and brow lifting (Viñas, Caviglia, Cortinas), PRS, 57:445, 1976
Antral-ethmoidal decompression in Graves' disease. Five-year experience (Calcaterra *et al*). West. J. Med., 124:87, 1976

Estlander Flap: See *Cross-Lip Flap*

ETTINGER, R. L.: Oral carcinoma in the aged edentulous patient. A review of seven case histories. Aust. Dent. J. 16:275, 1971
EUFINGER, H.: Surgical procedure in palpable lymph node hypertrophies. Chirurg., 44:163, 1973 (German)
EVANGELOU, G. *et al*: Treatment of 48 cases of postnatal pilonidal sinus by modified Fatey, Lord and Millar technique, PRS, 51:487, 1973. Acta chir. Hellenica, 44:684, 1972

EVANS, A. J.: Tube pedicle flap in cleft palate repair, PRS, 48:395, 1971. Proc. Roy. Soc. Med., 64:73, 1971
EVANS, A. J.: Treatment of burns today, PRS, 50:203, 1972. Proc. Roy. Soc. Med., 64:1295, 1971
EVANS, D., AND RENFREW, C.: Timing of primary cleft palate repair, PRS, 56:360, 1975. Scand. J. Plast. Reconstr. Surg., 8:153, 1974
EVANS, D. M.: Congenital ring-constriction of trunk. Brit. J. Plast. Surg., 26:340, 1973
EVANS, D. M.: Hypoglosso-facial anastomosis in treatment of facial palsy, PRS, 56:676, 1975. Brit. J. Plast. Surg., 27:251, 1974
EVANS, E. E.: Easy-to-make hand exerciser. Phys. Ther., 52:854, 1972
EVANS, E. M.: Treatment of chronic osteomyelitis by saucerization and skin grafting. Proc. Roy. Soc. Med., 64:1204, 1971
EVANS, J. G.: Silicones for medical application, PRS, 56:474, 1975. J. Polym. Med., 4:135, 1974
EVANS, J. N. *et al*: Blow-out fracture of the orbit. J. Laryng. & Otol., 85:1127, 1971
EVANS, J. N. *et al*: Laryngo-tracheoplasty. J. Leg. Med., 88:589, 1974
EVDOKIMOV, A. L. *et al*: Etiology and pathogenesis of the glossalgia syndrome. Stomatologiia (Mosk.), 53:12, 1974 (Russian)
EVERALL, J. D. *et al*: Treatment of primary melanoma by intralesional vaccinia before excision, PRS, 57:404, 1976. Lancet, 2:583, 1975
EVERETT, G. B. *et al*: Renal hemodynamic effects of general anesthesia in outpatients, PRS, 53:373, 1974. Anesth. Analg., Cleve., 52:470, 1973
EVERINGHAM, W. J., HORTON, C. E., AND DEVINE, C. J., JR.: Studies of urethral healing in dogs. PRS, 51:312, 1973
EVERSMANN, W., BURKHALTER, W., AND DUNN, C.: Transfer of the long flexor tendon of the index finger to the proximal phalanx of the long finger during index-ray amputation, PRS, 49:664, 1972. J. Bone & Joint Surg., 53:1343, 1971
EVERSOLE, L. R. *et al*: Mucoepidermoid carcinoma of minor salivary glands: report of 17 cases with follow-up. J. Oral Surg., 30:107, 1972
EVERSOLE, L. R. *et al*: Central and peripheral fibrogenic and neurogenic sarcoma of oral regions. Oral Surg., 36:49, 1973
EVRARD, J.: Osteoarticular infections of the hand. Ann. Chir., 28:267, 1974 (French)
EWING, M. R.: Significance of a single injury in the causation of basal-cell carcinoma of the skin. Aust. N. Z. J. Surg., 41:140, 1971

EXELBY, P. R.: Soft part sarcomas in children. Proc. Natl. Cancer Conf., *7*:619, 1973

Exophthalmos

Histiocytosis presenting as swelling of orbit and eyelid (Codling *et al*). Brit. J. Ophthalmol., *56*:517, 1972

Surgical decompression of the orbit for endocrine exophthalmos (Spira *et al*). Fortschr. Kiefer. Gesichtschir., *18*:35, 1974

Exstrophy: See *Bladder Exstrophy*

Extremities (See also *Burns; Contractures; Hands; Foot; Leg; Leg Ulcers; Lymphedema; War Injuries; Wringer Injuries*)

Extremity, upper, lipomas of (Phalen, Kendrick, Rodriquez), PRS, *48*:512, 1971. Am. J. Surg., *121*:298, 1971

Perfusion, isolation: adjunct to surgical excision in primary treatment of melanoma of extremities (Alrich, Manwaring, Horsley), PRS, *49*:473, 1972. Am. J. Surg., *121*:583, 1971

Serum enzymes in experimental ballistic injury to extremities (Lawson *et al*), PRS, *50*:423, 1972. Arch. Surg., *103*:741, 1971

Forearm, pitfalls in management of penetrating injuries of (Symonds *et al*), PRS, *49*:582, 1972. J. Trauma, *11*:47, 1971

Fibrosarcoma of thigh associated with prosthetic vascular graft (Herrmann *et al*), PRS, *48*:397, 1971. New England J. Med., *284*:91, 1971

Extremity, upper: bacteroides necrotizing fasciitis of (Rein, Cosman), PRS, *48*:592, 1971

Amputation alternative, freezing gangrenous extremity in poor risk patients (Niazmand, Miller, Barker), PRS, *52*:107, 1973. Am. J. Surg., *124*:701, 1972

Extremity, upper, causalgia and transthoracic sympathectomy (Buker *et al*), PRS, *52*:322, 1973. Am. J. Surg., *124*:724, 1972

Stereotaxic pinpointing of foreign bodies in limbs (McFadden), PRS, *50*:424, 1972. Ann. Surg., *175*:81, 1972

Limb ischemia and nerve injury (Lungborg), PRS, *51*:350, 1973. Arch. Surg., *104*:631, 1972

Extremities, injuries with severe skin avulsions; clinico-therapeutics aspects (Ionescu *et al*). Chirurgia (Bucur.), *21*:11, 1972 (Rumanian)

Dermotomy, decompression (Gaspard, Cohen, Gaspar), PRS, *50*:538, 1972. J.A.M.A., *220*:831, 1972

Humerus, fractured, radial nerve entrap-

Extremities — Cont.

ment in exuberant callus (Jackson *et al*), PRS, *51*:705, 1973. Mil. Med., *137*:203, 1972

Knee Pain and Disability. By Rene Cailliet. F. A. Davis Co., Philadelphia, 1973. PRS, *55*:86, 1975

Limb, shortened: dynamics of reparative regeneration after lengthening by method of distraction epiphysiolysis (Eydelshteyn, Udalova, Bochkarev), PRS, *54*:511, 1974. Acta chir. plast., *15*:149, 1973

Extremity, swollen, calculating volume changes from surface measurements (Lennihan, Mackereth), PRS, *54*:113, 1974. Am. J. Surg., *126*:649, 1973

Successful skin grafting in case of pemphigus vulgaris (Bertenyi *et al*). Brit. J. Plast. Surg., *26*:381, 1973

Extremity, sarcoma of soft tissue in (Suit, Russell, Martin), PRS, *54*:244, 1974. Cancer, *31*:1247, 1973

Extremity, tourniquet used on, instrument or weapon? (Sanders), PRS, *54*:236, 1974. Hand, *5*:119, 1973

Extremity, upper, posterior interosseous nerve syndrome secondary to rheumatoid synovitis (Millender, Nalebuff, Holdsworth), PRS, *52*:323, 1973. J. Bone & Joint Surg., *55A*:375, 1973

Lower extremity injuries, reconstructive surgery of (Cocke). J. Tenn. Med. Assoc., *66*:1039, 1973

Extremity, upper, household wringer injuries (McCullock, Boswick, Jonas), PRS, *52*:679, 1973. J. Trauma, *13*:1, 1973

Extremities, malignant tumors of, patients with, prosthesis on operating table after amputation in (Gur'ianova). Ortop. Travmatol. Protez., *34*:14, 1973 (Russian)

Extremity, upper, device for the continuous elevation of (Gardner), PRS, *51*:471, 1973

Electrical burns of upper extremity (Salisbury *et al*), PRS, *51*:648, 1973

Flaps, cross-leg, in children (Argamaso *et al*), PRS, *51*:662, 1973

Extremities, replanted: replantation surgery in China. American Replantation Mission, PRS, *52*:476, 1973

Limbs, use of tourniquet on, dangers and their prevention (Tubiana). Rev. Chir. Orthop., *59*:239, 1973 (French)

Open injuries of the lower extremity (Burkhalter). Surg. Clin. North Am., *53*:1439, 1973

Plastic surgery of skin in treatment of bone fractures of extremities with traumatic skin defects (Varavva). Vestn. Khir., *111*:97, 1973 (Russian)

Problems of primary treatment of large soft

Extremities – Cont.

tissue defects of lower limb combined with bone fractures (Jokic). Vojnosanit. Pregl., *30:*39, 1973 (Croatian)

Vein graft, saphenous, placing into upper arm – new cosmetic and rehabilitation method for patients under chronic hemodialysis (Lieschke *et al*). Z. Gesamte. Inn. Med., *28:*364, 1973 (German)

Extremity, lower, deep circular burns of (Ivanova), PRS, *52:*598, 1973. Zentralbl. Chir., *98:*331, 1973

Extremity salvage by small vessel revascularization (Jolly *et al*). Am. Surg., *40:*521, 1974

Extremity, lower, melanoma of, role of groin dissection in (McCarthy, Haagensen, Herter), PRS, *54:*237, 1974. Ann. Surg., *179:*156, 1974

Ring constriction of extremities (Vrebos), PRS, *56:*602, 1975. Brux. Med., *54:*693, 1974

Knee, medial compartment of, ligamentous injuries. Late reconstruction (Slocum *et al*). Clin. Orthop., *100:*23, 1974

Pain syndromes in upper extremity, chronic (Omer, Thomas), PRS, *56:*679, 1975. Clin. Orthop., *104:*37, 1974

Extremity, upper, nerve compression lesions of (Spinner, Spencer), PRS, *56:*679, 1975. Clin. Orthop., *104:*46, 1974

Surgical aspects of peripheral nerve trauma (Ducker *et al*). Curr. Probl. Surg., 1, Sept., 1974

Extremity, upper, war injuries of (Brara, Kathpalia, Char), PRS, *56:*228, 1975. Indian J. Surg., *36:*379, 1974

Dystrophy, reflex sympathetic, treated by continuous elevation by spica cast (Leach, Clawson, Caprio), PRS, *54:*502, 1974. J. Bone & Joint Surg., *56A:*416, 1974

Ischemia, limb, differential diagnosis and treatment in drug subculture (Kaufer *et al*), PRS, *57:*541, 1976. J. Trauma, *14:*853, 1974

Hands and feet, cartilaginous tumors of soft tissues (Dahlin, Salvador), PRS, *55:*385, 1975. Mayo Clin. Proc., *49:*721, 1974

Cellulitis: treatment of lymphedema (Bunchman, Lewis), PRS, *54:*64, 1974

Extremity, upper, fungal invasions secondary to large burns (Salisbury, Silverstein, Goodwin), PRS, *54:*654, 1974

Limbs, amputation or reconstruction? (Velez-Gutierrez), PRS, *55:*258, 1975. Rev. el Medico, *24:*19, 1974

Anomalies, multiple congenital, associated with teratogenic exposure (Nora, Nora), PRS, *56:*110, 1975. Arch. Environmental

Extremities – Cont.

Health, *30:*17, 1975

Vascular compartment syndromes (Fowler, Willis), PRS, *56:*597, 1975. Canad. J. Surg., *18:*157, 1975

Compartmental syndromes in which the skin is the limiting boundary (Gaspard *et al*). Clin. Orthop., *113:*65, 1975

Whirlpool therapy for fractures of extremities complicated by soft tissue wounds (Abraham *et al*), PRS, *55:*720, 1975. Orthop. Rev., *4:*47, 1975

Muscle and nerve injuries, differential diagnosis of; small, deep forearm lacerations (Schwager, Smith, Goulian), PRS, *55:*190, 1975

Extremities immobilized after skin grafting with inflatable splint (Schwager, Imber), PRS, *57:*523, 1976

EYDELSHTEYN, B. M., UDALOVA, N. F., AND BOCHKAREV, G. F.: Dynamics of reparative regeneration after lengthening by the method of distraction epiphysiolysis, PRS, *54:*511, 1974. Acta chir. plast., *15:*149, 1973

Eye (See also *Blepharoplasty, Ectropion, Entropion, Eyelids, Lagophthalmos*)

Ophthalmology, some plastic operations using sterilized homologous tissues (Tomilova, Czechova), PRS, *51:*486, 1973. Acta chir. plast., *13:*235, 1971

Oculocutaneous syndrome, three cases of new congenital (Morizane, Uemura, Shimizu), PRS, *49:*236, 1972. Acta Soc. Ophth. Japan, *75:*1316, 1971

System of Ophthalmology. Ed. by Sir Stewart Duke-Elder. Vol. XIV. Injuries. C. V. Mosby Co., St. Louis, 1972. PRS, *52:*571, 1973

Eye enucleation, use of homologous fascia for firm anchorate of homo- and allo-implants after (Kolen, Morozova), PRS, *53:*499, 1974. Acta chir. plast., *15:*46, 1973

Pediatric ophthalmology, outpatient anesthesia for (Nagel *et al*), PRS, *53:*373, 1974. Anesth. Analg., Cleve., *52:*558, 1973

Eye, the orbit (Trokel), PRS, *52:*451, 1973. Arch. Ophth., *89:*152, 1973

Eye, differential diagnosis in orbital injury (Smith, Wiggs), PRS, *53:*240, 1974. Arch. Ophth., *89:*484, 1973

Eye care in facial paralysis (Goren, Clemis), PRS, *52:*594, 1973. Arch. Otolaryng., *97:*227, 1973

Diplopia, injury to superior oblique muscle and trochlea and associated EOM imbalance (Harashina, Tajima), PRS, *53:*602, 1974. Jap. J. Plast. Reconstr. Surg., *16:*362, 1973

Eye — Cont.

Paracentesis: acute retrobulbar hemorrhage during elective blepharoplasty (Hartley, Lester, Schatten), PRS, *52:*8, 1973. Discussions by Lemoine, Rees, Newell, PRS, *52:*12, 1973

Ocular tissue damage, safety with lasers (Borland *et al*), PRS, *54:*383, 1974. Proc. Roy. Soc. Med., *66:*841, 1973

Stensen's duct transplantation, late results of. Vestn. Oftalmol., *5:*44, 1973 (Russian)

Transactions of the New Orleans Academy of Ophthalmology. By C. Beard *et al*. C. V. Mosby Co., St. Louis, 1974. PRS, *55:*355, 1975

Conjunctival sac reconstruction, modification of Csapody's method in complete obliteration of cavity (Morozov, Grechischlina), PRS, *56:*351, 1975. Acta chir. plast., *16:*209, 1974

Ophthalmic surgery, hyperthermia associated with (Beasley). Am. J. Ophth., *77:*76, 1974

Stensen's duct, extending to eyeball (Bascones *et al*). An. Esp. Odontoestomatol., *33:*9, 1974 (Spanish)

Eye abnormalities and skeletal deformities in Pierre Robin syndrome (Cosman, Keyser), PRS, *56:*109, 1975. Cleft Palate J., *11:*404, 1974

Eye, anterior segment, diseases of. Diagnosis and therapy (Nover *et al*). Fortschr. Med., *92:*233, 1974 (German)

Eye, orbicular muscle of, "fingerprint" inclusions in (Radnot). Ophthalmologica, *168:*282, 1974 (German)

Eye complications with blepharoplasty or other eyelid surgery (DeMere, Wood, Austin), PRS, *53:*634, 1974

Eye, dry, following blepharoplasty (Swartz, Schultz, Seaton), PRS, *54:*644, 1974

Retinal artery closure, central, during orbital hemorrhage from retrobulbar injection (Kraufhar, Seelenfreund, Froelich), PRS, *54:*382, 1974. Tr. Am. Acad. Ophth., *78:*65, 1974

Ocular protection shield (Horblass). Trans. Am. Acad. Ophthalmol. Otolaryngol., *78:*228, 1974

Polyglycolic acid sutures in ophthalmic surgery (White *et al*). Trans. Am. Acad. Ophthalmol. Otolaryngol., *78:*632, 1974

Ophthalmoplegia, progressive external, associated with retinal pigment epitheliopathy (Daniele, Cianchetti, Cao), PRS, *57:*755, 1976. Am. J. Ophth., *8:*585, 1975

Ocular compression and noncorticosteroidal anti-inflammatory agents (Obstbaum, Podos), PRS, *57:*113, 1976. Am. J. Ophth.,

Eye — Cont.

*79:*1008, 1975

Ophthalmoplegia, painful: the Tolosa-Hunt syndrome (Roca), PRS, *57:*256, 1976. Ann. Ophth., *7:*828, 1975

Carcinoma metastatic to anterior segment of eye (Ferry, Font), PRS, *57:*394, 1976. Arch. Ophth., *93:*472, 1975

Strabismus surgery, polyglycolic acid suture in (Blau *et al*), PRS, *57:*394, 1976. Arch. Ophth., *93:*538, 1975

The public face or psychological and legal complexities in plastic ophthalmic surgery (Lubkin). Brit. J. Ophthalmol., *59:*593, 1975

Pupils, fixed and dilated (Weinstock), PRS, *56:*104, 1975. Emerg. Med., *7:*123, 1975

Oculo-orbital injuries, severe (Dastoor), PRS, *56:*460, 1975. Internat. Surg., *60:*217, 1975

Eye trauma in childhood (Helveston), PRS, *57:*256, 1976. Pediatr. Clin. N. Am., *22:*501, 1975

"Dry eye" complication after blepharoplasty (Rees), PRS, *56:*375, 1975

Eye injuries in orbital fractures (Jabaley, Lerman, Sanders), PRS, *56:*410, 1975

Morphological aspects of xerophthalmia after transplantation of Stensen's duct into conjunctival cavity (Kurbanaeve *et al*). Vestn. Otfalmol., *2:*43, 1975 (Russian)

Eye, dry, keratoconjunctivitis sicca symptoms appearing after blepharoplasty (Graham, Messner, Miller), PRS, *57:*57, 1976

Eye, Burns of

Ocular complications associated with burns (Asch *et al*), PRS, *50:*205, 1972. J. Trauma, *11:*857, 1971

Eye, severely burned, early surgery of (Heinc). Cesk. Oftalmol., *28:*279, 1972 (Czechoslovakian)

Burns, eyelid deformities due to (Silverstein, Peterson), PRS, *51:*38, 1973

Early skin graft in the treatment of palpebral burns (Couderc *et al*). Bull. Soc. Ophthalmol. Fr., *74:*1159, 1974 (French)

Burns, 75% third degree, penetrating keratoplasty in patient with (Older, Allansmith), PRS, *56:*223, 1975. Ann. Ophth., *7:*309, 1975

Eye Socket (See also *Blepharoplasty, Blepharoptosis, Enophthalmos*)

Superior sulcus deformity and ptosis. Surgical correction (Spaeth). Int. Ophthalmol. Clin., *10:*791, 1971

Superior sulcus deformity. Prosthetic correction (Connelly). Int. Ophthalmol. Clin., *10:*799, 1971

Eye Socket—Cont.

Eye socket reconstruction with composite grafts (Orticochea), PRS, *48:*343, 1971

Reconstruction of eye socket for prosthesis (Van Clooster *et al*). Acta Stomatol. Belg., *69:*331, 1972 (Dutch)

Retinoblastomas, reconstruction of exenterated orbit in children (Murillo), PRS, *51:*346, 1973. Cir. cir. Mexico, *40:*76, 1972

Orbital lining, doughnut skin graft for (Hebert) (Follow-Up Clinic), PRS, *50:*402, 1972

Conjunctival melanoma in anophthalmic orbit (Scuderi *et al*). Ophthalmologica, *166:*172, 1973

Enucleation: correction of enophthalmos in the anophthalmic orbit (Iverson, Vistnes, Siegel), PRS, *51:*545, 1973

Anophthalmic orbit, surgical correction of lower eyelid ptosis (Vistnes, Iverson, Laub), PRS, *52:*346, 1973

Remote results of tunnel implants of phtoroplast into the orbital cavity after enucleation (Rubinchik). Oftalmol. Zh., *29:*288, 1974 (Russian)

Anophthalmos: surgical treatment of the contracted socket (Vistnes, Iverson), PRS, *53:*563, 1974

Experiences with movable bulbar implant of hydrophile gel methylacrylate Hydron, following enucleation (Olah). Z. Cesk. Oftalmol., *31:*180, 1975 (Slovakian)

Eye, Tumors of (See also *Eyelids, Neoplasms of; Melanoma, Eye and Orbit*)

Pterygium, inverse ungual (Caputo, Prandi), PRS, *57:*267, 1976. Arch. Dermat., *108:*817, 1973

Sarcoma, osteogenic, developing after radiotherapy for retinoblastoma (Shah, Arlen, Miller), PRS, *55:*255, 1975. Am. Surgeon, *40:*485, 1974

Meibomian gland carcinoma presenting as lacrimal gland tumor (Shields, Font), PRS, *55:*641, 1975. Arch. Ophth., *92:*304, 1974

Conjunctiva, invasive squamous cell carcinoma of (Iliff, Marback, Green), PRS, *56:*235, 1975. Arch. Ophth., *93:*119, 1975

Eye, carcinoma metastatic to anterior segment of (Ferry, Font), PRS, *57:*394, 1976. Arch. Ophth., *93:*472, 1975

Eyebrow transplantation (Van Droogenbroeck). Int. J. Lepr., *39:*629, 1971

Eyebrows (See also *Brow Lift; Leprosy*)

Eyebrows, reconstruction with free skin grafts (Yarchuk, Tertsionas), PRS, *52:*205, 1973. Acta chir. plast., *14:*82, 1972

Combination of 2 methods of restoration of the brows (Sukachev *et al*). Stomatologiia

Eyebrows—Cont.

(Mosk.), *51:*79, 1972 (Russian)

Eyebrow reconstruction with free transplantation of small grafts of hairy skin with subcutaneous fat layer (Limberg). Vestn. Khir., *106:*64, 1972 (Russian)

Eyebrows in leprous patients, correction of alopecia in (Guerrero-Santos, Matus, Vera-Strathmann (Follow-Up Clinic), PRS, *52:*183, 1973

Eyebrow reconstruction, buried graft method (Ausin Garcia, Bermudez Piernagorda), PRS, *56:*590, 1975. Rev. españ. cir. plast., *6:*97, 1973

Scope of plastic surgery in leprosy: a ten year progress report (Antia). Clin. Plast. Surg., *1:*69, 1974

Eyebrow, hemi-, reconstruction of, with temporoparietal flap (Mantero *et al*). Int. Surg., *59:*369, 1974

Eyebrow replacement, role of punch grafting in (Ranney). Lepr. Rev., *45:*153, 1974

Restoration of the eyebrows with hairy flaps of the chin using a Filatov tube flap (Arzhantsev). Voen. Med. Zh., *0:*38, 1974 (Russian)

Eyebrow reconstruction in the burned patient (Brent), PRS, *55:*312, 1975

Functional dermatochalasia (Carroll). Minn. Med., *59:*15, 1976

Eyelids (See also *Blepharoplasty; Blepharoptosis; Blepharospasm; Ectropion; Enophthalmos; Entropion; Epicanthus; Exophthalmos; Hypertelorism; Hypotelorism; Lacrimal Apparatus; Lagophthalmos*)

Partial eyelid autoplasty with one-stage mucosal or chondro-mucosal graft (Vandenbussche *et al*). Ann. chir. plast., *16:*322, 1971 (French)

Surgical treatment of trichiasis (Forough *et al*). Ann. Ocul. (Paris), *205:*1215, 1972 (French)

Eyelid edema and ecchymosis after corrective rhinoplasty, reducing the (Shehadi), PRS, *49:*508, 1972

Eyelids, lacrimal apparatus, and conjunctiva (Boniuk). Arch. Ophth., *90:*239, 1973

Cilia graft (English *et al*). Brit. J. Ophthalmol., *57:*763, 1973

Eyelid, lower, plastic surgery of, in partial defect or its absence (Gundrova). Oftalmol. Zh., *28:*483, 1973 (Russian)

Contemporary Oculoplastic Surgery. Ed. by P. Guibor and B. Smith. Grune & Stratton, Inc., New York, 1974

Eyelid, upper, total substitute (Alberth). Klin. Monatsbl. Augenheilkd., *165:*84,

Eyelids – Cont.

1974 (German)

Eyelid surgery, free total transplantation in (Neubauer). Klin. Monatsbl. Augenheilkd., *165*:86, 1974 (German)

Reconstructive and Plastic Surgery of the Eyelids. By Frank P. English and Warren A. Keats. Charles C Thomas, Springfield, Ill., 1975

Eyelid, metastatic gangrene of, in *Pseudomonas* septicemia (Treister *et al*), PRS, *57*:113, 1976. Ann. Ophth., 7:639, 1975

Atypical oculoplastic surgery in children (Neubauer). Klin. Monatsbl. Augenheilkd., *167*:199, 1975 (German)

Eyelids, Canthoplasty

Canthopexy; new approach (van der Meulen), PRS, *50*:474, 1972

Eyelash traction test to determine if the medial canthal ligament is detached (Furnas, Bircoll), PRS, *52*:315, 1973

New method for the fixation of the median palpebral ligament (Albano *et al*). Rev. Assoc. Med. Bras., *21*:291, 1975 (Portuguese)

Eyelids, Deformities, Acquired (See also *Blepharoplasty; Ectropion; Entropion; Lagophthalmos*)

Eyelid deformities, cosmetic, pinch technique for (Parkes). Arch. Ophth., *89*:324, 1973

Correction of blepharochalasis (Hollwich *et al*). Klin. Monatsbl. Augenheilkd., *166*:255, 1975 (German)

Eyelids, Deformities, Congenital (See also *Blepharoptosis*)

Congenital Anomalies of the Eyelids. By Ernesto P. Caronni. Minerva Medical Press, Turin, Italy, 1967. PRS, *50*:518, 1972

Schwartz's syndrome: malformation syndromes in human genetic disease (Nyhan), PRS, *52*:237, 1973

Eyelids, Epicanthus: See *Epicanthus*

Eyelids, Injuries of (See also *Eyelids, Reconstruction*)

Eyelid injuries, secondary plastic surgery of (Schmid). Klin. Monatsbl. Augenheilkd., *160*:581, 1972 (German)

Medial canthal ligament, eyelash traction test to determine if it is detached (Furnas, Bircoll), PRS, *52*:315, 1973

Eyelids, Neoplasms of (See also *Eyelids, Reconstruction*)

Partial eyelid autoplasty with one-stage mucosal or chondro-mucosal graft (Vanden-

Eyelids, Neoplasms of – Cont.

bussche *et al*). Ann. chir. plast., *16*:322, 1971 (French)

Plastic surgery for total lid defect due to resection of the cancer (Tajima *et al*). Folia Ophthalmol. Jap., *22*:949, 1971 (Japanese)

Plastic surgery of eyelid cancer (Ide *et al*). Ophthalmology (Tokyo), *13*:865, 1971 (Japanese)

Malignant tumors of eyelid (Leventhal, Messer), PRS, *52*:328, 1973. Am. J. Surg., *124*:522, 1972

Cancer of the eyelid – a cryosurgical approach (Zacarian). Ann. Ophth., *4*:473, 1972

Upper lid reconstruction (Fox). Arch. Ophth., *88*:46, 1972

Eyelids, lymphoid tumors of (Mortada). Bull. Ophthalmol. Soc. Egypt, *65*:529, 1972

Ear skin-cartilage plastic surgery for eyelid margin tumors (Hanselmayer *et al*). Opthalmologica, *165*:464, 1972 (German)

Pedicled skin grafts for eyelid cancer (Imaizumi *et al*). Ophthalmology (Tokyo), *14*:181, 1972 (Japanese)

Canthal region, medial, basal cell carcinoma of (Abraham, Jabaley, Hoopes), PRS, *53*:688, 1974. Am. J. Surg., *126*:492, 1973

Benign lymphocytic lymphoma of upper eyelid and left plica semilunaris (Tabor). Ann. Ophth., *5*:964, 1973

Carcinoma of eyelid, mucinous (adenocystic) (Rodrigues, Lubowitz, Shannon), PRS, *53*:601, 1974. Arch. Ophth., *89*:493, 1973

Eyelid margin, granular cell myoblastoma of (Friedman *et al*). Brit. J. Ophthalmol., *57*:757, 1973

Eyelids, voluminous pigmented basal cell epithelioma of (Henry *et al*). Bull. Soc. Ophtalmol. Fr., *73*:315, 1973 (French)

Carcinoma, lids and orbit, treatment of (Shannon). J. Med. Soc. N. J., *70*:914, 1973

Eyelids, tumors of, outcome of primary plastic surgery in (Zaikova *et al*). Oftalmol. Zh., *28*:485, 1973 (Russian)

Treatment of malignant disease of skin of orbital region (Lederman). Proc. Roy. Soc. Med., *66*:690, 1973

Infant, tumors of external canthus in (Hosxe *et al*). Rev. Stomatol. Chir. Maxillofac., *74*:483, 1973 (French)

Multicentric sebaceous adenocarcinoma of meibomian gland (Cavanagh *et al*). Am. J. Ophth., *77*:326, 1974

Pseudosarcomatous fasciitis (Meacham). Am. J. Ophth., *77*:747, 1974

Carcinoma, meibomian gland, presenting as lacrimal gland tumor (Shields, Font), PRS, *55*:641, 1975. Arch. Ophth., *92*:304, 1974

Full thickness graft from eyelid to eyelid

EZROKHIN, V. M.: Analysis of results of treatment of skin surface wounds after tattoo removal according to data of the Moscow Research Institute for Cosmetology for 1964–1970. Vestn. Dermatol. Venerol., *46:*61, 1972 (Russian)

EZROKHIN, V. M. *et al*: Treatment of skin wound surfaces with a collagen film after elimination of tattooing with a dermatome. Sov. Med., *34:*149, 1971 (Russian)

F

FABER, H.: Specifics of physical care after transsexual surgery. Am. J. Nurs., *73:*463, 1973

FABRE, L. AND CASTELNAU, J. L.: Rhinoplasty using Converse method. J. Fr. Otorhinolaryngol., *21:*938, 1972 (French)

FABREGA, HORACIO, JR.: *Disease and Social Behavior – An Interdisciplinary Perspective.* M. I. T. Press, Cambridge, Mass., 1974. PRS, *55:*699, 1975

FABRI, S. *et al*: Anatomical notes on the vascular and lymphatic structures of the hand. Ann. Osp. Maria Vittoria Torino, *17:*137, 1974 (Italian)

Face (See also *Facial*)

    Color Atlas of Oro-Facial Diseases. By M. A. Bedford. Year Book Medical Pub., Inc., Chicago, 1972.

    Practical method of skin sutures of the face (Kajima). Surg. Ther. (Osaka), *26:*532, 1972 (Japanese)

    Facial features, improvement (Huffstadt). Tijdschr. Ziekenverpl., *25:*994, 1972 (Dutch)

    Smile, the classification and criteria, applications in facial esthetics (Aboucaya). Acad. Rev., *2:*2611, 1973

    Facial scars and lymph outflow (Clodius). Praxis, *62:*336, 1973 (German)

    Facial skeleton, growth of, in guinea pigs after experimental fusion of premaxillo-maxillary suture (Letter to Editor). Proc. Finn. Dent. Soc., *69:*263, 1973

    Self-retaining midfacial retractor (Robbett). Trans. Am. Acad. Ophthalmol. Otolaryngol., *77:*1149, 1973

    "What's in a name?" (Beekhuis). Arch. Otolaryng., *100:*165, 1974

    Age and the face. Brit. Med. J., *2:*4, 1974

    Face, symmetry of, as pre- and postoperative consideration (Gorney, Harries), PRS, *54:*187, 1974

    Facial region, evolutive and embryological development (Sarrat), PRS, *57:*753, 1976.

Face – Cont.

    Cir. Plast. Ibero-Latino Am., *1:*7, 1975

    Face, principles in restoration of soft tissue damage (Tschopp). Helv. Chir. Acta, *42:*165, 1975 (German)

    Face growth in children after combined push-back and pharyngeal flap operations, cephalometric study of (Pearl, Kaplan), PRS, *57:*480, 1976

Face, Anatomy

    Facial artery branches (Mitz, Ricbourg, Lassau), PRS, *54:*500, 1974. Ann. chir. plast., *18:*339, 1973

    Face, development of (Stark), PRS, *53:*600, 1974. Surg. Gynec. & Obst., *137:*403, 1973

Face, Burns: See *Burns, Face*

Face, Congenital Deformities (See also *Cleft Lips; Facial Clefts; Hemifacial Atrophy; various specific deformities*)

    Clinical Delineation of Birth Defects. Ed. by Daniel Bergsma. Williams & Wilkins Co., Baltimore, 1971. PRS, *50:*79, 1972

    Congenital Malformations: Notes and Comments. By Joseph Warkany. Year Book Medical Publishers, Chicago, 1971. PRS, *52:*570, 1973

    Fissure of the lower lip, mandible, tongue associated with incomplete median cervical fissure (Kriens). ADM, *28:*57, 1971 (Spanish)

    Midfacial structures in rat, effect of lathyrogens on developing (Stivers, Steffek, Yarington), PRS, *49:*586, 1972. J. Surg. Res., *11:*415, 1971

    Melkersson-Rosenthal syndrome (Vistnes, Kernahan), PRS, *48:*126, 1971

    Maxillary retrusion, correction of prognathism associated with (Rusconi, Brusati), PRS, *48:*558, 1971

    Masticatory muscles, vascular hamartomata of (Azzolini, Nouvenne), PRS, *51:*107, 1973. Riv. ital. chir. plast., *3:*135, 1971

    Leprechaunism (Donohue's syndrome) in female infant (Poradovska, Jaworska, Hanc), PRS, *51:*233, 1973. Acta chir. plast., *14:*4, 1972

    Orofacial-digital syndrome, 11th case in same family (Vissain, Vaillaud), PRS, *51:*605, 1973. Ann. dermat. & syph., *99:*5, 1972

    Syndrome, Melkersson's: unusual case (Hawkins). J. Laryng. & Otol., *86:*943, 1972

    Facial teratoma in the newborn. Report of five cases (Gifford, MacCollum), PRS, *49:*616, 1972

Face, Congenital Deformities—Cont.

Functional dermatochalasia (Carroll). Minn. Med., *59:*15, 1976

Congenital deformity: frontonasal dysplasia with alar clefts in two sisters (Fox, Golden, Edgerton), PRS, *57:*553, 1976

Face, Infections of

Streptococcus gangrene of face, acute postoperative (Tschopp), PRS, *52:*204, 1973. Chir. Plast., *1:*244, 1972

Pyoderma, skin infections in Vietnam (Allen et al), PRS, *52:*103, 1973. Mil. Med., *137:*295, 1972

Trigeminal ganglions, human, recovery of herpes-simplex virus from (Baringer, Swoveland), PRS, *52:*321, 1973. New England J. Med., *288:*648, 1973

Infection, disseminated cytomegalovirus associated with death in patient with severe facial injuries (Constant, Davis, Maldonado), PRS, *51:*336, 1973

Pyoderma gangrenosum, facial, preceding ulcerative colitis (Decherd, Leyden, Holtzapple), PRS, *55:*645, 1975. Cutis, *14:*208, 1974

Infections, enhanced resistance to certain, in vitamin A-treated mice (Cohen, Elin), PRS, *54:*192, 1974

Pyoderma gangrenosum, hyperbaric oxygen therapy for (Thomas et al), PRS, *57:*405, 1976. Arch. Dermat., *110:*445, 1975

Cellulitis, synergistic necrotizing, clinicosurgical treatment of (Corrao, Beveraggi, Pietravello), PRS, *57:*764, 1976. Bol. y trab. soc. argent. cir., *36:*271, 1975

Cellulitis: Kaposi's varicelliform eruption complicating local facial trauma (Grossman, Berger, Hoehn), PRS, *55:*625, 1975

Face, Surgery of

Our experiences with regional skin flaps in the treatment of large defects of the head and neck region following tumor extirpation (Nagel). Arch. Klin. Exp. Ohren Nasen Kehlkopfheilkd., *199:*640, 1971 (German)

Flap, deltopectoral, to close extensive defects of face (Anderl), PRS, *53:*104, 1974. Chir. Plast., *1:*53, 1971

Reconstructive and plastic surgery of the face (Neuner). Schweiz. Monatsschr. Zahnheilkd., *81:*947, 1971 (German)

Postoperative maxillofacial surgeries, use of 1-phenyl-2-pyrrolidine-penthane in (Garlipp, Neder), PRS, *52:*331, 1973. A. Folha med. Brazil, *64:*947, 1972

Local skin flaps in treatment of cutaneous

Face, Surgery of—Cont.

contractures, sequelae of burns of the anterior and lateral sides of the neck (Janvier et al). Ann. chir. plast., *17:*26, 1972 (French)

Use of deltopectoral flap in cervicofacial restoration (Lejour et al). Ann. chir. plast., *17:*126, 1972 (French)

Face, acute postoperative streptococcus gangrene (Tschopp), PRS, *52:*204, 1973. Chir. Plast., *1:*244, 1972

Facial, jaw and oral surgery, analgesia with pentazocine following (Grasser). Med. Monatsschr., *26:*230, 1972 (German)

Maxillofacial and dental surgery, general anesthesia with association of gamma-OH (sodium 4-hydroxy-butyrate) and neuroleptoanalgesic drugs in (Antognini et al). Minerva Stomatol., *21:*255, 1972 (Italian)

Facial and dental anomalies, management of. Basic principles of orthodontic and plastic reconstruction (Demetriades et al). Odontostomatol. Proodos., *26:*151, 1972 (Greek)

Face, lower, extensive losses in, from war injuries, surgical rehabilitation after (Parsons, Beckwith, Thering), PRS, *49:*533, 1972

Newborn, facial teratoma in; report of 5 cases (Gifford, MacCollum), PRS, *49:*616, 1972

Face, plastic surgery of, principal false ideas and false friends in (Jost). Probl. Actuels Otorhinolaryngol., *357:*70, 1972 (French)

Maxillofacial and oral surgery coming of age in Puerto Rico (Valls). Rev. Odontol. P. R., *10:*31, 1972

Face, plastic and reparative surgery of, Maxillase 3000 in (Souyris et al). Rev. Odontostomatol. Midi Fr., *30:*57, 1972 (French)

Specificity of free skin graft of the face (Ito). Surg. Ther. (Osaka), *26:*515, 1972 (Japanese)

Progress in the technic of facial skin flap (Onizuka). Surg. Ther. (Osaka), *26:*519, 1972 (Japanese)

Pterygomaxillary fossa surgery for facial pain and some forms of epistaxis (Corvera, Somonte, Gonzalez-Romero), PRS, *52:*98, 1973. Tribuna Med. Mexico, *23:*3, 1972

Maxillofacial surgery, current methods of anesthesia (Mukovozov). Voen. Med. Zh., *6:*60, 1972 (Russian)

Face, corrective surgical office procedures of (Stough). Am. Fam. Physician, *7:*68, 1973

Maxillofacial surgery, trimethoprim-sulfamethoxazole combination (Eusaprim, in Stricker et al). J. Fr. Otorhinolaryngol., *22:*657, 1973 (French)

Maxillofacial surgery, extensive, cervical

Face, Surgery of — Cont.

neuromas following (Graham). J. Surg. Oncol., *5:*485, 1973

Face, skin defects of, reconstruction of (Kole). Langenbecks Arch. Chir., *334:*593, 1973 (German)

Tissues, soft, advancement of, to correct mild midfacial retrusion (O'Connor *et al*), PRS, *52:*42, 1973

Facial osteotomy. Surgical treatment of hypertelorism (Psillakis *et al*). Rev. Paul. Med., *82:*151, 1973 (Portuguese)

Plastic surgery of face — a medical problem? (Haas). Z. Laryngol. Rhinol. Otol., *52:*79, 1973 (German)

Facial incisions and approaches (Saad, Maisels), PRS, *54:*697, 1974. Brit. J. Surg., *61:*566, 1974

Facial surgery, use of rhomboid flap in (Cotton). Can. J. Otolaryngol., *3:*51, 1974

Facial defect, repair of, using free skin island flap with vascular anastomoses, case report. Chinese Med. J., *3:*163, 1974 (Chinese)

Combined orthopedic-plastic surgery of the jaws and face (Neuner). Fortschr. Kiefer. Gesichtschir., *18:*72, 1974 (German)

Photomontage in the planning of jaw and facial operations (Kriens). Fortschr. Kiefer. Gesichtschir.,*18:*101, 1974 (German)

Facial asymmetry, surgical orthodontic treatment of, using direct bonding plastic brackets (Kawamura *et al*). Int. J. Oral Surg., *3:*252, 1974

Combination of two products with antidepressive and tranquilizing actions. Their interest in an O. R. L. and facial surgery department (Pech *et al*). J. Fr. Otorhinolaryngol., *23:*267, 1974 (French)

Temperature, raised, after osteotomies (Tetsch), PRS, *55:*387, 1975. J. Maxillo-facial Surg., *2:*141, 1974

Facial asymmetry, treatment of, with Silastic implant (Sher *et al*). J. Oral Surg., *32:*460, 1974

Clinical success of distant transfer of free skin flap in head and neck regions by microvascular anastomoses (Fujino *et al*). Keio J. Med., *23:*47, 1974

Principles of reconstructive operations on the face using flaps and free grafts (Haas). Laryngol. Rhinol. Otol., *53:*371, 1974 (German)

Value of an original naso-tracheal catheter in maxillo-facial surgery and stomatology (Lachard *et al*). Rev. Stomatol. Chir. Maxillofac., *75:*1029, 1974 (French)

Amylase isoenzymes in serum after maxillo-facial surgery (Skude, Rothman), PRS,

Face, Surgery of — Cont.

*55:*120, 1975. Scand. J. Plast. Reconstr. Surg., *7:*105, 1974

Face and neck, operations on, correlations between some hemodynamic and blood coagulation indices in (Konobevtsev *et al*). Stomatologiia (Mosk.), *53:*23, 1974 (Russian)

Facial plastic surgery, anesthesia techniques and (Kean *et al*). Trans. Pa. Acad. Ophthalmol. Otolaryngol., *27:*45, 1974

Contour plastic surgery of traumatic facial disfigurements with EGMASS-12 and fluoroplast-4 plastics (Kabakov *et al*). Voen. Med. Zh., *2:*20, 1974 (Russian)

Face and neck, penetrating defects of, new developments in plastic operations to close, using Filatov's tube flap (Arzhantsev). Voen. Med. Zh., 27, July 1974 (Russian)

Forehead flap, modified non-delayed (Hamaker, Conley), PRS, *57:*680, 1976. Arch. Otolaryng., *101:*189, 1975

Facial contour defects, correction of, by precision-made silastic implants (Craig *et al*). Brit. J. Plast. Surg., *28:*67, 1975

Problems of plastic and reconstructive surgery in the face (Buschmann). Fortschr. Med., *93:*1691, 1975 (German)

Facial restoration (Diner). J. Arkansas Med. Soc., *71:*304, 1975

Surgical correction of facial asymmetry (Montandon). J. Genet. Hum.,*23:*123, 1975 (French)

Letters to the editor: what is maxillofacial surgery — who are maxillofacial surgeons? (Goldberg). J. Oral Surg., *33:*903, 1975

Facial reconstruction, dental, Proplast in (Kent *et al*), PRS, *56:*601, 1975. J. Oral Surg., *39:*347, 1975

Facial reconstruction, osteoneogenesis, new method for (Leake *et al*). J. Surg. Res., *18:*331, 1975

Facial contour reconstruction, room temperature vulcanizing silastic in (Wilkinson *et al*). J. Trauma, *15:*479, 1975

Blood loss and hypotensive anesthesia in oral-facial corrective surgery (Schaberg *et al*). J. Oral Surg., *34:*147, 1976

Alloplastic augmentation of middle-third facial deformities (Alexander). J. Oral Surg., *34:*165, 1976

Facial osteotomies, major, anesthetic management and intraoperative care of patients undergoing (Davies, Munro), PRS, *55:*50, 1975

Maxillofacial region, local use of corticosteroids in surgical interventions in (Shcherbatiuk). Stomatologiia (Mosk.),*54:*37, 1975 (Russian)

Face, Tumors of: See; *Face, Surgery of; Facial Neoplasms; also specific tumors*

FACER, G. W.: Management of nasal injury, PRS, *57:*257, 1976. Postgrad. Med., *57:*123, 1975

FACCINI, J. M. *et al*: Nasal chondroma. J. Laryng. & Otol., *87:*811, 1973

FACCINI, J. M. *et al*: Myxoma involving soft tissues of face. J. Laryng. & Otol., *87:*817, 1973

Facial Bones (See also *Craniofacial Surgery; Facial Injuries; Jaws, Fractures*)

Immediate treatment of complex injuries of the face (Petrolati *et al*). Minerva Chir., *26:*842, 1971 (Italian)

Frontal sinus fractures and injuries of the facial bones (Sibilly *et al*). Rev. Stomatol. Chir. Maxillofac., *72:*495, 1971 (French)

Bone development in angioma (Solovko). Vestn. Khir., *107:*123, 1971 (Russian)

Wire suture osteosynthesis in facial and skull traumatology (Rudert). Z. Laryngol. Rhinol. Otol., *50:*640, 1971 (German)

Statistical evaluation of 873 fractures of facial bones from the total number of 16324 patients treated at the Institute of Traumatology at Brno (Muska *et al*). Cesk. Stomatol., *72:*279, 1972 (Czechoslovakian)

Accidental injuries of facial bones (Fischer). Hippokrates, *43:*248, 1972 (German)

Facial bones in children, fractures of (Bales, Randall, Lehr), PRS, *52:*97, 1973. J. Trauma, *12:*56, 1972

External traction for depressed facial fractures (Lore *et al*). N.Y. State J. Med., *72:*490, 1972

Fractures, facial, in snowmobile injuries (Daniel, Midgley), PRS, *49:*38, 1972

Fractures of midface, precise method for determining displacement (Ferraro, Berggren), PRS, *50:*447, 1972

Fibrous dysplasia of facial bones (Biedermann *et al*). Radiobiol. Radiother. (Berl.), *13:*189, 1972 (German)

Dynamic study of fracture of the facial bones (Fuma). Shikwa Gakuho, *72:*534, 1972 (Japanese)

Four-years experience with surgical correction of deformities of the middle portion of the face (Kufner). Stomatologiia (Mosk.), *51:*49, 1972 (Russian)

Facial bones, tumors, diagnosis and treatment (Spiess *et al*). Ther. Umsch., *29:*664, 1972 (German)

Facial bones, holes especially for reconstruction of certain segments of (Peri *et al*). Ann. chir. plast., *18:*169, 1973 (French)

Facial Bones — Cont.

Facial bones, invasion of, by basal meningiomas (Kendall). Brit. J. Radiol., *46:*237, 1973

Fracture of frontal bone, unstable, depressed, extra-osseous Kirschner wire fixation for (Climo, Block, Alexander), PRS, *52:*200, 1973

Topographical anatomy of the total osteotomy of the midface (Matras *et al*). J. Maxillo-facial Surg., *3:*260, 1975

Middle-third facial osteotomies: their use in the correction of acquired and developmental dentofacial and craniofacial deformities (Epker *et al*). J. Oral Surg., *33:*491, 1975

Facial Clefts, (See also *Cleft Lip; various specific clefts*)

Cleft, total bilateral, regional ectodermal dysplasia with (Fara), PRS, *50:*308, 1972. Acta chir. plast., *13:*100, 1971

Facial clefting and its syndromes (Gorlin *et al*). Birth Defects, *7:*3, 1971

Unilateral transverse facial cleft — a method of surgical closure (Mansfield *et al*). Brit. J. Plast. Surg., *25:*29, 1972

Reconstruction of oblique facial clefts (Wilson *et al*). Cleft Palate J., *9:*109, 1972)

Ten-year survey of macrostomia (Ogo *et al*), PRS, *54:*106, 1974. Jap. J. Plast. Reconstr. Surg., *16:*431, 1973

Oro-ocular cleft, bilateral (Miller, Wood, Haq), PRS, *51:*590, 1973

Facial clefts, oblique (Dey), PRS, *52:*258, 1973

Congenital midline sinus of the upper lip (Bartels, Howard), PRS, *52:*665, 1973

Face, oblique clefts of (Kubacek, Penkava), PRS, *55:*638, 1975. Acta chir. plast., *16:*152, 1974

Oblique facial clefts (Penkava *et al*). Cesk. Stomatol., *74:*277, 1974 (Czech)

Clefts, facial, histochemical and light microscopic observations in hamsters (Ravindra, Chaudry), PRS, *55:*259, 1975. J. Anat., *117:*1, 1974

Clefts of face, rare (Schwenzer), PRS, *55:*720, 1975. J. Maxillo-facial Surg., *2:*224, 1974

Clefts of face in animal experiments (Pfeifer, Schlote, Van Kreybig), PRS, *55:*721, 1975. J. Maxillo-facial Surg., *2:*230, 1974

Cleft, first branchial, anomalies of (Dougall), PRS, *55:*252, 1975. J. Pediat. Surg., *9:*203, 1974

Clefting, facial, syndromes of (Gorlin, Cervenka), PRS, *56:*360, 1975. Scand. J. Plast. Reconstr. Surg., *8:*13, 1974

Clefts, monolateral facial, early bone deform-

Facial Clefts—Cont.
ities in (Psaume), PRS, *57:*762, 1976. Ann. chir. plast., *20:*299, 1975

Facial Deformity (See also *Face, Congenital Deformities; Facial Hypertrophy; Hemifacial Atrophy; Hypertelorism, etc.*)

Attempt at objective assessment of cosmetic damage. Application to several cases of facial scars (Danon *et al*). Ann. chir. plast., *17:*155, 1972 (French)

Scleroderma, linear form of, *coup de sabre,* repair of (Zamick, Weiss), PRS, *50:*520, 1972

Facial deformities, dermafat grafts in repair of (Spina, Ferreira, Psillakis), PRS, *52:*330, 1973. Rev. paulista med., *80:*19, 1972

Massive facial swelling associated with arteriovenous malformation (McCraw *et al*). Surg. Clin. North Am., *52:*415, 1972

Treatment of class II facial deformity. Orthodontic considerations (Orton). Brit. J. Oral Surg., *10:*243, 1973

Facial deformity, class II, treatment of. Segmental surgery (Barton). Brit. J. Oral Surg., *10:*265, 1973

Forehead, postoperative depressions on, plastic correction using alloplastic substances (Cerny *et al*). Cesk. Otolaryngol., *22:*277, 1973 (Czechoslovakian)

Oral-facial deformities, blood volume changes in surgical treatment of, preliminary report (Kelly, Terry). J. Oral Surg., *31:*90, 1973

Facial growth, influence on, of regeneration of the cartilaginous nasal septum in the rat, after resection (Kvinnsland, Breistein), PRS, *51:*190, 1973

Cartilage, growth potential of autografts from nasal septum in the rat (Kvinnsland), PRS, *52:*557, 1973

Facial deformity—surgical treatment (Pericots Ayats, Pericot). Trans. Congr. Int. Assoc. Oral Surg., *4:*345, 1973

Facial asymmetry, difficulties in and indications for treatment (Hovinga *et al*). Int. J. Oral Surg., *3:*234, 1974

Facial asymmetries, treatment by one-stage maxillary and mandibular bilateral osteotomies (Brami *et al*). Int. J. Oral Surg., *3:*239, 1974

Face, paraffinoma of (Bloem, Van der Waal), PRS, *56:*473, 1975. Oral Surg., *38:*675, 1974

Face, canine, altering the dimensions of, by induction of new bone formation (Calabrese, Winslow, Latham), PRS, *54:*467, 1974

Facial deformity, correcting (Tempest).

Facial Deformity—Cont.
Nurs. Times, *71:*1163, 1975

Impressions for metallic facial molds, direct wax method (Zini), PRS, *56:*115, 1975. Prosth. Dent., *33:*95, 1975

Facial reconstruction, new method: osteoneogenesis (Leake, Habal), PRS, *57:*125, 1976. Surg. Res., *18:*331, 1975

Children, cephalometric study of facial growth in, after combined pushback and pharyngeal flap operations (Pearl, Kaplan), PRS, *57:*480, 1976

Facial Deformity, Psychological Aspects

Psychiatrist joins surgery of appearance symposium—personal point of view (Edgell). Can. J. Otolaryngol., *2:*72, 1973

Suicide attempts related to congenital facial deformities (Berger), PRS, *51:*323, 1973

Facial disfigurements, minor, motivational mechanisms behind the wish for plastic surgery in persons with (Tyszka). Psychiatr. Pol., *7:*621, 1973 (Polish)

Prison surgery, 20 years of, evaluation (Lewison). Can. J. Otolaryngol., *3:*42, 1974

Facially disfigured, rehabilitation of (Editorial). M. J. Australia, *1:*28, 1974

Psychological considerations in corrective maxillary and midfacial surgery (Peterson *et al*). J. Oral Surg., *34:*157, 1976

Facial Hemiatrophy: See *Hemifacial Atrophy*

Facial Hypertrophy: See *Hemifacial Atrophy*

Facial Injuries (See also *Craniofacial Injuries; Jaw Fractures; Maxillary Fractures; Orbit, Fracture; Zygoma; etc.*)

Fractures of the Middle Third of the Facial Skeleton. Second edition. By H. C. Killey. John Wright & Sons, Ltd., Bristol., 1971. PRS, *51:*209, 1973

The Illness of Trauma. By Garrett Pipkin and Victor Buhler. Charles C Thomas, Springfield, Ill., 1971. PRS, *50:*519, 1972

Facial injuries associated with the battered child syndrome (Tate). Brit. J. Oral Surg., *9:*41, 1971

Biochemical sequelae to severe head and face trauma (Higgins). Brit. J. Oral Surg., *9:*79, 1971

Treatment of avoidable late sequelae of jaw and facial injuries (Lehnert). Chirurg., *42:*403, 1971 (German)

Temporomandibular joint damage in surgically treated maxillofacial injuries (Kraszewski *et al*). Czas. Stomatol., *24:*1043, 1971 (Polish)

Facio-frontal fractures (Kowalik *et al*). Czas.

Facial Injuries — Cont.

Stomatol., *24:*1137, 1971 (Polish)

Experiences in the treatment of complex mid-facial fractures (Dutescu *et al*). Dtsch. Stomatol., *21:*585, 1971 (German)

Complications in the surgical fixation of the mid-facial region (Schwenzer). Dtsch. Stomatol., *21:*592, 1971 (German)

Restoration of severe injuries in the frontal, nasal and ethmoidal region (Sanvenero-Rosselli). Dtsch. Zahn. Mund. Kiefer-heilkd., *57:*285, 1971 (Italian)

Fractures of skeleton of face, study of diagnosis and treatment based on 12 years' experience of over 600 major cases (Jurkiewicz, Nickell), PRS, *50:*199, 1972. J. Trauma, *11:*946, 1971

Ophthalmologic symptoms of basal orbital fractures (Friemel). Klin. Monatsbl. Augenheilkd., *159:*658, 1971 (German)

Fractures of central facial bones in their relation to skull base (Rehrmann *et al*). Langenbecks Arch. Chir. *329:*548, 1971 (German)

Current concepts in the treatment of fractures of the orbit (Hightower *et al*). Laryngoscope, *81:*725, 1971

Maxillofacial trauma patients, management; inside-out and bottom-up (Small). Mil. Med., *136:*553, 1971

Maxillofacial injuries, management of: medical viewpoint (De Fries), PRS, *49:*580, 1972. Mil. Med., *136:*558, 1971

Immediate treatment of complex injuries of the face (Petrolati *et al*). Minerva Chir., *26:*842, 1971 (Italian)

Naso-orbital fractures, complications and treatment (Beyer *et al*). Ophthalmologica, *163:*418, 1971

Fractures, vertical maxillary, transverse palatal wire for treatment of (Davis, Constant), PRS, *48:*191, 1971

Le Fort III fractures, sequelae of, total osteotomy of middle third of face for faciostenosis or (Tessier), PRS, *48:*533, 1971

Streptococcal wound infection with evidence of widespread tissue involvement (Haddow *et al*). Pediatrics, *48:*458, 1971

Facial injuries (Schneider). Praxis, *60:*1228, 1971 (German)

Facial injuries, treatment (Marques). Rev. Port. Estomatol. Cir. Maxillofac., *12:*45, 1971

Frontal sinus fractures and injuries of the facial bones (Sibilly *et al*). Rev. Stomatol. Chir. Maxillofac., *72:*495, 1971 (French)

Management of fresh facial fracture (Fukuda). Shujutsu, *25:*1173, 1971 (Japanese)

Repair of facial trauma (Igari *et al*). Shu-

Facial Injuries — Cont.

jutsu, *25:*1181, 1971

Management of fractures of the zygoma, orbital floor and maxilla (Makino). Shujutsu, *25:*1187, 1971 (Japanese)

Management of orbital fat herniation by facial injury (Saito *et al*). Shujutsu, *25:*1197, 1971 (Japanese)

Reconstructive and plastic surgery of the face (Neuner). Schweiz. Monatsschr. Zahnheilkd., *81:*947, 1971 (German)

Facial fractures in small children (White *et al*). South Med. J., *64:*1207, 1971

Severe injuries of the face (Makris *et al*). Stomatologia (Athenai), *28:*301, 1971 (Greek).

Collision injury, changing panorama of (Nahum, Siegel), PRS, *49:*671, 1972. Surg. Gynec. & Obst., *133:*783, 1971

Treatment of multiple facial traumata in Denmark (Glahn). Ugeskr. Laeger, *133:*2241, 1971 (Danish)

First management of combined injuries of bones and soft parts in the facial area (Meyer). Zentralbl. Chir., *96:*321, 1971 (German)

Clinical experiences in 2000 facial soft-tissue injuries (Schade). Zentralbl. Chir., *96:*1389, 1971 (German)

Head Injuries. Proceedings of an International Symposium, April, 1970. Williams & Wilkins Co., Baltimore, 1972. PRS, *51:*329, 1973

Maxillofacial surgeries, postoperative, use of 1-phenyl-2-pyrrolidine-penthane in (Garlipp, Neder), PRS, *52:*331, 1973. A. Folha med. Brazil., *64:*947, 1972

Facial trauma, early management (Yonkers *et al*). Am. Fam. Physician, *6:*68, 1972

Cerebrospinal rhinorrhea and frontal flap approach (Hosxe). Ann. chir. plast., *17:*191, 1972 (French)

Recent injuries of cranio-facial middle third (therapeutic attitudes). Ann. chir. plast., *17:*260, 1972 (French)

An approach to reconstruction of complex lower face injuries (Parsons *et al*). Brit. J. Plast. Surg., *25:*23, 1972

Dacryocystography in midfacial fractures (Stranc, Bunce), PRS, *52:*96, 1973. Brit. J. Plast. Surg., *25:*269, 1972

Unusual injuries of soft tissues of the lower lip during work (Veverka *et al*). Cesk. Stomatol., *72:*46, 1972 (Czechoslovakian)

Management of acute midfacial-orbital injuries (Georgiade). Clin. Neurosurg., *19:*301, 1972

Serum immunoglobulins in patients after use of preserved bovine tendon for anastomos-

Facial Injuries – Cont.

1974. Mil. Med., *138:*824, 1973

Maxillofacial injuries associated with snowmobiling (Karleen), PRS, *53:*682, 1974. Minn. Med., *Nov.:* 975, 1973

Primary treatment of lesions of soft facial parts in traffic accidents. I. General problems (Grellet). Nouv. Presse Med., *2:*2283, 1973 (French)

Primary treatment of injuries of facial soft parts in traffic accidents. II. Local problems (Grellet). Nouv. Presse Med., *2:*2343, 1973 (French)

Follow-up studies and results of Adam's method of intrafacial wire fixation of mandible (Zisser *et al*). Osterr. Z. Stomatol., *70:*310, 1973

Facial injuries, severe, disseminated cytomegalovirus infection associated with death in a patient with (Constant, Davis, Maldonado), PRS, *51:*336, 1973

Canthal ligament, medial, eyelash traction test to determine if it is detached (Furnas, Bricoll), PRS, *52:*315, 1973

Facial lacerations, findings in 300 patients (Koonin). PRS, *52:*525, 1973

Facial fractures, treatment of (Da Silva). Rev. Port. Estomatol. Cir. Maxillofac., *14:*99, 1973 (Portuguese)

Facial fractures, use of Kirschner wires in (Cadenat *et al*). Rev. Stomatol. Chir. Maxillofac., *74:*698, 1973 (French)

Fractures, facial, management of common (Schultz). Surg. Clin. North Am., *53:*3, 1973

Facial lacerations, basic plastic surgical techniques in repair of (Curtin). Surg. Clin. North Am., *53:*33, 1973

Facial injuries (Hoehn). Surg. Clin. North Am., *53:*1479, 1973

Facial fractures, naso-orbital-ethmoid, open surgical management of (Epker). Trans. Congr. Int. Assoc. Oral Surg., *4:*323, 1973

Maxillofacial surgery, tracheostomy in system of resuscitation and anesthesiological measures in (Dunaevskii *et al*). Tsitologiia, *15:*74, 1973 (Russian)

Fractures of face (Garanton, Benvenuto, Rodriguez de Lima), PRS, *55:*377, 1975. Venezuelana Cir., *27:*134, 1973

Facial Trauma and Concomitant Problems. Ed. by William B. Irby. C. V. Mosby Co., St. Louis, 1974. PRS, *55:*616, 1975

Immediate Care of the Acutely Ill and Injured. By Hugh Stephenson, Jr. C. V. Mosby Co., St. Louis, 1974. PRS, *57:*509, 1976

Surgical Treatment of Facial Injuries. 3rd edition. By John M. Converse. Williams &

Facial Injuries – Cont.

Wilkins Co., Baltimore, 1974

Face injuries involving loss, treatment of (Hasman), PRS, *54:*617, 1974. Acta chir., *53:*208, 1974

Surgical repair of intratemporal posttraumatic lesions of facial nerve (Hageman *et al*). Acta Chir. Belg., *73:*653, 1974 (Dutch)

Adams' cranial suspension method (Van Reck). Acta Stomatol. Belg., *71:*125, 1974 (French)

Nasotracheal intubation in maxillofacial surgery using bronchofibroscopy (Gille *et al*). Anesth. Analg. (Paris), *31:*551, 1974 (French)

Face, multiple dislocations of (Merville *et al*). Ann. chir. plast., *19:*105, 1974

Fractures, fronto-orbito-nasal (Bebain *et al*), PRS, *56:*353, 1975. Ann Otolaryng., *10:*545, 1974

Facial fractures, treatment in Hippocrates' time (De Moulin), PRS, *55:*718, 1975. Arch. chir. neerl., *26:*283, 1974

Facial bone fractures, main principles in treatment of (Satko). Cesk. Stomatol., *74:*46, 1974 (Slovakian)

Facial injuries (Dushoff), PRS, *55:*505, 1975. Emerg. Med., *6:*25, 1974

Facial injuries (mid-facial), cooperative care of. Specialized plastic and reconstructive surgery (Tiedemann *et al*). H.N.O., *22:*24, 1974 (German)

Maxillofacial injuries in war (Acharyya), PRS, *56:*225, 1975. Indian J. Surg., *36:*392, 1974

Seat belts and the eye (Taylor), PRS, *55:*727, 1975. Injury, *6:*3, 1974

Accidents, alcohol factor in (Karaharju, Stjernvoll), PRS, *55:*726, 1975. Injury, *6:*67, 1974

Face, soft tissue injuries, repair of (Letterman). J. Am. Med. Wom. Assoc., *29:*211, 1974

Maxillofacial injuries, bleeding from ear in (Martis, Karakasis), PRS, *55:*375, 1975. J. Maxillo-facial Surg., *2:*126, 1974

Fractures of middle third of facial skeleton (Smith), PRS, *55:*384, 1975. J. Maxillo-facial Surg., *2:*128, 1974

Facial skeleton, multiple dislocations of (Merville), PRS, *55:*715, 1975. J. Maxillofacial Surg., *2:*187, 1974

Alcoholism, acute, and craniofacial trauma: problem of differential diagnosis (Small), PRS, *54:*372, 1974. J. Oral Surg., *32:*275, 1974

Maxillofacial fractures, compound, comminuted, complex (Alling *et al*). J. Oral Surg., *32:*415, 1974

Facial Injuries — Cont.

mann), PRS, *56:*675, 1975. Acta chir. Austria, *7:*36, 1975

Face, fractures of middle third: technics of internal fixation (Berguer). An. Esp. Odontoestomatol., *34:*103, 1975

Face, fractures of lateral component of middle third (Oliveras Moreno). An. Esp. Odontoestomatol., *34:*199, 1975 (Spanish)

Maxillofacial trauma complication, inadvertent intracranial introduction of nasogastric tube (Seebacher, Nozik, Mathieu), PRS, *56:*238, 1975. Anesthesiology, *42:*100, 1975

Fixation of facial fractures. Current concepts (Banks). Brit. Dent. J., *138:*129, 1975

Maxillofacial injuries from vehicular accidents. Foreword (Schultz). Clin. Plast. Surg., *2:*1, 1975

Recurrent problems in emergency room management of maxillofacial injuries (Baker *et al*). Clin. Plast. Surg., *2:*65, 1975

Soft tissue facial injuries related to vehicular accidents (Seaton). Clin. Plast. Surg., *2:*79, 1975)

Frontal sinus and supraorbital fractures from vehicle accidents (Schultz). Clin. Plast. Surg., *2:*93, 1975

Medicolegal aspects of automobile injuries (Gorney). Clin. Plast. Surg., *2:*167, 1975

Midfacial fractures from vehicular accidents (Schultz *et al*). Clin. Plast. Surg., *2:*173, 1975

Errors in treatment of injuries of middle part of face (Stanko). Cesk. Stomatol., *75:*175, 1975 (Slovakian)

Plastic-surgical principles in the rehabilitation of severe mid-facial injuries (Tschopp). Fortschr. Kiefer. Gesichtschir., *19:*137, 1975 (German)

Surgical technic for the prevention of postoperative telecanthus in naso-ethmoidal fractures (Harle *et al*). Fortschr. Kiefer. Gesichtschir., *19:*147, 1975 (German)

Findings in the maxillary sinus following mid-facial fractures (Schwenzer). Fortschr. Kiefer. Gesichtschir., *19:*167, 1975 (German)

Results of primary orbital reconstructions in mid-facial fractures (Rolffs). Fortschr. Kiefer. Gesichtschir., *19:*184, 1975 (German)

Facial injuries (Nicoletis), PRS, *57:*256, 1976. J. Chir., *109:*495, 1975

Fractures, middle face, endoscopic findings of maxillary sinus after (Kreidler, Koch), PRS, *56:*463, 1975. J. Maxillo-facial Surg., *3:*10, 1975

Fracture, Le Fort, electrical pulp testing following (Tajima), PRS, *57:*259, 1976. J.

Facial Injuries — Cont.

Maxillo-facial Surg., *3:*74, 1975

Primary bone grafting in management of facial fractures (Bonanno *et al*). N.Y. State J. Med., *75:*710, 1975

Face, fractures of (Kelly, Harrigan), PRS, *57:*260, 1976. Oral Surg., *33:*146, 1975

Fractures, naso-orbital, primary treatment of (Van der Meulen, Ramselaar, Bloem), PRS, *55:*107, 1975

Facial cellulitis: Kaposi's varicelliform eruption complicating local facial trauma (Grossman, Berger, Hoehn), PRS, *55:*625, 1975

Fracture, facial, exposure through coronal incision for initial treatment (Shaw, Parsons), PRS *56:*254, 1975

Mandible, fractures of (Melmed, Koonin), PRS, *56:*323, 1975

Goalie mask for protection, confidence, PRS, *56:*104, 1975. Phys. & Sports Med., *3:*20, 1975

Face guards and mouth protectors, mandatory, case for (Heintz), PRS, *57:*406, 1976. Phys. & Sports Med., *3:*60, 1975

Hockey injuries, how, why, where, and when (Hayes), PRS, *55:*726, 1975. Phys. & Sports Med., *3:*61, 1975

Facial injuries, principles of primary management (Bartkowski). Pol. Przegl. Chir., *47:*529, 1975 (Polish)

Is there any possibility to technic of unilateral suspended fixation? (Muska). Stomatol. D.D.R., *25:*35, 1975 (German)

Treatment of comminuted fractures of the anterior sinus wall (Oppenheimer). Trans. Am. Acad. Ophthalmol. Otolaryngol., *80:*507, 1975

Maxillofacial surgery, new instrument for application of wires in (Tobin). Trans. Am. Ophthalmol. Otolaryngol., *80:*261, 1975

Diagnosis, clinical aspects and surgical treatment of traumatic curvature of the nose in the residual period of the injury (Martinkenas). Vestn. Otorinolaringol., *2:*49, 1975 (Russian)

Role of reconstructive surgery in treatment of early and late sequelae of injuries (Klemencic *et al*). Vojnosanit. Pregl., *32:*145, 1975

Early treatment of injuries of the soft facial tissues (Deutschmann). Zentralbl. Chir., *11:*641, 1975 (German)

Chain saw injury of the mandibulofacial region (Loe *et al*). J. Oral Surg., *34:*81, 1976

Facial Neoplasms

Facial hemangiomas, large, surgical removal of (Kufner, Petrovic), PRS, *50:*542, 1972.

Facial Neoplasms—Cont.

Acta chir. plast., *13:*152, 1971

Vascular tumors of the face (Stricker *et al*). Ann. chir. plast., *16:*220, 1971 (French)

Face and neck, neurogenous neoplasms of major nerves of (Katz, Passy, Kaplan), PRS, *49:*235, 1972. Arch. Surg., *103:*51, 1971

Significance of a single injury in the causation of basal-cell carcinoma of the skin (Ewing). Aust. N.Z. J. Surg., *41:*140, 1971

Reconstruction and reparation in radical surgery of tumors (Bergonzelli). Cancro, *24:*369, 1971 (Italian)

Plastic surgical treatment of facial skin cancer (Murray *et al*). J. Surg. Oncol., *3:*269, 1971

Basal cell carcinoma of the face. Problems of treatment and rehabilitation (Drepper). Minerva Stomatol., *20:*249, 1971 (German)

Face, malignant degeneration of basal cell carcinomas of; basal-squamous carcinoma (Stellmach, Rehrmann, Koch), PRS, *48:*471, 1971

Facial tumors and medical collaboration (Boleo-Tome). Rev. Port. Estomatol. Cir. Maxillofac., *12:*95, 1971 (Portuguese)

Facial plastic surgery with a rotation fat-cutaneous graft (Mukhin). Vestn. Khir., *107:*46, 1971 (Russian)

Cylindroma, 41 cases, results of catalogued examinations (Spiessl, Schuchardt), PRS, *51:*707, 1973. Adv. Jaw & Face Surg., Year Book, 1972

Metastatic basal cell epithelioma discovered by chemosurgery (Mikhail *et al*). Arch. Dermat., *105:*103, 1972

Chemosurgery for facial neoplasms (Mohs). Arch. Otolaryng., *95:*62, 1972

Facial tumors, repair of cutaneous defects around natural orifices (Garcia), PRS, *52:*603, 1973. Bol. Soc. Venezuelana Cir., *26:*351, 1972

Reconstruction and reparation in the radical surgery of tumors (Bergonzelli). Cancro, *24:*369, 1971 (Italian)

Face, nevi and hemangioma, indications for excision, limitations of excision, and suture technique (Kashima), PRS, *52:*687, 1973. Jap. J. Plast. Reconstr. Surg., *15:*346, 1972

Facial pachydermatocele in von Recklinghausen's disease (Bando), PRS, *52:*457, 1973. Jap. J. Plast. Reconstr. Surg., *15:*366, 1972

Plastic reconstitution of functional rehabilitation after greater surgical ablations in maxillofacial tumors (Popescu *et al*). J. Med. Lyon, *53:*303, 1972 (French)

Facial Neoplasms—Cont.

Face and scalp, benign and malignant tumors of, role of plastic surgery in treatment (Duverne). J. Med. Lyon, *53:*1063, 1972 (French)

Mesenchymoma, congenital malignant, of face (Ashbell *et al*), PRS, *49:*348, 1972

Remote results of epithelioma surgery and critical study of carcinologic results, apropos of 330 cases. Ann. chir. plast., *18:*44, 1973 (French)

Carcinoma of skin of face, nose, eyelids, and ears, electrocoagulation and curettage for (Whelan, Deckers), PRS, *52:*214, 1973. Cancer, *31:*159, 1973

Facial skull, eosinophilic granuloma in, clinical aspects and therapy of (Von Koppenfels *et al*). Dtsch. Zahnaerztl. Z., *28:*514, 1973

Face, fibrous dysplasia, further case, with misleading symptomatology (Cajgfinger *et al*). J. Fr. Otorhinolaryngol., *22:*67, 1973 (French)

Fibromatosis of face, juvenile, cranium bifidum occulta with (Bhatia *et al*). J. Laryng. & Otol., *87:*587, 1973

Face, myxoma involving soft tissues of (Faccini *et al*). J. Laryng. & Otol. *87:*817, 1973

Face, small defects of the, advantages of the bilobed flap for closure of (Morgan, Samiian), PRS, *52:*35, 1973

Change in function of adrenal cortex after operations in connection with malignant neoplasms in maxillofacial region (Shcherbtiuk). Stomatologiia (Mosk.), *52:*97, 1973 (Russian)

Indications and technique of hemimaxillectomy for treatment of advanced malignancy of the maxilla (Sammis). Trans. Int. Conf. Oral Surg., *4:*154, 1973

Facial tumors, malignant, full thickness skin graft for primary report of (Andra). Acta chir. plast. (Praha), *16:*85, 1974

Facial lesions, benign and malignant, minor surgery for (Dickinson *et al*) Am. Fam. Physician, *10:*102, 1974

Large flap plasty in otorhinolaryngology (Holub *et al*). Cesk. Otolaryngol., *23:*96, 1974 (Czech)

Fibroxanthoma resembling hemangioma of group of solitary blue rubber bleb nevus (Wasik *et al*). Dermatol. Monatsschr., *160:*35, 1974 (German)

Facial skin neoplasms, surgical-plastic treatment (Stolp). Dermatol. Monatsschr., *160:*387, 1974 (German)

Face, dermoid cysts of—recommendation for early excision (Pap). Eye, Ear, Nose, Throat Mon., *53:*239, 1974

Facial Neoplasms—Cont.

Incurable case in the area of facial surgery (Buschmann). Fortschr. Med., *92:*1063, 1974 (German)

Fibrosarcoma: problematic diagnosis in childhood (Gutjahr *et al*). H.N.O., *22:*181, 1974 (German)

Dermatological evaluation of amikacin (BB-K8) (Arata *et al*). Jpn. J. Antibiot., *27:*401, 1974 (Japanese)

Cryosurgical treatment of recurrent head and neck malignancies—a comparative study (Goode *et al*). Laryngoscope, *84:*1950, 1974

Head and neck, giant neurofibroma of (Mukherji), PRS, *53:*184, 1974

Face, hemangiomas of (Spina, Psillakis, Ferreira), PRS, *55:*723, 1975. Rev. paulista med., *83:*115, 1974

Our experience with chemotherapy in the treatment of orofacial cancers (Crepy). Rev. Stomatol. Chir. Maxillofac., *75:*166, 1974 (French)

Face, skin cancer of, reconstructive plastic surgery for (Piotti, Mascetti, Gambaro), PRS, *57:*670, 1976. Riv. ital. chir. plast., *6:*203, 1974

Advances in the surgical treatment of skin tumors (Wilflingseder). Wien. Med. Wochenschr., *124:*593, 1974 (German)

Localized neurofibromatosis of the right half of the face (Blemer *et al*). In *Plastische und Wiederherstellungs—Chirurgie,* ed. Hohler; pp. 357-61. Stuttgart Schattauer, 1975 (German)

Gallium-67 scintigraphy in the diagnosis of tumors in oromaxillofacial surgery (Maerker *et al*). Acta Stomatol. Belg., *72:*399, 1975 (German)

Problems of plastic and reconstructive surgery in the face (Buschmann). Fortschr. Med., *93:*1691, 1975 (German)

Face and neck, massive hemangioma of, combined treatment (Keaveny *et al*), PRS, *57:*256, 1976. J. Cardiovasc. Surg., *16:*159, 1975

Temporal or frontotemporal flap in cervicofacial oncology (Desaulty *et al*). J. Fr. Otorhinolaryngol., *24:*521, 1975 (French)

Extranasopharyngeal juvenile angiofibroma (Isherwood *et al*). J. Laryng. & Otol., *89:*535, 1975

Use of thermography to evaluate the optimum time for surgery after preoperative radiation (Scruggs *et al*). Laryngoscope, *85:*726, 1975

Immediate reconstruction in ablative head and neck surgery (Dinner *et al*). S. Afr. Med. J., *49:*1863, 1975

Facial Neoplasms—Cont.

Giant pilomantrixoma (Malherbe calcifying epithelioma) (Rothman *et al*). Arch. Surg., *111:*86, 1976

"Crown" excision of facial skin lesions (Robbins), PRS, *57:*251, 1976

Facial Nerve (See also *Facial Paralysis; Facial Spasm*)

Surgery of the facial nerve with anatomic and functional preservation of the ear (Chiossone Lares). Acta Otorinolaryngol. Iber. Am., *22:*599, 1971 (Spanish)

Surgery of the seventh cranial nerve (Beal *et al*). Alaska Med., *13:*137, 1971

Technic of approach to the 3d portion of the 7th nerve (Labayle *et al*). Ann. Otolaryngol. Chir. Cervicofac., *88:*363, 1971 (French)

Facial nerve decompression and grafting. A report of 8 cases (Karam). J. Med. Liban., *24:*505, 1971

Experimental observation on nerve regeneration after reconstructive surgery of the facial nerve (Tsukamoto). J. Otolaryngol. Jap., *74:*1340, 1971 (Japanese)

Facial nerve anastomosis—with special reference to the follow-up results (Nakamura *et al*). Otolaryngology (Tokyo), *43:*809, 1971 (Japanese)

Transplantation of the facial nerve (Kitamura). Otolaryngology (Tokyo), *43:*817, 1971 (Japanese)

Nerve, facial, management in parotid gland surgery (Beahrs, Chong), PRS, *51:*349, 1973. Am. J. Surg., *124:*473, 1972

Facial nerve homografts (Binns *et al*). Arch. Otolaryng., *95:*342, 1972

Selective facial nerve branch blocking (Totsuka *et al*). Arch. Otolaryng., *95:*360, 1972

Extratemporal facial nerve surgery (Kitamura *et al*). Arch. Otolaryng., *95:*369, 1972

Facial nerve tumors within the temporal bone (Farkashidy *et al*). Can. J. Otolaryngol., *1:*75, 1972

Five-year experience and results obtained in surgical treatment of ischemic lesions of 7th nerve (Steidl *et al*). Cas. Lek. Cesk., *111:*802, 1972 (Czechoslovakian)

Location relationship of N. facialis to parotid and N. auriculotemporalis (Schlums). Dtsch. Zahnaerztl. Z., *27:*917, 1972 German

Results of vidian neurectomy (Tsutsumi *et al*). J. Otolaryngol. Japan, *75:*1207, 1972 (Japanese)

Facial nerve injuries (McCabe). Laryngoscope, *82:*1891, 1972

Facial Nerve – Cont.

Facial nerve injuries, problems with, in oto-rhinolaryngologic practice. 2. On iatrogenic injuries of facial nerve, medico-legal situation of surgeon (Miehlke). Monatsschr. Ohrenheilkd. Laryngorhinol., *10:*461, 1972 (German)

Problems of the method of approach to the facial nerve canal – pointers on facial nerve surgery (Koike *et al*). Otolaryngology (Tokyo), *44:*345, 1972 (Japanese)

Facial nerve, neurofibroma of (Sellars). S. Afr. Med. J., *46:*1332, 1972

Auto-transplantation of motor nerves after surgery of parotid neoplasms with involvement of the facial nerve (Burlibasa *et al*). Stomatologia (Bucur.), *19:*81, 1972 (Rumanian)

Facial nerve repair, advances in (Smith). Surg. Clin. North Am., *52:*1287, 1972

Facial nerves, transected or resected, experiences in surgical care of (Lange). Arch. Klin. Exp. Ohren Nasen Kehlkopfheilkd., *205:*197, 1973 (German)

Facial nerves and periocular muscles, section of, in photosensitive Papio papio (Carlier *et al*). Electroencephalogr. Clin. Neurophysiol., *35:*13, 1973

Facial nerve, early nonsurgical decompression (Bryant). J. Louisiana M. Soc., *125:*85, 1973

Facial nerve, surgical anatomy of intraglandular portion (Celesnik), PRS, *53:*603, 1974. J. Maxillo-facial Surg., *1:*65, 1973

Facial nerve, peripheral part reconstruction of (Stricker). J. Maxillo-facial Surg., *1:*142, 1973

Facial nerve surgery (Naito *et al*). J. Otolaryngol. Jap., *76:*270, 1973 (Japanese)

Facial nerve, identification of, in parotid surgery (Maran). J. R. Coll. Surg. Edinb., *18:*58, 1973

Facial nerve, neurotization of peripheral branches of, during extirpation of parotid gland (Lur'e). Klin. Khir., *10:*73, 1973 (Russian)

Facial nerve anastomosis, protection of, with vein graft (Miglets *et al*). Laryngoscope, *83:*1027, 1973

Facial nerve anastomosis (Scaramella *et al*). Laryngoscope, *83:*1834, 1973

Facial nerve, neurilemmoma of (Lin *et al*). Neuroradiology, *6:*185, 1973

Facial nerve lesions, evaluation of surgical treatment, based on clinical and electromyographic findings (Emeryk *et al*). Neurol. Neurochir. Pol., *7:*467, 1973 (Polish)

Salivary gland disorders. I. Recognition, diagnosis, treatment (Schwartz, Friedman). New York J. Med., *73:*297, 1973

Facial Nerve – Cont.

Facial nerve, neurilemmoma of (Conley, Janecka), PRS, *52:*55, 1973

Facial nerve, surgical anatomy as related to ancillary operations in rhytidoplasty (Correia, Zani), PRS, *52:*549, 1973

Facial nerve and hypoglossal nerve, results of anastomoses between (Nisch). Psychiatr. Neurol. Med. Psychol. (Leipz.), *52:*488, 1973 (German)

Repair of the facial nerve using a deviant one-step intracranial nerve graft (Montaut *et al*). Rev. Otoneuroophtalmol., *45:*219, 1973 (French)

Facial nerve surgery (Nickman). Rocky Mt. Med. J., *70:*37, 1973

Funicular nerve grafting of the facial nerve (Apfelberg *et al*). Surg. Forum, *24:*513, 1973

Facial nerve, in monkeys, effects of cryosurgery on (Bagley *et al*). Surg. Forum, *24:*514, 1973

Facial nerve surgery, emergency case (Miehlke). Z. Laryngol. Rhinol. Otol., *52:*349, 1973 (German)

Facial nerve, reinnervation after resection of (Cerny *et al*). Acta Otolaryngol. (Stockh.), *77:*102, 1974

Facial nerve neuromas (Peytral *et al*), PRS, *56:*353, 1975. Ann. Otolaryng., *10:*555, 1974

Facial nerve, decompression in Melkersson's syndrome (Canale, Cox), PRS, *55:*715, 1975. Arch. Otolaryng., *100:*373, 1974

Facial nerve, protection in radical neck dissection (Ramsden, Maran), PRS, *54:*618, 1974. Brit. J. Surg., *61:*297, 1974

Anatomical landmarks useful in locating the facial nerve (Sylla *et al*). Bull. Soc. Med. Afr. Noire Lang. Fr., *19:*333, 1974 (French)

Surgical treatment of chronic migrainous neuralgia (Kunkel *et al*). Cleve. Clin. Q., *41:*189, 1974

Facial nerve decompression (McNeill). J. Laryng. & Otol. *88:*445, 1974

Facial nerve injuries in children (Kornbult). J. Laryng. & Otol., *88:*717, 1974

Facial nerve, Schwann cell tumors of (Conley *et al*). Laryngoscope, *84:*958, 1974

Hypoglossal-facial anastomosis (Hitselberger). Otolaryngol. Clin. North Am., *7:*545, 1974

Facial nerve dysfunction, electrophysiological testing in (Echternach). Phys. Ther., *54:*843, 1974

Facial trunk, personal technique for investigation of, in parotidectomy (Samengo), PRS, *54:*618, 1974. Prensa med. Argent., *50:*41, 1974

Transparotid approach in mandibular ameloblastoma recurrences (Gouiric *et al*). Rev.

Facial Nerve—Cont.

Stomatol. Chir. Maxillofac, *75:*58, 1974 (French)

Surgical anatomy of the neck (Jurkiewicz *et al*). Surg. Clin. North Am., *54:*1269, 1974

Neurotrophism in relation to muscle and nerve grafts in rats (Srour *et al*). Surg. Forum, *25:*508, 1974

Salivary Glands and the Facial Nerve. By John J. Conley. Grune & Stratton, New York, 1975. PRS, *57:*658, 1976

Surgical pathology of the peripheral nerve. Introduction (Noterman). Acta Chir. Belg. (Suppl), *1:*9, 1975 (French)

Facial nerve reconstruction and its prognosis (Sade). Ann. Otol. Rhin. & Laryng., *84:*695, 1975

Facial nerve branches, surgical repair of (Szal, Miller), PRS, *57:*395, 1976. Arch. Otolaryng., *101:*160, 1975

Facial nerve, aberrant course of (Griesen), PRS, *57:*259, 1976. Arch. Otolaryng., *101:*327, 1975

Nerve, facial, intraparotid neurilemmoma of (Aston, Sparks), PRS, *57:*116, 1976. Arch. Surg., *110:*757, 1975

Facial nerve, abnormalities of recovery of (Gagnon *et al*). Can. J. Otolaryngol., *4:*358, 1975

Proceedings: unusual reinnervation after resection of the facial nerve (Steidl *et al*). Electroencephalogr. Clin. Neurophysiol., *39:*547, 1975

Surgery of injuries of the facial nerve on the lateral region of the face (Haubrich). H.N.O., *23:*339, 1975 (German)

Facial nerve surgery (Rosen). Harefuah, *88:*416, 1975 (Hebrew)

Comparison of methods of extratemporal facial nerve repair (Ozsahinoglu *et al*). J. Laryng. & Otol., *89:*1085, 1975

Facial nerve injuries, traumatic, management of (Bowers). J. Natl. Med. Assoc., *67:*103, 1975

Proceedings: surgery for motor tics of the face and neck (Scoville). J. Neurol. Neurosurg. Psychiatry, *38:*408, 1975

Nerve, seventh, electric testing for injuries of (Kline), PRS, *57:*400, 1976. J. Oral Surg., *33:*215, 1975

Facial nerve, identification of, at secondary surgery (Janecka). Laryngoscope, *85:*896, 1975

Facial nerve, experimental funicular grafting of (Apfelberg, Gingrass), PRS, *55:*195, 1975

Facial Paralysis (See also *Facial Nerve*)

Facial paralysis, dynamic closure of eyelids in (G. H. Arion's procedure) (Muler *et al*).

Facial Paralysis—Cont.

Ann. Otolaryngol. Chir. Cervicofac., *87:*499, 1970 (French)

New gravity palpebral prosthesis in paralysis of the facial nerve. Advantages of the fenestrated prosthesis (Micheli Pellegrini). Arch. Ital. Otol., *81:*193, 1970 (Italian)

Facial palsy, surgical treatment (Serson Neto, Martins), PRS, *48:*88, 1971. Ars Curandi, *3:*62, 1970

Facial paralysis, essential, present surgical treatment of, our simplified technic (Martin *et al*). J. Med. Lyon, *51:*2001, 1970 (French)

Surgical and Microscopic Anatomy of the Temporal Bone. By Dorothy Wolff, Richard J. Bellucci, and Andrew A. Eggston. Hafner Publishing Co. Inc., New York, 1971. PRS, *49:*656, 1972

Surgery of the facial nerve with anatomic and functional preservation of the ear (Chiossone Lares). Acta Otorinolaryngol. Iber. Am., *22:*599, 1971 (Spanish)

Bell's palsy, bilateral pathology in (Safman), PRS, *51:*704, 1973. Arch. Otolaryng., *93:*55, 1971

Surgical treatment of traumatic facial paralysis with substance loss with tantalum thread (Martin *et al*). J. Fr. Otorhinolaryngol., *20:*1135, 1971 (French)

Paralysis, extratemporal facial nerve, treatment of (Togawa *et al*), PRS, *49:*233, 1972. J. Otol. Japan, *74:*122, 1971

Salivary flow: a prognostic test for facial paralysis (May, Harvey), PRS, *50:*537, 1972. Laryngoscope, *81:*179, 1971

Management of traumatic facial nerve paralysis (Graves *et al*). Laryngoscope, *81:*645, 1971

Surgical treatment of intratemporal facial nerve paralysis (Hazama *et al*). Otolaryngology (Tokyo), *43:*795, 1971 (Japanese)

Facial nerve anastomosis—with special reference to the follow-up results (Nakamura *et al*). Otolaryngology (Tokyo), *43:*809, 1971 (Japanese)

Plastic surgery of facial nerve paralysis (Kurata). Otolaryngology (Tokyo), *43:*847, 1971 (Japanese)

Dystrophy, progressive muscular, Landouzy-Dejerine, reconstruction in (Cocke, Davis), PRS, *48:*77, 1971

Nerve, seventh, case against primary repair of (DeMere) (Follow-Up Clinic), PRS, *48:*172, 1971

Facial paralysis, treatment by static suspension with dermal flaps (Guerrero-Santos, Ramierez, Espaillat), PRS, *48:*325, 1971

Surgical treatment of definitive facial paralysis (Meyer *et al*). Rev. Med. Suisse Ro-

Facial Paralysis — Cont.

mande., *91:*483, 1971 (French)

Facial paralysis, frigore. Surgical problems (De Sebastian). Acta Otorinolaryngol. Iber. Am., *23:*565, 1972 (Spanish)

Facial paralysis, results and indications of chordal neurolysis in (Chouard). Ann. Otolaryngol. Chir. Cervicofac., *89:*507, 1972 (French)

Selective facial nerve branch blocking (Totsuka *et al*). Arch. Otolaryng., *95:*360, 1972

Place of face lifting in the treatment of facial paralysis (Nicoletis). Cah. Med., *13:*379, 1972 (French)

Facial reanimation (Brody). Calif. Med., *116:*55, 1972

Facial paralyses (Gagnon *et al*). Can. J. Otolaryngol., *1:*21, 1972

Surgical therapy of irreparable paresis of facial nerve. Combination of static and dynamic hinges (Petrovic). Cesk. stomatol., *72:*410, 1972 (Slovakian)

Facial nerve, peripheral paralysis of, indications for surgical decompression in (Andreevski *et al*). God. Zb. Med. Fak. Skopje., *18:*215, 1972 (Serbian)

Palsy, facial, silicone mesh sheet as suspension material (Arai, Fukuda, Akiyama), PRS, *52:*463, 1973. Jap. J. Plast. Reconstr. Surg., *15:*447, 1972

Facial palsy, follow-up study of circumoral reconstruction (Tani), PRS, *52:*462, 1973. Jap. J. Plast. Reconstr. Surg., *15:*486, 1972

Bell's palsy — clinical survey (McCafferty). J. Otolaryngol. Soc. Aust., *3:*410, 1972

Bell's palsy: results of surgery, salivation test versus nerve excitability test as basis of treatment (May *et al*). Laryngoscope, *82:*1337, 1972

Facial paralysis, nerve decompression in (Decroix *et al*). Lille Med., *17:*1237, 1972 (French)

Palpebral spring in facial palsy (English *et al.*) M. J. Australia, *1:*223, 1972

Facial nerve lesions in otorhinolaryngological practice. 1. Problem diagnosis "Bell's palsy" (Miehlke). Monatsschr. Ohrenheilkd. Laryngorhinol., *106:*413, 1972

Acute peripheral facial nerve paralysis, prognostic criteria and value of surgical decompression (Poshumus Meyjes). Ned. Tijdschr. Geneeskd., *116:*319, 1972 (Dutch)

Early decompression of the facial nerve in Bell's palsy (Mechelse). Ned. Tijdschr. Geneeskd., *116:*1031, 1972 (Dutch)

Facial paralysis, facial reanimation in (Eberle). Otolaryngol. Clin. North Am., *5:*631, 1972

Facial nerve palsy, intratemporal, topodi-

Facial Paralysis — Cont.

agnosis of (Pietruski). Otolaryngol. Pol., *26:*619, 1972 (Polish)

Facial nerve paralysis, supplementary procedure for improvement (Curtin) (Follow-Up Clinic), PRS, *49:*84, 1972

Facial nerve paralysis, spontaneous, associated with ipsilateral benign parotid tumor (Cimorra, Ferreira, Martinez-Tello), PRS, *50:*523, 1972

Facial paralysis, traumatic, by damage of first portion. Total decompression of Fallopian acqueduct. Two successful cases (Garcin *et al*) Rev. Otoneuroophtalmol., *44:*305, 1972 (French)

Facial paralysis, plastic surgery on (Guerrero-Santos, Sandoval), PRS, *53:*108, 1974. Rev. San. Guadalajara, *5:*55, 1972

Primary myoplasty in removal of the parotid gland together with branches of the facial nerve (Naumov *et al*). Stomatologiia (Mosk.), *51:*30, 1972 (Russian)

Early plastic surgery of facial nerve (Salazkin *et al*). Vopr. Neirokhir., *36:*30, 1972 (Russian)

Syndrome, Melkersson-Rosenthal, surgical treatment of facial paralysis in (Cerny *et al*). Z. Laryngol. Rhinol. Otol., *51:*525, 1972 (German)

Surgery of the Facial Nerve. By Adolf Miehlke. W. B. Saunders Co., Philadelphia, 1973. PRS, *55:*85, 1975

Paralyzed face, correction of: muscle transposition (Stricker *et al*). Ann. chir. plast., *18:*213, 1973 (French)

Facial paralysis complicating cervico-cephalic zona with multiple localizations, successfully treated by surgery (Lallemant *et al*). Ann. Otolaryngol. Chir. Cervicofac., *90:*214, 1973 (French)

Facial paralysis, long-delayed surgery of. Apropos of two cases operated after seven and eight years (Natali *et al*). Ann. Otolaryngol. Chir. Cervicofac., *90:*378, 1973 (French)

Facial paralysis, means of fixing traction bands during palliative surgery of (Senechal *et al*). Ann. Otolaryngol Chir. Cervicofac., *90:*585, 1973 (French)

Facial paralysis, care of eye in (Goren, Clemis), PRS, *52:*544, 1973. Arch. Otolaryng., *97:*227, 1973

Facial palsy, peripheral, acute. Indications for surgical treatment (Stien *et al*). Arch. Otolaryng., *98:*187, 1973

Facial nerve paralysis following sagittal split mandibular osteotomy, case report (Dendy). Brit. J. Oral Surg., *11:*101, 1973

Facial paralysis, dynamic closing of eyelids

Facial Paralysis — Cont.

in (G. H. Arion's technic) (Muler). Cah. Med., *14:*333, 1973 (French)

Facial palsy, restoration of lid function with permanent magnets (Muehlbauer, Segeth, Viessmann), PRS, *53:*113, 1974. Chir. Plast., *1:*295, 1973

Facial paralysis, reconstruction of face through cross face nerve transplantation (Anderl), PRS, *53:*249, 1974. Chir. Plast., *2:*17, 1973

ENT practice, assessment of idiopathic and posttraumatic facial paralysis in: objective bases for surgery (Mundnich, Nessel). H.N.O., *21:*12, 1973 (German)

Bell's palsy: review of current treatment (Duncan). J. Am. Osteopath. Assoc., *73:*150, 1973

Facial nerve paralysis, traumatic, follow-up study of muscular function after surgery in (Morimitsu). J. Otolaryngol. Jap., *76:*1472, 1973 (Japanese)

Facial palsy: Bell's versus parotid vascular malformation, case report (May *et al*). Laryngoscope, *83:*2020, 1973

Facial paralysis, peripheral, current diagnostic problems and therapeutic indications in (Lazeanu *et al*). Otorinolaringologie, *18:*99, 1973 (Rumanian)

Facial paralysis after petro-mastoid evidement (functional recovery), free nerve graft in case of (Cadariu *et al*). Otorinolaringologie, *18:*121, 1973 (Rumanian)

Significance of decompression operation of facial nerve — based on changes in lymphatic flow in nerve (Kumagami *et al*). Otolaryngol. Jap., *76:*39, 1973 (Japanese)

Electrogustometry in diagnosis of facial nerve palsy (Pietruski). Otolaryngol. Pol., *27:*125, 1973 (Polish)

Bell's palsy, salivation test in diagnosis and prognosis (Pietruski *et al*). Otolaryngol. Pol., *27:*253, 1973 (Polish)

Facial paralysis, late reconstruction of lax oral sphincter in (Freeman), PRS, *51:*144, 1973

Leprosy, results of *temporalis* transfer in lagophthalmos due to (Ranney, Furness), PRS, *51:*301, 1973

Facial nerve division: surgical decisions in the treatment of major salivary gland tumors (Rankow), PRS, *51:*514, 1973

Facial paralysis, inferior, masseter muscle rotation in treatment of (Correia, Zani), PRS, *52:*370, 1973

Facial paralysis, peripheral, and post-parotidectomy, treatment with ACTH-GEL. Report of 17 cases (Banquer de Borello). Rev. Assoc. Odontol. Argent., *61:*5, 1973 (Span-

Facial Paralysis — Cont.

ish)

Facial paralysis with or without surgical treatment. Pre and postoperative neurophysiological control. Idiopathic facial paralysis. Electrophysiological patterns (Permuy Rodriguez *et al*). Rev. Esp. Otoneurooftalmol. Neurocir., *31:*333, 1973 (Spanish)

Facial paralysis, permanent, surgical treatment for. Rev. Stomatol. Chir. Maxillofac., *74:*499, 1973 (French)

Facial palsy, lid-load operation in (Perdikis). S. Afr. J. Surg., *11:*197, 1973

Facial nerve paralysis, some aspects. I. Introduction, etiology, applied anatomy and topognosis, and degree of paralysis (Potgieter). South African M. J., *47:*27, 1973

Facial nerve paralysis, some aspects. 3. Complications, prognosis and management (Potgieter). South African M. J., *47:*100, 1973

Facial paralysis (Morrissette). Vie Med. Can. Fr., *2:*534, 1973 (French)

The indications for facial nerve decompression (Helms). Wien. Klin. Wochenschr., *85:*95, 1973 (German)

Facial nerve paralysis, experimental; influence of decompression (Thane *et al*), PRS, *57:*530, 1976. Ann. Otol. Rhin. & Laryng., *83:*582, 1974

Facial nerve paralysis, experimental: influence of decompression (Green *et al*), PRS, *56:*462, 1975. Ann. Otol. Rhin & Laryng., *83:*582, 1974

Bell's paralysis, present status of therapy of: critical evaluation (Wolferman). Ann. Otol. Rhin. & Laryng., *83:* (sup.12), 1, 1974

Facial nerve, peripheral paresis of, problem of suitable time in indications for surgical management of (Jager *et al*). Bratisl. Lek. Listy., *61:*582, 1974 (Slovakian)

Facial palsy, hypoglosso-facial anastomosis in (Evans), PRS, *56:*676, 1975. Brit. J. Plast. Surg., *27:*251, 1974

Facial paralysis in children, problems of (Cajkova). Cesk. Pediatr., *29:*488, 1974 (Slovakian)

Surgical treatment of dysgnathia in Mobius' syndrome (Bunte). Fortschr. Kiefer. Gesichtschir., *18:*256, 1974 (German)

Facial paralysis, idiopathic, nonepidemic incidence (Adour, Wingerd), PRS, *54:*239, 1974. J.A.M.A., *227:*653, 1974

Syndrome, Hunt's; case report (Vogelgesang). J. Am. Osteopath. Assoc., *73:*762, 1974

Bell's palsy: diagnosis, management and results of treatment (Pulec). Laryngoscope,

Facial Paralysis – Cont.

84:2119, 1974

Facial paralysis in fractures of the petrous bone (Fisch). Laryngoscope, 84:2141, 1974

Long-standing facial paralysis rehabilitation (Copley et al). Laryngoscope, 84:2155, 1974

Facial palsy, diabetes mellitus causing (Bandtlow). Laryngol. Rhinol. Otol. (Stuttg.), 53:661, 1974 (German)

Facial paralysis as a problem of plastic surgery (Muhlbauer et al). Med. Klin., 69:1873, 1974 (German)

Muscle cross-reinnervation (Yellin). Nature, 249:596, 1974

Denervation in Bell's palsy. Evoked electromyographic study (Yanagihara et al). O.R.L., 36:361, 1974

Facial paralysis and herpes zoster oticus (Crabtree). Otolaryngol. Clin. North Am., 7:369, 1974

Extratemporal injury and repair of facial nerve (Miehlke). Otolaryngol. Clin. North Am., 7:467, 1974

Facial paralysis, experimental (Binns). Otolaryngol. Clin. North Am., 7:551, 1974

Facial palsy, technique for lid loading in management of lagophthalmos (Jobe), PRS, 53:29, 1974

Paralysis, facial, importance in treatment of, anatomy of smile (Rubin), PRS, 53:384, 1974

Facial nerve paralysis: 4 years experience with Morel-Fatio palpebral spring (Morgan, Rich), PRS, 53:404, 1974

Facial paralysis produced by combat wounds, treatment of (Morgan, Cramer), PRS, 53:647, 1974

Lagophthalmos, lid loading in management (Habal, Jobe) (Letter to the Editor), PRS, 54:211, 1974

Nerve, facial, paralyses coincident with, or subsequent to rhytidectomy (Castañares), PRS, 54:637, 1974

Current surgical treatment of the intratemporal facial palsy (Sprekelsen et al). Rev. Esp. Otoneurooftalmol. Neurocir., 32:149, 1974 (Spanish)

Two cases of late decompression in so-called frozen face paralysis (Ionesco et al). Rev. Laryngol. Otol. Rhinol. (Bord.), 95:775, 1974 (French)

Electromyographical studies of free autogenous muscle transplants in man (Hakelius et al). Scand. J. Plast. Reconstr. Surg., 8:211, 1974

Transplantation of free autogenous muscle in the treatment of facial paralysis. A clinical study (Hakelius). Scand. J. Plast. Reconstr. Surg., 8:220, 1974

Facial Paralysis – Cont.

Face, paralysis of, surgical correction (Salyer, Nickell), PRS, 55:634, 1975. South. M. J., 67:1166, 1974

Method of joining the ends of the damaged facial nerve in the posterior cranial fossa following total excision of neurinomas of the acoustic nerve (Zlotnik et al). Vopr. Neirokhir., 4:15, 1974 (Russian)

Neurititis of the facial nerve (Khondkarian et al). Zh. Nevropatol. Psikhiatr., 74:1637, 1974 (Russian)

Electrical examination and surgical indications in facial paralysis (Chouard). Ann. Otolaryngol. Chir. Cervicofac., 92:195, 1975 (French)

Minimum neurolysis in so-called frozen face paralysis (Bouche). Ann. Otolaryngol. Chir. Cervicofac., 92:203, 1975 (French)

Surgical treatment of traumatic facial paralysis (Charachon et al). Ann. Otolaryngol. Chir. Cervicofac., 92:213, 1975 (French)

Facial paralysis in children (Muler et al). Ann. Otolaryngol. Chir. Cervicofac., 92:229, 1975 (French)

Facial paralysis and tuberculous otitis. Significance of early neural decompression (Legent et al). Ann. Otolaryngol. Chir. Cervicofac., 92:235, 1975 (French)

Paralysis, facial, infectious mononucleosis, and mastoiditis (Michel, Pope, Patterson), PRS, 57:528, 1976. Arch. Otolaryng., 101:486, 1975

Abnormalities of recovery of the facial nerve (Gagnon et al). Can. J. Otolaryngol., 4:358, 1975 (French)

Surgery of otogenic facial paralysis (Moszynski). H.N.O., 23:313, 1975 (German)

Successful decompression of the facial nerve in facial spasm (Krmpotic-Nemanic et al). H.N.O., 23:376, 1975 (German)

Facial paralysis, peripheral, as asymmetry problem (Clodius). Helv. Chir. Acta, 42:157, 1975 (German)

Facial paralysis, idiopathic, herpes simplex virus in (Adar et al), PRS, 57:400, 1976. J.A.M.A., 233:527, 1975

Central functional changes after facial-spinal-accessory anastomosis in man and facial-hypoglossal anastomosis in the cat (Vera et al). J. Neurosurg., 43:181, 1975

Our experiences in the treatment of peripheral paralysis of the n. facialis (Jurisic et al). Med. Pregl., 28:487, 1975 (Serbian)

Editorial: the bell tolls for decompression? (Adour). New England J. Med., 292:748, 1975

Bell's palsy (Letter). New England J. Med. 293:360, 1975

Facial Paralysis — Cont.

Results of surgical and conservative treatment of peripheral facial nerve paralysis using our computational methods. A comparative study (Pietruski). Otolaryngol. Pol., 29:531, 1975 (Polish)

Birth trauma (Gresham), PRS, 57:681, 1976. Pediatr. Clin. N. Am., 22:317, 1975

Facial paralysis: tumors of salivary glands (Richardson et al), PRS, 55:131, 1975

Nerve, facial, experimental funicular grafting of (Apfelberg, Gingrass), PRS, 55:195, 1975

Transfer, platysma and *temporalis* muscle, surgical treatment of Moebius syndrome by (Edgerton, Tuerk, Fisher), PRS, 55:305, 1975

Lip, paralyzed lower, dynamic correction of (Puckett, Neale, Pickrell), PRS, 55:397, 1975

Lagophthalmos, lid-loading in management of (Micheli-Pellegrini) (Letter to the Editor), PRS, 55:482, 1975

Paralysis, facial, new technique to correct (Freilinger), PRS, 56:44, 1975

Cross-face-nerve transplantation for repair of paralyzed facial musculature (Anderl). In *Plastische und Wiederherstellungs-Chirurgie,* ed. by Hohler; pp. 137-42. Stuttgart, Schattauer, 1975 (German)

Clinical experience with dynamic reconstruction after facial paresis (Frellinger et al). In *Plastische und Wiederherstellungs-Chirurgie,* ed. by Hohler; pp. 151-6. Stuttgart; Schattauer, 1975 (German)

Facial paresis — the dynamic suspension of eyelid and the corner of the mouth to M. temporalis (Lemperle et al). In *Plastische und Wiederherstellungs-Chirurgie,* ed. by Hohler; pp. 143-50. Stuttgart; Schattauer, 1975 (German)

Repair of the facial nerve (Millesi et al). In *Plastische und Wiederherstellungs-Chirurgie,* ed. by Hohler; pp. 111-28. Stuttgart; Schattauer, 1975 (German)

Plastic surgery for facial paralysis (Muhlbauer et al). In *Plastische und Wiederherstellungs-Chirurgie,* ed. by Hohler; pp. 87-105. Stuttgart; Schattauer, 1975 (German)

Restoration of eyelid function in facial paresis by implantation of permanent magnets (Muhlbauer et al). In *Plastische und Wiederherstellungs-Chirurgie,* ed. by Hohler; pp. 157-64. Stuttgart; Schattauer, 1975

Ten years experience with alloplastics in facial paresis (Wilflingseder). In *Plastische und Wiederherstellungs-Chirurgie,* ed. by Hohler; pp. 107-9. Stuttgart; Schattauer,

Facial Paralysis — Cont.

1975 (German)

Facial paralysis, peripheral, primary, clinical and electrobiological basis for surgery in. Indications for emergency surgery (Castillo et al). Rev. Laryngol. Otol. Rhinol. (Bord.), 96:65, 1975

The point of view of the otologist in the treatment of essential facial paralysis (Martin). Rev. Otoneuroophtalmol., 47:53, 1975 (French)

Facial nerve paralysis, recent trends in treatment of (Kadry), PRS, 57:259, 1976. Thesis, Cairo Univ., 1975

Etiology, diagnosis and treatment of facial palsy of Bell's type (Najwer et al). Wiad. Lek., 28:32, 1975 (Polish)

Free Gracilis muscle transplantation, with microneurovascular anastomoses for the treatment of facial paralysis (Harii, Ohmori, Torii), PRS, 57:133, 1976

Transposition of lips for correction of facial paralysis (Pickrell, Puckett, Peters), PRS, 57:427, 1976.

Facial Spasm

Surgical treatment of essential blepharospasm (McCabe, Boles). Ann. Otol. Rhin. & Laryng., 81:611, 1972

Facial nerve block in the treatment of facial spasm (Wakasugi). Arch. Otolaryng., 95:356, 1972

Facial spasm and photosensitive epilepsy in Papio Papio (Naquet et al). Rev. Neurol. (Paris), 127:529, 1972 (French)

Complications in surgery for blepharospasm (Dortzbach). Am. J. Ophth., 75:142, 1973

Hemispasmus facialis, treatment of by scarification of nerve (Rosemann et al). Arch. Klin. Exp. Ohren Nasen Kehlkopfheilkd., 205:205, 1973 (German)

Hemifacial spasm: results of surgical treatment in 14 cases (Carvalho et al). Arq. Neuropsiquiatr., 31:91, 1973 (Portuguese)

Hemifacial spasm, idiopathic. New method of surgical treatment (Celis-Blaubach et al). Acta Otolaryngol. (Stockh.), 77:221, 1974

Facial nerve, hemi-facial spasm secondary to vascular compression of (Neagoy, Dohn), PRS, 56:676, 1975. Cleveland Clin. Quart., 41:205, 1974

Factitious Lesions

Cosmetic improvement of factitial defects (Orentreich et al). Med. Trial Tech. Q., 172:80, 1971

Factitious wounds: psychiatric and surgical dilemma (Drinker, Knorr, Edgerton), PRS, 50:458, 1972

248

FAGAN, M. J., JR.: Intramucosal insert: simplified technique for maxillary denture stabilization. Oral Implantol., *4:*504, 1974

FAUGER, B. *et al:* Use of cutaneous homografts in severely burned patients. Ann. Chir., *25:*919, 1971 (French)

FAHRER, M.: Considerations on the functional anatomy of the deep common flexor muscle of the fingers. Ann. Chir., *25:*945, 1971 (French)

FAHRER, M.: Observations of the origins of lumbrical muscles in the human hand. J. Anat., *110:*505, 1971

FAHRER, M.: Considerations on the origins of the lumbrical muscles: the digastric systems in the hand. Ann. Chir., *29:*979, 1975 (French)

FAHEY, D., AND MONROE, J. B.: Lingual thyroid, case report and review of literature, PRS, *57:*672, 1976. Arch. Otolaryng., *101:*574, 1975

FAIBISOFF, B.: Nerve gap: suture under tension *vs.* graft (with Terzis, Williams), PRS, *56:*166, 1975

FAIRBANKS, D. N. *et al:* Surgical management of large nasal septum perforations. Brit. J. Plast. Surg., *24:*382, 1971

FAIRBANKS, G. R., AND DINGMAN, R. O.: Restoration of the oral commissure, PRS, *49:*411, 1972

FAIRLEY, G. H.: Evidence for antigenicity in human tumors with reference both to melanoma and acute leukemia, PRS, *49:*473, 1972. Proc. Roy. Soc. Med., *64:*1044, 1971

FAIRLEY, G. H. *et al:* Detection of tumor specific immune reactions in human melanoma. Ann. N.Y. Acad. Sci., *177:*286, 1971

FAJARDO, L. F.: Platelet morphology after aspirin, PRS, *56:*474, 1975. Am. J. Clin. Path., *63:*554, 1975

FAJARDO, L. F.: Evaluation of cryosurgery for basal cell carcinoma (with Vistnes, Harris), PRS, *55:*71, 1975

FALABELLA, R.: Epidermal grafting, PRS, *50:*100, 1972. Arch. Dermat., *104:*592, 1971

FALARDEAU, M. *et al:* Case of giant cystosarcoma phylloides. Union Med. Can., *102:*1528, 1973 (French)

FALCES, E., AND GORNEY, M.: Use of ear cartilage grafts for nasal tip reconstructions, PRS, *50:*147, 1972

FALK, A. S.: Pharyngeal flap augmentation (with Cosman), PRS, *55:*149, 1975

FALK, D., AND LOOS, D. C.: Spongiocavernosum shunt in surgical treatment of idiopathic persistent priapism, PRS, *51:*233, 1973. J. Urol., *108:*101, 1972

FALK, MERVYN L.: *A Cleft Palate Team Addresses the Speech Clinician.* Charles C

Thomas, Springfield, Ill., 1971. PRS, *49:*568, 1972

FALTERMAN, K.: Lack of effect of skin cycle on survival of experimental skin flaps in rats (with Myers, Donovan), PRS, *57:*650, 1976

FANG, C. H. *et al:* Staged excision of eschars in extensive 3rd degree burns. Chinese Med. J., *4:*200, 1973

FANOUS, N. *et al:* Evaluation of forequarter amputation in malignant diseases. Surg. Gynec. & Obst., *142:*381, 1976

FARA, M.: Increase of biological value of pharyngeal flap by tubing its pedicle, PRS, *50:*201, 1972. Acta chir. plast., *13:*57, 1971

FARA, M.: Regional ectodermal dysplasia with total bilateral cleft, PRS, *50:*308, 1972. Acta chir. plast., *13:*100, 1971

FARA, M.: Importance of folding down muscle stumps in operation of unilateral clefts of lip, PRS, *50:*541, 1972. Acta chir. plast., *13:*162, 1971.

FARA, M.: Submucous cleft palates. Acta chir. plast. (Praha), *13:*221, 1971

FARA, M.: Experiences with eight operated rhynophyma patients, PRS, *51:*475, 1973. Acta chir. plast., *13:*254, 1971

FARA, M.: The importance of physiological reconstruction of the orbicularis oris muscle for esthetic and functional result in operations of unilateral cleft lip. Cesk. Stomatol., *71:*358, 1971 (Czech)

FARA, M.: Congenital defects in the hard palate, PRS, *48:*44, 1971

FARA, M.: Present state of cleft lip and palate treatment at Department of Plastic Surgery in Prague, PRS, *52:*682, 1973. Acta chir. plast., *14:*201, 1972

FARA, M.: Isolated clefts of the hard palate. Cas. Lek. Cesk., *111:*268, 1972 (Czech)

FARA, M.: Theory and empiricism in surgical treatment of orofacial clefts. Acta Univ. Carol. (Med. Mongr.) (Praha), *56:*31, 1973

FARA, M.: Muscles in cleft lip and palate and importance of their reconstruction for cosmetic and functional effect of treatment, PRS, *54:*623, 1974. Rozhl. chir., *53:*178, 1974

FARA, M.: Anatomy of a cleft lip. Clin. Plast. Surg., *2:*205, 1975

FARA, M., HRIVNAKOVA, J., AND BREJCHA, M.: Neurofibromatosis of the head, PRS, *48:*517, 1971. Acta chir. plast., *12:*141, 1970

FARA, M., HRIVNAKOVA, J., AND SEDLACKOVA, E.: Submucous cleft palates, PRS, *51:*481, 1973. Acta chir. plast., *13:*221, 1971

FARA, M., HRIVNAKOVA, J., AND KLASKOVA, O.: Incidence of clefts of palate with lip and palate alone in syndromes and atypical clefts, PRS, *51:*482, 1973. Acta chir. plast.,

*14:*13, 1972

FARA, M., VESELY, K., AND KAFKA, V.: Reconstruction of the vagina by thick skin graft, PRS, *52:*324, 1973. Acta chir. plast., *14:*127, 1972

FARA, M. *et al*: Substitute insertions of the velar muscles in clefts and their importance in reconstruction of the palate. Cesk. Otolaryngol., *21:*57, 1972 (Czech)

FARA, M. *et al*: Histology and electromyography of primary pharyngeal flaps. Cleft Palate J., *9:*64, 1972

FARA, M., HRIVNAKOVA, J., AND HORAK, I.: Middle ear complications in clefts. Results of stage I in long-term studies of hearing defects, considering type of cleft and age of the patient, PRS, *53:*607, 1974. Acta chir. plast., *15:*7, 1973

FARA, M., HRIVNAKOVA, J., AND DOBIAS, J.: Stenosing tendovaginitis of radial, dorsal, and volar compartments of the hand, PRS, *53:*606, 1974. Acta chir. plast., *15:*93, 1973

FARA, M., AND SMAHEL, J.: Human tail, PRS, *54:*512, 1974. Acta chir. plast., *15:*184, 1973

FARACI, R. P. *et al*: Radical treatment of recurrent cystosarcoma phylloides. Ann. Surg., *180:*796, 1974

FARACI, R. P., AND CHRETIEN, P. B.: Adneocarcinoma of the lacrimal gland with simultaneous pulmonary metastases, PRS, *55:*115, 1975. Arch. Surg., *109:*107, 1974

FARACI, R. P. *et al*: *in vitro* demonstration of cryosurgical augmentation of tumor immunity, PRS, *56:*599, 1975. Surgery, *77:*433, 1975

FARACO, MUNUERA, E.: Preprosthetic surgery in relation to oral anomalies. An. Est. Odontoestomatol., *34:*435, 1975 (Spanish)

FARAGO, G. *et al*: Availability of lipid for energy metabolism during hypovolemia, PRS, *49:*476, 1972. Surg. Forum, *22:*7, 1971

FARAH, R., AND RENO, G.: Congenital absence of penis, PRS, *50:*539, 1972. J. Urol., *107:*154, 1972

FARAH, R. *et al*: Penis tourniquet syndrome and penis amputation. Urology, *2:*310, 1973

FARBER, G. A., BURKS, J. W., AND SALINGER, C.: Hair transplants for male pattern baldness, PRS, *51:*475, 1973. South. M. J., *65:* 1380, 1972

FARINA, R.: Surgical treatment of hypospadias: experience in the treatment of 400 consecutive cases using Leveuf's technique. Brit. J. Plast. Surg., *25:*180, 1972

FARINA, R.: Arm flap repair of an extensive anterior thoracic wall defect, PRS, *54:*680, 1974

FARINA, R., AND VILLANO, J. B.: Follow-up of

bone grafts to the nose, PRS, *48:*251, 1971

FARINA, R. *et al*: Reduction mammaplasty with free grafting of nipple and areola. Brit. J. Plast. Surg., *25:*393, 1972

FARKAS, L. G.: Use of anthropometry in assessing cleft lip nose (with Lindsay), PRS, *49:*286, 1972

FARKAS, L. G. *et al*: Morphology of the orbital region in adults following the cleft lip-palate repair in childhood. Am. J. Phys. Anthropol., *37:*65, 1972

FARKAS, L. G. *et al*: Morphology of adult face after repair of isolated cleft palate in childhood. Cleft Palate J., *9:*132, 1972

FARKAS, L. G. *et al*: Replacement of a tracheal defect in the dog by a preformed composite graft, later report, PRS, *50:*238, 1972

FARKAS, L. G. *et al*: Ear morphology in cleft lip and palate anomaly. Arch. Otorhinolaryngol. (N.Y.), *206:*57, 1973

FARKAS, L. G. *et al*: Experimental study of the changes following Silastic rod preparation of a new tendon sheath and subsequent tendon grafting, PRS, *53:*614, 1974. J. Bone & Joint Surg., *55:*1149, 1973

FARKAS, L. G., AND LINDSAY, W. K.: Morphology of the adult face following repair of unilateral cleft lip and palate in childhood, PRS, *52:*652, 1973

FARKAS, L. G., THOMSON, H. G., AND MARTIN, R.: Some practical notes on the anatomy of the chicken toe for surgeon investigators, PRS, *54:*452, 1974

FARKASHIDY, J. *et al*: Facial nerve tumors within the temporal bone. Can. J. Otolaryngol., *1:*75, 1972

FARLEY, H. H.: Resection of rhabdomyosarcoma of the neck. An office procedure. Minn. Med., *59:*24, 1976

FARMAN, A. G. *et al*: Oral Kaposi's sarcoma. Oral Surg., *39:*288, 1975

FARNSWORTH, P. B. *et al*: Glossoptotic hypoxia and micrognathia—the Pierre Robin syndrome reviewed. Early recognition and prompt surgical treatment is important for survival. Clin. Pediatr. (Phila.), *10:*600, 1971

FARR, H. W.: Soft part sarcomas of the head and neck. Am. J. Surg., *122:*714, 1971

FARR, H. W., CARANDANG, C. M., AND HUVOS, A. G.: Malignant vascular tumors of head and neck, PRS, *48:*297, 1971. Am. J. Surg., *120:* 501, 1970

FARR, H. W., AND ARTHUR, K.: Epidermoid carcinoma of mouth and pharynx 1960-1964, PRS, *50:*97, 1972. Clin. Bull. Memorial Sloan-Kettering Cancer Ctr., *1:*130, 1971

FARRELL, M. F., *et al*: Study of lymphocyte depletion and serum complement perturbations following acute burn trauma, PRS, *52:*456, 1973. Surgery, *73:*697, 1973

FARRERA-ROJAS, R.: Radiological exploration of synovial cysts of the wrist, PRS, *53:*367, 1974. Cir. Avances Acad. Mexicana, *274:* 1972

FARRIOR, R. T.: Reconstructive surgery related to laryngology, PRS, *48:*196, 1971. Ann. Otol. Rhin. & Laryng., *79:*1061, 1970

FASANELLA, R. M.: Surgery for minimal ptosis: Fasanella-Servat operation, 1973. Trans. Ophthalmol. Soc. U.K., *93:*425, 1973

Fascia

Fasciitis, bacteroides necrotizing, of upper extremity (Rein, Cosman), PRS, *48:*592, 1971

Fascia lata, bank storage, comment on (Nemet *et al).* Arch. Ophth., *88:*695, 1972

Fascia lata grafts, simple method of obtaining (Drever), PRS, *50:*196, 1972

Fascia, homologous, used for firm anchorage of homo- and allo-implants after enucleation of eye (Kolen, Morozova), PRS, *53:*499, 1974. Acta chir. plast., *15:*46, 1973

Fascia lata: anophthalmic orbit. Surgical correction of lower eyelid ptosis (Vistnes, Iverson, Laub), PRS, *52:*346, 1973

Fascia lata, Cialit-stored and freeze-dried human, behavior in rats (McGregor, Lindop), PRS, *56:*683, 1975. Brit. J. Plast. Surg., *27:*155, 1974

Fingers in Dupuytren's contracture, patterns of diseased fascia in. Displacement of the neurovascular bundle (McFarlane), PRS, *54:*31, 1974

Fibromatosis, subcutaneous pseudosarcomatous (nodular fasciitis) (Lubritz, Ichinose), PRS, *56:*111, 1975. Cutis, *15:*43, 1975

Fat Grafts

Grafts, free adipodermal, in surgical treatment of progressive lipodystrophy (Sokolova), PRS, *52:*686, 1973. Acta chir. plast., *14:*157, 1972

Face, correction of contour defects of, with dermal and dermal-fat grafts (Leaf *et al).* Arch. Surg., *105:*715, 1972

Dermafat grafts in the repair of facial deformities (Spina, Ferreira, Psillakis), PRS, *52:*330, 1973. Rev. paulista med., *80:*19, 1972

Contour plastic surgery with adipose tissue (Shandalova). Vestn. Khir., *108:*62, 1972 (Russian)

Composite grafts of skin and fat (Sweeney). Brit. J. Plast. Surg., *26:*72, 1973

Calcification in dermofat grafts (Milward), PRS, *55:*119, 1975. Brit. J. Plast. Surg., *26:*179, 1973

Grafts, adipose tissue and dermo-adipose

Fat Grafts — Cont.

(Bocchiotti *et al).* Minerva Chir., *28:*1018, 1973 (Italian)

Experimental and clinical study of free grafts in skin-fat transplantation (Naumov *et al).* Stomatologiia (Mosk.), *52:*32, 1973 (Russian)

Grafts, adipodermal, for plasty of hypoplastic and aplastic breast (Bruckner, Lenz), PRS, *56:*355, 1975. Acta chir. plast., *16:*216, 1974

Adipose tissue graft in otorhinology (Tato). Arch. Otolaryng., *100:*467, 1974

Should free dermis-fat transplantation still be considered for use in face? (Walter). H.N.O., *22:*110, 1974 (German)

Repair of defects in the cheeks and lips (Haas). Laryngol. Rhinol. Otol. (Stuttg.), *53:*695, 1974 (German)

Surgical reconstruction of the breast (Kohnlein). Med. Klin., *69:*1647, 1974 (German)

Histological study of various aspects of the integration of dermo fat autografts (Horibe *et al).* Rev. Assoc. Med. Bras., *20:*312, 1974 (Portuguese)

Fatty tissue transplants, calcification of, in the mamma (Reinhardt). Roentgenblaetter, *27:*418, 1974

Free dermis fat transplantation as adjunct in the surgery of the parotid gland (Walter). Laryngol. Rhinol. Otol. (Stuttg.), *54:*435, 1975 (German)

Dermis fat graft for correction of the eyelid deformity of enophthalmos (Hawtof). Mich. Med., *74:*331, 1975

FAUBEL, W., AND FLACH, K.: Vascular status and function in paraplegics and tetraplegics, PRS, *54:*239, 1974. Ztschr. Orthop., *112:*111, 1974

FAVORSKALA, G. M.: Case of surgical intervention in maxillofacial area for 4th stage carcinoma of facial skin. Stomatologiia (Mosk.), *52:*84, 1973 (Russian)

FAVRET, P.: Course of diffuse congenital angiomatosis of the left lower limb. Phlebologie, *21:*355, 1968 (French)

FAY, R. *et al:* Surgical management of female congenital adrenal hyperplasia (adrenogenital syndrome). J. Urol., *112:*813, 1974

FAYE, I. *et al:* Two cases of Darier-Ferrand dermatofibrosarcoma. Bull. Soc. Med. Afr. Noire Lang. Fr., *18:*241, 1973 (French)

FAYEMI, A., AND TOKER, C.: Salivary duct carcinoma, PRS, *55:*116, 1975. Arch. Otolaryng., *99:*366, 1974

FAYEMI, A. O. *et al:* Malignant oncocytoma of parotid gland. Arch. Otolaryng., *99:*375, 1974

FAYOS, J. V.: Carcinoma of mandible. Result of radiation therapy. Acta Radiol. (Ther.) (Stockh.), *12:*378, 1973

FAYOS, J. V. *et al:* Therapeutic problem of metastatic neck adenopathy. Am. J. Roentgenol. Radium Ther. Nucl. Med., *114:*65, 1972

FAYOS, J. V., AND LAMPE, I.: Treatment of squamous cell carcinoma of oral cavity, PRS, *52:*102, 1973. Am. J. Surg., *124:*493, 1972

FEAGIN, J. A., AND WHITE, A. A.: Volkmann's ischemia treated by transfibular fasciotomy, PRS, *53:*110, 1974. Mil. Med., *138:*497, 1973

FEARON, B. *et al:* Subglottic stenosis in infants and children: clinical problem and experimental surgical correction. Can. J. Otolaryngol., *1:*281, 1972

FECHNER, R. E.: Benign breast disease in women on estrogen therapy, PRS, *50:*96, 1972. Cancer, *29:*273, 1972

FEDOROVSKII, A. A. *et al:* Restoration of lower extremity function after deep burns. Klin. Khir., *8:*1, 1972 (Russian)

FEEHAN, H. F., AND MANCUSI-UNGARO, A.: Use of cocaine as topical anesthetic in nasal surgery, PRS, *57:*62, 1975

FEGEN, J. P., BEEBE, D., AND PERSKY, L.: Basal cell carcinoma of penis, PRS, *49:*235, 1972. J. Urol., 104:864, 1970

FEIGIN, G. A.: *In vivo* staining of the cervical lymph nodes with Evans blue prior to cervical lymphadenomectomy. Zh. Ushn. Nos. Borl. Bolezn., *31:*115, 1971 (Russian)

FEIJO, W.: Surgical treatment of sequelae, PRS, *55:*722, 1975. Ars Curandi, 7:54, 1974

FEINBERG, T. *et al:* Questions that worry children with exstrophy. Pediatrics, *53:*242, 1974

FEINS, N. R.: Excision of giant nevus in newborn, PRS, *54:*380, 1974. J. Pediat. Surg., 8:825, 1973

FEINS, N. R.: Pediatric surgery. Current concepts. Pediatr. Clin. North Am., *21:*361, 1974

FEJERSKOV, O. *et al:* Primary malignant melanoma of hard palate: report of case. J. Oral Surg., *31:*53, 1973

FELDMANN, H.: Plastic management of nasal defects with special consideration of composite grafts. Laryngol. Rhinol. Otol. (Stuttg.), *53:*384, 1974 (German)

FELDSTEIN, M.: Skin clamps in cosmetic blepharoplasty. Arch. Ophth., *88:*659, 1972

FELDSTEIN, M.: Musculocutaneous flap technique in blepharoplasty. Arch. Otolaryng., *97:*294, 1973

FELLNER, C. H.: Organ donation, for whose sake? PRS, *54:*510, 1974. Ann. Int. Med., *79:*589, 1973

FELLNER, M. J.: Congenital unilateral benign papillomatosis of mouth. Arch. Dermat., *111:*769, 1975

FELLOWS, G. J. *et al:* Incomplete urethral duplication and urinary retention. Brit. J. Urol.,

*46:*449, 1974

FELT, J. L.: Undermining and redraping in rhinoplasty. Trans. Am. Acad. Ophthalmol. Otolaryngol., *80:*540, 1975

FELTRIN, G. *et al:* Nosographic classification of diseases caused by vibratory machines by means of angiographic examination. Minerva Cardioangiol., *18:*671, 1970 (Italian)

FENECH, F. F. *et al:* Holt-Oram syndrome in a Maltese family. Postgrad. Med. J., *47:*589, 1971

FENILI, P., AND FRANCESCONI, G.: Syndrome of Ehlers-Danlos, PRS, *53:*690, 1974. Minerva chir., *25:*1130, 1970

FEOFILOV, G. L. *et al:* Surgical treatment of funnel chest. Grudn. Khir., *16:*47, 1974 (Russian)

FEOKTISTOV, G. F.: Two cases of malignant synoviomas in children. Ortop. Travmatol. Protez., *31:*72, 1970 (Russian)

FERARU, F.: Wounds of neck. Treatment by prompt exploration. N.Y. State J. Med., *73:*1789, 1973

FERGUSON, J. W.: Central fibroma of the jaws. Brit. J. Oral Surg., *21:*205, 1974

FERGUSON-SMITH, M. A. *et al:* Multiple self-healing squamous epithelioma. Birth Defects, *7:*157, 1971

FERGUSSON, W.: Observations on cleft palate and on staphyloraphy (Classic Reprint), PRS, *48:*365, 1971

FERNANDES, M. *et al:* Two-stage urethroplasty. improved method for treating bulbomembranous strictures. Urology, *6:*568, 1975

FERNANDEZ, C. H. *et al:* Childhood rhabdomyosarcoma. Analysis of coordinated therapy and results. Am. J. Roentgenol. Radium Ther. Nucl. Med., *123:*588, 1975

FERNANDEZ, J. C.: Mammary reconstruction. Further experience with our technique, PRS, *51:*347, 1973. Bol. y trab. Acad. argent. cir., *56:*129, 1972

FERNANDEZ SABATA, A., AND YAYA HUAMAN, R.: The Gilliat and Wilson's test in carpal tunnel syndrome, PRS, *51:*232, 1973. Med. Clin., *46:*349, 1971

FERNANDEZ VILLORIA, J. M.: Versatility of tongue flap in oral reconstruction, PRS, *51:*602, 1973. Rev. españ. cir. plast., *2:*201, 1969

FERNANDEZ VILLORIA, J. M.: New method of elongation of corner of mouth, PRS, *49:*52, 1972

FERNANDEZ VILLORIA, J. M.: Study of the development of *orbicularis oris* muscle, PRS, *55:*205, 1975

FEROZE, R. M. *et al:* Vaginoplasty at the Chelsea hospital for women: a comparison of two techniques. Brit. J. Obstet. Gynaecol.,

82:536, 1975

FERRARO, J. W., AND BERGGREN, R. B.: Precise method for determination of the displacement in fractures of the midface, PRS, 50:447, 1972

FERRARO, J. W., AND BERGGREN, R. B.: Treatment of complex facial fractures, PRS, 53:683, 1974. J. Trauma, 13:783, 1973

FERREIRA, E. A.: Subtotal esophagoplasty by combined cervico-abdominal route; its possible use in megaesophagus. Rev. Paul. Med., 82:133, 1973 (Portuguese)

FERREIRA, M. C. et al: Surgical treatment of columellar losses. Rev. Paul. Med., 79:127, 1972 (Portuguese)

FERREIRA, M. C. et al: Case of cutis laxa with abnormal copper metabolism. Brit. J. Plast. Surg., 26:283, 1973

FERREIRA, M. C. et al: Cutis laxa: physiopathology and surgical treatment. Rev. Assoc. Med. Bras., 19:9, 1973 (Hungarian)

FERREIRA, M. C. et al: Hand replantation – experience of eight cases, PRS, 57:533, 1976. Rev. Assoc. med. bras., 21:149, 1975

FERRY, A., AND FONT, R.: Carcinoma metastatic to eye and orbit. II. Clinicopathological study of 26 patients with ca metastatic to anterior segment of eye, PRS, 57:394, 1976. Arch. Ophth., 93:472, 1975

FERRY, D. J., JR. et al: False aneurysm secondary to penetration of the brain through orbitofacial wounds. Report of two cases. J. Neurosurg., 36:503, 1972

FESTGE, O. A. et al: Urodynamic measurements following epispadias repair. Zentralbl. Chir., 99:337, 1974 (German)

FETROW, K. L.: Practical and important variations in sensory nerve supply to the hand. Hand, 2:178, 1970

FETROW, K. O.: Diagnosis and management of the severed flexor tendon of the hand. Surg. Clin. North Am., 54:923, 1974

FEUERSTEIN, S. S.: Revision techniques in otoplasty. Evaluation and management. Otolaryngol. Clin. North Am., 7:133, 1974

FEVRIER, J. C.: Surgical possibilities in the treatment of baldness. Bord. Med., 4:3255, 1971 (French)

FEYGELMAN, S. S.: Some questions of static tissue conservation theory, PRS, 55:725, 1975. Acta chir. plast., 16:113, 1974

FFOULKES-CRABBE, D. J., AND EMMA, E. E.: Tracheostomy in management of respiratory problems in developing country: study at Lagos University Teaching Hospital. Can. Anaesth. Soc. J., 19:478, 1972

FIALA, O., AND HEROUT, V.: Transplantation of homologous joints with partial replacement of homologous cancellous bone with autogenous marrow, PRS, 51:487, 1973. Acta chir. plast., 13:243, 1971

FIALA, O., AND HEROUT, V.: Transplantation of homogenous joints, PRS, 51:237, 1973. Acta chir. plast., 14:36, 1972

Fibroma

Nasopharyngeal fibroma with extrapharyngeal extensions (Gupta). Acta Otolaryngol. (Stockh.), 71:406, 1971

Case of ossifying fibroma of the maxillary sinus (Chiang). Otolaryngology (Tokyo), 43:367, 1971 (Japanese)

Nasopharyngeal fibroma (report of a case) (Gedosh). J. Arkansas Med. Soc., 68:410, 1972

Desmoid of the abdominal wall (Branzovsky). Rozhl. Chir., 51:87, 1972 (Czechoslovakian)

Cryosurgery in dermatologic office practice: special reference to dermatofibroma and mucous cyst of the lip (Spiller et al). South. Med. J., 68:157, 1975

Fibrosarcoma

Fibrosarcoma. Report of sixty-four cases (Bizer), PRS, 49:473, 1972. Am. J. Surg., 121:586, 1971

Fibrosarcoma of the mandible (Jochimsen et al). Minn. Med., 54:929, 1971

Dermatofibrosarcoma, Darier-Ferrand, with nasal localization (Moriame, Moriame, Ledoux-Corbusier). Arch. belges dermat. et syph., 28:167, 1972 (French)

Fibrosarcoma of mandible with pulmonary metastases: case report (MacFarlane). Brit. J. Oral Surg., 10:168, 1972

Surgical treatment of malignant soft-tissue tumors of the extremities in the adult (Burton et al). Clin. Orthop., 84:144, 1972

Dermatofibrosarcoma protuberans, unusual localization (Petkov, Andreev). Hautarzt, 23:508, 1972 (German)

Dermatofibrosarcoma protuberans (Srivastava, Bhargava). Indian J. Cancer, 9:257, 1972

Primary fibrosarcoma of the tongue: report of case (Ryan et al). J. Oral Surg., 30:135, 1972

Fibrosarcoma, massive, spontaneous cure (Berner) (Follow-Up Clinic), PRS, 50:77, 1972

Multiple tumors of arm (Burn). Proc. Roy. Soc. Med., 65:750, 1972

Two cases of dermatofibrosarcoma protuberans (Nagay et al). Wiad. Lek., 25:1025, 1972 (Polish)

Skin inflammation preceding recurrent fibro-

Fibrosarcoma—Cont.
    sarcoma (Welvaart, Polano), PRS, *52:*459, 1973. Arch. chir. neerl., *25:*35, 1973
    Extremities, fibrosarcoma of, surgical therapy (Castro, Hajdu, Fortner), PRS, *53:*371, 1974. Arch. Surg., *107:*284, 1973
    Retromammary tumors of pectoralis major muscle (Leggett). Aust. N.Z. J. Surg., *43:*37, 1973
    Dermatofibrosarcoma, Darier-Ferrand, two cases (Faye *et al*). Bull. Soc. Med. Afr. Noire Lang. Fr., *18:*241, 1973 (French)
    Fibrosarcoma of paranasal air sinuses (Cronin). J. Laryng. & Otol., *87:*667, 1973
    Fibrosarcoma in early infancy (Dahl *et al*). Pathol. Euro., *8:*193, 1973
    Fibrosarcoma of skin (Werner-Brzezinska, Dabska, Adamus). Polski tygodnik lek., *28:*102, 1973 (Polish)
    Dermatofibrosarcoma protuberans. (Report of case with multiple intrathoracic metastases and brief review of six others) (Bonnabeau *et al*). W. Va. Med. J., *69:*107, 1973
    Fibrosarcoma: problematic diagnosis in childhood (Gutjahr *et al*). H.N.O., *22:*181, 1974 (German)
    Tumors, minimal residual, active specific immunotherapy of: excision plus neuraminidase-treated tumor cells (Rios *et al*). Int. J. Cancer, *13:*71, 1974
    Cryosurgical treatment of recurrent head and neck malignancies—a comparative study (Goode *et al*). Laryngoscope, *84:*1950, 1974
    Dermatofibrosarcoma protuberans. Report of case with pulmonary metastasis and multiple intrathoracic recurrences (Bonnabeau *et al*). Oncology, *29:*1, 1974
    Dermatofibrosarcoma protuberans in parotid gland, case report (Junaid *et al*). Brit. J. Oral Surg., *12:*298, 1975

FICKLING, B. W.: Dentistry out of surgery—birth of specialty. Aust. Dent. J., *17:*178, 1972
FIDLER, I. J.: Immune stimulation—inhibition of experimental cancer metastasis, PRS, *54:*244, 1974. Cancer Res., *34:*491, 1974
FIDLER, J. P. *et al*: Carbon dioxide laser excision of acute burns with immediate autografting, PRS, *55:*253, 1975. J. Surg. Res., *17:*1, 1974
FIELD, P., AND VAN BOXEL, P.: Role of Linton flap procedure in management of stasis dermatitis and ulceration in lower limb, PRS, *49:*584, 1972. Surgery, *70:*920, 1971
FIELDHOUSE, J.: Bilateral temporomandibular joint ankylosis with associated micrognathia, case report. Brit. J. Oral Surg., *11:*213, 1974
FIELDING, I. R. *et al*: Lateral sinus thrombosis following radical neck dissection for malignant melanoma. Aust. N. Z. J. Surg., *43:*228, 1973

FIGALOVA, P., HAJNIS, K., AND SMAHEL, Z.: Interocular distance in children with cleft before operation, PRS, *55:*638, 1975. Acta chir. plast. *16:*65, 1974
FIGALOVA, P., AND SMAHEL, Z.: Cephalometric study of families with clefts, PRS, *56:*358, 1975. Acta chir. plast., *16:*247, 1974
FILICORI, R.: Histological aspects of dental pulp after resection of the inferior alveolar nerve in albino rats. Riv. Ital. Stomatol., *29:*37, 1974 (Italian)
FILIPOWICZ-BANACHOWA, A.: Report on II International symposium on lacrimal system. Klin. Oczna., *43:*340, 1973 (Polish)
FILIPOWICZ-BANACHOWA, A.: Surgical treatment of lacrimal duct obstruction in children. Klin. Oczna., *44:*789, 1974 (Polish)
FILIPOWICZ-BANACHOWA, A.: Reconstructive surgery of the lacrimal canaliculi obstruction. Klin. Oczna., *45:*35, 1975 (Polish)
FILIPOWICZOVA-BANACHOVA, A.: Treatment of lacrimal duct occlusions in children. Cesk. Oftalmol., *29:*105, 1973 (Czechoslovakian)
FILIPPI, B. *et al*: Congenital anomalies of hand, PRS, *49:*357, 1972. Rev. Ital. chir. plast., *3:*63, 1971
FILLER, R. M.: New method of fixation of silicone rubber catheters for long-term hyperalimentation, PRS, *53:*247, 1974. J. Pediat. Surg., *8:*395, 1973
FILLER, R. M. *et al*: Total intravenous nutrition—adjunct to management of infants with ruptured omphalocele, PRS, *48:*612, 1971. Am. J. Surg., *121:*454, 1971

Film Reviews
    Film, how to order, PRS, *50:*282, 1972; *55:*218, 1975
    Abdominoplasty. By I. Pitanguy, PRS, *50:*284, 1972
    Anatomy of the Hand. By R. Chase and W. L. White, PRS, *50:*284, 1972
    Areolar Approach to Augmentation Mammaplasty. By H. Jenny, PRS, *53:*344, 1974
    Areolar Approach with Silicone Gel Prosthesis. By J. W. Owsley, Jr., PRS, *55:*222, 1975
    Augmentation Mammaplasty as Office Procedure. By J. L. Baker, PRS, *53:*346, 1974
    Cervical Esophagostomy. By S. W. Hartwell and O. R. Cole, PRS, *50:*282, 1972
    Combined Breast and Abdominoplasty. By F. M. Grazer, PRS, *55:*219, 1975
    Complete Hand Replantation: Failure and Success. By J. F. Ely, PRS, *55:*221, 1975

Film Reviews—Cont.

Cosmetic Surgery of Face and Neck. By W. J. Pangman, PRS, *51:*202, 1973

Double Eyelid Blepharoplasty (Creation of a Superior Palpebral Fold). By R. S. Flowers, PRS, *55:*222, 1975

Esthetic Rhinoplasty. By G. C. Peck, PRS, *55:*218, 1975

Excision of Palmar Fascia (Dupuytren's Contracture) without Use of Tourniquet. By H. A. Johnson, PRS, *53:*347, 1974

Facial Fractures. By R. E. Straith, PRS, *50:*283, 1972

Gliding Mechanisms of Tendon and Tendon Grafts. By. J. W. Smith and H. Conway, PRS, *51:*204, 1973

Hypertrophy of Breast. By I. Pitanguy, PRS, *50:*285, 1972

Hypospadias: Technique of Penis Tunnelization. By D. U. Hinderer, PRS, *51:*201, 1973

Ketamine Anesthesia in Pediatric Plastic Surgery. By E. G. Zook, J. E. Bennett, and R. Roesch, PRS, *51:*203, 1973

Lateral Flap Cleft Lip Surgery. By S. K. Wynn, PRS, *51:*201, 1973

Management of Burns of the Upper Extremities. By R. E. Salisbury, N. S. Levine, and B. A. Pruitt, Jr., PRS, *55:*222, 1975

Management of Severe Burns in Children. By E. T. Boles, PRS, *51:*200, 1973

Microsurgery of Peripheral Nerves. By J. W. Smith, PRS, *51:*203, 1973

Obtaining a Healed Hand. By R. A. Heimburger, PRS, *55:*219, 1975

Homografts of Skin, .015 of an Inch. By J. Stein, B. Pruitt, and H. Pollock, PRS, *51:*203, 1973

Osteotomy and Advancement of Midface for Congenital Retrusion. By M. T. Edgerton, PRS, *55:*220, 1975

Prosthetic Replacement of MP Joints in Rheumatoid Finger. By A. E. Flatt, PRS, *50:*282, 1972

Radical Metacarpal Arthroplasty. By J. E. Adamson, H. H. Crawford, and C. E. Horton, *50:*285, 1972

Reduction Mammaplasty, Technical Refinements in Surgery. By J. W. Smith; and G. P. Craig, PRS, *53:*344, 1974

Reduction Mammaplasty Using a Lateral Wedge Resection. By W. E. Schatten, and J. H. Hartley, Jr., PRS, *55:*220, 1975

Reduction Mammaplasty with a Pedicle Dermal Flap. By P. K. McKissock, PRS, *53:*345, 1974

Replantation of Hand. By B. M. O'Brien, A. M. McLeod, and W. A. Morrison, PRS, *55:*224, 1975

Rhinoplasty, Saw Technique. By T. R.

Film Reviews—Cont.

Broadbent, R. M. Woolf, and E. Brown, PRS, *53:*344, 1974

Study Cases of Secondary Cleft Lip Care. By K. M. Marcks and A. E. Trevaskis, PRS, *51:*202, 1973

Subcutaneous Mastectomy with Immediate Prosthetic Reconstruction. By D. L. Weiner, and H. Volk, PRS, *55:*223, 1975

Surgical Correction of Open Bite. By J. Kufner, PRS, *50:*286, 1972

Surgical Correction of Sensitive Thumb. By H. A. Johnson, PRS, *53:*345, 1974

Surgical Treatment of Drooling. By T. F. Wilkie, PRS, *50:*283, 1972

Surgical Treatment of Hypernasality. By J. K. Chong, and L. M. Cramer, PRS, *55:*218, 1975

Surgical Treatment of Pressure Ulcers after Spinal Cord Injury. By B. Cannon *et al*, PRS, *53:*346, 1974

Technique of Flexible Implants. Resection Arthroplasty of MP Joints. By A. B. Swanson, PRS, *53:*347, 1974

Temporalis Muscle Transfer for Lagophthalmos. By D. W. Robinson, PRS, *55:*219, 1975

Thumb Reconstruction by Fifth Digit Transposition. By J. C. Kelleher, and J. G. Sullivan, PRS, *51:*200, 1973

Wound Healing, Secondary Intention. By H. Hayes, Jr., PRS, *53:*346, 1974

W-Plastic Scar Revision, W-Plastic Glabellar Rhytidectomy. By A. F. Borges, PRS, *51:*204, 1973

FINDLAY, I. A.: Ankylosis of coronoid to zygomatic bone. Brit. J. Oral Surg., *10:*30, 1972

FINDLAY, I. A.: Restriction of jaw movement due to abnormalities of coronoid process. Trans. Congr. Int. Assoc. Oral Surg., *4:*269, 1973

FINE, J.: Antero-inferior premaxillary approach to surgery of nasal septum. S. Afr. Med. J., *47:*49, 1973

FINE, J., WEISSMAN, J., AND FINESTONE, S. C.: Side effects after ketamine anesthesia: transient blindness, PRS, *54:*248, 1974. Anesth. & Analg., *53:*72, 1974

FINE, L., ROBINSON, J. E., AND BARNHART, G. W.: Absence or major loss of part of external ear, and correction, PRS, *54:*371, 1974. J. Prosth. Dent., *31:*313, 1974

FINE, R. N. *et al*: Renal transplantation in young children, PRS, *52:*680, 1973. Am. J. Surg., *125:*559, 1973

FINEGOLD, S. M.: Antimicrobial therapy of anaerobic infections, PRS, *57:*406, 1976. Postgrad. Med., *58:*72, 1975

Fingernails

Phalanx, distal, bone destroyed by periungual warts (Gardner, Acker), PRS, *52:*452, 1973. Arch. Dermat., *107:*275, 1973

Fingernail fold, reconstruction (Barfod), PRS, *52:*594, 1973. Rev. Latino Am. cir. plast., *17:*59, 1973

Fingernail, invisible glomus tumor of (Sibulkin, Healey), PRS, *55:*115, 1975. Arch. Surg., *109:*111, 1974

Fingernail fold reconstruction, one stage (Hayes), PRS, *54:*690, 1974. Hand, *6:*74, 1974

Acrylic resin material used to replace malformed fingernail (Bautista, Nery), PRS, *55:*234, 1975

Fingers, Amputations of (See also *Replantation*)

Index ray amputation, transfer of long flexor tendon of index finger to proximal phalanx of long finger (Eversmann, Burkhalter, Dunn), PRS, *49:*664, 1972. J. Bone & Joint Surg., *53:*1343, 1971

Finger joint amputations, retaining the articular cartilage (Whitaker *et al*), PRS, *49:*542, 1972

Fingertip amputations, Kutler repair (Freiberg, Manktelow), PRS, *50:*371, 1972

Digital amputations in diabetic patients (Sizer *et al*). Surgery, *72:*980, 1972

Finger, amputated, replacement of (Lendvay), PRS, *53:*685, 1974. Asian J. Med., *9:*249, 1973

Fingertip amputations, use of a volar flap for repair of (Snow) (Follow-Up Clinic), PRS, *52:*299, 1973

Finger amputations: flag flap (Iselin), PRS, *52:*374, 1973

Digits, replanted: replantation surgery in China (American Replantation Mission), PRS, *52:*476, 1973

Finger: clinical replantation of digits (O'Brien *et al*), PRS, *52:*490, 1973

Fingers, amputated: get in there and replant! (McDowell) (Editorial), PRS, *52:*562, 1973

Digit, surgical amputation through (Connolly, Goulston), PRS, *52:*595, 1973. Proc. Roy. Australasian Coll. Surgeons, *46:*241, 1973

Finger and thumb amputations, primary, critical review of results (Harvey, Harvey), PRS, *54:*690, 1974. Hand, *6:*157, 1974

Finger amputations and ability to work (Gruneberg, Spence), PRS, *56:*227, 1975. Hand, *6:*236, 1974

Amputation of thumb, rotation-transposition method for soft tissue replacement on dis-

Fingers, Amputations of — *Cont.*
tal segment (Argamaso), PRS, *54:*366, 1974

Phalanges, amputated, used to reconstruct thumb (De Macedo, Baroudi, Tozzi Netto), PRS, *57:*534, 1976. Cir. Plast. Ibero-Latino Am., *1:*97, 1975

Fingers, Baseball Injuries (See also *Fingers, Splints for*)

Thoughts on "mallet finger" (Huffstadt). Ned. tijdschr. geneeskd., *115:*1049, 1971 (Dutch)

Extensor: splints for mallet and boutonniere deformities (Elliott), PRS, *52:*282, 1973

Finger deformity, mallet, constructing an improved splint for (Snow), PRS, *52:*586, 1973

Fingers, Boutonniere Deformity

Surgical treatment of the "boutonniere" deformity. Experience with the I. Matev method (Buratti *et al*). Minerva Ortop., *23:*22, 1972 (Italian)

Boutonniere deformity, post-traumatic, reconstruction (Suzuki), PRS, *54:*375, 1974. Hand, *5:*145, 1973

Boutonniere and mallet deformities, splints for (Elliott), PRS, *52:*282, 1973

Problem of boutonniere deformity (Souter). Clin. Orthop., *0:*116, 1974

Boutonniere deformity (Chan *et al*). Ill. Med. J., *146:*532, 1974

Fingers, Burns (See also *Burns, Contractures*)

Fingers or toes, flexion contracture of, combined method of rotation flap and free skin graft (Morotomi *et al*), PRS, *50:*311, 1972. Jap. J. Plast. Reconstr. Surg., *14:*377, 1971

Scar contracture of fingers treated by temporary surgical syndactyly (Fittipaldi, Lanatta), PRS, *53:*243, 1974. Rev. españ. cir. plast., *5:*221, 1972

Fingers, Cysts

Finger, mucous cyst of, etiology and treatment of so-called (Kleinert *et al*), PRS, *51:*476, 1973. J. Bone & Joint Surg., *54A:*1455, 1972

Fingers, mucinous cysts and mucinous pseudocysts of (Dubin), PRS, *53:*611, 1974. Univ. Mich. M. J., *39:*78, 1973

Finger: mucous cysts: dorsal distal interphalangeal joint ganglion (Newmeyer, Kilgore, Graham), PRS, *53:*313, 1974

Fingers, bowenoid squamous cell carcinoma of (Gottlieb, Newman), PRS, *57:*679, 1976. Cutis, *16:*108, 1975

Fingers, Deformity: (See also *Fingers, Reconstructive Surgery; specific deformities; Syndactylism, etc.)*

Arthroplasty, flexible implant, for arthritic finger joints (Swanson), PRS, *51:*105, 1973. J. Bone & Joint Surg., *54A:*435, 1972

Mucous cyst of finger, so-called, etiology and treatment (Kleinert *et al*), PRS, *51:*476, 1973. J. Bone & Joint Surg., *54A:*1455, 1972

Capsulodesis and pulley advancement for correcton of claw finger deformity (Leddy *et al*), PRS, *51:*477, 1973. J. Bone & Joint Surg., *54A:*1465, 1972

Flexion contracture, dorsolateral flap from same finger to relieve (Joshi), PRS, *49:*186, 1972

Finger, bone destruction of distal phalanx caused by periungual warts (Gardner, Acker), PRS, *52:*452, 1973. Arch. Dermat., *107:*275, 1973

Fingers, supernumerary, rudimentary polydactyly (Shapiro, Juhlin, Brownstein), PRS, *54:*376, 1974. Arch. Dermat., *108:*223, 1973

Finger contractures and keloids in burn patients (Robitaille *et al*), PRS, *54:*113, 1974. Arch. Phys. Med., *54:*515, 1973

Clubbing, digital, objective assessment in caucasian, Negro, and oriental subjects (Sly *et al*), PRS, *54:*503, 1974. Chest, *64:*689, 1973

Mallet finger deformity, constructing improved splint for (Snow), PRS, *52:*586, 1973

Fingers, congenital broad constricting bands, use of cross-finger flap for treatment (Artz, Posch), PRS, *52:*645, 1973

Finger, little, progressive restriction of motion of metacarpophalangeal joint of, caused by traumatic entrapment of *extensor digiti minimi proprius* (Schultz), PRS, *54:*621, 1974. J. Bone & Joint Surg., *56A:*428, 1974

Joint, PIP, flexion contracture secondary to injury of anomalous ulnar lumbrical muscle insertion (Webber), PRS, *55:*226, 1975

Flexor and extensor mechanisms, method of studying relationships between the finger joints and (Snow, Switzer), PRS, *55:*242, 1975

Congenital absence of central slip of finger, reconstruction (Snow), PRS, *57:*455, 1976

Fingers, Dislocation

Sprains and dislocations of fingers (Pfeiffer), PRS, *50:*306, 1972. Ther. Umsch., *28:*815, 1971

Fingers, Dislocation – Cont.

Joint, metacarpophalangeal, complex dislocation (Green, Gerry), PRS, *54:*109, 1974. J. Bone & Joint Surg., *55A:*1480, 1973

Finger, index, dorsal dislocation of index MP joint (Cunningham, Schwarz), PRS, *56:*654, 1975

Fingers, Fractures

Metacarpals and phalanges, uncomplicated dislocated fractures of, treatment and prognosis (Bloem), PRS, *48:*392, 1971. Arch. chir. neerl., *23:*55, 1971

Fractures, finger, some unusual osteoarticular injuries (Soin), PRS, *53:*106, 1974. Proc. Roy. Australasian Coll. Surg., *46:*270, 1973

Finger fractures, treatment by immobilization on "plaster ball" (Bonvallet), PRS, *55:*249, 1975. Chirurgie, *100:*533, 1974

Fingers, distal fractures of, external osteosynthesis by reposition-fixation of fingernail (Belpomme), PRS, *57:*118, 1976. J. Internat. Surg., *60:*219, 1975

Phalanx, fracture, intraoperative reduction of (McMaster), PRS, *56:*671, 1975

Fingers, Infections: See *Hands, Infections*

Fingers, Injuries (See also *various categories*)

Digital epiphyseal necrosis, cold induced, in childhood (systemic ischemic necrosis) (Hakstian), PRS, *50:*631, 1972. Canad. J. Surg., *15:*168, 1972

Hair, human, constrictive digital injuries in infants, caused by (Beck, Wesser), PRS, *49:*420, 1972

Incisions, dorsal relaxation, in burst fingers (Joshi, Chaudhari), PRS, *54:*237, 1974. Hand, *5:*135, 1973

Fingers, degloved, treatment of (Frederiks), PRS, *54:*375, 1974. Hand, *5:*140, 1973

Flap, flag, use of for coverage of a small area on a finger or the palm (Vilain, Dupuis), PRS, *51:*397, 1973

Injury, soft tissue, by mercury from broken thermometer (Rachman), PRS, *54:*249, 1974. Am. J. Clin. Path., *61:*296, 1974

Index finger, replacement of soft tissue loss of distal phalanx (Bafna, Pande, Baid), PRS, *55:*379, 1975. Indian J. Plast. Surg., *7:*23, 1974

Fingers, trapped, and amputated fingertips in children (Illingworth), PRS, *56:*366, 1975. J. Pediat. Surg., *9:*853, 1974

Tendon repair, primary, purposeful delay, in cut flexor tendons in "some-man's-land" in children (Arons), PRS, *53:*638, 1974. Dis-

Fingers, Injuries — Cont.

cussion by Hartrampf, PRS, *54:*95, 1974

Fingers, prevention of adhesions in injury of extensor mechanism of (Parker, Wilkinson), PRS, *55:*109, 1975. South. M. J., *67:*796, 1974

Digital sheath, repair reaction of flexor tendon within (Matthews, Richards), PRS, *57:*261, 1976. Hand, *7:*27, 1975

Arthroplasty of proximal interphalangeal joint after trauma (Iselin), PRS, *57:*398, 1976. Hand, *7:*41, 1975

Angles of adjacent finger joints, simple, direct method for simultaneously measuring (Srinivasan), PRS, *57:*524, 1976

Islet grafts for the loss of pulp substance in the fingers (Bonnefous). Bull. Mem. Soc. Chir. Paris, *60:*411, 1970 (French)

Fingers, Paralysis: See *Hands, Nerve Injuries*

Fingers, Reconstructive Surgery (See also *Hands, Rheumatoid Disease of; Hands, Reconstructive Surgery; and Thumb*)

Digital surgery, avoiding postoperative pain in (Galinski). J. Am. Podiatry Assoc., *61:*23, 1971

Index finger pollicization, method and results in aplasia and hypoplasia of thumb (Buck-Gramcko), PRS, *50:*306, 1972. J. Bone & Joint Surg., *53:*1605, 1971

Finger joints, arthroplasty in rheumatoid arthritis with use of silicone rubber prostheses (Nienhuis *et al*), PRS, *49:*358, 1972. Nederl. tijdschr. geneesk., *115:*1889, 1971

Finger joint prosthesis for rheumatoid hand, new design (Nicolle), PRS, *53:*106, 1974. Ann. chir. plast., *17:*275, 1972

Finger joints, arthritic, flexible implant arthroplasty for (Swanson), PRS, *51:*105, 1973. J. Bone & Joint Surg., *54A:*435, 1972

Dorsolateral flap from same finger to relieve flexion contracture (Joshi). PRS, *49:*186, 1972

Finger reconstruction, roentgenological dynamics of reparative regeneration lengthening of metacarpals by distraction method (Ulitskyi, Malygin), PRS, *53:*487, 1974. Acta chir. plast., *15:*82, 1973

Joints, finger, technique for arthrodesis (Potenza), PRS, *54:*108, 1974. J. Bone & Joint Surg., *55A:*1534, 1973

Finger or palm, use of flag flap for coverage of small area on (Vilain, Dupuis). PRS, *51:*397, 1973

Finger, importance of not damaging volar

Fingers, Reconstructive Surgery — Cont.

digital arteries when using zig-zag incision on (Piggot, Black) (Letter to the Editor), PRS, *53:*80, 1974

Fingers, reconstruction of digital pulleys (Wray, Weeks). PRS, *53:*534, 1974

Digital reconstruction by neurosensitive tubular flap (Sancho), PRS, *57:*760, 1976. Rev. port. med. mil., *22:*212, 1974

Joint, proximal interphalangeal, arthroplasty after trauma (Iselin), PRS, *57:*398, 1976. Hand, *7:*41, 1975

Finger joint fusion, cortico-medullary peg for (Schetrumpf), PRS, *56:*596, 1975. Hand, *7:*81, 1975

Finger joints and flexor and extensor mechanisms, method of studying relationships between (Snow, Switzer). PRS, *55:*242, 1975

Finger, method for reconstruction of central slip of extensor tendon (Snow). PRS, *57:*455, 1976

Fingers, Ring Injuries

Lacerated wounds of fingers caused by rings (Major). Acta chir. plast. (Praha), *13:*117, 1971

Fingers, traumatic lesions caused by rings (Gonzalez Peirona, Martinez Sahuquillo), PRS, *56:*595, 1975. Rev. españ. cir. plast., *7:*157, 1974

Fingers, Splints for (See also *Fingers, Baseball Injuries*)

Finger-flexion device for flexor tendon injuries (Webber). PRS, *48:*284, 1971

Splint, internal wire, for adduction contracture of thumb (Araico, Valdes, Ortiz). PRS, *48:*339, 1971

Finger splint, dynamic, home-made (Thomson). PRS, *50:*302, 1972

Splints for mallet and boutonniere deformities (Elliott), PRS, *52:*282, 1973

Splint, improved, for mallet finger deformity, constructing (Snow). PRS, *52:*586, 1973

Fingers, Tendon Ruptures

Fingers, recent lesions of flexor tendons (Duparc *et al*), PRS, *53:*243, 1974. Ann. Chir., *27:*467, 1973

Flexor tendon injuries, alterations in finger growth following (Gaisford, Fleegler). PRS, *51:*164, 1973

Fracture, Colles', rupture of flexor tendons of index finger after (Southmayd *et al*), PRS, *57:*398, 1976. J. Bone & Joint Surg., *57A:*562, 1975

Fingers, Tendon Surgery (See also *Hands, Reconstructive Surgery*)

Long finger extensor tendon, traumatic dislocation of (Kettelkamp, Flatt, Moulds), PRS, *49:*664, 1972. J. Bone & Joint Surg., *53:*229, 1971

Fingers and thumb, flexor tendon grafts in. A study of factors influencing results in 1000 cases (Boyes, Stark), PRS, *50:*630, 1972. J. Bone & Joint Surg., *53:*1332, 1971

Finger, functional anatomy of extensor mechanism of (Harris, Rutledge), PRS, *51:*104, 1973. J. Bone & Joint Surg., *54A:*713, 1972

Fingers, tendon graft, evaluation of *flexor profundus* (Ojeda), PRS, *53:*606, 1974. Rev. Latino Am. cir. plast., *17:*57, 1973

Tenodesis, dynamic, of distal interphalangeal joint for use after severance of *profundus* alone (Kahn), PRS, *51:*536, 1973

PIP joint area, use of retrograde tendon flap in repairing severed extensor in (Snow). PRS, *51:*555, 1973

Digital flexor tendon mechanism: results of tenolysis, controlled evaluation in chickens (Hurst, McCain, Lindsay). PRS, *52:*171, 1973

Extensor digiti minimi, reconstruction of the transverse metacarpal arch in ulnar palsy by transfer of the (Ranney). PRS, *52:*406, 1973

Fingers: surgery of proximal pulley in injuries of *flexor longus* tendon (De la Caffiniere), PRS, *55:*511, 1975. Ann. chir. plast., *19:*201, 1974

Pulleys, digital, reconstruction (Wray, Weeks). PRS, *53:*534, 1974

Digital tendons, purposeful delay of primary repair of cut flexor tendons in "some-man's-land" in children (Arons), PRS, *53:*638, 1974. Discussion by Hartrampf, PRS, *54:*95, 1974

Intrinsics, attached, used to reconstruct central slip of extensor tendon of finger (Snow). PRS, *57:*455, 1976

Fingers, Transplantation (See also *Thumb*)

Digital transpositions (Blanco), PRS, *49:*103, 1972. Bull. Soc. Plast. Surg. Cordoba Argent., *1:*2, 1971

Digital transposition in injured hand (Harkins, Raffety), PRS, *51:*231, 1973. J. Bone & Joint Surg., *54A:*1064, 1972

Finger, ring, used for thumb reconstruction (Garcia-Velazco), PRS, *54:*109, 1974. Brit. J. Plast. Surg., *26:*406, 1973

Fingers, Vascular Injuries: See *Hands, Vascular Injuries*

Fingertips

Fingertip, amputated, reconstruction with triangular volar flap – new surgical procedure (Atasoy *et al*), PRS, *48:*512, 1971. J. Bone & Joint Surg., *52A:*921, 1970

Evaluation of reconstruction surgery of the finger tip with neuro-vascular island flap (Moroashi *et al*). Orthop. Surg. (Tokyo), *22:*951, 1971 (Japanese)

Fingertip injuries (Frazier *et al*). Pa. Med., *74:*51, 1971

Management of fingertip injuries (Demuth *et al*). Pa. Med., *74:*54, 1971

Treating acute fingertip injuries (Sandzen). Am. Fam. Physician, *5:*68, 1972

Fingertips, traumatically amputated, preservation (Weiner, Silver, Aiache). PRS, *49:*609, 1972

Kutler repair for fingertip amputations (Freiberg, Manktelow). PRS, *50:*371, 1972

Fingertip clubbing, objective assessment in caucasian, Negro, and oriental subjects (Sly *et al*), PRS, *54:*503, 1974. Chest, *64:*689, 1973

Fingertips, preservation of traumatically amputated (Gruber) (Letter to the Editor). PRS, *51:*328, 1973

Volar flap for repair of fingertip amputations (Snow) (Follow-Up Clinic). PRS, *52:*299, 1973

Fingertip amputations, neurovascular flap repair (Cole), PRS, *52:*595, 1973. Proc. Roy. Australasian Coll. Surgeons, *46:*399, 1973

Fingertip volar surface, lesions of, hypothenar region as donor area (Badim *et al*), PRS, *53:*498, 1974. Rev. brasil. cir., *62:*163, 1973

Fingertip injuries, partial-thickness grafting for (Nelson), PRS, *55:*510, 1975. Rev. Latino Am. cir. plast., *17:*47, 1973

Fingertip lesions, conservative treatment *versus* free skin grafting (Holm, Zachariae), PRS, *57:*261, 1976. Acta orthop. scandinav., *45:*382, 1974

Amputation of fingertip, surgical reconstruction (Tulli, Rusciani, Fabri), PRS, *56:*595, 1975. Chron. Dermat., *5:*2, 1974

Child, management of acute fingertip injury in (Sandzen), PRS, *56:*228, 1975. Hand, *6:*190, 1974

Fingertip injuries treated by thenar flap (Miller), PRS, *56:*465, 1975. Hand, *6:*311, 1974

Fingertips, amputated, in children (Illing-

Fingertips—Cont.
 worth), PRS, *56:*366, 1975. J. Pediat. Surg., *9:*853, 1974
 Fingertips and heels, innervated full-thickness skin graft to restore sensibility to (Maquieira). PRS, *53:*568, 1974
 Fingertip pulp, avulsion injury of, restoration of sensation using a local dorsolateral island flap (Joshi). PRS, *54:*175, 1974

FINK, G. H.: Use of a transverse carpal ligament window for the pulley in tendon transfers for median nerve palsy (with Snow). PRS, *48:*238, 1971
FINKEL, A. N. *et al*: Conservative treatment of large mandibular cyst, case report. N. Y. State Dent. J., *40:*353, 1974
FINLAY, B. *et al*: Electrosurgery burns resulting from use of miniature ECG electrodes, PRS, *55:*639, 1975. Anesthesiology, *41:*263, 1974
FINNEGAN, D. E.: Speech sound discrimination skills of 7 and 8 year old cleft palate males, PRS, *55:*382, 1975. Cleft Palate J., *11:*111, 1974
FINNEY, J. C. *et al*: Study of transsexuals seeking gender reassignment. Am. J. Psychiatry, *132:*962, 1975
FINSETH, F.: Plastic surgery in rural Ethiopia. PRS, *55:*545, 1975
FINSETH, F., CONSTABLE, J. D., AND CANNON, B.: Interfascicular nerve grafting: early experiences at Massachusetts General Hospital. PRS, *56:*492, 1975
FINSETH, F., KAVARANA, N., AND ANTIA, N.: Complications of free flap transfer to mouth region. PRS, *56:*652, 1975
FINSETH, K. A. *et al*: Health and disease in rural Ethiopia. Yale J. Biol. Med., *48:*105, 1975
FIRAT, T. *et al*: Two cases of aberrant lacrimal gland. Ann. Ophth., *3:*50, 1971
FIRAT, T. *et al*: Bilateral congenital entropion of upper eyelids. Brit. J. Ophthalmol., *57:*753, 1973
FIRICA, A. *et al*: Alleviation of experimental lymphedema by lymphovenous anastomosis in dogs. Am. Surg., *38:*409, 1972
FIRICA, D. *et al*: Re-operations in nasal hypoplasia. Otorinolaringologie, *16:*339, 1971 (Rumanian)
FIRICA, D. *et al*: Combined correction of the nasal pyramid and septum. Rev. Chir. (Otorinolaringol.), *20:*101, 1975 (Rumanian)
FIRICA, D. *et al*: Clinical and therapeutic aspects of nasal trauma. Rev. Chir. (Otorinolaringol.), *20:*199, 1975 (Rumanian)

FIRMIN, F., COCCARO, P. J., AND CONVERSE, J. M.: Cephalometric analysis in diagnosis and treatment planning of craniofacial dysostoses. PRS, *54:*300, 1974
FIRN, S.: Methoxyflurane analgesia for burns dressings and other painful ward procedures in children. Brit. J. Anaesth., *44:*517, 1972
FISCH, U.: Facial paralysis in fractures of the petrous bone. Laryngoscope, *84:*2141, 1974
FISHCHENKO, P. IA.: Tactics and methods of removing X-ray contrast foreign bodies from the soft tissues and joints of children. Khirurgiia (Mosk.), *48:*117, 1972 (Russian)
FISCHER, A.: Malgaigne's thoughts on autoplasty in the treatment of deforming scars. Riv. Stor. Med., *14:*60, 1970 (Italian)
FISCHER, H.: Accidental injuries of facial bones. Hippokrates, *43:*248, 1972 (German)
FISCHER, H.: Accidental injuries of the ears. Hippokrates, *43:*251, 1972 (German)
FISCHER, H.: Injuries due to compressor units. Hippokrates, *43:*254, 1972 (German)
FISCHER, H.: Therapy of gunshot wounds. Munch. Med. Wochenschr., *114:*1731, 1972
FISCHER, H. *et al*: Specific skin reactions in chronic congestive dermatoses. Dtsch. Med. J., *23:*381, 1972 (German)
FISCHER, R., AND KELLNER, G.: Osteosynthesis with splints in mandibular fractures. Osterr. Z. Stomatol., *70:*42, 1973 (German)
FISCHL, R. A.: Adhesives for primary closure of skin incisions (Follow-Up Clinic). PRS, *49:*333, 1972
FISCHL, R. A.: Hemifacial atrophy. Unusual cross-lip flap. New York J. Med., *73:*313, 1973
FISCHL, R. A.: Vertical abdominoplasty. PRS, *51:*139, 1973
FISCHL, R. A.: Retractor for use in breast augmentation. PRS, *57:*526, 1976
FISCHL, R. A., KAHN, S., AND SIMON, B. E.: Mondor's disease, unusual complication of mammaplasty. PRS, *56:*319, 1975
FISHER, A. A.: Allergic reactions due to metals used in dentistry, PRS, *56:*116, 1975. Cutis, *14:*797, 1974
FISHER, J. C.: Surgical treatment of Moebius syndrome by platysma and *temporalis* muscle transfers (with Edgerton, Tuerk). PRS, *55:*305, 1975
FISHER, J. C. *et al*: Development of a plastic surgical teaching service in a women's correctional institution. Am. J. Surg., *120:*269, 1975
FISHER, J. C. *et al*: Combined use of levator retrodisplacement and pharyngeal flap for congenital palate insufficiency. Cleft Palate J., *12:*270, 1975

FISHER, M., AND SCHNEIDER, R.: Congenital aplasia of cutis in 3 successive generations, PRS, *57:*267, 1976. Arch. Dermat., *108:*252, 1973

FISHER, R. H.: Bloodless field for tourniquet? Clin. Orthop., *0:*96, 1974

FISHER, S. J.: Preprosthetic surgery. J. Can. Dent. Assoc., *41:*297, 1975

FISHKIN, V. I. *et al*: Surgical correction of the Duchenne-Trendelenburg phenomenon. Ortop. Travmatol. Protez., *33:*6, 1972 (Russian)

FISHKIN, V. I. *et al*: Primary surgical treatment of open combined injuries of the hands and fingers according to the A. N. Syzganov-G. K. Tkachenko method. Ortop. Travmatol. Protez., *33:*48, 1972 (Russian)

FISK, G.R. *et al*: A casualty "hand" camera. Hand, 7:70,1975

FISK, N.: Rehabilitation program for gender dysphoria syndrome by surgical sex change (with Laub). PRS, *53:*388, 1974

FISK, N. M.: Gender dysphoria syndrome—indications for total gender reorientation and broadly based multi-dimensional rehabilitative regimen, PRS, *55:*260, 1975. West. J. Med., *120:*386, 1974

FISSETTE, J. *et al*: Surgery of the rheumatoid hand. Rev. Med. Liege, *26:*513, 1971 (French)

FISSETTE, J. *et al*: Decubitus ulcers in paraplegic. II. Surgical treatment. Rev. Med. Liege, *28:*475, 1973 (French)

FITTIPALDI, L.: Tracheotomy and tracheostomy in plastic surgery. Minerva Chir., *26:*1454, 1971 (Italian)

FITTIPALDI, L., AND LANATTA, H.: Temporary surgical syndactyly in treatment of cicatricial contracture of fingers, PRS, *53:*243, 1974. Rev. españ. cir. plast., *5:*221, 1972

FITZGERALD, D. M., AND HAMIT, H. F.: Variable significance of condylomata acuminata, PRS, *54:*504, 1974. Ann. Surg., *179:*328, 1974

FITZPATRICK, B.: Indications for surgery on the painful temporomandibular joint. Aust. Dent. J., *16:*355, 1971

FITZPATRICK, B.: Reconstruction of chin in cosmetic surgery, PRS, *57:*112, 1976. J. Oral Surg., *39:*522, 1975

FITZPATRICK, B. N.: Bone grafting in the body of the mandible. Report of cases. Aust. Dent. J., *16:*156, 1971

FITZPATRICK, B. N.: Genioplasty with reference to resorption and hinge sliding osteotomy. Int. J. Oral Surg., *3:*247, 1974

FITZPATRICK, M. B., BROWN, T. C., AND REID, J.: Malignant melanoma of head and neck, PRS, *50:*421, 1972. Canad. J. Surg., *15:*90, 1972

FIUMARA, N. J. *et al*: Gonorrhea and condyloma acuminata in male transsexual. Brit. J.

Vener. Dis., *49:*478, 1973

FLACH, A.: Therapy and prognosis of hypospadias? (Letter). Munch. Med. Wochenschr., *116:*1523, 1974 (German)

FLANDRE, O. *et al*: Study of the cicatrization of experimental burns in rats. Therapie, *26:*517, 1971 (French)

FLANIGAN, W. J. *et al*: Surgical significance of hyperosmolar coma, PRS, *48:*202, 1971. Am. J. Surg., *120:*652, 1970

FLANNAGAN, J.: View from within. J. Pract. Nurs., *24:*32, 1974

Flaps: See *Composite Flaps; Cross-Arm Flaps; Cross-Finger Flaps; Cross-Leg Flaps; Cross-Thigh Flaps; Free Flaps; Skin Flaps, etc.*

FLATT, ADRIAN E.: *The Care of Minor Hand Injuries*, Third Edition. C. V. Mosby Co., St. Louis, 1972. PRS, *51:*210, 1973

FLATT, ADRIAN E.: *The Care of the Rheumatoid Hand*, 3d Ed. C. V. Mosby Co., St. Louis, 1974. PRS, *56:*206, 1975

FLATT, A. E.: Tourniquet time in hand surgery, PRS, *50:*101, 1972. Arch. Surg., *104:*190, 1972

FLATT, A. E. *et al*: Restoration of rheumatoid finger joint function. 3. A follow-up note after fourteen years of experience with a metallic-hinge prosthesis. J. Bone & Joint Surg. (Am.), *54:*1317, 1972

FLAX, R. L. *et al*: Management of penetrating injuries of neck. Am. Surg., *39:*148, 1973

FLEEGLER, E. J.: Alterations in finger growth following flexor tendon injuries (with Gaisford). PRS, *51:*164, 1973

FLEISCHER, K. *et al*: Otorhinolaryngology. Rhinology. Munch. Med. Wochenschr., *116:*1791, 1974 (German)

FLEISCHMAN, E. V. *et al*: Comparative chromosome characteristics of reticulosarcomas and Hodgkin's disease. Neoplasma, *21:*51, 1974

FLEITZ, K. E. *et al*: Intraosseous malignant mixed tumor of maxilla; review of literature and case report. J. Oral Surg., *31:*927, 1973

FLEMING, P. M. *et al*: Silicone rubber drain in head and neck surgery. Trans. Am. Acad. Ophthalmol. Otolaryngol., *80:*254, 1975

FLEMING, W. B. *et al*: Results of radical excision of oral and oropharyngeal cancer requiring pedicle flap reconstruction. Aust. N. Z. J. Surg., *42:*148, 1972

FLEMMING, I.: Facial points in surgery of the aging face. H. N. O., *20:*88, 1972 (German)

FLEMMING, I. *et al*: Tracheal stenoses. Development and latest state of experimental surgery. O. R. L., *36:*179, 1974

FLETCHER, G. H. *et al*: Combination of radiation and surgery in oropharynx and laryngopharynx squamous cell carcinomas. Aktuel

Probl. Chir., *14:*347, 1970

FLETCHER, G. H. *et al:* Irradiation management of squamous cell carcinomas of oral cavity. Proc. Natl. Cancer Conf., *7:*137, 1973

FLEURY, A. F.: Use of prefolded flap to provide lining and cover in the repair of cervical fistulae (with Shapiro). PRS, *51:*319, 1973

FLIÉGER, S. *et al:* Contribution to the diagnosis and treatment of adamantinoma. Czas. Stomatol., *28:*1185, 1975 (Polish)

FLINTOFF, W. M., JR. *et al:* Increased homograft survival. Internal thoracic duct-esophageal shunt. Arch. Otolaryng., *97:*251, 1973

FLOERSHEIM, G. L. *et al:* Induction of tolerance to skin homografts with a methylhydrazine derivative. Synergism with antilymphocytic serum and morphologic responses of the lymphoid system. Agents Actions, *1:*115, 1970

FLORA, G. *et al:* Intraoperative injuries of carotid arteries and their surgical correction. Bruns Beitr. Klin. Chir., *219:*716, 1972 (German)

FLORA, G., AND SCHWAMBERGER, K.: Hyperhidrosis and its treatment by endoscopic-endotracheal sympathectomy, PRS, *52:*206, 1973. Chir. Praxis, *16:*19, 1972

FLORA, G., *et al:* Intraoperative injuries of carotid arteries and their surgical correction. Deutsch. Med. Wochenschr., *98:*716, 1973

FLORES DE JACOBY, L. *et al:* Electron microscopic studies in vestibuloplasty. Dtsch. Zahnaerztl. Z., *28:*1230, 1973 (German)

FLORES DE JACOBY, L. *et al:* Width of attached gingiva after use of gingival graft. Dtsch. Zahnaerztl. Z., *29:*492, 1974 (German)

FLORETTI, G. P. *et al:* Surgical problems in various urologic diseases in childhood. Pediatria (Napoli), *82:*398, 1974 (Italian)

FLOWERS, C. R. *et al:* Oral-pharyngeal movements during swallowing and speech. Cleft Palate J., *10:*181, 1973

FLOWERS, R. S.: Nasal augmentation by the intraoral route. PRS, *54:*570, 1974

FLUSSER, J.: Pathogenesis of club-like fingers. Vnitr. Lek., *16:*983, 1970 (Czechoslovakian)

FLUSSER, J. *et al:* Club-like fingers. Homeostatic response of the organism to long-term hyperemia of the arterial network. Cas. Lek. Cesk., *109:*1059, 1970 (Czechoslovakian)

FLUUR, E. *et al:* Unusual complication following surgically treated fracture of mandibular condyle. Int. J. Oral Surg., *2:*297, 1973

FLYNN, J. EDWARD: *Hand Surgery.* 2nd edition. Williams & Wilkins Co., Baltimore, 1975.

FLYNN, M. B., JESSE, R. H., AND LINDBERG, R. D.: Surgery and irradiation in treatment of squamous cell cancer of the supraglottic larynx, PRS, *52:*102, 1973. Am. J. Surg.,

*124:*477, 1972

FLYNN, M. B., MULLINS, F. X., AND MOORE, C.: Selection of treatment in squamous carcinoma of floor of mouth, PRS, *53:*497, 1974. Am. J. Surg., *126:*477, 1973

FLYNN, M. B., AND MOORE, C.: Marginal resection of mandible in management of squamous cancer of floor of mouth, PRS, *57:*540, 1976. Am. J. Surg., *128:*490, 1974

FOERSTER, D. W.: Silver nitrate cream treatment in burns, some interesting and unanticipated findings. J. Okla. State Med. Assoc., *65:*262, 1972

FOGH-ANDERSEN, P.: Epidemiology and etiology of clefts. Birth Defects, *7:*50, 1971

FOLESKY, H.: Chemical burns. Z. Aerztl. Fortbild. (Jena), *66:*365, 1972 (German)

FOLMAR, R. C., NELSON, C. L., AND PHALEN, G. S.: Ruptures of flexor tendons in hands of non-rheumatoid patients, PRS, *51:*106, 1973. J. Bone & Joint Surg., *54A:*579, 1972

FOMBEUR, J. P. *et al:* Palatal clefts and hearing. Ann. chir. plast., *20:*295, 1975 (French)

FOMBEUR, J. P. *et al:* Hearing disorders in children operated on for cleft palate. Ann. Otolaryngol. Chir. Cervicofac., *92:*436, 1975 (French)

FOMINA, L. I.: Comparative evaluation of the detoxification properties of different transfusion media during the treatment of burns. Voen. Med. Zh., *8:*35, 1971 (Russian)

FONKALSRUD, E. W.: Surgical management of congenital malformations of the lymphatic system, PRS, *56:*108, 1975. Am. J. Surg., *128:*152, 1974

FONKALSRUD, E. W. *et al:* Management of congenital lymphedema in infants and children. Ann. Surg., *177:*280, 1973

FONTAINE, C. J. *et al:* Perfusion in limb melanoma: indications and results. Proc. Roy. Soc. Med., *67:*99, 1974

FONTANA, A. M.: Method of osteo-cranioplasty with Silastic, PRS, *57:*767, 1976 (Italian). Riv. ital. chir. plast., *7:*539, 1975

FONTANA, A. M. *et al:* Cryotherapy in plastic surgery. Minerva Med., *65:*3677, 1974 (Italian)

FONTANA, A. M. *et al:* Some elective procedures for cranioplasty. Minerva Chir., *30:*665, 1975 (Italian)

FONTANA, D. *et al:* Surgical treatment of impotence by a silastic penile prosthesis. Minerva Urol., *24:*121, 1972 (Italian)

Foot (See also *Leg; Leprosy; Plantar Warts*)

Architecture of the epidermis in free autologous skin transplants on the human sole (Gloor *et al*). Dermatol. Monatsschr., *157:*812, 1971 (German)

Foot – Cont.

Restoration of the skin integument following frostbite of the heel (Klintsevich). Khirurgiia (Mosk.), *47:*34, 1971 (Russian)

Avulsive injuries to the heel (Stuckey). South. Med. J., *64:*1472, 1971

Plantar fibromatosis (Aviles, Arlen, Miller), PRS, *48:*295, 1971. Surgery, *69:*117, 1971

Perforating plantar ulcer in the course of diabetes (Grabowska *et al*). Wiad. Lek., *24:*1475, 1971

Initial management of severe open injuries and traumatic amputations of foot (Omer *et al*). Arch. Surg., *105:*696, 1972

Correction of a congenitally short fourth metatarsal (Johnson). Brit. J. Plast. Surg., *25:*201, 1972

Fibromatosis, differential diagnosis of soft tissue tumors, (Krieg, Puls), PRS, *51:*107, 1973. Bruns' Beitr. klin. Chir., *219:*450, 1972

Foot, leprotic paralysis of, evaluation of palliative surgery (Carayon, van Droogenbroeck, Girandeau). Med. trop., *32:*695, 1972 (French)

Foot, immersion, skin infections in Vietnam (Allen *et al*), PRS, *52:*103, 1973. Mil. Med., *137:*295, 1972

Silicone for immersion foot prophylaxis, where and how much to use (Douglas, Eby), PRS, *52:*97, 1973. Mil. Med., *137:*386, 1972

Lobster-claw feet, surgical correction (Weissman, Plaschkes). PRS, *49:*89, 1972

Footdrop, raumatic, new method for correction (Elsahy). PRS, *50:*614, 1972

Plantar fibromatosis, isolated (Warthan, Rudolph, Gross), PRS, *54:*379, 1974. Arch. Dermat., *108:*823, 1973

Foot-drop, anterior tibial compartment syndrome following muscle hernia repair (Wolfort, Mogelvang, Fitzer), PRS, *52:*452, 1973. Arch. Surg., *106:*97, 1973

Heel-ankle region, surgical management of soft tissue defects (Bennett, Kahn), PRS, *53:*113, 1974. J. Trauma, *12:*696, 1973

Foot, traumatic lesions of, free skin plasty in (Efimov *et al*). Klin. Khir., *10:*49, 1973

Metatarsal callus, chronic, painful, treatment by tendon transfer (Kiehn, Earle, Des Prez), PRS, *51:*154, 1973

Plantar warts, plantar calluses, and such (McDowell) (Editorial), PRS, *51:*196, 1973

Skin flap: distant transfer of island flap by microvascular anastomoses (Daniel, Taylor), PRS, *52:*111, 1973

Flap, island, successful transfer from the groin to the foot by microvascular anastomoses (O'Brien *et al*), PRS, *52:*271, 1973

Foot – Cont.

Feet, amputated: get in there and replant! (McDowell) (Editorial), PRS, *52:*562, 1973

Diabetic malum perforans, surgical treatment (Graber *et al*). Praxis, *62:*1405, 1973 (German)

Heel, functional graft of (Mir y Mir), PRS, *53:*498, 1974. Rev. español. cir. plast., *6:*89, 1973

Foot, degloving injuries of, reconstruction of plantar pad (McCabe, Kelly, Behan), PRS, *54:*109, 1974. Surg. Gynec. & Obst., *137:*971, 1973

Hallux valgus, use of Swanson's prosthesis for management of (Michon, Delagoutte, Jandeaux), PRS, *54:*627, 1974. Ann. chir. plast., *19:*13, 1974

Plantar ulcers, angiographic diagnosis and preventive surgery of (Frontera Vaca *et al*), PRS, *55:*109, 1975. Bol. Soc. cir. Plast. Reconstr. Cordoba, *5:*17, 1974

Toe, extra, case of true prehallux (Makino *et al*), PRS, *55:*380, 1975. Jap. J. Plast. Reconstr. Surg., *17:*252, 1974

Toe, fourth, lengthened with silicone block prosthesis (Ueba), PRS, *55:*380, 1975. Jap. J. Plast. Reconstr. Surg., *17:*296, 1974

Foot deformity in older patient with myelomeningocele, surgical correction of (Levitt *et al*). Orthop. Clin. North Am., *5:*19, 1974

Heels and fingertips, innervated full-thickness skin graft to restore sensibility to (Maquieira), PRS, *53:*568, 1974

Foot injury in frostbite (Holm, Vanggaard), PRS, *54:*544, 1974

Foot, macrodactyly of, surgical syndactyly after wedge resection (Diamond, Gould), PRS, *54:*691, 1974. South. M. J., *67:*645, 1974

Ankles, sprained, treated with oral proteolytic enzymes (Craig), PRS, *57:*262, 1976. Injury, *6:*313, 1975

Surgical management of neurotrophic ulcers in the diabetic foot (Martin *et al*). J. Am. Podiatry Assoc., *65:*365, 1975

Foot, puncture wounds of, gram negative osteomyelitis following (Miller *et al*), PRS, *57:*399, 1976. J. Bone & Joint Surg., *57A:*535, 1975

Heel, transfer of free groin flap to, by microvascular anastomosis (Rigg), PRS, *55:*36, 1975

Foot flap, *dorsalis pedis* arterialized flap (McCraw, Furlow), PRS, *55:*177, 1975

Plantar cross-foot flap (Taylor, Hopson), PRS, *55:*677, 1975. Discussion by Cannon, PRS, *56:*83, 1975

Heel, functional graft of (Mir y Mir) (Follow-Up Clinic), PRS, *55:*702, 1975

Foot—Cont.

Flat foot, longitudinal, surgical treatment (Hernandez-Carbajal *et al*), PRS, *57:*119, 1976. Rev. El Medico, *25:*20, 1975

Heel, ulcers of, surgical management of (Ger). Surg. Gynec. & Obst., *140:*909, 1975

Lobster claw feet, surgical correction (Onizuka), PRS, *57:*98, 1976

Foot and akle defects in children, cross-groin flap for coverage (Furnas), PRS, *57:*246, 1976

FOOTE, P. A., JR., AND CHANDLER, J. R.: Protection of carotid artery by fascia lata in head and neck surgery, PRS, *51:*351, 1973. South. M. J., *65:*1225, 1972

FORDHAM, S. D., AND SCHATZ, C. J.: Emergency sialography, PRS, *56:*593, 1975. Emergency Med., *7:*101, 1975

FORNAROLI, G.: Complication after alloplastic thigh augmentation, PRS, *56:*357, 1975. Polymers in Med., *4:*153, 1974

FOROUGH, M. *et al*: Surgical treatment of trichiasis. Ann. Ocul. (Paris), *205:*1215, 1972 (French)

FORRESTER, J. C. *et al*: Wolff's law in relation to healing skin wound, PRS, *48:*299, 1971. J. Trauma, *10:*770, 1970

FORSSELL, K. *et al*: Analysis of recurrence of odontogenic keratocysts. Proc. Finn. Dent. Soc., *70:*135, 1974

FORTNER, J. G. *et al*: Surgical treatment of recurrent melanoma, PRS, *55:*517, 1975. Surg. Clin. N. Am., *54:*865, 1974

FORTNER, J. G., SCHOTTENFELD, D., AND MACLEAN, B. J.: *En bloc* resection of primary melanoma with regional lymph node dissection, PRS, *56:*601, 1975. Arch. Surg., *110:*674, 1975

FORTNEY, H. D., ALCORN, R. W., AND MONACO, F.: Circumpalatal wires for stabilizing complete maxillary dentures or splints, PRS, *55:*375, 1975. J. Oral Surg., *32:*538, 1974

FORTUNATO, G.: Embryogenesis of primitive palate and cleft cyst of upper maxilla, PRS, *57:*401, 1976. Riv. ital. chir. plast., *6:*53, 1974

FOSSATI, G. *et al*: Cellular and humoral immunity against human malignant melanoma. Int. J. Cancer, *8:*185, 1971

FOTIN, A. V. *et al*: Removal of juvenile fibroma of the nasopharynx under endotracheal anesthesia with arterial hypotension. Vestn. Otorinolaringol., *33:*57, 1971 (Russian)

FOUAD, A. R.: Rare case of canaliculocele. Bull. Ophthalmol. Soc. Egypt, *65:*265, 1972

FOURNIER, P.: Survey of chemical peeling of the face (with Litton, Capinpin), PRS, *51:*645, 1973

FOURRIER, P., BERT, G., AND AUBIJOUX, J.: Traumatic lesions with respect to wearing seat belts in automobile accidents, PRS, *51:*110, 1973. Lyon chir., *68:*247, 1972

FOWLER, J. F.: Radiotherapy of next decade, PRS, *55:*644, 1975. Proc. Roy. Soc. Med., *67:*743, 1974

FOWLER, P. J., AND WILLIS, R. B.: Vascular compartment syndromes, PRS, *56:*597, 1975. Canad. J. Surg., *18:*157, 1975.

Fox, C. L.: Hypertonic balanced sodium solution in burn shock, PRS, *57:*401, 1976. Internat. Surg., *60:*348, 1975

Fox, DONNA RUSSELL, AND BLECHMAN, MARK: *Clinical Management of Voice Disorders.* Cliff Notes, Inc., Lincoln, Nebraska, 1975. PRS, *57:*657, 1976

Fox, G. L. *et al*: Mandibular retrognathia: a review of the literature and selected cases. J. Oral Surg., *34:*53, 1976

Fox, J. E. *et al*: Ameloblastoma of the maxilla. A report of two cases. Brit. Dent. J., *138:*61, 1975

Fox, J. L. *et al*: Fluorescein angiography in microvascular surgery: study using rodent artery. Stroke, *5:*196, 1974

Fox, J. W., IV: Plea for improved monitoring and use of cardiac assistance devices in gravely burned patient (Editorial), PRS, *56:*328, 1975

Fox, J. W., IV, GOLDEN, G. T., AND EDGERTON, M. T.: Surgical correction of absent nasal alae of Johanson-Blizzard syndrome, PRS, *57:*484, 1976

Fox, J. W., GOLDEN, G. T., AND EDGERTON, M. T.: Frontonasal dysplasia with alar clefts in two sisters; genetic considerations and surgical correction, PRS, *57:*553, 1976

Fox, S. A.: Surgery for progressive familial myopathic ptosis. Ann. Ophth., *3:*1033, 1971

Fox, S. A.: Downward displacement of medial canthus. Ann. Ophth., *3:*1082, 1971

Fox, S. A.: Lengthening and shortening palpebral fissure, PRS, *49:*356, 1972. Arch. Ophth., *86:*401, 1971

Fox, S. A.: Surgery of senile ectropion and entropion. Ann. Ophth., *4:*217, 1972

Fox, S. A.: Upper lid reconstruction. Arch. Ophth., *88:*46, 1972

Fox, S. A.: Palpebral dacryoadenectomy. Am. J. Ophth., *76:*314, 1973

Fox, S. A.: Simple levator resection operation, PRS, *56:*223, 1975. Ann. Ophth., *7:*315, 1975

Fox, S. A.: Modified Fasanella-Servat procedure for ptosis. Arch. Ophth., *93:*639, 1975

Fox, S. A.: Repair of nasocanthal malignancies by combined laissez-faire and chemosurgery techniques. Trans. Am. Acad. Ophthalmol. Otolaryngol., *79:*654, 1975

Fox, S. A.: Senile (atonic) entropion. Ann. Ophth., 8:167, 1976

Fox, S. A.: Repair of nasocanthal malignant neoplasms. Combined laissez-faire and chemosurgery techniques. Arch. Ophth., 94:278, 1976

Fox, Sidney A.: Ophthalmic Plastic Surgery, Fourth Edition. Grune & Stratton, New York, 1970. PRS, 48:174, 1971

Fox, Sidney A.: Lid Surgery, Current Concepts. Grune & Stratton, New York, 1972. PRS, 51:580, 1973

Frable, M. A.: Submaxillary gland excision, PRS, 48:294, 1971. Surg. Gynec. & Obst., 131:1155, 1970

Frable, M. A. et al: Hemorrhagic complications of facial fractures. Laryngoscope, 84:2051, 1974

Fradin, V. M.: Experience in the use of oxidized cellulose for hemostatic purposes. Zh. Ushn. Nos. Gorl. Bolezn. 82:1974 (Russian)

Fradkin, A. H.: Orbital floor fractures and ocular complications. Am. J. Ophth., 72:699, 1971

Fragiadakis, E. G.: Dupuytren's contracture, PRS, 50:94, 1972. Trans. 7th Panhellenic Cong. Surg. Soc., 1:241, 1971

Fragiadakis, E. G. et al: Tendon transfer in the hand. Use of the sublimis to reinforce the extensors. Int. Surg., 55:172, 1971

Fragiadakis, E. G. et al: Metastatic carcinoma of the hand. Hand, 4:268, 1972

Fragiadakis, E. G. et al: Sarcoma of tendon sheath. Hand, 5:71, 1973

Fraley, E. E., and Hutchens, H. C.: Radical ilioinguinal node dissection: skin bridge technique, PRS, 51:711, 1973. J. Urol., 108:279, 1972

Francesconi, G., and Fenili, O.: Considerations on complications following radium therapy of skin angiomas, PRS, 53:496, 1974. Bol. mal. orecch. gola naso, 88:215, 1970

Francesconi, G. et al: Methods of repair of the lower lip. G. Ital. Dermatol., 47:20, 1972 (Italian)

Francesconi, G., and Fenili, O.: Treatment of deflection of anterocaudal portion of nasal septum, PRS, 51:342, 1973

Francesconi, G. et al: Complications following abdominal dermolipectomies, PRS, 56:355, 1975. Riv. ital. chir. plast., 5:455, 1973

Francesconi, G. et al: Postoperative pharyngeal fistulas, PRS, 57:397, 1976. Riv. ital. chir. plast., 6:81, 1974

Franchebois, P.: How to improve surgical treatment of small cancerous lesions of lower lip. Union Med. Can., 102:1558, 1973 (French)

Franchebois, P.: Improved surgical treatment of cancer of lower lip, PRS, 56:461, 1975. Internat. Surg., 60:204, 1975

Franchebois, P. et al: Staphylorrhaphy with suture of the posterior pillars. Functional results. Rev. Laryngol. Otol. Rhinol. (Bord.), 91:698, 1970 (French)

Franciosi, R. V., Barney, E. J., and Kramer, M. F.: Surgical management of polydactyly, PRS, 57:760, 1976. Foot Surg., 14:103, 1975

Franco, A., Callejo, F., and Pedreno, F. J.: Skin necrosis following disseminated intravascular thrombotic syndrome, PRS, 54:693, 1974. Rev. españ. cir. plast., 7:55, 1974

Franco, P.: Cure of cleft lips in 1561 (Classic Reprint), PRS, 57:84, 1976

Franco, T.: Association of abdominoplasty to intracavitary surgeries, PRS, 50:638, 1972. Rev. Bras. Cir., 61:5, 1971

Franco Diaz, A., and Alonso Rosa, S.: Observations on clinical use of carbenicillin in extensive burns, PRS, 53:247, 1974. Rev. españ. cir. plast., 5:209, 1972

Franke, G. H. et al: Case of multiple primary carcinomas of the head and neck. Wis. Med. J., 70:242, 1971

Franke, K.: Typical sport lesions and sport injuries in the region of the hand. Z. Unfallmed. Berufskr., 67:176, 1974

Frankel, R. et al: Condylar growth in light of new experimental research results – literature survey. Dtsch. Stomatol., 23:452, 1973 (German)

Franklin, J. D., Reynolds, V. H., and Page, D. L.: Cutaneous melanoma: 20-year retrospective study with clinicopathologic correlation, PRS, 56:277, 1975

Franklyn, R. A.: Experience with acupuncture anesthesia in cosmetic plastic surgery. Am. J. Chin. Med., 2:345, 1974

Franks, A. S.: Oral rehabilitation following surgical treatment of mandibular malignancy. Proc. Roy. Soc. Med., 67:614, 1974

Franz, M. L. et al: Proportioned philtrum: a helpful measurement and ratio. Cleft Palate J., 9:143, 1972

Franzen, E.: Automatic intermittent insufflation of the tracheotomy tube cuff. Rev. Bras. Anestesiol., 21:103, 1971 (Portuguese)

Fraser, D. G., Bull, J. G., Jr, and Dunphy, E.: Malignant melanoma and coexisting malignant neoplasms, PRS, 49:109, 1972. Am. J. Surg., 122:169, 1971

Fraser, F. C.: Updating the genetics of cleft lip and palate. Birth Defects, 10:107, 1974

Fraser, F. C. et al: Relation of face shape to susceptibility to congenital cleft lip. A preliminary report. J. Med. Genet., 7:112, 1970

FRATIANNE, R. B.: Relationship of hematocrit levels to skin flap survival in the dog (with Earle, Nunez), PRS, *54:*341, 1974

FRAYSSE, E. *et al*: Treatment of a case of laterognathia associated with prognathism by the Trauner technic. Rev. Odontostomatol. Midi Fr., *28:*275, 1970 (French)

FRAZELL, E. L.: Review of the treatment of cancer of the mobile portion of the tongue. Cancer, *28:*1178, 1971

FRAZIER, CLAUDE A.: *Is it Moral to Modify Man?* Charles C Thomas, Springfield, Ill., 1974. PRS, *55:*356, 1975

FRAZIER, T. G. *et al*: Fingertip injuries. Pa. Med., *74:*51, 1971

FRECHE, C. *et al*: Bucco-sinusal communications. Ann. Chir., *28:*781, 1974 (French)

FRECKMAN, H. A.: Results in 169 patients with cancer of head and neck treated by intra-arterial infusion therapy, PRS, *52:*214, 1973. Am. J. Surg., *124:*501, 1972

FREDERIKS, E.: Vascular patterns in normal and cleft primary and secondary palate in human embryos, PRS, *52:*209, 1973. Brit. J. Plast. Surg., *25:*207, 1972

FREDERIKS, E.: Treatment of degloved fingers, PRS, *54:*375, 1974. Hand, *5:*140, 1973

FREDRICKS, S.: Tripod resection for "Pinocchio" nose deformity, PRS, *53:*531, 1974. Discussion by Peck, PRS, *53:*674, 1974

FREDRICKS, S.: Whither aesthetic surgery? PRS, *54:*387, 1974

FREDRICKS, S.: Lower rhytidectomy, PRS, *54:*537, 1974

FREDRICKSON, J. M.: Distant transfer of a free, living bone graft by microvascular anastomoses (with Ostrup), PRS, *54:*274, 1974

FREDRICKSON, J. M.: Reconstruction of mandibular defects after radiation, using a free, living bone graft transferred by microvascular anastomoses (with Ostrup), PRS, *55:*563, 1975

FREEDMAN, H. M. *et al*: Malignant melanoma of nasal cavity and paranasal sinuses, PRS, *52:*459, 1973. Arch. Otolaryng., *97:*322, 1973

FREEDMAN, P. D. *et al*: Calcifying odontogenic cyst. A review and analysis of seventy cases. Oral Surg., *40:*93, 1975

Free Flaps (See also *Bone Grafts, Free*)

Composite graft, free, problems of (Bando, Fukuda, Soeda), PRS, *52:*461, 1973. Jap. J. Plast. Reconstr. Surg., *15:*420, 1972

Omentum, autotransplant to large scalp defect with microsurgical revascularization (McLean, Buncke), PRS, *49:*268, 1972

Anastomoses, vascular, *vs* circulation across the junction, after transfer of the pedicle

Free Flaps—Cont.

(Hugo), PRS, *50:*216, 1972

Free flaps, dermo-epidermal, great omentum supporting, for treatment of radionecrosis of flexor folds, axilla, groin, neck (Kiricuta). Ann. chir. plast., *18:*65, 1973 (French)

Flap, free; composite tissue transfer by vascular anastomosis (Taylor, Daniel), PRS, *55:*642, 1975. Australian & New Zealand J. Surg., *43:*1, 1973

Flaps, composite free, experimental transfer with microvascular anastomoses (O'Brien, Shanmugan), PRS, *54:*117, 1974. Australian & New Zealand J. Surg., *43:*285, 1973

Omentum magnum in prethoracic transposition in breast plasties (Kiricuta, Popescu), PRS, *53:*242, 1974. Chir. Plast., *2:*47, 1973

Ankle-heel region, surgical management of soft tissue defects (Bennett, Kahn), PRS, *53:*113, 1974. J. Trauma, *12:*696, 1973

Microsurgical arterial repairs, use of Saran Wrap cuff in (McLean, Buncke), PRS, *51:*624, 1973

Anastomoses, microvascular, free transfer of skin flaps by (Daniel, Williams), PRS, *52:*16, 1973

Anastomoses, microvascular, distant transfer of an island flap by (Daniel, Taylor), PRS, *52:*111, 1973

Flap, island, first successful distant transfer of, in man (Buncke) (Editorial), PRS, *52:*178, 1973

Island flap, large, successful transfer from groin to foot by microvascular anastomoses (O'Brien *et al*), PRS, *52:*271, 1973

Cutaneous island flap, anatomical identification and transfer by microsurgical vascular anastomosis (Kaplan, Buncke, Murray), PRS, *52:*301, 1973

Gastroepiploic vessels as recipient or donor vessels in free transfer of composite flaps by microvascular anastomosis, use of (Harii, Ohmori), PRS, *52:*541, 1973

Microsutures, metallized, and new micro needle holder (O'Brien, Hayhurst), PRS, *52:*673, 1973

Stumps, faulty, of lower limb, free skin transplantation using "SITO" graft for (Serenkova), PRS, *54:*626, 1974. Acta chir. plast., *16:*16, 1974

Transfer by microanastomosis of scalp flap in case of cicatricial baldness (Baudet *et al*). Ann. chir. plast., *19:*313, 1974 (French)

Flap transfers, free, with microvascular anastomoses (O'Brien *et al*), PRS, *56:*683, 1975. Brit. J. Plast. Surg., *27:*220, 1974

Case of true prehallux (Makino *et al*), PRS,

Free Flaps—Cont.
57:338, 1976
Flaps, free groin, ten (Baudet, LeMaire, Guimberteau), PRS, 57:577, 1976
Flap, free, transfer, laryngeal reconstruction by (Nagahara, Hirose, Iwai), PRS, 57:604, 1976
Flaps, free, more—to publish or not to publish?—to use or not to use? (McDowell) (Editorial), PRS, 57:653, 1976
Groin flap, free, fourteen transfers (Serafin, Villarreal Rios, Georgiade), PRS, 57:707, 1976
Flap transfers, ten free: use of intra-arterial dye injection to outline a flap exactly (Boeckx, de Coninck, Vanderlinden), PRS, 57:716, 1976

FREEHAVER, A. A.: Tendon transfers to improve grasp in patients with cervical spinal cord injury. Paraplegia, 13:15, 1975
FREELAND, A. P. *et al*: Vascular supply of the cervical skin with reference to incision planning. Laryngoscope, 85:714, 1975
FREEMAN, B. S.: Results of epiphyseal transplants by flap and by free graft. (Follow-Up Clinic), PRS, 48:72, 1971
FREEMAN, B. S.: Immobilization of skin grafts by wide-mesh net (Follow-Up Clinic), PRS, 49:207, 1972
FREEMAN, B. S.: Whither subcutaneous mastectomy? (Editorial), PRS, 49:654, 1972
FREEMAN, B. S.: Successful treatment of some fibrous envelope contractures around breast implants, PRS, 50:107, 1972
FREEMAN, B. S.: Late reconstruction of the lax oral sphincter in facial paralysis, PRS, 51:144, 173
FREEMAN, B. S.: Subcutaneous mastectomy for central tumors of breast, with immediate reconstruction, PRS, 51:263, 1973. Discussions by Crile, Hutter, Snyderman, PRS, 51:445, 1973
FREEMAN, B. S.: Reconstruction of breast form by silastic gel from breast prostheses. Brit. J. Plast. Surg., 27:284, 1974
FREEMAN, B. S. *et al*: Analysis of suture withdrawal stress, PRS, 49:668, 1972. Surg. Gynec. & Obst., 131:441, 1970
FREEMAN, E. E. *et al*: New method for covering large surface area wounds with autografts. I. *In vitro* multiplication of rabbit-skin epithelial cells, PRS, 55:114, 1975. Arch. Surg., 108:721, 1974
FREEMAN, N. V.: Fenestrated tracheostomy tubes. Lancet, 1:259, 1973
FREEMAN, R. G., AND DUNCAN, W. C.: Recurrent skin cancer, PRS, 52:685, 1973. Arch. Dermat., 107:395, 1973

FREESTONE, J. T. *et al*: Intraoral mandibular resection for osteoradionecrosis. J. Oral Surg., 31:861, 1973
FREIBERG, A., AND MANKTELOW, R.: Kutler repair for fingertip amputations. PRS, 50:371, 1972
FREIDEL, C. *et al*: Resection of the mandible in children. Considerations on its reconstruction. Ann. chir. plast., 16:227, 1971 (French)
FREIDEL, C. *et al*: Critical study of Ward's technic in the treatment of temporo-mandibular ankylosis. Analysis of a homogenous series of 15 cases. Ann. chir. plast., 16:334, 1971 (French)
FREIDEL, M. *et al*: Early treatment of traumatic lesions of middle portion of face. J. Fr. Otorhinolaryngol., 21:917, 1972 (French)
FREIDEL, M. *et al*: Management of a multicular cystic image of the mandible. Rev. Stomatol. Chir. Maxillofac., 75:61, 1974 (French)
FREIDEL, M. *et al*: Post-traumatic telecanthus. Early treatment and secondary correction. Rev. Stomatol. Chir. Maxillofac., 75:266, 1974 (French)
FREIHOFER, H. P.: Results after mobilization of the mid-facial bone structure. Fortschr. Kiefer. Gesichtschir., 18:219, 1975 (German)
FREIHOFER, H. P., JR.: Results after midface-osteotomies. J. Maxillo-facial Surg., 1:30, 1973
FREIHOFER, H. P., JR. *et al*: Experiences with intraoral trans-osseous wiring of mandibular fractures. J. Maxillo-facial Surg., 1:248, 1973
FREIHOFER, H. P., JR. *et al*: Late results after advancing the mandible by sagittal splitting of the rami. J. Maxillo-facial Surg., 3:230, 1975
FREILINGER, G.: New technique to correct facial paralysis. PRS, 56:44, 1975
FREILINGER, G. *et al*: Clinical experience with dynamic reconstruction after facial paresis. In *Plastische und Wiederherstellungs-Chirurgie*, pp. 151-6., ed. Hohler; Stuttgart; Schattauer, 1975 (German)
FREITAG, V. *et al*: Bitemporal suspension as alternative method of craniofacial suspension. J. Maxillo-facial Surg., 1:154, 1973
FRENCH, W. E. AND BALE, G. F.: Midline cervical cleft of neck with associated branchial cyst. Am. J. Surg., 125:376, 1973
FRER, A. A. *et al*: Intraoral osteotomy of mandibular symphysis to correct bilateral lingual crossbite: report of case. J. Oral Surg., 30:754, 1972
FRESHWATER, M. F.: More about "B.L.," "Mr. Lucas," and Mr. Carpue (Letter to the Editor). PRS, 49:78, 1972
FRESHWATER, M. F.: Does the topical use of magnesium sulfate improve the results in

microvascular anastomoses? (Letter to the Editor). PRS, *55:*483, 1975

FRESHWATER, M. F.: Is arteriovenous shunting the correct explanation of the flap delay phenomenon? (Letter to the Editor). PRS, *55:*697, 1975

FRESHWATER, M. F.: Microirrigator (Letter to the Editor). PRS, *57:*508, 1976

FRESHWATER, M. F. *et al*: Skin grafting of burns: a centennial. A tribute to George David Pollock. J. Trauma, *11:*862, 1971

FRETILLERE, Y. *et al*: Dysembryoma of nasal fossa. Rev. Laryngol. Otol. Rhinol. (Bord.), *94:*569, 1973 (French)

FRETZIN, D., AND HELWIG, E.: Atypical fibroxanthoma of skin, PRS, *54:*243, 1974. Cancer, *31:*1541, 1973

FREYSS, G. *et al*: Ogura's technic in edematous exophthalmos. Bull. Soc. Ophtalmol. Fr., *73:*253, 1973 (French)

FRIED, M. P. *et al*: Cervical metastasis from an unknown primary. Ann. Otol. Rhin. & Laryng., *84:*152, 1975

FRIEDBERG, J. *et al*: Pediatric tracheotomy. Can. J. Otolaryngol., *3:*147, 1974

FRIEDBERG, S. A. *et al*: Tracheostome maintenance by obturator for prolonged or future needs. Ann. Otol. Rhin. & Laryng., *83:*520, 1974

FRIEDE, H.: Histology of the premaxillary-vomerine suture in a bilateral cleft case. Cleft Palate J., *10:*14, 1973

FRIEDE, H., AND PRUZANSKY, S.: Longitudinal study of growth in bilateral cleft lip and palate, from infancy to adolescence. PRS, *49:*392, 1972

FRIEDE, H., AND JOHANSON, B.: Follow-up study of cleft children treated with primary bone grafting, I. Orthodontic aspects, PRS, *56:*680, 1975. Scand. J. Plast. Reconstr. Surg., *8:*88, 1974

FRIEDEBOLD, G.: Reconstructive operations in cases of irreparable lesions of peripheral nerves, PRS *53:*369, 1974. Langenbecks Arch. Chir., *332:*363, 1972

FRIEDELL, M. T.: Editorial: surgery for obesity. Int. Surg., *60:*70, 1975

FRIEDENBERG, Z. B. *et al*: Bone reaction to varying amounts of direct current, PRS, *48:*95, 1971. Surg. Gynec. & Obst., *131:*894, 1970.

FRIEDENBERG, Z. B. *et al*: Stimulation of fracture healing by direct current in rabbit fibula, PRS, *50:*312, 1972. J. Bone & Joint Surg., *53:*1400, 1971

FRIEDERICH, H. C.: Case report on free transplantation of the mouth mucosa on the glans penis in humans. Hautarzt, *21:*84, 1970 (German)

FRIEDERICH, H. C.: Closing lower leg ulcers from the viewpoint of dermatologist. Z. Hautkr., *49:*377, 1974

FRIEDLAND, J. A., COCCARO, P. J., AND CONVERSE, J. M: Retrospective cephalometric analysis of mandibular bone absorption under silicone rubber chin implants. PRS, *57:*144, 1976

FRIEDLANDER, A. H.: Proteus vulgaris osteomyelitis of mandible. Case report. Oral Surg., *40:*39, 1975

FRIEDLANDER, A. H.: Modified lip stripping with reconstruction of a new vermilion border. N.Y. State Dent. J., *42:*27, 1976

FRIEDLANDER, A. H. *et al*: Peripheral ossifying fibroma: case report. J. Oral Surg., *31:*547, 1973

FRIEDLANDER, A. H. *et al*: Cheiloplasty for correction of microstomia secondary to untreated burn. J. Oral Surg., *32:*525, 1974

FRIEDLANDER, A. H. *et al*: Sclerosing hemangioma of the tongue: report of case. J. Oral Surg., *33:*212, 1975

FRIEDLANDER, A. H. *et al:* Treatment of massive dentigerous cysts of the mandible: a report of two cases. N.Y. State Dent. J., *42:*156, 1976

FRIEDMAN, E. *et al*: Central mucoepidermoid tumor of the mandible. Trans. Int. Conf. Oral Surg., *4:*129, 1973

FRIEDMAN, E. W., AND SCHWARTZ, A. E.: Diagnosis of salivary gland tumors, PRS, *55:*246, 1975. CA, *24:*266, 1974

FRIEDMAN, G.: Travase, effective enzyme for burn debridement (with Pennisi, Capozzi). PRS, *51:*371, 1973

FRIEDMAN, J. *et al*: Preliminary study of histological effects of three different types of electrosurgical currents. N.Y. State Dent. J., *40:*349, 1974

FRIEDMAN, J. M. *et al*: Cavernous hemangioma of oral cavity: review of literature and report of case. J. Oral Surg., *31:*617, 1973

FRIEDMAN, J. M. *et al:* Mixed tumors of oral cavity. Report of two cases. N.Y. State Dent. J., *41:*154, 1975

FRIEDMAN, W. H. *et al*: Brown tumor of maxilla in secondary hyperparathyroidism. Arch. Otolaryng., *100:*157, 1974

FRIEDMAN, W. H., BILLAR, H. F., AND SOM, M. L.: Repair of extended laryngotracheostenosis, PRS, *57:*759, 1976. Arch. Otolaryng., *101:*152, 1975

FRIEDMAN, Z. *et al*: Granular cell myoblastoma of eyelid margin. Brit. J. Ophthalmol., *57:*757, 1973

FRIEMEL, E.: Ophthalmologic symptoms of basal orbital fractures. Klin. Monatsbl. Augenheilkd., *159:*658, 1971 (German)

FRIEMEL, E.: Motility disorders of the eye in injuries of the osseous orbit (ophthalmologic report). Wien. Med. Wochenschr., *122:* Suppl 5:10, 1972 (German)

FRIES, I. B. *et al*: Contact dermatitis in surgeons from methylmethacrylate bone cement, PRS, *57:*406, 1976. J. Bone & Joint Surg., *57A:*547, 1975

FRIES, R.: Immediate and definite reconstruction after hemimandibulectomy. Minerva Stomatol., *20:*155, 1971

FRIES, R.: Advantages of basic concept in lip reconstruction after tumor resection, PRS, *52:*452, 1973. J. Maxillo-facial Surg., *1:*13, 1973

FRIES, R.: Technic and indication for the open axial medullary wiring in mandibular fractures. Fortschr. Kiefer. Gesichtschir., *19:*108, 1975 (German)

FRIES, R. *et al*: Systematic technic in the primary reconstruction of tissue loss in the mouth after excision of cancer. Acta Stomatol. Belg., *72:*443, 1975 (German)

FRILECK, S. P.: Mandibular vestibuloplasty with free graft of mucoperiosteal layer from hard palate (with Morgan, Gallegos). PRS, *51:*359, 1973

FRILEUX, C.: Leg ulcers of venous origin. Phlebologie, *27:*137, 1974 (French)

FRILEUX, C. *et al*: Good and bad feet in vascular pathology of the legs. Ann. Chir., *27:*308, 1973 (French)

FRISHBERG, I. A.: Surgery in aging of soft tissue of the face. Khirurgiia (Mosk.), *47:*43, 1971 (Russian)

FRITSCH, W. C. *et al*: Delayed purpuric reaction following superficial dermabrasion. Arch. Dermat., *112:*83, 1976

FRITSCHE, P.: Tracheotomy or long-term intubation? H.N.O., *21:*297, 1973 (German)

FRITSCHI, ERNEST P.: *Reconstructive Surgery in Leprosy.* Williams & Wilkins Co., Baltimore, 1971. PRS, *49:*567, 1972

FRITTSSHE, P. *et al*: Closure of large burn wounds in children. Vestn. Khir., *112:*103, 1974 (Russian)

FRITZ, G.: Treatment of injuries resulting from dog bites. Wien. Klin. Wochenschr., *84:*12, 1972 (German)

FRITZ, K.: Reconstructive surgery following total laryngectomy. Wien. Klin. Wochenschr., *86:*421, 1974 (German)

FROHLICH, J. *et al*: Frontobasal injuries in the neurosurgeon's competence. Rozhl. Chir., *53:*803, 1974 (Slovakian)

FROLMSON, A. I.: Hand reconstruction in arthritis mutilans. A case report. J. Bone & Joint Surg. (Am.), *53:*1377, 1971

FROMM, H., AND SCHAEFER, M.: Primary surgical management of frontal and fronto-basal cranio-cerebral injuries, PRS, *57:*396, 1976. Aktuel Chir., *10:*219, 1975

Frontal Bone (See also *Encephaloceles and Meningoceles*)

Frontal osteoplasty (Morales). Acta Otorinolaryngol. Iber. Am., *23:*849, 1972 (Spanish)

Acrylic implants for frontal bone defects (Blatt, Failla), PRS, *50:*543, 1972. Mil. Med., *137:*22, 1972

Frontal bone, osteoplastic, serious cosmetic complications of (Ward *et al*). Arch. Otolaryng., *98:* 389, 1973

Fronto-orbital epidermoid cyst (Ravault *et al*). Bull. Soc. Ophtalmol. Fr., *73:*793, 1973 (French)

Frontal bone defect, plastic surgery of, with special reference to tantalum (Zehm). H. N. O., *21:*79, 1973 (German)

Frontal cranial base, surgery of (Takahashi). J. Otolaryngol. Jap., *76:*1231, 1973 (Japanese)

Frontal bone, unstable depressed fracture of, extra-osseous Kirschner wire fixation for (Climo, Block, Alexander). PRS, *52:*200, 1973

Principles, methods and results of treatment of frontal bone defects (Bauer *et al*). Chirurg., *45:*514, 1974 (German)

Esthesioneuroblastoma: light and electron microscopic study (Kahn). Hum. Pathol., *5:*364, 1974

Extradural ossification following extradural hematoma, case report (Iwakuma *et al*). J. Neurosurg., *41:*104, 1974

Frontal skull fractures, depressed, including those involving sinus, orbit and cribriform plate, primary reconstruction of (Nadell *et al*). J. Neurosurg., *41:*200, 1974

Frontal bone, reconstruction of, following frontobasal fractures (Bauer *et al*). Z. Allgemeinmed, *50:*385, 1974 (German)

Correction of fronto-orbital defects (Schlondorff). Z. Laryngol. Rhinol. Otol., *53:*104, 1974 (German)

Tumors, frontonasal, diagnosis and management (Griffith). PRS, *57:*692, 1976

Frontal Sinus (See also *Paranasal Sinus Neoplasms*)

Giant frontal mucocele. Plastic surgery with acrylic resin (Ruch *et al*). Ann. Otolaryngol. Chir. Cervicofac., *88:*403, 1971 (French)

Reconstruction of the skull defect using dimethyl polysiloxan (DMPS) following surgery of bone tumor of the frontal sinus

Frontal Sinus—Cont.

(Sakurai *et al*). Otolaryngology (Tokyo), *43*:607, 1971 (Japanese)

Frontal sinus myxomas (Gryczynski). Pol. Tyg. Lek., *27*:1315, 1972 (Polish)

Frontal sinus defects, repair of, with methylmethacrylate (Komorn *et al*). South. Med. J., *65*:1432, 1972

Frontal sinus, osteoma, certain problems (Miller). Acta Otorhinolaryngol. Belg., *27*:171, 1973 (French)

Frontal sinus, fractures of: therapeutic procedure (Gaillard *et al*). Ann. Otolaryngol. Chir. Cervicofac., *90*:741, 1973 (French)

Frontal sinus, mucoceles of, causes and treatment (Bordley *et al*). Ann. Otol. Laryngol., *82*:696, 1973

Frontal sinus surgery, mucoperiosteal flap in Sewall-Boyden-McNaught operation (Baron *et al*). Laryngoscope, *83*:1266, 1973

Frontal sinus fractures, systematic evaluation and management of (Nichols *et al*). Trans. Am. Acad. Ophthalmol. Otolaryngol., *77*:1429, 1973

Frontal sinuses and ethmoid labyrinth, osteoma of (Gorshkov). Vestn. Otorinolaringol., *35*:86, 1973 (Russian)

Frontal sinus and nasal cavity, modification of drainage tube for formation of anastomosis between (Chernykh). Zh. Ushn. Nos. Gorl. Bolezn., *33*:82, 1973 (Russian)

Frontal sinus, large osteoma of, complex treatment (Pietruski *et al*). Otolaryngol. Pol., *28*:103, 1974 (Polish)

An isolated mucocele of the frontal sinus (Haberman *et al*). Acta Otorhinolaryngol. Belg., *29*:607, 1975 (French)

Frontal sinus and supraorbital fractures from vehicle accidents (Schultz). Clin. Plast. Surg., *2*:93, 1975

Unusual presentation of a frontal mucocele (Podoshin *et al*). Eye Ear Nose Throat Mon., *54*:69, 1975

Role of radiotherapy in the treatment of primary tumours of the frontal sinuses (Takacsi-Nagy *et al*). J. Laryng. & Otol., *90*:211, 1976

FRONTERA VACA, J.: Nerve homografts, PRS, *49*:105, 1972. Bull. Soc. Plast. Surg. Cordoba Argent., *1*:7, 1971

FRONTERA VACA, J. *et al*: Angiographic diagnosis and preventive surgery of plantar ulcers, PRS, *55*:109, 1975. Bol. Soc. cir. Plast. Reconstr. Cordoba, *5*:17, 1974

FRONTERA VACA, J. *et al*: Hansenian torpid ulcers, use of topical debridement, PRS, *55*:385, 1975. Tribuna Med. Argent., *19*:135, 1974

Frostbite (See also *War Injuries*)

Electrical and cold injuries of the hand (Brown). Orthop. Clin. North Am., *1*:321, 1970

Consequences of frostbite. Geriatrics, *26*:82, 1971 (Editorial)

Xenon-133 for prediction of tissue loss in human frostbite (Sumner *et al*), PRS, *48*:515, 1971. Surgery, *69*:899, 1971

Frostbite, experimental, in mouse, hyperbaric oxygen treatment of (Hardenbergh), PRS, *51*:354, 1973. J. Surg. Res., *12*:34, 1972

Cold injury, effect of sympathectomy on tissue loss after experimental frostbite of rabbit ear (Hardenbergh, Miles), PRS, *52*:99, 1973. J. Surg. Res., *13*:126, 1972

Primary reconstructive surgery on the hand following severe frostbite (Vodianov *et al*). Vestn. Khir., *107*:97, 1972 (Russian)

Hypothermia and injury due to exposure (Muhlbauer). Fortschr. Med., *91*:417, 1973 (German)

Hypothermia, profound, circulation in (Zarins, Skinner), PRS, *53*:115, 1974. J. Surg. Res., *14*:97, 1973

Dimethylsulfoxide, as preservative: preservation of structure and function in canine small intestinal autografts after freezing (LaRossa *et al*). PRS, *52*:174, 1973

Ears, frostbite of, treated with flurandrenolide ointment (Kobak), PRS, *57*:529, 1976. Eye, Ear, Nose & Throat Month., *54*:31, 1974

Frostbite of the hands (Welch *et al*). Hand, *6*:33, 1974

Clinical experiences in management of cold injuries: study of 110 cases (Kyosola). J. Trauma, *14*:32, 1974

Frostbite, human, host factors in (Sumner, Criblez, Doolittle), PRS, *54*:691, 1974. Mil. Med., *141*:454, 1974

Frostbite (Holm, Vanggaard). PRS, *54*:544, 1974

Frostbite, effects and prevention in wound healing (Butson), PRS, *56*:599, 1975. Canad. J. Surg., *18*:145, 1975

Changes in the soft tissue of the hands in chronic cold trauma—radiological and thermographical findings (Gavrilova *et al*). Radiol. Diagn. (Berl.), *16*:285, 1975 (German)

Frostbite, experimental, treated with intraarterial sympathetic blocking drugs (Snider, Porter), PRS, *57*:403, 1976. Surgery, *77*:557, 1975

FRUTTERO, F.: Problems of a corrective technic

for the lower cartilaginous arch of the nasal pyramid. Minerva Otorinolaringol., *21:*211, 1971 (Italian)

FRUTTERO, F.: Corrective techniques of deviations of septum and nasal pyramid, PRS, *56:*592, 1975. Nuovi Arch. Ital. Otol. Rinol. Laring., *2:*339, 1974

FRY, H. J. H.: Judicious turbinectomy for nasal obstruction, PRS, *52:*205, 1973. Australian & New Zealand J. Surg., *42:*291, 1973

FRY, H. J. H.: Radionecrosis of neck. Aust. N.Z. J. Surg., *43:*177, 1973

FRY, H. J. H.: Radionecrosis of neck, PRS, *52:*678, 1973. Proc. Roy. Australasian Coll. Surg., *46:*412, 1973

FRY, H. J. H: Principles of correction of old septal deformity after injury, PRS, *52:*677, 1973. Proc. Roy. Australasian Coll. Surg., *46:*418, 1973

FRYER, MINOT: Honorary degree for. PRS, *48:*520, 1971

FRYER, M. P.: Hemangiomas: role of plastic surgery in early treatment (Follow-Up Clinic), PRS, *50:*77, 1972

FRYER, M. P.: Subtotal nose reconstruction with direct cheek flap. PRS, *53:*436, 1974

FRYER, M. P. *et al:* Evaluation of internal wire pin fixation of mandibular fractures, PRS, *48:*294, 1971. Surg. Gynec. & Obst., *132:*9, 1971

FRYER, M. P. *et al:* Repair of trauma about the orbit. J. Trauma, *12:*290, 1972

FRYMOYER, J. W., AND BLAND, J.: Carpal tunnel syndrome in patients with myxedematous arthropathy, PRS, *52:*207, 1973. J. Bone & Joint Surg., *55A:*78, 1973

FU, K. K., STEWART, J. R., AND BAGSHAW, M. A.: Cervical node metastases from occult primary sites, PRS, *53:*604, 1974. Rocky Mountain M.J., *70:*31, 1973

FU, Y. S. *et al:* Non-epithelial tumors of nasal cavity, paranasal sinuses, and nasopharynx. Clinicopathologic study. 2. Osseous and fibro-osseous lesions, including osteoma, fibrous dysplasia, ossifying fibroma, osteoblastoma, giant cell tumor and osteosarcoma. Cancer, *33:*1289, 1974

FU, Y. S. *et al:* Non-epithelial tumors of nasal cavity, paranasal sinuses, and nasopharynx: clinicopathologic study. 3. Cartilaginous tumors (chondroma, chondrosarcoma). Cancer, *34:*453, 1974

FU, Y. S. *et al:* Malignant soft tissue tumors of probable histiocytic origin (malignant fibrous histiocytomas): general considerations and electron microscopic and tissue culture studies. Cancer, *35:*176, 1975

FUCHIHATA, H. *et al:* Radiotherapy of carci-

noma developed from leukoplakia. Oral Surg., *33:*137, 1972

FUCHS, J.: New method for surgery of xanthelasma. Klin. Monatsbl. Augenheilkd., *163:*324, 1973 (German)

FUENTE-DEL-CAMPO, A., BARRERA, G., AND ORTIZ-MONASTERIO, F.: Simple retractor for use in rhytidoplasties, PRS, *51:*696, 1973

FUENTES-AGUILAR, R.: Management of some tumors of soft tissues. PRS, *54:*380, 1974. Cir. Cir., *41:*175, 1973

FUJIKAMI, T. K. *et al:* Surgical orthodontic therapy for laterognathism and facial asymmetry. A.D.M., *30:*31, 1973 (Spanish)

FUJINO, T.: New method of dissection and use of expander in orbital reconstruction, PRS, *50:*312, 1972. Jap. J. Plast. Reconstr. Surg., *14:*507, 1971

FUJINO, T.: New reduction apparatus for zygoma and arch fractures, PRS, *51:*610, 1973. Jap. J. Plast. Reconstr. Surg., *15:*209, 1972

FUJINO, T.: Reconstructive rhinoplasty with auricular composite graft and forehead flap with periosteum. PRS, *50:*526, 1972

FUJINO, T.: Microvascular surgery in reconstructive plastic surgery. Keio J. Med., *23:*137, 1974

FUJINO, T.: Experimental "blowout" fracture of the orbit. PRS, *54:*81, 1974

FUJINO, T.: Is late severance of a pharyngeal flap feasible? (Letter to the Editor). PRS, *55:*483, 1975

FUJINO, T.: Reuse of dermatome tape (Letter to the Editor). PRS, *57:*738, 1976

FUJINO, T. *et al:* Reconstruction of the cervical esophagus using a deltopectoral flap. Jap. J. Plast. Reconstr. Surg., *15:*188, 1972 (Japanese)

FUJINO, T., HARASHINA, T., AND MIKATA, A.: Autogenous *en bloc* transplantation of mammary gland in dogs, using microsurgical technique. PRS, *50:*376, 1972

FUJINO, T. *et al:* Mechanism of orbital blowout fracture, PRS, *56:*352, 1975. Jap. J. Plast. Reconstr. Surg., *17:*427, 1974

FUJINO, T. *et al:* Clinical success of distant transfer of free skin flap in head and neck regions by microvascular anastomoses. Keio J. Med., *23:*47, 1974

FUJINO, T., AND AOYAGI, F.: Method of successive interrupted suturing in microvascular anastomoses. PRS, *55:*240, 1975

FUJINO, T., TANINO, R., AND SUGIMOTO, C.: Microvascular transfer of free deltopectoral dermal-fat flap. PRS, *55:*428, 1975

FUJINO, T., HARASHINA, T., AND AOYAGI, F.: Reconstruction for aplasia of breast and pectoral region by microvascular transfer of free flap from buttock, PRS, *56:*178, 1975. Discussion by Goldwyn, PRS, *56:*335, 1975

FUJINO, T., AND SAITO, S.: Repair of pharyngoesophageal fistula by microvascular transfer of free skin flap. PRS, *56:*549, 1975

FUJINO, T., HARASHINA, T., AND NAKAJIMA, T.: Free skin flap from the retroauricular region to the nose. PRS, *57:*338, 1976

FUJIWARA, A., *et al*: Functional reconstruction of the hand in cervical cord injury. Orthop. Surg. (Tokyo), *22:*874, 1971 (Japanese)

FUKAYA, M. *et al*: Correction of mandibular deformity with silicone implant. Aichi Gakuin J. Dent. Sci., *10:*150, 1972 (Japanese)

FUKUDA, O.: Management of fresh facial fracture. Shujutsu, *25:*1173, 1971 (Japanese)

FUKUDA, O.: Experience of reconstruction of the head with a giant jump flap. Jap. J. Plast. Reconstr. Surg., *15:*203, 1972 (Japanese)

FUKUDA, O.: Microtic ear: survey of 180 cases in 10 years. PRS, *53:*458, 1974

FUKUDA, O. *et al*: Open skin grafting for granulation wounds. Jap. J. Plast. Reconstr. Surg., *14:*183, 1971 (Japanese)

FUKUDA, O., AND ARAI, K.: Philtrum reconstruction in cleft lip repair, PRS, *53:*369, 1974. Jap. J. Plast. Reconstr. Surg., *16:*355, 1973

FUKUI, M. *et al*: Histologic study of healing process of mandibular condyle after unilateral condylotomy in rat. Jap. J. Oral Surg., *19:*16, 1973 (Japanese)

FULGOSI, A.: Diagnostical and therapeutic approach to disturbed excretory lacrimal ducts in infants and small children. Vojnosanit. Pregl., *32:*149, 1975 (Croatian)

FULLER, L. M., SULLIVAN, M. P., AND BUTLER, J. J.: Results of regional radiotherapy in localized Hodgkin's disease in children. PRS, *54:*699, 1974. Cancer, *32:*640, 1973

FULTON, J. E. JR.: Acne vulgaris. Postgrad. Med., *57:*157, 1975

FULTON, R. L., AND FISHER, R. P.: Pulmonary changes due to hemorrhagic shock; resuscitation with isotonic and hypertonic saline, PRS, *54:*624, 1974. Surgery, *75:*881, 1974

FUMA, Y.: Dynamic study of fracture of the facial bones. Shikwa Gakuho, *72:*534, 1972 (Japanese)

FUMAROLA, A.: Reconstruction of lower lip after extensive total amputation. Ann. chir. plast., *18:*79, 1973 (French)

FUNASAKA, S. *et al*: Actinomycosis of the zygomaticotemporal region and the study of its infectious route. Otolaryngology (Tokyo), *43:*923, 1971 (Japanese)

FUNG, E. H.: Fractures of zygoma, PRS, *50:*630, 1972. Asian J. Med., *8:*202, 1972

Funnel Chest

New procedure for the surgical treatment of pectus excavatum and pectus carinatum with a contribution of 26 case reports (Balchev). Nauchni. Tr. Vssh. Med. Inst. Sofiia, *50:*39, 1971

Our experience with the surgical treatment of pectus excavatum (Gaubert *et al*). Arch. Fr. Pediatr., *29:*449, 1972 (French)

Surgery of the funnel chest (Bauermeister). Bruns Beitr. Klin. Chir., *219:*241, 1972 (German)

Pectus excavatum – surgical management (DeNiord *et al*). Va. Med. Mon., *99:*614, 1972

Improved method for repair of pectus chest deformities (Shannon *et al*). Ann. Thorac. Surg., *16:*629, 1973

Funnel chest operation, early and late results (de Vivie *et al*), PRS, *53:*105, 1974. Bruns' Beitr. klin. Chir., *220:*284, 1973

Cardiomegaly and pectus excavatum (Hunt, Cole), PRS, *53:*604, 1974. Chest, *64:*511, 1973

Pectus excavatum, surgical treatment. Hemodynamic and functional findings and long-term results in 18 patients (Intonti *et al*). Minerva Chir., *28:*1347, 1973 (Italian)

Funnel chest, congenital, surgical treatment of patients with (Kondrashin). Ortop. Travmatol. Protez., *34:*34, 1973 (Russian)

Surgical treatment of congenital deformities of thoracic wall in children (Coman *et al*). Pediatria (Bucur.), *22:*543, 1973 (Rumanian)

Chondrosternal malformations (Venne). Union Med. Can., *102:*1352, 1973 (French)

Technical considerations in the surgical management of pectus excavatum and carinatum (Robicsek *et al*). Ann. Thorac. Surg., *18:*549, 1974

Surgical treatment of funnel chest and of pigeon breast in children (Perez *et al*). Bol. Med. Hosp. Infant Mex., *31:*117, 1974 (Spanish)

Funnel chest, simplified operation for correction of, indications and surgery (Geroulanos *et al*). Dtsch. Med. Wochenschr., *99:*57, 1974 (German)

Funnel chest, simplified corrective surgery of (Seling) (Letter). Dtsch. Med Wochenschr., *99:*479, 1974 (German)

Funnel chest, surgical treatment (Feofilov *et al*). Grudn. Khir., *16:*47, 1974 (Russian)

Funnel chest correction: indication, surgical procedure and results of a simplified and modified method (Geroulanos *et al*). Helv. Chir. Acta, *41:*101, 1974 (German)

Operative correction of pectus excavatum

Funnel Chest—Cont.
(Humphreys *et al*). J. Pediatr. Surg., 9:899, 1974

Chest deformities, physical development of children and adolescents following surgery for (Wodzinska-Balon *et al*). Pediatr. Pol., 49:713, 1974 (Polish)

Congenital malformations of the thoracic wall (Witz). Poumon Coeur, 30:35, 1974 (French)

Pectus excavatum, esthetic solution in female patients (Pinto), PRS, 56:678, 1975. Rev. brasil. cir., 64:136, 1974

Funnel chest, new surgical treatment (Kabelka). Rozhl. Chir., 53:700, 1974 (Czechoslovakian)

Late results of operative correction of funnel chest (Svend-Hansen). Ugeskr. Laeger, 136:2302, 1974 (Danish)

Diagnostic and surgical management of thoracic wall malformations (Mau). Z. Erkr. Atmungsorgane, 141:149, 1974 (German)

Funnel chest operation, results of, in pediatric surgical clinic in Bremen (Oelsnitz), PRS, 55:108, 1975. Ztschr. Kinderchir., 15:25, 1974

Indications and surgical technic for the correction of funnel chest and its results (Willital *et al*). Chirurg., 46:323, 1975 (German)

Surgical treatment of funnel chest. Surgical experience with 90 cases (Naef *et al*). Schweiz. Med. Wochenschr., 105:737, 1975 (French)

Surgical correction of pectus excavatum using a retrosternal bar (Sbokos *et al*). Thorax, 30:40, 1975

Surgical management of the funnel chest. Pedunculated inversionplasty (Jung *et al*). Ztschr. Orthop., 113:830, 1975 (German)

Chest, funnel, stabilization of chest wall after operation (Gross). PRS, 57:398, 1976. Ztschr. Kinderchir., 17:67, 1975

Surgical treatment of pectus excavatum: an experience with 90 operations (Naef). Ann. Thorac. Surg., 21:63, 1976

Letter: Does pectus excavatum cause functional disability? (Nolan *et al*). J. Thorac. Cardiovasc. Surg., 71:148, 1976

FUQUA, F.: Renaissance of urethroplasty: Belt technique of hypospadias repair, PRS, 50:200, 1972. J. Urol., 106:782, 1971

FURLOW, L. T., JR.: Cause and prevention of tourniquet ooze, PRS, 49:105, 1972. Surg. Gynec. & Obst., 32:1069, 1971

FURLOW, L. T., JR.: Simple test for nasal escape. PRS, 49:355, 1972

FURLOW, L. T., JR.: *Dorsalis pedis* arterialized

flap (with McCraw). PRS, 55:177, 1975

FURLOW, L. T., JR.: Role of tendon tissues in tendon healing. PRS, 57:39, 1976

FURMAN, E. B. *et al*: Specific therapy in water, electrolyte and blood-volume replacement during pediatric surgery, PRS, 56:237, 1975. Anesthesiology, 42:187, 1975

FURMAN, S.: On covering an exposed pacemaker (Letter to the Editor). PRS, 52:181, 1973

FURMANETS, A. I.: Rare case of congenital familial anomalous development of the hands. Ortop. Travmatol. Protez., 31:59, 1970 (Russian)

FURNAS, D. W.: Correction of prominent ears by conchamastoid sutures (Follow-Up Clinic). PRS, 52:434, 1973

FURNAS, D. W.: Intradiploic cranial screws and acrylic framework for reduction and external fixation of complex facial fractures. PRS, 54:169, 1974

FURNAS, D. W.: Straight-line repair followed by rotation advancement repair for wide unilateral lip clefts. Brit. J. Plast. Surg., 28:259, 1975

FURNAS, D. W.: Growth of homotransplanted ear cartilage in baby rabbits (with Allison, Achauer). PRS, 55:479, 1975

FURNAS, D. W.: Cross-groin flap for coverage of foot and ankle defects in children. PRS, 57:246, 1976

FURNAS, D. W.: Hand sandwich: adjacent flaps from opposing body surfaces (with Smith). PRS, 57:351, 1976

FURNAS, D. W., AND BIRCOLL, M. J.: Eyelash traction test to determine if the medial canthal ligament is detached. PRS, 52:315, 1973

FURNAS, D. W., HAQ, M. A., AND SOMERS, G.: One-stage reconstruction for exstrophy of the bladder in girls, PRS, 56:61, 1975. Discussion by Devine, PRS, 56:209, 1975

FURNESS, M. A.: Results of *temporalis* transfer in lagophthalmos due to leprosy (with Ranney). PRS, 51:301, 1973

FURSTOSS, J. A. *et al*: Composite nasal septal autografts of trachea. Ann. Otol. Rhin. & Laryng., 82:831, 1973

FURUKAWA, M.: Oriental rhinoplasty. Clin. Plast. Surg., 1:129, 1974

FUSTER, B. *et al*: An adjustable clamp for use in carotid ligation. Acta Neurol. Lat. Am., 16:224, 1970

FUSTER, B. *et al*: Circulation patterns during clamping of the carotid arteries as determined by cutaneous carotid photoplethysmography. Acta Neurol. Lat. Am., 17:273, 1971

FUTRELL, J. W., *et al*: Multiple primary sweat gland carcinomas, PRS, 49:473, 1972. Cancer, *28:*686, 1971

FUTRELL, J. W. *et al*: Carcinoma of sweat glands in adolescents, PRS, *51:*708, 1973. Am. J. Surg., *123:*594, 1972

FUTRELL, J. W., AND MYERS, G. H., JR.: Burn scar as immunologically privileged site, PRS, *52:*326, 1973. Surg. Forum, *23:*129, 1972

FUTRELL, J. W. *et al*: Physiologic and immunologic considerations of the lymphatic system in tumors and transplants. Surg. Gynec. & Obst., *140:*273, 1975

FUTRELL, J. W., AND IZANT, R. J., JR.: Migrating cervical mass. PRS, *57:*660, 1976

FUXA, G. *et al*: Contribution to Ehlers-Danlos syndrome. Klin. Monatsbl. Augenheilkd., *166:*247, 1975 (German)

G

GABAIDULINA, E. IA. *et al*: Barraker-Simmons disease. Stomatologiia (Mosk.), *51:*86, 1972 (Russian)

GABBIANI, G. *et al*: Granulation tissue as a contractile organ. A study of structure and function. J. Exp. Med., *135:*719, 1972

GABKA, J.: Neoplasty of the ascending ramus of the mandible for compensation of microgenia. Fortschr. Kiefer. Gesichtschir., *18:*179, 1974 (German)

GABKA, J.: Is it possible to prevent the occurrence of cleft lip and cleft palate? Zahnaerztl. Mitt., *65:*762, 1975 (German)

GABKA, J. *et al*: Histological studies of the soft tissue covering of the premaxilla in bilateral cleft lip and palate. Dtsch. Zahn. Mund. Kieferheilkd., *55:*106, 1970 (German)

GABRIEL, A.: Use of unlined skin flaps in repair of full-thickness cheek loss. Ceylon Med. J., *19:*28, 1974

GADRE, K. C.: Modification in technique of closure of nostrils. J. Laryng. & Otol., *58:*903, 1973

GADZALY, D.: Thermic hand lesions. Dtsch. Med. J., *21:*1398, 1970 (German)

GAFFNEY, T. W., AND CAMPBELL, R. P.: Feeding techniques for dysphagic patients, PRS, *56:*114, 1975. Am. J. Nursing, *74:*2194, 1975

GAGNON, N. B. *et al*: Facial paralyses. Can. J. Otolaryngol., *1:*21, 1972

GAGNON, N. B. *et al*: Abnormalities of recovery of the facial nerve. Can. J. Otolaryngol., *4:*358, 1975 (French)

GAILLARD, A.: Anterior traction of mandible during parotidectomy. Rev. Stomatol. Chir. Maxillofac., *73:*579, 1972 (French)

GAILLARD, J. *et al*: Fractures of frontal sinus: therapeutic procedure. Ann. Otolaryngol. Chir. Cervicofac., *90:*741, 1973 (French)

GAILLARD, J. *et al*: Fibromatous type ossifying

cervical tumor. J. Fr. Otorhinolaryngol., *22:*533, 1973 (French)

GAILLARD, J. *et al*: Diagnosis and management of unilateral parotid tumours (explorative parotidectomy). J. Fr. Otorhinolaryngol., *23:*77, 1974 (French)

GAILLARD, J. *et al*: Idiopathic tumoral hypertrophy of the masseter muscle. J. Fr. Otorhinolaryngol., *23:*561, 1974 (French)

GAILLARD, J. *et al*: Melanic tumor of nasal septum, 5-year course. J. Fr. Otorhinolaryngol., *23:*884, 1974 (French)

GAILLARD, J. *et al*: Carcinoma of external auditory canal. Extended exeresis of canal before irradiation. J. Fr. Otorhinolaryngol., *24:*137, 1975 (French)

GAISFORD, J. C.: Major resection of scalp and skull for cancer with immediate complete reconstruction of 14 cases (Follow-Up Clinic). PRS, *48:*369, 1971

GAISFORD, J. C: Midline forehead flap nasal reconstructions in patients with low browlines (with Richardson, Hanna). PRS, *49:*130, 1972

GAISFORD, J. C., AND FLEEGLER, E. J.: Alterations in finger growth following flexor tendon injuries. PRS, *51:*164, 1973

GAISFORD, J. C., AND ANDERSON, V. S.: First branchial cleft cysts and sinuses. PRS, *55:*299, 1975

GAJDA, Z.: Surgery for harelip in 19th century Cracow surgical clinic. Przegl. Lek., *26:*627, 1970 (Polish)

GALANTI, S. *et al*: Rhinoplasty from its beginning to the 19th century. Clin. Otorinolaringoiatr., *22:*339, 1970 (Italian)

GALDSTON, R.: The burning and the healing of children. Psychiatry, *35:*57, 1972

GALIL-OGLY, G. A. *et al*: Serous acinocellular salivary gland tumors. Arkh. Patol., *35:*47, 1973 (Russian)

GALINSKI, A. W.: Avoiding postoperative pain in digital surgery. J. Am. Podiatry Assoc., *61:*23, 1971

GALINSKI, A. W.: Neurofibromatosis – Von Recklinghausen's disease in podiatric medicine; review and report of two cases. J. Am. Podiatry Assoc., *64:*87, 1974

GALLAGHER, A. G.: Complications of circumcision. Brit. J. Urol., *44:*720, 1972

GALLARDO, M. H.: Reconstruction of maxillary vestibular sulcus. Pre and retropyromidal sulcus. Rev. Esp. Estomatol., *21:*30, 1973 (Spanish)

GALLEGOS, L. T.: Mandibular vestibuloplasty with free graft of mucoperiosteal layer from hard palate (with Morgan, Frileck). PRS, *51:*359, 1973

GALLETTI, G., CARLONI, M., AND DE FRANCHIS,

G.: Cryo-biological tissue preservation: experimental model, PRS, 55:117, 1975. Europ. Surg. Res., 6:90, 1974

GALLO, D.: Ground cartilage autograft, PRS, 50:99, 1972. Med. Colombiana, 42:17, 1971

GALLO, W. J. et al: Modification of the sagittal ramus – split osteotomy for retrognathia. J. Oral Surg., 34:178, 1976

GALLOWAY, D. V.: Abdominal panniculectomy after massive weight loss (with Kamper, Ashley). PRS, 50:441, 1972

GALLOZZI, E., BLANCATO, L. S., AND STARK, R. B.: Deliberate hypotension for blepharoplasty and rhytidectomy (Follow-Up Clinic). PRS, 49:453, 1972

GALLUS, S., HIRSH, J., AND TUTTLE, R. J.: Small subcutaneous doses of heparin in prevention of venous thrombosis, PRS, 52:331, 1973. New England J. Med., 288:545, 1973

GALSFORD, J. C.: Palliative surgery. J.A.M.A., 221:83, 1972

GALUSTOV, G. N.: Experience with active surgical treatment of patients with burns. Ortop. Travmatol. Protez., 34:49, 1973 (Russian)

GAMALEJA, N. F. et al: Experience of skin tumours treatment with laser radiation. Panminerva Med., 16:41, 1974

GAMEZ-ARAUJO, J. J. et al: Central hemangioma of mandible and maxilla: review of vascular lesion. Oral Surg., 37:230, 1974

GAMBARDELLA, R. J.: Kaposi's sarcoma and its oral manifestations, PRS, 56:364, 1975. Oral Surg., 38:591, 1974

GANGE, R. J. et al: Septopremaxillary attachment and midfacial growth. Experimental study on the albino rat. Am. J. Orthod., 66:71, 1974

Ganglions

Ganglia of wrist, multifunctional mesenchymal cells resembling smooth muscle cells in (Ghadially, Mehta), PRS, 48:397, 1971. Ann. Rheumat. Dis., 30:31, 1971

Arthrographic studies of wrist ganglions (Andren, Eiken), PRS, 49:663, 1972. J. Bone & Joint Surg., 53:299, 1971

Cysts, synovial, of wrist, radiological exploration of (Farrera-Rojas), PRS, 53:367, 1974. Cir. Avances Acad. Mexicana, 274:1972

Ganglions of wrist and hand (Nelson, Sawmiller, Phalen), PRS, 51:478, 1973. J. Bone & Joint Surg., 54A:1459, 1972

Radial artery occlusion by carpal ganglion (Kelly). PRS, 52:191, 1973

Ganglion, dorsal distal interphalangeal joint: mucous cysts (Newmeyer, Kilgore, Graham), PRS, 53:313, 1974

GANGULI, A. G., AND ROY, R. N.: Surgical management of pressure sores in paraplegics, PRS, 50:636, 1972. Indian J. Surg., 33:73, 1971

GANS, BENJAMIN J.: *Atlas of Oral Surgery*. C. V. Mosby Co., St. Louis, 1972

GANTSCHEV, M.: Mechanical-thermal lesions on the dorsal surface of the hand. Beitr. Orthop. Traumatol., 20:678, 1973 (German)

GANTZER, J.: Facial mutilations on ceramics of the Mochica culture. Med. Welt., 23:137, 1972 (German)

GANZ, H.: Experiments on cryosurgery of tumors of great blood vessels in neck. Minerva Med., 65:3645, 1974

GANZ, H. et al: Histological examinations on the hemostatic effect of freezing during surgical procedures in the head and neck. Laryngol. Rhinol. Otol. (Stuttg.), 54:328, 1975 (German)

GANZONI, N.: Intensive care of patients with burns – investment, costs and clinical aspects. Helv. Chir. Acta, 39:607, 1972 (German)

GANZONI, N. et al: Selection of transplantation thickness in free skin transplants. Helv. Chir. Acta, 40:267, 1973 (German)

GANZONI, N. et al: The excision of burns. Helv. Chir. Acta, 41:221, 1974 (German)

GAPANOVICH, V. I. et al: Combined tracheotomy tube. Zh. Ushn. Nos. Gorl. Bolezn., 33:113, 1973 (Russian)

GARANTON, J. A., BENVENUTO, R., AND RODRIGUEZ DE LIMA, A.: Fractures of face, PRS, 55:377, 1975. Bol. Soc. Venezuelana Cir., 27:134, 1973

GARAS, J. et al: Superficial parotidectomy for adenocarcinoma in 12-year-old girl, PRS, 51:483, 1973. Acta chir. Hellenica, 44:586, 1972

GARAS, J. et al: Neoplasms of parotid gland. Review of 185 operated cases. Int. Surg., 58:178, 1973

GARAS, J. et al: Papillary cystadenoma lymphomatosum (Warthin's tumor). Analysis of 14 operated cases. Minerva Med., 66:1683, 1975 (Italian)

GARAS, J. et al: Papillary cystadenoma lymphomatosum (Warthin's tumor). Review of 14 operated cases. Panminerva Med., 17:78, 1975

GARCES PARDO, R.: General norms for the treatment of burns in children. Rev. Sanid. Hig. Publica (Madr.), 43:379, 1969 (Spanish)

GARCEZ, J., SARAIVA, S., AND BRAGA, A., JR.: Keloid scars, PRS, 53:248, 1974. Folha Med. Brazil, 66:57, 1973

GARCIA, F. A., AND BLANDFORD, S. E.: Use of the three-tailed fascial sling with pull-out wires to correct blepharoptosis (Follow-Up Clinic). PRS, *50:*281, 1972

GARCIA, J. L. *et al*: Free gingival transplantations. An. Esp. Odontoestomatol., *31:*77, 1972 (Spanish)

GARCIA, L. G.: Repair of cutaneous defects around natural orifices, PRS, *52:*603, 1973. Bol. Soc. Venezuelana Cir., *26:*351, 1972

GARCIA, L. G., AND RODRIGUEZ DE LIMA, A.: Ankyloglossia associated with muscular dystrophy of Landouzy-Dejerine, PRS, *48:*195, 1971. Bol. Soc. Venezuelana Cir., *24:*995, 1970

GARCIA, L. G., AND MOROS, J. N.: Classification of cleft lip and palate, PRS, *52:*598, 1973. Bol. Soc. Venezuelana Cir., *26:*136, 1972

GARCIA, R. L., AND DAVIS, C. M.: PABA, more effective sunscreen, PRS, *53:*114, 1974. Mil. Med., *138:*331, 1973

GARCIA-VELAZCO, J.: Treatment of keloid scars with fluocynolone acetonide, PRS, *50:*637, 1972. Invest. Clin. Mexico, *10:*161, 1971

GARCIA-VELAZCO, J.: Nasal reconstructions after resection of cutaneous tumors, PRS, *50:*536, 1972. Invest. Clin. Mexico, *10:*229, 1971

GARCIA-VELAZCO, J.: Thumb reconstruction using ring finger, PRS, *54:*109, 1974. Brit. J. Plast. Surg., *26:*406, 1973

GARCIA-VELAZCO, J.: Half nose reconstruction, PRS, *54:*234, 1974. Brit. J. Plast. Surg., *26:*412, 1973

GARCIA-VELAZCO, J., AND ARAICO, J. L.: Double blind study on effect of oral proteolytic enzymes in postsurgical hand inflammation, PRS, *50:*632, 1972. Arch. Int. Med. Mex., *3:*7, 1972

GARCIN, M. *et al*: Traumatic facial paralysis by damage of first portion. Total decompression of Fallopian aqueduct. Two successful cases. Rev. Otoneuroophtalmol., *44:*305, 1972 (French)

GARDNER, L. W., AND ACKER, D. W.: Bone destruction of distal phalanx, caused by periungual warts, PRS, *52:*452, 1973. Arch. Dermat., *107:*275, 1973

GARDNER, R. C.: Device for continuous elevation of upper extremity. PRS, *51:*471, 1973

GARGIULO, E. A. *et al*: Use of titanium mesh and autogenous bone marrow in repair of nonunited mandibular fracture: report of case and review of literature. J. Oral Surg., *31:*371, 1973

GARLIPP, O. F., AND NEDER, A. C.: Use of 1-phenyl-2-pyrrolidine-penthane in postoperative maxillofacial surgeries, PRS, *52:*331, 1973. A. Folha Med. Brazil, *64:*947, 1972

GARNIER, M. J.: Tetanus in patients three years of age and up. A personal series of 230

consecutive patients. Am. J. Surg., *129:*459, 1975

GARRETT, W. S., JR.: Dog bite avulsions of lip, conservative concept (with Musgrave). PRS, *49:*294, 1972

GARRETT, W. S., JR.: Nasal gliomas (with Kubo, Musgrave). PRS, *52:*47, 1973

GARRIDO GARCIA, H. *et al*: Functional importance of the collaterals of the deep femoral artery in cases of obstruction of its orifice. Angiologia, *27:*45, 1975 (Spanish)

GARRISON, FIELDING H.: *An Introduction to the History of Medicine*. Fourth Edition, 1929. Reprinted by W. B. Saunders, Philadelphia, 1960. PRS, *57:*510, 1976

GARRISON, R. L. *et al*: Multiple facial trauma complicated by occlusion of the internal carotid artery. J. Oral Surg., *33:*131, 1975

GARRIZ, R. A. *et al*: Surgery of incontinence, PRS, *53:*107, 1974. Prensa Med. Argent., *60:*492, 1973

GARST, R. J.: Prosthetics in leprosy. Lepr. Rev., *42:*60, 1971

GARSTKA, J.: Use of brachial plexus anesthesia in hand surgery. Chir. Narzadow. Ruchu Ortop. Pol., *37:*599, 1972 (Polish)

GARTMANN, H.: Therapy of malignant melanoma, PRS, *51:*235, 1973. Deutsche Med. Wchnschr., *97:*1305, 1972

GARTMANN, H., AND TRITSCH, H.: Significance of histological findings in the prognosis of malignant melanoma, PRS, *51:*608, 1973. Deutsche med. Wchnschr., *97:*857, 1972

GARVAR, L. R., AND KRINGSTEIN, G. J.: Recurrent parotitis in childhood, PRS, *55:*246, 1975. J. Oral Surg., *32:*373, 1974

Gas Gangrene

Anaerobic streptococcal infections simulating gas gangrene (Anderson, Marr, Jaffe), PRS, *50:*422, 1972. Arch. Surg., *104:*196, 1972

Clostridial infection of paranasal sinuses (Saberman *et al*). Trans. Am. Acad. Ophthalmol. Otolaryngol., *76:*1356, 1972

Clostridial myonecrosis of abdominal wall (Eng, Casson, Berman), PRS, *52:*601, 1973. Am. J. Surg., *125:*367, 1973

Changes in evaluation and therapy of gas edema through administration of hyperbaric oxygenation. Clinical comparative study on 31 cases of gas edema (Zierott *et al*). Bruns Beitr. Klin. Chir., *220:*292, 1973 (German)

Gas gangrene, hyperbaric oxygen in management of clostridial myonecrosis (Jackson *et al*). Clin. Orthop., *96:*271, 1973

Gas infection of thigh (Editorial). Ill. Med.

Gas Gangrene — Cont.
  J., *144:*131, 1973
  Gas gangrene in New South Wales (Unsworth). M. J. Australia, *1:*1077, 1973
  Gas gangrene (Deveridge *et al*). M. J. Australia, *1:*1106, 1973
  Gas gangrene (Weinstein *et al*). New England J. Med., *289:*1129, 1973
  Clostridia (Weston, Kukral), PRS, *53:*691, 1974. Rocky Mountain M.J., *70:*43, 1973
  Gas gangrene, modern therapeutic approach (Van Zyl). S. Afr. J. Surg., *11:*181, 1973 (Afrikaans)
  Comparative study of experimental Clostridium perfringens infection in dogs treated with antibiotics, surgery, and hyperbaric oxygen (Demello *et al*). Surgery, *73:*936, 1973
  Gas gangrene, experiences with (Lerut *et al*), PRS, *56:*234, 1975. Acta chir. belg., *73:*35, 1974
  Clostridial myonecrosis of abdominal wall. Management after extensive resection (Phillips *et al*). Am. J. Surg., *128:*436, 1974
  Gas gangrene in diabetic population, incidence and significance of (Kahn). Angiology, *25:*462, 1974
  Gas gangrene, 24 cases. Value of combined surgical and hyperbaric oxygen therapy (Larcan *et al*). Ann. Chir., *28:*445, 1974 (French)
  Gas gangrene. Apropos of 32 cases (Vic-Dupont *et al*). Ann. Med. Interne (Paris), *125:*469, 1974 (French)
  Gas gangrene, classification, diagnosis and treatment (Schmauss *et al*). Bruns Beitr. Klin. Chir., *221:*134, 1974 (German)
  Gas gangrene, classification, diagnosis and therapy of (Zierott). Bruns Beitr. Klin. Chir., *221:*140, 1974 (German)
  Myonecrosis, clostridial, treatment of, with hyperbaric oxygen (Hart *et al*). J. Trauma, *14:*712, 1974
  Advantages of combining surgery with hyperbaric oxygen therapy (Larcan *et al*). Mater. Med. Pol., *6:*116, 1974
  Diagnosis and therapy of gas phlegmon (Bahr *et al*). Med. Klin., *69:*859, 1974 (German)
  Therapy of gas gangrene. Comparison of results of the standard and hyperbaric oxygen therapy (Sailer *et al*). Med. Klin., *69:*1620, 1974 (German)
  Gas gangrene of scrotum and perineum (Himal *et al*). Surg. Gynec. & Obst., *139:*176, 1974
  Hyperbaric oxygenation therapy of anaerobic wound infection (literature survey) (Berkutov). Vestn. Khir., *113:*92, 1974 (Rus-

Gas Gangrene — Cont.
  sian)
  Gas gangrene following intramuscular injections (Schmauss). Z. Aerztl. Fortbild. (Jena), *68:*41, 1974 (German)
  Gangrene and gas phlegmons, plastic surgery in sequelae of (Maler), PRS, *57:*676, 1976. Bol. y trab. soc. argent. cir., *36:*216, 1975
  Gas producing infection caused by Bacteroides (Ragnhildstveit *et al*). Tidsskr. Nor. Laegeforen, *96:*240, 1976 (Norwegian)

GASLOROWSKA, E.: Methods and indications of surgical treatment of hands in rheumatoid arthritis in the light of our personal records. Reumatologia, *11:*97, 1973 (Polish)
GASPAR FUENTES, A. *et al*: Comments of Peutz-Jeghers syndrome (observations of three personal cases). Rev. Esp. Enferm. Apar. Dig., *43:*261, 1974 (Spanish)
GASPARD, D. J., COHEN, J. L., AND GASPAR, M. R.: Decompression dermotomy, PRS, *50:*538, 1972. J.A.M.A., *220:*831, 1972
GASPARD, D. J. *et al*: Compartmental syndromes in which the skin is the limiting boundary. Clin. Orthop., *113:*65, 1975
GASPARINI, F. *et al*: Growth anomaly of tongue, its relation to jaw anomalies and its surgical treatment. Riv. Ital. Stomatol., *26:*160, 1971 (Italian)
GASSLER, R.: Physical therapy of the hand with special reference to splints and braces. Handchirurgie, *4:*11, 1972 (German)
GASTPAR, H.: Cervical lymphoma: topography, diagnosis, therapy. Munch. Med. Wochenschr., *116:*447, 1974 (German)
GATES, G. A.: Diagnosis and treatment of parotid tumors. Texas Med., *69:*74, 1973
GATOFF, A. M. *et al*: Surgical and orthodontic management of unerupted maxillary permanent incisor, case report. J. Am. Dent. Assoc., *89:*897, 1974
GAUBERT, J. *et al*: Our experience with the surgical treatment of pectus excavatum. Arch. Fr. Pediatr., *29:*449, 1972 (French)
GAUDENZ, R.: Hypertrophic breast. Praxis, *65:*164, 1976 (German)
GAUTIER, J. *et al*: Obstructive complications of assisted ventilation using prolonged tracheal intubation or tracheotomy. Prevention and supervision using systematic laryngoscopy; 185 cases. Sem. Hop. Paris, *49:*2779, 1973 (French)
GAUWERKEY, F. *et al*: Radiotherapy of epipharyngeal neoplasms. Strahlentherapie, *146:*125, 1973 (German)

GAVILAN ALONSO, C. *et al*: Cervical lymph node functional-radical dissection. Surgical anatomy. Technic and results. Acta Otorinolaryngol. Iber. Am., *23:*703, 1972 (Spanish)

GAVRELL, G. J.: Congenital curvature of the penis. J. Urol., *112:*489, 1974

GAVRILOVA, K. M. *et al*: Changes in the soft tissue of the hands in chronic cold trauma — radiological and thermographical findings. Radiol. Diagn. (Berl.), *16:*285, 1975 (German)

GAWRONSKI, M. *et al*: Rhabdomyoma in trigone of carotid artery. Patol. Pol., *26:*287, 1975 (Polish)

GAY, B.: Tuberculous hygroma of the hand. Beitr. Orthop. Traumatol., *18:*596, 1971 (German)

GAY, B. *et al*: Reconstructive surgery of the hand following burns. Beitr. Orthop. Traumatol., *19:*391, 1972 (German)

GAY, I. *et al*: Ossifying fibroma; case report. J. Oral Surg., *33:*368, 1975

GAY, R.: Synovectomy of flexors and flexor ruptures. Rev. Chir. Orthop., *58:*414, 1972 (French)

GAY, R. *et al*: Digital tenosynovectomy of flexor tendons in rheumatic involvement of the hand. Acta Orthop. Belg., *37:*470, 1971 (French)

GAYLIS, H. *et al*: Ulnar artery aneurysms of the hand. Surgery, *73:*478, 1973

GEDOSH, E. A.: Nasopharyngeal fibroma (report of a case). J. Arkansas Med. Soc., *68:*410, 1972

GEE, W., McROBERTS, J., AND ANSELL, J.: Penile prosthetic implant for treatment of organic impotence, PRS, *54:*111, 1974. Am. J. Surg., *126:*698, 1973

GEE, W. F. *et al*: Impotent patient: surgical treatment with penile prosthesis and psychiatric evaluation, PRS, *54:*505, 1974. J. Urol., *111:*41, 1974

GEELHOED, G. W. *et al*: Pseudomonas meningitis complicating radical resection for radiorecurrent cancer of paranasal sinuses: report of two patients successfully treated with intrathecal polymyxin. J. Surg. Oncol., *5:*365, 1973

GEERING, A.: Problems of prosthetic treatment of the edentulous mandible, especially before and after total plastic surgery of the floor of the mouth and the vestibulum by means of free skin flaps. Schweiz. Monatsschr. Zahnheilkd., *82:*263, 1972 (German)

GEERTS, M. L. *et al*: Generalized melanosis due to malignant melanoma. Arch. Belg. Dermatol. Syphiligr., *28:*395, 1972

GEHRING, G. G., VITENSON, J. H., AND WOODHEAD, D. M.: Congenital urethral perineal fistulas, PRS, *53:*245, 1974. J. Urol., *109:*419, 1973

GEHRKE, C. F. *et al*: Coagulation defects in burned patients, PRS, *49:*359, 1972. Surg. Gynec. & Obst., *133:*613, 1971

GEINE, G. O.: Plastic surgery of nose. Vestn. Otorinolaringol., *35:*3, 1973 (Russian)

GEISENHAINER, U.: Basal cell carcinoma of the lips. Occurrence, localization, sex and age distribution. Hautarzt, *21:*167, 1970 (German)

GELB, J.: Formula for Bonney's Blue skin marking ink (Letter to the Editor), PRS, *52:*425, 1973

GELBERMAN, R. H. *et al*: High-pressure injection injuries of the hand. J. Bone & Joint Surg. (Am.), *57:*935, 1975

GELBKE, H.: Plastic and reconstructive surgery. Langenbecks Arch. Chir., *332:*117, 1972 (German)

GELDMACHER, J.: Acute open hand injuries. Dtsch. Med. J., *21:*1383, 1970 (German)

GELDMACHER, J.: Fractures of the hand region — avoidance of failures. Chirurg., *43:*111, 1972 (German)

GELDMACHER, J.: Complications in wound healing following open hand injuries, PRS, *53:*367, 1974. Langenbecks Arch. Chir., *332:*479, 1972

GELDMACHER, J.: Proceedings: Pyogenic infection of hand and fingers. Langenbecks Arch. Chir., *334:*491, 1973 (German)

GELDMACHER, J. *et al*: Industrial accidents and hand injuries. Munch. Med. Wochenschr., *115:*1211, 1973 (German)

GELFAND, D. W. *et al*: Thymic hyperplasia in children recovering from thermal burns, PRS, *52:*327, 1973. J. Trauma, *12:*813, 1972

GELFAND, G. *et al*: Central cavernous hemangioma of mandible. J. Oral Surg., *33:*448, 1975

GELIN, L. E.: Reaction of body as whole to injury, PRS, *48:*96, 1971. J. Trauma, *10:*932, 1971

GELINAS, M. *et al*: Incidence and causes of local failure of irradiation in squamous cell carcinoma of faucial arch, tonsillar fossa and base of tongue. Radiology, *108:*383, 1973

GELLER, A. N.: Treatment of purulent diseases of the fingers and hands. Vestn. Khir., *108:*76, 1972 (Russian)

GELLMAN, A., BELLINGHAM, C., AND MALAMENT, M.: New spiral-flap urethroplasty, PRS, *54:*110, 1974. J. Urol., *110:*546, 1973

GELOT, R. *et al*: Primary oat-cell carcinoma of head and neck. Ann. Otol. Rhin. & Laryng., *84:*238, 1975

GELSINON, T. *et al*: Correction of mandibular nonunion and gross malocclusion: report of case. J. Oral Surg., *32:*855, 1974

Genetics (See also *Cleft Palate, Genetics of*)

Genetic factor in malignant melanoma (Wallace, Exton, McLeod), PRS, *48*:609, 1971. Cancer, *27*:1262, 1971

Epileptic women, children of, congenital malformations in, cleft lip and palate in particular (Elshove, Van Eck), PRS, *49*:359, 1972. Nederl. tijdschr. geneesk., *115*:1371, 1971

Genetic counseling of clefts, empirical recurrence risk figures for (Tolarova), PRS, *52*:683, 1973. Acta chir. plast., *14*:234, 1972

Syndrome, orofacial-digital, 11th case in same family (Vissain, Vaillaud), PRS, *51*:605, 1973. Ann dermat. & syph., *99*:5, 1972

Familial osteodysplasia (Anderson *et al*), PRS, *50*:633, 1972. J.A.M.A., *220*:1687, 1972

Congenital chordee with and without hypospadias in three brothers (Koraitim), PRS, *52*:98, 1973. J. Urol., *108*:976, 1972

Malaysians, cleft lips in (Sivaloganathan), PRS, *49*:176, 1972

Orofacial-digital syndrome (Perez Fernandez, Quetglas), PRS, *53*:116, 1974. Rev. españ. cir. plast., *5*:153, 1972

Familial malignant melanoma (Wallace, Beardmore, Exton), PRS, *52*:215, 1973. Ann. Surg., *177*:15, 1973

Congenital aplasia of cutis in 3 successive generations (Fisher, Schneider), PRS, *57*:267, 1976. Arch. Dermat., *108*:252, 1973

Genetic factors in natural history of marine leukemia virus infection (Rowe), PRS, *54*:242, 1974. Cancer Res., *33*:3061, 1973

Choanal atresia, familial, in rhinoplasty candidate (Parkes, Brennan), PRS, *53*:240, 1974. Eye, Ear, Nose & Throat Month., *52*:222, 1973

Congenital defects: malformation syndromes in human genetic disease (Nyhan). PRS, *52*:237, 1973

Syndrome, Gardner's: report of family (Koren *et al*), PRS, *55*:115, 1975. Ann. Surg., *180*:198, 1974

Family size, influence of combination of sexes of children on (Gray, Morrison), PRS, *57*:542, 1976. J. Heredity, *65*:169, 1974

One genetic system, in cleft lip and cleft palate (Chabora, Horowitz), PRS, *56*:231, 1975. Oral Surg., *38*:181, 1974

Genetic counseling in inborn and developmental defects (Tolarova), PRS, *54*:629, 1974. Rozhl. chir., *53*:151, 1974

Anthropology in genetic counseling (Smahel), PRS, *54*:629, 1974. Rozhl. chir., *53*:159, 1974

Genetics — Cont.

Congenital scalp defects in 4 generations (Weippl, Ader), PRS, *56*:460, 1975. Klin. Paediatr., *187*:84, 1975

Johanson-Blizzard syndrome, absent nasal alae of, surgical correction of (Fox, Golden, Edgerton). PRS, *57*:484, 1976

Genetic considerations and surgical correction of frontonasal dysplasia with alar clefts in two sisters (Fox, Golden, Edgerton). PRS, *57*:553, 1976

Genitalia (See also *Bladder Exstrophy; Epispadias; Hypospadias; Penis; Scrotum; Transsexual Surgery; Urethra; Vagina*)

Anorchism: definition of a clinical entity (Glenn, McPherson), PRS, *48*:514, 1971. J. Urol., *105*:265, 1971

Genito-perineal region, reparative surgery of (Savani *et al*). Minerva Chir., *26*:1474, 1971 (Italian)

Elephantias of female genitalia (Khanna, Joshi), PRS, *48*:379, 1971

Testicular prosthesis of plastic material (Molnar, Furka), PRS, *51*:106, 1973. Andrologia, *4*:141, 1972

Emasculation, self (Mendez, Kiely, Morrow), PRS, *51*:603, 1973. J. Urol., *107*:981, 1972

Sarcoma, Kaposi's, of external genitalia, conservative treatment for (Summers, Wilkerson, Wegryn), PRS, *51*:704, 1973. J. Urol., *108*:287, 1972

Genital skin, management of severe inflammatory and traumatic injuries to (Hawtrey, Culp, Hartford), PRS, *51*:349, 1973. J. Urol., *108*:431, 1972

Testicular prosthesis: new insertion operation (Solomon), PRS, *51*:348, 1973. J. Urol., *108*:435, 1972

Genital anomaly, bilateral scrotal testicular ectopia (Mininberg, Richman), PRS, *52*:324, 1973. J. Urol., *108*:652, 1972

Trauma and repair of external genital organs in men (Orlich, Gurdian-Morales), PRS, *50*:307, 1972. Rev. Latino Am. cir. plast., *15*:45, 1972

Micturition, neurogenic disorders of, plastic operation on urinary bladder in (Savchenko, Mokhort), PRS, *54*:504, 1974. Acta chir. plast., *15*:223, 1973

Genital reconstruction in female with adrenogenital syndrome (Spence *et al*). Brit. J. Urol., *45*:126, 1973

Testicles, artificial, in children, new Silastic gel testicular prosthesis (Puranik, Mencia, Gilbert), PRS, *52*:595, 1973. J. Urol., *109*:735, 1973

Noonan's syndrome and cryptorchidism (Redman), PRS, *52*:596, 1973. J. Urol.,

Genetics—Cont.
    *109:*909, 1973
    Testicular prosthesis, natural-feeling (Latti-mer *et al*), PRS, *53:*245, 1974. J. Urol., *110:*81, 1973
    Surgical correction of incomplete penoscrotal transposition (Glenn, Anderson), PRS, *54:*238, 1974. J. Urol., *110:*603, 1973
    Condylomata acuminata, variable significance of (Fitzgerald, Hamit), PRS, *54:*504, 1974. Ann. Surg., *179:*328, 1974
    Anomalies of male genitalia (Culp), PRS, *55:*250, 1975. Hum. Sexuality, *8:*126, 1974
    Clitoroplasty: experience during 19-year period (Kumar *et al*), PRS, *54:*504, 1974. J. Urol., *111:*81, 1974
    Cloaca, persistent, repair of genital defects associated with (Ambrose), PRS, *54:*504, 1974 J. Urol., *111:*256, 1974
    Genitalia, external, reconstruction of, in exstrophy of bladder: preliminary communication (Allen). J. Urol., *111:*830, 1974
    Clitoris hypertrophy in sexual anomalies, surgical treatment of (Mussinelli, Musio), PRS, *57:*674, 1976. Riv. ital. chir. plast., *6:*171, 1974
    Psychological repercussions of genital operations (Saucier). Union Med. Can., *103:*1233, 1974 (French)
    Genitalia of male children, timing of elective surgery on undescended testes and hypospadias. (Kelalis *et al*), PRS, *57:*400, 1976. Pediatrics, *56:*479, 1975
    Sexual organs, disturbed development of, in children (Anders *et al*), PRS, *57:*399, 1976. Stafleu's Wtnsch. Uitgevers. B.V., *93:* Monograph, 1975
    Scrotum and penis, syphilitic elephantiasis of (Elsahy). PRS, *57:*601, 1976

GENOVESI, E.: Suggestion for reducing hemorrhage in operations on lacrimal sac. Ophthalmologica, *166:*399, 1973
GENSSLER, W.: Malignant solid tumors in childhood, diagnosis and therapy. Z. Aerztl. Fortbild. (Jena), *67:*1021, 1973 (German)
GEORGE, G. C. AND BEUMONT, P. J.: Transsexualism in fourteen-year-old male. S. Afr. Med. J., *46:*1947, 1972
GEORGE, P. T., CREECH, B. J., AND BUNCKE, H. J.: Rapid new technique for microvascular anastomosis (loop technique). PRS, *55:*99, 1975
GEORGIADE, N. G.: Improved technique for one-stage repair of bilateral cleft lip. PRS, *48:*318, 1971
GEORGIADE, N. G.: Management of acute midfacial-orbital injuries. Clin. Neurosurg., *19:*301, 1972

GEORGIADE, N. G.: Breast reconstruction. N.C. Med. J., *33:*524, 1972
GEORGIADE, N. G.: Permanent section on plastic and reconstructive surgery in the American Medical Association (Letter to the Editor). PRS, *51:*579, 1973
GEORGIADE, N. G.: Fourteen free groin flap transfers (with Serafin, Villarreal Rios), PRS, *57:*707, 1976
GEORGIADE, N. G., KING, E. H., AND O'FALLON, W. M.: Enzyme analysis as test of skin viability. PRS, *53:*67, 1974
GEORGIADE, N. G., AND HARRIS, W. A.: Open and closed treatment of burns with povidone-iodine, PRS, *52:*640, 1973. Discussion by Pruitt, PRS, *53:*82, 1974
GEORGIADE, N. G., AND LATHAM, R. A.: Maxillary arch alignment in bilateral cleft lip and palate infant using pinned coaxial screw appliance. PRS, *56:*52, 1975
GEORGIADE, N. G., AND HYLAND, W.: Technique for subcutaneous mastectomy and immediate reconstruction in ptotic breast. PRS, *56:*121, 1975
GEORGIADE, NICHOLAS, AND HAGERTY, ROBERT: *Symposium on Management of Cleft Lip and Palate and Associated Deformities*, Vol. 8. C. V. Mosby Co., St. Louis, 1975. PRS, *56:*333, 1975
GEORGIADES, G. *et al*: Naso-orbito-ocular mucormycosis, apropos of a typical case. Ann. Ocul. (Paris), *205:*721, 1972 (French)
GEORGIADIS, N., AND KATSAS, A.: Topography of fat in sacroiliac region, PRS, *49:*110, 1972. Acta Chir. Hellenica, *18:*289, 1971
GEORGIEVA, E.: Glossodynia and its treatment. Vutr. Boles., *10:*63, 1971 (Bulgarian)
GER, R.: Operative treatment of advanced stasis ulcer using muscle transposition. Follow-up study, PRS, *49:*358, 1972. Am. J. Surg., *120:*376, 1970
GER, R.: Surgical management of decubitus ulcers by muscle transposition, PRS, *48:*298, 1971. Surgery, *69:*106, 1971
GER, R.: Surgical management of ulcerative lesions of the leg. Curr. Probl. Surg., *1:*52, 1972
GER, R.: Chronic ulceration of leg. Surg. Annu., *4:*123, 1972
GER, R.: Surgical management of ulcers of heel. Surg. Gynec. & Obst., *140:*909, 1975
GER, R. *et al*: Muscle transposition in deep localized burns. Arch. Surg., *104:*710, 1972
GERA, I.: Current views on periodontal surgery. I. Surgery of periodontal soft tissues. Fogorv. Sz., *68:*225, 1975 (Hungarian)
GERASHCHENKO, I. F. *et al*: Preliminary report. Alloplastic repair of bone defects in nose and anterior wall of frontal air sinus on primary

surgery of gunshot and other wounds (experimental study). Acta Chir. Plast. (Praha), *14:*166, 1972

GERHARD, U.: Surgical therapy of radiation-induced ulcer. Allgemeinmed., *49:*1699, 1973 (German)

GERMAN, J. C. *et al:* Porcine xenograft burn dressings, PRS, *50:*634, 1972. Arch. Surg., *104:*806, 1972

GERMAN, J. C., ALLYN, P. A., AND BARTLETT, R. H.: Pulmonary artery pressure monitoring in acute burn management, PRS, *53:*370, 1974. Arch. Surg., *106:*788, 1973

GERNER, R., JUDD, L., AND MANDELL, A.: Male transsexualism, PRS, *55:*259, 1975. West. J. Med., *120:*376, 1974

GERNER, R. E., AND MOORE, G. E.: Burn scar carcinoma and hypercalcemia, PRS, *55:*113, 1975. Erratum, PRS, *56:*241, 1975. Ann. Surg., *180:*95, 1974

GERNER, R. E. *et al:* Soft tissue sarcomas, PRS, *57:*404,1976. Ann. Surg., *181:*803, 1975

GEROULANOS, S. *et al:* Simplified operation for correction of funnel chest. Indications and surgery. Dtsch. Med. Wochenschr., *99:*57, 1974 (German)

GEROULANOS, S. *et al:* Funnel chest correction: indication, surgical procedure and results of a simplified and modified method. Helv. Chir. Acta, *41:*101, 1974 (German)

GEROULIS, A. J. *et al:* Internal maxillary artery ligation for posterior epistaxis. Surg. Forum, *26:*531, 1975

GEROW, F. J.: Modified Bonnacolto dacryocystorhinostomy (with Spira, Hardy), PRS, *52:*511, 1973

GEROW, F. J.: Complications of chemical face peeling (with Spira, Hardy), PRS, *54:*397, 1974

GEROW, F. J. *et al:* Fluid debridement of the burn wound. J. Trauma, *11:*1021, 1971

GEROW, F. J. *et al:* Plastic surgery application of synthetic implants. Med. Instrum., *7:*96, 1973

GEROW, F. J., SPIRA, M., AND HARDY, S. B.: Simplified design for reduction mammaplasty, PRS, *53:*271, 1974

GERSHEN, H. J.: Treatment of obstruction of the common canaliculus. Arch. Ophth., *88:*87, 1972

GERSHEN, H. J.: Modification of blepharoptosis clamp. Am. J. Ophth., *76:*589, 1973

GERSHEN, H. J.: Modification of approach to orbital fracture. Ann. Ophth., *5:*1123, 1973

GERSHKOVICH, S. M.: Primary closure of fresh injuries of the hand caught in rollers. Ortop. Travmatol. Protez., *7:*54, 1974 (Russian)

GERSHON, R. K.: Role of BCG vaccination in producing tumor immunity (with Ariyan).

PRS, *56:*430, 1975

GERTH, B.: Late results in synthetic nose chip implants. Z. Aerztl. Fortbild. (Jena), *67:*880, 1973 (German)

GERVAIS, C.: Plastic surgery of nose. Rev. Infirm., *23:*715, 1973

GET'MAN, I. I.: Case of congenital supernumerary nostril. Zh. Ushn. Nos. Gori. Bolezn., *33:*88, 1973 (Russian)

GETTER, L. *et al:* Biodegradable intraosseous appliance in the treatment of mandibular fractures. J. Oral Surg., *30:*344, 1972

GEVORKIAN, I. K.: Late effects of synthetic products used in surgery. Zh. Eksp. Klin. Med., *14:*35, 1974 (Russian)

GHADIALLY, F. N., AND MEHTA, P. N.: Multifunctional mesenchymal cells resembling smooth muscle cells in ganglia of wrist, PRS, *48:*397, 1971. Ann. Rheumat. Dis., *30:*31, 1971

GHALIOUNGI, P., AND EL-DAWAKHLY, Z.: Hesy or Hesy-re, PRS, *52:*603, 1973. Lebanese M. J., *25:*4, 1972

GHNASSIA, M. D. *et al:* Indications and limitation of ketamine anesthesia in plastic surgery. Ann. chir. plast., *17:*58, 1972 (French)

GHOSH, B. C. *et al:* Malignant schwannoma—clinicopathological study, PRS, *51:*708, 1973. Cancer, *31:*184, 1973

GHOSH, B. C. *et al:* Myxoma of jaw bones, PRS, *51:*707, 1973. Cancer, *31:*237, 1973

GHOSH, P.: Treatment of double nose. J. Laryng. & Otol., *87:*593, 1973

GHOSH, P. *et al:* An approach to palatopharyngeal incompetence. J. Laryng. & Otol., *86:*709, 1972

GIACOMELLI, V.: Concept of radical surgery of cancer. Tumori, *60:*445, 1974 (Italian)

GIACOMELLI, V.: Significance and methods of surgical treatment of lymphatic spread. Tumori, *60:*567, 1974 (Italian)

GIANASI, G. C. *et al:* Tracheotomy in resuscitation. Minerva Anestesiol., *39:*194, 1973 (Italian)

GIANNI, E.: Histopathological and prognostic considerations in 14 mixed tumors of salivary glands. Minerva Stomatol., *21:*173, 1972 (Italian)

GIANNOULOPOULOS, A. C.: Three cases of bone graft transplantation in mandible. Stomatologia (Athenai), *29:*427, 1972 (Greek)

GIARDINO, C. *et al:* Bone transplants in maxillofacial surgery. Arch. Stomatol. (Napoli), *11:*151, 1970 (Italian)

GIARELLI, L. *et al:* Heteroptic gastric mucosa in the tongue. Dtsch. Zahnaerztl. Z., *30:*823, 1975 (German)

GIBBS, J. R.: Letter: treatment of excessive axillary sweating. Lancet, *2:*654, 1974

GIBBS, R. C.: Keratosis of the palms and soles. J. Am. Podiatry Assoc., 60:423, 1970

GIBBS, S. L.: Dental aspects of surgical orthodontics. N.Y. State J. Med., 72:233, 1972

GIBRAIEL, E. A.: Open skin grafting in developing countries. Brit. J. Surg., 60:25, 1973

GIBSON, H. L.: Medical Photography. Eastman Kodak Co., Rochester, N. Y., 1973. PRS, 54:602, 1974

GIBSON, R. et al: Tracheotomy in neonates. Laryngoscope, 82:643, 1972

GIBSON, T.: Stratified squamous skin. Brit. J. Plast. Surg., 25:1, 1972

GIFFORD, G. H., JR.: Replantation of severed part of ear (Letter to the Editor). PRS, 49:202, 1972

GIFFORD, G. H., JR., AND MacCOLLUM, D. W.: Facial teratoma in newborn. Report of 5 cases. PRS, 49:616, 1972

GIFFORD, G. H., JR., SWANSON, L., AND MacCOLLUM, D. W.: Congenital absence of nose and anterior nasopharynx. PRS, 50:5, 1972

GIGNOUX, B. et al: Case of cystic lymphangioma of neck. J. Fr. Otorhinolaryngol., 21:519, 1972

GIGNOUX, M. et al: Value of the myotomy for the management of a cervical esophageal diverticulum. Ann. Chir., 29:847, 1975 (French)

GIGOVSKII, E. E.: 220 cases of surgery for the formation of an artificial vagina from the sigmoid intestine. Akush. Ginekol. (Mosk.), 45:64, 1969 (Russian)

GIGUERE, P.: Prognathism: surgical treatment. Can. J. Otolaryngol., 4:679, 1975 (French)

GILADI, A.: Use of water-insoluble papain (WIP) for debridement of burn eschar and necrotic tissue (with Shapira, Neuman). PRS, 52:279, 1973

GILADI, A. et al: Wide use of skin allografts. Harefuah, 80:594, 1971 (Hebrew)

GILBERT, A.: Vascular microsurgery. Ann. Chir., 29:1035, 1975 (French)

GILBERT, A. et al: Transfer to the hand of a sensitive free graft. Chirurgie, 101:691, 1975

GILBERT, H., AND KAGAN, R. A.: Recurrence patterns in squamous cell carcinoma of oral cavity, pharynx, and larynx, PRS, 56:363, 1975. J. Surg. Oncol., 6:357, 1974

GILBERT, H. D. et al: Congenital upper eyelid eversion and Down's syndrome. Am. J. Ophth., 75:469, 1973

GILBERTSEN, V. A., BEAN, S. F., AND FUSARO, R. M.: Palmar keratoses and visceral cancer, PRS, 50:205, 1972. Arch. Dermat., 105:222, 1972

GILCHREST, B.: Skin pigmentation, current concepts and relevance to plastic surgery (with Morgan, Goldwyn). PRS, 56:617, 1975

GILCHRIST, A. G.: Surgery of the nasal septum

and pyramid. J. Laryng. & Otol., 88:759, 1974

GILCHRIST, A. K.: Fatty type tumors of the foot – a report of two cases. J. Am. Podiatry Assoc., 65:142, 1975

GILDEN, D. H. et al: Central nervous system histoplasmosis after rhinoplasty. Neurology (Minneap.), 24:874, 1974

GILES, H. V.: Self-retaining retractor for buccal commissure. PRS, 49:230, 1972

GILIAZUMDINOVA, Z. S. et al: Reinnervation of mucous membrane of an artificial vagina. Akush. Ginekol. (Mosk.), 47:49, 1971 (Russian)

GILKES, J. J. H., AND BORRIE, P. F.: Morphoic basal cell carcinoma with invasion of orbit, PRS, 55:385, 1975. Proc. Roy. Soc. Med., 67:437, 1974

GILL, S. A.: Nursing the plastic surgery patient. A.O.R.N., 18:505, 1973

GILL, W., AND LONG, W. B.: Critical look at cryosurgery, PRS, 50:100, 1972. Internat. Surg., 56:344, 1971

GILL, W., LONG, W. B., AND MacLENNAN, W. D.: Hemangioma of mandible. J. Roy. Coll. Surg. Edinb., 18:52, 1973

GILLE, Y. D. et al: Nasotracheal intubation in maxillofacial surgery using bronchofibroscopy. Anesth. Analg. (Paris), 31:551, 1974 (French)

GILLETTE, W. B.: Effect of postmortem tissue fixation on tooth mobility and pocket depth in human beings. Oral Surg., 39:130, 1975

GILLISSEN, G.: Adhesion of homotransplants under treatment with histones. Langenbecks Arch. Chir., 327:278, 1970 (German)

GILSTON, A.: Prevention of ulceration during use of cuffed tracheostomy tube. Lancet, 1:1074, 1972

GIL-VERNET, J. M. et al: New surgical technique for balanitic hypospadias correction. J. Urol., 112:673, 1974

GIMENEZ, E. J.: Subtotal transbuccal osteotomy of face. Int. J. Orthod., 10:93, 1972

GIMENEZ, E. J.: Surgery of the smile. II. Rev. Assoc. Odontol. Argent., 60:59, 1972 (Spanish)

GIMENEZ, E. J.: Surgery for open bite, case report. Rev. Assoc. Odontol. Argent., 60:485, 1972

GIMENEZ, E. J.: Osteotomy of malar bone. Rev. Assoc. Odontol. Argent., 61:302, 1973 (Spanish)

GIMENEZ, E. et al: Transbuccal sagittal osteotomy of mandibular ascending ramus. Rev. Assoc. Odontol. Argent., 62:14, 1973 (Spanish)

GIMILLIO, G. G.: Treatment of hand injuries. Praxis, 62:385, 1973 (French)

Gingival Neoplasms (See also *Jaw Neoplasms; Mouth Neoplasms*)

Gingiva, cancers of, role of surgery in Fondation Curie (Durand *et al*). J. Radiol. Electrol. Med. Nucl., *53:*481, 1972 (French)

Gingival grafts (Lucchini). Actual Odontostomatol. (Paris), *27:*299, 1973

Multiple recurrent fibro-osseous epulides (Hayward). Int. J. Oral Surg., *2:*115, 1973

Gingival odontogenic epithelial hamartoma: case report (Baden *et al*). J. Oral Surg., *31:*932, 1973

Cancer of floor of mouth and gingiva (Landa *et al*). Surg. Clin.North Am., *53:*135, 1973

Gingival fibromatosis, idiopathic. Survey of literature and report of five cases (Winther *et al*). Tandlaegebladet, *77:*313, 1973 (Danish)

Place of surgery in the treatment of carcinomas of the oral cavity (Mendes da Costa *et al*). Acta chir. belg., *73:*529, 1974 (French)

Unusual presentation of rhabdomyosarcoma: a case report (Cove). Brit. J. Oral Surg., *12:*240, 1974

Pigmented neuroectodermal tumor of infancy: report of two cases (Ostrander *et al*). J. Oral Surg., *32:*626, 1974

Gingival graft, free, clinical assessment of use of, for correcting localized recession associated with frenal pull (Ward). J. Periodontol., *45:*78,1974

Papillary cystadenoma of ectopic minor salivary gland origin (Wilson *et al*). Oral Surg., *37:*915, 1974

Carcinoma, basal cell, and peripheral ameloblastoma (Simpson). Oral Surg., *38:*233, 1974

Gingiva, metastasis to (Perlmutter *et al*), PRS, *56:*364, 1975. Oral Surg., *38:*749, 1974

Treatment by excision and graft of split thickness skin in recurrent verrucous papillary carcinoma (Mayer *et al*). Rev. Stomatol. Chir. Maxillofac., *75:*98, 1974 (French)

Squamous cell carcinoma of the gingiva. Histological classification and grading of malignancy (Willen *et al*). Acta Otolaryngol. (Stockh.), *79:*146, 1975

Cancer of the mouth floor and gingiva (Guerrero Palacios). An. Esp. Odontoestomatol., *34:*421, 1975 (Spanish)

Primary malignant hemangioendothelioma of the gingiva. Report of a case and review of the literature (Wesley *et al*). Oral Surg., *39:*103, 1975

GINGOLD, N. *et al*: Problems of diagnosis in certain adenomegalies. Therapeutic implications. Rev. Roum. Med. Intern., *10:*295, 1973

(French)

GINGRASS, P., GRABB, W. C. AND GINGRASS, R. P.: Skin graft survival on avascular defects, PRS, *55:*65, 1975

GINGRASS, R. P.: Experimental funicular grafting of facial nerve (with Apfelberg), PRS, *55:*195, 1975

GINGRASS, R. P. *et al*: Complications with deltopectoral flap, PRS, *49:*501, 1972

GINGRASS, R. P., CUNNINGHAM, D. S., AND PALETTA, F. X.: Skin grafting of exposed arterial vein grafts: clinical and experimental study, PRS, *53:*689, 1974. J. Trauma, *13:*951, 1973

GIPSON, M.: Squamous cell carcinoma in epidermolysis bullosa dystrophica, PRS, *57:*760, 1976. Hand, *7:*179, 1975

GIPSON, M. *et al*: Incidence of schizophrenia and severe psychological disorders in patients 10 years after cosmetic rhinoplasty. Brit. J. Plast. Surg., *28:*155, 1975

GIRADET, R. E.: Technic of tracheostomy in adult. Am. J. Surg., *125:*372, 1973

GIRALT PRAT, P. M. *et al*: Technics of anesthesia and resuscitation in severely burned patients. Rev. Esp. Anestesiol. Reanim., *21:*539, 1974 (Spanish)

GIRAUD, F. *et al*: Holt-Oram syndrome (apropos of a familial case concerning 5 generations). Arch. Fr. Pediatr., *31:*765, 1974 (French)

GIRAUD, R. M. A., RIPPEY, J. J., AND RIPPEY, E.: Malignant melanoma of skin in black Africans, PRS, *57:*124, 1976. South African M. J., *49:*665, 1975

GIRGIS, I. H. *et al*: Method for assessment of nasal circulation, PRS, *56:*592, 1975. J. Laryng. & Otol., *88:*1149, 1974

GIRGIS, I. H. *et al*: Nasal circulation in certain pathological conditions, PRS, *56:*592, 1975. J. Laryng. & Otol., *88:*1159, 1974

GIRGIS, I. H. *et al*: Estimation of effect of drugs on nasal circulation, PRS, *56:*592, 1975. J. Laryng. & Otol., *88:*1163, 1974

GITTES, R. F. *et al*: Injection technique to induce penile erection. Urology, *4:*473, 1974

GLAHN, M.: Treatment of multiple facial traumata in Denmark. Ugeskr. Laeger, *133:*2241, 1971 (Danish)

GLAHN, M.: Surgical treatment of chronic osteomyelitis of mandible, PRS, *55:*717, 1975. J. Maxillo-facial Surg., *2:*238, 1974

GLANVILLE, H.: Future of powered hand prostheses. Hand, *3:*20, 1971

GLASER, A.: Salivary gland tumors—synopsis of 692 cases. Z. Aerztl. Fortbild. (Jena), *67:*915, 1973 (German)

GLASER, A. *et al*: Acinar cell tumors of salivary glands of head. Stomatol. D.D.R., *24:*110, 1974 (German)

GLASER, M. *et al*: Inhibitory effect of alpha-globulin on the second set allograft reaction. Proc. Soc. Exper. Biol. Med., *140:*996, 1972

GLASER, P., RADOMAN, V., AND CANONNE, O.: Prospective study of complications of subclavian vein catheterization, PRS, *53:*606, 1974. Ann. Chir., *27:*911, 1973

GLASGOLD, A. *et al*: Radical approach to advanced carcinoma of the head and neck by multi-disciplined team. J. Med. Soc. N. J., *72:*701, 1975

GLASS, A. J.: Midfacial fractures in a patient with cleft palate: report of case. J. Oral Surg., *30:*357, 1972

GLASS, R., AND PEREZ-MESA, C.: Management of inadequately excised epidermoid carcinoma, PRS, *54:*246, 1974. Arch. Surg., *108:*50, 1974

GLASS, T. G., JR.: Early debridement in pit viper bite. Surg. Gynec. & Obst., *136:*774, 1973

GLAUMANN, B. *et al*: Surgical treatment of pressure sores – study of results. Lakartidningen, *71:*493, 1974 (Swedish)

GLAZER, R. I. *et al*: Viral hepatitis: hazard to oral surgeons. J. Oral Surg., *31:*504, 1973

GLEASON, M. C.: Brow lifting through temporal scalp approach, PRS, *52:*141, 1973

GLENN, J.: Snakebitten hand (with Snyder, Straight), PRS, *49:*275, 1972

GLENN, J., AND ANDERSON, E.: Surgical correction of incomplete penoscrotal transposition, PRS, *54:*238, 1974. J. Urol., *110:*603, 1973

GLENN, J. F., AND MCPHERSON, A. T.: Anorchism: definition of clinical entity, PRS, *48:*514, 1971. J. Urol., *105:*265, 1971

GLICENSTEIN, J.: Net grafts in leg ulcers. Angieologie, *23:*151, 1971 (French)

GLICENSTEIN, J.: Difficulties of surgical treatment of abdominal dermodystrophies. Ann. chir. plast., *20:*147, 1975 (French)

GLICENSTEIN, J., PENNECOT, G. F., AND DUHAMEL, B.: Poland's syndrome, PRS, *54:*630, 1974. Ann. chir. plast., *19:*41, 1974

GLICENSTEIN, J. *et al*: Three-pronged plasty. Ann. chir. plast., *220:*257, 1975 (French)

GLINZ, W.: Measurement of pH in transplantation of skin autografts, PRS, *48:*518, 1971. Med. & Hygiene, *955:*437, 1971

GLINZ, W., AND CLODIUS, L.: Measurement of tissue pH for predicting viability in pedicle flaps: experimental studies in pigs, PRS, *52:*216, 1973. Brit. J. Plast. Surg., *25:*111, 1972

GLOBEVA, I. V. *et al*: Colpopoiesis operations in testicular forms of hermaphroditism, Probl. Endokrinol. (Mosk.), *19:*44, 1973 (Russian)

GLOGOFF, M. *et al*: Vestibular preparation for dentures. J. Mercer. Dent. Soc., *27:*14, 1973

Glomus Tumors

Multiple glomus tumours (Hollins). Proc. Roy. Soc. Med., *64:*806, 1971

Glomus tumor, multifocal, case report and review of literature (Hollingsworth, Ochsner), PRS, *51:*707, 1973. Am. Surgeon, *38:*161, 1972

Glomus tumors of hand (Carroll, Berman), PRS, *51:*104, 1973. J. Bone & Joint Surg., *54A:*691, 1972

Glomus tumors, subcutaneous (Anagnostou, Papademetrious, Toumazani), PRS, *52:*599, 1973. Surg. Gynec. & Obst., *136:*945, 1973

Tumor, glomus, invisible (Sibulkin, Healey), PRS, *55:*115, 1975. Arch. Surg., *109:*111, 1974

Glomus, nasal (Enfores, Herngren), PRS, *57:*670, 1976. J. Laryng. & Otol., *89:*863, 1975

Glomus tumors, bilateral subungual (Maley, MacDonald), PRS, *55:*488, 1975

GLOOBE, H.: Fibrotic arch around the deep branch of the ulnar nerve in the hand (with Lotem, Nathan), PRS, *52:*553, 1973. Discussion by Weeks, PRS, *52:*556, 1973

GLOOBE, H., AND LIBERTY, S.: Bilateral agenesis of *extensor carpi ulnaris*, PRS, *54:*376, 1974. Hand, *5:*175, 1973

GLOOR, M.: Secondary damage to hair follicles in full thickness skin autografts. Arch. Dermatol. Forsch., *249:*277, 1974

GLOOR, M. *et al*: Experimental studies on the blood supply of autologous, free full-skin transplants in the postoperative phase in man. Med. Welt., *21:*967, 1970 (German)

GLOOR, M. *et al*: Architecture of the epidermis in free autologous skin transplants on the human sole. Dermatol. Monatsschr., *157:*812, 1971 (German)

GLOOR, M. *et al*: Significance of the duration of pressure bandage for the result of autologous, free, full-skin transplantation. Experimental studies in guinea pigs. Dermatol. Monatsschr., *158:*190, 1972 (German)

GLOOR, M. *et al*: Revascularization of free full thickness skin autografts. Arch. Dermatol. Forsch., *246:*211, 1973

GLOOR, M. *et al*: Repair of skin defects with autologous skin homogenisate and wound contraction. Z. Hautkr., *48:*755, 1973

Glossectomy

Considerable incisor gaping treated by partial glossectomy (Lacour *et al*). Bull. Soc. Med. Afr. Noire Lang. Fr., *15:*332, 1970 (French)

Glossectomy — Cont.

Glossectomy rehabilitation by mandibular tongue prosthesis (Moore), PRS, *52:*332, 1973. J. Prosth. Dent., *28:*429, 1972

Changes in phonatory aspects of glossectomee intelligibility through vocal parameter manipulation (Skelly *et al*). J. Speech Hear. Disord., *37:*379, 1972

Role of total glossectomy in the management of cancer of the oral cavity (Myers). Otolaryngol. Clin. North Am., *5:*343, 1972

Glossectomy, partial discontinuous, and radical neck dissection for carcinoma of tongue (Spiro, Strong), PRS, *53:*602, 1974. Am. J. Surg., *126:*544, 1973

Glossectomy, total, for advanced carcinoma of base of tongue (Sessions *et al*). Laryngoscope, *83:*39, 1973

Glossectomy, total, use of pterygoid muscle sling to provide glossomimic function after (Washio). PRS, *51:*497, 1973

Glossectomy in mandibular prognathism (Pereira). Rev. Assoc. Paul. Cir. Dent., *27:*349, 1973 (Portuguese)

"Don't wave good-bye" (Daly). Am. J. Nurs., *74:*1641, 1974

Glossectomy, radical total (Kothary *et al*). Brit. J. Surg., *61:*209, 1974

Pretherapy speech intelligibility of a glossectomee (Riviere *et al*). J. Commun. Disord., *7:*357, 1974

Evaluation and rehabilitation of glossectomy speech behavior (Amerman *et al*). J. Commun. Disord., *7:*365, 1974

Glossectomy, total, and repair with amniotic membrane (Kothary). J. Indian Med. Assoc., *62:*87, 1974

E. N. T. case of the month (Miglets). Ohio State Med. J., *70:*37, 1974

Postoperative bronchopulmonary complications in malignant neoplasms of maxillofacial localization (Dunaevskii *et al*). Vestn. Khir., *113:*69, 1974

Report on the speech intelligibility of a glossectomee: perceptual and acoustic observations (LaRiviere *et al*). Folia Phoniatr. (Basel), *27:*201, 1975

Leiomyosarcoma of the head and neck: a review of the literature and report of two cases (Mindell *et al*). Laryngoscope, *85:*904, 1975

Swallowing and speech after radical total glossectomy with tongue prosthesis (De Souza *et al*). Oral Surg., *39:*356, 1975

Glossodynia: See *Tongue*

GLOVER, J. L.: Plasma scalpel excision of burns, PRS, *55:*657, 1975

GLUCKER, E., HIRSHOWITZ, B., AND GELLEI, B.:

Leiomyosarcoma of glans penis, PRS, *50:*406, 1972

GLUPE, J. *et al*: Combined cytostatic and irradiation treatment of head and neck tumors using the synchronization effect. H. N. O., *20:*18, 1972 (German)

GLYNN, P. J.: Use of surgery and local temperature elevation in myobacterium ulcerans infection. Aust. N.Z. J. Surg., *41:*312, 1972

GNANAPRAGASAM, A.: Fatal hemorrhage from the innominate artery complicating tracheostomy. J. Laryng. & Otol., *89:*853, 1975

GO, M. J. *et al*: Formation of metastases of basal cell epithelioma "basal cell carcinoma." Hautarzt, *24:*449, 1973 (German)

GOB, A.: Treatment of spastic thumbs in palm deformity. Reconstr. Surg. Traumatol., *13:*51, 1972

GODEAU, P. *et al*: Disseminated actinomycosis with cutaneous and osseous foci. Ann. Med. Interne (Paris), *122:*1129, 1971 (French)

GODUNOVA, G. S.: Operative treatment of congenital split hand. Ortop. Travmatol. Protez., *34:*47, 1973 (Russian)

GOEBEL, M. *et al*: Mechanical dermabrasion using a high-frequency polishing device. Hautarzt, *25:*570, 1974 (German)

GOEL, T. C., AND MISRA, S. C.: Omental transposition in treatment of tropical elephantiasis of lower limb, PRS, *53:*488, 1974. Indian J. Surg., *35:*381, 1973

GOEPFERT, H., JESSE, R. H., AND LINDBERG, R. D.: Arterial infusion and radiation therapy in treatment of advanced cancer of nasal cavity and paranasal sinuses, PRS, *53:*602, 1974. Am. J. Surg., *126:*464, 1973

GOEPFERT, H. *et al*: Squamous cell carcinoma of nasal vestibule. Arch. Otolaryng., *100:*8, 1974

GOEPFERT, H. *et al*: Cancer of the skin of the nose. Treatment by total skin excision and three-quarter thickness skin graft. Arch. Otolaryng., *102:*90, 1976

GOERTZ, E.: Exophytic bowenoid squamous cell carcinoma. Z. Hautkr., *50:*798, 1975 (German)

GOETE, D. K.: Erythroplasia of Queyrat treated with topically administered fluorouracil, PRS, *56:*680, 1975. Arch. Dermat., *110:*271, 1974

GOETTE, D. K., AND HELWIG, E. B.: Basal cell carcinomas and basal cell carcinoma-like changes overlying dermatofibromas, PRS, *57:*540, 1976. Arch. Dermat., *111:*589, 1975

GOFFINET, D. R. *et al*: Irradiation of clinically uninvolved cervical lymph nodes. Can. J. Otolaryngol., *4:*927, 1975

GOGAS, J. *et al*: Actinomycosis of the breast. Int. Surg., *57:*664, 1972

GOGAS, J., AND SKALKEAS, G.: Prognosis of mammary carcinoma in young women, PRS, 57:533, 1976. Surgery, 78:339, 1975

GOH, Y. S. et al: Failure of hand growth after x-ray therapy. Singapore Med. J., 14:19, 1973

GOHRBRANDT, E., GABKA, J., AND BERNDORFER, A.: Handbuch der Plastischen Chirurgie. Volume II, Chapters 21 and 22. Walter de Gruyter & Co., Berlin, 1973. PRS, 54:93, 1974

GOIN, J. M.: Silicone for facial furrows. J.A.M.A., 229:1581, 1974

GOIN, J. M.: On showing photographs preoperatively to patients (Letter to the Editor), PRS, 54:90, 1974

GOLA, R. et al: Use of tongue flaps in the treatment of sequelae of cleft lip and palate. Rev. Stomatol. Chir. Maxillofac., 74:626, 1973 (French)

GOLD, B. D. et al: Dermoid, epidermoid and teratomatous cysts of tongue and floor of mouth. J. Oral Surg., 32:107, 1974

GOLD, R. et al: Correction of dento-alveolar deformity by anterior alveolar osteotomy, case report. Bull. Monmouth Ocean Cty. Dent. Soc., 31:16, 1973

GOLDAN, S.: Bi-hinged chest-arm flap for lymphedema of upper limb (with Hirshowitz). PRS, 48:52, 1971

GOLDBERG, H. M. et al: Considerations in cosmetic plastic surgery. J. S.C. Med. Assoc., 72:7, 1976

GOLDBERG, M. H.: Letters to the editor: What is maxillofacial surgery—who are maxillofacial surgeons? J. Oral Surg., 33:903, 1975

GOLDBERG, M. H. et al: Oral orthopedics. Conn. Med., 37:615, 1973

GOLDBERG, M. H., MARCO, W., GOOGLE, F.: Parotid fistula: a complication of mandibular osteotomy. J. Oral Surg., 31:207, 1973

GOLDBERG, S.: Origin of the lumbrical muscles in the hand of the South African native. Hand, 2:168, 1970

GOLDBERG, S.: Rhytidectomy in men. Arch. Otolaryng., 97:497, 1973

GOLDBERG, S. et al: Spontaneous regression of an intraosseous vascular lesion after aspiration: report of case. J. Oral Surg., 30:734, 1972

GOLDBERG, S. J. et al: Ameloblastoma: review of the literature and report of case. J. Am. Dent. Assoc., 90:432, 1975

GOLDBERG, S. J. et al: Fractured mandible, from initial operation to removal of tantalum mesh. Report of a case. Oral Surg., 41:32, 1976

GOLDEN, G. T.: Surgical correction of absent nasal alae of Johanson-Blizzard syndrome (with Fox, Edgerton), PRS, 57:484, 1976

GOLDEN, G. T.: Frontonasal dysplasia with alar clefts in two sisters; genetic considerations and surgical correction (with Fox, Edgerton). PRS, 57:553, 1976

GOLDEN, G. T. et al: Current treatment of wringer injuries. Va. Med. Mon., 99:1073, 1972

GOLDEN, G. T. et al: Aesthetic excisional biopsy of nipple lesion. Am. J. Surg., 128:445, 1974

GOLDEN, G. T. et al: Areolar reconstruction for chronic subareolar abscess of breast. Surg. Gynec. & Obst., 138:609, 1974

GOLDEN, J. S.: Rhinoplasty in transsexuals, psychological considerations (with Trop), PRS, 55:593, 1975

GOLDIN, J. H.: Experimental tube pedicle lined with small bowel. Brit. J. Plast. Surg., 25:388, 1972

GOLDIN, J. H. et al: Case of familial dysautonomia: cutting skin grafts without anesthesia. Brit. J. Plast. Surg., 26:184, 1973

GOLDMAN, J. L. et al: High dosage preoperative radiation and surgery for carcinoma of larynx and laryngopharynx. Fourteen-year program. Laryngoscope, 82:1869, 1972

GOLDMAN, J. L. et al: Combined pre-operative irradiation and surgery for advanced cancer of the larynx and laryngopharynx. (A 14 year correlative statistical and histopathological study). Can. J. Otolaryngol., 4:251, 1975

GOLDMAN, L. et al: Laser systems and their applications in medicine and biology. Adv. Biomed. Eng. Med. Phys., 1:317, 1968

GOLDMAN, L. et al: High-power neodymium-YAG laser surgery. Acta Derm. Venereol. (Stockh.), 53:45, 1973

GOLDMAN L.: Effects of new laser systems on skin. Arch. Dermat., 108:385, 1973

GOLDMAN, L.: Status report on laser surgery, PRS, 53:247, 1974. Contemp. Surg., 3:18, 1973

GOLDMAN, L. D., AND GOLDWYN, R. M.: Some anatomical considerations of subcutaneous mastectomy, PRS, 51:501, 1973

GOLDMAN, R. J. et al: Appraisal of surgical correction in 130 cases of orbital floor fractures. Am. J. Ophth., 76:152, 1973

GOLDMAN, R. J. et al: Caldwell-Luc procedure to correct orbital floor fractures. Ann. Ophth., 5:1259, 1973

GOLDNER, J. L.: Hand surgery training. J. Bone & Joint Surg., (Am.), 52:1061, 1970

GOLDNER, J. L.: Tendon transfers in rheumatoid arthritis. Orthop. Clin. North Am., 5:425, 1974

GOLDNER, J. L., KAPLAN, I., AND KELLEHER, J. C.: Injured hand, PRS, 50:305, 1972. Arch. Surg., 103:691, 1971

GOLDNER J. L., AND URBANIAK, J. R.: Clinical experience with silicone Dacron metacarpal phalangeal and interphalangeal joint prostheses, PRS, *53:*372, 1974. J. Biomed. Mater. Res., *7:*137, 1973

GOLDSCHMIDT, E.: Treatment of ruptures and strictures of lacrimal ducts. Ugeskr. Laeger, *136:*1198, 1974 (Danish)

GOLDSMITH, H. S.: Long-term evaluation of omental transposition for chronic lymphedema, PRS, *55:*638, 1975. Ann. Surg., *180:*847, 1974

GOLDSMITH, H. S. *et al*: Malignant melanoma: current concepts of lymph node dissection. C.A., *22:*216,1972

GOLDSTEIN, B. H. *et al*: Actinomycosis of the maxilla: review of literature and report of case. J. Oral Surg., *30:*362, 1972

GOLDSTEIN, B. H. *et al*: Giant cell tumor of maxilla complicating Paget's disease of bone. J. Oral Surg., *32:*209, 1974

GOLDSTEIN, J. C.: Skin grafts in head and neck surgery. Otolaryngol. Clin. North Am., *5:*513, 1972

GOLDSTEIN, M.: Congenital urethral fistula with chordee, PRS, *57:*761, 1976. J. Urol., *113:*138, 1975

GOLDSTEIN, N.: Radon seed implants. Residual radioactivity after 33 years. Arch. Dermat., *111:*757, 1975

GOLDSTONE, A. I. *et al*: Should adenotonsillectomy be done in the cleft palate patient? Va. Med. Mon., *98:*133, 1971

GOLDWYN R. M.: George H. Monks, M.D.: neglected innovator, PRS, *48:*478, 1971

GOLDWYN, R. M.: Cosmetic surgery and the university hospital (Editorial). PRS, *49:*76, 1972

GOLDWYN, R. M.: Operating for the aging face. Psychiatry Med., *3:*187, 1972

GOLDWYN, R. M.: National Archives of Plastic Surgery (Editorial). PRS, *51:*436, 1973

GOLDWYN, R. M.: Some anatomical considerations of subcutaneous mastectomy (with Goldman). PRS, *51:*501, 1973

GOLDWYN, R. M.: Simon P. Hullihen: pioneer oral and plastic surgeon. PRS: *52:*250, 1973

GOLDWYN, R. M.: Discussion of "Z-plasty skin closure after lengthening the Achilles tendon," by Price and Ecker. PRS, *52:*431, 1973

GOLDWYN, R. M.: Pulmonary function and bilateral reduction mammaplasty, PRS, *53:*84, 1974

GOLDWYN, R. M.: Discussion of "Successful clinical transfer of ten free flaps by microvascular anastomoses," by Harii *et al*. PRS, *53:*469, 1974

GOLDWYN, R. M.: Plea for showing average result (Editorial). PRS, *54:*88, 1974

GOLDWYN, R. M.: Editorial: reconstruction after mastectomy. Arch. Surg., *110:*246, 1975

GOLDWYN, R. M.: Discussion of "Reconstruction for aplasia of breast and pectoral region by microvascular transfer of free flap from buttock," by Fujino, Harashina, Aoyagi. PRS, *56:*335, 1975

GOLDWYN, R. M.: Skin pigmentation, current concepts and relevance to plastic surgery (with Morgan, Gilchrest). PRS, *56:*617, 1975

GOLDWYN, R. M.: Editorial: the treatment of axillary hyperhidrosis. Arch. Surg., *111:*13, 1976

GOLDWYN, R. M.: Cryosurgery for large hemangiomas in adults (Follow-Up Clinic). PRS, *57:*512, 1976

GOLDWYN, ROBERT M.: *Physician Travelers.* Arno Press & The New York Times, New York, 1971. PRS, *50:*180, 1972

GOLDWYN, ROBERT M: *The Unfavorable Result in Plastic Surgery: Avoidance and Treatment.* Little, Brown & Co., Boston, 1972. PRS, *52:*186, 1973

GOLDWYN, ROBERT M.: *Plastic and Reconstructive Surgery of the Breast.* Little, Brown & Co., Boston, 1976.

GOLLIN, F. F. *et al*: Combined therapy in advanced head and neck cancer: a randomized study. Am. J. Roentgenol. Radium Ther. Nucl. Med., *114:*83, 1972

GOLOMB, F. M.: Perfusion of melanoma; 133 isolated perfusions in 114 patients. Panminerva Med., *18:*8, 1976

GOLOMB, H. M. *et al*: Cervical synovial sarcoma at the bifurcation of the carotid artery. Cancer, *35:*483, 1975

GOLOVATENKO, V. V.: Naso-tracheal fluorothane nitrous oxide anesthesia in uranoplasty. Stomatologiia (Mosk.), *51:*80, 1972 (Russian)

GOLUBEVA, I. V. *et al*: Colpopoiesis operations in testicular forms of hemaphroditism. Probl. Endokrinol. (Mosk.), *19:*44, 1973 (Russian)

GOMBOS, F. *et al*: Relationships between salivary and endocrine glands. 3. Immediate effects on testes and on the parotid glands of parotidectomy and castration of adult male rats. Arch. Stomatol. (Napoli), *10:*329, 1969 (Italian)

GOMENSORO, J. M.: Dermatology and cosmetology, PRS, *49:*362, 1972. Cir. plast. Uruguay, *11:*21, 1970

GOMEZ, L. S. *et al*: Effect of delayed lymphadenectomy on 239Pu)2 translocation in dogs. Health Phys., *27:*213, 1974

GONERT, H. J. *et al*: Silicone rubber for surgery of the hand. Ztschr. Orthop., *111:*664, 1973 (German)

GONZAGA PEREIRA, L.: Repositioning of a maxilla torn out during an automobile accident. Rev. Stomatol. Chir. Maxillofac., *72:*205, 1971 (French)

GONZALEZ, A. R., AND OJEDA, F. X.: Reconstruction of lips and buccal commissure after electrical burn, PRS, *49:*237, 1972. Semana med. Mexico, *68:*101, 1971

GONZALEZ, A. R., AND OJEDA, F. X.: Reconstruction of flexor profundus tendons with tendon grafts, PRS, *49:*582, 1972. Semana med. Mexico, *69:*147, 1971

GONZALEZ, G., MILLER, N., AND WASILEWSKI, V.: Progressive neuro-ototoxicity of kanamycin, PRS, *50:*312, 1972. Ann. Otol. Rhin. & Laryng., *81:*127, 1972

GONZALEZ, O. I.: General considerations of hand trauma, PRS, *48:*393, 1971. Cir. plast. Uruguaya, *11:*15, 1970

GONZALEZ PEIRONA, E., AND MARTINEZ SAHUQUILLO, A.: Traumatic lesions caused by rings, PRS, *56:*595, 1975. Rev. Españ. cir. plast., 7:157, 1974

GONZALEZ-ULLOA, M.: Building out malar prominences as addition to rhytidectomy, PRS, *53:*293, 1974. Discussion by Stark, PRS, *53:*469, 1974

GONZALEZ-ULLOA, M.: Ancillary effects of estrogen therapy after rhytidectomy (Letter to the Editor). PRS, *56:*203, 1975

GONZALEZ-ULLOA, M., AND FLORES, E. S.: Syndrome of obstetric remissness, PRS, *48:*95, 1971. Internat. Surg., *55:*63, 1971

GONZALEZ-ULLOA, M., AND STEVENS, E.: Ptosis E.: Sectional rhytidectomy, PRS, *50:*198, 1972. Internat. Surg., *56:*266, 1971

Gonzalez-ULLOA, M., AND STEVENS, E.: Ptosis of chin, witches' chin, PRS, *50:*54, 1972

GOODE, R. L.: Bone and cartilage grafts; current concepts. Otolaryngol. Clin. North Am., 5:447, 1972

GOODE, R. L.: Head and neck operations after radiation therapy. Oral Surg., *36:*170, 1973

GOODE, R. L. *et al*: Office cryotherapy for oral leukoplakia. Trans. Am. Acad. Ophthalmol. Otolaryngol., *75:*968, 1971

GOODE, R. L., LINEHAN, J. W., AND SHORAGO, G.: Recurrent mandibular dislocation, PRS, *53:*242, 1974. Arch. Otolaryng., *98:*97, 1973

GOODE, R. L. *et al*: Compression clamp for internal fixation of mandible. Arch. Otolaryng., *98:*377, 1973

GOODE, R. L. *et al*: Columellar advancement for nasal tip elevation. Laryngoscope, *83:*1123, 1973

GOODE, R. L. *et al*: Cryosurgical treatment of recurrent head and neck malignancies – a comparative study. Laryngoscope, *84:*1950, 1974

GOODMAN, M. L.: Middle ear and mastoid neoplasm, PRS, *49:*238, 1972. Ann. Otol. Rhin. & Laryng., *80:*419, 1971

GOODMAN, W. S.: External approach to rhino-

plasty. Can. J. Otolaryngol., *2:*207, 1973

GOODMAN, W. S. *et al*: Treatment of established antroalveolar fistulae. Can. J. Otolaryngol., *1:*97, 1972

GOODMAN, W. S. *et al*: External approach to rhinoplasty. Laryngoscope, *84:*2195, 1974

GOODSTEIN, D. B., COOPER, D., AND WALLACE, L.: Effect on speech of surgery for prognathism, PRS, *56:*354, 1975. Oral Surg., *37:*846, 1974

GOODWIN, M. N., JR.: Upper extremity fungal invasions secondary to large burns (with Salisbury, Silverstein), PRS, *54:*654, 1974

GOODWIN, M. R.: Variables in rhinoplasties in identical twins. Eye Ear Nose Throat Mon., *51:*109, 1972

GOONATILLAKE, H. D.: S. C. Paul Oration, 1971. Surgery of cancer of throat. Ceylon Med. J., *16:*69, 1971

GORACY, E., AND STRATIGOS, G. T.: Adenoameloblastoma: report of case. J. Am. Dent. Assoc., *86:*672, 1973

GORBAN, L.: Hygroma of the neck. Rev. Stomatol. Chir. Maxillofac., *75:*284, 1974 (French)

GORBUNOV, G. M.: Operation of cross autovenous shunting in post thrombophlebitic disease of the lower limbs. Vestn. Khir., *115:*57, 1975 (Russian)

GORBUSHINA, P. M. *et al*: Surgical treatment of progressive facial hemiatrophy (Romberg's disease). Stomatologiia (Mosk.), *54:*51, 1975 (Russian)

GORDON, D. S., AND BLAIR, G. A. S.: Titanium cranioplasty, PRS, *54:*688, 1974. Brit. Med. J., *2:*478, 1974

GORDON, H. L.: Our present technique for rhytidectomy (with Baker, Whitlow), PRS, *52:*232, 1973

GORDON, J. A.: Malignant melanoma – treatment of primary lesion. Cent. Afr. J. Med., *19:*76, 1973

GORDON, S. D.: "Button" skin repair of ear defect, PRS, *48:*190, 1971

GOREN, S. B., AND CLEMIS, J. D.: Care of eye in facial paralysis, PRS, *52:*594, 1973. Arch. Otolaryng., *97:*227, 1973

GORIS, J.: On the depth of burns and healing time in grade II thermal burns. Chirurgia (Bucur.), *20:*735, 1971 (Rumanian)

GORIS, J.: Simple method for continuous evaluation of urinary output in severely burned children, PRS, *49:*107, 1972. Surg. Gynec. & Obst., *132:*695, 1971

GORLIN, ROBERT J.: *Syndromes of the Head and Neck*. 2nd Ed. McGraw-Hill Co., New York, 1976

GORLIN, R. J., *et al*: Facial clefting and its syndromes. Birth Defects, 7:3, 1971

GORLIN, R. J., AND CERVENKA, J.: Syndromes

of facial clefting, PRS, *56:*360, 1975. Scand. J. Plast. Reconstr. Surg., *8:*13, 1974

GORMAN, J. B.: Rhinolalia aperta. Va. Med. Mon., *99:*1077, 1972

GORMAN, J. M.: Condylotomy for bilateral dislocation. Brit. J. Oral Surg., *12:*96, 1974

GORMLEY, J. W. *et al*: Epidermolysis bullosa and associated problems in oral surgical treatment. J. Oral Surg., *34:*45, 1976

GORMLEY, M. B. *et al*: Thermal trauma: a review of 22 electrical burns of the lip. J. Oral Surg., *30:*531, 1972

GORMLEY, M. B. *et al*: Odontogenic myxofibroma: report of two cases. J. Oral Surg., *33:*356, 1975

GORNEY, M.: Performance of cosmetic surgery by plastic surgery residents in city hospitals (Letter to the Editor), PRS, *48:*362, 1971

GORNEY, M.: Use of ear cartilage grafts for nasal tip reconstructions (with Falces), PRS, *50:*147, 1972

GORNEY, M.: Reconstruction of your self-image (Editorial), PRS, *51:*436, 1973

GORNEY, M.: Medicolegal aspects of automobile injuries. Clin. Plast. Surg., *2:*167, 1975

GORNEY, M., AND HARRIES, T.: Preoperative and postoperative consideration of natural facial asymmetry, PRS, *54:*187, 1974

GORSHKOV, S. Z.: Etiology, pathogenesis and treatment of elephantiasis of extremities. Klin. Med. (Mosk.), *50:*131, 1972 (Russian)

GORSHKOV, S. Z.: Vulval elephantiasis. Akush. Ginekol. (Mosk.), *2:*71, 1974 (Russian)

GORSHKOV, V. M.: Osteoma of frontal sinuses and the ethmoid labyrinth. Vestn. Otorinolaringol., *35:*86, 1973 (Russian)

GORSHKOV, V. V.: Restoration of missing portion of urethra in high hypospadias in children using modified Duplay method. Urol. Nefrol. (Mosk.), *38:*52, 1973 (Russian)

GORSKI, M.: Treatment of neoplastic tumors and neoplasm-like tumors of jaws in children. Czas. Stomatol., *25:*817, 1972 (Polish)

GORSKI, M. *et al*: Results of surgical treatment of jaw sarcoma. Dtsch. Zahn. Mund. Kieferheilkd., *58:*250, 1972 (German)

GOSHGARIAN, G., AND MILLER, T. A.: "Parachute" stent, PRS, *57:*530, 1976. Am. J. Surg., *130:*370, 1975

GOSLING, C. G.: Facial moulage technique for the plastic surgeon (with Thompson, Hayes), PRS, *49:*190, 1972

GOSSEREZ, M. *et al*: Indications for tongue-skin flap in reconstruction of oral tissue loss. J. Fr. Otorhinolaryngol., *22:*921, 1973 (French)

GOTTE, P.: Correction of maxillary retrognathism by partial osteotomy and transplantation of mandibular bone. Riv. Ital. Stomatol., *29:*59, 1974 (Italian)

GOTTE, P. *et al*: Subjective effects and personality changes in patients following surgical corrections of esthetic-functional malformations of the jaws. Riv. Ital. Stomatol., *26:*535, 1971 (Italian)

GOTTE, P. *et al*: Functional rehabilitation and esthetics of masticatory system in partially edentulous subjects with jaw abnormalities. Riv. Ital. Stomatol., *28:*259, 1973 (Italian)

GOTTLIEB, B., AND NEWMAN, B. A.: Bowenoid squamous cell carcinoma of digits, PRS, *57:*679, 1976. Cutis, *16:*108, 1975

GOTTLIEB, J. A., AND HILL, C. S., JR.: Chemotherapy of thyroid cancer with Adriamycin, PRS, *54:*373, 1974. New England J. Med., *290:*193, 1974

GÖTZ, H. *et al*: Experiments for developing fibroblastic endothelium on synthetic preparations, PRS, *54:*247, 1974. Bruns' Beitr. klin. Chir., *221:*142, 1974

GOUAZE, A. *et al*: Orbito-encephalic injuries. Neurochirurgie, *17:*291, 1971 (French)

GOUDSOUZIAN, N. G., MORRIS, R. H., AND RYAN, J. F.: Effects of warming blanket on maintenance of body temperature in anesthetized infants and children, PRS, *53:*687, 1974. Anesthesiology, *39:*351, 1973

GOUIRIC, R. *et al*: Transparotid approach in mandibular ameloblastoma recurrences. Rev. Stomatol. Chir. Maxillofac., *75:*58, 1974 (French)

GOULD, L. V. *et al*: Snowblower injuries. N. Y. State J. Med., *74:*887, 1974

GOULIAN, D.: Need for extensive undermining in face lifting operations. Brit. J. Plast. Surg., *26:*387, 1973

GOULIAN, D.: Use of bromphenol blue in the assay of rheomacrodex effects on flap viability (Follow-Up Clinic), PRS, *51:*206, 1973

GOULIAN, D.: Secondary surgery in transsexuals (with Bellinger), PRS, *51:*628, 1973

GOULIAN, D., JR.: Predicting extent of viability in flaps by measurement of gas tensions, using a mass spectrometer (with Guthrie, Cucin), PRS, *50:*385, 1972

GOULIAN, D., JR.: Small, deep forearm lacerations; differential diagnosis of muscle and nerve injuries (with Schwager, Smith), PRS, *55:*190, 1975

GOULIAN, D., JR., AND MCDIVITT, R. W.: Subcutaneous mastectomy with immediate reconstruction of breasts, using dermal mastopexy technique, PRS, *50:*211, 1972

GOUMAIN, A. J. *et al*: Our views on surgical treatment of ischiatic eschars. Ann. Chir., *26:*883, 1972 (French)

GOUMAIN, A. J. *et al*: Correction technic for mammary ptoses and hypertrophies. Ann. chir. plast., *17:*198, 1972 (French)

GOUMAIN, A. J. *et al*: Possibilities and limitations of surgery of the hand in 1972. Apropos of a case. Bord. Med., *5*:2041, 1972 (French)

GOUMAIN, A. J. *et al*: Spider flap in the treatment of cicatrix of burned fingers. Ann. chir. plast., *18*:275, 1973 (French)

GOUMAIN, A. J. M.: Cutting forceps for lateral osteotomy in rhinoplasty, PRS, *53*:358, 1974

GOUMAIN, A. J. M., BAUDET, J., AND MASSARD, J. F.: Surgical treatment of bedsores, PRS, *50*:422, 1972. J. Chir. Paris, *103*:237, 1972

GOURNET, C.: Bites, 84 cases. Ann. chir. plast., *18*:355, 1973 (French)

GOUZY, J. *et al*: Case of schwannoma of floor of mouth. J. Fr. Otorhinolaryngol., *21*:501, 1972 (French)

GRABB, W. C.: Management of nerve injuries in the forearm and hand. Orthop. Clin. North Am., *1*:419, 1970

GRABB, W. C.: Cart before the horse. Cleft Palate J., *9*:352, 1972

GRABB, W. C., AND DINGMAN, R. O.: Fate of amputated tissues of head and neck following replacement, PRS, *49*:28, 1972

GRABB, W. C.: Experimental method (Editorial), PRS, *49*:563, 1972

GRABB, W. C.: Intravenous fluorescein test as measure of skin flap viability (with Thorvaldsson), PRS, *53*:576, 1974

GRABB, W. C.: Skin graft survival on avascular defects (with Gingrass, Gingrass), PRS, *55*:65, 1975

GRABB, W. C.: Goodbye to the term "length-to-width ratio" (Letter to the Editor), PRS, *56*:330, 1975

GRABB, WILLIAM C., AND MYERS, M. BERT: *Skin Flaps*. Little, Brown & Co., Boston, 1976.

GRABB, WILLIAM C., AND SMITH, JAMES W.: *Plastic Surgery. A Concise Guide to Clinical Practice*. Little, Brown & Co., Boston, 1973. PRS, *54*:602, 1974

GRABB, WILLIAM C., ROSENSTEIN, SHELDON W., AND BZOCH, KENNETH R.: *Cleft Lip and Palate. Surgical, Dental, and Speech Aspects*. Little, Brown & Co., Boston, 1971. PRS, *49*:337, 1972

GRABER, W. *et al*: Surgical treatment of diabetic malum perforans. Praxis, *62*:1405, 1973 (German)

GRABOWSKA, H. *et al*: Perforating plantar ulcer in the course of diabetes. Wiad. Lek., *24*:1475, 1971 (Polish)

GRADY, A. D.: Treatment of recurrent carcinoma of female breast, PRS, *55*:719, 1975. Rocky Mountain M. J., *72*:24, 1972

GRAF-PINTHUS, B., AND BETTEX, M.: Long-term observation following presurgical orthopedic treatment in complete clefts of lip and palate, PRS, *55*:513, 1975. Cleft Palate J., *11*:253, 1974

Grafts: See *Bone Grafts; Cartilage Grafts; Composite Grafts; Dermal Grafts; Fascia Grafts; Fat Grafts; Homografts; Mucosal Grafts; Muscle Transplantation; Nerve Grafts; Skin Grafts; Tendon Grafts*

GRAHAM, P. W. *et al*: Tissue necrosis from vascular complications of upper extremity after arterial catheterization, PRS, *53*:487, 1974. Rev. Latino Am. cir. plast., *17*:37, 1973

GRAHAM, W. P., III: Incisions, amputations, and skin grafting in the hand. Orthop. Clin. North Am., *1*:213, 1970

GRAHAM, W. P., III: Explosion of strobe light unit (Letter to the Editor), PRS, *49*:331, 1972

GRAHAM, W. P., III: Cervical neuromas following extensive maxillofacial surgery. J. Surg. Oncol., *5*:485, 1973

GRAHAM, W. P., III: Variations of motor branch of median nerve at wrist, PRS, *51*:90, 1973

GRAHAM, W. P., III: Autotransfusion for blood loss in some major esthetic operations (with Noone, Royster), PRS, *51*:559, 1973

GRAHAM, W. P., III: Management of hand infections in narcotic addict (with Whitaker), PRS, *52*:384, 1973

GRAHAM, W. P., III: Mucous cysts: dorsal distal interphalangeal joint ganglion (with Newmeyer, Kilgore), PRS, *53*:313, 1974

GRAHAM, W. P., III: Teaching exercises for medical students in clinical aspects of wound healing, PRS, *53*:433, 1974

GRAHAM, W. P., III: Pericortical "compression" clamps for mandibular fixation (with Lung, Miller), PRS, *57*:487, 1976

GRAHAM, W. P., III *et al*: Simple reduction of zygomatic arch fractures, PRS, *48*:294, 1971. J. Trauma, *10*:874, 1970

GRAHAM, W. P., III *et al*: Symptomatic digital neuromas treated with local triamcinolone acetonide, PRS, *52*:97, 1973. Rev. Latino Am. cir. plast., *16*:13, 1972

GRAHAM, W. P., III *et al*: Complications following posterior pharyngeal flap surgery. Cleft Palate J., *10*:176, 1973

GRAHAM, W. P., III *et al*: Metastatic tumors of hand, PRS, *54*:376, 1974. Hand, *5*:177, 1973

GRAHAM, W. P., III *et al*: Transarticular joint amputations: value of preserving articular cartilage, PRS, *53*:495, 1974. J. Surg. Res., *14*:524, 1973

GRAHAM, W. P., III, AND ROYSTER, H.: Superior osteotomy: adjunct to osteoplastic nasal surgery, PRS, *53*:240, 1974. Rev. Latino Am. cir. plast., *17*:33, 1973

GRAHAM, W. P., III *et al*: Preventing hand disability from infection. Pa. Med., *78*:53,

1975

GRAHAM, W. P., III *et al*: Treating wringer injuries. Pa. Med., *78:*67, 1975

GRAHAM, W. P., III, MESSNER, K. H., AND MILLER, S. H.: Keratoconjunctivitis sicca symptoms appearing after blepharoplasty, PRS, *57:*57, 1976

GRAHAME, R. *et al*: Treatment of severe decubitus ulcers using Beaufort-Winchester water bed. Brit. J. Plast. Surg., *26:*75, 1973

GRAHN, E. C.: Power unit for functional hand splints. Bull. Prosthet. Res., *10:*52, 1970

GRAHNE, B.: Surgical treatment of severe traumatic and functional stenosis of larynx. H. N. O., *21:*234, 1973 (German)

GRAMMER, F. C. *et al*: Radioisotope study of vascular response to sagittal split osteotomy of mandibular ramus. J. Oral Surg., *32:*578, 1974

GRANATO, R. C.: Surgical approach to male transsexualism. Urology, *3:*792, 1974

GRANBERRY, W. M.: Gunshot wounds of the hand. Hand, *5:*220, 1973

GRAND, A. *et al*: Sino-carotid hyper-reflectivity (therapeutic value of intracavitary standby cardiac stimulation). Coer Med. Interne, *11:*265, 1972 (French)

GRANDVAL, C. M.: Lymphedema. Methods of study and therapeutic possibilities, PRS, *51:*479, 1973. Bol. y trab. Soc. argent cir., *56:*33, 1972

GRANITE, E. L.: Oronasal fistula following anterior maxillary osteotomy. J. Oral Surg., *33:*129, 1975

GRANT, D. A.: Treatment of asymmetry of the breasts. South. Med. J., *64:*1097, 1971

GRANT, G. H.: Editorial: The "intact" hand after crush and burn. J.A.M.A., *227:*1305, 1974

GRANTHAM, R. N. *et al*: Surgical treatment of lip cancer: recommendations for therapy in rural population. J. Okla. State Med. Assoc., *66:*451, 1973

Granulation Tissue (See also *Collagen; Wound Healing*)

Metabolic and blood flow changes in healing wounds: a measurement of microcirculatory development (Lim *et al*). Bibl. Anat., *10:*328, 1969

Handling of open wounds and granulation wounds (Tajima). Jap. J. Plast. Reconstr. Surg., *14:*135, 1971 (Japanese)

Treatments of the granulation wounds—therapeutic experience in extensive thermal burns (Kurata *et al*). Jap. J. Plast. Reconstr. Surg., *14:*150, 1971 (Japanese)

Management of wound surface and granulation wounds (Hiramoto *et al*). Jap. J. Plast.

Granulation Tissue—Cont.

Reconstr. Surg., *14:*158, 1971 (Japanese)

Treatment of trauma and granulation wounds (Hirayama). Jap. J. Plast. Reconstr. Surg., *14:*167, 1971 (Japanese)

Management of wounds, particularly granulation wounds (Uchida). Jap. J. Plast. Reconstr. Surg., *14:*174, 1971 (Japanese)

Open skin grafting for granulation wounds (Fukuda *et al*). Jap. J. Plast. Reconstr. Surg., *14:*183, 1971 (Japanese)

Fate of cutaneously and subcutaneously implanted trypsin purified dermal collagen in pig (Oliver). Brit. J. Exp. Pathol., *53:*540, 1972

Granulation tissue as a contractile organ. A study of structure and function (Gabbiani *et al*). J. Exp. Med., *135:*719, 1972

Granulation tissue, wound healing, of sialoadenectomized rats (Rulli). Rev. Fac. Odontol. Aracatuba, *2:*171, 1973 (Portuguese)

Granulation tissue, production of for skin grafting (Bertenyi). Z. Haut Geschlechtschr., *48:*153, 1973

Clinical use of porcine xenografts in conditions other than burns (State *et al*). Surg. Gynec. & Obst., *138:*13, 1974

Granuloma

Starch granulomas (Leonard), PRS, *52:*603, 1973. Arch. Dermat., *107:*101, 1973

GRAS ARTERO, M.: Influence of vitamin E in anomalous scar, PRS, *56:*363, 1975. Riv. ital. chir. plast., *5:*309, 1973

GRASSER, H.: Management of fractures of the orbital floor. Dtsch. Zahnaerztl. Z., *27:*120, 1972 (German)

GRASSER, H.: Analgesia with pentazocine following facial jaw and oral surgery. Med. Monatsschr., *26:*230, 1972 (German)

GRASSER, H.: Stable fixation in prognathism surgery. Z. W. R., *82:*1163, 1973

GRATE, M. R., AND HICKS, J. N.: Nasolabial subcutaneous pedicle flap, PRS, *53:*613, 1974. South. M. J., *66:*1234, 1973

GRATTAN, E.: Patterns, causes and prevention of facial injury in car occupants. Proc. Roy. Soc. Med., *65:*913, 1972

GRAUDINS, J., DUBEN, W., AND POPP, B.: Thrombosis with cava catheters, PRS, *52:*681, 1973. Zentralbl. Chir., *98:*274, 1973

GRAVES, C. L., McDERMOTT, R. W., AND BIDWAI, A.: Cardiovascular effects of isoflurane in surgical patients, PRS, *55:*727, 1975. Anesthesiology, *41:*486, 1974

GRAVES, T. A. *et al*: Management of traumatic facial nerve paralysis. Laryngoscope, *81:*645,

1971

GRAY, B. N.: Teratoma of neck. Aust. N.Z. J. Surg., *42*:294, 1973

GRAY, E., AND MORRISON, N. M.: Influence of combination of sexes of children on family size, PRS, *57*:542, 1976. J. Heredity, *65*:169, 1974

GRAY, F. B., GILLENWATER, J. Y., AND MULHOLLAND, S. G.: Perineal masses in male subjects, PRS, *50*:200, 1972. J. Urol., *106*:236, 1971

GRAY, F. J.: Infections of the hand. Papua New Guinea Med. J., *18*:113, 1975

GRAY, K. P.: Septal and associated cranial birth deformities: types, incidence and treatment. M. J. Australia, *1*:557, 1974

GRAZER, F. M.: Use of fiber optic bundles in plastic surgery, PRS, *48*:28, 1971

GRAZER, F. M.: Abdominoplasty, PRS, *51*:617, 1973

GRAZIANI, M.: Laterognathism, supraclusion and facial asymmetry from condylar hyperplasia. Oral Surg., *33*:884, 1972

GREAVES, M. W.: Introduction to pharmacology and physiology of itch, PRS, *57*:682, 1976. Proc. Roy. Soc. Med., *68*:529, 1975

GRECHUKHIN, V. P. *et al*: Clinical-experimental evaluation of long-acting penicillin preparations in treatment of anaerobic infections. Voen. Med. Zh., *4*:20, 1972 (Russian)

GRECO, J. *et al*: Cervico-temporo-frontal S-plasty for repair of cheek defects. Ann. chir. plast., *18*:319, 1973 (French)

GREELEY, P. W.: Influence of war on development of major subspecialty. Mil. Med., *138*:231, 1973

GREELEY, P. W.: Plastic surgical treatment of basal cell skin cancer. Mil. Med., *141*:443, 1974

GREEN, A. E. *et al*: An osteoma of the mandible. Brit. J. Oral Surg., *12*:225, 1974

GREEN, B. E., JR.: Use of modified head halter for Barton bandage, PRS, *49*:466, 1972

GREEN, B. F., JR.: Editorial: A philosophy of approach to treatment of hemangiomas. South. Med. J., *68*:383, 1975

GREEN, D. P.: True and false traumatic aneurysms in the hand. J. Bone & Joint Surg. (Am.), *55*:120, 1973

GREEN, D. P., AND GERRY, G. C.: Complex dislocation of metacarpophalangeal joint, PRS, *54*:109, 1974. J. Bone & Joint Surg., *55A*:1480, 1973

GREEN, D. P. *et al*: Extrication of the hand from a meat grinder. J. Trauma, *15*:32, 1975

GREEN, F. C.: Child abuse and neglect, priority problem for private physician, PRS, *57*:680, 1976. Pediatr. Clin. N. Am., *22*:329, 1975

GREEN, J. A. *et al*: Experimental facial nerve

paralysis: influence of decompression, PRS, *56*:462, 1975. Ann. Otol. Rhin. & Laryng., *83*:582, 1974

GREEN, J. R.: Results of various operations for sacrococcygeal pilonidal disease (with Sood, Parui), PRS, *56*:559, 1975

GREEN, M. F.: Lateral dermal sinus associated with an intradiploic cyst. Brit. J. Plast. Surg., *26*:202, 1973

GREEN, M. F., AND KADRI, S. W. M.: Acute closed-angle glaucoma, complication of blepharoplasty, PRS, *56*:676, 1975. Brit. J. Plast. Surg., *27*:25, 1974

GREEN, R. O., AND GOLDMAN, H.: Oral papillomas, PRS, *55*:506, 1975. Oral Surg., *38*:435, 1974

GREEN, W. L., AND NIEBAUER, J. J.: Results of primary and secondary flexor-tendon repairs in no-man's-land, PRS, *55*:509, 1975. J. Bone & Joint Surg., *56A:* 1216, 1974

GREENBLATT, D. J., AND KOCH-WESER, A. J.: Adverse reactions to intravenous diazepam (Valium): report from Boston Collaborative Drug Surveillance Program, PRS, *57*:541, 1976. Am. J. Med. Sci., *266*:261, 1973

GREENE, C. S.: The temporomandibular syndrome, PRS, *52*:678, 1973. J.A.M.A., *224*:622, 1973

GREENE, D. A.: Tracheostomy or not? J.A.M.A., *234*:1150, 1975

GREENE, N. M.: Insulin and anesthesia, PRS, *55*:259, 1975. Anesthesiology, *41*:75, 1974

GREENHALGH, R. M. *et al*: Single congenital arteriovenous fistula of the hand. Brit. J. Surg., *59*:76, 1972

GREENHOW, D. E.: Incorrect performance of Allen's test – ulnar artery flow erroneously presumed inadequate, PRS, *51*:603, 1973. Anesthesiology, *37*:356, 1972

GREENING, W. P.: Surgical treatment of thyroid tumors. Monogr. Neoplast. Dis. Var. Sites, *6*:231, 1970

GREENLEE, T. K., JR., AND PIKE, D.: Studies of tendon healing in rat, PRS, *48*:260, 1971

GREENTREE, L. B.: Acupuncture and American doctor in China, PRS, *56*:366, 1975. Surg. Gynec. & Obst., *139*:604, 1974

GREENWALD, H. S., JR. *et al*: Review of 128 patients with orbital fractures. Am. J. Ophth., *78*:655, 1974

GREENWAY, R. E.: Tracheostomy: surgical problems and complications. Int. Anesthesiol. Clin., *10*:151, 1972

GREER, D. M., JR.: Tongue flap for reconstruction of lips in electrical burns (with Zarem), PRS, *53*:310, 1974

GREER, D. M., JR.: Secondary correction of bilateral cleft lip deformities with Millard's midline muscular closure (with Oneal, Nobel), PRS, *54:*45, 1974

GREER, D. M., JR., MOORE, C. E., AND COLEMAN, P.: Orthoplast headcap for external fixation of facial fractures, PRS, *54:*614, 1974

GREER, D. M., JR., AND DIXON, J. L.: Drill for use in an inaccessible place, PRS, *57:*103, 1975

GREER, J. A. *et al*: Experimental facial nerve paralysis: influence of decompression. Ann. Otol. Rhin. & Laryng., *83:*582, 1974

GREGORIADES, G.: Chondrosarcoma of the hard palate. J. Laryng. & Otol., *86:*513, 1972

GREGORY-ROBERTS, F.: Resection and tucking of the fibrous tissue layers of the upper lid for correction of ptosis: a new operation. Trans. Aust. Coll. Ophthalmol., *2:*38, 1970

GRELLET, M.: Primary treatment of lesions of soft facial parts in traffic accidents. I. General problems. Nouv. Presse Med., *2:*2283, 1973

GRELLET, M.: Primary treatment of injuries of facial soft parts in traffic accidents. II. Local problems. Nouv. Presse Med., *2:*2343, 1973 (French)

GRELLET, M.: Mobile carcinoma of tongue. Rev. Stomatol. Chir. Maxillofac., *74:*111, 1973 (French)

GRELLET, M.: Mandibular osteosynthesis. Conclusion. Rev. Stomatol. Chir. Maxillofac., *74:*276, 1973 (French)

GRELLET, M. *et al*: Case of solitary mandibular cyst in a hemophilic. Rev. Stomatol. Chir. Maxillofac., *72:*734, 1971 (French)

GRELLET, M. *et al*: Case of basocellular nevomatosis. Rev. Stomatol. Chir. Maxillofac., *74:*97, 1973 (French)

GRELLET, M. *et al*: Reparative surgery on the mucosa of the floor of the mouth. Acta Stomatol. Belg., *72:*489, 1975 (French)

GRELLET, M. *et al*: Action of corticosteroids on cutaneous cicatrization. Use in maxillofacial surgery. Rev. Stomatol. Chir. Maxillofac., *76:*379, 1975 (French)

GREMINGER, R. F.: Correction of asymmetrical breasts (with Elliott, Hoehn). PRS, *56:*260, 1975

GRESHAM, E. L.: Birth trauma, PRS, *57:*681, 1976. Pediatr. Clin. N. Am., *22:*317, 1975

GRIBOR, P.: Surgical repair of congenital colobomas. Trans. Am. Acad. Ophthalmol. Otolaryngol., *79:*671, 1975

GRIESEN, O.: Aberrant course of facial nerve, PRS, *57:*259, 1976. Arch. Otolaryng., *101:*327, 1975

GRIFFIN, J. E., AND HAYES, H.: Congenital transposition of scrotum and penis. PRS, *55:*710, 1975

GRIFFIN, J. M.: Subcutaneous mastectomy; excess skin problem (with Hartley, Schatten).

PRS, *56:*5, 1975

GRIFFIN, J. M. *et al*: Visor flap reconstruction for massive oropharyngeal defect, PRS, *51:*457, 1973. Discussion by Edgerton, PRS, *51:*582, 1973

GRIFFITH, B. H.: Simplified technique for marking line of excision in rhytidectomy. Brit. J. Plast. Surg., *27:*276, 1974

GRIFFITH, B. H.: Frontonasal tumors: their diagnosis and management. PRS, *57:*692, 1976

GRIFFITH, B. H. *et al*: Von Recklinghausen's disease in children. PRS, *49:*647, 1972

GRIFFITH, B. H., AND McKINNEY, P.: Appraisal of treatment of basal cell carcinoma of skin. PRS, *51:*565, 1973

GRIFFITHS, D. A.: Functional anatomy of the hand. Med. Biol. Illus., *22:*150, 1972

GRIFFITHS, D. A., AND WEBB, A. J.: Surgical treatment of initial priapism and recurrent priapism, PRS, *54:*110, 1974. Proc. Roy. Soc. Med., *66:*1051, 1973

GRIFFITHS, J. C., AND HEYWOOD, O. B.: Biomechanical aspects of tourniquet, PRS, *54:*236, 1974. Hand, *5:*113, 1973

GRIFFITHS, M. V.: Recurrent facial swelling due to cavernous hemangioma. J. Laryng. & Otol., *88:*1135, 1974

GRIFFITHS, R. W. *et al*: Three years' experience of metacarpophalangeal joint replacement in the rheumatoid hand. Hand, *7:*275, 1975

GRIGNON, J. L.: Esthetic considerations of patient and surgeon: the nose-chin relationship. Actual Odontostomatol. (Paris), *26:*455, 1972

GRIGNON, J. L.: Plastic surgery and psychology: service rendered to patients, PRS, *57:*681, 1976. Ann. chir. plast., *20:*95, 1975

GRIGNON, J. L. *et al*: Nose burns in burned face: secondary treatment. Ann. chir. plast., *18:*161,1973

GRIGNON, J. L. *et al*: Mandibular osteosynthesis with cortical or transfixing steel wire: the "rubicon" of coherence. Rev. Stomatol. Chir. Maxillofac., *74:*222, 1973 (French)

GRIGNON, J. L. *et al*: Closure of orostomes and pharyngostomes in irradiated tissues requires respect of certain principles. Rev. Stomatol. Chir. Maxillofac., *75:*218, 1974 (French)

GROGONO, B. J.: Auger injuries. Injury, *4:*247, 1973

GRIGOR'EV, M. G.: Modern principles of therapy of patients with thermal burns. Ortop. Travmatol. Protez., *34:*1, 1973 (Russian)

GRIGOR'EV, M. G.: Methods of treatment of aftereffects of battle injuries in war invalids. Ortop. Travmatol. Protez., *34:*1, 1974 (Russian)

GRIGOR'EV, M. G. *et al*: Restoration of the function of the upper extremities in deformities following burns. Ortop. Travmatol. Protez., *32:*15, 1971 (Russian)

GRIGORIAN, A. V. *et al*: Enzyme therapy as a method of preparing trophic ulcers and protractedly nonhealing wounds for dermato-autoplasty. Klin. Khir., *9:*1, 1971 (Russian)

GRIGORIAN, A. V. *et al*: Treatment of phagedenic ulcers. Vestn. Khir., *106:*42, 1971 (Russian)

GRIGORIAN, A. V. *et al*: Treatment of trophic crural ulcers. Sov. Med., *10:*86, 1975 (Russian)

GRIGOROVITCH, G. A.: Danger of primary nerve sutures, PRS, *52:*208, 1973. Bull. Soc. Internat. Chir., *6:*495, 1972

GRILLO, H. C. *et al*: Low-pressure cuff for tracheostomy tubes to minimize tracheal injury. A comparative clinical trial. J. Thorac. Cardiovasc. Surg., *62:*898, 1971

GRIMES, J. H., NASHOLD, B. S., AND CURRIE, D. P.: Chronic electrical stimulation of paraplegic bladder, PRS, *52:*596, 1973. J. Urol., *109:*242, 1973

GRIMM, G.: Therapy of zygomatic fractures. Dtsch. Stomatol., *21:*605, 1971 (German)

GRIMM, G. *et al*: Surgical technic for malignant melanoma of the skin in the head and neck region. Dtsch. Zahn. Mund. Kieferheilkd., *57:*363, 1971 (German)

GRIMM, G. *et al*: Critical evaluation of surgical results in 101 cases of prognathism with special reference to Obwegeser-Dal Pont's method. Dtsch. Zahn. Mund. Kieferheilkd., *61:*295, 1973 (German)

GRISHIN, I. G.: Arthroplasty of metacarpo-phalangeal finger joints in patients with rheumatoid polyarthritis. Ortop. Travmatol. Protez., *35:*19, 1974 (Russian)

GRISOTTI, A., SAVOIA, A., AND TAIDELLI, G.: Statistical research of Curling's ulcer, PRS, *50:*308, 1972. Acta chir. plast., *13:*83, 1971

GRISWOLD, M. L., JR.: Series of skin burns with necrectomy immediately after electrolyte stabilization (Follow-Up Clinic), PRS, *49:*83, 1972

GRITSIUK, S. N.: Catheter-cannula for restoring the patency of the lacrimal ducts in children. Oftalmol. Zh., *26:*551, 1971 (Russian)

GROCOTT, J.: Maxillary osteotomies in cleft palate repairs. Br. J. Plast. Surg., *26:*261, 1973

GROGAN, J. B., AND MILLER, R. C.: Impaired function of polymorphonuclear leukocytes in patients with burns and other trauma, PRS, *53:*608, 1974. Surg. Gynec. & Obst., *137:*784, 1973

GROHMANN, W.: Open severance of carotid artery. Z. Aerztl. Fortbild., Jena, *66:*1031, 1972 (German)

GROMOV, M. W. *et al*: Primary plastic closure of

soft tissue defects in compound fractures of leg bones. Ortop. Travmatol. Protez., *33:*15, 1972 (Russian)

GRONERT, G. A., AND THEYE, R. A.: Pathophysiology of hyperkalemia induced by succinylcholine, PRS, *57:*263, 1976. Anesthesiology, *43:*89, 1975

GROSFELD, O.: Functional compensation of muscles after postoperative rehabilitation in reference to electromyographic analysis. Oral Surg., *38:*829, 1974

GROSHONG, L. E.: Technique for radical groin dissection. Surg. Gynec. & Obst., *136:*986, 1973

GROSS, A., CUTRIGHT, D. E., AND BHASKAR, S. N.: Effectiveness of pulsating water jet lavage in treatment of contaminated crush wounds, PRS, *51:*352, 1973. Am. J. Surg., *124:*373, 1972

GROSS, A. *et al*: Effect of antiseptic agents and pulsating jet lavage on contaminated wounds, PRS, *50:*542, 1972. Mil. Med., *137:*145, 1972

GROSS, A. *et al*: Evaluation of two antiseptic agents in surgical preparation of hands by new method, PRS, *53:*114, 1974. Am. J. Surg., *126:*49, 1973

GROSS, C. W. *et al*: Reconstruction following severe nasofrontal injuries. Otolaryngol. Clin. North Am., *5:*653, 1972

GROSS, C. W. *et al*: Malignant minor salivary gland tumors—report of 32 cases. Can. J. Otolaryngol., *3:*56, 1974

GROSS, M., ARNOLD, T. L., AND WATERHOUSE, K.: Fracture of penis: rationale of surgical management, PRS, *50:*95, 1972. J. Urol., *106:*708, 1971

GROSS, R.: Continuous subcutaneous sutures in surgical treatment of hypospadias. Pol. Przegl. Chir., *44:*111, 1972 (Polish)

GROSS, R.: Modification of stabilization of chest wall in funnel chest operation, PRS, *57:*398, 1976. Ztschr. Kinderchir., *17:*67, 1975

GROSS, R. *et al*: Treatment of Pierre Robin syndrome by Duhamel's method. Pediatr. Pol., *45:*1215, 1973 (Polish)

GROSSÀN, M.: Saccharin test of nasal mucociliary function, PRS, *57:*755, 1976. Eye, Ear, Nose & Throat Month., *54:*415, 1975

GROSSE, F. R.: Rabenhorst syndrome: a cardioacrofascial syndrome. Z. Kinderheilkd., *117:*109, 1974

GROSSHANS, E. *et al*: Woringer-Kolopp disease, epidermotropic cutaneous reticulosis, "Pagetoid reticulosis." Arch. Belg. Dermatol., *29:*195, 1973 (French)

GROSS-KIESELSTEIN, E. *et al*: Familial occurrence of the Freeman-Sheldon syndrome: craniocarpotarsal dysplasia. Pediatrics,

47:1064, 1971

GROSSMAN, A. R.: Sutilains ointment as topical debriding agent in burns. Internat. Surg., 58:93, 1973

GROSSMAN, A. R.: Current status of augmentation mammaplasty. PRS, 52:1, 1973

GROSSMAN, J., AND IZUNO, G.: Primary mucinous (adenocystic) carcinoma of skin, PRS, 55:257, 1975. Arch. Dermat., 110:275, 1974

GROSSMAN, J. A., BERGER, R., AND HOEHN, R. J.: Kaposi's varicelliform eruption complicating local facial trauma. PRS, 55:625, 1975

GROSSMAN, J. R., JR. et al: Intraoral junctional nevus: review of the literature and report of case. J. Oral Surg., 33:275, 1975

GROVER, F. L., NEWMAN, N. M., AND PATON, B. C.: Beneficial effect of pluronic F-68 on microcirculation in experimental hemorrhagic shock, PRS, 48:96, 1971. Surg. Forum, 21:30, 1970

GROVES, A. R., AND LAWRENCE, J. C.: Tangential excision of burns: experimental study using animal model, PRS, 49:359, 1972. Injury, 3:30, 1971

GROVES, R. J., AND GOLDNER, J. L.: Contracture of deltoid muscle in adult after intramuscular injections, PRS, 55:259, 1975. J. Bone & Joint Surg., 56A:817, 1974

GROWER, M. F. et al: Effect of water lavage on removal of tissue fragments from crush wounds. Oral Surg., 33:1031, 1972

GROZINGER, K. H.: Diagnosis and treatment of burns. Langenbecks Arch. Chir., 327:1197, 1970 (German)

GRUBER, R. P.: Preservation of traumatically amputated fingertips (Letter to the Editor), PRS, 51:328, 1973

GRUBER, R. P., KAPLAN, E. N., AND LUCAS, Z. J.: Skin homografts in rats compared to other organ transplantations. PRS, 53:64, 1974

GRUBER, R. P., LAUB, D. R., AND VISTNES, L. M.: Effect of hydrotherapy on clinical course and pH of experimental cutaneous chemical burns. PRS, 55:200, 1975

GRUBER, R. P., VISTNES, L., AND PARDOE, R.: Effect of commonly used antiseptics on wound healing. PRS, 55:472, 1975

GRUNDY, D. J.: Sjogren's disease with widespread lymphoid deposits. Proc. Roy. Soc. Med., 65:167, 1972

GRUNEBERG, R., AND SPENCE, A. J.: Finger amputations and ability to work, PRS, 56:227, 1975. Hand, 6:236, 1974

GRUNEBERG, V.: Preoperative cytostasis of extensive flat epithelial cancer of the tongue and floor of the mouth. Acta Stomatol. Belg., 72:437, 1975 (German)

GRUNER, O. P.: Skin grafting in ulcerating "cancer en cuirasse" – case report. Acta Chir.

Scand., 139:492, 1973

GRUSS, J. S.: Haemangioma of the mandible: a case report. Brit. J. Oral Surg., 12:24, 1974

GRUT, A.: Lesions caused by high pressure syringes. Ugeskr. Laeger., 136:934, 1974 (Danish)

GRYCZYNSKI, M.: Myxomas of frontal sinus. Pol. Tyg. Lek., 27:1315, 1972 (Polish)

GSCHWEND, N.: Results with silastic fingerprostheses in chronic progressive polyarthritis. Handchirurgie, 1:205, 1969 (German)

GSCHWEND, N. et al: Wrist joint of the patient with polyarthritis; problems in surgical treatment. Handchirurgie, 1:209, 1969 (German)

GSELL, F.: Reduction mammaplasty for extremely large breasts. PRS, 53:643, 1974

GUBA, A. M., JR., MULLIKEN, J. B., AND HOOPES, J. E.: Selection of antibiotics for human bites of hand. PRS, 56:538, 1975

GUCKIAN, J. C.: Complications of antimicrobial therapy, PRS, 53:374, 1974. Fam. Phys., 8:111, 1973

GUDURIC, A. et al: Analysis of bacteriological cultures in tracheostomized patients. Med. Pregl., 28:385, 1975 (Serbian)

GUERNSEY, L. H.: Free mucosal grafts in major reconstructive oral surgery. Trans. Int. Conf. Oral Surg., 4:198, 1973

GUERNSEY, L. H.: Stability of treatment results in class II malocclusion corrected by full mandibular advancement surgery. Oral Surg., 37:668, 1974

GUERRA, O. N.: Prosthetic management of surgically induced defects of the palate. Mo. Med., 71:690, 1974

GUERRERO PALACIOS, F.: Cancer of the mouth floor and gingiva. An. Esp. Odontoestomatol., 34:421, 1975 (Spanish)

GUERRERO-SANTOS, J.: Cosmetic repair of acute columellar-lip angle. PRS, 52:246, 1973

GUERRERO-SANTOS, J., AND RAMIREZ, M.: Cleft lip repair. Use of denuded vermilion flap, PRS, 48:197, 1971. Rev. Sanatorio Guadalajara, 3:125, 1970

GUERRERO-SANTOS, J., RAMIREZ, M., AND ESPAILLAT, L.: Treatment of facial paralysis by static suspension with dermal flaps. PRS, 48:325, 1971

GUERRERO-SANTOS, J. et al: Crossed denuded flap as complement to Millard technique in correction of cleft lip. PRS, 48:506, 1971

GUERRERO-SANTOS, J. et al: Surgical treatment of axillary hyperhidrosis, PRS, 49:588, 1972. Rev. San. Guadalajara, 4:49, 1971

GUERRERO-SANTOS, J. et al: Combined neurovascular pedicle and cross finger flap in thumb and index finger: a case report. J. Trauma, 12:440, 1972

GUERRERO-SANTOS, J., RAMIREZ, M., AND RI-
VERA, R.: Making permanent dimple in chin.
PRS, *50:*88, 1972

GUERRERO-SANTOS, J., RAMIREZ, M., AND ES-
PAILLAT, L.: Cervicofacial rhytidoplasty,
PRS, *51:*474, 1973. Rev. Latino Am. cir.
plast., *16:*31, 1972

GUERRERO-SANTOS, J., AND SANDOVAL, M.:
Plastic surgery on facial paralysis, PRS,
*53:*108, 1974. Rev. San. Guadalajara, *5:*55,
1972

GUERRERO-SANTOS, J. *et al*: Further experience
with tongue flap in cleft palate repair. Cleft
Palate J., *10:*192, 1973

GUERRERO-SANTOS, J., MATUS, R., AND VERA-
STRATHMANN, A.: Correction of alopecia of
eyebrows in leprous patients (Follow-up
Clinic). PRS, *52:*183, 1973

GUERRERO-SANTOS, J., ESPAILLAT, L., AND MO-
RALES, F.: Muscular lift in cervical rhytidoplasty. PRS, *54:*127, 1974

GUIBOR, P.: Lacrimal drain. Trans. Am. Acad.
Ophthalmol. Otolaryngol., *79:*OP417, 1975

GUIBOR, P.: Canaliculus intubation set. Trans.
Am. Acad. Ophthalmol. Otolaryngol.,
*79:*OP419, 1975

GUIBOR, P.: Surgical reconstruction of complications associated with fronto-ethmoid mucocele surgery. Trans. Am. Acad. Ophthalmol.
Otolaryngol., *80:*454, 1975

GUIBOR, P., AND SMITH, B.: *Contemporary
Oculoplastic Surgery*. Grune & Stratton Inc.,
New York, 1974

GUIBOR, P., AND SMITH, B.: Surgical correction
of severe cicatricial ectropion caused by
chickenpox, PRS, *55:*633, 1975. Arch. Ophth.,
*92:*307, 1974

GUIDA, C. A., PICCHI, A., AND INZIRILLO, S.:
Laparocele: advantages of lipectomy added to
laparocele's treatment, PRS, *56:*465, 1975.
Riv. ital. chir. plast., *5:*445, 1973

GUIDA, C. A., PICCHI, A., AND INZIRILLO, S.:
Areola and nipple reconstruction. PRS,
*56:*454, 1975

GUILLAMONDEGUI, O. M. *et al*: Aggressive surgery in treatment for parotid cancer: the role
of adjunctive postoperative radiotherapy.
Am. J. Roentgenol. Radium Ther. Nucl.
Med., *123:*49, 1975

GUILLEMIN, P., AND PARIETTI, R.: Presentation
of case of Fournier's disease with favorable
course, with cutaneous plasty. J. Urol. Nephrol. (Paris), *78:*703, 1972 (French)

GUIMARAES, S. B. *et al*: Thyroglossal duct remnants in infants and children. Mayo Clin.
Proc., *47:*117, 1972

GUIMBERTEAU, J-C.: Ten free groin flaps (with
Baudet, LeMaire). PRS, *57:*577, 1976

GUINEE, W. S.: Prolonged endotracheal intuba-

tion versus tracheostomy in infants and children. J. Arkansas Med. Soc., *68:*259, 1972

GULIAEV, G. V. *et al*: Effect of premedication
with droperidol, atropine, and promedol on
basic indices of blood circulation in patients
with tumors of the head and neck. Vestn.
Akad. Med. Nauk., *0:*65, 1974 (Russian)

GUMP, F. E., AND KINNEY, J. M.: Energy balance and weight loss in burned patients,
PRS, *49:*666, 1972. Arch. Surg., *103:*442, 1971

GUMPORT, S. L., AND HARRIS, M. N.: Results of
regional lymph node dissection for melanoma, PRS, *54:*243, 1974. Ann. Surg.,
*179:*105, 1974

GUNDROVA, R. A.: Plastic surgery of lower eyelid in partial defect or its absence. Oftalmol.
Zh., *28:*483, 1973 (Russian)

Gunshot Wounds

Ballistic injury to extremities, serum enzymes in experimental (Lawson *et al*),
PRS, *50:*423, 1972. Arch. Surg., *103:*741,
1971

Shotgun wounds, mechanism of (DeMuth),
PRS, *49:*475, 1972. J. Trauma, *11:*219, 1971

Facial injuries caused by shot wounds (Pons
et al). Rev. Stomatol. Chir. Maxillofac.,
*72:*743, 1971 (French)

Firearm wounds of the head and neck (Landeen). Eye Ear Nose Throat Mon., *51:* 222,
1972

Immediate management of facial gunshot
wounds: report of case (Cuttino *et al*). J.
Oral Surg., *30:*674, 1972

Gunshot wounds of face: initial care (Broadbent, Woolf), PRS, *52:*107, 1973. J.
Trauma, *12:*229, 1972

Gunshot wounds of face (Yao *et al*), PRS,
*52:*107, 1973. J. Trauma, *12:*523, 1972

Gunshot wounds, therapy of (Fischer).
Munch. Med. Wochenschr., *114:*1731, 1972

Shotgun wounds to extremities with vascular
injury treated with split thickness porcine
grafts (Ledgerwod, Lucas), PRS, *53:*249,
1974. Am. J. Surg., *125:*690, 1973

Head and neck, shotgun wounds to (May *et
al*). Arch. Otolaryng., *98:*373, 1973

Maxillofacial missile wounds, intermediate
and reconstructive care of (Osbon). J. Oral
Surg., *31:*429, 1973

Maxillofacial region, air-gun injuries in
(Matic *et al*). Vojnosanit. Pregl., *30:*561,
1973 (Serbian)

Maxillofacial injury, severe, suicidal gunshot
wounds resulting in (Nordenram *et al*).
Int. J. Oral Surg., *3:*29, 1974

Gunshot wounds of the face in peacetime
(Khomenko *et al*). Voen. Med. Zh., *2:*18,
1974 (Russian)

Gunshot Wounds — Cont.

Surgical therapy of gunshot and explosion injuries (Hammer *et al*). Fortschir. Kiefer. Gesichtschir., *19:*211, 1975 (German)

Management of shotgun wound of the symphysis (Lucas *et al*). J. Oral Surg., *33:*622, 1975

Shotgun injuries of face, surgical management (Kersten, McQuarrie), PRS, *56:*605, 1975. Surg. Gynec. & Obst., *140:*517, 1975

GUNTER, J. P.: Nasal reconstruction using pedicle skin flaps. Otolaryngol. Clin. North Am., *5:*457, 1972

GUNTER, J. P.: Revision of scars of head and neck. Otolaryngol. Clin. North Am., *7:*119, 1974

GUNTHER, H.: Combination injuries of the thumb. Handchirurgie, *2:*40, 1970 (German)

GUPTA, D. S.: Double palate, PRS, *57:*537, 1976. Oral Surg., *40:*53, 1975

GUPTA, O. P.: Nasopharyngeal fibroma with extrapharyngeal extensions. Acta Otolaryngol. (Stockh.), *71:*406, 1971

GUPTA, O. P. *et al*: Primary malignant melanoma of mouth. Indian J. Cancer, *8:*286, 1971

GUPTA, R. K., AND MORTON, D. L.: Suggestive evidence for *in vivo* binding of specific antitumor antibodies of human melanomas, PRS, *55:*641, 1975. Cancer Res., *35:*58, 1975

GUPTA, S. C.: Investigation into method for removal of dermal tattoos: report on animal and clinical experiments (Follow-Up Clinic). PRS, *50:*401, 1972

GUPTA, S. C. *et al*: Dermoid cyst of head, face, and neck, PRS, *54:*377, 1974. Indian M. Gaz., *12:*557, 1973

GURALNICK, WALTER C.: *Textbook of Oral Surgery*. Little, Brown & Co., Boston, 1968.

GURALNICK, W. C.: Letter: Who treats facial fractures? J. Trauma, *14:*990, 1974

GURALNICK, W. C.: Varaztad H. Kazanjian, M.D. New England J. Med., *292:*806, 1975

GURALNICK, W. C. *et al*: Myxoma of mandible: resection and immediate reconstruction. Brit. J. Oral Surg., *11:*217, 1974

GURDIN, M. M.: Honorary award of American Society for Aesthetic Plastic Surgery to Dr. Gustave Aufricht. PRS, *49:*70, 1972

GURDIN, M. M.: What's new in esthetic surgery? (Editorial). PRS, *49:*448, 1972

GURDIN, M. M.: Yesterday, today, and tomorrow (Presidential Address). PRS, *53:*255, 1974

GURDIN, M. M.: Should the subcutaneous tissue be plicated in a face lift? (Letter to the Editor). PRS, *55:*84, 1975

GUR'IANOVA, M. P.: Prosthesis on operating table after amputation in patients with ma-lignant tumors of extremities. Ortop. Travmatol. Protez., *34:*14, 1973 (Russian)

GUROVICDE CIOLA, E.: How to impede collapse of posterior mandibular resection, clinical case. Trib. Odontol. (B. Aires), *57:*318, 1973 (Spanish)

GURUCHARRI, V., HENZEL, J. H., AND MITCHELL, F. L.: Doppler flowmeter to monitor peripheral bloodflow during edema stage of snakebite. PRS, *53:*551, 1974

GUSAREV, V. F.: Plastic surgery of skin in treatment of cicatricial contractures and its morphological foundation. Ortop. Travmatol. Protez., *34:*61, 1973 (Russian)

GUSEV, E. P.: Simplified method of suturing in fractures of mandible. Stomatologiia (Mosk.), *51:*86, 1972 (Russian)

GUTHRIE, R. H., JR: Breast reconstruction after radical mastectomy. PRS, *57:*14, 1976

GUTHRIE, R. H., JR., GOULIAN, D., JR., AND CUCIN, R. L.: Predicting the extent of viability in flaps by measurement of gas tensions, using a mass spectrometer. PRS, *50:*385, 1972

GUTHRIE, R. H., JR. *et al*: Decubitus ulcers: prevention and treatment. Geriatrics, *28:*67, 1973

GUTHRIE, R. H., JR. *et al*: Pharyngostome repairs. Surg. Clin. North Am., *54:*767, 1974

GUTHRIE, R. H. *et al*: Silicone elastomer sheeting in development of pedicle flaps, PRS, *57:*404, 1976. Arch. Otolaryng., *101:*89, 1975

GUTJAHR, R. *et al*: Fibrosarcoma: problematic diagnosis in childhood. H.N.O., *22:*181, 1974 (German)

GUTMAN, D.: Mandibular bone grafting in trauma. Int. J. Oral Surg., *1:*103, 1972

GUTMAN, D. *et al*: Moebius' syndrome. Surgical management of case. Brit. J. Oral Surg., *11:*20, 1973

GUTMANN, J. *et al*: Angiomyoma of oral cavity. Oral Surg., *38:*269, 1974

GUTTENBERG, S. A.: Osteoradionecrosis of jaw, PRS, *54:*499, 1974. Am. J. Surg., *127:*326, 1974

GUTTERMAN, J. U. *et al*: Active immunotherapy with BCG for recurrent malignant melanoma. Lancet, *1:*1208, 1973

GUTTSCHES, O.: Functional anatomy of the forearm and the hand. Med. Klin., *66:*568, 1971 (German)

GUY, C. L.: Use of inflatable breast implants (with Rees, Coburn). PRS, *52:*609, 1973

GUZMAN FREIRE, J. E. *et al*: Arteriovenous fistula of anterior facial vessels: review of literature and report of case. J. Oral Surg., *32:*150, 1974

GWIEZDZINSKI, Z. *et al*: Squamous cell carcinoma in discoid lupus erythematosus. Przegl. Dermatol., *59:*37, 1972 (Polish)

Gynecomastia

H

Surgical enigma of gynecomastia (Walker). J. Natl. Med. Assoc., *63:*385, 1971

Gynecomastia (Badim *et al*), PRS, *51:*103, 1973. Rev. brasil. cir., *61:*141, 1971

Gynecomastia, prepubertal male (August, Chandra, Hung), PRS, *52:*679, 1973. J. Pediat., *80:*259, 1972

Gynecomastia, massive, surgical correction.(Letterman, Schurter). PRS, *49:*259, 1972

Gynecomastia, surgical treatment of (Barbarelli), PRS, *53:*242, 1974. Prensa med. argent., *59:*1188, 1972

Pathogenetic therapy of dyshormonal hyperplasia of male breast (Sidorenko *et al*). Vopr. Onkol., *18:*27, 1972 (Russian)

Gynecomastia, idiopathic, in seven preadolescent boys. Elevation of urinary estrogen excretion in two cases (Latorre *et al*). Am. J. Dis. Child., *126:*771, 1973

Gynecomastia, left-side idiopathic, in twenty-eight-month-old boy (Wiedemann *et al*). Helv. Paediatr. Acta, *28:*413, 1972 (German)

Gynecomastia, classification and surgical correction of (Simon, Hoffman, Kahn). PRS, *51:*48, 1973

Gynecomastia in puberty (Letter) (Bettex *et al*). Anaesthesiol. Intensivmed. Prax., *9:*114, 1974 (German)

Gynecomastia, extreme, correction of (Wray, Hoopes, Davis), PRS, *56:*677, 1975. Brit. J. Plast. Surg., *27:*39, 1974

Gynecomastia (Hussey). J.A.M.A., *228:*1423, 1974

Gynecomastia, significance of (Wehby, Salti), PRS, *56:*677, 1975. Lebanese M. J., *27:*719, 1974

Gynecomastia excisions, radial incision for (Eade), PRS, *54:*495, 1974

Surgical treatment of gynecomastia (Bretteville-Jensen). Brit. J. Plast. Surg., *28:*177, 1975

Gynecomastia (Hamer). Brit. J. Surg., *62:*326, 1975

Gynecomastia (Kabza *et al*). Wiad. Lek., *28:*1859, 1975 (Polish)

GYORY, G. *et al*: Morphologic changes and cytologically determined hormonal effects in the artificial vagina constructed from large intestine. Zentralbl. Gynekol., *93:*1121, 1971 (German)

GYURKO, G., AND CZEKELNIK, R.: Modified vascular anastomosis with invagination, PRS, *54:*622, 1974. Bruns' Beitr. klin. Chir., *221:*70, 1974

HAANAES, H. R.: Radiographic and clinical follow-up study of 150 oroantral communications. Int. J. Oral Surg., *3:*412, 1974

HAANAES, H. R. *et al*: Treatment of oroantral communication. Int. J. Oral Surg., *3:*124, 1974

HAANAES, H. R. *et al*: Oral antrostomy. Int. J. Oral Surg., *4:*55, 1975

HAAS, E.: Experiences with silastic in plastic surgery of the face. Z. Laryngol. Rhinol. Otol., *50:*751, 1971 (German)

HAAS, E.: Plastic surgery of face—a medical problem? Z. Laryngol. Rhinol. Otol., *52:*79, 1973 (German)

HAAS, E.: Esthetic, functional and anatomic viewpoint in rhinoplasties. Z. Laryngol. Rhinol. Otol., *52:*235, 1973 (German)

HAAS, E.: General points in rhinoplasty. Z. Laryngol. Rhinol. Otol., *52:*405, 1973 (German)

HAAS, E.: Correction of deformities of nasal bones; special care to avoid technical errors. Z. Laryngol. Rhinol. Otol., *52:*590, 1973 (German)

HAAS, E.: Problems particular to correction of bony or bony-chondral saddle nose. Z. Laryngol. Rhinol. Otol., *52:*866, 1973 (German)

HAAS, E.: Surgery of anomalies of position and shape of pinna. Laryngol. Rhinol. Otol. (Stuttg.), *53:*93, 1974 (German)

HAAS, E.: Suture techniques, scars and their correction. Laryngol. Rhinol. Otol. (Stuttg.), *53:*234, 1974 (German)

HAAS, E.: Principles of reconstructive operations on the face using flaps and free grafts. Laryngol. Rhinol. Otol., *53:*371, 1974 (German)

HAAS, E.: Reconstruction of nasal defects. Laryngol. Rhinol. Otol. (Stuttg.), *53:*530, 1974 (German)

HAAS, E.: Repair of defects in the cheeks and lips. Laryngol. Rhinol. Otol. (Stuttg.), *53:*695, 1974 (German)

HAAS, H. G.: Indications for intra-vital staining in surgery of the hand. Handchirurgie, *3:*135, 1971 (German)

HAAS, R. L.: Trigeminal neuralgia revisited. Trans. Int. Conf. Oral Surg., *4:*184, 1973

HABAL, M. B.: Further experiences with arytenoid-epiglottic flap for chronic aspiration pneumonia (with Vecchione, Murray), PRS, *55:*318, 1975

HABAL, M. B.: On the cutaneous porcine heterograft (Editorial), PRS, *57:*367, 1976

HABAL, M. B. *et al*: Mediastinal emphysema secondary to fracture of orbital floor. Am. J. Surg., *123:*606, 1972

HABAL, M. B., AND MURRAY, J. E.: Natural history of benign locally-invasive hemangioma of orbital region, PRS, *49:*209, 1972

HABAL, M. B., AND MURRAY, J. E.: Surgical treatment of life-endangering chronic aspiration pneumonia. Use of epiglottic flap to arytenoids, PRS, *49:*305, 1972

HABAL, M. B., SNYDER, H. H., JR., AND MURRAY, J.: Chondrosarcoma of hand, PRS, *53:*244, 1974. Am. J. Surg., *125:*775, 1973

HABAL, M. B. *et al*: Orbital reconstruction after radical resection. Ann. chir. plast., *18:*183, 1973 (French)

HABAL, M. B., AND MURRAY, J. E.: Orbital reconstruction after radical resection, PRS, *52:*205, 1973. Arch. Surg., *106:*353, 1973

HABAL, M. B., AND MURRAY, J. E.: Cranioorbital resection and neck dissection for recurrent mixed tumor of lacrimal gland, PRS, *51:*689, 1973

HABAL, M. B., AND MARDAM-BEY, O. H.: Noninvasive electrometric detection of nasal escape in patients with rhinophonia, PRS, *55:*386, 1975. Cleft Palate J., *11:*209, 1974

HABAL, M. B. *et al*: Experience with prefabricated silicone implants for reconstruction in facially deformed patients. J. Prosthet. Dent., *32:*292, 1974

HABAL, M. B., AND JOBE, R. P.: On lid loading in management of lagophthalmos (Letter to the Editor), PRS, *54:*211, 1974

HABAL, M. B., AND CHASET, R. B.: Infraciliary transconjunctival approach to orbital floor for correction of traumatic lesions, PRS, *55:*245, 1975. Surg. Gynec. & Obst., *139:*420, 1974

HABAL, M. B. *et al*: The "turban" nevoid basal cell syndrome. Current management with surgery, chemotherapy and immunotherapy. Int. Surg., *60:*493, 1975

HABERMAN, H. *et al*: An isolated mucocele of the frontal sinus. Acta Otorhinolaryngol. Belg., *29:*607, 1975 (French)

HACKETT, M. *et al*: Preliminary report on comparative use of lyophilized homograft and xenograft in closure of raw areas. Brit. J. Surg., *61:*427, 1974

HACKETT, M. E.: Cadaver homografts, PRS, *50:*202, 1972. Proc. Roy. Soc. Med., *64:*1291, 1971

HADDOW, J. E. *et al*: Streptococcal wound infection with evidence of widespread tissue involvement. Pediatrics, *48:*458, 1971

HAEGER, K.: Treatment of the post-thrombotic state in elderly patients. Zentralbl. Phlebol., *10:*178, 1971

HAFF, R. C. *et al*: Trends in current management of primary hyperparathyroidism. Surgery, *75:*715, 1974

HAGEMAN, R. *et al*: Surgical repair of intratem-

poral posttraumatic lesions of facial nerve. Acta Chir. Belg., *73:*653, 1974 (Dutch)

HAGERT, C. C.: New joint prosthesis in hand surgery. Nord. Med., *85:*513, 1971 (Swedish)

HAGERTY, R. F., AND MYLIN, W. K.: Cleft lip and palate, PRS, *53:*490, 1974. Contemp. Surg., *3:*44, 1973

HAGERTY, R. F. *et al*: Resection of massive abdominal pannicular adiposus, PRS, *55:*108, 1975. South. M. J., *67:*984, 1974

HAGERTY, R. F. *et al*: Advancement rotation flap for cancer of skin of nose. Surg. Gynec. & Obst., *138:*429, 1974

HAGOOD, C. O., JR., MOZERSKY, D. J., AND FITE, F. W.: Staged palliative resection of recurrent carcinoma of neck using extra anatomic carotid bypass, PRS, *56:*113, 1975. Surgery, *76:*671, 1974

HAGSTROM, W. J., JR.: Use of hemostatic agent as definitive dressing in management of donor sites in partial thickness skin grafting (Follow-Up Clinic), PRS, *51:*89, 1973

HAGSTROM, W. J., BROWN, J. V., AND LANDA, S. J. F.: Small tubed flap for cylindrical defects in leg, "cork" procedure, PRS, *49:*224, 1972

HAHN, M. J. *et al*: Hemangiopericytoma – ultrastructural study, PRS, *51:*707, 1973. Cancer, *31:*255, 1973

Hair (See also *Alopecia*)

Hair, gray, occurring after treatment with Vitamin E (Sehgal), PRS, *53:*502, 1974. Dermatologica, *145:*56, 1972

Hair patterning, scalp, as clue to early fetal brain development (Smith, Gong), PRS, *54:*370, 1974. J. Pediat., *83:*374, 1973

Hair transplantation to upper lip to create moustache (Vallis), PRS, *54:*606, 1974

Hair transplantation, tissue adhesive as an adjunct (Wilkinson, Iglesias), PRS, *56:*103, 1975. South. M. J., *67:*1408, 1974

Hair dyes, percutaneous penetration following use of (Maibach, Leaffer, Skinner), PRS, *57:*681, 1976. Arch. Dermat., *111:*1444, 1975

Sideburn relationship in male face-lift (Sturman), PRS, *57:*248, 1976

HAISOVA, L., AND MAZANEK, J.: Anesthesia with Ketalar in oral, jaw and facial surgery. Cesk. Stomatol., *73:*24, 1973 (Czechoslovakian)

HAISOVA, L. *et al*: Gerontology in mandibular and facial surgery. Cesk. Stomatol., *74:*42, 1974 (Czechoslovakian)

HAIT, M. R.: Microcrystalline collagen: new hemostatic agent, PRS, *48:*298, 1971. Am. J. Surg., *120:*330, 1970

HAJEK, S.: Values of LA 50 in patients with

burns of various age groups, PRS, *54:*506, 1974. Acta chir. plast., *15:*162, 1973

HAJEK, S. *et al*: Death causes after burns, PRS, *50:*201, 1972. Acta chir. plast., *12:*78, 1971

HAJEK, S., VRABEC, R., AND TOPINKA, H.: Fatal thermal accident in old people, PRS, *55:*639, 1975. Acta chir. plast., *16:*164, 1974

HAJNIS, K., AND FIGALOVA, P.: Shape of nose in cheilo-gnatho-palatoschisis unilateralis before operational repair, PRS, *53:*681, 1974. Acta chir. plast., *15:*11, 1973

HAJNIS, K. *et al*: Contribution to the assessment of the pre-operative condition of the nose in patients with palatoschisis. Acta chir. plast. (Praha), *16:*1, 1974

HAKELIUS, L.: Transplantation of free autogenous muscle in the treatment of facial paralysis. A clinical study. Scand. J. Plast. Reconstr. Surg., *8:*220, 1974

HAKELIUS, L. *et al*: Results of immediate and delayed surgical treatment of facial fractures with diplopia. J. Maxillo-facial Surg., *1:*150, 1973

HAKELIUS, L. *et al*: Electromyographical studies of free autogenous muscle transplants in man. Scand. J. Plast. Reconstr. Surg., *8:*211, 1974

HAKSTIAN, R. W.: Cold-induced digital epiphyseal necrosis in childhood (symmetric fecal ischemic necrosis), PRS, *50:*631, 1972. Canad. J. Surg., *15:*168, 1972

HAKSTIAN, R. W.: Perineural neurorrhaphy. Orthop. Clin. North Am., *4:*945, 1973

HAKSTIAN, R. W.: Microsurgery. Its role in surgery of the hand. Clin. Orthop., *0:*149, 1974

HAKSTIAN, R. W.: Vascular and neural microsurgery (applications to surgery of the hand). Union Med. Can., *103:*1750, 1974 (French)

HAKUBA, A.: Surgical treatment for a glomus jugulare tumor – report of a case growing extensively. A. Neurol. Surg. (Tokyo), *2:*403, 1974 (Japanese)

HALASA, A. H. *et al*: Tarsotomy for correction of cicatricial entropion. Ann. Ophth., *6:*837, 1974

HALL, B. D.: Aglossia-adactylia. Birth Defects, *7:*233, 1971

HALL, C. A.: Fiberoptic endoscopy in head and neck region (with Dellon, Chretien), PRS, *55:*466, 1975

HALL, H. D.: Vestibuloplasty, mucosal grafts (palatal and buccal). J. Oral Surg., *29:*786, 1971

HALL, H. D. *et al*: Treatment of maxillary alveolar hyperplasia by total maxillary alveolar osteotomy. J. Oral Surg., *33:*180, 1975

HALL, H. D. *et al*: Evaluation and refinement of intraoral vertical subcondylar osteotomy. J. Oral Surg., *33:*333, 1975

HALL, H. D. *et al*: Combined anterior and posterior maxillary osteotomy. J. Oral Surg., *34:*126, 1976

HALL, K. V.: Mortality and causes of death in burned patients treated by exposure method (with Sørensen), PRS, *51:*59, 1973

HALL, K. V., AND SØRENSEN, B.: Treatment of burn shock; comparative controlled trial of treatment by colloid infusion (Dextran-saline) and by exclusively electrolyte infusion (Ringer-lactate), PRS, *53:*491, 1974. Scand. J. Plast. Reconstr. Surg., 7:67, 1973

HALL, M. D.: Mandibular condylectomy with silicone rubber replacement (with Hartwell), PRS, *53:*440, 1974

HALL, ROBERT M.: *Facial, Oral, and Reconstructive Surgery.* Vol. 3. Springer-Verlag, New York, 1973

HALL, T.: Use of cancer chemotherapeutic agents in non-neoplastic diseases, PRS, *54:*114, 1974. Cancer, *31:*1256, 1973

HALLEN, O. *et al*: Suction flow drainage in head and neck surgery. New principle for postoperative suction drainage. Ann. Otol. Rhin. & Laryng., *82:*370, 1973

HALMOS, J.: Surgical treatment of progenia and associated open occlusion using technic of vertical osteotomy of ramus mandibulae. Cesk. Stomatol., *75:*83, 1975 (Slovakian)

HALVERSON, J. D. *et al*: Cystosarcoma phylloides of breast. Am. Surg., *40:*295, 1974

HALVOVA, M.: Experience with operations of maxillary cysts. Cesk. Stomatol., *73:*12, 1973 (Czechoslovakian)

HAM, F. J.: Free vascularized bone graft (with Taylor, Miller), PRS, *55:*533, 1975

HAM, F. J.: Free vascularized nerve graft (with Taylor), PRS, *57:*413, 1976

HAMAKER, R. C., AND CONLEY, J.: Modified non-delayed forehead flap, PRS, *57:*680, 1976. Arch. Otolaryng., *101:*189, 1975

HAMAL, P. B.: Leiomyosarcoma of penis – case report and review of literature, PRS, *57:*120, 1976. Brit. J. Urol., *47:*319, 1975

HAMATAKE, Y.: Clinical studies of congenital angiodysplasias in limbs. An analysis of 123 cases. Fukuoka Acta Med., *65:*833, 1974 (Japanese)

HAMBRAEUS, A. *et al*: Control by ventilation of airborne bacterial transfer between hospital patients, and its assessment by means of a particle tracer. 3. Studies with an airborne-particle tracer in an isolation ward for burned patients. J. Hyg. (Camb.), *70:*299, 1972

HAMBY, W. B.: Orbital decompression for exophthalmos. Clin. Neurosurg., *17:*18, 1970

HAMER, D. B.: Gynecomastia. Brit. J. Surg., *62:*326, 1975

HAMILTON, D. N. et al: Cell-mediated and humoral mechanisms in allograft and xenograft skin rejection. Brit. J. Surg., 58:858, 1971

HAMILTON, G. F.: Comprehensive management of the patient following hand injury and surgery. Prog. Phys. Ther., 1:176, 1970

HAMILTON, J. M.: Use of Webb bolt as space maintaining appliance in defects of mandible, PRS, 48:368, 1971

HAMILTON, J. M.: Rhytidectomy in the male, PRS, 53:629, 1974

HAMILTON, R., AND LaROSSA, D.: Method for repair of cleft earlobes, PRS, 55:99, 1975

HAMILTON, R. et al: Role of the lip adhesion procedure in cleft lip repair. Cleft Palate J., 8:1, 1971

HAMILTON, R. F., FOLEY, J. F., AND DAVIS, W. C.: Difficulties in diagnosing melanoma, PRS, 53:497, 1974. Contemp. Surg., 3:65, 1973

HAMILTON, W. C. et al: Osseous xanthoma and multiple hand tumors as a complication of hyperlipidemia. Report of a case. J. Bone & Joint Surg. (Am.), 57:551, 1975

HAMM, W. G.: Reduction mammaplasty by the Dufourmentel-Mouly method (with Schatten, Hartley), PRS, 48:306, 1971

HAMMER, U. et al: Surgical therapy of gunshot and explosion injuries. Fortschr. Kiefer. Gesichtschir. 19:211, 1975 (German)

HAMONET, C. et al: Myoelectric controlled orthosis for paralytic hand. Ann. Chir., 27:541, 1973 (French)

HAMONET, C. et al: Myoelectric-controlled orthosis, PRS, 56:596, 1975. Hand, 7:63, 1975

HAMPL, P. F. et al: Squamous cell carcinoma possibly arising from odontogenic cyst: report of case. J. Oral Surg., 31:359, 1973

HAMZA, K. N., AND DenBESTEN, L.: Bile salts producing stress ulcers during experimental shock, PRS, 50:100, 1972. Surgery, 71:161, 1972

HAN, S. H. et al: Prolonged survival of skin allografts in leprosy patients. Int. J. Lepr., 39:1, 1971

HANADA, K. et al: Longitudinal study of postoperative changes in the soft-tissue profile in bilateral cleft lip and palate from birth to 6 years. Am. J. Orthod., 67:363, 1975

Hands

Hand. By Guy Pulvertaft. Ed. by C. Rob and R. Smith. J. B. Lippincott Co., Philadelphia, 1970

Strength of the hand (Swanson et al). Bull. Prosthet. Res., 10:145, 1970

Education (Barron). Hand, 2:6, 1970

Anesthesia for hand surgery (Abadir). Orthop. Clin. North Am., 1:205, 1970

Hands – Cont.

Treatment of the stiff hand (Adamson). Orthop. Clin. North Am., 1:467, 1970

Hand: Pain and Impairment. By Rene Cailliet. F. A. Davis Co., Philadelphia, 1971. PRS, 49:452, 1972

The Hand. By Lee Milford, C. V. Mosby Co., St. Louis, 1971. PRS, 49:338, 1972

Symposium on the Hand, Volume III. Ed. by Lester M. Cramer and Robert A. Chase. C. V. Mosby Co., St. Louis, 1971. PRS, 50:610, 1972

Basic problems in the restoration of prehension (Rabischong). Ann. Chir., 25:927, 1971 (French)

Function of "normal" hand in stroke patients (Jebsen et al). Arch. Phys. Med. Rehabil., 52:170, 1971

Hand, in Maffuci syndrome (Howard, Lee), PRS, 50:307, 1972. Arch. Surg., 103:752, 1971

Note on skeletal lesions in scleroderma with three case reports (Campailla et al). Bull. Hosp. Joint Dis., 32:100, 1971

Editorial: the British Society for Surgery of the Hand (McKenzie). Hand, 3:7, 1971

Functional stimulation of disabled limbs (Chandler et al). Hand, 3:15, 1971

Fasciotomy, enzymic (Hueston), PRS, 48:512, 1971. Hand, 3:38, 1971

Hand table, useful (Prendiville), PRS, 48:519, 1971. Hand, 3:114, 1971

Long-acting conduction anesthesia in surgery of the hand (Achatzy). Handchirurgie, 3:119, 1971 (German)

Diabetic hand syndrome (Jung et al). Metabolism, 20:1008, 1971

How dextrous was Neanderthal man? (Musgrave). Nature (Lond.), 233:538, 1971

Bacteroides necrotizing fasciitis of upper extremity (Rein, Cosman), PRS, 48:592, 1971

Evaluation of Orenzyme in the prevention of swelling after hand surgery (Salisbury). Rev. Surg., 28:455, 1971

Motion, kinesiological recording with particular emphasis on electrogoniometers (Ebskov), PRS, 49:583, 1972. Scand. J. Plast. Reconstr. Surg., 5:96, 1971

Digital pain, hyperplastic Pacinian corpuscles cause of (Hart et al), PRS, 49:357, 1972. Surgery, 70:730, 1971

Influence of modern connective tissue biology upon surgery of the hand (Peacock). Surg. Annu., 3:249, 1971

Examination of the Hand. By George L. Lucas. Charles C Thomas, Springfield, Ill., 1972. PRS, 53:467, 1974

Cancer, visceral, palmar keratoses and (Gilbertsen, Bean, Fusaro), PRS, 50:205, 1972.

Hands — Cont.

Arch. Dermat., *105:*222, 1972

Occupational diseases of the milker's hand (Riboldi *et al*). Berufsdermatosen, *20:*166, 1972 (German)

Hand function — a practical method of assessment (Dickson *et al*). Brit. J. Surg., *59:*316, 1972

Use of brachial plexus anesthesia in hand surgery (Garstka). Chir. Narzadow. Ruchu Ortop. Pol., *37:*599, 1972 (Polish)

Fingers were made before forks (Moberg). Hand, *4:*201, 1972

Assessment of hand function. 1. Measurement of individual digits (Dickson *et al*). Hand, *4:*207, 1972

Findings of infrared thermography in hand surgery (Koob *et al*). Handchirurgie, *4:*123, 1972 (German)

Pathogenesis of extremity deformity in leprosy. A pathologic study on large sections of amputated extremities in relation to radiological appearance (Skinsnes *et al*). Int. J. Lepr., *40:*375, 1972

Nonsurgical aspects of surgery of hand (Kahn *et al*). N. Y. State J. Med., *72:*2201, 1972

Easy-to-make hand exerciser (Evans). Phys. Ther., *52:*854, 1972

Documentation of hand function with the use of office copying equipment (Metcalf *et al*). Phys. Ther., *52:*935, 1972

The Hand Book. By Moulton K. Johnson. Charles C Thomas, Springfield, Ill., 1973. PRS, *53:*343, 1974

Hand, radial, dorsal, and volar compartments, stenosing vaginitis of (Fara, Hrivnakova, Dobias), PRS, *53:*606, 1974. Acta chir. plast., *15:*93, 1973

Joints, artificial, in experiments (Barinka *et al*), PRS, *53:*500, 1974. Acta chir. plast., *15:*104, 1973

Use of an external tutor in hand surgery (Allieu *et al*). Acta Orthop. Belg., *39:*988, 1973 (French)

Positions for immobilization of the hand (Tubiana). Ann. Chir., *27:*459, 1973 (French)

Evaluation of hand function in children (Taylor *et al*). Arch. Phys. Med. Rehabil., *54:*378, 1973

Limb, upper, biomechanical aspects of tourniquet (Griffiths, Heywood), PRS, *54:*236, 1974. Hand, *5:*113, 1973

Calcinosis circumscripta of the hand in scleroderma (Schlenker *et al*). J. Bone & Joint Surg. (Am.), *55:*1051, 1973

Disabilities of hand under social security (Casesa). N. Y. State J. Med., *73:*2569,

Hands — Cont.

1973

Scleroderma hand: a reappraisal (Entin *et al*). Orthop. Clin. North Am., *4:*1031, 1973

Evaluation of the hand and its function (Brand). Orthop. Clin. North Am., *4:*1127, 1973

Plantaris, et Palmaris, keratosis (Kisner, Hendrix), PRS, *51:*424, 1973

Hand surgery under wrist block and local infiltration anesthesia, using upper arm tourniquet (Dupont *et al*), PRS, *50:*532, 1972; Letter to the Editor, PRS, *51:*685, 1973

Hand, and wrist, anomalous muscles and nerve entrapment in (Still, Kleinert), PRS, *52:*394, 1973

Hand surgery, upper arm tourniquet tolerance in (Bennett) (Letter to the Editor), PRS, *52:*660, 1973

The diabetic hand (Cochet). Praxis, *62:*1055, 1973 (French)

Therapeutic deductions (Allieu). Rev. Rhum. Mal. Osteoartic., *40:*203, 1973 (French)

Simple, inexpensive retractor for hand surgery (Khalil). South. Med. J., *66:*966, 1973

Conduction anesthesia in surgery of the hand (Oganesian). Vestn. Khir., *111:*111, 1973 (Russian)

Palmar Fascia. By H. B. Stack. Longman, London, 1974

Rehabilitation of the Hand. By C. B. W. Parry. 3rd Ed. Butterworth, London, 1974

Moto perpetuo — (Paganini). A theme for surgery of the hand (Bruner). Hand, *6:*115, 1974

Hand involvement in systemic lupus erythematosus (Bleifeld, Inglis), PRS, *55:*510, 1975. J. Bone & Joint Surg., *56A:*1207, 1974

Wire, barbed, use in surgery of hand (Meyrueis *et al*), PRS, *54:*502, 1974. J. chir., *107:*151, 1974

Simple technic for anesthesia of the hand and fingers (Winninger). Nouv. Presse Med., *3:*1303, 1974 (French)

Hand, clinical and functional assessment of, after metacarpophalangeal capsulotomy (Buch), PRS, *53:*452, 1974

Fingers: pure sign of lumbrical function (Aiache, Delagi), PRS, *54:*312, 1974

Palms, calcinosis of (Webb), PRS, *55:*719, 1975. Proc. Roy. Soc. Med., *67:*466, 1974

Study of 99mTc-polyphosphate as a joint imaging agent (Blake *et al*). S. Afr. Med. J., *48:*2292, 1974

Hand Pain & Impairment. 2nd edition. By Rene Cailliet. F. A. Davis Co., Philadelphia, 1975

Hands – Cont.

Hand, nontraumatic soft tissue afflictions of (Burton, Littler), PRS, *57*:534, 1976. Curr. Probl. Surg., *5*:56, 1975

Joints, proximal interphalangeal, of human hand, less known aspects (Kuczynski), PRS, *57*:398, 1976. Hand, 7:31, 1975

Some thoughts on examination of the hand (Parkes). Hand, 7:104, 1975

Metaplastic bone formation (myositis ossificans) in the soft tissues of the hand. Case report (Johnson *et al*). J. Bone & Joint Surg. (Am.), *57*:999, 1975

99mTc-polyphosphate scintigraphy of joints, xeroradiography and radiography of hands (Hermann *et al*). Nucl. Med. (Stuttg.), *13*:341, 1975 (German)

An evaluation of antiseptics used for hand disinfection in wards (Ojajarvi). J. Hyg. (Camb.), *76*:75, 1976

Measurementf angles of adjacent finger joints, simple, direct method for simultaneous (Srinivasan), PRS, *57*:524, 1976

Hemostasis in surgery of the hand (Johnson, Morain), PRS, *57*:666, 1976

Hands Amputation (See also *Hands, Prosthetic*)

Incisions, amputations, and skin grafting in the hand (Graham). Orthop. Clin. North Am., *1*:213, 1970

Amputation, physiological, and immediate prosthesis at University Hospital in Caracas (Sisiruca, Gonzales), PRS, *50*:538, 1972. Bol. Soc. Ven. Cir., *25*:1091, 1971

Some problems in the rehabilitation of patients with a partially amputated hand (Hees). Ned. tijdschr. geneeskd., *115*: 551, 1971 (Dutch)

Unusual indication for interthoracoscapular amputation (Slavik). Acta Chir. Orthop. Traumatol. Cech., *39*:164, 1972 (Czechoslovakian)

Prosthetic care of hand forearm amputation stumps (Schollner). Handchirurgie, *4*:139, 1972 (German)

Cartilage, articular, retaining in finger joint amputations (Whitaker *et al*), PRS, *49*:542, 1972

Amputations, transarticular joint, value of preserving articular cartilage (Graham *et al*), PRS, *53*:495, 1974. J. Surg. Res., *14*:524, 1973

Hands, amputated: get in there and replant! (McDowell) (Editorial), PRS, *52*:562, 1973

Hand grip: metacarpal hand (Michon, Jandeaux), PRS, *54*:620, 1974. Ann. chir. plast., *19*:97, 1974

Metacarpal hand (Michon, Dolich), PRS,

Hands Amputation – Cont.

57:119, 1976. Hand, *6*:285, 1974

Amputation or reconstruction (Velez- Gutierrez), PRS, *55*:258, 1975. Rev. el Medico., *24*:19, 1974

Hand replantation – experience with 8 cases (Ferreira *et al*), PRS, *57*:533, 1976. Rev. Assoc. med. bras., *21*:149, 1975

Hands, Anatomy

Lumbrical muscles of the hand. Remarks on their variation, normal and complementary functions (Winckler). Arch. Anat. Histol. Embryol. (Strasb.), *52*:379, 1969 (French)

Modifications in the musculus extensor digitorum lateralis in phylogenesis and in human ontogenesis (Kaneff *et al*). Acta Anat. (Basel), *77*:583, 1970 (German)

Variation in palmar creases (Alter). Am. J. Dis. Child., *120*:424, 1970

Fibro-aponeurotic formations of the palmar region (Kempf *et al*). Arch. Anat. Histol. Embryol. (Strasb.), *53*:353, 1970 (French)

Functional anatomy of the hand (Brown). Orthop. Clin. North Am., *1*:199, 1970

Structure and function of the skin of the hand (Barron). Hand, *2*:93, 1970

Hands of African patients (Walker). Hand, *2*:160, 1970

Tension in the lumbrical muscle (Stack). Hand, *2*:166, 1970

Origin of the lumbrical muscles in the hand of the South African native (Goldberg). Hand, *2*:168, 1970

Practical and important variations in sensory nerve supply to the hand (Fetrow). Hand, *2*:178, 1970

Intrinsic-extrinsic muscle control of the hand in power grip and precision handling. An electromyographic study (Long *et al*). J. Bone & Joint Surg. (Am.), *52*:853, 1970

Origin of the human hand (Marzke). Am. J. Phys. Anthropol., *34*:61, 1971

Pilot study of 198 normal children pinch strength and hand size in the growing hand (Weiss *et al*). Am. J. Occup. Ther., *25*:10, 1971

Considerations on the functional anatomy of the deep common flexor muscle of the fingers (Fahrer). Ann. Chir., *25*:945, 1971 (French)

Surgical anatomy, kinesiology and propedeutics of the hand (Calberg). Brux. Med., *51*:329, 1971 (French)

Form and size of the male hand (Kadanoff *et al*). Gegenbaurs. Morpho. Jahrb., *116*:293, 1971 (German)

Double anastomotic innervation of thenar

Hands, Anatomy — Cont.

mal interphalangeal joints of (Kuczynski), PRS, *57:*398, 1976. Hand, *7:*31, 1975

Anatomy of the metacarpo-phalangeal joints, with observations of the aetiology of ulnar drift (Wise). J. Bone & Joint Surg. (Br.), *57:*485, 1975

Extensor and flexor mechanisms, method of studying relationships between finger joints and (Snow, Switzer), PRS, *55:*242, 1975

Bundles, displaced neurovascular, in Dupuytren's contracture, Doppler ultrasound detection of (Elsahy), PRS, *57:*104, 1976

Hands, Burns, (See also *Burns; War Injuries*)

Application of fingernail hooks in splinting of burned hands (Von Prince *et al*). Am. J. Occup. Ther., *24:*556, 1970

Burned hand (Zellner). Chirurg., *41:*403, 1970 (German)

Thermic hand lesions (Gadzaly). Dtsch. Med. J., *21:*1398, 1970 (German)

Treatment of electrical burns (Muir). Hand, *2:*137, 1970

Problems in rehabilitation of the burnt hand (Parry). Hand, *2:*140, 1970

Full skin graft strips in plastic surgery to cover scar keloids of the hands following burns (Schonbauer). Handchirurgie, *2:*88, 1970 (German)

Bandage-free method for the covering of hand-burns (Brandt). Handchirurgie, *2:*203, 1970 (German)

Hand, hydrofluoric acid burns of (Dibbell *et al*), PRS, *48:*516, 1971. J. Bone & Joint Surg., *52A:*931, 1970

Treatment of burns of the hands (Brown). J. Okla. State Med. Assoc., *63:*141, 1970

Social readaptation of a patient after disabilitative electric burn of hands (Mattsson *et al*). Nord. Med., *84:*1381, 1970 (Swedish)

Management of the burned hand (Boswick). Orthop. Clin. North Am., *1:*311, 1970

Contact burn of the hand (Nanba *et al*). Orthop. Surg. (Tokyo), *21:*926, 1970 (Japanese)

Thermal injuries of the hand and their sequelae observed at the Department of Plastic Surgery, Tokyo Keisatsu Byoin (Omori *et al*). Orthop. Surg. (Tokyo), *21:*930, 1970 (Japanese)

Reconstructive surgery in severe deformation of the hand after deep burns (Dmitriev). Ortop. Travmatol. Protez., *31:*26, 1970 (Russian)

Surgery in cicatricial contractures of the hand and fingers after burns in children (Pakhomov). Ortop. Travmatol. Protez.,

Hands, Burns — Cont.

*31:*30, 1970 (Russian)

Principles of restorative-reconstructive surgery in burns of the hands (Biriukov). Vestn. Khir., *105:*80, 1970 (Russian)

Simplified method of treating burns of the hands (Slater *et al*). Brit. J. Plast. Surg., *24:*296, 1971

Burns of dorsum of hand (Barsky), PRS, *48:*396, 1971. Hand, *3:*88, 1971

Deep burns — burn contractures (Buchan). Hand, *3:*90, 1971

Maribor method of burns treatment. A report on the work of Janzekovic at Maribor, Yugoslavia (Barron). Hand, *3:*179, 1971

Surgery of scar contracture of the hands (Marumo *et al*). Jap. J. Plast. Reconstr. Surg., *14:*293, 1971 (Japanese)

Burned hand, management of (Whitson, Allen), PRS, *49:*106, 1972. J. Trauma, *11:*606, 1971

Mutilating injuries of the wrist (Bennett *et al*). J. Trauma, *11:*1008, 1971

Hand burns in children and their sequelae (Legal *et al*). Munch. Med. Wochenschr., *113:*572, 1971 (German)

Therapeutic experience in heat-press injury (Ishida *et al*). Orthop. Surg. (Tokyo), *22:*878, 1971 (Japanese)

Functional reconstruction of electric burn of the hand (Ishinada *et al*). Orthop. Surg. (Tokyo), *22:*882, 1971 (Japanese)

Reconstruction of the severely burned hand. 1. Transposition of the amputated finger (Murota *et al*). Orthop. Surg. (Tokyo), *22:*884, 1971 (Japanese)

Hand burns caused by a laundry press (Jakubik). Acta Chir. Orthop. Traumatol. Cech., *39:*49, 1972 (Czechoslovakian)

Case of dorsal burns of the hand. Tissue contracture. Grafts and flaps (Colson *et al*). Ann. chir. plast., *17:*34, 1972 (French)

Reconstructive surgery of the hand following burns (Gay *et al*). Beitr. Orthop. Traumatol., *19:*391, 1972 (German)

Management of deformities following electric fire burns (Craig). Hand, *4:*247, 1972

Heat-induced injuries of hand (Zellner), PRS, *51:*476, 1973. Langenbecks Arch. Chir., *332:*485, 1972

Palm, full-thickness burns, immediate or early excision and full-thickness grafting (Burkhardt), PRS, *49:*572, 1972

Radiographic changes in burns of the upper extremity (Schiele *et al*). Radiology, *104:*13, 1972

Application of "on top plasty" in severely burned hands (Murota). Shujutsu, *26:*35, 1972 (Japanese)

Hands, Burns — Cont.

al). Khirurgiia (Mosk.), *4:*36, 1975 (Russian)

Hands, burned (Huang, Larson, Lewis), PRS, *56:*21, 1975. Discussion by Bennett, PRS, *56:*442, 1975

Psychological reactions to facial and hand burns in young men. Can I see myself through your eyes? (Solnit *et al*). Psychoanal. Study Child., *30:*549, 1975

Treatment of contact burns of the palm in children (Chait). S. Afr. Med. J., *49:*1839, 1975

Burns of the Upper Extremity. By Roger E. Salisbury. W. B. Saunders Co., Philadelphia, 1976

Burn syndactyly, lateral-volar finger flap in treatment (MacDougal, Wray, Weeks), PRS, *57:*167, 1976

Hand, burned, severely, thumb reconstruction in (Pohl, Larson, Lewis), PRS, *57:*320, 1976

Hands, Congenital Anomalies (See also *Syndactylism*)

Hemodynamic aspects and diagnosis of angiodysplasias of the hand (Micall *et al*). Chir. Ital., *20:*1048, 1968 (Italian)

Congenital torsion of the hand (Luppis *et al*). Chir. Organi. Mov., *58:*134, 1969 (Italian)

Treatment of the cleft hand through syndactylization, a new simple method (Streli). Handchirurgie, *1:*104, 1969 (German)

Ear aplasia and forked hand. An association of these 2 congenital abnormalities (Plancq). Ann. chir. plast., *15:*229, 1970 (French)

Holt-Oram syndrome and hand malformations associated with congenital heart disease (Pernot *et al*). Arch. Mal. Coeur, *63:*1428, 1970 (French)

Treatment of congenital radial club hand (Define). Clin. Orthop., *73:*153, 1970

Lobster-claw deformities of the hand (Maisels). Hand, *2:*79, 1970

Five-fingered hand. One-stage pollicization of the radial finger (Kessler). Isr. J. Med. Sci., *6:*280, 1970

Radial meromelia. The deformity and its treatment (Bora *et al*). J. Bone & Joint Surg., (Am.), *52:*966, 1970

Apert's syndrome, hand and (Hoover, Flatt, Weiss), PRS, *49:*234, 1972. J. Bone & Joint Surg., *52A:*878, 1970

Anomalous muscle belly of the flexor digitorum superficialis. Report of a case (Vichare). J. Bone & Joint Surg. (Br.), *52:*757, 1970

Therapeutic experience in a case of extensive

Hands, Congenital Anomalies — Cont.

congenital skin defects in hands and feet (Iso). Orthop. Surg. (Tokyo), *21:*885, 1970 (Japanese)

Rare case of congenital familial anomalous development of the hands (Furmanets). Ortop. Travmatol. Protez., *31:*59, 1970 (Russian)

Polydactylism: disease or symptom? (Le Marec *et al*). Pediatrie, *25:*737, 1970 (French)

Hand, indications and therapy in congenital anomalies (Pernet, Pistelli), PRS, *50:*538, 1972. Rev. Latino Am. cir. plast., *14:*17, 1970

Skeleton of the hand in Down's syndrome (Janovec). Acta Chir. Orthop. Traumatol. Cech., *38:*106, 1971 (Czechoslovakian)

Split hand and foot anomaly in Macaca mulatta: a report of two cases (Morris *et al*). Am. J. Anat., *130:*481, 1971

Acrodysostosis. A syndrome of peripheral dysostosis, nasal hypoplasia, and mental retardation (Robinow *et al*). Am. J. Dis. Child., *121:*195, 1971

Functional evaluation of congenital hand anomalies (Skerik *et al*). Am. J. Occup. Ther., *25:*98, 1971

Symphalangism and deafness (McKusick). Birth Defects, *7:*124, 1971

Aglossia-adactylia (Hall). Birth Defects, *7:*233, 1971

Electrodactyly and cleft lip/palate (Jorgenson). Birth Defects, *7:*260, 1971

New syndrome manifested by mandibular hypoplasia, acroosteolysis, stiff joints and cutaneous atrophy (mandibuloacral dysplasia) in two unrelated boys (Young *et al*). Birth Defects, *7:*291, 1971

Treatment of central polydactyly (Wood). Clin. Orthop., *74:*196, 1971

Congenital triangular deformity of the tabular bones of hand and foot (Jaeger *et al*). Clin. Orthop., *81:*139, 1971

Plastic surgery in abnormalities of the hand (Millesi). Chirurg., *42:*60, 1971 (German)

Congenital abnormalities possibly induced by LSD-25. Review of the literature apropos of a personal case (Jeanbart *et al*). Gynecol. Obstet. (Paris), *70:*215, 1971 (French)

Immobilization of tiny hands (Brody). Hand, *3:*97, 1971

Genetics and malformations of the hand (Wynne-Davies). Hand, *3:*184, 1971

Congenital absence of the upper limb and hand. A review of the benefits in prehension and bimanual function by early prosthetic replacement (Lamb *et al*). Hand, *3:*193, 1971

Morphology and classification of symbrachy-

Hands, Congenital Anomalies – Cont.

dactylia (Blauth *et al*). Handchirurgie, *3:*123, 1971 (German)

Brachydactyly with absence of middle phalanges and hypoplastic nails. A new hereditary syndrome (Cuevas-Sosa *et al*). J. Bone & Joint Surg. (Br.), *53:*101, 1971

Bilateral aplasia of the tibia, polydactyly and absent thumb in father and daughter (Pashayan *et al*). J. Bone & Joint Surg. (Br.), *53:*495, 1971

Familial hand abnormality and sensorineural deafness: a new syndrome (Stewart *et al*). J. Pediatr., *78:*102, 1971

Unusual facies, cleft palate, mental retardation, and limb abnormalities in siblings – a new syndrome (Palant *et al*). J. Pediatr., *78:*686, 1971

Severe developmental failure with coarse facial features, distal limb hypoplasia, thickened palmar creases, bifid uvula, and ureteral stenosis: a previously unidentified familial disorder with lethal outcome (Rudiger *et al*). J. Pediatr., *79:*977, 1971

Short palmar muscle with a double insertion, including a fasciculus on the 5th metacarpal acting as an adductor (Comtet *et al*). Lyon Med., *225:*1161, 1971 (French)

Congenital abnormalities of the hands (Heybroek). Ned. tijdschr. geneeskd., *115:*1289, 1971 (Dutch)

Case of m. palmaris radialis (profundus) (Mattson). Nord. Med., *86:*1223, 1971 (Swedish)

Surgically treated case of brachydactylia of the metacarpal bone (Sano *et al*). Orthop. Surg. (Tokyo), *22:*146, 1971 (Japanese)

Nineteen cases of lobster hand (Nakamura *et al*). Orthop. Surg. (Tokyo), *22:*896, 1971 (Japanese)

Surgical treatment of congenital radial clubhand (Kuz'menko). Ortop. Travmatol. Protez., *32:*22, 1971 (Russian)

Familial occurrence of the Freeman-Sheldon syndrome: cranio-carpotarsal dysplasia (Gross-Kieselstein *et al*). Pediatrics, *47:*1064, 1971

Holt-Oram syndrome in a Maltese family (Fenech *et al*). Postgrad. Med. J., *47:*589, 1971

Hand, congenital anomalies of (Filippi *et al*), PRS, *49:*357, 1972. Rev. Ital. chir. plast., *3:*63, 1971

Hands of human embryos, prenatal development of tendon sheaths (Zauner, Nagel), PRS, *49:*664, 1972. Surg. Forum, *22:*430, 1971

Le Deformita Congenite Delle Mani ed il loro Trattamento. By A. Bonola and E. Morelli.

Hands, Congenital Anomalies – Cont.

Piccin Editore, Padua, Italy, 1972. PRS, *51:*443, 1973

Combined malformation of both hands (Matzen). Beitr. Orthop. Traumatol., *19:*251, 1972 (German)

Finger mutilation and polydactylia on prehistoric rock pictures in North America (Wellmann). Dtsch. Med. Wochenschr., *97:*527, 1972 (German)

Abnormalities of the hand associated with generalised developmental disorders of the skeleton (Chalmers). Hand, *4:*11, 1972

Treatment of radial club hand. Absent radius, aplasia of the radius, hypoplasia of the radius, radial paraxial hemimelia (Lamb). Hand, *4:*22, 1972

Operative treatment of congenital malformations of the hand (Buck-Gramcko). Hand, *4:*33, 1972

Classification of congenital malformations of the hand and upper extremity (Entin *et al*). Hand, *4:*215, 1972

Prostheses for children with unilateral congenital absence of the hand (Murray *et al*). J. Bone & Joint Surg. (Am.), *54:*1658, 1972

Hereditary syndrome of imperforate anus with hand, foot, and ear anomalies (Townes *et al*). J. Pediatr., *81:*321, 1972

Hands, congenital anomalies and their treatment (Bonola, Morelli), PRS, *51:*103, 1973. Piccin, Padua, 1972

Bilateral tibial aplasia with lobster-claw hands. A rare genetic entity (Kaloustian *et al*). Acta Paediatr. Scand., *62:*77, 1973

Congenital vascular malformations of the hand (Erikson *et al*). Acta Radiol. (Diagn.) (Stockh.), *14:*753, 1973

The facial-digital-genital (Aarskog) syndrome (Sugarman *et al*). Am. J. Dis. Child., *126:*248, 1973

Polydactyly, rudimentary (Shapiro, Juhlin, Brownstein), PRS, *54:*376, 1974. Arch. Dermat., *108:*223, 1973

Lobster claw defect with ectodermal defects, cleft lip-palate, tear duct anomaly and renal anomalies (Preus *et al*). Clin. Genet., *4:*369, 1973

Extensor carpi ulnaris, bilateral agenesis of (Gloobe, Liberty), PRS, *54:*376, 1974. Hand, *5:*175, 1973

Functional reconstruction of a congenital lobster-claw hand (Verdan). Handchirurgie, *5:*93, 1973 (German)

Symbrachydactylias (Blauth *et al*). Handchirurgie, *5:*121, 1973 (German)

Extensor digitorum brevis manus and hypertrophy of the synonym muscle of the feet (Koussouris). Handchirurgie, *5:*237, 1973

Hands, Deformities, Acquired — Cont.

PRS, *52:*679, 1973. J. Bone & Joint Surg., *54B:*499, 1972

Doigt en lorgnette and concentric bone atrophy associated with healed yaws osteitis. Report of two cases (Jones). J. Bone & Joint Surg. (Br.), *54:*341, 1972

Metacarpal hand (Michon). Acta Orthop. Belg., *39:*1182, 1973 (French)

Case report on Kirner's deformity (Himmel). Beitr. Orthop. Traumatol., *20:*221, 1973 (German)

Hand deformities: filling first intermetacarpal space in ulnar paralysis (Blanco, Aramburu, Maldonado), PRS, *54:*620, 1974. Bol. Sudamer. cir. Mano, *5:*38, 1973

Carpometacarpal boss (Artz, Posch), PRS, *53:*244, 1974. J. Bone & Joint Surg., *55A:*757, 1973

Hand, complex dislocation of metacarpophalangeal joint of (Green, Gerry), PRS, *54:*109, 1974. J. Bone & Joint Surg., *55A:*1480, 1973

Contractures: six-flap Z-plasty (Mir y Mir). PRS, *52:*625, 1973

Deformities of the fingers and thumb: surgical possibilities (Allieu). Rev. Rhum. Mal. Osteoartic., *40:*215, 1973 (French)

Failure of hand growth after X-ray therapy (Goh *et al*). Singapore Med. J., *14:*19, 1973

Skeletal growth disorders following radiotherapy and their treatment (Schulitz *et al*). Ztschr. Orthop., *111:*249, 1973 (German)

Surgical management of hand deformities in recessive dystrophic epidermolysis bullosa (Zarem *et al*). Brit. J. Plast. Surg., *27:*176, 1974

Mechanism of arch reversal in the surgically corrected claw hand (Ranney). Hand, *6:*266, 1974

Limb deformities in leprosy (Yadev). Indian J. Med. Sci., *28:*542, 1974

Surgical treatment of deformities of the hand and fingers with the aid of Volkov-Oganesian apparatus (Degtiareva *et al*). Ortop. Travmatol. Protez., *35:*24, 1974 (Russian)

Capsulotomy, metacarpophalangeal, clinical and functional assessment of the hand after (Buch). PRS, *53:*452, 1974

Synovial chondromatosis of hand (Constant, Harebottle, Davis). PRS, *54:*353, 1974

Elastic redressing-training devices in flexure contractures of the fingers (Codega *et al*). Polim. Med., *4:*189, 1974 (Polish)

Surgical treatment of deformations of the palm in the course of epidermolysis bullosa dystrophica (Kratochwil *et al*). Przegl. Dermatol., *61:*211, 1974 (Polish)

Hands, Deformities, Acquired — Cont.

Flexion contractures of the hand (Snow *et al*). J. Fla. Med. Assoc., *62:*19, 1975

Contraction of the hand in epidermolysis bullosa dystrophica and its surgical treatment (Arneri). Med. Pregl., *28:*451, 1975 (Serbian)

Joints, hand and finger, distortion of (Bloem), PRS, *57:*118, 1976. Nederl. tijdschr. geneesk., *119:*472, 1975

Letter: joint lesions in diabetes. New England J. Med., *292:*1033, 1975

Camptodactyly. Apropos of 25 cases (Dociu *et al*). Sem. Hop. Paris, *51:*1175, 1975 (French)

Hands, Dressings for

Evaluation of ice application with postoperative dressings (Omer *et al*). Clin. Orthop., *81:*117, 1971

Betadine and pHisoHex evaluated as antiseptic agents in surgical preparation of hands (Gross *et al*), PRS, *53:*114, 1974. Am. J. Surg., *126:*49, 1973

Silicone bag treatment of burned hands (Spira) (Follow-Up Clinic). PRS, *52:*80, 1973

Hands, Fractures

Tension strap osteosynthesis in unstable fractures of the metacarpal head (Adler). Monatsschr. Unfallheilkd., *72:*297, 1969 (German)

Hand fractures, complicated, management (Antoniadis, Papasoglou, Makris), PRS, *48:*393, 1971. Tr. 1st Panhellenic Cong. Orthop. Surg. & Traum., *1:*131, 1969

Surgery of fractures of the metacarpal bones and phalanges (Bogdanov *et al*). Vestn. Khir., *102:*84, 1969 (Russian)

Treatment of fractures in the area of the hand (Luther *et al*). Chirurg., *41:*222, 1970 (German)

Use of "A. O." plates in the hand (Simonetta). Hand, *2:*43, 1970

Dislocations, fractures and, upper extremity, intravenous lidocaine anesthesia for (Hawkins, Storey, Wells), PRS, *49:*234, 1972. J. Bone & Joint Surg., *52A:*1647, 1970

Fracture of carpal scaphoid in child aged 4 (Bloem), PRS, *48:*392, 1971. Arch. chir. neerl., *23:*91, 1971

Stable osteosynthesis in fractures of the hand bone (Wilhelm). Arch. Orthop. Unfallchir., *70:*275, 1971 (German)

Stable AO-osteosynthesis in open hand frac-

Hands, Fractures — Cont.

tures (Wilhelm). Arch. Orthop. Unfallchir., *71:*6, 1971 (German)

Treatment of fractures of the base of the first
metacarpal bones (Lascar). Bull. Mem.
Soc. Chir. Paris, *61:*267, 1971 (French)

Problems of fracture fixation in growing
hand bones (Segmuler *et al*). Handchirurgie, *3:*109, 1971 (German)

Hand, stable internal fixation of fractures of
(Rüedi, Burri, Pfeiffer), PRS, *49:*584, 1972.
J. Trauma, *11:*381, 1971

Experience with stable osteosynthesis in metacarpal fractures (Ruedi *et al*). Langenbecks Arch. Chir., *328:*285, 1971 (German)

Remote results of treatment of perilunar dislocations of the hand and dislocations of
the wrist similunar bone (Oleshko *et al*).
Ortop. Travmatol. Protez., *32:*27, 1971
(Russian)

Splint for treating fractures of the metacar-
pals and digital phalanges (Sukhorukov).
Ortop. Travmatol. Protez., *32:*76, 1971
(Russian)

Scaphoid fractures in child and their "specialties" (Dolling, Franke), PRS, *51:* 478, 1973.
Bruns' Beitr. klin Chir., *219:*462, 1972

Fractures of the hand region–avoidance of
failures (Geldmacher). Chirurg., *43:*111,
1972 (German)

Screw fixation and open reduction of fresh
fractures of scaphoid bone of hand (Pfeiffer), PRS, *51:*479, 1973. Helvet. chir. acta,
39: 471, 1972

Fractures of metacarpals and phalanges,
treatment of (Thevenin, Iselin), PRS,
*50:*419, 1972. J. Chir. Paris, *103:*251, 1972

Anterior approach for fractures of the dia-
physis and base of the first metacarpal
(Winninger). Nouv. Presse Med., *1:*1997,
1972 (French)

Position of osteosynthesis in the management of hand fractures (Pfeiffer). Ther.
Umsch., *29:*679, 1972 (German)

Navicular fractures in childhood (Napieralski). Zentralbl. Chir., *97:*542, 1972 (German)

Indications and limitations of conservation
management of bone fractures in the area
of the hand (Titze). Zentralbl. Chir.,
*97:*1723, 1972 (German)

*Operative Stabilization of the Hand Skele-
ton.* By Gottfried Segmuller. Verlag Hans
Huber, Bern, Stuttgart, Wien, 1973. PRS,
*55:*357, 1975

Indications and technics of AO osteosynthesis in the treatment of the fractures of
the hand (Helm). Acta Orthop. Belg.,
*39:*957, 1973 (French)

Hands, Fractures — Cont.

Osteosynthesis of the long bones of the hand
using the AO technic (Ramirez Gomez *et
al*). Acta Orthop. Belg., *39:*973, 1973
(French)

Indications and technic of osteosynthesis using a flexible screw (Thevenin). Acta Orthop. Belg., *39:*980, 1973 (French)

Fractures and dislocations of the hand. General conclusions (Van Wetter). Acta Orthop. Belg., *39:*1129, 1973) (French)

Results in the surgical treatment of pseu-
doarthroses of the carpal navicular bone
(Kral). Acta Chir. Orthop. Traumatol.
Cech., *40:*161, 1973 (Czechoslovakian)

Hamate bone, injuries of (Boin), PRS, *54:*374,
1974. Hand, *5:*235, 1973

Indications for the AO treatment of fractures
of the bones of the hand (Wilhelm *et al*).
Munch. Med. Wochenschr., *115:*371, 1973
(German)

Results of the treatment of dislocations of the
hand and carpal bones (Kuz'min). Ortop.
Travmatol. Protez., *34:*29, 1973 (Russian)

Intraosseous administration of olemorphocycline in the primary surgical treatment
of open fractures of the hand and foot
(Tkachenko *et al*). Vestn. Khir., *111:*103,
1973 (Russian)

New method for conservative treatment of
impacted metacarpo-phalangeal luxations
(Koncz). Arch. Orthop. Unfallchir., *79:*135,
1974 (German)

New technic of pressure osteosynthesis in the
hand (Bencivenga). Chirurg., *45:*327, 1974
(German)

Rigid fixation of bones of the hand using K
wires bonded with acrylic resin (Crockett).
Hand, *6:*106, 1974

Tourniquet, venous, acceleration of fracture
healing distal to (Kruse, Kelly), PRS,
*55:*387, 1975. J. Bone & Joint Surg., *56A:*
730, 1974

Fractures of the metacarpals and phalanges.
Their treatment by screws (Troques).
Nouv. Presse Med., *3:*1367, 1974 (French)

Osteosynthesis of the tubular bones of the
hand with metal plate (Paneva-Kholevich). Ortop. Travmatol. Protez., *35:*59,
1974 (Russian)

Abnormal callus in fractures of the long
bones of the hand (Lempereur). Rev. Med.
Liege, *29:*144, 1974 (French)

Flexion contracture in the interphalangeal
joints following splinting for simple metacarpal fractures (Vibild *et al*). Ugeskr.
Laeger, *136:*1439, 1974 (Danish)

Treatment of traumatic osteomyelitis of the
fingers and hand (Kosachev). Voen. Med.

Hands, Fractures—Cont.

Zh., *11:*64, 1974 (Russian)

Fractures of metacarpal bones, AO-osteosynthesis of (Hauer, Feldmeier, Wilhelm), PRS, *57:*119, 1976. Actuel. Chir., *10:*73, 1975

Internal fixation in fractures of the hand and fingers (Kenis *et al*). Acta Orthop. Belg., *41:*110, 1975

Proceedings: management of fracture of the hand (Lipscomb). J. Bone & Joint Surg. (Br.), *57:*257, 1975

Proceedings: Conservative or surgical treatment of hand fractures (Wilhelm). Munch. Med. Wochenschr., *117:*364, 1975 (German)

Transosseous osteosynthesis in fractures of the metacarpal bones (Chernavskii *et al*). Ortop. Travmatol. Protez., *1:*10, 1975 (Russian)

Primary treatment of fractures of metacarpal bones with reference to the functional capacity of the hand (Hrabovsky). Rozhl. Chir., *54:*80, 1975 (Czechoslovakian)

Hands, Grease Gun Injuries

High pressure injection injuries, the problems, pathogenesis and management (Kaufman). Hand, *2:*63, 1970

Hand injuries resulting from greaseguns and high pressure color injections (Hentschel). Handchirurgie, *2:*171, 1970 (German)

Injection gun injury of the hand with anticorrosive paint and paint solvent. A case report (Walton). Clin. Orthop., *74:*141, 1971

Airless paint gun injury of the hand. A surgical emergency (Remark *et al*). Mo. Med., *69:*196, 1972

High-pressure paint gun injuries of the hand: a report of two cases (Scher *et al*). Brit. J. Plast. Surg., *26:*167, 1973

Treatment of grease gun injuries (Baylor *et al*). J. Occup. Med., *15:*799, 1973

Treatment of high velocity paint gun injury of the hand (Wofford). South. Med. J., *66:*307, 1973

High pressure injection injuries of the hand: treatment by early mobilization (Palmieri). Bull. Hosp. Joint Dis., *35:*18, 1974

Injection injuries of hand, high velocity (Williams, Riordan), PRS, *54:*502, 1974. South. M. J., *67:*295, 1974

Hand injuries caused by high pressure syringes (Sougard). Ugeskr. Laeger, *136:*909, 1974 (Danish)

Lesions caused by high pressure syringes (Grut). Ugeskr. Laeger, *136:*934, 1974 (Danish)

Clinical picture and pathomorphology of traumatic high-pressure oil injections, the

Hands, Grease Gun Injuries—Cont.

so called "grease gun injury" (Kleinfeld *et al*). Chirurg., *46:*362, 1975 (German)

High pressure injection injuries of the hand (Lotem *et al*). Harefuah, *89:*213, 1975 (Hebrew)

Paint and grease gun injuries of hand (Mann), PRS *56:*230, 1975. J.A.M.A., *231:*933, 1975

Injection injury, high pressure: potential hazard of "enhanced recovery" (O'Reilly, Blatt), PRS, *57:*534, 1976. J.A.M.A., *233:*533, 1975

High-pressure injection injuries of the hand (Gelberman *et al*). J. Bone & Joint Surg. (Am.), *57:*935, 1975

High pressure injection injuries to the hand (DeCesare *et al*). J. Iowa Med. Soc., *65:*461, 1975

Accidental high-pressure injection-gun injuries of the hand; the role of the emergency radiologic examination (O'Reilly *et al*). J. Trauma, *15:*24, 1975

Hands, Infections

Hand onychomycosis (Zapater *et al*). Arch. Argent. Dermatol., *19:*183, 1969 (Spanish)

The Care of Hand Infection. By Joan Sneddon. Williams & Wilkins Co., Baltimore, 1970.

Sepsis in hand injuries (Sneddon). Hand, *2:*58, 1970

Diagnosis and therapy of soft tissue infections in the hand (Bohler). Hefte Unfallheilkd., *107:*221, 1970 (German)

Diagnosis and therapy of bone infections of the hand (Popkirov). Hefte Unfallheilkd., *107:*225, 1970 (German)

Evaluation of hand infections (Probst). Hefte Unfallheilkd., *107:*236, 1970 (German)

Therapy of severe hand phlegmons (Jussen *et al*). Hefte Unfallheilkd., *107:*248, 1970 (German)

Nocardia infection of the hand (Becton *et al*). J. Bone & Joint Surg. (Am.), *52:*1443, 1970

Infections of the hand (Carter *et al*). Orthop. Clin. North Am., *1:*455, 1970

Salmonella osteomyelitis of both hands and hand-foot syndrome (Constant, Green, Wagner), PRS, *48:*300, 1971. Arch. Surg., *102:*148, 1971

Auxiliary chemotherapy in bacterial infections of the hand (Brug *et al*). Arzneim. Forsch., *21:*586, 1971 (German)

Tuberculous hygroma of the hand (Gay). Beitr. Orthop. Traumatol., *18:*596, 1971 (German)

Wound infection in undressed sutured

Hands, Infections — Cont.

wounds of the hand (Wood). Brit. J. Surg., *58:*543, 1971

Pyogenic infections of the hand (Schink). Chirurg., *42:*356, 1971 (German)

Bacteriological analysis and chemo-therapeutic sequelae of purulent hand infections (Brug *et al*). Handchirurgie, *3:*93, 1971 (German)

Erysipeloid infection of digits (Lamphier). J. Fla. Med. Assoc., *58:*39, 1971

Whitlow trephine (Sharma *et al*). J. Indian Med. Assoc., *57:*209, 1971

Hand, minor infections, in Marine recruits: analysis of 100 consecutive cases (O'Donnell), PRS, *48:*93, 1971. Mil. Med., *136:*30, 1971

Paratuberculosis of hand (Bjornsson *et al*), PRS, *49:*584, 1972. Scand. J. Plast. Reconstr. Surg., *5:*156, 1971

Infections de la Main Chez l'Fnfant et l'Adulte. By R. Vilain and J. Michon. Masson & Cie, Paris, 1972. PRS, *52:*661, 1973

Tenosynovitis, tuberculous, chronic recurrent, of finger flexors (Anderl, Semenitz), PRS, *52:*206, 1973. Handsurg., *4:*3, 1972

Mycetoma of the hand. A report of three cases (Sethi *et al*). Indian J. Med. Sci., *26:*656, 1972

Histoplasmosis of the common palmar tendon sheath (Perlman *et al*). J. Bone & Joint Surg. (Am.), *54:*676, 1972

Treatment of suppurative diseases of the hand (Rykalin *et al*). Khirurgiia (Mosk.), *48:*94, 1972 (Russian)

Treatment of suppurative diseases of the fingers and hand (Demianiuk). Klin. Khir., *8:*56, 1972 (Russian)

Clinical course of tuberculous tenosynovitis of the hand (Kobayashi *et al*). Orthop. Surg. (Tokyo), *23:*122, 1972 (Japanese)

Current problems in the management of the septic hand (Kovalkovits *et al*). Orv. Hetil., *113:*1519, 1972 (Hungarian)

Maduromycosis of hand due to *Phialophora jeanselme* (Yongchiyud *et al*), PRS, *52:*97, 1973. Southeast Asian J. Trop. Med., *3:*138, 1972

Treatment of purulent diseases of the fingers and hands (Geller). Vestn. Khir., *108:*76, 1972 (Russian)

Treatment of suppurative diseases of the hand and fingers (Myslin *et al*). Voen. Med. Zh., *3:*34, 1972 (Russian)

Comparative evaluation of the efficacy of antibiotics in the treatment of purulent infections of soft tissues of hands and fingers (Babenko *et al*). Antibiotiki, *18:*844, 1973 (Russian)

Hands, Infections — Cont.

Coccidioidomycosis tenosynovitis in the hand (Iverson *et al*). J. Bone & Joint Surg., (Am.), *55:*413, 1973

Mycobacterium marinum (atypical acid-fast bacillus) infections of the hand (Williams *et al*). J. Bone & Joint Surg. (Am.), *55:*1042, 1973

Mycobacterium marinum infection of hand (Cortez, Panpey), PRS, *52:*322, 1973. J. Bone & Joint Surg., *55A:*363, 1973

Treatment of suppurative diseases of the fingers and hand (Shevkunov). Khirurgiia (Mosk.), *49:*19, 1973 (Russian)

Proceedings: pyogenic infection of hand and fingers (Geldmacher). Langenbecks Arch. Chir., *334:*491, 1973 (German)

Proceedings: acute suppurating infections of hands and fingers and their treatment (Reichmann). Langenbecks Arch. Chir., *334:*499, 1973 (German)

Hand infections in narcotic addict, management of (Whitaker, Graham). PRS, *52:*384, 1973

Drug addicts, soft tissue changes in the hands of (McCabe, Ditmars). PRS, *52:*538, 1973

Regional intraosseous infusion of morphocycline and oleomorphocycline in the treatment of severe forms of purulent infection of the hand and fingers (Kosachev). Vestn. Khir., *111:*63, 1973 (Russian)

Osteoarticular infections of the hand (Evrard). Ann. Chir., *28:*267, 1974 (French)

Valve of an external fixation device in the treatment of osteoarticular infections of the hand and fingers (Allieu *et al*). Ann. Chir., *28:*271, 1974 (French)

Phlegmon of the tendon sheaths (Michon). Ann. Chir., *28:*277, 1974 (French)

The classic. Infections of the hand (Kanavel). Clin. Orthop., *104:*3, 1974

Thermographic demonstration of tenosynovitis. A case report (Traycoff *et al*). Ohio State Med. J., *70:*632, 1974

Addicts, drug injection injuries of the hands and forearms (Ryan, Hoopes, Jabaley). PRS, *53:*445, 1974

Common and uncommon infections of the hand (Linscheid *et al*). Orthop. Clin. North Am., *6:*1063, 1975

Preventing hand disability from infection (Graham *et al*). Pa. Med., *78:*53, 1975

Infections of the hand (Gray). Papua New Guinea Med. J., *18:*113, 1975

Felon, acute monomyelocytic leukemia presenting as (Chang, Whitaker, LaRossa). PRS, *55:*623, 1975

Sheath, flexor digital, needle aspiration as

Hands, Infections — Cont.

aid in diagnosing tenosynovitis (Ryan, Hoopes). PRS, *56*:152, 1975

Hands, Injuries (See also Hands, Nerve Injuries; Hands; Reconstructive Surgery; Hands, Tendon Injuries; Hands, Vascular Injuries)

Fulminant Candida albicans sepsis with fatal clinical course beginning from a primary skin infection (Ketzan). Mykosen, *11*:699, 1968 (German)

Industry physician and accidents of the hand (Amphoux). Therapeutique, *44*:567, 1968 (French)

Initial management of hand wounds (Butler). Mil. Med., *134*:1, 1969

Hand injuries and rehabilitation (Blochin). Beitr. Orthop. Traumatol., *17*:586, 1970 (German)

Rehabilitation apparatus for hand injuries (Lambilliote). Bull. Mem. Soc. Chir. Paris, *60*:238, 1970 (French)

Post-traumatic algo-dystrophies (Voloir). Bull. Mem. Soc. Chir. Paris, *60*:293, 1970 (French)

Hand trauma, general considerations (Gonzalez), PRS, *48*:393, 1971. Cir. plast. Uruguaya, *11*:15, 1970

Acute closed hand injuries (Scharlzer). Dtsch. Med. J., *21*:1327, 1970 (German)

Treatment of glass injuries to the hand at work (Cameron). Hand, *2*:52, 1970

Assessment and management of the injured hand (James). Hand, *2*:97, 1970

Primary surgical treatment of extensive soft tissue defects of the hand (Willebrand et al). Handchirurgie, *2*:34, 1970 (German)

Combination injuries of the thumb (Gunther). Handchirurgie, *2*:40, 1970 (German)

Primary care for injured hands (Buck-Gramcko). Handchirurgie, *2*:47, 1970 (German)

Abnormal mental reactions of the injured (Iselin). Handchirurgie, *2*:61, 1970 (German)

Primary care for severe hand injuries. Handchirurgie, *2*:105, 1970 (German)

Interferences between the kind of injuries and wound healing in post-traumatic hand infections (Bilow et al). Hefte Unfallheilkd., *107*:249, 1970 (German)

Disastrous results in infected minor hand injuries (Rahmel). Hefte Unfallheilkd., *107*:251, 1970 (German)

Partially successful reimplantation of the hand (Roth). Helv. Chir. Acta, *37*:234, 1970 (German)

Delayed primary operation for open injuries

Hands, Injuries — Cont.

of the extremities, especially the hand (two-stage treatment) (Tophoj et al). Injury, *2*:51, 1970

Reconstruction after traumatic mutilations of the hand (Tubiana). Injury, *2*:127, 1970

Interphalangeal joint, proximal, athletic injuries requiring surgical treatment (McCue et al), PRS, *48*:511, 1971. J. Bone & Joint Surg., *52A*:937, 1970

An improved method of elevation of the injured hand (McMillan). J. R. Nav. Med. Serv., *56*:281, 1970

Expert opinion of hand injuries (Buck-Gramcko et al). Monatsschr. Unfallheilkd., *73*:474, 1970 (German)

Hand trauma (Bevin). N. C. Med. J., *31*:384, 1970

Closed crush injuries of the hand and forearm (Brown). Orthop. Clin. North Am., *1*:253, 1970

Measures for prevention of hand injuries and their results in industry (Takagishi et al). Orthop. Surg. (Tokyo), *21*:932, 1970 (Japanese)

Comprehensive management of the patient following hand injury and surgery (Hamilton). Prog. Phys. Ther., *1*:176, 1970

Aggressive combined management of the patient with hand injuries and hand surgery (Bevin). Prog. Phys. Ther., *1*:191, 1970

Hand, initial surgery of war wounds (Pires), PRS, *48*:94, 1971. Rev. port. Mil. Med., *18*:2, 1970

Joint Injuries of the Hand. By Richard G. Eaton. Charles C Thomas, Springfield, Ill., 1971. PRS, *49*:338, 1972

Osteo-Articular Injuries of the Hand. By Raymond Vilain et al. Expansion Scientifique Francaise, Paris, 1971. PRS, *49*:656, 1972

Peritendinous fibrosis of the dorsum of the hand (Bednarik et al). Acta Chir. Orthop. Traumatol., Cech., *38*:289, 1971 (Czechoslovakian)

Injuries of the extensors of the hand and fingers (analysis of 1000 cases) (Simun et al). Acta Chir. Orthop. Traumatol., Cech., *38*:298, 1971 (Slovakian)

Examination of the hand (Sherlock). Am. Surg., *37*:661, 1971

Functional restorations of hand mutilations caused by weapon explosions (Bourrel et al). Ann. chir. plast., *16*:215, 1971 (French)

Injured hand, panel by correspondence (Goldner, Kaplan, Kelleher), PRS, *50*:305, 1972. Arch. Surg., *103*:691, 1971

Deferred surgical procedures in crush injuries of the hand (Kus et al). Chir. Narza-

Hands, Injuries — Cont.

dow. Ruchu. Ortop Pol., *36:*413, 1971 (Polish)

"Card injuries of the hand" associated with multiple broken pins (Joshi). Hand, *3:*84, 1971

Nail-gun injury of the hand (Braun). J. Bone & Joint Surg., (Am.), *53:*383, 1971

Principles of early management in massive injuries of the hand (Wray). J. Indiana State Med. Assoc., *64:*1277, 1971

Hammering with the hands. Lancet, *1:*536, 1971 (Editorial)

Management of the acutely injured hand (Remark *et al*). Mo. Med., *68:*767, 1971

New device for the restoration of partially amputated hands (Dworecka *et al*). Mt. Sinai J. Med. N. Y., *38:*462, 1971

Hand injuries in skiing (Walcher). Munch. Med. Wochenschr., *113:*1573, 1971 (German)

Functional prognosis of contusion of the dorsal region of the hand (Iino *et al*). Orthop. Surg. (Tokyo), *22:*890, 1971 (Japanese)

Hand injury and underlying diseases (Ito *et al*). Orthop. Surg. (Tokyo), *22:*1007, 1971 (Japanese)

Our position with respect to anesthesia in reconstructive surgery of the wrist (Demichev *et al*). Ortop. Travmatol. Protez., *32:*19, 1971 (Russian)

Industrial injuries of the fingers and hands (Sartan). Ortop. Travmatol. Protez., *32:*65, 1971 (Russian)

Finger and hand injuries in workers in a glass factory (Iusufov). Ortop. Travmatol. Protez., *32:*73, 1971 (Russian)

Hand injuries, acute, early salvage in, with primary island flap (Chase), PRS, *48:*521, 1971

Present-day views on the management of hand injuries (Nagay *et al*). Pol. Przegl. Chir., *43:*645, 1971 (Polish)

What is the practical value of intravenous locoregional anesthesia in surgery of the hand? (Roucher). Presse Med., *79:*2330, 1971 (French)

Wrist and hand pathology related to sports (Torres-Baldo), PRS, *52:*323, 1973. Rev. Latino Am. cir. plast., *15:*17, 1971

Hand injuries: psychiatric considerations (Knorr *et al*). South. Med. J., *64:*1328, 1971

Management of fresh hand injuries (Spier). Ther. Ggw., *110:*1428, 1971 (German)

Hand injuries (Saeboe-Larssen). Tidsskr. Nor. Laegeforen, *91:*1886, 1971 (Norwegian)

Conduction anesthesia in hand and finger injuries (Skoblin *et al*). Vestn. Khir., *106:*96, 1971

Hands, Injuries — Cont.

"Spontaneous" and "post-traumatic" hand pressure edema, a model of typical but seldom timely recognized artifact (Schmauss *et al*). Z. Aerztl. Fortbild. (Jena), *65:*141, 1971 (German)

The Care of Minor Hand Injuries, Third Edition. By Adrian E. Flatt. C. V. Mosby Co., St. Louis, 1972. PRS, *51:*210, 1973

Value of an enzyme inhibitor in cicatrization (animal experimentation; application to hand surgery) (Comtet *et al*). Ann. chir. plast., *17:*145, 1972 (French)

Injury, blunt, thrombosis of ulnar artery of hand following (Luning), PRS, *51:*703, 1973; *52:*99, 1973. Arch. chir. neerl., *24:*289, 1972

Hand, corn picker injuries of (Melvin), PRS, *51:*231, 1973. Arch. Surg., *104:*26, 1972

Complications following the early treatment of hand injuries: an analysis of 100 cases (Conolly). Aust. N. Z. J. Surg., *42:*145, 1972

Topographic-anatomic tables for the graphical demonstration of diagnosis of open and covered hand injuries (Popstefanow *et al*). Beitr. Orthop. Traumatol., *19:*167, 1972 (German)

Possibilities and limitations of surgery of the hand in 1972. Apropos of a case (Goumain *et al*). Bord. Med., *5:*2041, 1972 (French)

An unusual mutilating injury of the hand (Reid). Brit. J. Plast. Surg., *25:*53, 1972

Laceration of hand. Can. Med. Assoc. J., *107:*1231, 1972

Restoration of work capacity in combined lesions of flexor tendons and nerves of the fingers (Rozowskaja *et al*). Chir. Narzadow. Ruchu Ortop. Pol., *37:*375, 1972 (Polish)

Surgical management of neglected cases of multiple flexor tendon and nerve injuries above the wrist (Strzyzewski). Chir. Narzadow. Ruchu Ortop. Pol., *37:*455, 1972 (Polish)

Infra-red thermography in hand surgery (Koob). Hand, *4:*65, 1972

Uses of occupational therapy in hand injuries (Nigst). Handchirurgie, *4:*3, 1972 (German)

Injuries due to compressor units (Fischer). Hippokrates, *43:*254, 1972 (German)

Hand, injured, digital transposition in (Harkins, Raffety), PRS, *51:*231, 1973. J. Bone & Joint Surg., *54A:*1064, 1972

Initial treatment of acute hand injuries (Williams). J. La. State Med. Soc., *124:*205, 1972

Tactics and methods of removing X-ray contrast foreign bodies from the soft tissues

Hands, Injuries – Cont.

and joints of children (Fishchenko). Khirurgiia (Mosk.), *48:*117, 1972 (Russian)

Hand, primary treatment of open injuries of (Millesi), PRS, *51:*478, 1973. Langenbecks Arch. Chir., *332:*469, 1972

Round-table discussion on the topic: acute hand injuries. Langenbecks Arch. Chir., *332:*501, 1972 (German)

Mercury as foreign body in the hand (Barabas *et al*). Magy. Traumatol. Orthop., *15:*299, 1972 (Hungarian)

Hypothenar hammer syndrome (Little *et al*). M. J. Australia, *1:*49, 1972

Hand injuries. M. J. Australia, *2:*522, 1972

Primary surgical treatment of open combined injuries of the hands and fingers according to the A. N. Syzganov-G. K. Tkachenko method (Fishkin *et al*). Ortop. Travmatol. Protez., *33:*48, 1972 (Russian)

Industrial injuries of the hand sustained in metallurgy plants (Diukov). Ortop. Travmatol. Protez., *33:*58, 1972 (Russian)

Hand injuries, severe compound dorsal, solution to (Millard, Cooley). PRS, *49:*215, 1972

Brake-produced hand injuries in farmers (Modrzewski *et al*). Pol Przegl. Chir., *44:*39, 1972 (Polish)

Surgical management of traumatic injuries of the hand (Kedra *et al*). Pol. Przegl. Chir., *44:*311, 1972 (Polish)

Hand injuries, delayed closure of (Quetglas), PRS, *51:*232, 1973. Rev. españ. cir. plast., *2:*193, 1972

Treatment of minor wounds of the hand in workers at Bryansk Machine-building Plant (Naumov). Sov. Med., *35:*139, 1972 (Russian)

Surgical emergencies of the hand (Schneewind). Surg. Clin. North Am., *52:*203, 1972

Injuries and diseases of the hand (Ivanova). Voen. Med. Zh., *3:*28, 1972 (Russian)

Hand and finger injuries (Bulaenko *et al*). Voen. Med. Zh., *3:*37, 1972 (Russian)

Management of Acute Hand Injuries. A Biological Approach. By Paul M. Weeks and R. Christie Wray. C. V. Mosby Co., St. Louis, 1973. PRS, *54:*216, 1974

Surgery of Repair as Applied to Hand Injuries. 4th Edition. By B. K. Rank, A. R. Wakefield, and J. T. Hueston. Williams & Wilkins Co., Baltimore, 1973. PRS, *53:*672, 1974

Hand injuries caused by blank cartridges (Emr). Acta Chir. Ortop. Traumatol. Cech., *40:*556, 1973 (Czechoslovakian)

Reflex algodystrophy and fractures of the hand (Bircher). Acta Orthop. Belg., *39:*1024, 1973 (French)

Emergencies with delayed operation in tropi-

Hands, Injuries – Cont.

cal countries (Kamel *et al*). Ann. Chir., *27:*531, 1973 (French)

Three hundred forty three injuries of fingers and hands treated in U. O. D. (Body *et al*). Ann. Chir., *27:*535, 1973 (French)

Early treatment of war wounds of the hand and forearm in Vietnam (Jabaley *et al*). Ann. Surg., *177:*167, 1973

Mucoid cysts and trauma (Civatte). Arch. Belg. Dermatol. Syphiligr., *29:*217, 1973 (French)

Hand, crush injury of, immediate interossei decompression following (Wolfort, Cochran, Fitzer), PRS, *53:*366, 1974. Arch. Surg., *106:*826, 1973

Treatment of open hand injuries (Henkert *et al*). Beitr. Orthop. Traumatol., *20:*378, 1973 (German)

Injuries to upper extremity inflicted by mechanical cornpicker (Louis *et al*). Clin. Orthop., *92:*231, 1973

Hand, grenade injury to, exostosis following (Lagundoye, Oluwasanmi), PRS, *54:*375, 1974. Hand, *5:*149, 1973

Gunshot wounds of the hand (Granberry). Hand, *5:*220, 1973

Proceedings: surgical reconstructive possibilities in severely mutilated hands (Verdan). Hefte Unfallheilkd., *114:*157, 1973 (German)

Auger injuries (Grogono). Injury, *4:*247, 1973

Hand, escalator injuries of (Reid), PRS, *54:*376, 1974. Injury, *5:*47, 1973

Hand injuries in childhood – a survey of fifty patients (Sharma *et al*). J. Ir. Med. Assoc., *66:*598, 1973

Examination and care of the acutely injured hand (Shadid). J. Okla. State Med. Assoc., *66:*139, 1973

Proceedings: complications of superficial infections of the hand (Buck-Gramcko). Langenbecks Arch. Chir., *334:*505, 1973 (German)

Diagnostic and therapeutic errors in the management of fresh hand injuries. Magy. Traumatol. Orthop., *16:*317, 1973 (Hungarian)

Saving the amputated digit and hand (O'Brien *et al*). M. J. Australia, *1:*558, 1973

Crush injuries of the hand and fingers. I. (Sandzen). Med. Trial Tech. Q., *19:*144, 1973

Crush injuries of the hand and fingers. 3. (Sandzen). Med. Trial Tech. Q., *19:*418, 1973

Industrial accidents and hand injuries (Geldmacher *et al*). Munch. Med. Wochenschr., *115:*1211, 1973 (German)

Injured hand (Stellbrink). Munch. Med.

Hands, Injuries — Cont.

Wochenschr., *115:*1959, 1973 (German)

Assessment of patients with injuries and surgical procedures of the hand (Bevin). N. C. Med. J., *34:*197, 1973

Common hand injuries in the athlete (Burton *et al*). Orthop. Clin. North Am., *4:*809, 1973

Reimplantation of amputated digits and hands (Kleinert *et al*). Orthop. Clin. North Am., *4:*957, 1973

Rehabilitation of the hand with motor and sensory impairment (Brand). Orthop. Clin. North Am., *4:*1135, 1973

Trauma and restorative surgery of the hand (Blokhin). Ortop. Travmatol. Protez., *34:*1, 1973 (Russian)

Microtrauma of the hand and fingers and its complications in the rural economy (Dem'ianiuk). Ortop. Travmatol. Protez., *34:*58, 1973 (Russian)

Primary blind suture in open combined injuries of the fingers and hand (Sartan). Ortop. Travmatol. Protez., *34:*59, 1973 (Russian)

Method of investigation of the function of the hand and fingers (Voitovich). Ortop. Travmatol. Protez., *34:*65, 1973 (Russian)

Thumb and index finger injuries, island pedicle flap in (Sullivan) (Follow-Up Clinic), PRS, *51:*208, 1973

Molten plastic injuries of hand (Baker) (Follow-Up Clinic), PRS, *52:*81, 1973

Hands of drug addicts, soft tissue changes in (McCabe, Ditmars). PRS, *52:*538, 1973

Occupation marks (Ronchese). Practitioner, *210:*507, 1973

Treatment of hand injuries (Gimillio). Praxis, *62:*385, 1973 (French)

Priorities in the treatment of acute hand injuries (Oberholzer). Proc. Mine. Med. Off. Assoc., *53:*2, 1973

Osteoarticular injuries of hand, unusual (Soin), PRS, *53:*106, 1974. Proc. Roy. Australasian Coll. Surg., *46:*270, 1973

An approach to the extensively injured hand (Staden). S. Afr. Med. J., *47:*380, 1973

Treatment of hand injuries (Kaplan). S. Afr. J. Surg., *11:*249, 1973

Ways of improving the results achieved by the treatment of open combined injuries of the hand (Kolontai *et al*). Sov. Med., *36:*87, 1973 (Russian)

Foreign body injuries of hands (Pompner). Zentralbl. Chir., *98:*1438, 1973 (German)

Treatment of Hand Injuries. Preservation and Restoration of Function. By Elden C. Weckesser. Year Book Medical Publishers, Chicago, 1974. PRS, *55:*700, 1975

Hands, Injuries — Cont.

Treating acute hand and finger injuries. 1. (Sandzen). Am. Fam. Physician, *9:*74, 1974

Treating acute hand and finger injuries (Sandzen). Am. Fam. Physician, *9:*100, 1974

Soft-tissue injury by mercury from a broken thermometer. A case report and review of the literature (Rachman). Am. J. Clin. Pathol., *61:*296, 1974

Hand trauma, Swanson's Silastic implants in (Michon, Delagoutte, Jandeaux), PRS, *54:*627, 1974. Ann. chir. plast., *19:*13, 1974

Low-velocity gunshot wounds of the hand (Duncan *et al*). Arch. Surg., *109:*395, 1974

Spontaneous healing of hand wounds (Conolly). Aust. N. Z. J. Surg. *44:*393, 1974

Time for surgery — urgency and delayed operation (Pohl). Beitr. Orthop. Traumatol., *21:*21, 1974 (German)

In a cultural mission of the People's Republic of China: reimplantation of limbs (Cesari). Chir. Organi. Mov., *61:*655, 1974 (Italian)

Hand wounds, soft tissue, spontaneous healing and wound contraction (Conolly), PRS, *54:*690, 1974. Hand, *6:*26, 1974

Hand, degloved mutilated, sensory flaps for (Joshi), PRS, *56:*229, 1975. Hand, *6:*247, 1974

Assessment and management of a plutonium contaminated wound case (Schofield *et al*). Health Phys., *26:*541, 1974

Editorial: The "intact" hand after crush and burn (Grant). J.A.M.A., *227:*1305, 1974

Hand arch, proximal carpal, disruption of (Primiano, Reep), PRS, *54:*503, 1974. J. Bone & Joint Surg., *56A:*328, 1974

Joint, fifth MP, progressive loss of motion caused by traumatic entrapment of *extensor digiti minimi proprius* (Schultz), PRS, *54:*621, 1974. J. Bone & Joint Surg., *56A:*428, 1974

Post-traumatic capillary hemangioma of the hand. A case report (Ben-Menachem *et al*). J. Bone & Joint Surg. (Am.), *56A:*1741, 1974

Treatment of open crushing type of industrial injuries of the hand and forearm: degloving, open circumferential, heat-press, and nail-bed injuries (Tajima). J. Trauma, *14:*995, 1974

Surgeons' injuries during operations (Veller *et al*). Klin. Khir., *8:*43, 1974 (Russian)

What is happening in hand surgery? (Carstam). Lakartidningen, *71:*2840, 1974 (Swedish)

Hand injury, psychological aspects of (Cone, Hueston), PRS, *54:*236, 1974. M. J. Aus-

Hands, Injuries — Cont.

Office and emergency room care of the injured hand (Peters *et al*). South. Med. J., *69:*53, 1976

Hands, Neoplasms (See also *Radiation Injuries*)

Tumors of the hand (Millesi *et al*). Handchirurgie, *1:*134, 1969 (German)

Treatment of malignant tumors in the region of the hand (Schink). Handchirurgie, *1:*154, 1969 (German)

Cutaneous radio-cancer of both hands (Papillon *et al*). J. Radiol. Electrol. Med. Nucl., *50:*750, 1969 (French)

Anglosarkoma (Tosovsky *et al*). Acta Chir. Orthop. Traumatol. Cech., *37:*281, 1970 (Czechoslovakian)

Cancer, extremities, results of radical surgery for (Miller). Aktuel Probl. Chir., *14:*689, 1970

Palm, nevoid basal cell carcinoma of (Tayler, Wilking), PRS, *49:*361, 1972. Arch. Dermat., *102:*654, 1970

Epitheloid sarcoma. A sarcoma simulating a granuloma or a carcinoma (Enzinger). Cancer, *26:*1029, 1970

Lipomas in the hand and wrist; diagnosis and treatment (Rodriguez *et al*). Clev. Clin. Q., *32:*201, 1970

Case report of multiple enchondroma (Sueyasu). Jap. J. Cancer Clin., *16:*947, 1970 (Japanese)

Keratosis of the palms and soles (Gibbs). J. Am. Podiatry Assoc., *60:*423, 1970

Two cases of malignant synoviomas in children (Feoktistov). Ortop. Travmatol. Protez., *31:*72, 1970 (Russian)

Malignant schwannomas of the hand: a review (Epstein). Bull. Hosp. Joint Dis., *32:*136, 1971

Late results following extirpation of melanosarcoma of the hand by superficial lymphangiectomy and lymphadenectomy (Reichmann). Handchirurgie, *3:*42, 1971 (German)

Bone tumors of the hand (Sattel *et al*). Handchirurgie, *3:*103, 1971

Juxtacortical chondrosarcoma of the hand (Jokl *et al*). J. Bone & Joint Surg. (Am.), *53:*1370, 1971

Solitary benign enchondroma of the long bones of the hand (Jewusiak *et al*). J. Bone & Joint Surg. (Am.), *53:*1587, 1971

Chondroma of the bones of the hand. A review of 110 cases (Takigawa). J. Bone & Joint Surg. (Am.), *53:*1591, 1971

Primary malignant tumors of the hand.

Hands, Neoplasms — Cont.

(Kendall *et al*). J. Kans. Med. Soc., *72:*376, 1971

Xanthomas of the hand (Huffstadt). Ned. tijdschr. geneeskd., *115:*1989, 1971 (Dutch)

Case of desmoid tumor of the 1st dorsal interosseous muscle (Hozumi). Orthop. Surg. (Tokyo), *22:*985, 1971 (Japanese)

Giant cell tumors of the tendon sheaths of the hand (Usol'tseva). Ortop. Travmatol. Protez., *32:*18, 1971 (Russian)

Aponeurotic sarcoma (Laskowski). Pol. Med. J., *10:*12, 1971

Sarcoma, parosteal (Soto), PRS, *49:*474, 1972. Rev. Latino Am. cir. plast., *15:*45, 1971

Tumors in the region of the hand (Schmidt). Zentralbl. Chir., *96:*1113, 1971 (German)

Palmar keratoses and visceral cancer (Gilbertsen, Bean, Fusaro), PRS, *50:*205, 1972. Arch. Dermat., *105:*222, 1972

Sweat gland carcinoma of the hand. A case report (Levitt *et al*). Clin. Orthop., *83:*95, 1972

Metastatic carcinoma of the hand (Fragiadakis *et al*). Hand, *4:*268, 1972

Chondromatous hamartomas arising from the volar digital plates. A case report (Heiple *et al*). J. Bone & Joint Surg. (Am.), *54:*393, 1972

Hand, glomus tumors of (Carroll, Berman), PRS, *51:*104, 1973. J. Bone & Joint Surg., *54A:*691, 1972

Lipomas of the hand. Including a case of lipoblastomatosis in a child (Paarlberg *et al*). Mayo Clin. Proc., *47:*121, 1972

Hand, eccrine poroma of (Mamoun *et al*), PRS, *50:*295, 1972

Cartilaginous tumors of the hand (Witwicki *et al*). Pol. Przegl. Radiol., *36:*307, 1972 (Polish)

Chondrosarcoma of the hand (Habal, Snyder, Murray), PRS, *53:*244, 1974. Am. J. Surg., *125:*775, 1973

Malignant giant cell tumor of the tendon sheath (Kahn). Arch. Pathol., *95:*203, 1973

Sarcoma of tendon sheath (Fragiadakis *et al*). Hand, *5:*71, 1973

Hamartoma in the hand — a simulator (Jeffery). Hand, *5:*79, 1973

Hand, metastatic tumors of (Graham *et al*), PRS, *54:*376, 1974. Hand, *5:* 177, 1973

Myxoma of the palm (Tolhurst). Hand, *5:*260, 1973

Rare tumors of the wrist joint and hand (Nigst). Handchirurgie, *5:*39, 1973 (German)

Hemangiomas of the hand — conservative treatment? (Huffstadt). Handchirurgie, *5:*115, 1973 (German)

Hands, Neoplasms — Cont.

Diagnosis of hand tumors (Segmuller). Helv. Chir. Acta, *40:*241, 1973 (German)

Hand neuromas and entrapped nerves, abdominal flap for (Brown, Flynn), PRS, *52:*595, 1973. J. Bone & Joint Surg., *55A:*575, 1973

Pigmented villonodular synovitis. Localized tumor on dorsum of hand (Burman). N.Y. State J. Med., *73:*2174, 1973

Sarcoma aponeuroticum (sarcoma of the aponeurosis) (Dabska *et al*). Pol. Tyg. Lek., *28:*99, 1973

Unusual histological appearance of a tumor of the palm of the hand (mixed tumor of the sweat glands?) (Auger *et al*). Union. Med. Can., *102:*373, 1973 (French)

Proceedings: epitheloid sarcoma (Kuchemann). Verh. Dtsch. Ges. Pathol., *57:*419, 1973 (German)

Benign tumors of the hand (Matton *et al*). Acta Orthop. Belg., *40:*172, 1974

Enchondromata of the hand bones (Noble *et al*). Ann. Chir., *28:*855, 1974 (French)

Embryonal rhabdomyosarcoma of the hand. A case report (McDowell *et al*). Clin. Orthop., *100:*238, 1974

Metastatic lesions of hand and forearm (Bryan *et al*), PRS, *56:*235, 1975. Clin. Orthop., *101:*167, 1974

Possibilities of dermatosurgery in neoplasms in the hand region (Petres *et al*). Fortschr. Med., *92:*1054, 1974 (German)

Sweat gland carcinoma of the hand (Lucas *et al*). Hand, *6:*98, 1974

Metacarpal bone, benign osteoblastoma of (Olbourne, Saad, Clement), PRS, *56:*229, 1975. Hand, *6:*198, 1974

Hand, enchondromata of bones of — review of 40 cases (Noble, Lamb), PRS, *56:*227, 1975. Hand, *6:*275, 1974

Primary epithelioid sarcoma of the hand and forearm. A review of thirteen cases (Bryan *et al*). J. Bone & Joint Surg. (Am.), *56:*458, 1974

Local gigantism of the hand associated with a plexiform neurofibroma of the ulnar nerve. Report of a case (Brihaye *et al*). J. Neurosurg. Sci., *18:*271, 1974

Tumors, cartilaginous, of soft tissues of hands and feet (Dahlin, Salvador), PRS, *55:*385, 1975. Mayo Clin. Proc., *49:*721, 1974

Liposarcoma of the hand (Sawhney *et al*). Am. Surg., *41:*117, 1975

Sarcomas, soft tissue (Gerner *et al*). PRS, *57:*404, 1976. Ann. Surg., *181:*803, 1975

Epithelioid sarcoma (Kuchemann). Beitr. Pathol., *155:*84, 1975

Hands, Neoplasms — Cont.

Malignant soft tissue tumors of probable histiocytic origin (malignant fibrous histiocytomas): general considerations and electron microscopic and tissue culture studies (Fu *et al*). Cancer, *35:*176, 1975

Metastatic malignancy of the hand (Basora *et al*). Clin. Orthop., *108:*182, 1975

Tumors of the hand (Bogumill *et al*). Clin. Orthop., *108:*214, 1975

Chondrosarcoma of the hand arising from a pre-existent benign solitary enchondroma (Culver *et al*). Clin. Orthop., *113:*128, 1975

Melanotic tumours of the hand (Banzet *et al*). Hand, *7:*183, 1975

Angiography in the diagnosis of osteoid-osteoma of the hand (O'Hara *et al*). J. Bone & Joint Surg. (Am.), *57:*163, 1975

Osseous xanthoma and multiple hand tumors as a complication of hyperlipidemia. Report of a case (Hamilton *et al*). J. Bone & Joint Surg. (Am.), *57:*551, 1975

Chondromas of the tendon sheath of the hand. Report of a case and review of the literature (Strong). J. Bone & Joint Surg. (Am.), *57:*1164, 1975

Metastases to the bones of the hand (Kumar). J. Natl. Med. Assoc., *67:*275, 1975

Hand, vascular leiomyoma of (Hauswald, Kasdan, Weiss), PRS, *55:*89, 1975

Tumor, malignant, of hand: acute monomyelocytic leukemia presenting as felon (Chang, Whitaker, LaRossa), PRS, *55:*623, 1975

Hand skeleton, parosteal osteogenic sarcoma of (Rombouts, Noel), PRS, *56:*465, 1975. Rev. chir. orthop., *61:*71, 1975

Juxtacortical osteogenic sarcoma localized in the hand. Presentation of 2 cases (Rombouts *et al*). Rev. Chir. Orthop., *61:*75, 1975 (French)

Hand, hemangiopericytoma of (Sen), PRS, *57:*746, 1976

Hands, Nerve Injuries (See also Hands, Injuries; Hands, Tendon Injuries; Leprosy)

Brand operation. Apropos of 12 personal cases (Bourrel). Ann. chir. plast., *13:*297, 1968

Treatment of paralysis of intrinsic muscles of the hand of leprous origin (Le Peltier *et al*). Maroc. Med., *49:*586, 1969 (French)

Sensory recovery after nerve repair (McQuillan). Hand, *2:*7, 1970

Zancolli capsulorrhaphy for ulnar claw hand — appraisal of 44 cases (Brown), PRS, *48:*512, 1971. J. Bone & Joint Surg., *52A:*868, 1970

Hands, Nerve Injuries—Cont.

(Welman). Ned. tijdschr. geneeskd., *116:*1029, 1972 (Dutch)

Anastomosis of the nerves of the upper limb and the problem of functonal restoration — a loss of tactile localization (Kobayashi *et al*). Orthop. Surg. (Tokyo), *23:*290, 1972 (Japanese)

Surgical treatment of deformities of the forearm and hand in patients with infantile cerebral palsy (Sedin). Ortop. Travmatol. Protez., *33:*53, 1972 (Russian)

Hand in quadriplegia (Lamb *et al*). Paraplegia, *9:*204, 1972

Treatment of spastic thumbs in palm deformity (Gob). Reconstr. Surg. Traumatol., *13:*51, 1972

Sensation loss in symptomatic digital neuromas; treatment with local triamcinolone acetonide (Graham *et al*), PRS, *52:*97, 1973. Rev. Latino Am. cir. plast., *16:*13, 1972

Hand, revival of sensation in transplantations and cutaneous grafts (Celli, Caroli), PRS, *51:*104, 1973. Riv. Chir. della Mano, *8:*23, 1972

Surgery of the hand in infants with cerebral palsy (Sarkin). S. Afr. Med. J., *45:*655, 1972

Hand, sensibility as opposed to sensation (Omer), PRS, *53:*108, 1974. Ann. Chir., *27:*479, 1973

Hand sensitivity restored by transfer of heterodigital skin transplant including its fascicular and nervous pedicle (Duparc, Roux), PRS, *53:*112, 1974. Ann. Chir., *27:*497, 1973

Myoelectric controlled orthesis for paralytic hand (Hamonet *et al*). Ann. Chir., *27:*541, 1973 (French)

Nerve function in hand, new simple test of (O'Riain), PRS, *53:*489, 1974. Brit. M.J., *3:*615, 1973

Brachial plexus, treatment of injuries to (Millesi, Meissl, Katzer), PRS, *53:*108, 1974. Bruns' Beitr. klin. Chir., *220:*429, 1973

Hand, motor disturbances, treatment of (Buck-Gramcko), PRS, *53:*367, 1974. Bruns' Beitr. klin. Chir., *220:*522, 1973

Hand surgery in infantile hemiplegia, technics–results (Cahuzac *et al*). Chirurgie, *99:*859, 1973 (French)

Hand in leprosy (Ranney). Hand, *5:*1, 1973

Temperature studies of the hand and its claw deformities due to peripheral nerve paralysis in leprosy (Enna *et al*). Hand, *5:*10, 1973

Paralytic claw fingers—a graft tenodesis operation (Parkes). Hand, *5:*192, 1973

Hands, Nerve Injuries—Cont.

Hand symptoms, uncommon causes of nerve compression with (Richmond), PRS, *54:*374, 1974. Hand, *5:*209, 1973

Extensor diversion graft operation for correction of intrinsic minus fingers in leprosy (Srinivasan). J. Bone & Joint Surg. (Br.), *55:*58, 1973

Opponensplasty, extensor indicis proprius (Burkhalter, Christensen, Brown), PRS, *53:*243, 1974. J. Bone & Joint Surg., *55A:*725, 1973

Operative treatment of spastic hand (Matev). Khirurgiia (Mosk.), *49:*14, 1973 (Russian)

Technique of nerve anastomosis (Kleinert *et al*). Orthop. Clin. North Am., *4:*907, 1973

Post-traumatic sympathetic dystrophy (Kleinert *et al*). Orthop. Clin. North Am., *4:*917, 1973

Perineural neurorrhaphy (Hakstian). Orthop. Clin. North Am., *4:*945, 1973

Mistakes in the treatment of injuries of nerves of the palm and fingers (Degtiareva *et al*). Ortop. Travmatol. Protez., *34:*24, 1973 (Russian)

Surgical reconstruction of prehensile function in tetraplegics (Zrubecky). Paraplegia, *11:*144, 1973

Nerve injuries of hand, thermograms after (Sokol, Berggren), PRS, *51:*449, 1973

Hand, paralytic claw, Fowler procedure for correction of (Enna, Riordan), PRS, *52:*352, 1973

Nerve entrapment in wrist and hand, anomalous muscles and (Still, Kleinert). PRS, *52:*394, 1973

Metacarpal arch, transverse, reconstruction of, in ulnar palsy by transfer of *extensor digiti minimi* (Ranney). PRS, *52:*406, 1973

Hand, fibrotic arch around deep branch of ulnar nerve in (Lotem, Gloobe, Nathan). PRS, *52:*553, 1973. Discussion by Weeks. PRS, *52:*556, 1973

Hemiplegic hand in children with cerebral palsy. Place of surgical treatment (Cahuzac *et al*). Rev. Chir. Orthop., *59:*321, 1973 (French)

The all-ulnar hand (Van Demark). S. D. J. Med., *26:*21, 1973

Reconstructive surgery of the hand in patients with leprosy (Briantseva *et al*). Vestn. Khir., *111:*67, 1973 (Russian)

Ninhydrin sweat test, protective sensation in hand and its co-relation to, following nerve laceration (Perry *et al*), PRS, *55:*248, 1975. Am. J. Phys. Med., *53:*113, 1974

Trauma-induced nerve sections without motor paralysis of the hand (Bourrel). Ann. Chir., *28:*831, 1974 (French)

Hands, Nerve Injuries—Cont.

Tourniquet paralysis (Middleton, Varian), PRS, *55:*385, 1975. Australian & New Zealand J. Surg., *44:*124, 1974

Flexor digitorum sublimis to profundus tendon transfer for flexion deformities in spastic paralysis (Yu *et al*). Can. J. Surg., *17:*225, 1974

Nerve compression lesions of upper extremity (Spinner, Spencer), PRS, *56:*679, 1975. Clin. Orthop., *104:*46, 1974

Sensation after nerve injury, tactile adherence for estimating loss of (Harrison), PRS, *56:*229, 1975. Hand, *6:*158, 1974

Sensation restored to degloved mutilated hand (Joshi), PRS, *56:*229, 1975. Hand, *6:*247, 1974

Preliminary experience with superficialis-to-profundus tendon transfer in the hemiplegic upper extremity (Braun *et al*). J. Bone & Joint Surg. (Am.), *56:*466, 1974

Tourniquet paralysis with prolonged conduction block. An electro-physiological study (Rudge). J. Bone & Joint Surg. (Br.), *56-B:*716, 1974

Fundamental principles of tendon transfer (Curtis). Orthop. Clin. North Am., *5:*231, 1974

Tendon transfers in the patient with spinal cord injury (Curtis). Orthop. Clin. North Am., *5:*415, 1974

Reeducation of sensation in hand after nerve injury and repair (Dellon, Curtis, Edgerton). PRS, *53:*297, 1974

Fascia in fingers in Dupuytren's contracture, patterns, placement of the neurovascular bundle (McFarlane). PRS, *54:*31, 1974

Flap, local dorsolateral island, to restore sensation after avulsion injury of fingertip pulp (Joshi). PRS, *54:*175, 1974

Injuries of brachial plexus, management of (Parry), PRS, *55:*719, 1975. Proc. Roy. Soc. Med., *67:*488, 1974

Paralysis, isolated, of *flexor pollicis longus* muscle (Krag), PRS, *56:*356, 1975. Scand. J. Plast. Reconstr. Surg., *8:*250, 1974

Improvement of function as a result of substitutive radialis operation because of radialis-paresis (Chakour *et al*). Ztschr. Orthop., *112:*341, 1974 (German)

A plea for rehabilitation in sensitivity alterations of the hand (Dardour *et al*). Ann. Chir., *29:*999, 1975 (French)

Causalgia (Sternschein *et al*), PRS, *56:*107, 1975. Arch. Phys. Med. & Rehab., *56:*58, 1975

Paralysis, brachial plexus, radiation-induced (Match), PRS, *56:*596, 1975. Arch. Surg., *110:*384, 1975

Hands, Nerve Injuries—Cont.

Surgery for the quadriplegic hand with active, strong wrist extension preserved. A study of 97 cases (Zancolli). Clin. Orthop., *112:*101, 1975

Sialography, emergency (Fordham, Schatz), PRS, *56:*593, 1975. Emergency Med., *7:*101, 1975

Hand, innervation of (Backhouse), PRS, *57:*760, 1976. Hand, *7:*107, 1975

Digital nerve, damaged (Wallace), PRS, *57:*760, 1976. Hand, *7:*139, 1975

Surgical treatment for absent single-hand grip and elbow extension in quadriplegia. Principles and preliminary experience (Moberg). J. Bone & Joint Surg. (Am.), *57:*196, 1975

Primary peripheral nerve repair in the hand and upper extremity (Holst). J. Trauma, *15:*909, 1975

Letter: longitudinal sliding of median nerve during hand movements: a contributory factor in entrapment neuropathy? (McLellan). Lancet, *1:*633, 1975

Letter: handlebar palsy (Small). New England J. Med., *292:*322, 1975

Nerve and muscle injuries, differential diagnosis; small, deep forearm lacerations (Schwager, Smith, Goulian). PRS, *55:*190, 1975

Suture, nerve, new technique, epineurium-anchoring funicular suture (Tsuge, Ikuta, Sakaue). PRS, *56:*496, 1975

Hand, median and ulnar nerve entrapment in, place of resection of hook of hamate in treatment of (Wissinger). PRS, *56:*501, 1975

Lumbrical plus syndrome (Baciu *et al*). Rev. Chir. Orthop., *61:*153, 1975 (French)

Pacinian corpuscle neuroma of digital nerves (Rhode *et al*). South. Med. J., *68:*86, 1975

Repair of nerves in the hand—when? where? how? (Becton). J. Med. Assoc. Ga., *65:*5, 1976

Forearm shunt procedure, vascular, median carpal tunnel syndrome following (Mancusi-Ungaro, Corres, Di Spaltro). PRS, *57:*96, 1976

Paralysis, median and ulnar nerve, use of *extensor pollicis longus* tendon as distal extension for *opponens* transfer (Kaplan, Dinner, Chait). PRS, *57:*186, 1976

Hand, anesthetic, restoration of sensation by free neuro-vascular flap from foot (Daniel, Terzis, Midgley). PRS, *57:*275, 1976

Diagnosis, intraoperative, for management of peripheral nerve lesions, using single fascicular recordings (Williams, Terzis), PRS, *57:*562, 1976. Discussion by Collins,

Hands, Nerve Injuries—Cont.
    PRS, *57:*744, 1976
    Corpuscles, pacinian, changes in primate, following volar pad excision and skin grafting (Miller, Rusenas). PRS, *57:*627, 1976

Hands, Prosthetic

Below-elbow control of an externally powered hand (Carlson). Bull. Prosthet. Res., *10:*43, 1970
Power unit for functional hand splints (Grahn). Bull. Prosthet. Res., *10:*52, 1970
Collins hand for arm amputees (Alfieri). Minerva Ortop., *21:*47, 1970 (Italian)
Some new thoughts on hand prosthesis (cosmetic movement) (Collins). Prog. Phys. Ther., *1:*244, 1970
Application of myoelectric hand prosthesis at different amputation levels below the elbow (Hierton *et al*). Scand. J. Rehabil. Med., *2:*23, 1970
Some new thoughts on hand prostheses (Collins). Hand, *3:*9, 1971
Gripping surfaces for artificial hands (Simpson). Hand, *3:*12, 1971
Future of powered hand prostheses (Glanville). Hand, *3:*20, 1971
External powered prostheses (Simpson). Hand, *3:*211, 1971
Hand prosthesis with adaptive internally powered fingers (Cool *et al*). Med. Biol. Eng., *9:*33, 1971
Electronic artificial limbs (Ichikawa). Surg. Ther. (Osaka), *24:*40, 1971 (Japanese)
Experimental results with the power-feedback system of an electrical hand prosthesis (Engelhardt *et al*). Biomed. Tech. (Stuttg.), *17:*238, 1972 (German)
Experiences with myo-electrical and reciprocal ortheses (Terbizan). Handchirurgie, *4:*81, 1972 (German)
Prosthetic replacement for irreparable hands (Rowland). Tex. Med., *68:*121, 1972
Functional prostheses for the mutilated hand (Paquin *et al*). Acta Orthop. Belg., *39:*1188, 1973 (French)
Hand prosthesis control via myoelectric patterns (Herberta *et al*). Acta Orthop. Scand., *44:*389, 1973
Hook, cosmetic hand cover for (Rubin, Gearhart), PRS, *53:*366, 1974. Bull. Prosthetics Res., *17:*83, 1973
An adaptive multi-functional hand prosthesis. (Codd *et al*). J. Physiol. (Lond.), *232:*55P, 1973
Prostheses and Rehabilitation after Arm Amputation. By Leonard F. Bender. Charles C Thomas, Springfield, Ill., 1974.

Hands, Prosthetic—Cont.
    PRS, *55:*487, 1975
    An artificial hand incorporating function and cosmesis (Kenworthy). Biomed. Eng., *9:*559, 1974
    Hand, prosthetic arthroplasty of (Urbaniak), PRS, *56:*679, 1975. Clin. Orthop., *104:*9, 1974
    Preliminary prosthesis for the partially amputated hand (Malick). Am. J. Occup. Ther., *29:*479, 1975
    Modern concepts in hand orthotics (McDougall). Hand, *7:*58, 1975
    Orthosis, myoelectric-controlled (Hamonet), PRS, *56:*596, 1975. Hand, *7:*63, 1975

Hands, Reconstructive Surgery (See also *Leprosy*)

Surgery of hand injuries. Short report. Langenbecks Arch. Chir., *322:*941, 1968 (German) (Editorial)
Reconstructive procedures after irreversible nerve damage in the upper extremity (Chase). Clin. Neurosurg., *17:*142, 1969
Immediate management of open hand injuries. Possible technical errors (Vangelista *et al*). Fracastoro, *62:*177, 1969 (Italian)
Experiences of a hand-surgeon in intravenous regional anesthesia (Solonen). Handchirurgie, *1:*132, 1969 (German)
Anatomy and surgery of the extensor tendon systems of the hand with reference to new surgical methods (Wilhelm). Hefte Unfallheilkd., *101:*1, 1969 (German)
Late results of ulnar head resection (Beck *et al*). Monatsschr. Unfallheilkd., *72:*432, 1969 (German)
Bunnell's Surgery of the Hand, Fifth Edition. By Joseph H. Boyes. J. B. Lippincott Co., Philadelphia, 1970. PRS, *48:*496, 1971
Acute open hand injuries (Geldmacher). Dtsch. Med. J., *21:*1383, 1970 (German)
Electromyography (EMG) in surgery of the hand (Leonard *et al*). Electromyography, *10:*239, 1970
Surgical restoration of the hand following infections (Koob). Hefte Unfallheilkd., *107:*230, 1970 (German)
First aid in fresh complex hand injuries (Bruchle). Hefte Unfallheilkd., *107:*241, 1970 (German)
Treatment of complex, wound infected hand injuries following the principle of the "urgency with postponed surgical treatment" of Iselin (Bongert). Hefte Unfallheilkd., *107:*243, 1970 (German)
Significance of postponed primary surgery in the treatment of infected hand injuries

Hands, Reconstructive Surgery—Cont.

(Krebs). Hefte Unfallheilkd., *107:*245, 1970 (German)

Hand surgery training (Goldner). J. Bone & Joint Surg., (Am.), *52:*1061, 1970

Capsulorrhaphy, Zancolli, for ulnar claw hand—appraisal of 44 cases (Brown), PRS, *48:*512, 1971. J. Bone & Joint Surg., *52A:*868, 1970

Errors in indications for plastic operations (Coerdt). Langenbecks Arch. Chir., *327:*652, 1970 (German)

Tendon transplantation and tendon replacement (Seiffert). Langenbecks Arch. Chir., *327:*1106, 1970 (German)

Repeated exploration with interfascicular neurolysis after primary repair of lesions of the nerves of the hand. Value in tropical practice (Bourrel). Med. Trop. (Mars.), *30:*672, 1970 (French)

An original technic for reconstruction of the extensor apparatus (De Albentiis *et al*). Minerva Chir., *25:*852, 1970 (Italian)

Current concepts of wound healing as applied to hand surgery (Madden). Orthop. Clin. North Am., *1:*325, 1970

Principles of tendon transfer (Beasley). Orthop. Clin. North Am., *1:*433, 1970

Experience and reflection on hand surgery in the past 15 years (Tsuge). Orthop. Surg. (Tokyo), *21:*882, 1970 (Japanese)

Sensory re-education of the hand (Salter). Prog. Phys. Ther., *1:*264, 1970

Management of hand injuries (Kaplan). S. Afr. Med. J., *44:*1011, 1970

Clinical experiences with estriol succinate in surgery of the hand (Berger *et al*). Wien. Klin. Wochenschr., *82:*582, 1970 (German)

Postponement of surgery of hand injuries. Experience of 100 cases (Helm). Z. Unfallmed. Berufskr., *63:*223, 1970 (German)

Phalangization of hand metacarpals (Karchinov), PRS, *50:*199, 1972. Acta chir. plast., *13:*47, 1971

Interphalangeal joint, stiff proximal, operative treatment (Rhode, Jennings), PRS, *48:*94, 1971. Am. Surgeon, *37:*44, 1971

Surgical correction of flexion deformities in hemophilia (Niemann). Am. Surg., *37:*685, 1971

Digit transpositions in children (Malek). Ann. Chir., *25:*1015, 1971 (French)

Use of Gosset's operation on the spastic hand (Peer *et al*). Beitr. Orthop. Traumatol., *18:*74, 1971 (German)

Silastic spacers in tendon grafting (Meulen). Brit. J. Plast. Surg., *24:*166, 1971

Surgical anatomy, kinesiology and propedeutics of the hand (Calberg). Brux. Med.,

Hands, Reconstructive Surgery—Cont.

*51:*329, 1971 (French)

An extension to an operating table for hand surgery (Ratliff *et al*). Hand, *3:*112, 1971

Dermal arthroplasty (Bailey). Hand, *3:*135, 1971

Indications for intra-vital staining in surgery of the hand (Haas). Handchirurgie, *3:*135, 1971 (German)

Tendon transfer in the hand. Use of the sublimis to reinforce the extensors (Fragiadakis *et al*). Int. Surg., *55:*172, 1971

Palmar nerve and tendon repair. J. A. M. A., *217:*1864, 1971 (Editorial)

Tourniquet ischemia, observations on effect of (Wilgis), PRS, *49:*664, 1972. J. Bone & Joint Surg., *53:*1343, 1971

Bloodless field. The situation of the surgeon facing acute ruptures of the hand and foot (Moberg). Lakartidningen, *68:*3015, 1971 (Swedish)

Hand injuries in patients with multiple injuries (Spler). Med. Welt., *5:*169, 1971 (German)

Experiences and rehabilitation results in single and repeated plastic surgery of flexor tendons (Pannike *et al*). Monatsschr. Unfallheilkd., *74:*211, 1971 (German)

Characteristics of treatment of hand and finger tendon injuries in patients of middle and old age (Demichev *et al*). Ortop. Travmatol. Protez., *32:*10, 1971 (Russian)

Carpal ligament, transverse, window for pulley in tendon transfers for median nerve palsy (Snow, Fink). PRS, *48:*238, 1971

Plasties of opposition by tendinous transplantation through the interosseous membrane (Duparc *et al*). Rev. Chir. Orthop., *57:*29, 1971 (French)

Trip to the U. S. A. for study of hand surgery (Mansat), Rev. Chir. Orthop., *57:* Suppl. *1:*237, 1971 (French)

Reconstruction of the severely mutilated hand (Pulvertaft). Rheumatol. Phys. Med., *11:*90, 1971

Kinesiological recording of motion with particular emphasis on electrogoniometers (Ebskov), PRS, *49:*583, 1972. Scand. J. Plast. Reconstr. Surg., *5:*96, 1971

Wrist joint, arthrodesis, follow-up of 60 cases (Rechnagel), PRS, *49:*583, 1972. Scand. J. Plast. Reconstr. Surg., *5:*120, 1971

Metacarpal transfer (Bevin). South. Med. J., *64:*1495, 1971

Cosmetic considerations in surgery of the hand (Beasley). Surg. Clin. North Am., *51:*471, 1971

Tourniquet ooze, cause and prevention (Furlow), PRS, *49:*105, 1972. Surg. Gynec. &

Hands, Reconstructive Surgery — Cont.
　Obst., *32:*1069, 1971
　Allgemeine und Spezielle Chirurgische Op-
　erationslehre: Die Operationen an der
　Hand. Ed. by W. Wachsmuth and A. Wil-
　helm. Springer-Verlag, Berlin, 1972. PRS,
　*51:*580, 1973
　Muscle Testing: Techniques of Manual Ex-
　amination, 3rd Edition. By Lucille Daniels
　and Catherine Worthingham. W. B. Saun-
　ders Co., Philadelphia, 1972. PRS, *53:*342,
　1974
　Clawed hand after injection of anesthetic.
　Anesth. Analg. (Cleve.), *51:*514, 1972
　Hand inflammation, postsurgical, double-
　blind study on the effect of oral proteolytic
　enzymes in (Garcia-Velazco, Araico), PRS,
　*50:*632, 1972. Arch. Int. Med. Mex., *3:*7,
　1972
　Hand surgery, tourniquet time in (Flatt),
　PRS, *50:*101, 1972. Arch. Surg., *104:*190,
　1972
　Some special technics in surgery of the hand
　(Lorthioir). Brux. Med., *52:*125, 1972
　(French)
　Restoration of the extensor tendons of the
　hand by flexors (Julliard). Bull. Mem. Soc.
　Chir. Paris, *62:*340, 1972 (French)
　Fifth metacarpal phalanx formation (Tub-
　iana *et al*). Chirurgie, *98:*68, 1972 (French)
　Some difficult situations in restorative sur-
　gery of the mutilated hand (Verdan). Chi-
　rurgie, *98:*295, 1972 (French)
　Homoosseous-cartilaginous arthroplasty of
　the small joints of the hand (Lazarov).
　Folia Med. (Plovdiv.), *14:*123, 1972
　Reconstruction of the nail fold (Barfod).
　Hand, *4:*85: 1972
　Silastic sheeting in hand surgery (Williams
　et al). Hand, *4:*273, 1972
　Table mounted magnifying glass (Micheli-
　nakis). Hand, *4:*277, 1972
　Tourniquet in reconstructive surgery of the
　hand (Wilgis). Handchirurgie, *4:*99, 1972
　Hand surgery, reconstructive, clinical effect
　of proteolytic enzymes after (McCue,
　Webster, Gieck), PRS, *51:*231, 1973. Inter-
　nat. Surg., *57:*479, 1972
　Transfer of the extensor digiti quinti to re-
　store pinch in ulnar palsy of the hand
　(Zweig *et al*). J. Bone & Joint Surg. (Am.),
　*54:*51, 1972
　Flexor muscle slide in the spastic hand: the
　Max Page operation (White). J. Bone &
　Joint Surg. (Br.), *54:*453, 1972
　Arthrodesis of the fingers (Santha *et al*).
　Magy. Traumatol. Orthop., *15:*161, 1972
　(Hungarian)
　Educational film: Zancolli's operation. Film

Hands, Reconstructive Surgery — Cont.
　commentary (Bourrel). Med. Trop.
　(Mars.), *32:*759, 1972 (French)
　New thought on hand surgery (Matev). Mod.
　Trends Orthop., *6:*95, 1972
　Hand surgery (in two parts) (Chase), PRS,
　*51:*477, 1973. New England J. Med.,
　*287:*1174, and 1227, 1972
　Arthroplasty of trapezio-metacarpal joint
　(Wilson). PRS, *49:*143, 1972
　Hand surgery, evaluations of oral trypsin-
　chymotrypsin for prevention of swelling
　after (Salisbury, Hunter). PRS, *49:*171,
　1972
　Flexor tendon repairs, complicated second-
　ary, use of pedicled tendon transfer with
　silicone rod in (Kessler). PRS, *49:*439, 1972
　Reconstruction surgery in hand dysfunction
　due to injuries of the volar side of the fore-
　arm (Miura *et al*). Shujutsu, *26:*62, 1972
　(Japanese)
　Reconstructive surgery on the hand (Spier).
　Ther. Ggw., *111:*684, 1972 (German)
　Atlas of Hand Surgery. By Robert A. Chase.
　W. B. Saunders Co., Philadelphia, 1973.
　PRS, *53:*586, 1974
　Distraction method of lengthening the meta-
　carpals (Ulitskyi, Malygin), PRS, *53:*487,
　1974. Acta chir. plast., *15:*82, 1973
　Surgical exposure of flexor tendons in the
　hand (Bruner). Ann. R. Coll. Surg. Engl.,
　*53:*84, 1973
　Synovitis of the extensors of the fingers asso-
　ciated with extensor digitorum brevis
　manus muscle. A case report (Riordan *et*
　al). Clin. Orthop., *95:*278, 1973
　Tourniquet pressure on upper limb, ischemic
　effects (Parkes), PRS, *54:*236, 1974. Hand,
　*5:*105, 1973
　Tourniquet, biomechanical aspects of (Grif-
　fiths, Heywood), PRS, *54:*236, 1974. Hand,
　*5:*113, 1973
　Tourniquet, instrument or weapon?
　(Sanders), PRS, *54:*236, 1974. Hand, *5:*119,
　1973
　Exsanguination of arm and hand (Burchell,
　Stack), PRS, *54:*236, 1974. Hand, *5:*124,
　1973
　Metacarpophalangeal flexor replacement for
　intrinsic-muscle paralysis (Burkhalter *et*
　al). J. Bone & Joint Surg. (Am.), *55:*1667,
　1973
　Arthrodesis of finger joints, technique for
　(Potenza), PRS, *54:*108, 1974. J. Bone &
　Joint Surg., *55A:*1534, 1973
　Twenty-five years of hand surgery. Personal
　reflections (Pulvertaft). J. Bone & Joint
　Surg., (Br.), *55:*32, 1973
　Distraction-compression method in recon-

Hands, Reconstructive Surgery – Cont.

structive surgery of the hand (Blokhin). Khirurgiia (Mosk.), *49:*10, 1973 (Russian)

Practical surgery of the hand. Foreword. Orthop. Clin. North Am., *4:*857, 1973

Rehabilitation of the hand with motor and sensory impairment (Brand). Orthop. Clin. North Am., *4:*1135, 1973

Profundus severance alone, dynamic tenodesis of distal interphalangeal joint, for use after (Kahn). PRS, *51:*536, 1973

Hand, nerve injuries in, thermograms after repair of (Sokol, Berggren). PRS, *51:*449, 1973

Hand Surgery: results of tenolysis, controlled evaluation in chickens (Hurst, McCain, Lindsay). PRS, *52:*171, 1973

Claw hand, paralytic, the Fowler procedure for correction of (Enna, Riordan). PRS, *52:*352, 1973

Hand surgery: flag flap (Iselin). PRS, *52:*374, 1973

Hand: reconstruction of transverse metacarpal arch in ulnar palsy by transfer of *extensor digiti minimi* (Ranney). PRS, *52:*406, 1973

Rehabilitation measures in the treatment of hand injuries and deformities (Blokhin *et al*). Sov. Med., *36:*125, 1973 (Russian)

Rehabilitation of the Hand. 3rd edition. By C. B. W. Parry. Butterworth & Co., Ltd., London and Toronto, 1974.

Symposium on Reconstructive Hand Surgery. (Plastic Surgery Symposia, Vol. 9) Ed. by J. William Littler *et al*. C. V. Mosby Co., St. Louis, 1974.

On the problem of operation treatment of spastic hand (Vlach *et al*). Acta Chir. Orthop. Traumatol. Cech., *41:*40, 1974 (Czechoslovakian)

Theoretical basis for surgery of the proximal pulley of flexor longus tendons in fingers (de la Caffiniere). Ann. chir. plast., *19:*201, 1974 (French)

Muscle grafts. Anatomical study and technic for the removal of extensor digitorum brevis and palmaris longus muscles (Dessapt *et al*). Ann. chir. plast., *19:*235, 1974 (French)

Multiple-angled incision on the volar surface of the hand (Becton *et al*). Arch. Surg., *109:*582, 1974

Paralysis, tourniquet (Middleton, Varian), PRS, *55:*385, 1975. Australian & New Zealand J. Surg., *44:*124, 1974

Functional palliative operations in the carpal region (Crasselt *et al*). Beitr. Orthop. Traumatol., *20:*399, 1974 (German)

Tendon sheath formation, experimental, out

Hands, Reconstructive Surgery – Cont.

of vasal tissue (Biro, Horvath, Herber), PRS, *55:*119, 1975. Bruns' Beitr. klin. Chir., *221:*319, 1974

New fixation plate for hand surgery (Kohnlein). Chirurg., *45:*482, 1974 (German)

Overview on new procedures in surgery of the hand (Jones *et al*). Clin. Orthop., *9:*154, 1974

Bloodless field for tourniquet? (Fisher). Clin. Orthop., *103:*96, 1974

Dynamic approach to problems of hand function using local anesthesia supplemented by intravenous fentanyl-droperidol (Hunter *et al*). Clin. Orthop., *104:*112, 1974

Microsurgery. Its role in surgery of the hand (Hakstian). Clin. Orthop., *104:*149, 1974

Microsurgery in hand surgery (Kleinert *et al*). Clin. Orthop., *104:*158, 1974

Corrective osteotomy in the hand (Reid). Hand, *6:*50, 1974

MP joints, screw fixation in Zancolli capsuloplasty (Reis), PRS, *56:*229, 1975. Hand, *6:*150, 1974

Instruments for hand surgery (Barron). Hand, *6:*211, 1974

Hand, metacarpal (Michon, Dolich), PRS, *57:*119, 1976. Hand, *6:*285, 1974

Post-traumatic interosseus-lumbrical adhesions. A cause of pain and disability in the hand (Watson *et al*). J. Bone & Joint Surg. (Am.), *56:*79, 1974

Phalangization of the first and fifth metacarpals. Indications, operative technique, and results (Tubiana *et al*). J. Bone & Joint Surg. (Am.), *56:*447, 1974

Hand surgery, use of barbed wire in (Meyrueis *et al*), PRS, *54:*502, 1974. J. chir., *107:*151, 1974

Postoperative instructions for hand surgery (Kasdan *et al*). J. Ky. Med. Assoc., *72:*32, 1974

Hand, selective peripheral nerve blocks for reconstructive surgery of (Connelly, Berry), PRS, *55:*109, 1975. M. J. Australia, *114:*94, 1974

Selective peripheral nerve blocks for reconstructive hand surgery (Conolly *et al*). M. J. Australia, *2:*94, 1974

Orthopedic problems of disordered function of the hand (Jager *et al*). Munch. Med. Wochenschr., *116:*247, 1974 (German)

Reconstructive surgery of the hand in contractures caused by epidermolysis bullosa (Bouman). Ned. tijdschr. geneeskd., *118:*993, 1974 (Dutch)

Rehabilitation and re-education in tendon transfers (Riordan). Orthop. Clin. North Am., *5:*445, 1974

Hands, Reconstructive Surgery—Cont.

Use of a surgical glove in treatment of edema in the hand (Perry). Phys. Ther., *54:*498, 1974

Arteries, volar digital, importance of not damaging, when using the zig-zag incision on a finger (Piggot, Black) (Letter to the Editor). PRS, *53:*80, 1974

Hand, reeducation of sensation after nerve injury and repair (Dellon, Curtis, Edgerton). PRS, *53:*297, 1974

Metacarpophalangeal capsulotomy, clinical and functional assessment of hand after (Buch). PRS, *53:*452, 1974

Hand surgery, self-retaining retractors for (Tegtmeier). PRS, *53:*485, 1974

Digital pulleys, reconstruction (Wray, Weeks). PRS, *53:*534, 1974

Muscle function: pure sign of lumbrical function (Aiache, Delagi). PRS, *54:*312, 1974

Chondromatosis, synovial, of the hand (Constant, Harebottle, Davis). PRS, *54:*353, 1974

Surgical treatment of clawhand. Metacarpophalangeal capsular shortening and advancement of the trochleae of the flexors (103 cases) (Bourrel *et al*). Rev. Chir. Orthop., *60* Suppl 2:243, 1974 (French)

Esthetics in surgery of the hand (Verdan *et al*). Rev. Med. Suisse Romande., *94:*989, 1974 (French)

Restoration of hand function. Rehabilitation of the injured hand (Parry). Trans. Med. Soc. Lond., *90:*101, 1974

Vascular and neural microsurgery (applications to surgery of the hand) (Hakstian). Union Med. Can., *103:*1750, 1974 (French)

Hand, reconstruction of, in epidermolysis bullosa (Bruckner). Zentralbl. Chir., *99:*328, 1974

Hand Surgery. 2nd edition. By J. Edward Flynn. Williams & Wilkins Co., Baltimore, 1975

Symposium on Hand Tendon Surgery. American Academy of Orthopaedic Surgeons. C. V. Mosby Co., St. Louis, 1975

Hand reconstruction (Tubiana). Acta Orthop. Scand., *46:*446, 1975

Capsulodesis versus proximal activation? (de Salamanca). Ann. Chir., *29:*987, 1975 (French)

Surgical treatment of flexion contracture of the hand by means of elongation-transfer of the flexor tendons (Mitroszewska *et al*). Chir. Narzadow. Ruchu Ortop. Pol., *40:*383, 1975 (Polish)

Post-operative complications in hand surgery (Reid). Hand, *7:*115, 1975

Hand table (Webb). Hand, *7:*187, 1975

Hands, Reconstructive Surgery—Cont.

Planning of surgical treatment (Tubiana). Hand, 7:223, 1975

Biodegradable tendon gliding device (Cutright *et al*). Hand, 7:228, 1975

Correction of ulnar subluxation of the extensor communis (Kilgore *et al*). Hand, 7:272, 1975

Reconstruction and replacement of the grip function in the maimed hand (Nigst). Langenbecks Arch. Chir., *339:*383, 1975 (German).

Wrist arthrodesis (Linclau, Hololtcheff), PRS, *57:*118, 1976. Nederl. tijdschr. geneesk., *119:*697, 1975

Preoperative and postoperative management: the role of allied health professionals (McCann *et al*). Orthop. Clin. North Am., *6:*881, 1975

Contracture, flexion, PIP joint, secondary to injury of anomalous ulnar lumbrical muscle insertion (Webber). PRS, *55:*226, 1975

Cancellous bone grafts from distal radius for use in hand surgery (MacCollum). PRS, *55:*477, 1975

Dislocation, dorsal, of index MP joint (Cunningham, Schwarz). PRS, *56:*654, 1975

Gerdox treatment in hand surgery (Domotor). Ther. Hung., *23:*27, 1975

Cartilage, articular, formation of, from free perichondrial grafts (Skoog, Johansson). PRS, *57:*1, 1976

Foot, free neurovascular flap from, to restore sensation to anesthetic hand (Daniel, Terzis, Midgley). PRS, *57:*275, 1976

Fingers, cross-hand digital transfer (Edgerton). PRS, *57:*281, 1976

Table, hand, inexpensive (MacDonald). PRS, *57:*392, 1976

Finger joints, angles of adjacent, simple, direct method for simultaneously measuring (Srinivasan). PRS, *57:*524, 1976

Hand surgery, hemostasis in (Johnson, Morain). PRS, *57:*666, 1976

Hands, Rheumatoid Disease of

Indications and possibilities of surgical intervention in chronic polyarthritis (Stellbrink). Handchirurgie, *1:*19, 1969 (German)

Rheumatic hand and its surgical treatment—main report (Stellbrink). Handchirurgie, *1:*182, 1969 (German)

Rheumatic hand and its surgical treatment. Orthopedic additional report (Tillman). Handchirurgie, *1:*197, 1969 (German)

Results with silastic finger-prostheses in chronic progressive polyarthritis

Hands, Rheumatoid Disease of – Cont.

(Gschwend). Handchirurgie, *1:*205, 1969 (German)

Wrist joint of the patient with polyarthritis; problems in surgical treatment (Gschwend *et al*). Handchirurgie, *1:*209, 1969 (German)

Surgical treatment of the rheumatic hand (Popelka). Handchirurgie, *1:*223, 1969 (German)

Indications and possibilities of surgery for "rheumatic hand" (Salvi). Reumatismo, *21:*57, 1969 (Italian)

Rheumatoid arthritis and surgical treatment (Arden, Harrison, Ansell), PRS, *48:*201, 1971. Brit. M. J., *4:*604, 1970

Assessment of function in the rheumatoid hand (MacBain). Can. J. Occup. Ther., *37:*95, 1970

Arthroplasty of the hand with silicone implants (Tubiana *et al*). Chirurgie, *96:*1000, 1970 (French)

Tenography in the rheumatoid hand (Brewerton). Hand, *2:*46, 1970

Distal profundus entrapment in rheumatoid disease (Hilal). Hand, *2:*48, 1970

Mutilating arthropathies in collagen diseases (Turcu *et al*). Med. Internat. (Bucur.), *22:*1135, 1970 (Rumanian)

Surgical treatment of the rheumatoid hand (Mastrorilli). Minerva Med., *61:*4071, 1970 (Italian)

Surgical treatment of the rheumatic hand (Jager). Munch. Med. Wochenschr., *112:*1875, 1970 (German)

Arthroplasty in traumatic arthritis of the joints of the hand (Swanson). Orthop. Clin. North Am., *1:*285, 1970

Evaluation of pinching strength in chronic rheumatoid arthritis (Yazuka *et al*). Orthop. Surg. (Tokyo), *21:*845, 1970 (Japanese)

Treatment of the rheumatoid hand. 1. Our therapeutic policy (Yamauchi *et al*). Orthop. Surg. (Tokyo), *21:*848, 1970 (Japanese)

Etiology of ulnar drift of the metacarpophalangeal joint in rheumatoid arthritis (Mitsuyasu *et al*). Orthop. Surg. (Tokyo), *21:*950, 1970 (Japanese)

Methods in the surgical treatment of chronic arthropathies of the hand (Salvi). Reumatismo, *22:*208, 1970 (Italian)

Metacarpophalangeal and interphalangeal joint reconstruction: use of silicone rubber-dacron prostheses for replacement of irreparable joints of the hand (Urbaniak *et al*). South. Med. J., *63:*1281, 1970

Surgery of Rheumatoid Arthritis. By Rich-

Hands, Rheumatoid Disease of – Cont.

ard L. Cruess and Nelson Mitchell. J. B. Lippincott Co., Philadelphia, 1971

Surgical reconstruction of the rheumatoid hand (Michon). Acta Orthop. Belg., *37:*459, 1971 (French)

Digital tenosynovectomy of flexor tendons in rheumatic involvement of the hand (Gay *et al*). Acta Orthop. Belg., *37:*470, 1971 (French)

Present status of rheumatoid hand surgery (Nalebuff). Am. J. Surg., *122:*304, 1971

Metacarpophalangeal arthroplasties with silicone implants (Rousso). Ann. Chir., *25:*951, 1971 (French)

Natural history of synovial hypertrophy in the rheumatoid hand (Kay). Ann. Rheum. Dis., *30:*98, 1971

Rheumatoid hand, prophylactic synovectomy of joints (Nicolle, Holt, Calnan), PRS, *49:*357, 1972. Ann. Rheumat. Dis., *30:*476, 1971

Lysosomal enzymes and inflammation with particular reference to rheumatoid diseases (Chayen, Bitensky), PRS, *49:*361, 1972. Ann. Rheumat. Dis., *30:*522, 1971

Inappropriate intrinsic muscle action in the rheumatoid hand (Swezey *et al*). Ann. Rheum. Dis., *30:*619, 1971

Connective tissue activation (Coster), PRS, *48:*398, 1971. Arth. & Rheum., *14:*41, 1971

Rapid method for evaluating the structure and function of the rheumatoid hand (Treuhaft *et al*). Arthritis Rheum., *14:*75, 1971

Synovectomy in the upper limbs. Indications and results (Stellbrink). Beitr. Orthop. Traumatol., *18:*117, 1971 (German)

Synovectomy in the upper limbs (Mohnig). Beitr. Orthop. Traumatol., *18:*129, 1971 (German)

Prophylactic synovectomy of the rheumatoid hand – a clinical trial with 5–8 year follow-up (Nicolle *et al*). Brit. J. Surg., *58:*305, 1971

Value of compression arthrodesis of finger joints (Strzyzewski *et al*). Chir. Narzadow. Ruchu Orthop. Pol., *36:*741, 1971 (Polish)

Functional assessment of the rheumatoid hand (Clawson *et al*). Clin. Orthop. 77:203, 1971

Zig-zag deformity in the rheumatoid hand (Stack *et al*). Hand, *3:*62, 1971

Trigger finger syndrome in rheumatoid arthritis not caused by flexor tendon nodules (Stellbrink). Hand, *3:*76, 1971

Proximal interphalangeal joint in rheumatoid arthritis (Harrison). Hand, *3:*125, 1971

Dermal arthroplasty (Bailey). Hand, *3:*135,

Hands, Rheumatoid Disease of—Cont.

1971

Deformities of the thumb in rheumatoid arthritis (Ratliff). Hand, *3:*138, 1971

Splintage in the rheumatoid hand (Souter). Hand, *3:*144, 1971

Synovectomy in juvenile rheumatoid arthritis (Eyring, Longert, Bass), PRS, *49:*663, 1972. J. Bone & Joint Surg., *53:*638, 1971

Rheumatoid disease, results of surgical synovectomy of digital joints (Ellison, Kelly, Flatt), PRS, *50:*631, 1972. J. Bone & Joint Surg., *53:*1041, 1971

Ulnar drift of the fingers in rheumatoid disease. Treatment by crossed intrinsic tendon transfer (Ellison *et al*). J. Bone & Joint Surg. (Am.), *53:*1061, 1971

Rheumatoid arthritis, arthrodesis of wrist for (Carroll, Dick), PRS, *50:*307, 1972. J. Bone & Joint Surg., *53:*1365, 1971

Hand reconstruction in arthritis mutilans. A case report (Frolmson). J. Bone & Joint Surg. (Am.), *53:*1377, 1971

Use of silastic in surgery of the hand. J. Chir (Paris), *101:*109, 1971 (French) (Editorial)

Rheumatic hand, surgical treatment of (Ceciliani, Tolu), PRS, *51:*104, 1973. Minerva ortop., *22:*175, 1971

Surgery of the hand in rheumatoid arthritis (Bailey *et al*). Mod. Trends Rheumatol., *2:*240, 1971

Arthroplasty of wrist joints in rheumatoid arthritis with use of silicone rubber prostheses (Nienhuis *et al*), PRS, *49:*358, 1972. Nederl. tijdschr. geneesk., *115:*1889, 1971

Surgery in rheumatoid arthritis of hand (Burns *et al*). N. Y. State J. Med., *71:*340, 1971

New joint prosthesis in hand surgery (Hagert). Nord. Med., *85:*513, 1971 (Swedish)

Rheumatoid hand repairs (Dobyns *et al*). Orthop. Clin. North Am., *2:*629, 1971

Rheumatoid arthritis of the wrist (Linscheid *et al*). Orthop. Clin. North Am., *2:*649, 1971

Treatment of arthrosis of the hands (Caruso). Prensa Med. Argent., *58:*629, 1971 (Spanish)

Arthroplasty, MP joint, for rheumatoid deformities in hand (Swanson), PRS, *52:*322, 1973. Rev. Latino Am. cir. plast., *15:*37, 1971

Surgery of the rheumatoid hand (Fissette *et al*). Rev. Med. Liege, *26:*513, 1971 (French)

Surgical treatment of the rheumatoid hand. The metacarpophalangeal joint (Kenesi). Rev. Rhum. Mal. Osteoartic., *38:*307, 1971 (French)

Carpometacarpal joint of thumb, surgical

Hands, Rheumatoid Disease of—Cont.

treatment of osteoarthritis of (Weilby), PRS, *49:*583, 1972. Scand. J. Plast. Reconstr. Surg., *5:*136, 1971

Surgery of rheumatoid hand and wrist (Marmor). Semin. Arthritis Rheum., *1:*7, 1971

Technic of plastic surgery of metacarpophalangeal joints in patients with chronic arthritis (Popelka). Acta Chir. Orthop. Traumatol. Cech., *39:*147, 1972 (Czechoslovakian)

Silicone implants in the hand (Bouwer). Acta Orthop. Belg., *58:*9, 1972

Aspects of rheumatoid hand surgery (Elken). Acta Orthop. Belg., *58:*9, 1972

Hand, rheumatoid, finger joint prosthesis for (Nicolle), PRS, *53:*106, 1974. Ann. chir. plast., *17:*275, 1972

Extensor expansion of the rheumatoid hand (Backhouse). Ann. Rheum. Dis., *31:*112, 1972

Silicone rubber-implants in hand surgery (Weigert *et al*). Arch. Orthop. Unfallchir., *73:*189, 1972 (German)

Chronic diseases of the synovial sheath (from hand surgery consulting hour) (Burkhardt). Beitr. Orthop. Traumatol., *19:*377, 1972 (German)

Functional efficiency of the hand following surgical treatment in severe ulnar deviation of fingers in rheumatoid arthritis (Strzyzewski *et al*). Chir. Narzadow. Ruchu Ortop. Pol., *37:*49, 1972 (Polish)

Hand function following tendon synovectomy at the wrist (Strzyzewski *et al*). Chir. Narzadow. Ruchu Ortop. Pol., *37:*381, 1972 (Polish)

Metacarpophalangeal joint surgery in rheumatoid arthritis: long-term results (Aptekar *et al*). Clin. Orthop., *83:*123, 1972

Quantitative results following implant arthroplasty of the proximal finger joints in the arthritic hand (Braun *et al*). Clin. Orthop., *83:*135, 1972

Variations in the insertion of the first dorsal interosseous muscle and their significance in the rheumatoid arthritis (Kuczynski). Hand, *4:*37, 1972

Flexible implant resection arthroplasty (Swanson). Hand, *4:*119, 1972

Treatment of prolapse and collapse of the proximal interphalangeal joint (Meulen). Hand, *4:*154, 1972

Flexible implant arthroplasty for arthritic finger joints: rationale, technique, and results of treatment (Swanson). J. Bone & Joint Surg. (Am.), *54:*435, 1972

Disabling arthritis at the base of the thumb: treatment by resection of the trapezium

Hands, Rheumatoid Disease of—Cont.

and flexible (silicone) implant arthroplasty (Swanson). J. Bone & Joint Surg. (Am.), *54:*456, 1972

Restoration of rheumatoid finger joint function. 3. A follow-up note after fourteen years of experience with a metallic-hinge prosthesis (Flatt *et al*). J. Bone & Joint Surg. (Am.), *54:*1317, 1972

Metacarpophalangeal joint of thumb, reconstruction in rheumatoid arthritis (Inglis *et al*), PRS, *51:*105, 1973. J. Bone & Joint Surg., *54A:*704, 1972

Natural history of the rheumatoid metacarpo-phalangeal joint (McMaster). J. Bone & Joint Surg. (Br.), *54:*637, 1972

Reconstruction of rheumatoid hands (Spivack). J. Med. Soc. N. J., *69:*547, 1972

Synovectomy of the rheumatoid hand. Lancet, *1:*131, 1972

Arthroplasty of the hand with silicone rubber prosthesis (Renner *et al*). Magy. Traumatol. Orthop., *15:*44, 1972 (Hungarian)

Surgery of the rheumatoid hand (Vainio). Mod. Trends Orthop., *5:*219, 1972

Pre-operative assessment of the hand, hip, and knee in rheumatoid arthritis (Bentley *et al*). Physiotherapy, *58:*83, 1972

"Swan-neck" deformity of the fingers in the rheumatoid hand: surgical correction (Rinaldi). Reumatismo, *24:*175, 1972 (Italian)

On the rheumatoid hand. Introduction (Tubiana). Rev. Chir. Orthop., *58:*399, 1972 (French)

Surgery of tenosynovitis of the extensors during chronic rheumatoid polyarthritis (Roullet). Rev. Chir. Orthop., *58:*407, 1972 (French)

Mechanism of finger deformities in the rheumatoid hand (Valentin). Rev. Chir. Orthop., *58:*445, 1972 (French)

Ulnar deviation. Arthroplasty of the metacarpophalangeal articulations (Allieu). Rev. Chir. Orthop., *58:*452, 1972 (French). Metacarpophalangeal tendinous reequilibrations in the rheumatoid hand. Rheumatoid thumb (Michon). Rev. Chir. Orthop., *58:*455, 1972 (French)

Correction of swan-neck deformities and rosette deformities in the rheumatoid hand (Achach). Rev. Chir. Orthop., *58:*461, 1972 (French)

Therapeutic indications in the rheumatoid hand (Tubiana). Rev. Chir. Orthop., *58:*464, 1972 (French)

Resorptive arthropathy and the opera-glass hand syndrome (Swezey *et al*). Semin. Arthritis Rheum., *2:*191, 1972–73

Hand, rheumatoid, reconstructive surgery

Hands, Rheumatoid Disease of—Cont.

of, early experience with Swanson silicone rubber prosthesis (McFarland), PRS, *51:*703, 1973. South M.J., *65:*1113, 1972

Erosive arthrosis (Kaludi). Union Med. Can., *101:*265, 1972 (French)

Characteristics of dynamic data of fingers in the healthy and rheumatoid hand (Seyfried). Z. Gesamte. Hyg., *18:*59, 1972 (German)

Synovial membrane and fluid, light and electron microscopic study, in joint involvement in progressive systemic sclerosis (scleroderma) (Schumacher), PRS, *53:*693, 1974. Am. J. Clin. Path., *60:*593, 1973

Arthritis, rheumatoid, synovial collagenase—regulation and metabolism of enzyme activity (Abe, Nagai), PRS, *53:*114, 1974. Asian M.J., *16:*155, 1973

Synovectomy for flexor tendon sheath involvement in rheumatoid arthritis (Jackson, Paton), PRS, *55:*109, 1975. Brit. J. Plast. Surg., *26:*122, 1973

Rheumatoid hand, functional results of excisional arthroplasty for (Robinson *et al*), PRS, *52:*688, 1973. Canad. M.A.J., *108:*1495, 1973

Pathogenesis of wind-mill wing position of fingers in primary chronic polyarthritis (Langloh). Fortschr. Med., *91:*313, 1973 (German)

Recent advances in the management of joint disease in the rheumatoid hand (Nicolle). Hand, *5:*91, 1973

Rheumatoid arthritis, mobility of metacarpophalangeal joints in (Loebl), PRS, *54:*376, 1974. Hand, *5:*165, 1973

Nerve conduction studies in resorptive arthropathies: opera-glass hand (Swezey *et al*). J Bone & Joint Surg. (Am.), *55:*1680, 1973

Synovitis, rheumatoid, posterior interosseous nerve syndrome secondary to (Millender, Nalebuff, Holdsworth), PRS, *52:*323, 1973. J. Bone & Joint Surg., *55A:*375, 1973

Role of surgery in the rheumatoid hand (Beckett *et al*). J. Ir. Med. Assoc., *66:*379, 1973

Surgical prevention and correction of deformities in the rheumatoid hand (Clark *et al*). Md. State Med. J., *22:*47, 1973

Implant arthroplasty in the hand. An introduction (Burton). Orthop. Clin. North Am., *4:*313, 1973

Pathogenesis and pathomechanics of rheumatoid deformities in the hand and wrist (Swanson *et al*). Orthop. Clin. North Am., *4:*1039, 1973

Hands, Rheumatoid Disease of—Cont.

Wrist and thumb in rheumatoid arthritis (Kleinert et al). Orthop. Clin. North Am., 4:1085, 1973

Intra-articular injection of radioisotopic beta emitters. Application to the treatment of the rheumatoid hand (Menkes et al). Orthop. Clin. North Am., 4:1113, 1973

Joint pain, degenerative arthritis of carpo-metacarpal joint of thumb (Lee), PRS, 53:106, 1974. Orthop. Rev., 2:45, 1973

Hand: efficacy of local steroid injection in treatment of stenosing tenovaginitis (Clark, Ricker, MacCollum). PRS, 51:179, 1973

Metacarpophalangeal subluxation in rheumatoid hand, role of intrinsic muscles in production of (Hueston, Wilson). PRS, 52:342, 1973

Synovectomy of the metacarpophalangeal joints in rheumatoid arthritis (Thompson et al). Proc. Roy. Soc. Med., 66:197, 1973

Diagnostic significance of tomography of the hand in rheumatoid arthritis (Eckhardt et al). Radiol. Diagn. (Berl.), 14:215, 1973 (German)

Methods and indications of surgical treatment of hands in rheumatoid arthritis in the light of our personal records (Gaslorowska). Reumatologia, 11:97, 1973 (Polish)

Synovectomy of the hand (Vainio). Rev. Rhum. Mal. Osteoartic., 40:205, 1973 (French)

Prosthesis and rehabilitation of the hand in chronic rheumatoid arthritis (Sany). Rev. Rhum. Mal. Osteoartic., 40:216, 1973 (French)

A new surgical procedure for correction of ulnar deviation of fingers in rheumatoid arthritis (Subhedar). Rheumatol. Phys. Med., 12:89, 1973

Treatment of chronic rheumatoid arthritis. 9. Treatment of tenosynovitis of the hand in chronic rheumatoid arthritis (Komatsubara et al). Ryumachi, 13:388, 1973 (Japanese)

Treatment of chronic rheumatoid arthritis. 10. Reconstruction of the hands in chronic rheumatoid arthritis (Inoue et al). Ryumachi, 13:390, 1973 (Japanese)

Conservative management of the wrist and hand in rheumatoid arthritis: the art of self-defense (Bennett). South. Med. J., 66:1267, 1973

Silicone rubber for surgery of the hand (Gonert et al). Ztschr. Orthop., 111:664, 1973 (German)

The Care of the Rheumatoid Hand, 3d Edi-

Hands, Rheumatoid Disease of—Cont.

tion. By Adrian E. Flatt. C. V. Mosby Co., St. Louis, 1974. PRS, 56:206, 1975

Arthroplasties of metacarpo-phalangeal joints with Swanson implants in the rheumatic hand. Critical appraisal of results (Allieu et al). Ann. Chir., 28:873, 1974 (French)

Deforming arthropathy in systemic lupus erythematosus (Russell et al). Ann. Rheum. Dis., 33:204, 1974

Results with the H-graft operation of Backdahl-Myrin in the treatment of ulnar deviation of the fingers (Jakob et al). Arch. Orthop. Unfallchir., 78:24, 1974 (German)

Exercise apparatus for patient with rheumatoid arthritis (Bens, Krewer), PRS, 55:519, 1975. Arch. Phys. Med., 53:477, 1974

Proceedings: deforming hand arthritis in systemic lupus erythematosus (Lawless et al). Arthritis Rheum., 17:323, 1974

Deforming non-erosive arthritis of the hand in systemic lupus erythematosus (Aptekar et al). Clin. Orthop., 100:120, 1974

Wrist, radial rotation in rheumatoid arthritis, tendon transfer for (Clayton, Ferlic), PRS, 55:637, 1975. Clin. Orthop., 100:176, 1974

Wrist, ulnar head resection in rheumatoid arthritis (Jackson et al), PRS, 56:228, 1975. Hand, 6:172, 1974

Oxyphenbutazone in plastic surgery (Chowdhury), PRS, 55:388, 1975. Indian J. Plast. Surg., 7:26, 1974

Dorsal tenosynovectomy and tendon transfer in the rheumatoid hand (Millender et al). J. Bone & Joint Surg. (Am.), 56:601, 1974

Loose vs. tight fitting of silastic prosthesis of the MP joint of the hand (Lewis). Med. Ann. D. C., 43:15, 1974

Tendon transfers in rheumatoid arthritis (Goldner). Orthop. Clin. North Am., 5:425, 1974

Arthroplasty of metacarpo-phalangeal finger joints in patients with rheumatoid polyarthritis (Grishin). Ortop. Travmatol. Protez., 35:19, 1974 (Russian)

Hand, synovial chondromatosis of (Constant, Harebottle, Davis). PRS, 54:353, 1974

Surgery of the rheumatoid arthritis of the hand (Prpic) Reumatizam, 21:167, 1974 (Croatian)

Arthroplasty by Swanson implants in the rheumatic hand. Experience from 100 cases, followed for more than 6 months (Kenesi et al). Rev. Rhum. Mal. Osteoartic., 41:271, 1974 (French)

Assessment of grip strength measurement in rheumatoid arthritis (Lee et al). Scand. J.

Hands, Rheumatoid Disease of—Cont.

Rheumatol., *3:*17, 1974

Synovectomy and articular cartilage (Schulitz), PRS, *54:*247, 1974. Ztschr. Orthop., *112:*118, 1974

Synovectomy of proximal interphalangeal joint in rheumatoid arthritis, 5-year follow-up (Ansell, Harrison), PRS, *56:*596, 1975. Hand, 7:34, 1975

Arthritis, rheumatoid, extra-articular causes of proximal joint stiffness in (Helal), PRS, *57:*119, 1976. Hand, 7:37, 1975

Three years' experience of metacarpophalangeal joint replacement in the rheumatoid hand (Griffiths *et al*). Hand, 7:275, 1975

Joints, MP, Silastic arthroplasty in rheumatoid arthritis (Mannerfelt *et al*), PRS, *57:*534, 1976. J. Bone & Joint Surg., *57A:*484, 1975

Principles of reconstructive surgery of the rheumatic hand (Wessinghage). Langenbecks Arch. Chir., *339:*395, 1975 (German)

Evaluation and treatment of early rheumatoid hand involvement (Millender *et al*). Orthop. Clin. North Am., *6:*697, 1975

Reconstructive surgery in the rheumatoid hand (Millender *et al*). Orthop. Clin. North Am., *6:*709, 1975

Surgical treatment of the swan-neck deformity in rheumatoid arthritis (Nalebuff *et al*). Orthop. Clin. North Am., *6:*733, 1975

Surgical treatment of the boutonniere deformity in rheumatoid arthritis (Nalebuff *et al*). Orthop. Clin. North Am., *6:*753, 1975

Rheumatoid nodules, benign (Simons, Schaller), PRS, *57:*123, 1976. Pediatrics, *56:*29, 1975

Hand injuries: needle aspiration of flexor digital sheath as aid in diagnosing tenosynovitis (Ryan, Hoopes). PRS, *56:*152, 1975

Regional intravenous administration of hydrocortisone in the treatment of the rheumatoid hand. I. Methods (Dabrowski). Reumatologia, *13:*301, 1975 (Polish)

Joint destruction in rheumatoid arthritis of hand (De la Caffiniere, Mozas, Achach), PRS, *56:*465, 1975. Rev. chir. orthop., *61:*61, 1975

Radiographic appearance of the rheumatoid hand (Schorn *et al*). S. Afr. Med. J., *49:*752, 1975

Hands, Skin Grafts and Flaps to

Tegumentary repair of lesions of the hand (Bajardi *et al*). Minerva Ortop., *20:*14, 1969 (Italian)

Treatment of wounds of the fingers and hand with preserved fetal membrane (Klassen *et al*). Vestn. Khir., *103:*89, 1969 (Russian)

Hands, Skin Grafts and Flaps to—Cont.

Principles of skin replacement in the hand (Harrison). Hand, *2:*106, 1970

Free graft (Cobbett). Hand, *2:*112, 1970

Use of skin flaps in hand injuries (Kinmonth). Hand, *2:*116, 1970

Degloving injuries (McGregor). Hand, *2:*130, 1970

Interpretation of skin loss and the preliminary treatment (Dawson). Hand, *2:*134, 1970

Millard "crane flap" for acute hand injuries (Crockett). Hand, *2:*156, 1970

Late results of island-flap plastic surgery (Zrubecky). Handchirurgie, *2:*129, 1970 (German)

Hand, use of tailored abdominal flap for surgical reconstruction (Kelleher *et al*), PRS, *49:*234, 1972. J. Bone & Joint Surg., *52A:*1552, 1970

Restoration of feeling in skin autotransplants transplanted to the hand and fingers (Matchin). Klin. Khir., *8:*57, 1970 (Russian)

Incisions, amputations, and skin grafting in the hand (Graham). Orthop. Clin. North Am., *1:*213, 1970

Local flaps for surgery of the hand (Beasley). Orthop. Clin. North Am., *1:*219, 1970

Problems in skin grafting of the palm in children (Ito). Orthop. Surg. (Tokyo), *21:*928, 1970 (Japanese)

Reconstructive surgery in severe deformation of the hand after deep burns (Dmitriev). Ortop. Travmatol. Protez., *31:*26, 1970 (Russian)

Indications for skin transplantation on a wide nourishing pedicle in injuries to the hand (Dmitrieva *et al*). Ortop. Travmatol. Protez., *31:*45, 1970 (Russian)

Principles of restorative-reconstructive surgery in burns of the hands (Biriukov). Vestn. Khir., *105:*80, 1970 (Russian)

Sub-clavicular tube flaps in reconstructive surgery of the hand (Dupart *et al*). Ann. Chir., *25:*1023, 1971 (French)

Use of flag-shaped flap in palmar defects (Vilain *et al*). Ann. Chir., *25:*1031, 1971 (French)

Surgical treatment of a case of dystrophic epidermolysis bullosa (Blauth). Handchirurgie, *3:*129, 1971 (German)

Hand injuries, skin cover in (Bailey), PRS, *48:*606, 1971. Injury, *2:*294, 1971

Hand skin tube constructor (Arai, Fukuda), PRS, *49:*240, 1972. Jap. J. Plast. Reconstr. Surg., *14:*330, 1971

Hand, cross finger flaps in (Johnson, Iverson), PRS, *49:*663, 1972. J. Bone & Joint

Hands, Skin Grafts and Flaps to – Cont.

ment for thumb web contracture (Hirshowitz *et al*). Hand, 7:291, 1975

Children, skin and soft tissue injuries of hand in (Bennett), PRS, *57:*261, 1976. Pediatr. Clin. N. Am., *22:*443, 1975

Hand tissue loss, adjacent flaps from opposing body surfaces (Smith, Furnas). PRS, *57:*351, 1976

Hands, Splints

New types of lively splints for peripheral nerve lesions affecting the hand (Parry *et al*). Hand, *2:*31, 1970

Modifications of the wrist-driven flexor hinge splint (McCluer *et al*). Arch. Phys. Med. Rehabil., *52:*233, 1971

Proportionally controlled externally powered hand splint (Patterson *et al*). Arch. Phys. Med. Rehabil., *52:*434, 1971

Physical therapy of the hand with special reference to splints and braces (Gassler). Handchirurgie, *4:*11, 1972 (German)

Polythene and Plastazote hand-resting splint (Sutcliffe *et al*). Physiotherapy, *58:*138, 1972

Farnham Park modular splint system (Ansell *et al*). Rheumatol. Phys. Med., *11:*334, 1972

Ratchet handsplint (McKenzie). Am. J. Occup. Ther., *27:*477, 1973

Traction hand splint (Wadsworth). Hand, *5:*268, 1973

Proceedings: plastic hand splints (Baumgartner). Hefte Unfallheilkd., *114:*297, 1973 (German)

Biological problems in the evolution of hand prostheses (Moberg). Orthop. Clin. North Am., *4:*1161, 1973

Adduction contracture of thumb, internal wire splint for (Araico, Valdes, Ortiz). PRS, *48:*339, 1973

Splinting, dynamic, for dorsal burns of hand (Salisbury, Palm). PRS, *51:*226, 1973

Hand splints made of plastics (Baumgartner). Z. Unfallmed. Berufskr., *66:*188, 1973 (German)

Hand: Principles of Splint Making. By N. R. Barr. Butterworth, London, 1974

Myoelectric hand splint (Silverstein *et al*). Am. J. Occup. Ther., *28:*99, 1974

A valuable splint for the rheumatoid hand (Nicolle *et al*). Hand, *7:*67, 1975

Ridged plaster volar slab (Varian). Hand, *7:*78, 1975

Splint, inflatable, to immobilize extremities after skin grafting (Schwager, Imber). PRS, *57:*523, 1976

Hands, Tendon Injuries (See also *Hands, Injuries; Hands, Nerve Injuries; Hands, Reconstructive Surgery*)

Management of flexor tendon injuries of the hand. The causes of primary suture failure (Buck-Gramcko). Monatsschr. Unfallheilkd., *72:*55, 1969 (German)

Tendon injuries of the hand (Wilhelm). Dtsch. Med. J., *21:*1391, 1970 (German)

Primary tendon repair (Bolton). Hand, *2:*56, 1970

Extensor tendon injuries of the back of the hand and wrist (Bruchle). Monatsschr. Unfallheilkd., *73:*503, 1970 (German)

Injuries to the extensor mechanism of the hand (Elliott). Orthop. Clin. North Am., *1:*335, 1970

Flexor tendon injuries (Potenza). Orthop. Clin. North Am., *1:*355, 1970

Physical therapy treatment following flexor tendon grafting (List). Prog. Phys. Ther., *1:*302, 1970

Biologic principles affecting repair of flexor tendons (Weiner *et al*). Adv. Surg., *5:*145, 1971

Flexor tendon, atraumatic retrieval (Kilgore *et al*), PRS, *49:*358, 1972. Am. J. Surg., *122:*430, 1971

Use of Jenning's barb wire in tendon sutures; absence of postoperative immobilization (Allieu *et al*). Ann. Chir., *25:*987, 1971 (French)

Tendon, flexor, repair, recent advances (Van Der Meulen), PRS, *49:*358, 1972. Arch. chir. neerl., *23:*129, 1971

Tendon lacerations of the hands (case P75) Can. Med. Assoc. J., *104:*415, 1971 (Editorial)

Tendon lacerations of the hands (case P75) (Percy). Can. Med. Assoc. J., *105:*635, 1971

Function of the hand following injuries of the flexor and extensor tendons (Zeyland-Malawka). Chir. Narzadow. Ruchu Ortop. Pol., *36:*33, 1971 (Polish)

Delayed primary suture in flexor tendon division (Salvi). Hand, *3:*181, 1971

Post-traumatic tenolysis in the hand (Nummi *et al*). Handchirurgie, *3:*11, 1971 (German)

Rehabilitation – conservative measures following surgical treatment of tendon injuries of the hand (Scharizer). Handchirurgie, *3:*99, 1971 (German)

Combined nerve and tendon injury in the palm (Rix). J.A.M.A., *217:*480, 1971

Hands, severely damaged, flexor tendon reconstruction (Hunter, Salisbury), PRS, *50:*632, 1972. J. Bone & Joint Surg., *53:*829, 1971

Hands, Tendon Injuries — Cont.

Flexor tendon injury of the hand — reconstructive surgery and evaluation (Suzuki). J. Jap. Orthop. Assoc., *45:*651, 1971

Injuries of the flexor tendon of the hand — free tendon graft following pedicle flap transfer (Suzuki *et al*). Orthop. Surg. (Tokyo), *22:*870, 1971 (Japanese)

Flexor tendon injuries, finger-flexion device for (Webber). PRS, *48:*284, 1971

Hand, treatment of flexor tendon lesions in (Schokkenbroek), PRS, *49:*358, 1972. Thesis, Univ. Utrecht, 1971

Treatment of injuries to the flexor tendons of the fingers at the level of the fibro-osseous canals (Tkachenko *et al*). Vestn. Khir., *107:*80, 1971 (Russian)

Results of treatment of injuries to the flexor tendons (Winston). Hand, *4:*45, 1972

Combined two-stage tenoplasty with silicone rods for multiple flexor tendon injuries in "no-man's-land" (Chong *et al*). J. Trauma, *12:*104, 1972

Hand, tendon injuries of (Schink), PRS, *51:*603, 1973. Langenbecks Arch. Chir., *332:*495, 1972

Early and late homoplasty in tendon injuries of the hand and fingers (Kolontai *et al*). Ortop. Travmatol. Protez., *33:*18, 1972 (Russian)

Avulsion injury of long flexor tendons (Chang, Thoms, White). PRS, *50:*260, 1972

Treatment of acute hand injuries (Chase). Proc. Mine. Med. Off. Assoc., *51:*9, 1972

Tendon injuries (Chase). Proc. Mine. Med. Off. Assoc., *51:*14, 1972

Indications for primary suture of the digital flexor tendons in injuries at the level of the synovial-aponeurotic sheath (Kornilov). Vestn. Khir., *108:*89, 1972 (Russian)

Late results of treating injuries to the flexor tendons of the fingers and hand (Dokish *et al*). Vestn. Khir., *108:*93, 1972 (Russian)

Tendons, flexor, recent lesions at finger level (Duparc *et al*), PRS, *53:*243, 1974. Ann. Chir., *27:*467, 1973

Hand, avulsion of the profundus tendon insertion in football players (Wenger), PRS, *52:*452, 1973. Arch. Surg., *106:*145, 1973

Hand, extensor tendon injuries of (McFarlane, Hampole), PRS, *53:*488, 1974. Canad. J. Surg., *16:*366, 1973

Philosophy of tendon repair (Entin). Orthop. Clin. North Am., *4:*859, 1973

Primary repair of flexor tendons (Kleinert *et al*). Orthop. Clin. North Am., *4:*865, 1973

Results and complications of flexor tendon grafting (Tubiana). Orthop. Clin. North Am., *4:*877, 1973

Hands, Tendon Injuries — Cont.

Treatment of patients with isolated injuries of tendons of the flexor digitorum profundus (Vodianov). Ortop. Travmatol. Protez., *34:*8, 1973 (Russian)

Flexor tendon injuries of the hand (Biro *et al*). Orv. Hetil., *114:*610, 1973 (Hungarian)

Extensor indicis proprius syndrome, clinical test (Spinner, Olshansky). PRS, *51:*134, 1973

Hand injuries: alterations in finger growth following flexor tendon injuries (Gaisford, Fleegler). PRS, *51:*164, 1973

Finger joints: dynamic tenodesis of distal interphalangeal joint, for use after severance of *profundus* alone (Kahn). PRS, *51:*536, 1973

Flap, retrograde tendon, use of in repairing severed extensor in PIP joint area (Snow). PRS, *51:*555, 1973

Tendon healing: results of tenolysis, controlled evaluation in chickens (Hurst, McCain, Lindsay). PRS, *52:*171, 1973

Tendon graft: evaluation of the *flexor profundus* of the fingers (Ojeda), PRS, *53:*606, 1974. Rev. Latino Am. cir. plast., *17:*57, 1973

Treatment of soft part deficiencies and tendon injuries of the hand (Spillner *et al*). Z. Allgemeinmed., *49:*68, 1973 (German)

Tendon, *flexor longus*, of fingers, surgery of proximal pulley in injuries (De la Caffiniere), PRS, *55:*511, 1975. Ann. chir. plast., *19:*201, 1974

In quest of the solution to severed flexor tendons (Kleinert *et al*). Clin Orthop., *104:*23, 1974

Tendon grafts for isolated injuries of the flexor digitorum profundus tendon (Wexler *et al*). Isr. J. Med. Sci., *10:*1448, 1974

Vascularization and the gliding mechanism of free flexor-tendon grafts inserted by the silicone-rod method (Urbaniak *et al*). J Bone & Joint Surg. (Am.), *56:*473, 1974

Hand, repair potential of digital flexor tendons (Matthews, Richards), PRS, *56:*679, 1975. J. Bone & Joint Surg., *56:*618, 1974

Initial care for lacerations of flexor tendons of the hand (Winslow *et al*). N. C. Med. J., *35:*38, 1974

Biomechanics of tendon transfer (Brand). Orthop. Clin. North Am., *5:*205, 1974

Children, cut flexor tendons in "some-man's-land," purposeful delay of primary repair (Arons), PRS, *53:*638, 1974. Discussion by Hartrampf, PRS, *54:*95, 1974

Diagnosis and management of the severed flexor tendon of the hand (Fetrow). Surg. Clin. North Am., *54:*923, 1974

Hands, Tendon Injuries — Cont.

Tendon sutures, tendon transplantations and tendon transfer on the hand (Wilhelm). Chirurg., *46*:301, 1975 (German)

Surgical exposure of the flexor pollicis longus tendon (Bruner). Hand, 7:241, 1975

Intra-tendinous tendon suture in the hand — a new technique (Tsuge *et al*). Hand, 7:250, 1975

Substitution of the tendon sheath by autologous vein in the "no-man's land" of the hand (Mihaly *et al*). Magy. Traumatol. Orthop., *18*:421, 1975 (Hungarian)

Injury of the tendons of the hand (Dubrov). Ortop. Travmatol. Protez., *5*:75, 1975 (Russian)

Laceration, should an incompletely severed tendon be sutured? (Reynolds, Wray, Weeks), PRS, *57*:36, 1976. Discussion by Kleinert, PRS, *57*:236, 1976

*Hands, Tendon Ruptures in (*See also *Hands, Rheumatoid Disease of)*

Unusual therapeutic method in extensor tendon rupture with bone involvement (Buck-Gramcko). Handchirurgie, *2*:210, 1970 (German)

Rupture of all digital flexor tendons in the wrist (Levin). Vestn. Khir., *105*:123, 1970 (Russian)

So-called spontaneous tendon ruptures in the rheumatoid hand (Luppino *et al*). Chir. Organi. Mov., *60*:661, 1971 (Italian)

Hands of non-rheumatoid patients, ruptures of flexor tendons in (Folmar, Nelson, Phalen), PRS, *51*:106, 1973. J. Bone & Joint Surg., *54A*:579, 1972

Synovectomy of flexors and flexor ruptures (Gay). Rev. Chir. Orthop., *58*:414, 1972 (French)

Rheumatoid arthritis, *flexor digitorum sublimis* transfer for multiple extensor tendon ruptures in (Nalebuff, Patel). PRS, *52*:530, 1973

Hands, Vascular Injuries

Acute disseminated lupus erythematosus with gangrene of the fingers of the hand (Raffi *et al*). Pediatrie, *23*:358, 1968 (French)

Circulatory diversion syndrome of the upper limb. Etio-pathogenic role of repeated micro-trauma (Langeron *et al*). Ann. Cardiol. Angiol. (Paris), *18*:235, 1969 (French)

Etiology and treatment of ischemic contractures of the forearm and hand (Duben). Handchirurgie, *1*:63, 1969 (German)

Fasciotomy in peripheral vascular surgery (Patman, Thompson), PRS, *49*:359, 1972.

Hands, Vascular Injuries — Cont.

Arch. Surg., *101*:663, 1970

Treatment of arterial injuries of the forearm and hand (Hentschel *et al*). Handchirurgie, *2*:18, 1970 (German)

Cases of severe vascular injury to the hand (Cameron). Hand, *2*:74, 1970

Angiography of the upper extremity (Rahmel). Handchirurgie, *2*:91, 1970 (German)

Anatomy of the arterial pattern of the palmar arch of the hand (Scharlzer). Handchirurgie, *2*:122, 1970 (German)

Examining the blood supply of the hand following injuries (Bruchie). Handchirurgie, *2*:147, 1970 (German)

Post-traumatic Raynaud's syndrome of the hand. Description of 2 cases (Tomasini). Med. Lav., *61*:378, 1970 (Italian)

Nosographic classification of diseases caused by vibratory machines by means of angiographic examination (Feltrin *et al*). Minerva Cardioangiol., *18*:671, 1970 (Italian)

Hand ischemia: hypothenar hammer syndrome (Conn *et al*). Proc. Inst. Med. Chic., *28*:83, 1970

Hypothenar hammer syndrome: posttraumatic digital ischemia (Conn *et al*). Surgery, *68*:1122, 1970

Accidental intra-arterial injection of promethazine HCl during general anesthesia: report of a case (Mostafavi *et al*). Anesthesiology, *35*:645, 1971

Hand, severe ischemia (Bergan, Conn, Trippel), PRS, *48*:94, 1971. Ann. Surg., *173*:301, 1971

Fasciotomy in massive venous thrombosis (Bialostozky *et al*). Arch. Inst. Cardiol. Mex., *41*:680, 1971 (Spanish)

Occupational true aneurysm of the ulnar artery in the palm (Mukerjea). Brit. J. Surg., *58*:934, 1971

Ischemia of the hand from using palm as hammer. Geriatrics, *26*:76, 1971 (Editorial)

Traumatic aneurysm of the radial artery in a 10-year-old child (Petrovic *et al*). Med. Pregl., *24*:517, 1971 (Serbian)

Arterial occlusion caused by jobs that are hard on the hands (Olin). Med. Times, *99*:178, 1971

Digitopalmar steal syndrome with peripheral arteriovenous fistula (De Pena Perez *et al*). Med. Welt., *15*:601, 1971 (German)

Patient with thrombosis of the ulnar artery in the hand caused by blunt trauma (Luning). Ned. Tijdschr. Geneeskd., *115*:1997, 1971 (Dutch)

Ulnar artery, false aneurysm after surgery employing tourniquet (Thio), PRS, *50*:540, 1972. Am. J. Surg., *123*:356, 1972

Hands, Vascular Injuries – Cont.

Hand, arterial aneurysms of (Poirier, Stansel), PRS, *51:*230, 1973. Am. J. Surg., *124:*72, 1972

Thrombosis of ulnar artery of hand following blunt injury (Luning), PRS, *51:*703, 1973; *52:*99, 1973. Arch. chir. neerl., *24:*289, 1972

Heroin addicts, necrotizing skin lesions in (Dunne, Johnson), PRS, *50:*538, 1972. Arch. Dermat., *105:*544, 1972

Results of the treatment of arteriovenous malformations of the extremities by means of muscle embolization. Preliminary report (Escobar Aldasoro *et al*). Arch. Inst. Cardiol. Mex., *42:*247, 1972 (Spanish)

Tourniquet time in hand surgery (Flatt), PRS, *50:*101, 1972. Arch. Surg., *104:*190, 1972

Incidence of the hypothenar hammer syndrome (Little *et al*). Arch. Surg., *104:*684, 1972

Trauma to the ulnar artery (Kettlekamp). Arch. Surg., *105:*682, 1972

Aneurysms and thromboses of the ulnar artery in the hand (Millender *et al*). Arch. Surg., *105:*686, 1972

Vascular complications of drug abuse (Maxwell, Olcott, Blaisdell), PRS, *51:*605, 1973. Arch. Surg., *105:*875, 1972

Single congenital arteriovenous fistula of the hand (Greenhalgh *et al*). Brit. J. Surg., *59:*76, 1972

Aneurysm of the ulnar artery. A case report (Kaplan *et al*). Bull. Hosp. Joint Dis., *33:*197, 1972

Symmetric ischemic necrosis – cold-induced digital epiphyseal necrosis in childhood (Hakstian), PRS, *50:*631, 1972. Canad. J. Surg., *15:*168, 1972

Digital nerve compression secondary to palmar aneurysm (O'Connor). Clin. Orthop., *83:*149, 1972

Significance of acral oscillography in functional circulation disorders caused by work with compressed-air tools (Oeser *et al*). Dtsch. Gesundheitsw., *27:*942, 1972 (German)

Drug addiction, puffy hand of; study of pathogenesis (Neviaser, Butterfield, Wieche), PRS, *51:*106, 1973. J. Bone & Joint Surg., *54A:*629, 1972

Hand, impending ischemic contracture; early diagnosis and management (Spinner *et al*). PRS, *50:*341, 1972

Angiography of the hand: guidelines for interpretation (Calenoff). Radiology, *102:*331, 1972

Ischemia of hand and fingers, method for assessing (Yao *et al*), PRS, *51:*348, 1973.

Hands, Vascular Injuries – Cont.

Surg. Gynec. & Obst., *135:*373, 1972

Extremity complications of drug abuse (Ritland, Butterfield), PRS, *54:*109, 1974. Am. J. Surg., *126:*639, 1973

Ultrasonic evaluation of the palmar circulation. A useful adjunct to radial artery cannulation (Mozersky *et al*). Am. J. Surg., *126:*810, 1973

Revascularization of the hand in a patient with complete interruption of the radial and ulnar arteries (Boyle *et al*). Arch. Phys. Med. Rehabil., *54:*229, 1973

Hand, aneurysms of (Kleinert, Burget, Morgan), PRS, *52:*595, 1973. Arch. Surg., *106:*554, 1973

Hand, acutely swollen, in drug user (Daniel), PRS, *53:*683, 1974. Arch. Surg., *107:*548, 1973

Circulatory patterns in the normal hand (Little *et al*). Brit. J. Surg., *60:*652, 1973

Main line accidental intra-arterial drug injection (Hawkins *et al*). Clin. Orthop., *94:*268, 1973

Limb, upper, ischemic effects of external and internal pressure on (Parkes), PRS, *54:*236, 1974. Hand, *5:*105, 1973

Hand problems, severe, in drug addicts (Petrie, Lamb), PRS, *54:*236, 1974. Hand, *5:*130, 1973

True and false traumatic aneurysms in the hand (Green). J. Bone & Joint Surg. (Am.), *55:*120, 1973

Tissue-viability assessment with the Doppler ultrasonic flowmeter in acute injuries of extremities (Scherr *et al*). J. Bone & Joint Surg. (Am.), *55:*157, 1973

Acute necrosis of the second interosseous compartment of the hand (Reid *et al*). J. Bone & Joint Surg. (Am.), *55:*1095, 1973

Hand ischemia, incidence of traumatic obstruction of superficial palmar arch (Bes, Descotes), PRS, *53:*107, 1974. J. Chir., *105:*261, 1973

Arterial occlusion: radial artery occlusion by a carpal ganglion (Kelly). PRS, *52:*191, 1973

Soft tissue changes in hands of drug addicts (McCabe, Ditmars). PRS, *52:*538, 1973

Arteries, ulnar, bilateral thrombosis of, in the hands (Eguro, Goldner). PRS, *52:*573, 1973

Catheterization, arterial, tissue necrosis from vascular complications of upper extremity after (Graham *et al*), PRS, *53:*487, 1974. Rev. Latino Am. cir. plast., *17:*37, 1973

Ulnar artery aneurysms of the hand (Gaylis *et al*). Surgery, *73:*478, 1973

Hands, Vascular Injuries—Cont.

Congenital arteriovenous fistula of the hand (Oschatz *et al*). Zentralbl. Chir., *98:*1783, 1973 (German)

Hand and energy. Arteriography in hand injuries, its symptomatology, its therapeutic implications (Mitz *et al*). Ann. Chir., *28:*835, 1974 (French)

Sympathectomy, upper limb (Koikkalainen *et al*). Ann. Chir. Gynaecol. Fenn., *63:*318, 1974

Hand, vascular lesions in (Neviaser, Adams), PRS, *55:*637, 1975. Clin. Orthop., *100:*111, 1974

Gangrene of the hand and forearm: a complication of radial artery cannulation (Katz *et al*). Crit. Care Med., *2:*270, 1974

Comparative angiographic investigations of the upper limb under local, regional and general anesthesia (Viehweger *et al*). Fortschr. Geb. Roentgenstr. Nuklearmed., *121:*303, 1974 (German)

Gangrene of the hand in a newborn child (Hoffman *et al*). Hand, *6:*70, 1974

Ischemic muscle contracture of the hand (Mittelmeier). Hefte Unfallheilkd., *0:*322, 1974 (German)

Hand, small-vessel flow in (Wilgis *et al*), PRS, *55:*509, 1975. J. Bone & Joint Surg., *56A:*1199, 1974

Drug subculture, orthopedic implications of (Kaufer *et al*), PRS, *57:*541, 1976. J. Trauma, *14:*853, 1974

Role of arteriography in the reconstruction of severe hand injuries (Salacz *et al*). Magy. Traumatol. Orthop., *17:*88, 1974 (Hungarian)

Loss of limb following intravenous diazepam (Schneider *et al*). Pediatrics, *53:*112, 1974

Drug injection injuries of hands and forearms in addicts (Ryan, Hoopes, Jabaley). PRS, *53:*445, 1974

Hand: patterns of diseased fascia in fingers in Dupuytren's contracture. Displacement of neurovascular bundles (McFarlane). PRS, *54:*31, 1974

Hand, aneurysm of (Carneiro). PRS, *54:*483, 1974

Aneurisms of the hand and fingers in children (Pous *et al*). Ann. Chir., *29:*1005, 1975 (French)

Intra-arterial injection of barbiturate (Nathan). Hand, *7:*175, 1975

Thrombosis of the ulnar artery in the hand (Herndon *et al*). J. Bone & Joint Surg. (Am.), *57:*994, 1975

Perforation of the deep palmar arch produced by surgical wire after tenorrhaphy. A case report and review of the literature (Diaz *et*

Hands, Vascular Injuries—Cont.

al). J. Bone & Joint Surg. (Am.), *57:*1150, 1975

Vascular disease, bull man's hand (Brady, O'Sullivan), PRS, *57:*262, 1976. J. Cardiovasc. Surg., *16:*157, 1975

Digital ischemia: hypothenar hammer syndrome (Pinkerton *et al*). J. Kans. Med. Soc., *76:*125, 1975

Effects of radial artery cannulation (Little *et al*). M. J. Australia, *2:*791, 1975

Raynaud's phenomenon, diagnosis and treatment (Porter *et al*), PRS, *56:*107, 1975. Surgery, *77:*11, 1975

Hand, ischemic contracture of intrinsic musculature of, presence of modified fibroblasts in (Madden, Carlson, Hines), PRS, *56:*595, 1975. Surg. Gynec. & Obst., *140:*509, 1975

Carpal tunnel syndrome, following vascular shunt procedure in the forearm (Mancusi-Ungaro, Corres, Di Spaltro). PRS, *57:*96, 1976

HANEKE, A. *et al*: Conservative surgical method for odontogenic maxillary sinus diseases. Observations on 113 patients. Z. W. R., *83:*20, 1974 (German)

HANEKE, E.: Psoriasis in autologous grafts. Dermatol. Monatsschr., *159:*227, 1973 (German)

HANLON, C. R.: Directors' memo (physician manpower), PRS, *56:*601, 1975. Bull. Am. Coll. Surg., *60:*30, 1975

HANNA, D. C.: Midline forehead flap nasal reconstructions in patients with low browlines (with Richardson, Gaisford). PRS, *49:*130, 1972

HANNA, M. *et al*: Histopathology of tumor regression after intra-lesional injection of *Mycobacterium bovis*. Development of immunity to tumor cells and BCG, PRS, *54:*509, 1974. J. Nat. Cancer Inst., *51:*1897, 1973

HANNA, M. K. *et al*: Genital function in males with vesical exstrophy and epispadias. Brit. J. Urol., *44:*169, 1972

HANQUET, M. *et al*: Hyperbaric oxygen therapy in a caisson using pure oxygen. Laval. Med., *42:*647, 1971 (French)

HANS, S. H., WEISER, R. S., AND KAU, S. T.: Prolonged survival of skin allografts in leprosy patients, PRS, *51:*611, 1973. Internat. J. Leprosy, *39:*1, 1971

HANSELMAYER, H.: Prognosis of injured canaliculi in relation to elapsed time until primary operation. Ophthalmologica, *166:*175, 1973

HANSELMAYER, H. *et al*: Injuries of lacrimal canaliculus: surgical technics and prognosis.

Klin. Monatsbl. Augenheilkd., *160:*572, 1972 (German)

HANSELMAYER, H. *et al:* Ear skin-cartilage plastic surgery for eyelid margin tumors. Ophthalmologica, *165:*464, 1972 (German)

HANSEN, A. *et al:* Vocalization via a cuffed tracheostomy tube. A new principle. Anaesthesia, *30:*878, 1975

HANSEN, J. E.: Cryosurgical therapy of benign lesions of skin and mucous membranes, PRS, *50:*424, 1972. Internat. Surg., *56:*403, 1971

HANSEN, L. S. *et al:* Traumatic bone cysts of jaws. Oral Surg., *37:*899, 1974

HANSEN, M. G., *et al:* Tumor thickness and lymphocytic infiltration in malignant melanoma of head and neck. Am. J. Surg., *128:*557, 1974

HAPPLE, R.: Malignant melanoma and L-dopa. Review of literature on the problem of causal relationship. Fortschr. Med., *92:*1065, 1974 (German)

HAPPLE, R. *et al:* Spontaneous regression and leukoderma in malignant melanoma. Hautarzt, *26:*120, 1975 (German)

HAQ, M. A.: One-stage reconstruction for exstrophy of the bladder in girls (with Furnas, Somers). PRS, *56:*61, 1975. Discussion by Devine. PRS, *56:*209, 1975

HARA, T., TSUYAMA, N., AND FURUSAWA, S.: Repair of sensation of median nerve by nerve crossing, PRS, *53:*369, 1974. Operation, *27:*551, 1973

HARAD, O., AND ISHII, H.: Condition of auditory ossicles in microtia. Findings in 57 middle ear operations. PRS, *50:*48, 1972

HARADA, N., AND SAWADA, A.: Surgical treatment for microphallus, PRS, *52:*207, 1973. J. Urol., *108:*594, 1972

HARADA, T.: Microspectrophotometric study of lactic dehydrogenase in experimental autotransplantation of skin to oral mucous membrane. J. Otolaryngol. Jap., *75:*1362, 1972 (Japanese)

HARADA, T., AND KUROZUMI, S.: Study of autologous skin graft in mucomembraneous floor by microspectrophotometry. J. Otolaryngol. Jap., *75:*1072, 1972 (Japanese)

HARADA, Y.: Scanning electron microscope study of microvascular anastomoses (with Servant, Ikuta). PRS, *57:*329, 1976

HARAMPIEV, K. *et al:* Rhinolithiasis associated with nasal polyposis. Srp. Arh. Celok. Lek., *101:*929, 1973 (Serbian)

HARASHINA, T.: Autogenous *en bloc* transplantation of mammary gland in dogs, using microsurgical technique (with Fujino, Mikata). PRS, *50:*376, 1972

HARASHINA, T.: Reconstruction for aplasia of breast and pectoral region by microvascular

transfer of free flap from buttock (with Fujino, Aoyagi), PRS, *56:*178, 1975. Discussion by Goldwyn, PRS, *56:*335, 1975

HARASHINA, T.: Free skin flap from retroauricular region to nose (with Fujino, Nakajima). PRS, *57:*338, 1976

HARASHINA, T., AND TAJIMA, S.: Injury to superior oblique muscle and trochlea and associated EOM imbalance, PRS, *53:*602, 1974. Jap. J. Plast. Reconstr. Surg., *16:*362, 1973

HARASHINA, T. *et al:* Rejection phenomena after homotransplantation of skin flaps in dogs by microvascular technique. PRS, *52:*390, 1973

HARASHINA, T., AND BUNCKE, H. J.: Study of washout solutions for microvascular replantation and transplantation. PRS, *56:*542, 1975

HARCOURT, F. L.: Pharyngo-esophagostomy. Eye, Ear, Nose, Throat, Mon., *52:*26, 1973

HARDAWAY, R. M.: Problem of acute severe trauma and shock, PRS, *49:*669, 1972. Surg. Gynec. & Obst., *133:*799, 1971

HARDENBERGH, E.: Hyperbaric oxygen treatment of experimental frostbite in mouse, PRS, *51:*354, 1973. J. Surg. Res., *12:*34, 1972

HARDENBERGH, E., AND MILES, J. A., JR.: Effect of sympathectomy on tissue loss after experimental frostbite of rabbit ear, PRS, *52:*99, 1973. J. Surg. Res., *13:*126, 1972

HARDILLIER, J.: Surgical treatment of varicose ulcers. Phlebologie, *27:*149, 1974 (French)

HARDIN, B.: Suggestion of George Bernard Shaw: adjunct in men's facelifting. PRS, *50:*416, 1972

HARDIN, J. C., JR.: Triple fractures of the mandible with flaring rami. Their treatment with lingual splints. Arch. Otolaryng., *98:*387, 1973

HARDIN, W. J.: Surgical management of malignant lesions of skin. Tex. Med., *69:*87, 1973

HARDING, R. L.: Replantation of mandible in cancer surgery (Follow-Up Clinic). PRS, *48:*586, 1971

HARDING, R. L.: Malignant ameloblastoma with pulmonary metastases, report of case and review of literature (with Herceg). PRS, *49:*456, 1972

HARDING, R. L.: Trainor blepharoplasty for ptosis (with Herceg). PRS, *49:*622, 1972

HARDING, R. L.: Obituary on Robert H. Ivy, M.D., PRS, *55:*122, 1974

HARDING, R. L.: Increasing complexities in world of plastic surgery. PRS, *56:*609, 1975

HARDING, R. L., AND MAZAHERI, M.: Growth and spatial changes in arch form in bilateral cleft lip and palate patients. PRS, *50:*591, 1972

HARDING, R. L. *et al:* Robert Henry Ivy 1881–

1974. Cleft Palate J., *11:*508, 1974

HARDMAN, F. G.: Keratocanthoma on the lips. Brit. J. Oral Surg., *9:*46, 1971

HARDNER, G. J. *et al:* Carcinoma of penis, PRS, *51:*349, 1973. J. Urol., *108:*428, 1972

HARDY, JAMES D.: *Human Organ Support and Replacement. Transplantation and Artificial Prostheses.* Charles C Thomas, Springfield Ill., 1971. PRS, *49:*81, 1972

HARDY, K. L.: Tracheostomy: indications, technics, and tubes, a reappraisal, PRS, *53:*105, 1974. Am. J. Surg., *126:*300, 1973

HARDY, R. W.: Current techniques in management of pain, PRS, *56:*602, 1975. Cleveland Clin. Quart., *41:*177, 1974

HARDY, S. B.: Electromyography in full thickness flaps rotated between upper and lower lips (Follow-Up Clinic). PRS, *48:*72, 1971

HARDY, S. B.: Modified Bonnacolto dacryocystorhinostomy (with Spira, Gerow). PRS, *52:*511, 1973

HARDY, S. B.: Simplified design for reduction mammaplasty (with Gerow, Spira). PRS, *53:*271, 1974

HARDY, S. B.: Complications of chemical face peeling (with Spira, Gerow). PRS, *54:*397, 1974

HARGISS, J. L.: Inferior aponeurosis *vs* orbital septum tucking for senile entropion. Arch. Ophth., *89:*210, 1973

HARGISS, J. L.: Anatomic approach to corrective surgery for blepharoptosis. Trans. Am. Acad. Ophthalmol. Otolaryngol., *79:*696, 1975

HARIHARAN, S.: Off-midline forehead flap for repair of small nasal defects (with Dhawan, Aggarwal). PRS, *53:*537, 1974

HARII, K.: Fundamental technique of microvascular surgery. Neurol. Surg. (Tokyo), *3:*889, 1975 (Japanese)

HARII, K., AND OHMORI, S.: Use of gastroepiploic vessels as recipient or donor vessels in free transfer of composite flaps by microvascular anastomoses. PRS, *52:*541, 1973

HARII, K., OHMORI, K., AND OHMORI, S.: Free deltopectoral skin flaps, PRS, *56:*678, 1975. Brit. J. Plast. Surg., *27:*231, 1974

HARII, K., OHMORI, K., AND MURAKAMI, F.: Hair transplantation with free scalp flap, PRS, *55:*374, 1975. Jap. J. Plast. Reconstr. Surg., *17:*381, 1974

HARII, K., OHMORI, K., AND OHMORI, S.: Successful clinical transfer of ten free flaps by microvascular anastomoses, PRS, *53:*259, 1974. Discussion by Goldwyn, PRS, *53:*469, 1974

HARII, K., OHMORI, K., AND OHMORI, S.: Hair transplantation with free scalp flaps. PRS, *53:*410, 1974

HARII, K., AND OHMORI, K.: Free groin flaps in children, PRS, *55:*588, 1975

HARII, K. *et al:* Free skin flap transfer. Clin. Plast. Surg., *3:*111, 1976

HARII, K., OHMORI, K., AND TORII, S.: Free *gracilis* muscle transplantation with microneurovascular anastomoses. PRS, *57:*133, 1976

HARII, K., OHMORI, K., AND SEKIGUCHI, J.: Free musculocutaneous flap, PRS, *57:*294, 1976. Discussion by Cannon, PRS, *57:*511, 1976

HARKINS, P. D., AND RAFFETY, J. E.: Digital transposition in the injured hand, PRS, *51:*231, 1973. J. Bone & Joint Surg., *54A:*1064, 1972

HARLE, F.: Primary, early secondary or late secondary osteoplasty in cleft surgery? Clinical and animal experimental study. Dtsch. Zahnaerztl. Z., *28:*612, 1973 (German)

HARLE, F.: Visor osteotomy to increase the absolute height of the atrophied mandible. A preliminary report. J. Maxillo-facial Surg., *3:*257, 1975

HARLE, F. *et al:* Problems and results of Eschler's dorsal masseter transposition for the treatment of Robin's syndrome. Dtsch. Zahnaerztl. Z., *27:*47, 1972 (German)

HARLE, F. *et al:* Experimental study on maxillary growth after bone grafting in clefts. J. Maxillo-facial Surg., *1:*194, 1973

HARLE, F. *et al:* Emergency situation following surgery for cleft palate in children with Robin syndrome and its therapy. Oster. Z. Stomatol., *70:*131, 1973 (German)

HARLE, F. *et al:* Pressure-plate osteosynthesis in zygomatic fractures. Dtsch. Zahnaerztl. Z., *30:*71, 1975 (German)

HARLE, F. *et al:* Surgical methods for the correction of malocclusion Angle II/1 with postoperative prosthetic rehabilitation. Dtsch. Zahnaerztl. Z., *30:*176, 1975 (German)

HARLE, F. *et al:* Surgical technic for the prevention of postoperative telecanthus in naso-ethmoidal fractures. Fortschr. Kiefer. Gesichtschir., *19:*147, 1975 (German)

HARNACK, K. *et al:* Endogenous eczema in a split-thickness skin graft. Dermatol. Monatsschr., *158:*28, 1972 (German)

HARNESS, D. *et al:* Double anastomotic innervation of thenar muscles. J. Anat., *109:*461, 1971

HARNESS, D. *et al:* Double motor innervation of the opponens pollicis muscles: an electromyographic study. J. Anat., *117:*329, 1974

HARPER, P. S.: Turban tumors (cylindromatosis). Birth Defects, *7:*338, 1971

HARPMAN, J. A.: Surgery of pterygoid fossa. Eye, Ear, Nose, Throat Mon., *53:*354, 1974

HARRELSON, J. M. *et al*: Hypertrophy of *flexor carpi ulnaris* as cause of ulnar nerve compression in distal part of forearm, PRS, 57:534, 1976. J. Bone & Joint Surg., 57A:554, 1975

HARRFELDT, H. P.: Problems of anesthesia in patients with burns. PRS, 50:203, 1972. Langenbecks Arch. Chir., 329:907, 1971

HARRFELDT, H. P.: General therapy and anesthesia of patients with burns. Monatsschr. Unfallheilkd., 75:103, 1972 (German)

HARRIES, T.: Preoperative and postoperative consideration of natural facial asymmetry (with Gorney). PRS, 54:187, 1974

HARRINGTON, P. C. *et al*: Effect of dermal grafts on the revascularization of skin flaps. Arch. Otolaryng., 95:58, 1972

HARRIS, A. W.: Adjustable clamp for use during plating and grafting procedures in mandible. Brit. J. Oral Surg., 10:220, 1972

HARRIS, C., AND RUTLEDGE, G. L.: Functional anatomy of extensor mechanism of finger, PRS, 51:104, 1973. J. Bone & Joint Surg., 54A:713, 1972

HARRIS, C. N., AND COURTEMANCHE, A. D.: Gastric mucosal cyst of tongue. PRS, 54:612, 1974

HARRIS, D. R.: Evaluation of cryosurgery for basal cell carcinoma (with Vistnes, Fajardo). PRS, 55:71, 1975

HARRIS, D. R., FILARSKI, S. A., JR., AND HECTOR, R. E.: Effect of Silastic sheet dressings on healing of split-skin graft donor sites. PRS, 52:189, 1973

HARRIS, J. A. *et al*: Attention, learning, and personality during ketamine emergence, PRS, 56:605, 1975. Anesth. Analg., Cleve., 54:169, 1975

HARRIS, J. J.: Clear cell hidradenoma presenting as a granuloma pyogenicum, PRS, 57:678, 1976. Cutis, 16:95, 1975

HARRIS, M.: Review of experimental work on dental cyst, PRS, 56:225, 1975. Proc. Roy. Soc. Med., 67:1259, 1974

HARRIS, M.: Psychosomatic disorders of mouth and face. Practitioner, 214:372, 1975

HARRIS, M. N. *et al*: Melanoma of the head and neck. Ann. Surg., 182:86, 1975

HARRIS, N. M. *et al*: Ilioinguinal lymph node dissection for melanomas, PRS, 52:215, 1973. Surg. Gynec. & Obst., 136:33, 1973

HARRIS, N. S. *et al*: Effect of Travase on wound healing. Tex. Rep. Biol. Med., 31:771, 1973

HARRIS, N. S., AND ABSTON, S.: Anti-porcine antibodies in xenografted burned patients, PRS, 55:113, 1975. J. Surg. Res., 16:599, 1974

HARRIS, T. R.: Respiration monitor for infants with tracheostomy. Lancet, 2:583, 1971

HARRIS, W. A.: Open and closed treatment of burns with povidone-iodine (with Georgiade), PRS, 52:640, 1973. Discussion by Pruitt, PRS, 53:82, 1974

HARRIS, W. A., AND DORTZBACH, R. K.: Levator tuck: simplified blepharoptosis procedure, PRS, 57:394, 1975. Ann. Ophth., 7:873, 1975

HARRIS, W. E.: Unusual response to treatment of a traumatic bone cyst: report of case. J. Am. Dent. Assoc., 84:632, 1972

HARRISON, A. M., GAISFORD, J. C., AND WECHSLER, R. L.: Gastric secretion in burned patient, PRS, 52:211, 1973. J. Trauma, 12:1041, 1973

HARRISON, D. F.: Surgical pathology of hypopharyngeal neoplasms. J. Laryng. & Otol., 85:1215, 1971

HARRISON, D. F.: Role of surgery in the management of postcricoid and cervical esophageal neoplasms. Ann. Otol. Rhin. & Laryng., 81:465, 1972

HARRISON, D. F.: Management of malignant tumors affecting the maxillary and ethmoidal sinuses. J. Laryng. & Otol., 87:749, 1973

HARRISON, D. F.: Should lymphadenectomy be discarded? 2. Cancer of the head and neck. J. R. Coll. Surg. Edinb., 18:357, 1973

HARRISON, D. F.: Intraoral malignancy with special reference to jaw replacement. Problems of reconstruction following preoperative radiotherapy. Proc. Roy. Soc. Med., 67:601, 1974

HARRISON, D. F. N.: Pathology and management of subglottic cancer, PRS, 48:200, 1971. Ann. Otol. Rhin. & Laryng., 80:6, 1971

HARRISON, H. N., BALES, H., AND JACOBY, F.: Behavior of mafenide acetate as basis for clinical use, PRS, 51:234, 1973. Arch. Surg., 103:449, 1971

HARRISON, H. N. *et al*: Absorption of C^{14}-labeled Sulfamylon acetate through burned skin. I. Experimental methods and initial observations, PRS, 53:492, 1974. J. Trauma, 12:986, 1972

HARRISON, H. N., BALES, H. W., AND JACOBY, F.: Absorption into burned skin of Sulfamylon acetate from 5% aqueous solution, PRS, 53:685, 1974. J. Trauma, 12:994, 1973

HARRISON, R. J. *et al*: Observations on hearing levels of preschool cleft palate children. J. Speech Hear. Disord., 36:252, 1971

HARRISON, S. G. *et al*: Reliable regional anesthesia of the upper limb: augmented axillary block allowing the shaving and overgrafting of multiple forearm tattoos. Brit. J. Plast. Surg., 25:195, 1972

HARRISON, S. H.: Proximal interphalangeal joint in rheumatoid arthritis. Hand, 3:125, 1971

HARRISON, S. H.: Pollicization in children.

Hand, *3:*204, 1971

HARRISON, S. H.: Pollicization for congenital deformities of hand, PRS, *53:*683, 1974. Proc. Roy. Soc. Med., *66:*634, 1973

HARRISON, S. H.: Tactile adherence for estimating loss of sensation after nerve injury, PRS, *56:*229, 1975. Hand, *6:*148, 1974

HARROLD, C. C., JR.: Management of cancer of floor of mouth, PRS, *51:*608, 1973. Am. J. Surg., *122:*487, 1971

HARROLD, M. W., CHAMPION, R. H., AND FORD, M. L.: Functional urethral construction in female epispadias, PRS, *50:*539, 1972. J. Urol., *107:*144, 1972

HARRY, R. D., KRUGER, R. L., AND MC-LAUGHLIN, C. W.: Elastofibroma dorsi, unusual soft tissue tumor simulating sarcoma, PRS, *53:*111, 1974. Am. J. Surg., *125:*773, 1973

HART, G. B.: Treatment of decompression illness and air embolism with hyperbaric oxygen, PRS, *56:*366, 1975. Aerospace Med., *45:*1190, 1974

HART, G. B. *et al:* Treatment of clostridial myonecrosis with hyperbaric oxygen. J. Trauma, *14:*712, 1974

HART, G. B. *et al:* Treatment of burns with hyperbaric oxygen. Surg. Gynec. & Obst., *139:*693, 1974

HART, G. D.: Hapsburg jaw, PRS, *48:*292, 1971. Canad. M. A. J., *104:*601, 1971

HART, W. R. *et al:* Hyperplastic Pacinian corpuscles: cause of digital pain, PRS, *49:*357, 1972. Surgery, *70:*730, 1971

HARTEL, P.: Ectropion after lower lid strain due to scar adherence. In *Plastische und Wiederherstellungs-Chirurgie,* ed. by Hohler; pp. 323–4. Schattauer, Stuttgart, 1975 (German)

HARTFALL, W. G. *et al:* Hyperhidrosis of the upper extremity and its treatment. Surg. Gynec. & Obst., *135:*586, 1972

HARTFORD, C. F. *et al:* Improved survival of burned aged patients treated with 0.5 percent silver nitrate. J. Am. Geriatr. Soc., *19:*833, 1971

HARTFORD, C. E. *et al:* Use of 0.5 percent silver nitrate in burns: results in 220 patients. J. Trauma, *12:*682, 1972

HARTFORD, C. E. *et al:* Use of multiple systemic antibiotics in treatment of patients with burns. Surg. Gynec. & Obst., *138:*837, 1974

HARTLEY, J. H., JR.: Reduction mammaplasty by Dufourmentel-Mouly method (with Schatten, Hamm). PRS, *48:*306, 1971

HARTLEY, J. H., JR.: A new face lift scissors. Brit. J. Plast. Surg., *27:*365, 1974

HARTLEY, J. H., JR., AND SCHATTEN, W. E.: Unilateral exophthalmos. PRS, *49:*576, 1972

HARTLEY, J. H., JR., AND SCHATTEN, W. E.:

Cavernous hemangioma of mandible. PRS, *50:*287, 1972

HARTLEY, J. H., JR., AND SCHATTEN, W. E.: Cervicofacial actinomycosis. PRS, *51:*44, 1973

HARTLEY, J. H., JR., LESTER, J. C., AND SCHATTEN, W. E.: Acute retrobulbar hemorrhage during elective blepharoplasty, PRS, *52:*8, 1973. Discussions by Lemoine, Rees, Newell, PRS, *52:*12, 1973

HARTLEY, J. H., JR., SCHATTEN, W. E., AND GRIFFIN, J. M.: Subcutaneous mastectomy: excess skin problem. PRS, *56:*5, 1975

HARTMAN, K. S.: Granular cell ameloblastoma. Oral Surg., *38:*241, 1974

HARTMANN, F., HARTUNG, C., AND ZEIDLER, H.: *Biopolymers and Biomechanics of Connective Tissue.* Springer-Verlag, New York, 1974. PRS, *57:*231, 1976

HARTRAMPF, C. R., JR.: Discussion of "Purposeful delay of cut flexor tendons in "some-man's land' in children," by Arons. PRS, *54:*95, 1974

HARTRAMPF, C. R., VASCONEZ, L. O., AND MATHES, S.: Construction of one good thumb from both parts of a congenitally bifid thumb. PRS, *54:*148, 1974

HARTUNG, B. *et al:* Malformations of the ear in cleft palate patients. J. Maxillo-facial. Surg., *1:*253, 1973

HARTWELL, S. W., JR., AND HALL, M. D.: Mandibular condylectomy with silicone rubber replacement. PRS, *53:*440, 1974

HARTWELL, S. W., JR. *et al:* Reconstruction of breast after mastectomy for cancer. PRS, *57:*152, 1976

HARTY, M.: The hand of man. Phys. Ther., *51:*777, 1971

HARVEY, F. J., AND HARVEY, P. M.: Critical review of results of primary finger and thumb amputations, PRS, *54:*690, 1974. Hand, *6:*157, 1974

HARVEY, J. P., JR. *et al:* Replantation of upper limb in 43-year-old woman, PRS, *56:*356, 1975. Clin. Orthop., *102:*167, 1974

HARVOLD, E. P.: Centric relation. Study of pressure and tension systems in bone modeling and mandibular positioning. Dent. Clin. North Am., *19:*473, 1975

HARWOOD-NASH, D.: Fate of infractured hamuli (with Thomson). PRS, *50:*354, 1972

HARY, M. *et al:* Diagnosis of glossodynia. Stomatologiia (Bucur.), *20:*355, 1973

HASEGAWA, A. *et al:* Open reduction at mandibular angle for correction of open bite caused by traffic injury. Jap. J. Oral Surg., *19:*52, 1973 (Japanese)

HASEGAWA, H.: Transverse abdominal flap for reconstruction after radical operations for recurrent breast cancer (with Tai). PRS, *53:*52, 1974

HASHAM, A. I.: Two-stage reconstruction of scrotum for tropical elephantiasis. J. Urol., *109:*659, 1973

HASHIMOTO, K. *et al*: Collagenolytic activities of squamous cell carcinoma of skin, PRS, *54:*116, 1974. Cancer Res., *33:*2790, 1973

HASHIMOTO, K., AND KANZAKI, T.: Cutis laxa, PRS, *57:*539, 1976. Arch. Dermat., *111:*861, 1975

HASMAN, L.: Treatment of injuries of face and head involving losses, PRS, *54:*617, 1974. Rozhl. chir., *53:*208, 1974

HASS, E.: Correction of deformities of nasal cartilage with special attention to sources of error. Z. Laryngol. Rhinol. Otol., *52:*699, 1973 (German)

HASTINGS, D. W.: Postsurgical adjustment of male transsexual patients. Clin. Plast. Surg., *1:*335, 1974

HATTOWSKA, H. *et al*: Neoplasms of large and small salivary glands. Czas. Stomatol., *28:*397, 1975 (Polish)

HATZIFOTIADIS, D. *et al*: Ameloblastic sarcoma in maxilla, case report. J. Maxillo-facial Surg., *1:*62, 1973

HAUBRICH, J.: Surgery of injuries of the facial nerve on the lateral region of the face. H. N. O., *23:*339, 1975 (German)

HAUER, G., FELDMEIER, C., AND WILHELM, K.: AO-osteosynthesis of fractures of metacarpal bones, PRS, *57:*119, 1976. Actuel. Chir., *10:*73, 1975

HAUSAMEN, J. E.: Cryosurgical therapy of oral leukoplakias. Dtsch. Zahnaerztl. Z., *28:*1032, 1973 (German)

HAUSAMEN, J. E.: Basis, technique, and indication for cryosurgery in tumors of oral cavity and face, PRS, *56:*470, 1975. J. Maxillo-facial Surg., *3:*41, 1975

HAUSAMEN, J. E. *et al*: Clinical aspects and therapy of bilateral temporomandibular joint ankylosis in chronic polyarthritis. Dtsch. Zahnaerztl. Z., *28:*493, 1973 (German)

HAUSAMEN, J. E., SAMII, M., AND SCHMID-SEDER, R.: Repair of mandibular nerve by autologous nerve grafting after resection of lower jaw, PRS, *53:*250, 1974. J. Maxillo-facial Surg., *1:*74, 1973

HAUSAMEN, J. E. *et al*: Animal experiments on the regeneration of the inferior alveolar nerve after injury during osteotomy of the lower jaw and microsurgery. Fortschr. Kiefer. Gesichtschir., *18:*93, 1974 (German)

HAUSAMEN, J. E., SAMII, M., AND SCHMID-SEDER, R.: Indication and technic for reconstruction of nerve defects in head and neck, PRS, *55:*720, 1975. J. Maxillo-facial Surg., *2:*159, 1974

HAUSAMEN, J. E., SAMII, M., AND SCHMID-

SEDER, R.: Restoring sensation to cut inferior alveolar nerve by direct anastomosis or by free autologous nerve grafting, experimental study in rabbits. PRS, *54:*83, 1974

HAUSAMEN, J. E. *et al*: Results of comparative animal experimental studies on controlled cryosurgical treatment of oral mucosa. Z. W. R., *83:*262, 1974 (German)

HAUSTEIN, U. F.: Healing prospects in the ulcus cruris. Dtsch. Gesundheitsw., *26:*264, 1971 (German)

HAUSTEIN, U. F.: Angioplastic sarcoma of scalp. Dermatol. Monatsschr., *160:*399, 1974 (German)

HAUSWALD, K. R., KASDAN, D. M., AND WEISS, D. L.: Vascular leiomyoma of hand. PRS, *55:*89, 1975

HAVEN, E. *et al*: Treatment of ulcers infected by Pseudomonas aeruginosa or pyocyanic bacilli. Phlebologie, *24:*349, 1971 (French)

HAVERLING, M.: Diagnosis of blow-out fractures of the orbit by tomography. Acta Radiol. (Diagn.) (Stockh.), *12:*347, 1972

HAW, C. S.: Pleomorphic adenoma of the parotid gland. A review of results of treatment. J. R. Coll. Surg. Edinb., *20:*25, 1975

HAWKINS, D. B.: Melkersson's syndrome: unusual case. J. Laryng. & Otol., *86:*943, 1972

HAWKINS, D. B. *et al*: Teratoma of pharynx and neck. Ann. Otol. Rhin. & Laryng., *81:*848, 1972

HAWKINS, D. B. *et al*: Bilateral macrostomia as isolated deformity. J. Laryng. & Otol., *87:*309, 1973

HAWKINS, D. B. *et al:* Micrognathia and glossoptosis in the newborn. Surgical tacking of the tongue in small jaw syndromes. Clin. Pediatr. (Phila.), *13:*1066, 1974

HAWKINS, D. B. *et al*: Endotracheal tube perforation of hypopharynx, PRS, *54:*373, 1974. West. J. Med., *120:*282, 1974

HAWKINS, L. G. *et al*: Main line accidental intraarterial drug injection. Clin. Orthop., *94:*268, 1973

HAWTOF, D. B.: Skin cleaning fluids for use with drum-type dermatomes (Letter to the Editor). PRS, *48:*171, 1971

HAWTOF, D.: Dermis fat graft for correction of the eyelid deformity of enophthalmos. Mich. Med., *74:*331, 1975

HAWTOF, D. B., RAM, S., AND ALANI, H.: Reconstruction of mammary hypoplasia associated with chest wall deformities. PRS, *57:*172, 1975

HAWTREY, C. E., CULP, D. A., AND HARTFORD, C. W.: Management of severe inflammatory and traumatic injuries to genital skin, PRS, *51:*349, 1973. J. Urol., *108:*431, 1972

HAY, S. *et al*: Twins with clefts: a descriptive

statistical analysis of selected variables. Cleft Palate J., 8:379, 1971

HAYES, B. W., JR.: Outpatient burns. Clin. Plast. Surg., 1:645, 1974

HAYES, C. W.: One stage nail fold reconstruction, PRS, 54:690, 1974. Hand, 6:74, 1974

HAYES, C. W., JR.: Anomalous flexor sublimis muscle with incipient carpal tunnel syndrome. PRS, 53:479, 1974

HAYES, D.: Hockey injuries: how, why, where, and when, PRS, 55:726, 1975. Phys. & Sports Med., 3:61, 1975

HAYES, J. E.: Facial moulage technique for the plastic surgeon (with Thompson, Gosling). PRS, 49:190, 1972

HAYES, P. A.: Correction of retrognathia by modified "C" osteotomy of ramus and sagittal osteotomy of mandibular body. J. Oral Surg., 31:682, 1973. Ariz. Dent. J., 20:22, 1974

HAYES, T., ATKINS, J., AND RAVENTOS, A.: Carcinoma of larynx—diagnosis and treatment by surgery or irradiation, PRS, 50:310, 1972. Ann. Otol. Rhin. & Laryng., 80:627, 1971

HAYHURST, J. W. et al: Experimental digital replantation after prolonged cooling, PRS, 56:227, 1975. Hand, 6:134, 1974

HAYNES, B. W.: Current problems in burns: perspective, PRS, 49:665, 1972. Arch. Surg., 103:454, 1971

HAYNES, B. W., JR.: Burn therapy—current appraisal. Surg. Annu., 3:125, 1971

HAYNES, B. W., JR.: Outpatient burns. Clin. Plast. Surg., 1:645, 1974

HAYNES, W. D. et al: Radiation treatment of carcinoma of nasal vestibule. Am. J. Roentgenol. Radium Ther. Nucl. Med., 120:595, 1974

HAYWARD, J. R.: Multiple recurrent fibro-osseous epulides. Int. J. Oral Surg., 2:115, 1973

HAYWARD, J. R.: Recurrent ameloblastoma 30 years after surgical treatment. J. Oral Surg., 31:368, 1973

HAYWARD, J. R.: Muscle closure in cleft palate repair. Trans. Int. Conf. Oral Surg., 4:74, 1973

HAYWARD, J. R. et al: Monostoic fibrous dysplasia of maxilla: report of cases. J. Oral Surg., 31:625, 1973

HAZAMA, H. et al: Surgical treatment of intratemporal facial nerve paralysis. Otolaryngology (Tokyo), 43:795, 1971 (Japanese)

HEANEY, T. G.: Reappraisal of environment, function and gingival specificity. J. Periodontol., 45:695, 1974

HEBERER, G., AND HEGEMANN, G.: Indication for Operation. Springer-Verlag, New York, 1974. PRS, 56:445, 1975

HÉBERT, J. G.: Advantages of doughnut skin graft for orbital lining (Follow-Up Clinic).

PRS, 50:402, 1972

HEBERT, P. W.: Treatment of urethral stricture: transurethral injection of triamcinolone, PRS, 51:603, 1973. J. Urol., 105:403, 1971

HECHT, A. et al: Blood volume lost during gingivectomy using two different anesthetic techniques. J. Periodontol., 45:9, 1974

HECKER, W. C.: Surgical correction in differentiation disorders of the urogenital sinus with clitoris hypertrophy (external female pseudohermaphroditism). Chirurg., 43:90, 1972 (German)

HEDDLE, S. B.: Increasing incidence of melanoma (with Cosman, Crikelair). PRS, 57:50, 1976

HEEB, M. A.: Deep soft tissue abscesses secondary to nonpenetrating trauma, PRS, 48:298, 1971. Surgery, 69:550, 1971

HEENEMAN, H.: On diagnosis and management of malignant oral tumors. Can. J. Otolaryngol., 3:168, 1974

HEENEMAN, H.: Identification of facial nerve in parotid surgery. Can. J. Otolaryngol., 4:145, 1975

HEERMANN, J.: Treatment of large septal perforations with skin-cartilage-skin grafts from pinna, packing for two weeks—picking off the skin. Laryngol. Rhinol. Otol. (Stuttg.), 53:935, 1974 (German)

HEES, J. W. VAN: Some problems in the rehabilitation of patients with a partially amputated hand. Ned. Tijdschr. Geneeskd., 115:551, 1971 (Dutch)

HEIDELBERGER, K. P. et al: Mucoepidermoid carcinoma of tongue. J. Laryng. & Otol., 87:1239, 1973

HEIDSIECK, C.: Intraosseous dermoid and epidermoid cysts in jaw region. Fortschr. Kiefer. Gesichtschir., 15:220, 1972 (German)

HEIKKINEN, E. S.: Treatment of burns in childhood. Duodecim, 90:262, 1974 (Finnish)

HEILQUIST, R.: Team work and clinical research in the treatment of cleft lip and palate. Sven. Tandlak. Tidskr., 66:145, 1973

HEIM, U., AND PFEIFFER, K. M.: Small Fragment Set Manual. Springer-Verlag, New York, 1974. PRS, 56:571, 1975

HEIMBURGER, R. A. et al: Burned feet in children, acute and reconstructive care, PRS, 52:684, 1973. Am. J. Surg., 125:575, 1973

HEINC, A.: Early surgery of severely burned eye. Cesk. Oftalmol., 28:279, 1972 (Czechoslovakian)

HEINIG, B.: Pleomorphic adenoma of parotid gland in child. Zentralbl. Chir., 98:249, 1973 (German)

HEINTZ, W. D.: Case for mandatory mouth protectors, PRS, 57:406, 1976. Phys. & Sports Med., 3:60, 1975

HEINZ, C.: Basis for the surgical treatment of patients with leprosy. Praxis, 62:1285, 1973 (German)

HEIPLE, K. G. et al: Chondromatous hamartomas arising from the volar digital plates. A case report. J. Bone & Joint Surg. (Am.), 54:393, 1972

HEISS, W. H.: Technique and results of tissue glueing, PRS, 52:216, 1973. Bull. Soc. Internat. Chir., 6:549, 1972

HEITE, H. J.: Prognosis based on death rate in relation to irritation, growth, and surface structure of primary focus in malignant melanoma. Arch. Dermatol. Forsch., 244:200, 1972 (German)

HEKNEBY, M.: Load of the temporomandibular joint: physical calculations and analyses, PRS, 54:372, 1974. J. Prosth. Dent., 31:303, 1974

HELAL, B. H.: Extra-articular causes of proximal interphalangeal joint stiffness in rheumatoid arthritis, PRS, 57:119, 1976. Hand, 7:37, 1975

HELBIG, D.: Surgical treatment of burns in childhood. Fortschr. Med., 91:982, 1973 (German)

HELFRICH, G. B. et al: Management of cancer of floor of mouth, PRS, 52:213, 1973. Am. J. Surg., 124:559, 1972

HELLER, A.: Pharyngoplasty through cross palatopharyngeal flaps, PRS, 57:117, 1976. J. Maxillo-facial Surg., 3:94, 1975

HELLMICH, S.: Preoperative assessment of risk factors in chip implants of nose. H. N. O., 20:218, 1972 (German)

HELLMICH, S.: Operative technique of rhinoplastic implants. Z. Laryngol. Rhinol. Otol., 51:298, 1972 (German)

HELLMICH, S.: Problem of cartilage bending in nose surgery (experimental and clinical aspects). H. N. O., 21:223, 1973 (German)

HELLMICH, S.: Treatment of the acute septal abscess. H. N. O., 22:278, 1974 (German)

HELLQUIST, R.: Early maxillary orthopedics in relation to maxillary cleft repair by periosteoplasty. Cleft Palate J., 8:36, 1971

HELLRIEGEL, W.: Indications for and results of percutaneous radiotherapy of malignant melanoma. Strahlentherapie, 149:1, 1975 (German)

HELM, U.: Indications and technics of AO osteosynthesis in the treatment of the fractures of the hand. Acta Orthop. Belg., 39:957, 1973 (French)

HELMAN, P. et al: Cancer of the floor of the mouth. S. Afr. J. Surg., 13:147, 1975

HELMIG, F. J.: Long-term results following operation for hypospadias. Klin. Paediatr., 186:421, 1974 (German)

HELMS, J.: Significance of early care of nose injuries for subsequent function. H. N. O., 21:77, 1973 (German)

HELMS, J.: The indications for facial nerve decompression. Wien. Klin. Wochenschr., 85:95, 1973 (German)

HELMUS, C. et al: Delirium tremens in head and neck surgery. Laryngoscope, 84:1479, 1974

HELPAP, B., AND CREMER, H.: Autoradiographic investigations of connective tissue proliferation in wounds of skin, PRS, 51:484, 1973. Res. Exper. Med., 157:289, 1972

HELPAP, B. et al: Tissue reaction after implantation of catgut sterilized by conventional methods and by radiation in parenchymatous organs, PRS, 53:114, 1974. Bruns' Beitr. klin. Chir., 220:323, 1973

HELSPER, J. T.: Problem stoma. J. Surg. Oncol., 6:151, 1974

HELSPER, J. T. et al: Cricopharyngeal achalasia. Am. J. Surg., 128:521, 1974

HELVESTON, E. M.: Eye trauma in childhood, PRS, 57:256, 1976. Pediatr. Clin. N. Am., 22:501, 1975

Hemangioma

Hemangiomas, large facial, surgical removal of (Kufner, Petrovič), PRS, 50:542, 1972. Acta chir. plast., 13:152, 1971

Vascular tumors of the face (Stricker et al). Ann. chir. plast., 16:220, 1971 (French)

Head and neck hemangiopericytoma (Walike, Bailey), PRS, 48:298, 1971. Arch. Otolaryng., 93:345, 1971

Maffucci syndrome, hand in (Howard, Lee), PRS, 50:307, 1972. Arch. Surg., 103:752, 1971

Hemangioma with petechial rash and treatment (Petechial angioma) (Kajima, Sai), PRS, 50:309, 1972. Jap. J. Plast. Reconstr. Surg., 14:411, 1971

Hemangioma, scrotal wall, in infant (Mininberg, Harley), PRS, 50:94, 1972. J. Urol., 106:789, 1971

Surgical treatment of hemangiomas (Makhov et al). Klin. Khir., 9:35, 1971 (Russian)

Port-wine stain, surgical tattooing of (Thomson, Wright). PRS, 48:113, 1971

Tuberous hemangioma of cheek skin (Spadafora, De Los Rios), PRS, 49:475, 1972. Prensa Univ. Arg., 5:6825, 1971

Rendu-Osler disease, adjuvant therapy in (Lapp et al). Rev. Med. Suisse Romande, 91:43, 1971 (French)

Radiation resistant angiomas of the jaws (surgical treatment—report of 3 cases) (Michelet et al). Rev. Odontostomatol. Midi Fr., 29:3, 1971 (French)

Hemangioma—Cont.

Hamartomata, vascular, of masticatory muscles (Azzolini, Nouvenne), PRS, *51:*107, 1973. Riv. ital. chir. plast., *3:*135, 1971

Radiologic patterns of hemangiopericytoma of leg (Hoeffel *et al*), PRS, *51:*704, 1973. Am. J. Surg., *123:*591, 1972

Hypoplasia, mammary, following radiation to infant breast (Skalkeas, Gogas, Pavlatos), PRS, *52:*679, 1973. Acta chir. plast., *14:*240, 1972

Angioma and fronto-orbital bone swelling: complete excision and immediate bone restoration (Marchac *et al*). Ann. chir. plast., *17:*73, 1972 (French)

Angiomatous lymphoid hamartomas: surgical implications (Block *et al*). Ann. Surg., *176:*620, 1972

Angiofibroma, invasive, surgical treatment (English *et al*). Arch. Otolaryng., *96:*312, 1972

Value of early detection by phlebography of venous abnormalities with voluminous angiomas in newborns and very young infants (Desmons *et al*). Bull. Soc. Fr. Dermatol. Syphiligr., *79:*523, 1972

Hemangiopericytoma, upper airway obstruction in newborn secondary to (Baden *et al*). Can. Med. Assoc. J., *107:*1202, 1972

Hemangioma treated by oral prednisone therapy (Boggio Robutti, Musio, Mazzola), PRS, *53:*111, 1974. Chir. Plast., *1:*95, 1972

Extremities, osteolytic hemangiomatosis of (Diaz-Ballesteros, Paramo-Diaz, and Lopez-Silva), PRS, *52:*454, 1973. Cir. y Cir., *40:*215, 1972

Hemangioma, congenital, of parotid gland in six-month-old child (Chaves, Oliveira), PRS, *53:*111, 1974. Folha Med. Brazil, *65:*385, 1972

Hemangiomas, cavernous, treatment by electrocoagulation using an elastic vein needle (Hiramoto), PRS, *51:*607, 1973. Jap. J. Plast. Reconstr. Surg., *15:*309, 1972

Hemangioma of face, indications for excision, limitations of excision, and suture technique (Kashima), PRS, *52:*687, 1973. Jap. J. Plast. Reconstr. Surg., *15:*346, 1972

Hemangioma of maxilla, central (Baum *et al*). J. Oral Surg., *30:*885, 1972

Vascular tumor, head and neck region, method of treatment (Ono *et al*). J. Otolaryngol. Japan, *75:*1091, 1972 (Japanese)

Hemangiopericytoma of child (Reich). Monatsschr. Kinderheilkd., *120:*430, 1972 (German)

Hemangioma of skin, pediatric aspects of treatment (Dorogi *et al*). Orv. Hetil., *113:*2522, 1972 (Hungarian)

Hemangioma—Cont.

Hemangioma, benign locally-invasive, of orbital region, natural history of (Habal, Murray). PRS, *49:*209, 1972

Hemangiomata, continuous compression treatment, evaluation in two cases (Mangus). PRS, *49:*490, 1972

Hemangiomas, role of plastic surgery in early treatment (Fryer) (Follow-Up Clinic). PRS, *50:*77, 1972

Arteriovenous fistulas in cavernous hemangiomas of face, treatment by muscle embolization (Bennett, Zook). PRS, *50:*84, 1972

Telangiectases within nasal skin graft, recurrence; management of epistaxis in Osler-Weber-Rendu disease (McCabe, Kelly). PRS, *50:*114, 1972

Hemangioma-thrombocytopenia syndrome (Paletta) (Follow-Up Clinic). PRS, *50:*183, 1972

Hemangioma, cavernous, of mandible (Hartley, Schatten). PRS, *50:*287, 1972

Hemangioma, facial, treatment by intravascular embolization with silicone spheres (Longacre, Benton, Unterthiner). PRS, *50:*618, 1972

Hemangiomas, cryosurgery in treatment of (Jarzab). Polski tygodnik lek., *27:*2025, 1972 (Polish)

Hemangiopericytoma of gum (Corenel *et al*). Rev. Stomatol. Chir. Maxillofac., *73:*295, 1972 (German)

Sturge-Weber syndrome, surgical therapy of typical and forme fruste variety of (Rasmussen, Mathieson, Le Blanc). Schweiz. Arch. Neurol. u. Psychiat., *111:*393, 1972

Hemangiomas, intraoral, use of cryotherapy in management of (Huang *et al*), PRS, *51:*707, 1973. South. M. J., *65:*1123, 1972

Prednisone therapy in management of large hemangiomas in infants and children (Brown, Neerhout, Fonkalsrud), PRS, *50:*96, 1972. Surgery, *71:*168, 1972

Cardiac alterations in case of Klippel-Trenaunay syndrome (Schmidt, Rastan), PRS, *51:*478, 1973. Ztschr. Kinderchir., *11:*468, 1972

Head and neck, congenital arteriovenous fistulas (Coleman), PRS, *53:*489, 1974. Am. J. Surg., *126:*557, 1973

Hemangiomas in children, steroid treatment of (Lasser, Stein), PRS, *53:*611, 1974. Arch. Dermat., *108:*565, 1973

Nasal bone, cavernous hemangioma of (Hirshowitz, Munk). Brit. J. Plast. Surg., *26:*81, 1973

Port wine stain, surgical tattooing for (Newton). Can. J. Otolaryngol., *2:*251, 1973

Hemangiopericytoma, ultrastructural study

Hemangioma — Cont.

(Hahn *et al*), PRS, *51:*707, 1973. Cancer, *31:*255, 1973

Hemangiomas — conservative approach (Huffstadt), PRS, *53:*111, 1974. Chir. Plast., *1:*305, 1973

Hemangiomas, corticoids in (Nasemann). Hautarzt, *24:*318, 1973 (German)

Syndrome, Maffucci's, functional and neoplastic significance (Lewis, Ketcham), PRS, *54:*116, 1974. J. Bone & Joint Surg., *55A:*1465, 1973

Hemangioma, cavernous, of oral cavity: review of literature and report of case (Friedman *et al*). J. Oral Surg., *31:*617, 1973

Hemangioma of mandible (Gill, Long, MacLennan). J. Roy. Coll. Surg. Edinb., *18:*52, 1973

Hemangiomas, cavernous, resolution of following prednisolone therapy (Zarem) (Follow-Up Clinic). PRS, *51:*207, 1973

Hemangiomas, intraoral, cryosurgery in treatment of (Kayhan *et al*). Rev. Laryngol. Otol. Rhinol. (Bord.), *94:*245, 1973

Hemangioma, cavernous, perimandibular (Sailer). Schweiz. Monatsschr. Zahnheilkd., *83:*1267, 1973 (German)

Hemangioma in childhood, treatment of, surgical therapy (Olivari *et al*). Z. Allgemeinmed., *49:*60, 1973 (German)

Hemangioma, sclerosing, ultrastructure of (Carstens, Schrodt), PRS, *57:*678, 1974. Am. J. Path., *77:*377, 1974

Hemangioma of bone (Davis *et al*). Arch. Otolaryng., *99:*443, 1974

Practical cryosurgery for oral lesions (Leopard *et al*). Brit. Dent. J., *136:*185, 1974

Haemangioma of the mandible: a case report (Gruss). Brit. J. Oral Surg., *12:*24, 1974

Hemangioma, orbital — clinical analysis of 79 cases (Shanghai First Medical College), PRS, *55:*633, 1975. Chinese M. J., *9:*162, 1974

Hemangioma of extremities (McNeill *et al*). Clin. Orthop., *101:*154, 1974

Angiography in surgical management of deep hemangiomas (McNeil *et al*), PRS, *56:*234, 1975. Clin. Orthop., *101:*176, 1974

Clinical studies of congenital angiodysplasias in limbs. An analysis of 123 cases (Hamatake). Fukuoka Acta Med., *65:*833, 1974 (Japanese)

Hemangioma, cutaneous, in children, management (Yaghnam), PRS, *56:*683, 1975. Jordan M. J., *9:*128, 1974

Hemangiopericytoma, metastatic, cured by radiotherapy (Dube, Paulson), PRS, *55:*388, 1975. J. Bone & Joint Surg., *56A:*833, 1974

Hemangioma — Cont.

Hemangioma, cavernous, recurrent facial swelling due to (Griffiths). J. Laryng. & Otol., *88:*1135, 1974

Hemangiomas, use of sodium morrhuate in management of (Morgan, Schow), PRS, *55:*255, 1975. J. Oral Surg., *32:*363, 1974

Cryosurgery in otolaryngology (Editorial). J. Otolaryngol. Jpn., *77:*799, 1974 (Japanese)

Experience with the treatment of angiomas and angiomatosis (Zelenin *et al*). Klin. Khir., *11:*75, 1974 (Russian)

Possible applications of lasers in surgery (Kaiser). Langenbecks Arch. Chir., *337:*671, 1974 (German)

Embolization, new technique (Djindjian), PRS, *54:*630, 1974. Nouvelle Presse Med., *3:*1475, 1974

Hemangioma, central, of mandible and maxilla: review of vascular lesion (Gamez-Araujo *et al*). Oral Surg., *37:*230, 1974

Hemangioma, central mandibular (Sanchez Torres *et al*). Oral Surg., *37:*509, 1974

Hemangioma involving maxillary sinus (Afshin, Sharmin), PRS, *56:*224, 1975. Oral Surg., *38:*204, 1974

Hemangioma, nasopharyngeal (Szlazak *et al*). Otolaryngol. Pol., *28:*329, 1974 (Polish)

Hemangioma, capillary, therapy of (Thormann). Paediatr. Grenzheb., *13:*109, 1974 (German)

Hemangiomas of face (Spina, Psillakis, Ferreira), PRS, *55:*723, 1975. Rev. paulista med., *83:*115, 1974

Surgical treatment of non-traumatic lower lip lesions with special reference to the step technique. A follow-up on 149 patients (Johanson *et al*). Scand. J. Plast. Reconstr. Surg., *8:*232, 1974

Anesthesia and resuscitation in operations for diseases and injuries of the tongue, and the floor of the mouth (Aleksandrov *et al*). Vestn. Khir., *112:*88, 1974 (Russian)

Hemangioendothelioma of the nose and accessory sinuses (Shchechkin). Vestn. Otorinolaringol., *4:*56, 1974 (Russian)

Mandibular deformities caused by benign tumors (Toman). Acta Stomatol. Belg., *72:*311, 1975 (German)

Treatment of hemangioma of the face (Slesinger). Acta Stomatol. Belg., *72:*495, 1975 (French)

Giant hemangioma (Varela-Irijoa *et al*). Angiologia, *27:*234, 1975 (Spanish)

Vascular sarcomas of the ethmoid sinus (hemangioendothelioma) (Pinel *et al*). Ann. Otolaryngol. Chir. Cervicofac., *92:*557, 1975 (French)

Haemangioma of the maxilla: a case report

Hemangioma – Cont.

(Tyldesley *et al*). Brit. J. Oral Surg., *13:*56, 1975

Intramuscular hemangioma in the head and neck (Clemis *et al*). Can. J. Otolaryngol., *4:*339, 1975

Hemangioma, massive, of neck and face, combined treatment (Keaveny *et al*), PRS, *57:*256, 1976. J. Cardiovasc. Surg., *16:*159, 1975

Hemangioma, cryosurgery for, clinical experience (Jarzab), PRS, *57:*539, 1976. J. Maxillo-facial Surg., *3:*146, 1975

Therapeutic percutaneous embolization for extra-axial vascular lesions of the head, neck, and spine (Hilal *et al*). J. Neurosurg., *43:*275, 1975

Sclerosing hemangioma of the tongue: report of case (Friedlander *et al*). J. Oral Surg., *33:*212, 1975

Central hemangioma of the mandible: intraoral resection and reconstruction (Piercell *et al*). J. Oral Surg., *33:*225, 1975

Hemangioma, central cavernous, of mandible (Gelfand *et al*). J. Oral Surg., *33:*448, 1975

Simple probe for cryosurgical therapy for hemangiomas (Hickory *et al*). J. Oral Surg., *33:*546, 1975

Central cavernous hemangioma of the mandible treated by an intraoral approach (Zalesin *et al*). J. Oral Surg., *33:*877, 1975

Hemangiomas, urinary tract, Klippel-Trenaunay syndrome associated with (Klein, Kaplan), PRS, *57:*675, 1976. J. Urol., *114:*596, 1975

Giant occipital hemangioendothelioma with thrombocytopenia, anemia and hypofibrinogenemia treated by total excision (Nagashima *et al*). Neurol. Surg. (Tokyo), *3:*547, 1975 (Japanese)

Primary malignant hemangioendothelioma of the gingiva. Report of a case and review of the literature (Wesley *et al*). Oral Surg., *39:*103, 1975

Muscle embolization: arteriovenous malformations of the mandible, graduated surgical management (Bryant, Maull), PRS, *55:*690, 1975. Discussion by Bennett, PRS, *56:*84, 1975

Hemangiomas of parotid gland in children (Williams). PRS, *56:*29, 1975

Cryosurgery for facial skin lesions (Leopard). Proc. Roy. Soc. Med., *68:*606, 1975

Cryosurgery of the oral mucous membranes (Poswillo). Proc. Roy. Soc. Med., *68:*608, 1975

Editorial: a philosophy of approach to treat-

Hemangioma – Cont.

ment of hemangiomas (Green). South. Med. J., *68:*383, 1975

Surgical treatment of cavernous hemangiomas of the face and neck (Kabakov). Stomatologiia (Mosk.), *54:*30, 1975 (Russian)

Hemangiomas of the skin in children (Kush *et al*). Vestn. Khir., *115:*65, 1975 (Russian)

Cryosurgery of supraglottic cavernous hemangioma (O'Neill *et al*). Arch. Otolaryng., *102:*55, 1976

Hemangioma of the nasal bones (Bridger). J. Laryng. & Otol., *90:*191, 1976

Hemangioma, "piecemeal principle," staged operations for better results (Weisman). PRS, *57:*570, 1976

Hemangioma, frontonasal tumors, diagnosis and management (Griffith). PRS, *57:*692, 1976

Hemangiopericytoma of hand (Sen). PRS, *57:*746, 1976

Argon laser management of cutaneous vascular deformities. A preliminary report (Apfelberg *et al*). West. J. Med., *124:*99, 1976

Hemifacial Atrophy

Progressive facial hemiatrophy with megalocornea, micropupil and central nebular dystrophy of the cornea (Collier). Acta Ophthalmol. (Kbh.), *49:*946, 1971 (French)

Hemifacial atrophy (Vickery). Brit. J. Oral Surg., *9:*102, 1971

Case of acute facial hemiatrophy (Parry-Romberg syndrome) (Nishikawa *et al*). Iryo, *25:*679, 1971 (Japanese)

Progressive right hemifacial atrophy with contralateral cerebral hemiatrophy (Kumar *et al*). J. Assoc. Physicians India, *19:*595, 1971

Hemifacial atrophy treated by buried de-epithelized flap, 20-year follow-up (Converse, Betson). PRS, *48:*278, 1971

Augmentation, soft tissue, experience with dimethyl-polysiloxane fluid in (Blocksma). PRS, *48:*564, 1971

Romberg-type hemiatrophy in a case of severe rheumatoid arthritis (Poniecki *et al*). Wiad. Lek., *24:*1313, 1971 (Polish)

Etiology of face asymmetry (Herrmann). Z.W. R., *80:*988, 1971 (German)

Facial hemiatrophy, progressive (O'Conor), PRS, *52:*688, 1973. Bol. y trab. Acad. argent. cir., *56:*543, 1972

Hypertrophy, primary hemifacial (Bergman), PRS, *52:*593, 1973. Arch. Otolaryng., *97:*490, 1973

Facial hemiatrophy. Unusual cross-lip flap

Hemifacial Atrophy—Cont.
(Fischl). New York J. Med., *73:*313, 1973
Injections, subcutaneous silicone, augmentation of surface contour by (Ashley, Thompson, Henderson). PRS, *51:*8, 1973
Hemifacial microsomia, first and second branchial arch syndrome (Converse *et al*). PRS, *51:*268, 1973
Facial atrophy, silicone fluid injections for (Rees, Ashley, Delgado). PRS, *52:*118, 1973
Microsomia, hemifacial, corrective treatment of skeletal asymmetry in (Converse *et al*). PRS, *52:*221, 1973
Progress in cosmetic surgery of bony facial profile (Schule). Zahnaerztl. Prax., *24:*371, 1973 (German)
Atrophy, hemifacial: repair with buried flap (Dey), PRS, *56:*590, 1975. Australian & New Zealand J. Surg., *44:*379, 1974
Hemifacial microsomia (dysostosis otomandibularis) (Converse *et al*). Fortschr. Kiefer. Gesichtschir., *18:*53, 1974
Facial microsomia, bilateral, diagnosis, classification, treatment (Converse *et al*). PRS, *54:*413, 1974
Surgical treatment of progressive facial hemiatrophy (Romberg's disease) (Gorbushina *et al*). Stomatologiia (Mosk.) *54:*51, 1975 (Russian)

HEMPEL, J.: Dermatofibrosarcoma protuberans of head and neck. H. N. O., *22:*176, 1974 (German)
HEMPEL, J. *et al*: Malignant melanoma of female genitalia. Z. Hautkr., *48:*711, 1973 (German)
HENDERSON, B. M., AND DUJON, E. B.: Snake bites in children, PRS, *54:*512, 1974. J. Pediat. Surg., *8:*729, 1973
HENDERSON, D.: Palatal island flap in the closure of oro-antral fistulae. Brit. J. Oral Surg., *12:*141, 1974
HENDERSON, D.: Assessment and management of bony deformities of middle and lower face. Brit. J. Plast. Surg., *27:*287, 1974
HENDERSON, D. *et al*: Combined cleft lip revision, anterior fistula closure and maxillary osteotomy; a one-stage procedure. Brit. J. Oral Surg., *13:*33, 1975
HENDERSON, J. W.: *Orbital Tumors.* W. B. Saunders Co., Philadelphia, 1973
HENDERSON, J. W. *et al*: Malignant melanoma primary in orbit: case report. Trans. Am. Acad. Ophthalmol. Otolaryngol., *76:*1487, 1972
HENDERSON, T.: Augmentation of surface contour by subcutaneous injections of silicone fluid (with Ashley, Thompson). PRS, *51:*8, 1973

HENDREN, W. H.: Nonrefluxing colon conduit for temporary or permanent urinary diversion in children. J. Pediatr. Surg., *10:*381, 1975
HENDREN, W. H.: Exstrophy of the bladder—an alternative method of management. J. Urol., *115:*195, 1976)
HENDREN, W. H. *et al*: Child with ambiguous genitalia. Curr. Probl. Surg., *1:*64, 1972
HENDRIX, J. H., JR.: Keratosis *palmaris et plantaris* (with Kisner). PRS, *51:*424, 1973
HENJYOJI, E. Y., AND LAUB, D. R.: Residency participation in out-of-country medical service, PRS, *53:*660, 1974
HENK, J. M.: Radiosensitivity of lymph node metastases, PRS, *56:*231, 1975. Proc. Roy. Soc. Med., *68:*85, 1975
HENKERT, K. *et al*: Treatment of open hand injuries. Beitr. Orthop. Traumatol., *20:*378, 1973 (German)
HENKES, H. E.: Lacrimal flow. Ned. Tijdschr. Geneeskd., *116:*465, 1972 (Dutch)
HENNS, R. J.: Canine eminence. Angle Orthod., *44:*326, 1974
HENRIK, H. *et al*: Surgical construction of vagina in primary agenesis and transsexualism. Tidsskr. Nor. Laegeforen, *93:*1042, 1973 (Norwegian)
HENRIK, H. *et al*: Surgical correction of breast deformities in young women. Tidsskr. Nor. Laegeforen., *93:*1044, 1973 (Norwegian)
HENRY, C. *et al*: Voluminous pigmented basal cell epithelioma of eyelids. Bull. Soc. Ophtalmol. Fr., *73:*315, 1973 (French)
HENSELL, V.: Causes and clinical signs of nerve damage, PRS, *51:*480, 1973. Langenbecks Arch. Chir., *332:*339, 1972
HENSON, R. E.: Ulcerations of lower extremities in the hospital patient. J. Am. Osteopath. Assoc., *73:*309, 1973
HENTSCHEL, M. *et al*: Treatment of arterial injuries of the forearm and hand. Handchirurgie, *2:*18, 1970 (German)
HENTZ, V. R. *et al*: Wound healing of skin flaps rotated into delayed or primary recipient sites, PRS, *52:*329, 1973. Surg. Forum, *23:*34, 1972
HENTZER, B. *et al*: Suction blister transplantation for leg ulcers. Acta Derm. Venerol. (Stockh.), *55:*207, 1975
HENZEL, J. H.: Doppler flowmeter to monitor peripheral bloodflow during the edema stage of snakebite (with Gurucharri, Mitchell). PRS, *53:*551, 1974
HENZEL, J. H., AND DEWEESE, M. S.: Morbid and mortal complications associated with prolonged central venous cannulation. Awareness, recognition, and prevention, PRS, *49:*477, 1972. Am. J. Surg., *121:*600,

1971

HEPLER, R. S., SUGIMURA, G. I., AND STRAATSMA, B. R.: Discussion of "Successful early relief of blindness occurring after blepharoplasty," by Hueston, Heinze, PRS, 57:233, 1976

HEPPENSTALL, R. B. et al: Gas tensions in healing tissues of traumatized patients, PRS, 54:625, 1974. Surgery, 75:874, 1974

HERAS PEREZ, J. M.: Complete vesical exstrophy, PRS, 56:231, 1975. Cir. Españ., 28:265, 1974

HERBERT, D. C.: Closure of a palatal fistula using a mucoperiosteal island flap. Brit. J. Plast. Surg., 27:332, 1974

HERBERT, D. C. et al: Harmless osteoporosis of the skull underlying basal cell carcinomas of the scalp. Brit. J. Plast. Surg., 27:248, 1974

HERBERTS, P. et al: Hand prosthesis control via myoelectric patterns. Acta Orthop. Scand., 44:389, 1973

HERBSMAN, H.: Experimental transplantation of free grafts of intestinal mucous membrane (Follow-Up Clinic). PRS, 49:207, 1972

HERCEG, S. J. et al: Surgical treatment of pressure sores. Pa. Med., 74:45, 1971

HERCEG, S. J., AND HARDING, R. L.: Grandenigo's syndrome following correction of posterior choanal atresia. PRS, 48:181, 1971

HERCEG, S. J., AND HARDING, R. L.: Malignant ameloblastoma with pulmonary metastases. Report of case and review of literature. PRS, 49:456, 1972

HERCEG, S. J., AND HARDING, R. L.: Trainor blepharoplasty for ptosis. PRS, 49:622, 1972

HERCEG, S. J., AND HARDING, R. L.: Squamous cell carcinoma arising in a mandibular cyst. PRS, 57:383, 1976

HERD, J. R.: Calcifying odontogenic cyst. Aust. Dent. J., 17:421, 1972

HERD, J. R.: Exostoses of the maxillary sinus wall. A diagnostic problem. Aust. Dent. J., 19:269, 1973

HEREDIA, L. et al: Mammary gland cancer in University Hospital of Caracas, PRS, 52:600, 1973. Biol. Soc. Venezuelana Cir., 26:295, 1972

Heredity: See *Genetics*

HEREFRATH, C. et al: Esophageal replacement with lyophilic dura in dogs, PRS, 54:619, 1974. Ztschr. Kinderchir., 14:146, 1974

HERGT, K.: Blood levels of thrombocytes in burned patients, observations on their behavior in relation to clinical condition of patient, PRS, 52:326, 1973. J. Trauma, 12:599, 1972

HERING, H. J.: Surgery of prognathism with osteotomy in the region of the 1st premolars. Fortschr. Kiefer. Gesichtschir., 18:129, 1974 (German)

HERMAN, C. M., MOQUIN, R. B., AND HORWITZ, D. L.: Coagulation changes of hemorrhagic shock in baboons, PRS, 50:311, 1972. Ann. Surg., 175:197, 1972

HERMAN, P. S. et al: Acquired (digital) fibrokeratomas. Complication of ingrown toenail. Acta Derm. Venereol. (Stockh.), 54:73, 1974

HERMAN, S., HOFFMAN, S., AND KAHN, S.: Revisional surgery after reduction mammaplasty. PRS, 55:422, 1975

HERMANN, H. J. et al: 99mTc-polyphosphate scintigraphy of joints, xeroradiography and radiography of hands. Nucl. Med. (Stuttg.), 13:341, 1975 (German)

HERMANN, J. B.: Tensile strength and knot security of surgical suture materials, PRS, 49:110, 1972. Am. Surgeon, 37:209, 1971

Hermaphroditism (See also *Hypospadias*)

Two pregnancies after later change of sex in a person with pseudohermaphroditism (Magre et al). Bull. Fed. Soc. Gynecol. Obstet. Lang. Fr., 23:513, 1971 (French)

Six cases of male pseudohermaphroditism treated by feminization surgery with special reference to their classification and prognosis (Tanaka et al). Clin. Endocrinol. (Tokyo), 19:467, 1971 (Japanese)

Results of treatment in cases of male hermaphroditism (Boczkowski). Ginekol. Pol., 42:1483, 1971 (Polish)

Case of male pseudo-hermaphroditism with mosaicism (Lofty et al). J. Egypt. Med. Assoc., 54:723, 1971

Hermaphroditism, true (Olsson et al), PRS, 48:514, 1971. J. Urol., 105:586, 1971

Intersex (Blelock). Proc. Mine. Med. Off. Assoc., 50:82, 1971

Hermaphroditism, true, and chimerism, case report (Benirschke et al). Trans. Pac. Coast Obstet. Gynecol. Soc., 39:17, 1971

Reconstructive surgery for vaginal pathology in girls (Kushch et al). Vestn. Khir., 107:114, 1971 (Russian)

Hermaphroditism, true, management of case with negative sex chromatin and an idiogram 46-XY (Barinka). Brit. J. Plast. Surg., 25:427, 1972

Surgical correction in differentiation disorders of the urogenital sinus with clitoris hypertrophy (external female pseudohermaphroditism) (Hecker). Chirurg., 43:90, 1972 (German)

Hermaphroditism, male, therapy in (Boczkowski). Ginekol. Pol., 44:353, 1973 (Pol-

Hermaphroditism — Cont.
   ish)
   Hermaphroditism, testicular forms of, colpo-poiesis operations in (Globeva *et al*). Probl. Endokrinol. Mosk. , *19:*44, 1973 (Russian)
   Hermaphroditism, true. Report of case and review of literature (Teixeira *et al*). Rev. Assoc. Med. Bras., *19:*231, 1973 (Portuguese)
   Surgical construction of the male external genitalia (Engel). Clin. Plast. Surg., *1:*229, 1974
   Surgical construction of female genitalia (Jones). Clin. Plast. Surg., *1:*255, 1974
   Sex determination: true hermaphroditism with XX/XY/XXY chromosome pattern (Broeders *et al*), PRS, *55:*387, 1975. Nederl. tijdschr. geneesk., *118:*726, 1974
   Vaginoplasty in intersexual status (Lodovici). Rev. Assoc. Med. Bras., *20:*405, 1974 (Portuguese)
   The management of paediatric hermaphroditism (Roux *et al*). S. Afr. Med. J., *48:*2088, 1974
   Hermaphroditism, authentic (Knoch *et al*). Zentralbl. Chir., *99:*662, 1974
   Aetiology and management of intersexuality (Dewhurst). Clin. Endocrinol. (Oxf.), *4:*625, 1975
   What should this patient's permanent sex be? Clin. Pediatr. (Phila.), *14:*297, 1975
   Problem of surgical treatment of megaclitoris in cases of female hermaphroditism (Arneri). Med. Pregl., *28:*459, 1975 (Serbian)
   Pregnancy and childbirth in a true hermaphrodite (Narita *et al*). Obstet. Gynecol., *45:*593, 1975
   Pseudohermaphroditism, male, operative treatment (Carl *et al*). Urologe (A)., *14:*178, 1975 (German)

HERMRECK, A. S., BERG, R. A., AND RUHLEN, J. R.: Polyuria of sepsis, PRS, *52:*330, 1973. Surg. Forum, *23:*53, 1972
HERNANDEZ, A. *et al*: Oncocytoma of parotid glands. Case presentation and review of literature. Del. Med. J., *45:*219, 1973
HERNANDEZ, B., AND BRAVO, P.: Diseases of nails, PRS, *48:*605, 1971. Dermat. Rev. Mexicana, *14:*335, 1970
HERNANDEZ, F. J.: Malignant blue nevus, PRS, *54:*380, 1974. Arch. Dermat., *107:*741, 1973
HERNANDEZ-CARBAJAL, B. *et al*: Surgical treatment of longitudinal flat foot, PRS, *57:*119, 1976. Rev. El Medico, *25:*20, 1975
HERNANDEZ-JAUREGUI, P., ESPERANZA-GARCIA, C., AND GONZALEZ-ANGULO, A.: Morphology of connective tissue grown in re-sponse to implanted silicone rubber: a light and electron microscopic study, PRS, *54:*510, 1974. Surgery, *75:*631, 1974
HERNDON, J. H., AND MORGAN, L. R.: Use of acrylic fiber in pressure dressing. PRS, *52:*591, 1973
HERNDON, W. A. *et al*: Thrombosis of the ulnar artery in the hand. J. Bone & Joint Surg. (Am.), *57:*994, 1975
HEROLD, H. Z., HURVITZ, A., AND TADMOR, A.: Saline cartilage extract for healing experimental long bone defects, PRS, *51:*487, 1973. Internat. Surg., *57:*246, 1972
HERR, N., AND GOULIAN, D.: Review of diastrophic dwarfism associated with cleft palate, PRS, *55:*383, 1975. Cleft Palate, J., *11:*229, 1974
HERRICK, P. C.: Repair of fractures of orbital floor using premolded Silastic prosthesis, PRS, *54:*105, 1974. New Zealand M. J., *78:*159, 1973
HERRMANN, J. B. *et al*: Fibrosarcoma of thigh associated with prosthetic vascular graft, PRS, *48:*397, 1971. New England J. Med., *284:*91, 1971
HERRMANN, M.: Etiology of face asymmetry. Z. W. R., *80:*988, 1971 (German)
HERRMANN, T. *et al*: Postoperative radiotherapy in intraocular malignant melanoblastoma. Radiobiol. Radiother. (Berl.), *15:*233, 1974 (German)
HERSHEY, F. B.: Operation for aneurysm of internal carotid artery high in neck; new and an old technique. Angiology, *25:*24, 1974
HERSHEY, H. G. *et al*: Soft tissue profile change associated with surgical correction of prognathic mandible. Am. J. Orthod., *65:*483, 1974
HERSHMAN, D. S. *et al*: Apertognathia — an interdisciplinary approach: report of case. J. Oral Surg., *30:*743, 1972
HERTZ, R. S.: Occurrence of verruca vulgaris on an intraoral skin graft. Unique growth with significant implications. Oral Surg., *34:*934, 1972
HERVOUET, F.: Unesthetic eyelid. Rev. Prat., *23:*3149, 1973 (French)
HERWERTH, M. *et al*: Observations of patients with late surgery for cleft palate. Fogorv. Sz., *68:*164, 1975 (Hungarian)
HERZOG, B.: Microangiographic observations of different kinds of colon anastomosis in rat, PRS, *48:*518, 1971. Helvet. chir. acta, *1:*179, 1971
HERZON, F. S. Bacteremia and local infections with nasal packing, PRS, *49:*580, 1972. Arch. Otolaryng., *94:*317, 1971
HESLOP, I. H.: Technique for division of condy-

lar neck of mandible. Brit. J. Oral Surg., *10:*16, 1972

HESS, D. A.: Effects of certain variables on speech of cleft palate persons. Cleft Palate J., *8:*387, 1971

HESTER, J. B.: Use of sodium nitroprusside as a hypotensive agent in plastic surgery. Postgrad. Med. J., *50:*582, 1974

HETTER, G. P.: Neck incisions relative to the cutaneous vasculature of the neck. Arch. Otolaryng., *95:*84, 1972

HETTICH, R., OTTEN, G., AND HENNE, W.: Positive effects of thrombolysis on superficial extent of standardized burns in animals, PRS, *50:*204, 1972. Langenbecks Arch. Chir., *329:*899, 1971

HEUGHAN, C., GRISLIS, G., AND HUNT, T.: Effect of anemia on wound healing, PRS, *54:*379, 1974. Ann. Surg., *179:*163, 1974

HEUGHAN, C., AND HUNT, T. K.: Some aspects of wound healing research: review, PRS, *56:*470, 1975. Canad. J. Surg., *18:*118, 1975

HEYBROEK, G.: Congenital abnormalities of the hands. Ned. tijdschr. geneeskd., *115:*1289, 1971 (Dutch)

HEYCOCK, M. H.: Field guide to cleft lip repair. Brit. J. Surg., *58:*567, 1971

HEYCOCK, M. H.: Use of X-ray image intensifier in management of nasal escape, PRS, *48:*394, 1971. Proc. Roy. Soc. Med., *64:*70, 1971

HEYMAN, L. S.: Prosthetic acids in blepharoptosis: shelf devices. Int. Ophthalmol. Clin., *10:*803, 1971

HEYN, G. *et al*: Diagnosis and therapy of ulcus cruris. Z. Aerztl. Fortbild. (Jena), *67:*662, 1973

HEYNER, S.: Antigenicity of cartilage grafts, PRS, *53:*613, 1974. Surg. Gynec. & Obst., *136:*298, 1973

HIBLER, N.: Motility disorders of the eye in injuries of the osseous orbit (rhinologic report). Wien. Med. Wochenschr., *122:*Suppl *5:*2, 1972 (German)

HICKORY, J. E. *et al*: Simple probe for cryosurgical therapy for hemangiomas. J. Oral Surg., *33:*546, 1975

HICKORY, J. E. *et al*: Conservative treatment of cysts of the jaws in nevoid basal cell carcinoma syndrome: report of a case. J. Oral Surg., *33:*693, 1975

HICKS, J. N. *et al*: Maxillofacial injuries. J. Med. Assoc. State Ala., *43:*319, 1973

HICKS, K. A. *et al*: Amyloidosis: report of case presenting with macroglossia. Brit. J. Plast. Surg., *26:*274, 1973

HICKS, K. A. *et al*: Method of fixation following the vertical midline split during the anterior

maxillary osteotomy. Brit. J. Oral Surg., *11:*265, 1974

Hidradenitis

Axillary hidradenitis suppurativa, simple and effective surgical technique (Pollock, Virnelli, Ryan). PRS, *49:*22, 1972

Hidradenitis suppurativa: pathologic study and use of skin flaps (Paletta) (Follow-Up Clinic). PRS, *49:*334, 1972

Hidradenitis suppurativa, treatment (Editorial). J.A.M.A., *223:*556, 1973

Axillary hidradenitis defects, closure with local triangular flaps (Lipshutz). PRS, *53:*677, 1974

Sweat glands, surgical treament of chronic suppurative hidradenitis (Borghouts), PRS, *55:*121, 1975. Arch. chir. neerl., *26:*201, 1974

Hidradenitis defects, axillary, closure with local triangular flaps (Lipshutz). PRS, *53:*677, 1974

Hidradenitis suppurativa of scrotum and perineum (Ward *et al*). Urology, *4:*463, 1974

Axillary hidradenitis (Anderson, Perry), PRS, *55:*726, 1975. Arch. Surg., *110:*69, 1975

Operative management of chronic hidradenitis suppurativa of the scrotum and perineum (Vickers). J. Urol., *114:*414, 1975

Hidradenitis suppurativea of axilla, surgical treatment of (Tasche, Angelats, Jayaram). PRS, *55:*559, 1975

HIETANEN, J. *et al*: Histology and ultrastructure of an ameloblastic fibroma, case report. Proc. Finn. Dent. Soc., *69:*129, 1973

HIGGINS, G.: Biochemical sequelae to severe head and face trauma. Brit. J. Oral Surg., *9:*79, 1971

HIGHT, D. W., AND ANDERTON, R. L.: Combined use of punch grafts and overlay sheet of split-skin graft for raw area in scalp. PRS, *52:*663, 1973

HIGHTOWER, D. R. *et al*: Current concepts in the treatment of fractures of the orbit. Laryngoscope, *81:*725, 1971

HILAL, S. K. *et al*: Therapeutic percutaneous embolization for extra-axial vascular lesions of the head, neck, and spine. J. Neurosurg., *43:*275, 1975

HILDESTAD, P.: Prosthetic reconstruction following maxillectomy. Prosthet. Dent., *30:*637, 1973

HILES, R. W.: Freeze-dried irradiated nerve homograft, PRS, *51:*480, 1973. Hand, *4:*79, 1972

HILES, R. W.: Should lymphadenectomy be discarded? 2. Malignant melanoma. J. R. Coll. Surg. Edinb., *18:*368, 1973

HILES, R. W.: Surgical treatment of malignant melanoma. Proc. Roy. Soc. Med., *67:*95, 1974

HILL, G. *et al:* Chemotherapy of malignant melanoma with dimethyl triazeno imidazole carboxamide (DITC) and nitrosourea derivatives (BCNU, CCNU), PRS, *55:*117, 1975. Ann. Surg., *180:*167, 1974

HILL, J. C. *et al:* Cicatricial ectropion in epidermolysis bullosa and in congenital icthyosis: its plastic repair. Can. J. Ophthalmol., *6:*89, 1971

HILLERUP, S.: Tattoo marking for registration of relapse after oral vestibuloplasty. Int. J. Oral Surg., *4:*65, 1975

HILLIS, R. E. *et al:* Fibrous histiocytoma of the lip: report of a case. J. Oral Med., *30:*81, 1975

HILLSKAMP, P., AND RAINONE, M. A.: Surgical plasty in postoperative eventrations in septic conditions. Use of nets of synthetic material, PRS, *55:*108, 1975. Bol. y trab. Acad. argent. cir., *58:*89, 1974

HIMAL, H. S. *et al:* Gas gangrene of scrotum and perineum. Surg. Gynec. & Obst., *139:*176, 1974

HIMMEL, D.: Case report on Kirner's deformity. Beitr. Orthop. Traumatol., *20:*221, 1973 (German)

HIMMELFARB, R. *et al:* Ameloblastoma treated by peripheral ostectomy. Ten-year follow-up. N. Y. State Dent. J., *38:*282, 1972

HIMMELFARB, R. *et al:* Myxoma treated by peripheral ostectomy. Six-year follow-up. N. Y. State Dent. J., *38:*612, 1972

HINDER, R. A. *et al:* Submandibular duct lithiasis associated with mixed salivary gland tumor. Case report. Brit. J. Surg., *60:*246, 1973

HINDERER, U. T.: Secondary repair of hypospadias failure, another use of penis tunnelization technique. PRS, *50:*13, 1972

HINDERER, U. T.: Hairbearing preauricular rotation flap and additional corrections in the treatment of the aging face. In *Plastische und Wiederherstellungs-Chirurgie,* ed. by Hohler; pp. 49–66. Schattauer, Stuttgart, 1975

HINDERER, U. T.: Dermolipectomy approach for augmentation mammaplasty. Clin. Plast. Surg., *2:*359, 1975

HINDERER, U. T.: Malar implants for improvement of facial appearance. PRS, *56:*157, 1975

HINDERER, U. T.: Blepharocanthoplasty with eyebrow lift, PRS, *56:*402, 1975

HINDERER, U. T.: Rhinoplasty and additional techniques of profiloplasty, PRS, *57:*756, 1976. Rev. Iber. Latinoamericana Cir. Plast., *1:*245, 1975

HINDS, E. C., HOMSY, C. A., AND KENT, J. N.: Use of biocompatible interface for combining tissues and prostheses in oral surgery. Trans. Congr. Int. Assoc. Oral Surg., *4:*210, 1973

HINDS, E., HONSY, C. A., AND KENT, J. N.: Use of biocompatible interface for binding tissues and prostheses in temporomandibular joint surgery, PRS, *56:*105, 1975. Oral Surg., *38:*512, 1974

HINES, EDWARD, AND KENT, JOHN: *Surgical Treatment of Developmental Jaw Deformities.* C. V. Mosby Co., St. Louis, 1972. PRS, *51:*580, 1973

HINMAN, F.: Surgical management of microphallus, PRS, *49:*585, 1972. J. Urol., *105:*901, 1971

HINMAN, F., JR.: Microphallus: characteristics and choice of treatment from study of 20 cases, PRS, *51:*604, 1973. J. Urol., *107:*499, 1972

HINMAN, F., JR.: One-stage reconstruction of external genitalia in female with exstrophy of bladder (with Owsley). PRS, *50:*227, 1972

HINSHAW, M. A. *et al:* New concept in tracheostomy balloon cuffs, PRS, *49:*669, 1972. Surg. Forum, *22:*194, 1971

HINTON, P. *et al:* Blood-volume changes and transfusion requirements of burned patients after the shock phase of injury. Lancet, *1:*913, 1972

HIRAMOTO, M.: Treatment of cavernous hemangiomas by electrocoagulation using elastic vein needle, PRS, *51:*607, 1973. Jap. J. Plast. Reconstr. Surg., *15:*309, 1972

HIRAMOTO, M. *et al:* Management of wound surface and granulation wounds. Jap. J. Plast. Reconstr. Surg., *14:*158, 1971 (Japanese)

HIRANANDANI, L. H.: Management of cervical metastasis in head and neck cancers. J. Laryng. & Otol., *85:*1097, 1971

HIRANANDANI, L. H.: Reconstructive surgery of oral cavity and pharynx following extensive resections in head and neck regions. J. Laryng. & Otol., *86:*991, 1972

HIRANO, M.: Cricopharyngeal myotomy for paralytic dysphagia. J. Fr. Otorhinolaryngol., *23:*732, 1974

HIRANO, M. *et al:* Results of treatment of maxillary cancer in our department and future problems. J. Otolaryngol. Jap., *75:*1088, 1972 (Japanese)

HIRASAWA, Y. *et al:* Peripheral nerve homografting, preliminary report, PRS, *56:*365, 1975. Acta chir. plast., *16:*222, 1974

HIRASAWA, Y. *et al:* Experimental study of regeneration of sympathetic nerve fibers after nerve homografting. PRS, *54:*671, 1974

History of Plastic Surgery—Cont.
tions of John Jones, M.D. (1729–1791) (Rogers), PRS, *49:*1, 1972

"B.L.," "Mr. Lucas," and Mr. Carpue, more about (Freshwater) (Letter to the Editor). PRS, *49:*78, 1972

Maliniac, Jacques: Special ASPRS Award to. PRS, *49:*242, 1972

Peer, Lyndon: Special Award of ASPRS to. PRS, *49:*243, 1972

Tanzer, R. C.: Ivy Society Award to. PRS, *49:*243, 1972

Dow Corning International Awards in Plastic Surgery: First (1971) Award to Dr. Frank McDowell, PRS, *49:*363, 1972; Second (1972) Award to Dr. Dean Hoskins, PRS, *51:*356, 1973; Third (1973) Award to Dr. Charles Horton, *53:*377, 1974; Final and Fourth (1974) Award to Dr. Milton Edgerton. PRS, *55:*391, 1975

McDowell, Frank: First (1971) Dow Corning Award to, PRS, *49:*363, 1972. Honorary Degree to, PRS, *53:*253, 1974

Crikelair, George: Kay-Kilner Prize to. PRS, *49:*592, 1972

Murray, Joseph: Modern Medicine Award to. PRS, *49:*592, 1972

Tycho Brahe and his sixteenth century nasal prosthesis (Lee). PRS, *50:*332, 1972

Webster, Jerome P., presentation of Honorary Award of American Association of Plastic Surgeons to (Edgerton). PRS, *50:*510, 1972

Horton, Charles E., Honored. PRS, *50:*546, 1972; Dow Corning Award to, *53:*377, 1974

Le Fort's papers on experimental study of fractures of the upper jaw, commentary on (Tessier), PRS, *50:*605, 1972

Le Fort, René, biographical sketch of (Tessier), PRS, *50:*606, 1972

Vrebos, Jacques: Award to. PRS, *49:*673, 1972

Development of reconstructive surgery in the Tadzhik S.S.R. (Pulatov). Vestn. Khir., *108:*6, 1972 (Russian)

Albucassis on Surgery and Instruments. By M. S. Spink and G. Lewis. University of California Press, Berkeley, 1973.

De Curtorum Chirurgia per Insitionem. By Gasparis Taliacotti. Ed. by Fernando Ortiz-Monasterio. Libreria Manuel Porrua, S. A., Mexico D. F., Mexico, 1973. PRS, *53:*466, 1974

Contributions of Sir Archibald McIndoe to surgery of the hand (Bruner). Ann. R. Coll. Surg. Engl., *53:*1, 1973

Wilfred Batten Lewis Trotter, 1872 to 1939. His legacy to pharyngeal surgeons (Whicker *et al*). Arch. Otolaryng., *97:*423,

History of Plastic Surgery—Cont.
1973

Webster, Jerome P., presentation of Academy plaque to (Humphreys). Bull. N.Y. Acad. Med., *49:*954, 1973

Rhinoplasty, history of (Snell). Can. J. Otolaryngol., *2:*224, 1973

Twenty-five years of hand surgery. Personal reflections (Pulvertaft). J. Bone & Joint Surg. (Br.), *55:*32, 1973

Billroth, Theodore; first laryngectomy for cancer (Weir). J. Laryng. & Otol., *87:*1161, 1973

Influence of war on development of major subspecialty (Greeley). Mil. Med., *138:*231, 1973

Hoskins, Dean: 1972 Dow Corning Award to, PRS, *51:*356, 1973

Ivy, Robert H., M.D., D.D.S. Tribute (Converse). PRS, *51:*411, 1973

Bruner, Jules: Presents McIndoe Lecture. PRS, *51:*717, 1973

DeMere, McCarthy: Chairman of Medical-Legal Committee, American Bar Association. PRS, *52:*219, 1973

Hullihen, Simon P., pioneer oral and plastic surgeon (Goldwyn). PRS, *52:*250, 1973

China, replantation surgery in (American Replantation Mission). PRS, *52:*476, 1973

Brown, Barrett, Prizes in Plastic Surgery: Announcements, PRS, *52:*605, 1973; PRS, *52:*659, 1973; Awarded to Dr. Rollin Daniel, PRS, *54:*634, 1974; Awarded to Dr. Paul Tessier, PRS, *56:*359, 1975. Awarded to Dr. Ian Taylor. PRS, *58:*399, 1976

Otolaryngology, impact of on world history. (Wilhelm, F., Clevland, G., Roosevelt, F.) (Lucente). Trans. Am. Acad. Ophthalmol. Otolaryngol., 77:1424, 1973

Plastic surgery, ophthalmic, review of early history (Spaeth). Trans. Pa. Acad. Ophthalmol. Otolaryngol., *26:*95, 1973

Burian, Frantisek, in Balkan Wars (Troshev), PRS, *55:*647, 1975. Acta chir. plast., *16:*193, 1974

"Andy Gump" (Steckler *et al*). Am J. Surg., *128:*545, 1974

Seventieth birthday of Prof. V. Karfik, D.Sc. (Peskova). Cas. Lek. Cesk, *113:*288, 1974 (Czech)

Bailey, Hamilton, contributions to surgery (Humphries). Int. Surg., *59:*203, 1974

Self-fulfilling prophecies: Reflections on the future of A.S.S.H. (Entin). J. Bone & Joint Surg. (Am.), *56:*1088, 1974

Plastic surgery of skin, rotational method of, history (priority of Dr. E. B. Eshe) (Varner *et al*). Khirurgiia (Mosk.), *50:*136, 1974 (Russian)

History of Plastic Surgery—Cont.

Durston, Will, "mammaplasty" (Letterman, Schurter). PRS, *53:*48, 1974

Larson, Duane: "Physician of the Year" Award. PRS, *53:*120, 1974

Lip repair (cheiloplasty) performed by new method (Stein) (Classic Reprint). PRS, *53:*332, 1974

Horton, Charles: 1973 Dow Corning Award to. PRS, *53:*377, 1974

Barsky, Arthur: Recipient of Special Honorary Citation of ASPRS, *53:*378, 1974: Barsky Society founded. PRS, *57:*273, 1976

Children's Medical Relief International, report on hospital in Saigon (Barsky) (Letter to the Editor). PRS, *53:*464, 1974

Davis, John Staige, advice to medical students (Murray) (Letter to the Editor). PRS, *53:*582, 1974

Establishment of Ralph Millard-Rudolph Light Chair of Plastic Surgery at University of Miami. PRS, *54:*123, 1974

Dingman, Reed: Honorary Degree to. PRS, *54:*124, 1974

Paré, Ambroise, opinion on mammaplasties (Montandon, Letterman) (Letter to the Editor). PRS, *54:*212, 1974

Cleveland, President, secret surgery (Rosenhouse), PRS, *55:*387, 1975. Private Practice, *6:*43, 1974

Valadier, Charles, forgotton pioneer in treatment of jaw injuries (Mcauley), PRS, *55:*635, 1975. Proc. Roy. Soc. Med., *67:*785, 1974

Seventieth birthday of Prof. Dr. V. Karfik, M.D., D.Sc. (Peskova). Rozhl. Chir., *53:*145, 1974 (Czechoslovakian)

Unhappy love affair of Johann Friedrich Dieffenbach (Skrobacki). Wiad. Lek., *27:*1121, 1974 (Polish)

The Healing Hand: Man and Wound in the Ancient World. By Guido Majno. Harvard University Press, Cambridge, 1975. PRS, *57:*230, 1976

Maurice Lisbonne. Ann. chir. plast., *20:*261, 1975 (French)

Paré, Ambroise, and evolution of surgical instrumentarium (Rogge), PRS, *57:*126, 1976. Arch. chir. neerl., *27:*1, 1975

Edgerton, Milton T.: 1974 Dow Corning Award to. PRS, *55:*391, 1975

Rank, Sir Benjamin: Honorary Fellow of American College of Surgeons. PRS, *55:*526, 1975

Lewis, John R.: Poet Laureate of Georgia. PRS, *55:*650, 1975

Marking ink, Bonney's blue (Johnson). PRS, *56:*155, 1975

History of Plastic Surgery—Cont.

History of American Society for Aesthetic Plastic Surgery (Crosby). PRS, *56:*506, 1975

Doctor George Goodfellow, the first civilian trauma surgeon (Trunkey). Surg. Gynec. & Obst., *141:*97, 1975

Editorial: reconstruction after mastectomy (Goldwyn). Arch. Surg., *110:*246, 1975

Cleft lips, cure of (Franco) (Classic Reprint). PRS, *57:*84, 1976

How patient experienced cleft lip operation in 1763 (Rintala). PRS, *57:*158, 1976

Lip, cleft, observations on (De la Faye) (Classic Reprint). PRS, *57:*216, 1976

Barsky Unit, end of chapter, end of story? (Mills) (Letter to the Editor). PRS, *57:*654, 1976

HITCHEN, J. E. *et al:* Unexpected obstruction of nasotracheal tube, case report. J. Oral Surg., *31:*722, 1973

HITSELBERGER, W. E.: Hypoglossal-facial anastomosis. Otolaryngol. Clin. North Am., *7:*545, 1974

HJORTING-HANSEN, E. *et al:* Acquired defects of the antrum. Trans. Int. Conf. Oral Surg., *4:*19, 1973

HLAVACEK, V.: Incidence of osseous giant-cell tumors in otorhinolaryngology. Cesk. Otolaryngol., *22:*77, 1973 (Czechoslovakian)

HNELESKI, I., S. JR. *et al:* Orbital floor implant. Am. J. Ophth., *76:*540, 1973

HO, C., KAUFMAN, R. L., AND MCALISTER, W. H.: Congenital malformations, PRS, *57:*762, 1976. Am. J. Dis. Child., *129:*714, 1975

HO, K. C., AND MARMOR, L.: Entrapment of ulnar nerve at elbow, PRS, *48:*606, 1971. Am. J. Surg., *121:*355, 1971

HO, L. C. Y.: Hypospadias: report on 193 treated cases (with Sykes). PRS, *50:*452, 1972

HO, L. C. Y., BAILEY, B. N., AND SYKES, P. J.: Composite reconstruction of mandible and temporomandibular joint, following hemimandibulectomy. PRS, *53:*414, 1974

HO, W. Y. *et al:* Acupuncture anesthesia, report of two cases. Am. J. Chin. Med., *1:*151, 1973

HOBBS, K. E. F.: Current status of subzero organ preservation, PRS, *57:*544, 1976. Proc. Roy. Soc. Med., *68:*290, 1975

HOBSLEY, M.: Amputation neuroma of great auricular nerve after parotidectomy. Brit. J. Surg., *59:*735, 1972

HOBSON, R. W., II, AND WRIGHT, C. B.: Peripheral side to side arteriovenous fistula. Hemodynamics and application in venous reconstruction, PRS, *53:*606, 1974. Am. J. Surg., *126:*411, 1973

HOCHLEITNER, H.: First aid in skin burns. Z. Allgemeinmed., *47:*1438, 1971 (German)

HOCHSTEIN, H. J.: Prosthetic or surgical therapy in congenital palatal defects in the adult. Dtsch. Stomatol., *21:*663, 1971 (German)

HOCHSTEIN, H. J.: Studies on the status of cleft surgery. Dtsch. Gesundheitsw., *27:*993, 1972 (German)

HOCHSTEIN, U. *et al:* Caries statistical studies in 1198 children with cleft lip and cleft palates. Dtsch. Zahn. Mund. Kieferheilkd., *55:*134, 1970 (German)

HODGINS, T. E., AND HANCOCK, R. A.: Hemangio-endothelial sarcoma of penis, PRS, *49:*235, 1972. J. Urol., *104:*867, 1970

HODOSH, M., POVAR, M., AND SHKLAR, G.: Development of self-supportive polymer tooth implant, PRS, *53:*372, 1974. J. Biomed. Mater. Res., *7:*205, 1973

HOEFFEL, J. C. *et al:* Radiologic patterns of hemangiopericytoma of leg, PRS, *51:*704, 1973. Am. J. Surg., *123:*591, 1972

HOEHLER, H.: Breast augmentation: axillary approach. Brit. J. Plast. Surg., *26:*373, 1973

HOEHN, J. G.: Use of commercial porcine skin for wound dressings (with Elliott). PRS, *52:*401, 1973

HOEHN, J. G.: Correction of asymmetrical breasts (with Elliott, Greminger). PRS, *56:*260, 1975

HOEHN, R., AND BINKERT, B.: Cholesteric liquid crystals; a new visual aid to study of flap circulation. PRS, *48:*209, 1971

HOEHN, R. J.: Facial injuries. Surg. Clin. North Am., *53:*1479, 1973

HOEKSEMA, P. E.: Decompression for "malignant" exophthalmos. Pract. Otorhinolaryngol. (Basel), *33:*356, 1971

HOENIG, J.: Management of transsexualism. Can. Psychiatr. Assoc. J., *19:*1, 1974

HOENIG, J. *et al:* Surgical treatment for transsexualism. Acta Psychiatr. Scand., *47:*106, 1971

HOFFBRAND, B. I., AND FORSYTH, R. P.: Hemodynamic consequences of moderate postoperative anemia in monkeys, PRS, *48:*400, 1971. Surg. Gynec. & Obst., *132:*61, 1971

HOFFMAN, D. E.: Carpal tunnel syndrome: importance of sensory nerve conduction studies in diagnosis, PRS, *57:*400, 1976. J.A.M.A., *233:*983, 1975

HOFFMAN, G. W.: Surgical correction of prognathism, PRS, *56:*105, 1975. South. M.J., *67:*1427, 1974

HOFFMAN, G. W. *et al:* Reduction mammoplasty. South. Med. J., *64:*1106, 1971

HOFFMAN, G. W. *et al:* Cosmetic surgery of breast. Clin. Obstet. Gynecol., *18:*253, 1975

HOFFMAN, S.: Correction of split nail deformity, PRS, *53:*685, 1974. Arch. Dermat., *108:*568, 1973

HOFFMAN, S.: Basal cell carcinoma of nail bed, PRS, *54:*380, 1974. Arch. Dermat., *108:*828, 1973

HOFFMAN, S.: Classification and surgical correction of gynecomastia (with Simon, Kahn). PRS, *51:*48, 1973

HOFFMAN, S.: Revisional surgery after reduction mammaplasty (with Herman, Kahn). PRS, *55:*422, 1975

HOFFMAN, S., SIFFERT, R. S., AND SIMON, B. E.: Experimental and clinical experiences in epiphyseal transplantation. PRS, *50:*58, 1972

HOFFMAN, S. *et al:* Gangrene of the hand in a newborn child. Hand, *6:*70, 1974

HOFFMAN, S., AND SIMON, B. E.: Experiences with Pitanguy method of correction of trochanteric lipodystrophy. PRS, *55:*551, 1975

HOFFMAN, W. W., AND HALL, W. V.: Modification of Spence's hood for one-stage surgical correction of distal shaft penile hypospadias, PRS, *53:*107, 1974. J. Urol., *109:*1017, 1973

HOFFMANN, E. *et al:* Treatment of esophageal diverticula. Zentralbl. Chir., *98:*1501, 1973 (German)

HOFMANN, H.: Rodent ulcer. Klin. Monatsbl. Augenheilkd., *159:*460, 1971 (German)

HOGAN, V. M.: Clarification of surgical goals in cleft palate speech and introduction of lateral port control (LPC) pharyngeal flap, PRS, *54:*505, 1974. Cleft Palate J., *10:*331, 1973

HOGAN, V. M.: A biased approach to the treatment of velopharyngeal incompetence. Clin. Plast. Surg., *2:*319, 1975

HOGEMAN, K. E. *et al:* One stage surgical and dental-orthopaedic correction of bimaxillary and craniofacial dysostoses. Dtsch. Zahn. Mund. Kieferheilkd., *57:*277, 1971

HOGEMAN, K. E. *et al:* Secondary bone grafting in cleft palate: a follow-up of 145 patients. Cleft Palate J., *9:*39, 1972

HOGEMAN, K. E. *et al:* One-stage surgical and dental-orthopedic correction of bimaxillary and craniofacial dysostosis. Fortschr. Kiefer. Gesichtschir., *18:*39, 1974

HOGEMAN, K. E. *et al:* On Le Fort III osteotomy for Crouzon's disease in children. Report of a four-year follow-up in one patient. Scand. J. Plast. Reconstr. Surg., *8:*169, 1974

HOGG, G. R.: Burn eschar, histopathological study (with Vistnes). PRS, *48:*56, 1971

HOGGINS, G. S. *et al:* Paget's disease of the maxilla. Brit. J. Oral Surg., *9:*122, 1971

HOGGINS, G. S., AND GRUNDY, M. C.: Melanotic

neuroectodermal tumor of infancy, PRS, 57:539, 1976. Oral Surg., 40:34, 1975

HOHLE, K. D. et al: Circumscribed deep burns of the hand. Burn degrees and their functional sequelae in conservative treatment. Monatsschr. Unfallheilkd., 76:108, 1973 (German)

HOHLE, K. D. et al: Split skin transplantation. Monatsschr. Unfallheilkd., 77:189, 1974 (German)

HOHLER, H.: Augmentation mammaplasty: axillary approach, PRS, 54:108, 1974. Langenbecks Arch. Chir., 334:981, 1973

HOHLER, H.: Facelifting and blepharoplasty. Surgical and suture techniques. In Plastische und Wiederherstellungs-Chirurgie, ed. by Hohler; pp. 35–47. Schattauer, Stuttgart, 1975 (German)

HOKI, A.: Cryogenic surgery of the head and neck. Saishin Igaku, 27:691, 1972 (Japanese)

HOLDAWAY, M. D.: Accidental burns and poisoning of children in the home. N.Z. Med. J., 75:280, 1972

HOLDCROFT, A. et al: Acceptability of swivel connectors. Brit. J. Anaesth., 46:298, 1974

HOLDCROFT, A. et al: Letter: swivel connections. Brit. J. Anaesth., 47:642, 1975

HOLDEN, H.: Indications and limitations of cryosurgery in head and neck neoplasia. Proc. Roy. Soc. Med., 67:76, 1974

HOLDEN, H. B.: Cryosurgery in treatment of head and neck neoplasia. Brit. J. Surg., 59:709, 1972

HOLDEN, H. B.: Practical Cryosurgery. Year Book Co., Chicago, 1976.

HOLDER, A. R.: Cosmetic breast surgery. J.A.M.A., 222:1101, 1972

HOLDER, I. A. et al: Enhanced survival in burned mice treated with antiserum prepared against normal and burned skin. J. Trauma, 11:1041, 1971

HOLEVICH, J., AND PANEVA-HOLEVICH, E.: Bipedicled island flaps, PRS, 50:307, 1972. Acta chir. plast., 13:106, 1971

HOLLANDER, L. et al: Management of cancer of parotid gland. Surg. Clin. North Am., 53:113, 1973

HOLLENDER, L. et al: Radiography of the temporomandibular joint after oblique sliding osteotomy of the mandibular rami. Scand. J. Dent. Res., 82:466, 1974

HOLLINGSWORTH, J. F., AND OCHSNER, J. L.: Multifocal glomus tumor: case report and review of literature, PRS, 51:707, 1973. Am. Surgeon, 38:161, 1972

HOLLINS, P. J.: Multiple glomus tumours. Proc. Roy. Soc. Med., 64:806, 1971

HOLLMANN, K.: Proceedings: early closure of the prolabium in piercing cleft lip, jaw and palate. Munch. Med. Wochenschr., 116:1064, 1974 (German)

HOLLOMAN, J. L.: Maxillary and mandibular osteotomy for maxillary and mandibular retrusion. Tex. Dent. J., 91:4, 1973

HOLLOWAY, J. P.: Transsexuals: legal considerations. Arch. Sex. Behav., 3:33, 1974

HOLLWICH, F. et al: Correction of blepharochalasis. Klin. Monatsbl. Augenheilkd., 166:255, 1975 (German)

HOLM, A., AND ZACHARIAE, L.: Fingertip lesions, conservative treatment versus free skin grafting, PRS, 57:261, 1976. Acta orthop. scandinav., 45:382, 1974

HOLM, P. C. A., AND VANGGAARD, L.: Frostbite. PRS, 54:544, 1974

HOLMES, E. C. et al: Regional lymph node metastases and the level of invasion of primary melanoma. Cancer, 37:199, 1976

HOLMES, L. B. et al: Phocomelia, flexion deformities and absent thumbs: a new hereditary upper limb malformation. Pediatrics, 54:461, 1974

HOLMES, OLIVER WENDELL: Our Hundred Days in Europe. Arno Press & The New York Times, New York, 1971. PRS, 57:373, 1976

HOLM-JENSEN, S.: Free skin grafting to male genitalia in case of lymphedema. Ugeskr. Laeger, 134:2160, 1972 (Danish)

HOLMLUND, D. E.: Knot properties of surgical suture materials, PRS, 56:366, 1975. Europ. Surg. Res., 6:65, 1974

HOLM-PEDERSEN, P., AND ZEDERFELDT, B.: Strength development of skin incisions in young and old rats, PRS, 48:610, 1971. Scand. J. Plast. Reconstr. Surg., 5:7, 1971

HOLM-PEDERSEN, P., AND ZEDERFELDT, B.: Granulation tissue formation in subcutaneously implanted cellulose sponges in young and old rats, PRS, 48:610, 1971. Scand. J. Plast. Reconstr. Surg., 5:13, 1971

HOLM-PEDERSEN, P., AND VIIDIK, A.: Maturation of collagen in healing wounds in young and old rats, PRS, 51:108, 1973. Scand. J. Plast. Reconstr. Surg., 6:16, 1972

HOLM-PEDERSEN, P., AND VIIDIK, A.: Tensile properties and morphology of healing wounds in young and old rats, PRS, 51:108, 1973. Scand. J. Plast. Reconstr. Surg., 6:24, 1972

HOLM-PEDERSEN, P., AND ZEDERFELDT, B.: Respiratory gas tensions and blood flow in wounds in young and old rats, PRS, 54:508, 1974. Scand. J. Plast. Reconstr. Surg., 7:91, 1973

HOLMSTROM, H.: Malignant melanoma – impressions from a study tour. Nord. Med., 86:1224, 1971 (Swedish)

HOLMSTRÖM, H.: Malignant melanoma – treatment and prognosis. Lakartidningen, 69:2425, 1972 (Swedish)

HOLMSTRÖM, H., AND JOHANSON, B.: Local radiation injury and its surgical treatment. Report of 170 cases. Scand. J. Plast. Reconstr. Surg., 6:156, 1972

HOLMSTROM, H. et al: Surgical treatment of eyelid cancer with special reference to tarso-conjuncival flaps. A follow-up on 193 patients. Scand. J. Plast. Reconstr. Surg., 9:107, 1975

HOLSCHNEIDER, A. M., AND LAHODA, F.: Electromyographic and electromanometric studies after *gracilis* transplantations following Pickrell's procedure, PRS, 54:631, 1974. Ztschr. Kinderchir., 14:288, 1974

HOLSCHNEIDER, A. M., AND HECKER, W. C.: Operative correction of recurrent rectovaginal and urethrovaginal fistulas, PRS, 57:761, 1976. Ztschr. Kinderchir., 17:227, 1975

HOLST, H. I.: Primary peripheral nerve repair in the hand and upper extremity. J. Trauma, 15:909, 1975

HOLT, J. A. G.: Cure of cancer – preliminary hypothesis, PRS, 55:116, 1975. Australasian Radiol., 18:15, 1974

HOLT, R. J. et al: Treatment of infected surface lesions with sulfamylon acetate cream. Arch. Dis. Child., 47:143, 1972

HOLTHUSEN, W.: Pierre Robin syndrome: unusual associated developmental defects. Ann. Radiol. (Paris), 15:253, 1972 (Multi-language)

HOLTJE, W. J. et al: Wave-line procedure in the repair of cleft lip. J. Maxillo-facial. Surg., 1:198, 1973

HOLTJE, W. J. et al: Indication, technic and clinical results of surgical treatment of open bite using Schuchardt's osteotomy of the lateral maxilla. Fortschr. Kiefer. Gesichtschir., 18:202, 1974 (German)

HOLTMANN, B.: Factors in production of inconspicuous scars (with Wray, Weeks). PRS, 56:86, 1975

HOLUB, M. et al: Large flap plasty in otorhinolaryngology. Cesk. Otolaryngol., 23:96, 1974 (Czech)

HOLUBEC, K.: Enormous elephantiasis of the scrotum, PRS, 52:681, 1973. Acta chir. plast., 14:191, 1972

Homografts (See also *Bone Homografts; Burns, Homografts for; Cartilage Homografts; Skin Grafts, Homografts and Heterografts*)

Cadaver kidneys, human, preservation for

Homografts – Cont.
transplantation (Kiser *et al*), PRS, 49:585, 1972. J. Urol., 105:779, 1971

Allografts, prevention of rejection by use of "Trasicor" (Ageeb *et al*), PRS, 52:463, 1973. Kasr el Fini J. Surg., 12:10, 1971

Cadaver homografts (Hackett), PRS, 50:202, 1972. Proc. Roy. Soc. Med., 64:1291, 1971

Allograft survival, effect of traumatic and nontraumatic shock on (Markley, Thorton, Smallman), PRS, 49:362, 1972. Surgery, 70:667, 1971

Allografts, rabbit skin, comparative effectiveness of corticosteroids applied topically as pretreatment (Klaue, Jolley), PRS, 49:362, 1972. Surgery, 70:718, 1971

Allografts and xenografts, appraisal as biological dressings for wounds and burns (Artz, Rittenburg, Yarbrough), PRS, 51:236, 1973. Ann. Surg., 175:934, 1972

Cadaver homografts, cutaneous, for early management of difficult wounds (Shuck, Bedeau, Thomas), PRS, 52:105, 1973. J. Trauma, 12:215, 1972

Cadaver kidneys, harvesting, preservation, and transportation of (Linke *et al*), PRS, 50:539, 1972. J. Urol., 107:184, 1972

Homografts, early application and coverage with tape, comparison of effects in healing of second degree burns (Miller, White). PRS, 49:552, 1972

Costal cartilage homografts preserved by radiation (Dingman) (Follow-Up Clinic). PRS, 50:516, 1972

Skin and subcutaneous tissue, study in rats of survival of composite homotransplants of, with microvascular anastomoses (Salyer, Kyger). PRS, 51:672, 1973

Eye, rabbit, anterior chamber, preparation of antilymphocyte serum by transplantation of lymphoid heterografts (White). PRS, 52:66, 1973

Homografts, composite, on antigenicity of immediately revascularized (Murray) (Letter to the Editor). PRS, 52:78, 1973

Rejection phenomena after homotransplantation of skin flaps in dogs by microvascular technique (Harashina *et al*). PRS, 52:390, 1973

Allografts, heart and skin, in inbred rats, factors responsible for the differential survival of (Warren, Lofgreen, Steinmuller), PRS, 53:689, 1974. Transplantation, 16:458, 1973

Transplantation, skin homografts in rats compared to other organs (Gruber, Kaplan, Lucas). PRS, 53:64, 1974

Homografts: reinnervation after orthotopic

Homografts — Cont.

grafting of peripheral nerve segments in inbred rats (Bucko, Steinmuller). PRS, *53:*326, 1974

Homografting, nerve, experimental study of the regeneration of sympathetic nerve fibers after (Hirasawa *et al*). PRS, *54:*671, 1974

Homograft, skin, survival prolonged with niridazole (Mandel, Mahmoud, Warren). PRS, *55:*76, 1975

Homograft skin, panniculectomy specimens as convenient and inexpensive source of (Swartz, Rueckert, Brown). PRS, *55:*628, 1975

HONEE, G. L. J. M., AND BLOEM, J. J. A. M.: Differential diagnosis of masseter muscle hypertrophy, PRS, *55:*715, 1975. J. Maxillo-facial Surg., *2:*246, 1974

HONEYCUTT, W. M., AND JANSEN, G. T.: Treatment of squamous cell carcinoma of the skin, PRS, *54:*380, 1974. Arch. Dermat., *108:*670, 1973

HONIGMANN, V. K.: The simultaneous surgical correction of lip and nose in unilateral cleft lip and cleft palate. Zahn. Mund. Kieferheilkd., *63:*246, 1975 (German)

HONJO, I. *et al*: Role of Passavant's ridge in cleft palate speech. Arch. Otorhinolaryngol. (N.Y.), *211:*203, 1975

HONJOW, I., ISSHIKI, N., AND MORIMOTO, M.: Pushback operation for complete unilateral cleft palate. PRS, *53:*306, 1974

HOOLEY, J. R. *et al*: Use of steroids in the prevention of some complications after traumatic oral surgery. J. Oral Surg., *32:*864, 1974

HOOPES, J. E.: Drug injection injuries of hands and forearms in addicts (with Ryan, Jabaley). PRS, *53:*445, 1974

HOOPES, J. E.: Gender dysphoria syndromes: position statement on so-called "transsexualism" (with Meyer). PRS, *54:*444, 1974

HOOPES, J. E.: W-epicanthoplasty (with Mulliken). PRS., *55:*435, 1975

HOOPES, J. E.: Needle aspiration of flexor digital sheath as aid in diagnosing tenosynovitis (with Ryan). PRS, *56:*152, 1975

HOOPES, J. E.: Where are we going? PRS, *56:*266, 1975

HOOPES, J. E.: Selection of antibiotics for human bites of hand (with Guba, Mulliken). PRS, *56:*538, 1975

HOOPES, J. E.: Effects of intralesional injection of triamcinolone on glucose-6-phosphate dehydrogenase and alanine aminotransferase activity in keloids (with Im, Mulliken). PRS, *56:*660, 1975

HOOPES, J. E. *et al*: Silver lactate burn cream, PRS, *49:*106, 1972. Surgery, *70:*29, 1971

HOOPES, J. E., AND IM, M. J. C.: Glycogen metabolism in epidermal wound healing, PRS, *56:*471, 1975. J. Surg. Oncol., *6:*408, 1974

HOOVER, B. B. *et al*: Electromyographic findings in high voltage electrical burns: two cases. South. Med. J., *64:*1392, 1971

HOOVER, G. H., FLATT, A. E., AND WEISS, M. W.: The hand and Apert's syndrome, PRS, *49:*234, 1972. J. Bone & Joint Surg., *52A:*878, 1970

HOPCROFT, S. C.: Axillary approach to brachial plexus anesthesia, PRS, *52:*331, 1973. Anesth. & Intens. Care, *1:*3, 1973

HOPKINS, R.: Fractures of the zygomatic complex. Ann. R. Coll. Surg. Engl., *49:*403, 1971

HOPKINS, R.: Some dental problems and the surgeon. Ann. R. Coll. Surg. Engl., *53:*95, 1973

HOPKINS, R.: Fractures of middle third of facial skeleton, PRS, *55:*377, 1975. Proc. Roy. Soc. Med., *67:*709, 1974

HOPKINS, R.: Injured face, PRS, *55:*633, 1975. Proc. Roy. Soc. Med., *67:*709, 1974

HOPKINS, R. *et al*: Two cases of Hunter's syndrome — anesthetic and operative difficulties in oral surgery. Brit. J. Oral Surg., *10:*286, 1973

HOPKINS, R. *et al*: Experience of pre-prosthetic surgery on the atrophic edentulous mandible. Brit. Dent. J., *137:*341, 1974

HOPKINS, R. *et al*: Use of a Le Fort I osteotomy as a surgical approach. Brit. J. Oral Surg., *13:*27, 1975

HOPKINS, R. E., AND CAMPBELL, W. A., III: One-stage hypospadias repair. Modification of Broadbent procedure, PRS, *57:*536, 1976. J. Urol., *112:*674, 1974

HOPSON, W. L. G.: Cross-foot flap (with Taylor), PRS, *55:*677, 1975. Discussion by Cannon. PRS, *56:*83, 1975

HOPSON, W. L. *et al*: Ameloblastoma with metastases to lung, ilium and soft tissues, case report. Brit. J. Plast. Surg., *25:*367, 1972

HOR, H. T.: Maxillo-facial injuries from the war in Cambodia. Rev. Stomatol. Chir. Maxillofac., *75:*1021, 1974 (French)

HORAK, V. F. *et al*: Traumatic facial aneurysm. Wien. Med. Wochenschr., *125:*222, 1975 (German)

HORBST, L. *et al*: 25 years experience with glottis widening surgery in our clinic. H.N.O., *23:*147, 1975 (German)

HORE, B. D. *et al*: Male transsexualism in England: sixteen cases with surgical intervention. Arch. Sex. Behav., *4:*81, 1975

HORIBE, K. *et al*: Histological study of various

aspects of the integration of dermo fat autografts. Rev. Assoc. Med. Bras., 20:312, 1974 (Portuguese)

HORIOT, J. C.: Cancer of mobile part of tongue. Therapeutic indications. J. Fr. Otorhinolaryngol., 22:875, 1973 (French)

HORMANN, D. et al: Late changes in urethras after perineal diversion in childhood. Z. Urol. Nephrol., 68:585, 1975 (German)

HORN, W.: Results of low-revolution skin grinding of seborrheic warts. Z. Hautkr., 48:971, 1973 (German)

HORNBLASS, A.: Ocular protection shield. Trans. Am. Acad. Ophthalmol. Otolaryngol., 78:228, 1974

HORNBLASS, A. et al: Oculofacial anomalies and corneal ulceration. Ann. Ophth., 6:575, 1974

HORNE, R. H., AND HORNE, J. H.: Fat embolization prophylaxis, use of hypertonic glucose, PRS, 54:624, 1974. Arch. Int. Med., 133:288, 1974

HORNER, R. L., WIEDEL, J. D., AND BRALLIAR, F.: Involvement of hand in epidermolysis bullosa, PRS, 49:663, 1972. J. Bone & Joint Surg., 53:1347, 1971

HORNOVA, J. et al: Correlation of clinical, surgical and histopathological findings in temporomandibular arthropathies. Cesk. Stomatol., 75:196, 1975 (Czechoslovakian)

HORNOVA, J. et al: Examination of the structure and surface of articular disc in surgically treated arthropathies. Cesk. Stomatol., 75:457, 1975 (Czechoslovakian)

HORNUNG, M. O., AND KREMENTZ, E. T.: Specific tissue and tumor responses of chimpanzees following immunization against human melanoma, PRS, 54:508, 1974. Surgery, 75:477, 1974

HOROVITZ, J. H., CARRICO, C. J., AND SHIRES, G. T.: Venous sampling sites for pulmonary shunt determinations in injured patient, PRS, 50:205, 1972. J. Trauma, 11:911, 1972

HOROWITZ, M. S.: Unusual tumors of ears and mandible. Arch. Klin. Exp. Ohren Nasen Kehlkopfheilkd., 205:203, 1973 (German)

HOROWITZ, S. L., AND MORISHIMA, A.: Palatal abnormalities in syndrome of gonadal dysgenesis and its variants and in Noonan's syndrome, PRS, 56:358, 1975. Oral Surg., 38:839, 1974

HORREE, W. A.: Adenoid cystic carcinoma of maxilla, PRS, 56:594, 1975. Arch. Otolaryng., 100:469, 1974

HORT, W. et al: Soft tissue tumours on the back of the knee. Ztschr. Orthop., 113:102, 1975 (German)

HORTON, C. E.: Growth of skin grafts, flaps and scars in young minipigs (with Baran).

PRS, 50:487, 1972

HORTON, Charles E.: Plastic and Reconstructive Surgery of the Genital Area. Little, Brown & Co., Boston, 1973. PRS, 54:601, 1974

HORTON, C. E.: Studies of urethral healing in dogs (with Everingham, Devine), 51:312, 1973

HORTON, C. E.: Discussion of "Achieving more nasal tip projection by use of small autogenous vomer or septal cartilage graft," by Sheen. PRS, 56:211, 1975

HORTON, C. E. et al: Use of vomerine flaps to cover raw area on nasal surface in cleft palate pushbacks. PRS, 51:421, 1973

HORTON, C. E., AND DEVINE, C. J., JR.: Plication of tunica albuginea to straighten curved penis. PRS, 52:32, 1973

HORTON, C. E., AND DEVINE, C. J., JR.: Peyronie's disease. PRS, 52:503, 1973

HORTON, C. E. et al: Vicryl, synthetic absorbable sutures, PRS, 56:363, 1975. Am. Surgeon, 40:729, 1974

HORTON, C. E. et al: Cosmetic surgery. Brit. Med. J., 3:566, 1974

HORTON, C. E. et al: Simple mastectomy with immediate reconstruction, PRS, 53:42, 1974

HORTON, C. E., AND GURSU, K. G.: Temporary suspension of lower lid after blepharoplasty. PRS, 55:371, 1975

HORTON, C. E., AND DEVINE, C. J., JR.: Secondary closures of penile skin incisions. PRS, 55:630, 1975

HORTON, C. E., AND SHARZER, L. A.: Simple method for determining limits of mandibular resection for carcinoma. PRS, 56:101, 1975

HORTON, J. E. et al: Healing of surgical defects in alveolar bone produced with ultrasonic instrumentation, chisel, and rotary bur, PRS, 57:257, 1976. J. Oral Surg., 39:536, 1975

HORWITZ, D. L. et al: Heparin treatment of live Escherichia coli bacteremia in rats, PRS, 52:106, 1973. J. Surg. Res., 13:120, 1972

HOSHI, S.: Management of avulsion injury—including degloving injury. Shujutsu, 26:53, 1972 (Japanese)

HOSNI, F. A. et al: Dacryocystorhinostomy—our experience with 100 cases. Eye, Ear, Nose, Throat Mon., 52:251, 1973

HOSXE, G.: Cerebrospinal rhinorrhea and frontal flap approach. Ann. chir. plast., 17:191, 1972 (French)

HOSXE, G.: Approach to temporomandibular joint. Rev. Stomatol. Chir. Maxillofac., 73:375, 1972

HOSXE, G. et al: Multiple facial injuries. Maroc Med., 52:732, 1972 (French)

HOSXE, G. et al: Recurrence of mandibular ameloblastoma previously treated by radiation. Rev. Stomatol. Chir. Maxillofac., *74:*135, 1973

HOSXE, G. *et al:* Tumors of external canthus in infant. Rev. Stomatol. Chir. Maxillofac., *74:*483, 1973 (French)

HOSXE, G. *et al:* Use of temporal aponeurosis for closing of periorbital tears during certain cases of diplopia. Rev. Stomatol. Chir. Maxillofac., *74:*393, 1974 (French)

HOSXE, G. *et al:* Advantage of the endo-oral approach for the treatment of malar fractures. Rev. Stomatol. Chir. Maxillofac., *75:*867, 1974 (French)

HOTZ, I.: Metastatic orbital tumors: case of orbital metastasis in malignant melanoma of skin. Klin. Monatsbl. Augenheilkd., *166:*176, 1975 (German)

HOTZ, M. M., AND PERKO, M.: Early management of bilateral total cleft lip and palate, PRS, *56:*467, 1975. Scand. J. Plast. Reconstr. Surg., *8:*104, 1974

HOTZ, R. *et al:* Therapy of tooth eruption disorders caused by cysts. Fortschr. Kieferorthop., *33:*19, 1972

HOTZ-JENNY, M. *et al:* Coordinated orthodontic and surgical treatment of cleft lip, jaw and palate. A contribution on the prevention of delayed adverse effects. Schweiz. Med. Wochenschr., *104:*718, 1974 (German)

HOUCK, W. S. *et al:* Carotid artery surgery and intermittent monocular blindness (amaurosis fugax). J. S. C. Med. Assoc., *68:*57, 1972

HOUSE, J. M. *et al:* Chemodectomas of nasopharynx. Arch. Otolaryng., *96:*138, 1972

HOVEY, L. M.: Transconjunctival lower lid blepharoplasty for removal of fat (with Tomlinson). PRS, *56:*314, 1975

HOVINGA, J. *et al:* Desmoplastic fibroma in mandible. Int. J. Oral Surg., *3:*41, 1974

HOVINGA, J. *et al:* Difficulties in and indication for treatment of facial asymmetry. Int. J. Oral Surg., *3:*234, 1974

HOWARD, F. M., AND LEE, R. E.: The hand in Maffucci syndrome, PRS, *50:*307, 1972. Arch. Surg., *103:*752, 1971

HOWARD, G. M.: Application of frozen sections to diagnosis of orbital tumors, PRS, *48:*509, 1971. Am. J. Ophth., *71:*221, 1971

HOWE, GEOFFREY L.: *Minor Oral Surgery.* Williams & Wilkins Co., Baltimore, 1971. PRS, *50:*180, 1972

HOWELL, A. *et al:* Chemodectomas of head and neck. Surg. Clin. North Am., *53:*175, 1973

HOWELL, J. B., AND FREEMAN, R. G.: Prominent inferior labial artery, PRS, *52:*678, 1973. Arch. Dermat., *107:*386, 1973

HOWELLS, C. H. L.: Infections in hospitals,

PRS, *56:*237, 1975. Proc. Roy. Soc. Med., *68:*95, 1975

HOWIE, C. C.: General anaesthesia in the adult burned patient. Postgrad. Med. J., *48:*152, 1972

HOZUMI, Y.: Case of desmoid tumor of the 1st dorsal interosseous muscle. Orthop. Surg. (Tokyo), *22:*985, 1971 (Japanese)

HRABOVSKY, J.: Primary treatment of fractures of metacarpal bones with reference to the functional capacity of the hand. Rozhl. chir., *54:*80, 1975 (Czechoslovakian)

HRIVNAKOVA, H., AND FARA, M.: Brevicollis (Klippel-Feil syndrome), PRS, *54:*628, 1974. Rozhl. chir., *53:*183, 1974

HRIVNAKOVA, J. *et al:* New method for the correction of nostril deformities in unilateral clefts. Rozhl. chir., *54:*437, 1975 (Czech)

HRIVOVA, E.: Therapy of upper eyelid ptosis at Ophthalmological Clinic on Olomouc. Cesk. Oftalmol., *29:*310, 1973 (Czechoslovakian)

HUANG, T. *et al:* Use of cryotherapy in management of intraoral hemangiomas, PRS, *51:*707, 1973. South, M. J., *65:*1123, 1972

HUANG, T. *et al:* Use of excisional therapy in management of snakebite, PRS, *55:*121, 1975. Ann. Surg., *179:*598, 1974

HUANG, T. T.: Adjustable razor dermatome: another efficient, economical, and portable dermatome, PRS, *57:*264, 1976. Surgery, *77:*703, 1975

HUANG, T. T., LARSON, D. L., AND LEWIS, S. R.: Burned hands, PRS, *56:*21, 1975. Discussion by Bennett, PRS, *56:*442, 1975

HUBER, C. J.: Hand and thermography. Ann. Chir., *29:*1025, 1975 (French)

HUBER, H. P.: Cosmetic evaluation of a new surgical technique for diagnostic skin biopsies and the excision of small skin tumours. Dermatologica, *148:*270, 1974 (German)

HUDDART, A. G. *et al:* Evaluation of arch form and occlusion in unilateral cleft palate subjects. Cleft Palate J., *9:*194, 1972

HUDSON, A. R. *et al:* Peripheral nerve autografts, PRS, *51:*349, 1973. J. Surg. Res., *12:*267, 1972

HUDSON, A. S.: Mirror-image unilateral condylar hyperplasia. Brit. J. Oral Surg., *10:*58, 1972

HUDSON, M. J.: Rupture of the corpus cavernosum of the penis. Brit. J. Clin. Pract., *29:*191, 1975

HUESTON, J. T.: Enzymic fasciotomy, PRS, *48:*512, 1971. Hand, *3:*38, 1971

HUESTON, J. T.: Z-closure. M. J. Australia, *1:*496, 1973

HUESTON, J. T. *et al:* Aetiology of trigger finger explained on the basis of intratendinous architecture. Hand, *4:*257, 1972

HUESTON, J. T., AND WILSON, W. F.: Role of intrinsic muscles in production of metacarpophalangeal subluxation in rheumatoid hand. PRS, *52:*342, 1973

HUESTON, J. T., AND TUBIANA, R.: *Dupuytren's Disease.* Grune & Stratton, New York, 1974. PRS, *57:*740, 1976

HUESTON, J. T., AND HEINZE, J. B.: Successful early relief of blindness occurring after blepharoplasty, PRS, *53:*588, 1974. Discussion by Hepler, Sugimura, Straatsma, PRS, *57:*233, 1976

HUFFMAN, A., AND STERIN, K.: Ten-year survival with multiple metastatic malignant melanoma: primary site unknown, PRS, *52:*459, 1973. Arch. Surg., *106:*234, 1973

HUFFMAN, G. G., AND LORSON, E. L.: Treatment of malocclusion in case of Treacher-Collins syndrome, PRS, *56:*105, 1975. J. Oral. Surg., *32:*612, 1974

HUFFMAN, G. G. *et al*: Ameloblastoma—the conservative surgical approach to treatment: report of four cases. J. Oral Surg., *32:*850, 1974

HUFFSTADT, A. J.: Thoughts on "mallet finger." Ned. tijdschr. geneeskd., *115:*1049, 1971 (Dutch)

HUFFSTADT, A. J.: Xanthomas of the hand. Ned. tijdschr. geneeskd., *115:*1989, 1971 (Dutch)

HUFFSTADT, A. J.: Skin avulsion of penis and scrotum. Ned. tijdschr. geneeskd., *116:*57, 1972 (Dutch)

HUFFSTADT, A. J.: Improvement of facial features. Tijdschr. Ziekenverpl., *25:*994, 1972 (Dutch)

HUFFSTADT, A. J.: Hemangiomas of the hand—conservative treatment? Handchirurgie, *5:*115, 1973 (German)

HUFFSTADT, A. J. C.: Hemangiomas—the conservative approach, PRS, *53:*111, 1974. Chir. Plast., *1:*305, 1973

HUFFSTADT, A. J. C.: Free skin grafting, PRS, *57:*125, 1976. Ned. tijdschr. geneesk., *119:*589, 1975

HUFFSTADT, A. J. C., KLASEN, H. J., AND EISMA, W. H.: Treatment of burned patients, PRS, *57:*263, 1976. Ned. tijdschr. geneesk., *119:*595, 1975

HUGER, W. E., JR: Avoidable pitfalls in augmentation mammaplasty. South. Med. J., *28:*703, 1975

HUGH, T. B.: Primary wound care in the casualty department. M. J. Australia, *2:*631, 1974

HUGHES, E. F. X. *et al*: Surgical work loads in community practice, PRS, *50:*206, 1972. Surgery, *71:*315, 1972

HUGHES, E. F. X., LEWITT, E. M., AND LORENZO, F. V.: Time utilization of population of general surgeons in community practice, PRS, *56:*606, 1975. Surgery, *77:*371, 1975

HUGHES, L. E.: Carcinoma of tongue. Brit. Med. J., *2:*768, 1972

HUGHES, L. E.: The place of frozen section in the practical management of melanoma. Brit. J. Surg., *62:*840, 1975

HUGHES, M. *et al*: Skin-lined tube as a complication of tracheostomy. Arch. Otolaryng., *94:*568, 1971

HUGHES, R. G.: Injured face, PRS, *55:*375, 1975. Proc. Roy. Soc. Med., *67:*712, 1974

HUGO, N. E.: Vascular anastomoses *vs.* circulation across junction after transfer of pedicle. PRS, *50:*216, 1972

HUGO, N. E. *et al*: Effect of primary wounding on tensile strength of secondary wounds, PRS, *48:*203, 1971. Surg. Gynec. & Obst., *131:*516, 1970

HUGO, N. E. *et al*: Repair of unilateral cleft lip nasal deformities. Cleft Palate J., *8:*257, 1971

HUGO, N. E. *et al*: Management of tumors of parotid gland. Surg. Clin. North Am., *53:*105, 1973

HUGO, N. E., AND STONE, E.: Anatomy for blepharoplasty. PRS, *53:*387, 1974. Discussion by Castañares. PRS, *53:*587, 1974

HUGUES, A. *et al*: Technic of cheiloplasty for extensive lip cancers. Presse Med., *79:*1690, 1971

HUININK, S. A. *et al*: Patient with complications after treatment of malignant melanoma. Ned. tijdschr. geneeskd., *116:*2046, 1972 (Dutch)

HULA, M.: Clear cell melanoblastoma. Dermatologica, *146:*86, 1973

HULA, M. *et al*: Recurrence of melanoblastoma in the mouth. Cesk. Stomatol., *71:*332, 1971 (Czechoslovakian)

HULAGU, C., EREZ, S., AND OCAK, V.: Congenital mandibular myoblastoma, PRS, *56:*222, 1975. Internat. Surg., *60:*46, 1975

HULL, M. J. *et al*: Retrognathic mandible—surgical correction. Oral Surg., *41:*2, 1976

Human Bite Injuries: See *Bites and Stings*

HUMMEL, R. P. *et al*: Inhibition of *Candida albicans* by *Escherichia coli in vitro* and in germfree mouse, PRS, *54:*118, 1974. J. Surg. Res., *15:*53, 1973

HUMMEL, R. P. *et al*: Continuing problem of sepsis following enzymatic debridement of burns. J. Trauma, *14:*572, 1974

HUMPHREY, L. J.: Discussion of "Skin testing for prognosis of therapy formulation in cancer patients: *caveat emptor*," by Mandel. PRS, *57:*743, 1976

HUMPHREY, L. J. *et al*: Restoration of immunologic memory in tumor-bearing mouse. J. Surg. Oncol., *6:*219, 1974

HUMPHREYS, G. H.: Presentation of Academy plaque to Jerome P. Webster, M.D. Bull. NY. Acad. Med., *49:*954, 1973

HUMPHREYS, G. H., II *et al*: Operative correction of pectus excavatum. J. Pediatr. Surg., *9:*899, 1974

HUMPHRIES, S. V.: Hamilton Bailey's contributions to surgery. Int. Surg., *59:*203, 1974

HUNG, M. *et al*: Bone grafting in temporomandibular ankylosis – preliminary report, PRS, *55:*634, 1975. Chinese M.J., *10:*610, 1973

HUNT, J. L. *et al*: Burn wound management. Heart, Lung, *2:*690, 1973

HUNT, K. K., JR., AND COLE, R.: Cardiomegaly and pectus excavatum, PRS, *53:*604, 1974. Chest, *64:*511, 1973

HUNT, T. K.: Standards for wound healing research, PRS, *52:*216, 1973. Surgery, *73:*153, 1973

HUNT, T. K. *et al*: Effect of differing ambient oxygen tensions on wound infections, PRS, *56:*599, 1975. Ann. Surg., *181:*35, 1975

HUNTER, J. M.: Evaluation of oral trypsin-chymotrypsin for prevention of swelling after hand surgery (with Salisbury). PRS, *49:*171, 1972

HUNTER, J. M., AND SALISBURY, R. E.: Flexor tendon reconstruction in severely damaged hands, PRS, *50:*632, 1972. J. Bone & Joint Surg., *53:*829, 1971

HUNTER, J. M. *et al*: Dynamic approach to problems of hand function using local anesthesia supplemented by intravenous fentanyl-droperidol. Clin. Orthop., *104:*112, 1974

HUOT, L. A.: Biopsy of cervical swelling. Can. J. Otolaryngol., *1:*310, 1972 (French)

HURIEZ, C. *et al*: Use of labelled idoquine in diagnosis of nevocarcinoma. Bul. Soc. Fr. Dermatol.Syphiligr., *79:*159, 1972 (French)

HURIEZ, C. *et al*: Arterial ulcers. Phlebologie, *25:*357, 1972 (French)

HURLEY, J. D.: Surgery and chemotherapy in head and neck tumors (Follow-Up Clinic). PRS, *48:*587, 1971

HURST, L. N., LINDSAY, W. K., AND LEE, J.: Viability of skin grafts stored in various media, PRS, *52:*687, 1973. Canad. J. Surg., *16:*206, 1973

HURST, L. N., MCCAIN, W. G., AND LINDSAY, W. K.: Results of tenolysis, controlled evaluation in chickens. PRS, *52:*171, 1973

HURWITZ, A. M.: Facelift patients. A.N.A. Clin. Sess., p. 185, 1972

HURWITZ, A.: Enhancing symbol of beauty – serious business of cosmetic mammaplasty. Aust. Nurses J., *3:*13, 1974

HURWITZ, J. J. *et al*: Role of intubation macrodacryocystography in management of problems of lacrimal system. Can. J. Ophthalmol., *10:*361, 1975

HURWITZ, P. J. *et al*: Microsurgical techniques and use of tissue adhesive in repair of peripheral nerves, PRS, *55:*512, 1975. Surg. Res., *17:*245, 1974

HUSSELS, I. E.: Progressive lipodystrophy. Birth Defects, *7:*299, 1971

HUSSEY, D. H. *et al*: Combined hydroxyurea and radiotherapy: a new dosage schedule. South Med. J., *65:*137, 1972

HUSSEY, H. H.: Gynecomastia. JAMA, *228:*1423, 1974

HUTCHER, N., AND HAYNES, B. W., JR.: Evans formula revisited, PRS, *52:*101, 1973. J. Trauma, *12:*453, 1972

HUTER, J. *et al*: Experiences with plastic surgery of the female breast (augmentation, reduction, lifting. Arch. Gynaekol., *219:*155, 1975 (German)

HUTTER, R. V. P.: Discussion of "Subcutaneous mastectomy for central tumors of breast with immediate reconstruction," by Freeman. PRS, *51:*445, 1973

HUVOS, A., SHAH, J., AND GOLDSMITH, H.: Clinicopathologic study of amelanotic melanoma, PRS, *51:*707, 1973. Surg. Gynec. & Obst., *135:*917, 1972

HUVOS, A. G., LEAMING, R. H., AND MOORE, O. S.: Clinicopathologic study of resected carotid artery; analysis of 64 cases, PRS, *53:*488, 1974. Am. J. Surg., *126:*570, 1973

HUVOS, A., AND GRABSTALD, H.: Urethral meatal and parameatal tumors in young men, clinicopathologic and electron microscopic study, PRS, *54:*110, 1974. J. Urol., *110:*688, 1973

HUVOS, A. G. *et al*: Prognostic factors in cutaneous malignant melanoma. Comparative study of long-term and short-term survivors. Hum. Pathol., *5:*347, 1974

HY, N. G. *et al*: Superficial and deep lymphadenectomy in cancer of penis, PRS, *54:*110, 1974. Asian J. Med., *9:*397, 1973

HYAMS, J. L. *et al*: Spindle cell carcinoma of the larynx. Can. J. Otolaryngol., *4:*307, 1975

HYBASEK, I.: A case of congenital bilateral choanal atresia treated surgically using the transpalatinal approach. Cesk. Otolaryngol., *24:*51, 1975 (Czechoslovakian)

HYBASEK, I. *et al*: Picture of tracheotomy in children. Cesk. Otolaryngol., *24:*351, 1975 (Czechoslovakian)

HYLAND, W.: Technique for subcutaneous mastectomy and immediate reconstruction in ptotic breast (with Georgiade). PRS, *56:*121, 1975

HYMES, A. C., SAFAVIAN, M. H., AND GUNTHER, T.: Influence of industrial surfactant, pluronic F-68, in treatment of hemorrhagic shock, PRS, *48:*612, 1971. J. Surg. Res., *11:*191, 1971

HYNIE, J. *et al*: Transsexual female. Cesk. Psychiatr., *71:*48, 1975 (Czechoslovakian)

Hyperbaric Oxygen (See also *Burns; Skin Flaps*)

Hyperbaric oxygen, tham, and antibiotics, effect on experimental burns in rats. (Bleser, Sztuka, Muller), PRS, *50:*95, 1972. Europ. Surg. Res., *3:*409, 1971

Hyperbaric oxygen treatment of experimental frostbite in mouse (Hardenbergh), PRS, *51:*354, 1973. J. Surg. Res., *12:*34, 1972

Hyperbaric oxygen therapy in injured subjects (Szekely *et al*). Injury, *4:*294, 1973

Decompresion illness and air embolism treated with hyperbaric oxygen (Hart), PRS, *56:*366, 1975. Aerospace Med., *45:*1190, 1974

Oxygen, hyperbaric, age of red blood cells destroyed by *in vivo* hyperoxia (Carolla), PRS, *56:*107, 1975. Aerospace Med., *45:*1273, 1974

Oxygen, hyperbaric, influence of treatment on survival of skin flaps (Jurell, Kaijser), PRS, *54:*701, 1974. Scand. J. Plast. Reconstr. Surg., *7:*25, 1974

Oxygen therapy, hyperbaric, for pyoderma gangrenosum (Thomas *et al*), PRS, *57:*405, 1976. Arch. Dermat., *110:*445, 1975

Oxygen, hyperbaric, treatment of osteoradionecrosis of mandible with (Mainous, Heart), PRS, *57:*758, 1976. Arch. Otolaryng., *101:*173, 1975

Oxygen therapy, hyperbaric, in replantation of severed limbs (Shanghai Sixth People's Hospital), PRS, *57:*763, 1976. Chinese M. J., *1:*197, 1975

Blood flow during 2-Torr exposures at different decompression rates (Cooke, Olson), PRS, *57:*120, 1976. J. Applied Physiol., *38:*643, 1975

Hyperhidrosis

Axillary hyperhidrosis, simple surgery for (Weaver, Copeman), PRS, *48:*606, 1971. Proc. Roy. Soc. Med., *64:*607, 1971

Axillary hyperhidrosis, surgical treatment of (Guerrero-Santos *et al*), PRS, *49:*588, 1972. Rev. San. Guadalajara, *4:*49, 1971

Hyperhidrosis — Cont.

Hyperhidrosis, axillary, surgical treatment of case of (Van Oost). Arch. Belg. Dermatol. Syphiligr., *28:*421, 1972 (French)

Hyperhidrosis and its treatment by endoscopic-endotracheal sympathectomy (Flora, Schwamberger), PRS, *52:*206, 1973. Chir. Praxis, *16:*19, 1972

Hyperhidrosis of the upper extremity and its treatment (Hartfall *et al*). Surg. Gynec. & Obst., *135:*586, 1972

Sweat gland, radical ablation for axillary hyperhidrosis (Bretteville-Jensen), PRS, *55:*114, 1975. Brit. J. Plast. Surg., *26:*158, 1973

Upper thoracic sympathectomy for palmar hyperhidrosis (Walden *et al*). Harefuah, *85:*357, 1973 (Hebrew)

Hyperhidrosis, axillary, surgical management (Letterman *et al*). J. Am. Med. Wom. Assoc., *28:*581, 1973

Hyperhidrosis, axillary, radical sweat gland ablation for (Bretteville-Jensen), PRS, *55:*114, 1975. Brit. J. Plast. Surg., *26:*158, 1973

Hyperhidrosis of upper limbs, thoracoscopic sympathectomy in treatment of (Kux), PRS, *53:*369, 1974. Rev. Asoc. med. Minas Gerais, Brazil, *23:*119, 1973

Sweat responses of a hyperhidrotic subject (Allen *et al*). Brit. J. Dermatol., *90:*277, 1974

Hyperhidrosis, axillary. Its quantification and surgical treatment (Munro *et al*). Brit. J. Dermatol., *90:*325, 1974

Hyperhidrosis, serious complication of operation for (Shaw). Brit. J. Plast. Surg., *27:*196, 1974

Axillary hyperhidrosis, surgical management of (Crutcher, Moschella), PRS, *55:*248, 1975. Cutis, *14:*367, 1974

Electroencephalogram in hyperhidrosis palmo-plantaris (Shafrir *et al*). Harefuah, *86:*238, 1974 (Hebrew)

Hyperhidrosis, axillary, tissue shaving for (Inaba *et al*), PRS, *55:*388, 1975. Jap. J. Plast. Reconstr. Surg., *17:*300, 1974

Prescription for perspiration. Lancet, *2:*90, 1974

Letter: Treatment of excessive axillary sweating (Gibbs). Lancet, *2:*654, 1974

Excessive axillary sweating (Sewell). Tex. Med., *70:*67, 1974

Surgical treatment of axillary hyperhidrosis using the Skoog and Thyresson method (Kristensen). Ugeskr. Laeger, *136:*2869, 1974 (Danish)

Surgical treatment of axillary hyperhidrosis

Hyperhidrosis — Cont.

in 123 patients (Bretteville-Jensen *et al*). Acta Derm. Venereol. (Stockh.), *55:*73, 1975

Hyperhidrosis, topical methenamine therapy for (Cullen), PRS, *57:*543, 1976. Arch. Dermat., *111:*1158, 1975

Letter: axillary hₗperhidrosis (Andersen *et al*). JAMA, *231:*1026, 1975

Surgical treatment of axillary hyperhidrosis (Bueno *et al*). J. Tenn. Med. Assoc., *68:*544, 1975

Hyperhidrosis and its surgical management (Ellis), PRS, *57:*538, 1976. Postgrad. Med., *58:*191, 1975

Hyperhidrosis, abrasio axillae in (Jemec), PRS, *57:*402, 1976. Scand. J. Plast. Reconstr. Surg., *9:*44, 1975

Editorial: The treatment of axillary hyperhidrosis (Goldwyn). Arch. Surg., *111:*13, 1976

Hypertelorism (See also *Craniofacial Surgery*)

Pseudohypertelorism, traumatic: eyelash traction test to determine if medial canthal ligament is detached (Furnas, Bircoll). PRS, *52:*315, 1973

Hypertelorism, analysis of twenty cases (Psillakis, Pereira, Ishida), PRS, *52:*451, 1973. Rev. bras. clin. terap., *2:*55, 1973

Orbital hypertelorism. II. Definite treatment of orbital hypertelorism (OR.H.) by extracranial osteotomies (Tessier *et al*). Scand. J. Plast. Surg., *7:*39, 1973

Hypertelorism, ocular, and craniofacial stenosis, craniofacial surgery for (Converse). Trans. Am. Acad. Ophthalmol. Otolaryngol., *77:*1352, 1973

Cleft children, interocular distance before operation (Figalova, Hajnis, Smahel), PRS, *55:*638, 1975. Acta chir. plast., *16:*65, 1974

Orbital hypertelorism (Tessier). Fortschr. Kiefer. Gesichtschir., *18:*14, 1974

Hypertelorism, surgical correction of (Schlondorff). Laryngol. Rhinol. Otol. (Stuttg.), *53:*98, 1974 (German)

Hypertelorism (Van der Meulen). Ned. tijdschr. geneeskd., *118:*451, 1974 (Dutch)

Orbital hypertelorism, experiences in treatment of (Tessier). PRS, *53:*1, 1974

Craniofacial osteotomies and reconstructions in infants and young children (Edgerton, Jane, Berry). PRS, *54:*13, 1974

Cephalometric analysis in diagnosis and treatment planning of craniofacial dysostoses (Firmin, Coccaro, Converse). PRS, *54:*300, 1974

Surgical treatment of hypertelorism. II: Craniofacial osteotomy (Psillakis *et al*).

Hypertelorism — Cont.

Rev. Paul. Med., *83:*129, 1974 (Portuguese)

Surgical correction of hypertelorism (Schlondorff). Z. Laryngol. Rhinol. Otol., *53:*98, 1974 (German)

Hypertelorism, craniofacial surgery (Ortiz-Monasterio *et al*), PRS, *57:*116, 1976. Bol. Med. Hosp. Infant., *32:*587, 1975

Correction of ocular hypertelorism (Epstein *et al*). Childs Brain, *1:*228, 1975

Intraoperative care, anesthetic management of patients undergoing major facial osteotomies (Davies, Munro). PRS, *55:*50, 1975

Hypertelorism: report on 50 craniofacial operations (Converse, Wood-Smith, McCarthy). PRS, *55:*283, 1975

Hypertrophic Scar: See *Scars, Hypertrophic*

Hypoglossal Nerve

Long-standing facial paralysis rehabilitation (Conley *et al*). Laryngoscope, *84:*2155, 1974

Central functional changes after facial-spinal-accessory anastomosis in man and facial-hypoglossal anastomosis in the cat (Vera *et al*). J. Neurosurg., *43:*181, 1975

Hypospadias (See also *Genitalia; Penis, Urethra*

Hypospadias, report on 325 cases (Kyrtatas, Vogiatzis), PRS, *53:*488, 1974. Tr. 7th Panhellenic Cong. Surg. *B:*889, 1970

One-stage surgical correction of hypospadias (Dettmar). Urologe, *9:*131, 1970 (German)

Hypospadias retractor (d'Assumpcao). Brit. J. Plast. Surg., *24:*417, 1971

Hypospadias, treatment of: ten year follow-up study (Tamir *et al*). Harefuah, *81:*370, 1971 (Hebrew)

Foreskin tube in one-stage correction of penile hypospadias (Ascopa *et al*), PRS, *49:*104, 1972. Internat. Surg., *55:*435, 1971

Fistula, recurrent, of penile urethra, repair of (Malament), PRS, *50:*200, 1972. J. Urol., *106:*704, 1971

Belt technique of hypospadias repair (Fuqua), PRS, *50:*200, 1972. J. Urol., *106:*782, 1971

Hypospadias: experience with a new one-stage repair (Hodgson urethroplasty) (Engel *et al*). Md. State Med. J., *20:*45, 1971

Hypospadias treatment (Cendron), PRS, *48:*607, 1971. Proc. Roy. Soc. Med., *64:*125, 1971

Hypospadias, two-stage repair (Broadbent, Woolf), PRS, *50:*539, 1972. Rocky Mountain M.J., *68:*37, 1971

Urethroplasty in hypospadias (Shakir-Al-

Hypospadias – Cont.

iev). Urol. Nefrol. (Mosk.), *36:*47, 1971 (Russian)

Treatment of hypospadias (Sladczyk). Z. Urol. Nephrol., *64:*823, 1971 (German)

Hypospadias, urethral reconstruction by flap from preputium (Maris), PRS *52:*324, 1973. Acta chir. plast., *14:*120, 1972

Surgical treatment of hypospadias: experience in the treatment of 400 consecutive cases using Leveuf's technique (Farina). Brit. J. Plast. Surg., *25:*180, 1972

Hypospadias (Berner). Calif. Med., *116:*56, 1972

Our experience in treatment of hypospadias. Surgical technics. Apropos of 195 cases (Cahuzac *et al*). Chirurgie, *98:*143, 1972 (French)

Child with ambiguous genitalia (Hendren *et al*). Curr. Probl. Surg., *1:*64, 1972

Chordee, webbed penis without (Perlmutter, Chamberlain), PRS, *50:*632, 1972. J. Urol., *107:*320, 1972

Rectal flap urethroplasty (Thompson *et al*). J. Urol., *107:*667, 1972

Hypospadias with double urethra, interurethral fenestration for (Durrani, Shah, Kakalia), PRS, *52:*98, 1973. J. Urol., *108:*586, 1972

Hypospadias, advancement of retracted urethral meatus following Cecil urethroplasty (Kahn, Simon, Hoffman), PRS, *52:*98, 1973. J. Urol., *108:*808, 1972

Hypospadias, congenital chordee with and without, in three brothers (Koraitim), PRS, *52:*98, 1973. J. Urol., *108:*976, 1972

Hypospadias in childhood, surgical treatment (Andreev *et al*). Khirurgiia (Sofia), *25:*304, 1972 (Bulgarian)

Hypospadias, treatment of (Mishev, Gikov). Khirurgiia, Sofia, *25:*387, 1972 (Bulgarian)

Treatment of hypospadias (Dey). M. J. Australia, *1:*110, 1972

Penis tunnelization technique in secondary repair of hypospadias failures (Hinderer), PRS, *50:*13, 1972

Hypospadias: report on 193 treated cases (Sykes, Ho). PRS, *50:*452, 1972

Continuous subcutaneous sutures in surgical treatment of hypospadias (Gross). Pol. Przegl. Chir., *44:*111, 1972 (Polish)

Penis incurvatum sine hypospadias, congenital shortness of urethra (Almendral Lucas, Martin Laborda), PRS, *53:*244, 1974. Rev. españ. Chir. plast., *5:*201, 1972

Urology, pediatric (King *et al*). Surg. Annu., *4:*391, 1972

Hypospadias, surgical correction (Spence). Tex. Med., *68:*47, 1972

Hypospadias – Cont.

Correction of hypospadias in infants (Able). Tex. Med., *68:*97, 1972

On the necessity and possibility of unification in the treatment of hypospadias (Savchenko *et al*). Urol. Nefrol. (Mosk.), *37:*69, 1972 (Russian)

Plastic and Reconstructive Surgery of the Genital Area. Ed. by Charles E. Horton. Little, Brown & Co., Boston, 1973. PRS, *54:*601, 1974

Catheter, Foley, use in perineal urethrostomy (Elsahy), PRS, *53:*488, 1974. Acta chir. plast., *15:*131, 1973

Hypospadias, penile forms of, single-stage correction of chordee and urethral plasty in (Podluzhniy). Acta chir. plast. (Praha), *15:*190, 1973

Penoscrotal hypospadias, new one-stage technique for repair (Sung), PRS, *52:*681, 1973. Australasian Coll. Surg., *46:*386, 1973

Hypospadiacs, reconstruction of urethra in, with the prepuce lobe (Maris). Bratisl. Lek. Listy., *59:*63, 1973 (Slovakian)

Hypospadias, use of free skin graft in correction of severe forms of (Maris). Bratisl. Lek. Listy., *59:*306, 1973 (Slovakian)

Hypospadias de-epithelialized overflap technique in repair of (Smith), PRS, *55:*110, 1975. Brit. J. Plast. Surg., *2:*106, 1973

Crypto-hypospadias – review of 38 cases (Dickie *et al*). Brit. J. Plast. Surg., *26:*227, 1973

Hypospadias procedures, plastic and reconstructive (Bischoff), PRS, *53:*244, 1974. Chir. Praxis, *16:*575, 1972; Part 2, 17:73, 1973

Hypospadias: results with Hodgson urethroplasty (Engel, Scott), PRS, *52:*208, 1973. J. Urol., *109:*115, 1973

Fistulas, congenital urethral perineal (Gehring, Vitenson, Woodhead), PRS, *53:*245, 1974. J. Urol., *109:*419, 1973

Hypospadias, penile, surgical correction by modification of Spence's hood (Hoffman, Hall), PRS, *53:*107, 1974. J. Urol., *109:*1017, 1973

Preputial blood supply, technique to preserve (Redman), PRS, *53:*110, 1974. J. Urol., *109:*1019, 1973

Hypospadias, dorsal tilt: embellishment to any operation for (Lattimer, Vakili, Smith), PRS, *53:*245, 1974. J. Urol., *109:*1035, 1973

Sex determination and its surgical correction in certain abnormalities of urogenital system in children (Kushch). Klin. Khir., *8:*39, 1973 (Russian)

Hypospadias – Cont.

Hypospadias repair by four layer sutures (Shishito, Shirai), PRS, *53:*368, 1974. Operation, *27:*559, 1973

Hypospadias: studies of urethral healing in dogs (Everingham, Horton, Devine), PRS, *51:*312, 1973

Hermaphroditism: management of intersexual anomalies (Theogaraj), PRS, *51:*632, 1973

Chordee: plication of the *tunica albuginea* to straighten the curved penis (Horton, Devine), PRS, *52:*32, 1973

Hypospadias, treatment of by Byars technique (Nosti, Davis), PRS, *52:*128, 1973

Hypospadias repair – elimination of fistulae (Smith), PRS, *52:*681, 1973. Proc. Roy. Australasian Coll. Surg., *46:*370, 1973

Hypospadias, penoscrotal, new one-stage technique for repair (Sung), PRS, *52:*681, 1973. Proc. Roy. Australasian Coll. Surg., *46:*386, 1973

Hypospadias treatment, our experience in (Ubiglia, Santoni Rugiu, Massei), PRS, *56:*358, 1975. Riv. ital. chir. plast., *5:*527, 1973

Hypospadias, high, in children, restoration of missing portion of urethra in, using modified Duplay method (Gorshkov). Urol. Nefrol. (Mosk.), *38:*52, 1973 (Russian)

Hypospadias, direct results of treatment (Krasulin *et al*). Urol. Nefrol. (Mosk.), *38:*57, 1973 (Russian)

Hypospadias repair with histoacrylic tissue adhesive and without indwelling catheter drainage (Vahlensieck). Urol. Res., *1:*2, 1973

Sex determination, tactics in, in children with anomalies in development of genital organs (Kushch *et al*). Vestn. Khir., *111:*80, 1973 (Russian)

Hypospadias, combined one stage urethroplasty for (Nwako), PRS, *55:*638, 1975. J. Pediat. Surg., *4:*467, 1974

Diaphragmatic hernia, three legs, two penises, and imperforate anus: complete salvage problem in newborn (Schwartz *et al*). J. Pediatr. Surg., *9:*525, 1974

Catheterization, intermittent, urologist's point of view (Perkash), PRS, *54:*504, 1974. J. Urol., *111:*356, 1974

Closure of fistula at penoscrotal junction of urethra (Kishev). J. Urol., *111:*774, 1974

Hypospadias, balanitic, correction, new surgical technique for (Gil-Vernet *et al*). J. Urol., *112:* 673, 1974

Hypospadias repair, one-stage (Hopkins, Campbell), PRS, *57:*536, 1976. J. Urol., *112:*674, 1974)

Hypospadias – Cont.

Hypospadias repair, one-stage, further experience with (Sadlowski *et al*). J. Urol., *112:*677, 1974

Hypospadias, treatment of, our experience in (Minkov *et al*). Khirurgiia (Sofiia), *27:*128, 1974 (Bulgarian)

Long-term results following operation for hypospadias (Helmig). Klin. Paediatr., *186:*421, 1974 (German)

Letter: testosterone cream: use or abuse? (Darby *et al*). Lancet, *2:*598, 1974

Hypospadias treatment (Mollard, Perrin), PRS, *56:*680, 1975. Lyon chir., *70:*402, 1974

Hypospadias incidence in Minnesota, etiologic factors (Sweet *et al*), PRS, *54:*238, 1974. Mayo Clin. Proc. Staff Meet., *49:*52, 1974

Hypospadias, plastic repair of (Caucci). Minerva Pediatr., *26:*1525, 1974 (Italian)

Hypospadias, therapy and prognosis of? (Letter) (Flach). Munch. Med. Wochenschr., *116:*1523, 1974 (German)

Hypospadias, critical assessment of management (Dickie, Williams), PRS, *54:*579, 1974

Neoplasty of female urethra (Sebek). Rozhl. Chir., *53:*47, 1974 (Czechoslovakian)

Cutaneous chordee, fact or fancy (Wettlauger). Urology, *4:*293, 1974

Surgical dressing for hypospadias repair (Redman *et al*). Urology, *4:*739, 1974

Hypospadias, surgical repair for. Urethroplasty by quadruple layer sutures (Shishito *et al*). Urol. Int. *29:*382, 1974

Treatment of hypospadias with a modification of the Duplay method (Bogdanova). Vestn. Khir., *112:*74, 1974 (Russian)

Complications in phallo- and urethroplasty (Mendel). Vestn. Khir., *113:*124, 1974 (Russian)

Value of supplementary measures for improvement of results in the hypospadias surgery (Wehnert *et al*). Z. Urol. Nephrol., *67:*595, 1974 (German)

Current problems in children's urology (Ecke). Z. Urol. Nephrol., *67:*623, 1974 (German)

Hypospadias, combination of plastic operations by Meyer-Burgdorff and Chocholka methods in one-stage surgical treatment (Wendt). Z. Urol. Nephrol., *67:*861, 1974 (German)

Hypospadias, mathematical planning for plastic surgery in (Murvanidze, Kocharova), PRS, *57:*761, 1976. Acta chir. plast., *17:*20, 1975

Silicone rubber casts of the distal urethra in studying fistula formation and other hypospadias problems (Townsend). Brit. J.

Hypospadias — Cont.

Plast. Surg., *28:*320, 1975

A long-term follow-up of hypospadias patients (Sommerlad). Brit. J. Plast. Surg., *28:*324, 1975

Surgical treatment of hypospadias and epispadias (Albrecht *et al*). Chirurg., *46:*503, 1975

Hypospadias: a general review (Keeton *et al*). J. Miss. State Med. Assoc., *16:*340, 1975

Fistula, congenital urethral, with chordee (Goldstein), PRS, *57:*761, 1976. J. Urol., *113:*138, 1975

Meatal advancement for distal hypospadias without chordee (Perlmutter *et al*). J. Urol., *113:*850, 1975

Distal hypospadias, chordee and torsion: the Allen-Spence procedure and new modifications (Klauber). J. Urol., *114:*765, 1975

Surgery of hypospadias (Buschmann). Langenbecks Arch. Chir., *339:*417, 1975 (German)

Hypospadias, timing of elective surgery (Kelalis *et al*), PRS, *57:*400, 1976. Pediatrics, *56:*479, 1975

Foley catheter modified for use in perineal urethrostomy (Tolhurst), PRS, *55:*503, 1975

Dehiscence, wound, secondary closure of penile skin incisions (Horton, Devine), PRS, *55:*630, 1975

Hypospadias: congenital transposition of scrotum and penis (Griffin, Hayes), PRS, *55:*710, 1975

The incidence of hypospadias in Sweden (Avellan). Scand. J. Plast. Reconstr. Surg., *9:*129, 1975

Indication, techniques and results of the operative correction of hypospadias using modification of the original Denis Browne technique (Marberger *et al*). Urologe. (A)., *14:*117, 1975 (German)

XX-male-syndrome. Pathogenesis and aspects of diagnostic pitfalls (Rehder *et al*). Urologe. (A)., *14:*182, 1975 (German)

Perineal corporeal compression: technique to evaluate chordee (Redman *et al*). Urology, *5:*351, 1975

Hypospadias, one-stage repair (Reddy). Urology, *5:*475, 1975

Urethroplasty, Devine inlay graft, experiences with (McKinney *et al*). Urology, *5:*487, 1975

Penis erection in hypospadias (Esch). Z. Urol. Nephrol., *68:*575, 1975 (German)

Treatment of hypospadias (Schubert *et al*). Z. Urol. Nephrol., *68:*579, 1975 (German)

Late changes in urethras after perineal diversion in childhood (Hormann *et al*). Z.

Hypospadias — Cont.

Urol. Nephrol., *68:*585, 1975 (German)

Rotation plasty in the surgical treatment of acquired penile urethral fistulas and abnormalities (Wandschneider). Z. Urol. Nephrol., *68:*727, 1975 (German)

Hypospadias, correlation with other congenital anomalies (Wehnert), PRS, *56:*466, 1975. Ztschr. Urol., *67:*857, 1975

Hypotelorism

Hypotelorism, orbital (Converse, McCarthy, Wood-Smith). PRS, *56:*389, 1975

I

IAKOVLEVA, I. A. *et al*: Angiofollicular hyperplasia lymph nodes. Vopr. Onkol., *19:*18, 1973 (Russian)

IAKUSHEV, S. I.: Active surgical treatment of burns. Ortop. Travmatol. Protez., *34:*51, 1973 (Russian)

IANNACCONE, P. R.: Multiple primary tumors. Four distinct head and neck tumors. Arch. Pathol., *99:*270, 1975

IARCHUK, N. I.: Restoration of pinna in congenital microtia. Zh. Ushn. Nos. Gorl. Belezn., *33:*46, 1973 (Russian)

IARCHUK, N. I.: Reconstruction of soft tissues of the nasal dorsum. Vestn. Khir., *113:*80, 1974 (Russian)

IBARRA-PEREZ, C. *et al*: Critical considerations on tracheotomy. Prensa Med. Mex., *36:*465, 1971 (Spanish)

ICHIKAWA, R.: Electronic artificial limbs. Surg. Ther. (Osaka), *24:*40, 1971 (Japanese)

IDE, A. *et al*: Plastic surgery of eyelid cancer. Ophthalmology (Tokyo), *13:*865, 1971 (Japanese)

IDE, A. *et al*: Problems concerning blow-out fractures in ophthalmology — with special reference to their etiology and classification. Ophthalmology (Tokyo), *14:*167, 1972 (Japanese)

IGARI, T. *et al*: Repair of facial trauma. Shujutsu, *25:*1181, 1971

IGEL, H. J. *et al*: New method for covering large surface area wounds with autografts. II. Surgical application of tissue culture expanded rabbit-skin autografts, PRS, *55:*114, 1975. Arch. Surg., *108:*724, 1974

IGLESIAS CENDON, J.: E.N.T. changes of atrophic polychondritis: report of a case. Acta Otolaryngol. Iber. Am., *22:*351, 1971 (Spanish)

IGNATOFF, J. M. *et al*: Incomplete exstrophy of bladder, PRS, *48:*514, 1971. J. Urol., *105:*579, 1971

IINO, R. *et al*: Functional prognosis of contusion of the dorsal region of the hand. Orthop. Surg. (Tokyo), *22:*890, 1971 (Japanese)

IKUTA, Y.: Improved instrument for small vessel anastomosis, PRS, *56:*358, 1975. Operation, *28:*1149, 1974

IKUTA, Y.: Autotransplant of omentum to cover large denudation of scalp. PRS, *55:*490, 1975

IKUTA, Y.: New technique for nerve suture, epineurium-anchoring funicular suture (with Tsuge, Sakaue). PRS, *56:*496, 1975

IKUTA, Y.: Scanning electron microscope study of microvascular anastomoses (with Servant, Harada). PRS, *57:*329, 1976

IKUTA, Y.: Free muscle transplantation in dogs by microneurovascular anastomoses (with Kubo, Tsuge). PRS, *57:*495, 1976

ILES, P. B. *et al*: Tuberculous lymphadenitis. Brit. Med. J., *1:*143, 1974

ILIADES, C. E. *et al*: Neurilemmoma of the pharynx. Laryngoscope, *82:*430, 1972

ILIFF, W., MARBACK, R., AND GREEN, R.: Invasive squamous cell carcinoma of conjunctiva, PRS, *56:*235, 1975. Arch. Ophth., *93:*119, 1975

ILLINGWORTH, C. M.: Trapped fingers and amputated fingertips in children, PRS, *56:*366, 1975. J. Pediat. Surg., *9:*853, 1974

IM, J. J. C., HOOPES, J. E., AND SOHN, Y. T.: Enzyme activities in regenerating epithelium during wound healing. I. Acid phosphatase, PRS, *52:*103, 1973; II. β-glucuronidase, *52:*104, 1973; III. β-galactosidase and β-glucosidase, *52:*104, 1973. J. Surg. Res., *12:*402, 406, 1972. IV. Amino transferases and NADP-dependent enzymes, PRS, *53:*611, 1974. J. Surg. Res., *15:*262, 1973

IM, M. J. C., MULLIKEN, J. B., AND HOOPES, J. E.: Effects of intralesional injection of triamcinolone on glucose-6-phosphate dehydrogenase and alanine aminotransferase activity in keloids. PRS, *56:*660, 1975

IMAGAWA, I.: Mechanism of recurrence of pigmented nevi following dermabrasion. Jap. J. Dermatol. (A)., *84:*273, 1974 (Japanese)

IMAI, M. *et al*: Experimental study of autologous transplantations of the skin to the oral mucosa. J. Otolaryngol. Jap., *74:*382, 1971 (Japanese)

IMAIZUMI, K. *et al*: Pedicled skin grafts for eyelid cancer. Ophthalmology (Tokyo), *14:*181, 1972 (Japanese)

IMAMALIEV, A. S., AND GASHIMOV, R. R.: Biological properties of bone tissue conserved in plastic material and sterilized with gamma rays, PRS, *55:*643, 1975. Acta chir. plast., *16:*129, 1974

IMAZATO, Y. *et al*: Case of normal speech recovery after pharyngeal flap operation. Jap. J.

Oral Surg., *19:*166, 1973 (Japanese)

IMBER, G., AND WILCOX, R. S.: Michel skin clips for rapid fixation of split-skin grafts to sharp edges of deep defects. PRS, *50:*534, 1972

IMBER, G. *et al*: Fibrous capsule formation after subcutaneous implantation of synthetic materials in experimental animals. PRS, *54:*183, 1974

IMMERGUT, M. *et al*: The local application of testosterone cream to prepubertal phallus, PRS, *49:*585, 1972. J. Urol., *105:*905, 1971

IMMERTREU, W.: Experiences with vestibuloplasty and plastic surgery on floor of mouth in edentulous mandibles. Quintessenz, *23:*15, 1972 (German)

IMMERTREU, W.: Reconstruction of floor of mouth and vestibule of edentulous mandible. Quintessence Int., *4:*9, 1973

Implantation Cysts (See also *Dermoid Cysts; Sebaceous Cysts*)

Epithelial implantation cysts, intra- and extraocular, deep lamellar resection of (Sugar). Am. J. Ophth., *76:*451, 1973

Epithelial regeneration in heterotopic connective tissue transplantations, experimental studies on (Plagmann *et al*). Dtsch. Zahnaerztl. Z., *29:*497, 1974 (German)

Implants (See also *anatomical area; Mammaplasty; Prostheses; Hands, Rheumatoid Disease of; Penis; Silicones; Devices, Medical; etc.*)

"Plastic" materials implantable in surgery (Lemaire *et al*). Acta Chir. Belg., *70:*156, 1971 (French)

Tolerance to synthetic material in plastic surgery (Lejour *et al*). Acta Chir. Belg., *70:*245, 1971 (French)

Granulation tissue formation in subcutaneously implanted cellulose sponges in young and old rats (Holm-Pedersen, Zederfeldt), PRS, *48:*610, 1971. Scand. J. Plast. Reconstr. Surg., *5:*13, 1971

Synthetic plastics, long-term reaction to (Rubin, Bromberg, Walden), PRS, *49:*110, 1972. Surg. Gynec. & Obst., *132:*603, 1971

Cryo-sterilization of plastic implants (Arit *et al*). Zentralbl. Chir., *96:*1131, 1971 (German)

Artificial Organs and Cardiopulmonary Support Systems. Ed. by Felix T. Rapaport and John P. Merrill. Grune & Stratton, New York, 1972. PRS, *51:*85, 1973

Plastic Materials in Surgery, Second Edition. By Bernard Bloch and Garth W. Hastings. Charles C Thomas, Springfield, Ill., 1972. PRS, *52:*83, 1973

Foreign bodies, metallic, electronic ausculta-

Implants — Cont.

tion of (Waller), PRS, *51:*610, 1973. Am. J. Surg., *123:*626, 1972

Nasal implants, fate of Silastic and vitrathene (Milward), PRS, *52:*217, 1973. Brit. J. Plast. Surg., *25:*276, 1972

Ureter, human, substitution of synthetic material (Wagenknect, Anvert), PRS, *51:*106, 1973. Chirurg, *43:*334, 1972

Symetroplast and its use in face and neck surgery (Roggendorf). Dtsch. Stomatol., *22:*845, 1972 (German)

Plastics, long-term effects of (Editorial). Food, Cosmet. Toxicol., *10:*567, 1972

Implants, acrylic, for frontal bone defects (Blatt, Failla), PRS, *50:*543, 1972. Mil. Med., *137:*22, 1972

Implants, alloplastic (Dickinson *et al*). Otolaryngol. Clin. North Am., *5:*481, 1972

Teflon string, treatment of cryptotia using (Ohmori, Matsumoto). PRS, *49:*33, 1972

Implants, Silastic breast, experiences with large series (Williams). PRS, *49:*253, 1972

Silastic ear implants, our experiences with (Lynch *et al*). PRS, *49:*283, 1972

Flexible Implant Resection Arthroplasty in the Hand and Extremities. By Alfred B. Swanson. C. V. Mosby Co., St. Louis, 1973. PRS, *54:*350, 1974

Implants in Surgery. By D. F. Williams and Robert Roaf. W. B. Saunders Co., London, Philadelphia, Toronto, 1973. PRS, *54:*480, 1974

Polymers, tissue reaction after implantation in thymectomized and non-thymectomized rats (Velikov, Papurov, Markov), PRS, *53:*614, 1974. Acta chir. plast., *15:*29, 1973

Transplantation of heterologous cartilage stored frozen and in 70° alcohol (Pankin, Chirkova), PRS, *54:*510, 1974. Acta chir. plast., *15:*155, 1973

Fibrin foam as filling material for defects in surgery of salivary gland. Animal experiments and clinical results (Jung *et al*). Arch. Klin. Exp. Ohren Nasen Kehlkopfheilkd., *204:*105, 1973 (German)

Implants, secondary intraorbital, insertion of (Soll). Arch. Ophth., *89:*214, 1973

Implants, plastic chin, avoiding bone resorption under (Parker), PRS, *53:*250, 1974. Arch. Otolaryng., *98:*100, 1973

Mesh, Dacron, used in original plastic procedure for inguinal hernia (Stoppa *et al*), PRS, *52:*463, 1973. Chirurgie, *99:*119, 1973

Implants, tooth, self supportive polymer (Hodosh, Povar, Shklar), PRS, *53:*372, 1974. J. Biomed. Mater. Res., *7:*205, 1973

Implants, poly (methyl methacrylate), experimental use of, in mandibular defects

Implants — Cont.

(Worley). J. Oral Surg., *31:*170, 1973

Impotence, erectile, penile implant for (Morales *et al*), PRS, *52:*596, 1973. J. Urol., *109:*641, 1973

Implants, synthetic, plastic surgery application of (Gerow *et al*). Med. Instrum., *7:*96, 1973

Implants, personally fabricated chin (Carlin). PRS, *51:*121, 1973

Implants, alloplastic, effect on bone (Jobe, Iverson, Vistnes); PRS, *51:*169, 1973. Discussions by Rees, Spira, PRS, *51:*174, 1973

Silicone bag, soft, for antral inflation (Bull). PRS, *51:*223, 1973

Retropharyngeal implantation of silicone gel pillows for velopharyngeal incompetence (Brauer). PRS, *51:*254, 1973

Prostheses: use of silicones in plastic surgery, retrospective view (Braley). PRS, *51:*280, 1973

Implants, compound silicone-bone, for mandibular reconstruction (Swanson *et al*). PRS, *51:*402, 1973

Implants, breast, silicone-gel, treatment of bilateral breast carcinomas in patient with (Benavent). PRS, *51:*588, 1973

Implants, silicone, fate of pseudosheath pocket around (Thomson). PRS, *51:*667, 1973

Mammaplasty, augmentation, current status of (Grossman). PRS, *52:*1, 1973

Buttock: gluteal augmentation (Cocke, Ricketson). PRS, *52:*93, 1973

Pacemaker, covering exposed (Furman) (Letter to the Editor). PRS, *52:*181, 1973

Kiel-bone implants to chin and nose (Penn) (Follow-Up Clinic). PRS, *52:*432, 1973

Transplants, bone, conserved in plastic material and sterilized with gamma rays (Imamaliev, Gashimov), PRS, *55:*643, 1975. Acta chir. plast., *16:*129, 1974

Transplants, homologous bone tissue, reaction of hemapoietic system to (Bruskina), PRS, *55:*643, 1975. Acta chir. plast., *16:*141, 1974

Implants, Swanson's Silastic, in hand traumatology (Michon, Delagoutte, Jandeaux), PRS, *54:*627, 1974. Ann. chir. plast., *19:*23, 1974

Synthetic preparations, experiments for developing a fibroblastic endothelium on (Götz *et al*), PRS, *54:*247, 1974. Bruns' Beitr. klin. Chir., *221:*142, 1974

Metacarpal heads, destroyed, new silicone implant to replace (Kessler), PRS, *56:*227, 1975. Hand, *6:*308, 1974

Implantable human parts, spare parts catalog — illustrated guide to rebuilding man,

Implants – Cont.

PRS, *55:*386, 1975. Modern Med., *42:*41, 1974

Implant, breast, new soft round silicone gel (Weiner, Aiache, Silver). PRS, *53:*174, 1974

Implants, new inflatable, for breast augmentation (Wise). PRS, *53:*360, 1974

Prosthesis, breast, planning augmentation mammaplasty (Snyder). PRS, *54:*132, 1974

Capsule, fibrous, formation after subcutaneous implantation of synthetic materials in experimental animals (Imber *et al*). PRS, *54:*183, 1974

Implants, inflatable breast (Rees, Guy, Coburn), PRS, *52:*609, 1973. Addendum, PRS, *54:*213, 1974

Mammaplasty, augmentation, with two different kinds of prostheses in same woman (Barney). PRS, *54:*265, 1974

Implantation of Dacron felt in bones of rabbits (Crouse, Campo, Kodsi). PRS, *54:*471, 1974

Complication after alloplastic thigh augmentation (Codega *et al*). Polim. Med., *4:*153, 1974

Calcification of implants, effect of structure of poly (glycolmethacrylate) gel on (Kopecek, Sppincl), PRS, *56:*365, 1975. Polymers in Med., *4:*129, 1974

Implants, silicone chin, for chin augmentation (Wray, Moore, Weeks), PRS, *54:*510, 1974. South. M.J., *67:*456, 1974

Tissue, connective, morphology in response to implanted silicone rubber (Hernandez-Jauregui, Esperanza-Garcia, Gonzalez-Angulo), PRS, *54:*510, 1974. Surgery, *75:*631, 1974

Transplants, free periosteal to reconstruct trachea (Kugan, Pasila), PRS, *55:*718, 1975. Ztschr. Kinderchir., *15:*371, 1974

Foreign body tumorigenesis, etiological factors, stages, and role of foreign body in (Brand *et al*), PRS, *56:*111, 1975. Cancer Res., *35:*279, 1975

Bone, incorporation of stainless steel, titanium, and Vitallium in (Linder, Lundskog), PRS, *57:*266, 1976. Injury, *6:*277, 1975

Corrosion of metallic orthopedic implants (Cahoon *et al*), PRS, *57:*266, 1976. J. Biomed. Mater. Res., 9:259, 1975

Dental facial reconstruction, Proplast in (Kent *et al*), PRS, *56:*601, 1975. J. Oral Surg., *39:*347, 1975

Infection: current use of prophylactic antibiotics in plastic and reconstructive surgery (Krizek, Koss, Robson). PRS, *55:*21, 1975

Implants – Cont.

Prosthesis, breast, used intracranially to temporarily stabilize reduction cranioplasty (Thomson, Hoffman). PRS, *55:*704, 1975

Implant, breast, exposed, treatment of by reimplantation behind posterior wall of capsule (Snyder). PRS, *5:*97, 1975

Implants, malar, for improvement of facial appearance (Hinderer). PRS, *56:*157, 1975

Implants, silicone, effect of hematoma on thickness of pseudosheaths around (Williams, Aston, Rees). PRS, *56:*194, 1975

Thoracic wall, repair of concavity of, with silicone elastomer implant (Baker, Mara, Douglas). PRS, *56:*212, 1975

Granuloma, foreign body reactions to polyurethane covers of some breast prostheses (Cocke, Leathers, Lynch), PRS, *56:*527, 1975

Implants, method of osteo-cranioplasty with Silastic (Fontana), PRS, *57:*767, 1976. (Italian) Riv. ital. chir. plast., 7:539, 1975

Implants, silicone breast, long-term study of reactions in rabbits (Lilla, Vistnes), PRS, *57:*637, 1976

IMRE, K.: Presence of foreign body in hand and foot, diagnosed too late. Magy. Traumatol. Orthop., *18:*277, 1975 (Hungarian)

INABA, M. *et al*: Subcutaneous tissue shaving method on osmidrosis axillae, PRS, *55:*388, 1975. Jap. J. Plast. Reconstr. Surg., *17:*300, 1974

INALSINGH, C. H.: Experience in treating 501 patients with keloids. Johns Hopkins Med. J., *134:*284, 1974

INDRESANO, A. T.: Simplified technique for wiring the condyloid process after intraoral vertical subcondylar osteotomy. J. Oral Surg., *33:*384, 1975

INGLIS, A. E. *et al*: Reconstruction of metacarpophalangeal joint of thumb in rheumatoid arthritis, PRS, *51:*105, 1973. J. Bone & Joint Surg., *54A:*704, 1972

INGLIS, F. G. *et al*: Subcutaneous mastectomy and immediate prosthetic implantation as alternative to simple mastectomy. Can. J. Surg., *17:*63, 1974

INNOCENZI, A. *et al*: Thoraco-brachial transposition of the greater omentum as a new surgical method in the treatment of postoperative lymphedema. Minerva Chir., *26:*947, 1971 (Italian)

INOUE, H. *et al*: Ulnar nerve paralysis of the carpal tunnel due to traumatic aneurysm of the ulnar artery. Orthop. Surg. (Tokyo), *22:*924, 1971 (Japanese)

INOUE, S. *et al*: Treatment of chronic rheumatoid arthritis. 10. Reconstruction of the hands in chronic rheumatoid arthritis. Ryumachi, *13*:390, 1973 (Japanese)

INOUE, T., SHIGEMATSU, Y., AND SATO, T.: Treatment of carcinoma of hypopharynx, PRS, *52*:460, 1973. Cancer, *31*:649, 1973

Instruments (See also *Devices, Medical*)

Cryo-bistoury and the electric bistoury in plastic surgery (Dogo). Cancro, *24*:337, 1971 (Italian)

Fiber optic bundles in plastic surgery, use of (Grazer). PRS, *48*:28, 1971

Skin cleansing fluids for use with drum-type dermatomes (Hawtof) (Letter to the Editor). PRS, *48*:171, 1971

Fiber-optic retractors for use in plastic surgery (Rosenberg). PRS, *48*:286, 1971

Dermabrader, simple and inexpensive (Rapperport). PRS, *48*:386, 1971

Forceps, bipolar, new, for electrocoagulation (Rosenberg). PRS, *48*:390, 1971

Retractor, self-retaining, for buccal commissure (Giles). PRS, *49*:230, 1972

Fiber-optic nasal septal retractors (Rosenberg). PRS, *49*:468, 1972

Wiring aid and intraoral elastic applicator, new (Marshall). PRS, *49*:579, 1972

Skin carrier for Padgett mesh dermatome (Doffing, Nelson, Kendall). PRS, *50*:299, 1972

Endotracheal tube holder and bite block (Randall, Padgett). PRS, *50*:412, 1972

Scalpels, on use of razor blade fragments as (Courtiss) (Letter to the Editor). PRS, *50*:608, 1972

Wire twister forceps, new (Natvig). PRS, *50*:626, 1972

Surgical instruments and operating room time, conserving (Johnson). PRS, *51*:96, 1973

Clamp, adjustable double, for use in microvascular surgery (Zirkle, Seidensricker). PRS, *51*:340, 1973

Dermatome, Padgett, effective safety devices for (Brent). PRS, *51*:467, 1973

Retractor, simple, for use in rhytidoplasties (Fuente-del-Campo, Barrera, Ortiz-Monasterio). PRS, *51*:696, 1973

Magnetic surgical instrument stand (Brent). PRS, *52*:318, 1973

Dermo-Jet, intralesional injection of keloids and hypertrophic scars with the (Vallis) (Follow-Up Clinic). PRS, *52*:434, 1973

Dermatome, drum, use of in reduction mammaplasty (De Wet). PRS, *52*:448, 1973

Mustarde suturing forceps (Carroll *et al*). Am. J. Ophth., *78*:860, 1974

New face lift scissors (Hartley). Brit. J.

Instruments – Cont.

Plast. Surg., *27*:365, 1974

Diathermy, bipolar (Robinson, Davies), PRS, *56*:116, 1975. Canad. J. Surg., *17*:287, 1974

Diamond knife for microsurgical repair of peripheral nerves (Terzis, Faibisoff, Williams). PRS, *53*:102, 1974

Disimpacting device for chisels, simple (Ortiz-Monasterio, Jaime). PRS, *53*:233, 1974

Steroids, injecting into scars, screw syringe for (Penoff). PRS, *53*:484, 1974

Retractors, self-retaining, for hand surgery (Tegtmeier). PRS, *53*:485, 1974

Doppler flowmeter to monitor peripheral bloodflow during edema stage of snakebite (Gurucharri, Henzel, Mitchell). PRS, *53*:551, 1974

Forceps, bipolar, new, fingertip-controlled, for electrocoagulation (Rosenberg). PRS, *54*:228, 1974

Tongue blade, reinforced, for Dingman mouth gag (Zook). PRS, *54*:682, 1974

Doppler flowmeter to detect small vessels for microsurgery (Aoyagi, Fujino, Ohshiro). PRS, *55*:372, 1975

Fiberoptic endoscopy in the head and neck region (Dellon, Hall, Chretien). PRS, *55*:466, 1975

Plasma scalpel excision of burns (Link, Zook, Glover). PRS, *55*:657, 1975

Doppler probe used for free transfer of groin flaps (Karkowski, Buncke), PRS, *55*:682, 1975. Discussion by Bingham. PRS, *56*:84, 1975

Bonney's blue marking ink (Johnson). PRS, *56*:155, 1975

Microirrigator (Rigg). PRS, *56*:349, 1975

Irrigation, automatic, bipolar jeweler's forceps, for coagulation in microsurgery (Dujovny, Vas, Osgood). PRS, *56*:585, 1975

Clamp, Babcock, for intraoperative reduction of phalangeal fractures (McMaster). PRS, *56*:671, 1975

Operatory unit, plastic surgery (Dingman, Pickens). PRS, *56*:673, 1975

Retractor, Caldwell Luc self-retaining (McCabe). Trans. Am. Acad. Ophthalmol. Otolaryngol., *80*:257, 1975

Dissector for transaxillary approach in augmentation mammaplasty (Agris, Dingman, Wilensky). PRS, *57*:10, 1976

Drill for use in an inaccessible place (Greer, Dixon). PRS, *57*:103, 1976

Doppler ultrasound detection of displaced neurovascular bundles in Dupuytren's contracture (Elsahy). PRS, *57*:104, 1976

Suction obturator, new, to control saliva after laryngopharyngectomy (Javor). PRS, *57*:106, 1976

Instruments — Cont.

Headlight, improved quartz-halogen (Kaye). PRS, *57:*110, 1976

Expansion of split-skin grafts, simple apparatus for (D'Hooghe). PRS, *57:*387,1976

Hand table, inexpensive (MacDonald). PRS, *57:*392, 1976

Compression clamps, pericortical, for mandibular fixation (Lung, Graham, Miller). PRS, *57:*487, 1976

Microirrigator (Freshwater) (Letter to the Editor). PRS, *57:*508, 1976

Retractor for use in breast augmentation (Fischl). PRS, *57:*526, 1976

Dermatome tape, reuse of (Fujino) (Letter to the Editor). PRS, *57:*738, 1976

INTERLANDI, G.: Surgical technic for treatment of pendulous abdomen complicated by suprapubic eventration. Minerva Chir., *29:*208, 1974 (Italian)

International Congresses of Plastic Surgery

International Congress of Plastic and Reconstructive Surgery, Sixth, PRS, *49:*672, 1972; *54:*122, 1974; *55:*650, 1975; *57:*411, 1976

Current trends observed at the International Confederation of Plastic and Reconstructive Surgery (Omori). Jap. J. Plast. Reconstr. Surg., *15:*24, 1972 (Japanese)

INTONTI, F. *et al:* Surgical treatment of pectus excavatum. Hemodynamic and functional findings and long-term results in 18 patients. Minerva Chir., *28:*1347, 1973 (Italian)

IOFFE, L. S.: Preoperative modeling of implant in plastic surgery using polymer mesh materials. Klin. Khir., *1:*56, 1974 (Russian)

IOFFE, N. S.: Retractor for tracheotomy. Zh. Ushn. Nos. Gorl. Bolezn., *3:*107, 1974 (Russian)

IONESCO, A. *et al:* Considerations on surgical treatment of deep burns (4th degree). Panminerva Med., *14:*237, 1972

IONESCO, R. *et al:* Two cases of late decompression in so-called frozen face paralysis. Rev. Laryngol. Otol. Rhinol. (Bord.), *95:*775, 1974 (French)

IONESCU, A. *et al:* Injuries with severe skin avulsions of extremities; clinico-therapeutic aspects. Chirurgia (Bucur.), *21:*11, 1972 (Rumanian)

IRBY, WILLIAM B.: *Current Advances in Oral Surgery,* Vol. 1. C. V. Mosby Co., St. Louis, 1974

IRBY, WILLIAM B.: *Facial Trauma and Concomitant Problems.* C. V. Mosby Co., St. Louis, 1974. PRS, *55:*616, 1975

IROSHNIKOVA, E. S.: Experience in the use of protective plates in resection of the maxilla. Stomatologiia (Mosk.), *50:*96, 1971 (Russian)

IRWIN, E. C. *et al:* Parents working with parents: the cleft palate program. Cleft Palate J., *10:*360, 1973

ISAEVA, R. I.: Orthodontic treatment of children with unilateral cleft palate before uranoplasty. Stomatologiia (Mosk.), *54:*54, 1975 (Russian)

ISAKOV, IU. V.: Unavoidable adverse sequelae of tracheostomy and possible ways of lessening them. Vestn. Khir., *107:*130, 1971 (Russian)

ISELIN, F.: Flag flap. PRS, *52:*374, 1973

ISELIN, F.: Arthroplasty of proximal interphalangeal joint after trauma, PRS, *57:*398, 1976. Hand, *7:*41, 1975

ISELIN, F. *et al:* Resensitization of the thumb with the Kuhn-Holevitch flap. Ann. chir. plast., *16:*295, 1971 (French)

ISELIN, M.: Abnormal mental reactions of the injured. Handchirurgie, *2:*61, 1970 (German)

ISELIN, M.: Surgical use of homologous tendon grafts preserved in cialit (Follow-Up Clinic). PRS, *49:*208, 1972

ISHERWOOD, I. *et al:* Extranasopharyngeal juvenile angiofibroma. J. Laryng. & Otol., *89:*535, 1975

ISHII, H.: Condition of auditory ossicles in microtia; findings in 57 middle ear operations (with Harada), PRS, *50:*48, 1972

ISHIDA, H. *et al:* Therapeutic experience in heat-press injury. Orthop. Surg. (Tokyo), *22:*878, 1971 (Japanese)

ISHINADA, Y. *et al:* Functional reconstruction of electric burn of the hand. Orthop. Surg. (Tokyo), *22:*882, 1971 (Japanese)

ISHRAT-HUSAIN, S.: Antro-oral fistula. Int. Surg., *58:*58, 1973

ISO, R.: Therapeutic experience in a case of extensive congenital skin defects in hands and feet. Orthop. Surg. (Tokyo), *21:*885, 1970 (Japanese)

ISO, R.: Growth of free grafted skin, PRS, *53:*371, 1974. Jap. J. Plast. Reconstr. Surg., *16:*265, 1973

ISSHIKI, N.: Pushback operation for complete unilateral cleft palate (with Honjow, Morimoto), PRS, *53:*306, 1974

ISSHIKI, N. *et al:* Indication and the results of pharyngeal flap operation. Arch. Klin. Exp. Ohren Nasen Kehlkopfheilkd., *200:*158, 1971

ISSHIKI, N., HONJO, I., AND SHIBA, M.: Operation of pharyngeal flap, postoperative progress. J. Otolaryngol. Jap., *75:*1063, 1972 (Japanese)

ISSHIKI, N., AND MORIMOTO, M.: New folded pharyngeal flap, PRS, *55:*461, 1975

ISTVAN, S.: Xenograft in the treatment of burns. Magy. Traumatol. Orthop., *18:*314, 1975 (Hungarian)

ITARUT, P. *et al*: Staphylococcal septicemia following removal of sebaceous cysts. Rocky Mt. Med. J., *71:*576, 1974

ITO, E.: Specificity of free skin graft of the face. Surg. Ther. (Osaka), *26:*515, 1972 (Japanese)

ITO, T.: Problems in skin grafting of the palm in children. Orthop. Surg. (Tokyo), *21:*928, 1970 (Japanese)

ITO, T. *et al*: Functional evaluation of the paralytic hand. Orthop. Surg. (Tokyo), *21:*952, 1970 (Japanese)

ITO, T. *et al*: Hand injury and underlying diseases. Orthop. Surg. (Tokyo), *22:*1007, 1971 (Japanese)

IUDENICH, V. V. *et al*: Amputation of the extremities in burns. Voen. Med. Zh., *10:*15, 1975 (Russian)

IUKHIN, L. S.: Osteonecrectomy and skin plasty in patients with deep burns. Ortop. Travmatol. Protez., *34:*18, 1973 (Russian)

IUKHIN, L. S. *et al*: Results of treatment of patients with deep burns. Vestn. Khir., *114:*78, 1975 (Russian)

IUPATOV, S. I. *et al*: Injury of the left common carotid artery. Vestn. Khir., *112:*105, 1974 (Russian)

IUPATOV, S. I. *et al*: Treatment of patients with trophic ulcers. Khirurgiia (Mosk.), *8:*52, 1975 (Russian)

IUSUFOV, G. G.: Finger and hand injuries in workers in a glass factory. Ortop. Travmatol. Protez., *32:*73, 1971 (Russian)

IVANKIEVICZ, D. *et al*: Mechanical measurement of tension after square and wedge excision on lower lip tumors. Z.W.R., *81:*176, 1972 (German)

IVANKIEVICZ, D. *et al*: Mechanical study of tension following quadrate- and wedge-excision of tumors of lower lip. Fogorv. Sz., *66:*164, 1973 (Hungarian)

IVANKIEVICZ, D. *et al*: Modification of surgical reposition of premaxilla in bilateral cleft lip, jaw and palate. Fogorv. Sz., *67:*161, 1974 (Hungarian)

IVANKIEVICZ, D. *et al*: Follow-up studies on hospitalized patients with sinus perforation. Fogorv. Sz., *67:*207, 1974

IVANOV, B. S.: Use of Kulikovsky's modified needle for suturing defects of mucosa of nasal septum. Vestn. Otorinolaringol., *34:*94, 1971 (Russian)

IVANOVA, L. A.: Injuries and diseases of the hand. Voen. Med. Zh., *3:*28, 1972 (Russian)

IVANOVA, M. N. *et al*: Period of detachment of burn scab in children and indications for autoplastic operations. Ortop. Travmatol. Pro-

tez., *35:*28, 1974 (Russian)

IVANOVA, N. P.: Treatment of deep circular burns of inferior extremities, PRS, *52:*598, 1973. Zentralbl. Chir., *98:*331, 1973

IVANOVA, N. P. *et al*: Treatment of severe deformities and contractures of lower extremities resulting from burns. Ortop. Travmatol. Protez., *34:*38, 1973 (Russian)

IVERSON, R. E.: Effective hemostasis with less epinephrine. Experimental and clinical study (with Siegel, Vistnes). PRS, *51:*129, 1973

IVERSON, R. E.: Bone deformation beneath alloplastic implants (with Jobe, Vistnes), PRS, *51:*169, 1973. Discussions by Rees, Spira. PRS, *51:*174, 1973

IVERSON, R. E.: Anophthalmic orbit. Surgical correction of lower eyelid ptosis (with Vistnes, Laub). PRS, *52:*346, 1973

IVERSON, R. E.: Surgical treatment of contracted socket (with Vistnes). PRS, *53:*563, 1974

IVERSON, R. E., LAUB, D. R., AND MADISON, M. S.: Hydrofluoric acid burns. PRS, *48:*107, 1971

IVERSON, R. E., AND VISTNES, L. M.: Keratoacanthoma is frequently dangerous diagnosis, PRS, *53:*687, 1974. Am. J. Surg., *126:*359, 1973

IVERSON, R. E. *et al*: Coccidioidomycosis tenosynovitis in the hand. J. Bone & Joint Surg., (Am.), *55:*413, 1973

IVERSON, R. E., VISTNES, L. M., AND SIEGEL, R. J.: Correction of enophthalmos in anophthalmic orbit. PRS, *51:*545, 1973

IVY, R. H.: Contributions of plastic surgery to other fields of surgical endeavor, PRS, *48:*400, 1971. Am. J. Surg., *95:*180, 1958

IVY, R. H.: Obituary on Harold R. Browne. PRS, *48:*406, 1971

IVY, ROBERT H.: Lectureship, PRS, *48:*410, 1971; PRS, *50:*431, 1972: Award to, PRS, *52:*605, 1973: Lecture given by at College of Physicians of Philadelphia, PRS *53:*696, 1974: Society, PRS, *49:*243, 1972; *50:*315, 546, 1972; *52:*692, 1973.

IVY, R. H.: Reminiscences of public health in Pennsylvania, cleft palate program, PRS, *48:*400, 1971. Tr. Coll. Physicians Phila., *38:*174, 1971

IVY, R. H.: Promotion of verbal and written communication of ideas to professional colleagues (Editorial), PRS, *49:*200, 1972

IVY, R. H.: Iliac bone graft to bridge mandibular defect, 49-year clinical and radiological follow-up, PRS, *50:*483, 1972

IVY, R. H.: Commentary on Mirault's Classic Reprint. PRS, *57:*506, 1976

IVY, R. H. AND EDGERTON, M. T.: Deformity is a

disease. Trans. Stud. Coll. Physicians Phila., 41:124, 1973

IWAI, H.: Limitations of conservation surgery in carcinoma involving the arytenois. Can. J. Otolaryngol., 4:434, 1975

IWAI, H.: Laryngeal reconstruction by free flap transfer (with Nagahara, Hirose). PRS, 57:604, 1976

IWAI, H. et al: Evaluation of total pharyngolaryngectomy for hypopharyngeal cancer. Arch. Otorhinolaryngol. (N.Y.), 209:223, 1975

IWAI, H. et al: Subtotal pharyngolaryngectomy conservation surgery for carcinoma of sinus pyriformis extending toward the larynx. Arch. Otorhinolaryngol. (N.Y.), 209:271, 1975

IWAI, H. et al: Centennial conference on laryngeal cancer papers. Primary laryngoplasty. Laryngoscope, 85:929, 1975

IWAKUMA, T. et al: Extradural ossification following an extradural hematoma, case report. J. Neurosurg., 41:104, 1974

IWAMURA, S. et al: Schwannoma of nasal cavity. Arch. Otolaryng., 96:176, 1972

IZUMI, A. K., AND ARNOLD, H. L.: Congenital annular bands (pseudoainhum): association with other congenital abnormalities, PRS, 55:519, 1975. J.A.M.A., 229:1208, 1974

J

JABALEY, M. E.: Drug injection injuries of hands and forearms in addicts (with Ryan, Hoopes), PRS, 53:445, 1974

JABALEY, M. E., NGUYEN, D. C., AND NGUYEN, T. L.: Use of local flap for burn contracture of neck, PRS, 48:288, 1971

JABALEY, M. F. et al: Early treatment of war wounds of the hand and forearm in Vietnam. Ann. Surg., 177:167, 1973

JABALEY, M. E., HOOPES, J. E., AND COCHRAN, T. C.: Transoral Silastic augmentation of the malar region, PRS, 56:676, 1975. Brit. J. Plast. Surg., 27:98, 1974

JABALEY, M. E., LERMAN, M., AND SANDERS, H. J.: Ocular injuries in orbital fractures, review of 119 cases, PRS, 56:410, 1975

JACKSON, C. E. et al: Hairy cutaneous malformations of palms and soles. A hereditary condition. Arch. Dermat., 111:1146, 1975

JACKSON, D.: Excision and closure of wound as applied to burns, PRS, 50:204, 1972. Proc. Roy. Soc. Med., 65:23, 1972

JACKSON, D., AND SIMPSON, H. E.: Primary melanoma of oral cavity, PRS, 57:264, 1976. J. Oral Surg., 39:553, 1975

JACKSON, D. M., AND STONE, P. A.: Tangential excision and grafting of burns. Method and

report of 50 consecutive cases, PRS, 52:210, 1973 Brit. J. Plast. Surg., 25:416, 1972

JACKSON, F. E. et al: Radial nerve entrapment in exuberant callus from fractured humerus: a case report, PRS, 51:705, 1973. Mil. Med., 137:203, 1972

JACKSON, I. T.: Delayed skin grafting in head and neck surgery, PRS, 50:99, 1972. Acta chir. plast., 13:16, 1971

JACKSON, I. T.: Closure of secondary palatal fistulae with intra-oral tissue and bone grafting, PRS, 52:100, 1973. Brit. J. Plast. Surg., 25:93, 1972

JACKSON, I. T.: Use of tongue flaps to resurface lip defects and close palatal fistulae in children, PRS, 49:537, 1972

JACKSON, I. T.: Recent advances in plastic surgery. Scott. Med. J., 17:153, 1972

JACKSON, I. T.: Method to keep dressings moist prior to delayed skin grafting, PRS, 56:347, 1975

JACKSON, I. T., AND LANG, W.: Secondary esophagoplasty after pharyngolaryngectomy, using modified deltopectoral flap, PRS, 48:155, 1971

JACKSON, I. T., AND PATON, K. C.: Extended approach to flexor tendon synovitis in rheumatoid arthitis, PRS, 55:109, 1975. Brit. J. Plast. Surg., 26:122, 1973

JACKSON, I. T. et al: Ulnar head resection in rheumatoid arthritis, PRS, 56:228, 1975. Hand, 6:172, 1974

JACKSON, P. D.: Parotid calculus. J. R. Nav. Med. Serv., 58:59, 1972

JACKSON, R.: Why do basal cell carcinomas recur (or not recur) following treatment? J. Surg. Oncol., 6:245, 1974

JACKSON, R. et al: Horrifying basal cell carcinoma: study of 33 cases and comparison with 435 non-horror cases and report on four metastatic cases. J. Surg. Oncol., 5:431, 1973

JACKSON, R. W. et al: Hyperbaric oxygen in management of clostridial myonecrosis (gas gangrene). Clin. Orthop., 96:271, 1973

JACOB, C. T., JR.: Teflon pharyngoplasty (with Sturim), PRS, 49:180, 1972

JACOBS, H. B.: Emergency percutaneous transtracheal catheter and ventilator, PRS, 52:106, 1973. J. Trauma, 12:50, 1972

JACOBS, H. B.: Skin knife – deep knife – ritual and practice of skin incisions, PRS, 54:241, 1974. Ann. Surg., 179:102, 1974

JACOBS, H. B. et al: Transtracheal catheter ventilation: clinical experiences in 36 patients. Chest, 65:36, 1974

JACOBS, H. G. et al: Treatment of lateral orbital fractures. Fortschr. Kiefer. Gesichtschir., 19:180, 1975 (German)

JACOBS, J. B. et al: Ultrastructure evidence for

destruction in halo nevus, PRS, *56:*112, 1975. Cancer Res., *35:*352, 1975

JACOBS, K. F., AND WALTER, C.: Reconstruction of nose after trauma, PRS, *57:*114, 1976. Actuel. Chir., *10:*157, 1975

JACOBS, L. A. *et al*: Synovial sarcoma of the head and neck. Am. J. Surg., *128:*527, 1974

JACOBS, R. L., AND RAY, D.: Effect of heat on bone healing: disadvantage in the use of power tools, PRS, *50:*638, 1972. Arch. Surg., *104:*687, 1972

JACOBS, S. C., AND McCULLOUGH, D. L.: Recurrent flail penis—unusual complication of penile prosthesis, PRS, *57:*536, 1976. J. Urol., *112:*768, 1974

JACOBSEN, K. *et al*: Dodd-Crockett operation. Analysis of long-term prognosis. Acta Chir. Scand., *140:*379, 1974

JACOBSON, A. *et al*: Mandibular prognathism. Am. J. Orthod., *66:*140, 1974

JACOBSSON, S.: Views on surgical treatment of malignant melanoma. Lakartidningen, *73:*530, 1976 (Swedish)

JACOBSSON, S. *et al*: Florid keratoacanthomas in a kidney transplant recipient. Case report. Scand. J. Plast. Reconstr. Surg., *8:*243, 1974

JACOBY, FLORENCE G.: *Nursing Care of the Patient with Burns*. C. V. Mosby Co., St. Louis, 1972

JAEGER, D. L.: Maintenance of function of the burn patient. Phys. Ther., *52:*627, 1972

JAEGER, M. *et al*: Congenital triangular deformity of the tabular bones of hand and foot. Clin. Orthop. *81:*139, 1971

JAEGER, M. *et al*: Orthopedic problems of disordered function of the hand. Munch. Med. Wochenschr., *116:*247, 1974 (German)

JAFEK, B., KREIGER, A., AND MORLEDGE, D.: Blindness following blepharoplasty, PRS, *54:*105, 1974. Arch. Otolaryng., *98:*366, 1973

JAFFE, B. F.: Diseases and surgery of nose. Clin. Symp., *26:*1, 1974

JAFFE, B. F., AND DeBLANC, C. B.: Sinusitis in children with cleft lip and palate, PRS, *49:*105, 1972. Arch. Otolaryng., *93:*479, 1971

JAFFE, N. *et al*: Rhabdomyosarcoma in children, improved outlook with multidisciplinary approach, PRS, *52:*600, 1973. Am. J. Surg., *125:*482, 1973

JAFFE, S. *et al*: Replantation of amputated extremities. Report of five cases. Ohio State Med. J., *71:*381, 1975

JAGER, M.: Surgical treatment of the rheumatic hand. Munch. Med. Wochenschr., *112:*1875, 1970 (German)

JAGER, M. *et al*: Problem of suitable time in indications for surgical management of peripheral paresis of facial nerve. Bratisl. Lek. Listy., *61:*582, 1974 (Slovakian)

JAGO, J. D.: Cleft lip and cleft palate. M. J. Australia, *2:*1045, 1970

JAHNKE, V.: Treatment of injuries to nasal base. Laryngol. Rhinol. Otol. (Stuttg.), *53:*657, 1974 (German)

JAIMOVICH, L., AND ABULAFIA, J.: Atypical fibroxanthoma with ganglial metastases, PRS, *57:*264, 1976. Med. Cut., *2:*15, 1973

JAISON, A. R.: Founding of the John Staige Davis Society of Plastic Surgeons of Maryland, Inc. Md. State Med. J., *20:*15, 1971

JAKOB, R. P. *et al*: Results with the H-graft operation of Backdahl-Myrin in the treatment of ulnar deviation of the fingers. Arch. Orthop. Unfallchir., *78:*24, 1974 (German)

JAKOBIEC, F. A. *et al*: Primary orbital melanoma. Am. J. Ophth., *78:*24, 1974

JAKOBSEN, A.: Rabbit anti-rat lymphocyte serum: *in vitro* antimacrophage activity of different types of antisera and relationship to immunosuppression. Acta Pathol. Microbiol. Scand., *81:*353, 1973

JACOBSSON, P. A. *et al*: Combined radiotherapy and surgery in treatment of carcinoma of tongue. Acta Otolaryngol. (Stockh.), *75:*321, 1973

JAKUBIK, J.: Hand burns caused by a laundry press. Acta Chir. Orthop. Traumatol. Cech., *39:*49, 1972 (Czechoslovakian)

JAKUBIK, J.: New knife for operation of prominent ears, PRS, *53:*601, 1974. Acta chir. plast., *15:*55, 1973

JAKUBIK, J., AND KUBACEK, V.: Injuries of hands during five-year period at Clinic of Plastic Surgery, PRS, *54:*621, 1974. Rozhl. chir., *53:*200, 1974

JAMES, CALNAN: *Recent Advances in Plastic Surgery, Number One*. Longman, Inc., New York, 1976.

JAMES, P.: Surgical treatment of mandibular joint disorders. Ann. R. Coll. Surg. Engl., *49:*310, 1971

JAMES, P. L. *et al*: Multiple neurofibromatosis associated with facial asymmetry. J. Oral Surg., *33:*439, 1975

JAMES, R. B. *et al*: Osteochondroma of mandibular coronoid process, case report. Oral Surg., *37:*189, 1974

JAMES, S., AND SALISBURY, A.: Facilitation of metastasis by antithymocyte globulin, PRS, *54:*244, 1974. Cancer Res., *34:*367, 1974

JAMRA, F. A.: Pedicle skin flaps in acute hand injuries. J. Med. Liban., *26:*59, 1973

JAMRA, F. A.: Cross-leg flaps. A review of eleven personal cases. Med. Liban., *27:*591, 1974

JANACKOVA, E.: On the problem of substitution of liquids after the operation on elephantiasis. Acta Chir. Orthop. Traumatol. Cech.,

*41:*564, 1974 (Czech)

JANE, J. A.: Craniofacial osteotomies and reconstructions in infants and young children (with Edgerton, Berry), PRS, *54:*13, 1974

JANE, J. A.: Radical reconstruction of complex cranioorbitofacial abnormalities. Birth Defects, *11:*341, 1975

JANE, J. A.: Surgery of craniofacial deformities. J. Neurol. Neurosurg. Psychiatry, *38:*409, 1975

JANECKA, I.: Neurilemmoma of facial nerve (with Conley), PRS, *52:*55, 1973

JANECKA, I. P.: Identification of facial nerve at secondary surgery. Laryngoscope, *85:*896, 1975

JANEKE, J. B., AND WRIGHT, W. K.: Studies on support of the nasal tip, PRS, *49:*102, 1972. Arch. Otolaryng., *93:*5, 1971

JANEKE, J. B. *et al*: Proplast in cavity obliteration and soft tissue augmentation. Arch. Otolaryng., *100:*24, 1974

JANOVEC, M.: Skeleton of the hand in Down's syndrome. Acta Chir. Orthop. Traumatol. Cech., *38:*106, 1971 (Czechoslovakian)

JANSEN, G. T.: Practical therapy for hyperkeratotic skin lesions. Geriatrics, *30:*71, 1975

JANSEN, G. T.: Treatment of basal cell epitheliomas and actinic keratoses. J.A.M.A., *235:*1152, 1976

JANSSENS, A.: Photoscanning of salivary glands, PRS, *48:*89, 1971. Acta Stomatol. belg., *67:*25, 1970

JANVIER, H. *et al*: Local skin flaps in treatment of cutaneous contractures, sequelae of burns of the anterior and lateral sides of the neck. Ann. chir. plast., *17:*26, 1972 (French)

JANVIER, H. *et al*: "Capital" LLL flap for extensive tissue loss of dorsal region. Ann. chir. plast., *17:*218, 1972 (French)

JANVIER, H. *et al*: Problems posed by restoration of labiomandibular areas in burn patients. Ann. chir. plast., *18:*255, 1973 (French)

JANVIER, H. *et al*: Special psychological aspect of the relation between client and surgeon in cosmetic surgery. Rev. Med. Suisse Romande., *94:*963, 1974 (French)

JANZEKOVIC, Z.: Early surgical treatment of the burned surface. Panminerva Med., *14:*228, 1972

JANZEKOVIC, Z.: Burn wound from the surgical point of view. J. Trauma, *15:*42, 1975

JANZEKOVIC, Z.: Past and present management burns. Magy. Traumatol. Orthop., *18:*260, 1975 (Hungarian)

JARRETT, J. F. *et al*: Local and regional skin flaps in head and neck surgery. Rocky Mt. Med. J., *70:*51, 1973

JARVIS, C. W. *et al*: Low voltage skin burns.

Pediatrics, *48:*831, 1971

JARZAB, G.: Cryosurgery in treatment of hemangiomas. Polski tygodnik lek., *27:*2025, 1972 (Polish)

JARZAB, G.: Clinical experience in cryosurgery of hemangioma, PRS, *57:*539, 1976. J. Maxillo-facial Surg., *3:*146, 1975

JARZEBSKI, J.: Congenital fistulas and cysts of the neck in our clinical material. Wiad. Lek., *25:*767, 1972 (Polish)

JASIENSKA, A. *et al*: Case of salivary gland ectopy to the suprahyoid region in a 4-year-old boy. Otolaryngol. Pol., *28:*705, 1974 (Polish)

JASTAK, J. T., AND GORETTA, C.: Ketamine HCl as continuous-drip anesthetic for outpatients, PRS, *53:*374, 1974. Anesth. Analg., Cleve., *52:*341, 1973

JAUSSERAN, M. *et al*: Current role of electrosurgery in treatment of cancers of oral cavity. J. Radiol. Electrol. Med. Nucl., *53:*471, 1972 (French)

JAVOR, P.: New suction obturator to control saliva after laryngopharyngectomy. PRS, *57:*106, 1976

Jaw, Ameloblastoma

Ameloblastomas in young people. Subperiosteal resections (Editorial). Rev. Stomatol. Chir. Maxillofac., *72:*667, 1971 (French)

Treatment of ameloblastoma of the mandible: resection via the intraoral route and simultaneous reconstruction by means of autogeneous bone transplant (Stea). Riv. Ital. Stomatol., *26:*395, 1971

Morphology and malignancy of adamantinomas (Spiessl, Prein), PRS, *51:*708, 1973. Adv. Jaw & Face Surg., Year Book, 1972

Ameloblastoma with metastases to lung, ilium and soft tissues, case report (Hopson *et al*). Brit. J. Plast. Surg., *25:*367, 1972

Mandibular cystic adamantinomas, two-stage surgery of (Rehrmann). Fortschr. Kiefer. Gesichtschir., *15:*195, 1972 (German)

Results of surgical therapy of adamantinomas (Koch). Fortschr. Kiefer. Gesichtschir., *15:*207, 1972 (German)

Ameloblastomas, 38, treatment and its results (Becker). Fortschr. Kiefer. Gesichtschir., *15:*211, 1972 (German)

Mandibular cystic neoplasia, adenoameloblastoma (Pinto *et al*), PRS, *53:*110, 1974. Gazeta sanit., *3:*127, 1972

Ameloblastoma treated by peripheral ostectomy. Ten-year follow-up (Himmelfarb *et al*). N. Y. State Dent. J., *38:*282, 1972

Papilliferous ameloblastic fibroma (Christ *et*

Jaw, Ameloblastoma – Cont.

al). Oral Surg., *34:*806, 1972

Ameloblastoma, malignant, with pulmonary metastases. Case report and review of the literature (Herceg, Harding). PRS, *49:*456, 1972

Ameloblastoma, treatment of (Pandya, Stuteville). PRS, *50:*242, 1972

Adenoameloblastoma (Martis, Karakasis). PRS, *50:*409, 1972

Mandible, ameloblastoma of, reconstruction of mental region by Millard's method in case of (Taen *et al*). Jap. J. Oral Surg., *19:*150, 1973 (Japanese)

Adenoameloblastoma: report of case (Goracy, Stratigos). J. Am. Dent. Assoc., *86:*672, 1973

Maxilla, ameloblastic sarcoma in, case report (Hatzifotiadis *et al*). J. Maxillo-facial Surg., *1:*62, 1973

Ameloblastoma originating in wall of primordial cyst: report of case (Byrd, Allen, Dunsworth). J. Oral Surg., *31:*301, 1973

Ameloblastoma, recurrent, 30 years after surgical treatment (Hayward). J. Oral Surg., *31:*368, 1973

Ameloblastoma, fibromatous, ultrastructure of (Csiba *et al*). Morphol. Igazsagugyi. Orv. Sz., *13;*183, 1973 (Hungarian)

Histology and ultrastructure of an ameloblastic fibroma, case report (Hietanen *et al*). Proc. Finn. Dent. Soc., *69:*129, 1973

Ameloblastoma, mandibular, recurrence, previously treated by radiation (Hosxe *et al*). Rev. Stomatol. Chir. Maxillofac., *74:*135, 1973

Ameloblastoma with regional and distant metastases (Byrne, Kosmala, Cunningham), PRS, *57:*540, 1976. Am. J. Surg., *128:*91, 1974

Ameloblastoma, radiological features of (McIvor). Clin. Radiol., *25:*237, 1974

Ameloblastoma of maxilla and mandible (Sehdev *et al*), PRS, *56:*225, 1975. Cancer, *33:*324, 1974

Mandible, gigantic ameloblastoma of, case report (Petriella *et al*). J. Oral Surg., *32:*44, 1974

Ameloblastic fibro-odontoma: case report (Sanders *et al*). J. Oral Surg., *32:*281, 1974

Mandibular resection and reconstruction for ameloblastoma in severe diabetic (Mason *et al*). J. Oral Surg., *32:*379, 1974

Ameloblastoma, report of two cases (Keaton *et al*). J. Oral Surg., *32:*382, 1974

Adenomatoid odontogenic tumor (adenoameloblastoma); case report (Meyer *et al*). J. Oral Surg., *32:*448, 1974

Ameloblastoma – the conservative surgical

Jaw, Ameloblastoma – Cont.

approach to treatment: report of four cases (Huffman *et al*). J. Oral Surg., *32:*850, 1974

Ameloblastoma (Tangen). Nor. Tannlaegeforen Tid., *84:*308, 1974 (Norwegian)

Ameloblastoma, granular cell (Hartman). Oral Surg., *38:*241, 1974

Adenoameloblastoma (Seymour, Funke, Irby), PRS, *56:*235, 1975. Oral Surg., *38:*860, 1974

Role of telecobalt therapy in the treatment of inoperable ameloblastomas (Takacsi-Nagy). Radiobiol. Radiother. (Berl.), *15:*453, 1974 (German)

Decalcified bone homotransplant used for repair of an extensive mandibular defect remaining after removal of recurrent ameloblastoma (Burlibasa *et al*). Rev. Chir. (Stomatol.), *21:*359, 1974 (Rumanian)

Ameloblastoma, recurrence, curetted and irradiated 16 years previously, hemimandibulectomy for (Bouez *et al*). Rev. Dent. Liban., *24:*1, 1974 (French)

Recurrences of ameloblastomas of the jaws. Statistical study; therapeutic indications (Cernea *et al*). Rev. Stomatol. Chir. Maxillofac., *75:*18, 1974 (French)

Several cases of primary or recurrent mandibular ameloblastomas treated by surgical curettage (Bataille *et al*). Rev. Stomatol. Chir. Maxillofac., *75:*33, 1974 (French)

Numerical data on the recurrence of ameloblastomas (Carlier *et al*). Rev. Stomatol. Chir. Maxillofac., *75:*37, 1974 (French)

Seven cases of ameloblastoma recurrence (Vilasco *et al*). Rev. Stomatol. Chir. Maxillofac., *75:*42, 1974 (French)

Radical therapy, without recurrence, of ameloblastic tumors of the jaws (Timosca). Rev. Stomatol. Chir. Maxillofac., *75:*47, 1974 (French)

Recurrences of ameloblastomas of the jaws (Plaza Carranza). Rev. Stomatol. Chir. Maxillofac., *75:*53, 1974 (French)

Transparotid approach in mandibular ameloblastoma recurrences (Gouiric *et al*). Rev. Stomatol. Chir. Maxillofac., *75:*58, 1974 (French)

Management of a mandibular ameloblastoma recurrence (Cadenat *et al*). Rev. Stomatol. Chir. Maxillofac., *75:*65, 1974 (French)

Hemimandibulectomy after recurrent ameloblastoma curetted and irradiated 16 years before (Bouez *et al*). Rev. Stomatol. Chir. Maxillofac., *75:*66, 1974 (French)

Ameloblastoma, gigantic, developing to size of infant's head, case (Tsutsui *et al*). Tokushima J. Exp. Med., *21:*69, 1974

Jaw, Ameloblastoma – Cont.

Ameloblastoma of the maxilla. A report of two cases (Fox *et al*). Brit. Dent. J., *138:*61, 1975

Contribution to the diagnosis and treatment of adamantinoma (Flieger *et al*). Czas. Stomatol., *28:*1185, 1975 (Polish)

Ameloblastoma: review of the literature and report of case (Goldberg *et al*). J. Am. Dent. Assoc., *90:*432, 1975

Ameloblastoma of upper jaw (Chaudhuri). J. Laryng & Otol., *89:*457, 1975

Ameloblastic odontoma in a very young child (Capitaine *et al*). Rev. Stomatol. Chir. Maxillofac., *76:*447, 1975 (French)

Jaw, Ankylosis, (See also *Temporomandibular Joint*)

Pseudoarthrosis of mandibular body treated by sliding bone graft (Merkx), PRS, *49:*662, 1972. Arch. chir. neerl., *23:*273, 1971

Ankylosis, temporomandibular, Sada's treatment for (Yoel), PRS, *49:*581, 1972. Bol. y trab. Acad. argent cir., *55:*375, 1971

Ankylosis of coronoid to zygomatic bone (Findlay). Brit. J. Oral Surg., *10:*30, 1972

Dental ankylosis, reversibility of surgically induced, in rats (Andreasen *et al*). Int. J. Oral Surg., *1:*98, 1972

Ankylosis, temporomandibular joint, bone grafting in (Hung *et al*), PRS, *55:*634, 1975. Chinese M. J., *10:*135, 1973

Mandible, pseudarthrosis, treatment of, using nonpedunculated bone suture grafting (Lehnert). Dtsch. Zahn. Mund. Kieferheilkd., *61:*45, 1973 (German)

Cancrum oris (noma), surgical repair of defects from (Durrani). PRS, *52:*629, 1973

Ankylosis, temporomandibular, use of silicone in (Alves Costa *et al*), PRS, *53:*365, 1974. Rev. brasil. cir., *63:*73, 1973

Coronoid process, restriction of jaw movement due to abnormalities of (Findlay). Trans. Congr. Int. Assoc. Oral Surg., *4:*269, 1973

Coronoid ostochondroma presenting as a coronozygomatic ankylosis. A case report (Cooper *et al*). Brit. Dent. J., *137:*99, 1974

Prevention of recurrence in surgery for ankylosis (Verbeck *et al*). Fortsch. Kiefer. Gesichtschir., *18:*241, 1974 (German)

Surgical mobilization of a clamped jaw following radiotherapy (Scheunemann *et al*). Fortschr. Kiefer. Gesichtschir., *18:*244, 1974 (German)

Mandibular ankylosis, surgical-orthodontic treatment (Snyder *et al*). J. Fla. Med. As-

Jaw, Ankylosis – Cont.

soc., *61:*569, 1974

Joint, temporomandibular, surgical treatment of ankylosis (El-Mofty), PRS, *55:*106, 1975. J. Oral Surg., *32:*202, 1974

Mandible, bilateral ankylosis of, in open position. Review of literature and report of case (Wallace *et al*). Oral Surg., *37:*179, 1974

Mandible, condylectomy with silicone rubber replacement (Hartwell, Hall). PRS, *53:*440, 1974

Jaw ankylosis, operative management (Roberts, Wright, Shamia), PRS, *55:*635, 1975. Trop. Doctor, *4:*121, 1974

Ankylosis of temporomandibular joint (Kameros, Himmelfarb), PRS, *57:*396, 1976. J. Oral Surg., *33:*282, 1975

Ankylosis, temporomandibular joint, unusual case of (Davis *et al*), PRS, *57:*758, 1976. Oral Surg., *40:*194, 1975

Ankylosis of mandible from *cancrum oris* (Oluwasanmi, Lagundoye, Akinyemi). PRS, *57:*342, 1976

Jaw, Bone Graft to

Bone transplants in maxillofacial surgery (Giardino *et al*). Arch. Stomatol. (Napoli), *11:*151, 1970 (Italian)

Iliac grafts in maxillofacial surgical pathology (Lourmet *et al*). Bull. Soc. Med. Afr. Noire Lang. Fr., *15:*343, 1970 (French)

Children, reconstructive operations on mandible in, clinico-experimental study (Kolesov *et al*), PRS, *51:*475, 1973. Acta chir. plast., *13:*203, 1971

Mandibular body, pseudoarthrosis of, treatment by sliding bone graft (Merkx), PRS, *49:*662, 1972. Arch. chir. neerl., *23:*273, 1971

Bone grafting in the body of the mandible. Report of cases (Fitzpatrick). Aust. Dent. J., *16:*156, 1971

Experimental approach to mandibular replacement: island vascular composite rib grafts (Strauch *et al*). Brit. J. Plast. Surg., *24:*334, 1971

Experimental homotransplantation in mandibular defects (Skaloud *et al*). Fogorv. Sz., *64:*305, 1971 (Hungarian)

Mandibular bone grafts (Bromberg, Walden, Rubin) (Follow-Up Clinic). PRS, *48:*172, 1971

Mandibular arch repair, anterior, bending iliac bone graft for (Millard, Deane, Garst). PRS, *48:*600, 1971

Overgrowth of a hypoplastic mandibular ramus after autoplastic bone grafting. An 18-year longitudinal radiographic study, us-

Jaw, Cysts — Cont.

Nasopalatine cyst, surgical removal, case report (Cardo *et al*). N. Y. State Dent. J., *39:*484, 1973

Cyst, radicular, extensive, of maxilla, case report (Sahyoun). Rev. Dent. Liban., *23:*83, 1973

Recurrences and multiplicity of cysts (Stoelinga). Trans. Int. Conf. Oral Surg., *4:*77, 1973

Marsupialization of large cysts of maxillas into maxillary sinus and/or nose. Followup investigation (Egyedi, Beyazit). Trans. Congr. Int. Assoc. Oral Surg., *4:*81, 1973

Dentigerous cysts (Prasanna *et al*). Can. J. Otolaryngol., *3:*625, 1974

Surgery of cysts from the nasal cavity: methods and results (Eskici). Dtsch. Zahnaerztl. Z., *29:*742, 1974 (Eng. Abstr.)

Mandibular cyst, large, conservative treatment of (Finkel *et al*). N. Y. State Dent. J., *40:*353, 1974

Jaws, traumatic bone cyst of: diagnosis, treatment and prognosis (Sapone *et al*). Oral Surg., *32:*127, 1974

Jaws, bone cyst of, traumatic (Hansen *et al*). Oral Surg., *37:*899, 1974

Several cases of primary or recurrent mandibular ameloblastomas treated by surgical curettage (Freidel *et al*). Rev. Stomatol. Chir. Maxillofac., *75:*33, 1974 (French)

Brephroplasty in the treatment of jaw cysts in children (Ruzin *et al*). Stomatologiia (Mosk.), *53:*44, 1974 (Russian)

Management of a multilocular cystic image of the mandible (Freidel *et al*). Rev. Stomatol. Chir. Maxillofac., *75:*61, 1974 (French)

Origin and development of large jaw cysts linked to the dental system (Deffez). Rev. Stomatol. Chir. Maxillofac., *75:*885, 1974 (French)

An unusual case of 'haemorrhagic' bone cyst (Vijayaraghavan *et al*). Brit. J. Oral Surg., *13:*64, 1975

Maxillary cysts, extensive, surgical management of (Jaworska). Czas. Stomatol., *28:*403, 1975 (Polish)

Impacted third molar embedded in dentigerous cyst (Kirstein). Dent. Radiogr. Photogr., *48:*39, 1975

Jaw cysts, study of biological chemistry on nature of (Suzuki), PRS, *57:*116, 1976. J. Maxillo-facial Surg., *3:*106, 1975

Mandibular cyst, median: review of literature and report of two cases (White *et al*). J. Oral Surg., *33:*372, 1975

Conservative treatment of cysts of the jaws in nevoid basal cell carcinoma syndrome: report of a case (Hickory *et al*). J. Oral Surg.,

Jaw, Cysts — Cont.

*33:*693, 1975

Retrosternal parathyroid adenomas manifesting in the form of a giant-cell "tumor" of the mandible (Akinoso *et al*). Oral Surg., *39:*724, 1975

Simple bone cyst, report of two cases (Ruprecht *et al*). Oral Surg., *39:*826, 1975

Cleidocranial dysostosis with mandibular cyst. Report of a case (Oatis *et al*). Oral Surg., *40:*62, 1975

Aspergillosis as a postoperative complication of a jaw cyst (Dolezalowa *et al*). Pol. Tyg. Lek., *30:*437, 1975 (Polish)

Jaw, cystic tumors of, results obtained with bone homograft in (Popescu *et al*). Rev. Odontostomatol. (Paris), *4:*51, 1975 (French)

Results after cystectomy connected with apicoectomy (Bohringer *et al*). Schweiz. Monatsschr. Zahnheilkd., *85:*186, 1975 (German)

Clinical characteristics and genetic identity of the basal cell nevus syndrome (Gorlin-Goltz syndrome) (Breytenbach *et al*). S. Afr. Med. J., *49:*544, 1975 (Afrikaans)

Treatment of massive dentigerous cysts of the mandible: a report of two cases (Friedlander *et al*). N. Y. State Dent. J., *42:*156, 1976

Nasolabial cyst (Renard, Morgan). PRS, *57:*240, 1976

Mandible, cyst of, squamous cell carcinoma arising in (Herceg, Harding). PRS, *57:*383, 1976

Jaw Deformities (See also *Cleft Palate; Craniofacial Surgery; Malocclusion; Prognathism; Retrognathism*)

Mandible in children, reconstructive operations (Kolesov *et al*), PRS, *51:*475, 1973. Acta chir. plast., *13:*203, 1971

Facial skeletal defects and methods of repair (Magonska-Oleszycka *et al*). Czas. Stomatol., *24:*1333, 1971 (Polish)

Subjective effects and personality changes in patients following surgical corrections of esthetic-functional malformations of the jaw (Gotte *et al*). Riv. Ital. Stomatol., *26:*535, 1971 (Italian)

Maxillary protrusion, surgical therapy of (Nordenram). Sven. Tandlak. Tidskr., *64:*339, 1971 (Swedish)

Maxillary protrusion, correction of, by posterior change of upper jaw (Nordenram). Sven. Tandlak. Tidskr., *64:*703, 1971 (Swedish)

Studies on variability (Michalek), PRS, *52:*321, 1973. Acta chir. plast., *14:*73, 1972

Jaw Deformities – Cont.

Mandibular deformity, correction of, with silicone implant (Fukaya *et al*). Aichi Gakuin J. Dent. Sci., *10:*150, 1972 (Japanese)

Secondary enlargement of the mandibular coronoid process (Bramley *et al*). Brit. J. Surg., *59:*426, 1972

Problems of laterognathism (Toman). Cesk. Stomatol., *72:*377, 1972

Mandibular hyperplasia, unilateral, surgical treatment of (Korzon *et al*). Czas. Stomatol., *25:*1081, 1972 (Polish)

Maxillary prognathism, surgical and prosthetic treatment of, case (Cataloglu). Dentoral (Istanbul), *4:*180, 1972 (Turkish)

Laterognathism, supraclusion and facial asymmetry from condylar hyperplasia (Graziani). Oral Surg., *33:*884, 1972

Maxillary prognathism. Surgical and prosthetic therapy (Diaz *et al*). Rev. Esc. Odontoal. Tucuman., *38:*43, 1972 (Spanish)

Jaw deformities, correction of, by surgical procedures on alveolar process (Piscevic *et al*). Stomatol. Glas. Srb., *205:*12, 1972 (Croatian)

Surgical treatment of excessive development of the mandible and of open bite by intercortical osteotomy of the mandible (Mitrofanov *et al*). Stomatologiia (Mosk.), *51:*48, 1972 (Russian)

Four years experience with surgical correction of deformities of the middle portion of the face (Kufner). Stomatologiia (Mosk.), *51:*49, 1972 (Russian)

Mandibular reconstruction: bone induction in alloplastic tray (Leake, Rappoport), PRS, *51:*236, 1973. Surgery, *72:*332, 1972

Surgical orthodontic therapy for laterognathism and facial asymmetry (Fujikami *et al*). A. D. M., *30:*31, 1973 (Spanish)

Maxillary protrusion in adults, combined orthodontic and surgical management of (Proffit *et al*). Am. J. Orthod., *64:*368, 1973

Maxillary prognathism, treatment planning in (Bishara). Am. J. Orthod., *64:*384, 1973

Jaw, enlargement of coronoid process of (Carraro *et al*), PRS, *54:*687, 1974. Bol. y trab. Acad. argent. cir., *57:*469, 1973

Premaxillary deformity, development and structure in bilateral cleft lip and palate (Latham), PRS, *54:*694, 1974. Brit. J. Plast. Surg., *26:*1, 1973

Mandible and mouth, reduplication (Davies, Morrison, Miller). Brit. J. Plast. Surg., *26:*84, 1973

Oral surgery procedures. II. Dysostosis mandibularis (Stellmach *et al*). Dent. Dienst., *25:*45, 1973 (German)

Unusually large torus mandibularis (Kopp *et*

Jaw Deformities – Cont.

al). Dent. Radiogr. Photogr., *46:*20, 1973

Mandibular deformities, open subcondylar osteotomy in treatment (Berenyi). Int. J. Oral Surg., *2:*81, 1973

Maxillo-mandibular surgery for correction of dentofacial deformities. 1. Preoperative evaluation (Weinberg *et al*). J. Can. Dent. Assoc., *39:*263, 1973

Orbital floor and maxilla, conjunctival approach in congenital malformation and trauma (Tessier), PRS, *53:*247, 1974. J. Maxillo-facial Surg., *1:*3, 1973

Simianism: surgical orthodontic correction of bimaxillary protrusion (Converse *et al*). J. Maxillo-facial Surg., *1:*8, 1973

Segmental alveolar osteotomy in the correction of maxillofacial malformations (Torrielli *et al*). Minerva Stomatol., *22:*218, 1973 (Italian)

Mandibular deformities, correction of (Neuner). Oral Surg., *36:*779, 1973

Maxillary protrusion, upper. Surgical treatment (Areinza *et al*). Ortodoncia, *37:*143, 1973 (Spanish)

Maxilla, protrusion of, osteotomy for (Costa *et al*), PRS, *54:*688, 1974. Rev. brasil cir., *63:*307, 1973

Jaw and dental deformities, surgical management of (Kay *et al*). Rev. Dent. Liban., *23:*61, 1973

Jaw abnormalities, partially edentulous subjects with, functional rehabilitation and esthetics of masticatory system in (Gotte *et al*). Riv. Ital. Stomatol., *28:*259, 1973 (Italian)

Jaw, lower, problem of osteoplasty (Plotnikov). Stomatologiia (Mosk.), *52:*43, 1973 (Russian)

Correction of anomalies of dento-maxillofacial system as method of treatment of arthropathies in adults (Uzhumetskene). Stomatologia (Mosk.), *52:*51, 1973 (Russian)

Maxillary and mandibular retrusion, maxillary and mandibular osteotomy for (Holloman). Tex. Dent. J., *91:*4, 1973

Mandibular asymmetry (Waite). Trans. Congr. Int. Assoc. Oral Surg., *4:*246, 1973

Facial deformity – surgical treatment (Pericots Ayats, Pericot). Trans. Congr. Int. Assoc. Oral Surg., *4:*345, 1973

Lip and jaw, upper, median cleft of (Penkava), PRS, *56:*358, 1975. Acta chir. plast., *16:*201, 1974

Mandible, pig, experimental surgical reduction of (Atherton *et al*). Am. J. Orthod., *65:*158, 1974

Symphysis, mandibular, used to correct asso-

Jaw Deformities — Cont.

ciated deformities (Michelet *et al*), PRS, *54:*619, 1974. Ann. chir. plast., *19:*69, 1974

Lip and jaw, middle cleft of (Penkava), PRS, *54:*506, 1974. Cesk. Stomatol., *2:*142, 1974

Jaw implant, metal-plastic, in repair of major mandibular defect after ameloblastoma resection (Wang, Li), PRS, *54:*701, 1974. Chinese M.J., *5:*84, 1974

Dystopia of lower molar in processus muscularis with genuine fusion with muscle (Benndorf). Dtsch. Zahn. Mund. Kieferheilkd., *62:*237, 1974 (German)

Possibilities of surgical treatment of unilateral mandibular dysostosis in adults (Stellmach). Fortschr. Kiefer. Gesichtschir., *18:*49, 1974 (German)

Results of follow-up examinations in orthopedic jaw operations (Trauner). Fortschr. Kiefer. Gesichtschir., *18:*64, 1974 (German)

Combined orthopedic-plastic surgery of the jaws and face (Neuner). Fortschr. Kiefer. Gesichtschir., *18:*72, 1974 (German)

Significance of functional dentition analysis for surgical-orthopedic procedures (Bock). Fortschr. Kiefer. Gesichtschir., *18:*99, 1974 (German)

Preoperative photography as an aid in orthopedic jaw surgery (Selle). Fortschr. Kiefer. Gesichtschir., *18:*106, 1974 (German)

Possible applications of stepwise osteotomy of the ascending ramus (Schwenzer). Fortschr. Kiefer. Gesichtschir., *18:*138, 1974 (German)

Behavior of the maxillary sinuses after orthopedic jaw operations (Perko). Fortschr. Kiefer. Gesichtschir., *18:*213, 1974 (German)

Indications, technic and results of block and segmental osteotomies of the maxilla and mandible in dysgnathias (Pfeifer). Fortschr. Kiefer. Gesichtschir., *18:*248, 1974 (German)

Surgical treatment of dysgnathia in Mobius' syndrome (Bunte). Fortschr. Kiefer. Gesichtschir., *18:*256, 1974 (German)

Mandible, congenital deformity, epignathus (Chander), PRS, *55:*636, 1975. Indian J. Surg., *36:*242, 1974

Cherubism (Schindel *et al*), PRS, *54:*689, 1974. Internat. Surg., *59:*225, 1974

Mandibular asymmetry (Erickson *et al*). J. Am. Dent. Assoc., *89:*1369, 1974

Binder's maxillo-nasal dysostosis. Apropos of 10 cases (Rival *et al*). J. Genet. Hum., *22:*263, 1974 (French)

Otomandibular anomalies: pathogenesis as guide to reconstruction (Poswillo). PRS,

Jaw Deformities — Cont.

*55:*378, 1975 J. Maxillo-facial Surg., *2:*64, 1974

Otomandibular dystosis, correction of (Obwegeser), PRS, *55:*378, 1975. J. Maxillo-facial Surg., *2:*73, 1974

Jaw, cleft upper, following primary osteoplasty and orthodontic treatment (Schmid *et al*), PRS, *55:*381, 1975. J. Maxillo-facial Surg., *2:*92, 1974

Defects, osseous contour, new alloplastic tray for (Leake), PRS, *55:*386, 1975. J. Maxillofacial Surg., *2:*146, 1974

Mandibular defects, extensive, use of allogenic bone and autogenous marrow in (Pike, Boyne), PRS, *55:*119, 1975. J. Oral Surg., *32:*177, 1974

Preoperative interview and psychological evaluation of orthognathic surgery patient (Peterson *et al*). J. Oral Surg., *32:*583, 1974

Maxillary defects, surgically acquired, speech intelligibility following prosthetic obturation of (Azia, Weinberg, Chalian), PRS, *55:*257, 1975. J. Prosth. Dent., *32:*87, 1974

Experience with prefabricated silicone implants for reconstruction in facially deformed patients (Habal *et al*). J. Prosthet. Dent., *32:*292, 1974

Mandible, anterior, Stafne defect of (Malkin *et al*). N. Y. State Dent. J., *40:*17, 1974

Multiple osteotomies in a single surgical stage (Curioni). Rev. Stomatol. Chir. Maxillofac., *75:*116, 1974 (French)

Partial bilateral anterior osteotomies of the upper jaw. Conditions for stability of the results (Landais). Rev. Stomatol. Chir. Maxillofac., *75:*118, 1974 (French)

Experiences and results in the treatment of malformations of the jaws by segmental osteotomies (Torrielli *et al*). Rev. Stomatol. Chir. Maxillofac., *75:*125, 1974 (French)

Maxillofacial orthopedic surgery. New methods (Meyer). Rev. Stomatol. Chir. Maxillofac., *75:*153, 1974 (French)

Subalveolar mandibular osteotomies in anteroposterior facial dysmorphism (Michelet *et al*). Rev. Stomatol. Chir. Maxillofac., *75:*156, 1974 (French)

Rhinoplasty and maxillary osteotomies (Aiach). Rev. Stomatol. Chir. Maxillofac., *75:*159, 1974 (French)

Maxillary retrognathism, correction of, by partial osteotomy and transplantation of mandibular bone (Gotte). Riv. Ital. Stomatol., *29:*59, 1974 (Italian)

Anomalies, orthodontic, and pseudoprognathism, incidence in patients with cleft lip, jaw, and palate (Mullerova, Brousi-

Jaw Deformities – Cont.

lova, Pasek), PRS, *54:*623, 1974. Rozhl. chir., *53:*164, 1974

Clefts of maxilla, maxillary growth after implantation of Surgicel (Thilander, Stenström), PRS, *56:*681, 1975. Scand. J. Plast. Reconstr. Surg., *8:*52, 1974

Maxillary arch, collapsed (Matthews), PRS, *56:*464, 1975. Scand. J. Plast. Reconstr. Surg., *8:*116, 1974

Classification of mandibular defects (Pavlov). Stomatologiia (Mosk.), *53:*43, 1974 (Russian)

Jaws, chewing efficiency before and after surgical correction of developmental deformities (Astrand). Sven. Tandlak. Tidskr., *67:*135, 1974

Diagnosis and treatment of maxillomandibular dysplasias (Converse *et al*). Am. J. Orthod., *68:*625, 1975

Process, coronoid, bilateral hypertrophy of (Shurman), *57:*117, 1976. Anesthesiology, *41:*491, 1975

Lingual mandibular bone concavity (Mainous *et al*). J. Am. Dent. Assoc., *90:*666, 1975

Jaw, trigonometric method of analysis of upper part of (Oblak), PRS, *57:*258, 1976. J. Maxillo-facial Surg., *3:*88, 1975

Maxillary deformities, Le Fort I osteotomy for correction of (Bell). J. Oral Surg., *33:*412, 1975

Dentofacial and craniofacial deformities, acquired and developmental, middle-third facial osteotomies, their use in correction of (Epker). J. Oral Surg., *33:*491, 1975

Total mandibular alveolar osteotomy in the management of skeletal (infantile) apertognathia (MacIntosh *et al*). J. Oral Surg., *33:*921, 1975

Maxillary exostoses. Surgical management of unusual case (Blakemore *et al*). Oral Surg., *40:*200, 1975

Surgical correction of jaw abnormalities causing severe facial deformities (Berenyi *et al*). Orv. Hetil., *116:*1767, 1975 (Hungarian)

Unilateral hyperplasia of the mandibular coronoid process. Case report (Kallioniemi *et al*). Proc. Finn. Dent. Soc., *71:*184, 1975

Experience with anesthesia in the surgical treatment of maxillofacial and dental deformities (Aleksandrov *et al*). Stomatologiia (Mosk.), *54:*30, 1975 (Russian)

Use of direct bonding materials for fixation and stabilization in the correction of facial deformities (Booth). J. Oral Surg., *34:*142, 1976

Jaw, Diseases (See also *Maxillary Diseases*)

Fibrous dysplasia of bone and primary hyperparathyroidism (Ehrig *et al*). Ann. Intern. Med., *77:*234, 1972

Spontaneous regression of an intraosseous vascular lesion after aspiration: report of case (Goldberg *et al*). J. Oral Surg., *30:*734, 1972

Spontaneous healing of large osteomyelitic defect in mandible, case report (Silbermann *et al*). J. Oral Surg., *30:*821, 1972

Trismus, plastic – difficult diagnostic problem (Maisels, Priestland), PRS, *55:*105, 1975. Brit. J. Plast. Surg., *26:*223, 1973

Maxilla, osteitis deformans of, report of atypical case (Kirby *et al*). J. Oral Surg., *31:*64, 1973

Aneurysmal bone cyst, case report (Oliver). Oral Surg., *35:*67, 1973

Two cases of coronoid process osteitis. Exceptional localization of mandibular osteitis (Delaire *et al*). Rev. Stomatol. Chir. Maxillofac., *74:*29, 1973 (French)

Case of pseudotumoral osteitis of mandibular angle in children (Delaire *et al*). Rev. Stomatol. Chir. Maxillofac., *74:*321, 1973 (French)

Wisdom teeth and inferior alveolar nerve. Tomographic localization (Crepy *et al*). Rev. Stomatol. Chir. Maxillofac., *74:*548, 1973 (French)

Therapy for central non-odontogenic lesions of the jaws (Bear). Trans. Int. Conf. Oral Surg., *4:*33, 1973

A simple treatment for localized alveolar osteitis (Coletti). Ann. Dent., *33:*46, 1974

Jaws, Paget's disease affecting, clinical problems in (McGowan). Brit. J. Oral Surg., *11:*230, 1974

Myositis ossificans: medial pterygoid muscle – a case report (Narang *et al*). Brit. J. Oral Surg., *12:*229, 1974

Large dental granuloma (? inflammatory pseudotumor) with unusual features, case report (Zegarelli *et al*). J. Am. Dent. Assoc, *89:*891, 1974

Eosinophilic granuloma of bone in childhood: report of case (Catalanotto). J. Dent. Child., *41:*33, 1974

Osteopetrosis: report of case (Boyko *et al*). J. Oral Surg., *32:*859, 1974

Bilateral nasolabial cyst (Brandao *et al*). Oral Surg., *37:*480, 1974

Osseous cryosurgery and its effects on adjacent pulpal tissues (Pollan *et al*). Oral Surg., *38:*668, 1974

Chronic necrotic osteitis of the jaw treated with cartilaginous graft (Krajnik *et al*).

Jaw Diseases — Cont.

Pol. Tyg. Lek., *30:*1879, 1975 (Polish)

Treatment of granulomas and cysts (discussion of their surgical treatment) (Drouillat). Rev. Odontostomatol. (Paris), *4:*123, 1975 (French)

Jaw, Dislocations (See also *Mandibular Condyle; Temporomandibular Joint)*

Jaw luxation, habitual, pathogenesis, clinical aspects and therapy of (Selle). Dtsch. Zahnaerztl. Z., *27:*831, 1972 (German)

Mandible, temporomandibular arthroplasty for chronic dislocation of (Sessions, Porubsky). Laryngoscope, *82:*2273, 1972

Mandibular dislocation, recurrent (Goode, Linehan, Shorago), PRS, *53:*242, 1974. Arch. Otolaryng., *98:*97, 1973

Jaw, forward traction in correction of retrodisplaced maxilla (Ciaburro *et al*), PRS, *52:*687, 1973. Canad. M. A. J., *108:*1511, 1973

Mandible, permanently dislocated, surgical correction of (Rawis *et al*). J. Oral Surg., *31:*385, 1973

Myotomy for management of recurrent and protracted mandibular dislocations (Laskin). Trans. Congr. Int. Assoc. Oral Surg., *4:*264, 1973

Mandible, prolonged traumatic dislocation of (Warren *et al*). J. Oral Surg., *32:*555, 1974

Jaw, Fibrous Dysplasia

Jaws, fibrous dysplastic lesions of, in Nigerians (Williams *et al*). Brit. J. Oral Surg., *11:*118, 1973

Jaws, fibrous dysplasia in, variations (Obwegesser, Freihofer, Horegs), PRS, *53:*603, 1974. J. Maxillo-facial Surg., *1:*161, 1973

Fibrous dysplasia of maxilla, monostoic; report of cases (Hayward *et al*). J. Oral Surg., *31:*625, 1973

Mandible, fibrous dysplasia of, radical operation with simultaneous reparative operation (Alichneiwicz *et al*). Czas. Stomatol., *27:*13, 1974

Mandible, fibrous dysplasia of (Quetglas *et al*), PRS, *57:*532, 1976. Cir. Plast. Ibero-Latino Am., *1:*25, 1975

Jaw Fractures (See also *Craniofacial Injuries; Facial Injuries; Maxillary Fractures)*

Severe compound comminuted fracture of the mandible (Bromige). Brit. J. Oral Surg., *9:*29, 1971

Difficulties in use of percutaneous osteosyn-

Jaw Fractures — Cont.

thesis in the mandible (Birke). Dtsch. Gesundheitsw., *26:*1379, 1971 (German)

Davidoff's craniofacial osteosynthesis and its indications (Davidoff). Dtsch. Stomatol., *21:*589, 1971 (German)

New method of fixation in mandibular fractures (Petz). Dtsch. Stomatol., *21:*653, 1971 (German)

Occlusion problems in functionally stable osteosynthesis of the mandible with teeth (Spiessl *et al*). Dtsch. Zahn. Mund. Kieferheilkd., *57:*293, 1971 (German)

Maxillary fractures, vertical, transverse palatal wire for treatment of (Davis, Constant). PRS, *48:*191, 1971

Mandible, precise immobilization of, simplified splint for (Baker, O'Malley). PRS, *48:*598, 1971

Surgical treatments of fractures of the corpus mandibulae without blockage, with diminutive screwed plates inserted via the endobuccal route (Michelet *et al*). Rev. Odontostomatol. Midi Fr., *29:*87, 1971 (French)

Use of Muller's plates (A–O technic) in mandibular fractures (Cadenat *et al*). Rev. Stomatol. Chir. Maxillofac., *72:*483, 1971 (French)

Surface osteosynthesis in osteoplasty of the mandible (Pavlov). Stomatologiia (Mosk.), *50:*86, 1971 (Russian)

Use of standard V.S. Vasiliev dental band bars in mandibular fractures (Vytrishchak). Stomatologiia (Mosk.), *50:*89, 1971 (Russian)

Mandibular fractures, evaluation of internal wire pin fixation (Fryer *et al*), PRS, *48:*294, 1971. Surg. Gynec. & Obst., *132:*9, 1971

Delayed results of osteoplasty of the mandible (Pavlov). Vestn. Khir., *107:*86, 1971 (Russian)

Mandibular external cortex osteosynthesis using intraoral approach (Peri *et al*). Ann. chir. plast., *17:*184, 1972 (French)

Osteosynthesis, percutaneous, local complications in, (Rostock model) of mandible (Birke). Beitr. Orthop. Traumatol., *19:*700, 1972 (German)

Adjustable locking plate for sectional metal cap splints. A further report (MacGregor). Brit. J. Oral Surg., *9:*251, 1972

Mandibular fractures in edentulous patient (Monteleone *et al*). Clin. Ortop., *23:*273, 1972 (Italian)

Evaluation of surgery of fractures in the temporomandibular joint region (Petz). Dtsch. Stomatol., *22:*411, 1972 (German)

Use of half-implanted splints in the reduction

Jaw Fractures — Cont.

of mandibular fractures (Kovari). Fogorv. Sz., *65:*555, 1972 (Hungarian)

Biodegradable intraosseous appliance in the treatment of mandibular fractures (Getter *et al*). J. Oral Surg., *30:*344, 1972

Use of wire sutures for fracture fixation (Mooney *et al*). Oral Surg., *34:*21, 1972

Evaluation of a compression intraosseous fixation device in mandibular fractures (Boyne *et al*). Oral Surg., *33:*696, 1972

Snowmobile injuries, facial fractures in (Daniel, Midgley). PRS, *49:*38, 1972

Mandible, simple technique for securing K-wire; wire, washer, nut (Mladick *et al*). PRS, *49:*228, 1972

Head halter, modified use for Barton bandage (Green). PRS, *49:*466, 1972

Mandible, Morris bi-phasic external bar splint for fixation (Baumgarten, DesPrez). PRS, *50:*66, 1972

Fractures of upper jaw, experimental study, Parts I and II (Le Fort) (Classic Reprint), PRS, *50:*497, 1972. Part III, PRS, *50:*600, 1972

Mandibular osteosynthesis, intraoral approach (Ciani). Rass. Int. Stomatol. Prat., *23:*163, 1972 (Italian)

Mandibular fractures treated by compression osteosynthesis (Luhr), PRS, *53:*241, 1974. Rev. espan. cir. plast., *5:*193, 1972

Mandibular fractures. Treatment by osteosynthesis by extraoral approach, case report (Dossantos *et al*). Rev. Fac. Odontol. Sao Jose dos Campos, *1:*15, 1972 (Spanish)

Injuries of medial vertical third of face (Pons *et al*). Rev. Fr. Odontostomatol., *19:*27, 1972 (French)

Present day assessment of osteosynthesis using a metal wire in the treatment of mandibular fractures (Bullens). Rev. Stomatol. Chir. Maxillofac, *73:*156, 1972 (French)

Osteosynthesis of fragments of the condyloid process of the mandible with suture placed by retromolar approach (Kozlov *et al*). Stomatologiia (Mosk.), *51:*24, 1972 (Russian)

Replantation as a method of treating high fractures of the neck of the mandibular condyle with dislocation of the articular head (Malyshev). Stomatologiia (Mosk.), *51:*25, 1972 (Russian)

Mandibular fractures, simplified method of suturing in (Gusev). Stomatologiia (Mosk.), *51:*86, 1972 (Russian)

Jaw, lower, rigid internal fixation of fractures of (Spiessl), PRS, *51:*476, 1973. Traum. Reconstr. Surg., *13:*124, 1972

Mandibular fractures, management in bush hospital (Wood, Miller), PRS, *51:*701, 1973.

Jaw Fractures — Cont.

Trop. Doctor, *2:*173, 1972

Surgical treatment of facial fractures (Birke, Sonnenburg). Zahntechnik (Berl.), *13:*443, 1972 (German)

Tissue tolerance and biomechanical questions of monomandibular wire fixation. Zentralbl. Chir., *97:*1008, 1972 (German)

Mandibular fractures, transoral reduction of (Rontal *et al*). Arch. Otolaryng., *97:*279, 1973

Maxilla, fracture of medial aspect. Diagnosis and treatment (May *et al*). Arch. Otolaryng., *97:*286, 1973

Mandible, compression clamp for internal fixation of (Goode *et al*). Arch. Otolaryng., *98:*377, 1973

Mandible, triple fractures with flaring rami. Their treatment with lingual splints (Hardin). Arch. Otolaryng., *98:*387, 1973

Methods for improving fragment adaptation in percutaneous osteosynthesis using plastic bridges (Birke). Dtsch. Stomatol., *23:*721, 1973 (German)

Jaw fractures, intermaxillary immobilization after, weight changes in patients with (Ritzau). Int. J. Oral Surg., *2:*122, 1973

Mandibular and maxillofacial fractures (Synder). J. Am. Osteopath. Assoc., *72:*637, 1973

Mandibular fractures, bilateral, open and closed reduction of, in a child (Kiley). J. Indianap. Dist. Dent. Soc., *27:*17, 1973

Fractures, facial, reduction and immobilization, osteosynthesis with miniaturized screwed plates (Michelet, Deymes, Dessus), PRS, *53:*241, 1974. J. Maxillo-facial Surg., *1:*79, 1973

Mandible, atrophic edentulous, fractures of, another way of treatment (Obwegeser *et al*). J. Maxillo-facial Surg., *1:*213, 1973

Mandibular fractures, experiences with intraoral transosseous wiring of (Freihofer *et al*). J. Maxillo-facial Surg., *1:*248, 1973

Skeletal relapse during intermaxillary fixation (McNeill, Hooley, Sundberg). J. Oral Surg., *31:*212, 1973

Mandibular fracture, nonunited, use of titanium mesh and autogenous bone marrow in repair of: report of case and review of literature (Gargiulo *et al*). J. Oral Surg., *31:*371, 1973

Surgical correction of malunited condylar fracture in child (Kwapis *et al*). J. Oral Surg., *31:*465, 1973

Corrosion of metal fracture fixation appliances (Byrne *et al*). J. Oral Surg., *31:*639, 1973

Percutaneous drilling technique for upper

Jaw Fractures – Cont.

border wiring of fractures of angle of mandible (Seldin). J. Oral Surg., *31:*720, 1973

Fractures, facial, complex, treatment of (Ferraro, Berggren), PRS, *53:*683, 1974. J. Trauma, *13:*783, 1973

Mouth and jaw injuries, care of (Schroder). Langenbecks Arch. Chir., *334:*445, 1973 (German)

Mandibular fractures, management of, in edentulous patients by intramedullary pinning (Bisi). Laryngoscope, *83:*22, 1973

Maxillary fractures, comprehensive care of bilateral (Stone). Laryngoscope, *83:*179, 1973

Mandibular fractures from civilian gunshot wounds: study of 20 cases (May *et al*). Laryngoscope, *83:*969, 1973

Fractures, mandibular, relationship to midface fractures (Linder), PRS, *53:*105, 1974. Mil. Med., *138:*487, 1973

Immobilization period for fractures of the mandibular body (Juniper, Awty), PRS, *54:*235, 1974. Oral Surg., *36:*157, 1973

Maxillary osteotomy, total, for correction of fracture malunion (Moncarz *et al*). Oral Surg., *36:*642, 1973

Osteosynthesis with splints in mandibular fractures (Fischer, Kellner).Osterr. Z. Stomatol., *70:*42, 1973 (German)

Mandible, edentulous, plate osteosynthesis in fractures of (Schroll). Osterr. Z. Stomatol., *70:*394, 1973 (German)

Mandibular fracture in course of labor in newborn infant (Jaworski *et al*). Pediatr. Pol., *48:*1501, 1973 (Polish)

Jaw fractures, replantation of avulsed anterior teeth in patients with (Lu), PRS, *51:*377, 1973

Outer mandibular plate osteosynthesis by endoral approach (Smatt). Rev. Dent. Liban., *23:*38, 1973

Osteosynthesis with steel wire. The "eversant" point in mandibular osteosynthesis (Palfer-Sollier *et al*). Rev. Stomatol. Chir. Maxillofac., *74:*214, 1973 (French)

Current attitudes towards fractures of the dentate portion of the mandible. 350 cases (Vallant *et al*). Rev. Stomatol. Chir. Maxillofac., *74:*216, 1973 (French)

Mandibular osteosynthesis with cortical or transfixing steel wire: the "rubicon" of coherence (Grignon *et al*). Rev. Stomatol. Chir. Maxillofac., *74:*222, 1973 (French)

Results of the use of Muller plates in mandibular osteosynthesis (Cadenat *et al*). Rev. Stomatol. Chir. Maxillofac., *74:*230, 1973 (French)

Mandibular osteosynthesis without blocking

Jaw Fractures – Cont.

by screwed minature stellite plates (Michelet *et al*). Rev. Stomatol. Chir. Maxillofac., *74:*239, 1973 (French)

Osteosynthesis with compression in the treatment of fractures of the lower jaw. Experimental basis and clinical results (Luhr *et al*). Rev. Stomatol. Chir. Maxillofac., *74:*264, 1973 (French)

Mandibular osteosynthesis. Conclusion (Grellet). Rev. Stomatol. Chir. Maxillofac., *74:*276, 1973 (French)

Mandibular fractures, excentric-dynamic compression plate; experimental study as contribution to a functionally stable osteosynthesis in (Schmoker *et al*). Schweiz. Monatsschr. Zahnheilkd., *83:*1496, 1973 (German)

Maxillary injury, accidental, rare case (Stanisavljevic). Srp. Arch. Celok. Lek., *101:*383, 1973 (Serbian)

Maxillary fractures, surgical method of fixation of, according to Adams (Bondar). Stomatologiia (Mosk.), *52:*91, 1973 (Russian)

Cranio-maxillary (mandibular) internal skeletal wiring with steel ligatures in jaw fractures (Nordenram, Hellem, Zettervall). Sven. Tandlak. Tidskr., *66:*81, 1973 (Swedish)

Corrective procedures to repair inadequately treated fractured mandibles and maxillae (Revzin). Trans. Int. Conf. Oral Surg., *4:*299, 1973

Lateral compression in the treatment of mandibular fractures (Kline). Trans. Int. Conf. Oral Surg., *4:*330, 1973

Use of the Morris splint in mandibular fractures (Seligman). Trans. Int. Conf. Oral Surg., *4:*333, 1973

Longstanding bilateral intracapsular fracture dislocation on the condyles treated by closed condylotomy (Canniff). Trans. Int. Conf. Oral Surg., *4:*336, 1973

Bone homoplasty in treatment of ununited fractures of lower jaw complicated by chronic osteomyelitis (Sysoliatin *et al*). Vestn. Khir., *111:*108, 1973

Study of fractures in general. 6. Reproduction of form and function (Schwenzer *et al*). Zahnaerztl. Prax., *24:*518, 1973 (German)

Study of fractures in general. 9. Surgical therapy (Schwenzer *et al*). Zahnaerztl. Prax., *24:*628, 1973 (German)

Small Fragment Set Manual. By U. Heim, and K. M. Pfeiffer. Springer-Verlag, New York, 1974. PRS, *56:*571, 1975

Stable compression plate fixation of mandibular fractures (Becker). Brit. J. Oral Surg., *12:*13, 1974

Jaw Fractures — Cont.

Mandibular process fractures, comparison of results of various therapeutic procedures in problems of (Muska). Cesk. Stomatol., *74:*198, 1974

Condyle, mandibular, unilateral hyperplasia of (Khanna *et al*), PRS, *55:*377, 1975. Indian J. Plast. Surg., *7:*11, 1974

Condylar process, mandibular, experimental study of fractures of (Da Fonseca), PRS, *55:*508, 1975. Internat. J. Oral Surg., *3:*89, 1974

Mandible, fractures of, absorbable synthetic suture material for internal fixation of (Roed-Petersen). Int. J. Oral Surg., *3:*133, 1974

Treatment of long standing bilateral fracture, non- and mal-union in atrophic edentulous mandibles (Boyne *et al*). Int. J. Oral Surg., *3:*213, 1974

Mandible, functionally stable osteosynthesis in (Schilli *et al*). Int. J. Oral Surg., *3:*349, 1974

Mandible, fracture of, external fixation with resin (Saitoh *et al*), PRS, *55:*378, 1975. Jap. J. Plast. Reconstr. Surg., *17:*225, 1974

Jaw fractures, method of internal suspension fixation (Mektubjian), PRS, *55:*379, 1975. J. Maxillo-facial Surg., *2:*134, 1974

Correction of mandibular nonunion and gross malocclusion: report of case (Gelsinon *et al*). J. Oral Surg., *32:*855, 1974

Biphase external fixation: technique and application (Rontal *et al*). Laryngoscope, *84:*1404, 1974

Fractures, maxillofacial, 168 treated at Naval Hospital (Mainous, Crowell, Smith), PRS, *54:*688, 1974. Mil. Med., *139:*278, 1974

Mandible, suppurative osteomyelitis of, secondary to fracture (Limongelli *et al*), PRS *56:*343, 1975. Oral Surg., *38:*850, 1974

Mandibular reductions, open, use of malleable metal mesh in. Report of 9 cases (Curry *et al*). Oral Surg., *38:*335, 1974

Fractures, mandibular, significance of persistent radiolucency of (Kappel *et al*). PRS, *53:*38, 1974

Mandible, experimental study of healing of fractures of membranous bone (Craft *et al*), PRS, *53:*321, 1974

Face, complex fractures of, reduction and fixation with intradiploic cranial screws and acrylic framework (Furnas), PRS, *54:*169, 1974

Fractures, mandibular: intermaxillary fixation using orthodontic brackets bonded to teeth (Minami, Morrill, Weber), PRS, *54:*492, 1974

Fractures, facial, fixation by Orthoplast

Jaw Fractures — Cont.

headcap (Greer, Moore, Coleman), PRS, *54:*614, 1974

Fractures, facial (Hopkins), PRS, *55:*633, 1975. Proc. Roy. Soc. Med., *67:*709, 1974

Jaw injuries, forgotten pioneer in treatment of, Charles Valadier (Mcauley), PRS, *55:*635, 1975. Proc. Roy. Soc. Med., *67:*785, 1974

Intermaxillary and internal wiring fixation. Review of techniques and report of cases (Barakat). Rev. Dent. Livan., *24:*39, 1974

Mandibular fracture, surgical-orthodontic therapy for. Modification of Black-Ivy procedure (Lucas Thomas *et al*). Rev. Esp. Estomatol., *22:*26, 1974 (Spanish)

Mandibular fracture, traumatic, related to radicular cyst, case (Schegg). Schweiz. Monatsschr. Zahnheilkd. *84:*291, 1974 (German)

Osteosynthesis of fractures of the mandible in children by using metal pins (Makienko *et al*). Stomatologiia (Mosk.), *53:*34, 1974 (Russian)

Osteosynthesis of the fractured mandible using homologous bone screws (Malevich *et al*). Stomatologiia (Mosk.), *53:*37, 1974 (Russian)

Treatment of mandibular fractures in the aged (Cherevatenko). Stomatologiia (Mosk.), *53:*46, 1974 (Russian)

Rehabilitation time in patients following restoration of the continuity of the fractured mandible (Ter-Asaturov *et al*). Stomatologiia (Mosk.), *53:*50, 1974 (Russian)

Mid-facial fractures: management and results (Khalil). W. Va. Med. J., *70:*153, 1974

Intra-oral fractures of toothless mandible, experimental studies and clinical experiences with plate osteosynthesis in (Schroll). Z. W. R., *83:*742, 1974 (German)

Experimental studies and clinical experiences with bone plate osteosynthesis in fractures of the edentulous mandible; IV (Schroll). Z. W. R., *83:*934, 1974 (German)

Experimental studies and clinical experiences with bone plate osteosynthesis in fractures of the edentulous mandible; V (Schroll). Z. W. R., *83:*1042, 1974 (German)

Mandibular fractures, surgical treatment. Special study of fractues. (3) (Schwenzer *et al*). Zahnaerztl. Prax., *25:*139, 1974

Fractures. By Charles A. Rockwood and David P. Green. J. B. Lippincott Co., Philadelphia, 1975. PRS, *57:*740, 1976

Fixation of facial fractures. Current concepts (Banks). Brit. Dent. J., *138:*129, 1975

New method of extraoral fixation by pressure (Muska). Cesk. Stomatol., *75:*67, 1975

Jaw Fractures – Cont.
(Czech)
Recurrent problems in emergency room management of maxillofacial injuries (Baker *et al*). Clin. Plast. Surg., *2*:65, 1975
Emergency care of severe facial injuries (Eade). Clin. Plast. Surg., *2*:73, 1975
Fractures of the mandible in motor vehicle accidents (Murray *et al*). Clin. Plast. Surg., *2*:131, 1975
Mandibular osteosynthesis by compression plates, clinical experience with (Tatrai). Forgorv. Sz., *68*:241, 1975 (Hungarian)
Mandibular fracture healing after surgical treatment (Prein *et al*). Fortschr. Kiefer. Gesichtschir., *19*:17, 1975 (German)
Experimental and histological studies in fracture healing on osteotomized rabbit mandibles after immobilization of the fragments by wire sutures and osteosynthesis plates (Schargus *et al*). Fortschr. Kiefer. Gesichtschir., *19*:21, 1975 (German)
Comparative scintigraphic studies following osteosynthesis (Wunderer). Fortschr. Kiefer. Gesichtschir., *19*:24, 1975 (German)
Biomechanics of osteosynthesis in the mandible (Rahn *et al*). Fortschr. Kiefer. Gesichtschir., *19*:37, 1975 (German)
Electronic measurements of biomechanics in mandibular osteosynthesis (Niederdellmann). Fortschr. Kiefer. Gesichtschir., *19*:42, 1975 (German)
Functionally stable osteosynthesis in mandibular fractures – problems and technic (Spiessl). Fortschr. Kiefer. Gesichtschir., *19*:68, 1975 (German)
Indication, technic and clinical results of compression osteosynthesis in mandibular fractures (5-year experience) (Schmitz *et al*). Fortschr. Kiefer. Gesichtschir., *19*:74, 1975 (German)
Report on results of the treatment of mandibular fractures with osteosynthesis plates (Scharf *et al*). Fortschr. Kiefer. Gesichtschir., *19*:82, 1975 (German)
Lingual splinting and interosseous fixation for early mobilization of mandibular symphysis/condyle fractures (Small). Fortschr. Kiefer. Gesichtschir., *19*:96, 1975 (German)
Surgical treatment of multiple mandibular fractures by means of wire osteosynthesis (Dieckmann *et al*). Fortschr. Kiefer. Gesichtshir., *19*:97, 1975 (German)
Technic and indication for the open axial medullary wiring in mandibular fractures (Fries). Fortschr. Kiefer. Gesichtschir., *19*:108, 1975 (German)
Clinical aspects of Fries' open and axial med-

Jaw Fractures – Cont.
ullary wiring in mandibular fractures (Langer *et al*). Fortschr. Kiefer. Gesichtschir., *19*:109, 1975 (German)
Relocation osteoplasty in pseudarthrosis of the mandible (Merkx). Fortschr. Kiefer. Gesichtschir., *19*:125, 1975 (German)
Importance of joint operative action in midfacial fractures and fractures of the frontal cranial base by the dental surgeon and the otolaryngologist (Langnickel *et al*). Fortschr. Kiefer. Gesichtschir., *19*:132, 1975 (German)
Surgical treatment of mandibular fractures during the age of growth (Kruger *et al*). Fortschr. Kiefer. Gesichtschir., *19*:201, 1975 (German)
Late results of osteosynthesis treatment in juvenile jaw fractures (Perko *et al*). Fortschr. Kiefer. Gesichtschir., *19*:206, 1975 (German)
Primary and secondary treatment in chin defect fractures (Reuther *et al*). Fortschr. Kiefer. Gesichtschir., *19*:215, 1975 (German)
Fractures, condylar, long-term results of functional treatment (Schettler, Rehrmann), PRS, *56*:463, 1975. J. Maxillo-facial Surg., *3*:14, 1975
Longitudinal study on electrical pulp testing following Le Fort type osteotomy and Le Fort type fracture (Tajima). J. Maxillo-facial Surg., *3*:74, 1975
Multiple facial trauma complicated by occlusion of the internal carotid artery (Garrison *et al*). J. Oral Surg., *33*:131, 1975
Occlusion of the internal carotid artery associated with mandibular fracture (Berman). J. Oral Surg., *33*:134, 1975
Use of Scialom pins for fracture fixation (Bahn). J. Oral Surg., *33*:268, 1975
Intraoral use of Kirschner pins (Reyes-Guerra). J. Oral Surg., *33*:304, 1975
Fractures, facial, survey of (Kelly, Harrigan), PRS, *57*:260, 1976. Oral Surg., *33*:146, 1975
Mandibular fractures, lateral compression clamp for (Norkus *et al*), PRS, *56*:598, 1975. Oral Surg., *39*:2, 1975
Mouth protectors, mandatory, case for (Heintz), PRS, *57*:406, 1976. Phys. & Sports Med., *3*:60, 1975
Fracture, maxillary, quick simple method for fixation of upper denture to maxilla (Bartels, Mara), PRS, *56*:221, 1975
Fractures of mandible (Melmed, Koonin), PRS, *56*:323, 1975
Functional treatment of fractures of the mandibular condyle and its neck (Delaire *et al*).

Jaw Fractures – Cont.

Rev. Stomatol. Chir. Maxillofac., *76:*331, 1975 (French)

Surgical treatment of a pseudoarthrosis of the mandible (Thomas *et al*). Rev. Stomatol. Chir. Maxillofac., *76:*489, 1975 (French)

Problems posed during surgical repair of a gunshot wound in the mandible (Roulaud *et al*). Rev. Stomatol. Chir. Maxillofac., *76:*493, 1975 (French)

Surgical treatment of mandibular fractures (Sonnenburg). Stomatol. D.D.R., *25:*673, 1975

Osteosynthesis of fragments of the mandible by homologous grafting of sections and ultrasonic coagulation (Petrov *et al*). Stomatologiia (Mosk.), *54:*29, 1975 (Russian)

Compression osteosynthesis by spikes with supports in fractures of the mental portion of the mandible (Zakharov *et al*). Stomatologiia (Mosk.), *54:*71, 1975 (Russian)

Comparative histological studies on various methods for osteosynthesis in the mandible (Bienengraber *et al*). Zahn. Mund. Kieferheilkd., *63:*668, 1975 (German)

Chain saw injury of the mandibulofacial region (Loe *et al*). J. Oral Surg., *34:*81, 1976

Dislocation of the condyle into the middle cranial fossa (Seymour *et al*). J. Oral Surg., *34:*180, 1976

Traumatic air embolism (Bowen *et al*). Med. Sci. Law, *16:*56, 1976

Fractured mandible, from initial operation to removal of tantalum mesh. Report of a case (Goldberg *et al*). Oral Surg., *41:*32, 1976

Technique for open reduction of subcondylar fractures (Peters *et al*). Oral Surg., *41:*273, 1976

Clamps, pericortical "compression" for mandibular fixation (Lung, Graham, Miller), PRS, *57:*487, 1976

Functionally stable osteosynthesis of the mandible by means of an excentric-dynamic compression plate. Results of a follow-up of 25 cases (Schmoker *et al*). Schweiz. Monatsschr. Zahnheilkd., *86:*167, 1976 (German)

Jaw Fractures in Children

Child, bilateral mandibular fractures in, open and closed reduction of (Kiley). J. Indianap. Dist. Dent. Soc., *27:*17, 1973

Fractures, mandibular, in young children, definitive treatment of (Leake *et al*), PRS, *54:*107, 1974. Oral Surg., *36:*164, 1973

Infant, newborn, mandibular fracture in, in course of labor (Jaworski *et al*). Pediatr. Pol., *48:*1501, 1973 (Polish)

Jaw, Infection of

Maxilla and mandible, chronic sclerosing osteomyelitis of; review of literature and case report (Towns). J. Oral Surg., *30:*903, 1972

Tooth extraction, fatal necrotizing fasciitis after (Crowson), PRS, *53:*602, 1974. Am. Surgeon, *39:*525, 1973

Current concepts in the treatment of acute and chronic osteomyelitis (Khosla). Trans. Int. Conf. Oral Surg., *4:*116, 1973

Maxillary osteomyelitis, isolation of Candida Tropicalis from orbital infection as complication of (Segal *et al*). Infection, *2:*111, 1974

Mandible, chronic osteomyelitis of, surgical treatment (Glahn), PRS, *55:*717, 1975. J. Maxillo-facial Surg., *2:*238, 1974

Jaw, mixed anaerobic infection of, case (Sharp *et al*). J. Oral Surg., *32:*457, 1974

Osteomyelitis, iatrogenic osteolysis, pathologic fracture and bone graft (Ellis *et al*). Oral Surg., *37:*364, 1974

Mandibular osteomyelitis in patient with chronic alcoholism: etiology, management, and statistical correlation (Silbermann *et al*). Oral Surg., *38:*530, 1974

Head and neck abscesses, conservative treatment of (Cosma, Popescu), PRS, *57:*670, 1976. J. Maxillo-facial Surg., *3:*198, 1975

Proteus vulgaris osteomyelitis of the mandible. Report of a case (Friedlander). Oral Surg., *40:*39, 1975

Condition of oxidation-reduction processes in patients with chronic osteomyelitis of the jaw and phlegmons of the maxillofacial area in connection with surgical intervention and anesthesia (Roznovan). Stomatologiia (Mosk.), *54:*33, 1975

Secondary sutures in the treatment of submandibular phlegmons (Kolodkin). Stomatologiia (Mosk.), *54:*86, 1975 (Russian)

Jaw, Micrognathia: See *Micrognathia*

Jaw Neoplasms (See also *Cancer, Head and Neck; Jaw, Ameloblastoma; Jaw, Fibrous Dysplasia; Jaw, Odontogenic Tumors; Maxillary Neoplasms*)

Mandible, periosteum and intraoral carcinoma (Marchetta, Sako, Murphy), PRS, *51:*608, 1973. Am. J. Surg., *122:*711, 1971

Osteogenic sarcoma of the facial and cranial bones. A review of forty-three cases (Caron *et al*). Am. J. Surg., *122:*719, 1971

Resection of the mandible in children. Considerations on its reconstruction (Freidel *et al*). Ann. chir. plast., *16:*227, 1971 (French)

Mandible, immediate functional restoration

Jaw Neoplasma – Cont.

after surgical treatment of advanced oral cancer (McQuarrie), PRS, *49:*103, 1972. Arch. Surg., *102:*447, 1971

Myxoma of mandible. Case report (Uthman *et al*). Brit. J. Oral Surg., *9:*151, 1971

Maxilla, chondrosarcomas of (Paddison, Hanks), PRS, *49:*474, 1972. Cancer, *28:*616, 1971

Prosthetic treatment after surgical removal of tumors in the jaw region (Schanewede). Dtsch. Stomatol., *21:*765, 1971 (German)

Clinical and histopathological study on chemotherapy of maxillary cancer with special reference to bleomycin (Takasaki). J. Otolaryngol. Jap., *74:*1129, 1971 (Japanese)

Fibrosarcoma of the mandible (Jochimsen *et al*). Minn. Med., *54:*929, 1971

Clinical remarks and considerations on preservation of the mandible in the Commando operation (Voena *et al*). Minerva Otorinolaringol., *21:*186, 1971 (Italian)

Surgery of retromaxillary space (Zehm). Monatsschr. Ohrenheilkd. Laryngorhinol., *105:*147, 1971 (German)

Mandible, defects of, Webb bolt as space maintaining appliance in (Hamilton) (Follow-Up Clinic), PRS, *48:*368, 1971

Mandible replantation in cancer surgery (Harding) (Follow-Up Clinic), PRS, *48:*586, 1971

Effect of hemimandibulectomy on the remaining temporomandibular joint (Schneider *et al*). Pract. Otorhinolaryngol. (Basel), *33:*1, 1971 (German)

Radiation resistant angiomas of the jaws (surgical treatment – report of 3 cases) (Michelet *et al*). Rev. Odontostomatol. Midi Fr., *29:*3, 1971 (French)

Mandible, chondrosarcoma of (Lanier, Rosenfeld, Wilkinson), PRS, *49:*109, 1972. South. M. J., *60:*711, 1971

Jaw, upper, case of giant osteochondroma of (Ozinkovskii *et al*). Zh. Ushn. Nos. Gori. Belezn., *31:*108, 1971 (Russian)

Mandible, osteosarcoma of, unusual case, diagnostic problems (Lathouwer). Acta Stomatol. Belg., *69:*429, 1972 (French)

Surgical management of premaxillary malignancy. Report of three cases (Tucker *et al*). Arch. Otolaryng., *95:*42, 1972

Mandibular resections (personal contribution to surgery of head and neck neoplasms). 1. Introduction (Editorial). Arq. Patol., *44:*5, 1972 (Portuguese)

Mandibular resection. 2. On cancer surgery (Editorial). Arq. Patol., *44:*9, 1972 (Portuguese)

Jaw Neoplasma – Cont.

Mandibular resections. 3. Surgical anatomy of mandible. Arq. Patol., *44:*21, 1972 (Portuguese)

Mandibular resections, 5. Arq. Patol., *44:*59, 1972 (Portuguese)

Mandible, myxoma of, with 35-year follow-up (Cawson). Brit. J. Oral Surg., *10:*59, 1972

Mandible, fibrosarcoma of, with pulmonary metastases: case report (MacFarlane). Brit. J. Oral Surg., *10:*168, 1972

Mandible, replacing, in oral cancer (Stark), PRS, *52:*327, 1973. Ca-A Cancer J. Clin., *22:*303, 1972

Immediate massive bone graft after block surgery of cancers of buccal cavity (Rodier *et al*). Chirurgie, *97:*785, 1972 (French)

Jaws, neoplastic tumors and neoplasm-like tumors of, in children, treatment (Gorski). Czas. Stomatol., *25:*817, 1972 (Polish)

Results of surgical treatment of jaw sarcoma (Gorski *et al*). Dtsch. Zahn. Mund. Kieferheilkd., *58:*250, 1972 (German)

Recurrent mandibular myxoma (Balogh *et al*). Forgorv. Sz., *65:*116, 1972 (Hungarian)

Maxillofacial region, cylindromas of (Stiebitz). Fortschr. Kiefer. Gesichtschir., *15:*60, 1972 (German)

Odontomaxillary surgery, adenomeloblastoma (Pinto *et al*), PRS, *53:*110, 1974. Gazeta sanit., *3:*127, 1972

Resection of the mandible in oral tumors (Rosemann). H.N.O., *20:*166, 1972 (German)

Mandibulectomy for malignant tumors, postoperative dysphagia after, clinical and cinefluorographic studies on (Ohhata). J. Jap. Stomatol. Soc., *39:*611, 1972 (Japanese)

Plastic reconstitution of functional rehabilitation after great surgical ablations in maxillofacial tumors (Popescu *et al*). J. Med. Lyon, *53:*303, 1972 (French)

Morphofunctional reconstitution of the mandible after extirpation of benign tumors or tumors with a local clinical malignancy (Timosca). J. Med. Lyon., *53:*353, 1972 (French)

Maxilla, leiomyosarcoma of, autopsy case (Takagi *et al*). J. Oral Pathol., *1:*125, 1972

Maxillary cancer, results of treatment of, in our department and future problems (Hirano *et al*). J. Otolaryngol. Jap., *75:*1088, 1972 (Japanese)

Cancers, pelvi-gingival, indications for surgery in (Richard *et al*). J. Radiol. Electrol. Med. Nucl., *53:*475, 1972 (French)

Maxillary tumors (Editorial). Monatsschr. Ohrenheilkd. Laryngorhinol., *106:*393, 1972 (German)

Jaw Neoplasma — Cont.

Maxillary tumors, radiotherapy of (Sala *et al*). Monatsschr. Ohrenheilkd. Laryngorhinol., *106:*396, 1972 (German)

Maxillary tumors, malignant, disease course and late results (Alajmo). Monatsschr. Ohrenheilkd. Laryngorhinol., *106:*398, 1972 (German)

Myxoma treated by peripheral ostectomy. Six-year follow-up (Himmelfarb *et al*). N. Y. State Dent. J., *38:*612, 1972

Maxilla, dysontegenic tumors of, in infancy (Deutschmann *et al*). Paediatr. Grenzgeb., *11:*141, 1972

Sarcoma of midface, resection of base of skull for (Dingman). Trans. Am. Acad. Ophthalmol. Otolaryngol., *76:*1371, 1972

Jaw tumors, surgery of (Davey), PRS, *50:*536, 1972. Trop. Doctor, *1:*170, 1972

Jaw resection, partial, in central giant cell granulomas (Mehnert *et al*). Zahnaerztl. Prax., *23:*433, 1972

Carcinoma, mandible, result of radiation therapy (Fayos). Acta Radiol. (Ther.) (Stockh.), *12:*378, 1973

Jaw preservation in one stage surgical repair of mandibular osteoradionecrosis (Nickell *et al*), PRS, *53:*682, 1974. Am. J. Surg., *126:*502, 1973

Maxilla, hemangioma of (Sawhney *et al*). Ann. Otol. Rhin. & Laryng., *82:*254, 1973

Mandible and ear, unusual tumors of (Horowitz). Arch. Klin. Exp. Ohren Nasen Kehlkopfheilkd., *205:*203, 1973 (German)

Some aspects of surgical treatment of tumors of head and neck which involve bone (Wilson, Westbury). Brit. J. Radiol., *46:*151, 1973

Alveolus, lower, carcinoma involving (Lee, Wilson), PRS, *52:*458, 1973. Brit. J. Surg., *60:*85, 1973

Jaw tumors in children (Deliner), PRS, *54:*235, 1974. Cancer, *32:*112, 1973

Jaw bones, myxoma of (Ghosh *et al*), PRS, *51:*707, 1973. Cancer, *31:*237, 1973

Incidence of osseous giant-cell tumors in otorhinolaryngology (Hlavacek). Cesk. Otolaryngol., *22:*77, 1973 (Czechoslovakian)

Mandible, osseous reconstruction following surgical resection (Boyne), PRS, *53:*365, 1974. J. Biomed. Mater. Res., *7:*195, 1973

Hodgkin's disease of maxilla (Tiwari). J. Laryng. & Otol., *87:*85, 1973

Maxilla, osteosarcoma and chondrosarcoma of (Wolfowitz). J. Laryng. & Otol., *87:*409, 1973

Maxilla, myxoma of, case report (Mostafa *et al*). J. Laryng. & Otol., *87:*1143, 1973

Jaw Neoplasma — Cont.

Jaw, radio-osteomyelitis of, recurrence of oral cancer in patients with (Nwokus), PRS, *53:*682, 1974. J. Maxillo-facial Surg., *1:*157, 1973

Mandible, central giant cell lesion in angle of; review of literature and report of case (Richter *et al*). J. Oral Surg., *31:*26, 1973

Mandible, osteogenic sarcoma of: review of literature and report of case (Wilcox *et al*). J. Oral Surg., *31:*49, 1973

Fibroma, giant cemento-ossifying, of maxilla: report of case and discussion (Small, Goodman). J. Oral Surg., *31:*113, 1973

Maxilla, myxoma of, report of case (Byrd, Kindrick, Dunsworth). J. Oral Surg., *31:*123, 1973

Mandibular canal, solitary intraosseous neurofibroma involving, case report (Singer, Gienger, Kullbom). J. Oral Surg., *31:*127, 1973

Squamous cell carcinoma arising in dentigerous cyst (Lapin *et al*). J. Oral Surg., *31:*354, 1973

Squamous cell carcinoma possibly arising from odontogenic cyst: report of case (Hampl *et al*). J. Oral Surg., *31:*359, 1973

Maxilla, metastatic bronchogenic carcinoma to: case report (Adler *et al*). J. Oral Surg., *31:*543, 1973

Fibroma, peripheral ossifying, report of case (Friedlander *et al*). J. Oral Surg., *31:*547, 1973

Eosinophilic granuloma of bone: case report (Snyder *et al*). J. Oral Surg., *31:*712, 1973

Mandible, eosinophilic granuloma of (Albers *et al*). J. Oral Surg., *31:*841, 1973

Intraosseous malignant mixed tumor of maxilla; review of literature and case report (Fleitz *et al*). J. Oral Surg., *31:*927, 1973

Mandible, hemangioma of (Gill, Long, MacLennan). J. Roy. Coll. Surg. Edinb., *18:*52, 1973

Mesenchymoma of mandible (Muldoon). J. Surg. Oncol., *5:*291, 1973

Anatomical and clinical features of mesenchymal tumors of the jaws (Odasso *et al*). Minerva Stomatol., *22:*269, 1973 (Italian)

Maxillofacial cancer, patients with. 1. Surgical treatment and nursing care (Welty *et al*). Nurs. Clin. North Am., *8:*137, 1973

Jaws, benign fibro-osseous lesions of: clinical-radiologic-histologic review of 65 cases (Waldron *et al*). Oral Surg., *35:*190, 1973

Carcinoma, squamous cell, of mandible, primary intra-alveolar. Report of a case (Sirsat, Sampat, Shrikhande). Oral Surg., *35:*366, 1973

Mandible, fibrosarcoma of, case report

Jaw Neoplasma — Cont.

(Wright *et al*). Oral Surg., *36:*16, 1973

Maxilla, central giant-cell lesion of: enucleation and immediate reconstruction (Pedersen). Oral Surg., *36:*790, 1973

Jaw, lower, myxoma of (Stewart *et al*). Oral Surg., *36:*800, 1973

Facial reconstruction: compound silicone-bone implants for mandibular reconstruction (Swanson *et al*), PRS, *51:*402, 1973

Case of basocellular nevomatosis (Grellet *et al*). Rev. Stomatol. Chir. Maxillofac., *74:*97, 1973

Maxillary fibromyxoma, massive, case (Vaillant *et al*). Rev. Stomatol. Chir. Maxillofac., *74:*473, 1973 (French)

Therapy and prognosis of malignant mesenchymal tumors in the mouth and jaw region (Mopert *et al*). Stomatol. D.D.R., *23:*525, 1973 (German)

Maxillofacial area, malignant neoplasms of, elimination of hazards in radical operations in (Malevich *et al*). Stomatologiia (Mosk.), *52:*24, 1973 (Russian)

Jaw, upper, malignant tumors of, treatment (Kavrokirov *et al*). Stomatologiia (Sofia), *55:*11, 1973 (Bulgarian)

Histopathology of some central non-odontogenic tumours and tumour-like conditions of the jaws (Kramer). Trans. Int. Conf. Oral Surg., *4:*28, 1973

Therapy for central non-odontogenic lesions of the jaws (Bear). Trans. Int. Conf. Oral Surg., *4:*33, 1973

Review of hyperparathyroidism and an interesting case presenting with a giant cell lesion (Chapnich). Trans. Int. Conf. Oral Surg., *4:*44, 1973

Central mucoepidermoid tumour of the mandible (Friedman *et al*). Trans. Int. Conf. Oral Surg., *4:*129, 1973

Secondary tumours of the maxilla (Towers). Trans. Int. Conf. Oral Surg., *4:*138, 1973

Bleomycin therapy of oral cancer (Watanabe *et al*). Trans. Int. Conf. Oral Surg., *4:*147, 1973

Hemimaxillectomy, indications and technique of, for treatment of advanced malignancy of maxilla (Sammis). Trans. Congr. Int. Assoc. Oral Surg., *4:*154, 1973

Two cases of osteogenic sarcoma of the mandible; indications for immediate reconstruction (De Lathouwer *et al*). Acta Chir. Belg., *73:*49, 1974 (French)

Extracardiac rhabdomyoma. Light and electron microscopic stdies of two cases in the mandibular area, with a review of previous reports (Albrechtsen *et al*). Acta Otolaryngol. (Stockh.), *78:*458, 1974

Jaw Neoplasma — Cont.

Jaw, osteoradionecrosis of (Guttenberg), PRS, *54:*499, 1974. Am. J. Surg., *127:*326, 1974

"Andy Gump." (Steckler *et al*). Am. J. Surg., *128:*545, 1974

Maxilla, carcinoma, surgical management (Som). Arch. Otolaryng., *99:*270, 1974

Maxilla, brown tumor of, in secondary hyperparathyroidism (Friedman *et al*). Arch. Otolaryng., *100:*157, 1974

Giant cell tumor of jaws associated with Paget disease of bone. Report of two cases and review of literature (Miller *et al*). Arch. Otolaryng., *100:*233, 1974

Maxilla, adenoid cystic carcinoma of (Horree), PRS, *56:*594, 1975. Arch Otolaryng., *100:*469, 1974

Mandible, myxoma of: resection and immediate reconstruction (Guralnick *et al*). Brit. J. Oral Surg., *11:*217, 1974

Haemangioma of the mandible: a case report (Gruss). Brit. J. Oral Surg., *12:*24, 1974

Central fibroma of the jaws (Ferguson). Brit. J. Oral Surg., *12:*205, 1974

Osteoma of the mandible (MacLennan *et al*). Brit. J. Oral Surg., *12:*219, 1974

An osteoma of the mandible (Green *et al*). Brit. J. Oral Surg., *12:*255, 1974

Desmoplastic fibroma of the mandible (Badger *et al*). Can. J. Otolaryngol., *3:*605, 1974

Mandibular tumors in primary hyperparathyroidism, diagnostic difficulties in (Rowinska *et al*). Czas. Stomatol., *27:*19, 1974 (Czechoslovakian)

Pterygoid fossa, surgery (Harpman). Eye, Ear, Nose, Throat Mon., *53:*354, 1974

Mandible, desmoplastic fibroma in (Hovinga *et al*). Int. J. Oral Surg., *3:*41, 1974

Mandible, neurilemmoma in, case (Sugimura *et al*). Int. J. Oral Surg., *3:*194, 1974

A hepatocarcinoma with osseous metastases (Muldoon). J. Laryng. & Otol., *88:*891, 1974

Maxilla, osteogenic sarcoma of (Madhavan *et al*). J. Laryng. & Otol., *88:*1125, 1974

Maxilla, chondrosarcoma of: surgery and reconstruction (Zehnder *et al*). J. La. State Med. Soc., *126:*243, 1974

Tumors of mandible, intraoral partial resection and reconstruction (Sailer), PRS, *55:*716, 1975. J. Maxillo-facial Surg., *2:*173, 1974

Jaws, osteosarcoma of, report of case and review of literature (Curtis *et al*). J. Oral Surg., *32:*125, 1974

Maxilla, giant cell tumor of, complicating Paget's disease of bone (Goldstein *et al*). J.

Jaw Neoplasma — Cont.

Oral Surg., *32:*209, 1974

Mandible, osteoradionecrosis of (Marciani, Plezia), PRS, *55:*247, 1975. J. Oral Surg., *32:*435, 1974

Mesenchymal chondrosarcoma, case report (Pittman *et al*). J. Oral Surg., *32:*443, 1974

Mandible, central mucoepidermoid tumor (carcinoma) (Alexander *et al*.). J. Oral Surg., *32:*541, 1974

Carcinoma, central mucoepidermoid, arising in maxillary odontogenic cyst (Marano, Hartman), PRS, *56:*363, 1975. J. Oral Surg., *32:*915, 1974

Premaxilla, angiosarcoma of (Karmody *et al*). Laryngoscope, *84:*560, 1974

Cryosurgical treatment of recurrent head and neck malignancies — a comparative study (Good *et al*). Laryngoscope, *84:*1950, 1974

Amputation and adriamycin in primary osteosarcoma (Cortes *et al*). New England J. Med., *29:*998, 1974

Mandible, primary osteogenic neoplasms of (Kulakowski *et al*). Nowotwory, *24:*23, 1974 (Polish)

Mandibular coronoid process, osteochondroma of, case report (James *et al*). Oral Surg., *37:*189, 1974

Mandible, osteochondroma of (Allan *et al*). Oral Surg., *37:*556, 1974

Benign osteoblastoma of the maxilla (Yip *et al*). Oral Surg., *38:*259, 1974

Jaw, metastatic malignant tumors of (Linkous, Welch), PRS, *56:*365, 1975. Oral Surg., *38:*703, 1974

Jaw replacement, intraoral malignancy with special reference to. Problems of reconstruction following preoperative radiotherapy (Harrison). Proc. Roy. Soc. Med., *67:*601, 1974

Mandibular malignancy, oral rehabilitation following surgical treatment of (Franks). Proc. Roy. Soc. Med., *67:*614, 1974

Maxillofacial surgery, malignant tumors in (Dos Reis *et al*). Rev. Port. Estomatol. Cir. Maxilofac., *15:*71, 1974

Management of a multilocular cystic image of the mandible (Freidel *et al*). Rev. Stomatol. Chir. Maxillofac., *75:*61, 1974 (French)

Pigmented tumor of the maxilla in the child (Mugnier *et al*). Rev. Stomatol. Chir. Maxillofac., *75:*771, 1974 (French)

Ewing's sarcoma localized to the mandible. 2 cases (Brocheriou *et al*). Rev. Stomatol. Chir. Maxillofac., *75:*877, 1974 (French)

Malignant mandibular schwannoma (Cernea *et al*). Rev. Stomatol. Chir. Maxillofac.,

Jaw Neoplasma — Cont.

*75:*1103, 1974 (French)

Jaw tumors, surgically removed, correction by stored allografts (Koumoura *et al*). Stomatologia (Athenai), *31:*197, 1974 (Greek)

Chondrosarcoma of the jaw (Martes *et al*). Stomatologia (Athenai), *31:*215, 1974 (Greek)

Use of preserved homologous embryonic bone in the reconstruction or restoration of defects following excision of cysts and benign tumors of the jaws (Zakharov *et al*). Stomatologiia (Mosk.), *53:*90, 1974 (Russian)

Diagnosis, surgical and radiotherapeutic treatment of malignant tumors of the upper jaw (Dimopoulos *et al*). Strahlentherapie, *147:*416, 1974

Lymphangioma of the maxilla in a newborn infant (Kspoian). Vestn. Khir., *112:*82, 1974 (Russian)

Postoperative bronchopulmonary complications in malignant neoplasms of maxillofacial localization (Dunaevskii *et al*). Vestn. Khir., *113:*69, 1974 (Russian)

Jaw, upper, intraoral complete resection (Shinbirev). Zdravookhr. Ross. Fed., *5:*106, 1974 (Russian)

Carcinoma, squamous cell, of gingiva. Histological classification and grading of malignancy (Willen *et al*). Acta Otolaryngol. (Stockh.), *79:*146, 1975

Gallium-67 scintigraphy in the diagnosis of tumors in oromaxillofacial surgery (Maerker *et al*). Acta Stomatol. Belg., *72:*399, 1975 (German)

Osteogenic sarcoma (osteosarcoma): results of therapy (Stein). Am. J. Roentgenol. Radium Ther. Nucl. Med., *123:*607, 1975

Desmoplastic fibroma of the mandible. A case report (Cunningham *et al*). Ann. Otol. Rhin. & Laryng., *84:*125, 1975

Surgical management of osteogenic sarcoma of the mandible (Pease *et al*). Arch. Otolaryng., *101:*761, 1975

Mandible, central angioma of, possible treatment (Monks), PRS, *57:*677, 1976. Brit. J. Oral Surg., *12:*296, 1975

Haemangioma of the maxilla: a case report (Tyldesley *et al*). Brit. J. Oral Surg., *13:*56, 1975

Jaws, eosinophilic granuloma with bilateral involvement (Ragab *et al*). Int. J. Oral Surg., *4:*73, 1975

Mandibular myoblastoma, congenital (Hulagu, Erez, Ocak), PRS, *56:*222, 1975. Internat. Surg., *60:*46, 1975

Maxilla, desmoplastic fibroma of (Sood *et al*). J. Laryng. & Otol., *89:*329, 1975

Jaw Neoplasma – Cont.

Carcinoma, squamous cell, of gums, prognosis of, with cytologically verified cervical lymph node metastases (Backstom *et al*). J. Laryng. & Otol., *89:*391, 1975

Central hemangioma of the mandible: intraoral resection and reconstruction (Piercell *et al*). J. Oral Surg., *33:*225, 1975

A "true giant cell tumor" in the mandible? (Small *et al*). J. Oral Surg., *33:*296, 1975

Mandibular condyle, myxoma of – surgical excision with immediate reconstruction (Colburn *et al*). J. Oral Surg., *33:*351, 1975

Fibroma, ossifying, case report (Gay *et al*). J. Oral Surg., *33:*368, 1975

Mandible, primary Ewing's sarcoma, case report (Blakemore *et al*). J. Oral Surg., *33:*376, 1975

Mandible, central cavernous hemangioma of (Gelfand *et al*). J. Oral Surg., *33:*448, 1975

Myxomatous tumors of the jaws (Kangur *et al*). J. Oral Surg., *33:*523, 1975

Histochemical studies of myxoma of the jaws (Mori *et al*). J. Oral Surg., *33:*529, 1975

Central cavernous hemangioma of the mandible treated by an intraoral approach (Zalesin *et al*). J. Oral Surg., *33:*877, 1975

Reconstruction of the oral cavity after extirpation of the malignant tumor of the oral floor and the mandible (Konno *et al*). J. Otolaryngol. Jpn., *78:*154, 1975 (Japanese)

Cervical-pectoral flaps in the treatment of advanced oral cancer (Shons *et al*). J. Surg. Oncol., *7:*213, 1975

Reticulosarcoma of the maxilla (Ristic *et al*). Med. Pregl., *28:*541, 1975 (Serbian)

Myxomas in jaw. Case of bilateral maxillary myxomas (Sveen *et al*). Nor. Tannlaegeforen Tid., *85:*230, 1975

Metastatic renal adenocarcinoma presenting as periapical pathosis in the maxilla. (Milobsky *et al*). Oral Surg., *39:*30, 1975

Primary malignant hemangioendothelioma of the gingiva. Report of a case and review of the literature (Wesley *et al*). Oral Surg., *39:*103, 1975

Multiple odontogenic tumors and other anomalies. An autosomal dominantly inherited syndrome (Schmidseder *et al*). Oral Surg., *39:*249, 1975

Benign osteoblastoma (Remagen *et al*). Oral Surg., *39:*279, 1975

Oral Kaposi's sarcoma (Farman *et al*). Oral Surg., *39:*288, 1975

Central adenocarcinoma of the mandible (Toth *et al*). Oral Surg., *39:*436, 1975

Central pacinian neurofibroma of the maxilla (Toth *et al*). Oral Surg., *39:*630, 1975

Jaw Neoplasma – Cont.

Ultrastructure of an odontogenic myxoma (Simes *et al*). Oral Surg., *39:*640, 1975

Paget's disease of bone, case report (Akin *et al*). Oral Surg., *39:*707, 1975

Central myxofibrosarcoma of the mandible treated by radical resection (Kummoona). Oral Surg., *39:*713, 1975

Retrosternal parathyroid adenomas manifesting in the form of a giant-cell "tumor" of the mandible (Akinoso *et al*). Oral Surg., *39:*724, 1975

Mandibular metastasis of osteogenic sarcoma, case report (Ohba *et al*). Oral Surg., *39:*821, 1975

Mandible, primary reticulum-cell sarcoma of. Review of literature and report of case (Campbell *et al*). Oral Surg., *39:*918, 1975

Melanotic neuroectodermal tumor of infancy. Report of a case (Hoggins *et al*). Oral Surg., *40:*34, 1975

Central mucoepidermoid tumors of the jaws. Report of nine cases and review of the literature (Browand *et al*). Oral Surg., *40:*631, 1975

Hemangioma: arteriovenous malformations of mandible, graduated surgical management (Bryant, Maull), PRS, *55:*690, 1975. Discussion by Bennett, PRS, *56:*84, 1975

Mandibular resection for carcinoma, simple method for determining limits (Horton, Sharzer), PRS, *56:*101, 1975

Orbito-maxillary resections for cancer, use of temporal muscle flap for reconstruction after (Bakamjian, Souther), PRS, *56:*171, 1975

Plombage with osseous homotransplants in some mandibular tumors (Popescu *et al*). Rev. Chir. (Stomatol.), *22:*209, 1975 (Rumanian)

Results obtained with bone homograft in cystic tumors of the jaw (Popescu *et al*). Rev. Odontostomatol. (Paris), *4:*51, 1975 (French)

Osseous desmoid fibroma of the mandible, apropos of 1 case (Rouchon *et al*). Rev. Stomatol. Chir. Maxillofac., *76:*527, 1975 (French)

Reconstruction of the defective mandible (Branemark *et al*). Scand. J. Plast. Reconstr. Surg., *9:*116, 1975

Osteochondroma of mandibular condyle (Wang-Norderud, Ragab), PRS, *57:*672, 1976. Scand. J. Plast. Reconstr. Surg., *9:*165, 1975

Rehabilitation needs of the cancer patient (Villanueva). South. Med. J., *68:*169, 1975

Myxoma of the jaw: clinical picture, diagno-

Jaw Neoplasma – Cont.

sis and treatment (Solov'ev *et al*). Stomatologiia (Mosk.), *54:*37, 1975 (Russian)

Hemangiopericytoma of the maxilla (Caldarelli *et al*). Arch. Otolaryng., *102:*49, 1976

Bilateral eosinophilic granuloma of the mandible (Storrs). Oral Surg., *41:*93, 1976

Cyst, mandibular, squamous cell carcinoma arising in (Herceg, Harding), PRS, *57:*383, 1976

Jaw, Odontogenic Tumors (See also *Jaw, Ameloblastoma*)

Odontoma, composite complex, with associated impaction and autogenous bone graft (Magnus *et al*). Mil. Med., *136:*373, 1971

Odontogenic calcifying epithelial tumor (Pindborg's tumor), case report (Ravisse *et al*). Ann. Anat. Pathol. (Paris), *18:*463, 1973 (French)

Familial congenital occurrence of multiple odontomas (Schmidseder *et al*). Dtsch. Zahnaerztl. Z., *28:*628, 1973 (German)

Odontogenic tumor, atypical, calcifying, containing "amyloid," light and electron microscopic study of (Mohamed *et al*). J. Oral Pathol., *2:*150, 1973

Maxilla, giant cemento-ossifying fibroma of: report of case and discussion (Small, Goodman). J. Oral Surg., *31:*113, 1973

Mandible, benign (true) cementoblastoma of (Curran *et al*). Oral Surg., *35:*168, 1973

Maxillary sinus, complex odontoma in (Caton *et al*). Oral Surg., *36:*658, 1973

Odontogenic tumor, rare variant of (Pons *et al*). Rev. Stomatol. Chir. Maxillofac., *74:*506, 1973 (French)

Jaw, edentulous, giant cell epulis in (Pajarola). Schweiz. Monatsschr. Zahnheilkd., *83:*1261, 1973 (German)

Tumor, odontogenic, calcifying epithelial (Pindborg tumor) (Wallace, MacDonald), PRS, *56:*683, 1975. Brit. J. Plast. Surg., *27:*23, 1974

Maxillary cementoblastoma, case report (Rolffs, *et al*). Dtsch. Zahnaerztl. Z., *29:*713, 1974 (German)

Case of gigantiform cementoma (Van Der Waal *et al*). Int. J. Oral Surg., *3:*440, 1974

Calcifying epithelial odontogenic tumor of the mandible of an 11-year-old child. Report of a case (Onishi *et al*). J. Jpn. Stomatol. Soc., *41:*286, 1974 (Japanese)

Mandible, cementifying fibroma of, case report (Albright *et al*). J. Oral Surg., *32:*294, 1974

Maxillary sinus fibro-odontoma in 12-year-old girl (Lepkowski). Otolaryngol. Pol.,

Jaw, Odontogenic Tumors – Cont.

*28:*239, 1974 (Polish)

Congenital epulis tumor (Bowe), PRS, *53:*227, 1974

Epulis, treatment (Lychak *et al*). Stomatologiia (Mosk.), *53:*83, 1974 (Russian)

Jaw tumors, odontogenic, results in therapy of (Schulz *et al*). Z. W. R., *83:*432, 1974 (German)

Cementoblastoma of the maxilla: report of case (Wiggins *et al*). J. Oral Surg., *33:*302, 1975

Odontogenic myxofibroma: report of two cases (Gormley *et· al*). J. Oral Surg., *33:*356, 1975

Mandible, cemento-ossifying fibroma of, case report (Martis *et al*). J. Oral Surg., *33:*364, 1975

Multiple odontogenic tumors and other anomalies. An autosomal dominantly inherited syndrome (Schmidseder *et al*). Oral Surg., *39:*249, 1975

Odontogenic myxoma. Clinical and ultrastructural study (White *et al*). Oral Surg., *39:*901, 1975

Benign cementoblastoma (true cementoma) (Anneroth *et al*). Oral Surg., *40:*141, 1975

Jaw, Prognathism: See *Prognathism*

Jaw Prostheses

Surgical treatment of common abnormalities in relation to oral prosthesis (Verne). J. Oral Surg., *29:*768, 1971

Reconstructive prosthesis in extensive resections of mandible for neoplasms (Cislaghi). Minerva Chir., *26:*1411, 1971 (Italian)

Instant prosthetic substitution after resection and disarticulation of mandible (Catania). Minerva Chir., *26:*1418, 1971 (Italian)

Webb bolt as space maintaining appliance in defects of the mandible (Hamilton) (Follow-Up Clinic), PRS, *48:*368, 1971

Silicone implants for reconstruction of flabby alveolar ridges (Bjorlin *et al*). Sven. Tandlak. Tidskr., *64:*789, 1971

Maxillectomy, presurgical maxillary prosthesis: analysis of speech intelligibility (Kipfmueller, Lang), PRS, *52:*204, 1973. J. Prosth. Dent., *28:*620, 1972

Jaw area, lower, reconstruction with bipedicled deltopectoral flap and Ticonium prosthesis (Wurlitzer, Ballantyne), PRS, *49:*220, 1972

K-wire to mandible, simple technique for securing, wire, washer, nut (Mladick *et al*), PRS, *49:*228, 1972

Mandibular prosthesis, universal internal

Jaw Prostheses — Cont.

immediate (De Rezende). Rev. Fac. Odontol. Sao Paulo, *10:*57, 1972

Maxillary resection, prostheses after, titanium blades for supporting (Cislaghi). Tumori, *58:*13, 1972 (Italian)

Maxillofacial prosthetics and reconstructive surgery, interrelated role (Salyer *et al*), PRS, *53:*692, 1974. Am. J. Surg., *126:*496, 1973

Maxillary surgery, immediate prosthetic replacement after completion of (Smatt). J. Med. Liban., *26:*73, 1973 (French)

Implant, preoperative modeling of, in plastic surgery, using polymer mesh materials (Ioffe). Klin. Khir., *1:*56, 1973 (Russian)

Mandibular reconstruction, compound silicone-bone implants for (Swanson *et al*), PRS, *51:*402, 1973

Maxillectomy, prosthetic reconstruction following (Hildestad). Prosthet. Dent., *30:*637, 1973

Custom fabricated silicone prostheses for mandibular replacement (Leake). Trans. Int. Conf. Oral Surg., *4:*159, 1973

New perspectives in prosthetic replacement of mandible after resection or disarticulation (Catania *et al*). Tumori, *59:*137, 1973 (Italian)

Two cases of osteogenic sarcoma of the mandible; indications for immediate reconstruction (De Lathouwer *et al*). Acta Chir. Belg., *73:*49, 1974 (French)

Mandible defect after ameloblastoma resection repaired by metal-plastic jaw implant (Wang, Li), PRS, *54:*701, 1974. Chinese M. J., *5:*84, 1974

Maxillary resection prosthesis with magnetic connection to eye epithesis (Ariely *et al*). Dtsch. Zahnaerztl. Z., *29:*819, 1974 (German)

Jaw implants, problems of (Baumann). H.N.O., *22:*191, 1974 (German)

Maxilla, combined fixed prosthesis and segmental osteotomy of, case report (Mansfield *et al*). J. Am. Dent. Assoc., *88:*603, 1974

Custom designing and fabricating silicone implants for mandibular defects (Chalian *et al*). J. Am. Dent. Assoc., *89:*1128, 1974

Bilateral free-end denture with consideration for simplified supplementation of anterior dentition (patient requested that natural mandibular anterior teeth be retained) (Ulmer). Quintessence Int., *5:*35, 1974

Head and neck defects, maxillofacial prostheses (Lepley), PRS, *55:*518, 1975. Surg. Clin. N. Am., *54:*787, 1974

Jaw Prostheses — Cont.

Primary reconstruction of mandible with wire mesh prosthesis (Terz *et al*). Surg. Gynec. & Obst., *139:*198, 1974

Maxillofacial prostheses, materials in (Schaaf), PRS, *57:*266, 1976. Dent. Clin. N. Am., *19:*347, 1975

Preprosthetic surgery in the front region of the mandible (Rosenquist). Int. J. Oral Surg., *4:*18, 1975

Chalmers J. Lyons memorial lecture: metal implants and the mandibular staple bone plate (Small). J. Oral Surg., *33:*571, 1975

Rehabilitating dentulous hemimandibulectomy patients (Moore *et al*). J. Prosthet. Dent., *35:*202, 1976

Mandibular replacements — a review of embedded implants (Williams *et al*). J. Prosthet. Dent., *35:*207, 1976

Jaw, Surgery (See also *Jaw, Bone Graft to; Jaw Deformities; Jaw, Neoplasms; Micrognathia; Prognathism*)

Surgical treatment of mandibular laterognathies (Delaire). Orthod. Fr., *41:*269, 1970 (French)

Mandible, reconstruction of (DeFries, Marble, Sell), PRS, *49:*102, 1972. Arch. Otolaryng., *93:*4, 1971

Mandibular reconstruction in Nigeria (Redpath). Brit. J. Oral Surg., *9:*85, 1971

Immediate intra-oral mandibular bone transplants (Torrielli). Minerva Stomatol., *20:*110, 1971 (Italian)

Immediate and definite reconstruction after hemimandibulectomy (Fries). Minerva Stomatol., *20:*155, 1971

Unilateral mandibular resection-disarticulation by an intraoral method and immediate reconstruction by bone and autograft (Bortot *et al*). Riv. Ital. Stomatol., *26:*605, 1971 (Italian)

Plastic repair of postoperative cavities of the jaw (Zagubeliuk). Stomatologiia (Mosk.), *50:*39, 1971 (Russian)

Mandibular osteotomy angle analyser (Johnasson *et al*). Sven. Tandlak. Tidskr., *64:*551, 1971

Delayed results of osteoplasty of the mandible (Pavlov). Vestn. Khir., *107:*86, 1971 (Russian)

Surgical interventions in the area of the temporomandibular joint (Arzhantsev). Voen. Med. Zh., *11:*23, 1971 (Russian)

Surgical Treatment of Developmental Jaw Deformities. By Edward Hines and John Kent. C. V. Mosby Co., St. Louis, 1972. PRS, *51:*580, 1973

Jaw, Surgery — Cont.

Mandible, segmental osteotomies of. Value in correction of facial profile abnormalities. Ann. chir. plast., *17:*173, 1972 (French)

Mandibular resections. 3. Surgical anatomy of mandible (Editorial). Arq. Patol., *44:*21, 1972 (Portuguese)

Mandibular resections, 5. (Editorial). Arq. Patol., *44:*59, 1972 (Portuguese)

Mandibular resections. 6. Mandibular resections followed by prosthesis (Editorial). Arq. Patol., *44:*69, 1972 (Portuguese)

Mandibular resections. 7. Mandibular resections with an immediate bone graft (Editorial). Arq. Patol., *44:*77, 1972 (Portuguese)

Mandibular resections. 8. Mandibular resections with other structures (Editorial). Arq. Patol., *44:*91, 1972 (Portuguese)

Mandibular resections. 9. Conclusions (Editorial). Arq. Patol., *44:*113, 1972 (Portuguese)

Maxilla, experiences with vertical osteotomy in (Wunderer). Dtsch. Zahn. Mund. Kieferheilkd., *59:*5, 1972 (German)

Surgical treatment of mandibular asymmetry: report of a case (Weinstein). J. Oral Surg., *30:*303, 1972

Posterior maxillary surgery — its place in the treatment of dentofacial deformities (West *et al*). J. Oral Surg., *30:*562, 1972

Syndrome, Guillain-Barre, after mandibular surgery, case report (Shuert *et al*). J. Oral Surg., *30:*913, 1972

Mandible, reconstruction (Alonso *et al*). Otolaryngol. Clin. North Am., *5:*501, 1972

Surgical correction of mandibular asymmetries (Zisser). Osterr. Z. Stomatol., *69:*304, 1972 (German)

Sectional osteotomies of the jaws. Their value in the correction of profile abnormalities (Merville *et al*). Rev. Fr. Odontostomatol., *18:*1094, 1971 (French)

Mandible, restoration of, following partial resection (Nahum *et al*). Trans. Am. Acad. Ophthalmol. Otolaryngol., *76:*957, 1972

Maxillary osteotomies, biologic basis for (Bell). Am. J. Phys. Anthropol., *38:*279, 1973

Mandibular bone and condyle, reconstruction of, after tumor surgery (Lahti *et al*). Ann. Chir. Gynaecol. Fenn., *62:*155, 1973

Mandibular resection, transbuccal subtotal, with immediate reconstruction (Pons *et al*). Ann. chir. plast., *18:*155, 1973 (French)

Regional composite-swivel flap in surgery (Conley). Arch. Klin. Exp. Ohren Nasen Kehlkopfheilkd., *205:*78, 1973 (German)

Maxillary nerve, resection of, in pterigopalatine fossa (Cerny). Cesk. Otolaryngol.,

Jaw, Surgery — Cont.

*22:*298, 1973 (Czechoslovakian)

Maxilla, interalveolar osteotomy in (Mehnert). Dtsch. Zahn. Mund. Kieferheilkd., *61:*289, 1973 (German)

Mandibular reconstruction, surgical, study on masticatory function with (Endo *et al*). Jap. J. Oral Surg., *19:*441, 1973 (Japanese)

Maxillo-mandibular surgery for correction of dentofacial deformities. 4. Maxillary retrusion (mandibular pseudoprognathism) (Weinberg *et al*). J. Can. Dent. Assoc., *39:*465, 1973

Mandibular reconstruction, immediate, following resection (Donohue). J. Can. Dent. Assoc., *39:*720, 1973

Maxillary defects, large, after tumor resection, late reconstruction of (Obwegeser). J. Maxillo-facial. Surg., *1:*19, 1973

Jaw, lower, repair of mandibular nerve by autologous nerve grafting after resection (Hausamen, Samii, Schmidseder), PRS, *53:*250, 1974. J. Maxillo-facial Surg., *1:*74, 1973

Maxillofacial surgery, osteosynthesis with miniaturized screwed plates (Michelet, Deymes, Dessus), PRS, *53:*241, 1974. J. Maxillo-facial Surg., *1:*79, 1973

Alveolar segmental osteotomy, tooth vitality after (Pepersack), PRS, *53:*251, 1974. J. Maxillo-facial Surg., *1:*85, 1973

Fixation, simplified method, after segmental orthodontic surgery (Cranin, Dennison). J. Oral Surg., *31:*109, 1973

Mandibular defects, experimental use of poly (methyl methacrylate) implants in (Worley). J. Oral Surg., *31:*170, 1973

Mandibular osteotomy, parotid fistula a complication of (Goldberg, Marco, Google). J. Oral Surg., *31:*207, 1973

Mandibular defects, experimental use of stainless steel wire mesh in (Bear *et al*). J. Oral Surg., *31:*348, 1973

Mandibular reconstruction (DeChamplain). J. Oral Surg., *31:*448, 1973

Maxillary diastemas, multiple, immediate surgical closure of (Peterson). J. Oral Surg., *31:*522, 1973

Maxillary osteotomy, total, nasal septum perforation following (Mainous *et al*). J. Oral Surg., *31:*869, 1973

Mandible, treatment of continuity defect (Worley *et al*). J. Oral Surg., *31:*942, 1973

Facial sling suspension of chin following resection of anterior mandible (Norante, McCabe). Laryngoscope, *83:*336, 1973

Mandible, prosthetic reconstruction of (Catania *et al*). Minerva med., *64:*3641, 1973 (Italian)

Jaw, Surgery – Cont.

Mandible, review of reconstruction (Bowerman). Proc. Roy. Soc. Med., *67:*610, 1974

Chromium-cobalt implants in dogs, effect of tissue on electrical properties of (Rusiniak). Protet. Stomatol., *24:*183, 1974 (Polish)

Our experience with mandibular resection by endobuccal approach and immediate transplantation of autologous bone (Stea). Rev. Stomatol. Chir. Maxillofac., *75:*55, 1974 (French)

Subalveolar mandibular osteotomies in anteroposterior facial dysmorphism (Michlet *et al*). Rev. Stomatol. Chir. Maxillofac., *75:*156, 1974 (French)

Maxillary bone and incisor in rabbit, development after operation when a few days old (Rosselli *et al*), PRS, *57:*395, 1976. Riv. ital. chir. plast., *6:*227, 1974

Maxillofacial surgery, amylase isoenzymes in serum after (Skude, Rothman), PRS, *55:*120, 1975. Scand. J. Plast. Reconstr. Surg., *7:*105, 1974

Kallocryl-K implantation, histological studies of rabbit jaw on tissue reaction following (Pinkert). Stomatol. D.D.R., *24:*342, 1974 (German)

Mandible, osteoplasty, our experience in (Nikandrov *et al*). Stomatologiia (Mosk.), *53:*22, 1974 (Russian)

Anesthesia and resuscitation in operations for diseases and injuries of the tongue, and the floor of the mouth (Aleksandrov *et al*). Vestn. Khir., *112:*88, 1974 (Russian)

Maxillectomy, rhinorrhea after (Clark, Weaver, Smith), PRS, *57:*395, 1976. Arch. Otolaryng., *101:*492, 1975

Method of localization and fixation for midfacial osteotomies (Banks *et al*). Brit. J. Oral Surg., *12:*263, 1975

Maxillary resection, partial, closure of defects after by means of mucosal flap obtained from mouth mucosa and upper lip (Korson *et al*). Czas. Stomatol., *28:*637, 1975 (Polish)

Mandibular positioning and bone modeling, study of pressure and tension systems in (Harvold). Dent. Clin. North Am., *19:*473, 1975

Osteotomy, Le Fort, longitudinal study on electrical pulp testing following (Tajima), PRS, *57:*259, 1976. J. Maxillo-facial Surg., *3:*74, 1975

Alveolar movement, segmental, after cortical osteotomy, experimental animal research (Duker), PRS, *57:*395, 1976. J. Maxillo-facial Surg., *3:*81, 1975

Condylotomy, clinical and experimental ap-

Jaw, Surgery – Cont.

praisal of surgical technique (Banks, Mackenzie), PRS, *57:*531, 1976. J. Maxillo-facial Surg., *3:*170, 1975

Maxillary alveolar hyperplasia, diagnosis and treatment planning (West *et al*). J. Maxillo-facial Surg., *3:*239, 1975

Maxilla, osteotomies of, complications (Westwood, Tilson), PRS, *57:*116, 1976. J. Oral Surg., *33:*104, 1975

Maxillary osteotomy, bone healing and revascularization after (Bell *et al*), PRS, *57:*531, 1976. J. Oral Surg., *33:*253, 1975

Mandibular ramus, osteotomies of, comparison of vertical and sagittal split (Wang, Waite), PRS, *57:*672, 1976. J. Oral Surg., *33:*596, 1975

Complete regeneration of body of ascending ramus and mandibular condyle in child after disarticulation (Anastassov *et al*). Rev. Odontostomatol. (Paris), *4:*43, 1975 (French)

Mandibular and maxillary osteotomy (Donald), PRS, *57:*673, 1976. West. J. Med., *123:*219, 1975

Reconstruction of the defective mandible (Branemark *et al*). Scand. J. Plast. Reconstr. Surg., *9:*116, 1975

JAWORSKA, L.: Surgical management of extensive maxillary cysts. Czas. Stomatol., *28:*403, 1975 (Polish)

JAWORSKA, M., AND DUDKIEWICZ, Z.: Goldenhar's syndrome, typical and atypical forms, PRS, *55:*646, 1975. Acta chir. plast., *16:*78, 1974

JAWORSKI, S.: Kenacort A in treatment of hypertrophic scars and keloids in children, PRS, *54:*624, 1974. Acta chir. plast., *15:*206, 1973

JAWORSKI, S. *et al*: Mandibular fracture in course of labor in newborn infant. Pediatr. Pol., *48:*1501, 1973 (Polish)

JAYARAM, B.: Surgical treatment of *hidradenitis suppurativa* of axilla (with Tasche, Angelats), PRS, *55:*559, 1975

JAZBI, B.: Nasal septum deformity in the newborn. Diagnosis and treatment. Clin. Pediatr. (Phila.), 13:953, 1974

JEANBART, P. *et al*: Congenital abnormalities possibly induced by LSD-25. Review of the literature apropos of a personal case. Gynecol. Obstet. (Paris), *70:* 215, 1971 (French)

JEBSEN, R. H. *et al*: Function of "normal" hand in stroke patients. Arch. Phys. Med. Rehabil., *52:*170, 1971

JEDRZEJEWSKA, T. *et al*: Evaluation of surgical treatment of labial frenum in prevention and treatment of periodontal diseases. Czas. Stomatol., *27:*413, 1974 (Polish)

JEEKEL, J. *et al*: Survival of mouse skin and heart heterografts in rats treated with xenogeneic hyperimmune antidonor serum. Transplantation, *17:*605, 1974

JEFFERY, C. C.: Hamartoma in the hand—a simulator. Hand, *5:*79, 1973

JEFFS, J. V. *et al*: Cone flap for resurfacing, reconstructing partial digits. Brit. J. Plast. Surg., *26:*163, 1973

JELENKO, C., III. *et al*: Effects of threshold burns on distant microcirculation. Surg. Forum, *22:*53, 1971

JELENKO, C., III, AND WHEELER, M. L.: Effects of antioxidants of long-term utility of ethyl linoleate as water-holding lipid for topical use postburn, PRS, *51:*350, 1973. J. Surg. Res., *12:*161, 1972

JELENKO, C., III, WHEELER, M. L., AND SCOTT, T. H., JR.: Studies in burns. X. Ethyl lineoleate: the water-holding lipid of skin. *A.* The evidence, PRS, *52:*210, 1973. *B.* Effects on *in vivo* burn eschar, PRS, *52:*211, 1973. J. Trauma, *12:*968, 974, 1972

JELENKO, C. *et al*: Threshold burning effects on distant microcirculation, PRS, *52:*456, 1973; *55:*113, 1975. Arch. Surg., *106:*317, 1973; Am. Surgeon, *40:*388, 1974

JELENKO, C. *et al*: Topical lipid protection of burned subjects and their wounds, PRS, *54:*623, 1974. Surgery, *75:*892, 1974

JELENKO, C., GARRISON, A. F., AND McKINLEY, J. C.: Respiratory problems complicating burn injury, PRS, *57:*538, 1976. Postgrad. Med., *58:*97, 1975

JELINEK, R., AND DOSTAL, M.: Role of mitotic activity in formation of secondary palate, PRS, *54:*628, 1974. Acta chir. plast., *15:*216, 1973

JEMEC, B.: Abrasio axillae in hyperhidrosis, PRS, *57:*402, 1976. Scand. J. Plast. Reconstr. Surg., *9:*44, 1975

JENNINGS, H. B., JR.: Plastic surgery in the Army, short historical account, PRS, *48:*413, 1971

JENNY, H.: Catastrophic results after silicone injections. In *Plastische und Wiederherstellungs Chirurgie*, ed. by Hohler; pp 331–4. Schattauer, Stuttgart, 1975

JENSEN, E. G., AND WEILBY, A.: Primary tendon suture in thumb and fingers, PRS, *56:*356, 1975. Hand, *6:*297, 1974

JENSEN, T. S. *et al*: Skin cancer. Ugeskr. Laeger, *134:*107, 1972 (Danish)

JEPPESEN, F. *et al*: Dislocation of the nasal septal cartilage in the newborn. Aetiology, spontaneous course and treatment. Acta Obstet. Gynecol. Scand., *51:*5, 1972

JEPPSON, P. H. *et al*: Carcinoma of external ear.

O.R.L., *35:*336, 1973

JEPPSSON, P. H. *et al*: Cancer of tongue. Acta Otolaryngol. (Stockh.), *75:*314, 1973

JEPPSSON, P. H. *et al*: Malignant tumors of oral cavity. O.R.L., *37:*109, 1975

JEPSEN, P. L.: Mafenide acetate in treatment of caustic chemical burns. Vet. Med. Small Anim. Clin., *67:*52, 1972

JEPSON, P. M., AND SILBER, I.: Urethral extrusion of penile prosthesis associated with urethritis, PRS, *53:*244, 1974. J. Urol., *109:*838, 1973

JEREMIAH, B. S.: Avulsion of scalp and its reconstruction, PRS, *48:*604, 1971. Internat. Surg., *55:*265, 1971

JERVIS, W. *et al*: Further applications of Limberg and Dufourmentel flaps, PRS, *54:*335, 1974

JESSE, R. H.: The treatment of oral cancer. C.A., *22:*209, 1972

JESSE, R. H. *et al*: Cancer of oral cavity. Is elective neck dissection beneficial?, PRS, *48:*297, 1971. Am. J. Surg., *120:*505, 1970

JESSE, R. H., LINDBERG, R. D., AND HORIOT, J. C.: Vocal cord cancer with commissure extension, choice of treatment, PRS, *51:*607, 1973. Am. J. Surg., *122:*437, 1971

JESSE, R. H. *et al*: Cervical lymph node metastasis: unknown primary cancer. Cancer, *31:*854, 1973

JESSE, R. H. *et al*: Squamous cell carcinoma of maxillary and ethmoid sinuses. Proc. Natl. Cancer Conf., *7:*193, 1973

JESSE, R. H. *et al*: Efficacy of combining radiation therapy with a surgical procedure in patients with cervical metastasis from squamous cancer of the oropharynx and hypopharynx. Cancer, *35:*1163, 1975

JETER, K., AND BLOOM, S.: Management of stomal complications following ileal or colonic conduit operations in children, PRS, *50:*200, 1972. J. Urol., *106:*425, 1971

JEWUSIAK, E. M. *et al*: Solitary benign enchondroma of the long bones of the hand. J. Bone & Joint Surg. (Am.), *53:*1587, 1971

JEZEK, M. *et al*: Complex treatment of poorly healing wounds of lower extremities. Rozhl. Chir., *53:*635, 1974 (Czechoslovakian)

JEZEQUEL, J. *et al*: Apparatus for reduction and fixation of complex fractures. Ann. Otolaryngol. Chir. Cervicofac., *90:*527, 1973 (French)

JIRAK, Z. *et al*: Correction factors in skin temperature measurement, PRS, *57:*127, 1976. J. Appl. Physiol., *38:*752, 1975

JIRASEK, J. E., AND ZWINGER, A.: Prenatally diagnosed Turner's syndrome, PRS, *54:*630, 1974. Časop. lék. česk., *113:*293, 1974

JOACHIMS, H. Z. *et al*: Invasive pleomorphic adenoma of hard palate. J. Laryng. & Otol.,

*87:*1147, 1973

JOBE, R.: Combined pharyngeal flap and palate pushback procedure: improvements in technique. Brit. J. Plast. Surg., *26:*384, 1973

JOBE, R. P.: Technique for lid loading in management of lagophthalmos of facial palsy, PRS, *53:*29, 1974

JOBE, R. P.: On lid loading in management of lagophthalmos (Letter to the Editor), PRS, *54:*211, 1974

JOBE, R. P., IVERSON, R., AND VISTNES, L.: Bone deformation beneath alloplastic implants, PRS, *51:*169, 1973. Discussions by Rees, Spira, PRS, *51:*174, 1973

JOCHIMSEN, P. R. *et al*: Fibrosarcoma of the mandible. Minn. Med., *54:*929, 1971

JOHANSEN, A. M., AND SORENSEN, B.: Treatment of donor sites, controlled trial with Fucidin gauze, PRS, *51:*109, 1973. Scand. J. Plast. Reconstr. Surg., *6:*47, 1972

JOHANSON, B. *et al*: Follow-up study of cleft lip and ₁palate patients treated with orthodontics, secondary bone grafting, and prosthetic rehabilitation. Scand. J. Plast. Reconstr. Surg., *8:*121, 1974

JOHANSON, B. *et al*: Surgical treatment of nontraumatic lower lip lesions with special reference to the step technique. A follow-up on 149 patients. Scand. J. Plast. Reconstr. Surg., *8:*232, 1974

JOHANSSON, C. F. *et al*: Mandibular osteotomy angle analyser. Sven. Tandlak. Tidskr., *64:*551, 1971

JOHANSSON, S. H.: Formation of articular cartilage from free perichondrial grafts (with Skoog), PRS, *57:*1, 1976

JOHNS, M. F. *et al*: Oncocytic and oncocytoid tumors of salivary glands. Laryngoscope, *83:*1940, 1973

JOHNSON, B. L. *et al*: Black orbital bone. Arch. Ophth., *88:*400, 1972

JOHNSON, C. C. *et al*: Oculopharyngeal muscular dystrophy. Am. J. Ophth., *77:*872, 1974

JOHNSON, C. F.: New technique for reduction mammaplasty (Letter to the Editor), PRS, *57:*372, 1976

JOHNSON, C. F. *et al*: Duplication of penis. Urology, *4:*722, 1974

JOHNSON, C. L.: Tracheostomy: emergency or elective? Ariz. Med., *32:*411, 1975

JOHNSON, H. A.: Simple method for the repair of minor post-operative cleft lip "whistling" deformity. Brit. J. Plast. Surg., *25:*152, 1972

JOHNSON, H. A.: Correction of a congenitally short fourth metatarsal. Brit. J. Plast. Surg., *25:*201, 1972

JOHNSON, H. A.: To magnify, or not to magnify (Letter to the Editor), PRS, *49:*331, 1972

JOHNSON, H. A.: Conserving surgical instruments and operating room time, PRS, *51:*96, 1973

JOHNSON, H. A.: Full-time plastic surgical research and sour grapes (Editorial), PRS, *51:*326, 1973

JOHNSON, H. A.: Possible dangers of using Fabricut as dermabrasive (Letter to the Editor), PRS, *51:*441, 1973

JOHNSON, H. A.: Facilitating suture removal in children, PRS, *55:*97, 1975

JOHNSON, H. A.: Another opinion on showing average result (Letter to the Editor), PRS, *55:*216, 1975

JOHNSON, H. A.: Bonney's blue marking ink, PRS, *56:*155, 1975

JOHNSON, H. C.: One-stage reconstruction of lacrimal apparatus (with Snow), PRS, *48:*453, 1971

JOHNSON, M., AND LLOYD, H. E. D.: Bilateral breast cancer 10 years after augmentation mammaplasty, PRS, *53:*88, 1974

JOHNSON, MOULTON K.: *The Hand Book.* Charles C Thomas, Springfield, Ill., 1973. PRS, *53:*343, 1974

JOHNSON, MOULTON K. AND COHEN, MYLES J.: *The Hand Atlas.* Charles C Thomas, Springfield, Ill., 1975

JOHNSON, M. K. *et al*: Metaplastic bone formation (myositis ossificans) in the soft tissues of the hand. Case report. J. Bone & Joint Surg. (Am.), *57:*999, 1975

JOHNSON, N. E. Secondary surgery of septum. Otolaryngol. Clin. North Am., *7:*75, 1974

JOHNSON, R. H., JR., HARRAH, J. D., AND KETCHUM, A. S.: Ill-advised biopsy, PRS, *51:*354, 1973. Am. Surgeon, *38:*357, 1972

JOHNSON, R. K., AND IVERSON, R. E.: Cross-finger pedicled flaps in hand, PRS, *49:*663, 1972. J. Bone & Joint Surg., *53:*913, 1971

JOHNSON, R. K., AND MORAIN, W. D.: Hemostasis in surgery of the hand, PRS, *57:*666, 1976

JOHNSTON, I. D.: The surgery of thyroid cancer. Brit. J. Surg., *62:*765, 1975

JOHNSTON, J. H.: Exstrophy of the bladder. Prog. Pediatr. Surg., *2:*147, 1971

JOHNSTON, J. H.: Lengthening of the congenital or acquired short penis. Brit. J. Urol., *46:*685, 1974

JOHNSTON, J. H.: Genital aspects of exstrophy. J. Urol., *113:*701, 1975

JOHNSTON, J. H. *et al*: Exstrophic anomalies and their surgical reconstruction. Curr. Probl. Surg., *1:*39, 1974

JOHNSTON, M. C. *et al*: Embryology of cleft lip and cleft palate. Clin. Plast. Surg., *2:*195, 1975

Joint Transplantation

Results of free transplanted toe joints in hand surgery (Zrubecky). Handchirurgie, *2:*67, 1970 (German)

Joint Transplantation – Cont.

Marrow, autogenous, to partially replace homologous bone when transplanting homologous joints (Fiala, Herout), PRS, *51:*487, 1973. Acta chir. plast., *13:*243, 1971

Temporomandibular joint, trial of sternoclavicular whole joint graft as substitute for (Snyder, Levine, Dingman), PRS, *48:*447, 1971

Joints, homogenous, transplantation of (Fiala, Herout), PRS, *51:*237, 1973. Acta chir. plast., *14:*36, 1972

Joint, formation of articular cartilage from free perichondrial grafts (Skoog, Johansson), PRS, *57:*1, 1976

JOKIC, N.: Problems of primary treatment of large soft tissue defects of lower limb combined with bone fractures. Vojnosanit. Pregl., *30:*39, 1973 (Croatian)

JOKINEN, K. *et al:* Endonasal dacryocystorhinostomy. Arch. Otolaryngl., *100:*41, 1974

JOKL, P. *et al:* Juxtacortical chondrosarcoma of the hand. J. Bone & Joint Surg. (Am.), *53:*1370, 1971

JOLLEYS, A., AND ROBERTSON, N. R. E.: Study of effects of early bone grafting in complete clefts of lip and palate, PRS, *52:*208, 1973. Brit. J. Plast. Surg., *25:*229, 1972

JOLLY, P. C. *et al:* Extremity salvage by small vessel revascularization. Am. Surg., *40:*521, 1974

JONDERKO, G. *et al:* Peutz-Jeghers-Touraine syndrome. Pol. Tyg. Lek., *29:*1669, 1974 (Polish)

JONECKO, A. *et al:* Case of painful Malherbe and Chenantais calcifying epithelioma. Wiad. Lek., *28:*673, 1975 (Polish)

JONECKO, A. *et al:* Surgical injuries and methemoglobinemia due to explosion of an oxidizing mixture. Wiad. Lek., *29:*158, 1976 (Polish)

JONES, A. C., JR.: Further experience with pharyngeal flap in the cleft palate patient. Trans. Pac. Coast Otoophthalmol. Soc., *55:*85, 1974

JONES, B. R.: Syndromes of lacrimal obstruction and their management. Trans. Ophthalmol. Soc. U.K., *93:*581, 1973

JONES, B. R.: Cautery to cure epiphora from punctal eversion. Trans. Ophthalmol. Soc. U.K., *93:*611, 1973

JONES, B. R.: Principles of lacrimal surgery. Trans. Ophthalmol. Soc. U.K., *93:*611, 1973

JONES, B. S.: Doigt en lorgnette and concentric bone atrophy associated with healed yaws osteitis. Report of two cases. J. Bone & Joint Surg. (Br.), *54:*341, 1972

JONES, F. R.: Relapsing polychondritis, PRS, *51:*331, 1973

JONES, F. R., AND TAURAS, A. P.: Periareolar incision for augmentation mammaplasty, PRS, *51:*641, 1973

JONES, H. W., JR.: Anomaly of external genitalia in female patients with exstrophy of bladder. Am. J. Obstet. Gynecol., *117:*748, 1973

JONES, H. W., JR.: Surgical construction of female genitalia. Clin. Plast. Surg., *1:*255, 1974

JONES, I. S.: Tumors of the lacrimal glands: their surgical management. South. Med. J., *64:*1503, 1971

JONES, K. G. *et al:* Overview on new procedures in surgery of the hand. Clin. Orthop., *9:*154, 1974

JONES, L. T. *et al:* Senile entropion. A new concept for correction. Am. J. Ophth., *74:*327, 1972

JONES, L. T. *et al:* Cure of ptosis by aponeurotic repair. Arch. Ophth., *93:*629, 1975

JONES, R. F. *et al:* Water bed in a spinal injury unit. M. J. Australia, *2:*1215, 1971

JONES, R. F., AND DICKINSON, W. E.: Total integumentectomy of leg for multiple "in-transit" metastases of melanoma, PRS, *51:*607, 1973. Am. J. Surg., *123:*588, 1972

JONES, R. G.: Short history of anaesthesia for harelip and cleft palate repair. Brit. J. Anaesth., *43:*796, 1971

JONES, S. A., BRENNAN, M., AND KUNDSIN, R. B.: *Candida* serology: aid in diagnosis of deep-organ candidiasis, PRS, *54:*119, 1974. J. Surg. Res., *14:*235, 1973

JOOB-FANCSALY, G.: Treatment of glossodynia with Ambosex. Forgorv. Sz., *66:*185, 1973 (Hungarian)

JOPLING, W. H.: Cubital tunnel external compression syndrome. Brit. Med. J., *2:*179, 1973

JORGENSEN, K. *et al:* Carcinoma of lip. Series of 869 patients. Acta Otolaryngol. (Stockh.), *75:*312, 1973

JORGENSEN, K. *et al:* Carcinoma of lip. Series of 869 cases. Acta Radiol. (Ther.) (Stockh.), *12:*177, 1973

JORGENSON, R. J.: Electrodactyly and cleft lip/palate. Birth Defects, *7:*260, 1971

JORTAY, A. M.: Metastatic tumors of oral cavity, pharynx and paranasal sinuses, PRS, *50:*635, 1972. Acta chir. belg., *70:*715, 1971

JORTAY, A.: Complications of radical neck dissection and their prevention, PRS, *55:*718, 1975. Arch. chir. belg., *73:*385, 1974

JOSEPH, D. L. *et al:* Risks of head and neck surgery in previously irradiated patients. Arch. Otolaryng., *97:*381, 1973

JOSHI, B. B.: "Card injuries of the hand" associated with multiple broken pins. Hand, *3:*84, 1971

JOSHI, B. B.: Dorsolateral flap from same finger

to relieve flexion contracture, PRS, *49:*186, 1972

JOSHI, B. B.: Sensory flaps for degloved mutilated hand, PRS, *56:*229, 1975. Hand, *6:*247, 1974

JOSHI, B. B.: Local dorsolateral island flap for restoration of sensation after avulsion injury of fingertip pulp, PRS, *54:*175, 1974

JOSHI, B. B., AND CHAUDHARI, S. S.: Dorsal relaxation incision in burst fingers, PRS, *54:*237, 1974. Hand, *5:*135, 1973

JOST, G.: Corrective surgery of facial skin ptoses. Probl. Actuels Otorhinolaryngol., *201:*10, 1970 (French)

JOST, G.: False primary truths, false friends in facial plastic surgery. Cah. Med., *12:*1275, 1971 (French)

JOST, G.: Harelips. Probl. Actuels Otorhinolaryngol., *223,* 1971 (French)

JOST, G. Correction of projection defect of tip of nose. Ann. chir. plast., *17:*245, 1972 (French)

JOST, G.: Principal false ideas and false friends in plastic surgery of face. Probl. Actuels Otorhinolaryngol., *357:*70, 1972 (French)

JOST, G.: Suture technics in rhinoplasty using the extramucosal technic. Ann. chir. plast., *18:*271, 1973 (French)

JOST, G.: Use of scissors in rhinoplasty. Ann. chir. plast., *18:*279, 1973 (French)

JOST, G. *et al*: Corbin's beaked nose. Ann. chir. plast., *17:*5, 1972 (French)

JOST, G. *et al*: Study of junction between the lateral cartilages of nose. Ann. chir. plast., *18:*175, 1973 (French)

JOST, G. *et al*: Choice of incision in mammaplasty. Ann. chir. plast., *19:*265, 1974 (French)

JOST, G., VERGNON, L., AND HADJEAN, E.: Postoperative nasal asymmetry, PRS, *57:*257, 1976. Ann. chir. plast., *20:*123, 1975

JOUGLARD, J. P.: Treatment of unilateral congenital hypoplasia or absence of breast (with Pierre), PRS, *56:*146, 1975

JU, D. M. C.: Etiology of cancer of lower lip, PRS, *52:*151, 1973

JULLIARD, A.: Restoration of the extensor tendons of the hand by flexors. Bull. Mem. Soc. Chir. Paris, *62:*340, 1972 (French)

JUNAID, T. A. *et al*: Dermatofibrosarcoma protuberans in parotid gland, case report. Brit. J. Oral Surg., *12:*298, 1975

JUNG, A. *et al*: Surgical management of the funnel chest. Pedunculated inversionplasty. Ztschr. Orthop., *113:*830, 1975 (German)

JUNG, E. G. *et al*: Chlorcolchicine in localized treatment of skin tumors. Schweiz. Med. Wochenschr., *104:*265, 1974 (German)

JUNG, H.: Differential diagnosis of "burning tongue." Fortschr. Med., *90:*1043, 1972 (German)

JUNG, H.: Malignant melanoma of the septum. Z. Laryngol. Rhinol. Otol., *51:*141, 1972 (German)

JUNG, H.: Intravital studies on the lymphdrainage from the nasopharyngeal roof in men. Laryngol. Rhinol. Otol. (Stuttg.), *53:*769, 1974 (German)

JUNG, H. *et al*: Fibrin foam as filling material for defects in surgery of salivary gland. Animal experiments and clinical results. Arch. Klin. Exp. Ohren Nasen Kehlkopfheilkd., *204:*105, 1973 (German)

JUNG, Y. *et al*: Diabetic hand syndrome. Metabolism, *20:*1008, 1971

JUNIEN-LAVILLAUROY, C. *et al*: Cervicofacial pseudoactinomycoses caused by corynebacteriae. J. Fr. Otorhinolaryngol., *20:*1115, 1971 (French)

JUNIEN-LAVILLAUROY, C. *et al*: Temporo-frontal flap. Its value in post-irradiation buccal-pharyngeal surgery. J. Fr. Otorhinolaryngol., *24:*763, 1975 (French)

JUNIPER, R. P., AND AWTY, M. D.: Immobilization period for fractures of mandibular body, PRS, *54:*235, 1974. Oral Surg., *36:*157, 1973

JURELL, G., AND KAIJSER, L.: Influence of varying pressure and duration of treatment with hyperbaric oxygen on survival of skin flaps, PRS, *54:*701, 1974. Scand. J. Plast. Reconstr. Surg., *7:*25, 1974

JURI, J.: Use of parieto-occipital flaps in surgical treatment of baldness, PRS, *55:*456, 1975

JURI, J., JURI, C., AND DE ANTUENO, J.: Modification of the Kapetansky technique for repair of whistling deformities of the upper lip, PRS, *57:*70, 1976

JURI, J., JURI, C., AND DE ANTUENO, J.: Reconstruction of sideburn for alopecia after rhytidectomy, PRS, *57:*304, 1976

JURISIC, A. *et al*: Our experiences in the treatment of peripheral paralysis of the n. facialis. Med. Pregl., *28:*487, 1975 (Serbian)

JURKIEWICZ, M. J.: to Emory University, PRS, *49:*364, 1972

JURKIEWICZ, M. J.: Discussion of "Investigation of bone changes in composite flaps after transfer to head and neck region," by Conley *et al*, PRS, *52:*79, 1973

JURKIEWICZ, M. J.: Treatment of macromastia in actively enlarging breast (with Mayl, Vasconez), PRS, *54:*6, 1974

JURKIEWICZ, M. J.: Transverse abdominal flaps and deep epigastric arcade (with Brown, Vasconez), PRS, *55:*416, 1975

JURKIEWICZ, M. J.: Basal cell carcinoma of medial canthal area (with Bostwick, Vasconez),

PRS, *55:*667, 1975

JURKIEWICZ, M. J., AND NICKELL, W. B.: Fractures of skeleton of face. Study of diagnosis and treatment based on 12 years' experience in treatment of over 600 major fractures of facial skeleton, PRS, *50:*199, 1972. J. Trauma, *11:*946, 1971

JURKIEWICZ, M. J. *et al*: Surgical anatomy of the neck. Surg. Clin. North Am., *54:*1269, 1974

JUSELIUS, H.: Dacryocystorhinostomy, PRS, *51:*701, 1973. Internat. Surg., *57:*883, 1972

JUSSEN, A. *et al*: Therapy of severe hand phlegmons. Hefte Unfallheilkd., *107:*248, 1970 (German)

JUSTUS, J. *et al*: Cellular immune defect: isolated immunocytic deficiency syndrome. Dtsch. Med. Wochenschr., *99:*936, 1974 (German)

JOURDAIN, J. C.: Study of clinical and histological criteria of prognosis of primary malignant melanomas. Ann. Dermatol. Syphiligr. (Paris), *101:*171, 1974 (French)

JUVARA, I., NECULA, T., AND MURGU, I.: Comparative study of vascular regeneration after different types of small bowel sutures, PRS, *54:*238, 1974. Lyon chir., *70:*52, 1974

K

KABAKOV, B. D.: Current status of the problem of treatment of maxillofacial wounds in field conditions. Voen. Med. Zh., *11:*16, 1971 (Russian)

KABAKOV, B. D.: Surgical treatment of cavernous hemangiomas of the face and neck. Stomatologiia (Mosk.), *54:*30, 1975 (Russian)

KABAKOV, B. D. *et al*: Contour plastic surgery of traumatic facial disfigurements with EG-MASS-12 and fluoroplast-4 plastics. Voen. Med. Zh., *2:*20, 1974 (Russian)

KABAKOV, V. D. *et al*: Correction of cicatricial deformations and defects of nose after deep facial burns. Vestn. Khir., *111:*91, 1973

KABELKA, M.: New surgical treatment of funnel chest. Rozhl. Chir., *53:*700, 1974 (Czechoslovakian)

KABZA, R., AND PASZ, S.: Plastubol spray in management of extensive surgical wounds, PRS, *56:*471, 1975. Wiad. Lek., *27:*1275, 1974

KABZA, R. *et al*: Gynecomastia. Wiad. Lek., *28:*1859, 1975 (Polish)

KACKER, S. K. *et al*: Hamartomas of ear and nose. J. Laryng. & Otol., *87:*801, 1973

KACZMARCZYK-STACHOWSKA, A. *et al*: Results of treatment of certain periodontal conditions by increasing depth of vestibule and widen-

ing gingival area. Czas. Stomatol., *26:*783, 1973 (Polish)

KADANOFF, D. *et al*: Form and size of the male hand. Gegenbaurs. Morpho. Jahrb., *116:*293, 1971 (German)

KADISH, S. P. *et al*: Treatment of minor salivary gland malignancies of upper food and air passage epithelium. A review of 87 cases. Cancer, *29:*1021, 1972

KADRY, M. K. M.: Anatomical, pathological, and clinical study of recent trends in treatment of facial nerve paralysis, PRS, *57:*259, 1976. Thesis, Cairo Univ., 1975

KAHN, L. B.: Malignant giant cell tumor of the tendon sheath. Arch. Pathol., *95:*203, 1973

KAHN, L. B.: Esthesioneuroblastoma: light and electron microscopic study. Hum. Pathol., *5:*364, 1974

KAHN, O.: Incidence and significance of gas gangrene in diabetic population. Angiology, *25:*462, 1974

KAHN, O. *et al*: Mortality of diabetic patients treated surgically for lower limb infection and/or gangrene. Diabetes, *23:*287, 1974

KAHN, S.: Classification and surgical correction of gynecomastia (with Simon, Hoffman), PRS, *51:*48, 1973

KAHN, S.: Dynamic tenodesis of distal interphalangeal joint, for use after severance of *profundus* alone, PRS, *51:*536, 1973

KAHN, S.: Newer textbooks: for reference or display? (Letter to the Editor), PRS, *54:*600, 1974

KAHN, S.: Mondor's disease, unusual complication of mammaplasty (With Fischl, Simon), PRS, *56:*319, 1975

KAHN, S.: Revisional surgery after reduction mammaplasty (with Herman, Hoffman), PRS, *55:*422, 1975

KAHN, S., STERN, H. D., AND RHODES, G. A.: Cutaneous and subcutaneous necrosis as complication of coumarin-congener therapy, PRS, *48:*160, 1971

KAHN, S., SIMON, B. E., AND HOFFMAN, S.: Advancement of retracted urethral meatus following Cecil urethroplasty for hypospadias, PRS, *52:*98, 1973. J. Urol., *108:*808, 1972

KAHN, S. *et al*: Nonsurgical aspects of surgery of hand. N. Y. State J. Med., *72:*2201, 1972

KAISER, N.: Possible applications of lasers in surgery. Langenbecks Arch. Chir., *337:*671, 1974 (German)

KAJIMA, H.: Practical method of skin sutures of the face. Surg. Ther. (Osaka), *26:*532, 1972

KAJIMA, H., AND SAI, S.: Hemangioma with petechial rash and treatment (Petechial angioma), PRS, *50:*309, 1972. Jap. J. Plast. Reconstr. Surg., *14:*411, 1971

KAKARAS, P.: Injuries of fingers, evaluation of treatment methods, PRS, *48:*393, 1971. Trans. 1st Panhellenic Cong. Orthop. Surg. & Traum., *1:*168, 1969

KALDEN, J. R., AND BUTHY, E. A.: Prolonged skin allograft survival in vitamin C-deficient guinea pigs, PRS, *51:*484, 1973. Europ. Surg. Res., *4:*114, 1972

KALIKO, I. M. *et al:* Physical therapy of chronic ulcers and torpidly granulating wounds. Vopr. Kurortol. Fizioter. Lech. Fiz. Kult., *36:*458, 1971 (Russian)

KALINICHENKO, N. I. *et al:* Case of total stripping of facial skin. Khirurgiia (Mosk.), *49:*122, 1972 (Russian)

KALKOFF, P., BAUMEISTER, L., AND GEHRING, D.: Endolymphatic radiotherapy in malignant melanoma of lower extremities. Arch. Derm. Forsch., *244:*250, 1972 (German)

KALLAY, F.: Reconstruction of nose deformities associated with unilateral cleft lip. Orv. Hetil., *115:*1946, 1974 (Hungarian)

KALLAY, F. *et al:* Complex treatment and care of children with cleft lip and palate. Orv. Hetil., *117:*3, 1976 (Hungarian)

KALLIONIEMI, H. *et al:* Unilateral hyperplasia of the mandibular coronoid process. Case report. Proc. Finn. Dent. Soc., *71:*184, 1975

KALOUSTIAN, V. M. DER *et al:* Bilateral tibial aplasia with lobster-claw hands. A rare genetic entity. Acta Paediatr. Scand., *62:*77, 1973

KALSBEEK, H. L.: Experience with the use of Teflon mesh in repair of incisional hernias, PRS, *54:*507, 1974. Arch. chir. neerl., *24:*71, 1974

KALTHOFF, P. G.: Hand muscle paralysis in leprosy and its surgical treatment. Handchirurgie, *3:*8, 1971

KALUDI, M.: Erosive arthrosis. Union. Med. Can., *101:*265, 1972 (French)

KAMAKURA, L.: Total reconstruction of ear in congenital microtia (with Spina, Psillakis), PRS, *48:*349, 1971

KAMAKURA, L.: New method for correction of prominent nasal tip (with Spina, Psillakis), PRS, *51:*416, 1973

KAMDAR, K. N. *et al:* Palatography. "A study of velopharyngeal closure." Australas. Radiol., *17:*26, 1973

KAMEL, E. J. *et al:* Emergencies with delayed operation in tropical countries. Ann. Chir., *27:*531, 1973 (French)

KAMER, F. M.: An absorbent, non-adherent nasal pack. Laryngoscope, *85:*384, 1975

KAMER, F. M. *et al:* Conservative management of the Negro nose. Laryngoscope, *85:*551, 1975

KAMER, F. M. *et al:* Two-stage concept of rhytidectomy. Trans. Am. Acad. Ophthalmol. Otolaryngol., *80:*546, 1975

KAMEROS, J., AND HIMMELFARB, R.: TMJ ankylosis, PRS, *57:*396, 1976. J. Oral Surg., *33:*282, 1975

KAMIENIEC, M. *et al:* Case of cervical lymphangioma. Otolaryngol. Pol., *28:*99, 1974 (Polish)

KAMINSKI, J. *et al:* Skin defects in fresh hand injuries. Pol. Przegl. Chir., *44:*31, 1972 (Polish)

KAMMER, G.: Replacement plastic surgery in subcutaneous mastectomy. Praxis, *61:*999, 1972 (German)

KAMPER, M. J., GALLOWAY, D. V., AND ASHLEY, F.: Abdominal panniculectomy after massive weight loss, PRS, *50:*441, 1972

KAMRASH, L. N. *et al:* Aerophoresis of penicillin in early postoperative period after skin autoplasty in patients with thermal trauma. Ortop. Travmatol. Protez, *34:*60, 1973 (Russian)

KANASUGI, K. *et al:* Malignant melanoma: 43 cases. Jap. J. Cancer Clin., *18:*380, 1972 (Japanese)

KANAVEL, A. B.: The classic. Infections of the hand. Clin. Orthop., *104:*3, 1974

KANDZARI, S. J. *et al:* Exstrophy of urinary bladder complicated by adenocarcinoma. Urology, *3:*496, 1974

KANE, A. M. *et al:* Meningoencephalocele of the paranasal sinuses. Laryngoscope, *85:*2087, 1975

KANE, E., KAPLAN, E. B., AND SPINNER, M.: Observations of course of ulnar nerve in arm, PRS, *53:*106, 1974. Ann. Chir., *27:*487, 1973

KANEFF, A. *et al:* Modifications in the musculus extensor digitorum lateralis in phylogenesis and in human ontogenesis. Acta Anat. (Basel), *77:*583, 1970 (German)

KANGUR, T. T. *et al:* Myxomatous tumors of the jaws. J. Oral Surg., *33:*523, 1975

KANTAWALA, S. A. *et al:* Fatal hemorrhage following tracheostomy. Case report. J. Postgrad. Med., *18:*156, 1972

KANTOROVA, V. I., AND TIMASHKEVICH, K. D.: Regeneration of cranial bones after implantation of preserved homologous bone shavings, PRS, *50:*206, 1972. Acta chir. plast., *13:*33, 1971

KAPETANSKY, D. I.: Surgical correction of blepharoptosis in myasthenia gravis. Am. J. Ophth., *74:*818, 1972

KAPETANSKY, D. I.: Bilateral transverse pharyngeal flap for repair of cleft palate, PRS, *52:*52, 1973

KAPETANSKY, D. I.: Animation and cosmetic balance in repair of congenital bilateral cleft lip; modified technique, PRS, *55:*383, 1975.

Cleft Palate J., *11*:219, 1974

KAPLAN, E. B. *et al*: Aneurysm of the ulnar artery. A case report. Bull. Hosp. Joint Dis., *33*:197, 1972

KAPLAN, E. N.: Use of combined palatal pushback and pharyngeal flap operation (Follow-Up Clinic on Buchholz *et al*), PRS, *51*:206, 1973

KAPLAN, E. N.: Skin homografts in rats compared to other organ transplantations (with Gruber, Lucas), PRS, *53*:64, 1974

KAPLAN, E. N.: Risk of malignancy in large congenital nevi, PRS, *53*:421, 1974

KAPLAN, E. N.: Malignant potential of large congenital nevi. West. J. Med., *121*:226, 1974

KAPLAN, E. N.: Soft palate repair by levator muscle reconstruction and buccal mucosal flap, PRS, *56*:129, 1975

KAPLAN, E. N.: Hearing acuity before and after pharyngeal flap procedure (Letter to the Editor), PRS, *56*:205, 1975

KAPLAN, E. N.: Cephalometric study of facial growth in children after combined pushback and pharyngeal flap operations (with Pearl), PRS, *57*:480, 1976

KAPLAN, E. N. *et al*: Craniofacial osteotomy. Calif. Med., *116*:53, 1972

KAPLAN E. N., BUNCKE, H. J., AND MURRAY, D. E.: Distant transfer of cutaneous island flaps in humans by microvascular anastomoses, PRS, *52*:301, 1973

KAPLAN, H. A. *et al*: Variations of cerebral dural sinuses at torcular herophili. Importance in radical neck dissection. Am. J. Surg., *124*:456, 1972

KAPLAN, I.: Management of hand injuries. S. Afr. Med. J., *44*:1011, 1970

KAPLAN, I.: Rapid method for constructing a functional sensitive penis. Brit. J. Plast. Surg., *24*:342, 1971

KAPLAN, I.: Scrotal flap in ischial decubitis. Brit. J. Plast. Surg., *25*:22, 1972

KAPLAN, I.: Reconstruction of the columella. Brit. J. Plast. Surg., *25*:37, 1972

KAPLAN, I.: Treatment of hand injuries. S. Afr. J. Surg., *11*:249, 1973

KAPLAN, I.: Management of injuries to the hand. Surg. Annual, *6*:283, 1974

KAPLAN, I. *et al*: Malignant melanomas in the South African Bantu. Brit. J. Plast. Surg., *25*:65, 1972

KAPLAN, I. *et al*: Partial mastectomy and mammaplasty performed with a CO 2 surgical laser. Comparative study. Brit. J. Plast. Surg., *26*:363, 1973

KAPLAN, I. *et al*: Carbon dioxide laser in head and neck surgery. Am. J. Surg., *128*:543, 1974

KAPLAN, I. *et al*: Simultaneous repair of cleft lip and palate in early infancy, PRS, *56*:681, 1975. Brit. J. Plast. Surg., *27*:134, 1974

KAPLAN, I., DINNER, M., AND CHAIT, L.: Use of *extensor pollicis longus* tendon as distal extension for *opponens* transfer, PRS, *57*:186, 1976

KAPLAN, J. M.: Rotation flaps, neck to cheek (with Stark), PRS, *50*:230, 1972

KAPLAN, J. M.: Development of cleft lip nose (with Stark), PRS, *51*:413, 1973

KAPPEL, D. A. *et al*: Significance of persistent radiolucency of mandibular fractures, PRS, *53*:38, 1974

KAPPESSER, H. J. *et al*: Asymmetric macrodactylia. Hautarzt, *26*:416, 1975 (German)

KARAHARJU, E. O., AND SJERNVOLL, L.: Alcohol factor in accidents, PRS, *55*:726, 1975. Injury, *6*:67, 1974

KARAKOUSIS, C. P., ELIAS, E. G., AND DOUGLASS, H. O.: Abdominal wall replacement with plastic mesh in ablative cancer surgery, PRS, *57*:533, 1976. Surgery, *78*:4, 1975

KARAM, F.: Facial nerve decompression and grafting. A report of 8 cases. J. Med. Liban., *24*:505, 1971

KARAPANDZIC, M.: Reconstruction of lip defects by local arterial flaps, PRS, *56*:676, 1975. Brit. J. Plast. Surg., *27*:93, 1974

KARCHINOV, K.: Phalangization of hand metacarpals, PRS, *50*:199, 1972. Acta chir. plast., *13*:47, 1971

KARCHINOV, K.: Radial polydactyly of the hand. Ortop. Travmatol. Protez., *35*:34, 1974 (Russian)

KARESEN, R.: Immune reactions against human malignant tumors. Tidssk. Nor. Laegeforen, *91*:2555, 1971 (Norwegian)

KARFIK, V.: Further development of congenital malformations influenced by surgical treatment. Acta Univ. Carol. (Med. Monogr.), (Praha), *56*:37, 1973

KARFIK, V.: In memory of Robert F. Ivy. Rozhl. Chir., *54*:661, 1975 (Czech)

KARFIK, V., AND SMAHEL, J.: Further experiences on free transfer of hairbearing skin, PRS, *48*:399, 1971. Acta chir. plast., *12*:227, 1970

KARJALAINEN, P., ALHAVA, E. M., AND VALTOLA, J.: Thenar muscle blood flow and bone mineral in forearms of lumberjacks, PRS, *57*:761, 1976. Brit. J. Indust. Med., *32*:11, 1975

KARKOWSKI, J., AND BUNCKE, H. J.: Simplified technique for free transfer of groin flaps, by use of Doppler probe, PRS, *55*:682, 1975. Discussion by Bingham, PRS, *56*:84, 1975

KARL, P. *et al*: Infrared thermometry in surgical flaps. Dtsch. Stomatol. *21*:657, 1971 (German)

KARLEEN, C. I.: Snowmobiling with associated maxillofacial injuries, PRS, *53:*682, 1974. Minn. Med., *Nov.:* 975, 1973

KARMODY, C. S. *et al*: Angiosarcoma of premaxilla. Laryngoscope, *84:*560, 1974

KAROBATH, H. *et al*: Electrocardiographic changes in a patient struck by lightning. Wien. Klin. Wochenschr., *84:*428, 1972 (German)

KARRING, T. *et al*: Conservation of tissue specificity after heterotopic transplantation of gingiva and alveolar mucosa. J. Periodont. Res., *6:*282, 1971

KARSELL, E. R.: Mammography at Mayo Clinic—a year's experience, PRS, *56:*106, 1975. Mayo Clin. Proc., *49:*954, 1974

KARTCH, M.: Correspondence: modified lacrimal probe. Arch. Ophth., *93:*163, 1975

KARTCH, M. C.: French-eye pigtail probe for lacrimal canaliculus repair. Am. J. Ophth., *72:*1145, 1971

KASAI, J.: Experience of manual myotomy for muscular torticollis in infants. Orthop. Surg. (Tokyo), *22:*1107, 1971 (Japanese)

KASDAN, M. L. *et al*: Postoperative instructions for hand surgery. J. Ky. Med. Assoc., *72:*32, 1974

KASHIMA, H.: Indications for excision, limitations of excision, and suture technique, PRS, *52:*687, 1973. Jap. J. Plast. Reconstr. Surg., *15:*346, 1972

KASPAROVA, N. N.: Foundations of planning of plastic operation of the upper lip in children with congenital complete bilateral cleft lip alveolar process and palate. Stomatologiia (Mosk.), *51:*52, 1972 (Russian)

KASTENBAUER, E. R.: Reconstruction of the nasal ala. Z. Laryngol. Rhinol. Otol., *52:*83, 1973 (German)

KASTENBAUER, E. R.: Suitability of tissue adhesive histoacryl in rhinoplasty. Z. Laryngol. Rhinol. Otol., *52:*240, 1973 (German)

KASTENBAUER, E.: External nose and nasal septum. Z. Laryngol. Rhinol. Otol., *52:*597, 1973 (German)

KASTENBAUER, E.: Rhinological aspects of lacrimal reconstruction. Laryngol. Rhinol. Otol. (Stuttg.), *53:*486, 1974 (German)

KASTENBAUER, E.: Rhinoplasty and nasal function. Munch. Med. Wochenschr., *116:*399, 1974 (German)

KATAYE, S.: Rhinoplasty. Ann. Otolaryngol. Chir. Cervicofac., *90:*123, 1973 (French)

KATAYE, S.: Fronto-ethmoidal anterior encephalocele (case report). Ann. Otolaryngol. Chir. Cervicofac., *92:*417, 1975 (French)

KATAYE, S. *et al*: Hydatid cyst of mouth floor, case. Ann. Otolaryngol. Chir. Cervicofac., *90:*727, 1973 (French)

KATO, T., AND KITAGAWA, S.: Congenital anomalies in rats and mice, produced by sulfonamides, PRS, *53:*607, 1974. Congen. Anom., *13:*7, 1973

KATOWITZ, J. A.: Silicone tubing in canalicular obstruction. Preliminary report. Arch. Ophth., *91:*459, 1974

KATOWITZ, J. A. *et al*: Ichthyosis congenita. Arch. Ophth., *91:*208, 1974

KATS, A. G.: Discussion on the right age for the surgical treatment of children with congenital cleft lip and palate. Stomatologiia (Mosk.), *50:*75, 1971 (Russian)

KATZ, A., AND LEWIS, J. S.: Nasal gliomas, PRS, *49:*587, 1972. Arch. Otolaryng., *94:*351, 1971

KATZ, A., AND HIRSCHI, S.: Giant cell reparative granuloma in temporal bone, PRS, *55:*723, 1975. Arch. Otolaryng., *100:*380, 1974

KATZ, A. D.: Midline dermoid tumors of neck, PRS, *55:*640, 1975. Arch. Surg., *109:*822, 1974

KATZ, A. D.: Unusual lesions of parotid gland. J. Surg. Oncol., *7:*219, 1975

KATZ, A. D., PASSY, V., AND KAPLAN, L.: Neurogenous neoplasms of major nerves of face and neck, PRS, *49:*235, 1972. Arch. Surg., *103:*51, 1971

KATZ, A. M. *et al*: Gangrene of the hand and forearm: a complication of radial artery cannulation. Crit. Care Med., *2:*270, 1974

KATZ, H. *et al*: Therapeutic challenge of premalignant and malignant skin lesions. Geriatrics, *30:*53, 1975

KATZ, J.: Survey of anesthetic choice among anesthesiologists, PRS, *53:*376, 1974. Anesth. Analg., Cleve., *52:*373, 1973

KAUFER, H. *et al*: Orthopedic implications of drug subculture, PRS, *57:*541, 1976. J. Trauma, *14:*853, 1974

KAUFMAN, G. *et al*: Ischemic necrosis of muscles of the buttock. A case report. J. Bone & Joint Surg. (Am.), *54:*1079, 1972

KAUFMAN, H. D.: High pressure injection injuries, the problems, pathogenesis and management. Hand, *2:*63, 1970

KAUFMAN, J. J., AND ROZ, S.: Use of implantable prostheses for treatment of urinary incontinence and impotence, PRS, *57:*675, 1976. Am. J. Surg., *130:*244, 1975

KAUFMAN, R. S.: Hearing loss in children with cleft palates. N.Y. State J. Med., *70:*2555, 1970

KAUFMANN, A. *et al*: Chronic lymphedema of extremities (problems of diagnosis and treatment). Chirurgia (Bucur.), *23:*249, 1974 (Rumanian)

KAUFMANN, J.: Surgical correction of male fertility disorders. Dtsch. Med. Wochenschr., *97:*1510, 1972 (German)

KAUL, B. K. *et al*: Hemangiosarcoma in children: two case reports. Am. Surg., *40:*643, 1974

KAUSHIK, S. P. *et al*: Electrical burn of abdomen, case report. Aust. N. Z. J. Surg., *43:*186, 1973

KAVARANA, N.: Complications of free flap transfers to mouth region (with Finseth, Antia). PRS, *56:*652, 1975

KAVARANA, N. M.: Use of folded forehead flap for reconstruction after large excision of full thickness of cheek. PRS, *56:*629, 1975

KAVKA, S. J.: Basal cell adenomas. Arch. Otolaryng., *100:*247, 1974

KAVROKIROV, V. *et al*: Treatment of malignant tumors of upper jaw. Stomatologiia (Sofia), *55:*11, 1973 (Bulgarian)

KAWAI, T. *et al*: Auricular composite graft in nasal reconstruction: report of 3 cases. Jap. J. Oral Surg., *19:*95, 1973 (Japanese)

KAWAMURA, J. *et al*: Prognosis in muscular torticollis. Orthop. Surg. (Tokyo), *23:*44, 1972 (Japanese)

KAWAMURA, M. *et al*: Surgical orthodontic treatment of facial asymmetry using direct bonding plastic brackets. Int. J. Oral Surg., *3:*252, 1974

KAWIAK, H.: Evaluation of the surgical treatment of 175 children with cleft of secondary palate. Probl. Med. Wieku. Rozwoj., *3:*193, 1973 (Polish)

KAY, A. G.: Natural history of synovial hypertrophy in the rheumatoid hand. Ann. Rheum. Dis., *30:*98, 1971

KAY, J. H.: Letter: skin grafts and leg ulcers. N. Z. Med. J., *82:*317, 1975

KAY, L. W.: Differential diagnosis of cysts of jaws, PRS, *49:*470, 1972. Proc. Roy. Soc. Med., *64:*550, 1971

KAY, L. W. *et al*: Surgical management of dental and jaw deformities. Rev. Dent. Liban., *23:*61, 1973

KAY, N. R. *et al*: Management of electrical injuries of extremities. Surg. Clin. North Am., *53:*1459, 1973

KAYA, U. *et al*: Total extirpation of invasive glomus jugular tumors, PRS, *56:*464, 1975. Ann. oto-laryng. Chir. Cervicofac., *91:*595, 1974

KAYE, B. L.: Neurologic changes with excessively large breasts, PRS, *50:*305, 1972. South. M. J., *65:*177, 1972

KAYE, B. L.: Simplified method for correcting prominent ear (Follow-Up Clinic). PRS, *52:*184, 1973

KAYE, B. L.: "Home-made" suction drain for small areas. PRS, *52:*447, 1973

KAYE, B. L.: Axillary breasts. PRS, *53:*61, 1974

KAYE, B. L.: Axillary breasts. An aesthetic deformity of the trunk. Clin. Plast. Surg., *2:*397, 1975

KAYE, B. L.: Improved quartz-halogen headlight. PRS, *57:*110, 1976

KAYE, B. L., AND LOTUACO, G. G.: Simplified technique for congenital lop ear. PRS, *54:*667, 1974

KAYHAN, V. *et al*: Cryosurgery in treatment of intraoral hemangiomas. Rev. Laryngol. Otol. Rhinol. (Bord.), *94:*245, 1973

KAZANDZHIEV, R.: Correction of mammary gland hypoplasia by H. G. Arion's retroglandular balloon prosthesis. Khirurgiia (Sofiia), *26:*339, 1973 (Bulgarian)

KAZANJIAN, V. H., AND CONVERSE, JOHN M.: *Surgical Treatment of Facial Injuries*. 3rd Ed. Williams & Wilkins Co., Baltimore, 1974

KEAN, H.: One stage repair of the twisted nose. Eye, Ear, Nose, Throat Mon., *52:*502, 1974

KEAN, H. *et al*: Anesthesia techniques and facial plastic surgery. Trans. Pa. Acad. Ophthalmol. Otolaryngol., *27:*45, 1974

KEATON, W. M. *et al*: Ameloblastoma, report of two cases. J. Oral Surg., *32:*382, 1974

KEAVENY, T. V. *et al*: Combined treatment of massive hemangioma of neck and face, PRS, *57:*256, 1976. J. Cardiovasc. Surg., *16:*159, 1975

KEDRA, H. *et al*: Surgical management of traumatic injuries of the hand. Pol. Przegl. Chir., *44:*311, 1972 (Polish)

KEELER, L. L. *et al*: Chronic lymphedema of scrotum and penis. J. Med. Soc. N.J., *71:*575, 1974

KEEN, R. R.: Orbital fractures treated with teflon implants. Trans. Int. Conf. Oral Surg., *4:*311, 1973

KEETON, J. E. *et al*: Hypospadias: a general review. J. Miss. State Med. Assoc., *16:*340, 1975

KEIER, A. N.: Separation of short stumps of shoulders from the cicatricial adhesion to skin of chest. Ortop. Travmatol. Protez., *4:*67, 1975 (Russian)

KEISER, H. R.: Disruption of healed scars in scurvy—result of disequilibrium in collagen metabolism (with Cohen), PRS, *57:*213, 1976. Discussion by Chvapil, PRS, *57:*376, 1976

KEITER, J., BAKOWSKI, M. J., AND WEEKS, P. M.: Byssal thread formation: collagen-glycosaminoglycan interaction, PRS, *52:*328, 1973. Surg. Forum, *23:*27, 1972

KEKELIDZE, A. A.: Case of acute nasal bleeding requiring unilateral ligation of the external carotid artery. Vestn. Otorinolaringol., *33:*108, 1971 (Russian)

KELALIS, P. P.: Urinary diversion in children by sigmoid conduit: its advantages and limitations. J. Urol., *112:*666, 1974

KELALIS, P. *et al*: Timing of elective surgery on genitalia of male children with particular reference to undescended testes and hypospadias, PRS, *57:*400, 1976. Pediatrics, *56:*479, 1975

KELIKIAN, H.: *Congenital Deformities of the Hand and Forearm.* W. B. Saunders Co., Philadelphia, 1974. PRS, *56:*445, 1975

KELLER, E. E. *et al*: Orthognathic surgery. Review of mandibular body procedures. Mayo Clin. Proc., *51:*117, 1976

KELLEY, J. H. *et al*: Procedure for lengthening the phallus in boys with exstrophy of the bladder. J. Pediatr. Surg., *6:*645, 1971

KELLY, A. P., JR.: Management of epistaxis in Osler-Weber-Rendu disease; recurrence of telangiectases within nasal skin graft (with McCabe), PRS, *50:*114, 1972

KELLY, D. E., AND HARRIGAN, W. F.: Survey of facial fractures, PRS, *57:*260, 1976. Oral Surg., *33:*146, 1975

KELLY, D. E., AND KLEIN, K. M.: Lip reconstruction following resection for unusual basal cell carcinoma, PRS, *57:*539, 1976. Oral Surg., *40:*19, 1975

KELLY, D. R. *et al*: Benign lymphoepithelial lesions of the salivary glands. Arch. Otolaryng., *101:*71, 1975

KELLY, E. E.: Feeding cleft palate babies — today's babies, today's methods. Cleft Palate J., *8:*61, 1971

KELLY, G. L.: Radial artery occlusion by carpal ganglion. PRS, *52:*191, 1973

KELLY, J. F., AND TERRY, B. C.: Blood volume changes in surgical treatment of oral-facial deformities: preliminary report. J. Oral Surg., *31:*90, 1973

KELLY, J. F. *et al*: Technetium-99m radionuclide bone imaging for evaluating mandibular osseous allografts. J. Oral Surg., *33:*11, 1975

KELLOGG, R. H. *et al*: Chloramphenicol as an adjunct in the topical treatment of burns. Am. J. Hosp. Pharm., *29:*386, 1972

Keloid (See also *Scars, Hypertrophic*)

Corticoid intralesional injections with dermojet in treatment of hypertrophic scars and keloids (Henel, Pinto), PRS, *48:*519, 1971. A Folha Med., *61:*337, 1970

Keloids and hypertrophic scars, biologic basis for treatment (Peacock, Madden, Trier), PRS, *51:*709, 1973. South. M. J., *63:*755, 1970

Keloid scars, treatment with fluocinolone acetonide (Garcia-Velazco), PRS, *50:*637, 1972. Invest. Clin. Mexico, *10:*161, 1971

Keloids and hypertrophic scars, follow-up treatment with triamcinolone (Ketchum,

Keloid — Cont.

Robinson, Masters). PRS, *48:*256, 1971

Keloids, management by surgical excision and local injections of steroid (Singleton, Gross), PRS, *52:*331, 1973. South. M. J., *64:*1377, 1971

Keloid and hypertrophic scar, human, collagen synthesis in (Cohen, Keiser, Sjoerdsma), PRS, *50:*205, 1972. Surg. Forum, *22:*488, 1971

Keloid scars, treatment of, by subtotal excision and graft (14 cases) (Bourrel *et al*). Ann. chir. plast., *17:*304, 1972 (French)

Keloid scars, 15, pathological and clinical study of (Prévost-Thiériot *et al*), PRS, *51:*608, 1973. Ann. dermat. & syph., *99:*269, 1972

Keloid, monstrous (Duperrat, *et al*). Bull. Soc. Fr. Dermatol. Syphiligr., *79:*210, 1972 (French)

Keloids and scars, treatment of (Sugimoto), PRS, *51:*610, 1973. Jap. J. Plast. Reconstr. Surg., *15:*157, 1972

Collagen synthesis: inhibition of scar formation by proline analog cis-hydroxyproline (Lane *et al*), PRS, *52:*104, 1973. J. Surg. Res., *13:*135, 1972

Keloids, current concepts in management of (Strahan *et al*). Otolaryngol. Clin. North Am., *5:*521, 1972

Triamcinolone acetonide solution, intradermal injection with excision and skin grafting, in eradication of large auricular keloids (Converse, Stallings). PRS, *49:*461, 1972

Keloid recurrence, correlation with completeness of local excision; a negative report (Cosman, Wolff). PRS, *50:*163, 1972

Keloid and hypertrophic scar, histamine and collagen synthesis in (Cohen *et al*), PRS, *51:*709, 1973. Surg. Forum, *23:*509, 1972

Kenacort A to treat hypertrophic scars and keloids in children (Jaworski), PRS, *54:*624, 1974. Acta chir. plast., *15:*206, 1973

Keloids and finger contractures, correction in burn patients (Robitaille *et al*), PRS, *54:*113, 1974. Arch. Phys. Med., *54:*515, 1973

Keloids, use of homografts in (Snyder). Brit. J. Plast. Surg., *26:*32, 1973

Keloids, radiotherapy in treatment of, in East Africa (Edsmyr *et al*). East Afr. Med. J., *50:*457, 1973

Keloid scars (Garcez, Saraiva, Braga), PRS, *53:*248, 1974. Folha Med. Brazil, *66:*57, 1973

Keloids, radiation therapy of (Asakura *et al*), PRS, *54:*118, 1974. Jap. J. Plast. Reconstr. Surg., *16:*496, 1973

Keloid — Cont.

Triamcinolone, inhibition of mature ³H-collagen destruction by (Rudolph, Klein), PRS, *53:*692, 1974. J. Surg. Res., *14:*435, 1973

Keloid, origin of hypertrophic scar (Linares *et al*), PRS, *53:*495, 1974. J. Trauma, *13:*70, 1973

Vaccination scars in deltoid area, pitfall of surgical excision of (Musgrave) (Letter to the Editor). PRS, *51:*198, 1973

Keloids and hypertrophic scars, intralesional injection of, with Dermo-Jet (Vallis) (Follow-Up Clinic), PRS. *52:*434, 1973

Keloids, modifying evolution of (Linares), PRS, *55:*517, 1975. Rev. Latino Am. cir. plast., *17:*51, 1973

Keloids, therapy with corticosteroids (Kyrtatas), PRS, *53:*502, 1974. Tr. 28th Panhellenic Cong. Medicosurg. Soc., *1:*242, 1973

Keloid, treatment with lemon juice in prevention of recurrences (Reuter). Zentralbl. Chir., *98:*604, 1973 (German)

Keloids, treatment with triamcinolone acetonide (Martinova). Acta Chir. Orthop. Traumatol. Cech., *41:*136, 1974 (Czechoslovakian)

Keloids, lobule, button compression for (Snyder). Brit. J. Plast. Surg., *27:*186, 1974

Keloids and X-rays (Editorial). Brit. Med. J., *3:*592, 1974

Keloids in the African (Oluwasanmi). Clin. Plast. Surg., *1:*179, 1974

Keloids, experience treating 501 patients with (Amar Inalsingh), PRS, *57:*764, 1976. Johns Hopkins Med. J., *134:*284, 1974

Keloids and hypertrophic scars, cryosurgery for. Preliminary report (Pierce). J. Natl. Med. Assoc., *66:*174, 1974

Dermatofibrosarcoma protuberans or keloid — a warning (Manalan, Cohen, Theogaraj). PRS, *53:*96, 1974

Keloids and hypertrophic scars (Ketchum, Cohen, Masters). PRS, *53:*140, 1974

Keloids, study of 1,000 patients in South India (Ramakrishnan, Thomas, Sundararajan). PRS, *53:*276, 1974

Keloids, bilateral earlobe (Cosman, Wolff). PRS, *53:*540, 1974

Keloid scars after cutiplastic operations in children, prevention and treatment (Troshkov *et al*). Vestn. Khir., *113:*73, 1974 (Russian)

Recurrent keloid in the pedicle skin graft of the concha auriculae (Arbuzov). Zdravookhr. Ross. Fed., *5:*111, 1974 (Russian)

Facial scars resulting from vehicular accidents (Lewis). Clin. Plast. Surg., *2:*143, 1975

Keloid management and present status

Keloid — Cont.

(Doyle, Passey), PRS, *57:*123, 1976. Eye, Ear, Nose & Throat Month., *54:*239, 1975

Keloids, effects of intralesional injection of triamcinolone on glucose-6-phosphate dehydrogenase and alanine aminotransferase activity in (Im, Mulliken, Hoopes). PRS, *56:*660, 1975

Treatment of auricular keloids (Kulcynski *et al*). Otolaryngol. Pol., *29:*137, 1975 (Polish)

Keloid growth, presumptive evidence of effect of pregnancy estrogens on (Moustafa, Abdel-Fattah). PRS, *56:*450, 1975

Clinical evaluation of X-ray therapy in the treatment of keloid as compared with other therapeutic methods (Kik). Przegl. Chir., *47:*1173, 1975 (Polish)

Action of corticosteroids on cutaneous cicatrization. Use in maxillofacial surgery (Grellet *et al*). Rev. Stomatol. Chir. Maxillofac., *76:*379, 1975 (French)

Tumors of connective tissue of skin (Ariel). Rev. Surg., *32:*153, 1975

Keloid and normal tissue, cell size and growth characteristics of cultured fibroblasts isolated from (Russell, Witt). PRS, *57:*207, 1976

Keloids: reappraisal of shaving and skin grafting for hypertrophic burn scars (Moustafa, Abdel-Fattah). PRS, *57:*463, 1976

Indications for surgical treatment of keloids and correlation of various therapeutic methods (Kik). Pol. Przegl. Chir., *48:*69, 1976 (Polish)

KELSH, J. M.: Cystosarcoma phylloides in twelve-year-old girl. N. C. Med. J., *35:*295, 1974

KEMBLE, J. V.: Importance of nasal septum in facial development. J. Laryng. & Otol., *87:*379, 1973

KEMP, W. A. *et al*: Treatment of severe decubitus ulcers using the Beaufort-Winchester flotation bed. Rheumatol. Phys. Med., *11:*401, 1972

KEMPF, I. *et al*: Fibro-aponeurotic formations of the palmar region. Arch. Anat. Histol. Embryol. (Strasb.), *53:*353, 1970 (French)

KEMPFLE, B. *et al*: Surgical treatment of large jaw cysts by cystectomy (part II) with autohemocomplement. Med. Hyg. (Geneve), *30:*1472, 1972 (French)

KEMSLEY, G. M.: Transmission of hepatitis B virus in dermabrasion? (Letter to the Editor). PRS, *56:*440, 1975

KENDALL, B.: Invasion of facial bones by basal meningiomas. Brit. J. Radiol., *46:*237, 1973

KENDALL, T. E. *et al*: Primary malignant tumors of the hand. J. Kans. Med. Soc., 72:376, 1971

KENEDI, R. M. et al: Tissue mechanics. Phys. Med. Biol., 20:699, 1975

KENEFICK, J. S.: Some aspects of salivary gland disorders, PRS, 57:395, 1976. Proc. Roy. Soc. Med., 68:283, 1975

KENEFICK, T. C.: Retropharyngeal lipoma. J. Laryng. & Otol., 88:805, 1974

KENEPP, N. et al: Evaluation of maxillary antrostomy in treatment of fractures of middle third of face. J. Trauma, 13:884, 1973

KENERMAN, R. P.: Experience with plasty using double Filatov flap for treatment of large tissue defects in one or both legs and feet, PRS, 53:689, 1974. Acta chir. plast., 15:120, 1973

KENESI, C.: Surgical treatment of the rheumatoid hand. The metacarpophalangeal joint. Rev. Rhum. Mal. Osteoartic., 38:307, 1971 (French)

KENESI, C. et al: Arthroplasty by Swanson implants in the rheumatic hand. Experience from 100 cases, followed for more than 6 months. Rev. Rhum. Mal. Osteoartic., 41:271, 1974 (French)

KENIS, M. et al: Internal fixation in fractures of the hand and fingers. Acta Orthop. Belg., 41:110, 1975

KENNEDY, R. E.: Marsupialization of inoperable orbital dermoids. Trans. Am. Ophthalmol. Soc., 68:146, 1970

KENNEDY, T. L. et al: Surgery of violence. 1. Civilian bomb injuries. Brit. Med. J., 1:382, 1975

KENNET, S.: Premalignant lesions of mouth, PRS, 53:105, 1974. Contemp. Surg., 2:55, 1973

KENNETT, S.: Temporomandibular joint ankylosis: rationale for grafting in young patient. J. Oral Surg., 31:744, 1973

KENNETT, S. et al: Mandibular micrognathia: etiology and surgical management. J. Oral Surg., 31:8, 1973

KENT, J. N. et al: Condylar reconstruction: treatment planning. Oral Surg., 37:489, 1974

KENT, J. N. et al: Proplast in dental facial reconstruction, PRS, 56:601, 1975. J. Oral Surg., 39:347, 1975

KENWORTHY, G.: An artificial hand incorporating function and cosmesis. Biomed. Eng., 9:559, 1974

KEPES, E. R., AND FOLDES, E. F.: Transient abducens paralysis following nerve blocks of head and neck, PRS, 53:246, 1974. Anesthesiology, 38:893, 1973

KEPPKE, E. M.: Abdominoplasty (with Baroudi, Netto). PRS, 54:161, 1974

Keratoacanthoma (See also *Cancer, Squamous Cell*)

Keratoacanthomas: diagnostic pitfall in skin tumor pathology. Rational therapeutic attitude (Vandenbussche et al). Ann. chir. plast., 17:289, 1972 (French)

Keratoacanthoma, unusual case report (Brown, Leuy), PRS, 52:327, 1973. Cutis, 8:585, 1972

Keratoacanthoma, review of 57 cases (Cohen et al). PRS, 49:138, 1972

Keratoacanthoma is frequently dangerous diagnosis (Iverson, Vistnes), PRS, 53:687, 1974. Am. J. Surg., 126:359, 1973

Keratoacanthoma, immunological reaction in (Brown, Tan), PRS, 53:496, 1974. Cancer Res., 33:2030, 1973

Keratoacanthoma, solitary, in child (Price et al). Am. J. Dis. Child., 128:110, 1974

Pseudorecidivism of irradiated basal cell carcinoma (Poyzer et al). Australas. J. Dermatol., 15:77, 1974

Keratoacanthoma, squamous cell carcinoma diagnosed as (Mikhail), 54:381, 1974. Cutis, 13:378, 1974

Keratoacanthoma, strange tumor (Noble). Nouv. Presse Med., 3:535, 1974 (French)

Keratoacanthoma, solitary intraoral (Scofield, Werning, Shukes), PRS, 55:106, 1975. Oral Surg., 37:889, 1974

Keratoacanthoma of lower lip (Azaz, Lustman), PRS, 56:234, 1975. Oral Surg., 38:918, 1974

Surgical treatment of non-traumatic lower lip lesions with special reference to the step technique. A follow-up on 149 patients (Johanson et al). Scand. J. Plast. Reconstr. Surg., 8:232, 1974

Florid keratoacanthomas in a kidney transplant recipient. Case report (Jacobsson et al). Scand. J. Plast. Reconstr. Surg., 8:243, 1974

Giant keratoacanthoma of the nose (Rapaport). Arch. Dermat., 111:73, 1975

Treatment of keratoacanthoma (Ebner et al). Wien. Med. Wochenschr., 125:91, 1975 (German)

Keratosis

Comparison of chemical peeling, dermabrasion and 5-fluorouracil in cancer prophylaxis (Spira et al). J. Surg. Oncol., 3:367, 1971

Keratoses, palmar, and visceral cancer (Gilbertsen, Bean, Fusaro). PRS, 50:205, 1972. Arch. Dermat., 105:222, 1972

Surgical treatment of familial plantar hyperkeratosis (Swenson et al). Nebr. Med. J.,

Keratosis — Cont.
57:377, 1972
Keratosis, intractable plantar (Mann *et al*). Orthop. Clin. North Am., *4*:67, 1972
Acquired (digital) fibrokeratomas. Complication of ingrown toenail (Herman *et al*). Acta Derm. Venereol. (Stockh.), *54*:73, 1974
Practical cryosurgery for oral lesions (Leopard *et al*). Brit. Dent. J., *136*:185, 1974
Experience of skin tumours treatment with laser radiation (Gamaleja *et al*). Panminerva Med., *16*:41, 1974
Surgical treatment of non-traumatic lower lip lesions with special reference to the step technique. A follow-up on 149 patients (Johanson *et al*). Scand. J. Plast. Reconstr. Surg., *8*:232, 1974
Practical therapy for hyperkeratotic skin lesions (Jansen). Geriatrics, *30*:71, 1975
Cryosurgery in dermatologic office practice: special reference to dermatofibroma and mucous cyst of the lip (Spiller *et al*). South. Med. J., *68*:157, 1975

KERN, E. B.: Nose structure and function, PRS, *57*:257, 1976. Postgrad. Med., *57*:101, 1975
KERN, F. B., AND BINNS, J. H.: Subcutaneous mastectomy and reconstruction in large breasts. PRS, *54*:648, 1974
KERNAHAN, D. A.: Melkersson-Rosenthal syndrome (with Vistnes). PRS, *48*:126, 1971
KERNAHAN, D. A.: Cleft lip and palate classification (Letter to the Editor). PRS, *51*:578, 1973
KERNERMAN, R. P.: Experience with plasty using double Filatov flap for treatment of large tissue defects in one or both legs and feet. Acta chir. plast. (Praha), *15*:120, 1973
KERR, N. W.: Life and work of dental surgeon and oral surgeon in Peoples Republic of China. Brit. J. Oral Surg., *11*:36, 1973
KERRY, R. L. *et al*: Effects of 5-fluorouracil on skin graft survival. Ohio State Med. J., *67*:1093, 1971
KERSTELL, J.: Pathogenesis of post-traumatic fat embolism, PRS, *49*:671, 1972. Am. J. Surg., *121*:712, 1971
KERSTEN, T. E., AND McQUARRIE, D. G.: Surgical management of shotgun injuries of face, PRS, *56*:605, 1975. Surg. Gynec. & Obst., *140*:517, 1975
KERTH, J. D. *et al*: Radical neck dissection in carcinoma of head and neck. Surg. Clin. North Am., *53*:179, 1973
KERTH, J. D. *et al*: Revision in unsuccessful rhinoplasty. Otolaryngol. Clin. North Am., *7*:65, 1974

KESSELRING, U. K.: Reduction mammaplasty with L-shaped suture line (with Meyer). PRS, *55*:139, 1975
KESSLER, F. B.: Use of pedicled tendon transfer with silicone rod in complicated secondary flexor tendon repairs. PRS, *49*:439, 1972
KESSLER, F. B.: Pedicled tendon transfer (Letter to the Editor). PRS, *50*:398, 1972
KESSLER, I.: Five-fingered hand. One-stage pollicization of the radial finger. Isr. J. Med. Sci., *6*:280, 1970
KESSLER, I.: Aetiology and management of adduction contracture of thumb in rheumatoid arthritis, PRS, *54*:376, 1974. Hand *5*:170, 1973
KESSLER, I.: New silicone implant for replacement of destroyed metacarpal heads, PRS, *56*:227, 1975. Hand, *6*: 308, 1974
KESSLER, W. O. *et al*: Agenesis of penis. Embryology and management. Urology, *1*:226, 1973
KETCHAM, A. S.: Modern trends in prevention of cancer recurrence. Aktuel Probl. Chir., *14*:183, 1970
KETCHAM, A. S. *et al*: Ethmoid sinuses: re-evaluation of surgical resection. Am. J. Surg., *126*:469, 1973
KETCHUM, L. D.: Experimental use of Pluronic F68 in microvascular surgery (Letter to the Editor). PRS, *54*:478, 1974
KETCHUM, L. D., ROBINSON, D. W., AND MASTERS, F. W.: Follow-up on treatment of hypertrophic scars and keloids with triamcinolone. PRS, *48*:256, 1971
KETCHUM, L. D., ROBINSON, D. W., AND MASTERS, F. W.: Dupuytren's contracture, PRS, *51*:348, 1973. J. Kansas M. Soc., *73*:108, 1972
KETCHUM, L. D., COHEN, I. K., AND MASTERS, F. W.: Hypertrophic scars and keloids. PRS, *53*:140, 1974
KETCHUM, L. D. *et al*: Experimental use of Pluronic F68 in microvascular surgery. PRS, *53*:288, 1974
KETCHUM, L. D., MASTERS, F. W., AND ROBINSON, D. W.: Mandibular reconstruction using a composite island rib flap. PRS, *53*:471, 1974
KETTLEKAMP, D. B.: Trauma to the ulnar artery. Arch. Surg., *105*:682, 1972
KETTLEKAMP, D., FLATT, A., AND MOULDS, R.: Traumatic dislocation of the long-finger extensor tendon, PRS, *49*:664, 1972. J. Bone & Joint Surg., *53*:229, 1971
KETTY, N. *et al*: Ankyloglossia with psychological implications. J. Dent. Child., *41*:43, 1974
KETZAN, I.: Fulminant Candida albicans sepsis with fatal clinical course beginning from a primary skin infection. Mykosen, *11*:699, 1968 (German)

KHADZHLEV, I. I.: New urinary bladder made from rectum. Khirurgiia (Sofiia), *26:*168, 1973 (Bulgarian)

KHAFIF, R. A. *et al*: Plunging ranula. J. Oral Surg., *33:*537, 1975

KHAIKIN, G. I.: Treatment of face bites. Vestn. Khir., *109:*95, 1973 (Russian)

KHALIL, G. A.: Simple, inexpensive retractor for hand surgery. South. Med. J., *66:*966, 1973

KHALIL, G. A.: Mid-facial fractures: management and results. W. Va. Med. J., *70:*153, 1974

KHAMAPIRAD, B. *et al*: Microsurgery of lacrimal sac. Trans. Ophthalmol. Soc. N.Z., *25:*144, 1973

KHANIN, A. A. *et al*: Derivative neoformation in reparative regeneration of skin. Zh. Eksp. Klin. Med., *13:*8, 1973 (Russian)

KHANNA, N. N.: Technique for epispadias repair. PRS, *52:*365, 1973

KHANNA, N. N., AND JOSHI, G. K.: Elephantiasis of female genitalia. PRS, *48:*379, 1971

KHANNA, N. N. *et al*: Unilateral hyperplasia of mandibular condyle, PRS, *55:*377, 1975. Indian J. Plast. Surg., *7:*11, 1974

KHITERER, M. G.: Operative treatment of retention cysts by the method of coagulation. Stomatologiia (Mosk.), *50:*84, 1971 (Russian)

KHITROV, F. M.: Development of method for reconstruction of nasal defects using Filatov's graft. Stomatologiia (Mosk.), *52:*36, 1973 (Russian)

KHITROV, F. M. *et al*: Technic of joining an artificial esophagus and the pharynx. Vestn. Khir., *113:*105, 1974 (Russian)

KHODADAD, G.: Long-term results of microvascular repair and replacement, PRS, *48:*198, 1971. Surgery, *69:*397, 1971

KHOMENKO, N. M. *et al*: Gunshot wounds of the face in peacetime. Voen. Med. Zh., *2:*18, 1974 (Russian)

KHONDKARIAN, O. A. *et al*: Neuritis of the facial nerve. Zh. Nevropatol. Psikhiatr., *74:*1637, 1974 (Russian)

KHOSLA, V. M.: Current concepts in the treatment of acute and chronic osteomyelitis. Trans. Int. Conf. Oral Surg., *4:*116, 1973

KHOSLA, V. M. *et al*: Unilateral oblique osteotomy for correction of open bite after multiple facial fractures: report of case. J. Oral Surg., *29:*821, 1971

KHRINENKO, V. P.: Surgical treatment of ptosis complicated by blepharophimosis and epicanthus. Oftalmol. Zh., *26:*433, 1971 (Russian)

KHRINENKO, V. P.: Correction of congenital ptosis by method of levator shortening. Oftalmol. Zh., *30:*304, 1975 (Russian)

KHRISTICH, A. D. *et al*: Dermatoplasty. Khirurgiia (Mosk.), *49:*122, 1973 (Russian)

KHROMOV, B. M.: Surgery of lymphatic system; review of the literature. Khirurgiia (Mosk.), *49:*122, 1973 (Russian)

KHROMOV, B. M. *et al*: New data on use of lasers in surgery (literature survey). Khirurgiia (Mosk.), *9:*134, 1974 (Russian)

KIA-NOURY, M.: Common carotid kinking and cerebral insufficiency, PRS, *54:*239, 1974. Internat. Surg., *58:*9, 1973

KIEHN, C. L.: Regional block of thigh: uses in plastic surgery (with Earle, DesPrez). PRS, *49:*134, 1972

KIEHN, C. L.: Use of angiography in outlining solitary solid tumors of head and neck (with Mandel, Sykora). PRS, *52:*61, 1973

KIEHN, C. L.: Prognostic significance of delayed cutaneous reactivity in head and neck cancer patients (with Mandel). PRS, *53:*72, 1974

KIEHN, C. L.: Discussion of "Surgical correction of lesions of the temporomandibular joints" by Dingman, Dingman, and Lawrence. PRS, *55:*484, 1975

KIEHN, C. L.: Valvular obstruction of nasal airway (with DesPrez), PRS, *56:*307, 1975

KIEHN, C. L. *et al*: Temporal muscle transfers to incompetent soft palate, PRS, *48:*335, 1971

KIEHN, C. L., DESPREZ, J. D., AND BENSON, J. W.: Significance of radio-phosphorus uptake by metastatic head and neck neoplastic cell (Follow-Up Clinic). PRS, *50:*183, 1972

KIEHN, C. L., EARLE, A. S., AND DESPREZ, J. D.: Treatment of chronic, painful metatarsal callus by tendon transfer. PRS, *51:*154, 1973

KIEHN, C. L., DESPREZ, J. D., AND CONVERSE, C. F.: New procedure for total temporomandibular joint replacement. PRS, *53:*221, 1974

KIEHN, C. L. *et al*: One-stage correction of pendulous flap. PRS, *55:*33, 1975

KIELAR, R. A.: Sebaceous carcinoma of the caruncle. South. Med. J., *68:*347, 1975

KIELY, J., TITUS, J., AND ORIVS, A.: Thorotrast-induced hepatoma presenting as hyperparathyroidism, PRS, *54:*235, 1974. Cancer, *31:*1312, 1973

KIELY, P. E. *et al*: Unusual tumor of neck and superior mediastinum. J. Ir. Med. Assoc., *67:*306, 1974

KIENE, S. *et al*: Surgical treatment of ulcus cruris venosum permagnum. Zentralbl. Chir., *98:*1350, 1973 (German)

KIK, A.: Radiation ulcer following X-ray therapy of skin neoplasms. Przegl. Dermatol., *58:*755, 1971 (Polish)

KIK, A.: Clinical evaluation of X-ray therapy in the treatment of keloid as compared with other therapeutic methods. Przegl. Chir., 47:1173, 1975 (Polish)

KIK, A.: Indications for surgical treatment of keloids and correlation of various therapeutic methods. Pol. Przegl. Chir., 48:69, 1976 (Polish)

KILEY, G. G.: Open and closed reduction of bilateral mandibular fractures in a child. J. Indianap. Dist. Dent. Soc., 27:17, 1973

KILGORE, E. S., JR. et al: Atraumatic flexor tendon retrieval, PRS, 49:358, 1972. Am. J. Surg., 122:430, 1971

KILGORE, E. S., JR.: Mucous cysts: dorsal distal interphalangeal joint ganglion (with Newmeyer, Graham). PRS, 53:313, 1974

KILGORE, E. S. et al: Correction of ulnar subluxation of the extensor communis. Hand, 7:272, 1975

KILLEY, H. C.: Fractures of the Middle Third of the Facial Skeleton, Second Edition. John Wright & Sons, Ltd., Bristol, 1971. PRS, 51:209, 1973

KILLEY, H. C.: Surgical treatment of oro-antral fistula (a report on 362 cases of oro-antral fistula treated by the buccal flap operation). Minerva Stomatol., 20:166, 1971

KILLEY, H. C.: Bilateral fibrous hyperplasia of the palate. Int. J. Oral Surg., 3:302, 1974

KILLEY, H. C. et al: An Outline of Oral Surgery, Part 1 & 2. Williams & Wilkins Co., Baltimore, 1971

KILLEY, H. C., SEWARD, G. R., AND KAY, L. W.: An Outline in Oral Surgery, Part II. John Wright & Sons, Ltd., Bristol, 1971. PRS, 51:209, 1973

KILLEY, H. C. et al: Observations based on the surgical closure of 362 oro-antral fistulas. Int. Surg., 57:545, 1972

KILMAN, J. W. et al: Reasonable surgery for rhabdomyosarcoma, PRS, 53:612, 1974. Ann. Surg., 178:346, 1973

KIM, Z. W., AND ROSENTHAL, S. P.: Effect of orally administered zinc sulphate ($ZNSO_2$) on healing incised wounds, PRS, 48:96, 1971. J. Surg. Res., 10:597, 1970

KIM, Z. W. et al: Effect of homograft rejection on wound healing, PRS, 48:202, 1971. Surg. Gynec. & Obst., 131:495, 1970

KIMCHE, D. et al: Treatment of exstrophy of the bladder. Harefuah, 80:375, 1971 (Hebrew)

KING, D., KARKOWSKI, J., AND MILLER, S. H.: Plantar lichen planus—treatment by excision and skin grafting, PRS, 56:668, 1975

KING, E. H.: Enzyme analysis as test of skin viability (with Georgiade, O'Fallon). PRS, 53:67, 1974

KING, G. D.: Transoral resection for cancer of the oral cavity. Otolaryngol. Clin. North Am., 5:321, 1972

KING, H. C.: Otolaryngological evaluation of the cleft palate patient. Laryngoscope, 82:276, 1972

KING, JOHN HARRY, AND WADSWORTH, JOSEPH A. C.: An Atlas of Ophthalmic Surgery, Second Edition. J. B. Lippincott Co., Philadelphia, 1970. PRS, 49:204, 1972

KING, L. R. et al: Pediatric urology. Surg. Annu., 4:391, 1972

KINMONTH, J. B., AND NEGUS, D.: Arteriovenous fistulae in management of lower limb discrepancy, PRS, 55:249, 1975. J. Cardiovasc. Surg., 15:447, 1974

KINMONTH, M. H.: Use of skin flaps in hand injuries. Hand, 2:116, 1970

KIPFMUELLER, L. J., AND LANG, B. R.: Presurgical maxillary prosthesis: analysis of speech intelligibility, PRS, 52:204, 1973. J. Prosth. Dent., 28:620, 1972

KIPIKASA, A.: Surgical treatment of complications after irradiation for malignant facial neoplasms. Rozhl. Chir., 54:427, 1975 (Slovakian)

KIPIKASA, A., AND GREGOROVA, I.: Task of sex and age in formation of Dupuytren's contracture, PRS, 48:513, 1971. Acta chir. plast., 12:166, 1970

KIPIKASA, A. et al: Late sequelae to traumatic scalpation of penis and scrotum, PRS, 52:680, 1973. Acta chir. plast., 14:255, 1972

KIPIKASA, A. et al: Review of treatment of malignant skin neoplasms during the past 10 years at clinical Center for Plastic Surgery in Kosice. Rozhl. Chir., 54:416, 1975 (Slovakian)

KIPP, D. C.: Obituary on James Theodore Mills, M.D. PRS, 54:251, 1974

KIRBY, J. W. et al: Osteitis deformans of maxilla, report of atypical case. J. Oral Surg., 31:64, 1973

KIRCHHOFF, H.: Vaginal aplasia. Fortschr. Med., 92:495, 1974 (German)

KIRCHNER, J. A.: Tracheal reconstruction with autogenous mucochondrial graft (with Krizek). PRS, 50:123, 1972

KIRCHNER, J. A.: Pyriform sinus cancer: a clinical and laboratory study. Ann. Otol. Rhin. & Laryng., 84:793, 1975

KIRCHNER, J. A. et al: Fusion of vocal cords following intubation and tracheostomy. Trans. Am. Acad. Ophthalmol. Otolaryngol., 77:188, 1973

KIRIANFF, T. G.: Volume measurements of unequal breasts. PRS, 54:616, 1974

KIR'IANOVA, M. G. et al: Plastic surgery of postoperative defects of lower jaw by boiled bone reimplantation (experimental study). Stomatologiia (Mosk.), *51*:80, 1972 (Russian)

KIRICHENKO, G. D. *et al*: Primary multiple malignant neoplasms of the organs of the digestive system. Khirurgiia (Mosk.), *48*:54, 1972 (Russian)

KIRICUTA, I.: Treatment of radionecrosis of flexor folds, axilla, groin, neck, using the great omentum supporting dermo-epidermal free flaps. Ann. chir. plast., *18*:65, 1973 (French)

KIRICUTA, I., AND POPESCU, V.: Breast plasties with omentum magnum in prethoracic transposition, PRS, *53*:242, 1974. Chir. Plast., *2*:47, 1973

KIRICUTA, I., AND POPESCU, V.: Reconstructive surgery for radionecrosis of hand: omentum graft with autologous free skin transplants, PRS, *55*:511, 1975. Ann. chir. plast., *19*:243, 1974

KIRICUTA, I., POPESCU, V., AND SUCEAVA, I.: Treatment for huge esopharyngostomas appearing after total laryngectomy for irradiated laryngeal cancer, PRS, *56*:464, 1975. Ann. oto-laryng., *91*:585, 1974

KIRMAN, C.: Letter: Collagenases: human and bacterial. New England J. Med., *291*:1363, 1974

KIRPATOVSKII, I. D. *et al*: Transplantation of multiple skin flaps of haired part of head in alopecia. Khirurgiia (Mosk.), *49*:112, 1973 (Russian)

KIRPATOVSKII, I. D. *et al*: Replantation of limb and certain principles of restoration of blood and lymph circulation. Ortop. Travmatol. Protez., *4*:58, 1975

KIRSCH, N.: Malignant melanoma developing in a tattoo. Int. J. Dermatol., *11*:16, 1972

KIRSCHNER, H. *et al*: Ceramic implantations in the maxillary bone. Bull. Group Eur. Rech. Sci. Stomatol. Odontol., *17*:123, 1974 (French)

KIRSCHNER, R. A. *et al*: Rhinophyma – cold knife and contour dermabrasion. Eye, Ear, Nose, Throat Mon., *53*:421, 1974

KIRSTEIN, W.: Impacted third molar embedded in dentigerous cyst. Dent. Radiogr. Photogr., *48*:39, 1975

KISER, W. S. *et al*: Preservation of human cadaver kidneys for transplantation, PRS, *49*:585, 1972. J. Urol., *105*:779, 1971

KISH, R. S., AND SRIVASTOVA, D. C.: Iatrogenic dislocation of corpora cavernosa, PRS, *50*:200, 1972. J. Urol., *106*:711, 1971

KISHAEV, E. V.: Surgery in radiation-induced ulcers undergoing malignization. Med. Radiol. (Mosk.), *16*:48, 1971 (Russian)

KISHEV, S. V.: Closure of fistula at penoscrotal junction of urethra. J. Urol., *111*:774, 1974

KISHEV, S. V.: "Thumb" urethroplasty. A modi-

fication and comparative study. Urology, *4*:320, 1974

KISLOV, R.: Surgical correction of cupped ear. PRS, *48*:121, 1971

KISNER, W. H.: Reply to "Keratosis *palmaris et plantaris* – some prospective thoughts" (Letter to the Editor). PRS, *52*:568, 1973

KISNER, W. H., AND HENDRIX, J. H., JR.: Keratosis *palmaris et plantaris*. PRS, *51*:424, 1973

KIS'OV, D. I.: Intranasal incision of maxillary sinus through inferior nasal passage. Vestn. Otorinolaringol. *35*:56, 1973 (Russian)

KISSIN, B. *et al*: Head and neck cancer in alcoholics, PRS, *52*:685, 1973. J.A.M.A., *224*:1174, 1973

KISSLING, M. *et al*: Evaluation of antilymphocyte serum: comparison of skin allograft survival and rosette inhibition. Experientia, *29*:105, 1973

KITAMURA, T.: Transplantation of the facial nerve. Otolaryngology (Tokyo), *43*:817, 1971

KITAMURA, T. *et al*: Extratemporal facial nerve surgery. Arch. Otolaryng., *95*:369, 1972

KITANO, F. *et al*: Successfully operated case of cervical teratoma in a newborn infant. Surg. Ther. (Osaka), *26*:236, 1972 (Japanese)

KITSERA, A. E. *et al*: Rhinoseptoplasty. Vestn. Otorinolaringol., *4*:31, 1974 (Russian)

KIVISAARI, J., AND NIINIKOSKI, J.: Use of Silastic tube and capillary sampling technique in measurement of tissue PO_2 and PCO_2, PRS, *52*:688, 1973. Am. J. Surg., *125*:623, 1973

KIWERSKI, J.: Transplantation of the musculocutaneous nerve on the median nerve in an attempt at improving the function of the hand of a tetraplegic. Chir. Narzadow. Ruchu Ortop. Pol., *40*:173, 1975 (Polish)

KLAINER, A. S. *et al*: Surface alterations due to endotracheal intubations. Am. J. Med., *58*:674, 1975

KIZHAEV, E. V.: Surgery in radiation-induced ulcers undergoing malignization. Med. Radiol. (Mosk.), *16*:48, 1971 (Russian)

KLAMMT, J.: Keratocyst of jaws. Dtsch. Stomatol., *22*:501, 1972 (German)

KLASEN, H. J.: Too thick lips and double lips, PRS, *48*:195, 1971. Nederl. tijdschr. geneesk., *115*:408, 1971

KLASEN, H. J.: Cold water treatment as first aid in burned patients, PRS, *57*:122, 1976. Nederl. tijdschr. geneesk., *119*:601, 1975

KLÁSKOVÁ-BURIÁNOVÁ, O.: Epidemiological study of cleft lip and palate in Bohemia, PRS, *54*:505, 1974. Acta chir. plast., *15*:258, 1973

KLASSEN, G. IA. *et al*: Treatment of wounds of the fingers and hand with preserved fetal membrane. Vestn. Khir., *103*:89, 1969 (Russian)

KLASSEN, G. IA. *et al*: Skin transplantation

under ambulatory conditions. Ortop. Travmatol. Protez., *33:*15, 1972 (Russian)

KLAUBER, G. T.: Distal hypospadias, chordee and torsion; the Allen-Spence procedure and new modifications. J. Urol., *114:*765, 1975

KLAUBER, G. T., AND WILLIAMS, D. I.: Epispadias with incontinence, PRS, *54:*504, 1974. J. Urol., *111:*110, 1974

KLAUBER, G. T. *et al*: Preputial skin-bridging. Complication of circumcision. Urology, *3:*722, 1974

KLAUE, P.: Successful pretreatment of rabbit-skin allotransplants with triamcinolone acetonide, PRS, *55:*117, 1975. Bruns' Beitr. klin. Chir., *221:*313, 1974

KLAUE, P., AND JOLLEY, W. B.: Comparative effectiveness of corticosteroids applied topically as pretreatment of rabbit skin allografts, PRS, *49:*362, 1972. Surgery, *70:*718, 1971

KLEBANOFF, G.: Early clinical experience with a disposable unit for intraoperative salvage and reinfusion of blood loss (intraoperative autotransfusion), PRS, *48:*202, 1971. Am. J. Surg., *120:*718, 1970

KLEBER, M. *et al*: Preliminary results of deepening of the vestibulum by means of Edlan's and Mejachar's methods. Stomatol. D.D.R., *24:*670, 1974 (German)

KLEIN, A. *et al*: Cystosarcoma phylloides of breast—conservative procedures or amputation? Pol. Tyg. Lek., *27:*1401, 1972 (Polish)

KLEIN, D. R.: Sculptured ear. South. Med. J., *64:*1150, 1971

KLEIN, E., CASE, R. W., AND BURGESS, G. H.: Chemotherapy of skin cancer, PRS, *53:*250, 1974. Cancer, *23:*228, 1973

KLEIN, L., AND RUDOLPH, R.: ³H-collagen turnover in skin grafts, PRS, *51:*352, 1973. Surg. Gynec. & Obst., *135:*49, 1972

KLEIN, L. A., HALL, R. L., AND SMITH, R. B.: Surgical treatment of priapism: note on heparin-induced priapism, PRS, *51:*233, 1973. J. Urol., *108:*104, 1972

KLEIN, P.: Chronic skin wound. New method for treatment. Hefte Unfallheilkd., *114:*162, 1973 (German)

KLEIN, P.: Skin culture for treatment of leg ulcer. Z. Hautkr., *49:*433, 1974 (German)

KLEIN, P., AND KOHLER, J.: First clinical results following treatment of chronic and acute skin defects with an autologous skin homogenizate, PRS, *52:*461, 1973. Bruns' Beitr. klin. Chir., *220:*214, 1973

KLEIN, T. W., AND KAPLAN, G. W.: Klippel-Trenaunay syndrome associated with urinary tract hemangiomas, PRS, *57:*675, 1976. J. Urol., *114:*596, 1975

KLEINE-NATROP, H. E.: Treatment of recurrent basalioma. Arch. Geschwulstforsch., *43:*75, 1974 (German)

KLEINE-NATROP, H. E. *et al*: Basalioma therapy from dermatologist's viewpoint. Dermatol. Monatsschr., *158:*884, 1972 (German)

KLEINERT, H. E.: Anomalous muscles and nerve entrapment in the wrist and hand (with Still), PRS, *52:*394, 1973

KLEINERT, H. E.: Discussion of "Should an incompletely severed tendon be sutured?" by Reynolds, Wray, Weeks, PRS, *57:*236, 1976

KLEINERT, H. E. *et al*: Etiology and treatment of so-called mucous cyst of finger, PRS, *51:*476, 1973. J. Bone & Joint Surg., *54A:*1455, 1972

KLEINERT, H. E., BURGET, G. C., AND MORGAN, J. A.: Aneurysms of hand, PRS, *52:*595, 1973. Arch. Surg., *106:*554, 1973

KLEINERT, H. E. *et al*: Primary repair of flexor tendons. Orthop. Clin. North Am., *4:*865, 1973

KLEINERT, H. E. *et al*: Technique of nerve anastomosis. Orthop. Clin. North Am., *4:*907, 1973

KLEINERT, H. E. *et al*: Post-traumatic sympathetic dystrophy. Orthop. Clin. North Am., *4:*917, 1973

KLEINERT, H. E. *et al*: Place of microsurgery in hand surgery. Orthop. Clin. North Am., *4:*929, 1973

KLEINERT, H. E. *et al*: Reimplantation of amputated digits and hands. Orthop. Clin. North Am., *4:*957, 1973

KLEINERT, H. E. *et al*: Wrist and thumb in rheumatoid arthritis. Orthop. Clin. North Am., *4:*1085, 1973

KLEINERT, H. E. *et al*: In quest of the solution to severed flexor tendons. Clin. Orthop., *104:*23, 1974

KLEINERT. H. E. *et al*: Microsurgery in hand surgery. Clin. Orthop., *104:*158, 1974

KLEINFELD, F. *et al*: Clinical picture and pathomorphology of traumatic high-pressure oil injections, the so called "grease gun injury." Chirurg., *46:*362, 1975 (German)

KLEINFELDT, D.: Results with Cottle's method of septum surgery. Dtsch. Gesundheitsw., *27:*362, 1972 (German)

KLEINFELDT, D. *et al*: Results of plastic surgery of the ear using the McEvitt, Joseph and Converse methods. Dtsch. Gesundheitsw., *26:*1840, 1971 (German)

KLEMENCIC, H.: Malignant potentials of basal cell carcinoma. Chir. Maxillofac. Plast., *7:*99, 1970 (Croatian)

KLEMENCIC, H. *et al*: Role of reconstructive surgery in treatment of early and late sequelae of injuries. Vojnosanit. Pregl., *32:*145, 1975

KLEMENTOV, A. V. *et al*: Anesthesia for operations on the parotid gland. Stomatologiia (Mosk.), *53*:97, 1974 (Russian)

KLIMENKO, L. F. *et al*: Characteristics of treatment of thermal burns in children. Klin. Khir., *3*:38, 1975 (Russian)

KLINE, D. G. *et al*: Effect of mobilization on blood supply and regeneration of injured nerves, PRS, *51*:349, 1973. J. Surg. Res., *12*:254, 1972

KLINE, D. G. *et al*: Neuroma in continuity. Its preoperative and operative management. Surg. Clin. North Am., *52*:1189, 1972

KLINE, D. G., AND HACKETT, E. R.: Reappraisal of timing for exploration of civilian peripheral nerve injuries, PRS, *57*:120, 1976. Surgery, *78*:54, 1975

KLINE, R. L. *et al*: Pressure-dependent factors in edema formation in canine forelimbs, PRS, *56*:603, 1975. J. Pharmacol. Exp. Ther., *193*:452, 1975

KLINE, S. N.: Lateral compression in the treatment of mandibular fractures. Trans. Int. Conf. Oral Surg., *4*:330, 1973

KLINE, S. N.: Electric testing for injuries of seventh nerve, PRS, *57*:400, 1976. J. Oral Surg., *33*:215, 1975

KLINGENSMITH, W. C., III: Resolution of increased splenic size and uptake of 99mTc-sulfur colloid. J. Nucl. Med., *15*:1203, 1974

KLINTSEVICH, G. N.: Restoration of the skin integument following frostbite of the heel. Khirurgiia (Mosk.), *47*:34, 1971 (Russian)

KLOSE, R. *et al*: Clinical studies on single-drug anesthesia using ketamine in patients with burns. Anaesthesist, *22*:121, 1973 (German)

KLUSENER, R.: Making intranasal operations easier. Z. Laryngol. Rhinol. Otol., *52*:93, 1973 (German)

KLUZAK, R.: Transplantation of rib growth cartilages. Experimental study and possible use in primary cleft lip repairs. PRS, *49*:61, 1972

KLUZAK, R.: Autotransplantation of rib growth cartilage, histological findings, PRS, *53*:499, 1974. Acta Chir. orthop. Trauma cech., *40*:89, 1973

KLUZAK, R.: Is radical neck dissection of value in patients with advanced metastasizing melanoblastoma of head and neck? PRS, *54*:619, 1974. Rozhl. chir., *53*:204, 1974

KNEAFSEY, D. V. *et al*: Laryngostomy instead of tracheostomy. Ir. Med. J., *68*:279, 1975

KNEZEVIC, G. *et al*: Surgical-orthodontic treatment of diastema mediana with hypertrophican frenulum. Acta Stomatol. Croat., *7*:173, 1972–73 (Croatian)

KNIESER, M. R.: "De-epithelization" of the dermal pedicle in reduction mammaplasty (with Parsons). PRS, *57*:619, 1976

KNIGHTLY, J. J., SWAMINATHAN, A. P., AND RUSH, B. F., JR.: Management of penetrating wounds of neck, PRS, *53*:495, 1974. Am. J. Surg., *126*:575, 1973

KNIZE, D. M.: Influence of periosteum and calcitonin on onlay bone graft survival. PRS, *53*:190, 1974

KNOCH, H. G. *et al*: Advantages and disadvantages of tracheotomy. Follow-up results. Z. Aerztl. Fortbild. (Jena), *66*:675, 1972 (German)

KNOCH, H. G. *et al*: Authentic hermaphroditism. Zentralbl. Chir., *99*:662, 1974 (German)

KNORR, N. J.: Motivational patterns of patients seeking cosmetic (esthetic) surgery (with Edgerton), PRS, *48*:551, 1971

KNORR, N. J.: Feminine loss of identity in rhinoplasty. Arch. Otolaryng., *96*:11, 1972

KNORR, N. J.: Factitious wounds; psychiatric and surgical dilemma (With Drinker, Edgerton), PRS, *50*:458, 1972

KNORR, N. J. *et al*: Hand injuries: psychiatric considerations. South. Med. J., *64*:1328, 1971

KNOTEK, J. *et al*: Salivary gland neoplasms in records of Slovak Institute of Oncology in years 1960 to 1969. Nowotwory, *22*:245, 1972 (Polish)

KNOWLES, P. W.: Common childhood accidents, PRS, *54*:383, 1974. Hospital Med., *10*:48, 1974

KNUTSON, C. O. *et al*: Melanoma. Curr. Probl. Surg., *3*:55, 1971

KNUTSON, C. O., HORI, J. M., AND WATSON, F. R.: Melanoma of head and neck, PRS, *52*:214, 1973. Am. J. Surg., *124*:543, 1972

KNYSH, I. T. *et al*: Evaluation of methods of treating patients with malignant tumors of soft tissue. Khirurgiia (Mosk.), *48*:96, 1972 (Russian)

KOATZ, M.: Emergency tracheotomy. A new technical variant. Prensa med. Argent., *58*:1666, 1971 (Spanish)

KOB, D. *et al*: Results of therapy of lip neoplasms from a radiotherapeutic point of view. Zahn. Mund. Kieferheilkd., *63*:473, 1975 (German)

KOBAK, M. W.: Possible efficacy of treatment of frostbite of ears with flurandrenolide ointment, PRS, *57*:529, 1976. Eye, Ear, Nose & Throat Month., *54*:31, 1974

KOBAYASHI, M. *et al*: Clinical course of tuberculous tenosynovitis of the hand. Orthop. Surg. (Tokyo), *23*:122, 1972 (Japanese)

KOBAYASHI, S. *et al*: Anastomosis of the nerves of the upper limb and the problem of functional restoration – a loss of tactile localization. Orthop. Surg. (Tokyo), *23*:290, 1972 (Japanese)

KOBERG, W.: Single-step correction of mandibular prognathism and habitual jaw luxation.

Fortschr. Kiefer. Gesichtschir., *18:*234, 1974 (German)

KOBERG, W., AND KOBLIN, I.: Speech development and maxillary growth in relation to technique and timing of palatoplasty, PRS, *52:*455, 1973. J. Maxillo-facial Surg., *1:*44, 1973

KOBERG, W. R.: Present view on bone grafting in cleft palate (a review of the literature). J. Maxillo-facial Surg., *1:*185, 1973

KOBIELA-KRZYSTKOWA, K. *et al*: Diagnosis and surgical treatment of syndrome of unilateral paralysis of eyeball-elevating muscles. Klin. Oczna., *43:*1197, 1973 (Polish)

KOBLIN, I. *et al*: Sensitivity of the lower lip after protection or resection of the inferior alveolar nerve in progenia operations. Fortschr. Kiefer. Gescihtschir., *18:*151, 1974 (German)

KOBLIN, I., AND KOCH, H.: On nature of muco-epidermoid tumors of major and minor salivary glands, PRS, *54:*499, 1974. J. Maxillo-facial Surg., *2:*19, 1974

KOBLIN, I., AND REICH, B.: Changes in facial skeleton in cases of neurofibromatosis, PRS, *56:*463, 1975. J. Maxillo-facial Surg., *3:*23, 1975

KOBURG, E.: Simple method for plastic closure of wide septum perforation. Arch. Klin. Exp. Ohren Nasen Kehlkopfheilkd., *205:*289, 1973 (German)

KOBUS, K. Effect of various methods of postoperative procedures aiming at healing of skin grafts. Pol. Przegl. Chir., *46:*723, 1974 (Polish)

KOBUS, K. *et al*: Z-plasty in treatment of contractures of extremities following burns. Chir. Narzadow. Ruchu Ortop. Pol., *37:*529, 1972 (Polish)

KOBUS, K. *et al*: Personal experiences in treatment of late periods of burns. Pol. Tyg. Lek., *28:*1811, 1973 (Polish)

KOBUS, K. *et al*: Results of treatment of infected ulcerations of lower extremities. Wiad. Lek., *27:*233, 1974 (Polish)

KOCH, H.: Results of surgical therapy of adamantinomas. Fortschr. Kiefer. Gesichtschir., *15:*207, 1972 (German)

KOCH, H.: Statistical evaluation of tumors of head and neck in infancy and childhood, PRS, *54:*628, 1974. J. Maxillo-facial Surg., *2:*26, 1974

KOCH, H. *et al*: Prevention of hearing damage in cleft palate patients. Dtsch. Stomatol., *23:*816, 1973 (German)

KOCH, H., PFEIFLE, K., AND KREIDLER, J.: Biological behavior of basaliomas, PRS, *56:*472, 1975. J. Maxillo-facial Surg., *3:*35, 1975

KOCH, J. A.: Two stage surgery for cleft lip, jaw, palate and velum. Dtsch. Stomatol., *21:*635, 1971 (German)

KOCH, J. A.: Surgical closure of cleft palate. Zentralbl. Chir., *96:*447, 1971 (German)

KODAIRA, T.: Prosthetic management of oral defects limited to the hard palate and caused by surgical treatment of tumor. Shikwa Gakuho, *72:*69, 1972 (Japanese)

KODSI, M. S.: Incorporation and tolerance of Dacron felt in bones of rabbits (with Crouse, Campo). PRS, *54:*471, 1974

KOECHLIN, C.: Abdominal plastic surgery. Rev. Med. Suisse Romande, *94:*981, 1974 (French)

KOEHNLEIN, H. E.: Effects of various hemostyptic drugs in rats. PRS, *50:*462, 1972

KOEHNLEIN, H. E., HARTWIG, J., AND HARTUNG, H.: Experiences in treatment of severe burns, PRS, *53:*370, 1974. Bruns' Beitr. Klin. Chir., *220:*643, 1973

KOGGE, J., AND KOCH, H.: Mortality following operations of head and neck, PRS, *54:*625, 1974. J. Maxillo-facial Surg., *2:*32, 1974

KOHNLEIN, H. E.: Skin transplantation and skin substitutes. Langenbecks Arch. Chir., *327:*1090, 1970 (German)

KOHNLEIN, H. E.: Experimental principles of local therapy for burns. I. Monatsschr. Unfallheilkd., *74:*464, 1971 (German)

KOHNLEIN, H. E.: Experimental basis of typical treatment of burns. II. Monatsschr. Unfallheilkd., *74:*507, 1971 (German)

KOHNLEIN, H. E.: Current possibilities of plastic surgery. Z. Allgemeinmed., *49:*45, 1973 (German)

KOHNLEIN, H. E.: New fixation plate for hand surgery. Chirurg., *45:*482, 1974 (German)

KOHNLEIN, H. E.: Surgical reconstruction of the breast. Med. Klin., *69:*1647, 1974 (German)

KÖHNLEIN, H. E., AND BREHMER, U.: Application of acrylate and bakelite adhesive in surgery, PRS, *50:*422, 1972. Bruns' Beitr. klin. Chir., *219:*159, 1972

KÖHNLEIN, H. E., AND DIETRICH, F.: Experiments in local burn treatment, PRS, *52:*212, 1973. Chir. Plast., *1:*207, 1972

KÖHNLEIN, H. E., AND LEMPERLE, G.: Experiments and clinical observations on cold water treatment of fresh burns, PRS, *52:*212, 1973. Chir. Plast., *1:*216, 1972

KÖHNLEIN, H. E., AND ILG, A. M.: Experiments on control and measurement of blood supply in flaps, PRS, *52:*597, 1973. Bruns' Beitr. klin. Chir., *220:*313, 1973

KÖHNLEIN, H. E., LEMPERLE, G., AND SCHERER, M.: Attempts at interference with phagocytosis of RES, PRS, *53:*376, 1974. Bruns' Beitr. klin. Chir., *220:*643, 1973

KÖHNLEIN, H. E. *et al*: Problems in the surgical

treatment of malignant melanomas. Chirurg., *45*:356, 1974 (German)

KOIKE, Y. *et al*: Therapeutic methods in angiogenic tumor of the head and neck. Otolaryngology (Tokyo), *44*:93, 1972 (Japanese)

KOIKE, Y. *et al*: Problems of the method of approach to the facial nerve canal — pointers on facial nerve surgery. Otolaryngology (Tokyo), *44*:345, 1972 (Japanese)

KOIKKALAINEN, K. *et al*: Upper limb sympathectomy. Ann. Chir. Gynaecol. Fenn., *63*:318, 1974

KOJIMA, K., AND ONIZUKA, T.: Simplified mesh dermatome, PRS, *49*:239, 1972. Jap. J. Plast. Reconstr. Surg., *14*:269, 1971

KOJIMA, K., ICHINOSE, M., AND ONITSUKA, T.: Bilateral cross thigh flap, case report, PRS, *51*:609, 1973. Operation, Japan, *26*:1065, 1972

KOJIMA, T. *et al*: Case of carpal tunnel syndrome due to lumbricalis anomaly. Orthop. Surg. (Tokyo), *22*:746, 1971 (Japanese)

KOKOSCHKA, E. M. *et al*: Epitheliomas of external ear. Z. Haut. Geschlechtskr., *47*:779, 1972 (German)

KOK-VAN ALPHEN, C. C. *et al*: Microphthalmos and orbital cyst. Ophthalmologica, *167*:389, 1973

KOLÄR, J. *et al*: Gastrointestinal complications in burns. Med. Klin., *66*:1617, 1971 (German)

KOLÄR, J., *et al*: Systemic effects of burns on bone mineral metabolism, PRS, *50*:541, 1972. Acta chir. plast., *13*:133, 1971. II. Influence of general anesthesia, PRS, *57*:763, 1976. Acta chir. plast., *17*:56, 1975

KOLCZUN, M. C. *et al*: Antibiotic concentrations in human bone, PRS, *54*:507, 1974. J. Bone & Joint Surg., *56A*:305, 1974

KOLE, H.: Reconstruction of skin defects on face. Langenbecks Arch. Chir., *334*:593, 1973 (German)

KOLE, H.: Surgical treatment of maxillary protrusion and retrognathism. Fortschr. Kiefer. Gesichtschir., *18*:46, 1974 (German)

KOLEN, A. A., AND MOROZOVA, O. D.: Employment of homologous fascia for firm anchorage of homo- and allo-implants used after enucleation of eye, PRS, *53*:499, 1974. Acta chir. plast., *15*:46, 1973

KOLESOV, A. A. *et al*: Reconstructive operations on mandible in children: clinico-experimental study, PRS, *51*:475, 1973. Acta chir. plast., *13*:203, 1971

KOLESOV, A. A. *et al*: Use of preserved homologous bone in plastic surgery of the mandible in children. Stomatologiia (Mosk.), *51*:49, 1972 (Russian)

KOLIN, I. S.: Psychosexual dynamics of patients undergoing mammary augmentation (with Baker, Bartlett), PRS, *53*:652, 1974

KOLIN, I. S., BAKER, J. L., AND BARTLETT, E. S.: Psychosexual aspects of mammary augmentation, PRS, *55*:636, 1975. Human Sexuality, *8*:88, 1974

KOLIV, L., WIEBERDINK, J., AND RENEMAN, S.: Anticoagulation in microvascular surgery, PRS, *52*:208, 1973. Europ. Surg. Res., *5*:52, 1973

KOLKER, I. I. *et al*: Bacteremia in burned patients. Khirurgiia (Mosk.), *48*:31, 1972 (Russian)

KOLODKIN, A. V.: Secondary sutures in the treatment of submandibular phlegmons. Stomatologiia (Mosk.), *54*:86, 1975 (Russian)

KOLONTAI, Iu. Iu. *et al*: Early and late homoplasty in tendon injuries of the hand and fingers. Ortop. Travmatol. Protez., *33*:18, 1972 (Russian)

KOLONTAI, Iu. Iu. *et al*: Ways for improving the results achieved by the treatment of open combined injuries of the hand. Sov. Med., *36*:87, 1973 (Russian)

KOLOS, D. *et al*: Replantation of a hand severed through the palm. M. J. Australia, *2*:559, 1974

KOMATSUBARA, Y. *et al*: Treatment of chronic rheumatoid arthritis. 9. Treatment of tenosynovitis of the hand in chronic rheumatoid arthritis. Ryumachi, *13*:388, 1973 (Japanese)

KOMINOS, S. D. *et al*: Mode of transmission of *Pseudomonas aeruginosa* in a burn unit and an intensive care unit in a general hospital. Appl. Microbiol., *23*:309, 1972

KOMORN, R. M.: Management of vascular tumors of the head and neck. South. Med. J., *65*:1106, 1972

KOMORN, R. M.: Regional flaps in head and neck surgery. Tex. Med., *70*:70, 1974

KOMORN, R. M. *et al*: Repair of frontal sinus defects with methyl-methacrylate. South. Med. J., *65*:1432, 1972

KONCZ, M.: New method for conservative treatment of impacted metacarpo-phalangeal luxations. Arch. Orthop. Unfallchir., *79*:135, 1974 (German)

KONDO, A. *et al*: Incomplete subsymphyseal epispadias. Jap. J. Urol., *64*:412, 1973 (Japanese)

KONDO, A. *et al*: Priapism as a surgical emergency. Jap. J. Urol., *65*:189, 1974 (Japanese)

KONDRASHIN, N. I.: Surgical treatment of patients with congenital funnel chest. Ortop. Travmatol. Protez., *34*:34, 1973 (Russian)

KONICKOVA, Z., MATEJICEK, V., AND VRABEC, R.: Methodic experience with determination of endotoxin in serum, PRS, *54*:506, 1974. Acta chir. plast., *15*:170, 1973

KONIGOVA, R.: In memory of A. B. Wallace. Rozhl. Chir., *54*:420, 1975 (Czechoslovakian)

KONIGOVA, R. *et al*: Shortcomings in the treatment of burns in the shock period. Rozhl. Chir., *50:*600, 1971 (Czechoslovakian)

KONNO, A. *et al*: Reconstruction of oral cavity after extirpation of malignant tumor of oral floor and mandible. J. Otolaryngol. Jap., *78:*154, 1975 (Japanese)

KONOBEVTSEV, O. F. *et al*: Correlations between some hemodynamic and blood coagulation indices in operations on face and neck. Stomatologiia (Mosk.), *53:*23, 1974 (Russian)

KONONENKO, N. G. *et al*: Extent of operation in skin neoplasm metastases into the inguinal-femoral lymphatic nodes. Klin. Khir., *10:*48, 1974 (Russian)

KONSTANTINOVA, K. V.: Modification of plastic repair of bladder exstrophy. Urol. Nefrol. (Mosk.), *32:*43, 1974 (Russian)

KONTOR, E.: Technic of isolated veloplasty. Magy. Traumatol. Orthop., *16:*215, 1973 (Hungarian)

KONTOR, E. *et al*: 3 years experience in the early orthodontic management and subsequent surgery of cleft lip and palate in children. Orv. Hetil., *112:*1957, 1971 (Hungarian)

KONZ, B.: Surgical mesh technic for covering large skin defects. Hautarzt, *26:*277, 1975 (German)

KONZ, B.: Dermatome excision of multiple basaliomas of the trunk skin. Hautarzt, *26:*647, 1975 (German)

KOOB, E.: Surgical restoration of the hand following infections. Hefte Unfallheilkd., *107:*230, 1970 (German)

KOOB, E.: Infra-red thermography in hand surgery. Hand, *4:*65, 1972

KOOB, E. *et al*: Findings of infrared thermography in hand surgery. Handchirurgie, *4:*123, 1972 (German)

KOONIN, A. J.: Findings in 300 patients with facial lacerations, PRS, *52:*525, 1973

KOONIN, A. J.: Fractures of mandible (with Melmed), PRS, *56:*323, 1975

KOONIN, A. J., AND MELMED, E. P.: Painless donor sites, PRS, *54:*697, 1974. South African M. J., *47:*2241, 1973

KOONTZ, W. W. JR. *et al*: Cloacal exstrophy with the potential for urinary control; an unusual presentation. J. Urol., *112:*828, 1974

KOOTSTRA, G., HUFFSTADT, A. J. C., AND KAUER, J. M. G.: Styloid bone, clinical and embryological study, PRS, *56:*228, 1975. Hand, *6:*185, 1974

KOPECEK, J., AND SPPINCL, L.: Effect of structure of poly (glycolmethacrylate) gel on calcification of implants, PRS, *56:*365, 1975. Polymers in Med., *4:*129, 1974

KOPIK, I. I.: Function of the external respiration in children suffering from congenital cleft lip and cleft palate. Stomatologiia (Mosk.), *49:*50, 1970 (Russian)

KOPP, F. H.: Mowlem-Jackson auto-homologous grafts in large surface burns. Monatsschr. Unfallheilkd., *75:*268, 1972 (German)

KOPP, W. K. *et al*: Unusually large torus mandibularis. Dent. Radiogr. Photogr., *46:*20, 1973

KOPTA, J. A.: Evaluating teaching methods, PRS, *50:*638, 1972. Surgery, *71:*793, 1972

KORAITIM, M.: Congenital chordee with and without hypospadias in three brothers, PRS, *52:*98, 1973. J. Urol., *108:*976, 1972

KORCHIN, L.: Dermoid cyst with lingual sinus tract, case report. Oral Surg., *37:*175, 1974

KORCHMAROS, I.: Contralateral rhinostomy for dacryocystitis due to facial malformations. Acta Ophthalmol (Kbh.), *50:*399, 1972

KOREN, E. *et al*: Gardner's syndrome: report of family, PRS, *55:*115, 1975. Ann. Surg., *180:*198, 1974

KORKHOV, S. I. *et al*: Topical application of anti-staphylococcal plasma in the complex treatment of burns. Voen. Med. Zh., *8:*39, 1971 (Russian)

KÖRLOF, B. *et al*: Radiation-sterilized split skin: new type of biological wound dressing. Preliminary report. Scand. J. Plast. Reconstr. Surg., *6:*126, 1972

KÖRLOF, B. *et al*: Resection of thoracic wall and local flap repair for recurrences of mammary carcinoma. Brit. J. Plast. Surg., *26:*322, 1973

KÖRLOF, B., NYLEN, B., AND RIETZ, K. A.: Bone grafting of skull defects, PRS, *52:*378, 1973

KORMFALT, S. A., OKMIAN, L., AND JONSSON, N.: Everted anastomoses in esophagus of piglet, PRS, *53:*683, 1974. Ztschr. Kinderchir., *13:*306, 1973

KORN, M. B.: Micro-angiography of the skin veins in the lower limbs. Bibl. Anat., *10:*168, 1969

KORNBERG, J. *et al*: Ultra thin silicone polymer membrane: a new synthetic skin substitute. Trans. Am. Soc. Artif. Intern. Organs, *18:*39, 1972

KORNBERG, R., AND ACKERMAN, A. B.: Pseudomelanoma, recurrent melanocytic nevus following partial surgical removal, PRS, *57:*765, 1976. Arch. Dermat., *111:*1588, 1975

KORNBLUT, A. D.: Facial nerve injuries in children. J. Laryng. & Otol., *88:*717, 1974

KORNBLUT, A. D. *et al*: Complications of head and neck surgery. Arch. Otolaryng., *94:*246, 1971

KORNBLUT, A. D. *et al*: Rhinophyma and intranasal carcinoma. J. Laryng. & Otol., *87:*1137, 1973

KORNBLUT, A. D. *et al*: Parotid lymphangioma:

congenital tumor. O. R. L., *35:*303, 1973

KORNBLUT, A. D. *et al*: Effectiveness of sterno-mastoid muscle flap in preventing post-paro-tidectomy occurrence of Frey syndrome. Acta Otolaryngol. (Stockh.), *77:*378, 1974

KORNBLUT, A. D. *et al*: Scintiscanning with gallium citrate 67. Diagnosis of head and neck malignant neoplasms. Arch. Otolar-yng., *100:*201, 1974

KORNFALT, R. *et al*: Fibrinolysis in lymphan-gioma. Acta Paediatr. Scand., *62:*538, 1973

KORNILOV, N. V.: Indications for primary su-ture of the digital flexor tendons in injuries at the level of the synovial-aponeurotic sheath. Vestn. Khir., *108:*89, 1972 (Russian)

KORNITZER, G. D. *et al*: Methods of urinary diversion. Geriatrics, *29:*85, 1974

KOROLEV, L. F. *et al*: Evaluation of biochemical changes in blood of patients with severe burns during reconstructive operation on the skin. Sov. Med., *8:*149, 1975 (Russian)

KORSAN-BENGSTEN, M. *et al*: Follow-up study of cleft children treated with primary bone grafting. II. Audiological aspects. Scand. J. Plast. Reconstr. Surg., *8:*161, 1974

KORYTOWSKI, J. *et al*: Plasmocytoma of the na-sal cavity and sphenoid sinus. Otolaryngol. Pol., *25:*347, 1971 (Polish)

KORZON, T. *et al*: Surgical treatment of unilat-eral mandibular hyperplasia. Czas. Stoma-tol., *25:*1081, 1972 (Polish)

KORZON, T. *et al*: Closure of defects after partial maxillary resection by means of mucosal flap obtained from mouth mucosa and upper lip. Czas. Stomatol., *28:*637, 1975 (Polish)

KOSACHEV, A. N. *et al*: Electromyographic characteristics of the muscles of the perioral region in residual deformities of the nose and upper lip following elimination of unilateral congenital cleft. Stomatologiia (Mosk.), *54:*42, 1975 (Russian)

KOSACHEV, I. D.: Regional intraosseous infu-sion of morphocycline and oleomorphocyline in the treatment of severe forms of purulent infection of the hand and fingers. Vestn. Khir., *111:*63, 1973 (Russian)

KOSACHEV, I. D.: Treatment of traumatic osteo-myelitis of the fingers and hand. Voen. Med. Zh., *11:*64, 1974 (Russian)

KOSENOW, W.: Side effects of drugs in children, PRS, *53:*115, 1974. Chir. Praxis, *16:*143, 1972

KOSHELEV, V. N. *et al*: Destruction of mela-noma metastases with a laser. Vopr. Onkol., *21:*98, 1975 (Russian)

KOSLOSKE, A. M. *et al*: Giant "bathing trunk" nevus with malignant melanoma treated by excision and split thickness skin grafting. J. Pediatr. Surg., *10:*823, 1975

KOSOKOVIC, F. *et al*: Surgery of benign and mixed parotid gland neoplasms. Rad. Med. Fak. Zagrebu., *20:*239, 1972 (Croatian)

Koss, K. G. *et al*: Small cell (oat cell) carcinoma of minor salivary gland origin. Cancer, *30:*737, 1972

Koss, N.: Current use of prophylactic antibiot-ics in plastic and reconstructive surgery (with Krizek, Robson), PRS, *55:*21, 1975

Koss, N., ROBSON, M. C., AND KRIZEK, R. J.: Scalping injury, PRS, *55:*439, 1975

KOSTER, H. D. *et al*: Comparative study of mu-cosal grafts and lyophilized dura. Dtsch. Zah-naerztl. Z., *28:*1229, 1973 (German)

KOSTLER, J. *et al*: Surgery of melanocytoblas-toma of the skin. Zentralbl. Chir., *97:*601, 1972 (German)

KOSTOWIECKI, M. *et al*: Elastic fibers around sebaceous glands in the human lips. Z. Mik-rosk. Anat. Forsch., *84:*385, 1971

KOSTYLEV, M. V. Reconstruction of the cuta-neocartilaginous part of the nasal septum by grafting an auricular transplant. Vestn. Khir., *107:*84, 1971 (Russian)

KOSTYSHIN, A. T.: Resection of the nasal sep-tum with reimplantation of autocartilage. Vestn. Otorinolaringol., *3:*93, 1975 (Russian)

KOTHARI, D. R. *et al*: Implantable fluid transfer system for treatment of impotence. J. Bio-mech., *5:*567, 1972

KOTHARY, P. M.: Total glossectomy and repair with amniotic membrane. J. Indian Med. As-soc., *62:*87, 1974

KOTHARY, P. M., POTDAR, G. G., AND DE SOUZA, L. J.: Observations on voice tunnels in laryngectomies, PRS, *52:*97, 1973. Am. J. Surg., *124:*535, 1972

KOTHARY, P. M. *et al*: Radical total glossec-tomy. Brit. J. Surg., *61:*209, 1974

KOTTON, R.: Odontogenic keratocyst of maxilla. J. Laryng. & Otol., *86:*1169, 1972

KOTYZA, F.: Surgical treatment of lower lip and commissure cancer. Cesk. Otolaryngol., *22:*100, 1973 (Czechoslovakian)

KOUMANS, R. K.: Transplantation and burns. Lancet, *1:*1190, 1975

KOUMOURA, F.: Case of large calculus of the submandibular gland. Stomatologia (Ath-enai), *32:*157, 1975 (Greek)

KOUMOURA, F. *et al*: Correction of surgically removed jaw tumors by stored allografts. Sto-matologia (Athenai), *31:*197, 1974 (Greek)

KOUSSOURIS, P.: Extensor digitorum brevis manus and hypertrophy of the synonym mus-cle of the feet. Handchirurgie, *5:*237, 1973

KOVALENKO, A. F. *et al*: Nursing of children with congenital cleft lip and palate during the first year of life. Stomatologiia (Mosk.), *53:*41, 1974 (Russian)

KOVALENKO, P. P., AND DEMICHEV, N. P.: Homologous tendon plasty of hand and finger flexor tendons, PRS, *51*:603, 1973. Acta chir. plast., *14*:60, 1972

KOVALKOVITS, I.: Organization of centralized patient care in hand injuries. Orv. Hetil., *115*:2737, 1974 (Hungarian)

KOVALKOVITS, I. *et al*: Current problems in the management of the septic hand. Orv. Hetil., *113*:1519, 1972 (Hungarian)

KOVANOV, V. V. *et al*: Plastic closure of different skeletal segments with formalinized bone homotransplant. Eksp. Khir. Anesteziol., *2*:4, 1974 (Russian)

KOVARI, F.: Use of half-implanted splints in the reduction of mandibular fractures. Fogorv. Sz., *65*:555, 1972 (Hungarian)

KOVINSKII, I. T. *et al*: Method of "transfers" in free skin transplantation on granulating wound. Ortop. Travmatol. Protez., *35*:85, 1974 (Russian)

KOVLENKO, P. P. *et al*: External ear reconstruction using skin from the retroauricular area and preserved cartilage. Vestn. Khir., *103*:114, 1972

KOWALIK, S.: Functional disorders following resection of the tongue and floor of the mouth. Czas. Stomatol., *25*:369, 1972 (Polish)

KOWALIK, S.: Removal of salivary glands. Czas. Stomatol., *26*:1069, 1973 (Polish)

KOWALIK, S.: Surgical treatment of advanced carcinoma of lower lip. Wiad. Lek., *27*:273, 1974 (Polish)

KOWALIK, S. *et al*: Facio-frontal fractures. Czas. Stomatol., *24*:1137, 1971 (Polish)

KOWALIK, S. *et al*: Serum immunoglobulins in patients after use of preserved bovine tendon for anastomosing facial bones. Czas. Stomatol., *25*:1087, 1972 (Polish)

KOWALIK, S. *et al*: Use of bone grafts. Czas. Stomatol., *27*:161, 1974 (Polish)

KOWALSKA-KULESZA, K.: Actinomycosis of the parotid gland. Otolaryngol. Pol., *25*:455, 1971 (Polish)

KOWALSKI, M. *et al*: Evaluation of speech in patients with cleft palate in the light of late results of surgical treatment. Otolaryngol. Pol., *26*:107, 1972 (Polish)

KOZIN, I. A.: Chondroplasty of pyriform-aperture margin in residual deformities of unilateral cleft lip, PRS, *50*:95, 1972. Acta chir. plast., *13*:7, 1971

KOZIN, I. A.: Rare nasal deformity similar to unilateral cleft lip nose but without cleft lip, PRS, *52*:682, 1973. Acta chir. plast., *14*:210, 1972

KOZIN, I. A.: Primary cheiloplasty in congenital unilateral cleft lip and palate by the modified Millard method. Stomatologiia (Mosk.), *53*:40, 1974 (Russian)

KOZLOV, A. L. *et al*: Treatment of experimental tumors with laser beams in combination with fast electrons. Vopr. Onkol., *19*:93, 1973 (Russian)

KOZLOV, A. P.: Antitumor effect of laser radiation. Acta Radiol. (Ther.) (Stockh.), *12*:241, 1973

KOZLOV, L. A.: Free dermatoplasty in correction of vaginal defects. Akush. Ginekol. (Mosk.), *48*:57, 1972 (Russian)

KOZLOV, V. A. *et al*: Osteosynthesis of fragments of the condyloid process of the mandible with suture placed by retromolar approach. Stomatologiia (Mosk.), *51*:24, 1972 (Russian)

KOZLOV, V. A. *et al*: Surgical correction of the open bite by a 2-stage mobilization of the lateral portions of the maxilla. Stomatologiia (Mosk.), *54*:29, 1975 (Russian)

KOZLOWSKI, K. *et al*: Metachondromatosis: report of a case in a 6 year old boy. Aust. Paediatr. J., *11*:42, 1975

KRAAIJENHAGEN, H. A.: Technique for parotid biopsy. J. Oral Surg., *33*:328, 1975

KRACMER, M. *et al*: Surgical treatment of burns. Rozhl. Chir., *50*:595, 1971 (Czechoslovakian)

KRAG, C.: Isolated paralysis of *flexor pollicis longus* muscle, PRS, *56*:356, 1975. Scand. J. Plast. Reconstr. Surg., *8*:250, 1974

KRAHULEC, I. *et al*: Changes of resonance during speech after surgical interventions in the meso- and epipharynx. Cesk. Otolaryngol., *23*:363, 1974 (Slovakian)

KRAJINA, Z.: Histological base of functional surgery of septum and external nasal pyramid. Laryngol. Rhinol. Otol. (Stuttg.), *53*:895, 1974 (German)

KRAJNIK, J. *et al*: Treatment of cleft hard palate using lyophilized cartilage plate. Preliminary communication. Czas. Stomatol., *27*:711, 1974 (Polish)

KRAJNIK, J. *et al*: Evaluation of therapeutic results in the surgical treatment of cleft palate using lyophilized plates of xenogenous cartilage. Czas. Stomatol., *28*:497, 1975 (Polish)

KRAJNIK, J. *et al*: Chronic necrotic osteitis of the jaw treated with cartilaginous graft. Pol. Tyg. Lek., *30*:1879, 1975 (Polish)

KRAKOVIC, M.: Malignant tumors of male mammary gland, report of 16 cases. Bruns Beitr. Klin. Chir., *221*:35, 1974 (German)

KRAL, J.: Results in the surgical treatment of pseudoarthroses of the carpal navicular bone. Acta Chir. Orthop. Traumatol. Cech., *40*:161, 1973 (Czechoslovakian)

KRAL, J. G.: Surgical reduction of adipose tissue hypercellularity in man. Scand. J. Plast.

Reconstr. Surg., *9:*140, 1975

KRAMER, I. R.: Histopathology of some central non-odontogenic tumours and tumour-like conditions of the jaws. Trans. Int. Conf. Oral Surg., *4:*28, 1973

KRAMER, I. R. *et al*: Use of exfoliative cytology and protein estimations in preoperative diagnosis of odontogenic keratocysts. Int. J. Oral Surg., *2:*143, 1973

KRAMMER, E. B. *et al*: Juxtaoral organ: the importance of knowledge of this organ in oral pathology and surgery. Wien. Klin. Wochenschr., *86:*639, 1974 (German)

KRANZL, B. *et al*: Investigation into the applicability of cytodiagnosis in the early detection of oral cavity cancer at the department of oral surgery. Wien. Klin. Wochenschr., *86:*647, 1974 (German)

KRASULIN, V. V. *et al*: Direct results of treatment of hypospadias. Urol. Nefrol. (Mosk.), *38:*57, 1973 (Russian)

KRASULIN, V. V. *et al*: Subcutaneous splinting of the penis with two lateral polyethylene prostheses as a method of treatment of impotence. Urol. Nefrol. (Mosk.), *39:*42, 1974 (Russian)

KRASZEWSKI, J.: Selected diagnostic methods and treatment of dysfunction of temporomandibular joints applying the method of temporal myoplasties in soldiers. Czas. Stomatol., *26:*601, 1973 (Polish)

KRASZEWSKI, J. *et al*: Temporomandibular joint damage in surgically treated maxillofacial injuries. Czas. Stomatol., *24:*1043, 1971 (Polish)

KRATOCHWIL, Z.: Hair loss: a rare complication of facelift. In *Plastische und Wiederherstellungs-Chirurgie*, ed. by Hohler; pp. 321–2. Schattauer, Stuttgart, 1975 (German)

KRATOCHWIL, Z. *et al*: Surgical treatment of deformations of the palm in the course of epidermolysis bullosa dystrophica. Przegl. Dermatol., *61:*211, 1974 (Polish)

KRATZ, R. C.: Repair of septal perforations with composite grafts. Arch. Otolaryng., *98:*380, 1973

KRAUFHAR, M. F., SEELENFREUND, M. H., AND FROELICH, D. B.: Central retinal artery closure during orbital hemorrhage from retrobulbar injection, PRS, *54:*382, 1974. Tr. Am. Acad. Ophth., *78:*65, 1974

KRAUSE, C. J.: Forehead island flap in oral cavity reconstruction. Arch. Otolaryng., *97:*283, 1973

KRAUSE, C. J. *et al*: Complications associated with combined therapy of oral and pharyngeal neoplasms. Ann. Otol. Rhin. & Laryng., *81:*496, 1972

KRAUSE, C. J. *et al*: Carcinoma of oral cavity.

Arch. Otolaryng., *97:*354, 1973

KRAUSE, C. J. *et al*: Aging face. J. Iowa Med. Soc., *64:*242, 1973

KRAUSE, C. J. *et al*: Palatoplasty: a comparative study. Trans. Am. Acad. Ophthalmol. Otolaryngol. *80:*551, 1975

KRAUSE, C. J. *et al*: Comparative study of results of the von Langenbeck and the V-Y pushback palatoplasties. Cleft Palate J., *13:*11, 1976

KRAUSEN, A. S. *et al*: Pilomatrixoma masquerading as parotid mass. Laryngoscope, *84:*528, 1974

KRAUSE-SENTIES, L.: Surgical treatment of carotid body tumors, PRS, *49:*237, 1972. Arch. Inv. Med. Mex., *2:*25, 1971

KRAUSS, M. *et al*: Experience in treatment of lymphedema of lower extremities. Mater. Med. Pol., *5:*271, 1973

KRAWCZUK-HERMANOWICZOWA, O. *et al*: Case of elevated cellular nevus of the eyelid edge. Klin. Oczna., *44:*69, 1974 (Polish)

KRAWCZYKOWA, Z. *et al*: Malignant exophthalmos of both eyes. Klin. Oczna., *43:*835, 1973 (Polish)

KREBS, H.: Significance of postponed primary surgery in the treatment of infected hand injuries. Hefte Unfallheilkd., *107:*245, 1970 (German)

KREBS, H.: Surgical treatment of radiation injuries of the skin. Bruns Beitr. Klin. Chir., *218:*665, 1971 (German)

KREIDER, J. W. AND BENJAMIN, S. A.: Tumor immunity and the mechanism of polyinosinic-polycytidylic acid inhibition of tumor growth. J. Natl. Cancer Inst., *49:*1303, 1972

KREIDLER, J.: Field of activity of pediatric nurse in mouth, jaw and plastic surgery as illustrated in West German jaw hospital. Dtsch. Krankenpflegez, *26:*127, 1973 (German)

KREIDLER, J.: Median mandibular cyst, case report. Dtsch. Zahnaerztl. Z., *29:*633, 1973 (German)

KREIDLER, J. F., AND KOCH, H.: Endoscopic findings of maxillary sinus after middle face fractures, PRS, *56:*463, 1975. J. Maxillo-facial Surg., *3:*10, 1975

KREKELER, G.: Using lyophilized dura in open vestibuloplasty. Z. W. R., *83:*639, 1974 (German)

KREMENTZ, E. T. *et al*: Chemotherapy of melanoma of the extremities of perfusion: fourteen years clinical experience. Ann. Surg., *175:*900, 1972

KREMMYDAS, B. *et al*: Evaluation of prophylactic antibiotics in orthopedics and traumatology, PRS, *56:*471, 1975. Tr. 8th Panhel. Cong. Surg. Soc., *A:* 308, 1973

KRENAR, J. *et al*: Surgery or irradiation of skin neoplasms? Rozhl. Chir., *54:*421, 1975 (Czechoslovakian)

KRESBERG, H.: Histiocytosis X – a case report. Trans. Int. Conf. Oral Surg., *4:*40, 1973

KRIEG, H., AND PULS, C.: Differential diagnosis of fibromatosis of soft tissue tumors, PRS, *51:*107, 1973. Bruns' Beitr. klin. Chir., *219:*450, 1972

KRIEGER, K.: Subcutaneous ligation of varicose veins. Z. Hautkr., *49:*383, 1974 (German)

KRIENS, O.: Fissure of the lower lip, mandible, tongue associated with incomplete median cervical fissure. ADM, *28:*57, 1971 (Spanish)

KRIENS, O.: Development of intravelar veloplasty at the Nordwestdeutsche Kieferklinik. Dtsch. Zahn. Mund. Kieferheilkd., *57:*393, 1971 (German)

KRIENS, O.: Indirect fossa arthroplasty in temporomandibular joint ankylosis. Preliminary report. Dtsch. Zahnaerztl. Z., *28:*433, 1973 (German)

KRIENS, O.: Photomontage in the planning of jaw and facial operations. Fortschr. Kiefer. Gesichtschir., *18:*101, 1974 (German)

KRIENS, O.: Maxillary osteotomy in early childhood, PRS, *55:*378, 1975. J. Maxillo-facial Surg., *2:*150, 1974

KRIENS, O: Functional anatomic findings in cleft velum and correction by intravelar plastic operation, PRS, *55:*111, 1975. Ztschr. Kinderchir., *15:*21, 1974

KRIKUN, L. A.: Clinical features of median cleft of nose, PRS, *52:*682, 1973. Acta chir. plast., *14:*137, 1972

KRINITZ, K. *et al*: Malignant melanoma and hairy nevus. Dermatol. Monatsschr., *158:*130, 1972 (German)

KRISCH, A.: Modern methods of partial nasal reconstruction. Laryngol. Rhinol. Otol. (Stuttg.), *54:*424, 1975 (German)

KRISCHER, J. P. *et al*: Changing cleft widths: a problem revisited. Am. J. Orthod., *67:*647, 1975

KRISTENSEN, H. S.: Editorial: complications after tracheostomy. Ugeskr. Laeger., *136:*2255, 1974 (Danish)

KRISTENSEN, J. K.: Surgical treatment of axillary hyperhidrosis using the Skoog and Thyresson method. Ugeskr. Laeger, *136:*2869, 1974 (Danish)

KRITSKII, A. V.: Role of sound spectrography in the evaluation of cleft palate speech. Stomatologiia (Mosk.), *51:*90, 1972 (Russian)

KRIVOSIC-HORBER, R., TEMPE, D., GAUTHIER-LAFAYE, J. P.: Can we rehabilitate children exposed to prolonged intubation? Anesth. Analg. (Paris), *29:*411, 1972 (French)

KRIZEK, T. J.: Evaluation of topical povidone-iodine ointment in experimental burn wound sepsis (with Robson, Schaerf), PRS, *54:*328, 1974

KRIZEK, T. J.: Tropical ulcers (with Ariyan), PRS, *55:*324, 1975

KRIZEK, T. J.: Scalping injury (with Koss, Robson), PRS, *55:*439, 1975

KRIZEK, T. J., AND COSSMAN, D. V.: Experimental burn wound sepsis: variations in response to topical agents, PRS, *52:*325, 1973. J. Trauma, *12:*553, 1972

KRIZEK, T. J., AND KIRCHNER, J. A.: Tracheal reconstruction with autogenous mucochondrial graft, PRS, *50:*123, 1972

KRIZEK, T. J., AND ROBSON, M. C.: Potential pitfalls in use of deltopectoral flap, PRS, *50:*326, 1972

KRIZEK, T. J., AND ROBSON, M.: Deltopectoral flap for reconstruction of irradiated cancer of head and neck, PRS, *52:*105, 1973. Surg. Gynec. & Obst., *135:*787, 1972

KRIZEK, T. J., AND ROBSON, M. C.: Split flap in head and neck reconstruction, PRS, *53:*613, 1974. Am. J. Surg., *126:*488, 1973

KRIZEK, T. J., AND ARIYAN, S.: Severe acute radiation injuries of hands, PRS, *51:*14, 1973

KRIZEK, T. J. *et al*: Delayed primary excision and skin grafting of burned hands, PRS, *51:*524, 1973

KRIZEK, T. J., ROBSON, M. C., AND GROSKIN, M. G.: Experimental burn sepsis – evaluation of enzymatic debridement, PRS, *55:*515, 1975. J. Surg. Res., *17:*219, 1974

KRIZEK, T. J., KOSS, N., AND ROBSON, M. C.: Current use of prophylactic antibiotics in plastic and reconstructive surgery, PRS, *55:*21, 1975

KRMPOTIC-NEMANIC, J. *et al*: Successful decompression of the facial nerve in facial spasm. H.N.O., *23:*376, 1975 (German)

KROESEN, G. *et al*: Tracheotomy in intensive therapy. Z. Allgemeinmed., *50:*285, 1974 (German)

KROGH, K.: Plastic surgical treatment of radiation scars after plantar warts. Ugeskr. Laeger, *134:*2155, 1972 (Danish)

KROGH, L.: Lymphovenous shunt. S. Afr. Med. J., *47:*1389, 1973

KROGMAN, W. M. *et al*: Longitudinal study of the craniofacial growth pattern in children with clefts as compared to normal, birth to six years. Cleft Palate J., *12:*59, 1975

KRUCHINSKI, G. V.: New method of palate defect repair, PRS, *51:*234, 1973. Acta chir. plast., *14:*23, 1972

KRUCHINSKI, G. V.: Classification of auricular anomalies and significance for their surgical treatment, PRS, *52:*677, 1973. Acta chir. plast., *14:*225, 1972

KRUCHINSKI, G. V.: Auricle reconstruction using reinforced auricular cartilage, PRS, 53:601, 1974. Acta chir. plast., 15:72, 1973

KRUCHINSKI, G. V. et al: Correction of partial defects of the pinna. Vestn. Otorinolaringol., 3:10, 1975 (Russian)

KRUEGER, J. L. et al: Acrocephalosyndactyly (Apert's syndrome). Ann. Ophth., 6:787, 1974

KRUGER, E.: Surgical treatment of open bite using 3-part osteotomy of the maxilla. Fortschr. Kiefer. Gesichtschir., 18:211, 1974 (German)

KRUGER, E.: Surgical treatment of retrognathia and bird face. Quintessenz, 25:25, 1974 (German)

KRUGER, E.: Preprosthetic surgery. Z.W.R., 83:8, 1974 (German)

KRUGER, E. et al: Surgical treatment of mandibular fractures during the age of growth. Fortschr. Kiefer. Gesichtschir., 19:201, 1975 (German)

KRUGER, GUSTAV O.: Textbook of Oral Surgery. 4th edition. C. V. Mosby Co., St. Louis, 1974

KRUGER, G. O.: Sialolithotomy. Am. Fam. Physician, 5:116, 1972

KRUGMAN, M. F. et al: Synovial sarcoma of head and neck. Arch. Otolaryng., 98:53, 1973

KRUGMAN, M. E. et al: Maxillectomy cavity care with a pulsating stream irrigator. Eye, Ear, Nose Throat Mon., 54:104, 1975

KRUK-ZAGAJEWSKA, A. et al: Limited cavernous lymphangioma of neck. Otolaryngol. Pol., 27:233, 1973 (Polish)

KRUK-ZAGAJEWSKA, A. et al: Pharyngocervical neuroma. Wiad. Lek., 27:1893, 1974 (Polish)

KRUPP, S.: Operative treatment of pressure sores in paraplegics. Reconstr. Surg. Traumatol., 13:159, 1972

KRUPP, S., AND RUFLI, T.: Therapy of badly-healing or non-healing leg ulcers by repeated application of homografts, PRS, 55:257, 1975. Schweiz. med. Wchnschr., 104:1148, 1974

KRUSE, C. G. et al: Benign and malignant schwannomas of facial nerve simulating parotid neoplasms. H.N.O., 21:107, 1973 (German)

KRUSE, C. G. et al: Indications for salivary gland tumor surgery. H.N.O., 22:55, 1974 (German)

KRUSE, R. L., AND KELLY, P. J.: Acceleration of fracture healing distal to venous tourniquet, PRS, 55:387, 1975. J. Bone & Joint Surg., 56A:730, 1974

KRUSZCYNSKI, T. et al: Difficulties in diagnosing malignant melanoma in young persons. Klin. Oczna., 42:921, 1972 (Polish)

KSANDER, G. A.: Skin tension lines in domestic pig (with Rose, Vistnes), PRS, 57:729, 1976

KSPOIAN, T. S.: Lymphangioma of the maxilla in a newborn infant. Vestn. Khir., 112:82, 1974 (Russian)

KUBACEK, V., AND PENKAVA, J.: Oblique clefts of face, PRS, 55:638, 1975. Acta chir. plast., 16:152, 1974

KUBACEK, V. et al: Lactation after the implantation of a gel-prosthesis into hypoplastic breasts. Cesk. Gynekol., 40:606, 1975 (Czech)

KUBO, K., GARRETT, W. S., JR., AND MUSGRAVE, R. H.: Nasal gliomas, PRS, 52:47, 1973

KUBO, M. et al: Pierre Robin syndrome—case report and statistical study. Iryo, 25:311, 1971 (Japanese)

KUBO, T., IKUTA, Y., AND TSUGE, K.: Free muscle transplantation in dogs by microneurovascular anastomoses, PRS, 57:495, 1976

KUCHARSKI, A. et al: Cystosarcoma phylloides of the mammary gland. Pol. Przegl. Chir., 43:1791, 1971 (Polish)

KUCHARSKI, S.: Surgical-prosthetic management of partially edentulous adult with malocclusion. Protet. Stomatol., 24:217, 1974 (Polish)

KUCHEMANN, K.: Proceedings: epithelioid sarcoma. Verh. Dtsch. Ges. Pathol., 57:419, 1973 (German)

KUCHEMANN, K.: Epithelioid sarcoma. Beitr. Pathol., 155:84, 1975

KUCZYNSKI, K.: Variations in the insertion of the first dorsal interosseous muscle and their significance in the rheumatoid arthritis. Hand, 4:37, 1972

KUCZYNSKI, K.: Functional micro-anatomy of peripheral nerve trunks, PRS, 54:693, 1974. Hand, 6:1, 1974

KUCZYNSKI, K.: Flexor digitorum superficialis tendon in fingers of human hand, PRS, 56:227, 1975. Hand, 6:121, 1974

KUCZYNSKI, K.: Carpometacarpal joint of human thumb, PRS, 56:229, 1975. J. Anat., 118:119, 1974

KUCZYNSKI, K.: Less known aspects of proximal interphalangeal joints of human hand, PRS, 57:398, 1976. Hand, 7:31, 1975

KUEHN, P. G. et al: Surgical treatment of stomal recurrences in cancer of the larynx. Am. J. Surg., 122:445, 1971

KUFFER, R., AND SOUBIRAN, J. M.: Use of thin skin grafts in the therapy of some buccal mucosa lesions. Bull. Soc. franc. dermat. et syph., 78:632, 1971 (French)

KUFNER, I.: Four years experience with surgical correction of deformities of the middle portion of the face. Stomatologiia (Mosk.), 51:49, 1972 (Russian)

KUFNER, J.: Effect of burns on development of jaws and teeth. Cesk. Stomatol., 74:172,

1974. (Czechoslovakian)

KUFNER, J., AND PETROVIC, S.: Surgical removal of large facial hemangiomas, PRS, 50:542, 1972. Acta chir. plast., 13:152, 1971

KUGAN, T., AND PASILA, M.: Free periosteal transplants in tracheal reconstruction, PRS, 55:718, 1975. Ztschr. Kinderchir., 15:371, 1974

KUGLER, S.: Surgical experiences with stitchless wound closure. Fortschr. Med., 92:621, 1974 (German)

KUHL, M.: Fraising and abrading. Arch. Dermatol. Forsch., 244:159, 1972 (German)

KUIPER, D. H.: Silicone granulomatous disease of breast simulating cancer, PRS, 52:452, 1973. Mich. Med., 72:215, 1973

KUIPER, J. S.: Skin disinfection with ethanol, without and with additives, PRS, 54:511, 1974. Arch. chir. neerl., 24:15, 1974

KUISK, H. et al: Opacification of the "paralymphatic system" during lymphography. Minn. Med., 58:443, 1975

KULAKOWSKI, A. et al: Primary osteogenic neoplasms of mandible. Nowotwory, 24:23, 1974 (Polish)

KULAKOWSKI, A. et al: Extensive cornifying carcinoma of lower lip—special clinical form. Nowotwory, 24:201, 1974 (Polish)

KULBER, H. et al: Tracheostomy closure and scar revisions. Arch. Otolaryng., 96:22, 1972

KULCZYNSKI, B.: Midline cysts and fistulas of the neck. Otolaryngol. Pol., 26:49, 1972 (Polish)

KULCZYNSKI, B. et al: Treatment of auricular keloids. Otolaryngol. Pol., 29:137, 1975 (Polish)

KUMAGAMI, H. et al: Significance of decompression operation of facial nerve—based on changes in lymphatic flow in nerve. Otolaryngol. Jap., 76:39, 1973 (Japanese)

KUMAR, H. et al: Clitoroplasty: experience during 19-year period, PRS, 54:504, 1974. J. Urol., 111:81, 1974

KUMAR, P. et al: Progressive right hemifacial atrophy with contralateral cerebral hemiatrophy. J. Assoc. Physicians India, 19:595, 1971

KUMAR, P. P.: Metastases to the bones of the hand. J. Natl. Med. Assoc., 67:275, 1975

KUMMOONA, R.: Central myxofibrosarcoma of the mandible treated by radical resection. Oral Surg., 39:713, 1975

KUMMOONA, R.: Chrome cobalt and gold implant for the reconstruction of a traumatized orbital floor. Oral Surg., 41:293, 1976

KUNE, G. A.: Carcinoma in a pharyngeal pouch: five-year survival after resection. Aust. N.Z.J. Surg., 41:249, 1972

KUNERT, P. et al: Clinical and histological results after extensive split skin transplantation. In Plastische und Wiederherstellungs-Chirurgie, ed. by Hohler; pp. 251-7. Stuttgart; Schattauer, 1975 (German)

KUNKEL, R. S. et al: Surgical treatment of chronic migrainous neuralgia. Cleve. Clin. Q., 41:189, 1974

KUNSMAN, J.: Nursing care after primary excision. R.N., 37:25, 1974

KUO, T. P.: Electrical injuries: clinical experience of 100 cases, PRS, 53:490, 1974. Riv. ital. chir. plast., 4:51, 1973

KUPCHIK, B. M. et al: Treatment of extensive turban tumor of scalp (single observation). Vopr. Onkol., 19:77, 1973 (Russian)

KURATA, K.: Plastic surgery of facial nerve paralysis. Otolaryngology (Tokyo), 43:847, 1971 (Japanese)

KURATA, K. et al: Treatments of the granulation wounds—therapeutic experience in extensive thermal burns. Jap. J. Plast. Reconstr. Surg., 14:150, 1971 (Japanese)

KURBANAEVA, E. S. et al: Morphological aspects of xerophthalmia after transplantation of Stensen's duct into the conjunctival cavity. Vestn. Oftalmol., 2:43, 1975 (Russian)

KURBANAEVA, F. S.: Late results of Stensen's duct transplantation. Vestn. Oftalmol., 5:44, 1973 (Russian)

KURILIN, I. A.: Use of alloplastic materials for reconstructive surgery of nose, larynx and trachea. Zh. Ushn. Nos. Gorl. Bolezn., 31:46, 1971 (Russian)

KUROHARA, S. S. et al: Role of radiation therapy and of surgery in the management of localized epidermoid carcinoma of the maxillary sinus. Am. J. Roentgenol. Radium Ther. Nucl. Med., 114:35, 1972

KURSAR, G. H.: Dacryocystorhinostomy: microsurgical approach. J. Am. Osteopath. Assoc., 73:387, 1974

KURZ, M.: Reconstruction of a lacrimal ductule through the implantation of a vein from the back of the hand. Klin. Monatsbl. Augenheilkd., 160:307, 1972 (German)

KUS, H. et al: Deferred surgical procedures in crush injuries of the hand. Chir. Narzadow. Ruchu Ortop. Pol., 36:413, 1971 (Polish)

KUS, H. et al: Acquired complicated elephantiasis of lower extremity. Pol. Przegl. Chir., 44:1743, 1972 (Polish)

KUSH, N. L. et al: Hemangiomas of the skin in children. Vestn. Khir., 115:65, 1975 (Russian)

KUSHCH, N. L.: Sex determination and its surgical correction in certain abnormalities of urogenital system in children. Klin. Khir., 8:39, 1973 (Russian)

KUSHCH, N. L. et al: Reconstructive surgery for

vaginal pathology in girls. Vestn. Khir., *107:*114, 1971 (Russian)

KUSHCH, N. L. *et al:* Tactics in sex determination in children with anomalies in development of genital organs. Vestn. Khir., *111:*80, 1973 (Russian)

KUSHNER, J. *et al:* Crouzon's disease (craniofacial dysostosis). Modern diagnosis and treatment. J. Neurosurg., *37:*434, 1972

KUTZ, C. M.: Surgical treatment of stasis ulcers. Angiology, *23:*665, 1972

KUX, P.: Thoracoscopic sympathectomy in treatment of hyperhidrosis of upper limbs, PRS, *53:*369, 1974. Rev. Asoc. med. Minas Gerais, Brazil, *23:*119, 1973

KUZ'MENKO, V. F.: Peculiarities in the clinical picture, diagnosis and treatment of actinomycosis of the jaws. Stomatologiia (Mosk.), *51:*77, 1972 (Russian)

KUZ'MENKO, V. V.: Surgical treatment of congenital radial clubhand. Ortop. Travmatol. Protez., *32:*22, 1971 (Russian)

KUZ'MIN, K. P.: Results of the treatment of dislocations of the hand and carpal bones. Ortop. Travmatol. Protez., *34:*29, 1973

KUZNETSOVA, I. L.: Rare anomaly of nose. Vestn. Otorinolaringol., *34:*94, 1972 (Russian)

KVINNSLAND, S.: Growth in height of autotransplanted nasal septum in rat. Its correlation to increase in height of upper face. Acta Odontol. Scand., *31:*317, 1973

KVINNSLAND, S.: Growth potential of autografts of cartilage from nasal septum in rat, PRS, *52:*557, 1973

KVINNSLAND, S.: Partial resection of cartilaginous nasal septum in rats: its influence on growth. Angle. Orthod., *44:*135, 1974

KVINNSLAND, S.: Autogenous transplantation of the nasal septum cartilage in the rat. Arch. Oral Biol., *19:*767, 1974

KVINNSLAND, S., AND BREISTEIN, L.: Regeneration of cartilaginous nasal septum in rat, after resection. Its influence on facial growth. PRS, *51:*190, 1973

KWAAN, H. C., AND SILVERMAN, S.: Fibrinolytic activity in lesions of hereditary hemorrhagic telangiectasia, PRS, *52:*597, 1973. Arch. Dermat., *107:*571, 1973

KWANGCHOW, CHUNG SHAN MEDICAL COLLEGE: Experience in replantation of severed fingers, PRS, *55:*248, 1975. Chinese M.J., *6:*71, 1973

KWANGCHOW CHUNG SHAN MEDICAL COLLEGE: Experimental study of effect of ilex pubescens on vessels of isolated organs, with report on clinical use in limb replantation, PRS, *55:*250, 1975. Chinese M.J., *2:*28, 1974

KWAPIS, B. W. *et al:* Surgical correction of mal-

united condylar fracture in child. J. Oral Surg., *31:*465, 1973

KWART, L.: Polyester implants in comprehensive treatment of maxillofacial deformities. Czas. Stomatol., *25:*37, 1972 (Polish)

KWIATKOWSKI, J. *et al:* Nasal abruption. Otolaryngol. Pol., *28:*703, 1974 (Polish)

KYGER, E. R., III: Studies in rats of survival of composite homotransplants of skin and subcutaneous tissue, with microvascular anastomoses (with Salyer), PRS, *51:*672, 1973

KYOSOLA, K.: Clinical experiences in management of cold injuries: study of 110 cases. J. Trauma, *14:*32, 1974

KYRTATAS, J. D., AND VOGIATZIS, N.: Hypospadias report on 325 cases, PRS, *53:*488, 1974. Tr. 7th Panhellenic Cong. Surg., *B:* 889, 1970

KYRTATAS, J. D.: Therapy of keloids by corticosteroids, PRS, *53:*502, 1974. Tr. 28th Panhellenic Cong. Medicosurg. Soc., *1:*242, 1973

L

LABAYLE, J. *et al:* Technic of approach to the 3rd portion of the 7th nerve. Ann. Otolaryngol. Chir. Cervicofac., *88:*363, 1971 (French)

Labial Frenum

Frenectomy in dental practice (Werelds *et al*). Acta Stomatol. Belg., *68:*475, 1971 (Dutch)

High attachment of lower lip frenum. Its consequence and therapy (Zabrodsky *et al*). Cesk. Stomatol., *72:*86, 1972 (Czech)

Anterior Z-plasty ridge extension (Prowler). Oral Surg., *33:*172, 1972

Effect of superior labial frenectomy in cases with midline diastema (Bergstrom *et al*). Am. J. Orthod., *63:*633, 1973

Muco-gingival surgery. New technic for frenectomy and bridectomy (Lascala *et al*). Rev. Assoc. Paul. Cir. Dent., *27:*135, 1973 (Portuguese)

Labial frenum, usefulness of surgical diathermy for removal of abnormal attachment of (Banach). Czas. Stomatol., *27:*405, 1974

Labial frenum, evaluation of surgical treatment of, in prevention and treatment of periodontal diseases (Jedrzejewska *et al*). Czas. Stomatol., *27:*413, 1974 (Polish)

An oral contraceptive drug and gingival enlargement; the relationship between local and systemic factors (Pearlman). J. Clin. Periodontol., *1:*47, 1974

Orthodontically corrected midline diastemas. A histologic study and surgical procedure

Labial Frenum — Cont.

(Campbell *et al*). Am. J. Orthod., *67*:139, 1975

LACCOURREYE, H. *et al*: Assessment of a year's systematic use in cancer of otorhinolaryngological area of new antimitotic: bleomycin. Study of 209 patients. Ann. Otolaryngol. Chir. Cervicofac., *89*:219, 1972 (French)

LACCOURREYE, H. *et al*: Pharyngotomy for colonic anastomosis during total esophagoplasty. J. Chir., *107*:83, 1974 (French)

LACERDA ABREU, C.: Wrinkles, etiopathogenic theory, PRS, *50*:417, 1972. Rev. paulista med. Brazil, *78*:93, 1971

LACHARD, J. *et al*: Mixed tumors of buccal cavity. Rev. Stomatol. Chir. Maxillofac., *73*:216, 1972 (French)

LACHARD, J. *et al*: Parotidectomy for inflammatory lesions. Rev. Stomatol. Chir. Maxillofac., *73*:235, 1972 (French)

LACHARD, J. AND VITTON, J.: Treatment of mandibular retrognathism using retrocondylar cartilage graft (Trauner procedure). Ann. chir. plast., *18*:50, 1973 (French)

LACHARD, J. *et al*: Treatment of perforations of the roof of the mouth. Alveolar buccosinusal communications. Rev. Stomatol. Chir. Maxillofac., *75*:208, 1974 (French)

LACHARD, J. *et al*: Value of an originale nasotracheal catheter in maxillo-facial surgery and stomatology. Rev. Stomatol. chir. Maxillofac., *75*:1029, 1974 (French)

LACHARD, J. *et al*: Cervical lymph node excision. Conservative technics. Acta Stomatol. Belg., *72*:393, 1975 (French)

LACHARD, J. *et al*: Surgical treatment of maxillary sequelae of labio-palatine clefts. Pterygo-maxillary disjunction. Rev. Stomatol. Chir. Maxillofac., *75*:77, 1974 (French)

LACOUR, J. *et al*: Treatment of malignant tumors of salivary glands at Gustave-Roussy institute. Aktuel Probl. Chir., *14*:389, 1970

LACOUR, M. *et al*: Considerable incisor gaping treated by partial glossectomy. Bull. Soc. Med. Afr. Noire Lang. Fr., *15*:332, 1970

Lacrimal Apparatus (See also *Dacryocystorhinostomy*)

Carcinoma of lacrimal canaliculi and lacrimal sac (Paxton, Davidorf, Makley), PRS, *48*:293, 1971. Arch. Ophth., *84*:749, 1970

Lacrimal gland, aberrant, in orbit (Baldridge), PRS, *48*:293, 1971. Arch. Ophth., *84*:758, 1970

Technic of lacrimal intubation (Editorial). Bull. Soc. Ophtalmol. Fr., *70*:1149, 1970 (French)

Conjunctive-rhinostomy (Trivedi *et al*). J. All

Lacrimal Apparatus

India. Ophthalmol. Soc., *18*:170, 1970

Canaliculo-dacryocysto-rhinostomy. A simple technique (Saxena). J. All India Ophthalmol. Soc., *18*:173, 1970

Modified technique of external dacryocystorhinostomy (Pico). Am. J. Ophth., *72*:679, 1971

Technique for conjunctivo-dacryocystorhinostomy (Cox). Am. J. Ophth., *72*:931, 1971

French-eye pigtail probe for lacrimal canaliculus repair (Kartch). Am. J. Ophth., *72*:1145, 1971

Restoration of the lacrimal apparatus. Value of venous grafts (Stricker *et al*). Ann. chir. plast., *16*:314, 1971 (French)

Lacrimal gland, aberrant, two cases (Firat *et al*). Ann. Ophth., *3*:50, 1971

Downward displacement of medial canthus (Fox). Ann. Ophth., *3*:1082, 1971

Wound closure after lacrimal sac surgery (Sisler). Ann. Ophth., *3*:1357, 1971

Lacrimal apparatus, surgery of, in children, remarks (Worst). Annee Ther. Clin. Ophtalmol., *22*:187, 1971 (French)

Use of the pigtail catheter in reconstruction of the lacrimal ducts (Dereume-de Corte). Bull. Soc. Belge. Ophtalmol., *159*:590, 1971 (French)

Restoration of lacrimal canaliculi by means of a pigtail probe (Bernard *et al*). Bull. Soc. Ophtalmol. Fr., *71*:419, 1971 (French)

Dacryorhinostomy operation: some technical procedures (Thomas *et al*). Bull. Soc. Ophtalmol. Fr., *71*:468, 1971 (French)

Results of surgery activating the upper lacrimal duct by P. A. Erlyshev's method in reflex lacrimation (Sultanov *et al*). Oftalmol. Zh., *26*:391, 1971 (Russian)

Catheter-cannula for restoring the patency of the lacrimal ducts in children (Gritsiuk). Oftalmol. Zh., *26*:551, 1971 (Russian)

Reconstructive surgery of the nasolacrimal duct and its variations (Miyake). Ophthalmology (Tokyo), *13*:1027, 1971 (Japanese)

Three cases of dacryocytorhinostomy (Takayama *et al*). Otolaryngology (Tokyo), *43*:673, 1971 (Japanese)

Lacrimal apparatus, one-stage reconstruction of (Snow, Johnson), PRS, *48*:453, 1971

Tumors of the lacrimal glands: their surgical management (Jones). South. Med. J., *64*:1503, 1971

Developments in lacrimal canalicular surgery (Maquire *et al*). Trans. Ophthalmol. Soc. U.K., *91*:923, 1971

Comparative evaluation of hammerless methods of forming openings in the bone (Sultanov). Vestn. Oftalmol., *3*:83, 1971

Lacrimal Apparatus – Cont.

(Russian)

Ten years of experiences with Falk's lacrimal sac surgery (Schondorf). Z. Laryngol. Rhinol. Otol., *50:*194, 1971 (German)

Contralateral rhinostomy for dacryocystitis due to facial malformation (Korchmaros). Acta Ophthalmol. (Kbh.), *50:*390, 1972

Lacrimal sac, endoscopic observations on internal surface of, following dacryocystorhinostomy (Tajima, Maruyama, Ikegami). Acta Soc. Ophthalmol. Japan, *76:*1242, 1972

New use of the Bowman probe in dacryocystorhinostomy (Delman). Ann. Ophth., *4:*505, 1972

Lacrimal canaliculus, hard to repair severed (Meacham), PRS, *50:*304, 1972. Arch. Ophth., *87:*406, 1972

Treatment of obstruction of the common canaliculus (Gershen). Arch. Ophth., *88:*87, 1972

Surgical treatment of lacrimal duct obstructions (Bernard). Arch. Ophtalmol. (Paris), *32:*177, 1972 (French)

Implantation of small lacrimal tube for improved drainage of aqueous humor into subconjunctival space (Stark). Ber. Dtsch. Ophthalmol. Ges., *71:*647, 1972

Intubation macrodacryocystography (Lloyd *et al*). Brit. J. Ophth., *56:*600, 1972

Lacrimal sac operations, self-retaining retractor for (Lyall). Brit. J. Ophth., *56:*636, 1972

Imperforate puncta with blocked nasolacrimal duct (Aggarwal). Brit. J. Ophth., *56:*788, 1972

Nasolacrimal duct, polyethylene intubation of, in chronic dacryocystitis, review of 40 cases with one-year follow up (Singh, Garg). Brit. J. Ophth., *56:*914, 1972

Lacrimal sac, dacryocystography in midfacial fractures (Stranc, Bunce), PRS, *52:*96, 1973. Brit. J. Plast. Surg., *25:*269, 1972

Rare case of canaliculocele (Fouad). Bull. Ophthalmol. Soc. Egypt, *65:*265, 1972

Surgery of lacrimal duct injuries (Struplova *et al*). Cesk. Oftalmol., *28:*237, 1972 (Czech)

Nasolacrimal duct stenosis, surgical care following middle face fractures (Domke). Dtsch. Gesundheitsw., *27:*2141, 1972 (German)

Nasolacrimal duct, intubation of, with polythene tube (Mukherjee *et al*). Indian J. Ophthalmol., *20:*16, 1972

Dacryocystorhinostomy (Juselius), PRS, *51:*701, 1973. Internat. Surg., *57:*883, 1972

Three flaps dacryocystorhinostomy (Mostafa

Lacrimal Apparatus – Cont.

et al) J. Laryng. & Otol., *86:*829, 1972

Reconstruction of lacrimal ductule through the implantation of a vein from the back of the hand (Kurz). Klin. Monatsbl. Augenheilkd., *160:*307, 1972 (German)

Lacrimal canaliculus, injuries of, surgical technics and prognosis (Hanselmayer *et al*). Klin. Monatsbl. Augenheilkd., *160:*572, 1972 (German)

Lacrimal flow (Henkes). Ned. Tijdschr. Geneeskd., *116:*465, 1972 (Dutch)

Lacrimostomy with permanent intubation (Zakharov). Oftal. zhur., *27:*297, 1972 (Russian)

Lacrimal drainage (Rosengren). Ophthalmologica, *164:*409, 1972

Lacrimal gland, malignant mixed tumor of (Sperling, Krimmer), PRS, *50:*81, 1972

Late bilateral naso-orbital fracture and dacryostenosis (Smith). Trans. Am. Acad. Ophthalmol. Otolaryngol., *76:*1378, 1972

Palpebral dacryoadenectomy (Talara *et al*). Am. J. Ophth., *75:*461, 1973

Tycron for canalicular repair (White). Am. J. Ophth., *75:*731, 1973

Palpebral dacryoadenectomy (Fox). Am. J. Ophth., *76:*314, 1973

Lacrimal canaliculi, traumatic section of, therapeutical attitudes and results (Caravel). Ann. chir. plast., *18:*371, 1973 (French)

Weeping without stenosis of the lacrimal ducts (Medrano *et al*). Annee. Ther. Clin. Ophtalmol., *24:*409, 1973 (French)

Lacrimal tubes, silicone rubber, conjunctivodacryocystorhinostomy using (Carroll, Beyer). Arch. Ophth., *89:*113, 1973

Lacrimal apparatus, canalicular blockage (Chang). Aust. J. Ophthalmol., *1:*58, 1973

Test for spontaneous canalicular functioning (Murube). Aust. J. Ophthalmol., *1:*61, 1973

Bicanalicular annular intubation in lacrimal canaliculi sections (Murube). Bull. Mem. Soc. Fr. Ophtalmol., *86:*223, 1973 (French)

Lacrimal sac, inverted papilloma of (Lavergne *et al*). Bull. Soc. Belge. Ophtalmol., *165:*323, 1973 (French)

Technic and results of treatment of traumatic canalicular sections using Worst's "pig tail" sound (Bronner *et al*). Bull. Soc. Ophtalmol. Fr., *73:*939, 1973 (French)

Lacrimal sac, carcinoma of (Schindler *et al*). Can. J. Ophthalmol., *8:*161, 1973

Lacrimal duct occlusions in children, treatment of (Filipowiczova-Banachova). Cesk. Oftalmol., *29:*105, 1973 (Czechoslovakian)

Hypotension anaesthesia in dacryocystorhinostomy (Zohairy *et al*). Eye, Ear, Nose,

Lacrimal Apparatus — Cont.

Surv. Ophthalmol., *19:*57, 1974

Lacrimal ducts, ruptures and strictures of, treatment (Goldschmidt). Ugeskr. Laeger, *136:*1198, 1974 (Danish)

Indications for endonasal dacryocystorhinostomy (Egorov *et al*). Vestn. Oftalmol., *5:*75, 1974 (Russian)

Modifications of dacryocystorhinostomy (Bakin). Vestn. Oftalmol., *6:*69, 1974 (Russian)

Dacryocystorhinostomy procedure, modifications of (Chandler), PRS, *57:*754, 1976. Am. J. Ophth., *80:*522, 1975

Letter: pyrex tubes in conjunctivodacryocystorhinostomy (Baylis *et al*). Am. J. Ophth., *79:*887, 1975

Lacrimal drainage following repair of inferior canaliculus (Ortiz, Kraushar), PRS, *57:*113, 1976. Ann. Ophth., *7:*739, 1975

Correspondence: modified lacrimal probe (Kartch). Arch. Ophth., *93:*163, 1975

Lacrimal gland removal, keratoconjunctivitis sicca after (Scherz, Dohlman), PRS, *56:*460, 1975. Arch. Ophth., *93:*281, 1975

Role of intubation macro-dacryocystography in management of problems of the lacrimal system (Hurwitz *et al*). Can. J. Ophthalmol., *10:*361, 1975

Lateral anastomosis of the lacrimal apparatus and lacrimal ductules (Wang). Chin. Med. J. (Engl.), *6:*424, 1975 (Chinese)

Deformities of the midface resulting from malunited orbital and naso-orbital fractures (Converse *et al*). Clin. Plast. Surg., *2:*107, 1975

Technic and results in tear duct reconstruction in facial injuries (Nwoku *et al*). Fortschr. Kiefer. Gesichtschir., *19:*148, 1975 (German)

Falk's lacrimal sac surgical technique for stenosis (Mootz *et al*). H.N.O., *23:*358, 1975 (German)

Contributions to the surgical technique of external dacryocystorhinostomy (Menezo *et al*). Klin. Monatsbl. Augenheilkd., *166:*108, 1975 (German)

Contributions to the therapy of epiphora (Brandt). Klin. Monatsbl. Augenheilkd., *167:*105, 1975 (German)

Reconstructive surgery of lacrimal canaliculi obstruction (Filipowicz-Banachowa). Klin. Oczna., *45:*35, 1975 (Polish)

Size and localization of bone aperture in external dacryocystorhinostomy (Volkov *et al.*) Oftalmol. Zh., *30:*179, 1975 (Russian)

Technic of activation of the lower lacrimal point (Boishtian). Oftalmol. Zh., *30:*309, 1975 (Russian)

Lacrimal Apparatus — Cont.

Dacryocystorhinostomy with nasolacrimal duct prosthesis (Thorton *et al*). Ophthalmic Surg., *6:*50, 1975

Sjögren's syndrome (Akin, Kreller, Walters), PRS, *56:*462, 1975. Oral Surg., *33:*27, 1975

Technical variant of autograft for lacrimal duct obstruction (Munteanu *et al*). Rev. Chir. Oftalmol. *19:*151, 1975 (Rumanian)

Possibilities of ensuring lacrimal drainage by permeabilization of the obstructed nasolacrimal duct (Popa *et al*). Rev. Chir. Oftalmol., *19:*307, 1975 (Rumanian)

Lacrimal drain (Guibor). Trans. Am. Acad. Ophthalmol. Otolaryngol., *79:*417, 1975

Canaliculus intubation set (Guibor). Trans. Am. Acad. Ophthalmol. Otolaryngol. *79:*OP419, 1975

Repair of nasocanthal malignancies by combined laissez-faire and chemosurgery techniques (Fox). Trans. Am. Acad. Ophthalmol. Otolaryngol., *79:*654, 1975

Comparative evaluation of the effectiveness of 3 modifications of external dacryocystorhinostomy (Sultanov). Vestn. Oftalmol., *3:*77, 1975 (Russian)

Diagnostical and therapeutic approach to disturbed excretory lacrimal ducts in infants and small children (Fulgosi). Vojnosanit. Pregl., *32:*149, 1975 (Croatian)

Lacrimal function, keratoconjunctivitis sicca symptoms appearing after blepharoplasty (Graham, Messner, Miller), PRS, *57:*57, 1976

LAFFOLE, P. *et al*: Historical form of cancer of the lower lip. Ann. Otolaryngol. Chir. Cervicofac., *91:*325, 1974 (French)

LAFON, H.: Inverted papillomas. J. Fr. Otorhinolaryngol., *23:*507, 1974 (French)

Lagophthalmos (See also *Facial Paralysis; Leprosy*)

Temporalis transplantation procedure for paralytic lagophthalmos (Sen), PRS, *50:*304, 1972. Internat. Surg., *56:*410, 1971

Orbicularis muscle paralysis, dynamic closure of lids in (Arion), PRS, *50:*629, 1972. Internat. Surg., *57:*48, 1972

Eyelid function, restoration in facial palsy with permanent magnets (Muehlbauer, Segeth, Viessmann), PRS, *53:*113, 1974. Chir. Plast., *1:*295, 1973

Lid loading technique in management of lagophthalmos of facial palsy (Jobe), PRS, *53:*29, 1974

Lagophthalmos: four years' experience with Morel-Fatio palpebral spring (Morgan, Rich). PRS, *53:*404, 1974

Lagophthalmos – Cont.

Lid loading in management of lagophthalmos (Habal, Jobe) (Letter to the Editor), PRS, 54:211, 1974

Lid loading in management of lagophthalmos (Micheli-Pellegrini) (Letter to the Editor). PRS, 55:482, 1975

LAGROT, F.: Causes and prevention of occupational radiodermatitis of the hands in physicians. Bull. Acad. Natl. Med. (Paris), 155:806, 1971 (French)

LAGROT, F., MICHEAU, P., AND COSTAGLIOLA, M.: Role of skin grafts in organ grafting, PRS, 48:613, 1971. Rev. españ. cir. plast., 4:57, 1971

LAGROT, F. *et al*: Value of excision-homograft in burned patients. Ann. Chir., 27:191, 1973 (French)

LAGROT, F. *et al*: Series of 104 operated cases of radiodermatitis of hand (179 hands). Ann. chir. plast., 18:233, 1973 (French)

LAGUNDOYE, S. B.: Ankylosis of mandible from *cancrum oris* (with Oluwasanmi, Akinyemi). PRS, 57:342, 1976

LAGUNDOYE, S. B., AND OLUWASANMI, J. O.: Exostosis following grenade injury to the hand, PRS, 54:375, 1974. Hand, 5:149, 1973

LAGUNOVA, I. G. *et al:* Possibility of treating metastases of melanoma with laser irradiation. Eksp. Khir. Anesteziol. 16:50, 1971 (Russian)

LAHOTI, R. K., AND SHARMA, H. S. D.: Study of lymphocyte depletion and hypogamma-globulinemia on survival of skin homografts: experimental study in albino rats, PRS, 53:497, 1974. Indian J. Surg., 35:375, 1973

LAHTI, A. *et al*: Circulatory changes in the premaxilla during treatment for bilateral complete cleft lip and palate. Scand. J. Plast. Reconstr. Surg., 6:132, 1972

LAHTI, A. *et al*: Reconstruction of the mandibular bone and the condyle after tumor surgery. Ann. Chir. Gynaecol. Fenn., 62:155, 1973

LAHTI, A., RINTALA, A., AND SOIVIO, A. I.: Educational level of patients with cleft lip and palate, PRS, 55:252, 1975. Cleft Palate J., 11:36, 1974

LAING, J. E., AND HARVEY, J.: *The Management & Nursing of Burns*. 2nd Ed. Medical Examination Pub. Co., Inc., Flushing, N.Y., 1971

LAIRD, S. M. *et al*: Effect of methoxyflurane analgesia on renal function in burned patients: an investigation. Postgrad. Med. J., 48:133, 1972

LAITINEN, J.: Treatment of cervical syndrome by acupuncture, PRS, 57:768, 1976. Scand. J. Rehab. Med., 7:114, 1975

LAKE, C. F.: Problems of septal areas, PRS, 57:114, 1976. Postgrad. M. J., 57:108, 1975

LALARDRIE, J. P., AND JOUGLARD, J. P.: *Plasties Mammaires pour Hypertrophie et Ptose*. Masson & Cie., Paris, 1973. PRS, 53:673, 1974

LALARDRIE, J. P., AND JOUGLARD, J. P.: *Chirurgie Plastique de Sein*. Masson et Cie, Paris, 1974.

LALARDRIE, J. P., AND MITZ, V.: Plastic operation for reducing size of breast by so-called skin-vault technique, PRS, 56:106, 1975. J. chir., 108:57, 1974

LALARDRIE, J. P. *et al*: Dermo-dermal uniting: an experimental study, PRS, 57:268, 1976. Ann. chir. plast., 20:183, 1975

LALLEMANT, Y. *et al*: Cervico-cephalic zona with multiple localizations, complicated by facial paralysis, successfully treated by surgery. Ann. Otolaryngol. Chir. Cervicofac., 90:214, 1973 (French)

LALLEMANT, Y. *et al*: Papillary cystadenolymphoma of parotid gland associated with cervical lymph node tuberculosis. Ann. Otolaryngol. Chir. Cervicofac., 90:224, 1973 (French)

LALLEMANT, Y. *et al*: Aphagia following traumatic coma. Attempts at physiopathogenic interpretation. Treatment. Ann. Otolaryngol. Chir. Cervicofac., 90:329, 1973 (French)

LALLEMANT, Y. *et al*: Jugomandibular complex radionecrosis. Therapeutic problems. Ann. Otolaryngol. Chir. Cervicofac., 90:763, 1973 (French)

LALLEMANT, Y. *et al*: Nasopharyngeal fibroma. Significance of super-selective angiography and embolization. Ann. Otolaryngol. Chir. Cervicofac., 92:127, 1975 (French)

LAM, S. J.: Modified technique for stabilising the spastic thumb. J. Bone & Joint Surg. (Br.), 54:522, 1972

LAM, W. K. *et al*: Tissue reaction to cuffed tube materials. Anaesth. Intensive Care, 2:260, 1974

LAMB, D. W.: Treatment of radial club hand. Absent radius, aplasia of the radius, hypoplasia of the radius, radial paraxial hemimelia. Hand, 4:22, 1972

LAMB, D. W. *et al*: Hand in quadriplegia. Hand, 3:31, 1971

LAMB, D. W. *et al*: Congenital absence of the upper limb and hand. A review of the benefits in prehension and bimanual function by early prosthetic replacement. Hand, 3:193, 1971

LAMB, D. W. *et al*: Hand in quadriplegia. Paraplegia, 9:204, 1972

LAMB, F. S., SILVA, Y. J., AND WALT, A. J.: Thomas Blizzard Curling – man and ulcer, PRS, 48:296, 1971. Surgery, 69:646, 1971

LAMB, M. M. *et al*: The intellectual function of cleft palate children compared on the basis of cleft type and sex. Cleft Palate J., *10:*367, 1973

LAMBERT, J. A.: Parotid gland tumors, PRS, *48:*518, 1971. Mil. Med., *136:*484, 1971

LAMBILLIOTE, P.: Rehabilitation apparatus for hand injuries. Bull. Mem. Soc. Chir. Paris, *60:*238, 1970 (French)

LAMBRECHT, W.: Congenital bifid sternum, PRS, *57:*760, 1976. Ztschr. Kinderchir., *17:*128, 1975

LAMKE, L. O.: Evaporative water loss from burns under different environmental conditions. Scand. J. Plast. Reconstr. Surg., *5:*77, 1971

LAMKE, L. O.: Influence of different "skin grafts" on the evaporative water loss from burns. Scand. J. Plast. Reconstr. Surg., *5:*82, 1971

LAMKE, L. O.: Evaporative water loss from normal and burnt skin, PRS, *49:*665, 1972. Thesis, Dept. Surg., Linkoping Univ., Sweden, 1971

LAMMLI, K. *et al*: Reconstruction surgery of the esophagus with delto-pectoral flap. Pract. Otorhinolaryngol. (Basel), *33:*11, 1971 (German)

LAMONT, E.: Congenital inversion of nipple in identical twins. Brit. J. Plast. Surg., *26:*178, 1973

LAMONT, E.: On nasal tip projection (Letter to the Editor). PRS, *57:*228, 1976

LAMP, J. C.: Conjunctival approach for exploration of orbital floor (with Lynch, Royster). PRS, *54:*153, 1974

LAMPE, C. E.: 3 cases of fibromatosis. Nord. Med., *85:*291, 1971 (Danish)

LAMPHIER, T. A.: Erysipeloid infection of digits. J. Fla. Med. Assoc., *58:*39, 1971

LANCHOW GENERAL HOSPITAL: Reconstruction of missing thumbs with improved "cocked hat" operation, PRS, *55:*637, 1975. Chinese M. J., *10:*177, 1974

LAND, R. E.: Anatomic relationships of right subclavian vein, PRS, *48:*197, 1971. Arch. Surg., *102:*178, 1971

LANDA, S. J. *et al*: Cancer of floor of mouth and gingiva. Surg. Clin. North Am., *53:*135, 1973

LANDA, S. J. *et al*: Advances in the surgical treatment of pressure sores. Rev. Surg., *33:*1, 1976

LANDA, S. J. F., AND LESAVOY, M. A.: Subclavian artery in head and neck surgery, PRS, *55:*376, 1975. J. Maxillo-facial Surg., *2:*104, 1974

LANDAIS, H.: Various methods for the closure of bucco-nasal communications. Rev. Stomatol. Chir. Maxillofac., *74:*642, 1973 (French)

LANDAIS, H.: Partial bilateral anterior osteotomies of the upper jaw. Conditions for stability of the results. Rev. Stomatol. Chir. Maxillofac., *75:*118, 1974 (French)

LANDAIS, H.: Our experience with 107 buccosinusal communications without failure of closure. Rev. Stomatol. Chir. Maxillofac., *75:*186, 1974 (French)

LANDAIS, H. *et al*: Case of maxillary malignant melanoma with 6-year recovery. J. Fr. Otorhinolaryngol., *21:*638, 1972 (French)

LANDAZURI, H., FLORES, R. F., AND LINO, R. B.: Maximum lethal dose of propanidide, PRS, *53:*692, 1974. Rev. Latino Am. cir. plast., *17:*69, 1973

LANDE, J. L. VAN DE *et al*: Hypoplasia of the breast, a psychosocial disease. Ned. tijdschr. geneeskd., *116:*428, 1972 (Dutch)

LANDEEN, J. M.: Firearm wounds of the head and neck. Eye Ear Nose Throat Mon., *51:*222, 1972

LANDESMAN, H. M. *et al*: Patient survey of denture tolerance before and after mandibular vestibuloplasty with skin grafting. J. Am. Dent. Assoc., *90:*806, 1975

LANDOLT, A. M. *et al*: Pathogenesis of cerebral infarction secondary to mechanical carotid artery occlusion. Stroke, *1:*52, 1970

LANDSMEER, J. E. F.: *Atlas of Anatomy of Hand*. Longman, London, 1975.

LANE, J. M. *et al*: Inhibition of scar formation by proline analog cis-hydroxyproline, PRS, *52:*104, 1973. J. Surg. Res., *13:*135, 1972

LANFRANCHI, R. *et al*: Surgical treatment of scar retractions of the palm of the hands. Arch. Putti. Chir. Organi. Mov., *24:*233, 1969 (Italian)

LANG, B.: Treatment of pressure sores in handicapped children, PRS, *57:*683, 1976. Cutis, *16:*158, 1975

LANG, W.: Secondary esophagoplasty after pharyngolaryngectomy, using modified deltopectoral flap (with Jackson), PRS, *48:*155, 1971

LANGAUER-LEWOWICKA, H. *et al*: Pneumoencephalocele as a complication of nasal septum resection. Neurol. Neurochir. Pol., *5:*583, 1971 (Polish)

LANGE, D. *et al*: Malignant tumours in the ENR-region. IV. Tumours of the parotid gland. Arch. Geschwulstforsch, *42:*358, 1973 (German)

LANGE, G.: Experiences in surgical care of transected or resected facial nerves. Arch. Klin. Exp. Ohren Nasen Kehlkopfheilkd., *205:*197, 1973 (German)

LANGE, M. J.: Fenestrated tracheostomy tubes. Lancet, *2:*444, 1973

LANGENBECK, B.: New method for operation on

complete congenital cleft of hard palate (Classic Reprint). PRS, *49:*323, 1972

LANGENBECK, B.: Uranoplasty by means of raising mucoperiosteal flaps (Classic Reprint). PRS, *49:*326, 1972

LANGER, F. AND GROSS, A.: Immunogenicity of allograft articular cartilage, PRS, *54:*507, 1974. J. Bone & Joint Surg., *56A:*297, 1974

LANGER, H. *et al*: Clinical aspects of Fries' open and axial medullary wiring in mandibular fractures. Fortschr. Kiefer. Gesichtschir., *19:*109, 1975 (German)

LANGERON, P.: Possibilities and indications for surgery in sequelae of phlebitis. Chirurgie, *98:*708, 1972 (French)

LANGERON, P. *et al*: Circulatory diversion syndrome of the upper limb. Etio-pathogenic role of repeated micro-trauma. Ann. Cardiol. Angeiol. (Paris), *18:*235, 1969 (French)

LANGEZAAL, O. A. *et al*: Malignant epithelial tumors of parotid gland. Classification, staging and treatment. Arch. chir. neerl., *25:*441, 1973

LANGLOH, N.: Pathogenesis of wind-mill wing position of fingers in primary chronic polyarthritis. Fortschr. Med., *91:*313, 1973 (German)

LANGLOIS, P., WILLIAMS, H. B., AND GURD, F. N.: Effect of elemental diet on mortality rates and gastrointestinal lesions in experimental burns, PRS, *52:*211, 1973. J. Trauma, *12:*771, 1972

LANGNICKEL, R. *et al*: Importance of joint operative action in mid-facial fractures and fractures of the frontal cranial base by the dental surgeon and the otolaryngologist. Fortschr. Kiefer. Gesichtschir., *19:*132, 1975 (German)

LANIER, V. C., JR.: Surgical treatment of exophthalmos. PRS, *55:*56, 1975

LANIER, V. C., ROSENFELD, L., AND WILKINSON, H. A.: Chondrosarcoma of mandible, PRS, *49:*109, 1972. South. M. J., *60:*711, 1971

LANIER, V. C., JR. *et al*: Mixed tumors of salivary glands: 44-year study. South. Med. J., *65:*1485, 1972

LANIER, V. C., JR., AND NEALE, H. W.: Necrosis of penis with decubitus ulcer: debridement and closure with scrotal flap. PRS, *54:*609, 1974

LANIER, V. C., JR: Surgical treatment of exophthalmos. A review. PRS, *55:*56, 1975

LANSIGAN, N. C., JR. *et al*: Renal carcinoma presenting as metastasis to uvula. Urology, *2:*449, 1973

LANSKY, S. B. *et al*: School phobia in children with malignant neoplasms, PRS, *57:*766, 1976. Am. J. Dis. Child., *129:*42, 1975

LANZ, O.: Die Transplantation Betreffend (Classic Reprint). PRS, *50:*395, 1972

LAPA, F.: Surgical correction of midfacial retrusion (nasomaxillary hypoplasia), in presence of normal dental occlusion (with Psillakis, Spina). PRS, *51:*67, 1973

LAPAYOWKER, M. S. *et al*: Pigmented villonodular synovitis of temporomandibular joint. Radiology, *108:*313, 1973

LAPAYOWKER, M. S., AND RONIS, M. L.: Problems in tumors of ethmoid and sphenoid sinuses, PRS, *56:*677, 1975. Adv. Oto-rhinolaryngol., *21:*19, 1974

LAPCHENKO, S. N. *et al*: Allo-, homo- and autografts of supporting skeleton of concha auriculae (comparative results). Zh. Ushn. Nos. Gori. Bolezn., *33:*48, 1973 (Russian)

LAPEYROLERIE, F. M. *et al*: Pseudoankylosis from fusion of coronoid process and zygomatic arch. J. Oral Surg., *31:*788, 1973

LAPIDOT, A. *et al*: Dorsum of tongue pedicle flap replacing the epiglottis: an experimental study. Arch. Otolaryng., *94:*197, 1971

LAPIDOT, A. *et al*: Innervated partial hemitongue pseudoepiglottis: experimental study. Laryngoscope, *83:*1841, 1973

LAPIDOT, A., AND BEN-HUR, N.: Fastening base of tongue forward to hyoid for relief of respiratory distress in Pierre Robin syndrome. PRS, *56:*89, 1975

LAPIERE, C. M.: Biology and pathology at molecular level of connective tissue fibrous proteins, PRS, *51:*609, 1973. Arch. belges dermat. et syph., *28:*15, 1972

LAPIN, R. *et al*: Squamous cell carcinoma arising in dentigerous cyst. J. Oral Surg., *31:*354, 1973

LAPORTE, G. *et al*: The hand of "pelote" players. A model of traumatic pathology. Ann. Chir., *29:*499, 1975 (French)

LAPP, R. *et al*: Adjuvant therapy in Rendu-Osler disease. Rev. Med. Suisse Romande, *91:*43, 1971 (French)

LARCAN, A. *et al*: Gas gangrene, 24 cases. Value of combined surgical and hyperbaric oxygen therapy. Ann. Chir., *28:*445, 1974 (French)

LARCAN, A. *et al*: Advantages of combining surgery with hyperbaric oxygen therapy. Mater. Med. Pol., *6:*116, 1974

LARENG, L. *et al*: Emergency aid and transport of seriously burnt patients. Cah. Anesthesiol., *19:*1049, 1971 (French)

LARGIADER, F.: Cryosurgery of inoperable malignant tumors, PRS, *53:*371, 1974. Bull. Soc. Internat. Chir., *32:*466, 1973

LA RIVIERE, C. *et al*: Report on the speech intelligibility of a glossectomee: perceptual and acoustic observations. Folia Phoniatr. (Basel), *27:*201, 1975

LARK, C.: Nurses' reactions to transsexual surgery, PRS, *57:*767, 1976. AORN, *22:*743, 1975

LARKIN, J. M. *et al:* Tetanus following minor burn. J. Trauma, *15:*546, 1975

LARNDER, D. A. *et al:* Fate of the phagocyte in dermabrasion of tattoos with table salt. Australas. J. Dermatol., *15:*110, 1974

LAROSSA, D.: Importance of muscle reconstruction in primary and secondary cleft lip repair (with Randall, Whitaker). PRS, *54:*316, 1974

LAROSSA, D. *et al:* Preservation of structure and function in canine small intestinal autografts after freezing, PRS, *52:*174, 1973

LARRARD, J. DE *et al:* Role of trauma in etiology of Dupuytren's contracture. Arch. Mal. Prof., *31:*721, 1969 (French)

LARSEN, J., AND PLESS, J.: Replantation of severed ear parts, PRS, *57:*176, 1976. Discussion by Mladick, PRS, *57:*375, 1976

LARSEN, O. A. *et al:* Treatment of chronic gangrenous skin lesions with measures increasing distal blood pressure with special regard to induced moderate hypertension. Scand. J. Clin. Lab. Invest., *31:*213, 1973

LARSEN, R. R., HILL, G. J., II, AND ROTZER, E. R.: Reticulum cell sarcoma in head and neck surgery, PRS, *50:*421, 1972. Am. J. Surg., *123:*338, 1972

LARSON, D. L.: Burned hands (with Huang, Lewis), PRS, *56:*21, 1975. Discussion by Bennett, PRS, *56:*442, 1975

LARSON, D. L.: Thumb reconstruction in the severely burned hand (with Pohl, Lewis). PRS, *57:*320, 1976

LARSON, D. L. *et al:* Techniques for decreasing scar formation and contractures in burned patient, PRS, *49:*586, 1972. J. Trauma, *11:*807, 1971

LARSON, P. C., JR. *et al:* Effects of anesthetics on cerebral, renal, and splanchnic circulations, PRS, *55:*645, 1975. Anesthesiology, *41:*169, 1974

LARSON, R. R., AND HILL, G. J., II: Improved systemic chemotherapy for malignant melanoma, PRS, *49:*667, 1972. Am. J. Surg., *122:*36, 1971

LARSON, S. J.: Dynamic anatomy of ulnar nerve at elbow (with Apfelberg). PRS. *51:*76,1973

LA RUFFA, H.: Reconstruction in pharyngostome with fibroscopic study of its interior lumen, PRS, *53:*683, 1974. Bol. y trab. Soc. argent. cir., *34:*263, 1973

LA RUFFA, H.: Indications and contraindications of orbital reconstructive surgery, PRS, *53:*601, 1974. Bol. y trab. Soc. argent. cir., *34:*294, 1973

Laryngeal Neoplasms

Laryngectomy, extensive, due to cancer, new method of plastic operation for pharyngo-

Laryngeal Neoplasms – Cont.

esophageal tract (Lukovsky, Tytar), PRS, *48:*511, 1971. Acta chir. plast., *12:*157, 1970

Laryngeal preservation, tracheal resection with (Lawrence, Creech, Terz), PRS, *48:*604, 1971. Am. J. Surg., *120:*482, 1970

Laryngectomy, hyposmia after paranasal sinus exenteration or (Hoye, Ketcham, Henkin), PRS, *48:*391, 1971. Am. J. Surg., *120:*485, 1970

Carcinoma *in situ* of larynx. Twenty-year study of results of its management (Miller), PRS, *48:*397, 1971. Am. J. Surg., *120:*492, 1970

Surgery, reconstructive, related to laryngology (Farrior), PRS, *48:*196, 1971. Ann. Otol. Rhin. & Laryng., *79:*1061, 1970

Hemilaryngectomy, reconstructive (Cabrear Trigo), PRS, *48:*294, 1971. Prensa méd. argent., *57:*1946, 1970

Vocal cord cancer with commissure extension (Jesse, Lindberg, Horiot), PRS, *51:*607, 1973. Am. J. Surg., *122:*437, 1971

Carcinoma of larynx – diagnosis and treatment by surgery or irradiation (Hayes, Atkins, Raventos), PRS, *50:*310, 1972. Ann. Otol. Rhin. & Laryng., *80:*627, 1971

Carcinoma of larynx, post-irradiation (Baker, Weisman), PRS, *50:*310, 1972. Ann. Otol. Rhin. & Laryng., *80:*634, 1971

Cancers, pharyngeal and laryngeal, elective neck dissection for; evaluation (Ogura, Biller, Wette), PRS, *50:*309, 1972. Ann. Otol. Rhin. & Laryng., *80:*646, 1971

Cancer, pharyngeal and laryngeal, *in vivo* staining of (Shedd, Gaeta), PRS, *49:*108, 1972. Arch. Surg., *102:*442, 1971

Laryngectomees, vocal rehabilitation (Taub, Spiro), PRS, *51:*236, 1973. Am. J. Surg., *124:*87, 1972

Larynx, supraglottic, squamous cell cancer, surgery and radiation in treatment (Flynn, Jesse, Lindberg), PRS, *52:*102, 1973. Am. J. Surg., *124:*477, 1972

Laryngectomy, reed-fistula method of speech rehabilitation after (Shedd *et al*), PRS, *52:*107, 1973. Am. J. Surg., *124:*510, 1972

Laryngectomies, observations on voice tunnels in (Kothary, Potdar, De Souza), PRS, *52:*97, 1973. Am. J. Surg., *124:*535, 1972

Carcinoma of supraglottis and pyriform sinus, combined radiation therapy and surgery for (Wang, Schultz, Miller), PRS, *52:*213, 1973. Am. J. Surg., *124:*551, 1972

Larynx, fibrous xanthoma of (Rolander *et al*). Arch. Otolaryng., *96:*168, 1972

Larynx and laryngopharynx, carcinoma of, high dosage preoperative radiation and surgery for. Fourteen-year program (Gold-

Laryngeal Neoplasms — Cont.

man *et al*). Laryngoscope, *82:*1869, 1972

Laryngectomy and pharyngectomy, defects of upper esophagus and pharynx following, plastic surgery in cases of (Pasnikowski). Otolaryngol. Pol., *26:*439, 1972 (Polish)

Laryngectomy, radiological appearance of lower pharynx following, and management of tissue defect by modified method of Messerklinger (Wazny, Czerwonka). Otolaryngol. Pol., *26:*681, 1972 (Polish)

Laryngectomy and radical neck dissection (Bjarnason). Timarit. Hjukrunarfil. Isl., *48:*84, 1972 (Icelandic)

Larynx and pharynx, selection of patients for conservation surgery of (Ogura). Trans. Am. Acad. Ophthalmol. Otolaryngol., *76:*741, 1972

Hemilaryngectomy: deglutition evaluation and rehabilitation (Schoenrock *et al*). Trans. Am. Acad. Ophthalmol. Otolaryngol. *76:*752, 1972

Larynx and hypopharynx, cancers of, chemotherapy of (Leroux-Robert). Acta Otorhinolaryngol. Belg., *27:*883, 1973 (French)

Larynx and hypopharynx, cancer of, functionally-oriented partial surgery in. Introductory discussion (Leroux-Robert). Acta Otorhinolaryngol. Belg., *27:*938, 1973 (French)

Laryngeal cancer, salvage surgery in (Lerinck *et al*). Acta Otorhinolaryngol. Belg., *27:*993, 1973 (French)

Laryngectomy and pharyngolaryngectomy, salvage, after cancericidal cobalt therapy (Poncet). Acta Otorhinolaryngol. Belg., *27:*1005, 1973 (French)

Laryngectomees, vocal rehabilitation with air bypass voice prosthesis (Taub, Bergner), PRS, *53:*114, 1974. Am. J. Surg., *125:*748, 1973

Laryngectomy for carcinoma, first (Stell). Arch. Otolaryng., *98:*293, 1973

Larynx and hypopharynx, conservation surgery of — selection of patients and results (Ogura *et al*). Can. J. Otolaryngol., *2:*11, 1973

Laryngopharynx, neurofibromatosis of (Morris). Can. J. Otolaryngol., *2:*17, 1973

Cancer, first laryngectomy for: Theodore Billroth (Weir). J. Laryng. & Otol., *87:*1161, 1973

Larynx and hypopharynx, conservation surgery of (Schechter, McLarey), PRS, *53:*683, 1974. Mil. Med., *138:*639, 1973

Cancer, laryngeal, irradiated, treatment for huge esopharyngostomas appearing after total laryngectomy for (Kiricuta, Popescu, Suceava), PRS, *56:*464, 1975. Ann. oto-lar-

Laryngeal Neoplasms — Cont.

yng., *91:*585, 1974

Subtotal reconstructive surgery in the treatment of laryngeal cancers (Piquet *et al*). Ann. Otolaryngol. Chir. Cervicofac., *91:*311, 1974 (French)

Laryngotracheal autograft for postcricoid carcinoma, reevaluation (Som). Ann. Otol. Rhin. & Laryng., *83:*481, 1974

Laryngectomies in dogs, everting closure of pharyngoesophageal defects (Sobol, Tucker, Tucker), PRS, *55:*107, 1975. Arch. Otolaryng., *100:*148, 1974

Larynx, cancer of, changes in voice production during radiotherapy for (Murray, Bone, Essen), PRS, *56:*105, 1975. J. Speech & Hearing Disorders, *39:*194, 1974

Laryngectomized patient, speech and vocational rehabilitation of (Sako *et al*), PRS, *57:*532, 1976. J. Surg. Oncol., *6:*197, 1974

Carcinoma, post-cricoid, some aspects of dysphagia (Thomas), PRS, *55:*718, 1975. Proc. Roy. Soc. Med., *67:*477, 1974

Laryngectomy, total, reconstructive surgery following (Fritz). Wien. Klin. Wochenschr., *86:*421, 1974 (German)

Laryngectomy, voice rehabilitation after — results with hypopharyngeal prosthesis (Sisson *et al*), PRS, *57:*396, 1976. Arch. Otolaryng., *101:*178, 1975

Combined pre-operative irradiation and surgery for advanced cancer of the larynx and laryngopharynx. A 14 year correlative statistical and histopathological study. (Goldman *et al*). Can. J. Otolaryngol., *4:*251, 1975

Treatment of adenocarcinomas of the larynx (Eschwege *et al*). Can. J. Otolaryngol., *4:*290, 1975

Spindle cell carcinoma of the larynx (Hyams). Can. J. Otolaryngol., *4:*307, 1975

Limitations of conservation surgery in carcinoma involving the arytenoid (Iwai). Can. J. Otolaryngol., *4:*434, 1975

Significance of positive margins in hemilaryngectomy specimens (Bauer *et al*). Laryngoscope, *85:*1, 1975

Spontaneous pharyngeal fistula and wound infection following laryngectomy (Briant). Laryngoscope, *85:*829, 1975

Centennial conference on laryngeal cancer papers. Primary laryngoplasty (Iwai *et al*). Laryngoscope, *85:*929, 1975

Regional skin flaps in partial laryngectomy (Conley). Laryngoscope, *85:*942, 1975

Conservation surgery for epidermoid carcinoma of the marginal area (aryepiglottic fold extension) (Ogura *et al*). Laryngoscope, *85:*1801, 1975

Laryngeal Neoplasms — Cont.

Conservation surgery for epidermoid carcinoma of the supraglottic larynx (Ogura *et al*). Laryngoscope, *85:*1808, 1975

Carcinoma of larynx presenting with cervical lymph nodes (Maw), PRS, *56:*226, 1975. Proc. Roy. Soc. Med., *68:*80, 1975

Obturator, suction, new, to control saliva after laryngopharyngectomy (Javor). PRS, *57:*106, 1976

Larynx

Laryngology, reconstructive surgery related to (Farrior), PRS, *48:*196, 1971. Ann. Otol. Rhin. & Laryng., *79:*1061, 1970

Laryngeal injuries, acute, blunt, treatment of (Olson, Miles), PRS *50:*305, 1972. Ann. Otol. Rhin. & Laryng., *80:*704, 1971

Laryngeal fractures, experimental, acute treatment of (Miles, Olson, Rodriquez), PRS, *50:*419, 1972. Ann. Otol. Rhin. & Laryng., *80:*710, 1971

Larynx and cervical trachea, penetrating wounds of (LeMay), PRS, *49:*670, 1972. Arch. Otolaryng., *94:*558, 1971

Laryngo-pharynx and cervical esophagus, repair after radiation (Shaw), PRS, *49:*238, 1972. Proc. Roy. Soc. Med., *64:*734, 1971

Auscultation, electronic, of metallic foreign bodies (Waller), PRS, *51:*610, 1973. Am. J. Surg., *123:*626, 1972

Laryngotracheal trauma, minibikes new factor in (Alonso *et al*). Ann. Otol. Rhin. & Laryng., *82:*800, 1973

Larynx, severe traumatic and functional stenosis of, surgical treatment (Grahne). H.N.O., *21:*234, 1973

Laryngeal stenosis, postintubation, oral mucosal free graft in glottic reconstruction for (Neumann). H.N.O., *22:*215, 1974 (German)

Auditory function, relation to esophageal speech proficiency (Martian, Hoops), PRS, *56:*594, 1975. J. Speech & Hearing Res., *17:*80, 1974

Laryngo-tracheal stenoses, reconstructive possibilities in (Naumann). Munch. Med. Wochenschr., *116:*465, 1974 (German)

Clinical Management of Voice Disorders. By Donna Russell Fox and Mark Blechman. Cliff Notes, Inc., Lincoln, Nebraska, 1975. PRS, *57:*657, 1976

Larynx, modified Tokyo (Nelson, Parkin, Potter), PRS, *57:*396, 1976. Arch. Otolaryng., *101:*107, 1975

Chondroplasty, laryngeal, for appearance (Wolfort, Parry). PRS, *56:*371, 1975

Larynx, reconstruction of, by free flap trans-

Larynx — Cont.

fer (Nagahara, Hirose, Iwai). PRS, *57:*604, 1976

Lascala, N. T. *et al*: Muco-gingival surgery. New technic for frenectomy and bridectomy. Rev. Assoc. Paul. Cir. Dent., *27:*135, 1973 (Portuguese)

Lascar, R.: Treatment of fractures of the base of the first metacarpal bone. Bull. Mem. Soc. Chir. Paris, *61:*267, 1971 (French)

Laser Surgery

Effect of laser rays on wound healing (Mester *et al*). Am. J. Surg., *122:*532, 1971

Laser radiation, intercellular transfer of toxic components after (May, Rounds, Cone), PRS, *48:*297, 1971. J. Nat. Cancer Inst., *46:*655, 1971

Laser surgery in aerodigestive tract (Strong *et al*), PRS, *53:*486, 1974. Am. J. Surg., *126:*529, 1973

Laser surgery, status report (Goldman), PRS, *53:*247, 1974. Contemp. Surg., *3:*18, 1973

Laser excision of acute third degree burns, followed by immediate autografting (Stellar *et al*), PRS, *53:*685, 1974. J. Trauma, *13:*45, 1973

Lasers, safety with (Borland *et al*), PRS, *54:*383, 1974. Proc. Roy. Soc. Med., *66:*841, 1973

Tumors, experimental, treatment with laser beams in combination with fast electrons (Kozlov *et al*). Vopr. Onkol., *19:*93, 1973 (Russian)

Carbon dioxide laser, possibilities in surgery (Verschueren, Koudstaal, Oldhoff), PRS, *56:*362, 1975. Acta chir. belg., *73:*197, 1974

Head and neck surgery, carbon dioxide laser in (Kaplan *et al*). Am. J. Surg., *128:*543, 1974

Laser, carbon dioxide, debridement of decubitus ulcers, followed by immediate rotation flap or skin graft closure (Stellar *et al*), PRS, *54:*242, 1974. Ann. Surg., *179:*230, 1974

Use of carbon dioxide laser for debridement of third degree burns (Levine *et al*), PRS, *54:*240, 1974. Ann. Surg., *179:*246, 1974

Excision of deep burns with the carbon dioxide laser (Bowen *et al*). Brit. J. Plast. Surg., *27:*322, 1974

Carbon dioxide laser excision of acute burns with immediate autografting (Fidler *et al*), PRS, *55:*253, 1975. J. Surg. Res., *17:*1, 1974

Lasers in surgery, new data on use of (literature survey) (Khromov *et al*). Khirurgiia

Laser Surgery — Cont.
(Mosk.), *9:*134, 1974 (Russian)
Laser, carbon dioxide, experimental surgery with, on Cloudman S91 melanoma (Oosterhuis, Verschueren, Oldhoff), PRS, *57:*680, 1976. Acta chir. belg., *74:*422, 1975
Carbon dioxide laser, surgical uses (Peled, Kaplan, Stephenson), PRS, *57:*123, 1976. Folha Med. Brazil, *70:*5, 1975

LASKIN, D. M.: Myotomy for the management of recurrent and protracted mandibular dislocations. Trans. Int. Conf. Oral Surg., *4:*264, 1973
LASKIN, D. M.: Letter: survey of surgical privileges: a study in futility. J. Trauma, *14:*990, 1974
LASKIN, D. M.: Editorial: The art and science of orthognathic surgery. J. Oral Surg., *33:*905, 1975
LASKOWSKI, J.: Aponeurotic sarcoma. Pol. Med. J., *10:*12, 1971
LASS, N. J. *et al*: Exposure of medical and dental students to the disorder of cleft palate. Cleft Palate J., *10:*306, 1973
LASSER, A. E., AND STEIN, A. F.: Steroid treatment of hemangiomas in children, PRS, *53:*611, 1974. Arch. Dermat., *108:*565, 1973
LASSERRE, J.: Apropos of the technic of ureterointestinal anastomosis. Ann. Chir. Infant., *12:*460, 1971 (French)
LASSUS, C.: One stage correction of the sequelae of unilateral harelip. Rev. Stomatol. Chir. Maxillofac., *72:*323, 1971 (French)

Lateral Cervical Fistula (See also Branchial Cysts)

Congenital lateral fistulae of the neck. Clinical and therapeutic aspects (De Campora *et al*). Valsalva, *43:*97, 1967 (Italian)
Case of resection of a full congenital lateral fistula of the neck with simultaneous tonsillectomy (Chizhikov *et al*). Zh. Ushn. Nos. Gorl. Bolezn., *32:*101, 1972 (Russian)
Neck, congenital medial and lateral cysts and fistulae of, experience in surgical treatment of (Aminev *et al*). Stomatologiia (Mosk.), *52:*83, 1973 (Russian)

LATHAM, R. A.: Growth mechanism of the human face with special reference to cleft lip and palate conditions. Ann. R. Coll. Surg. Engl., *48:*30, 1971
LATHAM, R. A.: Development and structure of premaxillary deformity in bilateral cleft lip and palate, PRS, *54:*694, 1974. Brit. J. Plast. Surg., *26:*1, 1973
LATHAM, R. A.: Altering the dimensions of the

canine face by induction of new bone formation (with Calabrese, Winslow). PRS, *54:*467, 1974
LATHAM, R. A.: Maxillary arch alignment in bilateral cleft lip and palate infant using pinned coaxial screw appliance (with Georgiade). PRS, *56:*52, 1975
LATHAM, R. A. *et al*: Problem of tissue deficiency in cleft palate: an experiment in mobilising the palatine bones of cleft dogs. Brit. J. Plast. Surg., *26:*252, 1973
LATHAM, R. A. *et al*: Induction of new palatal growth as an aid to cleft closure in dogs: neopalate formation. Brit. J. Plast. Surg., *27:*264, 1974
LATHAM, R. A. *et al*: A question of the role of the vomer in the growth of the premaxillary segment. Cleft Palate J., *12:*351, 1975
LATHAM, W. D.: Restoring the overhang of the upper lip in repairs of oral commissure (with Wall, Cameron). PRS, *49:*626, 1972
LATHAM, W. D.: Reconstructions of nose and upper lip with nasolabial flaps (with Cameron, Dowling). PRS, *52:*145, 1973
LATHOUWER, C. DE: Unusual case of osteosarcoma of mandible: diagnostic problems. Acta Stomatol. Belg., *69:*429, 1972 (French)
LATINA, J. A.: Incidence of postoperative wound infections during Vietnam conflict, PRS, *57:*677, 1976. Mil. Med., *140:*354, 1975
LATORRE, H. *et al*: Idiopathic gynecomastia in seven preadolescent boys. Elevation of urinary estrogen excretion in two cases. Am. J. Dis. Child., *126:*771, 1973
LATTIMER, J. K.: Surgical antireflux procedure for scarred or exstrophic bladders, variation of technique. Urology, *3:*508, 1974
LATTIMER, J. K., VAKILI, B., AND SMITH, A. M.: Dorsal tilt: embellishment to any operation for hypospadias, PRS, *53:*245, 1974. J. Urol. *109:*1035, 1973
LATTIMER, J. K. *et al*: Natural-feeling testicular prosthesis, PRS, *53:*245, 1974. J. Urol., *110:*81, 1973
LAUB, D. R.: Hydrofluoric acid burns (with Iverson, Madison). PRS, *48:*107, 1971
LAUB, D. R.: Use of water bed for prevention of pressure sores (with Siegel, Vistnes). PRS, *51:*31, 1973
LAUB, D. R.: Anophthalmic orbit, surgical correction of lower eyelid ptosis (with Vistnes, Iverson). PRS, *52:*346, 1973
LAUB, D. R.: Discussion of "A variation of the rotation-advancement operation for repair of wide unilateral cleft lips," by Asensio. PRS, *53:*341, 1974
LAUB, D. R.: Surgical construction of male genitalia for female-to-male transsexual (with

Noe, Birdsell). PRS, *53:*511, 1974

LAUB, D. R.: Residency participation in out-of-country medical service (with Henjyoji). PRS, *53:*660, 1974

LAUB, D. R.: Effect of hydrotherapy on clinical course and pH of experimental cutaneous chemical burns, (with Gruber, Vistnes). PRS, *55:*200, 1975

LAUB, D. R. *et al:* Median cerebrofacial dysgenesis. Calif. Med., *112:*19, 1970

LAUB, D. R., AND FISK, N.: Rehabilitation program for gender dysphoria syndrome by surgical sex change. PRS, *53:*388, 1974

LAUBE, J. *et al:* Treatment of scalping. Zentralbl. Chir., *95:*994, 1970 (German)

LAUDENBACH, P. *et al:* Preoperative diagnosis of cystadenolymphomas by sialography and radioisotope scanning. Rev. Stomatol. Chir. Maxillofac., *75:*759, 1974 (French)

LAUFER, D. *et al:* Patient motivation and response to surgical correction of prognathism. Oral Surg., *41:*309, 1976

LAURENCET, F. L. *et al:* Clinical development of three patients bitten by a viper. Schweiz. Med. Wochenschr., *102:*981, 1972 (French)

LAURENCON, M. *et al:* Electric burns and neurologic manifestations. Ann. chir. plast., *17:*54, 1972 (French)

LAURENCON, M. *et al:* Value of "tissue circulation" treatment in plastic and reconstructive surgery. Results with Hydrosarpan 711. Comparison with placebo. Ann. chir. plast., *17:*221, 1972 (French)

LAURENTACCI, G., AND DIOGUARDI, D.: System of heterophile antibody serum in rabbits with skin allografts, PRS, *57:*680, 1976. Riv. ital. chir. plast., *6:*111, 1974

LAURING, L.: Jaw-winking blepharoptosis. Am. J. Ophth., *76:*604, 1973

LAURO, R. *et al:* On a case of median cleft of the lower lip. Acta Chir. Ital., *25:*307, 1969 (Italian)

LAVERGNE, G. *et al:* Inverted papilloma of lacrimal sac. Bull. Soc. Belge. Ophtalmol., *165:*323, 1973 (French)

LAVRISCHEVA, G. I., GRIGORIEV, M. G., AND ABAKOV, A. A.: Comparable aspects of use of solid and split homotransplants in bridging large segmental defects in long bones, PRS, *57:*767, 1976. Acta chir. plast., *17:*27, 1975

LAW, E. J., HOEFER, R. W., AND MACMILLAN, B. G.: Clinical experience with axillary burns in children, PRS, *52:*101, 1973. J. Trauma, *12:*34, 1972

LAW, E. J. *et al:* Experience with systemic candidiasis in burned patient, PRS, *52:*326, 1973. J. Trauma, *12:*543, 1972

LAW, E. J. *et al:* Prospective upper gastrointestinal series in evaluation of burned children,

PRS, *53:*491, 1974. Am. J. Surg., *126:*366, 1973

LAWHORN, T. I. *et al:* Oral zinc therapy in thermal burns. South. Med. J., *64:*1538, 1971

LAWLESS, C. A.: Helping patients with endotracheal and tracheostomy tubes communicate. Am. J. Nurs. *75:*2151, 1975

LAWLESS, O. J. *et al:* Proceedings: Deforming hand arthritis in systemic lupus erythematosus. Arthritis Rheum., *17:*323, 1974

LAWRENCE, G. A.: Cystosarcoma phylloides. Indian J. Cancer, *9:*231, 1972

LAWRENCE, J. C., AND CARNEY, S. A.: Tangential excision of burns. Studies of metabolic activity of recipient areas for skin grafts, PRS, *54:*695, 1974. Brit. J. Plast. Surg., *26:*93, 1973

LAWRENCE, J. C., AND STONE, P. A.: Protection of damaged tissue by skin cover, PRS, *54:*696, 1974. Brit. J. Plast. Surg., *26:*101, 1973

LAWRENCE, R. A.: Surgical correction of lesions of temporomandibular joints (with Dingman, Dingman), PRS, *55:*335, 1975. Discussion by Kiehn, PRS, *55:*484, 1975

LAWRENCE, R. A. *et al:* Reconstruction of burned ear. Otolaryngol. Clin. North Am., *5:*667, 1972

LAWRENCE, W., JR.: Management of malignant melanoma. Am. Surg., *38:*93, 1972

LAWRENCE, W., JR.: Operative treatment of malignant melanoma of the limb (a point of view). Va. Med. Mon., *102:*141, 1975

LAWRENCE, W., JR., CREECH, H. B., AND TERZ, J. J.: Tracheal resection with laryngeal preservation, PRS, *48:*604, 1971. Am. J. Surg., *120:*482, 1970

LAWRENCE, W., JR. *et al:* Preoperative irradiation for head and neck cancer: prospective study. Cancer, *33:*318, 1974

LAWSON, L. I.: Re-do pharyngeal flap (with Owsley, Chierici), PRS, *57:*180, 1976

LAWSON, N. S. *et al:* Serum enzymes in experimental ballistic injury to extremities, PRS, *50:*423, 1972. Arch. Surg., *103:*741, 1971

LAWTON, R. L. *et al:* Intra-arterial infusion. A seven-year study. Oncology, *26:*259, 1972

LAZAREV, I. R. *et al:* Use of lasers for treatment of skin neoplasms. Klin. Khir., *11:*36, 1973 (Russian)

LAZAROV, G.: Homoosseous-cartilaginous arthroplasty of the small joints of the hand. Folia Med. Plovdiv., *14:*123, 1972

LAZEANU, M. *et al:* Current diagnostic problems and therapeutic indications in peripheral facial paralysis. Otorinolaringologie, *18:*99, 1973 (Rumanian)

LEACH, R. E., CLAWSON, D. K., AND CAPRIO, A.: Continuous elevation by spica cast in treatment of reflex sympathetic dystrophy, PRS, *54:*502, 1974. J. Bone & Joint Surg., *56A:*416, 1974

LEAF, N. *et al:* Correction of contour defects of face with dermal and dermal-fat grafts. Arch. Surg., *105:*715, 1972

LEAFSTEDT, S. W. *et al:* Adenoid cystic carcinoma of major and minor salivary glands, PRS, *51:*608, 1973. Am. J. Surg., *122:*756, 1971

LEAKE, D.: Custom fabricated silicone prostheses for mandibular replacement. Trans. Int. Conf. Oral Surg., *4:*159, 1973

LEAKE, D. L.: Interim report on osseous contour reconstruction using alloplastic materials and particulate bone grafting. Int. J. Oral Surg., *3:*286, 1974

LEAKE, D. L.: New alloplastic tray for osseous contour defects, PRS, *55:*386, 1975. J. Maxillo-facial Surg., *2:*146, 1974

LEAKE, D. L.: Mandibular reconstruction with a new type of alloplastic tray: preliminary report. J. Oral Surg., *32:*23, 1974

LEAKE, D. L., AND RAPPOPORT, M.: Mandibular reconstruction: bone induction alloplastic tray, PRS, *51:*236, 1973. Surgery, *72:*332, 1972

LEAKE, D. L. *et al:* Definitive treatment of mandibular fractures in young children, PRS, *54:*107, 1974. Oral Surg., *36:*164, 1973

LEAKE, D. L. *et al:* Correction of discontinuity defect of maxilla by bone grafting. J. Oral Surg., *32:*467, 1974

LEAKE, D. L., AND HABAL, M. B.: Osteoneogenesis: new method for facial reconstruction, PRS, *57:*125, 1976. Surg. Res., *18:*331, 1975

LEANDERSON, R. *et al:* Age factor and reduction of open nasality following superiorly based velopharyngeal flap operation in 124 cases, PRS, *56:*681, 1975. Scand. J. Plast. Reconstr. Surg., *8:*156, 1974

LEAPE, L. L.: Urgency of fluid administration in resuscitation of burn shock. J. Surg. Res., *11:*513, 1971

LEAPE, L. L.: Kinetics of burn edema formation in primates, PRS, *51:*706, 1973. Ann. Surg., *176:*223, 1972

LEATHERS, H. K.: Foreign body reactions to polyurethane covers of some breast prostheses (with Cocke, Lynch). PRS, *56:*527, 1975

LEBAN, S. G. *et al:* Benign lymphoepithelial sialoadenopathies. The Mikulicz/Sjogren controversy. Oral Surg., *38:*735, 1974

LEBEDEVA, T. M.: Treatment of an electric burn of the face. Stomatologiia (Mosk.), *51:*77, 1972 (Russian)

LEBOURG, L.: Note of lingual mutilations and their possible surgical repair. Rev. Stomatol.

Chir. Maxillofac., *76:*311, 1975 (French)

LEBOVITZ, S. S., MILER, O. F., AND DICKEY, R. F.: Subungual exostosis, PRS, *54:*375, 1974. Cutis, *13:*426, 1974

LEDDY, J. P. *et al:* Capsulodesis and pulley advancement for correction of claw-finger deformity, PRS, *51:*477, 1973. J. Bone & Joint Surg., *54A:*1465, 1972

LEDERER, F. L.: Symposium on reconstructive plastic surgery of head and neck. Rehabilitative responsibilities and philosophies. Otolaryngol. Clin. North Am., *5:*405, 1973

LEDERMAN, D. A.: Lateral periodontal cyst: report of a case. J. Oral Med., *30:*62 1975

LEDERMAN, M.: Treatment of malignant disease of skin of orbital region. Proc. Roy. Soc. Med., *66:*690, 1973

LEDGERWOOD, A., AND LUCAS, C. E.: Split-thickness porcine graft in treatment of close-range shotgun wounds to extremities with vascular injury, PRS, *53:*249, 1974. Am. J. Surg., *125:*690, 1973

LEDGERWOOD, A. M., AND LUCAS, C. E.: Massive thigh injuries with vascular disruption: role of porcine skin grafting of exposed arterial vein grafts, PRS, *53:*368, 1974. Arch. Surg., *107:*201, 1973

LEE, B. S.: Degenerative arthritis of carpometacarpal joint of thumb, PRS, *53:*106, 1974. Orthop. Rev., *2:*45, 1973

LEE, C. M. *et al:* Priapism: treatment by corpus cavernosum-saphenous vein anastomosis. Ann. Surg., *175:*279, 1972

LEE, C. M., AND YEAKEL, A. E.: Patient refusal of surgery following Innovar premedication, PRS, *56:*604, 1975. Anesth. Analg., Cleve., *54:*224, 1975

LEE, D. C.: Tycho Brahe and his sixteenth century prosthesis, PRS, *50:*332, 1972

LEE, E. S., AND WILSON, J. S. P.: Carcinoma involving the lower alveolus, PRS, *52:*458, 1973. Brit. J. Surg., *60:*85, 1973

LEE, J. G.: Detection of residual carcinoma of oral cavity, oropharynx, hypopharynx, and larynx: study of surgical margins. Trans. Am. Acad. Ophthalmol. Otolaryngol., *78:*149, 1974

LEE, J. G. *et al:* Occult regional metastasis: carcinoma of oral tongue. Laryngoscope, *82:*1273, 1972

LEE, J. G. *et al:* Radical neck dissection: elective, therapeutic and secondary. Arch. Otolaryng., *101:*656, 1975

LEE, P. *et al:* Assessment of grip strength measurement in rheumatoid arthritis. Scand. J. Rheumatol., *3:*17, 1974

LEE, S. M. *et al:* Synovial sarcoma in children. Surg. Gynec. & Obst., *138:*701, 1974

LEE, Y. C.: Early heterografting of partial

thickness burns. J. Trauma, *12:*818, 1972

LEE, Y. C.: Expanding hematoma after rhytidectomy, retrospective study (with Rees, Coburn). PRS, *51:*149, 1973

LEEMING, D. W.: Gravitational edema of the lungs observed during assisted respiration, PRS, *54:*502, 1974. Chest, *64:*719, 1973

LEFFERT, R. D., WEISS, C., AND ATHANASOULIS, C. A.: Vincula with particular reference to their vessels and nerves, PRS, *55:*510, 1975. J. Bone & Joint Surg., *56A:*1191, 1974

LE FORT, R.: Experimental study of fractures of upper jaw. (Classic Reprint), Parts I and II, PRS, *50:*497, 1972. Part III, PRS, *50:*600, 1972

LeFort Fractures: See *Craniofacial Injuries; Facial Injuries; Jaw Fractures*

Leg (See also *Cross-Leg Flaps; Extremities; Leg Ulcer*)

Angiography in venous dysplasias of the limbs (Thomas *et al*). Am. J. Roentgenol. Radium Ther. Nucl. Med., *113:*722, 1971

Congenital constriction bands of the lower extremity (Srivastava *et al*). Indian J. Pediatr., *38:*76, 1971

Remote results of nerve suture performed following traumatic lesions of the peripheral nerves of the lower limbs (Danilewicz). Pol. Przegl. Chir., *43:*1369, 1971 (Polish)

Avulsive injuries to the heel (Stuckey). South. Med. J., *64:*1472, 1971

Application of a combined flat pedicled graft for plastic surgery of trophic ulcers of the leg and foot (Bondar'). Vestn. Khir., *107:*116, 1971 (Russian)

Venous dynamics, lower limb, in normal persons and children of patients with varicose veins (Reagan, Folse), PRS, *48:*92, 1971. Surg. Gynec. & Obst., *132:*15, 1971

Skin carcinomas in the region of the lower extremities (Ebner *et al*). Wien. Klin. Wochenschr., *83:*459, 1971 (German)

Integumentectomy, total, of leg for multiple "in-transit" metastases of melanoma (Jones, Dickinson), PRS, *51:*607, 1973. Am. J. Surg., *123:*588, 1972

Leg, radiologic patterns of hemangiopericytoma of (Hoeffel *et al*), PRS, *51:*704, 1973. Am. J. Surg., *123:*591, 1972

Freezing gangrenous extremity in poor risk patients (Niazmand, Miller, Barker), PRS, *52:*107, 1973. Am. J. Surg., *124:*701, 1972

Is there still a place for plastic and reconstructive surgery in treatment of open leg fractures? (Allieu *et al*). Ann. chir. plast., *17:*212, 1972

Chemotherapy of melanoma of the extremities by perfusion: fourteen years clinical

Leg — Cont.

experience (Krementz *et al*). Ann. Surg., *175:*900, 1972

Phlebography (Thomas). Arch. Surg., *104:*145, 1972

Diagnosis of lower limb venous thrombosis by Doppler ultrasound technique (Sigel *et al*). Arch. Surg., *104:*174, 1972

Ultrasonic velocity detector in the diagnosis of thrombophlebitis (Strandness *et al*). Arch. Surg., *104:*180, 1972

Lymphangiosarcoma arising in chronic lymphedematous extremities (Woodward *et al*). Cancer, *30:*562, 1972

Leg, results of exploratory fasciotomy of, in predominantly venous edema (Atanasescu *et al*). Chirurgia (Bucur.), *21:*429, 1972 (Rumanian)

Reinnervation of the denervated muscles by nerve transplantation (Sakellarides *et al*). Clin. Orthop., *83:*195, 1972

Subcutaneous fasciotome. An instrument for relief of compression in anterior, lateral and posterior compartments of the leg from trauma and other causes (Bate). Clin. Orthop., *83:*235, 1972

Two cases of neurofibromatosis with giant lower extremity (Miyake *et al*). Orthop. Surg., (Tokyo), *23:*221, 1972 (Japanese)

"Cork" procedure, small tubed flap for cylindrical defects in the leg (Hagstrom, Brown, Landa). PRS, *49:*224, 1972

Calf of leg, atrophic, successful filling of, with dermal-fat graft (Crocenzi). PRS, *49:*351, 1972

Limb, lower, reconstruction with Mustardé flap (Milke), PRS, *53:*368, 1974. Rev. Soc. Med. Cir. San Jose, *5:*83, 1972

Micro-circulation of the skin of the normal leg, in varicose veins and in the postthrombotic syndrome (Allan). S. Afr. J. Surg., *10:*29, 1972

Avulsion of skin of lower limb, extensive traumatic (Lejour *et al*), PRS, *54:*238, 1974. Acta chir. belg., *72:*456, 1973

Legs and feet, large tissue defects in one or both, experience with plasty using double Filatov flap for treatment of (Kernerman). Acta. chir. plast. (Praha), *15:*120, 1973

Muscle hernia repair, anterior tibial compartment syndrome following (Wolfort, Mogelvang, Fitzer), PRS, *52:*452, 1973. Arch. Surg., *106:*97, 1973

Amputation, major, for recurrent melanoma of extremity (Turnbull, Shah, Fortner), PRS, *52:*599, 1973. Arch. Surg., *106:*496, 1973

Pretibial lacerations (Tandon *et al*). Brit. J. Plast. Surg., *26:*172, 1973

Leg – Cont.

Treatment of chronic gangrenous skin lesions with measures increasing distal blood pressure with special regard to induced moderate hypertension (Larsen *et al*). Scand. J. Clin. Lab. Invest., *31:*213, 1973

Leg, surgical management of arterial occlusion following percutaneous femoral angiography (Yellin, Shore), PRS, *52:*453, 1973. Surgery, *73:*772, 1973

Pelvectomy – indications, technic and results of hemipelvectomy in 4 cases (Eliopoulos), PRS, *56:*473, 1975. Tr. 8th Panhellenic Cong. Surg. Soc., *A:*263, 1973

Leg, lower, unusual injury of, surgical procedure (Schuhr). Zentralbl. Chir., *98:*1708, 1973 (German)

Amputation stumps of lower limb, faulty, free skin transplantation using "SITO" graft (Serenkova), PRS, *54:*626, 1974. Acta chir. plast., *16:*16, 1974

Band, constriction, congenital, of thigh (Owen-Smith), PRS, *54:*503, 1974. Australian & New Zealand J. Surg., *44:*57, 1974

Band, ischiopedic bilateral congenital (Boucher), PRS, *55:*119, 1975. Bol. Soc. cir. Plast. y Reconstr. Cordoba, *5:*21, 1974

Leg flaps, local delayed (Bowen, Meares), PRS, *56:*683, 1975. Brit. J. Plast. Surg., *27:*167, 1974

Congenital lower limb amputee, conservative management of (Varma *et al*), PRS, *55:*249, 1975. Indian J. Surg., *36:*193, 1974

Leg, chronically swollen painful, etiological factors (Stallworth *et al*), PRS, *54:*690, 1974. J.A.M.A., *228:*1656, 1974

Bands, congenital annular (Pseudoainhum) associated with other congenital abnormalities (Izumi, Arnold), PRS, *55:*519, 1975. J.A.M.A., *229:*1208, 1974

Fistulae, arteriovenous, in management of lower limb discrepancy (Kinmonth, Negus), PRS, *55:*249, 1975. J. Cardiovasc. Surg., *15:*447, 1974

Lower extremity venous trauma, repair of (Rich *et al*), PRS, *57:*535, 1976. J. Trauma, *14:*639, 1974

Degloving, cutaneous, of lower limbs run over by vehicle (Roucher, Mallard, Latreille), PRS, *55:*511, 1975. Lyon chir., *70:*312, 1974

Necrosis: knee-to-knee syndrome (Carlin). PRS, *53:*353, 1974

Complication after alloplastic thigh augmentation (Codega *et al*). Polymers in Med., *4:*153, 1974

Thigh augmentation, alloplastic, complication after (Fornaroli), PRS, *56:*357, 1975.

Leg – Cont.

Polymers in Med., *4:*153, 1974

Limb, regional cutaneous metastases in melanoma of (Cox), PRS, *55:*257, 1975. Surg. Gynec. & Obst., *139:*385, 1974

Muscle flaps applied to leg (Amar, Aubaniac, Bureau), PRS, *56:*230, 1975. Ann. chir. plast., *20:*61, 1975

Military surgical team in Belfast (Boyd). Ann. R. Coll. Surg., Engl., *56:*15, 1975

Lower limbs, lymphedema of, operations for (Chilvers, Kinmonth), PRS, *57:*262, 1976. J. Cardiovasc. Surg., *16:*115, 1975

Amputation stump management – use of shrink plastic film as surgical dressing (Dowie), PRS, *57:*122, 1976. M. J. Australia, *2:*187, 1975

Anomaly, congenital web (pterygium) of popliteal area, surgical treatment of (Tuerk, Edgerton). PRS, *56:*339, 1975

Soft tissue tumours on the back of the knee (Hort *et al*). Ztschr. Orthop., *113:*102, 1975 (German)

Leg defects repaired with fascio-muscle flaps (Robbins). PRS, *57:*460, 1976

Leg Ulcer

Ulcer, stasis, advanced, operative treatment using muscle transposition (Ger), PRS, *49:*358, 1972. Am. J. Surg., *120:*376, 1970

Vitamin B6 deficiency in patients with leg ulcers and in their family members (Wolfram *et al*). Hautarzt, *21:*75, 1970 (German)

Ulcers, stasis, of leg, pathophysiology and treatment of (Myers, Cherry), PRS, *49:*104, 1972. Am. Surgeon, *37:*167, 1971

Tissue repair in atonic ulcerations of the lower limbs (Calas). Angeiologie, *23:*143, 1971 (French)

Net grafts in leg ulcers (Glicenstein). Angeiologie, *23:*151, 1971 (French)

Stasis ulcer and "fibrinogen Baltimore" (Smith *et al*). Arch. Dermat., *104:*221, 1971

Ulcer, refractory postphlebitic, surgical treatment (Silver *et al*), PRS, *49:*584, 1972. Arch. Surg., *103:*554, 1971

Mesh graft plastic in the therapy of leg ulcers (Diabal *et al*). Cesk. Dermatol., *46:*267, 1971 (Czechoslovakian)

Healing prospects in the ulcus cruris (Haustein). Dtsch. Gesundheitsw., *26:*264, 1971 (German)

Remote results of the surgical treatment of the post-thrombophlebitic syndrome (Dauderis). Khirurgiia (Mosk.), *47:*55, 1971 (Russian)

Lower limbs, surgical repair of ulcer due to venous stasis in (Damiani *et al*). Minerva Chir., *26:*1471, 1971 (Italian)

Leg Ulcer – Cont.

Follow-up study of skin transplantation in leg ulcer (Ponten). Nord. Med., *88:*1221, 1971 (Swedish)

Treatment of ulcers infected by *Pseudomonas aeruginosa* or pyocyanic bacilli (Haven *et al*). Phlebologie, *24:*349, 1971 (French)

Pinch grafts for cutaneous ulcers (Smith *et al*). South. Med. J., *64:*1166, 1971

Linton flap procedure, role in management of stasis dermatitis and ulceration in lower limb (Field, Van Boxel), PRS, *49:*584, 1972. Surgery, *70:*920, 1971

Varicose veins, lower limb venous dynamics in normal persons and children of patients with (Reagan, Folse), PRS, *48:*92, 1971. Surg. Gynec. & Obst., *132:*15, 1971

Treatment of varicose ulcers and their preparation for skin plastic surgery using bacteriostatic hemopaste (Sin'kevich). Vestn. Khir., *106:*37, 1971 (Russian)

Use of embryonal tissue for therapeutic purposes (Batrak). Vrach. Delo., *10:*127, 1971 (Russian)

Free full skin transplantation by the Corachan method (Anke *et al*). Zentralbl. Chir., *96:*799, 1971 (German)

Treatment of the post-thrombotic state in elderly patients (Haeger). Zentralbl. Phlebol., *10:*178, 1971

Ulcers, stasis, of legs, relationship between edema and healing rate of (Myers, Rightor, Cherry), PRS, *51:*605, 1973. Am. J. Surg., *124:*666, 1972

Surgical treatment of stasis ulcers (Kutz). Angiology, *23:*665, 1972

Venous leg ulcers, surgical treatment of (Volder, Oosterwijk), PRS, *51:*704, 1973. Arch. chir. neerl., *24:*245, 1972

Use of bipedicled flaps in the management of pretibial skin defects (el-Falaky). Aust. N. Z. J. Surg., *41:*253, 1972

Use of surgery and local temperature elevation in Mycobacterium ulcerans infection (Glynn). Aust. N. Z. J. Surg., *41:*312, 1972

Bairnsdale ulcer (Alsop). Aust. N. Z. J. Surg., *41:*317, 1972

Possibilities and indications for surgery in sequelae of phlebitis (Langeron). Chirurgie, *98:*708, 1972 (French)

Surgical management of ulcerative lesions of the leg (Ger). Curr. Probl. Surg., *1:*52, 1972

Leg ulcers, Thiersch's graft used for shortening the healing process of (Arma-Szlachcic *et al*). Dermatologica, *145:*92, 1972 (German)

Specific skin reactions in chronic congestive dermatoses (Fischer *et al*). Dtsch. Med. J., *23:*381, 1972 (German)

Leg Ulcer – Cont.

Therapy of the ulcus cruris (Walther). Munch. Med. Wochenschr., *114:*1069, 1972 (German)

Ulcers and hypodermitis (Vigoni). Phlebologie, *25:*353, 1972 (French)

Plastic surgery treatment of chronic venous ulcers of the leg (Ponten). Scand. J. Plast. Reconstr. Surg., *6:*74, 1972

Immediate and remote results of treatment of trophic leg ulcers at the Vangou health resort (D'iakanov). Sov. Med., *35:*140, 1972 (Russian)

Leg, chronic ulceration of (Ger). Surg. Annu., *4:*123, 1972

Flap surgery in sickle cell anemia, exchange transfusion for (Ashbell), PRS, *51:*705, 1973. Surg. Forum, *23:*517, 1972

Use of a quantum generator (laser) in the treatment of wounds (Shchur *et al*). Vestn. Khir., *108:*85, 1972 (Russian)

New local therapy of leg ulcer (Noack *et al*). Z. Aerztl. Fortbild. (Jena), *66:*368, 1972 (German)

Leg ulcers due to disordered venous and arterial hemodynamics in lower extremities, surgery of (Tschirkov *et al*). Z. Haut. Geschlechtskr., *47:*911, 1972 (German)

Good and bad feet in vascular pathology of legs (Frileux *et al*). Ann. Chir., *27:*308, 1973 (French)

Werner's syndrome. Familial ulcerous scleroderma with cataracts and diabetes (Vandaele). Arch. Belg. Dermatol., *29:*251, 1973 (French)

Lower extremities, ulcerations of, in the hospital patient (Henson). J. Am. Osteopath. Assoc., *73:*309, 1973

Ulcer of ankle-heel region, surgical management (Bennett, Kahn), PRS, *53:*113, 1974. J. Trauma, *12:*696, 1973

Varicose ulcers, crural, surgical tactics in (Tarapon *et al*). Klin. Khir., *12:*49, 1973 (Russian)

Ulcers, stasis (Phelps), PRS, *53:*373, 1974. Lahey Clin. Bull., *22:*54, 1973

Varicose ulcers, large, use of cutaneous homografts in surgical treatment of (Brunner *et al*). Phlebologie, *26:*249, 1973 (French)

Arterial ulcers (Huriez *et al*). Phlebologie, *25:*357, 1973

Varicose ulcers, crural, combined treatment of (Noczynski *et al*). Pol. Przegl. Chir., *45:*431, 1973 (Polish)

Varicose ulcers, crural, surgical treatment by Babcock-Linton method (Witek). Pol. Przegl. Chir., *45:*1209, 1973 (Polish)

Clofazimine ointment in treatment of trophic ulcers (Ellis, Taube). South African M. J.,

Leg Ulcer – Cont.

47:378, 1973

Foot and shin, persistently unhealing wounds and ulcers of, plastic surgery of skin with A. K. Tychinkina's modification of treatment (Zarivchatskii). Vestn. Khir., 111:80, 1973 (Russian)

Ulcus cruris, diagnosis and therapy of (Heyn et al). Z. Aerztl. Fortbild. (Jena), 67:662, 1973 (German)

Surgical treatment of ulcus cruris venosum permagnum (Kiene et al). Zentralbl. Chir., 98:1350, 1973 (German)

Leg ulcer, Dodd-Crockett operation. Analysis of long-term prognosis (Jacobsen et al). Acta Chir. Scand., 140:379, 1974

Arterial below knee bypass grafts. Experience with modified bovine heterograft (Slovin). Am. J. Surg., 128:58, 1974

Leg ulceration in sickle cell anemia (Serjeant), PRS, 54:503, 1974. Arch. Intern. Med., 133:681, 1974

Leg ulceration in sickle anemia (Serjeant). Arch. Intern. Med., 133:690, 1974

Varicose ulcers and eczema, management of. Diseases of skin (Ryan). Brit. Med. J., 1:192, 1974

Edema, vertical drainage in treatment of leg ulcers (Bourne), PRS, 57:535, 1976. Brit. M. J., 2:581, 1974

Methods of surgical treatment of post-thrombophlebitic syndrome (Cristian). Chirurgia (Bucur.), 23:31, 1974 (Rumanian)

Leg ulcer, surgical treatment of post-thrombophlebitic syndrome in ulceration stage (Cristian). Chirurgia (Bucur.), 23:223, 1974 (Rumanian)

Diabetic patients, mortality of, treated surgically for lower limb infection and/or gangrene (Kahn et al). Diabetes, 23:287, 1974

Treatment of arterial circulation disorders. Clinical results after lumbar sympathectomy (Sunkat et al). Fortschr. Med., 92:694, 1974 (German)

Cast, spica, for continuous elevation in treatment of reflex sympathetic dystrophy (Leach, Clawson, Caprio), PRS, 54:502, 1974. J. Bone & Joint Surg., 56A:416, 1974

Cross-leg flaps. A review of eleven personal cases (Jamra). J. Med. Liban., 27:591, 1974

Pathogenesis and surgical treatment of post-thrombophlebitic and varicose leg ulcers (Pokrovskli et al). Khirurgiia (Mosk.), 11:73, 1974 (Russian)

Surgical creation of fascial "stocking" in patients with postthrombotic syndrome of the lower limbs (Makhov et al). Khirurgiia (Mosk.), 5:46, 1974 (Russian)

Leg, chronic ulcer of venous origin

Leg Ulcer – Cont.

(Roucher), PRS, 57:119, 1976. Lyon chir., 70:388, 1974

Peridural anesthesia in arterial diseases of lower limbs (Caminiti). Minerva Anestesiol., 40:313, 1974

Stasis ulcer (Lofgren), PRS, 54:237, 1974. Minnesota Med., 57:135, 1974

Leg ulcers of venous origin (Frileux). Phlebologie, 27:137, 1974 (French)

Study of 1,000 ulcers treated in a non-hospitalized clientele (Cantegrel). Phlebologie, 27:141, 1974 (French)

Surgical treatment of varicose ulcers (Hardillier). Phlebologie, 27:149, 1974 (French)

Malignant transformation of leg ulcers. Apropos of 3 cases (Nguyen et al). Phlebologie, 27:215, 1974 (French)

Ulcers, venous stasis treated by dermal overgrafting, substitute for skin flap repairs in some injuries of extremities (Thompson, Ell). PRS, 54:290, 1974

Leg ulcers, badly-healing or non-healing, repeated application of homografts (Krupp, Rufli), PRS, 55:257, 1975. Schweiz. med. Wchnschr., 104:1148, 1974

Results of treatment of infected ulcerations of lower extremities (Kobus et al). Wiad. Lek., 27:233, 1974 (Polish)

Latest studies on the effect of laser beams on wound healing. Clinical and electronoptic experiences (Mester et al). Z. Exp. Chir., 7:9, 1974 (German)

Leg ulcers, lower, closing, from viewpoint of dermatologist (Friederich). Z. Hautkr., 49:377, 1974

Varicose veins, subcutaneous ligation of (Krieger). Z. Hautkr., 49:383, 1974 (German)

Leg ulcer, skin culture for treatment of (Klein). Z. Hautkr., 49:433, 1974 (German)

Femoropopliteal and femorotibial arterial reconstructive surgery. Special reference to the autogenous venous bypass procedure using unreversed vein after eversion valvectomy (Vanttinen et al). Acta Chir. Scand., 141:341, 1975

Suction blister transplantation for leg ulcers (Hentzer et al). Acta Derm. Venereol. Stockh., 55:207, 1975

Subfascial ligation (Linton operation) of the perforating leg veins to treat post-thrombophlebitic syndrome (Bowen). Am. Surg., 41:148, 1975

Functional importance of the collaterals of the deep femoral artery in cases of obstruction of its orifice (Garrido Garcia et al). Angiologia, 27:45, 1975 (Spanish)

Muscle flaps in the repair of skin defects over

Leg Ulcer – Cont.

the exposed tibia (McHugh *et al*). Brit. J. Plast. Surg., *28:*205, 1975

Surgical treatment of ulcus cruris venosum (Muller). Helv. Chir. Acta, *42:*169, 1975 (German)

Surgical treatment of livedo reticularis (Aldasoro *et al*). Int. Surg., *60:*44, 1975

Competition between collateral vessels in femoro-popliteal by-pass grafting (Mason *et al*). J. Cardiovasc. Surg. (Torino), *16:*373, 1975

Current status of thermography in peripheral vascular disease (Spence *et al*). J. Cardiovasc. Surg. (Torino), *16:*572, 1975

Management of leg ulcers (Lewis *et al*). J. Tenn. Med. Assoc., *68:*289, 1975

Treatment of patients with trophic ulcers (Iupatov *et al*). Khirurgiia (Mosk.), *8:*52, 1975 (Russian)

Surgical treatment of superficial varicose veins of the lower limbs (Prokopyshin). Klin. Khir., *1:*5, 1975 (Russian)

Surgical treatment of the post-phlebitis syndrome. I. (Villa *et al*). Minerva Chir., *30:*16, 1975 (Italian)

Surgical treatment of the post-phlebitis syndrome. II. (Villa *et al*). Minerva Chir., *30:*21, 1975 (Italian)

Letter: skin grafts and leg ulcers (Kay). N. Z. Med. J., *82:*317, 1975

Varicose ulcer, etiopathology and treatment (Bialostozky *et al*). Prensa Med. Mex., *40:*92, 1975 (Spanish)

Varicose ulcers (Eriksson *et al*). Scand. J. Soc. Med., *3:*13, 1975

Treatment of trophic crural ulcers (Grigorian *et al*). Sov. Med., *10:*86, 1975 (Russian)

Sympathectomy revisited: dodo or phoenix? (Takats). Surgery, *78:*644, 1975

Letter: Venous stasis (Cranley). Surgery, *77:*370, 1975

Treatment of ulcus venosum cruris (Bjordal). Tidsskr. Nor. Laegeforen, *95:*1809, 1975 (Norwegian)

Use of "catgut ligatures" in treatment of trophic ulcers of the lower limbs (Sashikova). Vestn. Khir., *115:*57, 1975 (Russian)

Operation of cross autovenous shunting in post thrombophlebitic disease of the lower limbs (Gorbunov). Vestn. Khir., *115:*57, 1975 (Russian)

Varicose symptom complex, limits of conservative and surgical treatment of (Schulze-Bergmann). Z. Hautkr., *50:*147, 1975 (German)

Legal Aspects

Plastic surgery, damages for unsuccessful (Editorial). J. Kans. Med. Soc., *75:*55,

Legal Aspects – Cont.

1974

Liabilities engendered in emergency department (Stevens), PRS *54:*383, 1974. J. Legal Med., *2:*17, 1974

Medico-legal experiences in allegations of inadequate explanation and negligence (Becker). Laryngol. Rhinol. Otol. Stuttg., *53:*75, 1974 (German)

Limitations of the role of social insurance, especially disability insurance, in cases of esthetic damage (Viret). Rev. Med. Suisse Romande., *94:*1005, 1974 (French)

Protection against malpractice litigation (Bergen). Arch. Otolaryng., *101:*182, 1975

The public face or psychological and legal complexities in plastic ophthalmic surgery (Lubkin). Brit. J. Ophthalmol., *59:*593, 1975

Malpractice: positive steps for plastic surgeons (Dorner). Mich. Med., *74:*298, 1975

LEGAL, H. *et al*: Hand burns in children and their sequelae. Munch. Med. Wochenschr., *113:*572, 1971 (German)

LEGENT, F. *et al*: Facial paralysis and tuberculous otitis. Significance of early neural decompression. Ann. Otolaryngol. Chir. Cervicofac., *92:*235, 1975 (French)

LEGGETT, C. A.: Retromammary tumors of pectoralis major muscle. Aust. N. Z. J. Surg., *43:*37, 1973

LEHMAN, J. A., JR.: Silastic cranioplasty. Ohio State Med. J., *69:*441, 1973

LEHMAN, J. A., JR. *et al*: Plastic surgery in prison. An apparently negative result. Ohio State Med. J., *69:*893, 1973

LEHMAN, J. A., AND CUDDAPAH, S.: True hare lip – case report, PRS, *56:*109, 1975. Cleft Palate J., *11:*497, 1974

LEHMANN, C. *et al*: Tracheotomy in the multi-injured. Cah. Anesthesiol., *19:*335, 1971 (French)

LEHMANN, J. F. *et al*: Therapeutic heat and cold, PRS, *56:*475, 1975. Clin. Orthop., *99:*207, 1974

LEHMANN, W. B.: Bilateral pneumothorax five days after tracheotomy decannulation. Ann. Otol. Rhin. & Laryng., *83:*128, 1974

LEHNERT, S.: Treatment of avoidable late sequelae of jaw and facial injuries. Chirurg., *42:*403, 1971 (German)

LEHNERT, S.: Treatment of pseudarthrosis of mandible using non-pedunculated bone suture grafting. Dtsch. Zahn. Mund. Kieferheilkd., *61:*45, 1973 (German)

LEHNERT, S.: Primary treatment of orbital fractures by means of cartilage transplantation. Fortschr. Kiefer. Gesichtschir., *19:*185, 1975

(German)

LEHR, H. B.: Cancer of tongue; results of treatment in 258 consecutive cases (with Whitaker, Askovitz). PRS, 50:363, 1972

LEHRMAN, A.: Reconstruction of hand for peripheral nerve injuries. N. Y. State J. Med., 72:2401, 1971

LEHTINEN, R. et al: Unilateral hyperplasia of mandibular condyle. Suom. Hammaslaak. Toim., 68:253, 1972 (Finnish)

LEHV, M. S.: Aid to meshed skin grafting. PRS, 56:584, 1975

LEIBERT, P. S., AND STOOL, S. E.: Rhabdomyosarcoma of tongue in infant: results of combined radiation and chemotherapy. PRS, 53:681, 1974. Ann. Surg., 178:621, 1973

LEIFER, C. et al: Spindle-cell carcinoma of oral mucosa. Light and electron microscopic study of apparent sarcomatous metastasis to cervical lymph nodes. Cancer, 34:597, 1974

LEIGHEB, G. et al: Cryosurgery and basal cell epitheliomas. Clinical and histological study. Minerva Med., 65:3676, 1974

LEIS, H. P.: Breast cancer, a surgical dilemma. Ann. Chir., 29:852, 1975

LEIS, S. N. et al: Skin grafting: contemporary concepts and applications. J. Am. Osteopath. Assoc., 74:631, 1975

LEIVY, D. M. AND TOVI, D.: Autogenous bone cranioplasty, PRS, 49:239, 1972. Acta chir. scandinav., 136:385, 1970

LEJEUNE, F. J. et al: Malignant cervicofacial melanoma. Review of 78 cases. Bull. Cancer (Paris), 59:255, 1972 (French)

LEJOUR, M.: Indications for Aries-Pitanguy technique in mammary gland ptosis, PRS, 50:199, 1972. Acta chir. belg., 70:5, 1971

LEJOUR, M.: One stage reconstruction of nasal skin defects with local flaps, PRS, 52:205, 1973. Chir. Plast., 1:254, 1972

LEJOUR, M.: Reconstruction of skin defects of cheek with large island flap, PRS, 56:473, 1975. Acta chir. belg., 74:183, 1975

LEJOUR, M. et al: Tolerance to synthetic material in plastic surgery. Acta chir. belg., 70:245, 1971 (French)

LEJOUR, M. et al: Use of deltopectoral flap in cervicofacial restoration. Ann. chir. plast., 17:126, 1972 (French)

LEJOUR, M. et al: Extensive traumatic avulsion of skin of lower limb, PRS, 54:238, 1974. Acta chir. belg., 72:456, 1973

LEJOUR, M. et al: Problems involving skin in open fractures of tibia, PRS, 54:110, 1974. Acta chir. belg., 72:472, 1973

LEJOUR, M., LORIAUX, C., AND HARDY, A.: Surgical and hormonal management of grossly hypertrophied breast in puberty, PRS, 55:636, 1975. Ann. chir. plast., 19:347, 1974

LEJOUR, M., AND LECOCQ, C.: Psychological im-

plications of cosmetic surgery, PRS, 56:603, 1975. Acta chir. belg., 74:5, 1975

LEMAIRE, J-M., Ten free groin flaps (with Baudet, Guimberteau). PRS, 57:577, 1976

LEMAIRE, R. et al: "Plastic" materials implantable in surgery. Acta chir. belg., 70:156, 1971 (French)

LE MAREC, B. et al: Polydactylism: disease or symptom? Pediatrie, 25:737, 1970 (French)

LeMAY, S. R.: Penetrating wounds of larynx and cervical trachea, PRS, 49:670, 1972. Arch. Otolaryng., 94:558, 1971

LEMOINE, A. N., JR.: Discussion of "Acute retrobulbar hemorrhage during elective blepharoplasty," by Hartley et al. PRS, 52:12, 1973

LE MOUEL, C. et al: Rational tube for nasal tracheal intubation in buccal and oropharyngeal surgery. Ann. Otolaryngol. Chir. Cervicofac., 90:775, 1973 (French)

LEMPEREUR, L.: Abnormal callus in fractures of the long bones of the hand. Rev. Med. Liege, 29:144, 1974 (French)

LEMPERLE, G., KOHNLEIN, H. E., AND VON KANNEN, W.: Cold water treatment of fresh burns, PRS, 50:204, 1972. Langenbecks Arch. Chir., 329:898, 1971

LEMPERLE, G. et al: Facial paresis—the dynamic suspension of eyelid and the corner of the mouth to M. temporalis. In Plastische und Wiederherstellungs-Chirurgie, ed. by Hohler; pp. 143–50. Schattauer, Stuttgart, 1975 (German)

LEMPERLE, G. et al: Granuloma after subcutaneous injection of facial wrinkles with Teflon paste. In Plastische und Wiederherstellungs-Chirurgie, ed by Hohler; pp. 335-9. Schattauer, Stuttgart, 1975 (German)

LENCO, W., McKNIGHT, M., AND MacDONALD, A. S.: Effects of cortisone acetate, methylprednisolone and medroxyprogesterone on wound contracture and epithelialization in rabbits, PRS, 56:470, 1975. Ann. Surg., 181:67, 1975

LENCZYK, J. M. et al: Surgery in cancer of head and neck. Use of posterior cervical flap. N. Y. State J. Med., 72:239, 1972

LENDVAY, P. G.: Replacement of amputated finger, PRS, 53:685, 1974. Asian J. Med., 9:249, 1973

LENGYEL, E. et al: Giant fibroadenoma of breast in young. Orv. Hetil., 114:2545, 1973 (Hungarian)

LENHARD, V. et al: Retro-orbital fibrosis in Ormond's disease. Dtsch. Med. Wochenschr., 99:2286, 1974 (German)

LENIHAN, JOHN: Human Engineering. The Body Re-Examined. George Brazillier Inc., New York, 1974. PRS, 56:572, 1975

LENNARD, E. S. et al: Immunologic and nutritional evaluation of burn neutrophil function. J. Surg. Res., *16:*286, 1974

LENNIHAN, R., JR., AND MACKERETH, M.: Calculating volume changes in swollen extremity from surface measurements, PRS, *54:*113, 1974. Am. J. Surg., *126:*649, 1973

LENQUIST, S. *et al*: Significance of local malignant lesions of the neck diagnosed accidentally during parathyroid exploration. Acta Chir. Scand., *141:*721, 1975

LENTINI, G. *et al*: Clinical observations on postoperative reflex syndromes of the cervical autonomic nervous sytem. Clin. Otorinolaringoiatr., *22:*104, 1970 (Italian)

LENTRODT, J.: Rare case of pleomorphic rhabdomyosarcoma of the lower lip. Dtsch. Mund. Kieferheilkd., *57:*97, 1971 (German)

LENTRODT, J.: Malignant degeneration of mixed parotid gland tumors. Fortschr. Kiefer. Gesichtschir., *15:*101, 1972 (German)

LENTRODT, J.: Diagnosis and therapy of fractures of floor of orbit. Dtsch. Zahn. Mund. Kieferheilkd., *60:*232, 1973 (German)

LENTRODT, J.: Contribution to reconstruction of lower lip after tumor resection combined with neck dissection, PRS, *57:*529, 1976. J. Maxillo-facial Surg., *3:*139, 1975

LENTRODT, J. *et al*: Radiographic and surgical report difference in fractures of the orbital margin. Dtsch. Zahnaerztl. Z., *26:*1232, 1971 (German)

LENTRODT, J., AND LUHR, H. G.: Reconstruction of lower lip after tumor resection combined with radical neck dissection. PRS, *48:*579, 1971

LENTRODT, J. *et al*: Indications for surgical or conservative treatment of mandibular fractures. Fortschr. Kiefer. Gesichtschir., *19:*65, 1974 (German)

LENZ, P. *et al*: Possibilities of prosthetic treatment of malocclusion Angle II/1 with and without surgical preparation. Dtsch. Zahnaerztl. Z., *30:*179, 1975 (German)

LEONARD, D. D.: Starch granulomas, PRS, *52:*603, 1973. Arch. Dermat., *107:*101, 1973

LEONARD, J. R., AND HASS, A. C.: Management of cancer of the oral cavity. Trend toward combined radiotherapy and surgery, PRS, *48:*398, 1971. Am. J. Surg., *120:*514, 1970

LEONARD, M. H. *et al*: Electromyography (EMG) in surgery of the hand. Electromyography, *10:*239, 1970

LEONE, C. R., JR.: Mucous membrane grafting for cicatricial entropion. Ophthalmic Surg., *5:*24, 1974

LEONE, C. R., JR.: Internal tarsus *orbicularis* resection for senile spastic entropion, PRS, *57:*257, 1976. Ann. Ophth., *7:*1004, 1975

LEONE, C. R., JR.: Repair of cicatricial ectro-

pion by horizontal shortening and pedicle flap. Ophthalmic Surg., *6:*47, 1975

LEONE, C. R., JR. *et al*: Bilateral blowout fractures. Ann. Ophth., *4:*495, 1972

LEONI, P.: Rhinoplasty, some errors and difficulties. Acta Otorinolaryngol. Iber. Am., *22:*139, 1971 (Italian)

LEOPARD, P. J.: Cryosurgery and its application to oral surgery. Brit. J. Oral Surg., *13:*128, 1975

LEOPARD, P. J.: Cryosurgery for facial skin lesions. Proc. Roy. Soc. Med., *68:*606, 1975

LEOPARD, P. J. *et al*: Practical cryosurgery for oral lesions. Brit. Dent. J., *136:*185, 1974

LEPAW, M. I.: Inexpensive method for cooling skin grafts, PRS, *55:*18, 1975. Cutis, *14:*595, 1974

LE PELTIER, P. *et al*: Treatment of paralysis of intrinsic muscles of the hand of leprous origin. Maroc. Med., *49:*586, 1969 (French)

LEPKOWSKI, A.: Maxillary sinus fibro-odontoma in 12-year-old girl. Otolaryngol. Pol., *28:*239, 1974 (Polish)

LEPLEY, J. B.: Current practices in maxillofacial prosthetics, PRS, *55:*518, 1975. Surg. Clin. N. Am., *54:*787, 1974

LEPLEY, J. B. *et al*: Functional and cosmetic restoration of massive orofacial defect. J. Prosthet. Dent., *30:*635, 1973

LEPPARD, M. B.: Epidermoid cysts and polyposis coli, PRS, *55:*640, 1975. Proc. Roy. Soc. Med., *67:*1036, 1974

Leprosy (see also *Facial Paralysis; Hands, Nerve; Lagophthalmos*)

Treatment of paralysis of intrinsic muscles of the hand of leprous origin (Le Peltier *et al*). Maroc. Med., *49:*586, 1969 (French)

Leporine nose (Pardina, Frontera Vaca), PRS *48:*394, 1971. Bull. Plast. Reconstr. Surg. Argent., *1:*12, 1970

Reconstructive Surgery in Leprosy, By Ernest P. Fritschi. John Wright & Sons, Bristol, 1971. PRS, *49:*567, 1972

Leprosy, prolonged survival of skin allografts in (Hans, Weiser, Kau), PRS, *51:*611, 1973. Internat. J. Leprosy, *39:*1, 1971

Review of surgery in leprosy (Antia). Int. J. Lepr., *39:*616, 1971

Subcutaneous Achilles tenotomy in the treatment of perforating ulcer of the foot in leprosy (Yosipovitch *et al*). Int. J. Lepr., *39:*631, 1971

Reconstructive surgery in leprosy deformities (Selvapandian). Int. J. Lepr., *39:*660, 1971

Prosthetics in leprosy (Garst). Lepr. Rev., *42:*60, 1971

Intravenous regional analgesia for hand surgery in leprosy (Thangaraj). Lepr. Rev.,

Leprosy—Cont.

42:266, 1971

Clinico-surgical treatment of a case of lepromatous cubital neuritis (Mangeon *et al*). Rev. Bras. Med., *28:*263, 1971 (Portuguese)

Leprous disfigurement of face, reconstructive operations (Daykhes), PRS, *52:*321, 1973. Acta chir. plast., *14:*101, 1972

Management of the foot in leprosy (White *et al*). Clin. Orthop., *85:*115, 1972

Pathogenesis of extremity deformity in leprosy. A pathologic study of large sections of amputated extremities in relation to radiological appearance. (Skinsnes *et al*). Int. J. Lepr., *40:*375, 1972

Leprosy, radical metatarsectomy for intractable plantar ulceration in (Bhasin *et al*). Lepr. Rev., *43:*53, 1972

Peripheral nerve surgery in leprous neuritis (technics, value and respective indications of procedures) (Carayon *et al*). Med. Trop. (Mars.), *32:*23, 1972 (French)

Leprosy, selection of cases and results of direct surgery of 535 mixed nerves in (Carayon *et al*). Med. Trop. (Mars.), *32:*157, 1972 (French)

Leprotic paralysis of foot, evaluation of palliative surgery in (Carayon, van Droogenbroeck, Girandeau). Med. trop., *32:*695, 1972 (French)

Leprosy, summary of recent abstracts, #8 (Browne). Trop. Dis. Bull., *69:*863, 1972

Leprosy, internal anatomy of nerve trunks in relation to neural lesions of. Observations on pathology, symptomatology and treatment (Sunderland). Brain, *96:*875, 1973

Cubital tunnel external compression syndrome (Jopling). Brit. Med. J., *2:*179, 1973

Leprosy in mouth, jaws, and facial region (Werner). Dtsch. Zahnaerztl. Z., *28:*64, 1973 (German)

Leprosy, surgery and (Editorial). Lepr. Rev., *43:*119, 1973

Temporalis transfer in lagophthalmos due to leprosy (Ranney, Furness). PRS, *51:*301, 1973

Alopecia of eyebrows in leprous patients, correction of (Guerrero-Santos, Matus, Vera-Strathmann) (Follow-Up Clinic), PRS, *52:*183, 1973

Nose, prefabricated silicone implants (Antia *et al*). PRS, *52:*264, 1973

Paralytic claw hand, Fowler procedure for correction of (Enna, Riordan). PRS, *52:*352, 1973

Leprosy, basis for the surgical treatment of patients with (Heinz). Praxis, *62:*1285, 1973 (German)

Leprosy patients, rehabilitation of, by correc-

Leprosy—Cont.

tion of nasal deformities. New ways in correction of the saddle-nose. Praxis, *62:*1305, 1973 (German)

Graft, buried, to reconstruct eyebrows (Ausin Garcia, Bermudez Piernagorda), PRS, *56:*590, 1975. Rev. españ. cir. plast., *6:*97, 1973

Leprosy for Practitioners. By S. J. Yawalkar. Popular Prakashan, Ltd., Bombay, India, 1974. PRS, *55:*616, 1975

Surgical Rehabilitation in Leprosy. Ed. by Frank McDowell and Carl Enna. Williams & Wilkins Co., Baltimore, 1974.

Current treatment of leprosy in the Malta pavilion of the Hopital Saint-Louis (Pennec). Ann. Med. Interne (Paris), *125:*561, 1974 (French)

Leprosy, plantar ulcers in, angiographic diagnosis and preventive surgery of (Frontera Vaca *et al*), PRS, *55:*109, 1975. Bol. Soc. cir. Plast. y Reconstr. Cordoba, *5:*17, 1974

Scope of plastic surgery in leprosy: a ten year progress report (Antia). Clin. Plast. Surg., *1:*69, 1974

Limb deformities in leprosy (Yadev). Indian J. Med. Sci., *28:*542, 1974

A clinical assessment of neurolysis for leprous involvement of the ulnar nerve (Enna *et al*). Int. J. Lepr., *42:*162, 1974

Leprosy, lepromatous, redundant and wrinkled facial skin in. Correlation of clinical and histopathological findings (Enna *et al*). Int. J. Lepr., *42:*297, 1974

Leprosy, neurolysis and transposition of ulnar nerve in (Enna). J. Neurosurg., *40:*734, 1974

Leprosy, lepromatous, pathologic changes in soft palate (Reichart), PRS, *56:*593, 1975. Oral Surg., *38:*898, 1974

Leprosy, significance of nerve involvement in (Antia). PRS, *54:*55, 1974

Skin, dartos, and nerve biopsies as aids to diagnosis in leprosy (Pandya), PRS, *54:*70, 1974. Discussion by Brand, PRS, *54:*218, 1974

Plastic surgery of the face in leoprosy (Maillard *et al*). Rev. Med. Suisse Romande, *94:*729, 1974 (French)

Surgical therapy for venous stasis (De Palma). Surgery, *76:*910, 1974

Debridement of Hansenian torpid ulcers (Frontera Vaca *et al*), PRS, *55:*385, 1975. Tribuna Med. Argent., *19:*135, 1974

Leprosy, chronic ulceration in patient with (Noe, Barber), PRS, *55:*727, 1975. West. J. Med., *121:*430, 1974

Nerve grafting in leprosy (McLeod *et al*).

Leprosy — Cont.

Brain, *98:*203, 1975

Letter: nerve grafting in leprosy (Crawford). Lancet, *2:*326, 1975

Leprous face, plastic surgery of (Maillard *et al*). Helv. Chir. Acta, *42:*161, 1975 (French)

Hansen's disease: a podiatrist's experience (Cooper). J. Am. Podiatry Assoc., *65:*300, 1975

Leprosy, opponensplasty in intrinsic muscle paralysis of thumb in (Palande *et al*), PRS, *57:*674, 1976. J. Bone & Joint Surg., *57A:*489, 1975

Transverse metatarsal head resection — a radical approach to the problems of forefoot ulceration (Andersen). Lepr. Rev., *46:*191, 1975

Leprosy, correction of facial profile in (Teixeira), PRS, *57:*113, 1976. Rev. Assoc. med. Bras., *21:*124, 1975

Letter: nerve grafting in leprosy (McLeod *et al*). Lancet, *1:*95, 1976

LERF, B.: Graft conditioning with non-specific ribonucleic acid, PRS, *52:*463, 1973. Bruns' Beitr. klin. Chir., *220:*206, 1973

LERINCK, P. L. *et al*: Salvage surgery in laryngeal cancer. Acta Otorhinolaryngol. Belg., *27:*993, 1973 (French)

LERMAN, M.: Ocular injuries in orbital fractures, review of 119 cases (with Jabaley, Sanders), PRS, *56:*410, 1975

LERMAN, R., AND PITCOCK, J.: Frozen section experience in 3,249 specimens, PRS, *51:*712, 1973. Surg. Gynec. & Obst., *135:*930, 1972

LeROUX, P., AND JONES, S. H.: Total permanent removal of wrinkles from forehead, PRS, *56:*675, 1975. Brit. J. Plast. Surg., *27:*359, 1974

LEROUX-ROBERT, J. *et al*: Statistical study of 148 cases of cancer of buccal floor treated for more than 5 years. Ann. Otolaryngol. Chir. Cervicofac., *89:*477, 1972 (French)

LEROUX-ROBERT, J. *et al*: Tumoral process developed in cicatrix of thyroglossal tract cyst. J. Fr. Otorinolaryngol., *21:*617, 1972 (French)

LEROUX-ROBERT, J.: Chemotherapy of cancers of larynx and hypopharynx. Acta Otorhinolaryngol. Belg., *27:*883, 1973 (French)

LEROUX-ROBERT, J.: Functionally-oriented partial surgery in cancer of larynx and hypopharynx. Introductory discussion. Acta Otorhinolaryngol. Belg., *27:*938, 1973 (French)

LEROUX-ROBERT, J. *et al*: Cherubism (apropos of case). Ann. Otolaryngol. Chir. Cervicofac., *90:*95, 1973 (French)

LEROUX-ROBERT, J. *et al*: Gardner's syndrome. Apropos of two familial cases. Ann. Otolaryngol. Chir. Cervicofac., *90:*161, 1973

LERUT, T. *et al*: Experiences with treatment of gas gangrene, PRS, *56:*234, 1975. Acta chir. belg., *73:*35, 1974

LESICA, A. *et al*: Atypical fibroxanthoma of ethmoid sinus. Arch. Otolaryng., *101:*506, 1975

LESOINE, W.: Current views on the surgery of tongue carcinomas. Z. Laryngol. Rhinol. Otol., *49:*242, 1970 (German)

LESOVAIA, N. D.: Significance of the anatomical structure of the submandibular salivary gland in salivary calculi. Stomatologiia (Mosk.), *53:*25, 1974 (Russian)

LESSA, S. F. *et al*: Revascularization of skin autografts, PRS, *53:*112, 1974. Folha Med. Brazil, *66:*17, 1973

LESSA, S., AND CARREIRAO, S.: Ankyloglossia, PRS, *57:*258, 1976. Folha Med. Brazil, *70:*295, 1975

LESSLER, M. A. *et al*: Effect of cryostorage on oxygen uptake and autograft viability of rat skin. Cryobiology, *10:*185, 1973

LESTER, J. C.: Acute retrobulbar hemorrhage during elective blepharoplasty (with Hartley, Schatten), PRS, *52:*8, 1973. Discussions by Lemoine, Rees, Newell, PRS, *52:*12, 1973

L'ESTRANGE, P. R. *et al*: A variation in subperiosteal implant design. A case report. Brit. Dent. J., *138:*141, 1975

LETH, A.: Cell swelling, factor in ischemic tissue, PRS, *53:*501, 1974. Circulation, *48:*455, 1973

LETSON, J. A., JR. *et al*: Septal dermoplasty for von Willebrand's disease in children. Laryngoscope, *83:*1078, 1973

LETTERMAN, G.: Obituary on Robert E. Moran, M.D., PRS, *51:*493, 193

LETTERMAN, G.: Suggested anatomical nomenclature for the nose (with Schurter), PRS, *57:*490, 1976

LETTERMAN, G.: SCHURTER, M., AND SENDI, H.: Surgery of syndactyly, PRS, *48:*93, 1971. Woman Physician, *25:*763, 1970

LETTERMAN, G., AND SCHURTER, M.: Surgical correction of gynecomastia, PRS, *49:*259, 1972

LETTERMAN, G. *et al*: Surgical management of axillary hyperhidrosis. J. Am. Med. Wom. Assoc., *28:*581, 1973

LETTERMAN, G., AND SCHURTER, M.: Pattern for postauricular incision in rhytidectomy, PRS, *51:*697, 1973

LETTERMAN, G. *et al*: Repair of soft tissue injuries of face. J. Am. Med. Wom. Assoc., *29:*211, 1974

LETTERMAN, G., AND SCHURTER, M.: Will Durston's "mammaplasty," PRS, *53:*48, 1974

LETTERMAN, G., AND SCHURTER, M.: Inframammary-based dermofat flaps in mammary reconstruction following subcutaneous mastectomy, PRS, *55:*156, 1975

LETTERMAN, G. S.: Surgical correction of exophthalmos, history, technique, and long-term follow-up (with Moran, Schurter), PRS, *49:*595, 1972

LETTERMAN, G. S.: Ambroise Paré's opinion on mammaplasties (Letter to the Editor), PRS, *54:*212, 1974

Leukoplakia

Tobacco chewing in English coal miners. A preliminary report (Tyldesley). Brit. J. Oral Surg., *9:*21, 1971

Diffuse recurring leukoplakia of the buccal cavity, with epitheliomatous degeneration (Basset *et al*). Bull. Soc. Fr. Dermatol. Syphiligr., *78:*160, 1971 (French)

Leukoplakia of tongue treated by vermilionectomy (Barakat). Rev. Dent. Liban., *21:*47, 1971

Office cryotherapy for oral leukoplakia (Goode *et al*). Trans. Am. Acad. Ophthalmol. Otolaryngol., *75:*968, 1971

Leukoplakia, intraoral, cryotherapy of (Sako, Marchetta, Hayes), PRS, *52:*102, 1973. Am. J. Surg., *124:*482, 1972

Comparative study of the clinical picture and histopathologic structure of oral leukoplakia (Banoczy *et al*). Cancer, *29:*1230, 1972

Radiotherapy of carcinoma developed from leukoplakia (Fuchihata *et al*). Oral Surg., *33:*137, 1972

Presence of Candida in 723 oral leukoplakias among Indian villagers (Daftary *et al*). Scand. J. Dent. Res., *80:*75, 1972

Leukoplakia, intraoral, clinical picture and therapy of (Esser *et al*). Dtsch. Zahn. Mund. Keiferheilkd., *60:*378, 1973 (German)

Leukoplakias, oral, cryosurgical therapy of (Hausamen). Dtsch. Zahnaerztl. Z., *28:*1032, 1973 (German)

Leukoplakias, oral, snuff-induced, Danish, study of (Roed-Petersen *et al*). J. Oral Pathol., *2:*301, 1973

Leukoplakia of lip: acquired *cheilitis glandularis simplex* (Epinette, Hurwitz), PRS, *51:*334, 1973

Practical cryosurgery for oral lesions (Leopard *et al*). Brit. Dent. J., *136:*185, 1974

Surgery in premalignant lesions (Som). Can. J. Otolaryngol., *3:*551, 1974

Surgical treatment of non-traumatic lower lip lesions with special reference to the step technique. A follow-up on 149 patients (Johanson *et al*). Scand. J. Plast. Reconstr. Surg., *8:*232, 1974

Cryosurgery and its application to oral sur-

Leukoplakia – Cont.

gery (Leopard). Brit. J. Oral Surg., *13:*128, 1975

Therapeutic challenge of premalignant and malignant skin lesions (Katz *et al*). Geriatrics, *30:*53, 1975

Leukoplakia, oral (Srivastava), PRS, *56:*224, 1975. Internat. Surg., *58:*614, 1975

DNA content of leukoplakia cells of oral mucosa (Pfitzer, Pape), PRS, *57:*115, 1976. J. Maxillo-facial Surg., *3:*119, 1975

Evaluation, surveillance and treatment of panoral leukoplakia (Poswillo). J. Maxillofacial. Surg., *3:*205, 1975

Leukoplakia buccalis, an enigma (Cooke), PRS, *57:*258, 1976. Proc. Roy. Soc. Med., *68:*337, 1975

Cryosurgery of the oral mucous membranes (Poswillo). Proc. Roy. Soc. Med., *68:*608, 1975

Leukoplakia, snuff-induced, (snuff dippers keratosis) (Raque *et al*). South. Med. J., *68:*565, 1975

LEUZ, C. A.: Conservative program for managing cleft palates without use of mucoperiosteal flaps (with Blocksma, Mellerstig), PRS, *55:*160, 1975

LEVANT, B. A.: Experience with Levant frame for cranio-maxillary fixation. Brit. J. Oral Surg., *11:*30, 1973

LEVEEN, H. H. *et al*: Chemical acidification of wounds, adjuvant to healing and unfavorable action of alkalinity and ammonia, PRS, *54:*114, 1974. Ann. Surg., *178:*745, 1973

LEVEN, B. *et al*: Location and prognosis of iatrogenic nerve lesions. Munch. Med. Wochenschr., *115:*1956, 1973 (German)

LEVENE, A.: Treatment of malignant melanoma. Brit. Med. J., *1:*545, 1973

LEVENSON, S. M. *et al*: Chemical debridement of burns, PRS, *55:*514, 1975. Ann. Surg., *180:*670, 1974

LEVENTHAL, H. H., AND MESSER, R. J.: Malignant tumors of eyelid, PRS, *52:*328, 1973. Am. J. Surg., *124:*522, 1972

LEVERMENT, J. N. *et al*: Tracheal size following tracheostomy with cuffed tracheostomy tubes: an experimental study. Thorax, *30:*271, 1975

LEVIGNAC, J.: Reconstruction of large perioral defects and correction of stenosis and distortion due to extensive burns of face. J. Maxillo-facial Surg., *1:*129, 1973

LEVIN, A. O. *et al*: Hematological and biochemical indices after the comprehensive treatment of melanoblastomas of the lower extremities. Vopr. Onkol., *20:*39, 1974 (Russian)

LEVIN, J. M., AND BORNSTEIN, L. A.: Initial burn experience in recent Middle East conflict, PRS, *54:*432, 1974

LEVIN, J. M., ROBINSON, D. W., AND LIN, F.: Acinic cell carcinoma, PRS, *55:*724, 1975. Arch. Surg. *110:*64, 1975

LEVIN, J. M., AND MASTERS, F. W.: Simple method for changing bolus dressings, PRS, *55:*500, 1975

LEVIN, L. L.: Rupture of all digital flexor tendons in the wrist. Vestn. Khir., *105:*123, 1970 (Russian)

LEVIN, M. P. *et al*: Comparison of iliac marrow and biodegradable ceramic in periodontal defects, PRS, *57:*114, 1976. J. Bio-Med. Mater., *9:*183, 1975

LEVINE, M. R. *et al*: Complications of blepharoplasty. Ophthalmic Surg., *6:*53, 1975

LEVINE, N., SEIFTER, E., AND LEVENSON, S. M.: Enzymatic debridement of burns, PRS, *49:*665, 1972. Surg. Forum, *22:*57, 1971

LEVINE, N. *et al*: Debridement of experimental skin burns of pigs with bromelain, pineapple stem enzyme, PRS, *52:*413, 1973

LEVINE, N., SEIFTER, E., AND LEVENSON, S. M.: Enzymatic debridement of burns. Rev. Surg., *30:*72, 1973

LEVINE, N. *et al*: Use of carbon dioxide laser for debridement of third degree burns, PRS, *54:*240, 1974. Ann. Surg., *179:*246, 1974

LEVINE, N. S. *et al*: Spinal cord injury following electrical accidents: case reports. J. Trauma, *15:*459, 1975

LEVINE, N. S. *et al*: Laser, scalpel, electrosurgical, and tangential excisions of third degree burns, PRS, *56:*286, 1975

LEVINE, N. S., SALISBURY, R. E., AND MASON, A. D., JR.: Effect of early surgical excision and homografting on survival of burned rats and of intraperitoneally-infected burned rats, PRS, *56:*423, 1975

LEVINE, P. H.: Acute effect of cigarette smoking on platelet function; possible link between smoking and arterial thrombosis, PRS, *53:*489, 1974. Circulation, *48:*619, 1973

LEWIS, W. R. *et al*: Topical immunotherapy of basal cell carcinomas with dinitrochlorobenzene, PRS, *54:*245, 1974. Cancer Res., *33:*3036, 1974

LEVITT, R. L. *et ai*: Sweat gland carcinoma of the hand. A case report. Clin. Orthop., *83:*95, 1972

LEVITT, R. L. *et al*: Surgical correction of foot deformity in the older patient with myelomeningocele. Orthop. Clin. North Am., *5:*19, 1974

LEVY, A.: Bleeding in central nervous system, severe complication of therapy with anticoagulants, PRS, *50:*95, 1972. Ther. Umsch., *28:*821, 1971

LEVY, D. M., AND APFELBERG, D. B.: Results by anterior transposition for ulnar neuropathy at elbow, PRS, *50:*419, 1972. Am. J. Surg., *123:*304, 1972

LEVY, L. F.: Peripheral nerve injuries. S. Afr. J. Surg., *11:*255, 1973

LEVY, M.: Severe injury due to shark bite. Harefuah, *87:*258, 1974 (Hebrew)

LEVY, N. B., AND WYNBRANDT, G. D.: Quality of life on maintenance hemodialysis, PRS, *57:*675, 1976. Lancet, *6:*1328, 1975

LEWANDOWSKI, L.: Analysis and therapeutic results in odontogenic cysts bulging into maxillary sinuses. Czas. Stomatol., *28:*649, 1975 (Polish)

LEWIN, M. L. *et al*: Midface osteotomies for correction of facial deformities (craniofacial dysostosis and maxillary hypoplasia). Trans. Am. Acad. Ophthalmol. Otolaryngol., *76:*946, 1972

LEWIN, M. L. *et al*: Speech results after Millard island flap repair in cleft palate and other velopharyngeal insufficiencies. Cleft Palate J., *12:*263, 1975

LEWINN, L. R., GUTHRIE, R. H., AND KOVACHEV, D.: One-stage coverage of large chest wall defect with giant bipedicled flap, PRS, *56:*336, 1975

LEWIS, C. E., JR., MUELLER, C., AND EDWARDS, W. S.: Venous stasis on the operating table, PRS, *52:*99, 1973. Am. J. Surg., *124:*780, 1972

LEWIS, J. A.: Loose *vs.* tight fitting of silastic prosthesis of the MP joint of the hand. Med. Ann. D. C., *43:*15, 1974

LEWIS, J. E. *et al*: Le Fort III osteotomy to correct dish-face deformity resulting from facial trauma. S. Afr. Med. J., *49:*1915, 1975

LEWIS, JOHN R., JR.: *Atlas of Aesthetic Plastic Surgery.* Little, Brown & Co., Boston, 1973. PRS, *53:*673, 1974

LEWIS, J. R., JR.: Facial scars resulting from vehicular accidents. Clin. Plast. Surg., *2:*143, 197

LEWIS, J. R., JR.: Segmental approach to rhitidectomy, PRS, *56:*297, 1975

LEWIS, J. S.: Squamous carcinoma of ear, PRS, *52:*600, 1973. Arch. Otolaryng., *97:*41, 1973

LEWIS, M. G. *et al*: Halo naevus — a frustrated malignant melanoma. Brit. Med. J., *2:*47, 1972

LEWIS, M. R. *et al*: Management of leg ulcers. J. Tenn. Med. Assoc., *68:*289, 1975

LEWIS, R. J., AND KETCHAM, A.: Maffucci's syndrome, functional and neoplastic significance, PRS, *54:*116, 1974. J. Bone & Joint Surg., *55A:*1465, 1973

LEWIS, R. J., AND QUINBY, W. C.: Electrosurgical excision of full-thickness burn, PRS,

*56:*233, 1975. Arch. Surg., *110:*191, 1975

LEWIS, S. R.: Treatment of lymphedema (with Bunchman), PRS, *54:*64, 1974

LEWIS, S. R.: Burned hands (with Huang, Larson), PRS, *56:*21, 1975. Discussion by Bennett, PRS, *56:*442, 1975

LEWIS, S. R.: Thumb reconstruction in the severely burned hand (with Pohl, Larson), PRS, *57:*320, 1976

LEWISON, E.: Twenty years of prison surgery, evaluation. Can. J. Otolaryngol., *3:*42, 1974

LEWISON, E. F.: Breast cancer surgery from Halsted to 1972. Proc. Natl. Cancer Conf., *7:*275, 1973

LEWORTHY, G. W., AND SCHLIESSER, H.: Hearing acuity before and after pharyngeal flap procedure, PRS, *56:*49, 1975

LEY, R.: Digestive complications in patients with severe burns, PRS, *57:*263, 1976. Acta chir. belg., *74:*277, 1975

LI, C. S. *et al*: Primary application of one-stage abdominal tubed pedicle, PRS, *51:*232, 1973. Hand, *4:*184, 1972

LIACOPOULOS-BRIOT, M. *et al*: Comparison of skin allograft rejection and cytotoxic antibody production in two lines of mice genetically selected for "high" and "low" antibody synthesis. Transplantation, *14:*590, 1972

LIAN, E. C. Y.: Iatrogenic platelet dysfunction: emerging peril (with Wolfe), PRS, *55:*602, 1975

LIANDE, V. S.: Modern concepts of indications for tracheotomy. Zh. Ushn. Nos. Gorl. Bolezn., *33:*69, 1973 (Russian)

LICHSTEIN, E. *et al*: Diagonal earlobe crease: prevalence and implications as coronary risk factor, PRS, *54:*371, 1974. New England J. Med., *290:*615, 1974

LICHTFELD, P. L. M., AND SNOW, G. B.: Reconstruction by skin flaps in head and neck region, PRS, *54:*117, 1974. Arch. chir. neerl., *25:*379, 1973

LICHTI, E. L. *et al*: Wound fluid zinc levels during tissue repair. Sequential determination by surgically implanted Teflon cylinders, PRS, *49:*588, 1972. Am. J. Surg., *121:*665, 1971

LICHTI, E. L., SCHILLING, J. A., AND SHURLEY, H. M.: Wound fluid and plasma zinc levels in rats during tissue repair, PRS, *50:*422, 1972. Am. J. Surg., *123:*253, 1972

LICHTI, E. L., AND ERICKSON, T. G.: Traumatic arteriovenous fistula. Clinical evaluation and intraoperative monitoring with Doppler ultrasonic flowmeter, PRS, *54:*505, 1974. Am. J. Surg., *127:*333, 1974

LICHTIGER, B., MACKAY, B., AND TESSEMER, C. F.: Spindle-cell variant of squamous carcinoma, PRS, *48:*199, 1971. Cancer, *26:*1311,

1970

LICHTVELD, P. L. M., AND SNOW, G. B.: Reconstruction by skin flaps in head and neck region, PRS, *54:*117, 1974. Arch. chir. neerl., *25:*379, 1973

LIE, J. T., GORDON, L. P., AND TITUS, J. L.: Juvenile temporal arteritis, PRS, *57:*757, 1976. J.A.M.A., *234:*496, 1975

LIESCHKE, H. J. *et al*: Placing saphenous vein graft into upper arm — new cosmetic and rehabilitation method for patients under chronic hemodialysis. Z. Gesamte. Inn. Med., *28:*364, 1973 (German)

LIEVANO, A.: Neurovascular island flap, PRS, *49:*471, 1972. Rev. Latino Am. cir. plast., *15:*33, 1971

LIGHTERMAN, I.: Silicone granuloma of penis, PRS, *57:*517, 1976

LILDHOLDT, T., AND SOGAARD, H.: Metastasizing basal cell carcinoma, PRS, *57:*678, 1976. Scand. J. Plast. Reconstr. Surg., *9:*170, 1975

LILJEDAHL, S. O.: Treatment of burns at Karolinska Hospital. Int. J. Vitam. Nutr. Res., *12:*184, 1972 (German)

LILJEDAHL, S. O., FRIS, A., AND WICKMAN, K.: Successful treatment of candida septicemia in severely burned patients with new antimycotic, Clotrimazole (Bay b 5097), PRS, *52:*101, 1973. Injury, *4:*157, 1972

LILLA, J. A., AND VISTNES, L. M.: Long-term study of reactions to various silicone breast implants in rabbits, PRS, *57:*637, 1976

LILLY, J. R., AND PECK, C. A.: Immediate heterografting of burns in children, PRS, *55:*252, 1975. J. Pediat. Surg., *9:*335, 1974

LILY, N. R.: Re-vascularization of a free skin autograft. Acta Chir. Acad. Sci. Hung., *12:*181, 1971

LILY, N. R.: Re-innervation of a free skin autograft. Acta Chir. Acad. Sci. Hung., *12:*237, 1971

LIM, R. C. *et al*: Platelet response and coagulation changes following massive blood replacement, PRS, *53:*690, 1974. J. Trauma, *13:*577, 1973

LIMB REPLANTATION RESEARCH GROUP, FIRST TEACHING HOSPITAL, HUMAN MEDICAL COLLEGE: Autotransplantation of amputated finger, PRS, *53:*487, 1974. Chinese M.J., *8:*110, 1973

LIMBERG, A. A.: Eyebrow reconstruction with free transplantation of small grafts of hairy skin with subcutaneous fat layer. Vestn. Khir., *106:*64, 1972 (Russian)

LIMBERG, A. A. *et al*: Results of the complex treatment of facial deformities, bite disorders after congenital unilateral cleft lip and palate, and surgery. Vestn. Khir., *111:*105, 1973

LIMONGELLI, W. A. *et al*: Suppurative osteomyelitis of mandible secondary to fracture, PRS, *56:*353, 1975. Oral Surg., *38:*850, 1974

LIN, S. R. *et al:* Neurilemmoma of facial nerve. Neuroradiology, *6:*185, 1973

LINARES, H. A.: Is it possible to modify evolution of hypertrophic scars? PRS, *55:*517, 1975. Rev. Latino Am. cir. plast., *17:*51, 1973

LINARES, H. A. *et al:* Origin of hypertrophic scar, PRS, *53:*495, 1974. J. Trauma, *13:*70, 1973

LINCLAU, L. A., AND HOLOLTCHEFF, I. J.: Wrist arthrodesis: indication and result, PRS, *57:*118, 1976. Nederl. tijdschr. geneesk., *119:*697, 1975

LIND, B.: Tracheotomy material. Tidsskr. Nor. Laegeforen, *93:*2380, 1973 (Norwegian)

LINDAHL, F.: Papillary thyroid carcinoma in Denmark 1943–68. II. Treatment and survival. Acta Chir. Scand., *14:*504, 1975

LINDAU, M.: Unusual case in ambulatory practice. Dtsch. Stomatol., *23:*861, 1973 (German)

LINDBERG, R. D. *et al:* Surgery and postoperative radiotherapy in the treatment of soft tissue sarcomas in adults. Am. J. Roentgenol. Radium Ther. Nucl. Med., *123:*123, 1975

LINDENAUER, S. M.: Congenital arteriovenous fistula and Klippel-Trenaunay syndrome, PRS, *50:*200, 1972. Ann. Surg., *174:*248, 1971

LINDER, L., AND LUNDSKOG, J.: Incorporation of stainless steel, titanium and Vitallium in bone, PRS, *57:*266, 1976. Injury, *6:*277, 1975

LINDER, L. E.: Relationship of midface fractures to mandibular fractures in various forms of trauma: study of 4,015 cases, PRS, *53:*105, 1974. Mil. Med., *138:*487, 1973

LINDFORS, O. *et al:* Exstrophy of the bladder. Fifty years' survival following cystosigmoidostomy. Case report. Scand. J. Urol. Nephrol., *9:*282, 1975

LINDGREN, T. W. *et al:* Body image scale for evaluating transsexuals. Arch. Sex. Behav., *4:*639, 1975

LINDGREN, V. V., AND CARLIN, G. A.: Preventing pulled-down or deformed earlobe in rhytidectomies, PRS, *51:*598, 1973

LINDHOLM, H.: Phoniatric speech evaluation after velopharyngoplasty. A clinical study of 82 cleft palate patients. Scand. J. Plast. Reconstr. Surg., *5:*47, 1971

LINDORF, H. H.: Wound closure of skin incisions using tissue adhesives. Dtsch. Zahnaerztl. Z., *28:*1131, 1973 (German)

LINDORF, H. H.: New incision technics for apicoectomy. Zahnaerztl. Z., *29:*1036, 1974 (German)

LINDSAY, W. K.: Forces and directions in future of plastic surgery, PRS, *48:*303, 1971

LINDSAY, W. K.: Evaluation of adults with re-

paired bilateral cleft lips and palates (with Birch), PRS, *48:*457, 1971

LINDSAY, W. K.: Results of tenolysis, controlled evaluation in chickens (with Hurst, McCain), PRS, *52:*171, 1973

LINDSAY, W. K.: Discussion of "Treatment of respiratory obstruction in micrognathia by use of nasogastric tube," by McEvitt, PRS, *52:*306, 1973

LINDSAY, W. K.: Morphology of adult face following repair of unilateral cleft lip and palate in childhood (with Farkas), PRS, *52:*652, 1973

LINDSAY, W. K.: Surgical repair of cleft palate. Clin. Plast. Surg., *2:*309, 1975

LINDSAY, W. K., AND FARKAS, L. G.: Use of anthropometry in assessing cleft-lip nose, PRS, *49:*286, 1972

LINDSTROM, J. *et al:* Long-term treatment and prognosis of malignant tumors of nasopharynx. O.R.L., *37:*103, 1975

LINK, W. J. *et al:* Wound healing of mouse skin incised with plasma scalpel, PRS, *54:*113, 1974. J. Surg. Res., *14:*505, 1973

LINK, W. J., ZOOK, E. G., AND GLOVER, J. L.: Plasma scalpel excision of burns, PRS, *55:*657, 1975

LINKE, C. A. *et al:* Harvesting, preservation and transportation of cadaver kidneys, PRS, *50:*539, 1972. J. Urol., *107:*184, 1972

LINKNER, L. M. *et al:* Prevention of bacterial growth and local infection in burn wounds. J. Pediatr. Surg., *7:*310, 1972

LINKOUS, C. M., AND WELCH, J. T.: Metastatic malignant tumors of jaw, PRS, *56:*365, 1975. Oral Surg., *38:*703, 1974

LINKOW, L. I.: Pterygoid extension implant for totally and partially edentulous maxillae. Int. J. Orthod., *12:*9, 1974

LINSCHEID, R. L. *et al:* Rheumatoid arthritis of the wrist. Orthop. Clin. North Am., *2:*649, 1971

LINSCHEID, R. L. *et al:* Common and uncommon infections of the hand. Orthop. Clin. North Am., *6:*1063, 1975

LINZ, A. M. *et al:* Blow-in fracture of the lateral wall of the orbit. Trans. Int. Conf. Oral Surg., *4:*306, 1973

Lipodystrophy (See also *Esthetic Surgery*)

Fat in the sacroiliac region, topography of (Georgiadis, Katsas), PRS, *49:*110, 1972. Acta Chir. Hellenica, *18:*289, 1971

Progressive lipodystrophy (Hussels). Birth Defects, *7:*299, 1971

Inguinocrural cutaneous flaccidity (Spadafora, Toledo Rios, De Los Rios), PRS, *49:*233, 1972. Prensa med. argent., *58:*1393, 1971

Lipodystrophy, progressive, free adipodermal

Lipodystrophy – Cont.

grafts in surgical treatment of (Sokolova), PRS, *52:*686, 1973. Acta chir. plast., *14:*157, 1972

Dermolipectomies crurales (Pitanguy). Ann. chir. plast., *17:*40, 1972 (French)

Dermolipectomies, crural, technic and indications for (Ducourtioux). Ann. chir. plast., *17:*204, 1972 (French)

Lipodystrophy, generalized, failure of hypophysectomy in (Mabry *et al.*) J. Pediatr., *81:*990, 1972

Barraker-Simmons disease (Gubaidulina *et al*). Stomatologiia (Mosk.), *51:*86, 1972 (Russian)

Cruro-femoro-gluteal or circumgluteal plasty (Delerm, Cirotteau). Ann. chir. plast., *18:*31, 1973 (French)

Lipodystrophy, partial, silicone treatment of (Rees, Coburn), PRS, *55:*505, 1975. J.A.M.A., *230:*868, 1974

Lipomatosis and lipodystrophy, nosography of, in light of present criticism (Lupo *et al*), PRS, *57:*683, 1976. Riv. ital. chir. plast., *6:*135, 1974

Technic and indications for crural dermolipectomies (Ducourtioux). Ann. chir. plast., *17:*204, 1975 (French)

Treatment of steatomery in the female: theory and practice (Vilain). Ann. chir. plast., *20:*135, 1975 (French)

Abdominal lipectomy (Pitanguy). Clin. Plast. Surg., *2:*401, 1975

Abdominal dermolipectomies (Regnault). Clin. Plast. Surg., *2:*411, 1975

Some considerations in surgical alteration of the feminine silhouette (Vilain). Clin. Plast. Surg., *2:*449, 1975

Surgical correction of steatomeries (Vilain). Clin. Plast. Surg., *2:*467, 1975

Correction of lipodystrophy of the lateral thoracic aspect and inner side of the arm and elbow dermosenescence (Pitanguy). Clin. Plast. Surg., *2:*477, 1975

Pitanguy method of correction of trochanteric lipodystrophy, experience with (Hoffman, Simon), PRS, *55:*551, 1975

Lipoma

Lipomas of upper extremity (Phalen, Kendrick, Rodriquez), PRS, *48:*512, 1971. Am. J. Surg., *121:*298, 1971

Extensor tendon rupture, Madelung's deformity with (Schulstad), PRS, *49:*583, 1972. Scand. J. Plast. Reconstr. Surg., *5:*153, 1971

Lipomatosis, benign, symmetrical (Szabo *et al*). Orv. Hetil., *113:*2652, 1972 (Hungarian)

Lipoma – Cont.

Launois-Bensaude adenolipomatosis (Springer, Whitehouse), PRS, *50:*291, 1972

Advanced laryngeal compression due to diffuse symmetric lipomatosis (Madelung's disease) (Birnholz *et al*). Brit. J. Radiol., *46:*245, 1973

Lipoma, unusual case in ambulatory practice (Lindau). Dtsch. Stomatol., *23:*861, 1973 (German)

Lipoma, giant, of back and neck (Hirshowitz, Goldan), PRS, *52:*312, 1973

Adenolipomatosis, symmetrical. Two cases (Vaillant *et al*). Rev. Stomatol. Chir. Maxillofac., *74:*125, 1973 (French)

Lipoid proteinosis, successful surgical treatment of (Buchan *et al*). Brit. J. Dermatol., *90:*561, 1974

Fibrolipoma of the palate: report of two cases (Stewart *et al*). N.Y. State Dent. J., *40:*603, 1974

Lipomas: axillary breasts (Kaye), PRS, *53:*61, 1974

Lipoma, cause of paralysis of deep radial (posterior interosseous) nerve (Wu, Jordan, Eckert), PRS, *54:*508, 1974. Surgery, *75:*790, 1974

Case report on lipomatosis dolorosa (dercum) (Schwerdtner). Z. Gesamte Inn. Med., *29:*726, 1974 (German)

Oral lipofibromas (Dybkowska-Klos). Czas. Stomatol., *28:*987, 1975 (Polish)

Madelung's disease, benign symmetrical lipomatosis (Schuler, Graham, Horton). PRS, *57:*663, 1976

Lip Pits, Congenital

Lip pits with cleft lip and palate (Palubis *et al*). Birth Defects, *7:*254, 1971

Congenital lip pits with cleft lip or palate (Tan *et al*). J. Singapore Paediatr. Soc., *13:*75, 1971

Sinuses, congenital lower lip, surgical repair (Bowers). PRS, *49:*632, 1972

Lips (See also Lips, Deformity of; Lips, Neoplasms, etc.)

Method of primary reconstruction of nose and upper lip (Zehm). Arch. Klin. Exp. Ohren Nasen Kehlkopfheilkd., *199:*638, 1971 (German)

Theory and practice of free composite graft (Soeda). Jap. J. Plast. Reconstr. Surg., *14:*97, 1971 (Japanese)

Congenital lip sinuses of the lower lip: report of case (Zallen). J. Oral Surg., *29:*732, 1971

Congenital lip pits with cleft lip or palate (Tan *et al*). J. Singapore Paediatr. Soc., *13:*75, 1971

Lips — Cont.

Microscopic observations on the course of muscles and the construction of the upper lip of man (Plenk *et al*). Verh. Anat. Ges., *65:*341, 1971 (German)

Elastic fibers around sebaceous glands in the human lips (Kostowiecki *et al*). Z. Mikrosk. Anat. Forsch., *84:*385, 1971

Electric burns of the mouth in children (Mladick). Arch. Dermat., *105:*296, 1972

Further applications of the rotation advancement technique (Saad *et al*). Brit. J. Plast. Surg., *25:*116, 1972

Naso-labial full thickness graft (Beare *et al*). Brit. J. Plast. Surg., *25:*315, 1972

Foreign objects in the lip (Pavek). Cesk. Stomatol., *72:*41, 1972 (Czech)

Unusual injuries of soft tissues of the lower lip during work (Veverka *et al*). Cesk. Stomatol., *72:*46, 1972 (Czech)

Proportioned philtrum: a helpful measurement and ratio (Franz *et al*). Cleft Palate J., *9:*143, 1972

Electrosurgical correction of maxillary double lip (Peterson). Dent. Dig., *78:*182, 1972

Nasolabial flap in reconstruction of the nose (Burnam). J. Fla. Med. Assoc., *59:*32, 1972

Thermal trauma: a review of 22 electrical burns of the lip (Gormley *et al*). J. Oral Surg., *30:*531, 1972

Lip incompetency and its treatment (Miller). N.Y. State Dent. J., *38:*210, 1972

Lip, dog bite avulsions of, conservative concept (Musgrave, Garrett). PRS, *49:*294, 1972

Hair lip, traumatic, or complications of moustache (Shepard, Melvin, Kleinert). PRS, *49:*346, 1972

Upper lip, restoring the overhang in repairs to oral commissure (Wall, Cameron, Latham), PRS, *49:*626, 1972

Lip, lower, total reconstruction with bilateral Estlander flaps (Murray). PRS, *49:*658, 1972

Lip defects, lower, double-V excision for better repair (Hirshowitz). PRS, *50:*153, 1972

Labial flap for reconstruction of the anterior oral cavity (Schwartz *et al*). Surg. Gynec. & Obst., *135:*276, 1972

Lip and palate, acquired fissures of (Pitanguy, Lessa, Garcia), PRS, *54:*687, 1974. Rev. brasil. cir., *63:*317, 1973

Cheiloplasty (lip repair) performed by new method (Stein) (Classic Reprint). PRS, *53:*332, 1974

Reconstitution of lip, tongue and glottis function (Schmid). Acta Stomatol. Belg., *72:*301, 1975 (German)

Cheiloplasty of thin lips. Proposal of a tech-

Lips — Cont.

nic (Delerm *et al*). Ann. chir. plast., *20:*243, 1975 (French)

Lateral congenital sinus of the upper lip (Mahler *et al*). Brit. J. Plast. Surg., *28:*203, 1975

Orbicularis oris muscle, study of development (Fernandez Villoria). PRS, *55:*205, 1975

Lips, patulous: serious implications of multiple mucosal neuromata (Bowers). PRS, *56:*554, 1975

Cryosurgery in dermatologic office practice: special reference to dermatofibroma and mucous cyst of the lip (Spiller *et al*). South. Med. J., *68:*157, 1975

Modified lip stripping with reconstruction of a new vermilion border (Friedlander). N.Y. State Dent. J., *42:*27, 1976

Lips, Cross-Lip Flap: See *Cross-Lip Flap*

Lips, Deformity of (See also *Cleft Lip; Facial Clefts*)

Lip defects, lower, bipedicled V-Y flap technique for primary repair of (Hollmann), PRS, *48:*391, 1971. Acta chir. plast., *12:*223, 1970

Lip, lower, plastic reconstruction following neoplastic exeresis (Bocchiotti, Colonna, Fumarola). Cancro, *24:*197, 1971 (Italian)

Corner of mouth, new method of elongating (Fernandez Villoria). PRS, *49:*52, 1972

Angle of mouth, *orbicularis* advancement flap for restoration of (Converse). PRS, *49:*99, 1972

Lip, lower, congenital sinuses, surgical repair of (Bowers). PRS, *49:*632, 1972

Lip, lower, reconstruction after extensive total amputation (Fumarola). Ann. chir. plast., *18:*79, 1973 (French)

Lip, lower, prominent inferior labial artery (Howell, Freeman), PRS, *52:*678, 1973. Arch. Dermat., *107:*386, 1973

Lip, lower, one-stage reconstruction of whole (Olivari). Brit. J. Plast. Surg., *26:*66, 1973

Lip, lower, reconstruction of after central excisions (Bretteville-Jensen). Brit. J. Plast. Surg., *26:*247, 1973

Lip, defects of vermilion border of, innervated muco-muscular flap for correction of (Watson). Brit. J. Plast. Surg., *26:*355, 1973

Surgical correction of labium duplex by W-plasty (Czeti). Fogorv. Sz., *66:*186, 1973 (Hungarian)

Lips: acquired *cheilitis glandularis simplex* (Epinette, Hurwitz). PRS, *51:*334, 1973

Lip, upper, congenital midline sinus of (Bar-

Lips, Deformity of—Cont.

tels, Howard). PRS, *52:*665, 1973

Lip, lower, and chin, immediate reconstruction of, following total resection for extensive cancer (Bullens). Acta Stomatol. Belg., *71:*63, 1974 (Dutch)

Cheilitis granulomatosa. Melkersson-Rosenthal syndrome (Rintala *et al*), PRS, *54:*687, 1974. Scand. J. Plast. Reconstr. Surg., *7:*130, 1974

Lips, transposition of, for correction of facial paralysis (Pickrell, Puckett, Peters). PRS, *57:*427, 1976

Lips, Esthetic Surgery of

Lips, too thick and double (Klasen), PRS, *48:*195, 1971. Nederl. tijdschr. geneesk., *115:*408, 1971

Lip, surgical procedures for improvement of esthetics (Stellmach). Zahnaerztl. Prax., *24:*237, 1973 (German)

Lips, Neoplasms

Carcinoma of lips—reparative plasties (O'Conor), PRS, *48:*194, 1971. Bull. Acad. Argent. Cir., *54:*542, 1970

Basal cell carcinoma of the lips. Occurrence, localization, sex and age distribution (Geisenhainer). Hautarzt, *21:*167, 1970 (German)

Unusual clinical course of squamous cell carcinoma of the lower lip (Mordovtsev). Vestn. Dermatol. Venerol., *44:*66, 1970 (Russian)

Lip, upper, malignant tumors of, and perialar semilunar excision (De Dulanto *et al*). Actas Dermosifiliogr., *62:*371, 1971 (Spanish)

Epidermoid carcinoma of the lip after renal transplantation. Report of two cases (Berger *et al*). Arch. Intern. Med., *128:*609, 1971

Lip reconstruction employing lingual flap (Carvalhal Franca), PRS, *49:*102, 1972. Assoc. med. Brasil, *17:*123, 1971

Oral carcinoma in the aged edentulous patient. A review of seven case histories (Ettinger). Aust. Dent. J., *16:*275, 1971

Keratoacanthoma on the lips (Hardman). Brit. J. Oral Surg., *9:*46, 1971

Lip, lower, plastic reconstruction following neoplastic exeresis (Bocchiotti, Colonna, Fumarola). Cancro, *24:*197, 1971 (Italian)

Rare case of pleomorphic rhabdomyosarcoma of the lower lip (Lentrodt). Dtsch. Zahn. Mund. Kieferheilkd., *57:*97, 1971 (German)

Actinic chronic cheilitis and its relations to epitheliomas of the lower lip (Serra). G.

Lips, Neoplasms—Cont.

Ital. Dermatol., *46:*397, 1971 (Italian)

On two cases of Spitz-Allen juvenile melanoma (Mariotti *et al*). G. Ital. Dermatol., *46:*497, 1971 (Italian)

Precancerous states of the vermilion border of the lower lip. Value of preventive vermilionectomy (Marchac *et al*). J. Fr. Otorhinolaryngol., *20:*1029, 1971 (French)

Lip, lower, reconstruction after tumor resection combined with radical neck dissection (Lentrodt, Luhr), PRS, *48:*579, 1971

Technic of cheiloplasty for extensive lip cancers (Hugues *et al*). Presse Med., *79:*1690, 1971 (French)

Cancer, lip, lower, cheiloplasty after surgical excision of (Timosca *et al*). Rev. Med. Chir. Soc. Med. Nat. Iasi., *75:*909, 1971 (Rumanian)

De novo malignant tumors in organ transplant recipients (Penn *et al*). Transplant Proc., *3:*773, 1971

Late results of low-voltage roentgen therapy and spontaneous regression of cutaneous hemangiomas in children (Svistunova *et al*). Vopr. Onkol., *17:*99, 1971 (Russian)

Vermilionectomy (Soubiran). Actual Odontostomatol. (Paris), *26:*501, 1972

Surgical management of premaxillary malignancy. Report of three cases (Tucker *et al*). Arch. Otolaryng., *95:*42, 1972

Cancer of the lip at risk (Wilson *et al*). Brit. J. Oral Surg., *9:*186, 1972

Cancer, extensive, lower lip, simple total and partial cheiloplasty for (Mrovec). Cesk. Otolaryngol., *21:*296, 1972 (Czechoslovakian)

Lip carcinoma, clinical studies on (Buder, Pape). Deutsche Stomatol., *22:*746, 1972 (German)

Methods of repair of the lower lip (Francesconi *et al*). G. Ital. Dermatol., *47:*20, 1972 (Italian)

Lip tumors, role of surgery in treatment of, 32 cases (Abbes *et al*). J. Fr. Otorhinolaryngol., *21:*640, 1972 (French)

Adenoid squamous cell carcinoma of the lip: report of cases (Tomich *et al*). J. Oral Surg., *30:*592, 1972

Primary multiple malignant neoplasms of the organs of the digestive system (Kirichenko *et al*). Khirurgiia (Mosk.), *48:*54, 1972 (Russian)

Cancer of the lip (Yonkers *et al*). Laryngoscope, *82:*625, 1972

Acinic cell adenocarcinoma of minor salivary gland origin (Trodahl). Mil. Med., *137:*234, 1972

Cancer, lip, problem of metastases (Durkov-

Lips, Neoplasms – Cont.

sky *et al*). Neoplasma, *19:*653, 1972

Distant cutaneous metastases in a patient with squamous-cell carcinoma of the lip (Bordin *et al*). Oral Surg., *34:*445, 1972

Double-V excision for better repair of lower lip defects (Hirshowitz), PRS, *50:*153, 1972

Squamous cell carcinoma in discoid lupus erythematosus (Gwiezdzinski *et al*). Przegl. Dermatol., *59:*37, 1972 (Polish)

Case of labio-mental hemangiopericytoma (Cadenat *et al*). Rev. Stomatol. Chir. Maxillofac., *73:*49, 1972 (French)

Diagnostic errors in lip neoplasms (Volkov). Sov. Med., *35:*142, 1972 (Russian)

Lips, cancer of, surgical treatment (Makres *et al*). Stomatologia (Athenai), *29:*321, 1972 (Greek)

Mechanical measurement of tension after square and wedge excision on lower lip tumors (Ivankievicz *et al*). Z.W.R., *81:*176, 1972 (German)

Carcinoma, lip. Series of 869 patients (Jorgensen). Acta Otolaryngol. (Stockh.), *75:*312, 1973

Lip carcinoma. Series of 869 cases (Jorgensen *et al*). Acta Radiol. (Ther.) (Stockh.)., *12:*177, 1973

Surgical treatment of lower lip and commissure cancer (Kotyza). Cesk. Otolaryngol., *22:*100, 1973 (Czechoslovakian)

Tumor of lower lip, technique for immediate reconstruction after ablation (Meyer, Shapiro), PRS, *53:*241, 1974. Chir. Plast., *2:*1, 1973

Lower lip tumors, mechanical study of tension following quadrate- and wedge-excision of (Ivankievicz *et al*). Fogorv. Sz., *66:*164, 1973 (Hungarian)

Lip reconstruction after tumor resection, advantages of basic concept (Fries), PRS, *52:*452, 1973. J. Maxillo-facial Surg., *1:*13, 1973

Cancer, lip, surgical treatment: recommendations for therapy in rural population (Grantham *et al*). J. Okla. State Med. Assoc., *66:*451, 1973

Lip, bilateral granular cell myoblastoma of, case report (Slavkin *et al*). J. Oral Surg., *31:*848, 1973

Lip, upper, basal cell adenoma of. Report of case (Bollinger *et al*). Oral Surg., *35:*600, 1973

Cancer of lower lip, on etiology of (Ju), PRS, *52:*151, 1973

Cancer, lip, lower, new surgical method for removal of (Shaaban). Syria Dent. J., *9:*7, 1973 (Arabic)

Lip cancer (Rygard *et al*). Ugeskr. Laeger,

Lips, Neoplasms – Cont.

*135:*1866, 1973 (Danish)

Lip, lower, small cancerous lesions of, how to improve surgical treatment of (Franchebois). Union Med. Can., *102:*1558, 1973 (French)

Clinical aspects and treatment of precancerous state in lower lips (Schonberger *et al*). Z. Aerztl. Fortbild. (Jena), *67:*69, 1973 (German)

Place of surgery in the treatment of carcinomas of the oral cavity (Mendes da Costa *et al*). Acta Chir. Belg., *73:*529, 1974 (French)

Lip cancer: surgical management (Beckman *et al*). Am. J. Surg., *128:*732, 1974

Historical form of cancer of the lower lip (Laffole *et al*). Ann. Otolaryngol. Chir. Cervicofac., *91:*325, 1974 (French)

Carcinoma, lip plug, consideration of aetiology of, with special reference to local geographical tumor incidence (Cubey). Brit. J. Cancer, *30:*95, 1974

Radical neck dissection in advanced tumors of the head and neck. Considerations on 52 cases (Caldarola *et al*). Cancro, *27:*187, 1974 (Italian)

Surgical grand rounds. Carcinoma of lip (Beal). Ill. Med. J., *146:*462, 1974

Basal cell adenoma of intraoral minor salivary gland origin (Strychalski). J. Oral Surg., *32:*595, 1974

Lip tumors, cryosurgery of (Trushkevich *et al*). Klin. Khir., *10:*54, 1974 (Russian)

Repair of defects in the cheeks and lips (Haas). Laryngol. Rhinol. Otol. (Stuttg.), *53:*695, 1974 (German)

Causes of recurrences of lip cancer and their treatment (Svistunov). Med. Radiol. (Mosk.), *19:*67, 1974 (Russian)

Carcinoma, lower lip, extensive cornifying, special clinical form (Kulakowski *et al*). Nowotwory, *24:*201, 1974 (Polish)

Carcinoma, lip. Analysis of material of 25 years (Molnar *et al*). Oncology, *29:*101, 1974

Carcinoma, squamous cell, adenoid, of lower lip vermilion mucosa (Weitzner). Oral Surg., *37:*589, 1974

Lip, lower, keratoacanthoma of (Azaz, Lustman), PRS, *56:*234, 1975. Oral Surg., *38:*918, 1974

Lip: reconstruction of philtrum with auricular composite grafts (Psillakis, Kamakura, Spina), PRS, *56:*676, 1975. Rev. Asoc. med. Brasil, *20:*297, 1974

Lip, lower, immediate reconstruction in primary tumors of (Silla), PRS, *57:*671, 1976. Riv. ital. chir. plast., *6:*257, 1974

Surgical treatment of non-traumatic lower

Lips, Neoplasms – Cont.

lip lesions with special reference to the step technique. A follow-up on 149 patients (Johanson *et al*). Scand. J. Plast. Reconstr. Surg., *8:*232, 1974

Carcinoma of lip (Creely, Peterson), PRS, *55:*106, 1975. South. M. J., *67:*779, 1974

The so-called eosinophilic soft-tissue granuloma (Castrup *et al*). Strahlentherapie, *148:*139, 1974 (German)

Surgical treatment of advanced carcinoma of the lower lip (Kowalik). Wiad. Lek., *27:*1974 (Polish)

Cancer, lower lip, in initial stages, treatment of (Protopopov *et al*). Vopr. Onkol., *20:*96, 1974 (Russian)

Lip, lower, reconstruction of corners of mouth after resection of (Manuylenko), PRS, *57:*756, 1976. Acta chir. plast., *17:*38, 1975

Systematic technic in the primary reconstruction of tissue loss in the mouth after excision of cancer (Fries *et al*). Acta Stomatol. Belg., *72:*443, 1975 (German)

Head and neck cancer manpower study (Strong *et al*). Am. J. Surg., *129:*273, 1975

Analysis of mortality and morbidity in 100 composite resections for oral carcinoma (Robins *et al*). Am. J. Surg., *130:*178, 1975

Cancer, lip, electroneurophysiology in control of reparative surgery of (Cocero *et al*). Arch. Neurobiol. (Madr.), *37:*31, 1974 (Spanish)

Carcinoma, lip-plug, and its management by modified Abbe flap (Cubey). Brit. J. Plast. Surg., *28:*80, 1975

Surgical treatment of lower lip carcinoma with simultaneous plastic reconstruction of tissue defect (Soltan). Czas. Stomatol., *28:*1089, 1975 (Polish)

Cancer of lower lip, improved surgical treatment of (Franchebois), PRS, *56:*461, 1975. Internat. Surg., *60:*204, 1975

Lip, lower, reconstruction after tumor resection combined with neck dissection (Lentrodt), PRS, *57:*529, 1976. J. Maxillo-facial Surg., *3:*139, 1975

Contribution to the primary reconstruction of the upper lip and labial commissure following tumour excision (Zisser). J. Maxillofacial Surg., *3:*211, 1975

Fibrous histiocytoma of the lip: report of a case (Hillis *et al*). J. Oral Med., *30:*81, 1975

Simple probe for cryosurgical therapy for hemangiomas (Hickory *et al*). J. Oral Surg., *33:*546, 1975

Congenital granular-cell myoblastoma (Cussen, Mahon), PRS, *56:*472, 1975. J. Pediat. Surg., *10:*249, 1975

Lips, Neoplasms – Cont.

Cervical-pectoral flaps in the treatment of advanced oral cancer (Shons *et al*). J. Surg. Oncol., *7:*213, 1975

Mixed tumors of oral cavity. Report of two cases (Friedman *et al*). N.Y. State Dent. J., *41:*154, 1975

Basal-cell carcinoma of the vermilion mucosa and skin of the lip (Weitzner). Oral Surg., *39:*634, 1975

Lip reconstruction following resection for unusual basal cell carcinoma (Kelly, Klein), PRS, *57:*539, 1976. Oral Surg., *40:*19, 1975

An original method of plastic surgery after treatment of cancer of the lower lip by resection (Urtila). Rev. Stomatol. Chir. Maxillofac., *76:*579, 1975 (French)

Lip, lower, reconstruction through chin flap (Tomasoni), PRS, *57:*756, 1976 (Italian). Riv. ital. chir. plast., *7:*403, 1975

Carcinoma of the lower lip (Brozman). Rozhl. Chir., *54:*430, 1975 (Slovakian)

Clinical assessment of final results in the treatment of metastases of cancer of the lower lip (Tazuev). Stomatologiia (Mosk.), *54:*40, 1975 (Russian)

Recurrences and metastases of cancer of the lower lip (Protopopov *et al*). Vopr. Onkol., *21:*83, 1975 (Russian)

Results of therapy of lip neoplasms from a radiotherapeutic point of view (Kob *et al*). Zahn. Mund. Kieferheilkd., *63:*473, 1975 (German)

Technic and direct results of cryosurgery of lip cancer (Trushkevich *et al*). Stomatologiia (Mosk.), *55:*37, 1976 (Russian)

Lips, Paralysis of (See also *Facial Paralysis*)

Sphincter, lax oral, in facial paralysis, late reconstruction of (Freeman). PRS, *51:*144, 1973

Masseter muscle rotation in treatment of inferior facial paralysis (Correia, Zani). PRS, *52:*370, 1973

Paralysis, unilateral, of lower lip, dynamic correction of (Puckett, Neale, Pickrell). PRS, *55:*397, 1975

Mouth, corner of, "over and out" flap for restoration of (Converse). PRS, *56:*575, 1975

Face, paralysis of, transposition of lips for correction of (Pickrell, Puckett, Peters). PRS, *57:*427, 1976

Lips, Reconstruction of (See also *Cross-Lip Flap; Lips, Neoplasms*)

Lingual flap for lip reconstruction (Carvalhal Franca), PRS, *49:*102, 1972. Assoc. med. Brasil, *17:*123, 1971

Tumor resection combined with radical neck

Plast. Surg., *27:*59, 1974

LISTON, R.: Closure of cleft palate (Classic Reprint). PRS, *48:*167, 1971

LISTON, R.: Cleft palate – velosynthesis (Classic Reprint). PRS, *48:*366, 1971

LITTENBERG, R. L. *et al*: Gallium 76 for localization of septic lesions, PRS, *54:*512, 1974. Ann. Int. Med., *77:*403, 1973

LITTLE, J. H. *et al*: Frozen section diagnosis of suspected malignant melanoma of the skin. Cancer, *34:*1163, 1974

LITTLE, J. M. *et al*: Incidence of the hypothenar hammer syndrome. Arch. Surg., *104:*684, 1972

LITTLE, J. M. *et al*: Hypothenar hammer syndrome. M. J. Australia, *1:*49, 1972

LITTLE, J. M. *et al*: Circulatory patterns in the normal hand. Brit. J. Surg., *60:*652, 1973

LITTLE, J. M. *et al*: Effects of radial artery cannulation. M. J. Australia, *2:*791, 1975

LITTLER, J. W.: On the adaptability of man's hand (with reference to the equiangular curve). Hand, *5:*187, 1973

LITTLER, J. William: *Symposium on Reconstructive Hand Surgery*. C. V. Mosby Co., St. Louis, 1974

LITTLEWOOD, M., AND MURRAY, D. S.: Clinical trial of cutaneous malignancies, PRS, *55:*116, 1975. Brit. J. Plast. Surg. *26:*140, 1973

LITTON, C., FOURNIER, P., AND CAPINPIN, A.: Survey of chemical peeling of face, PRS, *51:*645, 1973

LITTON, W. B. *et al*: Surgical management of carcinoma of the oral cavity. Otolaryngol. Clin. North Am., *5:*303, 1972

LITWILLER, O. B.: Globulomaxillary cyst treated by marsupialization. Dent. Radiogr. Photogr., *48:*42, 1975

LITWIN, M. S.: Comparison of effects of dextran 70 and dextran 40 in postoperative animals, PRS, *50:*100, 1972. Surgery, *71:*295, 1972

LITWIN, M. S.: Laser photocoagulation. Panminerva Med., *16:*29, 1974

LIVERSEDGE, R. L.: Oral malignant melanoma, PRS, *57:*678, 1976. Brit. J. Oral Surg., *13:*40, 1975

LIVINGSTON, R. J. *et al*: Treatment of orbital fractures by infraorbital-transantral approach. J. Oral Surg., *33:*586, 1975

LiVOLSI, V. A. *et al*: Carcinoma arising in median ectopic thyroid (including thyroglossal duct tissue). Cancer, *34:*1303, 1974

LLADO OLIVAR, B.: Mucosal and cutaneous fistulas of dental and salivary origin. An. Esp. Odontoestomatol., *33:*385, 1974 (Spanish)

LLOYD, G. A. *et al*: Intubation macrodacryocystography. Brit. J. Ophthalmol., *56:*600, 1972

LLOYD, G. A. *et al*: Subtraction macrodacryocystography. Brit. J. Radiol., *47:*379, 1974

LLOYD, J. R.: Improved management of skin graft donor sites. Arch. Surg., *108:*561, 1974

LLOYD, L. A.: Craniofacial reconstruction: ocular management of orbital hypertelorism. Trans. Am. Ophthalmol. Soc., *73:*123, 1976

LO, C. J.: Reconstruction of severed ears by implanting cartilage. Chinese Med. J., *54:*714, 1974 (Chinese)

LOCKWOOD, H.: A planning technique for segmental osteotomies. Brit. J. Oral Surg., *12:*102, 1974

LODHA, S. C.: Treatment of pilonidal sinus by "Z" plasty. J. Indian Med. Assoc., *62:*307, 1974

LODOVICI, O.: Congenital anomalies of vagina, PRS, *48:*514, 1971. Rev. Latino Am. cir. plast., *13:*80, 1969

LODOVICI, O.: New reduction mastoplasty technic by bilateral adenomastectomy in treatment of breast hypertrophy. Rev. Assoc. Med. Bras., *20:*240, 1974 (Portuguese)

LODOVICI, O.: Vaginoplasty in intersexual status. Rev. Assoc. Med. Bras., *20:*405, 1974 (Portuguese)

LODOVICI, O.: Indication for the technics of reduction mammoplasties according to the physiopathology of breast hypertrophy. Rev. Hosp. Clin. Fac. Med. Sao Paulo, *29:*300, 1974 (Portuguese)

LODOVICI, O. *et al*: Unusual case of congenital abnormality of the urogenital apparatus associated with exstrophy of the bladder in a female patient. Rev. Assoc. Med. Bras., *20:*374, 1974 (Portuguese)

LOE, F. A. *et al*: Chain saw injury of the mandibulofacial region. J. Oral Surg., *34:*81, 1976

LOEB, R.: Earlobe tailoring during facial rhytidoplasties, PRS, *49:*485, 1972

LOEBL, E. C., BAXTER, C. R., AND CURRERI, W. P.: Mechanisms of erythrocyte destruction in early postburn period, PRS, *54:*112, 1974. Ann. Surg., *178:*681, 1973

LOEBL, E. C. *et al*: Use of quantitative biopsy cultures in bacteriologic monitoring of burn patients, PRS, *55:*114, 1975. J. Surg. Res., *16:*1, 1974

LOEBL, E. C. *et al*: Erythrocyte survival following thermal injury, PRS, *55:*252, 1975. J. Surg. Res., *16:*96, 1974

LOEBL, W. Y.: Mobility of metacarpophalangeal joints in rheumatoid arthritis, PRS, *54:*376, 1974. Hand, *5:*165, 1973

LOERS, F. J. *et al*: Induced hypotension for E. N. T. surgery. Z. Prakt. Anaesth., *8:*232, 1973 (German)

LOEW, D., LANGER, P., AND BOCHUM, K.: Quantitative and qualitative behavior of thrombocytes during scalding shock in rabbit, PRS, *53:*607, 1974. Langenbecks Arch.

Chir., *333:*71, 1973

LOFGREN, K. A.: Stasis ulcer, PRS, *54:*237, 1974. Minnesota Med., *57:*135, 1974

LOFGREN, R. H.: Surgery of the pterygomaxillary fossa. Arch. Otolaryng., *94:*516, 1971

LOGINOV, L. P. *et al*: Dermatomic autoplasty in deep burns. Sov. Med., *34:*52, 1971 (Russian)

LOKICH, J. J., AND FREI, E., III: Phase II study of concurrent methotrexate and bleomycin chemotherapy, PRS, *55:*256, 1975. Cancer Res., *34:*2240, 1974

LOMAKIN, B. N. *et al*: Plastic surgery in burns in the middle-aged and elderly. Khirurgiia, *49:*17, 1972

LOMBARD, J. P.: Benign hypertrophy of masseter muscles, PRS, *56:*593, 1975. Rev. Esp. Estomatogia, *17:*23, 1969

LOMOV-OPPOKOV, Iu. G. *et al*: Salivary calculi in the minor salivary glands. Stomatologiia (Mosk.), *53:*91, 1974 (Russian)

LONG, C., II *et al*: Intrinsic-extrinsic muscle control of the hand in power grip and precision handling. An electromyographic study. J. Bone & Joint Surg. (Am.), *52:*853, 1970

LONG, J. C., AND ELLIS, P. P.: Total unilateral visual loss following orbital surgery, PRS, *49:*662, 1972. Am. J. Ophth., *71:*218, 1971

LONGACRE, J. J.: *Cleft Palate Deformation.* Charles C Thomas, Springfield, Ill., 1970. PRS, *48:*275, 1971

LONGACRE, J. J.: *Scar Tissue, its Use and Abuse: The Surgical Correction of Deformation Due to Hypertrophic Scar and the Prevention of its Formation.* Charles C Thomas, Springfield, Ill., 1972. PRS, *52:*187, 1973

LONGACRE, J. J.: *Rehabilitation of the Facially Disfigured. Prevention of Irreversible Psychic Trauma by Early Reconstruction.* Charles C Thomas Co., Springfield, Ill., 1973. PRS, *54:*93, 1974

LONGACRE, J. J. *et al*: Influence of selecting the time for staphylorraphia upon maxillary and facial growth. Ann. chir. plast., *13:*241, 1968 (French)

LONGACRE, J. J. *et al*: Influence of time selection for palate reflection on phonation development. Ann. chir. plast., *13:*249, 1968 (French)

LONGACRE, J. J., BENTON, C., AND UNTERTHINER, A.: Treatment of facial hemangioma by intravascular embolization with silicone spheres, PRS, *50:*618, 1972

LONGHURST, P.: Submandibular sialolithiasis in child. Brit. Dent. J., *135:*291, 1973

LOPEZ, E. M., AND ARANHA, G. V.: Value of sinography in management of decubitus ulcers, PRS, *53:*208, 1974

LOPEZ, O.: Employment of carica papaya endopeptidase associated with benzidamine in plastic surgery, PRS, *52:*104, 1973. Tribuna Med. Argent., *15:*611, 1972

LOPEZ-ENGELKING, R.: Various aspects of pathology of penis, PRS, *55:*638, 1975. Cir. Cir., *42:*169, 1975

LOPEZ-MAS, J. *et al*: Skin graft pigmentation, new approach to prevention, PRS, *49:*18, 1972

LORD, G. *et al*: Subungual glomus tumors. Nouv. Presse Med., *3:*445, 1974 (French)

LORD, I. J.: Comparison of preoperative and primary radiotherapy in treatment of carcinoma of hypopharynx. Brit. J. Radiol., *46:*175, 1973

LORE, JOHN M., JR.: *An Atlas of Head and Neck Surgery,* Second Edition. W. B. Saunders Co., Philadelphia, 1973. PRS, *54:*94, 1974

LORE, J. M., JR.: Total reconstruction of hypopharynx with tongue flap and dermal graft. Ann. Otol. Rhin. & Laryng., *83:*476, 1974

LORE, J. M., JR.: Partial and radical maxillectomy. Otolaryngol. Clin. North Am., *9:*255, 1976

LORE, J. M., JR., AND ZINGAPAN, E. G.: Deltopectoral flap, PRS, *49:*477, 1972. Arch. Otolaryng., *94:*13, 1971

LORE, J. M., JR. *et al*: External traction for depressed facial fractures. N.Y. State J. Med., *72:*490, 1972

LORTHIOIR, J.: Some special technics in surgery of the hand. Brux. Med., *52:*125, 1972 (French)

LO RUSSO, .D.: Techniques to repair nasal septum perforations, PRS, *53:*681, 1974. Bol. Mal. orecch. gola naso, *88:*184, 1970

LOSCH, G. M.: Proceedings: repair of skin defects in hand injuries. Langenbecks Arch. Chir., *334:*599, 1973 (German)

LOSCH, G. M., AND DUNCKER, H. R.: Anatomy and surgical treatment of syndactylism, PRS, *50:*167, 1972

LOSKEN, H. W., DAVIES, D., AND GORDON, W.: Coverage of scalp and skull defect in patient with systemic form of scleroderma, PRS, *51:*212, 1973

LOTEM, M., GLOOBE, H., AND NATHAN, H.: Fibrotic arch around deep branch of ulnar nerve in hand, PRS, *52:*553, 1973. Discussion by Weeks, PRS, *52:*556, 1973

LOTEM, M. *et al*: High pressure injection injuries of the hand. Harefuah, *89:*213, 1975 (Hebrew)

LOTFY, A. H. *et al*: Case of male pseudo-hermaphroditism with mosaicism. J. Egypt. Med. Assoc., *54:*723, 1971

LOTSMANOV, I. A. *et al*: Lymphocytoma of external nose. Vestn. Otorinolaringol., *35:*97, 1973 (Russian)

Lotuaco, G. G.: Simplified technique for correction of congenital lop ear (with Kaye), PRS, 54:667, 1974

Louhimo, I. et al: Acquired laryngotracheal stenosis in children. J. Pediatr. Surg., 6:730, 1971

Louis, D. S. et al: Injuries to upper extremity inflicted by mechanical cornpicker. Clin. Orthop., 92:231, 1973

Lourmet, J. et al: Iliac grafts in maxillofacial surgical pathology. Bull. Soc. Med. Afr. Noire Lang. Fr., 15:343, 1970 (French)

Love, R. T., Jr.: Nutrition in the burned patient. J. Miss. State Med. Assoc., 13:391, 1972

Lovely, F. W.: Surgical correction of deformities of the facial skeleton. N. S. Med. Bull., 51:55, 1972

Lovo, F. G. et al: Thermographic aspects of radionecrosis following radiological treatments of neoplasia, PRS, 57:402, 1976. Riv. ital. chir. plast., 6:125, 1974

Lowbury, E. J.: Infection associated with burns. Postgrad. Med. J., 48:338, 1972

Lowbury, E. J. et al: Topical chemoprophylaxis for burns: trials of creams containing silver sulphadiazine and trimethoprim. Injury, 3:18, 1971

Lowbury, E. J. et al: Protective isolation in a burns unit: the use of plastic isolators and air curtains. J. Hyg. (Camb.), 69:529, 1971

Lowbury, E. J. et al: Alternative forms of local treatment for burns. Lancet, 2:1105, 1971

Lowbury, E. J. L.: Prevention and treatment of sepsis in burns, PRS, 50:202, 1972. Proc. Roy. Soc. Med., 65:23, 1972

Lowbury, E. J. L. et al: Alternative forms of local treatment for burns, PRS, 50:420, 1972. Lancet, 2:7734, 1972

Lowe, J. T., Jr. et al: Submaxillary gland tumors. Laryngoscope, 84:542, 1974

Lowry, J. C.: Some economic aspects of oral surgery. Brit. J. Oral Surg., 11:249, 1974

Lowry, L. D., Billings, B. L., and Leonard, J. D.: Otolaryngic findings in cleft palate population, PRS, 55:251, 1975. Cleft Palate J., 11:62, 1974

Lowry, R. B., Courtemanche, A. D., and MacDonald, C.: Submucous cleft palate and general practitioner, PRS, 53:489, 1974. Canad. M.A.J., 109:995, 1973

Loynoz, G. C., and Bricano, L.: Neck tumors and fistulae in children, PRS, 48:196, 1971. Bol. Soc. Venezuelana Cir., 24:955, 1970

Lu, M.: Replantation of avulsed anterior teeth in patients with jaw fractures, PRS, 51:377, 1973

Lubkin, V.: The public face or psychological and legal complexities in plastic ophthalmic surgery. Brit. J. Ophthalmol., 59:593, 1975

Lubowe, I. I.: Treatment of the aging skin by dermatologic methods. J. Am. Geriatr. Soc., 24:25, 1976

Lubritz, R. R., and Ichinose, H.: Nodular fasciitis, PRS, 56:111, 1975. Cutis, 15:43, 1975

Lucas, C. S. et al: Vaginal reconstruction after extensive perineal resection. A case report. Obstet. Gynecol., 39:73, 1972

Lucas, George L.: Examination of the Hand. Charles C Thomas, Springfield, Ill., 1972. PRS, 53:467, 1974

Lucas, G. L. et al: Sweat gland carcinoma of the hand. Hand, 6:98, 1974

Lucas, J. W. et al: Management of shotgun wound of symphysis. J. Oral Surg., 33:622, 1975

Lucas, Thomas M. et al: Surgical-orthodontic therapy for mandibular fracture. Modification of Black-Ivy procedure. Rev. Esp. Estomatol., 22:26, 1974 (Spanish)

Lucas, Z. J.: Skin homografts in rats compared to other organ transplantations (with Gruber, Kaplan), PRS, 53:64, 1974

Lucchini, J. P.: Gingival grafts. Actual. Odontostomatol. (Paris), 27:299, 1973 (French)

Luce, E. A., and Hoopes, J. E.: Electrical burn of scalp and skull, PRS, 54:359, 1974

Lucente, F. E.: Psychological problems in otolaryngology. Laryngoscope, 83:1684, 1973

Lucente, F. E.: Impact of otolaryngology on world history. (Wilhelm, F.), (Cleveland, G.), (Roosevelt, F.). Trans. Am. Acad. Ophthalmol. Otolaryngol., 77:1424, 1973

Lucente, F. E.: Sex and the otolaryngologist, PRS, 57:671, 1976. Eye, Ear, Nose & Throat Month., 54:338, 1975

Ludewig, R. M., Rudolf, L. E., and Wangensteen, S. L.: Reduction of experimental wound infection with iodized gut sutures, PRS, 49:670, 1972. Surg. Gynec. & Obst., 133:946, 1971

Ludin, E. N. et al: Chemical face peeling. Conn. Med., 38:353, 1974

Luger, A.: First aid and local therapy of burns. Wien. Klin. Wochenschr., 82:169, 1970 (German)

Luhr, H. G.: Primary reconstruction of orbital floor defects following injury and neoplasm surgery. Dtsch. Zahn. Mund. Kieferheilkd., 57:1, 1971 (German)

Luhr, H. G.: Reconstruction of lower lip after tumor resection combined with radical neck dissection (with Lentrodt), PRS, 48:579, 1971

Luhr, H. G.: Treatment of mandibular fractures by compression osteosynthesis, PRS, 53:241, 1974. Rev. españ. cir. plast., 5:193, 1972

Luhr, H. G.: Surgical correction of posttraumatic occlusion disorders. Fortschr. Kiefer.

Gesichtschir., *18:*227, 1974 (German)

LUHR, H. G. *et al*: Diagnosis and therapy of tumors and pseudotumors of the temporomandibular joint. Dtsch. Zahnaerztl. Z., *28:*505, 1973 (German)

LUHR, H. G. *et al*: Osteosynthesis with compression in the treatment of fractures of the lower jaw. Experimental basis and clinical results. Rev. Stomatol. Chir. Maxillofac., *74:*264, 1973 (French)

LUHR, H. G. *et al*: Transplantation of homologous dura in reconstruction of the orbital floor. The results of five years experience. Trans. Int. Conf. Oral Surg., *4:*340, 1973

LUKOVSKYI, L. A., AND TYTAR, G. M.: New method of plastic operation for pharyngoesophageal tract in case of extensive laryngectomy due to cancer, PRS, *48:*511, 1971. Acta chir. plast., *12:*157, 1970

LULENSKI, G. C. *et al*: Tracheal incision as a contributing factor to tracheal stenosis. An experimental study. Ann. Otol. Rhin. & Laryng., *84:*781, 1975

LUMERMAN, H. *et al*: Synchronous malignant mucoepidermoid tumor of parotid gland and Warthin's tumor in adjacent lymph node. Oral Surg., *39:*953, 1975

LUND, B. A. *et al*: Chin. Mayo Clin. Proc., *48:*417, 1973

LUND, K. *et al*: Overgrowth of a hypoplastic mandibular ramus after autoplastic bone grafting. An 18-year longitudinal radiographic study, using metallic implants. Trandaegebladet, *75:*1279, 1971

LUND, O. E.: Blepharo-oculo-cranial dysplasia — a so far unknown syndrome? Med. Klin., *69:*1715, 1974 (German)

LUND, P. C., CWIK, J. C., AND PAGDANGANAN, R. T.: Etidocaine — new long-acting local anesthetic agent: clinical evaluation, PRS, *53:*372, 1974. Anesth. & Analg., Cleve., *52:*482, 1973

LUNDBERG, C. *et al*: Penicillin treatment in oral surgery in patients with coagulation disorders. Int. J. Oral Surg., *4:*198, 1975

LUNDBERG, M. *et al*: Changes in masticatory function after surgical treatment of mandibular prognathism. Cineradiographic study of bolus position. Acta Odontol. Scand., *32:*39, 1974

LUNDBORG, G.: Microcirculation in rabbit tendon, PRS, *57:*261, 1976. Hand, 7:1, 1975

LUNDGREN, D.: Influence of estrogen and progesterone on exudation, inflammatory cell migration and granulation tissue formation in preformed cavities, PRS, *54:*697, 1974. Scand. J. Plast. Reconstr. Surg., 7:20, 1973

LUNDGREN, D.: Influence of estrogen and progesterone on vascularization of granulation

tissue in preformed cavities, PRS, *54:*698, 1974. Scand. J. Plast. Reconstr. Surg., 7:85, 1973

LUNDGREN, D., AND LINDHE, J.: Exudation, inflammatory cell migration and granulation tissue formation in preformed cavities, PRS, *54:*698, 1974. Scand. J. Plast. Reconstr. Surg., 7:1, 1973

LUNG, R. J., GRAHAM, W. P., III, AND MILLER, S. H.: Pericortical "compression" clamps for mandibular fixation, PRS, *57:*487, 1976

LUNGBORG, G.: Limb ischemia and nerve injury, PRS, *51:*350, 1973. Arch. Surg., *104:*631, 1972

LUNING, P.: Patient with thrombosis of the ulnar artery in the hand caused by blunt trauma. Ned. tijdschr. geneeskd., *115:*1997, 1971 (Dutch)

LUNING, P.: Patient with thrombosis of ulnar artery of hand following blunt injury, PRS, *51:*703, 1973; *52:*99, 1973. Arch. chir. neerl., *24:*289, 1972

LUPO, G., AND BOGGIO-ROBUTTI, G.: Plastic surgery of breast and of mammarian region, PRS, *49:*357, 1972. Minerva med., Italy, Monograph, 1971

LUPO, G. *et al*: Nosography of lipomatosis and lipodystrophy in light of present criticism, PRS, *57:*683, 1976. Riv. ital. chir. plast., 6:135, 1974

LUPPINO, T. *et al*: So-called spontaneous tendon ruptures in the rheumatoid hand. Chir. Organi. Mov., *60:*661, 1971 (Italian)

LUPPINO, T. *et al*: Dissociated paralysis of median nerve in forearm caused by compression of anterior interosseous nerve (Kiloh-Nevin syndrome). Chir. Organi. Mov., *61:*89, 1972 (Italian)

LUPPIS, F. *et al*: Congenital torsion of the hand. Chir. Organi. Mov., *58:*134, 1969 (Italian)

Lupus

Skin grafting in systemic lupus erythematosus patients who are on steroids (Tuerk), PRS, *50:*382, 1972

Lupus erythematosus, systemic, Sjögren's syndrome in (Alarcon-Segovia, Velazquez-Forero, Gonzalez-Jimenez), PRS, *56:*237, 1975. Ann. Int. Med., *81:*577, 1974

LUR'E, A. S.: Neurotization of peripheral branches of facial nerve during extirpation of parotid gland. Klin. Khir., *10:*73, 1973 (Russian)

LUSSKIN, R. *et al*: Peripheral surgery after stroke. An orthopedic-rehabilitative effort. Geriatrics, *26:*65, 1971

LUTHER, R. *et al*: Treatment of fractures in the area of the hand. Chirurg., *41:*222, 1970 (German)

Lutman, G. B.: Epithelial nests in intraoral sensory nerve endings simulating perineural invasion in patients with oral carcinoma, PRS, *54:*234, 1974. Am. J. Clin. Path., *61:*275, 1974

Lutz, L. A.: Secretary-patient relationship (Letter to the Editor), PRS, *53:*81, 1974

Luxenberg, M. N.: Repair of drooping brow and upper eyelid, secondary to facial nerve palsy. Trans. Am. Acad. Ophthalmol. Otolaryngol., *77:*721, 1973

Lyall, M.: Self-retaining retractor for lacrimal sac operations. Brit. J. Ophthalmol., *56:*636, 1972

Lychak, V. S. *et al:* Treatment of epulis. Stomatologiia (Mosk.), *53:*83, 1974 (Russian)

Lymph Nodes

Head and neck, lymphoma masquerading as carcinoma (Elias, Mittelman), PRS, *49:*360, 1972. Am. J. Surg., *122:*424, 1971

Lymph node spread, regional, in cancer of tongue (Saxena), PRS, *48:*199, 1971. Cancer, *27:*38, 1971

Lymphographic diagnosis of malignancy (Macdonald). Proc. Roy. Soc. Med., *65:*719, 1972

Lymphoma, Burkitt's, in West Malaysia (Ramanathan), PRS, *52:*103, 1973. Southeast Asian J. Trop. Med., *3:*249, 1972

Reticuloendothelial system, phagocytosis of, attempts at interference with (Köhnlein, Lemperle, Scherer), PRS, *53:*376, 1974. Bruns' Beitr. klin. Chir., *220:*643, 1973

Hodgkin's disease, after care in (pathology) (Eder). Fortschr. Geb. Roentgenstr. Nuklearmed., *Suppl:* 116–7, 1973 (German)

Lymphographic observations following surgery of cervical lymphatic system (Adamus). Otolaryngol. Pol., *27:*451, 1973 (Polish)

Prognostic significance of lymph node reactions in malignant melanoma (Mioudzewska). Nowotwory, *23:*89, 1973 (Polish)

Lymph nodes, angiofollicular hyperplasia of (Iakovleva *et al*). Vopr. Onkol., *19:*18, 1973 (Russian)

Tuberculous cervical lymphadenitis (Ord, Matz), PRS, *54:*687, 1974. Arch. Otolaryng., *99:*327, 1974

Lymphadenitis, tuberculous (Iles, *et al*). Brit. Med. J., *1:*143, 1974

Active enhancement of mouse skin allografts: effect of Bordetella pertussis and regional lymphadenectomy (Clark *et al*). Brit. J. Surg., *61:*325, 1974

Lymph node sectioning, probability in (Wilkinson *et al*). Cancer, *33:*1269, 1974

Lymph Nodes – Cont.

Histopathology of lymph node toxoplasmosis (Peychl *et al*). Cas. Lek. Cesk., *113:*392, 1974 (Czech)

Lymphadenitis, toxoplasmatic, demonstration of parasites in (Peychl). Cesk. Patol., *10:*86, 1974 (Czechoslovakian)

Biopsy of enlarged superficial lymph nodes (Sinclair, Beckman, Ellman), PRS, *54:*694, 1974. J.A.M.A., *228:*602, 1974

Current status of endolymphatic therapy with radionuclides (Peters *et al*). Lymphology, *7:*49, 1974

Lymphoscintigraphy in lymph node metastases from oral cancer (Quintarelli). Minerva Stomatol., *23:*147, 1974 (Italian)

Lymphoma, cervical. Topography, diagnosis, therapy (Gastpar). Munch. Med. Wochenschr., *116:*447, 1974

Hodgkin's disease, reticulosarcomas and, comparative chromosome characteristics of (Fleischman *et al*). Neoplasma, *21:*51, 1974

Lymphography in case of combined toxoplasmosis of lymph nodes and stationary Hodgkin's disease (Bottcher). Roentgenblaetter, *27:*257, 1974 (German)

Surgical anatomy of the neck (Jurkiewicz *et al*). Surg. Clin. North Am., *54:*1269, 1974

Opacification of the "para-lymphatic system" during lymphography (Kuisk *et al*). Minn. Med., *58:*443, 1975

Lymph nodes, cervical, management in head and neck cancer (Stell), PRS, *56:*226, 1975. Proc. Roy. Soc. Med., *68:*83, 1975

Lymph node metastases, radiosensitivity of (Henk), PRS, *56:*231, 1975. Proc. Roy. Soc. Med., *68:*85, 1975

Physiologic and immunologic considerations of the lymphatic system in tumors and transplants (Futrell *et al*). Surg. Gynec. & Obst., *140:*273, 1975

Lymph Nodes, Excision (See also *Neck Dissections*)

Lymph nodes, barrier function of. Review of experimental studies and their implications for cancer surgery (Strauli). Aktuel Probl. Chir., *14:*161, 1970

Groin dissection, protection of femoral vessels after (Schweitzer), PRS, *49:*109, 1972. Am. J. Surg., *122:*223, 1971

Complete axillary node dissection with preservation of the pectoralis major muscle (Sanders). Arch. Surg., *103:*518, 1971

Node, regional dissection in treatment of malignant melanoma (Paglia, Knapper, Fortner), PRS, *50:*98, 1972. Clin. Bull. Memorial Sloan-Kettering Cancer Center, *1:*136, 1971

Lymph Nodes, Excision – Cont.

Lymphography for determining the radicality of regional lymph node removal in malignant neoplasms of the skin of the extremities (Trishkin). Vopr. Onkol., *17:*3, 1971 (Russian)

Biopsy, ill-advised (Johnson, Harrah, Ketchum), PRS, *51:*354, 1973. Am. Surgeon, *38:*357, 1972

Groin dissection, modified technique (Van der Ploez, Koops), PRS, *51:*479, 1973. Arch. chir. neerl., *24:*31, 1972

Skin bridge technique, new procedure in radical ilioinguinal node dissection (Fraley, Hutchens), PRS, *51:*711, 1973. J. Urol., *108:*279, 1972

Lymphadenectomy, regional, effect of on development of concomitant immunity (Soloway *et al*). Surg. Forum, *23:*101, 1972

Axillary metastases from unknown primary sites (Copeland). Ann. Surg., *178:*25, 1973

Hodgkin's disease in children (Schnitzer *et al*), PRS, *52:*458, 1973. Cancer, *31:*560, 1973

Hodgkin's disease in children, localized, results of regional radiotherapy in (Fuller, Sullivan, Butler), PRS, *54:*699, 1974. Cancer, *32:*640, 1973

Lymphadenectomy, lymphographic findings following. Contribution to problem of lymph vessel regeneration (Wolf). Fortschr. Geb. Roentgenstr. Nuklearmed., *119:*35, 1973 (German)

Lymphadenectomy, should be discarded? 1. Immunological considerations (Baum). J. R. Coll. Surg. Edinb., *18:*351, 1973

Effects of immune depression on chemical carcinogenesis in rat. I. Regional lymphadenectomy (Bolton). Oncology, *27:*430, 1973

Lymph nodes, axillary, radical dissection for malignant melanoma (Milton, McCarthy), PRS, *53:*112, 1974. Proc. Roy. Australasian Coll. Surg., *46:*694, 1973

Ilioinguinal lymph node dissection for melanomas (Harris *et al*), PRS, *52:*215, 1973. Surg. Gynec. & Obst., *136:*33, 1973

Technique for radical groin dissection (Groshong). Surg. Gynec. & Obst., *136:*986, 1973

Surgical management of malignant lesions of skin (Hardin). Tex. Med., *69:*87, 1973

Lymph node dissection, radical groin (Papaioannou, Critselis, Yamalakis), PRS, *56:*473, 1975. Tr. 8th Panhellenic Cong. Surg. Soc., A: 276, 1973

Lymph node dissection, regional, for melanoma (Gumport, Harris), PRS, *54:*243, 1974. Ann. Surg., *179:*105, 1974

Lymph node dissection, regional, "prophylactic" (Polk *et al*). Ann. Surg., *180:*257, 1974

Lymph Nodes, Excision – Cont.

Cellular immune defect: isolated immunocytic deficiency syndrome (Justus *et al*). Dtsch. Med. Wochenschr., *99:*936, 1974

Effect of delayed lymphadenectomy on 239Pu02 translocation in dogs (Gomez *et al*). Health Phys., *27:*213, 1974

Extent of operation in skin neoplasm metastases into inguinal-femoral lymphatic nodes (Knonenko *et al*). Klin. Khir., *10:*48, 1974 (Russian)

Synovial sarcoma in children (Lee *et al*). Surg. Gynec. & Obst., *138:*701, 1974

Results of treating malignant melanoma intralymphatically with radioactive isotopes (Ariel). Surg. Gynec. & Obst., *139:*726, 1974

Concept of radical surgery of cancer (Giacomelli). Tumori, *60:*445, 1974 (Italian)

Significance and methods of surgical treatment of lymphatic spread (Giacomelli). Tumori, *60:*567, 1974 (Italian)

Indications for regional lymphadenectomy in melanoblastoma of the skin of the extremities (Vagner *et al*). Vopr. Onkol., *20:*33, 1974 (Russian)

Hematological and biochemical indices after the comprehensive treatment of melanoblastomas of the lower extremities (Levin *et al*). Vopr. Onkol., *20:*39, 1974 (Russian)

Regional lymphadenectomy and tumor curability. Experimental observations in a murine lymphosarcoma (Perez *et al*). Am. J. Roentgenol. Radium Ther. Nucl. Med., *123:*621, 1975

Proceedings: effect of lymphadenectomy on neoplasm immunity (Oikawa *et al*). Hokkaido J. Med. Sci., *50:*84, 1975 (Japanese)

Metastases, lymph node, radiosensitivity of (Henk), PRS, *56:*231, 1975. Proc. Roy. Soc. Med., *68:*85, 1975

Regional lymphadenectomy and varied tumor antigenicity (Ziegler *et al*). Surg. Forum, *26:*170, 1975

Regional lymphadenectomy and tumor immunity (Pendergrast *et al*). Surg. Gynec. & Obst., *142:*385, 1976

Lymphangioma (See also *Cystic Hygroma*)

Rare vascular tumor of the neck: cystic hygroma of the neck (Stefanovic *et al*). Srp. Arh. Celok. Lek., *98:*1065, 1970 (Serbian)

Late results of radical surgery for extensive racemose lymphangioma of the arm (Reichmann). Handchirurgie, *3:*1971 (German)

Lymphangiomas, cystic, in children: report of 32 cases including lesions at rare sites (Singh, Baboo, Pathak), PRS, *48:*517, 1971.

Lymphangioma — Cont.

Surgery, *69:*947, 1971

Lymphangiography and surgery in lymphangioma of the skin (Edwards *et al*). Brit. J. Surg., *59:*36, 1972

Lymphangioma cavernosum palati molli et uvulae (Sylwanowicz *et al*). Otolaryngol. Pol., *26:*467, 1972 (Polish)

Primary tumors and injuries of lymphatic system (Overbeck *et al*). Chirurg., *44:*107, 1973

Lymphatic system, surgery of (review of the literature) (Khromov). Khirurgiia (Mosk.), *49:*122, 1973 (Russian)

Lymphatic malformations, control by resection (Fonkalsrud), PRS, *56:*108, 1975. Am. J. Surg., *128:*152, 1974

Anaesthesia for cystic hygroma in a neonate (Weller). Anaesthesia, *29:*588, 1974

Anesthetic problems in surgery for varying levels of respiratory obstruction in infants and children (Wilson *et al*). Anesth. Analg. (Cleve.), *53:*878, 1974

Practical cryosurgery for oral lesions (Leopard *et al*). Brit. Dent. J., *136:*185, 1974

Lymphangioma of the maxilla in a newborn infant (Kspoian). Vestn. Khir., *112:*82, 1974 (Russian)

Identification of facial nerve at secondary surgery (Janecka). Laryngoscope, *85:*896, 1975

Lymphangioma, long-term follow-up study (Saijo, Munro, Mancer), PRS, *56:*642, 1975

Lymphedema

Lymphedema, post-mastectomy, of arm, surgical management (Clodius), PRS, *49:*585, 1972. Chir. Praxis, *15:*273, 1971

Indications and technic of creating a lymphovenous anastomosis in lymphedema of the extremities (Pokrovskii *et al*). Klin. Khir., *9:*11, 1971 (Russian)

Thoraco-brachial transposition of the greater omentum as a new surgical method in the treatment of postoperative lymphedema (Innocenzi *et al*). Minerva Chir., *26:*947, 1971 (Italian)

Surgical treatment of lymphedema of the lower limb (current orientations) (Elbaz). Phlebologie, *24:*253, 1971 (French)

Lymphedema of upper limb, bi-hinged chest-arm flap for (Hirshowitz, Goldan), PRS, *48:*52, 1971

Female genitalia, elephantiasis of (Khanna, Joshi), PRS, *48:*379, 1971

Lymphangiography of neck, direct magnifying (Nonyama *et al*), PRS, *50:*312, 1972. Pract. Otologia Kyoto, *64:*871, 1971

Edemas, surgical, diffusion factor for (Appi-

Lymphedema — Cont.

ani Sotomayor *et al*), PRS, *49:*585, 1972. Tribuna méd. argent., *13:*B22, 1971

Alleviation of experimental lymphedema by lymphovenous anastomosis in dogs (Firica *et al*). Am. Surg., *38:*409, 1972

Adenolympho-saphenous anastomosis using the Nielubowicz-Olszewski-Sakolowski method (Moreno Gonzalez *et al*). Angiologia, *24:*5, 1972 (Spanish)

Transposition of the greater omentum in lymphedema caused by chronic venous insufficiency (Alcocer Andalon *et al*). Arch. Inst. Cardiol. Mex., *42:*444, 1972 (Spanish)

Treatment of severe lymphedema of the extremities by venous-lymphatic anastomosis (Cossu *et al*). Atti. Accad. Med. Lomb., *27:*55, 1972 (Italian)

Lymphedema, methods of study and therapeutic possibilities (Grandval), PRS, *51:*479, 1973. Bol. y trab. Soc. argent cir., *56:*33, 1972

Lymphedema, operation for (Beal). Ill. Med. J., *142:*494, 1972

Lymphedema, scrotal and penile, as complication of testicular prosthesis (Elsahy), PRS, *52:*207, 1973. J. Urol., *108:*595, 1972

Lymphogenic edema, acquired, of extremities (Beshlei *et al*). Klin. Khir., *10:*52, 1972 (Russian)

Elephantiasis of extremities, etiology, pathogenesis and treatment of (Gorshkov). Klin. Med. (Mosk.), *50:*131, 1972 (Russian)

Treatment by nylon setons of lymphoedema of the arm following radical mastectomy (O'Reilly). M. J. Australia, *1:*1269, 1972

Lymphscrotum of filarial origin. Surgical treatment by lymphatico-venous fistula (Arrighi *et al*). Med. Trop. (Mars.), *32:*305, 1972 (French)

Lymphedema, treatment of. Thompson's operation (David *et al*). Nouv. Presse Med., *1:*2327, 1972 (French)

Trypsin-chymotrypsin, oral, for prevention of swelling after hand surgery, evaluation of (Salisbury, Hunter), PRS, *49:*171, 1972

Lymphedema, appropriate surgical procedures in (Smith) (Follow-Up Clinic), PRS, *49:*334, 1972

Primary lymphatic edema of lower limbs. 1. Lymphographic and histologic examination of vessels and lymph nodes in primary lymphedema (Olszewski *et al*). Pol. Przegl. Chir., *44:*657, 1972 (Polish)

Acquired complicated elephantiasis of lower extremity (Kus *et al*). Pol. Przegl. Chir., *44:*1743, 1972 (Polish)

Lymphovenous anastomosis in the treatment of the lymphedema of the lower extremities

Lymphedema — Cont.

(Moreno Gonzalez). Rev. Clin. Esp., *124:*503, 1972 (Spanish)

Treatment of patients having undergone surgery for venous lymphatic diseases of the limbs at the Sochi-Matsesta resort (Aleksandrova). Sov. Med., *35:*137, 1972 (Russian)

Lymphedema (Stone *et al*). Surg. Gynec. & Obst., *135:*625, 1972

Lymphedema and its treatment; with special reference to edema of the arm after a radical operation for breast cancer (Masuda *et al*). Surg. Ther. (Osaka), *26:*308, 1972 (Japanese)

Lymphedema, free skin grafting to male genitalia in case of (Holm-Jensen). Ugeskr. Laeger, *134:*2160, 1972 (Danish)

Experiences with Goldsmith's omental transposition (Buri). Vasa, *1:*45, 1972 (German)

Volume changes in swollen extremity, calculating from surface measurements (Lennihan, Mackereth), PRS, *54:*113, 1974. Am. J. Surg., *126:*649, 1973

Treatment of lymphatic and venous edema of lower extremities (Mayall). Angiologia, *25:*177, 1973 (Spanish)

Lymphedema, congenital, in infants and children, management of (Fonkalsrud *et al*). Ann. Surg., *177:*280, 1973

Nodular subepidermal fibrosis in non-filarial endemic elephantiasis of legs (Price) Brit. J. Dermatol., *89:*451, 1973

Leg, swollen (Dale). Curr. Probl. Surg., *1:*66, 1973

Surgical treatment of lymphedema of the arm after breast amputation (Bohmert). Fortschr. Med., *91:*228, 1973 (German)

Arm, secondary lymphedema of (Clodius, Uhlschmid, Madritsch), PRS, *53:*605, 1974. Helvet. chir. acta, *40:*659, 1973

Elephantasis of lower limb, omental transposition in treatment of (Goel, Misra), PRS, *53:*488, 1974. Indian J. Surg., *35:*381, 1973

Late results of lymphovenous anastomosis (Nielubowicz *et al*). J. Cardiovasc. Surg. (Torino), Spec. No.: 113, 1973

Surgical treatment of postmastectomy lymphedema of the upper limb (Cordeiro *et al*). J. Cardiovasc. Surg. (Torino), Spec. No.: 125, 1973

Unsolved problem of peripheral lymphedema (Tosatti). Lymphology, *6:*167, 1973

Lymphedema, chronic, after treatment for cancer of breast (Mayer *et al*), PRS, *54:*111, 1974. Lyon chir., *69:*401, 1973

Lymphedema of lower extremities, experience in treatment of (Krauss *et al*). Mater. Med. Pol., *5:*271, 1973

Lymphedema — Cont.

Lymphovenous shunt (Krogh). S. Afr. Med. J., *47:*1389, 1973

Plastic surgery on elephantiasis of legs: case report (Sivaloganathan *et al*). Southeast Asian J. Trop. Med. Public Health, *4:*279, 1973

Lymphedema, management by staged subcutaneous excision (Miller, Harper, Longmire), PRS, *52:*453, 1973. Surg. Gynec. & Obst., *136:*586, 1973

Surgical treatment of lymphedema and its indications (Mindikoglu *et al*). Turk. Tip. Dern. Derg., *39:*426, 1973 (Turkish)

Present state of surgical treatment of lymphedemas of lower extremities (Barinka). Acta Chir. Orthop. Traumatol. Cech., *41:*557, 1974 (Czech)

On the problem of substitution of liquids after the operation on elephantiasis (Janackova). Acta Chir. Orthop. Traumatol. Cech., *41:*564, 1974 (Czech)

Vulval elephantiasis (Gorshkov). Akush. Ginekol. (Mosk.), *2:*71, 1974 (Russian)

Lymphedema, chronic, omental transposition for, longterm evaluation of (Goldsmith), PRS, *55:*638, 1975. Ann. Surg., *180:*847, 1974

Lymphedema of limbs, evaluation of Thompson's buried dermal flap operation for (Sawhney), PRS, *56:*680, 1975. Brit. J. Plast. Surg., *27:*278, 1974

Lymphedema praecox, staged treatment (Tilley *et al*). Can. Med. Assoc. J., *110:*309, 1974

Lymphedema of extremities, chronic (problems of diagnosis and treatment) (Kaufmann *et al*). Chirurgia (Bucur.), *23:*249, 1974 (Rumanian)

Filarial elephantiasis of the leg (Mukherji *et al*). Clin. Plast. Surg., *1:*83, 1974

Extremity, lower, chronically swollen painful, etiological factors (Stallworth *et al*), PRS, *54:*690, 1974. J.A.M.A., *228:*1656, 1974

Lymphedema of scrotum and penis, chronic (Keeler *et al*). J. Med. Soc., *71:*575, 1974

Preservation and autotransplantation of skin in elephantiasis of extremities (Zaboloskii *et al*). Klin. Khir., *3:*45, 1974 (Russian)

Milroy's disease, thrombocytosis, and strokes (Sturm *et al*). Minn. Med., *57:*689, 1974

Lymphedema, physiopathology and treatment of (Pflug). Phlebologie, *27:*393, 1974 (French)

Lymphedema, treatment of (Bunchman, Lewis), PRS, *54:*64, 1974

Vulvar elephantiasis (Cardinal), PRS, *54:*377, 1974. Rev. Medico, *24:*43, 1974

Lymphedema — Cont.

Lymphedema, management of, with modified Thompson's method (Bohmert *et al*). Ther. Ggw., *113:*842, 1974 (German)

Lymphedema, new technique of drainage of subcutaneous tissue of limbs with nylon net for treatment (Degni). Vasa, *3:*329, 1974

Surgical treatment of gigantic elephantiasis of the lower extremities in children (Mateshuk *et al*). Vestn. Khir., *112:*83, 1974 (Russian)

Factitious lymphedema of the hand (Smith). J. Bone & Joint Surg. (Am.), *57:*89, 1975

Lymphedema of lower limbs, operations for (Chilvers, Kinmonth), PRS, *57:*262, 1976. J. Cardiovasc. Surg., *16:*115, 1975

Lymphedema, recent evaluations on treatment of (Cariati *et al*), PRS, *57:*399, 1976. J. Cardiovasc. Surg., *16:*192, 1975

Pressure dependent factors in edema formation in canine forelimbs (Kline *et al*), PRS, *56:*603, 1975. J. Pharmacol. Exp. Ther., *193:*452, 1975

Lymphedema, scrotal and penile, surgical management (Vaught, Litvok, McRoberts), PRS, *57:*761, 1976. J. Urol., *113:*204, 1975

Diagnosis and treatment of lymphangiosarcoma in the presence of lymphostasis of the upper extremity following mastectomy (Oshmianskaia *et al*). Khirurgiia (Mosk.), *2:*23, 1975 (Russian)

Lymphedema, chronic, condition of reimplanted skin after operative treatment of (Belogliadova). Klin. Khir., *3:*63, 1975 (Russian)

Phlebo-lymphatic surgery in treatment of post-phlebitic syndrome (Battezzati *et al*). Minerva Chir., *30:*410, 1975 (Italian)

Lymphedema of extremity, Thompson's operation on (Sakaguchi *et al*), PRS, *56:*466, 1975. Operation, *29:*211, 1975

Lymphedema, clinical review and follow-up study (Saijo, Munro, Mancer), PRS, *56:*513, 1975

Lymphedema of extremity, surgical management (Miller), PRS, *56:*633, 1975

Lymphatics, lymphedema and lymphangiosarcoma (Deigert). Rocky Mt. Med. J., *72:*210, 1975

Management of endemic (non-filarial) elephantiasis of lower legs (Price). Trop. Doct., *5:*70, 1975

Surgical treatment of elephantiasis of the upper extremities (Zabolotskil). Vestn. Khir., *115:*67, 1975 (Russian)

Elephantiasis, syphilitic, of penis and scrotum (Elsahy), PRS, *57:*601, 1976

LYNCH, D. J., LAMP, J. C., AND ROYSTER, H. P.: Conjunctival approach for exploration of orbital floor, PRS, *54:*153, 1974

LYNCH, JOHN B., AND LEWIS, STEPHEN R.: *Symposium on the Treatment of Burns*, Volume 5. C. V. Mosby Co., St. Louis, 1973. PRS, *53:*585, 1974

LYNCH, J. B.: Foreign body reactions to polyurethane covers of some breast prostheses (with Cocke, Leathers), PRS, *56:*527, 1975

LYNCH, J. B. *et al*: Changing patterns of mortality in burns, PRS, *48:*329, 1971

LYNCH, J. B. *et al*: Our experiences with Silastic ear implants, PRS, *49:*283, 1972

LYONS, G. D.: Wharton duct problem. J. La. State Med. Soc., *123:*348, 1971

LYONS, J. H., JR.: Cervical pharyngostomy. Safe alternative for gastrointestinal decompression. Am. J. Surg., *127:*387, 1974

M

MABRY, C. C. *et al*: Failure of hypophysectomy in generalized lipodystrophy. J. Pediatr., *81:*990, 1972

MABRY, C. C. *et al*: Trismus pseudocamptodactyly syndrome: Dutch-Kentucky syndrome. J. Pediatr., *85:*503, 1974

MABRY, R. L. *et al*: Extended lateral rhinotomy for resection of malignant melanoma. South. Med. J., *67:*65, 1974

MACALISTER, A. D.: Dislocating jaw. Trans. Int. Conf. Oral Surg., *4:*259, 1973

MACARTHUR, J. D., AND MOORE, F. D.: Epidemiology of burns: burn-prone patient, PRS, *56:*233, 1975. J.A.M.A., *231:*259, 1975

MACCARTY, C. S.: Acoustic neuroma and suboccipital approach (1967–1972), PRS, *56:*111, 1975. Mayo Clin. Proc., *50:*15, 1975

MACCOLLUM, D. W.: Facial teratoma in newborn, report of 5 cases (with Gifford), PRS, *49:*616, 1972

MACCOLLUM, D. W.: Congenital absence of nose and anterior nasopharynx; report of two cases (with Gifford, Swanson), PRS, *50:*5, 1972

MACCOLLUM, M. S.: Efficacy of local steroid injection in treatment of stenosing tenovaginitis (with Clark, Ricker), PRS, *51:*179, 1973

MACCOLLUM, M. S.: Cancellous bone grafts from distal radius for use in hand surgery, PRS, *55:*477, 1975

MACCOMB, W. S.: Diagnosis and treatment of metastatic cervical cancerous nodes from unknown primary site, PRS, *51:*351, 1973. Am. J. Surg., *124:*441, 1972

MACDONALD, C. J.: Inexpensive hand table, PRS, *57:*392, 1976

MacDonald, D. M.: Thyroglossal cysts and fistulae. Int. J. Oral Surg., *3:*342, 1974

MacDonald, G. B. *et al*: Treatent of minimal prognathism by midline mandibular ostectomy. J. Oral Surg., *33:*386, 1975

MacDonald, J. S.: Lymphographic diagnosis of malignancy. Proc. Roy. Soc. Med., *65:*719, 1972

MacDougal, B. A. *et al*: Reduction mammaplasty: comparison of techniques. J. Okla. State Med. Assoc., *67:*82, 1974

MacDougal, B., Wray, R. C., Jr., and Weeks, P. M.: Lateral-volar finger flap for treatment of burn syndactyly, PRS, *57:*167, 1976

MacDougal, B. A., Weeks, P. M., and Wray, R. C., Jr.: Spontaneous regression of primary lesion of metastatic malignant melanoma, PRS, *57:*355, 1976

MacFarlane, W. I.: Fibrosarcoma of mandible with pulmonary metastases: case report. Brit. J. Oral Surg., *10:*168, 1972

MacGregor, A. J.: Adjustable locking plate for sectional metal cap splints. A further report. Brit. J. Oral Surg., *9:*251, 1972

Machacek, E.: Paget's disease in inverted nasal papilloma. Arch. Otorhinolaryngol. (N.Y.), *206:*17, 1973 (German)

Machtens, E., Karwetzky, R., and Meisel, H. H.: Corticotomy and wedge-shaped tongue excision as supporting therapy in late orthodontic cases. Z.W.R., *81:*1070, 1972 (German)

Maciejczyk, S. *et al*: Treatment of polydactylia in the light of our records. Chir. Narzadow. Ruchu Ortop. Pol., *40:*229, 1975 (Polish)

Maciejczyk, S. *et al*: Our experience in the treatment of hand scarring contracture following burns. Chir. Narzadow. Ruchu Ortop. Pol., *40:*377, 1975 (Polish)

MacIntosh, R. B.: Total mandibular alveolar osteotomy, PRS, *55:*715, 1975. J. Maxillo-facial Surg., *2:*210, 1974

MacIntosh, R. *et al*: Total mandibular alveolar osteotomy in the management of skeletal (infantile) apertognathia. J. Oral Surg., *33:*921, 1975

Mackenzie, D.: History of sutures, PRS, *53:*502, 1974. Med. Hist., *17:*158, 1973

Mackeprang, M. *et al*: Observations on congenital heart disease in a mortality study of children with cleft lip and palate. J. Chronic Dis., *24:*39, 1971

Mackie, R. M.: Malignant melanomata: aid to preoperative diagnosis. Brit. J. Surg., *59:*632, 1972

Mackie, R. M. *et al*: Cell-mediated immunity in patients with malignant melanoma. Brit. J. Dermatol., *87:*523, 1972

Mackie, R. M. *et al*: Assessment of prognosis in patients with malignant melanoma. Lancet, *2:*455, 1972

MacLean, L. D.: Prophylactic antibiotic therapy in surgery, PRS, *57:*405, 1976. Canad. J. Surg., *18:*243, 1975

MacLennan, W. D. *et al*: Osteoma of the mandible. Brit. J. Oral Surg., *12:*219, 1974

MacLeod, P. *et al*: Whistling face syndrome — craniocarpo-tarsal dysplasia. Report of a case and a survey of the literature. Clin. Pediatr. (Phila.), *13:*184, 1974

MacMillan, B., Law, E. J., and Holder, A.: Experience with *candida* infections in burn patient, PRS, *50:*634, 1972. Arch. Surg., *104:*509, 1972

MacMillan, B. C. *et al*: Epidemiology of *Pseudomonas* in burn intensive care unit, PRS, *54:*378, 1974. J. Trauma, *13:*627, 1973

MacMillan, B. G.: Ecology of bacteria colonizing the burned patient given topical and systemic gentamicin therapy: a five-year study. J. Infect. Dis., *124:*278, 1971 Suppl

MacMillan, B. G.: Burns in children. Clin. Plast. Surg., *1:*633, 1974

MacMillan, B. G.: Burns in children. Clin. Plast. Surg., *1:*645, 1974

Macomber, W. B., and Wang, M. K. H.: Congenital neoplasms of nose (Follow-Up Clinic). PRS, *50:*77, 1972

Macon, W. L., and Pories, W. J.: Effect of iron deficiency anemia on wound healing, PRS, *48:*399, 1971. Surgery, *69:*792, 1971

Macroglossia

Tongue excision, wedge-shaped, and corticotomy as supporting therapy in late orthodontic cases (Machtens, Karwetzky, Meisel). Z. W. R., *81:*1070, 1972 (German)

Amyloidosis: report of case presenting with macroglossia (Hicks *et al*). Brit. J. Plast. Surg., *26:*274, 1973

Exomphalos-macroglossia-gigantism syndrome from surgical viewpoint (EMG-syndrome) (Reuter). Zentralbl. Chir., *99:*668, 1974 (German)

Macrostomia

Macrostomia, ten-year survey of (Ogo *et al*), PRS, *54:*106, 1974. Jap. J. Plast. Reconstr. Surg., *16:*431, 1973

Macrostomia, bilateral, as isolated deformity (Hawkins *et al*). J. Laryng. & Otol., *87:*309, 1973

Macrostomia, clinical aspects and therapy of (Shetty *et al*). Zahn. Mund. Kieferheilkd., *62:*745, 1974

MacWilliams, P., and Noojin, R. O.: Vesicular metastatic melanoma, PRS, *56:*112, 1975.

South. M. J., *67*:1365, 1974

MADDEN, J. W.: Current concept of wound healing as applied to hand surgery. Orthop. Clin. North Am., *1*:325, 1970

MADDEN, J. W.: On "The contractile fibroblast" (Editorial). PRS, *52*:291, 1973

MADDEN, J. W.: Plastic surgery and burns. Surg. Gynec. & Obst., *142*:213, 1976

MADDEN, J. W., AND PEACOCK, E. E., JR.: Studies on the biology of collagen during wound healing: III. Dynamic metabolism of scar collagen and remodeling of dermal wounds, PRS, *51*:235, 1973. Ann. Surg., *174*:511, 1971

MADDEN, J. W., AND PEACOCK, E. E.: Some thoughts on repair of peripheral nerves, PRS, *48*:91, 1971. South. M. J., *64*:17, 1971

MADDEN, J. W., CARLSON, E., AND HINES, J.: Presence of modified fibroblasts in ischemic contracture of intrinsic musculature of hand, PRS, *56*:595, 1975. Surg. Gynec. & Obst., *140*:509, 1975

MADDOX, W. A. *et al*: Cancer of the tongue: review of thirteen-year experience — 1955-1968. Am. Surg., *37*:624, 1971

Madelung's Disease: See *Lipoma*

MADHAVAN, M. *et al*: Osteogenic sarcoma of maxilla. J. Laryng. & Otol., *88*:1125, 1974

MADISON, M. S.: Hydrofluoric acid burns (with Iverson, Laub). PRS, *48*:107, 1971

MADYKENOV, O. M. *et al*: Use of heterogenous peritoneum for treating skin donor sites. Khirurgiia (Mosk.), *49*:28, 1972 (Russian)

MAER, P. *et al*: Iatrogenic Volkmann's ischemia result of pressure due to transfusion, PRS, *51*:231, 1973. Internat. Surg., *57*:415, 1972

MAERKER, R. *et al*: Gallium-67 scintigraphy in the diagnosis of tumors in oromaxillofacial surgery. Acta Stomatol. Belg., *72*:399, 1975 (German)

MAES, J., AND STARK, R. B.: Unusual cleft lip deformity (Letter to the Editor). PRS, *54*:346, 1974

MAGEE, P. N.: Carcinogens in environment, PRS, *55*:644, 1975. Proc. Roy. Soc. Med., *67*:741, 1974

MAGIERSKI, M.: Topical refrigeration analgesia for skin transplantation in patients with burns. Anaesth. Resusc. Intensive Ther., *2*:77, 1974

MAGNUS, W. W.: Initial care and assessment of maxillofacial injuries. Am. Fam. Physician, *8*:116, 1973

MAGNUS, W. W. *et al*: Composite complex odontoma with associated impaction and autogenous bone graft, case report. Mil. Med., *136*:373, 1971

MAGNUSON, R. H.: Simple office procedure for the repair of senile entropion. Ophthalmic Surg., *6*:83, 1975

MAGONSKA-OLESZYCKA, A. *et al*: Facial skeletal defects and methods of repair. Czas. Stomatol., *24*:1333, 1971 (Polish)

MAGOVERN, G. J. *et al*: Clinical and experimental evaluation of controlled-pressure intratracheal cuff. J. Thorac. Cardiovasc. Surg., *64*:747, 1972

MAGRE, J. *et al*: Two pregnancies after late change of sex in a person with pseudohermaphroditism. Bull. Fed. Soc. Gynecol. Obstet. Lang. Fr., *23*:513, 1971 (French)

MAGUIRE, A. J. *et al*: Anterior pharyngeal pouch. Can. J. Otolaryngol., *3*:225, 1974

MAHE, E., AND CAMBLIN, J.: Frontal hairline in treatment of male pattern baldness, PRS, *54*:617, 1974. Ann. chir. plast., *19*:61, 1974

MAHE, E. *et al*: Musculus depressor septi nasi. Study of its action and the role played in its resection during the post-operative course of cosmetic rhinoplasties. Ann. chir. plast., *19*:257, 1974 (French)

MAHE, E. *et al*: Resection of the depressor muscle of the tip in esthetic rhinoplasties. Ann. Otolaryngol. Chir. Cervicofac., *92*:381, 1975 (French)

MAHLER, D. *et al*: Haifa dressing for burns. Brit. J. Plast. Surg., *25*:58, 1972

MAHLER, D. *et al*: Colorimetric estimation of blood loss during surgery of burns. Brit. J. Plast. Surg., *25*:130, 1972

MAHLER, D. *et al*: Use of preserved skin for resurfacing of burns. Harefuah, *82*:122, 1972 (Hebrew)

MAHLER, D. *et al*: Resurfacing of burns with preserved skin. Isr. J. Med. Sci., *8*:141, 1972

MAHLER, D., AND KAUFMAN, T.: Asymptomatic rhinolith in rhinoplasty. PRS, *54*:490, 1974

MAHLER, D. *et al*: Tangential excision and grafting for burns of the hand. Brit. J. Plast. Surg., *28*:189, 1975

MAHLER, D. L., AND FORREST, W. H., JR.: Relative analgesic potencies of morphine and hydromorphone in postoperative pain, PRS, *57*:267, 1976. Anesthesiology, *42*:602, 1975

MAHLER, D. M. *et al*: Lateral congenital sinus of the upper lip. Brit. J. Plast. Surg., *28*:203, 1975

MAHMOUD, A. F.: Marked prolongation of skin homograft survival with niridazole (with Mandel, Warren). PRS, *55*:76, 1975

MAIBACH, H. I., AND ROVEE, D. T.: *Epidermal Wound Healing.* Year Book Medical Publishers, Chicago, 1972. PRS, *52*:429, 1973

MAIBACH, H. I., LEAFFER, M. A., AND SKINNER, W. A.: Percutaneous penetration following use of hair dyes, PRS, *57*:681, 1976. Arch. Dermat., *111*:1444, 1975

MAILLARD, G. F. et al: Plastic surgery of the face in leprosy. Rev. Med. Suisse Romande, 94:729, 1974 (French)

MAILLARD, G. F. et al: Plastic surgery of leprous face. Helv. Chir. Acta, 42:161, 1975 (French)

MAILLARD, G. F., OTTO, R., AND CLODIUS, L.: Xeroradiography examinations in orbito-nasal surgery. PRS, 55:664, 1975

MAINOUS, E., AND HAMMER, D.: Surgical closure of oroantral fistula using gold foil technique, PRS, 55:375, 1975. J. Oral Surg., 32:528, 1974

MAINOUS, E. G. et al: Nasal septum perforation following total maxillary osteotomy, case report. J. Oral Surg., 31:869, 1973

MAINOUS, E. G. et al: Restoration of resected mandible by grafting with combination of mandible homograft and autogenous iliac marrow, and postoperative treatment with hyperbaric oxygenation. Oral Surg., 35:13, 1973

MAINOUS, E. G., CROWELL, N. T., AND SMITH, G. L.: Review of 168 maxillofacial fractures treated at Naval Hospital, PRS, 54:688, 1974. Mil. Med., 139:278, 1974

MAINOUS, E. G., AND HEART, G. B.: Osteoradionecrosis of mandible—treatment with hyperbaric oxygen, PRS, 57:758, 1976. Arch. Otolaryng., 101:173, 1975

MAINOUS, E. G. et al: Lingual mandibular bone concavity. J. Am. Dent. Assoc., 90:666, 1975

MAISELS, D. O.: Lobster-claw deformities of the hand. Hand, 2:79, 1970

MAISELS, D. O.: Timing and choice of operation for primary repairs of clefts of the lip and palate. Ann. R. Coll. Surg. Engl., 48:32, 1971

MAISELS, D. O.: Surgery of abnormalities of external ear excluding agenesis, PRS, 55:714, 1975. Proc. Roy. Soc. Med., 67:1201, 1974

MAISELS, D. O., AND PRIESTLAND, H. A.: Plastic trismus—difficult diagnostic problem, PRS, 55:105, 1975. Brit. J. Plast. Surg., 26:223, 1973

MAJEWSKA, E.: Calcifying epithelioma of Malherbe in parotid gland region in a 6-year-old girl. Pol. Tyg. Lek., 29:1997, 1974 (Polish)

MAJNO, GUIDO: The Healing Hand: Man and Wound in the Ancient World. Harvard University Press, Cambridge, 1975. PRS, 57:230, 1976

MAJOR, A.: Lacerated wounds of fingers caused by rings. Acta Chir. Plast. (Praha), 13:117, 1971

MAKAREVICH, V. T. et al: Preparation of burn wounds for autodermatoplasty. Voen. Med. Zh., 1:31, 1973 (Russian)

MAKHANI, J. S.: Dribbling of saliva in children with cerebral palsy and its management. Indian J. Pediatr., 41:272, 1974

MAKHOV, N. I. et al: Surgical treatment of hemangiomas. Klin. Khir., 9:35, 1971 (Russian)

MAKHOV, N. I. et al: Surgical creation of fascial "stocking" in patients with postthrombotic syndrome of the lower limbs. Khirurgiia (Mosk.), 5:46, 1974 (Russian)

MAKHOVSKII, V. Z.: Replacement of circular skin defect of penis. Vestn. Khir., 111:99, 1973 (Russian)

MAKIENKO, M. A. et al: Osteosynthesis of fractures of the mandible in children by using metal pins. Stomatologiia (Mosk.), 53:34, 1974 (Russian)

MAKINO, K.: Management of fractures of the zygoma, orbital floor and maxilla. Shujutsu, 25:1187, 1971 (Japanese)

MAKINO, K. et al: Case of true prehallux, PRS, 55:380, 1975. Jap. J. Plast. Reconstr. Surg., 17:252, 1974

MAKINO, M. et al: Case of the winging hand. Orthop. Surg. (Tokyo), 22:992, 1971 (Japanese)

MAKISHIMA, K. et al: Alveolar rhabdomyosarcoma of the ethmoid sinus. Laryngoscope, 85:400, 1975

MAKOSKI, H. B. et al: Tabular and case demonstrations of 100 malignant melanomas treated by endolymphatic therapy. Med. Welt., 25:1042, 1974 (German)

MAKRES, G. et al: Surgical treatment of cancer of lips. Stomatologia (Athenai), 29:321, 1972 (Greek)

MAKRIS, G. et al: Severe injuries of the face. Stomatologia (Athenai), 28:301, 1971 (Greek)

MALAMENT, I. B., DUNN, M. E., AND DAVIS, R.: Pressure sores, operant conditioning approach to prevention, PRS, 56:470, 1975. Arch. Phys. Med. & Rehab., 56:161, 1975

MALAMENT, M.: Repair of recurrent fistula of the penile urethra, PRS, 50:200, 1972. J. Urol., 106:704, 1971

Malar: See Cheek; Orbit; Zygoma

MALATSKII, S. I. et al: Successful resuscitation in injuries caused by electric current. Ortop. Travmatol. Protez., 32:72, 1971 (Russian)

MALBEC, E. F., QUAIFE, J. V., AND ARCE GONZALEZ, C.: Wrinkles of face, PRS, 50:198, 1972. El Dia Medico Argent., 44:15, 1972

MALEK, R.: Digit transpositions in children. Ann. Chir., 25:1015, 1971 (French)

MALEK, R.: Nasal deformities and their treatment in secondary cleft lip patients, PRS, 56:461, 1975. Scand. J. Plast. Reconstr. Surg., 8:136, 1974

MALEK, R. *et al*: Pollicization of the index finger in children. Ann. chir. plast., *16:*198, 1971 (French)

MALER, L.: Plastic surgery in sequelae of gangrene and gas phlegmons, PRS, *57:*676, 1976. Bol. y trab. soc. argent. cir., *36:*216, 1975

MALEVICH, E. S. *et al*: Elimination of hazards in radical operations in malignant neoplasms of maxillofacial area. Stomatologiia (Mosk.), *52:*24, 1973 (Russian)

MALEVICH, E. S. *et al*: Osteosynthesis of the fractured mandible using homologous bone screws. Stomatologiia (Mosk.), *53:*37, 1974 (Russian)

MALEY, E. D., AND MacDONALD, C. J.: Bilateral subungual glomus tumors. PRS, *55:*488, 1975

MALGAIGNE, J. F.: Du bec-de-lièvre (Classic Reprint). PRS, *57:*359, 1976

MALHERBE, W. D.: Injuries to the skin of the male external genitalia in Southern Africa. S. Afr. Med. J., *49:*147, 1975

MALHERBE, W. D., AND VAN DER WALT, J. J.: Mid-dermis graft, experimental study, PRS, *53:*113, 1974. Arch. chir. neerl., *25:*91, 1973

MALICK, M. H.: Preliminary prosthesis for the partially amputated hand. Am. J. Occup. Ther., *29:*479, 1975

MALINIAC, JACQUES W.: *Breast Deformities and their Repair*. Waverly Press, Baltimore, 1950. Reissued by Krieger Publishing Co., Huntington, N. Y., 1971. PRS, *49:*568, 1972

MALINOWSKI, J.: Evaluation of therapeutic methods in prognathism. Czas. Stomatol., *25:*1227, 1972 (Polish)

MALINOWSKI, J.: Anterior nasal spina as source for autogenous bone grafts, preliminary report. Czas. Stomatol., *26:*881, 1973 (Polish)

MALINOWSKI, J. *et al*: Surgical treatment of prognathism. Otolaryngol. Pol., *29:*481, 1975 (Polish)

MALKIN, M. *et al*: Stafne defect of anterior mandible. N. Y. State Dent. J., *40:*17, 1974

MALKIN, R. B. *et al*: Scrotal skin recession phalloplasty. J. Urol., *113:*343, 1975

MALLEN, R. W.: Otoplasty. Can. J. Otolaryngol., *3:*74, 1974

MALLEN, R. W. *et al*: Dorsal rhinotomy approach to nasal gliomas. Can. J. Otolaryngol., *3:*187, 1974

MALLEN, R. W. *et al*: Chylous fistula following right radical neck dissection. Can. J. Otolaryngol., *4:*177, 1975

MALLIAKAS, S. *et al*: Femoral nerve paralysis caused by traumatic hematoma of iliopsoas muscle, PRS, *57:*537, 1976. Ann. chir., *29:*591, 1975

MALM, O. J.: Treatment of serious burns.

Tidsskr. Nor. Laegeforen, *91:*2033, 1971 (Norwegian)

Malocclusion (See also *Jaw Deformities; Micrognathia; Prognathism*)

Surgical treatment of mandibular laterognathies (Delaire). Orthod. Fr., *41:*269, 1970 (French)

Technic for partial segment osteotomy of the upper maxillary (Parant *et al*). Orthod. Fr., *41:*325, 1970 (French)

Corticotomy, a surgical-orthodontical method (Tenebaum). Ortodoncia, *34:*162, 1970 (Spanish)

Treatment of a case of laterognathia associated with prognathism by the Trauner technic (Fraysse *et al*). Rev. Odontostomatol. Midi Fr., *28:*275, 1970 (French)

Surgery or orthodontics – a philosophy of approach (Walker *et al*). Dent. Clin. North Am., *15:*771, 1971

Planning pre- and postoperative treatment in orthodontic surgical procedures (Spiessl *et al*). Dtsch. Stomatol., *21:*734, 1971 (German)

Surgical shifting of the lateral lower jaw alveolar process for correction of cross bite and crowding (Zisser). Dtsch. Zahnaerztl. Z., *26:*956, 1971 (German)

Surgical treatment of severe dento-maxillary irregularities (Popescu *et al*). Int. Dent. J., *21:*346, 1971

Correction of skeletal type of anterior open bite (Bell). J. Oral Surg., *29:*706, 1971

Unilateral oblique osteotomy for correction of open bite after multiple facial fractures: report of case (Khosla *et al*). J. Oral Surg., *29:*821, 1971

Laterognathism of mandible supported by calcified residue of Meckel's cartilage (Mangiante), PRS, *51:*102, 1973. Riv. ital. chir. plast., *3:*233, 1971

Oral surgery in orthodontic practice (Briche *et al*). Stomatologia (Athenai), *28:*259, 1971

Surgical-orthodontic treatment of diastema mediana with hypertrophican frenulum. Acta Stomatol. Croat., *7:*173, 1972–73 (Croatian)

An appraisal of surgical orthodontics (Salzmann). Am. J. Orthod., *61:*105, 1972

Cephalometric prediction for orthodontic surgery (McNeill *et al*). Angle Orthod., *42:*154, 1972

Skeletal open bite associated with bimaxillary dento-alveolar protrusion, evaluation and treatment (Silbermann *et al*). Brit. J. Oral Surg., *10:*223, 1972

Surgical and orthodontic cooperation as a

Malocclusion — Cont.

basis for optimal therapeutic success in special jaw anomalies (Muska *et al*). Dtsch. Stomatol., *22:*128, 1972 (German)

Surgical possibilities and limits of surgery of the deep bite (Schwenzer). Dtsch. Zahnaerztl. Z., *27:*549, 1972 (German)

Surgical correction of deep bite and open bite (Mehnert). Dtsch. Zahn. Mund. Kieferheilkd, *59:*13, 1972 (German)

Surgical correction of alveolar malposition (Zisser). Dtsch. Zahn. Mund. Kieferheilkd., *59:*68, 1972 (German)

Subtotal transbuccal osteotomy of face (Gimenez). Int. J. Orthod., *10:*93, 1972

Maxillary midline diastema, closure of, with frenectomy and corticotomy (Massey). J. Ga. Dent. Assoc., *46:*26, 1972

Maxillary osteotomy — surgical orthodontics (Daniel). J. Ky. Dent. Assoc., *24:*13, 1972

Total maxillary osteotomy and repositioning of the maxilla: report of case (Cruickshank *et al*). J. Oral Surg., *30:*586, 1972

Apertognathia — an interdisciplinary approach: report of case (Hershman *et al*). J. Oral Surg., *30:*743, 1972

Intraoral osteotomy of mandibular symphysis to correct bilateral lingual crossbite: report of case (Frer *et al*). J. Oral Surg., *30:*754, 1972

Surgical correction of mandibular asymmetries (Zisser). Osterr. Z. Stomatol., *69:*304, 1972 (German)

Surgery of the smile. II. (Gimenez). Rev. Asoc. Odontol. Argent., *60:*59, 1972 (Spanish)

Surgery for open bite, case report (Gimenez). Rev. Asoc. Odontol. Argent., *60:*485, 1972 (Spanish)

Segmented osteotomies of the upper jaw (Souyris *et al*). Rev. Stomatol. Chir. Maxillofac., *73:*43, 1972 (French)

Surgical treatment of excessive development of the mandible and of open bite by intercortical osteotomy of the mandible (Mitrofanov *et al*). Stomatologiia (Mosk.), *51:*48, 1972 (Russian)

Bite, vertically open, surgical treatment of (Petrovic), PRS, *53:*682, 1974. Acta chir. plast., *15:*39, 1973

Malocclusion, open-bite, surgical-orthodontic correction of, case report (McNeill). Am. J. Orthod., *64:*38, 1973

Multidisciplinary responsibilities in orthopedic-occlusal rehabilitation (Rutrick *et al*). Am. J. Orthod., *64:*491, 1973

Treatment of class II facial deformity. Maxillary operations (Seward). Brit. J. Oral Surg., *10:*254, 1973

Malocclusion — Cont.

Correction of dento-alveolar deformity by anterior alveolar osteotomy, case report (Gold *et al*). Bull. Monmouth Ocean Cty. Dent. Soc., *31:*16, 1973

Oral orthopedics (Goldberg *et al*). Conn. Med., *37:*615, 1973

Immediate surgical repositioning of one- and two-tooth dento-osseous segments (Bell). Int. J. Oral Surg., *2:*265, 1973

Malocclusions, skeletal, orthodontic surgery important part of treatment. Case presentation (Elias *et al*). Int. J. Orthod., *11:*75, 1973

Open reduction at mandibular angle for correction of open bite caused by traffic injury (Hasegawa *et al*). Jap. J. Oral Surg., *19:*52, 1973 (Japanese)

Maxillo-mandibular surgery for correction of dentofacial deformities. 3. Maxillary protrusion (Weinberg *et al*). J. Can. Dent. Assoc., *39:*416, 1973

Maxillo-mandibular surgery for correction of dentofacial deformities. 6. Apertognathia (open bite) (Weinberg *et al*). J. Can. Dent. Assoc., *39:*623, 1973

Open bite, contribution to surgical treatment of (Schroll). J. Maxillo-facial Surg., *1:*203, 1973

In vitro studies on lines of osteotomy in pterygoid region (Wikkeling *et al*). J. Maxillofacial Surg., *1:*209, 1973

Orthodontic surgery, segmental, simplified method of fixation after (Cranin, Dennison). J. Oral Surg., *31:*109, 1973

Orthodontist's view of surgical orthodontics (Rosenstein). J. Oral Surg., *31:*177, 1973

Correction of maxillary protrusion with severe vertical dysplasia — multidisciplinary approach (Tarsitano *et al*). J. Oral Surg., *31:*675, 1973

Segmental alveolar osteotomy in the correction of maxillofacial malformations (Torrielli *et al*). Minerva Stomatol., *22:*218, 1973 (Italian)

Corrective operation for laterognathism (Papadopoulos). Odontostomatol. Proodos., *27:*161, 1973 (Greek)

Severe deep bite corrected by surgery and prosthodontics (Tamas *et al*). Orv. Hetil., *114:*2911, 1973 (Hungarian)

Indication for surgical orthodontic interventions — results and failures (Wunderer). Osterr. Z. Stomatol., *70:*382, 1973 (German)

Alveolar segment recession: maxillary recession for bucktooth deformity (Russell, Beason). PRS, *51:*220, 1973

Case of forced straightening (Burkle). Quin-

Malocclusion — Cont.
tessenz, *24:*91, 1973 (German)

Surgical correction of tooth malposition (Scartascini *et al*). Trib. Odontol. (B. Aires), *57:*40, 1973

Cross bite, frontal (Reychler *et al*). Acta Stomatol. Belg., *71:*91, 1974 (Dutch)

Canine eminence (Henns). Angle Orthod., *44:*326, 1974

Anterior maxillary osteotomy, method of fixation following vertical split during (Hicks *et al*). Brit. J. Oral Surg., *11:*265, 1974

Reversed occlusions in frontal region of teeth treated by corticotomy (Subrtova *et al*). Cesk. Stomatol., *74:*206, 1974 (Czechoslovakian)

Malocclusion, late results of separation of raphe palati in (Dyras *et al*). Czas. Stomatol., *27:*635, 1974 (Polish)

Results of surgical treatment of lateral occlusion by way of mandibular ramus osteotomy (Baranczak *et al*). Czas. Stomatol., *27:*1199, 1974 (Polish)

Malocclusion, three-phase surgery for, is taped for training (Editorial). Dent. Surv., *50:*78, 1974

Changes in the soft tissues after corrective osteotomies in the jaw region (Steinhauser). Dtsch. Zahnaerztl. Z., *29:*1065, 1974 (German)

Possible applications of stepwise osteotomy of the ascending ramus (Schwenzer). Fortschr. Kiefer. Gesichtschir., *18:*138, 1974 (German)

Treatment of the gnathic open bite (Steinhardt *et al*). Fortschr. Kiefer. Gesichtschir., *18:*199, 1974 (German)

Indication, technic and clinical results of surgical treatment of open bite using Schuchardt's osteotomy of the lateral maxilla (Holtje *et al*). Fortschr. Kiefer. Gesichtschir., *18:*202, 1974 (German)

Single-step higher repositioning of the alveolar process in the treatment of open bite due to rickets (Erwig *et al*). Fortschr. Kiefer. Gesichtschir., *18:*207, 1974 (German)

Results of surgical correction of open bite using Schuchardt's method (Nwoku). Fortschr. Kiefer. Gesichtschir., *18:*209, 1974 (German)

Surgical treatment of open bite using 3-part osteotomy of the maxilla (Kruger). Fortschr. Kiefer. Gesichtschir., *18:*211, 1974 (German)

Results of surgical correction of open bite using Kole's method (Aarnes). Fortschr. Kiefer. Gesichtschir, *18:*217, 1974 (German)

Reconstruction of individual occlusion after

Malocclusion — Cont.
faulty facial bone fracture healing (Matras). Fortschr. Kiefer. Gesichtschir., *18:*223, 1974 (German)

Surgical correction of posttraumatic occlusion disorders (Luhr). Fortschr. Kiefer. Gesichtschir., *18:*227, 1974 (German)

Tongue asymmetries, influence of, on development of jaws and position of teeth (Austermann *et al*). Int. J. Oral Surg., *3:*261, 1974

Mandibular alveolar osteotomy, total (MacIntosh), PRS, *55:*715, 1975. J. Maxillo-facial Surg., *2:*210, 1974

Malocclusion, zygomatic complex fracture with an avulsed tooth causing, case report (Dunsworth). J. Oral Surg., *32:*131, 1974

Malocclusion, treatment in case of Treacher-Collins syndrome (Huffman, Lorson), PRS, *56:*105, 1975. J. Oral Surg., *32:*612, 1974

Surgical correction of posterior crossbite (Bell *et al*). J. Oral Surg., *32:*811, 1974

Correction of mandibular nonunion and gross malocclusion: report of case (Gelsinon *et al*). J. Oral Surg., *32:*855, 1974

Open-bite, skeletal, new dynamic functional method in surgical treatment of (Curioni *et al*). Minerva Stomatol., *23:*175, 1974

Evaluation of surgical procedure of sagittal split osteotomy of mandibular ramus (Wang *et al*). Oral Surg., *38:*167, 1974

Patient treated by surgical orthodontics, 44-month evaluation of, case report (Palomo *et al*). Oral Surg., *38:*520, 1974

Malocclusion, class II, corrected by full mandibular advancement surgery, stability of treatment results in (Guernsey). Oral Surg., *37:*668, 1974

Maxillary osteotomy, simplifying Le Fort I type (Dupont, Ciaburro, Prévost). PRS, *54:*142, 1974

Malocclusion, partially edentulous adult with, surgical-prosthetic management of (Kucharski). Protet. Stomatol., *24:*217, 1974 (Polish)

Case of forced positional change (redressement force) (Burkle). Quintessence Int., *5:*39, 1974

Discussion of indications for alveolar segmental osteotomy of the jaws (Cros *et al*). Rev. Stomatol. Chir. Maxillofac., *75:*107, 1974 (French)

Surgical treatment of upper incisive protrusions in adolescents (Deffez *et al*). Rev. Stomatol. Chir. Maxillofac., *75:*111, 1974 (French)

Segmental osteotomies of the jaws in orthodontic disorders (Souyris *et al*). Rev. Stomatol. Chir. Maxillofac., *75:*122, 1974

Malocclusion – Cont.

(French)

Maxillary alveolar protrusions (Piscevic *et al*). Rev. Stomatol. Chir. Maxillofac., *75:*128, 1974 (French)

Partial corticotomies and osteotomies (Del Hoyo *et al*). Rev. Stomatol. Chir. Maxillofac., *75:*131, 1974 (French)

Complementary orthopedic treatments after surgical treatment of upper incisor protrusion in adolescents (Deffez *et al*). Rev. Stomatol. Chir. Maxillofac., *75:*134, 1974 (French)

Surgery of laterognathism of articular origin (Toman). Rev. Stomatol. Chir. Maxillofac., *75:*148, 1974 (French)

Indications and techniques for surgical treatment of superior proalveolia (Michelet *et al*). Rev. Stomatol. Chir. Maxillofac., *75:*1093, 1974 (French)

Bite anomalies in adults, combined forms, surgical treatment of (Arzhantsev *et al*). Stomatologiia (Mosk.), *53:*38, 1974 (Russian)

Use of a Le Fort I osteotomy as a surgical approach (Hopkins *et al*). Brit. J. Oral Surg., *13:*27, 1975

Surgical methods for the correction of malocclusion Angle II/1 with postoperative prosthetic rehabilitation (Harle *et al*). Dtsch. Zahnaerztl. Z., *30:*176, 1975 (German)

Possibilities of prosthetic treatment of malocclusion Angle II/1 with and without surgical preparation (Lenz *et al*). Dtsch. Zahnaerztl. Z., *30:*179, 1975 (German)

Orthosurgical teamwork. (Olson *et al*). J. Am. Dent. Assoc., *90:*998, 1975

Teamwork approach to correct a severe prosthodontic problem (Belinfante *et al*). J. Am. Dent. Assoc., *91:*357, 1975

Combined anterior and posterior maxillary ostectomy: a new technique (Wolford *et al*). J. Oral Surg., *33:*842, 1975

Editorial: The art and science of orthognathic surgery (Laskin). J. Oral Surg., *33:*905, 1975

Research on orthognathic surgery – an NIDR state-of-the-art workshop (Editorial). J. Oral Surg., *33:*907, 1975

Correction of severe open-bite associated with muscular disease. Report of a case (Steinhauser *et al*). Oral Surg., *39:*509, 1975

Dentofacial orthopedics and orthopedic surgery (Benoist *et al*). Rev. Stomatol. Chir. Maxillofac., *76:*175, 1975 (French)

Surgical correction of the open bite by a 2-stage mobilization of the lateral portions of the maxilla (Kozlov *et al*). Stomatologiia

Malocclusion – Cont.

(Mosk.), *54:*29, 1975 (Russian)

Surgical orthodontic treatment planning: profile analysis and mandibular surgery (Worms *et al*). Angle Orthod., *46:*1, 1976

Interdental osteotomy for immediate repositioning of dental-osseus elements (Merrill *et al*). J. Oral Surg., *34:*118, 1976

Combined anterior and posterior maxillary osteotomy (Hall *et al*). J. Oral Surg., *34:*126, 1976

MALONEY, M. L.: Submucosal frenotomy, PRS, *55:*507, 1975. Oral Surg., *38:*23, 1974

MALONEY, P. L. *et al*: Free buccal mucosal grafts for vestibuloplasty. J. Oral Surg., *30:*716, 1972

MALONEY, P. L., SHEPHERD, N. S., AND DOKU, H. C.: Immediate vestibuloplasy with free mucosal grafts, PRS, *55:*246, 1975. J. Oral Surg., *32:*343, 1974

MALONEY, P. L. *et al*: Mucosal grafting in oral reconstructive surgery. J. Oral Surg., *32:*705, 1974

MALONEY, P. L. *et al*: Asutural maxillary vestibuloplasty. Oral Surg., *37:*858, 1974

MALT, R. A. AND McDOWELL, F.: Cable from Cathay. New England J. Med., *288:*1353, 1973

MALTZ, R. *et al*: Carcinoma of the tonsil: results of combined therapy. Laryngoscope, *84:*2172, 1974

MALYSHEV, V. A.: Replantation as a method of treating high fractures of the neck of the mandibular condyle with dislocation of the articular head. Stomatologiia (Mosk.), *51:*25, 1972 (Russian)

MAMATTAH, H. J. *et al*: Bacteremia in burned patient. J. Clin. Pathol., *26:*388, 1973

Mammaplasty (See also *Breasts*)

Breast Deformities and their Repair. By Jacques W. Maliniac. Waverly Press, Baltimore, 1950. Reissued by Krieger Publishing Co., Huntington, N. Y., 1971. PRS, *49:*568, 1972

Plasties Mammaires pour Hypertrophie et Ptose. By J. P. Lalardrie and J. P. Jouglard. Masson & Cie., Paris, 1973. PRS, *53:*673, 1974

Chirurgie Plastique de Sein (Plastic Surgery of the Breast). By J. P. Lalardrie and J. P. Jouglard. Masson et Cie, Paris, 1974.

Plastic and Reconstructive Surgery of the Breast. By Robert M. Goldwyn. Little, Brown & Co., Boston, 1976

Mammarian region, plastic surgery of breast and (Lupo, Boggio-Robutti), PRS, *49:*357, 1972. Minerva med., Italy, Monograph, 1971

Mammaplasty—Cont.

Breast surgery, suction drainage in (Editorial). Brit. Med. J., *3:*554, 1973

Breast surgery—as office procedure (Richards). Can. Med. Assoc. J., *109:*305, 1973

Mammaplasty with omentum magnum in prethoracic transposition (Kiricuta, Popescu), PRS, *53:*242, 1974. Chir. Plast., *2:*47, 1973

Mammaplasty (Dion). Infirm. Can., *15:*21, 1973 (French)

Breast, the beauty, the beast, and (Danilevicius). J.A.M.A., *223:*683, 1973

Mammaplasty: value of mammography in cosmetic surgery of breasts (Perras, Papillon. PRS, *52:*132, 1973

Mammaplasty, technique of inferior flap (Robertson) (Follow-Up Clinic). PRS, *52:*433, 1973

Breast, and esthetics (Vilain), PRS, *54:*620, 1974. Ann. chir. plast., *19:*1, 1974

Mammaplasty with reduced blood loss: effect of noradrenalin (Bretteville-Jensen), PRS, *56:*677, 1975. Brit. J. Plast. Surg., *27:*31, 1974

Breasts, modifications to (Editorial). Brit. Med. J., *3:*135, 1974

Psychological aspects in plastic surgery of the breast (Eicher *et al*). Fortschr. Med., *92:*1407, 1974 (German)

Mammaplasty, evaluation of techniques in municipal teaching hospital (Bromberg, Song, Norwitz). PRS, *53:*33, 1974

Axillary breasts (Kaye). PRS, *53:*61, 1974

Mammaplasties, Ambroise Paré's opinion on (Montandon, Letterman) (Letter to the Editor). PRS, *54:*212, 1974

Mammaplasty with J-shaped scar (Elbaz), PRS, *57:*260, 1976. Ann. chir. plast., *20:*101, 1975

Experiences with plastic surgery of the female breast (augmentation, reduction, lifting) (Huter *et al*). Arch. Gynaekol., *219:*155, 1975 (German)

Proceedings: Psychological aspects in augmentation and reduction plasties (Eicher *et al*). Arch. Gynaekol., *219:*157, 1975 (German)

Cosmetic surgery of the breast (Hoffman *et al*). Clin. Obstet. Gynecol., *18:*253, 1975

Mammary asymmetry (Rees). Clin. Plast. Surg., *2:*371, 1975

Some considerations in surgical alteration of the feminine silhouette (Vilain). Clin. Plast. Surg., *2:*449, 1975

Esthetic-surgical breast enlargement, exchange mastectomy, and breast reconstruction following mamma amputation. New clinical and radiographic findings

Mammaplasty—Cont.

(von Lutzki *et al*). Med. Welt., *26:*381, 1975 (German)

Mammaplasty, factors in production of inconspicuous scars (Wray, Holtmann, Weeks). PRS, *56:*86, 1975

Mammaplasty, causes of failure in (Piotti), PRS, *57:*759, 1976 (Italian). Riv. ital. chir. plast., *7:*447, 1975

Body sculpturing (Tearston *et al*). Surg. Clin. North Am., *55:*151, 1975

Errors and dangers of mammaplasty (Bruckner). Zentralbl. Chir., *100:*1266, 1975

Mammaplasty, Augmentation

Mammary prostheses, personal experience and critical study of (Vrebos), PRS, *50:*199, 1972. Acta chir. belg., *70:*300, 1971

Personal and clinical experience with mammary prosthesis implantations (Vrebos). Ann. chir. plast., *17:*114, 1972 (French)

Breast prosthesis, folded: new clinical and radiological entity (Slonim *et al*). Australas. Radiol., *16:*159, 1972

Breast, long-term effects of plastics on (Editorial). Food, Cosmet. Toxicol., *10:*567, 1972

Silastic breast implants, experiences with large series (Williams). PRS, *49:*253, 1972

Prosthesis, natural-Y breast, further studies (Ashley). PRS, *49:*414, 1972

Mammaplasty, augmentation, treating complications (Silver). PRS, *49:*637, 1972

Breast implants, successful treatment of some fibrous envelope contractures around (Freeman). PRS, *50:*107, 1972

Prosthesis, mammary, new inflatable, clinical trial and evaluation (Regnault *et al*). PRS, *50:*220, 1972

Mammarian hypotrophies, some considerations concerning application of liquid silicone in (Roa-Roa). PRS, *50:*419, 1972. Rev. Latino Am. Cir. Plast., *15:*17, 1972

Breast prosthesis, critical study of, and attempt at definition of ideal prosthesis (Nicoletis). Ann. chir. plast., *18:*239, 1973 (French)

Breast augmentation prostheses. Critical study of results (Pollet). Ann. chir. plast., *18:*301, 1973 (French)

Mammary silicone granuloma. Migration of silicone fluid to abdominal wall and inguinal region (Delage *et al*). Arch. Dermat., *108:*105, 1973

Breast augmentation: axillary approach. Brit. J. Plast. Surg., *26:*373, 1973

Nice adventure for a woman (Brown). Infirm. Can., *15:*24, 1973 (French)

Correction of mammary gland hypoplasia by

Mammaplasty, Augmentation — Cont.

Mammary asymmetry (Rees). Clin. Plast. Surg., 2:371, 1975

Ultrasonic diagnosis of breast prosthesis implanted after operative treatment of tumors or augmentation plastic of the breast (Audretsch). Geburtshilfe Frauenheilkd., 35:853, 1975 (German)

Breast augmentation, psychosexual aspects (Kolin, Baker, Bartlett), PRS, 55:636, 1975. Human Sexuality, 8:88, 1974

Breast augmentation, when patients inquire about (Bryant), PRS, 55:508, 1975. Human Sexuality, 8:127, 1974

Letter: Breast prostheses (Marchant). Lancet, 2:187, 1975

Letter: Breast prostheses (Watts). Lancet, 2:280, 1975

Letter: Breast prosthesis (Burns). Lancet, 2:1259, 1975

Breast-halving incision for subcutaneous mastectomy (Corso, Zubiri). PRS, 56:1, 1975

Exposed breast implant, treatment of by reimplantation behind posterior wall of capsule (Snyder). PRS, 56:97, 1975

Congenital hypoplasia, unilateral, or absence of breast (Pierre, Jouglard). PRS, 56:146, 1975

Flap from buttock, microvascular transfer for aplasia of breast and pectoral region (Fujino, Harashina, Aoyagi), PRS, 56:178, 1975. Discussion by Goldwyn, PRS, 56:335, 1975

Mammaplasty, augmentation, effect of hematoma on thickness of pseudosheaths around silicone implants (Williams, Aston, Rees). PRS, 56:194, 1975

Prostheses, breast, foreign body reaction to polyurethane covers of some (Cocke, Leathers, Lynch). PRS, 56:527, 1975

Mammaplasty, augmentation, and simultaneous reduction of areola, through periareolar incision (Bartels, Mara). PRS, 56:588, 1975

Breast augmentation, transareolar incision for (Pitanguy, Carreirao, Garcia), PRS, 54:501, 1974. Rev. brasil. chir., 63:301, 1973

Breast prostheses, capsular retraction in (Planas *et al*), PRS, 56:594, 1975. Rev. españ. cir. plast., 7:206, 1974

Augmentation mammaplasty, avoidable pitfalls in (Huger). South. Med. J., 68:703, 1975

Augmentation mammaplasty through a circumareolar incision using a solid, gel-filled implant (Norman *et al*). South. Med. J.,

Mammaplasty, Augmentation — Cont.

68:1456, 1975

Letter: Breast prostheses (Watts). Lancet, 1:145, 1976

Letter: Breast prostheses (Marchant). Lancet, 1:360, 1976

Letter: Breast prostheses (Snyderman). Lancet, 1:494, 1976

Augmentation mammaplasty, dissector for transaxillary approach (Agris, Dingman, Wilensky). PRS, 57:10, 1976

Breast augmentation, cushioned, after subcutaneous mastectomy (Rubin). PRS, 57:23, 1976

Steroids, soluble, use within inflatable breast prostheses (Perrin). PRS, 57:163, 1976

Breast hypoplasia associated with chest wall deformities, reconstruction of (Hawtof, Ram, Alani). PRS, 57:172, 1976

Mammaplasty, augmentation, failure of steroid instillation to prevent capsular contracture after (Price) (Letter to the Editor). PRS, 57:371, 1976

Breast implants introduced through abdominal route (Planas). PRS, 57:434, 1976

Breast augmentation, retractor for use in (Fischl). PRS, 57:526, 1976

Breast implants, silicone, long-term study of reactions in rabbits (Lilla, Vistnes). PRS, 57:637, 1976

Mammaplasty, correction of asymmetries of breasts (Elsahy). PRS, 57:700, 1976

Aplasia of breast, unilateral, giant implant for (Marchac, Alkhatib). PRS, 57:749, 1976

External gel-filled prosthesis of the breast (Prosnak). Pol. Przegl. Chir., 48:81, 1976 (Polish)

Mammaplasty, Complications

Breasts, management of patients with complications from injections of foreign materials (Ortiz-Monasterio, Trigos). PRS, 50:42, 1972

Contractures, fibrous envelope around breast implants, successful treatment of some (Freeman). PRS, 50:107, 1972

Mammary silicone granuloma (Delage, Shane, Johnson), PRS, 54:373, 1974. Arch. Dermat., 108:105, 1973

Anti-estrogen, use of an, after a reduction mammaplasty to prevent recurrence of virginal hypertrophy of breasts (Sperling, Gold). PRS, 52:439, 1973

Cancer, bilateral breast, 10 years after an augmentation mammaplasty (Johnson, Lloyd). PRS, 53:88, 1974

Scarring, circumferential capsular, in aug-

Mammaplasty, Complications — Cont.

mentation mammaplasty, role of steroids in prevention (Peterson, Burt). PRS, *54:*28, 1974

Pharyngitis as source of postoperative infection around a breast implant (Smith) (Letter to the Editor). PRS, *54:*347, 1974

Revisional surgery after reduction mammaplasty (Herman, Hoffman, Kahn). PRS, *55:*422, 1975

Breasts, large, subcutaneous mastectomy, excess skin problem with (Hartley, Schatten, Griffin). PRS, *56:*5, 1975

Breast implant, exposed, treatment of by reimplantation behind posterior wall of capsule (Snyder). PRS, *56:*97, 1975

Hematoma, effect on thickness of pseudo-sheaths around silicone implants (Williams, Aston, Rees). PRS, *56:*194, 1975

Mammaplasty complication, Mondor's disease (Fischl, Kahn, Simon). PRS, *56:*319, 1975

Breast, method for recontouring domed nipple (Vecchione). PRS, *57:*30, 1976

Contracture, capsular, after augmentation mammaplasty, failure of steroid instillation to prevent (Price) (Letter to the Editor). PRS, *57:*371, 1976

Mammaplasty, Dermal Pedicle (See also *Mammaplasty, Reduction*)

Dermal flap, vertical, reduction mammaplasty with (McKissock). PRS, *49:*245, 1972

Mastectomy, subcutaneous, reduction mammaplasty, or mastopexy, single dermal pedicle for nipple transposition in (Weiner *et al*). PRS, *51:*115, 1973

Mastoplasty with safety pedicle (Ribeiro, Backer), PRS, *53:*486, 1974. Rev. españ. cir. plast., *6:*223, 1973

Strömbeck's mammaplasty, late results of (Müller). PRS, *54:*664, 1974

Superomedial dermal pedicle for nipple transposition (Orlando *et al*). Brit. J. Plast. Surg., *28:*42, 1975

"Dermal pedicle," so-called, used in certain types of reduction mammaplasties, what is really in the (McDowell) (Editorial). PRS, *56:*201, 1975

"De-epithelization" of dermal pedicle in reduction mammaplasty (Parsons, Knieser), PRS, *57:*619, 1976

Mammaplasty, Mastopexy (See also *Mammaplasty, Reduction*)

Aries-Pitanguy technique in mammary gland ptosis, indications of (Lejour), PRS, *50:*199, 1972. Acta chir. belg., *70:*5, 1971

Mastopexy technique, dermal, subcutaneous mastectomy with immediate reconstruc-

Mammaplasty, Mastopexy — Cont.

tion of breasts using (Goulian, McDivitt). PRS, *50:*211, 1972

Mastopexy, subcutaneous mastectomy, or reduction mammaplasty, single dermal pedicle for nipple transposition in (Weiner *et al*). PRS, *51:*115, 1973

Breast, pendulous, surgery for (Andreeva *et al*). Vestn. Khir., *111:*50, 1973 (Russian)

Mastopexy: evaluation of mammaplasty techniques in municipal teaching hospital (Bromberg, Song, Norwitz). PRS, *53:*33, 1974

Mastopexy: surgical rehabilitation after massive weight reduction (McCraw). PRS, *53:*349, 1974

Mastopexy operation, new, for mild or moderate breast ptosis (Bartels, Strickland, Douglas). PRS, *57:*687, 1976

Mammaplasty, Nipple Operations: See *Breasts, Nipple Operations*

Mammaplasty, Reduction (See also *Breasts, Cystosarcoma Phylloides; Mammaplasty, Mastopexy*)

Mammary gland ptosis, indications for Aries-Pitanguy technique in (Lejour), PRS, *50:*199, 1972. Acta chir. belg., *70:*5, 1971

Mammaplasty, reduction, by Dufourmentel-Mouly method (Schatten, Hartley, Hamm). PRS, *48:*306, 1971

Reduction mammaplasty (Hoffman *et al*). South. Med. J., *64:*1106, 1971

Mammary ptoses and hypertrophies, correction technic (Goumain *et al*). Ann. chir. plast., *17:*198, 1972

Breast plastic surgery, L-form cicatrix in (Elbaz *et al*). Ann. chir. plast., *17:*283, 1972

Breast reduction: is it an aid to cancer detection? (Rees *et al*). Brit. J. Plast. Surg., *25:*144, 1972

Mammaplasty, reduction, with free grafting of nipple and areola (Farina *et al*). Brit. J. Plas. Surg., *25:*393, 1972

Mammaplasty, reduction, basic rules and problems in light of personal experience (Winkler), PRS, *51:*230, 1973. Chir. Plast., *1:*85, 1972

Breast, cosmetic surgery (Holder). J.A.M.A., *222:*1101, 1972

Mammaplasty, reduction, with vertical dermal flap (McKissock). PRS, *49:*245, 1972

Mammaplasty, surgical treatment of gynecomastia (Barbarelli). PRS, *53:*242, 1974. Prensa med. argent., *59:*1188, 1972

Mammaplasty, reduction, based on vertical bipedicle and "tennis ball" assembly (Pers, Bretteville-Jensen), PRS, *51:*103, 1973.

Mammaplasty, Reduction – Cont.

Mammaplasty, reduction, new technique (Ribeiro). PRS, *55:*330, 1975

Reduction mammaplasty, revisional surgery after (Herman, Hoffman, Kahn). PRS, *55:*422, 1975

Mammaplasty, reduction, variation of Biesenberger technique (Carlsen, Tershakowec). PRS, *55:*653, 1975

Mammaplasties, reduction, what is really in so-called "dermal pedicle" used in certain types of? (McDowell) (Editorial). PRS, *56:*201, 1975

Breast, cords around (Mondor's disease), unusual complication of mammaplasty (Fischl, Kahn, Simon). PRS, *56:*319, 1975

Mammaplasty, reduction, new technique (Johnson) (Letter to the Editor). PRS, *57:*372, 1976

Mammaplasty with curved incisions (Cardoso de Castro). PRS, *57:*596, 1976

Mammaplasty, reduction, "de-epithelization" of dermal pedicle in (Parsons, Knieser). PRS, *57:*619, 1976

MAMOUN, S. M. *et al*: Eccrine poroma of hand. PRS, *50:*295, 1972

MAN, K., AND TOLMEYER, J. A.: Operative treatment of dislocation of temporomandibular joint, PRS, *57:*396, 1976. Nederl. tijdschr. geneesk., *119:*1498, 1975

MANAKOV, P. M. *et al*: Simultaneous plastic surgery of brachial artery and median nerve in their complete intersection. Ortop. Travmatol. Protez., *35:*60, 1974 (Russian)

MANALAN, S. S., COHEN, I. K., AND THEOGARAJ, S. D.: *Dermatofibrosarcoma protuberans* or keloid – warning. PRS, *53:*96, 1974

MANCER, K.: Lymphedema, clinical review and follow-up study (with Saijo, Munro). PRS, *56:*513, 1975

MANCER, K.: Lymphangioma, long-term follow-up study (with Saijo, Munro). PRS, *56:*642, 1975

MANCHESTER, G. H.: Tattoo removal. New simple technique. California Med., *118:*10, 1973

MANCHESTER, G. H.: Comment on "Simple method for emergency orotracheal intubation" (Letter to the Editor). PRS, *51:*83, 1973

MANCHESTER, G. H.: Removal of commercial tattoos by abrasion with table salt. PRS, *53:*517, 1974

MANCHESTER, G. H., MANI, M. M., AND MASTERS, F. W.: Simple method for emergency orotracheal intubation. PRS, *49:*312, 1972

MANCHESTER, W. M.: Some technical improvements in reconstruction of mandible and temporomandibular joint. PRS, *50:*249, 1972

MANCUSI-UNGARO, A.: Use of cocaine as topical anesthetic in nasal surgery (with Feehan). PRS, *57:*62, 1975

MANCUSI-UNGARO, A., CORRES, J. J., AND DISPALTRO, F.: Median carpal tunnel syndrome following a vascular shunt procedure in the forearm. PRS, *57:*96, 1976

MANDEL, L., AND BAURMASH, H.: Role of sialography in extraparotid disease, PRS, *48:*195, 1971. Oral Surg., *31:*164, 1971

MANDEL, M., DVORAK, K., AND DeCOSSE, J.: Salivary immunoglobulins in patients with oropharyngeal and bronchopulmonary carcinoma, PRS, *54:*108, 1974. Cancer, *31:*1408, 1973

MANDEL, M. A.: Skin testing for prognosis or therapy formulation in cancer patients: *caveat emptor,* PRS, *57:*621, 1976. Discussion by Humphrey, PRS, *57:*743, 1976

MANDEL, M. A.: Synergistic effect of salicylates on methotrexate toxicity. PRS, *57:*733, 1976

MANDEL, M. A. *et al*: Cystosarcoma phylloides. Treatment by subcutaneous mastectomy with immediate prosthetic implantation, PRS, *50:*630, 1972. Am. J. Surg., *123:*718, 1972

MANDEL, M. A., DVORAK, K., AND DeCOSSE, J. J.: Secretory immunoglobulin levels in cancer patients, PRS, *51:*708, 1973. Surg. Forum, *23:*513, 1972

MANDEL, M. A., KIEHN, C. L., AND SYKORA, G. F.: Use of angiography in outlining solitary solid tumors of head and neck. PRS, *52:*61, 1973

MANDEL, M. A., AND KIEHN, C. L.: Prognostic significance of delayed cutaneous reactivity in head and neck cancer patients. PRS, *53:*72, 1974

MANDEL, M. A., MAHMOUD, A. F., AND WARREN, K. S.: Marked prolongation of skin homograft survival with niridazole. PRS, *55:*76, 1975

MANDELCORN, M. S. *et al*: Orbital blast injury, case report. Can. J. Ophthalmol., *8:*597, 1973

MANDELSON, J. A.: Selection of plasma volume expanders for resuscitation following trauma, PRS, *57:*676, 1976. Mil. Med., *140:*258, 1975

Mandible (See also *Jaw*)

Mandible, lever effects on. 4. Lever lengths of mandible in dogs following experimental exclusion of masticatory muscles (Ehler *et al*). Anat. Anz., *134:*425, 1973 (German)

Coronoid process of jaw, enlargement of (Carraro *et al*), PRS, *54:*687, 1974. Bol. y trab. Acad. argent cir., *57:*469, 1973

Mandible, massive osteolysis of: attempt at reconstruction (Booth *et al*). J. Oral Surg., *32:*787, 1974

Mandible — Cont.

Mandibulectomy patient, bilateral, occlusion effect in (Schweitzer). J. Speech, Hear. Disord., *39:*360, 1974

Reactive changes in mandibular tissues after reimplantation of boiled bone sections. Stomatologiia (Mosk.), *53:*80, 1974 (Russian)

Coronoid processes, bilateral hypertrophy of (Shurman), PRS, *57:*117, 1976. Anesthesiology, *41:*491, 1975

Metal implants and mandibular staple bone plate (Small). J. Oral Surg., *33:*571, 1975

Mandible, arteriovenous malformations of, graduated surgical management (Bryant, Maull), PRS, *55:*690, 1975. Discussion by Bennett, PRS, *56:*84, 1975

Complete regeneration of the body of the ascending ramus and mandibular condyle in a child after disarticulation (Anastassov *et al*). Rev. Odontostomatol. (Paris), *4:*43, 1975 (French)

Reconstruction and rehabilitation of the mandible in unilateral agenesis of the articular process (Stellmach). Z. W. R., *85:*74, 1976 (German)

Mandible, Ankylosis: See *Jaw, Ankylosis*

Mandible, Bone Grafting: See *Jaw, Bone Graft to*

Mandible, Cancer: See *Jaw Neoplasms*

Mandible Cysts: See *Jaw, Cysts*

Mandible Deformities: See *Jaw, Deformities; Micrognathia; Prognathism; Retrognathism; etc.*

Mandible Dislocation: See *Jaw, Dislocations*

Mandible Fractures: See *Jaw Fractures*

Mandible, Resection of: See *Jaw Neoplasms; Jaw Prostheses; Jaw, Surgery*

Mandibular Condyle (See also *Jaw, Ankylosis; Temporomandibular Joint*)

Effect of early postnatal condylectomy on the growth of the mandible (Pimenidis *et al*). Am. J. Orthod., *62:*42, 1972

Facial skeletal changes after mandibular condylectomy in growing and adult monkeys (Sarnat *et al*). Am. J. Orthod., *62:*428, 1972

Mandible, condylar neck of, technique for division (Heslop). Brit. J. Oral Surg., *10:*16, 1972

Condylar hyperplasia, mirror-image unilateral (Hudson). Brit. J. Oral Surg., *10:*58, 1972

Mandibular Condyle — Cont.

Condylectomy, electromyographic activities of jaw muscles before and after (Tsukamoto *et al*). Brit. J. Oral Surg., *10:*78, 1972

Condylectomy, intra-oral, applied to unilateral condylar hyperplasia (Sear). Brit. J. Oral Surg., *10:*143, 1972

Late effects of mandibular condylectomy (Poswillo). Oral Surg., *33:*500, 1972

Teflon implantation in temporomandibular arthroplasty (Cook). Oral Surg., *33:*706, 1972

Role of condylotomy with interpositional silicone rubber in temporomandibular joint ankylosis (Estabrooks *et al*). Oral Surg., *34:*2, 1972

Marlex 50 to replace mandibular condyle (Pennisi) (Follow-Up Clinic). PRS, *49:*565, 1972

Clinico-roentgenological characteristics of arthroplasty by lyophilized bone homograft in ankylosis of the temporomandibular joint (Tkachenko). Stomatologiia (Mosk.), *51:*84, 1972 (Russian)

Mandibular condyle, unilateral hyperplasia (Lehtinen *et al*). Suom. Hammaslaak. Toim., *68:*253, 1972 (Finnish)

Role of condyle in postnatal growth of mandible (Meikle). Am. J. Orthod., *64:*50, 1973

Condylar growth in light of new experimental research results — literature survey (Frankel *et al*). Dtsch. Stomatol., *23:*452, 1973 (German)

Surgical management of condyloid process fractures (Muska *et al*). Dtsch. Stomatol., *23:*897, 1973

Mandibular condyle, surgically treated fracture, unusual complication following (Fluur *et al*). Int. J. Oral Surg., *2:*297, 1973

Mandibular condyle after unilateral condylotomy in rat, histologic study of healing process of (Fukui *et al*). Jap. J. Oral Surg., *19:*16, 1973 (Japanese)

Roentgenological assessment of reconstruction of articular end of lyophilized jaw transplanted into defect of lower jaw following its resection with exarticulation (Plotnikov *et al*). Stomatologiia (Mosk.), *52:*35, 1973 (Russian)

Mandibular condyle, fractures of, surgical method of treatment (Mushka *et al*). Stomatologiia (Mosk.), *52:*89, 1973 (Russian)

Use of biocompatible interface for combining tissues and protheses in oral surgery. (Hinds *et al*). Trans. Int. Conf. Oral Surg., *4:*210, 1973

Mandibular asymmetry (Waite). Trans. Int. Conf. Oral Surg., *4:*246, 1973

Dislocating jaw (Macalister). Trans. Int.

Mandibular Condyle – Cont.

Conf. Oral Surg., *4:*259, 1973

Condylotomy, closed, longstanding bilateral intracapsular fracture dislocation on the condyles treated by (Canniff). Trans. Congr. Int. Assoc. Oral Surg., *4:*336, 1973

Condylotomy for bilateral dislocation (Gorman). Brit. J. Oral Surg., *12:*96, 1974

Osteoma of the mandible (MacLennan *et al*). Brit. J. Oral Surg., *12:*219, 1974

Indications for surgical or conservative treatment of mandibular fractures (Lentrodt *et al*). Fortschr. Kiefer. Gesichtschir., *19:*65, 1974 (German)

Mandibular condyle, unilateral hyperplasia of (Khanna *et al*), PRS, *55:*377, 1975. Indian J. Plast. Surg., *7:*11, 1974

Bilateral hyperplasia of coronoid processes, symmetrical, restricted opening of mouth from (Rusconi *et al*). J. Oral Surg., *32:*452, 1974

Condylar reconstruction: treatment planning (Kent *et al*). Oral Surg., *37:*489, 1974

Condylectomy, mandibular, with silicone rubber replacement (Hartwell, Hall). PRS, *53:*440, 1974

Experimental study on the role of the condyle in mandibular growth (Vitton). Rev. Stomatol. Chir. Maxillofac., *75:*1001, 1974 (French)

Condylar fractures, long-term results of functional treatment of (Schettler, Rehrmann), PRS, *56:*463, 1975. J. Maxillo-facial Surg., *3:*14, 1975

Experience with intraoral vertical subcondylar osteotomy (Akin *et al*). J. Oral Surg., *33:*324, 1975

Evaluation and refinement of intraoral vertical subcondylar osteotomy (Hall *et al*). J. Oral Surg., *33:*333, 1975

Simplified technique for wiring the condyloid process after intraoral vertical subcondylar osteotomy (Indresano). J. Oral Surg., *33:*384, 1975

Joint, temporomandibular, surgical correction of lesions of (Dingman, Dingman, Lawrence), PRS, *55:*335, 1975. Discussion by Kiehn, PRS, *55:*484, 1975

Criteria for condylotomy: a clinical appraisal of 211 cases (Banks *et al*). Proc. Roy Soc. Med., *68:*601, 1975

Condyle, mandibular, osteocartilaginous exostosis of (Wang-Norderud, Ragab), PRS, *57:*672, 1976. Scand. J. Plast. Reconstr. Surg., *9:*165, 1975

Mandibular Nerve

Changes in dentition of guinea-pig following partial section of inferior alveolar nerve

Mandibular Nerve – Cont.

(Ronning *et al*). Arch. Oral Biol., *18:*1059, 1973

Related maxillary sinus problem: diagnosis and treatment of second division trigeminal neuralgia (Cogan). Trans. Int. Conf. Oral Surg., *4:*179, 1973

Trigeminal neuralgia revisited (Haas). Trans. Int. Conf. Oral Surg., *4:*184, 1973

Animal experiments on the regeneration of the inferior alveolar nerve after injury during osteotomy of the lower jaw and microsurgery (Hausamen *et al*). Fortschr. Kiefer. Gesichtschir., *18:*93, 1974 (German)

Inferior alveolar nerve, regeneration of, histological study of (Choukas *et al*). J. Oral Surg., *32:*347, 1974

Alveolar nerve, inferior, cut, restoring sensation by direct anastomosis or by free autologous nerve grafting (Hausamen, Samii, Schmidseder). PRS, *53:*83, 1974

Histological aspects of dental pulp after resection of inferior alveolar nerve in albino rats (Filicori). Riv. Ital. Stomatol., *29:*37, 1973 (Italian)

Mandibular canal, postoperative defects of, comparative study of results of autologous grafting of, using minced muscle tissue and coagulated blood (Solomennyi). Stomatologiia (Mosk.), *53:*82, 1974 (Russian)

Trigeminal neuralgia: treatment by repetitive peripheral neurectomy. Supplemental report (Quinn *et al*). J. Oral Surg., *33:*591, 1975

MANDRES, G. *et al*: Complete traumatic avulsion of skin of penis and scrotum. Bull. Soc. Sci. Med. Grand Duche. Luxemb., *110:*69, 1973 (French)

MANDYBUR, T. I.: Melanotic nerve sheath tumors. J. Neurosurg., *41:*187, 1974

MANGEON, G. *et al*: Clinico-surgical treatment of a case of lepromatous cubital neuritis. Rev. Bras. Med., *28:*263, 1971 (Portuguese)

MANGIANTE, P.: Case of laterognathism of mandible supported by calcified residue of Meckel's cartilage, PRS, *51:*102, 1973. Riv. ital. chir. plast., *3:*233, 1971

MANGUS, D. J.: Continuous compression treatment of hemangiomata. PRS, *49:*490, 1972

MANGUS, D. J.: *Flexor pollicis longus* tendon transfer for restoration of opposition of thumb. PRS, *52:*155, 1973

MANGUS, D. J. *et al*: Tendon repairs with nylon and modified pull-out technique. PRS, *48:*32, 1971

MANI, M. M.: Simple method for emergency orotracheal intubation (with Manchester, Masters). PRS, *49:*312, 1972

MANIGAND, G. *et al*: Hamartomas of cervical region. Ann. Med. Interne (Paris), *124:*433, 1973 (French)

MANISCALCO, J. E. *et al*: Cranioplasty: method of prefabricating alloplastic plates. Surg. Neurol., *2:*339, 1974

MANITZ, U.: Surgical treatment and after care in muscular torticollis. Beitr. Orthop. Traumatol., *21:*376, 1974 (German)

MANKTELOW, R.: Kutler repair for fingertip amputations (with Freiberg). PRS, *50:*371, 1972

MANN, R. A. *et al*: Intractable plantar keratosis. Orthop. Clin. North Am., *4:*67, 1972

MANN, R. J.: Paint and grease gun injuries of hand, PRS, *56:*230, 1975. J.A.M.A., *231:*933, 1975

MANN, S. G.: Kaposi's sarcoma. Experience with ten cases. Am. J. Roentgenol. Radium Ther. Nucl. Med., *121:*793, 1974

MANNERFELT, L. *et al*: Silastic arthroplasty of metacarpophalangeal joints in rheumatoid arthritis, PRS, *57:*534, 1976. J. Bone & Joint Surg., *57A:*484, 1975

MANNHEIM, R. W.: Factor XIII concentrate in osteotomies and cystectomies with heterologous bone implantation. Z.W.R., *83:*323, 1974 (German)

MANNY, J., HARUZI, I., AND YOSIPOVITCH, Z.: Osteomyelitis of clavicle following subclavian vein catheterization, PRS, *52:*454, 1973. Arch. Surg., *106:*342, 1973

MANNY, N. *et al*: Hazard of immunosuppressive therapy. Brit. Med. J., *2:*291, 1972

MANSAT, M.: Trip to the U.S.A. for study of hand surgery. Rev. Chir. Orthop., *57:*(Suppl. 1) 237, 1971 (French)

MANSBERGER, A. R., JR., AND KANG, J. S.: New method for repair of full-thickness defects of abdominal wall, PRS, *54:*247, 1974. Am. Surgeon, *40:*117, 1974

MANSCHOT, W. A.: Therapy of conjunctival melanoma. Ned. tijdschr. geneeskd., *118:*1109, 1974 (Dutch)

MANSELL, P. W. A. *et al*: Delayed hypersensitivity to 5-fluorouracil following topical chemotherapy of cutaneous cancers, PRS, *56:*600, 1975. Cancer Res., *35:*1288, 1975

MANSELL, P. W. A. *et al*: Macrophage-mediated destruction of human malignant cells *in vivo*, PRS, *56:*472, 1975. J. Nat. Cancer Inst., *54:*471, 1975

MANSFIELD, M. J. *et al*: Combined fixed prosthesis and segmental osteotomy of maxilla, case report. J. Am. Dent. Assoc., *88:*603,1974

MANSFIELD, O. T. *et al*: Unilateral transverse facial cleft – a method of surgical closure. Br. J. Plast. Surg., *25:*29, 1972

MANSONE, A. Y.: Rare case of congenital mid-face underdevelopment (*dysgenesis cerebro-facialis mediana*), PRS, *54:*617, 1974. Acta chir. plast., *15:*201, 1973

MANSOURY, A. T., MOUSTAFA, F., AND BURHAN, A.: New classification of cleft lip and cleft palate, PRS, *53:*490, 1974. Bull. Alexandria Fac. Med., *7:*30, 1973

MANTEL, K. *et al*: Tracheotomy or long-term intubation in acute respiratory insufficiency? Langenbecks Arch. Chir., *327:*906, 1970

MANTERO, R. *et al*: Reconstruction of hemi-eyebrow with temporoparietal flap. Int. Surg., *59:*369, 1974

MANTZ, J. M. *et al*: Tracheal stenosis and sterilization of tracheotomy cannulas with ethylene oxide. Sem. Hop. Paris, *48:*3367, 1972 (French)

MANUEL LOPEZ, R., AND FERNANDEZ JARDON, L.: Utility of POR-8 used topically in plastic surgery, PRS, *53:*614, 1974. Rev. españ. cir. plast., *5:*249, 1973

MANUILENKO, B. A.: Restorative operations in the surgical treatment of the external integuments. Vopr. Onkol., *20:*3, 1974 (Russian)

MANUYLENKO, B. A.: Reconstruction of corners of mouth after resection of lower lip, PRS, *57:*756, 1976. Acta chir. plast., *17:*38, 1975

MANZANO, J. L. *et al*: Decannulation of tracheostomised children. An. Esp. Pediatr., *8:* 297, 1975 (Spanish)

MANZANO, J. L. *et al*: Care and complications of tracheotomy. Rev. Esp. Anestesiol. Reanim., *22:*490, 1975 (Spanish)

MAPES, A. H. *et al*: Longitudinal analysis of maxillary growth increments in cleft lip and palate patients, PRS, *56:*109, 1975. Cleft Palate J., *11:*450, 1974

MAQUIEIRA, N. O.: Innervated full-thickness skin graft to restore sensibility to fingertips and heels. PRS, *53:*568, 1974

MAQUIEIRA, N. O. *et al*: Reimplantation of limbs, experimental study, PRS, *51:*354, 1973. Rev. argent. cir., *22:*66, 1972

MAQUIRE, C. J. *et al*: Developments in lacrimal canalicular surgery. Trans. Ophthalmol. Soc. U.K., *91:*923, 1971

MARAN, A. G.: Septoplasty. J. Laryng. & Otol., *87:*196, 1973

MARAN, A. G.: Identification of facial nerve in parotid surgery. J. R. Coll. Surg. Edinb., *18:*58, 1973

MARAN, A. G., AND STEWART, I. A.: Bizarre nasal injury. PRS, *55:*498, 1975

MARANO, P. D., AND HARTMAN, K. S.: Central mucoepidermoid carcinoma arising in maxillary odontogenic cyst, PRS, *56:*363, 1975. J. Oral Surg., *32:*915, 1974

MARBERGER, H. *et al*: Indication, techniques and results of operative correction of hypospadias using modification of original Denis Browne technique. Urologe (A)., *14*:117, 1975 (German)

MARBLE, H. B., JR., *et al*: Precise technique for restoration of bony facial contour deficiencies with silicone rubber implants: report of cases. J. Oral Surg., *30*:737, 1972

MARCHAC, D.: Cutaneous epitheliomas in patients less than 40 years old. Nouvelle Presse Med., *1*:3035, 1972 (French)

MARCHAC, D.: Extensive superficial vulvectomy with primary skin grafting for premalignant lesions, PRS, *54*:691, 1974. Brit. J. Plast., Surg., *26*:40, 1973

MARCHAC, D.: Post-traumatic repositional osteotomies. Rev. Stomatol. Chir. Maxillofac., *75*:262, 1974 (French)

MARCHAC, D. *et al*: Precancerous state of the vermilion border of the lower lip. Value of preventative vermilionectomy. J. Fr. Otorhinolaryngol., *20*:1029, 1971 (French)

MARCHAC, D. *et al*: Angioma and fronto-orbital bone swelling: complete excision and immediate bone restoration. Ann. chir. plast., *17*:73, 1972 (French)

MARCHAC, D. *et al*: Repair of orbital roof by duplication of frontal bone flap. Nouv. Presse Med., *2*:2413, 1973 (French)

MARCHAC, D. *et al*: Repair of severe frontoorbital lesion by repositioning or osteotomy and bone grafting, PRS, *55*:375, 1975. Ann. chir. plast., *19*:41, 1974

MARCHAC, D., AND COPHIGNON, J.: Technique for embedding split ribs in cranioplasty. PRS, *55*:237, 1975

MARCHAC, D., AND ALKHATIB, B.: Giant breast implant for unilateral aplasia. PRS, *57*:749, 1976

MARCHAND, J. *et al*: Limited epitheliomas of nasal fossae and sinuses. Probl. Actuels Otorhinolaryngol., *125*:52, 1970 (French)

MARCHANT, J.: Letter: Breast prostheses. Lancet, *2*:187, 1975

MARCHANT, J.: Letter: Breast prostheses. Lancet *1*:360, 1976

MARCHETTA, F. C.: Carcinoma of oral cavity — general principles of therapy. J. Surg. Oncol., *6*:349, 1974

MARCHETTA, F. C.: Carcinoma of the thyroid gland: current therapy. J. Surg. Oncol., *6*:401, 1974

MARCHETTA, F. C., SAKO, K., AND MATSURA, H.: Modified neck dissection for carcinoma of thyroid gland, PRS, *48*:199, 1971. Am. J. Surg., *120*:452, 1970

MARCHETTA, F. C., SAKO, K., AND MURPHY, J. B.: Periosteum of mandible and intraoral carcinoma, PRS, *51*:608, 1973. Am. J. Surg., *122*:711, 1971

MARCHIORO, T. L. *et al*: Ureteroileostomy in renal transplant patients. Urology, *3*:171, 1974

MARCIANI, R. D., AND PLEZIA, R. A.: Osteoradionecrosis of mandible, PRS, *55*:247, 1975. J. Oral Surg., *32*:435, 1974

MARCIANI, R. D. *et al*: Reimplantation of freeze-treated mandibular bone. J. Oral Surg., *33*:261, 1975

MARCIANI, R. D. *et al*: Postoperative sequelae of cryosurgery. J. Oral Surg., *33*:485, 1975

MARCONDES, A. O., AND RUFATTO, L. A.: Hospital burn units, PRS, *55*:721, 1975. Ars Curandi, *7*:64, 1974

MARECHAL, R.: Seborrheic alopecia. Surgical treatment by ligature of the scalp arteries. Nouv. Presse Med., *1*:257, 1972 (French)

MARECHAL, R.: New osteoclast. Ann. Otolaryngol. Chir. Cervicofac., *91*:537, 1974 (French)

MARGOLIN, V. L.: Comparative evaluation of certain methods of skin preservation. Ortop. Travmatol. Protez., *35*:26, 1974 (Russian)

MARIANI, U.: Use of healed superficial burns as donor site for split-skin grafts, PRS, *57*:191, 1976

MARIN, ARIAS, G.: Giant hemangioma of head and face, PRS, *49*:474, 1972. Rev. Latino Am. cir. plast., *14*:41, 1970

MARINO, A.: Reconstructive surgery of nasal septum perforation. Considerations and personal technic. Valsalva, *43*:114, 1967 (Italian)

MARINO, E.: Immediate repair after adenomastectomy, PRS, *49*:582, 1972. Rev. argent. cir., *20*:120, 1971

MARIOTTI, F. *et al*: On two cases of Spitz-Allen juvenile melanoma. G. Ital. Dermatol., *46*:497, 1971 (Italian)

MARIS, F.: Our method of repairing "shell" ear deformity, PRS, *51*:475, 1973. Acta chir. plast., *14*:47, 1972

MARIS, F.: Urethral reconstruction in hypospadias by flap from preputium, PRS, *52*:324, 1973. Acta chir. plast., *14*:120, 1972

MARIS, F.: Reconstruction of urethra in hypospadiacs with the prepuce lobe. Bratisl. Lek. Listy, *59*:63, 1973 (Slovakian)

MARIS, F.: Use of free skin graft in correction of severe forms of hypospadias. Bratisl. Lek. Listy, *59*:306, 1973 (Slovakian)

Marjolin Ulcer: See Burns, Cancer in

MARKEY, J. C., JR. *et al*: Penetrating neck wounds: a review of 218 cases. Am. Surg., *41*:77, 1975

MARKLAND, C., AND MERRILL, D.: Accidental penile gangrene, PRS, *51*:348, 1973. J. Urol., *108*:494, 1972

MARKLAND, C. *et al*: Management of infants

with cloacal exstrophy. J. Urol., *109:*740, 1973

MARKLAND, C., AND HASTINGS, D.: Vaginal construction using cecal and sigmoid bowel segments in transsexual patients, PRS, *54:*622, 1974. J. Urol., *111:*217, 1974

MARKLEY, K., THORTON, S. W., AND SMALL-MAN, E.: Effect of traumatic and nontraumatic shock on allograft survival, PRS, *49:*362, 1972. Surgery, *70:*667, 1971

MARLOWE, F. I.: Acquired atresia of external auditory canal. Arch. Otolaryng., *96:*380, 1972

MARLOWE, F. I.: Survey of blepharoplasty. Trans. Pa. Acad. Ophthalmol. Otolaryngol., *26:*114, 1973

MARLOWE, F. I. *et al*: Tumors of salivary glands. Trans. Pa. Acad. Ophthalmol. Otolaryngol., *26:*36, 1973

MARMOR, L.: Surgery of rheumatoid hand and wrist. Semin. Arthritis Rheum., *1:*7, 1971

MARQUES, L.: Treatment of facial injuries. Rev. Port. Estomatol. Cir. Maxillofac., *12:*45, 1971 (Portuguese)

MARRA, L. *et al*: Iatrogenic ankylosis of temporomandibular joint. Report of case. Oral. Surg., *35:*596, 1973

MARSHALL, J. H.: New intraoral elastic applicator and wiring aid, PRS, *49:*579, 1972

MARSHALL, J. H. *et al*: Fatal tetanus complicating a small partial-thickness burn. J. Trauma, *12:*91, 1972

MARSHALL, M. A. *et al*: Analgesia for burns dressing using methoxyflurane. Brit. J. Anaesth., *44:*80, 1972

MARSHALL, V. C.: Skin tumors in immunosuppressed patients, PRS, *54:*115, 1974. Australian & New Zealand J. Surg., *43:*214, 1973

MARSHALL, V. C.: "Transplant leg," skin flap avulsion of leg due to minor trauma after renal transplantation, PRS, *54:*116, 1974. Australian & New Zealand J. Surg., *43:*223, 1973

MARSHALL, V. F.: Notes on Boyce-Vest operation for exstrophy of bladder. J. Urol., *109:*111, 1973

MARSHALL, V. F., AND SPELLMAN, R. M.: Free grafts to mucosa from the urinary bladder: I. For construction of urethra in humans; II. For production of bone in dogs (Follow-Up Clinic), PRS, *48:*369, 1971

MARSHIN, I. N. *et al*: Inspired air humidifier in tracheostomy. Voen. Med. Zh., *4:*80, 1974 (Russian)

MARSICANO, A. R., JR., HUTTON, J. J., AND BRYANT, W. M.: Fatal hemolysis from mafenide treatment of burns in patient with glucose-6-phosphate dehydrogenase deficiency, PRS, *52:*197, 1973

MARTEL, P. G.: Case study of transsexual male. Can. Psychiatr. Assoc. J., *19:*13, 1974 (French)

MARTES, C. *et al*: Preprosthetic surgery of jaw anomalies. Odontiatrike, *213:*8, 1973 (Greek)

MARTES, C. *et al*: Chondrosarcoma of the jaw. Stomatologia (Athenai), *31:*215, 1974 (Greek)

MARTIAN, D. E., AND HOOPS, H. R.: Relationship between esophageal speech proficiency and selected measure of auditory function, PRS, *56:*594, 1975. J. Speech & Hearing Res., *17:*80, 1974

MARTIN, C. *et al*: Case of cystic lymphangioma of neck. J. Fr. Otorhinolaryngol., *23:*255, 1974 (French)

MARTIN, C. E., ROSENFELD, L., AND McSWAIN, B.: Carotid body tumors: 16-year follow-up of 7 malignant cases, PRS, *53:*612, 1974. South. M. J., *66:*1236, 1973

MARTIN, F. F. *et al*: Treatment of radionecrosis of the wrist using a great omentum flap and skin graft. Ann. chir. plast., *19:*247, 1974 (French)

MARTIN, H.: The point of view of the otologist in the treatment of essential facial paralysis. Rev. Otoneuroophtalmol., *47:*53, 1975 (French)

MARTIN, H. *et al*: Present surgical treatment of essential facial paralysis. Our simplified technic. J. Med. Lyon, *51:*2001, 1970 (French)

MARTIN, H. *et al*: Surgical treatment of traumatic facial paralysis with substance loss with tantalum thread. J. Fr. Otorhinolaryngol., *20:*1135, 1971 (French)

MARTIN, R.: Some practical notes on anatomy of chicken toe for surgeon investigators (with Farkas, Thomson), PRS, *54:*452, 1974

MARTIN, W. J. *et al*: Surgical management of neurotrophic ulcers in the diabetic foot. J. Am. Podiatry Assoc., *65:*365, 1975

MARTINEZ, M. G., JR. *et al*: Primary neurogenic sarcomas of the oral region: a report of two cases. Ala. J. Med. Sci., *13:*32, 1976

MARTINEZ, S. A. *et al*: Elective carotid artery resection. Arch. Otolaryng., *101:*744, 1975

MARTINEZ ANDRES, J.: Selective compressor for pharyngostomas. Acta Otorinolaryngol. Iber. Am., *24:*87, 1973 (Polish)

MARTINEZ-GARCIA, W. R.: Surgical correction of recurrent bony ankylosis of the temporomandibular joint. Brit. J. Oral Surg., *9:*110, 1971

MARTINEZ-MORA, J., BOIX-OCHOA, J., AND TRESSERA, L.: Vascular tumors of parotid region in children, PRS, *50:*96, 1972. Surg. Gynec. & Obst., *133:*973, 1971

MARTINEZ SAHUQUILLO, A., MORALES LUPIANEZ, F., AND CONEJO GARCIA, E.: First branchial arch syndrome, PRS, *53:*109, 1974. Rev. españ. cir. plast., *3:*185, 1970

MARTINEZ SAHUQUILLO, A., AND MORALES LUPIANES, F.: Poland's syndrome, PRS, *54:*630, 1974. Rev. españ. cir. plast., *7:*1, 1974

MARTINEZ-TELLO, F. *et al*: Nasal glioma in relation to fronto-ethmoidal encephalocele. Z. Laryngol. Rhinol. Otol., *51:*591, 1972 (German)

MARTINEZ TRENS, M. *et al*: Use of ketamine chloride in anesthesia of the burn patient. Rev. Esp. Anestesiol. Reanim., *19:*144, 1972 (Spanish)

MARTINKENAS, L. V.: Diagnosis, clinical aspects and surgical treatment of traumatic curvature of nose in residual period of injury. Vestn. Otorinolaringol., *2:*49, 1975 (Russian)

MARTINOT, M. P.: Palpebro-conjunctival melanotic tumor. Bull. Soc. Ophtalmol. Fr., *74:*457, 1974 (French)

MARTINOVA, M.: Treatment of keloids with triamcinolone acetonide. Acta Chir. Orthop. Traumatol. Cech., *41:*136, 1974 (Czechoslovakian)

MARTINS, A. M.: Immediate internal mandibular restoration. Modification of Benoist's prosthesis fixation method. Rev. Fac. Odontol. Sao Paulo, *11:*407, 1973 (Portuguese)

MARTINS, L. C.: Surgical treatment of alar cartilages. Rev. Assoc. Med. Bras., *21:*55, 1975 (Portuguese)

MARTIS, C., AND KARAKASIS, D.: Bleeding from ear in maxillofacial injuries, PRS, *55:*375, 1975. J. Maxillo-facial Surg., *2:*126, 1974

MARTIS, C. *et al*: Cemento-ossifying fibroma of mandible, case report. J. Oral Surg., *33:*364, 1975

MARTIS, C. S., AND KARAKASIS, D. T.: Adenoameloblastoma, PRS, *50:*409, 1972

MARTIS, C. S. *et al*: Ankylosis of temporomandibular joint caused by Still's disease. Oral Surg., *35:*462, 1973

MARTIS, C. S. *et al*: Prophylactic neck dissection in oral carcinoma. Int. J. Oral Surg., *3:*293, 1974

MARUMO, E. *et al:* Surgery of scar contracture of the hands. Jap. J. Plast. Reconstr. Surg., *14:*293, 1971 (Japanese)

MARUMO, E. *et al*: Rare congenital deformity of hand, PRS, *55:*380, 1975. Jap. J. Plast. Reconstr. Surg., *17:*217, 1974

MARUSIAK, D. F.: Epidermal cyst of the external acoustic canal. Vestn. Otorinolaringol., *3:*102, 1975 (Russian)

MARX, W. L. *et al*: Mammography, accuracy, clinical value and limitations, PRS, *51:*103, 1973. Arch. chir. neerl., *23:*315, 1971

MARYNEN, L.: Use of ketamine in subjects with burns. Anesth. Analg. (Paris), *30:*1043, 1973

MARZKE, M. W.: Origin of the human hand. Am. J. Phys. Anthropol., *34:*61, 1971

MASHBERG, A., MORRISSEY, J. B., AND GARFINKLE, L.: Next time a patient says "aah," PRS, *56:*105, 1975. Emerg. Med., *7:*43, 1975

MASHIH, B. K. *et al*: Webbed penis. J. Urol., *111:*690, 1974

MASING, H.: Treatment of nose stenoses. Arch. Klin. Exp. Ohren Nasen Kehlkopfheilkd., *199:*352, 1971 (German)

MASIUKOVA, E. M. *et al*: Reconstruction of a subcutaneous artificial esophagus into a retrosternal one. Vestn. Khir., *112:*113, 1974 (Russian)

MASON, A. D., JR.: Effect of early surgical excision and homografting on survival of burned rats and of intraperitoneally-infected burned rats (with Levine, Salisbury), PRS, *56:*423, 1975

MASON, A. Y.: Conservative surgical treatment of carcinoma of breast, PRS, *55:*719, 1975. Proc. Roy. Soc. Med., *67:*473, 1974

MASON, B. A. *et al*: Mandibular resection and reconstruction for ameloblastoma in severe diabetic. J. Oral Surg., *32:*379, 1974

MASON, C. L. *et al*: Use of thin skin grafts in preprosthetic surgery (lower and upper jaws). Ann. Odontostomatol. (Lyon), *27:*131, 1970 (French)

MASON, D., AND LINDBERG, R. B.: Macronumbers of microorganisms, PRS, *55:*113, 1975. Lancet, *2:*292, 1974

MASON, D. A.: Verrucous carcinoma of mouth. Brit. J. Oral Surg., *10:*64, 1972

MASON, D. K., AND CHISHOLM, D. M.: *Salivary Glands in Health and Disease.* C. V. Mosby Co., St. Louis, 1975

MASON, J. R. *et al*: Competition between collateral vessels in femoro-popliteal by-pass grafting. J. Cardiovasc. Surg. (Torino), *16:*373, 1975

MASSENGILL, R. JR. *et al:* Lingual flaps: effect on speech articulation and physiology. Ann. Otol. Rhin. & Laryng., *79:*853, 1970

MASSENGILL, R., JR. *et al*: Lingual positions of cleft palate patients with and without velopharyngeal closure. Folia Phoniatr. (Basel), *22:*185, 1970

MASSENGILL, R., QUINN, G., AND PICKRELL, K.: Use of palatal stimulant to decrease velopharyngeal gap, PRS, *48:*296, 1971. Ann. Otol. Rhin. & Laryng., *80:*135, 1971

MASSENGILL, R., JR., PICKRELL, K., AND ROBINSON, M.: Results of pushback operations in treatment of submucous cleft palate, PRS, *51:*432, 1973

MASSENGILL, R., AND QUINN, G.: Adenoidal atrophy, velopharyngeal incompetence and sucking exercises, PRS, *55:*376, 1975. Cleft

Palate J., *11:*196, 1974

MASSENGILL, R., AND GEORGIADE, N.: Results obtained from using new anteriorly superiorly based pharyngeal flap, PRS, *55:*512, 1975. Cleft Palate J., *11:*333, 1974

Masseter Muscle, Hypertrophy of

Masseter muscles, benign hypertrophy of (Lombard), PRS, *56:*593, 1975. Rev. Esp. Estomatogia, *17:*23, 1969

Masseter muscles and mandibular angles, benign hypertrophy of (Waldhart, Lynch), PRS, *48:*294, 1971. Arch. Surg., *102:*115, 1971

Masseter muscle and mandibular angle, bilateral hypertrophy of, surgical correction (Waldhart). Osterr. Z. Stomatol., *68:*462, 1971 (German)

Idiopathic tumoral hypertrophy of the masseter muscle (Gaillard *et al*). J. Fr. Otorhinolaryngol., *23:*561, 1974 (French)

Masseter muscle hypertrophy, differential diagnosis (Honee, Bloem), PRS, *55:*715, 1975. J. Maxillo-facial Surg., *2:*246, 1974

MASSEY, G. B. *et al*: Intraoral oblique osteotomy of the mandibular ramus. J. Oral Surg., *32:*755, 1974

MASSEY, W. R.: Closure of maxillary midline diastema with frenectomy and corticotomy. J. Ga. Dent. Assoc., *46:*26, 1972

MASSIHA, H., AND MONAFO, W. W.: Dermal ischemia in thermal injury: importance of venous occlusion, PRS, *57:*538, 1976. J. Trauma, *14:*705, 1974

MASSLER, M.: Tooth replantation, PRS, *55:*506, 1975. Dent. Clin. N. Am., *18:*2, 1974

MASSON, J. K.: Simple island flap for reconstruction of concha-helix defects. Brit. J. Plast. Surg., *25:*399, 1972

Mastectomy, Subcutaneous

Adenomastectomy, immediate repair after (Marino), PRS, *49:*582, 1972. Rev. argent. cir., *20:*120, 1971

Mastectomy, subcutaneous, with immediate prosthetic implantation, in cystosarcoma phylloides (Mandel *et al*), PRS, *50:*630, 1972. Am. J. Surg., *123:*718, 1972

Mammectomy, subcutaneous, new hope for benign breast disease (Allen). J. Arkansas Med. Soc., *69:*153, 1972

Mastectomy, subcutaneous (Weiner) (Editorial), PRS, *49:*654, 1972

Mastectomy, whither subcutaneous? (Freeman) (Editorial), PRS, *49:*654, 1972

Mastectomy, subcutaneous, with immediate reconstruction of breasts, using dermal mastopexy technique (Goulian, McDivitt), PRS, *50:*211, 1972

Mastectomy, Subcutaneous — Cont.

Mastectomy, subcutaneous, replacement plastic surgery in (Kammer). Praxis, *61:*999, 1972 (German)

Mammaplasty, reduction, subcutaneous mastectomy, or mastopexy, single dermal pedicle for nipple transposition in (Weiner *et al*), PRS, *51:*115, 1973

Mastectomy, subcutaneous, for central tumors of breast, with immediate reconstruction (Freeman), PRS, *51:*264, 1973. Discussions by Crile, Hutter, Snyderman, PRS, *51:*445, 1973

Breast: some anatomical considerations of subcutaneous mastectomy (Goldman, Goldwyn), PRS, *51:*501, 1973

Mastectomy, subcutaneous, syntax, and seat belts (McDowell) (Editorial), PRS, *51:*575, 1973

Carcinoma of breast and chronic cystic disease treated by subcutaneous mastectomy (Pennisi, Capozzi), PRS, *52:*520, 1973

Mastectomy, subcutaneous, with reconstruction (Stallings). Am. Fam. Physician, *10:*184, 1974

Mastectomy, subcutaneous, reconstruction of breast after (Bouman), PRS, *55:*719, 1975. Arch. chir. neerl., *26:*343, 1974

Mastectomy, subcutaneous, and immediate prosthetic implantation as alternative to simple mastectomy (Inglis *et al*). Can. J. Surg., *17:*63, 1974

Subcutaneous mastectomy (Molenaar). Clin. Plast. Surg., *1:*427, 1974

Subcutaneous mastectomy with immediate reconstruction (Horton *et al*), PRS, *53:*42, 1974

Subcutaneous mastectomy with immediate prosthetic reconstruction — operation in search of patients (Snyderman) (Letter to the Editor), PRS, *53:*582, 1974

Mastectomy, subcutaneous, and reconstruction in large breasts (Kern, Binns), PRS, *54:*648, 1974

Mastectomy, breast reconstruction after, indications (Van Dongen, Lichtveld), PRS, *57:*397, 1976. Nederl. tijdschr. geneesk., *119:*997, 1975

Mastectomy, subcutaneous, inframammary-based dermofat flaps in mammary reconstruction following (Letterman, Schurter), PRS, *55:*156, 1975

Mastectomy, subcutaneous, case against; biological basis for management of benign disease of breast (Peacock), PRS, *55:*14, 1975. Discussion by Watson, PRS, *55:*225, 1975

Mastectomy, subcutaneous, breast-halving incision for (Corso, Zubiri), PRS, *56:*1, 1975

Mastectomy, Subcutaneous — Cont.

Mastectomy, subcutaneous; excess skin problem (Hartley, Schatten, Griffin), PRS, *56:*5, 1975

Mastectomy, subcutaneous, incidence of obscure carcinoma in (Pennisi, Capozzi), PRS, *56:*9, 1975. Discussion by Snyderman, PRS, *56:*208, 1975

Mastectomy, subcutaneous, and immediate reconstruction in ptotic breast (Georgiade, Hyland), PRS, *56:*121, 1975

Augmentation, cushioned, after subcutaneous mastectomy (Rubin), PRS, *57:*23, 1976

MASTERS, F. W.: Simple method for emergency orotracheal intubation (with Manchester, Mani), PRS, *49:*312, 1972

MASTERS, F. W.: Hypertrophic scars and keloids (with Ketchum, Cohen), PRS, *53:*140, 1974

MASTERS, FRANK W., AND LEWIS, JOHN R. JR.: *Symposium on Aesthetic Surgery of the Face, Eyelid, and Breast,* Vol. IV. C. V. Mosby Co., St. Louis, 1972. PRS, *51:*687, 1973

MASTERS, FRANK W., AND LEWIS, JOHN R. JR.: *Symposium on Aesthetic Surgery of the Nose, Ears, and Chin.* C. V. Mosby Co., St. Louis, 1973. PRS, *54:*479, 1974

Mastopexy: See *Mammaplasty, Mastopexy*

MASTRANGELO, M. *et al:* Clinical and histologic correlation of melanoma regression after intralesional BCG therapy, case report, PRS, *54:*381, 1974. J. Nat. Cancer Inst., *52:*19, 1974

MASTRANGELO, M. J. *et al:* Malignant melanoma. Pa. Med., *75:*43, 1972

MASTROCOLA, R., AND ZITER, W. D.: Resins in oral surgery, PRS, *57:*266, 1976. Dent. Clin. N. Am., *19:*407, 1975

MASTRORILLI, A.: Surgical treatment of the rheumatoid hand. Minerva Med., *61:*4071, 1970 (Italian)

MASUDA, K. *et al:* Lymphedema and its treatment; with special reference to edema of the arm after a radical operation of breast cancer. Surg. Ther. (Osaka), *26:*308, 1972 (Japanese)

MASUHARA, K., TAMAI, S., AND SASAUCHI, N.: Muscle autotransplantation using microsurgical technique, PRS, *53:*110, 1974. Asian M. J., *15:*45, 1972

MATAR, J. H. *et al:* Carcinoma of tonsil and nasopharynx; 20-year results. Am. J. Roent. Radium Ther., *117:*517, 1973

MATCH, R. M.: Radiation-induced brachial plexus paralysis, PRS, *56:*596, 1975. Arch. Surg., *110:*384, 1975

MATCHIN, A. A.: Restoration of feeling in skin autotransplants transplanted to the hand and fingers. Klin. Khir., *8:*57, 1970 (Russian)

MATCHIN, E. N.: Restoration of integument in severely burned patients. Ortop. Travmatol. Protez., *34:*53, 1973 (Russian)

MATCHIN, E. N.: Skeletal suspension in treatment of burns. Vestn. Khir., *111:*79, 1973 (Russian)

MATEJICEK, V. *et al:* Septic shock in burn illness, PRS, *54:*507, 1974. Acta chir. plast., *15:*263, 1973

MATERSON, R. S., AND LOTZ, J. W.: Cloran telescoping oral orthosis, PRS, *57:*543, 1976. Arch. Phys. Med. Rehabil., *56:*409, 1975

MATESHUK, R. V. *et al:* Surgical treatment of gigantic elephantiasis of the lower extremities in children. Vestn. Khir., *112:*83, 1974 (Russian)

MATEV, I.: Operative treatment of spastic hand. Khirurgiia (Mosk.), *49:*14, 1973 (Russian)

MATEV, I.: Traumatic skin defects of the hand. Acta Chir. Plast. (Praha), *17:*77, 1975

MATEV, I. B.: New thought on hand surgery. Mod. Trends Orthop., *6:*95, 1972

MATHE, G. *et al:* Embryonic sarcomas of the mouth. Rev. Stomatol. Chir. Maxillofac., *75:*170, 1974 (French)

MATHES, S.: Construction of one good thumb from both parts of congenitally bifid thumb (with Hartrampf, Vasconez), PRS, *54:*148, 1974

MATHIAS, D.: Skin and homograft cartilage reconstruction, PRS, *57:*125, 1976. Arch. Otol., *101:*301, 1975

MATHIEU, A. *et al:* Expanding aneurysm of radial artery after frequent puncture, PRS, *53:*245, 1974. Anesthesiology, *38:*401, 1973

MATHIEU, H. *et al:* Ionic disorders in uro-ileal shunts. Arch. Fr. Pediatr., *31:*241, 1974 (French)

MATHOG, R. H.: Scar revision. Minn. Med., *57:*31, 1974

MATIASHIN, I. M. *et al:* Surgical tactics in severe electrical burn with injury of sacrum and rectum. Klin. Khir., *10:*68, 1974 (Russian)

MATIC, V. *et al:* Air-gun injuries in maxillofacial region. Vojnosanit. Pregl., *30:*561, 1973 (Serbian)

MATOUSEK, V. *et al:* Analysis of relative contributions by donor and recipient to variation in time taken for rejection of skin grafts in weak histocompatibility systems. Folia Biol. (Praha), *19:*402, 1973

MATRAS, H.: Reconstruction of individual occlusion after faulty facial bone fracture healing. Fortschr. Kiefer. Gesichtschir., *18:*223, 1974 (German)

MATRAS, H. *et al:* Non-sutured nerve transplantation, report on animal experiments, PRS, *52:*453, 1973. J. Maxillo-facial Surg., *1:*37, 1973

MATRAS, H., AND HOLLMANN, K.: Problems of soft tissue injuries of face, PRS, *56:*675, 1975. Acta chir. Austria, *7:*36, 1975

MATRAS, H. *et al:* Topographical anatomy of the total osteotomy of the midface. J. Maxillo-facial Surg., *3:*260, 1975

MATSUMOTO, A. *et al:* Tension releasing graft to extensive burn scar on face, PRS, *53:*607, 1974. J. Jap. Accident Med. Assoc., *21:*329, 1973

MATSUMOTO, K.: Follow-up study on reconstruction of microtia with silicone framework (with Ohmori, Nakai), PRS, *53:*555, 1974

MATSUMOTO, T., DE LAURENTIS, D. A., AND MORELLO, D. C.: Use of tissue adhesive spray in skin grafting, PRS, *53:*113, 1974. Internat. Surg., *57:*978, 1972

MATSUMURA, M., KUBO, R., AND ONO, M.: Surgical results in cancer of tongue. J. Otolaryngol. Jap., *75:*1086, 1972 (Japanese)

MATSUO, T. *et al:* A method of intermaxillary fixation for repair of mandibular prognathism with resin postcrowns. J. Jpn. Stomatol. Soc., *41:*151, 1974 (Japanese)

MATSUURA, H., KAWABE, Y., AND KONDO, T.: Indication for modified neck dissection. J. Otolaryngol. Japan, *75:*1083, 1972 (Japanese)

MATSUYA, T., MIYAZAKI, T., AND YAMAOKA, M.: Fibrescopic examination of velopharyngeal closure in normal individuals, PRS, *55:*514, 1975. Cleft Palate J., *11:*286, 1974

MATTER, P., BARCLAY, T. L., AND KONICKOVA, Z.: *Research in Burns.* Hans Huber Publishers, Bern, Stuttgart, Vienna, 1971. PRS, *50:*79, 1972

MATTHES, H.: Problems of anesthesia in treatment of maxillo-facial injuries. Langenbecks Arch. Chir., *334:*415, 1973 (German)

MATTHEWS, D.: Obituary. Gustavo Sanvenero Rosselli – 1887-1974. Brit. J. Plast. Surg., *27:*297, 1974

MATTHEWS, D.: Collapsed maxillary arch, PRS, *56:*464, 1975. Scand. J. Plast. Reconstr. Surg., *8:*116, 1974

MATTHEWS, D.: Rapid expansion in clefts, PRS, *56:*396, 1975

MATTHEWS, D. N.: Reconstruction in head and neck surgery, PRS, *49:*240, 1972. Proc. Roy. Soc. Med., *64:*731, 1971

MATTHEWS, G. J. *et al:* Painful traumatic neuromas. Surg. Clin. North Am., *52:*1313, 1972

MATTHEWS, L. S., AND HIRSCH, C.: Temperature measured in human cortical bone when drilling, PRS, *50:*312, 1972. J. Bone & Joint Surg., *54:*297, 1972

MATTHEWS, P., AND RICHARDS, H.: Repair potential of digital flexor tendons, PRS, *56:*679, 1975. J. Bone & Joint Surg., *56:*618, 1974

MATTHEWS, P., AND RICHARDS, H.: Repair reaction of flexor tendon within digital sheath, PRS, *57:*261, 1976. Hand, *7:*27, 1975

MATTON, G.: Esthetic blepharoplasty, PRS, *57:*529, 1976. Acta chir. belg., *74:*358, 1975

MATTON, G. *et al:* Surgical treatment. Acta chir. belg., *73:*189, 1974 (French)

MATTON, G., AND D'HOOGHE, P.: Reconstructive surgery in radionecrosis of breast and thoracic wall, PRS, *56:*226, 1975. Acta chir. belg., *73:*301, 1974

MATTON, G. *et al:* Benign tumors of the hand. Acta Orthop. Belg., *40:*172, 1974

MATTSON, H. S.: Case of m. palmaris radialis (profundus). Nord. Med., *86:*1223, 1971 (Swedish)

MATTSSON, H. S. *et al:* Social readaptation of a patient after disabilitative electric burn of hands. Nord. Med., *84:*1381, 1970 (Swedish)

MATUSIS, Z. E. *et al:* Immunologic reactivity in burned patients and autoplasty. Khirurgiia (Mosk.), *48:*36, 1972 (Russian)

MATVEEV, V. F. *et al:* Effect of surgical treatment on psychic readaptation of patients with congenital and acquired defects of the face. Stomatologiia (Mosk.), *51:*54, 1972 (Russian)

MATZEN, P. F., JR.: Combined malformation of both hands. Beitr. Orthop. Traumatol., *19:*251, 1972 (German)

MAU, H.: Diagnostic and surgical management of thoracic wall malformations. Z. Erkr. Atmungsorgane, *141:*149, 1974 (German)

MAUGERY, J. *et al:* Cancerous exophthalmos caused by intraorbital melanoma. Bull. Soc. Ophtalmol. Fr., *71:*258, 1971 (French)

MAULL, K. I.: Arteriovenous malformations of the mandible, graduated surgical management (with Bryant), PRS, *55:*690, 1975. Discussion by Bennett, PRS, *56:*84, 1975

MAW, A. R.: Assessment of treatment methods for carcinoma of larynx presenting with cervical lymph nodes, PRS, *56:*226, 1975. Proc. Roy. Soc. Med., *68:*80, 1975

MAW, R. B. *et al:* Scarification of temporal tendon for treatment of chronic subluxation of temporomandibular joint. J. Oral Surg., *31:*22, 1973

Maxilla (See also *Jaw*)

Technic for partial segment osteotomy of the

Maxilla — Cont.

upper maxillary (Parant *et al*). Orthod. Fr., *41:*325, 1970 (French)

Surgical treatment of upper prognathism (Dautrey *et al*). Acta Stomatol. Belg., *68:*335, 1971 (French)

Restoration of maxillary cleft using periosteum flaps in the case of complete labiopalatine cleft (Santoni-Rugiu *et al*). Ann. chir. plast., *16:*326, 1971 (French)

Transoral and transverse incision for excision of the maxillary sinus (Rush *et al*). J. Surg. Oncol., *3:*53, 1971

Infratemporal approach to the orbit and pterygopalatine fossa (Denecke). Monatsschr. Ohrenheilkd. Laryngorhinol., *105:*150, 1971 (German)

Significance of periosteum in bone regeneration in the maxilla-premaxilla after bone resection (surgical experimental and histological study in growing rabbits). 2 (Engdahl). Nord. Med., *86:*1221, 1971 (Swedish)

Maxilla, variability, studies of (Michalek), PRS, *52:*321, 1973. Acta chir. plast., *14:*73, 1972

Lateral alveolo-maxillary osteotomies. Revascularization studies (Rontal *et al*). Arch. Otolaryng. *95:*18, 1972

Anterior maxillary osteotomy: a retrospective evaluation of sinus health, patient acceptance, and relapses (Young *et al*). J. Oral Surg., *30:*69, 1972

Midline splitting of the maxilla for correction of malocclusion (Steinhauser). J. Oral Surg., *30:*413, 1972

Posterior maxillary surgery, its place in the treatment of dentofacial deformities (West *et al*). J. Oral Surg., *30:*562, 1972

Horizontal osteotomy for correction of maxillary retrusion: report of case (Pedersen). J. Oral Surg., *30:*581, 1972

Total maxillary osteotomy and retrepositioning of the maxilla: report of case (Cruickshank *et al*). J. Oral Surg., *30:*586, 1972

Revascularization and bone healing after maxillary corticotomies (Bell *et al*). J. Oral Surg., *30:*640, 1972

Necrosis of the anterior maxilla following osteotomy (Parnes *et al*). Oral Surg., *33:*326, 1972

Surgical correction of retrognathism by forward movement of a part of the maxilla with simultaneous bone transplantation (Zisser). Osterr. Z. Stomatol., *69:*143, 1972 (German)

Segmental osteotomies of the upper jaw (Souyris *et al*). Rev. Stomatol. Chir. Maxillofac., *73:*43, 1972 (French)

Use of free periosteum for bone formation in

Maxilla — Cont.

congenital clefts of the maxilla. A preliminary report (Ritsila *et al*). Scand. J. Plast. Reconstr. Surg., *6:*57, 1972

Prosthetic management of oral defects limited to the hard palate and caused by surgical treatment of tumor (Kodaira). Shikwa Gakuho, *72:*69, 1972 (Japanese)

Maxilla, retrodisplaced, forward traction to correct (Ciaburro *et al*), PRS, *52:*687, 1973. Canad. M.A.J., *108:*1511, 1973

Maxillary growth and speech development in relation to technique and timing of palatoplasty (Koberg, Koblin), PRS, *52:*455, 1973. J. Maxillo-facial Surg., *1:*44, 1973

Maxillary recession for bucktooth deformity (Russell, Beason), PRS, *51:*220, 1973

Growth of facial skeleton in guinea pigs after experimental fusion of premaxillo-maxillary suture (Letter to Editor). Proc. Finn. Dent. Soc., *69:*263, 1973

Preoperative prosthesis in hemi-resections of the maxillary bone (Cadenat *et al*). Rev. Stomatol. Chir. Maxillofac., *74:*682, 1973 (French)

A planning technique for segmental osteotomies (Lockwood) Brit. J. Oral Surg., *12:*102, 1974

Ceramic implantations in the maxillary bone (Kirschner *et al*). Bull. Group Eur. Rech. Sci. Stomatol. Odontol., *17:*123, 1974 (French)

Maxillary growth inhibition in rats, surgically induced (Serals, Biggs), PRS, *55:*247, 1975. Cleft Palate J., *11:*1, 1974

Contribution to the construction of resection prostheses in cases of limited oral aperture (Ehricht). Dtsch. Zahnaerztl. Z., *29:*948, 1974 (German)

Surgical correction of the skeleton in the area of the orbit and maxilla (Schmid). Fortschr. Kiefer. Gesichtschir., *18:*28, 1974 (German)

Maxillary anterior segmentary osteotomy: experimental research on vascular supply of osteotomized segment (Brusati *et al*). Fortschr. Kiefer. Gesichtschir., *18:*90, 1974

Midline splitting of the maxilla for correction of dental-facial disharmonies (Steinhuser). Fortschr. Kiefer. Gesichtschir., *18:*189, 1974

Behavior of the maxillary sinuses after orthopedic jaw operations (Perko). Fortschr. Kiefer. Gesichtschir., *18:*213, 1974 (German)

Maxillae, totally and partially edentulous, pterygoid extension implant for (Linkow). Int. J. Orthod., *12:*9, 1974

Maxilla, dentures or splints for, stabilized by

Maxilla — Cont.

circumpalatal wires (Fortney, Alcorn, Monaco), PRS, *55:*375, 1975. J. Oral Surg., *32:*538, 1974

Surgical correction of posterior crossbite (Bell *et al*). J. Oral Surg., *32:*811, 1974

Medical correction of maxillary and mandibular prognathism (Van Put). Rev. Belge. Med. Dent., *29:*465, 1974 (Dutch)

Multiple osteotomies in a single surgical stage (Curioni). Rev. Stomatol. Chir. Maxillofac., *75:*116, 1974 (French)

Partial bilateral anterior osteotomies of the upper jaw. Conditions for stability of the results (Landais). Rev. Stomatol. Chir. Maxillofac., *75:*118, 1974 (French)

Rhinoplasty and maxillary osteotomies (Aiach). Rev. Stomatol. Chir. Maxillofac., *75:*159, 1974 (French)

Value of an original naso-tracheal catheter in maxillo-facial surgery and stomatology (Lachard *et al*). Rev. Stomatol. Chir. Maxillofac., *75:*1029, 1974 (French)

Techniques and indications for superior maxillary osteotomies (Dupuis *et al*). Rev. Stomatol. Chir. Maxillofac., *75:*1055, 1974 (French)

Maxilla, upper, cleft cyst of, and primitive palate, embryogenesis of (Fortunato), PRS, *57:*401, 1976. Riv. ital. chir. plast., *6:*53, 1974

Bone development, maxillary, in rabbit operated when few days old (Rosselli *et al*), PRS, *57:*395, 1976. Riv. ital. chir. plast., *6:*227, 1974

Maxilla, growth in width studied by implant method (Bjork, Skieller), PRS, *56:*354, 1975. Scand. J. Plast. Reconstr. Surg., *8:*25, 1974

Neurotrophism in relation to muscle and nerve grafts in rats (Srour *et al*). Surg. Forum, *25:*508, 1974

Intraoral complete resection of the upper jaw (Shinbirev). Zdravookhr. Ross. Fed., *5:*106, 1974 (Russian)

Diagnosis and treatment of maxillomandibular dysplasias (Converse *et al*). Am. J. Orthod., *68:*625, 1975

Postmaxillectomy rhinorrhea: corrected by transposition of parotid duct opening (Clark *et al*). Arch. Otolaryng., *101:*492, 1975

Kartagener's syndrome in childhood. Report of 2 cases (Shubich *et al*). Bol. Med. Hosp. Infant Mex., *32:*493, 1975 (Spanish)

Maxillectomy cavity care with a pulsating stream irrigator (Krugman *et al*). Eye Ear Nose Throat Mon., *54:*104, 1975

Surgical anatomy of the pterygopalatine

Maxilla — Cont.

fossa (Wentges). J. Laryng. & Otol., *89:*35, 1975

Topographical anatomy of the total osteotomy of the midface (Matras *et al*). J. Maxillo-facial Surg., *3:*260, 1975

Middle-third facial osteotomies: their use in the correction of acquired and developmental dentofacial and craniofacial deformities (Epker *et al*). J. Oral Surg., *33:*491, 1975

Combined anterior and posterior maxillary ostectomy: a new technique (Wolford *et al*). J. Oral Surg., *33:*842, 1975

Maxillary exostoses. Surgical management of an unusual case (Blakemore *et al*). Oral Surg., *40:*200, 1975

Soft tissue changes associated with total maxillary advancement: a preliminary study (Dann *et al*). J. Oral Surg., *34:*19, 1976

Partial and radical maxillectomy (Lore). Otolaryngol. Clin. North Am., *9:*255, 1976

Maxilla, advancement of, preservation of posterior pharyngeal flap during (Ruberg, Randall, Whitaker). PRS, *57:*335, 1976

Maxillary Artery

Arteriovenous fistula of anterior facial vessels: review of literature and report of case (Guzman Freire *et al*). J. Oral Surg., *32:*150, 1974

Traumatic facial aneurysm (Horak *et al*). Wien. Med. Wochenschr., *125:*222, 1975 (German)

Maxillary Diseases (See also *Jaw, Diseases*)

Paget's disease of the maxilla (Hoggins *et al*). Brit. J. Oral Surg., *9:*122, 1971

Unilateral hypertrophy of the facial bones (Pilar-Svoboda). Chir. Maxillofac. Plast., *8:*3, 1971 (Croatian)

Surgery of retromaxillary space (Zehm). Monatsschr. Ohrenheilkd. Laryngorhinol., *105:*147, 1971 (German)

Maxillary cyst (Dickson). Proc. Mine. Med. Off. Assoc., *50:*81, 1971

Median palatal cyst: report of case (Thornton *et al*). J. Oral Surg., *30:*661, 1972

Aneurysmal bone cyst of the maxilla (Ellis *et al*). Oral Surg., *34:*26, 1972

Marsupialization of large cysts of the maxillas into the maxillary sinus and/or nose. A follow-up investigation (Egyedi *et al*). Trans. Int. Conf. Oral Surg., *4:*81, 1973

Osteitis fibros (brown tumor) of the maxilla (Bedard *et al*). Laryngoscope, *84:*2093, 1974

Keratinizing squamous epithelial cysts (keratocysts) in the jaws (Stiebitz *et al*). Wien.

Maxillary Sinus — Cont.
& Otol., *88:*281, 1974

Immunological aspects of maxillary sinusitis (Zeromska), PRS, *55:*726, 1975. J. Maxillo-facial Surg., *2:*242, 1974

Vidian neurectomy — some technical remarks (Nomura). Laryngoscope, *84:*578, 1974

Maxillary sinus, foreign bodies in (Svenn). Nor. Tannlaegeforen Tid., *84:*152, 1974 (Norwegian)

Sinus, maxillary, hemangioma involving (Afshin, Sharmin), PRS, *56:*224, 1975. Oral Surg., *38:*204, 1974

Antral packing (Cheesman), PRS, *55:*634, 1975. Proc. Roy. Soc. Med., *67:*716, 1974

Critical study of the surgical approach to the maxillary sinus, using an osteoplastic flap (Obreja *et al*). Rev. Chir. (Otorinolarin-gol.), *19:*335, 1974 (Rumanian)

Maxillary antrum sinus and odontogenic cyst, differential diagnosis of, in dental X-ray film (Bethmann *et al*). Stomatol. D.D.R., *24:*126, 1974 (German)

Maxillary sinus diseases, odontogenic, con-servative surgical method for. Observa-tions on 113 patients (Haneke *et al*). Z. W. R., *83:*20, 1974 (German)

Emergency care of severe facial injuries (Eade). Clin. Plast. Surg., *2:*73, 1975

Findings in the maxillary sinus following mid-facial fractures (Schwenzer). Fortschr. Kiefer. Gesichtschir., *19:*167, 1975 (Ger-man)

An operation for the relief of chronic nasal obstruction (Williams). J. Laryng. & Otol., *89:*527, 1975

Endoscopic findings of maxillary sinus after middle face fractures (Kreidler, Koch), PRS, *56:*463, 1975. J. Maxillo-facial Surg., *3:*10, 1975

Complex odontoma of the maxillary sinus: report of case (Curreri *et al*). J. Oral Surg., *33:*45, 1975

Treatment of orbital fractures by an infraor-bital-transantral approach (Livingston *et al*). J. Oral Surg., *33:*586, 1975

Malignant disease, maxillary sinusitis mim-icking (Towers, McAndrews), PRS, *57:*126, 1976. J. Oral Surg., *39:*718, 1975

Meningoencephalocele of the paranasal si-nuses (Kane *et al*). Laryngoscope, *85:*2087, 1975

Our experience with the joining of tissues using cyacrin (Volkov *et al*). Vestn. Otori-nolaringol., *2:*81, 1975 (Russian)

Maxillofacial Deformities: See *Jaw, Deformities (also specific deformities)*

Maxillofacial Injuries: See *Craniofacial Injuries; Facial Injuries; Jaw Fractures; Maxillary Fractures; etc.*

Maxillofacial Prostheses: See *Jaw Prostheses; Prostheses*

Maxillofacial Surgery: See *Face, Surgery; Facial Injuries; Jaws, Fractures; Jaws, Surgery; Nose, Fractures; Orbit, Fracture; War Injuries; Zygoma; etc.*

MAXWELL, J. A., KEPES, J. J., AND KETCHUM, L. D.: Acute carpal tunnel syndrome second-ary to thrombosis of persistent median ar-tery, PRS, *53:*368, 1974. J. Neurosurg., *38:*774, 1973

MAXWELL, T. M., OLCOTT, C., AND BLAISDELL, F. W.: Vascular complications of drug abuse, PRS, *51:*605, 1973. Arch. Surg., *105:*875, 1972

MAY, HANS: *Plastic and Reconstructive Sur-gery*, Third Edition. F. A. Davis Co., Phila-delphia, 1971. PRS, *48:*589, 1971

MAY, J. F., ROUNDS, D. E., AND CONE, C. D.: Intercellular transfer of toxic components after laser radiation, PRS, *48:*297, 1971. J. Nat. Cancer Inst., *46:*655, 1971

MAY, M., AND HARVEY, J. E.: Salivary flow: prognostic test for facial paralysis, PRS, *50:*537, 1972. Laryngoscope, *81:*179, 1971

MAY, M., AND LUCENTE, E. F.: "Bell's palsy" caused by basal cell carcinomas, PRS, *50:*635, 1972. J.A.M.A., *220:*159, 1972

MAY, M. *et al*: Bell's palsy: results of surgery, salivation test versus nerve excitability test as basis of treatment. Laryngoscope, *82:*1337, 1972

MAY, M. *et al*: Fracture of medial aspect of maxilla. Diagnosis and treatment. Arch. Otolaryng., *97:*286, 1973

MAY, M. *et al*: Shotgun wounds to head and neck. Arch. Otolaryng., *98:*373, 1973

MAY, M. *et al*: Mandibular fractures from civil-ian gunshot wounds: study of 20 cases. Lar-yngoscope, *83:*969, 1973

MAY, M. *et al*: Facial palsy: Bell's versus pa-rotid vascular malformation, case report. Laryngoscope, *83:*2020, 1973

MAY, M. *et al*: Penetrating neck wounds: selec-tive exploration. Laryngoscope, *85:*57, 1975

MAYALL, R. C.: Treatment of lymphatic and venous edema of lower extremities. Angiolo-gia, *25:*177, 1973 (Spanish)

MAYALL, M. F.: Nasal fractures. Their occur-rence, management and some late results. J. R. Coll. Surg. Edinb., *18:*31, 1973

MAYER, A. H., AND RIJSCOSCH, J. K. C.: Sweat gland carcinoma with regional lymph node metastases, PRS, *57:*404, 1976. Arch. chir. neerl., *27:*77, 1975

MAYER, M. *et al*: Chronic lymphedema after treatment for cancer of breast without recurrence, results of lymphatic drainage as used by Thompson, PRS, *54:*111, 1974. Lyon chir., *69:*401, 1973

MAYER, R.: Surgical treatment of mandibular prognathism. Acta Stomatol. Belg., *68:*383, 1971 (French)

MAYER, R. *et al*: Treatment by excision and graft of split thickness skin in recurrent verrucous papillary carcinoma. Rev. Stomatol. Chir. Maxillofac., *75:*98, 1974 (French)

MAYL, N., VASCONEZ, L. O., AND JURKIEWICZ, M. J.: Treatment of macromastia in actively enlarging breast, PRS, *54:*6, 1974

MAYNARD, J.: Historical and pathological curiosities of parotid disease. Guys Hosp. Rep., *121:*45, 1972

MAYS, H. B.: Epispadias: plan of treatment, PRS, *50:*632, 1972. J. Urol., *107:*251, 1972

MAZAHERI, M.: Growth and spatial changes in arch form in bilateral cleft palate (with Harding), PRS, *50:*591, 1972

MAZAURIC, F. X. *et al*: Historical mixed tumor of soft palate? (Or mixed tumor of pharyngeal extension of parotid gland.) J. Fr. Otorhinolaryngol., *21:*515, 1972 (French)

MAZAURIC, F. X. *et al*: Repair of partial loss of skin substance from the nasal pyramid. J. Fr. Otorhinolaryngol., *22:*815, 1973 (French)

MAZAURIC, F. X. *et al*: Cutaneous plastic surgery of the nose. Rieger's flap. J. Fr. Otorhinolaryngol., *23:*513, 1974 (French)

MAZZOLA, R., ANTONELLI, A., AND CIOCCARELLI, M.: Autogenous muscle grafts in men, PRS, *57:*683, 1976. Riv. ital. chir. plast., *6:*161, 1974

MAZZONI, G. *et al*: Effect of porcine renal retransplantation into new recipient after 1–3 days of residence in allogenic situation, PRS, *53:*613, 1974. Europ. Surg. Res., *5:*129, 1973

MCAULEY, J. E.: Charles Valadier: forgotten pioneer in treatment of jaw injuries, PRS, *55:*635, 1975. Proc. Roy. Soc. Med., *67:*785, 1974

MCBRIDE, C. M.: Diagnosis and management of malignant melanoma: some current approaches and controversies. Proc. Natl. Cancer Conf., *7:*581, 1973

MCBRIDE, C. M.: Management of malignant melanoma. Adv. Surg., *8:*129, 1974

MCBRIDE, C. M., BOWEN, J. M., AND DMOCHOWSKI, L. L.: Antinucleolar antibodies in sera of patients with malignant melanoma, PRS, *52:*328, 1973. Surg. Forum, *23:*92, 1972

MCBRIDE, M. E., DUNCAN, W. C., AND KNOX, J. M.: Evaluation of surgical scrub brushes,

PRS, *53:*615, 1974. Surg. Gynec. & Obst., *137:*934, 1973

MCCABE, B. F.: Injuries to facial nerve. Laryngoscope, *82:*1891, 1972

MCCABE, B. F.: Caldwell Luc self-retaining retractor. Trans. Am. Acad. Ophthalmol. Otolaryngol., *80:*257, 1975

MCCABE, B. F., AND BOLES, R.: Surgical treatment of essential blepharospasm. Ann. Otol. Rhin. & Laryng., *81:*611, 1972

MCCABE, W. P., AND KELLY, A. P., JR.: Management of epistaxis in Osler-Weber-Rendu disease, recurrence of telangiectases within skin graft, PRS, *50:*114, 1972

MCCABE, W. P., REBUCK, J. W., AND KELLY, A. P.: Leukocytic response as monitor of immunodepression in burn patients, PRS, *52:*456, 1973. Arch. Surg., *106:*155, 1973

MCCABE, W. P. *et al*: Cellular immune response of humans to pigskin, PRS, *51:*181, 1973

MCCABE, W. P., AND DITMARS, D. M., JR.: Soft tissue changes in hands of drug addicts, PRS, *52:*538, 1973

MCCABE, W. P., KELLY, A. P., AND BEHAN, F. C.: Reconstruction of plantar pad after degloving injuries of foot, PRS, *54:*109, 1974. Surg. Gynec. & Obst., *137:*971, 1973

MCCABE, W. P. *et al*: Soft tissue defects in Weber-Christian disease. Brit. J. Plast. Surg., *27:*107, 1974

MCCABE, W. P. *et al*: Panniculectomy following intestinal bypass. Brit. J. Plast. Surg., *27:* 346, 1974

MCCAFFERTY, G. J.: Bell's palsy—clinical survey. J. Otolaryngol. Soc. Aust., *3:*410, 1972

MCCAIN, W. G.: Results of tenolysis, controlled evaluation in chickens (with Hurst, Lindsay), PRS, *52:*171, 1973

MCCALLUM, D. I. *et al*: Intra-epidermal carcinoma of the eyelid margin. Brit. J. Dermatol., *93:*239, 1975

MCCANN, V. H. *et al*: Preoperative and postoperative management: the role of allied health professionals. Orthop. Clin. North Am., *6:*881, 1975

MCCARTHY, J. G.: Role of the groin dissection in the management of patients with melanoma of the lower extremity. Rev. Surg., *28:*374, 1971

MCCARTHY, J. G.: Report on 50 craniofacial operations (with Converse, Wood-Smith), PRS, *55:*283, 1975

MCCARTHY, J. G.: Orbital hypotelorism (with Converse, Wood-Smith), PRS, *56:*389, 1975

MCCARTHY, J. G., HAAGENSEN, C. D., AND HERTER, F. P.: Role of groin dissection in management of melanoma of lower extremity, PRS, *54:*237, 1974. Ann. Surg., *179:*156,

PRS, *49:*77, 1972

McDOWELL, F.: Intermezzo regarding Langenbeck, PRS, *49:*325, 1972; Commentary on Langenbeck, PRS, *49:*330, 1972

McDOWELL, F.: Commentary on Dorrance's Classic Reprint, PRS, *50:*277, 1972

McDOWELL, F.: Voice of polite dissent (Editorial), PRS, *50:*507, 1972

McDOWELL, F.: Department of negative results (Editorial), PRS, *50:*507, 1972

McDOWELL, F.: Editorial addendum to Classic Reprint of René Le Fort, PRS, *50:*607, 1972

McDOWELL, F.: Plantar warts, plantar calluses, and such (Editorial), PRS, *51:*196, 1973

McDOWELL, F.: Sagging surgeons, swing shift, and so on (Editorial), PRS, *51:*327, 1973

McDOWELL, F.: Subcutaneous mastectomy, syntax, and seat belts (Editorial), PRS, *51:*575, 1973

McDOWELL, F.: What happens to all those tears? (Editorial), PRS, *51:*682, 1973

McDOWELL, F.: Will a wider flap have a greater viable length? (Editorial), PRS, *52:*76, 1973

McDOWELL, F.: Productive and counterproductive efforts: parthenogenesis of great medical center (Editorial), PRS, *52:*178, 1973

McDOWELL, F.: Discussion of "Treatment of respiratory obstruction in micrognathia by use of nasogastric tube," by McEvitt, PRS, *52:*306, 1973

McDOWELL, F.: Get in there and replant! (Editorial), PRS, *52:*562, 1973

McDOWELL, F.: Authors, editors, and style manual (Editorial), PRS, *52:*658, 1973

McDOWELL, F.: Dedication of this issue to Dr. Robert H. Ivy (Editorial), PRS, *53:*579, 1974

McDOWELL, F.: Tattoo erasing (Editorial), PRS, *53:*580, 1974

McDOWELL, F.: Early relief of blindness occurring after blepharoplasty (Editorial), PRS, *53:*581, 1974

McDOWELL, F.: On breast tonometry (Editorial), PRS, *54:*88, 1974

McDOWELL, F.: Success in healing and saving lives in patients with enormous, deep burns (Editorial), PRS, *54:*209, 1974

McDOWELL, F.: Note on history of this journal (Editorial), PRS, *54:*676, 1974

McDOWELL, F.: Rare, inexorable, lethal "benign mixed tumor" of parotid (Editorial), PRS, *55:*214, 1975

McDOWELL, F.: Free, living bone graft (Editorial), PRS, *55:*612, 1975

McDOWELL, F.: What is really in so-called "dermal pedicle" used in certain types of reduction mammaplasties? (Editorial), PRS, *56:*201, 1975

McDOWELL, F.: Polonius revisited (Editorial),

PRS, *56:*568, 1975

McDOWELL, F.: Commentary on Franco's Classic Reprint, PRS, *57:*84, 1976

McDOWELL, F.: Commentary on de la Faye's Classic Reprint, PRS, *57:*221, 1976

McDOWELL, F.: Commentary on Malgaigne's "Du bec-de-lièvre" Classic Reprint, PRS, *57:*364, 1976

McDOWELL, F.: Misery of the burned child (Editorial), PRS, *57:*369, 1976

McDOWELL, F.: More free flaps – to publish or not to publish? – to use or not to use? (Editorial), PRS, *57:*653, 1976

McDOWELL, F., AND ENNA, C. D.: *Surgical Rehabilitation in Leprosy.* Williams & Wilkins Co., Baltimore, 1974

McEVITT, W. G.: Conversion of inferiorly-based pharyngeal flap to superiorly-based position, PRS, *48:*36, 1971

McEVITT, W. G.: Treatment of respiratory obstruction in micrognathia by use of nasogastric tube, PRS, *52:*138, 1973. Discussions by Lindsay, McDowell, Randall, PRS, *52:*306, 1973

McFADDEN, J. T.: Stereotaxic pinpointing of foreign bodies in limbs, PRS, *50:*424, 1972. Ann. Surg., *175:*81, 1972

McFARLAND, G. B., JR.: Early experience with silicone rubber prosthesis (Swanson) in reconstructive surgery of rheumatoid hand, PRS, *51:*703, 1973. South. M. J., *65:*1113, 1972

McFARLAND, G. B., JR. *et al*: Paralysis of the intrinsic muscles of the hand secondary to lipoma in Guyon's tunnel. J. Bone & Joint Surg. (Am.), *53:*375, 1971

McFARLAND, G. E., III: Otolaryngologist's role in catastrophe surgery. Laryngoscope, *83:*1048, 1973

McFARLAND, G. E., III: Reconstructive flaps in otolaryngology. Laryngoscope, *84:*1267, 1974

McFARLANE, M. W. *et al*: Dentinal dysplasia: report of a family. J. Oral Surg., *32:*867, 1974

McFARLANE, R.: Patterns of diseased fascia in fingers in Dupuytren's contracture, displacement of neurovascular bundle, PRS, *54:*31, 1974

McFARLANE, R. M., AND HAMPOLE, M. K.: Treatment of extensor tendon injuries of hand, PRS, *53:*488, 1974. Canad. J. Surg., *16:*366, 1973

McGIBBON, B. M., AND PALETTA, F. X.: Further concepts in gustatory sweating, PRS, *49:*639, 1972

McGIBBON, B. M. *et al*: Thermal regulation in patients after healing of large deep burns, PRS, *52:*164, 1973

McGINNIS, T. B. *et al*: High bilateral funiculoorchiectomy: secondary to avulsion injury.

Urology, *4:*596, 1974

McGOWAN, D. A.: Clinical problems in Paget's disease affecting jaws. Brit. J. Oral Surg., *11:*230, 1974

McGRAIL, J. S.: Management of maxillary fractures. Otolaryngol. Clin. North Am., *9:*223, 1976

McGREGOR, IAN A.: *Fundamental Techniques of Plastic Surgery and their Surgical Applications.* 5th edition. Williams & Wilkins Co., Baltimore, 1972. PRS, *53:*342, 1974

McGREGOR, IAN A.: *Fundamental Techniques of Plastic Surgery.* 6th edition. Longman, Inc., New York, 1975.

McGREGOR, I. A.: Degloving injuries. Hand, *2:*130, 1970

McGREGOR, I. A.: Eyelid reconstruction following subtotal resection of upper or lower lid. Brit. J. Plast. Surg., *26:*346, 1973

McGREGOR, I. A., AND Jackson, I. T.: Groin flap, PRS, *52:*217, 1973. Brit. J. Plast. Surg., *25:*3, 1972

McGREGOR, I. A., AND MORGAN, G.: Axial and random pattern flaps, PRS, *55:*118, 1975. Brit. J. Plast. Surg., *26:*202, 1973

McGREGOR, J. C., AND LINDOP, G. B. M.: Behavior of Cialit-stored and freeze-dried human *fascia lata* in rats, PRS, *56:*683, 1975. Brit. J. Plast. Surg., *27:*155, 1974

McGREGOR, M. W.: Report from American Board of Plastic Surgery, PRS, *49:*73, 1972; *50:*513, 1972

McGREGOR, M., AND STEISS, C.: Obituary on Gerald B. O'Connor, M.D., PRS, *51:*612, 1973

McGUIRE, E., AND WEISS, R.: Scrotal flap urethroplasty for strictures of deep urethra in infants and children, PRS, *54:*110, 1974. J. Urol., *110:*599, 1973

McHUGH, M. *et al:* Muscle flaps in the repair of skin defects over the exposed tibia. Brit. J. Plast. Surg., *28:*205, 1975

McIVOR, J.: Radiological features of ameloblastoma. Clin. Radiol. *25:*237, 1974

McIVOR, M.: Radiological features of odontogenic keratocysts. Brit. J. Oral Surg., *10:*116, 1972

McKAY, D. L., JR.: Balanitis xerotica obliterans in children. J. Urol., *114:*773, 1975

McKEE, D. M.: Temporal island flap for replacement of oral and pharyngeal mucosa. South. Med. J., *66:*534, 1973

McKEE, P.: Grafts: some intraoral uses. J. Contra Costa Dent. Soc., *16:*16, 1972

McKELVIE, P.: Metastatic routes in the neck. Can. J. Otolaryngol., *3:*473, 1974

McKELVIE, P.: Assessment of cryotherapy in otorhinolaryngology. Proc. Roy. Soc. Med., *67:*78, 1974

McKENZIE, D. S.: Editorial: the British Society for Surgery of the hand. Hand, *3:*7, 1971

McKENZIE, I. F. *et al:* Evidence for adaptation of skin grafts in enhanced irradiated mice. Transplantation, *14:*661, 1972

McKENZIE, I. F. *et al:* Immunogenicity and enhancement for private specificities H-2, 12, 16, 20 and 21. Transplantation, *17:*328, 1974

McKENZIE, M. W.: Ratchet handsplint. Am. J. Occup. Ther., *27:*477, 1973

McKINNEY, D. E. *et al:* Experiences with Devine inlay graft urethroplasty. Urology, *5:*487, 1975

McKINNEY, P.: Appraisal of treatment of basal cell carcinoma of skin (with Griffith), PRS, *51:*565, 1973

McKINNEY, P., AND MONN, L. N.: Comfortable mattress for outpatient surgery, PRS, *52:*446, 1973

McKINNEY, P. *et al:* Augmentation mammaplasty using non-inflatable prosthesis through circum-areola incision. Brit. J. Plast. Surg., *27:*35, 1974

McKINNEY, P. *et al:* Nasal xeroradiography. Brit. J. Plast. Surg., *27:*352, 1974

McKISSOCK, P. K.: Reduction mammaplasty with vertical dermal flap., PRS, *49:*245, 1972

McKUSICK, V. A.: Symphalangism and deafness. Birth Defects, *7:*124, 1971

McLAREN, K. R.: Surgery of external ear. J. Laryng. & Otol., *88:*23, 1974

McLAUGHLIN, A. P., III *et al:* Fate of methylcholanthrene tumor cells in bone: analysis of immune factors in host resistance, PRS, *53:*688, 1974. J. Surg. Res., *14:*186, 1973

McLAUGHLIN, C. W.: Here dwells our strength, PRS, *55:*518, 1975. Bull. Am. Coll. Surgeons, *59:*7, 1974

McLEAN, D. H., AND BUNCKE, H. J., JR.: Autotransplant of omentum to large scalp defect with microsurgical revascularization, PRS, *49:*268, 1972

McLEAN, D. H., AND BUNCKE, H. J., JR.: Use of Saran Wrap cuff in microsurgical arterial repairs, PRS, *51:*624, 1973

McLELLAN, D. L.: Letter: longitudinal sliding of median nerve during hand movements: a contributory factor in entrapment neuropathy? Lancet, *1:*633, 1975

McLEOD, J. G. *et al:* Nerve grafting in leprosy. Brain, *98:*203, 1975

McLEOD, J. G. *et al:* Nerve grafting in leprosy. Lancet, *1:*95, 1976

McMAHON, R. E. *et al:* Skeletal models as adjunct to jaw surgery. J. Oral Surg., *31:*340, 1973

McMANUS, W. F., EURENIUS, K., AND PRUITT, B. A.: Disseminated intravascular coagulation in burned patients, PRS, *53:*492, 1974. J. Trauma, *13:*416, 1973

McMASTER, M.: Natural history of the rheumatoid metacarpo-phalangeal joint. J. Bone & Joint Surg. (Br.), *54:*637, 1972

McMASTER, P.: Massive hemorrhage in elephantiasis neurofibroma. Brit. J. Surg., *59:*984, 1972

McMASTER, W. C.: Treatment of dog bite injuries, especially those of face (with Schultz), PRS, *49:*494, 1972

McMASTER, W. C.: Intraoperative reduction of phalangeal fractures, PRS, *56:*671, 1975

McMILLAN, G. H.: An improved method of elevation of the injured hand. J. R. Nav. Med. Serv., *56:*281, 1970

McNAMARA, J. J. *et al*: Clinical fat embolism in combat casualties, PRS, *51:*711, 1973. Ann. Surg., *176:*54, 1972

McNAMARA, J. J. *et al*: Effect of hypertonic glucose in hypovolemic shock in man, PRS, *51:*710, 1973. Ann. Surg., *176:*247, 1972

McNEIL, T. W. *et al*: Value of angiography in surgical management of deep hemangiomas, PRS, *56:*234, 1975. Clin. Orthop., *101:*176, 1974

McNEILL, R.: Facial nerve decompression. J. Laryng. & Otol., *88:*445, 1974

McNEILL, R. W.: Surgical-orthodontic correction of open-bite malocclusion, case report. Am. J. Orthod., *64:*38, 1973

McNEILL, R. W. *et al*: Cephalometric prediction for orthodontic surgery. Angle Orthod., *42:*154, 1972

McNEILL, R. W., HOOLEY, H. R., AND SUNDBERG, R. J.: Skeletal relapse during intermaxillary fixation. J. Oral Surg., *31:*212, 1973

McNEILL, T. W. *et al*: Hemangioma of extremities. Clin. Orthop., *101:*154, 1974

McPEAK, C. J.: Intralymphatic therapy with immune lymphocytes. Cancer, *28:*1126, 1971

McPHEDRAN, N. T. *et al*: Study of surgical practice in Alberta for 1970. Can. J. Surg., *16:*77, 1973

McQUARRIE, D. G.: Immediate functional restoration of mandible after surgical treatment of advanced oral cancer, PRS, *49:*103, 1972. Arch. Surg., *102:*447, 1971

McQUARRIE, D. G.: Safe replacement of tracheostomy tubes. Surg. Gynec. & Obst., *140:*769, 1975

McQUILLAN, W.: Sensory recovery after nerve repair. Hand, *2:*7, 1970

McQUILLAN, W. M. *et al*: Sensory evaluation after median nerve repair. Hand, *3:*101, 1971

McWILLIAMS, A. R. *et al*: Effect on protrusive tongue force of detachment of genioglossus muscle. J. Am. Dent. Assoc., *86:*1310, 1973

McWILLIAMS, B. J.: Clinical use of Peabody picture vocabulary test with cleft palate preschoolers, PRS, *56:*110, 1975. Cleft Palate J., *11:*439, 1974

McWILLIAMS, B. J. *et al*: Educational, occupational, and marital status of cleft palate adults. Cleft Palate J., *10:*223, 1973

MEACHAM, C. T.: The hard to repair severed lacrimal canaliculus, PRS, *50:*304, 1972. Arch. Ophth., *87:*406, 1972

MEACHAM, C. T.: Pseudosarcomatous fasciitis. Am. J. Ophth., *77:*747, 1974

MEADE, R. J.: Composite ear grafts for construction of columella (Follow-Up Clinic), PRS, *48:*73, 1971

MEAKINS, J. L.: Body's response to infection, PRS, *57:*264, 1976. AORN, *22:*37, 1975

MECHELSE, K.: Early decompression of the facial nerve in Bell's palsy. Ned. tijdschr. geneeskd., *116:*1031, 1972 (Dutch)

MEDGYESI, S.: Repair of large incisional hernias with pedicle skin flaps, PRS, *51:*486, 1973. Scand. J. Plast. Reconstr. Surg., *6:*69, 1972

MEDGYESI, S.: Photoelectric oscillometry. I. Physiological and technical study factors in measurement of skin circulation, PRS, *53:*501, 1074. Scand. J. Plast. Reconstr. Surg., *7:*29, 1973

MEDGYESI, S.: Observations on pedicle bone grafts in goats. Vascular connections between soft tissues and bones, PRS, *54:*509, 1974. Scand. J. Plast. Reconstr. Surg., *7:*110, 1973

Medical Education

Medical students, on appearance and attire of (Pickrell) (Editorial), PRS, *51:*438, 1973

Medical center, parthenogenesis of great, productive and counterproductive efforts. (McDowell) (Editorial), PRS, *52:*178, 1973

Style manual, authors, editors, and (McDowell) (Editorial), PRS, *52:*658, 1973

Educational Program, Jacksonville Hospital, Oral and Maxillofacial Surgery Department, University of Florida Affiliate (Editorial). J. Oral Surg., *32:*541, 1974

Role of pediatric surgery in general surgical education (Tunnell). J. Pediatr. Surg., *9:*743, 1974

Medical education, bridging gap between premedical and (Snyder *et al*) (Editorial), PRS, *53:*214, 1974

Teaching "core" knowledge in surgery, use of student-written programmed texts (Ryan, Coleman), PRS, *53:*429, 1974

Teaching exercises for medical students in clinical aspects of wound healing (Graham), PRS, *53:*433, 1974

Development of a plastic surgical teaching service in a women's correctional institu-

Medical Education – Cont.

   tion (Fisher *et al*). Am. J. Surg., *129:*269, 1975

   Education, continuing, and plastic surgery (Broadbent) (Editorial), PRS, *57:*88, 1976

Medical Ethics

   Fee entitlement in failed cosmetic surgery (Rieger). Dtsch. Med. Wochenschr., *99:*2068, 1974 (German)

   Esthetic surgery: plastic surgeon s obligations to the emotionally disturbed patient (Edgerton) (Editorial), PRS, *55:*81, 1975

   Ethics, medical practice, some current trends in (Owsley) (Editorial), PRS, *56:*567, 1975

   Ethics, medical, Polonius revisited (McDowell) (Editorial), PRS, *56:*568, 1975

MEDINA, E. A.: New technique for post-surgical fistulas, PRS, *50:*424, 1972. Rev. Latino Am. cir. plast., *15:*25, 1972

MEDOFF, G.: Current concepts in treatment of osteomyelitis, PRS, *57:*405, 1976. Postgrad. Med., *58:*157, 1975

MEDRANO, C. *et al*: Weeping without stenosis of the lacrimal ducts. Annee. Ther. Clin. Ophtalmol., *24:*409, 1973 (French)

MEGALLI, M., AND LATTIMER, J. K.: Review of management of 140 cases of exstrophy of bladder, PRS, *52:*597, 1973. J. Urol., *109:*246, 1973

MEGGITT, B. F. *et al*: Battered buttock syndrome – fat fractures. A report on a group of traumatic lipomata. Brit. J. Surg., *59:*165, 1972

MEGUID, M. M. *et al*: Long free-flowing scarf – a new health hazard to children. Pediatrics, *49:*290, 1972

MEHDIRATTA, K. S. *et al*: Extensive postoperative surgical emphysema with pneumomediastinum and pneumothorax. Int. Surg., *57:*666, 1972

MEHLER, J. *et al*: Therapy of large defects of hair-covered scalp. Langenbecks Arch. Chir., *331:*265, 1972 (German)

MEHNERT, H.: Surgical correction of deep bite and open bite. Dtsch. Zahn. Mund. Kieferheilkd., *59:*13, 1972 (German)

MEHNERT, H.: Interalveolar osteotomy in maxilla. Dtsch. Zahn. Mund. Kieferheilkd., *61:*289, 1973 (German)

MEHNERT, H. *et al*: First aid in jaw and craniofacial injuries. Z. Allgemeinmed., *47:*1436, 1971 (German)

MEHNERT, H. *et al*: Partial jaw resection in central giant cell granulomas. Zahnaerztl. Prax., *23:*433, 1972

MEHREGAN, A. H.: Effect of 1-tri-iodothyronine on marginal scars of skin grafted burns in rats (with Zamick), PRS, *51:*71, 1973

MEHTA, D. N. *et al*: Myxoma of antrum. J. Laryng. & Otol., *88:*281, 1974

MEIJER, A. H. *et al*: Sweat gland carcinoma with regional lymph node metastasis. Arch. chir. neerl., *27:*77, 1975

MEIJER, R.: When your patient asks about plastic surgery. Med. Times, *99:*117, 1971

MEIJER, R.: Modified Aufricht reduction mammaplasty, PRS, *53:*129, 1974. Discussion by Aufricht, PRS, *53:*132, 1974

MEIKLE, M. C.: Role of condyle in postnatal growth of mandible. Am. J. Orthod., *64:*50, 1973

MEIKLE, M. C. *In vivo* transplantation of mandibular joint of rat; and autoradiographic investigation into cellular changes at condyle. Arch. Oral Biol., *18:*1011, 1973

MEISTER, R. *et al*: Topographical and applied anatomy of the temporomandibular joint of various domestic animals with special reference to resection of the articular disc. 2. Calf (Bos taurus). Z. Exp. Chir., *5:*271, 1972 (German)

MEISTER, R. *et al*: Topographic and applied anatomy of temporomandibular joint (articulatio temporomandibularis) of various domestic animals with special reference to resection possibilities of discus articularis. 4. Swine (Sus srofa domesticus). Z. Exp. Chir., *6:*437, 1973 (German)

MEKTUBJIAN, S. R.: Method of internal suspension fixation in jaw fractures – general considerations, PRS, *55:*379, 1975. J. Maxillo-facial Surg., *2:*134, 1974

MEKTUBJIAN, S. R.: Internal indirect fixation with hooks as possible procedure in orbital fracture treatment, PRS, *57:*394, 1976. J. Maxillo-facial Surg., *3:*132, 1975

Melanoma

   Melanomas, hemangiomas with clinical appearance of (Gomez-Orbaneja), PRS, *51:*607, 1973. Actas dermo-sif. Madrid, *12:*379, 1969

   Melanoma, malignant, current concepts on (Das Gupta). Surg. Annu., *2:*183, 1970

   Malignant melanomas of the maxillary sinus (Tret'iak). Zh. Ushn. Nos. Gorl. Bolezn., *30:*98, 1970 (Russian)

   Melanoma, malignant, and coexisting malignant neoplasms (Fraser, Bull, Dunphy), PRS, *49:*109, 1972. Am. J. Surg., *122:*169, 1971

   Melanoma, desmoplastic malignant (a rare variant of spindle cell melanoma) (Conley, Lattes, Orr), PRS, *49:*587, 1972. Cancer, *28:*914, 1971

   Melanoma (Knutson *et al*). Curr. Probl.

Melanoma—Cont.

Surg., *3:*55, 1971

Dubreuilh's melanosis in cervicofacial carcinology: precancerous state or in-situ cancer? (Cesarini *et al*). J. Fr. Otorhinolaryngol., *20:*1037, 1971 (French)

Malignant melanoma (Pilleron). Laval. Med., *42:*933, 1971 (French)

Malignant melanoma—impressions from a study tour (Holmstrom). Nord. Med., *86:*1224, 1971 (Swedish)

Brief notes on malignant melanomas (Cellerino). Prensa Med. Argent., *58:*1601, 1971 (Spanish)

Melanoma, malignant (Moore, Gerner), PRS, *49:*108, 1972. Surg. Gynec. & Obst., *132:*427, 1971

Malignant melanoma of head and neck (Simons), PRS, *52:*102,˙1973. Am. J. Surg., *124:*485, 1972

Head and neck melanoma (Knutson, Hori, Watson), PRS, *52:*214, 1973. Am. J. Surg., *124:*543, 1972

Melanosis, Dubreuilh's: therapeutic paradox (Vandenbussche *et al*). Ann. chir. plast., *17:*289, 1972 (French)

Melanoma, malignant, generalized melanosis due to (Geerts *et al*). Arch. Belg. Dermatol. Syphiligr., *28:*395, 1972

Melanomata, malignant: aid to preoperative diagnosis (Mackie). Brit. J. Surg., *59:*632, 1972

Halo naevus—a frustrated malignant melanoma (Lewis *et al*). Brit. Med. J., *2:*47, 1972

Melanoma, malignant cervicofacial. Review of 78 cases (Lejeune *et al*). Bull. Cancer (Paris), *59:*255, 1972

Melanoma, malignant, value of iodinated vector: 7-Iodoquinoleine-I 131 in diagnosis and care of (Moretti *et al*). Bull. Soc. Fr. Dermatol. Syphiligr., *79:*155, 1972 (French)

Use of labelled iodoquine in diagnosis of nevocarcinoma (Huriez *et al*). Bull. Soc. Fr. Dermatol. Syphiligr., *79:*159, 1972 (French)

Melanoma, isotopic examination of, with labelled iodoquine (Delisle *et al*). Bull. Soc. Fr. Dermatol. Syphiligr., *79:*163, 1972 (French)

Topographic diagnosis of nevocarcinoma and their metastases, using labelled bleomycin (Robert *et al*). Bull. Soc. Fr. Dermatol. Syphiligr., *79:*166, 1972 (French)

Successive nevocarcinomas complicating Dubreuilh's melanosis evolving over period of 38 years (Castelain). Bull. Soc. Fr. Dermatol. Syphiligr., *79:*276, 1972 (French)

Head and neck, malignant melanoma (Fitz-

Melanoma—Cont.

patrick, Brown, Reid), PRS, *50:*421, 1972. Canad. J. Surg., *15:*90, 1972

Malignant melanoma and hairy nevus (Krinitz *et al*). Dermatol. Monatsschr., *158:*130, 1972 (German)

Malignant melanoma developing in a tattoo (Kirsch). Int. J. Dermatol., *11:*16, 1972

Malignant melanoma: 43 cases (Kanasugi *et al*). Jap. J. Cancer Clin., *18:*380, 1972 (Japanese)

Difficulties in diagnosing malignant melanoma in young persons (Kruszcynski *et al*). Klin. Oczna., *42:*921, 1972 (Polish)

Melanoma, malignant (Mastrangelo *et al*). Pa. Med., *75:*43, 1972

Melanoma and trauma. A clinical study of Zulu feet under conditions of persistent and gross trauma (Bentley-Phillips *et al*). S. Afr. Med. J., *46:*535, 1972

Melanoma, amelanotic, clinicopathologic study of (Huvos, Shah, Goldsmith), PRS, *51:*707, 1973. Surg. Gynec. & Obst., *135:*917, 1972

Melanoma, malignant, lymphographic evaluation of 116 cases of (Musumeci *et al*). Tumori, *58:*1, 1972

Malignant melanoma of the septum (Jung). Z. Laryngol. Rhinol. Otol., *51:*141, 1972 (German)

Melanoma, juvenile, and spindle cell nevi (Coskey, Mehregan), PRS, *53:*611, 1974. Arch. Dermat., *108:*535, 1973

Melanoma, malignant, of nasal cavity and paranasal sinuses (Freedman *et al*), PRS, *52:*459, 1973. Arch. Otolaryng., *97:*322, 1973

Moles, pigmented, development and elimination of, anatomical distribution of primary malignant melanoma (Nicholls), PRS, *54:*116, 1974. Cancer, *32:*191, 1973

Melanoma, difficulties in diagnosing (Hamilton, Foley, Davis), PRS, *53:*497, 1974. Contemp. Surg., *3:*65, 1973

Melanoblastoma, clear cell (Hula). Dermatologica, *146:*86, 1973

Malignancy of melanocytoblastoma. Analysis of malignant skin melanomas of head and neck region (Eneroth *et al*). H.N.O., *21:*208, 1973 (German)

Head and neck, malignant melanoma (Salem, Travezan), PRS, *54:*115, 1974. Internat. Surg., *58:*790, 1973

Melanoma and halo nevi (Epstein *et al*), PRS, *53:*248, 1974. J.A.M.A., *225:*373, 1973

Melanoma, malignant, infiltrating, of heel: case report (Routsaw). J. Am. Podiatry Assoc., *63:*319, 1973

Newborn, excision of giant nevus in (Feins),

Melanoma – Cont.

PRS, *54:*380, 1974. J. Pediat. Surg., *8:*825, 1973

Association of malignant melanoma and malignant lymphoma (Tashima). Lancet, *1:*266, 1973

Melanoma, malignant, lymphangiographic studies in series of 55 patients with (De Roo). Lymphology, *6:*6, 1973

Melanoma, malignant, spontaneous regression (Doyle *et al*). M. J. Australia, *2:*551, 1973

Melanoma, malignant, and pregnancy and the puerperium (Bergamaschi *et al*). Minerva Ginecol., *25:*623, 1973 (Italian)

Melanoma, malignant, in children: report of two cases (Wojnerowicz *et al*). Nowotwory, *23:*227, 1973 (Polish)

Melanoma, malignant. Survey of 232 cases (Biran *et al*). Oncology, *28:*331, 1973

Melanoma, malignant, diagnosis and management of: some current approaches and controversies (McBride). Proc. Natl. Cancer Conf., *7:*581, 1973

Melanoma, nasal cavity (Boutin *et al*). Union Med. Can. *102:*1872, 1973

Melanoma, malignant, of head and neck, tumor thickness and lymphocytic infiltration in (Hansen *et al*). Am. J. Surg., *128:*557, 1974

Head and neck, melanoma of mucous membranes of (Conley, Pack), PRS, *54:*699, 1974. Arch. Otolaryng., *99:*315, 1974

Melanoma, clinical experience in 77 patients (Pilheu), PRS, *56:*112, 1975. Bol. y Trab. Acad. argent. cir., *58:*392, 1974

Superficial melanoma in a tattoo (Wolfort *et al*). Brit. J. Plast. Surg., *27:*303, 1974

Melanoma, malignant, role of frozen section in diagnosis and management (Davis, Little), PRS, *54:*700, 1974. Brit. J. Surg., *61:*505, 1974

Malignant melanoma and L-dopa. Review of literature on the problem of causal relationship (Happle). Fortschr. Med., *92:*1065, 1974 (German)

Letter: further risk with bleomycin (Pandeya *et al*). J. Am. Osteopath. Assoc., *74:*260, 1974

Melanotic tumor of nasal septum, 5-year course (Gaillard *et al*). J. Fr. Otorhinolaryngol., *23:*884, 1974 (French)

Melanotic nerve sheath tumors (Mandybur). J. Neurosurg., *41:*187, 1974

Malignancy, risk of, in large congenital nevi (Kaplan), PRS, *53:*421, 1974

Pigmented tumor of the maxilla in the child (Mugnier *et al*). Rev. Stomatol. Chir. Maxillofac., *75:*771, 1974 (French)

Melanoma, malignant, suspected early pri-

Melanoma – Cont.

mary (Redman). Rocky Mt. Med. J., *71:*161, 1974

Melanoma, use of lymphangiography in (Ariel), PRS, *56:*113, 1975. Surgery, *76:*654, 1974

Melanomas, development of two, in same patient within 16 year period (Lischka *et al*). Z. Hautkr., *49:*129, 1974 (German)

Melanoma of the head and neck (Harris *et al*). Ann. Surg., *182:*86, 1975

Pseudomelanoma, recurrent melanocytic nevus following partial surgical removal (Kornberg, Ackerman), PRS, *57:*765, 1976. Arch. Dermat., *111:*1588, 1975

Malignant melanoma: the patient with an unknown site of primary origin (Baab *et al*). Arch. Surg., *110:*896, 1975

Juvenile melanoma disseminatum (Capetanakis). Brit. J. Dermatol., *92:*207, 1975

The place of frozen section in the practical management of melanoma (Hughes). Brit. J. Surg., *62:*840, 1975

Melanomas, human, melanogenesis in (Chen, Chavin), PRS, *56:*112, 1975. Cancer Res., *35:*606, 1975

Melanoma, malignant, suspected early primary (Redman), PRS, *56:*113, 1975. Cutis, *15:*98, 1975

Melanoma, benign juvenile: clinicopathological study of 51 lesions (Andrade Malabehar), PRS, *57:*677, 1976. Grac. Med. Mex., *110:*181, 1975

Melanoma, malignant, spontaneous regression and leukoderma in (Happle *et al*). Hautarzt, *26:*120, 1975 (German)

Melanoma, malignant, during treatment with levodopa (Pelfrene). Nouv. Presse Med., *4:*1365, 1975 (French)

Amelanotic melanoma (Shah). Prog. Clin. Cancer, *6:*195, 1975

Melanoma, Congenital

Malignant melanoma developing in intrauterine life (Conu *et al*). Rom. Med. Rev., *15:*41, 1971

Congenital malignant melanoma (Mompoint *et al*). N. Y. State J. Med., *72:*1629, 1972

Melanotic neuroectodermal tumor of infancy. Case report and review (Elomaa *et al*). Proc. Finn. Dent. Soc., *69:*227, 1973

Melanotic neuroectodermal tumour of infancy (Oldhoff *et al*). Trans. Int. Conf. Oral Surg., *4:*55, 1973

Malignant melanoma in childhood (Olbourne *et al*). Brit. J. Plast. Surg., *27:*305, 1974

Melanotic neuroectodermal tumor of infancy (Hoggins, Grundy), PRS, *57:*539, 1976. Oral Surg., *40:*34, 1975

Melanoma, Mouth – Cont.

Melanosis, gingival, surgical treatment of (Sierra). Rev. Fed. Odontol. Colomb., *22:*51, 1973 (Spanish)

Oral mucous membrane, primary melanoma in (Anneroth *et al*). Sven. Tandlak. Tidskr., *66:*27, 1973

Melanoma of mucous membranes of head and neck (Conley, Pack), PRS, *54:*699, 1974. Arch. Otolaryng., *99:*315, 1974

Melanoma, primary malignant, of oral cavity in Indians (Soman, Sirsat), PRS, *56:*224, 1975. Oral Surg., *38:*426, 1974

Melanoma, oral malignant (Liversedge), PRS, *57:*678, 1976. Brit. J. Oral Surg., *13:*40, 1975

Melanoma, primary, of oral cavity (Jackson, Simpson), PRS, *57:*264, 1976. J. Oral Surg., *39:*553, 1975

Mucosal melanomas of the head and neck (Barton). Laryngoscope, *85:*93, 1975

Melanoma, Prognosis in

Therapeutic planning and prognosis in cutaneous malignant melanoma (Veronesi *et al*). Arch. Ital. Chir., *95:*607, 1969 (Italian)

Effect of biopsy on the prognosis of melanoma (Epstein). J. Surg. Oncol., *3:*251, 1971

Malignant melanoma. Clinico-pathological study of 92 patients in a 20-year period (Abbud Ochoa *et al*). Prensa Med. Mex., *36:*284, 1971 (German)

Melanoma, malignant, prognosis in relation to clinical presentation (Shah, Goldsmith), PRS, *50:*309, 1972. Am. J. Surg., *123:*286, 1972

Primary focus in malignant melanoma, prognosis based on death rate in relation to irritation, growth, and surface structure of (Heite). Arch. Dermatol. Forsch., *244:*200, 1972 (German)

Cures achieved in patients with metastatic malignant melanoma of the skin (Conrad). Cancer, *30:*144, 1972

Melanoma, malignant, significance of histological findings in prognosis (Gartmann, Tritsch), PRS, *51:*608, 1973. Deutsche med. Wchnschr., *97:*857, 1972

Clinical diagnosis and biological behavior of cutaneous malignant melanoma (Sumrall). J. Natl. Med. Assoc., *64:*359, 1972

Analysis of the survival of patients with pigmented neoplasms (Shevchenko *et al*). Klin. Khir., *1:*36, 1972 (Russian)

Malignant melanoma – treatment and prognosis (Holmstrom). Lakartidningen, *69:*2425, 1972 (Swedish)

Assessment of prognosis in patients with malignant melanoma (Mackie *et al*). Lancet,

Melanoma, Prognosis in – Cont.

*2:*455, 1972

Prognostic significance of clinical factors in malignant melanoma of the skin (Mioduszewska *et al*). Nowotwory, *22:*15, 1972 (Polish)

Prognostic value of histological criteria in malignant melanoma of the skin (Mioduszewska *et al*). Nowotwory, *22:*113, 1972 (Polish)

Melanoma, malignant, prognosis in (Weidner). Med. Klin., *68:*419, 1973 (German)

Survival with melanoma (Cox), PRS, *52:*685, 1973. Proc. Roy. Australasian Coll. Surg., *46:*630, 1973

Melanomas, malignant, primary, study of clinical and histological criteria of prognosis of (Jourdain). Ann. Dermatol. Syphiligr. (Paris), *101:*171, 1974 (French)

Prognosis of cutaneous malignant melanoma (Sinha, Buntine), PRS, *56:*113, 1975. Canad. J. Surg., *17:*328, 1974

Melanoma, malignant, cutaneous, prognostic factors in. Comparative study of long-term and short-term survivors (Huvos *et al*). Hum. Pathol., *5:*347, 1974

Melanomas, malignant, of Lille, 1967–1972; comparison between "histoprognosis" and actual outcome (Vandenbussche *et al*), PRS, *57:*680, 1976. Acta chir. belg., *74:*406, 1975

Melanoma, salvage in (Editorial). Brit. Med. J., *2:*353, 1975

Malignant melanoma of the extremities: a clinocopathologic study using levels of invasion (microstage) (Wanebo *et al*). Cancer, *35:*666, 1975

Melanoma, cutaneous: 20-year retrospective study with clinicopathologic correlation (Franklin, Reynolds, Page), PRS, *56:*277, 1975

Melanoma, clinical experience with 77 patients (Pilheu), PRS, *57:*124, 1976. Prensa med. argent., *62:*97, 1975

Melanoma, Skin

Melanoma, malignant, of skin of head and neck (Ballantyne), PRS, *48:*200, 1971. Am. J. Surg., *120:*425, 1970

Malignant melanoma and vitiligo (Milton *et al*). Australas. J. Dermatol., *12:*131, 1971

Malignant melanomas of the face (Romieu *et al*). J. Fr. Otorhinolaryngol., *20:*1121, 1971 (French)

Melanomas, cutaneous malignant, clinical diagnosis, classification and histogenetic concepts of early stages of (Mihm, Clark, From), PRS, *49:*667, 1972. New England J. Med., *284:*1078, 1971

Melanoma, Treatment – Laser – Cont.

surgery with carbon dioxide laser (Oosterhuis, Verschueren, Oldhoff), PRS, *57:*680, 1976. Acta chir. belg., *74:*422, 1975

Laser therapy of human benign and malignant neoplasms of the skin (Wagner *et al*). Acta Radiol. (Ther.) (Stockh.), *14:*417, 1975

Destruction of melanoma metastases with a laser (Koshelev *et al*). Vopr. Onkol., *21:*98, 1975 (Russian)

Melanoma Treatment – Lymph Node Dissections

Melanoma, selective regional lymphadenectomy for, mathematical aid to clinical judgment (Polk, Linn), PRS, *50:*97, 1972. Ann. Surg., *174:*402, 1971

A new approach to radical retroperitoneal iliac and femoral node dissection (Wagner *et al*). Arch. Surg., *103:*681, 1971

Elective lymph-node dissection for melanoma (Davis *et al*). Brit. J. Surg., *58:*820, 1971

Melanoma, malignant, regional node dissection in treatment of (Paglia, Knapper, Fortner), PRS, *50:*98, 1972. Clin. Bull. Memorial Sloan-Kettering Cancer Center, *1:*136, 1971

Prophylactic regional lymph node excision in malignant melanoma (Abu-Dalu *et al*). Harefuah, *80:*129, 1971 (Hebrew)

Role of the groin dissection in the management of patients with melanoma of the lower extremity (McCarthy). Rev. Surg., *28:*374, 1971

Melanomas of lower extremity, extended radical groin dissection for (Ariel), PRS, *48:*200, 1971. Surg. Gynec. & Obst., *132:*116, 1971

Ilio-inguinal lymphadenectomy in the treatment of regional metastases of cutaneous melanoblastomas of the lower extremities (Vagner *et al*). Vestn. Khir., *107:*55, 1971 (Russian)

Melanoma, malignant, treatment by wide excision alone *versus* lymphadenectomy (Conrad), PRS, *50:*636, 1972. Arch. Surg., *104:*587, 1972

Malignant melanoma: current concepts of lymph node dissection (Goldsmith *et al*). C. A., *22:*216, 1972

Melanoma, malignant. Should lymphadenectomy be discarded? (Hiles). J. R. Coll. Surg. Edinb., *18:*368, 1973

Malignant melanoma, radical dissection of axillary lymph nodes (Milton, McCarthy), PRS, *53:*112, 1974. Proc. Roy. Australasian Coll. Surg., *46:*694, 1973

Melanomas, ilioinguinal lymph node dissection for (Harris *et al*), PRS, *52:*215, 1973. Surg. Gynec. & Obst., *136:*33, 1973

Melanoma Treatment – Lymph Node Dissections – Cont.

Melanoma, regional lymph node dissection for (Gumport, Harris), PRS, *54:*243, 1974. Ann. Surg., *179:*105, 1974

Melanoma of lower extremity, role of groin dissection in management (McCarthy, Haagensen, Herter), PRS, *54:*237, 1974. Ann. Surg., *179:*156, 1974

Radical neck dissection in advanced tumors of the head and neck. Considerations on 52 cases (Caldarola *et al*). Cancro, *27:*187, 1974 (Italian)

Indications for regional lymphadenectomy in melanoblastoma of the skin of the extremities (Vagner *et al*). Vopr. Onkol., *20:*33, 1974 (Russian)

Tumor thickness, level of invasion and node dissection in stage I cutaneous melanoma (Breslow). Ann. Surg., *182:*572, 1975

Melanoma, primary, *en bloc* resection with regional lymph node dissection (Fortner, Schottenfeld, Maclean), PRS, *56:*601, 1975. Arch. Surg., *110:*674, 1975

Regional lymph nodes in malignant melanoma: is routine excision indicated? (Davis). Prog. Clin. Cancer, *6:*183, 1975

Malignant melanoma. Role of node dissection reappraised (Southwick). Cancer, *37:*202, 1976

Melanoma Treatment – Miscellaneous or Mixed

Clinical aspects and theray of malignant melanoma (Storck). Hautarzt, *21:*187, 1970 (German)

Treatment of advanced or recurrent malignant melanoma (Pettavel *et al*). Schweiz. Med. Wochenschr., *100:*988, 1970 (French)

Melanoma, malignant, improved systemic chemotherapy for (Larson, Hill), PRS, *49:*667, 1972. Am. J. Surg., *122:*36, 1971

Surgical technic for malignant melanoma of the skin in the head and neck region (Grimm *et al*). Dtsch. Zahn. Mund. Kieferheilkd., *57:*363, 1971 (German)

Treatment of malignant melanomas of the skin (Palmer). Laval. Med., *42:*926, 1971

Melanoma, malignant, surgical treatment (Lissaios *et al*), PRS, *51:*483, 1973. Acta chir. Hellenica, *44:*619, 1972

Melanoma, multiple "in-transit" metastases of, total integumentectomy of leg for (Jones, Dickinson), PRS, *51:*607, 1973. Am. J. Surg., *123:*588, 1972

Management of malignant melanoma (Lawrence). Am. Surg., *38:*93, 1972

Melanoma, malignant, therapy of (Gartman), PRS, *51:*235, 1973. Deutsche med.

Melanoma Treatment—Miscellaneous or Mixed—Cont.

Wchnschr., *97:*1305, 1972

Melanoma, malignant maxillary, case with 6-year recovery (Landais *et al*). J. Fr. Otorhinolaryngol., *21:*638, 1972 (French)

Surgical approach to the treatment of melanoma (Wuester). J. Med. Soc. N. J., *69:*235, 1972

Melanoma, primary, surgery of: problems and practice (Davis *et al*). M. J. Australia, *2:*778, 1972

Melanoma, malignant, patient with complications after treatment of (Huinink *et al*). Ned. tijdschr. geneeskd., *116:*2046, 1972 (Dutch)

Melanoma, malignant: surgical aspects of treatment (Edwards). Proc. Roy. Soc. Med., *65:*140, 1972

Intracranial metastatic malignant melanoma: long-term survival following subtotal resection (Bauman *et al*). South. Med. J., *65:*344, 1972

Melanomas, malignant, of skin, clinical features and results of surgical treatment of (Putnik *et al*). Vojnosanit. Pregl., *29:*401, 1972

Surgery of melanocytoblastoma of the skin (Kostler *et al*). Zentralbl. Chir., *97:*601, 1972 (German)

Melanoma, Stage I, surgical treatment of (Dellon, Ketcham), PRS, *53:*370, 1974. Arch. Surg., *106:*738, 1973

Melanoma, Stage I, surgical treatment of (Conrad). Arch. Surg., *106:*740, 1973

Melanoma, malignant, treatment of (Levene). Brit. Med. J., *1:*545, 1973

Melanoma, malignant—treatment of primary lesion (Gordon). Cent. Afr. J. Med., *19:*76, 1973

Melanomas, malignant, new radiological-surgical concepts in primary treatment of (Scherer *et al*). Fortschr. Geb. Roentgenstr. Nuklearmed., *118:*174, 1973 (German)

Melanoma, malignant, place of surgery in treatment of (Pettavel). Schweiz. Med. Wochenschr., *103:*1424, 1973 (French)

Melanoma, malignant, management of (McBride). Adv. Surg., *8:*129, 1974

Melanoma, malignant, chemotherapy of, with dimethyl triazeno imidazole carboxamide (DITC) and nitrosourea derivatives (BCNU, CCNU) (Hill *et al*), PRS, *55:*117, 1975. Ann. Surg., *180:*167, 1974

Practical cryosurgery for oral lesions (Leopard *et al*). Brit. Dent. J., *136:*185, 1974

Combination therapy: some concepts and results (Skipper). Cancer Chemother. Rep. (Suppl.), *4:*137, 1974

Melanoma Treatment—Miscellaneous or Mixed—Cont.

Melanoma, advanced metastatic malignant, prognostic correlations and response to treatment in (Einhorn *et al*), PRS, *55:*115, 1975. Cancer Res., *34:*1995, 1974

Integration of chemotherapy into combined modality therapy of solid tumors. IV. Malignant melanoma (Comis *et al*). Cancer Treat. Rev., *1:*285, 1974

Problems in the surgical treatment of malignant melanomas (Kohnlein *et al*). Chirurg., *45:*356, 1974 (German)

Treatment of malignant melanoma (Editorial). Lancet, *2:*1119, 1974

Melanoma, malignant, head and neck, surgical treatment for (Nagel). Laryngol. Rhinol. Otol. (Stuttg.), *53:*241, 1974

Cryosurgical treatment of recurrent head and neck malignancies—a comparative study (Goode *et al*). Laryngoscope, *84:*1950, 1974

Melanoma, malignant, surgical treatment (Hiles). Proc. Roy. Soc. Med., *67:*95, 1974

Melanoma, malignant, extended lateral rhinotomy for resection of (Mabry *et al*). South. Med. J., *67:*65, 1974

Metastasis, surgical treatment of recurrent melanoma (Fortner *et al*), PRS, *55:*517, 1975. Surg. Clin. N. Am., *54:*865, 1974

Tridimensional resection of primary malignant melanoma (Ariel). Surg. Gynec. & Obst., *139:*601, 1974

Metastatic melanoma treated in a pregnant woman: pre- and postnatal implications (Toussi *et al*). Union Med. Can., *103:*1968, 1974 (French)

Advances in the surgical treatment of skin tumors (Wilflingseder). Wien. Med. Wochenschr., *124:*593, 1974 (German)

Present concepts of the treatment of malignant melanoma (Banzet *et al*). Acta Chir. Belg., *74:*395, 1975 (French)

Contemporary treatment of malignant melanoma (Cady *et al*). Am. J. Surg., *129:*472, 1975

Staging laparotomy in the treatment of metastatic melanoma of the lower extremities (Cohen *et al*). Ann. Surg., *182:*710, 1975

Resection, *en bloc*, of primary melanoma with regional lymph node dissection (Fortner, Schottenfeld, Maclean), PRS, *56:*601, 1975. Arch. Surg., *110:*674, 1975

Delayed exposed skin grafting in surgery for breast cancer and melanoma (Rees *et al*). Clin. Oncol., *1:*131, 1975

Giant "bathing trunk" nevus with malignant melanoma treated by excision and split thickness skin grafting (Kosloske *et al*). J.

Melanoma Treatment – Miscellaneous or Mixed – Cont.

Pediatr. Surg., *10:*823, 1975

Surgical treatment of skin melanoma (Bazhenova). Khirurgiia (Mosk.), *11:*26, 1975 (Russian)

Some of our views on the surgical treatment of malignant melanoma (Bogdanov *et al*). Med. Pregl., *28:*481, 1975 (Serbian)

Surgical management of melanoma metastatic to the lung: problems in diagnosis and management (Cahan). Prog. Clin. Cancer, *6:*205, 1975

On therapy planning in malignant melanoma (Baldauf *et al*). Radiobiol. Radiother. (Berl.), *16:*51, 1975 (German)

Operative treatment of malignant melanoma of the limb (a point of view) (Lawrence). Va. Med. Mon., *102:*141, 1975

Views on surgical treatment of malignant melanoma (Jacobsson). Lakartidningen, *73:*530, 1976 (Swedish)

Management of malignant tumors of the maxillary sinus (Birt *et al*). Otolaryngol. Clin. North Am., *9:*249, 1976

Melanoma Treatment – Perfusion

Melanoma, limb, perfusion in: indications and results (Fontaine *et al*). Proc. Roy. Soc. Med., *67:*99, 1974

Isolated regional perfusion in the treatment of malignant melanomas of the extremities (Schraffordt Koops *et al*). Arch. chir. neerl., *27:*237, 1975

Survival after regional perfusion for limb melanoma (Cox). Aust. N. Z. J. Surg., *45:*32, 1975

Salvage procedures for locally advanced malignant melanoma of the lower limb (with special reference to the role of isolated limb perfusion and radical lymphadenectomy) (Weaver *et al*). Clin. Oncol., *1:*45, 1975

Results of hyperthermic perfusion for melanoma of the extremities (Stehlin *et al*). Surg. Gynec. & Obst., *140:*339, 1975

Survival and regional disease control after isolation-perfusion for invasive stage I melanoma of the extremities (Sugarbaker *et al*). Cancer, *37:*188, 1976

Perfusion of melanoma. 133 isolated perfusions in 114 patients (Golomb). Panminerva Med., *18:*8, 1976

Melanoma Treatment – Radiation

Melanoma, malignant, of lower extremities, endolymphatic radiotherapy in (Kalkoff, Baumeister, Gehring). Arch. Derm. Forsch., *244:*250, 1972 (German)

Usefulness of radiotherapy in the treatment

Melanoma Treatment – Radiation – Cont.

of cutaneous melanoma (Reignier). Acta Chir. Belg., *73:*237, 1974 (French)

Radiotherapy of malignant melanoma (Lissner *et al*). Chirurg., *45:*362, 1974 (German)

Current status of endolymphatic therapy with radionuclides (Peters *et al*). Lymphology, 7:49, 1974

Melanoma, malignant, radiotherapy in (Pearson). Proc. Roy. Soc. Med., *67:*96, 1974

Results of treating malignant melanoma intralymphatically with radioactive isotopes (Ariel). Surg. Gynec. & Obst., *139:*726, 1974

Indications for and results of percutaneous radiotherapy of malignant melanoma (Hellriegel). Strahlentherapie, *149:*1, 1975 (German)

MELEGA, J. M.: Treatment of necrotic scab in deep burns, PRS, *55:*721, 1975. Ars Curandi, 7:42, 1974

MELEGA, J. M.: What's new in treatment of burns? PRS, *55:*721, 1975. Ars Curandi, 7:68, 1974

MELEGA, J. M. *et al*: Overall treatment of severe burn patient, PRS, *55:*722, 1975. Ars Curandi, 7:10, 1974

MELI: Transsigmoid cutaneous ureterostomies. Ann. Chir. Infant., *12:*450, 1971 (French)

MELIKOV, A. M. *et al*: Teratoma of neck in children. Pediatriia, *3:*78, 1974 (Russian)

MELLIERE, D. *et al*: Our attitude towards the treatment of thyroid cancer (a report of 50 cases). Ann. Endocrinol. (Paris), *35:*285, 1974 (French)

MELLERSTIG, K. E.: Conservative program for managing cleft palates without use of mucoperiosteal flaps (with Blocksma, Leuz). PRS, *55:*160, 1975

MELMAN, E. *et al*: Regional anesthesia in children, PRS *57:*405, 1976. Anesth. Analg. Cleve., *54:*387, 1975

MELMED, E. P.: Fractures of zygomatic-malar complex. S. Afr. Med. J., *46:*569, 1972

MELMED, E. P.: Breast reduction. S. Afr. Med. J., *46:*1518, 1972

MELMED, E. P., AND KOONIN, A. J.: Fractures of mandible, review of 909 cases. PRS, *56:*323, 1975

MEL'NIK, A. K. *et al*: Clinical use of a 10 percent solution of placental albumin. Probl. Gematol. Pereliv. Krovi., *16:*7, 1971 (Russian)

Meloplasty: See *Rhytidectomy*

MELROSE, R. J. *et al*: Mucoepidermoid tumors of intraoral minor salivary glands: clinicopathologic study of 54 cases. J. Oral Pathol., 2:314, 1973

MELSOM, M. A.: Surgical experiences in Nepal. Ann. R. Coll. Surg. Engl., 57:268, 1975

MELVIN, P. M.: Corn picker injuries of the hand, PRS 51:231, 1973. Arch. Surg., 104:26, 1972

MENARD, Y.: Transposition of greater omentum for reconstruction of chest wall (with Dupont). PRS 49:263, 1972

MENDEL, A. K.: Complications in phallo- and urethroplasty. Vestn. Khir., 113:124, 1974 (Russian)

MENDELSON, J. A.: Letters to editor: laser excision of burns. J. Trauma, 13:575, 1973

MENDES DA COSTA, P. et al: The place of surgery in the treatment of carcinomas of the oral cavity. Acta Chir. Belg., 73:529, 1974 (French)

MENDEX V. et al: Lymphangioma of tongue associated with cervical cystic hygroma and anterior open bite, PRS, 57:757, 1976. O Medico, 79:199, 1975

MENDEZ, R., KIELY, W. F., AND MORROW, J. W.: Self-emasculation, PRS, 51:603, 1973. J. Urol., 107:981, 1972

MENEZO, J. L. et al: Contributions to the surgical technique of external dacryocystorhinostomy. Klin. Monatsbl. Augenheilkd., 166:108, 1975 (German)

Meningocele: See *Encephalocele and Meningocele*

MENKES, C. J. et al: Intra-articular injection of radioisotopic beta emitters. Application to the treatment of the rheumatoid hand. Orthop. Clin. North Am., 4:1113, 1973

MENN, H.: Current management of cancer of skin. Postgrad. Med., 52:161, 1972

MENNIG: Rhino-surgical tasks in orbit. Arch. Otorhinolaryngol. (N.Y.), 207:285, 1974 (German)

MENNING, H.: Problems of face and neck surgery near the orbital base of the skull. Z. Aerztl. Fortbild. (Jena.), 69:949, 1975 (German)

MENZOIAN, J. O. et al: Bilateral hip disarticulation with total thigh flaps for extensive decubitus ulcers: a case report. R. I. Med. J., 55:251, 1972

MERCER, C. W., AND LOGIC, L. R.: Cardiac arrest due to hyperkalemia following intravenous penicillin administration, PRS 53:609, 1974. Chest, 64:358, 1973

MERCIER, P.: Inner osseous architecture and sagittal splitting of ascending ramus of the mandible. J. Maxillo-facial Surg., 1:171, 1973

MERGUET, H.: Complete traumatic transection of external and internal carotid arteries. Thorax chirurgie, 22:68, 1974 (German)

MERKX, C. A.: Treatment of pseudo-arthrosis of mandibular body by sliding bone graft, PRS, 49:662, 1972. Arch. chir. neerl., 23:273, 1971

MERKX, C. A.: Relocation osteoplasty in pseudarthrosis of the mandible. Fortschr. Kiefer. Gesichtschir., 19:125, 1975 (German)

MERLINI, C. et al: Closure of buccosinusal communications with double pedicle flaps. Rev. Stomatol. Chir. Maxillofac., 75:199, 1974 (French)

MERLINI, C. et al: Closing orosinusal communication with double flap. Riv. Ital. Stomatol., 29:73, 1974 (Italian)

MERLO, G.: Surgical treatment of metastatic cancer in elderly patients. Vopr. Onkol., 19:57, 1973 (Russian)

MERRILL, R. G. et al: Interdental osteotomy for immediate repositioning of dental-osseous elements. J. Oral Surg., 34:118, 1976

MERVILLE, L.: Segmental osteotomies of mandible. Value in correction of facial profile abnormalities. Ann. chir. plast., 17:173, 1972 (French)

MERVILLE, L.: Multiple dislocations of facial skeleton, PRS, 55:715, 1975. J. Maxillo-facial Surg., 2:187, 1974

MERVILLE, L. et al: Sectional osteotomies of the jaws. Their value in the correction of profile abnormalities. Rev. Fr. Odontostomatol., 18:1094, 1971 (French)

MERVILLE, L. C. et al: Multiple dislocations of face. Ann. chir. plast., 19:105, 1974 (French)

MESKHIA, N. S. et al: Biological material for bridging *dura mater* defects, PRS, 53:692, 1974. Acta chir. plast., 15:33, 1973

MESSINA, C.: Abnormalities of the innervation of the muscles of the thenar eminence in 2 cases of carpal tunnel syndrome. Riv. Patol. Nerv. Ment., 89:455, 1968 (Italian)

MESSINA, V. M. et al: State of the maxilla and mandible in children with different forms of congenital clefts before operation on the palate. Stomatologiia (Mosk.), 49:48, 1970 (Russian)

MESSNER, K. H.: Keratoconjunctivitis sicca symptoms appearing after blepharoplasty (with Graham, Miller). PRS, 57:57, 1976

MESTDAGH, C. et al: Acute accidental radiodermatitis. Arch. Belg. Dermatol. Syphilligr., 24:73, 1968 (French)

MESTER, E. et al: Experimental and clinical observations with laser rays. Langenbecks Arch. Chir., 327:310, 1970 (German)

MESTER, E. et al: Effect of laser rays on wound healing. Am. J. Surg., 122:532, 1971

MESTER, E. et al: Effect of laser radiation on

wound healing. Z. Exp. Chir., 4:307, 1971 (German)

MESTER, E. et al: Stimulation of wound healing by laser rays. Acta Chir. Acad. Sci. Hung., 13:315, 1972

MESTER, E. et al: Stimulation of wound healing by means of laser rays. Clinical and electron microscopical study. Acta Chir. Acad. Sci. Hung., 14:347, 1973

MESTER, E., et al: Laser in the locoregional treatment of tumors. Panminerva Med., 16:36, 1974

MESTER, E. et al: Latest studies on the effect of laser beams on wound healing. Clinical and electronoptic experiences. Z. Exp. Chir., 7:9, 1974 (German)

METCALF, V. A. et al: Documentation of hand function with the use of office copying equipment. Phys. Ther., 52:935, 1972

METCALF, W.: Analysis of cancer survival as exponential phenomenon, PRS, 55:256, 1975. Surg. Gynec. & Obst. 139:731, 1974

Metric System

Metric system, standardization of measurements in medicine by conversion to (Buren, Ryan). PRS, 54:459, 1974

METTAUER, J. P.: On staphylorraphy (Classic Reprint). PRS, 48:364, 1971

METZ, H. H.: Mandibular staple implant for an atrophic mandibular ridge: solving retention difficulties of a denture. J. Prosthet. Dent., 32:572, 1974

METZ, H. S. et al: Saccadic velocity and active force studies in blow-out fractures of the orbit. Am. J. Ophth., 78:665, 1974

MEULEMANS, G.: Trauma and fractures of orbital region. Rev. Stomatol. Chir. Maxillofac., 73:569, 1972 (French)

MEULEMANS, G. et al: Lipoma of oral cavity. Acta Stomatol. Belg., 70:431, 1973 (French)

MEULEN, J. C. VAN DER: Silastic spacers in tendon grafting. Brit. J. Plast. Surg., 24:166, 1971

MEULEN, J. C. VAN DER: Causes of prolapse and collapse of the proximal interphalangeal joint. Hand, 4:147, 1972

MEULEN, J. C. VAN DER: Treatment of prolapse and collapse of the proximal interphalangeal joint. Hand, 4:154, 1972

MEYER, F. U.: Models for improvement of split skin transplantation. Dtsch. Zahn. Mund. Kieferheilkd., 58:328, 1972 (German)

MEYER, H.: Articulotemporal syndrome. Report of 4 cases. Monastsschr. Ohrenheilkd. Laryngorhinol., 104:413, 1970 (German)

MEYER, I. et al: Adenomatoid odontogenic tumor (adenoameloblastoma); case report. J. Oral Surg., 32:488, 1974

MEYER, J.: First management of combined injuries of bones and soft parts in the facial area. Zentralbl. Chir., 96:321, 1971 (German)

MEYER, J. K.: Psychiatric considerations in the sexual reassignment of non-intersex individuals. Clin. Plast. Surg., 1:275, 1974

MEYER, J. K. et al: Is plastic surgery effective in rehabilitation of deformed delinquent adolescents? PRS, 51:53, 1973

MEYER, J. K., AND HOOPES, J. E.: Gender dysphoria syndromes: position statement on so-called "transsexualism." PRS 54:444, 1974

MEYER, JON K.: *Clinical Management of Sexual Disorders.* Williams & Wilkins Co., Baltimore, 1976

MEYER, R.: Plastic reconstruction after disfiguring operation of face and neck. Aktuel. Probl. Chir., 14:367, 1970

MEYER, R.: Reconstruction of columella of nasal septum. O.R.L., 34:170, 1972 (French)

MEYER, R: Rhinoplasty today. Rev. Med. Suisse Romande., 94:971, 1974 (French)

MEYER, R. et al: Surgical treatment of definitive facial paralysis. Rev. Med. Suisse Romande., 91:483, 1971 (French)

MEYER, R., AND SHAPIRO, M. A.: Technique for immediate reconstruction of lower lip after ablation of tumor, PRS, 53:241, 1974. Chir. Plast., 2:1, 1973

MEYER, R. et al: New aspects in corrective rhinoplasty. H.N.O., 22:154, 1974 (German)

MEYER, R. et al: Malformations of head. Rev. Otoneuroophtalmol., 46:447, 1974 (French)

MEYER, R., AND KESSELRING, U. K.: Reduction mammaplasty with L-shaped suture line. PRS, 55:139, 1975

MEYER, R. A.: Mandibular symphysis as donor site in bone grafting for surgical correction of open bite: report of case. J. Oral Surg., 30:125, 1972

MEYER, W.: Delayed corrections of labio-maxillary clefts: nose and upper lip. Rev. Stomatol. Chir. Maxillofac., 75:74, 1974 (French)

MEYER, W.: Maxillofacial orthopedic surgery. New methods. Rev. Stomatol. Chir. Maxillofac., 75:153, 1974 (French)

MEYERHOFF, W. et al: Gold foil closure of oroantral fistula. Laryngoscope, 83:940, 1973

MEYEROWITZ, B. R. et al: Massive abdominal panniculectomy. J.A.M.A., 225:408, 1973

MEYEROWITZ, B. R. et al: From massive weight loss to abdominal panniculectomy. R.N., 37:1, 1974

MEYERS, A.: Fibrin split products in the severely burned patient, PRS, 51:606, 1973. Arch. Surg., 105:404, 1972

MEYERS, E. N.: Role of total glossectomy in the management of cancer of the oral cavity. Otolaryngol. Clin. North Am., 5:343, 1972

MEYERS, E. N. et al: Management of chylous

fistulas. Laryngoscope, *85:*835, 1975

MEYRUEIS, J. P. *et al*: Use of barbed wire in surgery of hand, PRS, *54:*502, 1974. J. chir., *107:*151, 1974

MIAN, E., FRANCESCONI, G., AND CRUDELI, F.: Experiences in methodical aphoresis, PRS, *53:*692, 1974. Minerva dermat., *47:*8, 1972

MICALL, G. *et al*: Hemodynamic aspects and diagnosis of angiodysplasias of the hand. Chir. Ital., *20:*1048, 1968 (Italian)

MICALI, G. *et al*: Clinical and therapeutic consideration on vaginal agenesis. Minerva Chir., *26:*1480, 1971 (Italian)

MICALI, G., AND SCUDERI, N.: Amino acid composition of normal and pathologic skin., PRS, *56:*367, 1975. Riv. ital. chir. plast., *5:*573, 1973

MICHAEL, E.: Place of accessory nerve repair in neck dissection. H.N.O., *21:*360, 1973 (German)

MICHAELI, D., AND MEDINI, E.: Treatment of *Pseudomonas pyocyaneus* infections with combined carbenicillin and gentamycin, PRS, *50:*637, 1972. Harefuah, *72:*312, 1972

MICHAL, V. *et al*: Direct arterial anastomosis on corpora cavernosa penis in therapy of erective impotence. Rozhl. Chir., *52:*587, 1973 (Czechoslovakian)

MICHAL, V. *et al*: Femoro-pudendal by-pass, internal iliac thromboendarterectomy and direct arterial anastomosis to the cavernous body in the treatment of erectile impotence. Bull. Soc. Int. Chir., *33:* 343, 1974

MICHALEK, V.: Studies on variability of maxilla, PRS, *52:*321, 1973. Acta chir. plast., *14:*73, 1972

MICHAUD, B. *et al*: Four cases of peno-scrotal avulsions. J. Urol. Nephrol. (Paris), *81:*558, 1975 (French)

MICHEAU, C.: Mixed parotid tumor with tyrosine crystals. Ann. Anat. Pathol. (Paris), *18:*469, 1973 (French)

MICHEL, R. G., POPE, T. H., AND PATTERSON, C. N.: Infectious mononucleosis, mastoiditis, and facial paralysis, PRS, *57:*528, 1976. Arch. Otolaryng., *101:*486, 1975

MICHELET, A. *et al*: Osteosynthesis with screwed plates in maxillofacial surgery. Experience with 500 satellite plates. Int. Surg., *58:*249, 1973

MICHELET, F. X. *et al*: Radiation resistant angiomas of the jaws (surgical treatment – report of 3 cases). Rev. Odontostomatol. Midi Fr., *29:* 3, 1971 (French)

MICHELET, F. X. *et al*: Surgical treatments of fractures of the corpus mandibulae without blockage, with diminutive screwed plate inserted via the endobuccal route. Rev. Odontostomatol. Midi Fr., *29:*87, 1971 (French)

MICHELET, F. X. *et al*: Long-term evolution of

some cases of Robin's syndrome of the newborn. Rev. Stomatol. Chir. Maxillofac., *73:*77, 1972 (French)

MICHELET, F. X. *et al*: Treatment of face fractures by external fixation with divergent nail bundles. Rev. Stomatol. Chir. Maxillofac., *73:*177, 1972 (French)

MICHELET, F. X., DEYMES, J., AND DESSUS, B.: Osteosynthesis with miniaturized screwed plates in maxillofacial surgery, PRS, *53:*241, 1974. J. Maxillo-facial Surg., *1:*79, 1973

MICHELET, F. X. *et al*: Mandibular osteosynthesis without blocking by screwed miniature stellite plates. Rev. Stomatol. Chir. Maxillofac., *74:*239, 1973 (French)

MICHELET, F. X. *et al*: Complete prosthesis of temporo-mandibular joints. Rev. Stomatol. Chir. Maxillofac., *74:*647, 1973 (French)

MICHELET, F. X. *et al:* Utilization of mandibular symphysis, PRS, *54:*619, 1974. Ann. chir. plast., *19:*69, 1974

MICHELET, F. X. *et al*: Repositioning and surgical retention of the median tubercle in the sequelae of bilateral labio-maxillary cleft. Rev. Stomatol. Chir. Maxillofac., *75:*83, 1974 (French)

MICHELET, F. X. *et al*: Subalveolar mandibular osteotomies in anteroposterior facial dysmorphism. Rev. Stomatol. Chir. Maxillofac., *75:*156, 1974 (French)

MICHELET, F. X. *et al*: Depressed fractures of the upper part of the face. Rev. Stomatol. Chir. Maxillofac., *75:*243, 1974 (French)

MICHELET, F. X. *et al*: Indications and techniques for surgical treatment of superior proalveolia. Rev. Stomatol. Chir. Maxillofac., *75:*1093, 1974 (French)

MICHELI-PELLEGRINI, V.: New gravity palpebral prosthesis in paralysis of the facial nerve. Advantages of the fenestrated prosthesis. Arch. Ital. Otol., *81:* 193, 1970 (Italian)

MICHELI-PELLEGRINI, V.: More on lid-loading in the management of lagophthalmos (Letter to the Editor). PRS, *55:*482, 1975

MICHELI-PELLEGRINI, V., FRANCESCONI, G., AND FENILI, O.: Plastic surgery and malignant oncology of teguments, PRS, *57:*766, 1976 (Italian). Riv. ital. chir. plast., *7:*197, 1975

MICHELINAKIS, E.: Table mounted magnifying glass. Hand, *4:*277, 1972

MICHON, J.: Surgical reconstruction of the rheumatoid hand. Acta Orthop. Belg., *37:*459, 1971 (French)

MICHON, J.: Metacarpophalangeal tendinous reequilibrations in the rheumatoid hand. Rheumatoid thumb. Rev. Chir. Orthop., *58:*455, 1972 (French)

MICHON, J.: Metacarpal hand. Acta Orthop.

Belg., *39:*1182, 1973 (French)

MICHON, J.: Phlegmon of the tendon sheaths. Ann. Chir., *28:*277, 1974 (French)

MICHON, J., DELAGOUTTE, J. P., AND JANDEAUX, M.: Swanson's Silastic implants in hand traumatology, PRS, *54:*627, 1974. Ann. chir. plast., *19:*13, 1974

MICHON, J., DELAGOUTTE, J. P., AND JANDEAUX, J. P.: Use of Swanson's prosthesis for management of hallux valgus, PRS, *54:*627, 1974. Ann. chir. plast., *19:*23, 1974

MICHON, J., AND JANDEAUX, M.: Metacarpal hand, PRS, *54:*620, 1974. Ann. chir. plast., *19:*97, 1974

MICHON, J., AND DOLICH, B. H.: Metacarpal hand, PRS, *57:*119, 1976. Hand, *6:*285, 1974

Micrognathia (See also *Chin; Pierre-Robin Syndrome: Retrognathism)*

Micrognathia, Z-shaped sliding osteotomy for advancing mandible in (Min *et al*). J. Korean Dent. Assoc., *10:*379, 1972

Micrognathism, surgical correction of case (Cavina). Minerva Stomatol., *21:*211, 1972 (Italian)

Micrognathia, treatment in neonatal period; report of 65 cases (Monroe, Ogo). PRS, *50:*317, 1972

Mandibular hypoplasia and late development of glossopharyngeal airway obstruction (Cosman, Crikelair). PRS, *50:*573 1972

Mandibular micrognathia: etiology and surgical management (Kennett *et al*). J. Oral Surg., *31:*8, 1973

Mandible advancement by sagittal ramus split and suprahyoid myotomy (Steinhauser). J. Oral Surg., *31:*516, 1973

Mandibular lengthening by gradual distraction (Snyder *et al*). PRS, *51:*506, 1973

Respiratory obstruction in micrognathia, treatment of, by use of nasogastric tube (McEvitt), PRS, *52:*138, 1973. Discussions by Lindsay, McDowell, Randall. PRS, *52:*306, 1973

Micrognathism, surgical treatment of (Zisser). Z.W.R., *82:*831, 1973 (German)

Growing jaw during and after orthopedic-surgical extension in children with congenital microgenia (Schettler *et al*). Fortschr. Kiefer. Gesichtschir., *18:*166, 1974 (German)

Microgenia and its treatment (Schroder). Fortschr. Kiefer. Gesichtschir., *18:*169, 1974 (German)

Neoplasty of the ascending ramus of the mandible for compensation of microgenia (Gabka). Fortschr. Kiefer. Gesichtschir., *18:*179, 1974 (German)

Surgical treatment of microgenia without in-

Micrognathia – Cont.
terruption of continuity (Neuner *et al*). Fortschr. Kiefer. Gesichtschir., *18:*183, 1974 (German)

Neurologic disorders following surgical correction of progenia and microgenia (Niederdellmann *et al*). Fortschr. Kiefer. Gesichtschir., *18:*186, 1974 (German)

Micrognathia in Hanhart's syndrome (Wexler, Novark), PRS, *54:*99, 1974

Diagnosis and treatment of maxillomandibular dysplasias (Converse *et al*). Am. J. Orthod., *68:*625, 1975

Visor osteotomy to increase the absolute height of the atrophied mandible. A preliminary report (Harle). J. Maxillo-facial Surg., *3:*257, 1975

Micrognathia, relief of respiratory obstruction by use of large nasogastric tube (Benfield) (Letter to the Editor). PRS *56:*570, 1975

Retrognathic mandible – surgical correction (Hull *et al*). Oral Surg., *41:*2, 1976

Implants, silicone rubber chin, mandibular bone absorption under, retrospective cephalometric analysis (Friedland, Coccaro, Converse). PRS, *57:*144, 1976

Microsurgery (See also *Free Flaps; Replantation)*

Microangiographic observations of different kinds of colon anastomosis in rat (Herzog), PRS, *48:*518, 1971. Helvet. chir. acta, *1:*179, 1971

Microvascular repair and replacement, long-term results (Khodadad). PRS, *48:*198, 1971. Surgery, *69:*397, 1971

Anticoagulants, bleeding in central nervous system, severe complication of therapy with (Levy), PRS, *50:*95, 1972. Ther. Umsch., *28:*821, 1971

Precise management of heparin therapy (Boden *et al*), PRS, *52:*332, 1973. Am. J. Surg., *124:*777, 1972

Microsurgical technique, muscle autotransplantation using (Masuhara, Tamai, Sasauchi), PRS, *53:*110, 1974. Asian M. J., *15:*45, 1972

Microvascular surgery in orthopedics and traumatology (Tamai *et al*), PRS, *51:*705, 1973. J. Bone & Joint Surg., *54B:*637, 1972

Groin flap (McGregor, Jackson), PRS, *52:*217, 1973. Brit. J. Plast. Surg., *25:*3, 1972

Microsurgical revascularization, autotransplant of omentum to large scalp defect (McLean, Buncke). PRS, *49:*268, 1972

Mammary gland in dogs, autogenous *en bloc*

Microsurgery—Cont.

transplantation using microsurgical technique (Fujino, Harashina, Mikata). PRS, *50:*376, 1972

Microsurgical techniques for neurosurgery, laboratory training in (De Klerk *et al*). S. Afr. Med. J., *46:*1972

Microvascular anastomosis, signs of patency (Acland), PRS, *52:*325, 1973. Surgery, *72:*744, 1972)

Rhinobasis, microsurgery of, in injuries (Osterwald). Arch. Klin. Exp. Ohren Nasen Kehlkopfhelkd., *205:*213, 1973 (German)

Microsurgery: free flap, composite tissue transfer by vascular anastomosis (Taylor, Daniel), PRS, *55:*642, 1975. Australian & New Zealand J. Surg., *43:*1, 1973

Microvascular repair in traumatic amputations of upper limb (Miller), PRS, *53:*367, 1974. Australian & New Zealand J. Surg., *43:*19, 1973

Microsurgery for experimental transfer of composite free flaps (O'Brien, Shanmugan), PRS, *54:*117, 1974. Australian & New Zealand J. Surg., *43:*285, 1973

Microvascular anastomosis, great toe transplantation in thumb replacement (Buncke *et al*), PRS, *55:*109, 1975. Brit. J. Plast. Surg., *26:*194, 1973

Anticoagulation in microvascular surgery (Koliv, Wieberdink, Reneman), PRS *52:*208, 1973. Europ. Surg. Res., *5:*52, 1973

Microsurgery of peripheral nerves (Millesi), PRS, *54:*375, 1974. Hand, *5:*157, 1973

Place of microsurgery in hand surgery (Kleinert *et al*). Orthop. Clin. North Am., *4:*929, 1973

Saran Wrap cuff in microsurgical arterial repairs, use of (McLean, Buncke). PRS, *51:*624, 1973

Microvascular anastomoses, study in rats of survival of composite homotransplants of skin and subcutaneous tissue, with (Salyer, Kyger). PRS, *51:*672, 1973

Microvascular anastomoses, free transfer of skin flaps by (Daniel, Williams). PRS, *52:*16, 1973

Microvascular anastomoses, distant transfer of island flap by (Daniel, Taylor). PRS, *52;*111, 1973

Microvascular anastomoses for successful transfer of large island flap from groin to foot (O'Brien *et al*). PRS, *52:*271, 1973

Microvascular surgery, cutaneous island flaps, anatomical identification and transfer by microsurgical vascular anastomosis (Kaplan, Buncke, Murray). PRS, *52:*301, 1973

Microsurgery—Cont.

Microsurgery: rejection phenomena after homotransplantation of skin flaps in dogs by microvascular technique (Harashina *et al*). PRS, *52:*390, 1973

Microsurgery, clinical replantation of digits O'Brien *et al*). PRS, *52:*490, 1973

Microvascular anastomoses, use of gastroepiploic vessels as recipient or donor vessels in free transfer of composite flaps by (Harii, Ohmori). PRS, *52:*541, 1973

Leg, amputated: get in there and replant! (McDowell) (Editorial). PRS, *52:*562, 1973

Hand, replantation of completely amputated distal thumb without venous anastomosis (Serafin, Kutz, Kleinert), PRS, *52:*579, 1973. Commentary by Buncke, *52:*581, 1973

Microsurgery, metallized microsutures and new micro needle holder (O'Brien, Hayhurst). PRS *52:*673, 1973

Thrombus formation in microvascular surgery, experimental study of effects of surgical trauma (Acland), PRS, *52:*454, 1973. Surgery, *73:*766, 1973

Microvascular anastomoses, free flap transfers with (O'Brien *et al*), PRS *56:*683, 1975. Brit. J. Plast. Surg., *27:*220, 1974

Microvascular surgery: modified vascular anastomosis with invagination (Gyurko, Czekelnik), PRS, *54:*622, 1974. Bruns' Beitr. klin. Chir., *221:*70, 1974

Microvascular surgery, small vessel anastomosis—effect of anticoagulant therapy on patency rate (Shanghai First Medical College), PRS, *54:*239, 1974. Chinese M.J., *1:*6, 1974

Nerve trunks, functional micro-anatomy of (Kuczynski), PRS, *54:*693, 1974. Hand, *6:*1, 1974

Microvascular anastomosis, improved instrument for (Ikuta), PRS, *56:*358, 1975. Operation, *28:*1149, 1974

Microsurgical repair of peripheral nerves, diamond knife for (Terzis, Faibisoff, Williams). PRS, *53:*102, 1974

Microvascular anastomoses, successful clinical transfer of ten free flaps by (Harii, Ohmori, Ohmori), PRS, *53:*259, 1974. Discussion by Goldwyn, PRS, *53:*469, 1974

Microvascular surgery, experimental use of Pluronic F68 (Ketchum *et al*). PRS, *53:*288, 1974

Microsurgical revascularization: hair transplantation with free scalp flaps (Harii, Ohmori, Ohmori). PRS, *53:*410, 1974

Polyethylene bag background in microsurgical repair of peripheral nerves (Terzis, Faibisoff, Williams). PRS, *53:*596, 1974

Microsurgery – Cont.

Magnesium sulfate and silicone rubber vascular cuff used to improve patency rates in microvascular surgery (Nomoto, Buncke, Chater). PRS, *54:*157, 1974

Microvascular anastomoses, distant transfer of free living bone graft (Östrup, Fredrickson). PRS, *54:*274, 1974

Microvascular surgery, experimental use of Pluronic F68 in (Ketchum) (Letter to the Editor). PRS, *54:*478, 1974

Rhinorrhea, cerebrospinal, microsurgical treatment of (Baumberger *et al*). Schweiz. Med. Wochenschr., *104:*521, 1974 (German)

Microvascular surgery, fluorescein angiography in: study using rodent artery (Fox *et al*). Stroke, *5:*196, 1974

Microsurgical techniques and use of tissue adhesive in repair of peripheral nerves (Hurwitz *et al*), PRS, *55:*512, 1975. Surg. Res., *17:*245, 1974

Grafting of ureter, autologous free, with dogs (Esch), PRS, *57:*120, 1976. Acta chir. Austria, *7:*43, 1975

Nerve, peripheral, interfascicular dissection with surgical microscope (Noterman), PRS, *56:*466, 1975. Acta chir. belg., *74:*192, 1975

Vascular microsurgery (Gilbert). Ann. Chir., *29:*1035, 1975 (French)

Microvascular surgery, superficial temporal artery in (Ricbourg, Mitz, Lassau), PRS, *57:*262, 1976. Ann. chir. plast., *20:*197, 1975

Nerve, facial, surgical repair of branches (Szal, Miller), PRS, *57:*395, 1976. Arch. Otolaryng., *101:*160, 1975

Microvascular surgery, experimental and clinical application of (Tsai), PRS, *56:*605, 1975. Ann. Surg., *181:*169, 1975

Microvascular anastomoses, transfer of free groin flap to heel (Rigg). PRS, *55:*36, 1975

Grafting, experimental funicular, of the facial nerve (Apfelberg, Gingrass). PRS, *55:*195, 1975

Microvascular anastomoses, method of successive interrupted suturing in (Fujino, Aoyagi). PRS, *55:*240, 1975

Microsurgery, detection of small vessels by Doppler flowmeter (Aoyagi, Fujino, Ohshiro). PRS, *55:*372, 1975

Microvascular transfer of free deltopectoral dermal-fat flap (Fujino, Tanino, Sugimoto). PRS, *55:*428, 1975

Microvascular anastomoses, does topical use of magnesium sulfate improve results? (Freshwater) (Letter to the Editor). PRS,

Microsurgery – Cont.

*55:*483, 1975

Microsurgery, autotransplant of omentum to cover large denudation of scalp (Ikuta). PRS, *55:*490, 1975

Microvascular surgery, free vascularized bone graft (Taylor, Miller, Ham). PRS, *55:*533, 1975

Microvascular anastomoses, reconstruction of mandibular defects after radiation, using free living bone graft (Östrup, Fredrickson). PRS, *55:*563, 1975

Microvascular surgery, free groin flaps in children (Harii, Ohmori). PRS, *55:*588, 1975

Microvascular surgery, small artery anastomosis using cuff of *dura mater* and tissue adhesive (Tschopp). PRS, *55:*606, 1975

Microvascular anastomoses, experimental effects of heparin or magnesium sulfate on patency of (Engrav *et al*). PRS, *55:*618, 1975

Microsurgery: neurovascular free flaps (Daniel, Terzis, Schwarz). PRS, *56:*13, 1975

Microsurgery: rapid loop technique for microvascular anastomosis (George, Creech, Buncke). PRS, *56:*99, 1975

Microvascular transfer of free flap from buttock for aplasia of breast and pectoral region (Fujino, Harashina, Aoyagi), PRS, *56:*178, 1975. Discussion by Goldwyn, PRS, *56:*335, 1975

Microvascular surgery, anatomy of several free flap donor sites (Taylor, Daniel). PRS, *56:*243, 1975

Irrigation of vessels: microirrigator (Rigg). PRS, *56:*349, 1975

Microsurgery, interfascicular nerve grafting: early experiences at Massachusetts General Hospital (Finseth, Constable, Cannon). PRS, *56:*492, 1975

Microsurgery, new technique for nerve suture, epineurium-anchoring funicular suture (Tsuge, Ikuta, Sakaue). PRS, *56:*496, 1975

Microvascular replantation and transplantation, study of washout solutions for (Harashina, Buncke). PRS, *56:*542, 1975

Microvascular transfer of free skin flap to repair pharyngoesophageal fistula (Fujino, Saito). PRS, *56:*549, 1975

Microsurgery, bipolar jeweler's forceps with automatic irrigation for coagulation in (Dujovny, Vas, Osgood). PRS, *56:*585, 1975

Fire hazard during CO_2 laser microsurgery on the larynx and trachea (Snow *et al*). Anesth. Analg. (Cleve.), *55:*146, 1976

Microsurgery—Cont.

Microneurovascular anastomoses, free *gracilis* muscle transplantation with, for treatment of facial paralysis (Harii, Ohmori, Torii). PRS, *57:*133, 1976

Microclamps, damage caused by: scanning electron microscopy study of micro-arterial damage and repair (Thurston *et al*). PRS, *57:*197, 1976

Microsurgery: restoration of sensation to anesthetic hand by free neurovascular flap from foot (Daniel, Terzis, Midgley). PRS, *57:*275, 1976

Digital transfer, cross-hand (Edgerton). PRS, *57:*281, 1976

Flap, free musculocutaneous (Harii, Ohmori, Sekiguchi), PRS, *57:*294, 1976. Discussion by Cannon, PRS, *57:*511, 1976

Microvascular anastomoses, scanning electron microscope study of (Servant, Ikuta, Harada). PRS, *57:*329, 1976

Microvascular surgery, free skin flap from retroauricular region to nose (Fujino, Harashina, Nakajima). PRS, *57:*338, 1976

Microvascular surgery: free vascularized nerve graft (Taylor, Ham). PRS, *57:*413, 1976

Microneurovascular anastomoses, free muscle transplantation in dogs by (Kubo, Ikuta, Tsuge). PRS, *57:*495, 1976

Microvascular surgery: ten free groin flaps (Baudet, LeMaire, Guimberteau). PRS, *57:*577, 1976

Microvascular surgery, laryngeal reconstruction by free flap transfer (Nagahara, Hirose, Iwai). PRS, *57:*604, 1976

Microsurgery, fourteen free groin flap transfers (Serafin, Villarreal Rios, Georgiade). PRS, *57:*707, 1976

Microvascular surgery: ten free flap transfers: use of intra-arterial dye injection to outline a flap exactly (Boeckx, de Coninck, Vanderlinden). PRS, *57:*716, 1976

Microtia: See *Ear Deformities, Congenital*

MIDDENDORP, U. G.: Tracheal stenosis following tracheotomy. Helv. Chir. Acta, *39:*555, 1972 (German)

MIDDLETON, D. S.: Clinical approach to derangement of mandicular joint. J. R. Coll. Surg. Edinb., *17:*287, 1972

MIDDLETON, R. W. D., AND VARIAN, J. P.: Tourniquet paralysis, PRS, *55:*385, 1975. Australian & New Zealand J. Surg., *44:*124, 1974

MIDGLEY, R. D.: Restoration of sensation to anesthetic hand by free neurovascular flap

from foot (with Daniel, Terzis). PRS, *57:*275, 1976

Midline Lethal Granuloma

Face and jaw pains, due to Wegener's granuloma (Von Damarus). Z. Laryngol. Rhinol. Otol., *52:*901, 1973 (German)

Granuloma of face, malignant midline, curative treatment (Calatrava), PRS, *57:*539, 1976. J. Maxillo-facial Surg., *3:*160, 1975

Progressive lethal ulceration of the nose (Kraus-Chatellier) (Stefani *et al*). Klin. Monatsbl. Augenheilkd., *167:*110, 1975 (German)

Wegener's granuloma, residual nasal deformity after (Domarus). PRS, *56:*216, 1975

Midfacial necrosis: apropos of 2 cases and review of the literature (Steenberghe *et al*). Rev. Stomatol. Chir. Maxillofac., *76:*509, 1975 (French)

MIEHLKE, ADOLF: *Surgery of the Facial Nerve.* W. B. Saunders Co., Philadelphia, 1973. PRS, *55:*85, 1975

MIEHLKE, A.: Facial nerve lesions in otorhinolaryngological practice. 1. Problem diagnosis "Bell's palsy." Monatsschr. Ohrenheilkd. Laryngorhinol., *106:*413, 1972

MIEHLKE, A.: Problems with facial nerve injuries in otorhinolaryngologic practice. 2. On iatrogenic injuries of facial nerve, medicolegal situation of surgeon. Monatsschr. Ohrenheilkd. Laryngorhinol., *106:*461, 1972 (German)

MIEHLKE, A.: Editorial on contribution: position on development of regional plastic and rehabilitation surgery. By H. L. Wullstein. H.N.O., *21:*21, 1973 (German)

MIEHLKE, A.: Emergency case in facial nerve surgery. Z. Laryngol. Rhinol. Otol., *52:*349, 1973 (German)

MIEHLKE, A.: Extratemporal injury and repair of facial nerve. Otolaryngol. Clin. North Am., *7:*467, 1974

MIEHLKE, A. *et al*: Regeneration of peripheral nerve after effect of ionizing radiation. O.R.L., *34:*88, 1972 (German)

MIGLETS, A. W., JR.: Nasal squamous papillomas. Ohio State Med. J., *69:*829, 1973

MIGLETS, A. W., JR.: E.N.T. case of the month. Ohio State Med. J., *70:*37, 1974

MIGLETS, A. W., JR.: Proptosis caused by paranasal sinus neoplasm. Ohio State Med. J., *70:*171, 1974

MIGLETS, A. W. *et al*: Protection of facial nerve anastomosis with vein graft. Laryngoscope, *83:*1027, 1973

MIHALY, F. *et al*: Substitution of the tendon sheath by autologous vein in the "no-man's land" of the hand. Magy. Traumatol. Orthop., *18:*421, 1975 (Hungarian)

MIHM, M. C., CLARK, W. H., AND FROM, L.: Clinical diagnosis, classification and histogenetic concepts of early stages of cutaneous malignant melanomas, PRS, *49:*667, 1972. New England J. Med., *284:*1078, 1971

MIHM, M. C., JR. *et al*: Early detection of primary cutaneous malignant melanoma, PRS, *54:*380, 1974. New England J. Med., *289:*989, 1973

MIKATA, A.: Autogenous *en bloc* transplantation of mammary gland in dogs, using microsurgical technique (with Fujino, Harashina). PRS, *50:*376, 1972

MIKHAIL, G. R.: Bowen's disease and squamous cell carcinoma of nail bed, PRS, *55:*256, 1975. Arch. Dermat., *110:*267, 1974

MIKHAIL, G. R.: Squamous cell carcinoma diagnosed as keratoacanthoma, PRS, *54:*381, 1974. Cutis, *13:* 378, 1974

MIKHAIL, G. R.: Chemosurgery in treatment of cancer. Int. J. Dermatol., *14:*33, 1975

MIKHAIL, G. R. *et al*: Metastatic basal cell epithelioma discovered by chemosurgery. Arch. Dermat., *105:*103, 1972

MIKOLJI, V.: Congenital clefts associated with other malformations. Chir. Maxillofac. Plast., *7:*55, 1970 (Croation)

MIKULICKOVA, H. *et al*: Pneumocephalus as a rare complication of mid-facial fractures. Cesk. Stomatol., *72:*285, 1972 (Czechoslovakian)

Mikulicz' Disease

Benign lymphoepithelial sialoadenopathies. The Mikulicz/Sjögren controversy (Leban *et al*). Oral Surg., *38:*735, 1974

Benign lymphoepithelial lesions of the salivary glands (Kelly *et al*). Arch. Otolaryng., *101:*71, 1975

MIKUNI, M. *et al*: Diagnosis and treatment of blowout fractures. Ophthalmology (Tokyo), *14:*261, 1972 (Japanese)

MILDE, H. *et al*: Mixed tumors of soft tissues of mouth. Fortschr. Kiefer. Gesichtschir., *15:*56, 1972 (German)

MILDENBERGER, H., AND SCHWEIZER, P.: Congenital polyps of urethra in children, PRS, *53:*368,1974. Ztschr.Kinderchir., *13:*240, 1973

MILES, W. K., OLSON, N. R., AND RODRIQUEZ, A.: Acute treatment of experimental laryngeal fractures, PRS, *50:*419, 1972. Ann. Otol. Rhin. & Laryng., *80:*710, 1971

MILFORD, LEE: *The Hand*. C. V. Mosby Co., St. Louis, 1971. PRS, *49:*338, 1972

Military Surgery: See *War Injuries*

MILKE, A.: Mustardé flap in reconstruction of inferior limb, PRS, *53:*368, 1974. Rev. Soc. Med. Cir. San Jose, *5:*83, 1972

MILKOVSKA-DIMITROVA, T., AND ILIEF, I. V.: Possibilities of surgical treatment in femoral dislocation in Ehlers-Danlos syndrome, PRS, *54:*511, 1974. Lyon chir., *70:*38, 1974

MILLAR, H. S. *et al*: Combined intracranial and facial approach for excision and repair of cancer of ethmoid sinuses. Aust. N.Z. J. Surg., *43:*179, 1973

MILLAR, R.: Management of the child with a burned hand. J. Ir. Med. Assoc., *66:*604, 1973

MILLARD, C. *et al*: Keloidal cicatrices encountered during surgery of protruding ears. Ann. Otolaryngol. Chir. Cervicofac., *92:*432, 1975 (French)

MILLARD, D. RALPH: *Cleft Craft: Unilateral Cleft Lip*. Vol. 1. Little, Brown & Co., Boston, 1976.

MILLARD, D. R.: Congenital nasal tip retrusion and three little composite ear grafts. PRS, *48:*501, 1971

MILLARD, D. R.: Versatility of chondromucosal flap in nasal vestibule, PRS, *50:*580, 1972

MILLARD, D. R., JR.: Gillies Memorial Lecture. Jousting with the first knight of plastic surgery. Brit. J. Plast. Surg., *25:*73, 1972

MILLARD, D. R., JR.: Nipple and areola reconstruction by split-skin graft from the normal side. PRS, *50:*350, 1972

MILLARD, D. R., JR.: More on "no-dressing" technique (Letter to the Editor). PRS, *51:*577, 1973

MILLARD, D. R., JR.: Reconstructive rhinoplasty for lower half of a nose. PRS, *53:*133, 1974

MILLARD, D. R., JR.: Discussion of "A variation of rotation-advancement operation for repair of wide unilateral cleft lips," by Asensio. PRS, *53:*340, 1974

MILLARD, D. R., JR.: Reconstructive rhinoplasty for lower two-thirds of the nose. PRS, *57:*722, 1976

MILLARD, D. R., JR. *et al*: Breast reconstruction: a plea for saving the uninvolved nipple. Am. J. Surg., *122:*763, 1971

MILLARD, D. R., JR. *et al*: Median cleft of the lower lip and mandible: a case report. Brit. J. Plast. Surg. *24:*391, 1971

MILLARD, D. R., JR., DEANE, M., AND GARST, W. P.: Bending iliac bone graft for anterior mandibular arch repair. PRS, *48:*600, 1971

MILLARD, D. R., AND COOLEY, S. G. E.: Solution to coverage in severe compound dorsal hand injuries. PRS, *49:*215, 1972

MILLARD, D. R., JR. *et al*: Submental and submandibular lipectomy in conjunction with face lift, in male and female. PRS, *49:*385, 1972

MILLENDER, L. H. *et al*: Aneurysms and thromboses of the ulnar artery in the hand. Arch. Surg., *105:*686, 1972

MILLENDER, L. H.; NALEBUFF, E. A., AND HOLDSWORTH, D. E.: Posterior interosseous nerve syndrome secondary to rheumatoid synovitis, PRS, *52:*323, 1973. J. Bone & Joint Surg., *55A:*375, 1973

MILLENDER, L. H., ALBIN, R. E., AND NALEBUFF, E. A.: Delayed volar advancement flap for thumb tip injuries. PRS, *52:*635, 1973

MILLENDER, L. H. *et al*: Dorsal tenosynovectomy and tendon transfer in the rheumatoid hand. J.Bone & Joint Surg.(Am.),*56:*601,1974

MILLENDER, L. H. *et al*: Evaluation and treatment of early rheumatoid hand involvement. Orthop. Clin. North Am., *6:*697, 1975

MILLENDER, L. W. *et al*: Reconstructive surgery in the rheumatoid hand. Orthop. Clin. North. Am., *6:*709, 1975

MILLER, A. H.: Carcinoma *in situ* of larynx, 20-year study of results of management, PRS, *48:*397, 1971. Am. J. Surg., *120:*492, 1970

MILLER, A. J.: Single fingertip injuries treated by thenar flap, PRS, *56:*465, 1975. Hand, *6:*311, 1974

MILLER, A. S. *et al*: Giant cell tumor of jaws associated with Paget disease of bone. Report of two cases and review of literature. Arch. Otolaryng., *100:*233, 1974

MILLER, D.: Cryosurgery for the treatment of neoplasms of the oral cavity. Otolaryngol. Clin. North Am., *5:*377, 1972

MILLER, D.: Management of keratosis and carcinoma *in situ* with cryosurgery. Can. Otolaryngol., *3:*557, 1974

MILLER, D.: Cryosurgery as therapeutic modality in treatment of tumors of head and neck. Proc. Roy. Soc. Med., *67:*69, 1974

MILLER, D., AND BERGSTROM, L.: Vascular complications of head and neck surgery, PRS, *55:*107, 1975. Arch. Otolaryng., *100:*136, 1974

MILLER, E. H. *et al*: Gram-negative osteomyelitis following puncture wounds of foot, PRS, *57:*399, 1976. J. Bone & Joint Surg., *57A:*535, 1975

MILLER, E. L.: Preprosthetic surgery from the viewpoint of the prosthodontist. J. Oral Surg., *29:*760, 1971

MILLER, G. D. H.: Assessment of place of microvascular repair in traumatic amputations of upper limb, PRS, *53:*367, 1974. Australian & New Zealand J. Surg., *43:*19, 1973

MILLER, G. D. H.: Free vascularized bone graft (with Taylor, Miller). PRS, *55:*533, 1975

MILLER, H.: Lip incompetency and its treatment. N.Y. State Dent. J., *38:*210, 1972

MILLER, J. M. *et al*: Cystic hygroma colli in adult. Johns Hopkins Med. J., *134:*233, 1974

MILLER, M.: Osteoma of frontal sinus, certain problems. Acta Otorhinolaryngol. Belg., *27:*171, 1973 (French)

MILLER, S. H.: Keratoconjunctivitis sicca symptoms appearing after blepharoplasty (with Graham, Messner). PRS, *57:*57, 1976

MILLER, S. H.: Pericortical "compression" clamps for mandibular fixation (with Lung, Graham). PRS, *57:*487, 1976

MILLER, S. H., AND MORRIS, W. J.: Current concepts in diagnosis and management of fractures of orbital floor, PRS, *50:*629, 1972. Am. J. Surg., *123:*560, 1972

MILLER, S. H., WOOD, A. M., AND HAQ, M. A.: Bilateral oro-ocular cleft. PRS, *51:*590, 1973

MILLER, S. H. *et al*: Breast reconstruction after radical mastectomy. Am. Fam. Physician, *11:*97, 1975

MILLER, S. H., AND RUSENAS, I.: Changes in primate pacinian corpuscles following volar pad excision and skin grafting. PRS, *57:*627, 1976

MILLER, T., HARPER, J., AND LONGMIRE, W. P.: Management of lymphedema by staged subcutaneous excision, PRS, *52:*453, 1973. Surg. Gynec. & Obst., *136:*586, 1973

MILLER, T. A.: Deleterious effect of split-skin homograft coverage on split-skin graft donor sites. PRS, *53:*316, 1974

MILLER, T. A.: Surgical management of lymphedema of extremity. PRS, *56:*633, 1975

MILLER, T. A.: Blister and the second degree burn in guinea pigs: effect of exposure (with Wheeler). PRS, *57:*74, 1976

MILLER, T. A., AND WHITE, W. L.: Healing of second degree burns, comparison of effects of early application of homografts and coverage with tape. PRS, *49:*552, 1972

MILLER, T. R.: Results of radical surgery for cancer of extremities. Aktuel Probl. Chir., *14:* 689, 1970

MILLER, T. R.: 100 cases of hemipelvectomy: a personal experience. Surg. Clin. North Am., *54:*905, 1974

MILLESI, H.: Plastic surgery in abnormalities of the hand. Chirurg., *42:*60, 1971 (German)

MILLESI, H.: Nerve injuries of the hand. Dtsch. Med. J., *22:*82, 1971 (German)

MILLESI, H.: Breast reconstruction after breast amputation. Dtsch. Med. Wochenschr., *97:*785, 1972 (German)

MILLESI, H.: Operative repair of transected peripheral nerves, PRS, *51:*481, 1973. Langenbecks Arch. Chir., *332*:347, 1972

MILLESI, H.: Primary treatment of open injuries of hand, PRS, *51*:478, 1973. Langenbecks Arch. Chir., *332*:469, 1972

MILLESI, H.: Reconstruction of thumb by transfer of toe tissue, PRS, *53*:107, 1974. Chir. Plast., *1*:347, 1973

MILLESI, H.: Microsurgery of peripheral nerves, PRS, *54*:375, 1974. Hand, *5*:157, 1973

MILLESI, H. *et al*: Tumors of the hand. Handchirurgie, *1*:134, 1969 (German)

MILLESI, H., MEISSL, G., AND BERGER, A.: Interfascicular nerve-grafting of median and ulnar nerves, PRS, *51*:233, 1973. J. Bone & Joint Surg., *54B*:727, 1972

MILLESI, H., MEISSL, G., AND KATZER, H.: Treatment of injuries to brachial plexus, PRS, *53*:108, 1974. Bruns' Beitr. klin. Chir., *220*:429, 1973

MILLESI, H. *et al:* Repair of the facial nerve. In *Plastische und Wiederherstellungs-Chirurgie,* ed. by Hohler; pp, 111–28. Schattauer, Stuttgart, 1975 (German)

MILLION, R. R.: Elective neck irradiation for TXNO squamous carcinoma of oral tongue and floor of mouth. Cancer, *34*:149, 1974

MILLS, N. L. *et al*: One-stage operation for cervico-mediastinal cystic hygroma in infancy. J. Thorac. Cardiovasc. Surg., *65*:608, 1973

MILLS, R. L.: Barsky Unit: end of chapter, end of story? (Letter to the Editor). PRS, *57*:654, 1976

MILOBSKY, S. A. *et al*: Metastatic renal adenocarcinoma presenting as periapical pathosis in the maxilla. Oral Surg., *39*:30, 1975

MILSTONE, E. B., AND HELWIG, E. G.: Basal cell carcinoma in children, PRS, *53*:688, 1974. Arch. Dermat., *108*:523, 1973

MILTON, G. W. *et al*: Malignant melanoma and vitiligo. Australas. J. Dermatol., *12*:131, 1971

MILTON, G. W., AND MCCARTHY, W. H.: Radical dissection of axillary lymph nodes for malignant melanoma, PRS, *53*:112, 1974. Proc. Roy. Australasian Coll. Surg., *46*:694, 1973

MILTON, S. G.: Experimental studies on island flaps. I. Surviving length, PRS, *48*:574, 1971; II. Ischemia and delay, PRS, *49*:444, 1972

MILWARD, T. M.: Treatment of burns. 2. Skin replacement in burns. Nurs. Times, *67*:1468, 1971

MILWARD, T. M.: Fate of Silastic and vitrathene nasal implants, PRS, *52*: 217, 1973. Brit. J. Plast. Surg., *25*: 276, 1972

MILWARD, T. M.: Calcification in dermofat grafts, PRS, *55*: 119, 1975. Brit. J. Plast. Surg., *26*: 179, 1973

MIN, B. *et al:* L-shaped osteotomy performed for prognathism and right displacement with open bite of mandible. J. Korean Dent. Assoc., *10*:373, 1972 (Korean)

MIN, B. *et al:* Z-shaped sliding osteotomy for advancing mandible in micrognathia. J. Korean Dent. Assoc., *10*:379, 1972 (Korean)

MINAMI, R. T., HOLDERNESS, H., AND VISTNES, L. M.: Tie-over dressing, with polyurethane foam. PRS, *52*:672, 1973

MINAMI, R. T., TSANG, D., AND HABER, S.: Osteochondromatous choristoma of esophagus. PRS, *53*:94, 197⁴

MINAMI, R. T., JAFEK, B. W., AND COOPER, S.: Spontaneous arteriovenous fistula arising from external carotid artery during pregnancy. PRS, *53*:230, 1974

MINAMI, R. T., MORRILL, L. R., AND WEBER, J., JR.: Intermaxillary fixation using orthodontic brackets bonded to teeth. PRS, *54*:492, 1974

MINAMI, R. T. *et al:* Velopharyngeal incompetence without overt cleft palate, collective review and experience with 98 patients. PRS, *55*:573, 1975

MINCEY, D. L. *et al:* Simplified exercise for temporomandibular joint following condylotomy. Oral Surg., *39*:844, 1975

MINDELL, R. S. *et al:* Leiomyosarcoma of head and neck: review of literature and report of two cases. Laryngoscope, *85*:904, 1975

MINDIKOGLU, A. N. *et al:* Surgical treatment of lymphedema and its indications. Turk. Tip. Dern. Derg., *39*:426, 1973 (Turkish)

MINDIKOGLU, N.: Principles of regional treatment of burns. Turk. Tip. Cemiy. Mecm., *37*:107, 1971 (Turkish)

MINERVINI, F.: Duhamel procedure for treatment of Pierre Robin syndrome (Letter to the Editor). PRS, *51*:686, 1973

MINEV, M. *et al:* Matching of compatible blood in burn patients treated with multiple blood transfusions. Khirurgiia (Sofiia), *26*:113, 1973 (Bulgarian)

MININBERG, D. T., AND HARLEY, D. P.: Scrotal wall hemangioma in infant, PRS, *50*:94, 1972. J. Urol., *106*:789, 1971

MININBERG, D. T., AND RICHMAN, A.: Bilateral scrotal testicular ectopia, PRS, *52*:324, 1973. J. Urol., *108*:652, 1972

MININBERG, D. T. *et al:* Subcellular muscle studies in the prune belly syndrome, PRS, *52*:597, 1973. J. Urol., *109*:524, 1973

MINKOV, N. *et al:* Our experience in treatment of hypospadias. Khirurgiia (Sofiia), *27*:128, 1974 (Bulgarian)

MINKOW, F. V., AND STEIN, F.: Phalangization of thumb, PRS, *54*:375, 1974. J. Trauma, *13*:649, 1973

MINTON, J. P.: Mumps virus and BCG vaccine in metastatic melanoma, PRS, 52:600, 1973. Arch. Surg., 106:503, 1973

MIODUSZEWSKA, O.: Prognostic significance of lymph node reactions in malignant melanoma. Nowotwory, 23:89, 1973 (Polish)

MIODUSZEWSKA, O. et al: Prognostic significance of clinical factors in malignant melanoma of the skin. Nowotwory, 22:15, 1972 (Polish)

MIODUSZEWSKA, O. et al: Prognostic value of histological criteria in malignant melanoma of the skin. Nowotwory, 22:113, 1972 (Polish)

MIRABILE, J. C., PAWL, R. P., AND HART, C. R.: Delayed infection following tantalum cranioplasty, PRS, 54:702, 1974. Mil. Med., 140:398, 1974

MIR Y MIR, L.: Four-flap Z-plasty (Letter to the Editor). PRS, 50:509, 1972

MIR Y MIR, L.: Six-flap Z-plasty. PRS, 52:625, 1973

MIR Y MIR, L.: Possibilities of functional graft of heel, PRS, 53:498, 1974. Rev. españ. cir. plast., 6:89, 1973

MIR Y MIR, L.: Fractures in rhinoplasty, PRS, 54:499, 1974. Acta chir. plast., 16:48, 1974

MIR Y MIR, L.: New biological indication for mesh skin grafting, PRS, 54:246, 1974. Rev. españ. cir. plast., 7:25, 1974

MIR Y MIR, L.: Functional graft of heel (Follow-Up Clinic). PRS, 55:702, 1975

MIRANDA, F. R.: Cleft lip and palate: therapy. ADM, 27:423, 1970 (Spanish)

MIRAULT, G.: Lettre sur l'operation du bec-de-lièvre (Classic Reprint). PRS, 57:502, 1976

MIRCEVSKI, M. et al: Cooperation of a neurosurgeon and plastic surgeon during the surgical treatment of an encephalocele sincipitalis. Med. Pregl., 28:529, 1975 (Serbian)

MIROV, L. B.: Age changes in the forehead area and a surgical method of treating them. Vestn. Dermatol. Venerol., 45:74, 1971 (Russian)

MIROV, L. B.: Correction of the postburn deformity of the left breast. Vestn. Khir., 114:85, 1975 (Russian)

MIRSKIF, M. B.: Studies made by Russian scientists on skin transplantation. Horm. Metab. Res., 1:67, 1969 (Russian)

MIRSKII, M. B.: History of rhinoplasty in Russia. Vestn. Khir., 108:132, 1972 (Russian)

MIRSKII, M. B.: Problem of bone transplantation in studies of Russian surgeons at beginning of 20th century. Vestn. Khir., 111:141, 1973 (Russian)

MISHEV, P. AND GIKOV, D.: Treatment of hypospadias. Khirurgiia, Sofia, 25:387, 1972 (Bulgarian)

MISTERKA, S.: Late results of one-step excision of an esophageal diverticulum. Wiad. Lek., 27: 15, 1974 (Polish)

MITAGVARIIA, N. P. et al: Divided tracheotomy tube for registering respiration, introducing gas mixtures and connection to an artificial respiration apparatus. Patol. Fiziol. Fksp. Ter., 15:86, 1971 (Russian)

MITCHELL, F. L.: Doppler flowmeter to monitor peripheral bloodflow during the edema stage of snakebite (with Gurucharri, Henzel). PRS, 53:551, 1974

MITCHELL, J. H. et al: Malignant melanoma in Gippsland, Victoria: incidence and study of 65 cases. M. J. Australia, 1: 1352, 1972

MITCHELL, W. E., JR. et al: Particulate marrow graft for restoration of mandibular symphysis. Oral Surg., 37:196, 1974

MITCHERLING, J. J. et al: Synovial sarcoma of the neck: report of case. J. Oral Surg., 34:64, 1976

MITROFANOV, G. G. et al: Surgical treatment of excessive development of the mandible and of open bite by intercortical osteotomy of the mandible. Stomatologiia (Mosk.), 51:48, 1972 (Russian)

MITROSZEWSKA, H. et al: Surgical treatment of flexion contracture of the hand by means of elongation-transfer of the flexor tendons. Chir. Narzadow. Ruchu Ortop. Pol., 40:383, 1975 (Polish)

MITROVIC, M. et al: 2 cases of unusual tumors of the ear. Med. Glas., 25:86, 1971 (Croatian)

MITSUYASU, M. et al.: Etiology of ulnar drift of the metacarpophalangeal joint in rheumatoid arthritis. Orthop. Surg. (Tokyo), 21:950, 1970 (Japanese)

MITTELMEIER, H.: Ischemic muscle contracture of the hand. Hefte Unfallheilkd., 0:322, 1974 (German)

MITZ, V.: New data on surgery of breast hypertrophy and ptosis, PRS, 55:248, 1975. J. chir., 107:595, 1974

MITZ, V., RICBOURG, B., AND LASSAU, J. P.: Branches of facial artery, PRS, 54:500, 1974. Ann. chir. plast., 18:339, 1973

MITZ, V. et al: Hand and energy. Arteriography in hand injuries, its symptomatology, its therapeutic implications. Ann. Chir., 28:835, 1974 (French)

MITZ, V., ELBAZ, J. S., AND VILDE, F.: Study of dermal elastic fibers during plastic surgery of truncus, PRS, 56:233, 1975. Ann. chir. plast., 20:31, 1975

MITZ, V. et al: Use of the flag shaped flap to cover losses of substance of the third phalanx. Ann. chir. plast., 20:337, 1975 (French)

MIURA, T.: Thumb reconstruction using radial

innervated cross-finger pedicled graft, PRS, *52:*595, 1973. J. Bone & Joint Surg., *55A:*563, 1973

MIURA, T. *et al:* Reconstruction surgery in hand dysfunction due to injuries of the volar side of the forearm. Shujutsu, *26:*62, 1972 (Japanese)

MIURA, T., AND NAKAMURA, R.: Use of paired flaps to simultaneously cover dorsal and volar surfaces of raw hand. PRS, *54:*286, 1974

Mixed Salivary Gland Tumor: See Parotid Neoplasms; Salivary Gland Neoplasms

MIYAKE, I.: Reconstruction of the eyelid with oral mucosal lining: experience in 2 cases. Jap. J. Plast. Reconstr. Surg., *15:*182, 1972 (Japanese)

MIYAKE, M.: Reconstructive surgery of the nasolacrimal duct and its variations. Ophthalmology (Tokyo), *13:*1027, 1971 (Japanese)

MIYAKE, M. *et al:* Two cases of neurofibromatosis with giant lower extremity. Orthop. Surg. (Tokyo), *23:*221, 1972 (Japanese)

MIYAMOTO, R. *et al:* Hypernephroma metastatic to head and neck. Laryngoscope, *83:*898, 1973

MLADENOVIC, Z. *et al:* Ankylosis of the temporomandibular joint. Med. Pregl., *28:*491, 1975 (Serbian)

MLADICK, R. A.: Electric burns of the mouth in children. Arch. Dermat., *105:*296, 1972

MLADICK, R. A.: Discussion of "Replantation of severed ear parts," by Larsen, Pless. PRS, *57:*375, 1976

MLADICK, R. A. *et al:* Pocket principle, new technique for reattachment of severed ear part. PRS, *48:*219, 1971

MLADICK, R. A. *et al:* Simple technique for securing K-wire to mandible. PRS, *49:*228, 1972

MLADICK, R. A. *et al:* Management of catastrophic postoperative breakdown after massive oropharyngeal cancer surgery. PRS, *49:*316, 1972

MLADICK, R. A. *et al:* Head and neck cancer; comprehensive team approach. Med. Trial Tech. Q., *177:*82, 1973

MLADICK, R. A., AND CARRAWAY, J. H.: Ear reattachment by modified pocket principle. PRS, *51:*584, 1973

MLADICK, R. A. *et al:* Core resection, composite regional ear resection. PRS, *53:*281, 1974

MLECHIN, B. M. *et al:* Diagnosis and surgical tactics in rhinogenic intraocular complications. Vestn. Otorinolaringol., *2:*32, 1974 (Russian)

MOBERG, E.: Bloodless field. The situation of the surgeon facing acute ruptures of the hand

and foot. Lakartidningen, *68:*3015, 1971 (Swedish)

MOBERG, E.: Fingers were made before forks. Hand, *4:* 201, 1972

MOBERG, E.: Biological problems in the evolution of hand prostheses. Orthop. Clin. North Am., *4:*1161, 1973

MOBERG, E.: Surgical treatment for absent single-hand grip and elbow extension in quadriplegia. Principles and preliminary experience. J. Bone & Joint Surg. (Am.), *57:*196, 1975

MOBINI, J. *et al:* Squamous cell carcinoma arising in thyroglossal duct cyst. Am. Surg., *40:*290, 1974

MOBLEY, J. E.: Congenital torsion of the penis, PRS, *52:*596, 1973. J. Urol., *109:*517, 1973

MOCAVERO. G. *et al:* Pre-. intra-, and postoperative problems in new therapeutic trend in Pierre Robin syndrome. Minerva Anestesiol., *41:*294, 1975 (Italian)

MOCERI, L. M. *et al:* Electromyographic verification of viable muscle tissue following a double-pendulum flap procedure for surgical repair of bilateral cleft lip. Cleft Palate J., *12:*405, 1975

MODAN, B. *et al:* Radiation induced head and neck tumors, PRS, *54:*498, 1974. Lancet, *1:*227, 1974

MODREZEWSKI, K. *et al:* Brake-produced hand injuries in farmers. Pol. Przegl. Chir., *44:*39, 1972 (Polish)

MOEHLENBECK, F. W.: Pilomatrixoma (calcifying epithelioma), PRS, *53:*687, 1973. Arch. Dermat., *108:*532, 1973

MOENCH, H. C., AND PHILLIPS, T. L.: Carcinoma of nasopharynx, review of 146 patients with emphasis on radiation dose and time factors. PRS, *52:*102, 1973. Am. J. Surg., *124:* 515, 1972

MOGUILEVSKY, L., BARBARELLI, J., AND ZANNIELLO, M. A.: Lipophagic granuloma of female breast, PRS, *57:*397, 1976. Bol. y trab. Soc. argent cir., *35:*581, 1974

MOHAMED, A. H. *et al:* Light and electron microscopic study of atypical calcifying odontogenic tumor containing "amyloid." J. Oral Pathol., *2:*150, 1973

MOHNIG, W.: Synovectomy in the upper limbs. Beitr. Orthop. Traumatol., *18:*129, 1971

MOHS, F. E.: Chemosurgery for the microscopically controlled excision of skin cancer. J. Surg. Oncol., *3:*257, 1971

MOHS, F. E.: Chemosurgery for facial neoplasms. Arch. Otolaryng., *95:*62, 1972

MOLENAAR, A.: Esthetic operations of the eyelids. Ned. tijdschr. geneeskd., *116:*68, 1972 (Dutch)

MOLENAR, A.: Subcutaneous mastectomy. Clin.

Plast. Surg., *1:*427, 1974

MOLINARI, R.: Indications, limitations and results of traditional latero-cervical lymph node excision. Tumori, *60:*573, 1974 (Italian)

MOLLARD, P.: Treatment of bladder exstrophy. Bladder reconstruction. Dry repair. Ann. Chir. Infant., *12:*385, 1971 (French)

MOLLARD, P.: Treatment of bladder exstrophy. 1. Bladder reconstruction. Extension plasties. Ann. Chir. Infant., *12:*386, 1971 (French)

MOLLARD, P.: Treatment of bladder exstrophy. Internal shunt. Vesicorectal implantations. Ann. Chir. Infant., *12:*391, 1971 (French)

MOLLARD, P.: Ureterosigmoidostomy. Introduction. Ann. Chir. Infant., *12:*393, 1971 (French)

MOLLARD, P.: Treatment of bladder exstrophy. External shunt. Nephrostomy, ureterostomy, trigonostomy. Ann. Chir. Infant., *12:*445, 1971 (French)

MOLLARD, P.: Treatment of bladder exstrophy. Urinary results of the different methods. Ann. Chir. Infant., *12:*467, 1971 (French)

MOLLARD, P., AND PERRIN, P.: Treatment of hypospadias, PRS, *56:*680, 1975. Lyon chir., *70:*402, 1974

MOLLER: Ear pathology and hearing loss in cleft palate. Treatment of cleft palate in Bergen. Tidsskr. Nor. Laegeforen, *94:*2078, 1974 (Norwegian)

MOLLER, G.: Progressive facial hemiatrophy, PRS, *48:*195, 1971. Cir. Plast. Uruguay, *10:*52, 1969

MOLLER, GORAN: *Transplantation Reviews.* Vol. 7. *Immunological Surveillance Against Neoplasia.* Williams & Wilkins Co., Baltimore, 1971. PRS, *51:*86, 1973

MOLLER, J. F. *et al:* Histologic follow-up study of free autogenous skin grafts to alveolar ridge in humans. Int. J. Oral Surg., *1:*283, 1972

MOLLER, R., NIELSEN, A., AND REYMANN, F.: Multiple basal cell carcinoma and internal malignant tumors, PRS, *57:*679, 1976. Arch. Dermat., *111:*585, 1975

MOLLOWITZ, D.: *The Accident Man.* Joh. Ambrosius Barth, Frankfurt, 1974. PRS, *56:*333, 1975

MOLNAR, J., AND FURKA, I.: Testicular prosthesis of plastic material, PRS, *51:*106, 1973 Andrologia, *4:*141, 1972

MOLNAR, L.: Our experience with the intermediary flap plastic of Blair-Kettesy. Klin. Monatsbl. Augenheilkd., *163:*590, 1973 (Polish)

MOLNAR, L. *et al:* Carcinoma of lip. Analysis of material of 25 years. Oncology, *29:*101, 1974

MOLTENO, A. C. *et al:* "Physiological" orbital implant. Brit. J. Ophthalmol., *57:*615, 1973

MOMMA, W. C., KOBERG, W., AND MAI, W.: Indications for and results of Abbe flap operation, PRS. *56:*352, 1975. Scand. J. Plast. Reconstr. Surg., *8:*142, 1974

MOMMA, W. G. *et al:* Late results after therapy of temporomandibular joint luxation using the so-called bridle operation. Dtsch. Zahnaerztl. Z., *27:*838, 1972 (German)

MOMPOINT, O. *et al:* Congenital malignant melanoma. N. Y. State J. Med., *72:*1629, 1972

MONACO, A. P. *et al:* Survey of the current status of the clinical uses of antilymphocyte serum. Surg. Gynec. & Obst., *142:*417, 1976

MONACO, V. *et al:* Clinical significance of functional residual capacity in post-injury state, PRS, *49:*588, 1972. Surg. Forum, *22:*42, 1971

MONAFO, W., CHUNTRASAKUL, C., AND AYVOZIAN, V.: Hypertonic sodium solutions in treatment of burn shock, PRS, *54:*241, 1974. Am. J. Surg., *126:*778, 1973

MONAFO, W. W.: New concepts in burn shock efficacy of hypertonic lactated saline solution, PRS, *54:*240, 1974. Rev. Latino Am. cir. plast., *17:*65, 1973

MONAFO, W. W.: Tangential excision. Clin. Plast. Surg., *1:*591, 1974

MONAFO, W. W., AULENBACHER, C. E., AND PAPPALARDO, C.: Early tangential excision of the eschars of major burns, PRS, *50:*634, 1972. Arch. Surg., *104:*503, 1972

MONAFO, WILLIAM W.: *The Treatment of Burns.* Warren H. Green, Inc., St. Louis, Mo., 1970. PRS, *48:*496, 1971

MONCARZ, V. *et al:* Total maxillary osteotomy for correction of fracture malunion. Oral Surg., *36:*642, 1973

MONCRIEF, J. A.: Development of topical therapy, PRS, *50:*96, 1972. J. Trauma, *11:*906, 1971

MONCRIEF, J. A.: Burn formulae. J. Trauma, *12:*538, 1972

MONCRIEF, J. A.: Burns. New England J. Med., *288:*444, 1973

MONELL, C. M.: Hair transplant, PRS, *57:*669, 1976. West. J. M., *123:*220, 1975

MONET, P., AND GOSSET, J.: Post-traumatic stiffening of thumb in adduction, PRS, *57:*674, 1976. Chirurgie, *101:*402, 1975

MONEY, J.: Sex reassignment therapy in gender identity disorders. Int. Psychiatry Clin., *8:*197, 1971

MONEY, J.: Long-term psychologic follow-up of intersexed patients. Clin. Plast. Surg., *1:*271, 1974

Money, J. et al: Families of seven male-to-female transsexuals after 5–7 years: Sociological sexology. Arch. Sex. Behav., 4:187, 1975

Money, John, and Ehrhardt, Anke A.: *Man and Woman, Boy and Girl.* Johns Hopkins University Press, Baltimore, 1972. PRS, 52:295, 1973

Monks, F. T.: Central angioma of mandible, a possible treatment, PRS, 57:677, 1976. Brit. J. Oral Surg., 12:296, 1975

Monks, G. H.: Correction, by operation, of some nasal deformities and disfigurements (Classic Reprint), PRS, 48:485, 1971

Monroe, C. W.: Our experiences with silicone ear framework, report of 17 ears in 15 patients, PRS, 49:428, 1972

Monroe, C. W: Plea for balance, presidential address, PRS, 52:471, 1973

Monroe, C. W.: Recession of premaxilla in bilateral cleft lip and palate (Follow-Up Clinic), PRS, 54:482, 1974

Monroe, C. W., and Ogo, K.: Treatment of micrognathia in neonatal period, report of 65 cases, PRS, 50:317, 1972

Monroe, J. B., and Fahey, D.: Lingual thyroid, PRS, 57:530, 1976. Arch. Otolaryng., 101:574, 1975

Monroy, D. et al: Functional lymph node neck dissection. Acta Otorinolaryngol. Iber. Am., 23:19, 1972 (Spanish)

Montague, D. K.: Transsexualism. Urology, 2:1, 1973

Montanana, J., Codina, J., and Rodes, A.: Pollicization in congenital anomalies of thumb, PRS, 54:621, 1974. Rev. españ. cir. plast., 7:63, 1974

Montandon, D.: Treatment of partial loss of substance of nose. Rev. Med. Suisse Romande., 93:769, 1973 (French)

Montandon, D.: Surgical correction of facial asymmetry. J. Genet. Hum., 23:123, 1975 (French)

Montandon, D. et al: Contractile fibroblast, its relevance in plastic surgery. PRS, 52:286, 1973

Montandon, D., and Letterman, G. S.: Ambroise Paré's opinion on mammaplasties (Letter to the Editor). PRS, 54:212, 1974

Montandon, D. et al: Plastic surgery in benign mastopathy. Helv. Chir. Acta, 42:173, 1975 (French)

Montano, R. R.: Surgical approach to problem lower denture. J. Conn. State Dent. Assoc., 47:95, 1973

Montaut, J. et al: Repair of the facial nerve using a deviant one-step intracranial nerve graft. Rev. Otoneuroophtalmol., 45:219, 1973 (French)

Monteil, R. et al: Experimentation with a new

wound healing agent combining a catalase and an antiseptic agent in the local treatment of burns. Therapie, 26:535, 1971 (French)

Monteleone, M. et al: Mandibular fractures in edentulous patient. Clin. Ortop., 23:273, 1972 (Italian)

Montes, L. F. et al: Punch excision technique for removing basal cell epithelioma. Geriatrics, 30:65, 1975

Montgomery, W. W.: Facial fractures related to orbit. Laryngoscope, 82:1897, 1972

Montgomery, W. W.: Ossifying cementoma (cementifying fibroma). Trans. Am. Acad. Ophthalmol. Otolaryngol., 76:1380, 1972

Montgomery, W. W.: Silicone tracheal T-tube. Ann. Otol. Rhin. & Laryng., 83:71, 1974

Montgomery, W. W.: Surgery to prevent aspiration. Arch. Otolaryng., 101:679, 1975

Montgomery, William Wayne: *Surgery of the Upper Respiratory System.* Lea & Febiger, Philadelphia, 1971. PRS, 49:205, 1972

Monti, A. E. et al: Preventive retention after mandibular surgery for prognathism. Ortodoncia, 36:151, 1972

Montorsi, W.: Surgical treatment of severe obesity. Minerva Med., 66:2629, 1975 (Italian)

Monty, C. P.: Clinical evaluation of "reinforced" split-skin grafts. Brit. J. Surg., 58:917, 1971

Mooney, C. S. et al: Simultaneous bilateral radical neck dissection following high-level radiation therapy. J. Surg. Oncol., 1:335, 1969

Mooney, J. W. et al: Use of wire sutures for fracture fixation. Oral Surg., 34:21, 1972

Moore, C.: Cigarette smoking and cancer of mouth, pharynx and larynx, PRS, 49:473, 1972. J.A.M.A., 218:553, 1971

Moore, C., Mullins, F., and Scott, R. M.: Preoperative irradiation in cancer of head and neck, PRS, 52:213, 1973. Am. J. Surg., 124:555, 1972

Moore, C. et al: Sebaceous cyst extraction through mini-incisions. Brit. J. Plast. Surg., 28:307, 1975

Moore, D. J.: Glossectomy rehabilitation by mandibular tongue prosthesis, PRS, 52:332, 1973. J. Prosth. Dent., 28:429, 1972

Moore, D. J. et al: Rehabilitating dentulous hemimandibulectomy patients. J. Prosthet. Dent., 35:202, 1976

Moore, Francis D.: *Transplant: The Give and Take of Tissue Transplantation.* Simon and Schuster, New York, 1972. PRS, 51:84, 1973

Moore, G. E., and Gerner, R. E.: Cancer immunity — hypothesis and clinical trial of lymphocytotherapy for malignant diseases, PRS,

*48:*398, 1971. Ann. Surg., *172:*733, 1970

MOORE, G. E., AND GERNER, R. E.: Malignant melanoma, PRS, *49:*108, 1972. Surg. Gynec. & Obst., *132:*427, 1971

MOORE, J. E., AND RUSSELL, J. G.: Geniohyoid and genioglossus muscles, PRS, *55:*506, 1975. J. Oral Surg., *38:*2, 1974

MORE, S. W. *et al:* Epitheloid sarcoma masquerading as Peyronie's disease. Cancer, *35:*1706, 1975

MOORE, W. S.: Practicable classification of injured for computer simulation studies, PRS, *49:*361, 1972. Mil. Med., *135:*752, 1970

MOOSE, S. M.: An original procedure for closing large oroantral openings where conventional procedures have failed. Trans. Int. Conf. Oral Surg., *4:*175, 1973

MOOSE, S. M.: Transoral surgical removal of a sialolith in the submandibular gland. Int. J. Oral Surg., *3:*318, 1974

MOOTZ, W. *et al:* Hemangiopericytoma of the nose. Z. Laryngol. Rhinol. Otol., *49:*257, 1970 (German)

MOOTZ, W. *et al:* Falk's lacrimal sac surgical technique for stenosis. H. N. O., *23:*358, 1975 (German)

MOPERT, S. *et al:* Therapy and prognosis of malignant mesenchymal tumors in the mouth and jaw region. Stomatol. DDR, *23:*525, 1973 (German)

MORAG, B. *et al:* Value of tomography of the sternoclavicular region. Clin. Radiol., *26:*57, 1975

MORAIN, W. D.: Postoperative hypertension as etiological factor in hematoma after rhytidectomy, prevention with chlorpromazine (with Berner, Noe), PRS, *57:*314, 1976

MORALES, F.: Muscular lift in cervical rhytidoplasty (with Guerrero-Santos, Espaillat), PRS, *54:*127, 1974

MORALES, K.: Frontal osteoplasty. Acta Otorinolaryngol. Iber. Am., *23:*849, 1972 (Spanish)

MORALES, P. A. *et al:* Penile implant for erectile impotence, PRS, *52:*596, 1973. J. Urol., *109:*641, 1973

MORALES LUPIANEZ, F. *et al:* Surgical abrasion in chemical burns (report of a case). Actas Dermosifiliogr., *61:*25, 1970 (Spanish)

MORAN, R. E., LETTERMAN, G. S., AND SCHURTER, M. A.: Surgical correction of exophthalmos. PRS, *49:*595, 1972

MORDOVTSEV, V. N.: Unusual clinical course of squamous cell carcinoma of the lower lip. Vestn. Dermatol. Verenol., *44:*66, 1970 (Russian)

MOREL-FATIO, D. *et al:* Corrections of nostril deformations in sequelae of cleft lip. Ann. chir. plast., *13:*252, 1968 (French)

MOREL-FATIO, D. *et al:* Use of human skin pre-

served in cialit in plastic surgery. Ann. chir. plast., *18:*101, 1973 (French)

MORENO GONZALEZ, E. *et al:* Adenolympho-saphenous anastomosis using the Nielubowicz-Olszewski-Sakolowski method. Angiologia, *24:*5, 1972 (Spanish)

MORENO-GONZALEZ, E.: Lymphovenous anastomosis in the treatment of the lymphedema of the lower extremities. Rev. Clin. Esp., *124:*503, 1972 (Spanish)

MORETTI, *et al:* Value of an iodinated vector: 7-Iodoquinoleine-I 131 in diagnosis and care of malignant melanoma. Bull. Soc. Fr. Dermatol. Syphiligr., *79:*155, 1972 (French)

MORGAN, B. D.: Tattoos. Brit. Med. J., *2:*34, 1974

MORGAN, B. L.: Aftercare of rhytidectomies with "no-dressing" technique (Letter to the Editor). PRS, *51:*576, 1973

MORGAN, B. L., AND SAMIIAN, M. R.: Advantages of bilobed flap for closure of small defects of face. PRS, *52:*35, 1973

MORGAN, D. H.: Temporomandibular joint surgery. Correction of pain, tinnitus, and vertigo. Dent. Radiogr. Photogr., *46:*27, 1973

MORGAN, J. E., GILCHREST, B., AND GOLDWYN, R. M.: Skin pigmentation, current concepts and relevance to plastic surgery. PRS, *56:*617, 1975

MORGAN, J. R., AND SCHOW, C. E.: Use of sodium morrhuate in management of hemangiomas, PRS, *55:*255, 1975. J. Oral Surg., *32:*363, 1974

MORGAN, L. R., AND STEIN, F.: Method for rapid and good thumb reconstruction. PRS, *50:*131, 1972

MORGAN, L. R., GALLEGOS, L. T., AND FRILECK, S. P.: Mandibular vestibuloplasty with free graft of mucoperiosteal layer from hard palate, PRS, *51:*359, 1973

MORGAN, L. R., AND RICH, A. M.: Four years' experience with the Morel-Fatio palpebral spring. PRS, *53:*404, 1974

MORGAN, L. R., AND CRAMER, L. M.: Treatment of facial paralysis produced by combat wounds. PRS, *53:*647, 1974

MORGAN, R. G.: Fibre light attachment for the Dott cleft palate gag. Brit. J. Plast Surg., *25:*199, 1972

MORGAN, S. C., AND ZBYLSKI, J. R.: Repair of massive soft tissue defects by open jump flaps. PRS, *50:*265, 1972

MORGAN, A. *et al:* Hearing problems in velar insufficiency. J. Fr. Otorhinolaryngol., *21:*891, 1972 (French)

MORI, M. *et al:* Histochemical studies of myxoma of the jaws. J. Oral Surg., *33:* 529, 1975

MORIAME, N., MORIAME, G., AND LEDOUX-

CORBUSIER, M.: Darier-Ferrand dermato-fibrosarcoma with nasal localization. Arch. belges dermat. et syph., 28:167, 1972 (French)

MORIARTY, M. et al: Skin carcinoma – a 13-year follow-up of 514 cases treated in 1960. Ir. Med. J., 67:638, 1974

MORIKE, K. D.: Tendon connections of musculus flexor digitorum profundus of the human hand. Gegenbaurs. Morphol. Jahrb., 119:809, 1973 (German)

MORIMITSU, T.: Follow-up study of muscular function after surgery in traumatic facial nerve paralysis. J. Otolaryngol. Jap., 76:1472, 1973 (Japanese)

MORIMOTO, M.: Pushback operation for complete unilateral cleft palate (with Honjow, Isshiki). PRS, 53:306, 1974

MORIMOTO, M.: New folded pharyngeal flap (with Isshiki). PRS, 55:461, 1975

MORITSCH, E.: Successful late management of a severed nose tip. Monatsschr. Ohrenheilkd. Laryngorhinol., 104:365, 1970 (German)

MORIZANE, H., UEMURA, Y., AND SHIMIZU, K.: Three cases of a new congenital oculocutaneous syndrome, PRS, 49:236, 1972. Acta Soc. Ophth. Japan, 75:1316, 1971

MORLEY, G. W. et al: Vaginal reconstruction following pelvic exenteration: surgical and psychological considerations. Am. J. Obstet. Gynecol., 116:996, 1973

MORLEY, MURIEL E.: Cleft Palate & Speech. 7th Ed. Longman, Inc., New York, 1971

MOROASHI, M. et al: Evaluation of reconstruction surgery of the finger tip with neurovascular island flap. Orthop. Surg. (Tokyo), 22:951, 1971 (Japanese)

MOROTOMI, T. et al: A combined method of rotation flap and free skin graft to flexion contracture of fingers or toes, PRS, 50:311, 1972. Jap. J. Plast. Reconstr. Surg., 14:377, 1971

MOROTOMI, T. et al: Follow-up study on mesh skin grafts, PRS, 53:371, 1974. Jap. J. Plast. Reconstr. Surg., 16:258, 1973

MOROZOV, V. I., AND GRECHISCHLINA, V. A.: Modification of Csapody's method on conjunctival sac reconstruction in complete obliteration of cavity, PRS, 56:351, 1975. Acta chir. plast., 16:209, 1974

MORRELL, S. G. et al: An aseptic tracheostomy suction catheter. Lancet, 1:76, 1972

MORRILL, L. R. et al: Surgical correction of mandibular prognathism. I. Cephalometric report. Am. J. Orthod., 65:503, 1974

MORRIS, H. D.: Neurofibromatosis of laryngopharynx. Can. J. Otolaryngol., 2:17, 1973

MORRIS, H. L.: Velopharyngeal competence and primary cleft palate surgery, 1960–1971; a critical review. Cleft Palate J., 10:62, 1973

MORRIS, L. N. et al: Split hand and foot anomaly in Macaca mulatta: a report of two cases.

Am. J. Anat., 130:481, 1971

MORRISON, R.: Preoperative radiotherapy in carcinoma of hypopharynx. Brit. J. Radiol., 46:646, 1973

MORRISON, R. B. et al: Wound sepsis in plastic surgery unit. Brit. J. Plast. Surg., 25:435, 1972

MORRISON, W. A. et al: Long term nerve function in replantation surgery of the hand and digits. Ann. Chir., 29:1041, 1975 (French) (English)

MORRISSETTE, Y.: Facial paralysis. Vie Med. Can. Fr., 2:534, 1973 (French)

MORROW, L. M. et al: Mandibular vestibuloplasty utilizing a skin graft. J. Ky. Dent. Assoc., 25:13, 1973

MORSE, N., AND SMITH, P. C.: Ketamine anesthesia in hydranencephalic infant, PRS, 55:120, 1975. Anesthesiology, 40:407, 1974

MORSE, T. S.: Editorial on talking to bereaved burned children, PRS, 49:586, 1972. J. Trauma, 11:894, 1971

MORTADA, A.: Injuries to the orbit and eye adnexa in Egypt. Bull. Ophthalmol. Soc. Egypt, 63:41, 1970

MORTADA, A.: Results of levator resection advancement operation for simple congenital ptosis with absent levator palpebrae muscle action. Bull. Ophthalmol. Soc. Egypt, 63:243, 1970

MORTADA, A.: Lymphoid tymors of eyelids. Bull. Ophthalmol. Soc. Egypt, 65:529, 1972

MORTADA, A. et al: Modified blepharoplasty for malignant lid tumours. Bull. Ophthalmol. Soc. Egypt, 63:421, 1970

MORTON, D., JR., MADDEN, J. W., AND PEACOCK, E. E.: Effect of local smooth muscle antagonist on wound contraction, PRS, 51:709, 1973. Surg. Forum, 23:511, 1972

MORTON, D. L. et al: BCG immunotherapy of malignant melanoma: summary of 7-year experience, PRS, 55:515, 1975. Ann. Surg., 180:635, 1974

MOSADOMI, A: Neurilemmoma of the tongue. J. Oral Med., 30:44, 1975

MOSAVY, S. H. et al: Split hands and feet. S. Afr. Med. J., 49:1842, 1975

MOSBY, E. L. et al: Improved splint in anterior osteotomies. J. Oral Surg., 32:225, 1974

MOSBY, E. L. et al: Compound dermoid cyst of floor of mouth. J. Oral Surg., 32:601, 1974

MOSELEY, H. S., AND PORTER, J. M.: Femoral-axillary artery bypass for arm ischemia, PRS, 52:454, 1973. Arch. Surg., 106:347, 1973

MOSER, M. H., DIPIRRO, E., AND McCOY, F. J.: Sudden blindness following blepharoplasty. PRS, 51:364, 1973

MOSEROVA, J., AND PROUZAS, Z: Standard non-contact burn. Subcutaneous temperature-dynamics during thermal injury, PRS,

*54:*506, 1974. Acta chir. plast., *15:*247, 1973

MOSEROVA, J. *et al:* Experimental use of collagenase in the debridement of thermally damaged skin. J. Hyg. Epidemiol. Microbiol. Immunol. (Praha), *18:*494, 1974

MOSEROVA, J. *et al:* Method of collection and storage of dermoepidermal grafts from pigs, PRS, *54:*626, 1974. Rozhl. chir., *53:*190, 1974.

MOSEROVA, J. *et al:* Bacteriological control of dermoepidermal transplants from pig's carcasses. Rozhl. Chir., *53:*631, 1974 (Czechoslovakian)

MOSIMAN, R.: Lymphangiosarcoma, brawny arm complication after mastectomy. Helv. Chir. Acta, *40:*651, 1973 (French)

MOSKALIK, K. G. *et al:* Use of optical quantum generators (lasers) in oncology. Vopr. Onkol., *18:*97, 1972 (Russian)

MOSS, G. S. *et al:* Decline in pancreatic insulin release during hemorrhagic shock in baboons, PRS, *50:*423, 1972. Ann. Surg., *175:*210, 1972

MOSS, G. S., NEWSON, B., AND DAS GUPTA, T. K.: Normal electron histochemistry and effect of hemorrhagic shock on pulmonary surfactant system, PRS, *56:*469, 1975. Surg. Gynec. & Obst., *140:*53, 1975

MOSTAFA, H. M. *et al:* Three flaps dacryocystorhinostomy. J. Laryng. & Otol., *86:*829, 1972

MOSTAFA, H. M. *et al:* Myxoma of maxilla, case report. J. Laryng. & Otol., *87:*1143, 1973

MOSTAFAVI, H. *et al:* Accidental intra-arterial injection of promethazine HCl during general anesthesia: report of a case. Anesthesiology, *35:*645, 1971

MOSTARDI, R. A. *et al:* Chronic cannulation for intermittent intravenous fluid administration, PRS, *57:*127, 1976. J. Appl. Physiol., *38:*750, 1975

MOSTOVOI, S. I. *et al:* Device for irrigation of the margins of pharyngostomas stimulating healing of the preparations. Zh. Ushn. Nos. Gorl. Bolezn., *6:*97, 1974 (Russian)

MOSZYNSKI, B.: Surgery of otogenic facial paralysis. H. N. O., *23:*313, 1975 (German)

MOTAMED, H. A.: *Color Anatomy and Kinesiology of the Hand.* Hosein A. Motamed, Chicago, 1973. PRS, *55:*699, 1975

MOTOJI, T. *et al:* Cross species immunosuppressive effects of antilymphocyte serum in mice and rats. Transplantation, *14:*536, 1972

MOTSAY, G. J. *et al:* Pulmonary microcirculation in endotoxin-shocked dogs: effect of phenoxybenzamine and methylprednisolone on precapillary and postcapillary resistances, PRS, *53:*609, 1974. J. Surg. Res., *14:*406, 1973

MOTTA, G. *et al:* Surgical excision of the submandibular salivary glands in diabetic retinitis. Surv. Ophthalmol., *19:*63, 1974

MOULY, R.: Addendum to article on Dr. Suzanne Noël. PRS, *48:*138, 1971

MOUNIER-KUHN, P. *et al:* Clinical trial of C. 05 in practical otorhinolaryngology and cervicofacial surgery. J. Fr. Otorhinolaryngol., *20:*865, 1971 (French)

MOUSSAVI, H. *et al:* Synovial sarcoma of the tongue, report of a case. J. Laryng. & Otol., *88:*795, 1974

MOUSSEAU, M. *et al:* One-step bilateral excision of cervical lymph nodes. J. Chir. (Paris), *104:*279, 1972 (French)

MOUSTAFA, F., AND GHAZALY, M. I.: Surgical treatment of rodent ulcer, clinical report on 131 cases, PRS, *53:*494, 1974. Bull. Alexandria Fac. Med., *8:*24, 1973

MOUSTAFA, M. F. H., AND ABDEL-FATTAH, A. M. A.: Presumptive evidence of effect of pregnancy estrogens on keloid growth. PRS, *56:*450, 1975

MOUSTAFA, M. F. H., AND ABDEL-FATTAH, A. M. A.: Reappraisal of shaving and skin grafting for hypertrophic burn scars. PRS, *57:*463, 1976

Mouth

Buccal mucosa lesions, use of thin skin grafts in therapy of some (Kuffer, Soubiran). Bull. Soc. franc. dermat. et syph., *78:*632, 1971 (French)

Intraoral sebaceous gland adenoma (Epker, Henny), PRS, *48:*609, 1971. Cancer, *27:*987, 1971

Experimental study of autologous transplantation of the skin to the oral mucosa (Imai *et al*). J. Otolaryngol. Jap., *74:*382, 1971 (Japanese)

Ileal or colonic conduit operations in children, management of stomal complications following (Jeter, Bloom), PRS, *50:*200, 1972. J. Urol., *106:*425, 1971

Transbuccal flaps for reconstruction of floor of mouth (Cohen, Edgerton). PRS, *48:*8, 1971

Free skin transplantation in oral cavity (Schwenzer). Z.W.R., *80:*523, 1971 (German)

Oral leukoplakia, cryotherapy of (Sako, Marchetta, Hayes), PRS, *52:*102, 1973. Am. J. Surg., *124:*482, 1972

Grafts: some intraoral uses (McKee). J. Contra Costa Dent. Soc., *16:*16, 1972

Study of autologous skin graft in mucomembranous floor by microspectrophotometry (Harada, Kurozumi). J. Otolaryngol. Jap., *75:*1072, 1972 (Japanese)

Microspectrophotometric study of lactic dehydrogenase in experimental auto-transplantation of skin to oral mucous membrane

Mouth—Cont.

(Harada). J. Otolaryngol. Jap., *75*:1362, 1972 (Japanese)

Mouth, corner of, new method of elongating (Fernandez Villoria). PRS, *49*:52, 1972

Orbicularis advancement flap for restoration of angle of mouth (Converse). PRS, *49*:99, 1972

Buccal commissure, self-retaining retractor for (Giles). PRS, *49*:230, 1972

Oral commissure, restoring the overhang of upper lip in repairs of (Wall, Cameron, Latham). PRS, *49*:626, 1972

Labial flap for reconstruction of the anterior oral cavity (Schwartz *et al*). Surg. Gynec. & Obst., *135*:276, 1972

Atlas of Diseases of Oral Mucosa. By J. J. Pindborg. 2nd Ed. W. B. Saunders Co., Philadelphia, 1973.

Oral mucosa, lymphoid hyperplasia in (Adkins). Aust. Dent. J. *18*:38, 1973

Oral lesions, premalignant (Kennet), PRS, *53*: 105, 1974. Contemp. Surg., *2*:55, 1973

Oral precancerous conditions in 407 Malaysians—with correlation to oral habits (Ramanathan *et al*), PRS, *52*:458, 1973. Med. J. Malaya, *27*:173, 1973

Cheilitis glandularis simplex, acquired (Epinette, Hurwitz). PRS, *51*:334, 1973

Thermometer, broken, soft tissue injury by mercury from (Rachman), PRS, *54*:249, 1974. Am. J. Clin. Path., *61*:296, 1974

Irrigation device, oral, bacteremia after use of (Berger *et al*), PRS, *55*:260, 1975. Ann. Int. Med., *80*:570, 1974

Allergy to metals used in dentistry (Fisher), PRS, *56*:116, 1975. Cutis, *14*:797, 1974

Cytological studies after autotransplantation in the oral cavity (Rolling *et al*). Dtsch. Zahnaertztl. Z., *29*:875, 1974 (Eng. Abstr.) (German)

Late results of periodontal surgical interventions (Banoczy *et al*). Fogorv. Sz., *67*:321, 1974 (Hungarian)

Dentures or splints, maxillary, circumpalatal wires for stabilizing (Fortney, Alcorn, Monaco), PRS, *55*:375, 1975. J. Oral Surg., *32*:538, 1974

Etiology and management of hypermobile mucosa overlying the residual alveolar ridge (Desjardins *et al*). J. Prosthet. Dent., *32*:619, 1974

Oral papillomas (Green, Goldman), PRS, *55*:506, 1975. Oral Surg., *38*:435, 1974

Oral manifestations of Kaposi's sarcoma (Gambardella), PRS, *56*:364, 1975. Oral Surg., *38*:591, 1974

Oral mucosa, blue nevus of (Teles, Cardoso, Goncalves), PRS, *56*:234, 1975. Oral Surg.,

Mouth—Cont.

38:905, 1974

Oral submucous fibrosis (O'Riordan), PRS, *55*:723, 1975. Proc. Roy. Soc. Med., *67*:877, 1974

Indications for skin grafts in chronic diseases of the mouth (Soubiran *et al*). Rev. Stomatol. Chir. Maxillofac., *75*:103, 1974 (French)

Phlogosol therapy in inflammations of the oral mucosa (Balogh). Ther. Hung., *22*:83, 1974

New incision technics for apicocectomy (Lindorf). Zahnaerztl Z., *29*:1036, 1974 (German)

Mouth, congenital unilateral benign papillomatosis of (Fellner). Arch. Dermat., *111*:769, 1975

Cryosurgery and its application to oral surgery (Leopard). Brit. J. Oral Surg., *13*:128, 1975

Mouth and throat examinations: next time a patient says "aah" (Mashberg, Morrissey, Garfinkle), PRS, *56*:105, 1975. Emerg. Med., *7*:43, 1975

Mouth, electrical burns of (Wagner, Schwartz), PRS, *56*:232, 1975. Emerg. Med., *7*:275, 1975

Penicillin treatment in oral surgery in patients with coagulation disorders (Lundberg *et al*). Int. J. Oral Surg., *4*:198, 1975

Oral leukoplakia (Srivastava), PRS, *56*:224, 1975. Internat. Surg., *58*:614, 1975

Mouth cavity, upper part, trigonometric method of analysis, (Oblak), PRS, *57*:258, 1976. J. Maxillo-facial Surg., *3*:88, 1975

Mouth: clinical and histological late findings on pedicled skin flaps in oral cavity (Rehrmann, Blessing, Reil), PRS, *57*:540, 1976. J. Maxillo-facial Surg., *3*:155, 1975

Periadenitis mucosa necrotica recurrens (Nicholas, Bays, Lyon), PRS, *56*:593, 1975. J. Oral Surg., *33*:65, 1975

Soft tissue closure of unilateral congenital maxillary alveolar cleft (Christensen *et al*). J. Oral Surg., *33*:872, 1975

Metaplasia of adult oral mucous membrane (Sweeny *et al*). J. Surg. Res., *19*:303, 1975

Fistula of tongue, congenital midline (Samant *et al*), PRS, *56*:597, 1975. Oral Surg., *39*:34, 1975

Mouth: study of development of *orbicularis oris* muscle (Fernandez Villoria). PRS, *55*:205, 1975

Flap, "over and out," for restoration of corner of mouth (Converse). PRS, *56*:575, 1975

Mouth, leukoplakia buccalis (Cooke), PRS, *57*:258, 1976. Proc. Roy. Soc. Med., *68*:337, 1975

Mouth – Cont.

Advantages and disadvantages of various mucosal incisions (Perko). Schweiz. Monatsschr. Zahnheilkd., *85:*167, 1975 (German)

A case of buccal hemangiopericytoma (Wllodarkiewicz *et al*). Czas. Stomatol., *29:*159, 1976 (Polish)

Epidermolysis bullosa and associated problems in oral surgical treatment (Gormley *et al*). J. Oral Surg., *34:*45, 1976

Mouth Deformities (See also *Lips, Deformity of; Jaw, Deformities*)

Stomal stenosis, new concept in treatment (Richardson, Linton, Leadbetter), PRS, *51:*236, 1973. J. Urol., *108:*159, 1972

Commisure, oral, restoration of (Fairbanks, Dingman). PRS, *49:*411, 1972

Mouth and mandible, reduplication (Davies, Morrison, Miller). Brit. J. Plast. Surg., *26:*84, 1973

Bucktooth deformity, maxillary recession for (Russell, Beason). PRS, *51:*220, 1973

Repair of defects in the cheeks and lips (Haas). Laryngol. Rhinol. Otol. (Stuttg.), *53:*695, 1974 (German)

Buccopharyngeal membrane, persistent (Chandra, Yadava, Sharma). PRS, *54:*678, 1974

Repair with Filatov's flap in defects and deformations of the oral region (Shipacheva). Vestn. Khir., *113:*65, 1974 (Eng. Abstr.) (Russian)

Congenital deformity, double palate (Gupta) PRS, *57:*537, 1976. Oral Surg., *40:*53, 1975

Experience with anesthesia in the surgical treatment of maxillofacial and dental deformities (Aleksandrov *et al*). Stomatologiia (Mosk.), *54:*30, 1975

Plastic closure of extensive defects of the maxillofacial area following extensive surgical operations for cancer (Shental *et al*). Stomatologiia (Mosk.), *54:*36, 1975 (Russian)

Mouth Floor (See also *Mouth, Neoplasms; Ranula*)

Mouth, reconstruction of floor of, transbuccal flaps for (Cohen, Edgerton). PRS, *48:*8, 1971

Epitheliomas, floor of mouth, primary localization, respective indications for radiation and surgery in treatment of (Dulac). J. Radiol. Electrol. Med. Nucl., *53:*467, 1972 (French)

Mouth, floor of, anterior tumors, surgical treatment (Auriat *et al*). Ann. Otolaryngol. Chir. Cervicofac., *90:*648, 1973

Mouth Floor – Cont.

(French)

Mouth, floor, hydatid cyst of, case (Kataye *et al*). Ann. Otolaryngol. Chir. Cervicofac., *90:*727, 1973 (French)

Multiple sublingual dermoid cysts (Akinosi). Brit. J. Oral Surg., *12:*235, 1974

Management of fistulae of the head and neck after radical surgery (Stell *et al*). J. Laryng. & Otol., *8:*819, 1974

Mouth, floor, compound dermoid cyst of (Mosby *et al*). J. Oral Surg., *32:*601, 1974

Use of steroids in the prevention of some complications after traumatic oral surgery (Hooley *et al*). J. Oral Surg., *32:*864, 1974

Triangular cervical flap in primary reconstruction of buccopharyngeal cavity (Poisson *et al*). Union Med. Can., *103:*1420, 1974

Anesthesia and resuscitation in operations for diseases and injuries of the tongue, and the floor of the mouth (Alexsandrov *et al*). Vestn. Khir., *112:*88, 1974 (Russian)

Postoperative bronchopulmonary complications in malignant neoplasms of maxillofacial localization (Dunaevskii *et al*). Vestn. Khir., *113:*69, 1974 (Russian)

Electrocoagulation of epitheliomas of the mouth floor. Study of 254 cases (Cernea *et al*). Acta Stomatol. Belg., *72:*221, 1975 (French)

Preoperative cytostasis of extensive flat epithelial cancer of the tongue and floor of the mouth (Gruneberg). Acta Stomatol. Belg., *72:*437, 1975 (German)

Primary reconstruction of the floor of the mouth following radical surgery of cancer (Zisser). Acta Stomatol Belg., *72:*457, 1975 (German)

Reparative surgery on the mucosa of the floor of the mouth (Grellet *et al*). Acta Stomatol. Belg., *72:*489, 1975 (French)

Technique for closure of the floor of the mouth in monobloc resection (Barton *et al*) Arch. Otolaryng., *101:*50, 1975

Mouth, floor of, dermoid cyst of (Oatis *et al*), PRS, *56:*597, 1975. J. Oral Surg., *39:*192, 1975

Sarcoidosis and ranula of sublingual gland (Narang, Dixon), PRS, *57:*258, 1976. J. Oral Surg., *39:*376, 1975

Mouth Infections: See *Jaw, Infections*

Mouth Neoplasms (See also *Cancer, Head and Neck; Jaw Neoplasms; Tongue Neoplasms, etc.*)

Cancer of mouth, early diagnosis of (Borcbakan), PRS, *57:*123, 1976. J. Fac. M. Univ. Ankara, *22:*469, 1969

Mouth Neoplasms – Cont.

Carcinoma, oral, response to preoperative methotrexate infuson therapy (DesPrez *et al*), PRS, *48:*199, 1971. Am. J. Surg., 120:461, 1970

Cancer of oral cavity. Is elective neck dissection beneficial? (Jesse *et al*), PRS, *48:*297, 1971. Am. J. Surg., *120:*505, 1970

Oral cavity cancer, trend toward combined radiotherapy and surgery in management (Leonard, Hass), PRS, *48:*398, 1971. Am. J. Surg., *120:*514, 1970

Surgery of the mandible and transmandibular surgery of the bucco-pharyngeal cavity tumors (Richard). Cancro, *23:*301, 1970 (French)

Metastatic tumors of oral cavity, pharynx, and paranasal sinuses (Jortay), PRS, *50:*635, 1972. Acta chir. belg., *70:*715, 1971

Oral floor cancer, comparison of operative repairs of (Papaioannou, Critselis, Giamalakis), PRS, *49:*474, 1972. Acta chir. Hellenica, *18:*376, 1971

Cancer of floor of mouth, management of (Harrold), PRS, *51:*608, 1973. Am. J. Surg., *122:*487, 1971

Carcinoma, intraoral, periosteum of mandible and (Marchetta, Sako, Murphy), PRS, *51:*608, 1973. Am. J. Surg., *122:*711, 1971

Cancer, subglottic, pathology and management of (Harrison), PRS, *48:*200, 1971. Ann. Otol. Rhin. & Laryng., *80:*6, 1971

Oral cancer, advanced, immediate functional restoration of mandible after surgical treatment (McQuarrie), PRS, *49:*103, 1972. Arch. Surg., *102:*447, 1971

Cryosurgery and electrosurgery compared in the treatment of experimentally induced oral carcinoma (Poswillo). Brit. Dent. J., *131:*347, 1971

Buccal mucosa lesions, use of thin skin grafts in therapy (Kuffer, Soubiran). Bull. Soc. franc. dermat. et syph., *78:*632, 1971 (French)

Mouth and pharynx, epidermoid carcinoma of, 1960–1964 (Farr, Arthur), PRS, *50:*97, 1972. Clin. Bull. Memorial Sloan-Kettering Cancer Ctr., *1:*130, 1971

Cancer of mouth, larynx, and pharynx, cigarette smoking and (Moore), PRS, *49:*473, 1972. J.A.M.A., *218:*553, 1971

Experience in indwelling aspiration by a tube drain following surgery of cervical metastases of malignant oral cancer (Shimizu). J. Jap. Stomatol. Soc., *38:*574, 1971 (Japanese)

Therapy of malignant tumor of the head and neck region (Takayama *et al*). J. Otolaryngol. Jap., *74:*422, 1971 (Japanese)

Mouth Neoplasms – Cont.

Integrated radiation and operation in the treatment of carcinoma of the head and neck: experience in 101 patients (Rush *et al*). J. Surg. Oncol., *3:*151, 1971

Buccal pouch cancer, advanced, surgical management of patients with (Sivaloganathan), PRS, *51:*108, 1973. Med. J. Malaya, *26:*116, 1971

Clinical remarks and considerations on preservation of the mandible in the Commando operation (Voena *et al*). Minerva Otorinolaringol., *21:*186, 1971 (Italian)

Effect of hemimandibulectomy on the remaining temporo-mandibular joint (Schneider *et al*). Pract. Otorhinolaryngol. (Basel), *33:*1, 1971 (German)

Current status of mouth cancer treatment (Pilheu *et al*). Prensa Med. Argent., *58:*1812, 1971 (Spanish)

Carcinoma of mouth and jaw, treatment using chemotherapy-surgery combination (Routledge), PRS, *49:*238, 1972. Proc. Roy. Soc. Med., *64:*737, 1971

Cryosurgery in the management of tumors of the head and neck (Chandler *et al*). South. Med. J., *64:*1440, 1971

Management of metastatic adenopathies in cancer of the mouth (Dutescu *et al*). Stomatologia (Bucur)., *18:*425, 1971 (Rumanian)

Surgical treatment of carcinoma of the floor of the mouth (Barton). Surg. Gynec. & Obst., *133:*971, 1971

Oral cavity tumors, management of (Schlegel). Zahnaerztl Prax., *22:*76, 1971 (German)

Planned preoperative irradiation and surgery for advanced cancer of the oral cavity, pharynx and larynx (Roswit *et al*). Am. J. Roentgenol. Radium Ther. Nucl. Med., *114:*59, 1972

Combined therapy in advanced head and neck cancer: a randomized study (Gollin *et al*). Am. J. Roentgenol. Radium Ther. Nucl. Med., *114:*83, 1972

Tonsillar fossa, cervical lymph node metastases in squamous cell carcinoma (Barkley *et al*), *52:*103, 1973. Am. J. Surg., *124:*462, 1972

Mouth and pharynx, epidermoid carcinoma, prognostic significance of histologic grade (Arthur, Farr), PRS, *52:*102, 1973. Am. J. Surg., *124:*489, 1972

Oral cavity squamous cell carcinoma, treatment of (Fayos, Lampe), PRS, *52:*102, 1973. Am. J. Surg., *124:*493, 1972

Cancer of floor of mouth (Helfrich *et al*), PRS, *52:*213, 1973. Am. J. Surg., *124:*559, 1972

Cancer, otorhinolaryngological area, assess-

Mouth Neoplasms—Cont.

ment of a year's systematic use of new antimitotic: bleomycin. Study of 209 patients (Laccourreye *et al*). Ann. Otolaryngol. Chir. Cervicofac., *89:*219, 1972 (French)

Cancer, buccal floor, statistical study of 148 cases of, treated for more than 5 years (Leroux-Robert *et al*). Ann. Otolaryngol. Chir. Cervicofac., *89:*477, 1972 (French)

Complications associated with combined therapy of oral and pharyngeal neoplasms (Krause *et al*). Ann. Otol. Rhin. & Laryng., *81:*496, 1972

Use of scalp flaps following resection of oral cancer (Dhawan *et al*). Aust. N. Z. J. Surg., *41:*363, 1972

Cancer, oral and oropharyngeal, requiring pedicle flap reconstruction, results of radical excision of (Fleming *et al*). Aust. N. Z. J. Surg., *42:*148, 1972

Carcinoma, verrucous, of mouth (Mason). Brit. J. Oral Surg., *10:*64, 1972

Treatment of oral cancer (Jesse). CA., *22:*209, 1972

Cancer, oral, reconstruction and rehabilitation (Stark). CA., *22:*303, 1972

Oral cancer, reconstruction and rehabilitation (Stark), PRS, *52:*327, 1973. Ca-A Cancer J. Clin., *22:*303, 1972

Treatment of minor salivary gland malignancies of upper food and air passage epithelium. A review of 87 cases (Kadish *et al*). Cancer, *29:*1021, 1972

Treatment of cancer of mouth and pharynx (Muldoon). Cent. Afr. J. Med., *18:*57, 1972

Immediate massive bone graft block surgery of cancers of the buccal cavity (Rodier *et al*). Chirurgie, *97:*785, 1972 (French)

Functional disorders following resection of the tongue and floor of the mouth (Kowalik). Czas. Stomatol., *25:*369, 1972 (Polish)

Oral cavity, lipomas of (Stelinska *et al*). Czas. Stomatol., *25:*931, 1972 (Polish)

Resection of the mandible in oral tumours (Rosemann). H.N.O., *20:*166, 1972 (German)

Mouth, schwannoma of floor, case (Gouzy *et al*). J. Fr. Otorhinolaryngol., *21:*501, 1972 (French)

Oral cavity and pharynx, reconstructive surgery following extensive resections in head and neck regions (Hiranandani). J. Laryng. & Otol., *86:*991, 1972

Plastic reconstitution of functional rehabilitation after great surgical ablations in maxillofacial tumors (Popescu *et al*). J. Med. Lyon, *53:*303, 1972

Segmental sagittal splitting of the mandible

Mouth Neoplasms—Cont.

in the surgical treatment of carcinoma of the floor of the mouth (Perl). J. Oral Surg., *30:*656, 1972

Reconstructive surgery of head and neck cancer (Takeda *et al*). J. Otolaryngol. Jap., *75:*1085, 1972 (Japanese)

Cancer, floor of mouth, results of treatment of, in Warsaw Oncological Institute (Danczak). J. Radiol. Electrol. Med. Nucl., *53:*470, 1972 (French)

Cancers, oral cavity, current role of electrosurgery in treatment of (Jausseran *et al*). J. Radiol. Electrol. Med. Nucl., *53:*471, 1972

Cancers, floor of mouth, role of surgery in treatment of (Durand *et al*). J. Radiol. Electrol. Med. Nucl., *53:*473, 1972 (French)

Surgery in cancer of head and neck. Use of posterior cervical flap (Lenczyk *et al*). N.Y. State J. Med., *72:*239, 1972

Topical treatment of carcinoma of the mouth floor (Danczak). Nowotwory, *22:*139, 1972 (Polish)

Carcinoma, oral cavity (Schroll). Osterr. Z. Erforsch. Bekaempf. Krebskr., *27:*261, 1972 (German)

Primary reconstructive surgery using a pedicled flap in head and neck tumors. 1. The use of forehead skin flap in malignant oral tumor (Murakami *et al*). Otolaryngology (Tokyo), *44:*85, 1972 (Japanese)

Surgical management of carcinoma of the oral cavity (Litton *et al*). Otolaryngol. Clin. North Am., *5:*303, 1972

Transoral resection for cancer of the oral cavity (King). Otolaryngol. Clin. North Am., *5:*321, 1972

Role of total glossectomy in the management of cancer of the oral cavity (Meyers). Otolaryngol. Clin. North Am., *5:*343, 1972

Cryosurgery for the treatment of neoplasms of the, oral cavity (Miller). Otolaryngol. Clin. North Am., *5:*377, 1972

Buccal cavity, mixed tumors of (Lachard *et al*). Rev. Stomatol. Chir. Maxillofac., *73:*216, 1972 (French)

Advanced neoplasms of head and neck. Treatment with combined radiation and chemotherapy (Cammack *et al*). Rocky Mt. Med. J., *69:*54, 1972

Therapy of oral neoplasms (Zuppinger *et al*). Schweiz. Med. Wochenschr., *102:*657, 1972 (German)

Neoplasms of the floor of the mouth. Analysis of 70 cases (Bachelot *et al*). Sem. Hop. Paris, *48:*1413, 1972 (French)

Oral tumors, Burkitt's lymphoma in West Malaysia (Ramanathan), PRS, *52:*103,

Mouth Neoplasms—Cont.

1973. Southeast Asian J. Trop. Med., *3:*249, 1972

Oral cancer, immediate reconstruction of major defects following surgery for, based on arterial skin flaps (Zampakos *et al*). Stomatologia (Athenai), *29:*347, 1972 (Greek)

Labial flap for reconstruction of the anterior oral cavity (Schwartz *et al*). Surg. Gynec. & Obst., *135:*276, 1972

Mouth cancer—concepts of treatment (Pizer *et al*). Va. Med. Mon., *99:*148, 1972

Carcinoma, oral, use of tubed flaps in reconstructing defects (Trichilis), PRS, *52:*450, 1973. Acta chir. hellenica, *45:*99, 1973

Mandibular arch, simple technic for immediate reconstruction of, after surgery for cancer exeresis: importance of stainless steel pins. Acta Stomatol. Belg., *70:*315, 1973 (French)

Oral cavity, lipoma of (Meulemans *et al*). Acta Stomatol. Belg., *70:*431, 1973 (French)

Tonsil, carcinoma of (and nasopharynx); 20-year results (Matar). Am. J. Roent. Radium Ther., *117:*517, 1973

Mouth, floor of, squamous carcinoma of (Flynn, Mullins, Moore), PRS, *53:*497, 1974. Am. J. Surg., *126:*477, 1973

Cancer, oral, reconstruction after surgery, using a frozen autogenous mandibular stent graft (Weaver, Smith), PRS, *53:*499, 1974. Am. J. Surg., *126:*505, 1973

Mouth cancer, management (Williams). Ann. Roy. Coll. Surgeons England, *52:*49, 1973

Oral cavity, forehead island flap in reconstruction of (Krause). Arch. Otolaryng., *97:*283, 1973

Carcinoma, oral cavity, cryosurgery for recurrent (Chandler). Arch. Otolaryng., *97:*319, 1973

Squamous cell cancer of buccal mucosa (Conley *et al*). Arch. Otolaryng., *97:*330, 1973

Oral cavity, carcinoma of (Krause *et al*). Arch. Otolaryng., *97:*354, 1973

Carcinoma involving lower alveolus (Lee, Wilson), PRS, *52:*458, 1973. Brit. J. Surg., *60:*85, 1973

Carcinoma, verrucous, perineural invasion and anaplastic transformation of (Demian, Buskin, Echevarria), PRS, *54:*245, 1974. Cancer, *32:*395, 1973

Premalignant lesions of mouth (Kennet), PRS, *53:*105, 1974. Contemp. Surg., *2:*55, 1973

Cancer, oral, recurrence in patients with radio-osteomyelitis of jaw (Nwokus), PRS, *53:*682, 1974. J. Maxillo-facial Surg., *1:*157,

Mouth Neoplasms—Cont.

1973

Oral cavity, fibrous tumor originating in, in infancy, case report (Takagi *et al*). J. Oral Pathol., *2:*293, 1973

Cancer, surgery for oral, pharyngeal and laryngeal, prophylactic antibiotics in (double-blind study) (Dor *et al*). Laryngoscope, *83:*1992, 1973

Malaysians' mouths, oral precancerous conditions correlated to oral habits (Ramanathan *et al*), PRS, *52:*458, 1973. Med. J. Malaya, *27:*173, 1973

Chinese female, oral carcinoma in (Ramanathan, Lakshimi), PRS, *55:*245, 1975. M. J. Malaysia, *28:*84, 1973

Oral cavity, leiomyomas of. Review of literature and clinicopathologic study of 7 new cases (Cherrick *et al*). Oral Surg., *35:*54, 1973

Oral regions, sarcoma of, central and peripheral fibrogenic and neurogenic (Eversole *et al*). Oral Surg., *36:*49, 1973

Oral surgery and patient who has had radiation therapy for head and neck cancer (Carl *et al*). Oral Surg., *36:*651, 1973

Flap, prefolded, to provide lining and cover in repair of cervical fistulae (Shapiro, Fleury). PRS, *51:*319, 1973

Facial defect: visor flap reconstruction for a massive oropharyngeal defect (Griffin *et al*), PRS, *51:*457, 1973. Discussion by Edgerton, PRS, *51:*582, 1973

Denture, folded, making an intraoral prosthesis or, for insertion into a small mouth (Corso, Schachter). PRS, *52:*94, 1973

Cancer, oral, surgical management of (Baker). Proc. Natl. Cancer Conf., *7:*133, 1973

Carcinomas, squamous cell, of oral cavity, irradiation management of (Fletcher *et al*). Proc. Natl. Cancer Conf., *7:*137, 1973

Cancer, oral, management of teeth related to treatment of (Daly *et al*). Proc. Natl. Cancer Conf., *7:*147, 1973

Oral cavity, rehabilitation of, by plastic surgery after cancer resections (Edgerton). Proc. Natl. Cancer Conf., *7:*199, 1973

Oral neoplastic lesions and their prevention (Pena *et al*). Rev. Port. Estomatol. Chir. Maxilofac., *14:*5, 1973 (Portuguese)

Mucoepidermoid tumors, two cases (Bataille *et al*). Rev. Stomatol. Chir. Maxillofac., *74:*148, 1973 (French)

Therapy and prognosis of malignant mesenchymal tumors in the mouth and jaw region (Mopert *et al*). Stomatol. D.D.R., *23:*525, 1973 (German)

Cancer, floor of mouth and gingiva (Landa).

Mouth Neoplasms – Cont.

Surg. Clin. N. Am., *53:*135, 1973

Cancer, mouth, advanced, primary rehabilitation after total glossectomy and laryngectomy with mandibulectomy (Terz, King, Lawrence). Surg. Gynec. & Obst., *136:*276, 1973

Mouth, helpful maneuver for excision of intraoral malignant tumors (Vasconez, Jurkiewicz, Tyras), PRS, *52:*601, 1973. Surg. Gynec. & Obst., *136:*985, 1973

Bleomycin therapy of oral cancer (Watanabe *et al*). Trans. Int. Conf. Oral Surg., *4:*147, 1973

Place of surgery in the treatment of carcinomas of the oral cavity (Mendes da Costa *et al*). Acta Chir. Belg., *73:*529, 1974 (French)

Carcinoma, oral, epithelial nests in intraoral sensory nerve endings simulating perineural invasion in (Lutman), PRS, *54:*234, 1974. Am. J. Clin. Path., *61:*275, 1974

Carcinoma, soft palate and uvula (Seydel *et al*). Am. J. Roentgenol. Radium Ther. Nucl. Med., *120:*603, 1974

Mouth, floor of, squamous cancer of, marginal resection of mandible in management of (Flynn, Moore), PRS, *57:*540, 1976. Am. J. Surg., *128:*490, 1974

Reconstructive experience with the medially based deltopectoral flap (Park *et al*). Am. J. Surg., *128:*545, 1974

Chinese male, oral carcinoma in (Ramanathan, Lakshimi), PRS, *54:*246, 1974. Asian J. Med., *10:*3, 1974

Malay female, oral carcinoma in (Ramanathan, Lakshimi), PRS, *55:*642, 1975. Asian J. Med., *10:*129, 1974

Practical cryosurgery for oral lesions (Leopard *et al*). Brit. Dent. J., *136:*185, 1974

Oral tumors, malignant, on diagnosis and management of (Heeneman). Can. J. Otolaryngol., *3:*168, 1974

Cancer, oropharyngeal, primary, and hypercalcemia (Terz *et al*). Cancer, *33:*334, 1974

Carcinoma, spindle-cell, of oral mucosa. Light and electron microscopic study of apparent sarcomatous metastasis to cervical lymph nodes. Cancer, *34:*597, 1974

Radical neck dissection in advanced tumors of the head and neck. Considerations on 52 cases (Caldarola *et al*). Cancro, *27:*187, 1974 (Italian)

Oral cavity, gestational tumor of (Sobotkowska). Czas. Stomatol., *27:*895, 1974 (Polish)

Mandibular arch, preservation of, in floor of mouth carcinoma employing temporary pharyngostome (Cummings). J. Laryng. & Otol., *88:*329, 1974

Mouth Neoplasms – Cont.

Carcinoma, epidermoid, of oral cavity, immunity suppression by bleomycin-methotrexate combined treatment (Bitter), PRS, *54:*508, 1974. J. Maxillo-facial Surg., *2:*35, 1974

Cancers, primary oral, cell-mediated and humoral immune responses to (Cannell), PRS, *55:*385, 1975. J. Maxillo-facial Surg., *2:*108, 1974

Neoplasms, multiple primary, in blacks compared to whites; further cancers in patients with cancer of buccal cavity and pharynx (Newell, Kremeutz, Roberts), PRS, *54:*700, 1974. J. Nat. Cancer Inst., *52:*639, 1974

Role of radiotherapy in the treatment of oral cancer (Vermund *et al*). J. Oral Surg., *32:*690, 1974

Philosophy of head and neck cancer surgery (Steckler *et al*). J. Prosthet. Dent., *32:*307, 1974

Cancers, cheek, surgical management of (Bakamjian). J. Surg. Oncol., *6:*255, 1974

Head and neck cancer, recurrence patterns in squamous cell carcinoma of oral cavity, pharynx, and larynx (Gilbert, Kagan), PRS, *56:*363, 1975. J. Surg. Oncol., *6:*257, 1974

Carcinoma, oral cavity – general principles of therapy (Marchetta). J. Surg. Oncol., *6:*349, 1974

Carcinoma, squamous cell, of tonsil, surgical treatment (Whicker *et al*). Laryngoscope, *84:*90, 1974

Lymphoscintigraphy in lymph node metastases from oral cancer (Quintarelli). Minerva Stomatol., *23:*147, 1974 (Italian)

Carcinoma, oral cavity, microinvasive, case (Zerbinati *et al*). Minerva Stomatol., *23:*211, 1974 (Italian)

Tumors of oral cavity, cryosurgery for (Bekke, Snow), PRS, *55:*376, 1975. Nederl. tijdschr. geneesk., *118:*1359, 1974

Intraoral submucosal pseudosarcomatous fibromatosis (Solomon *et al*). Oral Surg., *38:*264, 1974

Oral cavity, angiomyoma of (Gutmann *et al*). Oral Surg., *38:*269, 1974

Intraoral condyloma acuminatum (Summers *et al*). Oral Surg., *38:*273, 1974

Rhabdomyosarcoma of oral cavity in children, dental complications in treatment (Carl, Sako, Schaff), PRS, *56:*223, 1975. Oral Surg., *38:*367, 1974

Mouth, malignant melanoma of, in Indians (Soman, Sirsat), PRS, *56:*224, 1975. Oral Surg., *38:*426, 1974

Sarcoma, Kaposi's, oral manifestations (Gambardella), PRS, *56:*364, 1975. Oral

Mouth Neoplasms – Cont.

Surg., *38:*591, 1974

Bleeding as initial sign of carcinoma of tonsil (Suh *et al*), *56:*355, 1975. Oral Surg., *38:*695, 1974

Metastasis to gingiva (Perlmutter *et al*), PRS, *56:*364, 1975. Oral Surg., *38:*749, 1974

Cancer, oral, lymph node metastases in; correlation of histopathology with survival (Noone *et al*), PRS, *53:*158, 1974

Tumor, epulis, congenital (Bowe). PRS, *53:*227, 1974

Our experience with chemotherapy in the treatment of orofacial cancers (Crepy). Rev. Stomatol. Chir. Maxillofac., *75:*166, 1974 (French)

Embryonic sarcomas of the mouth (Mathe *et al*). Rev. Stomatol. Chir. Maxillofac., *75:*170, 1974

Buccal mucosa, verrucous carcinoma of (Dame, Schuh, Hull), PRS, *55:*517, 1975. South. M.J., *67:*1070, 1974

Carcinoma, intraoral, interstitial radiotherapy for (Ochsner, Collins), PRS, *55:*642, 1975. South. M.J., *67:*1150, 1974

Oral surgical care in the Rostock district – a pilot study (Andrä *et al*). Stomatol. D.D.R., *24:*582, 1974 (German)

Experience with surgical treatment of malignant mouth tumors in the aged with special reference to pre- and postoperative treatment (Muller *et al*). Stomatol. D.D.R., *24:*791, 1974 (German)

Oral, laryngeal and pharyngeal cancers, deglutition after resection of (Doberneck *et al*). Surgery, *75:*87, 1974

Carcinoma, oral cavity, oropharynx, hypopharynx, and larynx, detection of residual: study of surgical margins (Lee). Trans. Am. Acad. Ophthalmol. Otolaryngol., *78:*149, 1974

Lingual flap reconstruction after resection for cancer (DeSanto). Trans. Am. Acad. Ophthalmol. Otolaryngol., *78:*1135, 1974

Postoperative bronchopulmonary complications in malignant neoplasms of maxillofacial localization (Dunaevskii *et al*). Vestn. Khir., *113:*69, 1974 (Russian)

Investigation into the applicability of cytodiagnosis in the early detection of oral cavity cancer at the department of oral surgery (Kränzl *et al*). Wien. Klin. Wochenschr., *86:*647, 1974 (German)

Pull-through surgery in mouth floor-tongue neoplasms (Scheunemann). Acta Stomatol. Belg., *72:*229, 1975 (German)

Surgical technic in combined treatment of cancer of the tongue and mouth floor (Becker). Acta Stomatol. Belg., *72:*247,

Mouth Neoplasms–Cont.

1975 (German)

Technical possibilities of destruction and reconstruction in surgery of cancer of the tongue and mouth floor (Torrielli *et al*). Acta Stomatol. Belg., *72:*259, 1975 (French)

Carcinoma of the mouth floor. Possibilities and limitations of surgical treatment (Schwenzer). Acta Stomatol. Belg., *72:*277, 1975 (French)

Reconstitution of lip, tongue and glottis function (Schmid). Acta Stomatol. Belg., *72:*301, 1975 (German)

Head and neck cancer manpower study (Strong *et al*). Am. J. Surg., *129:*273, 1975

Analysis of mortality and morbidity in 100 composite resections for oral carcinoma (Robins *et al*). Am. J. Surg., *130:*178, 1975

Combined chemotherapy and cryosurgery for oral cancer (Benson). Am. J. Surg., *130:*596, 1975

Report on a partial necrosis of the tongue caused by an endotracheal tube (Bagenyi *et al*). Anaesthesist, *24:*136, 1975 (German)

Cancer of the mouth floor and gingiva (Guerrero Palacios). An. Est. Odontoestomatol., *34:*421, 1975 (Spanish)

Carcinoma of the oral cavity. An analysis of 478 cases (Hirata *et al*). Ann. Surg., *182:*98, 1975

Technique for closure of the floor of the mouth in monobloc resection (Barton *et al*). Arch. Otolaryng., *101:*50, 1975

Cancer of oral cavity, tongue flap reconstruction (Sessions, Dedo, Ogura), PRS, *57:*395, 1976. Arch. Otolaryng., *101:*166, 1975

Mandibular osteotomy and lingual flaps. Use in patients with cancer of the tonsil area and tongue base (DeSanto *et al*). Arch. Otolaryng., *101:*652, 1975

Immunosuppression and cancer. Importance in head and neck surgery (Penn). Arch. Otolaryng., *101:*667, 1975

Use of a tongue flap for the repair of defects following radical surgery of the head and neck (Robertson). Aust. N.Z. J. Surg., *45:*395, 1975

Mouth, malignant melanoma of (Liversedge), PRS, *57:*678, 1976. Brit. J. Oral Surg., *13:*40, 1975

Cryosurgery and its application to oral surgery (Leopard). Brit. J. Oral Surg., *13:*128, 1975

Intravenous hyperalimentation in patients with head and neck cancer (Copeland *et al*). Cancer, *35:*606, 1975

Combination of radiotherapy and surgery in the treatment of head and neck cancers

Mouth Neoplasms—Cont.

(Cachin *et al*). Cancer Treat. Rev., *2*:177, 1975

Cancer excision, reconstruction of extensive full-thickness of oral walls following (De la Plaza), PRS, *57*:530, 1976. Cir. Plast. Ibero-Latino Am., *1*:35, 1975

Oral lipofibromas (Dybkowska-Klos). Czas. Stomatol., *28*:987, 1975 (Polish)

Mesenchymal tumors of the mouth (Takacsi Nagy). Dtsch. Zahnaerztl. Z., *30*:827, 1975 (German)

Carcinoma, early squamous cell, in mouth: next time a patient says "aah" (Mashberg, Morrissey, Garfinkle), PRS, *56*:105, 1975. Emerg. Med., *7*:43, 1975

Surgical treatment of 150 cases of squamous cell carcinoma of the mouth (Caracciolo). Int. Surg., *60*:546, 1975

Initial mismanagement and delay in diagnosis of oral cancer (Shafer). J. Am. Dent. Assoc., *90*:1262, 1975

Temporo-frontal flap. Its value in post-irradiation buccal-pharyngeal surgery (Junien-Lavillauroy *et al*). J. Fr. Otorhinolaryngol., *24*:763, 1975 (French)

Tumors of oral cavity and face, basis, technique and indication for cryosurgery in (Hausamen), PRS, *56*:470, 1975. J. Maxillo-facial Surg., *3*:41, 1975

Radical approach to advanced carcinoma of the head and neck by multi-disciplined team (Glasgold *et al*). J. Med. Soc. N.J., *72*:701, 1975

Carcinoma of floor of mouth, squamous cell, with extensive mandibular involvement (Rubin *et al*), PRS, *56*:600, 1975. J. Oral Surg., *39*:184, 1975

Mouth, primary melanoma of (Jackson, Simpson), PRS, *57*:264, 1976. J. Oral Surg., *39*:553, 1975

Reconstruction of the oral cavity after extirpation of the malignant tumor of the oral floor and the mandible (Konno *et al*). J. Otolaryngol. Jpn., *78*:154, 1975 (Japanese)

Cervical-pectoral flaps in the treatment of advanced oral cancer (Shons *et al*). J. Surg. Oncol., *7*:213, 1975

Mucosal melanomas of the head and neck (Barton). Laryngoscope, *85*:93, 1975

Cryo-irrigator (Murinets-Markevich *et al*). Med. Tekh., *3*:37, 1975 (Russian)

Development of an oral cancer detection program in a hospital (Wasserman). N.Y. State Dent. J., *41*:77, 1975

Mixed tumors of the oral cavity. Report of two cases (Friedman *et al*). N.Y. State Dent. J., *41*:154, 1975

Oral cavity, malignant tumors of (Jeppsson

Mouth Neoplasms—Cont.

et al). O.R.L., *37*:109, 1975

Trichinosis associated with oral squamous cell carcinoma (Bruce), PRS, *57*:265, 1976. Oral Surg., *33*:136, 1975

Oral Kaposi's sarcoma (Garman *et al*). Oral Surg., *39*:288, 1975

Osteomas, extra-abdominal manifestations of Gardner's syndrome (Neale, Pickrell, Quinn). PRS, *56*:92, 1975

Pheochromocytoma in "multiple mucosal neuromata syndrome" (Bowers). PRS, *56*:554, 1975

Cheek, large excision of full thickness of, use of folded forehead flap for reconstruction after (Kavarana). PRS, *56*:629, 1975

Cancer of the floor of the mouth (Helman *et al*). S. Afr. J. Surg., *13*:147, 1975

Management of oral and pharyngeal cancer: a multidisciplinary approach (El-Domeiri *et al*). Surg. Clin. North Am., *55*:107, 1975

Primary neurogenic sarcomas of the oral region: a report of two cases (Martinez *et al*). Ala. J. Med. Sci., *13*:32, 1976

Neurilemmomas of the face and oral cavity (Partyka *et al*). Czas. Stomatol., *29*:147, 1976 (Polish)

Mouth, Surgery of (See also Jaw, Surgery; Mouth Neoplasms; Oral Surgery; Tongue; etc.)

Oral reconstruction, versatility of tongue flap in (Fernandez Villoria), PRS, *51*:602, 1973. Rev. españ. cir. plast., *2*:201, 1969

Oral cavity, reconstruction (Myers). Otolaryngol. Clin. North Am., *5*:413, 1972

Mouth, use of tubed flaps in reconstructing defects of the oral cavity (Trichilis), PRS, *52*:450, 1973. Acta chir. hellenica, *45*:99, 1973

Mouth, reconstruction after cancer surgery, use of frozen autogenous mandibular stent graft (Weaver, Smith), PRS, *53*:499, 1974. Am. J. Surg., 126:505, 1973

Mouth, reconstruction of corners of, after resection of lower lip (Manuylenko), PRS, *57*:756, 1976. Acta chir. plast., *17*:38, 1975

Thyroid, lingual, case report and review of literature (Fahey, Monroe), PRS *57*:672, 1976. Arch. Otolaryng., *101*:574, 1975

Mouth: reconstruction of extensive full-thickness defects of oral walls, following cancer excision (De la Plaza), PRS, *57*:530, 1976. Cir. Plast. Ibero-Latino Am., 1:35 1975

Mouth region, complications of free flap transfer to (Finseth, Kavarana, Antia), PRS, *56*:652, 1975

MOYEN, E. N. *et al:* Pyocyanic infection in

burned patients. Immunitary protection. Nouv. Presse Med., *1:*947, 1972 (French)

MOYER, D. G.: Pilonidal cyst of the scalp.Arch. Dermat., *105:*578, 1972

MOYLAND, J. A., JR. *et al:* Circulatory changes following circumferential extremity burns evaluated by the ultrasonic flowmeter: an analysis of 60 thermally injured limbs. J. Trauma, *11:*763, 1971

MOYLAN, J. A., JR., RECKLER, J. M., and MA-SON, A. D., JR.: Hypertonic lactate saline resuscitation in thermal injury, PRS, *49:*665, 1972. Surg. Forum, *22:*49, 1971

MOYLAN, J. A., JR. *et al:* Tracheostomy in thermally injured patients: a review of five years' experience. Am. Surg., *38:*119, 1972

MOYLAN, J. A., JR., RECKLER, J. M., AND MA-SON, A. D., JR.: Resuscitation with hypertonic lactate saline in thermal injury, PRS, *52:*598, 1973. Am. J. Surg., *125:*580, 1973

MOYLAN, J. A., ADIB, K., AND BIRNBAUM, M.: Fiberoptic bronchoscopy following thermal injury, PRS, *56:*598, 1975. Surg. Gynec. & Obst., *140:*541, 1975

MOYNAHAN, E. J.: Skin wrinkling in cystic fibrosis, PRS, *56:*356, 1975. Lancet, *10:*907, 1974

MOYSE, P. *et al:* Lymph node invasion in cancers of mobile portion of tongue. Bull. Cancer (Paris), *59:*161, 1972 (French)

MOYSE, P. *et al:* Local and lymph node treatment of epitheliomas of the mobile part of the tongue. Rev. Stomatol. Chir. Maxillofac., *74:*574, 1973 (French)

MOZERSKY, D. J. *et al:* Ultrasonic evaluation of the palmar circulation. A useful adjunct to radial artery cannulation. Am. J. Surg., *126:*810, 1973

MOZOLEWSKI, F. *et al:* Treatment of acquired choanal atresia. Arch. Otolaryng., *94:*276, 1971

MROVEC, J.: Simple total and partial cheiloplasty for extensive cancer of lower lip. Cesk. Otolaryngol., *21:*296, 1972. (Czechoslovakian)

Mucosal Grafts

Case report on free transplantation of the mouth mucosa on the glans penis in humans (Friederich). Hautarzt, *21:*84, 1970 (German)

Partial eyelid autoplasty with one-stage mucosal or chondro-mucosal graft (Vandenbussche *et al*). Ann. chir. plast., *16:*322, 1971 (French)

Treatment of gingival fibrosis by free mucous membrane transplantation (Muller *et al*). Dtsch. Zahn. Mund. Kieferheilkd., *57:*8, 1971) (German)

Mucosal Grafts—Cont.

Vestibuloplasty, mucosal grafts (palatal and buccal) (Hall). J. Oral Surg., *29:*786, 1971

Experimental study of autologous transplantation of the skin to the oral mucosa (Imai *et al*). J. Otolaryngol. Jap., *74:*382, 1971 (Japanese)

Mucosa, gingival and alveolar, heterotopic transplantation of, conservation of tissue specificity after (Karring *et al*). J. Periodont. Res., *6:*282, 1971

Bladder, urinary, free grafts of mucosa from: I: For construction of a urethra in humans; II: For production of bone in dogs (Marshall) (Follow-Up Clinic), PRS, *48:*369, 1971

Free gingival transplantations (Garcia *et al*). An. Esp. Odontoestomatol., *31:*77, 1972 (Spanish)

Free gingival grafts—clinical aspects and cytology of healing (Bernimoulin *et al*). Dtsch. Zahnaerztl. Z., *27:*357, 1972 (German)

Reconstruction of the eyelid with oral mucosal lining: experience in 2 cases (Miyake). Jap. J. Plast. Reconstr. Surg., *15:*182, 1972 (Japanese)

Free buccal mucosal grafts for vestibuloplasty (Maloney *et al*). J. Oral Surg., *30:*716, 1972

Anterior Z-plasty ridge extension (Prowler). Oral Surg., *33:*172, 1972

Mucous membrane, intestinal, experimental transplantation of (Herbsman) (Follow-Up Clinic), PRS, *49:*207, 1972

Surgical research with mucous grafts (Quarner *et al*), PRS, *50:*99, 1972. Tribuna Med. Mexico, *21:*3, 1972

Problems and results of free mucosa transplantation in the oral cavity (Nwoku). Z.W.R., *81:*586, 1972 (German)

Mouth mucosa transplantation, free, within the scope of diagnostic and therapeutic laryngeal fissure (Neumann *et al*). Arch. Klin. Exp. Ohren Nasen Kehlkopfheilkd., *205:*371, 1973 (German)

Mucosal grafts and lyophilized dura, comparative study of (Koster *et al*). Dtsch. Zahnaerztl. Z., *28:*1229, 1973

Mucosal graft from cheek, free, used in preprosthetic surgery, histologic study of (Dekker *et al*). Int. J. Oral Surg., *2:*284, 1973

Mucosal grafts, split-thickness, expanded (Shepherd, *et al*). J. Oral Surg., *31:*687, 1973

Mucosa, masticatory, free grafts of, clinical and histologic studies of donor tissues utilized for (Soehren *et al*). J. Periodontol.,

Mucosal Grafts—Cont.

44:727, 1973

Mucosa grafts, free palatal. Evaluation in 26 cases (Wiggins *et al*). Oral Surg., *35:*35, 1973

Graft, free, of mucoperiosteal layer from hard palate for mandibular vestibuloplasty (Morgan, Gallegos, Frileck), PRS, *51:*359, 1973

Oral surgery, free mucosal grafts in major reconstructive (Guernsey). Trans. Congr. Int. Assoc. Oral Surg., *4:*198, 1973

Width of attached gingiva after use of gingival graft (Flores de Jacoby *et al*). Dtsch. Zahnaerztl. Z., *29:*492, 1974 (German)

Grafts, free mucosal, immediate vestibuloplasty with (Maloney, Shepherd, Doku), PRS, *55:*246, 1975. J. Oral Surg., *32:*343, 1974

Oral reconstructive surgery, mucosal grafting in (Maloney *et al*). J. Oral Surg., *32:*705, 1974

Significant differences and advantages between full thickness and split thickness flaps (Staffileno). J. Periodontol., *45:*421, 1974

Reappraisal of environment, function, and gingival specificity (Heaney). J. Periodontol., *45:*695, 1974

Formation of attached mucosa in cases of periodontolysis. II. Free autografts of attached mucosa (Nicolas *et al*). Rev. Belge Med. Dent., *28:*417, 1974 (French)

Complications of free grafts of oral mucosa (Brasher *et al*). J. Periodontol., *46:*133, 1975

Mucosal graft, contiguous (Sternlicht). J. Periodontol., *46:*221, 1975

Technic of free autologous mucosal grafts (Busschop *et al*). Rev. Belge Med. Dent., *30:*215, 1975

Mucous Membrane

Oral mucous membrane, microspectrophotometric study of lactic dehydrogenase in experimental autotransplantation of skin to (Harada). J. Otolaryngol. Jap., *75:*1362, 1972 (Japanese)

Topical cocaine and general anaesthesia: an investigation of the efficacy and side effects of cocaine on the nasal mucosae (Anderton *et al*). Anaesthesia, *30:*809, 1975

Lidocaine topical film strip for oral mucosal biopsies (Roller *et al*). J. Oral Med., *30:*55, 1975

MUEHLBAUER, W. D., SEGETH, H., AND VIESSMANN, A.: Restoration of lid function in facial palsy with permanent magnets, PRS,

*53:*113, 1974. Chir. Plast., *1:*295, 1973

MUELLER, C. F. *et al*: Roentgenologic appearance of chest following radical neck dissection. Am. J. Roentgenol. Radium Ther. Nucl. Med., *117:*840, 1973

MUGNIER, A. *et al*: Pigmented tumor of the maxilla in the child. Rev. Stomatol. Chir. Maxillofac., *75:*771, 1974 (French)

MÜHLBAUER, D.: Successful replantation of subtotally separated ear using local hypothermia. Chirurg, *44:*85, 1973 (German)

MUHLBAUER, W. *et al*: Facial paralysis as a problem of plastic surgery. Med. Klin., *69:*1873, 1974 (German)

MUHLBAUER, W. D.: Simple and physiologic method to correct protruding ears, PRS, *51:*229, 1973. Chir. Plastica, *1:*126, 1972

MUHLBAUER, W. D.: Hypothermia and injury due to exposure. Fortschr. Med., *91:*417, 1973 (German)

MUHLBAUER, W. D.: Plastic surgery in treatment of obesity. Munch. Med. Wochenschr., *117:*747, 1975 (German)

MUHLBAUER, W. D. *et al*: Long-term behaviour of preserved homologous rib cartilage in the correction of saddle nose deformity. Brit. J. Plast. Surg., *24:*325, 1971

MUHLBAUER, W. D. *et al*: Plastic surgery for facial paralysis. In *Plastische und Wiederherstellungs-Chirurgie*, ed. by Hohler; pp. 87–105. Schattauer, Stuttgart, 1975 (German)

MUHLBAUER, W. D. *et al*: Restoration of eyelid function in facial paresis by implantation of permanent magnets. In *Plastische und Wiederherstellungs-Chirurgie*, ed. by Hohler; pp. 157–64. Schattauer, Stuttgart, 1975 (German)

MUHLBERGER, G. *et al*: Value of plate thermography in the diagnosis of the breast. Munch. Med. Wochenschr., *116:*2047, 1974 (German)

MUHLER, G.: Tonsillectomy in patients with cleft palate. Z. Laryngol. Rhinol. Otol., *51:*806, 1972 (German)

MUHLER, G. *et al*: Problems of tonsillectomy and adenotomy in patients with cleft palate. Fogorv. Sz., *67:*310, 1974 (Hungarian)

MUIR, I. F.: Treatment of electrical burns. Hand, *2:*137, 1970

MUIR, I. F.: Treatment of severe burns. Drugs, *1:*429, 1971

MUIR, I. F.: Aspects of plastic surgery. Cleft lip and palate—general. Brit. Med. J., *3:*107, 1974

MUIR, I. F.: Aspects of plastic surgery. Cleft lip and palate—management. Brit. Med. J., *3:*162, 1974

MUKERJEA, S. K.: Occupational true aneurysm of the ulnar artery in the palm. Brit. J.

1974. Rozhl. chir., *53:*164, 1974

MULLIKEN, J. B.: Large frontoethmoidal encephalomeningocele, PRS, *51:*592, 1973

MULLIKEN, J. B.: Selection of antibiotics for human bites of hand (with Guba, Hoopes), PRS, *56:*538, 1975

MULLIKEN, J. B.: Effects of intralesional injection of triamcinolone on glucose-y-phosphate dehydrogenase and alanine aminotransferase activity in keloids (with Im, Hoopes), PRS, *56:*660, 1975

MULLIKEN, J. B., AND HOOPES, J. E.: W-epicanthoplasty, PRS, *55:*435, 1975

MUNCHHOFF, C.: Treatment of burns. Schwest. Rev., *12:*26, 1974 (German)

MUNCHHOFF, C.: Denudation of frontal and parietal bones after burn. In *Plastische und Wiederherstellungs-Chirurgie,* ed. by Hohler; pp. 317-20. Schattauer, Stuttgart, 1975 (German)

MUNDNICH, K.: Dysplasias of middle and inner ear in different types of malformation, PRS, *56:*352, 1975. Proc. Roy. Soc. Med., *67:*1197, 1974

MUNDNICH, K. AND NESSEL, E.: Assessment of idiopathic and post-traumatic facial paralysis in ENT practice: objective bases for surgery. H.N.O., *21:*12, 1973 (German)

MUNRO, D. D. *et al:* Axillary hyperhidrosis. Its quantification and surgical treatment. Brit. J. Dermatol., *90:*325, 1974

MUNRO, I. R.: Anesthetic management and intraoperative care of patients undergoing major facial osteotomies (with Davies), PRS, *55:*50, 1975

MUNRO, I. R.: Orbito-cranio-facial surgery: team approach, PRS, *55:*170, 1975

MUNRO, I. R.: Lymphedema, clinical review and follow-up study (with Saijo, Mancer), PRS, *56:*513, 1975

MUNRO, I. R.: Lymphangioma, long-term follow-up study (with Saijo, Mancer), PRS, *56:*642, 1975

MUNSON, E. S., AND WAGMAN, I.: Diazepam treatment of local anesthetic induced seizures, PRS, *51:*610, 1973. Anesthesiology, *27:*523, 1972

MUNSTER, A. M.: New horizons in surgical immunobiology. Host defence mechanisms in burns. Ann. R. Coll. Surg. Engl., *51:*69, 1972

MUNSTER, A. M.: Lymphocytotherapy in experimental *Pseudomonas* sepsis, PRS, *52:*329, 1973. Surg. Forum, *23:*42, 1972

MUNSTER, A. M.: Trouble with I-V in long run, PRS, *56:*597, 1975. Emergency Med., *7:*230, 1975

MUNSTER, A. M., GOODWIN, M. N., AND PRUITT, N. A., JR.: Acalculous cholecystitis in burned patients, PRS, *50:*541, 1972. Am. J.

Surg., *122:*591, 1971

MUNSTER, A. M. *et al*: Heterotopic calcification following burns: prospective study, PRS, *52:*210, 1973. J. Trauma, *12:*968, 1972

MUNSTER, A. M. *et al*: Use of immunological enhancement in skin transplantation in burns. Surg. Forum, *24:*48, 1973

MUNTEANU, G. *et al*: Technical variant of autograft for lacrimal duct obstruction. Rev. Chir. Oftalmol, *19:*151, 1975 (Rumanian)

MUNTENESCU, M. *et al*: On our septo-rhinoplastic method of re-calibration of the nasal fossae in surgical treatment of ozena. Otorinolaringologie, *16:*271, 1971 (Rumanian)

MUNTENESCU, M. *et al*: Reflections on corrective or modeling rhinoplasty. Otorinolaringologie, *17:*419, 1972 (Rumanian)

MURAKAMI, Y. *et al*: Primary reconstructive surgery using a pedicled flap in head and neck tumors. 1. The use of forehead skin flap in malignant oral tumor. Otolaryngology (Tokyo), *44:*85, 1972 (Japanese)

MURAKAMI, Y. *et al*: Primary reconstructive surgery of head and neck tumors with pedicle flaps. II. Application of a pedicle flap of the anterior chest wall to partially pharyngectomized cases. Otolaryngology (Tokyo), *44:*289, 1972 (Japanese)

MURAZIAN, R. I.: Transfusion of whole blood in burn shock. Khirurgiia (Mosk.), *48:*23, 1972 (Russian)

MURILLO, R.: Reconstruction of exenterated orbit in children due to retinoblastomas, PRS, *51:*346, 1973. Cir. cir. Mexico, *40:*76, 1972

MURINETS-MARKEVICH, B. N. *et al*: Cryo-irrigator. Med. Tekh., *3:*37, 1975 (Russian)

MURKEN, R. E. *et al*: Hypothyroidism following combined therapy in carcinoma of laryngopharynx. Laryngoscope, *82:*1306, 1972

MUROTA, K.: Application of "on top plasty" severely burned hands. Shujutsu, *26:* 35, 1972 (Japanese)

MUROTA, K. *et al:* Reconstruction of the severely burned hand. 1. Transposition of the amputated finger. Orthop. Surg. Tokyo, *22:*884, 1971

MURRAY, D. S. *et al*: Simple technique of primary excision of full thickness burns in children. J. R. Coll. Surg. Edinb., *18:*176, 1973

MURRAY, J. E.: Plastic surgery (Letter to Editor). Ann. Surg., *176:*258, 1972

MURRAY, J. E.: Annual discourse – organ replacement, facial deformity, and plastic surgery. New England J. Med., *287:*1069, 1972

MURRAY, J. E.: Natural history of benign locally-invasive hemangioma of orbital region (with Habal), PRS, *49:*209, 1972

MURRAY, J. E.: Surgical treatment of life-endangering chronic aspiration pneumonia, use of epiglottic flap to arytenoids (with Habal), PRS, *49:*305, 1972

MURRAY, J. E.: On antigenicity of immediately vascularized composite homografts (Letter to the Editor), PRS, *52:*78, 1973

MURRAY, J. E.: Advice of John Staige Davis to medical students (Letter to the Editor), PRS, *53:*582, 1974

MURRAY, J. E.: Letter: Procedures to prevent chronic aspiration. New England J. Med., *293:*561, 1975

MURRAY, J. E.: Further experiences with arytenoid-epiglottic flap for chronic aspiration pneumonia (with Vecchione, Habal), PRS, *55:*318, 1975

MURRAY, J. E. *et al:* Plastic surgical treatment of facial skin cancer. J. Surg. Oncol., *3:*269, 1971

MURRAY, J. E. *et al:* Regional cranio-orbital resection for recurrent tumors, with delayed reconstruction, PRS, *50:*97, 1972. Surg. Gynec. & Obst., *134:*437, 1972

MURRAY, J. F.: Total reconstruction of lower lip with bilateral Estlander flaps, PRS, *49:*658, 1972

MURRAY, J. F.: History of analgesia in burns. Postgrad. Med. J., *48:*124, 1972

MURRAY, J. F. *et al:* Prostheses for children with unilateral congenital absence of the hand. J. Bone & Joint Surg. Am., *54:*1658, 1972

MURRAY, J. F. *et al:* Fractures of the mandible in motor vehicle accidents. Clin. Plast. Surg., *2:*131, 1975

MURRAY, T., BONE, R., AND ESSEN, C.: Changes in voice production during radiotherapy for laryngeal cancer, PRS, *56:*105, 1975. J. Speech & Hearing Disorders, *39:*194, 1974

MURTHY, C. P. *et al:* Effects of estrogen on wound healing—experimental study, PRS, *55:*254, 1975. Indian J. Surg., *36:*1, 1974

MURUBE, J.: Test for spontaneous canalicular functioning. Aust. J. Ophthalmol., *1:*61, 1973

MURUBE, J.: Bicanalicular annular intubation in lacrimal canaliculi sections. Bull. Mem. Soc. Fr. Ophtalmol., *86:*223, 1973 (French)

MURVANIDZE, D. D.: Vesicosigmo-anastomosis using Maydl method in exstrophy of urinary bladder. Bratisl. Lek. Listy, *61:*396, 1974 (Slovakian)

MURVANIDZE, D. D., AND KOCHAROVA, S. Y.: Mathematical planning for plastic surgery in hypospadias, PRS, *57:*761, 1976. Acta chir. plast., *17:*20, 1975

Muscle Grafts, Free

Skeletal muscle, autogenous free grafts of. Preliminary experimental study (Thomp-

Muscle Grafts, Free—Cont.
son), PRS, *48:*11, 1971

Skeletal muscle, autogenous free grafts in dog, investigation with report on successful free graft of skeletal muscle in man (Thompson), PRS, *50:*423, 1972. Transplantation, *12:*353, 1971

Muscle autotransplantation using microsurgical technique (Masuhara, Tamai, Sasauchi), PRS, *53:*110, 1974. Asian M.J., *15:*45, 1972

Muscle, skeletal, transplanted as free autograft in new pharyngoplasty (Thompson), PRS, *56:*355, 1975. Riv. ital. chir. plast., *5:*495, 1973

Sphincter, dynamic muscle, of pharynx, indications and convenient surgical moment (Orticochea), PRS, *54:*619, 1974. Ann. chir. plast., *19:*5, 1974

Grafts, muscle. Anatomical study and technic for removal of extensor digitorum brevis and palmaris longus muscles (Dessapt *et al*). Ann. chir. plast., *19:*235, 1974 (French)

Muscle transplant, *palmaris longus*, pharyngo-palatoplasty (Song, Bromberg), PRS, *56:*677, 1975. Brit. J. Plast. Surg., *27:*337, 1974

Muscle grafts in men, autogenous (Mazzola, Antonelli, Cioccarelli), PRS, *57:*683, 1976. Riv. ital. chir. plast., *6:*161, 1974

Transplantation, free gracilis muscle, with microneurovascular anastomoses for the treatment of facial paralysis (Harii, Ohmori, Torii), PRS, *57:*133, 1976

Muscle transplantation, free, in dogs, by microneurovascular anastomoses (Kubo, Ikuta, Tsuge), PRS, *57:*495, 1976

Muscle, Transposition of

Muscle transposition in operative treatment of advanced stasis ulcer, follow-up study (Ger), PRS, *49:*358, 1972. Am. J. Surg., *120:*376, 1970

Landouzy-Dejerine progressive muscular dystrophy, reconstruction in (Cocke, Davis), PRS, *48:*77, 1971

Muscle transposition in surgical management of decubitus ulcers (Ger), PRS, *48:*298, 1971. Surgery, *69:*106, 1971

Myoplastic closure of fistulae of osteomyelitis origin (Popkirov), PRS, *51:*610, 1973. Bruns' Beitr. klin. Chir., *219:*658, 1972

Mouth angle, *orbicularis* advancement flap for restoration of (Converse), PRS, *49:*99, 1972

Pedicle muscle flaps and their applications in the surgery of repair (Pers *et al*). Brit. J. Plast. Surg., *26:*313, 1973

Muscle Transposition of—Cont.

Latissimus dorsi transfer to restore elbow flexion (Zancolli, Mitre), PRS, *53:*684, 1974. J. Bone & Joint Surg., *55:*1265, 1973

Muscle transfer: results of *temporalis* transfer in lagophthalmos due to leprosy (Ranney, Furness), PRS, *51:*301, 1973

Muscle rotation, masseter, in treatment of inferior facial paralysis (Correia, Zani), PRS, *52:*370, 1973

Muscle transposition and skin grafting to cover exposed bone (Vasconez, Bostwick, McCraw), PRS, *53:*526, 1974

Flap, turnover island, of *gluteus maximus* muscle for repair of sacral decubitus ulcer (Stallings, Delgado, Converse), PRS, *54:*52, 1974

Muscle transposition in treatment of severe wounds (Dalton), PRS, *55:*640, 1975. South. M.J., *67:*1203, 1974

Muscle flaps, pedicled, function in diaphragmatic defects (Brandesky), PRS, *54:*620, 1974. Ztschr. Kinderchir., *14:*260, 1974

Electromyographic and electromanometric studies after *gracilis* transplantations following Pickrell's procedure (Holschneider, Lahoda), PRS, *54:*631, 1974. Ztschr. Kinderchir., *14:*288, 1974

Flaps, muscle, applied to leg (Amar, Aubaniac, Bureau), PRS, *56:*230, 1975. Ann. chir. plast., *20:*61, 1975

Temporalis and platysma muscle transfers, surgical treatment of Moebius syndrome by (Edgerton, Tuerk, Fisher), PRS, *55:*305, 1975

Orbicularis oris transfer to correct unilateral paralysis of lower lip (Puckett, Neale, Pickrell), PRS, *55:*397, 1975

Muscle transplants to correct facial paralysis (Freilinger), PRS, *56:*44, 1975

MUSGRAVE, J. H.: How dextrous was Neanderthal man? Nature (Lond.), *233:*538, 1971

MUSGRAVE, K. S.: A cephalometric radiographic evaluation of pharyngeal flap surgery for correction of palatopharyngeal incompetence. Cleft Palate J., *8:*118, 1971

MUSGRAVE, R. H.: Pitfall of surgical excision of vaccination scars in deltoid area (Letter to the Editor), PRS, *51:*198, 1973

MUSGRAVE, R. H.: Nasal gliomas (with Kubo, Garrett), PRS, *52:*47, 1973

MUSGRAVE, R. H., AND GARRETT, W. S., JR.: Dog bite avulsions of lip, conservative concept, PRS, *49:*294, 1972

MUSGRAVE, R. H. *et al:* Review of the results of two different surgical procedures for the repair of clefts of the soft palate only. Cleft Palate J., *12:*281, 1975

MUSHKA, K.: Modified fixation of bone fragments in the treatment of prognathism. Stomatologiia (Mosk.), *50:*78, 1971 (Russian)

MUSHKA, K. *et al:* Combined treatment of fracture of facial bones concomitant with affections of other organs by oral surgeon and anesthesiologist. Stomatologiia (Mosk.), *51:*83, 1972

MUSHKA, K. *et al:* Surgical method of treatment of fractures of mandibular condyle. Stomatologiia (Mosk.), *52:*89, 1973 (Russian)

MUSIEROWICZ, A. *et al:* Considerations on malignant transformation of congenital exstrophic bladder. Wiad. Lek., *29:*153, 1976 (Polish)

MUSKA, K.: Can the turning of the upper fragment in operations for progeny by Kostecka technic be prevented? Sb. Ved. Pr. Lek. Fak. Karlovy. Univ., *14:*337, 1971 (Czech)

MUSKA, K.: Comparison of results of various therapeutic procedures in problems of mandibular process fractures. Cesk. Stomatol., *74:*198, 1974 (Czechoslovakian)

MUSKA, K.: New method of extraoral fixation by pressure. Cesk. Stomatol., *75:*67, 1975 (Czech)

MUSKA, K. *et al:* Statistical evaluation of 873 fractures of facial bones from the total number of 16,324 patients treated at the Institute of Traumatology at Brno. Cesk. Stomatol., *72:*279, 1972 (Czechoslovakian)

MUSKA K. *et al:* Surgical and orthodontic cooperation as a basis for optimal therapeutic success in special jaw anomalies. Dtsch. Stomatol., *22:*128, 1972 (German)

MUSKA, K. *et al:* Piercing injuries of the face caused by wooden foreign bodies. Z. Aerztl. Fortbild. (Jena), *66:*400, 1972 (German)

MUSKA, K. *et al:* Surgical management of condyloid process fractures. Dtsch. Stomatol., *23:*897, 1973

MUSKA, V. K.: Is there any possibility to technic of unilateral suspended fixation? Stomatol. D.D.R., *25:*35, 1975 (German)

MUSSINELLI, F., AND MUSIO, L.: Surgical treatment of clitoris hypertrophy in sexual anomalies, PRS, *57:*674, 1976. Riv. ital. chir. plast., *6:*171, 1974

MUSTARD, R. A.: Role of surgery in the management of thyroid cancer. Can. Med. Assoc. J., *113:*109, 1975

MUSTARDÉ, JOHN CLARKE: *Plastic Surgery in Infancy and Childhood.* F. &. S. Livingstone, Edinburgh, 1971. PRS, *49:*451, 1972

MUSTARDÉ, J. C.: Fresh look at Le Mesurier: the problem of the drifting ala. Brit. J. Plast. Surg., *24:*258, 1971

MUSTARDÉ, J. C.: Congenital deformities in the orbital region. Proc. Roy. Soc. Med., *64:*1121,

1971

Mustardé, J. C.: Problems in eyelid reconstruction. Ann. Ophthalmol., *4:*883, 1972

Mustardé, J. C.: Problems and possibilities in ptosis surgery, PRS, *56:*381, 1975

Musto, P. *et al*: Considerations on use of ketamine anesthesia alone in surgical treatment, PRS, *56:*367, 1975. Riv. ital. chir. plast., *5:*585, 1973

Musumeci, R. *et al*: Lymphographic evaluation of 116 cases of malignant melanoma. Tumori, *58:*1, 1972 (Italian)

Mutou, W. D. *et al*: Intradermal double eyelid operation and its follow-up results. Brit. J. Plast. Surg., *25:*285, 1972

Mutou, Y.: Complications of augmentation rhinoplasty in orientals. Brit. J. Plast. Surg., *28:*160, 1975

Mutz, H. *et al*: Skin transplantation in childhood burns. Z. Aerztl. Fortbild. (Jena), *66:*922, 1972

Myerowitz, P. D. *et al*: Tracheostomy cuff designed to prevent suffocation. J. Surg., *122:*835, 1971

Myers, B.: Effect of local anesthesia with epinephrine on skin flap survival (with Reinisch), PRS, *54:*324, 1974

Myers, B., Donovan, W., and Falterman, K.: Lack of effect of skin cycle on survival of experimental skin flaps in rats, PRS, *57:*650, 1976

Myers, E. N.: Management of pharyngocutaneous fistula. Arch. Otolaryng., *95:*10, 1972

Myers, E. N.: Role of total glossectomy in the management of cancer of the oral cavity. Otolaryngol. Clin. North Am., *5:*343, 1972

Myers, E. N.: Reconstruction of oral cavity. Otolaryngol. Clin. North Am., *5:*413, 1972

Myers, E. N. *et al*: Management of chylous fistulas. Laryngoscope, *85:*835, 1975

Myers, M. B.: Vascularization of porcine skin heterografts (with Toranto, Salyer), PRS, *54:*195, 1974. Discussion by Ben-Hur, PRS, *54:*352, 1974

Myers, M. B., and Cherry, G.: Pathophysiology and treatment of stasis ulcers of leg, PRS, *49:*104, 1972. Am. Surgeon, 37:167, 1971

Myers, M. B., and Cherry, G.: Blood supply of healing wounds: functional and angiographic, PRS, *48:*299, 1971; *51:*708, 1973. Arch. Surg., *102:*49, 1971

Myers, M. B., and Cherry, G.: Augmentation of survival in pedicle skin flaps by chemical production of ischemia, PRS, *49:*669, 1972. Surg. Forum, *22:*485, 1971

Myers, M. B., Rightor, M., and Cherry, G.: Relationship between edema and healing rate of stasis ulcers of legs, PRS, *51:*605, 1973. Am. J. Surg., *124:*666, 1972

Myers, M. B., Cherry, G., and Milton, S.: Tissue gas levels as index of adequacy of circulation: relation between ischemia and development of collateral circulation (delay phenomenon), PRS, *50:*101, 1972. Surgery, *71:*15, 1972

Myers, M. B., Cherry, G., and Bombet, R.: On lack of any effect of gravity on survival of tubed flaps, PRS, *51:*428, 1973

Myers, M. B., and Wolf, M.: Vascularization of healing wounds, PRS, *56:*471, 1975. Am. Surgeon, *12:*716, 1974

Myers, M. B., and Rightor, M.: Augmentation of wound strength by pretreatment with epinephrine, PRS, *54:*202, 1974. Discussion by Weeks, PRS, *54:*351, 1974

Myers, M. Bert (with William C. Grabb): *Skin Flaps*. Little, Brown & Co., Boston, 1976

Myers, R. P., and Kelalis, P. P.: Penile gangrene successfully treated by debridement and scrotal skin bridge, case report, PRS, *52:*596, 1973. J. Urol., *109:*733, 1973

Myers, R. T. *et al*: Useful and inexpensive carrier for split thickness meshed skin grafts. Am. Surg., *39:*238, 1973

Myslin, A. N. *et al*: Treatment of suppurative diseases of the hand and fingers. Voen. Med. Zh., *3:*34, 1972 (Russian)

Mysliwiec, L.: Case of maxillary sarcoidosis. Czas. Stomatol. *28:*303, 1975 (Polish)

N

Nade, S.: Osteogenesis after bone transplantation, graft, cell, and indicative phenomena, PRS, *52:*686, 1973. Proc. Roy. Australasian Coll. Surg., *46:*261, 1973

Nadell, J. *et al*: Primary reconstruction of depressed frontal skull fractures including those involving sinus, orbit and cribriform plate. J. Neurosurg., *41:*200, 1974

Naef, A. P.: Surgical treatment of pectus excavatum: an experience with 90 operations. Ann. Thorac. Surg., *21:*63, 1976

Naef, A. P. *et al*: Surgical treatment of funnel chest. Surgical experience with 90 cases. Schweiz. Med. Wochenschr., *105:*737, 1975 (French)

Nagahara, K., Hirose, A., and Iwai, H.: Laryngeal reconstruction by free flap transfer, PRS, *57:*604, 1976

Nagashima, C. *et al*: Giant occipital hemangioendothelioma with thrombocytopenia, anemia and hypofibrinogenemia treated by total excision. Neurol. Surg. (Tokyo), *3:*547, 1975

Nagathan, M. K., and Krishnamurthy, K. R.: Melanoameloblastoma, PRS, *54:*381,

1974. J. Pediat. Surg., *8:*977, 1973

NAGAY, B. *et al:* Present-day views on the management of hand injuries. Pol. Przegl. Chir., *43:*645, 1971 (Polish)

NAGAY, B. *et al:* Two cases of dermatofibrosarcoma protuberans. Wiad. Lek., *25:*1025, 1972 (Polish)

NAGEL, E. L. *et al:* Outpatient anesthesia for pediatric ophthalmology, PRS, *53:*373, 1974. Anesth. Analg., Cleve., *52:*558, 1973

NAGEL, F.: Correcture of the saddle nose. Z. Laryngol. Rhinol. Otol., *49:*250, 1970 (German)

NAGEL, F: Our experiences with regional skin flaps in the treatment of large defects of the head and neck region following tumor extirpation. Arch. Klin. Exp. Ohren Nasen Kehlkopfheilkd., *199:*640, 1971 (German)

NAGEL, F.: Practical course of regional, plastic and constructive surgery. I. Free, primary skin transplantation in head and neck surgery. Basic considerations, technique and indication. H.N.O., *20:*319, 1972 (German)

NAGEL, F.: Reconstruction of partial auricular loss, PRS, *49:*340, 1972

NAGEL, F.: Reconstruction of human external ear in animal experiments. Arch. Klin. Exp. Ohren Nasen Kehlkopfheilkd., *205:*166, 1973 (German)

NAGEL, F.: Surgical treatment of malignant melanoma of head and neck. Laryngol. Rhinol. Otol. (Stuttg.), *53:*241, 1974 (German)

NAGEL, G. A.: Evidence for tumor immunity in human malignant melanoma. Schweiz. Med. Wochenschr., *100:*995, 1970 (German)

NAGY, E., AND ZINGG, W.: Simple standardized method for studying tensile strength of healing incisions in animals, PRS, *48:*202, 1971. Canad. J. Surg., *14:*136, 1971

NAGY, L. T.: Fibrosarcoma of tongue. Int. J. Oral Surg., *2:*303, 1973

NAHUM, A. M., AND SIEGEL, A. W.: Changing panorama of collision injury, PRS, *49:*671, 1972. Surg. Gynec. & Obst., *133:*783, 1971

NAHUM, A. M. *et al:* Restoration of mandible following partial resection. Trans. Am. Acad. Ophthalmol. Otolaryngol., *76:*957, 1972

NAIDR, J.: Noma in African children. Cesk. Pediatr., *27:*366, 1972 (Czechoslovakian)

Nails

Nails, diseases of (Hernandez, Bravo), PRS, *48:*605, 1971. Dermat. Rev. Mexicana, *14:*335, 1970

Subungual hematoma, painless evacuation. (Wee, Shieber), PRS, *48:*200, 1971. Surg. Gynec. & Obst., *131:*531, 1970

Split nail deformity, correction of (Hoffman),

Nails—Cont.

PRS, *53:*685, 1974. Arch. Dermat., *108:*568, 1973

Ungual pterygium, inverse (Caputo, Prandi), PRS, *57:*267, 1976. Arch. Dermat., *108:*817, 1973

Nail bed, basal cell carcinoma of (Hoffman), PRS, *54:*380, 1974. Arch. Dermat., *108:*828, 1973

Nail disorders, abrasion in treatment of (Behl). Indian J. Dermatol., *18:*77, 1973

Nail fold reconstruction (Barfod), PRS, *52:*594, 1973. Rev. Latino Am. cir. plast., *17:*59, 1973

Nail bed, Bowen's disease and squamous cell carcinoma of (Mikhail), PRS, *55:*256, 1975. Arch. Dermat., *110:*267, 1974

Subungual exostosis (Lebovitz, Miler, Dickey), PRS, *54:*375, 1974. Cutis, *13:*426, 1974

Nail fold reconstruction, one stage (Hayes), PRS, *54:*690, 1974. Hand, *6:*74, 1974

Subungual glomus tumors (Lord *et al*). Nouv. Presse Med., *3:*445, 1974 (French)

Illustrated technique for the complete removal of nail matrix and hyponychium without skin incisions. Suppan nail technique no. 2. (Weisfeld). J. Am. Podiatry Assoc., *65:*481, 1975

NAIRN, R. C. *et al:* Anti-tumor immunoreactivity in patients with malignant melanoma. M. J. Australia, *1:*397, 1972

NAITO, H. *et al:* Neurosurgeons' interest in exophthalmos. 1. Diagnosis of exophthalmos. Keio J. Med., *22:*85, 1973

NAITO, H. *et al:* Neurosurgeon's interest in exophthalmos. 2. Surgical approach. Keio J. Med., *22:*93, 1973

NAITO, H. *et al:* Skin and rectal temperatures during ether and halothane anesthesia in infants and children, PRS, *55:*644, 1975. Anesthesiology, *41:*237, 1974

NAITO, T. *et al:* Surgery of facial nerve. J. Otolaryngol. Jap., *76:*270, 1973 (Japanese)

NAJWER, K. *et al:* Etiology, diagnosis and treatment of facial palsy of Bell's type. Wiad. Lek., *28:*32, 1975 (Polish)

NAKAI, H.: Follow-up study on reconstruction of microtia with silicone framework (with Ohmori, Matsumoto), PRS, *53:*555, 1974

NAKAJIMA, K.: Early bone grafting in clefts of the lip, maxilla and palate. Acta Med. (Fukuoka), *44:*17, 1974 (Japanese)

NAKAJIMA, T.: Free skin flap from retroauricular region to nose (with Fujino, Harashina), PRS, *57:*338, 1976

NAKAMURA, J. *et al:* 19 cases of lobster hand. Orthop. Surg. (Tokyo), *22:*896, 1971 (Japanese)

NAKAMURA, N. *et al*: Facial nerve anastomosis – with special reference to the follow-up results. Otolaryngology (Tokyo), *43:*809, 1971 (Japanese)

NAKAMURA, R.: Use of paired flaps to simultaneously cover dorsal and volar surfaces of raw hand (with Miura), PRS, *54:*286, 1974

NAKAMURA, S. *et al*: Facial growth of children with cleft lip and/or palate. Cleft Palate J., *9:*119, 1972

NAKAMURA, T. *et al*: Facial fractures. Analysis of five years of experience. Arch. Otolaryng., *97:*288, 1973

NAKAMURA, Y. *et al*: Inspired oxygen concentrations using a humidifier-tracheostomy T-piece system. Brit. J. Anaesth., *44:*61, 1972

NALEBUFF, E. A.: Present status of rheumatoid hand surgery. Am. J. Surg., *122:*304, 1971

NALEBUFF, E. A.: Delayed volar advancement flap for thumb tip injuries (with Millender, Albin), PRS, *52:*635, 1973

NALEBUFF, E. A., AND PATEL, M. R.: Flexor digitorum sublimis transfer for multiple extensor tendon ruptures in rheumatoid arthritis, PRS, *52:*530, 1973

NALEBUFF, E. A. *et al*: Surgical treatment of the swan-neck deformity in rheumatoid arthritis. Orthop. Clin. North Am., *6:*733, 1975

NALEBUFF, E. A. *et al*: Surgical treatment of the boutonniere deformity in rheumatoid arthritis. Orthop. Clin. North Am., *6:*753, 1975

NALTO, H. *et al*: Atypical intermittent exophthalmos due to hyperplasia of lacrimal gland associated with dacryolithiasis. Surg. Neurol., *1:*84, 1973

NAM, I. W.: Clinico-roentgenographic studies on application of bone grafts in dentistry. J. Korean Dent. Assoc., *10:*351, 1972 (Korean)

NAMBA, K.: Sensation in grafted skin, and factors which influence long-term result: indication of skin graft (part 2), PRS, *53:*612, 1974. Jap. J. Plast. Reconstr. Surg., *16:*338, 1973

NAMBA, K., UCHIDA, T., AND DATE, S.: Experimental studies of resurfacing effects of autograft, homograft, heterograft, fibrin membrane and P.V.F. for large skin defect in rats, PRS, *54:*382, 1974. Jap. J. Plast. Reconstr. Surg., *16:*375, 1973

NAMBA, K., YANASE, K., AND HORIUCHI, H.: Scar tissue carcinoma – experience in 24 cases, PRS, *54:*115, 1974. Jap. J. Plast. Reconstr. Surg., *16:*549, 1973

NAMBIAR, R. *et al*: Giant fibro-adenoma (cystosarcoma phylloides) in adolescent females: clinicopathological study. Brit. J. Surg., *61:*113, 1974

NANBA, K.: Treatment of scar contracture of the perineal region. Jap. J. Plast. Reconstr. Surg., *14:*382, 1971 (Japanese)

NANBA, T. *et al*: Contact burn of the hand. Orthop. Surg. (Tokyo), *21:*926, 1970 (Japanese)

NANCE, F. C. *et al*: Aggressive outpatient care of burns. J. Trauma, *12:*144, 1972

NANDA, R.: Effect of Vitamin A on potentiality of rat palatal processes to fuse *in vivo* and *in vitro*, PRS, *55:*383, 1975. Cleft Palate J., *11:*123, 1974

NAPIERALSKI, K.: Navicular fractures in childhood. Zentralbl. Chir., *97:*542, 1972 (German)

NAQUET, R. *et al*: Facial spasm and photosensitive epilepsy in Papio Papio. Rev. Neurol. (Paris), *127:*529, 1972 (French)

NARA, T. *et al*: Facial reconstruction with tubed pedicle flaps in extensive soft tissue loss after a bear bite. Jap. J. Plast. Reconstr. Surg., *14:*502, 1971 (Japanese)

NARANG, R. AND WELLS, H.: Decalcified bone matrix implantation in bone defects. Trans. Congr. Int. Assoc. Oral Surg., *4:*64, 1973

NARANG. R. *et al*: Myositis ossificans: medial pterygoid muscle – a case report. Brit. J. Oral Surg., *12:*229, 1974

NARANG, R., AND WELLS, H.: Experimental osteogenesis with decalcified allogenic bone matrix in palatal defects, PRS, *55:*118, 1975. Oral Surg., *37:*153, 1974

NARANG, R., AND DIXON, R. A.: Sarcoidosis and ranula of sublingual gland, PRS, *57:*258, 1976. J. Oral Surg., *39:*376, 1975

NARANG, R., AND DIXON, R. A., JR.: Temporomandibular joint arthroplasty with *fascia lata*, PRS, *57:*117, 1976. Oral Surg., *39:*45, 1975

NARAYANAN, M.: New-variation of cheek reconstruction with bipolar scalp flap (Letter to the Editor), PRS, *48:*274, 1971

NARITA, O. *et al*: Pregnancy and childbirth in a true hermaphrodite. Obstet. Gynecol., *45:*593, 1975

Nasal Septum

Reconstructive surgery of nasal septum perforation. Considerations and personal technic (Marino). Valsalva, *43:*114, 1967 (Italian)

Nasal septum, surgical management of perforations (Spina, Haro Hernandes), PRS, *48:*510, 1971; *52:*321, 1973. Rev. Latino Am. cir. plast., *13:*54, 1969

Nasal septum perforations, techniques to repair (Lo Russo), PRS, *53:*681, 1974. Bol. Mal. orecch. gola naso, *88:*184, 1970

Surgical repair of perforations of the nasal septum (Zini *et al*). Boll. Mal. orecch. gola naso, *88:*278, 1970 (Italian)

Nasal Septum – Cont.

Importance of corrective plastic surgery of the septum in the treatment of cartilaginous deviated nose (Muller). Z. Aerztl. Fortbild. (Jena), *64:*349, 1970 (German)

Repositioning of the nasal septum without mucosal dissection (Neveu). Ann. chir. plast., *16:*231, 1971 (French)

Surgical management of large nasal septum perforations (Fairbanks *et al*). Brit. J. Plast. Surg., *24:*382, 1971

Initial experiences with Cottle's nasal septum reconstruction (Salus *et al*). H.N.O., *19:*311, 1971 (German)

Septoplasty or reposition of the nasal septum, basic element of rhinoplasty (its functional and esthetic value) (Cajgfinger *et al*). J. Med. Lyon, *52:*1513, 1971 (French)

Nasal septum: experimental and clinical correlation of surgery or injury (Wexler). Laryngoscope, *81:*1409, 1971

Pneumoencephalocele as a complication of nasal septum resection (Langauer-Lewowicka *et al*). Neurol. Neurochir. Pol., *5:*583, 1971 (Polish)

On our septo-rhinoplastic method of re-calibration of the nasal fossae in surgical treatment of ozena (Muntenescu *et al*). Otorinolaringologie, *16:*271, 1971 (Rumanian)

Nasal obstruction, views of plastic surgeon concerning nasal obstructions (Pollet). Probl. Actuels Otorhinolaryngol., *203:*22, 1971 (French)

Reconstruction of the cutaneocartilaginous part of the nasal septum by grafting an auricular transplant (Kostylev). Vestn. Khir., *107:*84, 1971 (Russian)

Nasal septum, defects of mucosa of, use of Kulikovsky's modified needle for suturing (Ivanov). Vestn. Otorinolaringol., *34:*94, 1971 (Russian)

Dislocation of the nasal septal cartilage in the newborn. Aetiology, spontaneous course and treatment (Jeppesen *et al*). Acta Obstet. Gynecol. Scand., *51:*5, 1972

Contralateral rhinostomy for dacryocystitis due to facial malformations (Korchmaros). Acta Ophthalmol. (Kbh.), *50:*399, 1972

Results with Cottle's method of septum surgery (Kleinfeldt). Dtsch. Gesundheitsw., *27:*362, 1972 (German)

Correction of the nasal septum deviation: a new conservative technique (Papangelou). J. Laryng. & Otol., *86:*83, 1972

Rhinoplasty. 2. Plea for discontinuance of submucous resection of septum operation (Blomfield). J. Otolaryngol. Soc. Aust., *3:*422, 1972

Nasal Septum – Cont.

Septum, nasal, reconstruction of columella of (Meyer). O.R.L., *34:*170, 1972 (French)

Defects, surgically created in the septal cartilages of young guinea pigs, healing of (Stenström, Thilander), PRS, *49:*194, 1972

Nasal septal retractors, fiber-optic (Rosenberg), PRS, *49:*468, 1972

Nasal pyramid and septum, surgery in one stage, combined rhinoplasty (Barletta), PRS, *50:*418, 1972. Prensa méd. argent., *59:*112, 1972

Nasal septum, autotransplanted, in rat, growth in height of. Its correlation to increase in height of upper face (Kvinnsland). Acta Odontol. Scand., *31:*317, 1973

Nasal septum, submucosal resection of; its current status (Sedee *et al*). Acta otorhinolaryngol. Belg., *27:*539, 1973

Septal perforations and rhinoplasty (Senechal *et al*). Ann. Otolaryngol. Chir. Cervicofac., *90:*659, 1973 (French)

Nasal septum, wide perforation, simple method for plastic closure (Koburg). Arch. Klin. Exp. Ohren Nasen Kehlkopfheilkd., *205:*289, 1973 (German)

Nasal septum, homograft reconstruction of (Roper). Arch. Otolaryng., *97:*235, 1973

Nasal septal cartilage, early submucous resection of, pilot study in canine pups (Bernstein). Arch. Otolaryng., *97:*273, 1973

Septal perforations, repair with composite grafts (Kratz). Arch. Otolaryng., *98:*380, 1973

Nasal spina, anterior, as source for autogenous bone grafts, preliminary report (Malinowski). Czas. Stomatol., *26:*881, 1973 (Polish)

Septal surgery: high septal transfixion (Brennan, Parkes), PRS, *54:*234, 1974. Internat. Surg., *58:*732, 1973

Nasal septum, cartilaginous, dislocation of, in newborn infants (Cajgfinger *et al*). J. Fr. Otorhinolaryngol., *22:*62, 1973 (French)

Nasal obstruction, place of septal replacement operation in treatment of (Siegler). J. Laryng. & Otol., *87:*153, 1973

Septoplasty (Maran). J. Laryng. & Otol., *87:*196, 1973

Nasal septum, importance of, in facial development (Kemble). J. Laryng. & Otol., *87:*379, 1973

Nasal septum in repairing surgical defects of palate (Clifford). J. Laryng. & Otol., *87:*655, 1973

Nasal septum perforation following total maxillary osteotomy, case report (Mainous *et al*). J. Oral Surg., *31:*869, 1973

Nasal septum defects, our method of closing

Nasal Septum — Cont.

Child abuse, loss of columella and septum from unusual form of (Orton), PRS, *56:*345, 1975

Resection, submucous, use of cocaine as topical anesthetic in (Feehan, Mancusi-Ungaro), PRS, *57:*62, 1975

Nasal obstruction, problems of septal areas (Lake), PRS, *57:*114, 1976. Postgrad. M. J., *57:*108, 1975

Combined correction of the nasal pyramid and septum (Firica *et al*). Rev. Chir. (Otorinolaringol.), *20:*101, 1975 (Rumanian)

Our experience with the joining of tissues using cyacrin (Volkov *et al*). Vestn. Otorinolaringol., *2:*81, 1975 (Russian)

Resection of the nasal septum with reimplantation of autocartilage (Kostyshin). Vestn. Otorinolaringol., *3:*93, 1975 (Russian)

Mechanisms of early maxillary growth — implications for surgery (Siegel). J. Oral Surg., *34:*106, 1976

Late complications after septum surgery (Sloth *et al*). Ugeskr. Laeger, *138:*88, 1976 (Danish)

Nasal Splints

Adhesive backing to nasal splints, addition of (Singer), PRS, *48:*505, 1971

NASEMANN, T.: Corticoids in hemangiomas. Hautarzt, *24:*318, 1973 (German)

NASH, G., AND MOYLAN, J.: Paradoxical catheter embolism, PRS, *48:*198, 1971. Arch. Surg., *102:*213, 1971

NASHIMURA, T., TAGAGI, M., AND KOTANI, Y.: Identification and serological typing of *Pseudomonas aeruginosa* by fluorescent antibody technique, PRS, *52:*687, 1973. Japan J. Exp. Med., *43:*43, 1973

NASHOLD, B. S. *et al:* Electromicturition in paraplegia: implication of spinal neuro-prosthesis, PRS, *50:*419, 1972. Arch. Surg., *104:*195, 1972

NASILOWSKI, W.: Simplified formula for calculating fluid requirements in severely burned patients. Pol. Tyg. Lek., *26:*1950, 1971 (Polish)

NASILOWSKI, W.: Allogenic skin grafting in treatment of burns. Pol. Tyg. Lek., *27:*509, 1972 (Polish)

NASJLETI, C. E., CASTELLI, W. A., AND BLANKENSHIP, J. R.: Storage of teeth before reimplantation in monkeys, PRS, *57:*115, 1976. Oral Surg., *39:*20, 1975

Nasopharynx (See also *Pharynx*)

Angiofibromas, juvenile nasopharyngeal, radiological treatment of (Briant, Fitzpa-

Nasopharynx — Cont.

trick, Book), PRS, *48:*198, 1971. Ann. Otol. Rhin. & Laryng., *79:*1108, 1970

Nasopharyngeal fibroma with extrapharyngeal extensions (Gupta). Acta Otolaryngol. (Stock.), *71:*406, 1971

Nasopharyngeal fibroma (Muler). Ann. Otolaryngol. Chir. Cervicofac., *88:*455, 1971 (French)

Surgical treatment of juvenile nasopharyngeal angiofibroma (Thomsen). Arch. Otolaryng., *94:*191, 1971

Treatment of acquired choanal atresia (Mozolewski *et al*). Arch. Otolaryng., *94:*276, 1971

Epignathus: basicranial teratoma. A case report and review of the literature (Tuson). Brit. J. Surg., *58:*935, 1971

Cryosurgery in the management of tumors of the head and neck (Chandler *et al*). South. Med. J., *64:*1440, 1971

Removal of juvenile fibroma of the nasopharynx under endotracheal anesthesia with arterial hypotension (Fotin *et al*). Vestn. Otorinolaringol., *33:*57, 1971 (Russian)

Carcinoma of nasopharynx, review of 146 patients with emphasis on radiation dose and time factors (Moench, Phillips), PRS, *52:*102, 1973. Am. J. Surg., *124:*515, 1972

Nasopharynx, chemodectomas of (House *et al*). Arch. Otolaryng., *96:*138, 1972

Nasopharyngeal fibroma. Report of a case (Gedosh). J. Arkansas Med. Soc., *68:*410, 1972

Presurgical internal maxillary artery embolization in juvenile angiofibroma (Roberson *et al*). Laryngoscope, *82:*1524, 1972

Removal of a large shell fragment from the nasopharynx (Awty). Oral Surg., *33:*513, 1972

Nose and anterior nasopharynx, congenital absence; report on two cases (Gifford, Swanson, MacCollum), PRS, *50:*5, 1972

Facial pain and some forms of epistaxis, treatment by surgery in pterygomaxillary fossa (Corvera, Somonte, Gonzalez-Romero), PRS, *52:*98, 1973. Tribuna Med. Mexico, *23:*3, 1972

Juvenile angiofibroma (Neel *et al*), PRS, *53:*496, 1974. Am. J. Surg., *126:*547, 1973

Nasopharyngeal stenosis following tonsillectomy and adenoidectomy. Report of 6 cases and their repair (McDonald *et al*). Arch. Otolaryng., *98:*38, 1973

Angiofibroma, juvenile, case of (Parker), PRS, *53:*248, 1974. Arch. Otolaryng., *98:*129, 1973

Nasopharyngeal angiofibroma, juvenile (Duvall *et al*). Minn. Med., *56:*283, 1973

Nasopharynx — Cont.

Osseous metastasis: its relationship to primary carcinoma of the head and neck (Arlen *et al*). Am. J. Surg., *128:*566, 1974

Rhabdomyosarcoma of the head and neck (Smith). Can. J. Otolaryngol., *3:*618, 1974

Non-epithelial tumors of nasal cavity, paranasal sinuses, and nasopharynx: clinicopathologic study. 3. Cartilaginous tumors (chondroma, chondrosarcoma) (Fu *et al*). Cancer, *34:*453, 1974

Nasopharyngeal angiofibroma, treatment of 44 cases (Editorial). Chinese Med. J., *6:*371, 1974 (Chinese)

Intravital studies on the lymph-drainage from the nasopharyngeal roof in men (Jung). Laryngol. Rhinol. Otol. (Stuttg.), *53:*769, 1974 (German)

Angiofibroma: treatment approach (Biller *et al*). Laryngoscope, *84:*695, 1974

Juvenile angiofibroma: a more rational therapeutic approach based upon clinical and experimental evidence (Ward *et al*). Laryngoscope, *84:*2181, 1974

Glandular (seromucinous) hamartoma of the nasopharynx (Baillie *et al*). Oral Surg., *38:*760, 1974

Fibromas, juvenile (Pasnikowski *et al*). Otolaryngol. Pol., *28:*245, 1974 (Polish)

Nasopharyngeal angiofibroma, juvenile (Christiansen *et al*). Trans. Am. Acad. Ophthalmol. Otolaryngol., *78:*1140, 1974

Juvenile fibroma with atypical course (Sopek *et al*). Wiad. Lek., *27:*915, 1974

Nasopharyngeal fibroma. Significance of super-selective angiography and embolization (Lallemant *et al*). Ann. Otolaryngol. Chir. Cervicofac., *92:*127, 1975 (French)

Nasopharyngeal fibroma and embolization (Muler *et al*). Ann. Otolaryngol. Chir. Cervicofac., *92:*332, 1975 (French)

Preoperative embolization of juvenile angiofibromas of the nasopharynx (Pletcher *et al*). Ann. Otol. Rhin. & Laryng., *84:*740, 1975

A case of congenital bilateral choanal atresia treated surgically using the transpalatinal approach (Hybasek). Cesk. Otolaryngol., *24:*51, 1975 (Czechoslovakian)

Non-chromaffin paraganglioma of the nasopharynx (Scoppa *et al*). J. Laryng. & Otol., *89:*653, 1975

Combined approach for massive nasopharyngeal fibroma (Rege *et al*). J. Laryng. & Otol., *89:*1219, 1975

Nasopharyngeal angiofibroma in the elderly: report of a case (Pradillo *et al*). Laryngoscope, *85:*1063, 1975

Nasopharynx, malignant tumors of, long-

Nasopharynx — Cont.

term treatment and prognosis (Lindstrom *et al*). O. R. L., *37:*103, 1975

Endoscopy, fiberoptic, in head and neck region (Dellon, Hall, Chretien), PRS, *55:*466, 1975

NASSERI, M. *et al:* Successful replantation of severed extremities. Langenbecks Arch. Chir., *327:*771, 1970 (German)

NATALI, R. *et al:* Long-delayed surgery of facial paralysis. Apropos of two cases operated after seven and eight years. Ann. Otolaryngol. Chir. Cervicofac., *90:*378, 1973 (French)

NATHAN, H.: Search for ideal suture, PRS, *50:*637, 1972. Internat. Surg., *57:*26, 1972

NATHAN, H.: Fibrotic arch around deep branch of ulnar nerve in hand (with Lotem, Gloobe), PRS, *52:*553, 1973. Discussion by Weeks, PRS, *52:*556, 1973

NATHAN, P.: Intra-arterial injection of barbiturate. Hand, *7:*175, 1975

NATHAN, P. *et al:* Effect of synthetic dressing formed on burn wound in rats: comparison of allografts, collagen sheets, and polyhydroxyethylmethacrylate in control of wound infection. Appl. Microbiol., *28:*465, 1974

NATHANSON, S. E., AND JACKSON, R. T.: Blood flow measurements in skin flaps, PRS, *57:*265, 1976. Arch. Otolaryng., *101:*354, 1975

NATIELLA, J. R. *et al:* Tissue response to cryosurgery of oral cavity in rhesus monkeys. Arch. Pathol., *98:*183, 1974

NATVIG, P.: New surgical wire twister forceps, PRS, *50:*626, 1972

NATVIG, P. *et al:* Anatomical details of osseous-cartilaginous framework of nose, PRS, *48:*528, 1971

NAUMANN, H. H.: Reconstructive possibilities in laryngo-tracheal stenoses. Munch. Med. Wochenschr., *116:*465, 1974 (German)

NAUMANN, W. H.: Methods of correcting exophthalmus. Laryngol. Rhinol. Otol. (Stuttg.), *53:*469, 1974 (German)

NAUMOV, IU. V.: Treatment of minor wounds of the hand in workers at Bryansk Machine-building Plant. Sov. Med., *35:*139, 1972 (Russian)

NAUMOV, P. V. *et al:* Primary myoplasty in removal of the parotid gland together with branches of the facial nerve. Stomatologiia (Mosk.), *51:*30, 1972 (Russian)

NAUMOV, P. V. *et al:* Experimental and clinical study of free grafts in skin-fat transplantation. Stomatologiia (Mosk.), *52:*32, 1973 (Russian)

NAVA, B. E. *et al:* Study of cerebral electric activity in dog head transplant. Arch. Neurobiol. (Madr.), *36:*471, 1973 (Spanish)

NAVA, B. E. *et al*: Head implants in dogs. I. Surgical problems. Rev. Clin. Esp., *129:*443, 1973 (Spanish)

NAVA, B. E. *et al*: Head implants in dogs. II. Neurologic and electroencephalographic studies. Rev. Clin. Esp., *130:*301, 1973 (Spanish)

NAVARRETE, F. *et al*: Lingual cysticercosis. Bol. Med. Hosp. Infant. Mex., *31:*101, 1974 (Spanish)

NAYLOR, A. *et al*: Primary skin-grafting in the treatment of chronic osteomyelitis. Brit. J. Surg., *59:*117, 1972

NAZIF, M.: Hypodontia, anomalies of the extremities, and associated stenosis of lacrimal ducts: report of case. J. Dent. Child., *40:*479, 1973

NEAGOY, D. R., AND DOHN, D. F.: Hemi-facial spasm secondary to vascular compression of facial nerve, PRS, *56:*676, 1975. Cleveland Clin. Quart., *41:*205, 1974

NEALE, H.: Construction of perineal body in female (with Pickrell, Peters), PRS, *55:*529, 1975

NEALE, H. W.: Use of nonexpanded mesh graft. J. Trauma, *14:*247, 1974

NEALE, H. W.: Dynamic correction of unilateral paralysis of lower lip (with Puckett, Pickrell), PRS, *55:*397, 1975

NEALE, H. W., PICKRELL, K. L., AND QUINN, G. W.: Extra-abdominal manifestations of Gardner's syndrome, PRS, *56:*92, 1975

Neck

Thyroid nodules in children, hazards in diagnosis and management (Block, Horn, Miller), PRS, *48:*198, 1971. Am. J. Surg., *120:*447, 1970

Paralysis of accessory nerve after minor surgery on the triangle of neck side (Paul). Zentralbl. Chir., *95:*1298, 1970 (German)

Neck, penetrating wounds, re-emphasis of need for prompt exploration (Ashworth, Williams, Byrne), PRS, *48:*612, 1971. Am. J. Surg., *121:*387, 1971

Our experinces with regional skin flaps in the treatment of large defects of the head and neck region following tumor extirpation (Nagel). Arch. Klin. Exp. Ohren Nasen Kehlkopfheilkd., *199:*640, 1971 (German)

Clinical trial of C.05 in practical otorhinolaryngology and cervico-facial surgery (Mounier-Kuhn *et al*). J. Fr. Otorhinolaryngol., *20:*865, 1971 (French)

Neck, penetrating injuries, treatment of (Weil, Steichen), PRS, *49:*110, 1972. J. Trauma, *11:*590, 1971

Turner's syndrome (gonadal dysgenesis),

Neck — Cont.

genitourinary tract abnormalities (Persky, Owens), PRS, *48:*514, 1971. J. Urol., *105:*309, 1971

Neck, burn contracture of, use of local flap for (Jabaley, Nguyen, Nguyen), PRS, *48:*288, 1971

Neck, direct magnifying lymphangiography of (Nonyama *et al*), PRS, *50:*312, 1972. Pract. Otologia Kyoto, *64:*871, 1971

Wounds, penetrating, of neck, management (Weaver *et al*), PRS, *49:*241, 1972. Surg. Gynec. & Obst., *133:*49, 1971

Use of deltopectoral flap in cervicofacial restoration (Lejour *et al*). Ann. chir. plast., *17:*126, 1972 (French)

Neck incisions relative to the cutaneous vasculature of the neck (Hetter). Arch. Otolaryng., *95:*84, 1972

Neck, nape, and anterior chest, switch flaps from (Briant). Can. J. Otolaryngol., *1:*299, 1972

Neck contractures resulting from burn injuries, management of (Pap), PRS, *51:*351, 1973. Internat. Surg., *57:*413, 1972

Neck, penetrating injury of (unusual automobile accident) (Abrol, Kapur, Raveendran). J. Laryng. & Otol., *86:*1253, 1972

Conservation in head and neck surgery (Tobin). J. Maine Med. Assoc., *63:*137, 1972

Cryosurgery of the head and neck (Von Leden). Tex. Med., *68:*108, 1972

Neck, midline cervical cleft of, with associated branchial cyst (French, Bale). Am. J. Surg., *125:*376, 1973

Neck, penetrating wounds of, management (Knightly, Swaminathan, Rush), PRS, *53:*495, 1974. Am. J. Surg., *126:*575, 1973

Neck, penetrating injuries of, management (Flax *et al*). Am. Surg., *39:*148, 1973

Klippel-Feil syndrome and associated hearing loss (Stark, Borton), PRS, *52:*682, 1973. Arch. Otolaryng., *97:*415, 1973

Neck, wounds of. Treatment by prompt exploration (Feraru). N.Y. State J. Med., *73:*1789, 1973

Bronchogenic cyst of the suprasternal area (Constant, Davis, Edminster), PRS, *52:*88, 1973

Neck, radionecrosis of (Fry), PRS, *52:*678, 1973. Proc. Roy. Australasian Coll. Surg., *46:*412, 1973

Neck, lipomatosis at prevailing cervical localization (Visentini, Mazzoleni, Linda), PRS, *56:*363, 1975. Riv. ital. chir. plast., *5:*483, 1973

Neck, penetrating injuries of, experience in operative management (Enker *et al*). Surg. Clin. North Am., *53:*87, 1973

Neck Dissection—Cont.

Laryng. & Otol., *85*:1097, 1971

Delayed contralateral cervical metastases with laryngeal and laryngopharyngeal cancers (Biller *et al*). Laryngoscope, *81*:1499, 1971

Neck dissection, radical, combined with tumor resection, reconstruction of lower lip after (Lentrodt, Luhr), PRS, *48*:579, 1971

Esthetic approach for neck dissection (Appiani Sotomayor), PRS, *49:* 581, 1972. Prensa med. argent., *58:*1436, 1971

Management of metastatic adenopathies in cancer of the mouth (Dutescu *et al*). Stomatologia (Bucur.), *18:*425, 1971 (Rumanian)

Prophylactic removal of lymph nodes and cellular tissue of the neck in patients with laryngeal and laryngopharyngeal cancer (Baradulina *et al*). Vestn. Otorinolaringol., *33:*55, 1971 (Russian)

In vivo staining of the cervical lymph nodes with Evans blue prior to cervical lymphadenomectomy (Feigin). Zh. Ushn. Nos. Borl. Bolezn., *31:*115, 1971 (Russian)

Functional lymph node neck dissection (Monroy *et al*). Acta Otorinolaryngol. Iber. Am., *23:*19, 1972 (Spanish)

Cervical lymph node functional-radical dissection. Surgical anatomy. Technic and results (Gavilan Alonso *et al*. Acta Otorinolaryngol. Iber. Am., *23:*703, 1972 (Spanish)

Therapeutic problem of metastatic neck adenopathy (Fayos *et al*). Am. J. Roentgenol. Radium Ther. Nucl. Med., *114:*65, 1972

Head and neck surgery, reticulum cell sarcoma in (Larsen, Hill, Rotzer), PRS, *50:*421, 1972. Am. J. Surg., *123:*338, 1972

Cancerous nodes, metastatic cervical, from unknown primary site, diagnosis and treatment of (MacComb), PRS, *51:*351, 1973. Am. J. Surg., *124:*441, 1972

Metastatic cervical lymph nodes in cutaneous melanoma of head and neck (Donnellan *et al*), PRS, *52:*103, 1973. Am. J. Surg., *124:*450, 1972

Neck dissection, radical, importance of variations of cerebral dural sinuses at torcular herophili (Kaplan *et al*). Am. J. Surg., *124:*456, 1972

Metastases, cervical lymph node, in squamous cell carcinoma of tonsillar fossa, base of tongue, supraglottic larynx and hypopharynx (Barkley *et al*), PRS, *52:*103, 1973. Am. J. Surg., *124:*462, 1972

Operations on residual or recurrent cervical adenopathies following curative doses of cobalt therapy (Poncet). Ann. Otolaryngol. Chir. Cervicofac., *89:*405, 1972 (French)

Neck Dissection—Cont.

Neck dissection, unilateral, unilateral cerebral circulation decrease following (Ristow *et al*). Arch. Klin. Exp. Ohren Nasen Kehlkopfheilkd., *202:*523, 1972 (German)

Head and neck cancer, composite operation (commando procedure), (Yonemoto *et al*), PRS, *51:*235, 1973. Arch. Surg., *104:*809, 1972

Neck dissection, radical, unilateral, direct cervical microlymphography as method of checking patients after (Piragine). Ateneo. Parmense (Acta Biomed.), *1:*3, 1972 (Italian)

Sino-carotid hyper-reflectivity (therapeutic value of intracavitary standby cardiac stimulation) (Grand *et al*). Coer Med. Interne, *11:*265, 1972 (French)

Surgical consequences in cylindroma of submandibular gland with invasion of common carotid artery (Stellmach). Fortschr. Kiefer. Gesichtschir., *15:*97, 1972 (German)

One step bilateral excision of cervical lymph nodes (Mousseau *et al*). J. Chir. (Paris), *104:*279, 1972 (French)

Neck dissection, indication for modified (Matsuura, Kawabe, Kondo). J. Otolaryngol. Japan, *75:*1083, 1972 (Japanese)

Increased cerebrospinal fluid pressure following unilateral radical neck dissection (Tobin). Laryngoscope, *82:*817, 1972

Head and neck, lymphatic cannulation of (Smith) (Follow-Up Clinic), PRS, *49:*454, 1972

Value of the autogenous dermal graft for carotid artery protection (Curutchet *et al*). Surgery, *71:*876, 1972

Neck dissection, radical, roentgenologic appearance of chest following (Mueller *et al*). Am. J. Roentgenol. Radium Ther. Nucl. Med., *117:*840, 1973

Mortality and morbidity rates in head and neck surgery, factors minimizing (Beahrs), PRS, *53:*692, 1974. Am. J. Surg., *126:*443, 1973

Neck dissection and discontinuous partial glossectomy for epidermoid carcinoma of tongue (Spiro, Strong), PRS, *53:*602, 1974. Am. J. Surg., *126:*544, 1973

Neck dissection, significance of jugular vein invasion by metastatic carcinoma (Djalilian *et al*), PRS, *53:*604, 1974. Am. J. Surg., *126:*566, 1973

Technic of conservative cervical lymphadenectomy (Pech, Cannoni, Lisbonnis). Ann. chir. plast., *18:*37, 1973 (French)

Cancers, lower lip, lymph node problem in treatment of (Dargent *et al*). Ann. Otolar-

Neck Dissection—Cont.

yngol. Chir. Cervicofac., *90:*609, 1973 (French)

Neck dissection, radical. Mortality and morbidity (Yarington *et al*). Arch. Otolaryng., *97:*306, 1973

Neck dissection, simultaneous bilateral radical. Preservation of external jugular vein (Weingarten). Arch. Otolaryng., *97:*309, 1973

Surgical treatment of carcinoma of pyriform sinus (Barton). Arch. Otolaryng., *97:*337, 1973

Cancer, head and neck, composite operation (commando procedure) (Yonemoto *et al*), PRS, *51:*235, 1973. Arch. Surg., *104:*809, 1973

Neck dissection; radical, elective *vs.* therapeutic, as treatment for epidermoid carcinoma of oral cavity and oropharynx (Spiro *et al*). Arch. Surg., *107:*382, 1973

Neck dissection, radical, lateral sinus thrombosis following, for malignant melanoma (Fielding *et al*). Aust. N.Z. J. Surg., *43:*228, 1973

Cervical lymph node metastasis: unknown primary cancer (Jesse *et al*). Cancer, *31:*854, 1973

Neck dissection for malignant oral and maxillofacial tumors; clinicopathological analysis of 419 cases. Chinese Med. J., *10:*596, 1973 (Chinese)

Surgical procedure in palpable lymph node hypertrophies (Eufinger). Chirurg., *44:*163, 1973 (German)

Neck dissection, pain syndromes as late sequelae of (Pfeifle *et al*). Dtsch. Zahnaerztl. Z., *28:*968, 1973 (German)

Dosage-controlled cryotherapy in inoperable, exulcerating recurrent tumor over carotid artery (Neumann *et al*). H. N. O., *21:*195, 1973 (German)

Neck dissection, place of accessory nerve repair in (Michael). H. N. O., *21:*360, 1973 (German)

Morphological changes in lymph node deposits of oral squamous carcinoma (Shear *et al*). Int. J. Oral Surg., *2:*1, 1973

Review of surgical treatment of 90 cases of cancer of thyroid (Caracciolo). Int. Surg., *58:*402, 1973

Neck dissection, radical, postoperative management with continuous suction drainage (Sekiyama *et al*). Jap. J. Oral Surg., *19:*276, 1973 (Japanese)

Conservative curettage of neck. Practical management (Perrin *et al*). J. Fr. Otorhinolaryngol., *22:*229, 1973 (French)

Neck dissection, bilateral, simultaneous

Neck Dissection—Cont.

blindness following (Chutkow, Sharbrough, Riley), PRS, *53:*374, 1974. Mayo Clin. Proc., *48:*713, 1973

Neck dissection, radical, objectives and standards in care of patient with (O'Dell). Nurs. Clin. North Am., *8:*159, 1973

Lymphographic observations following surgery of cervical lymphatic system (Adamus). Otolaryngol. Pol., *27:*451, 1973

Mixed tumor, recurrent, of lacrimal gland, cranio-orbital resection and neck dissection for (Habal, Murray), PRS, *51:*689, 1973

Approaches used in E. N. T. oncological surgery (Baron *et al*). Rev. Laryngol. Otol. Rhinol. (Bord.), *94:*521, 1973 (French)

Tumors of parapharyngeal region. II. Neural tumors, chemodectomas chordemas, branchial cysts. Surgical treatment. Conclusions (De Padua Bertelli *et al*). Rev. Paul. Med., *82:*103, 1973 (Portuguese)

Metastases, cervical node, from occult primary sites (Fu, Stewart, Bagshaw), PRS, *53:*604, 1974. Rocky Mountain M.J., *70:*31, 1973

Wound complications after neck dissection and composite resection (Doberneck), PRS, *52:*322, 1973. Surgery, *73:*261, 1973

Carcinoma, head and neck, radical neck dissection in (Kerth *et al*). Surg. Clin. North Am., *53:*179, 1973

Hemorrhage from internal jugular vein controlled by a balloon catheter (Cohen, Chretien), PRS, *52:*462, 1973. Surg. Gynec. & Obst., *136:*791, 1973

Neck dissection, elective, for carcinoma of tongue and floor of mouth (Som). Trans. Am. Acad. Ophthalmol. Otolaryngol., *77:*182, 1973

Head and neck cancer, advanced, surgical management (Vrachnos, Paraskevas, Stylogiannis), PRS, *56:*473, 1975. Tr. 8th Panhellenic Cong. Surg. Soc., *A:* 190, 1973

Place of surgery in the treatment of carcinomas of the oral cavity (Mendes da Costa *et al*). Acta chir. belg., *73:*529, 1974 (French)

Epidermoid carcinoma of the supraglottic larynx. Role of neck dissection in initial surgical treatment (Shah *et al*). Am. J. Surg., *128:*494, 1974

Adenoid cystic carcinoma of salivary origin. A clinico-pathologic study of 242 cases. (Spiro *et al*). Am. J. Surg., *128:*512, 1974

Cervical node metastasis from epidermoid carcinoma of the oral cavity and oropharynx. A critical assessment of current staging (Spiro *et al*). Am. J. Surg., *128:*562, 1974

Neck Dissection — Cont.

Results of high dose radiation and surgery in the treatment of advanced cancer of the head and neck (Carlfi *et al*). Am. J. Surg., *128:*580, 1974

Our attitude towards the treatment of thyroid cancer (a report of 50 cases) (Melliere *et al*). Ann. Endocrinol. (Paris), *35:*285, 1974 (French)

Neck dissection, bilateral, recurrent postoperative cerebral edema in patient seven years following, case history. Anesth. Analg. (Cleve.), *53:*254, 1974

Head and neck cancer, complications of radical neck dissection and their prevention (Jortay), PRS, *55:*718, 1975. Arch. chir. belg., *73:*385, 1974

Nodal metatases in T₂ supraglottic carcinoma, incidence (Cummings). Arch. Otolaryng., *99:*268, 1974

Neck, dissection radical, protection of facial nerve in (Ramsden, Maran), PRS, *54:*618, 1974. Brit. J. Surg., *61:*297, 1974

Metastatic routes in the neck (McKelvie). Can. J. Otolaryngol., *3:*473, 1974

Elective neck irradiation for TXNO squamous carcinoma of oral tongue and floor of mouth (Million). Cancer, *34:*149, 1974

Radical neck dissection in advanced tumors of the head and neck. Considerations on 52 cases (Caldarola *et al*). Cancro, *27:*187, 1974 (Italian)

Prophylactic neck dissection in oral carcinoma (Martis *et al*). Int. J. Oral Surg., *3:*293, 1974

Elective tracheostomy in head and neck tumour surgery (Shaw *et al*). J. Laryng. & Otol., *88:*599, 1974

Neck dissection, pseudotumors of clavicle following (Pfeifle *et al*), PRS, *54:*502, 1974. J. Maxillo-facial Surg., *2:*14, 1974

Mortality in head and neck operations (Kogge, Koch), PRS, *54:*625, 1974. J. Maxillo-facial Surg., *2:*32, 1974

Anomalies of subclavian artery in head and neck surgery (Landa, Lesavoy), PRS, *55:*376, 1975. J. Maxillo-facial Surg., *2:*104, 1974

Laryngectomized patient, speech and vocational rehabilitation of (Sako *et al*). J. Surg. Oncol., *6:*197, 1974

Tumors of submandibular gland (Trail *et al*). Laryngoscope, *84:*1225, 1974

Delirium tremens in head and neck surgery (Helmus *et al*). Laryngoscope, *84:*1479, 1974

Carcinoma of the tonsil: results of combined therapy (Maltz *et al*). Laryngoscope, *84:*2172, 1974

Neck Dissection — Cont.

Surgical technique (Sedgwick). Major Probl. Clin. Surg., *15:*170, 1974

Neck dissection and laryngectomy, incisions for (Snow). O. R. L., *36:*61, 1974

Immune response: prognostic significance of delayed cutaneous reactivity in head and neck cancer patients (Mandel, Kiehn), PRS, *53:*72, 1974

Lymph node metastases in oral carcinoma, correlation of histopathology with survival (Noone *et al*), PRS, *53:*158, 1974

Neck dissection, radical, value in patients with advanced metastasizing melanoblastoma of head and neck (Kluzak), PRS, *54:*619, 1974. Rozhl. chir., *53:*204, 1974

Carcinoma, recurrent, of neck, staged palliative resection using extra anatomic carotid bypass (Hagood, Mozersky, Fite), PRS, *56:*113, 1975. Surgery, *76:*671, 1974

Surgical anatomy of the neck (Jurkiewicz *et al*). Surg. Clin. North Am., *54:*1269, 1974

Anesthesiological problems in head and neck surgery (Emanuelli *et al*). Tumori, *60:*491, 1974 (Italian)

Significance and methods of surgical treatment of lymphatic spread (Giacomelli). Tumori, *60:*567, 1974 (Italian)

Indications, limitations and results of traditional latero-cervical lymph node excision (Molinari). Tumori, *60:*573, 1974 (Italian)

Indications, limits and results of functional latero-cervical lymph node excision (Pignataro). Tumori, *60:*585, 1974 (Italian)

Cancer of the Head and Neck. By R. G. Chambers *et al*. Excerpta Medica Co., Amsterdam, 1975

Papillary thyroid carcinoma in Denmark 1943–68. II. Treatment and survival (Lindahl). Acta Chir. Scand., *14:*504, 1975

Cervical lymph node excision. Conservative technics (Lachard *et al*). Acta Stomatol. Belg., *72:*393, 1975 (French)

Epidermoid carcinoma with sebaceous differentiation in the vallecula. Report of a case (Assor). Am. J. Clin. Pathol., *63:*891, 1975

Control by irradiation alone of nonfixed clinically positive lymph nodes from squamous cell carcinoma of the oral cavity, oropharynx, supraglottic larynx, and hypopharynx (Schneider *et al*). Am. J. Roentgenol. Radium Ther. Nucl. Med., *123:*42, 1975

Chylothorax complicating radical neck dissection (Cavallo *et al*). Am. Surg., *41:*266, 1975

Comparison of long-term carcinologic results between radical and conservative cervical surgery (Andre *et al*). Ann. Otolaryngol. Chir. Cervicofac., *92:*113, 1975 (French)

Neck Dissection — Cont.

Cervical metastasis from an unknown primary (Fried *et al*). Ann. Otol. Rhin. & Laryng., *84:*152, 1975

Primary oat-cell carcinoma of head and neck (Gelot *et al*). Ann. Otol. Rhin. & Laryng., *84:*238, 1975

Rehabilitation of the shoulder after radical neck dissection (Saunders *et al*). Ann. Otol. Rhin. & Laryng., *84:*812, 1975

Transsternal radical neck dissection. Postoperative complications and management (Sisson *et al*). Arch. Otolaryng., *101:*46, 1975

Complications of dermal graft protection of carotid artery (Dedo *et al*). Arch. Otolaryng., *101:*649, 1975

Radical neck dissection: elective, therapeutic and secondary (Lee *et al*). Arch. Otolaryng., *101:*656, 1975

Elective carotid artery resection (Martinez *et al*). Arch. Otolaryng., *101:*744, 1975

Multiple primary tumors. Four distinct head and neck tumors (Iannaccone). Arch. Pathol., *99:*270, 1975

Combined radiation therapy and surgery in the treatment of advanced head and neck cancer (Rossman). Ariz. Med., *32:*869, 1975

The surgery of thyroid cancer (Johnston). Brit. J. Surg., *62:*765, 1975

Neck dissection, radical, right, chylous fistula following (Mallen *et al*). Can. J. Otolaryngol., *4:*177, 1975

Limitations of surgery in the treatment of head and neck cancer (Stell). Can. J. Otolaryngol., *4:*508, 1975

Irradiation of clinically uninvolved cervical lymph nodes (Goffinet *et al*). Can. J. Otolaryngol., *4:*927, 1975

Combination of radiotherapy and surgery in the treatment of head and neck cancers (Cachin *et al*). Cancer Treat. Rev., *2:*177, 1975

Value of tomography of the sterno-clavicular region (Morag *et al*). Clin. Radiol., *26:*57, 1975

Covering of defects in the lateral head and neck regions with shoulder flaps (Schaupp *et al*). H.N.O., *23:*160, 1975 (German)

Treatment of cancerous adenopathies of the neck (Andre). J. Fr. Otorhinolaryngol., *24:*223, 1975 (French)

Diagnostic and therapeutic regime for reducing mortality after resection of tumors in head and neck (Reil *et al*). J. Maxillo-facial Surg., *3:*54, 1975

Tumor resection combined with neck dissection, reconstruction of lower lip after (Lentrodt), PRS, *57:*529, 1976. J. Maxillo-facial

Neck Dissection — Cont.

Surg., *3:*139, 1975

Chylothorax, postoperative. Six cases in 2,500 operations, with survey of world literature (Cevese *et al*). J. Thorac. Cardiovasc. Surg., *69:*966, 1975

Regional neck lymph nodes and primary tumors. 1. Neck lymph node metastases (Simon). Laryngol. Rhinol. Otol. (Stuttg.), *54:*997, 1975 (German)

Use of thermography to evaluate the optimum time for surgery after preoperative radiation (Scruggs *et al*). Laryngoscope, *85:*726, 1975

Management of chylous fistulas (Meyers *et al*). Laryngoscope, *85:*835, 1975

Muscle and fascial grafts in carotid artery protection (Sadoyama). Laryngoscope, *85:*841, 1975

Planned pharyngostome (de Souza *et al*). Laryngoscope, *85:*848, 1975

The problem of advanced supraglottic carcinoma (Siirala *et al*). Laryngoscope, *85:*1633, 1975

Surgical therapy of thyroid malignoma (Pichimaier *et al*). Med. Klin., *70:*158, 1975 (German)

Bronchiolar obstruction, further experiences with the arytenoid-epiglottic flap for chronic aspiration pneumonia (Vecchione, Habal, Murray), PRS, *55:*318, 1975

Neck dissection, radical, stress fracture of clavicle after (Cummings, First), PRS, *55:*366, 1975

Neck lump, patient has (Devine), PRS, *57:*118, 1976. Postgrad. Med., *57:*131, 1975

Nodes, metastatic lymph, in neck, significance and management of (Burge), PRS, *56:*464, 1975. Proc. Roy. Soc. Med., *68:*77, 1975

An original method of plastic surgery after treatment of cancer of the lower lip by resection (Urtila). Rev. Stomatol. Chir. Maxillofac., *76:*579, 1975 (French)

Use of double transverse incision with radical block dissection of the neck (van Zyl *et al*). S. Afr. J. Surg., *13:*43, 1975 (Afrikaans)

Rehabilitation needs of the cancer patient (Villanueva). South. Med. J., *68:*169, 1975

Hearing impairment following radical neck dissection (Young *et al*). Trans. Pa. Acad. Ophthalmol. Otolaryngol., *28:*155, 1975

Posterior triangle in radical neck surgery (Skolnik *et al*). Arch. Otolaryng., *102:*1, 1976

Synovial sarcoma of the neck: report of case (Mitcherling *et al*). J. Oral Surg., *34:*64, 1976

Neck Dissection – Cont.

Tumors, skin testing for prognosis or therapy formulation in cancer patients: *caveat emptor* (Mandel), PRS, *57:*621, 1976. Discussion by Humphrey, PRS, *57:*743, 1976

Resection and immediate reconstruction for patients with "inoperable" recurrent head and neck cancer (Robson). Surg. Clin. North Am., *56:*111, 1976

Neck Neoplasms (See also *Neck Dissections*)

Surgery, radiological and combined treatment of latero-cervical metastases (Cherubino *et al*). Arch. Ital. Otol., *80:*297, 1969 (Italian)

Neck tumors and fistulae in children (Loynoz, Bricano), PRS, *48:*196, 1971. Bol. Soc. Venezuelana Cir., *24:*955, 1970

Clinical observations on postoperative reflex syndromes of the cervical autonomic nervous system (Lentini *et al*). Clin. Otorinolaringoiatr. *22:*104, 1970 (Italian)

Two unusual cases of neck tumors (Disleiev *et al*). Khirurgiia (Sofiia), *23:*408, 1970 (Bulgarian)

Thyroid tumors, surgical treatment of (Greening). Monogr. Neoplast. Dis. Var. Sites, *6:*231, 1970

Rare vascular tumor of the neck: cystic hygroma of the neck (Stefanovic *et al*). Srp. Arh. Celok. Lek., *98:*1065, 1970 (Serbian)

Head and neck surgery: the pursuit of excellence (Baker). Am. J. Surg., *122:*433, 1971

Soft part sarcomas of the head and neck (Farr). Am. J. Surg., *122:*714, 1971

Major cervico-facial surgery and geriatrics (Andre *et al*). Ann. Otolaryngol. Chir. Cervicofac., *88:*295, 1971 (French)

Complications of head and neck surgery (Kornblut *et al*). Arch. Otolaryng., *94:*246, 1971

Neurogenous neoplasms of major nerves of face and neck (Katz, Passy, Kaplan), PRS, *49:*235, 1972. Arch. Surg., *103:*51, 1971

Tumor therapy with high frequency hyperthermia (decimeter-waves). Animal experiments (Dietzel *et al*). Biomed. Tech. (Stuttg.), *16:*213, 1971 (German)

Surgical technic for malignant melanoma of the skin in the head and neck region (Grimm *et al*). Dtsch. Zahn. Mund. Kieferheilkd., *57:*363, 1971 (German)

Experience in indwelling aspiration by a tube drain following surgery of cervical metastases of malignant oral cancer (Shimizu). J. Jap. Stomatol. Soc., *38:*574, 1971 (Japanese)

Development in the Japan Society of Cancer Research of the Head and Neck Region in

Neck Neoplasms – Cont.

the last few years (Sakai). J. Otolaryngol. Jap., *74:*550, 1971 (Japanese)

Diagnosis and treatment of neurogenic tumors of the neck (Afrapetian). Khirurgiia (Mosk.), *47:*53, 1971 (Russian)

Case of successfully operated thyroid cancer infiltrating great vessels on the left side of the neck (Dobrev *et al*). Khirurgiia (Sofiia), *24:*214, 1971 (Bulgarian)

Cryosurgery in the management of tumors of the head and neck (Chandler *et al*). South. Med. J., *64:*1440, 1971

Case of multiple primary carcinomas of the head and neck (Franke *et al*). Wis. Med. J., *70:*242, 1971

Neck and head, cutaneous melanoma of, clinicopathologic study (Donnellan *et al*), PRS, *52:*103, 1973. Am. J. Surg., *124:*450, 1972

Neck, malignant melanoma of (Simons), PRS, *52:*102, 1973. Am. J. Surg., *124:*485, 1972

Neck, cancer of, preoperative irradiation in (Moore, Mullins; Scott), PRS, *52:*213, 1973. Am. J. Surg., *124:*555, 1972

Neck chemodectomas, selective management (Westbrook *et al*), PRS, *52:*102, 1973. Am. J. Surg., *124:*760, 1972

Role of surgery in the management of postcricoid and cervical esophageal neoplasms (Harrison). Ann. Otol. Rhin. & Laryng., *81:*465, 1972

Operability of metastatic neck cancer (Shaw). Brit. J. Clin. Pract., *26:*187, 1972

Biopsy of cervical swelling (Huot). Can. J. Otolaryngol., *1:*310, 1972 (French)

Treatment of head and neck cancer with intra-arterial cytotoxic drugs and radiotherapy (Sealy *et al*). Cancer, *30:*187, 1972

Clinical and therapeutical problems in metastases of the cervical lymph nodes (Bohndorf). Fortschr. Geb. Roentgenstr. Nuklearmed., *116:*246, 1972 (German)

Combined cytostatic and irradiation treatment of head and neck tumors using the synchronization effect (Glupe *et al*). H. N. O., *20:*18, 1972 (German)

Cervical teratoma (Rickham). Helv. Pediatr. Acta, *27:*549, 1972 (German)

Teratoma, cervical neonatal, case report (Singh *et al*). Indian Pediatr., *9:*229, 1972

Palliative surgery (Galsford). J.A.M.A., *221:*83, 1972

Cryosurgery of malignant neoplasms of the head and neck (Chandler). J.A.M.A., *221:*387, 1972

Skin flaps in head and neck surgery (Stell *et al*). J. Laryng. & Otol., *86:*419, 1972

Value of preoperative angiography in the

Neck Neoplasms – Cont.

surgical management of cervical hourglass neurofibroma. Case report (Rinaldi). J. Neurosurg., 36:97, 1972

Neck, malignant tumors of, combined therapy for (Oshmianskaia). Med. Radiol. (Mosk.), 17:78, 1972

Neurogenic tumor of the neck in the newborn, report of a case healed with only surgical treatment (Bonamico et al). Minerva Pediatr., 24:266, 1972 (Italian)

Surgery in cancer of head and neck. Use of posterior cervical flap (Lenczyk et al). N. Y. State J. Med., 72:239, 1972

Intra-arterial infusion. A seven-year study (Lawton et al). Oncology, 26:259, 1972

Therapeutic methods in angiotenic tumor of the head and neck (Koike et al). Otolaryngology (Tokyo), 44:93, 1972 (Japanese)

Advanced neoplasms of head and neck. Treatment with combined radiation and chemotherapy (Cammack et al). Rocky Mt. Med. J., 69:54, 1972

Burkitt's lymphoma in West Malaysia (Ramanathan), PRS, 52:103, 1973. Southeast Asian J. Trop. Med., 3:249, 1972

Management of vascular tumors of the head and neck (Komorn). South. Med. J., 65:1106, 1972

Surgery, reconstructive, newer concepts in patients with head and neck cancer (Salyer, Nickell), PRS, 51:485, 1973. South. M.J., 65:1364, 1972

Successfully operated case of cervical teratoma in a newborn infant (Kitano et al). Surg. Ther. (Osaka), 26:236, 1972 (Japanese)

Indications for surgical treatment of cervical chemodectomas (Viturin et al). Vestn. Khir., 108:3, 1972 (Russian)

Neurilemmoma of cervical portion of vagus nerve (Reddick, Myers), PRS, 53:111, 1974. Am. J. Surg., 125:744, 1973

Cure and palliation by surgery in advanced cancer of head and neck (Bakamjian et al), PRS, 53:688, 1974. Am. J. Surg., 126:482, 1973

Hamartomas of cervical region (Manigand et al). Ann. Med. Interne (Paris), 124:433, 1973 (French)

Schwannoma, latero-cervical, remarks on case (Cinca et al). Ann. Otolaryngol. Chir. Cervicofac., 90:307, 1973 (French)

Malignancy, metastatic cervical, occult primary (Winegar, Griffin), PRS, 54:501, 1974. Arch. Otolaryng., 98:159, 1973

Neck, teratoma of (Gray). Aust. N.Z. J. Surg., 42:294, 1973

Neck, giant cystic hygroma, treatment

Neck Neoplasms – Cont.

(Crawford, Vivakananthan), PRS, 54:697, 1974. Brit. J. Plast. Surg., 26:69, 1973

Parathyroid carcinoma (Schantz, Castleman), PRS, 52:458, 1973. Cancer, 31:600, 1973

Fibromatous type ossifying cervical tumor (Gaillard et al). J. Fr. Otorhinolaryngol., 22:533, 1973 (French)

Intercarotid glomus and its glomic tumor (Taillens). J. Fr. Otorhinolaryngol., 22:595, 1973 (French)

Hypernephroma metastatic to head and neck (Miyamoto et al). Laryngoscope, 83:898, 1973

Carotid body tumors – idiosyncracies (Pollack). Oncology, 27:81, 1973

Lipoma of submandibular space with osseous metaplasia (Dutescu et al). Oral Surg., 35:611, 1973

Tumor of neck: giant lipoma of back and neck (Hirshowitz, Goldan), PRS, 52:312, 1973

Lipomatosis at prevailing cervical localization (Visentini, Mazzoleni, Linda), PRS, 56:363, 1975. Riv. ital. chir. plast., 5:483, 1973

Malignant carotid body tumors, 16-year follow-up of 7 cases (Martin, Rosenfeld, McSwain), PRS, 53:612, 1974. South. M.J., 66:1236, 1973

Chemodectomas of head and neck (Howell et al). Surg. Clin. North Am., 53:175, 1973

Neurofibromatosis of cervico-occipital region (Smirnitskii). Vestn. Khir., 110:124, 1973 (Russian)

Thyroid neoplasms, treatment of, following radiotherapy, surgical aspects of (Balazs et al). Zentralbl. Chir., 98:1842, 1973 (German)

Surgical treatment for a glomus jugulare tumor – report of a case growing extensively (Hakuba). A. Neurol. Surg. (Tokyo), 2:403, 1974 (Japanese)

Neck, solitary mass in, diagnosis and treatment (Doberneck). Am. Surg., 40:181, 1974

Tumors, invasive glomus jugular, total extirpation of (Kaya et al), PRS, 56:464, 1975. Ann. oto-laryng., 91:595, 1974

Tumors of neck, midline dermoid (Katz), PRS, 55:640, 1975. Arch. Surg., 109:822, 1974

Cancer, thyroid, in young patients in Great Britain (Richardson et al). Brit. J. Surg., 61:85, 1974

Metastatic routes in the neck (McKelvie). Can. J. Otolaryngol., 3:473, 1974

Rhabdomyosarcoma of the head and neck (Smith). Can. J. Otolaryngol., 3:618, 1974

Large flap plasty in otorhinolaryngology

Neck Neoplasms — Cont.

(Holub *et al*). Cesk. Otolaryngol., *23:*96, 1974 (Czech)

Neck and superior mediastinum, unusual tumor of (Kiely *et al*). J. Ir. Med. Assoc., *67:*306, 1974

Teratomas, multiple, of head and neck (Dudgeon *et al*). J. Pediatr., *85:*139, 1974

Carcinoma of the thyroid gland: current therapy (Marchetta). J. Surg. Oncol., *6:*401, 1974

Neck, tumors of great blood vessels in, experiments on cryosurgery of (Ganz). Minerva Med., *65:*3645, 1974

Adriamycin as chemotherapy for thyroid cancer (Gottlieb, Hill), PRS, *54:*373, 1974. New England J. Med., *290:*193, 1974

Neck, teratoma of, in children (Melikov *et al*). Pediatriia, *3:*78, 1974 (Russian)

Hygroma of the neck (Gorban). Rev. Stomatol. Chir. Maxillofac., *75:*284 1974 (French)

Hyperparathyroidism, primary, trends in current management (Haff *et al*). Surgery, *75:*715, 1974

Neck carcinoma, recurrent, staged palliative resection using extra anatomic carotid bypass (Hagood, Mozersky, Fite), PRS, *56:*113, 1975. Surgery, *76:*671, 1974

Branchiogenic carcinoma (Betkowski). Wiad. Lek., *27:*1671, 1974 (Polish)

Pharyngocervical neuroma (Kruk-Zagajewska *et al*). Wiad. Lek., *27:*1893, 1974 (Polish)

Surgery and postoperative radiotherapy in the treatment of soft tissue sarcomas in adults (Lindberg *et al*). Am. J. Roentgenol. Radium Ther. Nucl. Med., *123:*123, 1975

Childhood rhabdomyosarcoma. Analysis of coordinated therapy and results (Fernandez *et al*). Am. J. Roentgenol. Radium Ther. Nucl. Med., *123:*588, 1975

Head and neck cancer manpower study (Strong *et al*). Am. J. Surg., *129:*273, 1975

Thyroid cancer, childhood, a lethal disease? (Buckwalter *et al*). Ann. Surg., *18:*632, 1975

Carcinoid tumor metastatic to neck (Welling, Taggart), PRS, *55:*724, 1975. Arch. Surg., *110:*111, 1975

Role of surgery in the management of thyroid cancer (Mustard). Can. Med. Assoc. J., *113:*109, 1975

Cervical synovial sarcoma at the bifurcation of the carotid artery (Golomb *et al*). Cancer, *35:*483, 1975

Cervical thymoma (Bothra *et al*). Int. Surg., *60:*301, 1975

Glomus jugulare tumours (a series of 21 cases) (Thomsen *et al*). J. Laryng. & Otol.,

Neck Neoplasms — Cont.

*89:*1113, 1975

Use of thermography to evaluate the optimum time for surgery after preoperative radiation (Scruggs *et al*). Laryngoscope, *85:*726, 1975

Carcinoma, medullary, of thyroid gland in "multiple mucosal neuromata syndrome" (Bowers), PRS, *56:*554, 1975

Neck, metastatic lymph nodes in, significance and management (Burge), PRS, *56:*464, 1975. Proc. Roy. Soc. Med., *68:*77, 1975

Cancer from remnants of thyrolingual duct (Valdina *et al*). Vopr. Onkol., *21:*16, 1975 (Russian)

Synovial sarcoma of the neck: report of case (Mitcherling *et al*). J. Oral Surg., *34:*64, 1976

Neck, migrating cervical mass (Futrell, Izant), PRS, *57:*660, 1976

Methotrexate toxicity, synergistic effect of salicylates on (Mandel), PRS, *57:*733, 1976

Neck Surgery (See also *Cancer, Head and Neck; Neck Dissections*)

Thyroidectomy in pediatric patient, indications for (Sanfelippo, Beahrs, Hayles), PRS, *51:*702, 1973. Am. J. Surg., *122:*472, 1971

Head and Neck Surgery. By P. M. Stell and A. G. D. Maran. J. B. Lippincott Co., Philadelphia, 1972. PRS, *52:*295, 1973

Cancer, head and neck, preoperative irradiation in (Moore *et al*). Am. J. Surg., *124:*555, 1972

Cancer, head and neck, reconstructive surgery of (Takeda *et al*). J. Otolaryngol. Jap., *75:*1085, 1972 (Japanese)

Epiglottic flap to the arytenoids in surgical treatment of life-endangering chronic aspiration pneumonia (Habal, Murray), PRS, *49:*305, 1972

Cancer, head and neck, irradiated, deltopectoral flap for reconstruction of (Krizek *et al*). Surg. Gynec. & Obst., *135:*787, 1972

Neck, cervical pharyngoesophageal reconstruction, prefabrication techniques in (Bakamjian, Holbrook), PRS, *55:*107, 1975. Brit. J. Plast. Surg., *26:*214, 1973

Cancer, head and neck, mortality in surgery for (Williams *et al*). J. Laryng. & Otol., *87:*431, 1973

Vein, internal jugular, hemorrhage controlled by balloon catheter (Cohen, Chretien), PRS, *52:*462, 1973. Surg. Gynec. & Obst., *136:*791, 1973

Neck, treatment of injuries involving loss (Hasman), PRS, *54:*617, 1974. Acta chir.,

Neck Surgery – Cont.
53:208, 1974
Neck operations, certain, characteristics of anesthesiological care in (Aleksandrov *et al*). Klin. Khir., *10:*23, 1974 (Russian)
Cancer, head and neck, recurrent, surgical management (Som *et al*). Otolaryngol. Clin. North Am., *7:*163, 1974
Cancer, head and neck, recurrent, cryosurgery for (Chandler). Otolaryngol. Clin. North Am., *7:*193, 1974
Paralysis, trapezius, after minor surgical procedures in posterior cervical triangle (Dunn). South. Med. J., *67:*312, 1974
Success rate of cervical exploration for hyperparathyroidism (Satava *et al*). Arch. Surg., *110:*625, 1975
Cancer, head and neck, management of recurrent (Editorial). Brit. Med. J., *2:*54, 1975
Flap, arytenoid-epiglottic, for chronic aspiration pneumonia, further experiences with (Vecchione, Habal Murray), PRS, *55:*318, 1975

NEDELEC, M. *et al*: Neo-bladder made from the rectum in surgical care of uro-genital malformations. J. Urol. Nephrol. (Paris), *81:*481, 1975
NEEL, H. B., III: Cryosurgery for tumors of head and neck. Experimental and clinical considerations. Minn. Med., *55:*886, 1972
NEEL, H. B., III, KETCHAM, A. S., AND HAMMOND, W. G.: Requisites for successful cryogenic surgery of cancer, PRS, *48:*398, 1971. Arch. Surg., *102:*45, 1971
NEEL, H. B., III *et al*: Juvenile angiofibroma, PRS, *53:*496, 1974. Am. J. Surg., *126:*547, 1973
NEELY, M. G.: Lung transplantation, PRS, *52:*688, 1973. Proc. Roy. Australasian Coll. Surg., *46:*152, 1973
NEFF, G.: Occupational therapeutic measures before and after surgical correction of hands with congenital malformations. Handchirurgie, *7:*99, 1975 (German)
NEIMAN, G. S. *et al*: Delayed pharyngeal flap success: report of a case. Cleft Palate J., *12:*244, 1975
NELSON, C. L., SAWMILLER, S., AND PHALEN, G. S.: Ganglions of wrist and hand, PRS, *51:*478, 1973. J. Bone & Joint Surg., *54A:*1459, 1972
NELSON, I. W., PARKIN, J. L., AND POTTER, J. F.: Modified Tokyo larynx, PRS, *57:*396, 1976. Arch. Otolaryng., *101:*107, 1975
NELSON, P.: Partial-thickness grafting in cases of fingertip injuries, PRS, *55:*510, 1975. Rev. Latino Am. cir. plast., *17:*47, 1973

NELMET, P. *et al*: Comment on bank storage of fascia lata. Arch. Ophth., *88:*695, 1972

Neoplasms, Miscellaneous

Neoplasia, epithelial, possible role of riboflavin deficiency in. II. Effect on skin tumor development (Wynder, Chan), PRS, *48:*93, 1971. Cancer, *26:*1221, 1970
Meningioma, parapharyngeal, with special reference to cell of origin (Shuangshoti, Netzky, Fitz-Hugh), PRS, *49:*237, 1972. Ann. Otol. Rhin. & Laryng., *80:*464, 1971
Parosteal sarcoma (Sota), PRS, *49:*474, 1972. Rev. Latino Am. cir. plast., *15:*45, 1971
Tumor excisions, repair of cutaneous defects around natural orifices (Garcia), PRS, *52:*603, 1973. Bol. Soc. Venezuelana Cir., *26:*351, 1972
Complications of chemosurgery (Aronsohn). Eye Ear Nose Throat Mon., *51:*48, 1972
Frozen section experience in 3,249 specimens (Lerman, Pitcock), PRS, *51:*712, 1973. Surg. Gynec. & Obst., *135:*930, 1972
Tumors, visceral, spreading to skin (Brownstein, Helwig), PRS, *52:*460, 1973. Arch. Dermat., *107:*80, 1973
Ectopic meningiomas (Shuangshoti *et al*). Arch. Otolaryng., *98:*102, 1973
Tumor, occult primary (Winegar, Griffin), PRS, *54:*501, 1974. Arch. Otolaryng., *98:*159, 1973
Leukemia virus infection, marine, genetic factors in (Rowe), PRS, *54:*242, 1974. Cancer Res., *33:*3061, 1973
Tumors of soft tissues, management of some (Fuentes-Aguilar), PRS, *54:*380, 1974. Cir. Cir., *41:*175, 1973
Tumor cells in bone, methylcholanthrene, fate of: analysis of immune factors in host resistance (McLaughlin *et al*), PRS, *53:*688, 1974. J. Surg. Res., *14:*186, 1973
Gliomas, nasal (Kubo, Garrett, Musgrave), PRS, *52:*47, 1973
Neurilemmoma of facial nerve (Conley, Janecka), PRS, *52:*55, 1973
Sarcomas, soft part, in children (Exelby). Proc. Natl. Cancer Conf., *7:*619, 1973
Adenomegalies, problems of diagnosis in certain (Gingold *et al*). Rev. Roum. Med. Intern., *10:*295, 1973 (French)
Sarcomas, soft tissue, management of (Das Gupta). Surg. Gynec. & Obst., *137:*1012, 1973
Hemipelvectomy – indications, technic, and results on 4 cases (Eliopoulos *et al*), PRS, *56:*473, 1975. Tr. 8th Panhellenic Cong. Surg. Soc., *A:*263, 1973
Tumors, malignant, solid, in childhood, diag-

Nerve, Median (See also *Leprosy*)

Neurovascular cutaneous island pedicles for deficient median nerve sensibility. New technique and results of serial functional tests (Omer *et al*), PRS, *49:*104, 1972. J. Bone & Joint Surg., *52A:*1181, 1970

Median nerve palsy, use of transverse carpal ligament window for pulley in tendon transfers for (Snow, Fink), PRS, *48:*238, 1971

Hamartomas of median nerve, treatment of (Paletta, Rybka), PRS, *51:*705, PRS, *51:*705, 1973. Ann. Surg., *176:*217, 1972

Syndrome, Kiloh-Nevin. Dissociated paralysis of median nerve in forearm caused by compression of anterior interosseous nerve (Luppino *et al*). Chir. Organi. Mov., *61:*89, 1972 (Italian)

Median and ulnar nerves, interfascicular nerve grafting of (Millesi, Meissl, Berger), PRS, *51:*233, 1973. J. Bone & Joint Surg., *54B:*727, 1972

Nerve, median in carpal tunnel, neurolysis as surgical treatment of Kienbock's disease (Codega, Codega, Kus), PRS, *53:*246, 1974. Internat. Surg., *58:*378, 1973

Carpal tunnel, palmar cutaneous branch of the median nerve and the approach to (Taleisnik), PRS, *53:*684, 1974. J. Bone & Joint Surg., *55:*1212, 1973

Struthers' ligament: source of median nerve compression above elbow (Smith, Fisher), PRS, *53:*366, 1974. J. Neurosurg., *38:*778, 1973

Paralyzed median nerve, repair of sensation by nerve crossing (Hara, Tsuyama, Furusawa), PRS, *53:*369, 1974. Operation, *27:*551, 1973

Median nerve at wrist, variations of motor branch of (Graham), PRS, *51:*90, 1973

Anastomosis to restore median nerve function after destructive lesions which preclude end-to-end repair (Sunderland), PRS, *57:*537, 1976. Brain, *97:*1, 1974

Simultaneous plastic surgery of brachial artery and median nerve in their complete intersection (Manakov *et al*). Ortop. Travmatol. Protez., *35:*60, 1974 (Russian)

Thrombophlebitis-induced median neuropathy (Oh, Kim), PRS, *55:*510, 1975. South. M.J., *67:*1041, 1974)

Nerve, Radial (See also *Leprosy*)

Radial tunnel syndrome (Roles, Maudsley), PRS, *52:*679, 1973. J. Bone & Joint Surg., *54B:*499, 1972

Radial nerve entrapment in exuberant callus from fractured humerus (Jackson *et al*),

Nerve, Radial—Cont.

PRS, *51:*705, 1973. Mil. Med., *137:*203, 1972

Radial nerve innervated cross finger flap to reconstruct thumb (Wilkinson), PRS, *51:*476, 1973. South. M.J., *65:*992, 1972

Nerve, radial, compressed in patients with rheumatoid arthritis (Millender, Nalebuff, Holdsworth), PRS, *52:*323, 1973. J. Bone & Joint Surg., *55A:*375, 1973

Paralysis of deep radial (posterior interosseous) nerve caused by lipoma (Wu, Jordan, Eckert), PRS, *54:*508, 1974. Surgery, *75:*790, 1974

Nerve, Transplantation (See also *Nerve Grafts*)

Spinal cord, transplantations of nerves and roots of (Petrov). Reconstr. Surg., Traumatol., *12:*250, 1971

Nerve transplants, treatment of injuries to brachial plexus (Millesi, Meissl, Katzer), PRS, *53:*108, 1974. Bruns' Beitr. klin. Chir., *220:*429, 1973

Nerve transplantation, cross-face, reconstruction of face in facial paralysis (Anderl), PRS, *53:*249, 1974. Chir. Plast., *2:*17, 1973

Adhesives for nerve transplantation, report on animal experiments (Matras *et al*), PRS, *52:*453, 1973. J. Maxillo-facial Surg., *1:*37, 1973

Nerve defects in head and neck, reconstruction of (Hausamen, Samii, Schmidseder), PRS, *55:*720, 1975. J. Maxillo-facial Surg., *2:*159, 1974

Nerve homografting, experimental study of regeneration of sympathetic nerve fibers after (Hirasawa *et al*). PRS, *54:*671, 1974

Nerve, Ulnar (See also *Leprosy*)

Ulnar nerve, entrapment at elbow (Ho, Marmor), PRS, *48:*606, 1971. Am. J. Surg., *121:*355, 1971

Ulnar neuropathy at elbow, results of anterior transposition for (Levy, Apfelberg), PRS, *50:*419, 1972. Am. J. Surg., *123:*304, 1972

Arm, course of ulnar nerve in (Kane, Kaplan, Spinner), PRS, *53:*106, 1974. Ann. Chir., *27:*487, 1973

Ulnar nerve, effect of graded compression on nerve conduction velocity (Rainer *et al*), PRS, *53:*684, 1974. Arch. Surg., *107:*719, 1973

Paralysis, ulnar, filling first intermetacarpal space (Blanco, Aramburu, Maldonado), PRS, *54:*620, 1974. Bol. Sudamer. cir. Mano, *5:*38, 1973

Palsy, ulnar nerve, 16 cases treated by de-

Nerve, Ulnar — Cont.

compression without transposition (Wilson, Krout), PRS, *53:*366, 1974. J. Neurosurg., *38:*780, 1973

Ulnar neuropathy: dynamic anatomy of the ulnar nerve at elbow (Apfelberg, Larson). PRS, *51:*76, 1973

Arch, transverse metacarpal, reconstruction of, in ulnar palsy by transfer of the *extensor digiti minimi* (Ranney). PRS, *52:*406, 1973

Ulnar nerve in hand, fibrotic arch around deep branch of (Lotem, Gloobe, Nathan), PRS, *52:*553, 1973. Discussion by Weeks, PRS, *52:*556, 1973

Forearm, ulnar nerve compression in distal part of, hypertrophy of *flexor carpi ulnaris* as cause of (Harrelson *et al*), PRS, *57:*534, 1976. J. Bone & Joint Surg., *57A:* 554, 1975

Nerves, Injuries of (See also *Facial Paralysis*)

Peripheral nerve and root disturbances following active immunization against smallpox and tetanus (Deliyannakis), PRS, *48:*608, 1971. Mil. Med., *136:*458, 1971

Peripheral nerves, some thoughts on repair of (Madden, Peacock), PRS, *48:*91, 1971. South. M. J., *64:*17, 1971

Surgical Disorders of the Peripheral Nerve. By Sir Herbert Seddon. Williams & Wilkins Co., Baltimore, 1971. PRS, *52:*82, 1973

Nerve injury, limb ischemia and (Lungborg), PRS, *51:*350, 1973. Arch. Surg., *104:*631, 1972

Nerve sutures, primary, danger of (Grigorovitch), PRS, *52:*208, 1973. Bull. Soc. Internat. Chir., *6:*495, 1972

Neurectomy, vidian, results of (Tsutsumi *et al*). J. Otolaryngol. Japan, *75:*1207, 1972 (Japanese)

Nerves, injured, effect of mobilization on blood supply (Kline *et al*), PRS, *51:*349, 1973. J. Surg. Res., *12:*254, 1972

Nerves, injured, operative surgical restitution of (Samii), PRS, *51:*480, 1973. Langenbecks Arch. Chir., *332:*255, 1972

Nerve damage, causes and clinical signs of (Hensell), PRS, *51:*480, 1973. Langenbecks Arch. Chir., *332:*339, 1972

Nerves, peripheral transected, operative repair of (Millesi), PRS, *51:*481, 1973. Langenbecks Arch. Chir., *332:*347, 1972

Peripheral nerve lesions, reconstructive operations for (Friedebold), PRS, *53:*369, 1974. Langenbecks Arch. Chir., *332:*363, 1972

Nerve conduction velocity, effect of graded compression on (Rainer *et al*), PRS, *53:*684, 1974. Arch. Surg., *107:*719, 1973

Nerves, Injuries of — Cont.

Nerves, peripheral, microsurgery of (Millesi), PRS, *54:*375, 1974. Hand, *5:*157, 1973

Muscle fibers, skeletal, denervation of different types of (Tomanek, Lund), PRS, *55:*258, 1975. J. Anat., *116:*395, 1973

Nerve lesions, iatrogenic, location and prognosis (Leven *et al*). Munch. Med. Wochenschr., *115:*1956, 1973 (German)

Ganglions, human trigeminal, recovery of herpes-simplex virus from (Baringer, Swoveland), PRS, *52:*321, 1973. New England J. Med., *288:*648, 1973

Nerve injuries, peripheral (Levy). S. Afr. J. Surg., *11:*255, 1973

Nerve injuries, peripheral (Ellis), PRS, *56:*230, 1975. Hand, *6:*142, 1974

Nerve injury, estimating loss of sensation after by tactile adherence (Harrison), PRS, *56:*229, 1975. Hand, *6:*148, 1974

Nerves, peripheral, effect of cryosurgery on (Beazley, Bagley, Ketcham), PRS, *54:*687, 1974. J. Surg. Res., *16:*231, 1974

Microsurgery, restoring sensation to cut inferior alveolar nerve by direct anastomosis or by free autologous nerve grafting (Hausamen, Samii, Schmidseder). PRS, *53:*83, 1974

Nerves, peripheral, diamond knife for microsurgical repair of (Terzis, Faibisoff, Williams). PRS, *53:*102, 1974

Nerves, peripheral, polyethylene bag background in microsurgical repair of (Terzis, Faibisoff, Williams). PRS, *53:*596, 1974

Nerve involvement in leprosy, significance of (Antia). PRS, *54:*55, 1974

Nerves, peripheral, posttraumatic lesions of (Petrolati, Diara), PRS, *57:*675, 1976. Riv. ital. chir. plast., *6:*185, 1974

Tissue adhesive with microsurgical techniques in repair of peripheral nerves (Hurwitz *et al*), PRS, *55:*512, 1975. Surg. Res., *17:*245, 1974

Nerve paralysis, femoral, caused by traumatic hematoma of iliopsoas muscle (Malliakas *et al*), PRS, *57:*537, 1976. Ann. chir., *29:*591, 1975

Nerve gap, suture under tension *vs.* graft (Terzis, Faibisoff, Williams), PRS, *56:*166, 1975

Denervation of Meissner corpuscle, sequential histological study after nerve division in rhesus monkey (Dellon, Witebsky, Terrill). PRS, *56:*182, 1975

Nerve suture, new technique, epineurium-anchoring funicular suture (Tsuge, Ikuta, Sakaue), PRS, *56:*496, 1975

Nerve injuries, civilian peripheral, reappraisal of timing for exploration (Kline,

Nerves, Injuries of – Cont.
Hackett), PRS, *57:*120, 1976. Surgery, *78:*54, 1975

Nerves lesions, peripheral, single fascicular recordings as intraoperative tool for management of (Williams, Terzis), PRS, *57:*562, 1976. Discussion by Collins, PRS, *57:*744, 1976

Pacinian corpuscles, primate, changes in, following volar pad excision and skin grafting (Miller, Rusenas). PRS, *57:*627, 1976

NETTO, F. T.: Abdominoplasty (with Baroudi, Keppke), PRS, *54:*161, 1974

NEUBAUER, H.: Free total transplantation in lid surgery. Klin. Monatsbl. Augenheilkd., *165:*86, 1974

NEUBAUER, H.: Atypical oculoplastic surgery in children. Klin. Monatsbl. Augenheilkd., *167:*199, 1975 (German)

NEUMAN, Z.: Complications of sulfamylon treatment of burns. Harefuah, *81:*518, 1971 (Hebrew)

NEUMAN, Z.: Reconstruction of cleft lip and palate. Harefuah, *81:*563, 1971 (Hebrew)

NEUMAN, Z.: Use of water-insoluble papain (WIP) for debridement of burn eschar and necrotic tissue (with Shapira, Giladi), PRS, *52:*279, 1973

NEUMAN, Z.: Early treatment of burns of dorsum of hand by tangential excision and skin grafting (with Wexler, Yeschua). PRS, *54:*268, 1974

NEUMANN, O. G.: Oral mucosal free graft in glottic reconstruction for postintubation laryngeal stenosis. H.N.O., *22:*215, 1974 (German)

NEUMANN, O. G. *et al:* Free mouth mucosa transplantation within the scope of diagnostic and therapeutic laryngeal fissure. Arch Klin. Exp. Ohren Nasen Kehkopfheilkd., *205:*371, 1973 (German)

NEUMANN, O. G. *et al:* Dosage-controlled cryotherapy in inoperable exulcerating recurrent tumor over carotid artery. H. N. O., *21:*195, 1973 (German)

NEUNER, O.: Simple procedure for correction of the hump nose. Brit. J. Plast. Surg., *24:*375, 1971

NEUNER, O.: Reconstructive and plastic surgery of the face. Schweiz. Monatsschr. Zahnheilkd., *81:*947, 1971 (German)

NEUNER, O.: New surgical method in habitual temporomandibular joint luxation and subluxation. Dtsch. Zahnaerztl. Z., *28:*935, 1973 (German)

NEUNER, O.: Corrective plastic surgery of cleft nose, PRS, *52:*451, 1973. J. Maxillo-facial Surg., *1:*50, 1973

NEUNER, O.: Correction of mandibular deformities. Oral Surg., *36:*779, 1973

NEUNER, O.: Author's own therapeutic method for habitual temporomandibular joint luxation and subluxation. Schweiz. Monatsschr. Zahnheilkd., *83:*61, 1973 (German)

NEUNER, O.: Combined orthopedic-plastic surgery of the jaws and face. Fortschr. Kiefer. Gesichtschir., *81:*72, 1974 (German)

NEUNER, O. *et al:* New pathways in surgical treatment of fibromatosis gingivae. Schweiz. Monatsschr. Zahnheilkd., *83:*1327, 1973 (German)

NEUNER, O. *et al:* Surgical treatment of microgenia without interruption of continuity. Fortschr. Kiefer. Gesichtschir., *18:*183, 1974 (German)

NEUNER, O. *et al:* Single-jaw splinting following orthopedic jaw surgery. Fortschr. Kiefer. Gesichtschir., *18:*276, 1974 (German)

NEUNER, O. *et al:* Delayed corrections of labiomaxillary clefts: soft palate. Rev. Stomatol. Chir. Maxillofac., *75:*68, 1974 (French)

NEUPOKOEV, N. I.: Tissue respiration of Filatov's pedicled graft at various stages of plastic operations. Stomatologiia (Mosk.), *51:*11, 1972 (Russian)

Neurofibromas

Neurofibromatosis of head (Fára, Hrivnáková, Brejcha), PRS *48:*517, 1971. Acta chir. plast., *12:*141, 1970

Gastrointestinal bleeding as manifestation of von Rècklinghausen's disease of skin (Wilkerson), PRS, *49:*108, 1972. Am. Surgeon, *37:*298, 1971

Neoplasms, neurogenous, of major nerves of face and neck (Katz, Passy, Kaplan), PRS, *49:*235, 1972. Arch. Surg., *103:*51, 1971

Carotid neurofibroma in a child (Slim *et al*). Am. J. Surg., *123:*343, 1972

Von Recklinghausen's disease: clinicopathological study (Brasfield, Gupta), PRS, *50:*309, 1972. Ann. Surg., *175:*86, 1972

Neurofibroma, elephantiasis, massive hemorrhage in (McMaster). Brit. J. Surg., *59:*984, 1972

Surgical treatment of malignant soft-tissue tumors of the extremities in the adult (Burton *et al*). Clin. Orthop., *84:*144, 1972

Pachydermatocele in von Recklinghausen's disease (Bando), PRS, *52:*457, 1973. Jap. J. Plast. Reconstr. Surg., *15:*366, 1972

Value of preoperative angiography in the surgical management of cervical hourglass neurofibroma. Case report (Rinaldi). J. Neurosurg., *36:*97, 1972

Evaluation of methods of treating patients with malignant tumors of soft tissue

Neurofibromas – Cont.

(Knysh *et al*). Khirurgiia (Mosk.), *48:*96, 1972 (Russian)

Isolated neurofibroma of the orbit (Chwirot). Klin. Oczna., *42:*781, 1972 (Polish)

Von Recklinghausen's disease in children (Griffith *et al*). PRS, *49:*647, 1972

Facial nerve, benign and malignant schwannomas of, simulating parotid neoplasms (Kruse *et al*). H.N.O., *21:*107, 1973 (German)

Neurofibrosarcoma of tongue (Rapoport *et al*), PRS, *54:*234, 1974. Internat. Surg., *58:*738, 1973

Neurofibroma, intraosseous, solitary, involving mandibular canal: case report (Singer, Gienger, Kullbom). J. Oral Surg., *31:*127, 1973

Neurofibromatosis – Von Recklinghausen's disease in podiatric medicine; review and report of two cases (Galinski). J. Am. Podiatry Assoc., *64:*87, 1974

Nerve growth stimulating activity in disseminated neurofibromatosis (Schenkein *et al*), PRS, *54:*377, 1974. New England J. Med., *290:*613, 1974

Neurofibroma, giant, of head and neck (Mukherji). PRS, *53:*184, 1974

Neurofibromatosis, changes in facial skeleton in (Koblin, Reich), PRS, *56:*463, 1975. J. Maxillo-facial Surg., *3:*23, 1975

Clinical-pathological conference: Case 10, part 2. Neurofibrosarcoma (Carpenter *et al*). J. Oral Surg., *33:*38, 1975

Multiple neurofibromatosis associated with facial asymmetry (James *et al*). J. Oral Surg., *33:*439, 1975

Primary neurogenic sarcomas of the oral region: a report of two cases (Martinez *et al*). Ala. J. Med. Sci., *13:*32, 1976

Neurofibromas, frontonasal tumors, diagnosis and management (Griffith). PRS, *57:*692, 1976

Neuromas

Neuroma, amputation, of great auricular nerve after parotidectomy (Hobsley). Brit. J. Surg., *59:*735, 1972

Triamcinolone acetonide treatment for symptomatic digital neuromas (Graham *et al*), PRS, *52:*97, 1973. Rev. Latino Am. cir. plast., *16:*13, 1972

Neuroma in continuity. Its preoperative and operative management (Kline *et al*). Surg. Clin. North Am., *52:*1189, 1972

Neuromas, painful traumatic (Mathews *et al*). Surg. Clin. North Am., *52:*1313, 1972

Neuromas, hand, abdominal flap for (Brown, Flynn), PRS, *52:*595, 1973. J. Bone & Joint

Neuromas – Cont.

Surg., *55A:*575, 1973

Triamcinolone acetonide to treat terminal neuromas (Pataky, Graham, Munger), PRS, *53:*607, 1974. J. Surg. Res., *14:*36, 1973

Neuromas, facial nerve (Peytral *et al*), PRS, *56:*353, 1975. Ann. Otolaryng., *10:*555, 1974

Neuroma, Morton's (Telesynski *et al*). Chir. Narzadow. Ruchu Ortop. Pol., *39:*199, 1974

Nerve tumors of the foot: diagnosis and treatment (Berlin *et al*). J. Am. Podiatry Assoc., *65:*157, 1975

Neuroma, acoustic, and suboccipital approach (MacCarty), PRS, *56:*111, 1975. Mayo Clin. Proc., *50:*15, 1975

Neuromata, multiple mucosal, serious implications of (Bowers). PRS, *56:*554, 1975

Neuroma, single fascicular recordings, intraoperative tool for management of peripheral nerve lesions (Williams, Terzis), PRS, *57:*562, 1976. Discussion by Collins, PRS, *57:*744, 1976

Fingertip avulsions, changes in primate pacinian corpuscles following volar pad excision and skin grafting (Miller, Rusenas). PRS, *57:*627, 1976

NEVEU, M.: Repositioning of the nasal septum without mucosal dissection. Ann. chir. plast., *16:*231, 1971 (French)

Nevi (See also Skin Neoplasms)

Nevi and nevus-similar syndrome (Wiskemann), PRS, *53:*111, 1974. Chir. Praxis, *16:*629, 1972

Premalignant nature of sebaceous nevus of Jadassohn (Constant, Davis). PRS, *50:*257, 1972

Spitz's nevus (Dobbelaere *et al*). Arch. Belg. Dermatol., *29:*339, 1973 (French)

Nevus, spindle cell, in adults and children (Coskey, Mehregan), PRS, *53:*611, 1974. Arch. Dermat., *108:*535, 1973

Nevus, giant, excision in newborn (Feins), PRS, *54:*380, 1974. J. Pediat. Surg., *8:*825, 1973

Z-closure (Hueston). M. J. Australia, *1:*496, 1973

Therapeutic possibilities in nevobasalioma (Scholz *et al*). Dermatol. Monatsschr., *160:*1016, 1974 (German)

Benign juvenile melanoma (Spitz) (Thormann). Paediatr. Grenzgeb., *13:*91, 1974 (German)

Nevus sebaceous of Jadassohn (Baker), PRS, *57:*403, 1976. Arch. Otolaryng., *101:*515, 1975

Nevi – Cont.

Nevus, halo, ultrastructure evidence for destruction in (Jacobs *et al*), PRS, *56:*112, 1975. Cancer Res., *35:*352, 1975

Epidermal and other congenital organoid nevi (Solomon *et al*). Curr. Probl. Pediatr., *6:*1, 1975

Nevus of Ota (Yeschua, Wexler, Neuman). PRS, *55:*229, 1975

Cryosurgery for facial skin lesions (Leopard). Proc. Roy. Soc. Med., *68:*606, 1975

Nevi, Giant

Giant pigmented nevus (Rudolph, Wood), PRS, *55:*641, 1975. Cutis, *14:*223, 1974

Malignant potential of large congenital nevi (Kaplan). West. J. Med., *121:*226, 1974

Nevus, giant, "piecemeal principle," staged operations for better results (Weisman). PRS, *57:*570, 1976

Nevus, giant pigmented, defining malignant potential of (Dellon, Edelson, Chretien). PRS, *57:*611, 1976

Nevi, Pigmented

Nevi, benign pigmented, histologic artifacts of (Sagebiel), PRS, *51:*483, 1973. Arch. Dermat., *106:*691, 1972

Nevus, giant pigmented (Rudolph, Wood), PRS, *55:*641, 1975. Cutis, *14:*223, 1974

Surgical therapy of extended skin tumors of the torso (Petres *et al*). Hautarzt, *25:*566, 1974 (German)

Case of elevated cellular nevus of the eyelid edge (Krawczuk-Hermanowiczowa *et al*). Klin. Oczna., *44:*69, 1974 (Polish)

Nevus, blue, of oral mucosa (Teles, Cardoso, Goncalves), PRS, *56:*234, 1975. Oral Surg., *38:*905, 1974

Experience of skin tumours treatment with laser radiation (Gamaleja *et al*). Panminerva Med., *16:*41, 1974

Advances in the surgical treatment of skin tumors (Wilflingseder). Wien. Med. Wochenschr., *124:*593, 1974 (German)

Melanocytic nevus, recurrent, following partial surgical removal (Kornberg, Ackerman), PRS, *57:*765, 1976. Arch. Dermat., *111:*1588, 1975

Benign juvenile melanoma. A study of 51 lesions (Andrade). Mod. Probl. Paediatr., *17:*212, 1975

Nevi, Pigmented, Malignancy in (See also *Melanoma; Nevi, Giant*)

Nevus, malignant blue (Hernandez), PRS, *54:*380, 1974. Arch. Dermat., *107:*741, 1973

Nevi, halo, and melanoma (Epstein *et al*),

Nevi, Pigmented, Malignancy in – Cont.

PRS, *53:*248, 1974. J.A.M.A., *225:*373, 1973

Nevus, intradermal, malignant melanoma developing from (Okun *et al*), PRS, *57:*264, 1976. Arch. Dermat., *110:*599, 1974

Nevi, large congenital, risk of malignancy (Kaplan). PRS, *53:*421, 1974

Melanoma, defining malignant potential of giant pigmented nevus (Dellon, Edelson, Chretien). PRS, *57:*611, 1976

NEVIASER, R. J.: *Flexor digitorum superficialis indicis* and carpal tunnel syndrome, PRS, *56:*230, 1975. Hand, *6:*155, 1974

NEVIASER, R. J., WILSON, J. N., AND LIEVANO, A.: Rupture of ulnar collateral ligament of thumb (gamekeeper's thumb). Correction by dynamic repair, PRS, *50:*306, 1972. J. Bone & Joint Surg., *53:*1357, 1971

NEVIASER, R. J., BUTTERFIELD, W. C., AND WIECHE, D. R.: Puffy hand of drug addiction, study of pathogenesis, PRS, *51:*106, 1973. J. Bone & Joint Surg., *54A:*629, 1972

NEVIASER, R. J., AND ADAMS, J. P.: Vascular lesions in hand, PRS, *55:*637, 1975. Clin. Orthop., *100:*111, 1974

NEVILLE, A. P.: Early detection of cancer, PRS, *55:*642, 1975. Proc. Roy. Soc. Med., *67:*743, 1974

NEWELL, F. W.: Discussion of "Acute retrobulbar hemorrhage during elective blepharoplasty," by Hartley *et al.* PRS, *52:*12, 1973

NEWELL, R., KREMEUTZ, E., AND ROBERTS, T.: Multiple primary neoplasms in blacks compared to whites. II. Further cancers in patients with cancer of buccal cavity and pharynx, PRS, *54:*700, 1974. J. Nat. Cancer Inst., *52:*639, 1974

NEWMAN, L. F. *et al*: Nontranssexual men who seek sex reassignment. Am. J. Psychiatry, *131:*437, 1974

NEWMEYER, W. L., KILGORE, E. S., JR., AND GRAHAM, W. P., III: Mucous cysts, dorsal distal interphalangeal joint ganglion. PRS, *53:*313, 1974

NEWSOME, M. W. *et al*: Use of an air-fluidized bed in the care of patients with extensive burns. Am. J. Surg., *124:*52, 1972

NEWSOME, T. W., CURRERI, W., AND EURENIUS, K.: Visceral injuries: unusual complication of electrical burn, PRS, *51:*606, 1973. Arch. Surg., *105:*494, 1972

NEWSOME, T. W., AND EURENIUS, K.: Suppression of granulocyte and platelet production by *Pseudomonas* burn wound infection, PRS, *52:*209, 1973. Surg. Gynec. & Obst., *136:*373, 1973

NEWTON, N. C. *et al*: Adenoid cystic carcinoma of head and neck, PRS, *52:*600, 1973. Proc.

Roy. Australasian Coll. Surgeons, *46:*720, 1973

NEWTON, R. A.: Mentoplasty. Can. J. Otolaryngol., *2:*235, 1973

NEWTON, R. A.: Surgical tattooing for port wine stain. Can. J. Otolaryngol., *2:*251, 1973

NGUYEN, M. C. *et al*: Malignant transformation of leg ulcers. Apropos of three cases. Phlebologie, *27:*215, 1974 (French)

NIARCHOS, A. P. *et al*: Association of Wolff-Parkinson-White syndrome with congenital abnormalities of hands and feet. Brit. Heart J., *36:*409, 1974

NIAZMAND, R., MILLER, T., AND BARKER, W. F.: Improved technic for freezing the gangrenous extremity in poor risk patients, PRS, *52:*107, 1973. Am. J. Surg., *124:*701, 1972

NICHOL, T. D. *et al*: Management of soft tissue injuries of face to reduce scar formation. J. Ky. Med. Assoc., *71:*495, 1973

NICHOLAS, G. G., NOONE, R. B., AND GRAHAM, W. P.: Carpal tunnel syndrome in pregnancy, PRS, *48:*513, 1971. Hand, *3:*80, 1971

NICHOLAS, K. C., BAYS, R. A., AND LYON, E. D.: *Periadenitis mucosa necrotica recurrens*, PRS, *56:*593, 1975. J. Oral Surg., *33:*65, 1975

NICHOLLS, E. M.: Development and elimination of pigmented moles and anatomical distribution of primary malignant melanoma, PRS, *54:*116, 1974. Cancer, *32:*191, 1973

NICHOLS, H. M.: Dilemma of intact *superficialis* tendon, PRS, *56:*596, 1975. Hand, *7:*85, 1975

NICHOLS, H. M.: Editorial: Emergency treatment of hand injuries. Mil. Med., *140:*358, 1975

NICHOLS, R. D. *et al*: Systematic evaluation and management of fractures of frontal sinus. Trans. Am. Acad. Ophthalmol. Otolaryngol., *77:*1429, 1973

NICHOLSON, D. H., AND GUZAK, S. V.: Visual loss complicating repair of orbital floor fractures, PRS, *49:*356, 1972. Arch. Ophth., *86:*369, 1971

NICKELL, W. B.: Special considerations in resurfacing hand injuries with groin flap, PRS, *54:*690, 1974. South. M. J., *67:*567, 1974

NICKELL, W. B., JURKIEWICZ, M. J., AND SALYER, K. E.: Repair of skull defects with autogenous bone, PRS, *51:*353, 1973. Arch. Surg., *105:*431, 1972

NICKELL, W. B. *et al*: One stage surgical repair of mandibular osteoradionecrosis with jaw preservation, PRS, *53:*682, 1974. Am. J. Surg., *126:*502, 1973

NICKELL, W. B., SALYER, K. E., AND VARGAS, M. A.: Practical variations in use of deltopectoral flap, PRS, *54:*700, 1974. South. M. J., *67:*697, 1974

NICKMAN, N. J.: Surgery of facial nerve. Rocky Mt. Med. J., *70:*37, 1973

NICOLAS, G. *et al*: Formation of attached mucosa in cases of periodontolysis. II. Free autografts of attached mucosa. Rev. Belge. Med. Dent., *28:*417, 1974 (French)

NICOLETIS, C.: Place of face lifting in the treatment of facial paralysis. Cah. Med., *13:*379, 1972 (French)

NICOLETIS, C.: Critical study of breast prosthesis and attempt at definition of ideal prosthesis. Ann. chir. plast., *18:*239, 1973 (French)

NICOLETIS, C.: Facial injuries, PRS, *57:*256, 1976. J. chir., *109:*495, 1975

NICOLIS, G., CAPETANAKIS, J., AND PANAS, E.: Intraepidermic epithelioma of Borst and Jadassohn, PRS, *49:*473, 1972. Ann. Dermat. et Syph., *98:*161, 1971

NICOLLE, F. V.: New design of finger joint prosthesis for rheumatoid hand, PRS, *53:*106, 1974. Ann. chir. plast., *17:*275, 1972

NICOLLE, F. V.: Recent advances in the management of joint disease in the rheumatoid hand. Hand, *5:*91, 1973

NICOLLE, F. V., HOLT, P. J. L., AND CALNAN, J. S.: Prophylactic synovectomy of joints of rheumatic hand, PRS, *49:*357, 1972. Ann. Rheum. Dis., *30:*476, 1971

NICOLLE, F. V. *et al*: Prophylactic synovectomy of the rheumatoid hand – a clinical trial with 5–8 year follow-up. Brit. J. Surg., *58:*305, 1971

NICOLLAE, F. V. *et al*: A valuable splint for the rheumatoid hand. Hand, *7:*67, 1975

NIEDERDELLMAN, H.: Electronic measurements of biomechanics in mandibular osteosynthesis. Fortschr. Kiefer. Gesichtschir., *19:*42, 1975 (German)

NIEDERDELLMANN, H. *et al*: Neurologic disorders following surgical correction of progenia and microgenia. Fortschr. Kiefer. Gesichtschir., *18:*186, 1974 (German)

NIEDERDELLMANN, H., MUNKER, G., AND LANGE, G.: Reconstruction of defect of orbital floor with rotated flap from nasal wall, PRS, *55:*375, 1975. J. Maxillo-facial Surg., *2:*153, 1974

NIELUBOWICZ, J. *et al*: Late results of lymphovenous anastomosis. J. Cardiovasc. Surg. (Torino), Spec. No.: 113, 1973

NIEMANN, K. M.: Surgical correction of flexion deformities in hemophilia. Am. Surg., *37:*685, 1971

NIENHUIS, R. L. F. *et al*: Arthroplasty of finger joints in rheumatoid arthritis with use of silicone rubber prostheses, PRS, *49:*358, 1972. Nederl. tijdschr. geneesk., *115:*1889, 1971

NIGST, H.: Dupuytren's contracture, PRS, *50:*306, 1972. Ther. Umsch., *28:*818, 1971

NIGST, H.: Uses of occupational therapy in hand injuries. Handchirurgie, *4:*3, 1972 (German)

NIGST, H.: Rare tumors of the wrist joint and hand. Handchirurgie, *5:*39, 1973 (German)

NIGST, H.: Reconstruction and replacement of the grip function in the maimed hand. Langenbecks Arch. Chir., *339:*383, 1975 (German)

NIIMURA, M.: Fibrosarcoma in burn scar, PRS, *52:*457, 1973. Saigai Igaku, Disaster Med., *15:*366, 1972

NIINIKOSKI, J., HUNT, T. K., AND DUNPHY, J. E.: Oxygen supply in healing tissue, PRS, *50:*422, 1972. Am. J. Surg., *123:*247, 1972

NIINIKOSKI, J., AND HUNT, T. K.: Measurement of wound oxygen with implanted Silastic tube, PRS, *50:*98, 1972. Surgery, *71:*22, 1972

NIKANDROV, A. M. *et al*: Our experience in osteoplasty of mandible. Stomatologiia (Mosk.), *53:*22, 1974 (Russian)

NIKITIN, V. V.: Chemico-biological properties of low molecular silicone polymers and employment in conserving homologous tissues of mesenchymal origin, PRS, *50:*206, 1972. Acta chir. plast., *13:*61, 1971

NIKOL'SKII, A. D. *et al*: Sapheno-cavernous anastomosis as a method of treatment of priapism. Urol. Nefrol. (Mosk.), *1:*58, 1975 (Russian)

NILGES, T. C., AND NORTHERN, J. L.: Iatrogenic ototoxic hearing loss, PRS, *49:*240, 1972. Ann. Surg., *173:*281, 1971

NIMBERG, R. B. *et al*: Isolation of immunosuppressive peptide fraction from the serum of cancer patients, PRS, *56:*600, 1975. Cancer Res., *35:*1489, 1975

NINH, T. N., AND NINH, T. X.: Cystic hygroma in children. Report of 126 cases, PRS, *55:*252, 1975. J. Pediat. Surg., *9:*191, 1974

NINI, W. *et al*: Epidermoid cyst after a total skin graft for eventration. Chirurgie, *98:*50, 1972 (French)

NIRMUL, G. *et al*: Cyclophosphamide-induced immunologic tolerance to skin homografts. Surg. Forum, *22:*287, 1971

NISCH, G.: Results of anastomoses between facial and hypoglossal nerve. Psychiatr. Neurol. Med. Psychol. (Leipz.), *25:*488, 1973 (German)

NISHIKAWA, K. *et al*: Case of acute facial hemiatrophy (Parry-Romberg syndrome). Iryo, *25:*679, 1971 (Japanese)

NISHIOKA, K. AND NANJOH, B.: Biological reactivity of pedicled skin to passive cutaneous anaphylaxis, PRS, *49:*239, 1972. Jap. J. Plast. Reconstr. Surg., *14:*333, 1971

NISHIOKA, K. *et al*: Histochemical study of pedicle skin flaps; approach to the microcirculation of the flaps. Jap. J. Plast. Reconstr. Surg., *15:*210, 1972 (Japanese)

NISONSON, I., AND LATTIMER, J. K.: How well can exstrophied bladder work? PRS, *51:*604, 1973. J. Urol., *107:*664, 1972

NISWANDER, J. D. *et al*: Sex ratio and cleft lip with or without cleft palate. Lancet, *2:*858, 1972

NIZOLEK, J. A.: Tourniquet difficulty during intravenous regional anesthesia, PRS, *52:*323, 1973. South. M. J., *64:*1411, 1971

NOACK, W. *et al*: New local therapy of leg ulcer. Z. Aerztl. Fortbild. (Jena), *66:*368, 1972 (German)

NOBEL, G. L.: Secondary correction of bilateral cleft lip deformities with Millard's midline muscular closure (with Oneal, Greer). PRS, *54:*45, 1974

NOBLE, H. B., AND LYNE, E. D.: *Candida* osteomyelitis and arthritis from hyperalimentation therapy, PRS, *55:*259, 1975. J. Bone & Joint Surg., *56A:*825, 1974

NOBLE, J. *et al*: Enchondromata of the hand bones. Ann. Chir., *28:*855, 1974 (French)

NOBLE, J., AND LAMB, D. W.: Enchondromata of bones of hand—review of 40 cases, PRS, *56:*227, 1975. Hand, *6:*275, 1974

NOBLE, J. P.: Strange tumor. Nouv. Presse Med., *3:*535, 1974 (French)

NOCZYNSKI, L. *et al*: Combined treatment of crural varicose ulcers. Pol. Przegl. Chir., *45:*431, 1973 (Polish)

NODL, F.: Micrometastases in malignant melanoma. Arch. Derm. Forsch., *244:*239, 1972 (German)

NOE, J. M.: Postoperative hypertension as etiological factor in hematoma after rhytidectomy, prevention with chlorpromazine (with Berner, Morain). PRS, *57:*314, 1976

NOE, J. M., AND CONSTABLE, J. D.: New approach to pulmonary burns, PRS, *53:*686, 1974. J. Trauma, *13:*1015, 1973

NOE, J. M., BIRDSELL, D., AND LAUB, D. R.: Surgical construction of male genitalia for female-to-male transsexual. PRS, *53:*511, 1974

NOE, J. M., AND BARBER, J.: Chronic ulceration in patient with leprosy, PRS, *55:*727, 1975. West. J. Med., *121:*430, 1974

NOE, J. M. *et al*: Advantages of double releases in axillary, antecubital and popliteal contractures. J. Trauma, *15:*762, 1975

NOLAN, J. O.: Cryosurgical treatment of rhinophyma. PRS, *52:*437, 1973

NOLAN, S. P. *et al*: Letter: Does pectus excavatum cause functional disability? J. Thorac. Cardiovasc. Surg., *71:*148, 1976

Noma

Lagrot's operation and Rizzali-Esmach operation in the treatment of temporomaxillary ankylosis, sequelae of noma (Diop *et al*). Bull. Soc. Med. Afr. Noire Lang. Fr., *15*:263, 1970 (French)

An exceptional form of noma (Diop *et al*). Bull. Soc. Med. Afr. Noire Lang. Fr., *16*:599, 1971 (French)

Noma in African children (Naidr). Cesk. Pediatr., *27*:366, 1972 (Czechoslovakian)

Cancrum oris (Tempest), PRS, *50*:535, 1972. Trop. Doctor, *1*:164, 1972

Noma (*cancrum oris*), surgical repair of defects from (Durrani). PRS, *52*:629, 1973

Noma (*cancrum oris*), ankylosis of mandible from (Oluwasanmi, Lagundoye, Akinyemi). PRS, *57*:342, 1976

NOMOTO, H., BUNCKE, H. J., AND CHATER, N. L.: Improved patency rates in microvascular surgery when using magnesium sulfate and silicone rubber vascular cuff. PRS, *54*:157, 1974

NOMURA, Y.: Vidian neurectomy – some technical remarks. Laryngoscope, *84*:578, 1974

NONYAMA, J. *et al*: Direct magnifying lymphangiography of neck, PRS, *50*:312, 1972. Pract. Otologia Kyoto, *64*:871, 1971

NOONE, R. B. *et al*: Effect on middle ear disease of fracture of the pterygoid hamulus during palatoplasty. Cleft Palate J., *10*:23, 1973

NOONE, R. B., GRAHAM, W. P., III, AND ROYSTER, H. P.: Autotransfusion for blood loss in some major esthetic operations, PRS, *51*:559, 1973

NOONE, R. B. *et al*: Nutritional care after head and neck surgery. Postgrad. Med., *53*:80, 1973

NOONE, R. B. *et al*: Lymph node metastases in oral carcinoma, correlation of histopathology with survival, PRS, *53*:158, 1974

NOORDHOFF, M. S.: Control and prevention of hypertrophic scarring and contracture. Clin. Plast. Surg., *1*:49, 1974

NORA, A. H., AND NORA, J. J.: Syndrome of multiple congenital anomalies associated with teratogenic exposure, PRS, *56*:110, 1975. Arch. Environmental Health, *30*:17, 1975

NORANTE, J. D. AND McCABE, B. F.: Fascial sling suspension of chin following resection of anterior mandible. Laryngoscope, *83*:336, 1973

NORDENRAM, A.: Surgical therapy of maxillary protrusion. Sven. Tandlak. Tidskr., *64*:339, 1971 (Swedish)

NORDENRAM, A.: Correction of maxillary protrusion by posterior change of upper jaw. Sven. Tandlak. Tidskr., *64*:703, 1971 (Swedish)

NORDENRAM, A. *et al*: Clinical-radiographical investigation of operation material of jaw cysts. Nor. Tannlaegeforen Tid., *82*:455, 1972 (Norwegian)

NORDENRAM, A., HELLEM, S., AND ZETTERVALL, R.: Cranio-maxillary (mandibular) internal skeletal wiring with steel ligatures in jaw fractures. Sven. Tandlak. Tidskr., *66*:81, 1973 (Swedish)

NORDENRAM, A. *et al*: Suicidal gunshot wounds resulting in severe maxillofacial injury. Int. J. Oral Surg., *3*:29, 1974

NORDENRAM, A. *et al*: Mandibular retrusion surgically corrected by bilateral subcondylar ramus osteotomy and bone transplantation. Nor. Tannlaegeforen Tid., *84*:52, 1974 (Norwegian)

NORDGAARD, J. O.: Persistent sensory disturbances and diplopia following fractures of the zygoma. Arch. Otolaryng., *102*:80, 1976

NORKUS, R. G. *et al*: Application of lateral compression clamp in management of mandibular fractures, PRS, *56*:598, 1975. Oral Surg., *39*:2, 1975

NORMAN, J. D. *et al*: Augmentation mammaplasty through a circumareolar incision using a solid, gel-filled implant. South. Med. J., *68*:1456, 1975

NORMAN, J. L., CUNNINGHAM, P. J., AND CLEVELAND, B. R.: Skin and subcutaneous metastases from gastrointestinal carcinoid tumors, PRS, *50*:421, 1972. Arch. Surg., *103*:767, 1971

NORRIS, C. W. *et al*: Head and neck pain: T-M joint syndrome. Laryngoscope, *84*:1466, 1974

NORTH, J. F.: Mammary hyperinvolution and ptosis. Brit. J. Plast. Surg., *28*:310, 1975

NORTON, L. A. *et al*: Consideration of chin in surgical-orthodontic procedures. Isr. J. Dent. Med., *22*:124, 1973

NORWITZ, S.: Evaluation of mammaplasty techniques in municipal teaching hospital (with Bromberg, Song), PRS, *53*:33, 1974

NORWOOD, O. T.: Male pattern baldness: classification and incidence, PRS, *57*:753, 1976. South. M. J., *68*:1359, 1975

NORWOOD, O'TAR T.: *Hair Transplant Surgery*. Charles C Thomas, Springfield, Ill., 1974. PRS, *54*:349, 1974

Nose (See also *Nasal Septum; Rhinoplasty*)

Surgery of the Upper Respiratory System. By William Wayne Montgomery. Lea & Febiger, Philadelphia, 1971. PRS, *49*:205, 1972

Photoelastic analysis of nasal support (Clark), PRS, *49*:101, 1972. Arch. Otolaryng., *93*:3, 1971

Nose – Cont.

Anatomical details of the osseous-cartilaginous framework of the nose (Natvig *et al*), PRS, *48:*528, 1971

Nose in man, on development of primary palate and (Azzolini, Mangiante), PRS, *49:*359, 1972. Rev. Ital. chir. plast., *3:*1, 1971

Experiences with upper lateral nasal cartilage in reconstruction of the lower eyelid (Lipshutz). Am. J. Ophth., *73:*592, 1972

Nasal entomophthorosis. Preliminary immunopathological study of new case (Andrade *et al*). Am. J. Trop. Med. Hyg., *22:*361, 1972

Nasal prosthesis, Tycho Brahe and his sixteenth century (Lee). PRS, *50:*332, 1972

Turbinectomy, judicious, for nasal obstruction (Fry), PRS, *52:*205, 1973. Australian & New Zealand J. Surg., *42:*291, 1973

Nasal turbinate function (Cole). Can. J. Otolaryngol., *2:*259, 1973

Rhinolith (Dutta). J. Oral Surg., *31:*876, 1973

Nose, the mature (Parkes, Kamer). Laryngoscope, *83:*157, 1973

Rhinolithiasis associated with nasal polyposis (Harampiev *et al*). Srp. Arh. Celok. Lek., *101:*929, 1973 (Serbian)

Biopsy, nasal and mucous membrane, Sjögren's syndrome (Powell, Larson, Hankin), PRS, *55:*246, 1975. Ann. Int. Med., *81:*25, 1974

Nasal lesions in electroplate workers, clinical manifestations of chromic acid toxicity (Cohen, Davis, Kramkowski), PRS, *54:*371, 1974. Cutis, *13:*558, 1974

Surgical suture materials and suture techniques in oto-rhino-laryngology (Schenke). H.N.O., *22:*356, 1974 (German)

Nasal circulation, method of assessment (Girgis *et al*), PRS, *56:*592, 1975. J. Laryng. & Otol., *88:*1149, 1974

Nasal circulation in certain pathological conditions (Girgis *et al*), PRS, *56:*592, 1975. J. Laryng. & Otol., *88:*1159, 1974

Nasal circulation, estimation of effect of drugs on (Girgis *et al*), PRS, *56:*592, 1975. J. Laryng. & Otol., *88:*1163, 1974

Nasal abruption (Kwiatkowski *et al*). Otolaryngol. Pol., *28:*703, 1974 (Polish)

Calculus, nasal: asymptomatic rhinolith in rhinoplasty. (Mahler, Kaufman). PRS, *54:*490, 1974

Experience in the use of oxidized cellulose for hemostatic purposes (Fradin). Zh. Ushn. Nos. Gorl. Bolezn., *6:*82, 1974 (Russian)

Nasal allergy, some aspects of (Taub), PRS, *57:*671, 1976. Eye, Ear, Nose & Throat Month., *54:*326, 1975

Nose – Cont.

Saccharin test of nasal mucociliary function (Grossan), PRS, *57:*755, 1976. Eye, Ear, Nose & Throat Month., *54:*415, 1975

An absorbent, non-adherent nasal pack (Kamer *et al*). Laryngoscope, *85:*384, 1975

Airway, nasal, valvular obstruction of (DesPrez, Kiehn). PRS, *56:*307, 1975

Nose structure and function (Kern), PRS, *57:*257, 1976. Postgrad. Med., *57:*101, 1975

Nose: recent advances in pathology of olfaction (Douek *et al*), PRS, *57:*682, 1976. Proc. Roy. Soc. Med., *68:*467, 1975

Anatomy of nose, suggested nomenclature for (Schurter, Letterman). PRS, *57:*490, 1976

Nose, Anterior Atresia (See also Nose, Choanal Atresia)

Nostril stenosis and atresia. Dilator tube (Vergnon *et al*). Ann. Otolaryngol. Chir. Cervicofac., *88:*675, 1971 (French)

Treatment of nose stenoses (Masing). Arch. Klin. Exp. Ohren Nasen Kehlkopfheilkd., *199:*352, 1971 (German)

Nasal atresia with breathing impairment in an infant (Champy *et al*). Ann. chir. plast., *19:*189, 1974 (French)

Use of extra-mucosal dissection in the treatment of certain vestibular stenoses (Alach). Ann. chir. plast., *19:*273, 1974 (French)

Nose, Bone and Cartilage Autografts to

Nasal tip cartilage, use in correction of saddle nose deformity (Penkava), PRS, *50:*94, 1972. Acta chir. plast., *13:*25, 1971

Bone grafts to the nose, follow-up of (Farina, Villano). PRS, *48:*251, 1971

Nasal pyramid, lower portion, reconstruction with composite auricular grafts (Dufourmentel, Le Pesteur), PRS, *54:*499, 1974. Ann. chir. plast., *18:*199, 1973

Grafts, osteoperiosteal, to reconstruct dorsum nasi (Ditroi), PRS, *55:*634, 1975. Acta chir. plast., *16:*171, 1974

Graft, autogenous vomer or septal cartilage, small, to achieve more nasal tip projection (Sheen), PRS, *56:*35, 1975. Discussion by Horton, PRS, *56:*211, 1975

Nasal tip, absorption of small bone graft in (Sheen) (Letter to the Editor), PRS, *56:*332, 1975

Nose, Choanal Atresia

Gradenigo's syndrome following correction of posterior choanal atresia (Herceg, Harding). PRS, *48:*181, 1971

Nose – Cont.

Choanal atresia in newborn, bilateral. Two case reports (Tuncer *et al*). Turk. J. Pediatr., *13:*147, 1971

Rhinoplasty candidate, familial choanal atresia in (Parkes, Brennan), PRS, *53:*240, 1974. Eye, Ear, Nose & Throat Month., *52:*222, 1973

Choanal atresia, complete bilateral bony (Lipshutz) (Follow-Up Clinic). PRS, *51:*207, 1973

Choanal atresia, congenital (Trail *et al*). South. Med. J., *66:*470, 1973

A case of congenital bilateral choanal atresia treated surgically using the transpalatinal approach (Hybasek). Cesk. Otolaryngol., *24:*51, 1975 (Czechoslovakian)

Congenital choanal atresia – a technique for surgical correction (Smith *et al*). Trans. Am. Acad. Ophthalmol. Otolaryngol., *80:*527, 1975

Nose, Cleft Lip Deformities (See also *Cleft Lip, Secondary Deformity*)

Nose, leporine (Pardina, Frontera Vaca), PRS, *48:*394, 1971. Bull. Plast. Reconstr. Surg. Argent., *1:*12, 1970

Cleft of nose, median (Krikun), PRS, *52:*682, 1973. Acta chir. plast., *14:*137, 1972

Nose, rare nasal deformity similar to unilateral cleft lip nose but without cleft lip (Kozin), PRS, *52:*682, 1973. Acta chir. plast., *14:*210, 1972

Repair of columella base deformity in unilateral cleft lip (Onizuka). Brit. J. Plast. Surg., *25:*33, 1972

Nose, cleft-lip, use of anthropometry in assessing (Lindsay, Farkas). PRS, *49:*286, 1972

Nose, shape of, in cheilo-gnatho-palatoschisis unilateralis before operational repair (Hajnis, Figalova), PRS, *53:*681, 1974. Acta chir. plast., *15:*11, 1973

Cleft nose, corrective plastic surgery (Neuner), PRS, *52:*451, 1973. J. Maxillo-facial Surg., *1:*50, 1973

Noses associated with clefts of lip and palate, correction of (Schwenzer), PRS, *53:*240, 1974. J. Maxillo-facial Surg., *1:*91, 1973

Nose, development of cleft lip (Stark, Kaplan). PRS, *51:*413, 1973

Alar wing procedure, crossed, for correction of late deformity in the unilateral cleft lip nose (Whitlow, Constable). PRS, *52:*38, 1973

Nasal deformities, cleft lip, new method for correcting (Elsahy), PRS, *55:*383, 1975. Cleft Palate J., *11:*214, 1974

Lip, cleft, and nose, primary simultaneous

Nose, Cleft Lip Deformities – Cont.

correction, in unilateral cleft lip (Velazquez, Ortiz-Monasterio), PRS, *54:*558, 1974

Nasal deformities and their treatment in secondary repair of cleft lip patients (Malek), PRS, *56:*461, 1975. Scand. J. Plast. Reconstr. Surg., *8:*136, 1974

Alar cartilage and nasal deformity in unilateral cleft lip (Stenström) (Follow-Up Clinic). PRS, *55:*359, 1975

Nose, unilateral cleft lip, treatment of (McComb). PRS, *55:*596, 1975

Nose, Deformities of

Deformity due to heroin (Apton). Proc. Rudolph Virchow Med. Soc. City N.Y., *27:*19, 1968–69

Nose, middle clefts of, osseous changes in (Brejcha, Fara), PRS, *50:*633, 1972. Acta chir. plast., *13:*141, 1971

Nasal deformities and disfigurements, correction by operation of some (Monks) (Classic Reprint). PRS, *48:*485, 1971

Use of free transplantation of previously coded auricles of the external ear and local plastic surgery to replace defects in the nasal dorsum, apex, alae and septum (Balon). Vestn. Khir., *106:*63, 1971 (Russian)

Use of alloplastic materials for reconstructive surgery of nose, larynx and trachea (Kurilin). Zh. Ushn. Nos. Gorl. Bolezn., *31:*46, 1971 (Russian)

Nose, median cleft of (Krikun), PRS, *52:*682, 1973. Acta chir. plast., *14:*137, 1972

Corbin's beaked nose (Jost *et al*). Ann. chir. plast., *17:*5, 1972 (French)

Reconstruction of the columella (Kaplan). Brit. J. Plast. Surg., *25:*37, 1972

On the etiopathogenesis of congenital lateral nasal clefts (Mulfay *et al*). Otorinolaringologie, *17:*9, 1972 (Rumanian)

Nostril, supernumerary (Onizuka, Tai). PRS, *50:*403, 1972

Deformities of the middle 3rd of the face: naso-maxillary hypoplasia (Psillakis *et al*). Rev. Asoc. Med. Bras., *18:*185, 1972 (Portuguese)

Nasal deformities caused by inadequate posture during sleep (Abreu), PRS, *51:*475, 1973. Rev. brasil. clin. terapeut., *1:*633, 1972

Rare anomaly of nose (Kuznetsova). Vestn. Otorinolaringol., *34:*94, 1972 (Russian)

Treatment of double nose (Ghosh). J. Laryng. & Otol., *87:*593, 1973

Nose, cleft, corrective plastic surgery (Neuner), PRS, *52:*451, 1973. J. Maxillo-facial Surg., *1:*50, 1973

Nose, Deformities of – Cont.

Nasal septum, cartilaginous in rat, regeneration in, after resection, influence on facial growth (Kvinnsland, Breistein). PRS, *51:*190, 1973

Deformities of nose, ear, and hand: relapsing polychondritis (Jones), PRS, *51:*331, 1973

Nostril, case of congenital supernumerary (Get'man). Zh. Ushn. Nos. Gorl. Bolezn., *33:*88, 1973

Septal and associated cranial birth deformities: types, incidence and treatment (Gray). M. J. Australia, *1:*557, 1974

Nose deformities from trauma (Winston), PRS, *55:*375, 1975. Proc. Roy. Soc. Med., *67:*713, 1974

Congenital double columella (Rawat *et al*). Brit. J. Plast. Surg., *28:*153, 1975

An ideal donor site for the auricular composite graft (Argamaso). Brit. J. Plast. Surg., *28:*219, 1975

Atrophic rhinitis: proplast as an implant material in surgical treatment (Whitehead). Can. J. Otolaryngol., *4:*505, 1975

Deformities of the midface resulting from malunited orbital and naso-orbital fractures (Converse *et al*). Clin. Plast. Surg., *2:*107, 1975

Long-term experience with poly (glycol-monomethacrylate) gel in plastic operations of the nose (Voldrich *et al*). J. Biomed. Mater. Res., *9:*675, 1975

Deformities, cosmetic nasal, complicating prolonged nasotracheal intubation in critically ill newborn infants (Baxter *et al*), PRS, *57:*114, 1976. Pediatrics, *55:*884, 1975

Proboscis lateralis (D'Assumpção). PRS, *55:*494, 1975

Nasal deformity, residual, after Egener's granuloma (Domarus). PRS, *56:*216, 1975

Nose deformity, surgical correction of absent nasal alae of Johanson-Blizzard syndrome (Fox, Golden, Edgerton). PRS, *57:*484, 1976

Nose, Dermoid Cyst

Fistula of dorsum of nose (Brownstein, Shapiro, Slevin), PRS, *54:*377, 1974. Arch. Dermat., *109:*227, 1974

Nose, nasolabial cyst (Renard, Morgan). PRS, *57:*240, 1976

Nose, Diseases

Nose, destructive lesions of (Damiani *et al*). Minerva Chir., *26:*1429, 1971 (Italian)

Rhinotomy, hemilateral, in treatment of hereditary hemorrhagic telangiectasis (Whicker *et al*). Arch. Otolaryng., *96:*319, 1972

Nose, Diseases – Cont.

Osler-Weber-Rendu disease, management of epistaxis in; recurrence of telangiectases within nasal skin graft (McCabe, Kelly). PRS, *50:*114, 1972

Nose and throat, iatrogenic disorders of (Chignell). Proc. Roy. Soc. Med., *65:*679, 1972

Nasal and sinus therapy, potential complications of (Schmidt). J. Med. Trial Tech. Q., *20:*75, 1973

Partial or total closure of nostrils in atrophic rhinitis (Shah *et al*). Arch. Otolaryng., *100:*196, 1974

Nose, diseases and surgery of (Jaffe). Clin. Symp., *26:*1, 1974

Rhinolith, asymptomatic, in rhinoplasty (Mahler, Kaufman). PRS, *54:*490, 1974

Nose, Fractures of (See also *Facial Injuries; Nose, Injuries of*)

Nasal fractures, anterior ethmoid nerve block for treatment of (Seitchick). PRS, *48:*187, 1971

Fractures, nasal. Their occurrence, management and some late results (Mayell). J. R. Coll. Surg., Edinb., *18:*31, 1973

Submucous resection, acute (Adamson) (Follow-Up Clinic). PRS, *52:*432, 1973

Open surgical management of naso-orbital-ethmoid facial fractures (Epker). Trans. Int. Conf. Oral Surg., *4:*323, 1973

Nose and orbit fractures, primary treatment (Van der Meulen, Ramselaar, Bloem), PRS, *55:*107, 1975. Nederl. tijdschr. geneesk., *118:*841, 1974

Xeroradiography examinations in orbitonasal surgery (Maillard, Otto, Clodius). PRS, *55:*664, 1975

Clinical and therapeutic aspects of nasal trauma (Firica *et al*). Rev. Chir. (Otorinolaringol.), *20:*199, 1975 (Rumanian)

Nose, Infections of

Bacteremia and local infections with nasal packing (Herzon), PRS, *49:*580, 1972. Arch. Otolaryng., *94:*317, 1971

Naso-orbito-ocular mucormycosis, apropos of typical case (Georgiades *et al*). Ann. Ocul. (Paris), *205:*721, 1972 (French)

Mucormycosis, rhinocerebral (Berger, Disque, Topazian), PRS, *57:*671, 1976. Oral Surg., *40:*27, 1975

Nose, Injuries of

Preliminary report. Alloplastic repair of bone defects in nose and anterior wall of frontal air sinus on primary surgery of gunshot

Nose Injuries of—Cont.

and other wounds (experimental study) (Gerashchenko *et al*). Acta chir. plast. (Praha), *14:*166, 1972

Nasal trauma, penetrating: report of unusual case and discussion of management (Apfelberg *et al*). J. Trauma, *12:*821, 1972

Nasofrontal injuries, severe, reconstruction following (Gross *et al*). Otolaryngol. Clin. North Am., *5:*653, 1972

Nasal ala, loss of, from dog bite, immediate composite graft to (Wynn), PRS, *50:*188, 1972

Nasal necrosis; complication of nasotracheal intubation (Zwillich, Pierson), PRS, *53:*681, 1974. Chest, *64:*376, 1973

Nose injuries, significance of early care of, for subsequent function (Helms). H. N. O., *21:*77, 1973 (German)

Nasal fractures, their diagnoses, complications and treatment (Stoksted *et al*). H. N. O., *21:*304, 1973 (German)

Filling of traumatic notch at base of nose using eyebrow incision (Perrin). J. Fr. Otorhinolaryngol., *22:*242, 1973

Nasal fractures. Their occurrence, management and some late results (Mayell). J. R. Coll. Surg., Edinb., *18:*31, 1973

Nasal injuries in newborn infants (Cvetnic *et al*). Lijec. Vjesn., *95:*693, 1973 (Croatian)

Replantation, nasal tip (Cort), PRS, *52:*194, 1973

Nose, principles of correction of old septal deformity after injury (Fry), PRS, *52:*677, 1973. Proc. Roy. Australasian Coll. Surg., *46:*418, 1973

Naso-orbital-ethmoid facial fractures, open surgical management of (Epker). Trans. Congr. Int. Assoc. Oral Surg., *4:*323, 1973

Nasal trauma, acute, in children (Pirsig). Z. Laryngol. Rhinol. Otol., *52:*265, 1973 (German)

Nose, dog bite of, replantation of composite graft of nasal ala (Elsahy), PRS, *55:*633, 1975. Acta chir. plast., *16:*124, 1974

Degloving the nose (Egyedi), PRS, *55:* 375, 1975. J. Maxillo-facial Surg., *2:*101, 1974

Treatment of injuries to the nasal base (Jahnke). Laryngol. Rhinol. Otol. (Stuttg.), *53:*657, 1974 (German)

Nose and auricles, management of injuries to (Biskupska-Wiedo *et al*). Pol. Przegl. Chir., *46:*619, 1974 (Polish)

Trauma, nose deformity from (Winston), PRS, *55:*375, 1975. Proc. Roy. Soc. Med., *67:*713, 1974

Nose reconstruction after trauma (Jacobs, Walter), PRS, *57:*114, 1976. Actuel. Chir., *10:*157, 1975

Nose Injuries of—Cont.

Nose, leading with (Donald), PRS, *57:*755, 1976. Emerg. Med., *7:*27, 1975

Nasal injury, bizarre (Maran). PRS, *55:*498, 1975

Columella and septum, loss of, from unusual form of child abuse (Orton). PRS, *56:*345, 1975

Nose injury, management of (Facer), PRS, *57:*257, 1976. Postgrad. Med., *57:*123, 1975

Nose, Leprosy of: See *Leprosy*

Nose Neoplasms

Oncological surgery, nasal reconstruction of losses: 15 years' experience (Barrera, Serrano-Rebeil, Ortiz-Monasterio), PRS, *48:*89, 1971. Mem. V Cong. Mexicano Dermat., *5:*541, 1970

Epitheliomas, limited, of nasal fossae and sinuses (Marchand *et al*). Probl. Actuels Otorhinolaryngol., *125:*52, 1970 (French)

Hemangiopericytoma of the nose (Mootz *et al*). Z. Laryngol. Rhinol. Otol., *49:*257, 1970 (German)

Nasal gliomas (Katz, Lewis), PRS, *49:*587, 1972. Arch. Otolaryng., *94:*351, 1971

Plasmocytoma of the nasal cavity and sphenoid sinus (Korytowski *et al*). Otolaryngol. Pol., *25:*347, 1971 (Polish)

Giant-cell tumor of nasal bones (Sgouras, Georgiades). PRS, *48:*184, 1971

Plastic surgery in basalioma of the nose (Soares *et al*). Rev. Bras. Med., *28:*269, 1971 (Portuguese)

Darier-Ferrand dermatofibrosarcoma with nasal localization (Moriame, Moriame, Ledoux-Corbusier). Arch. belges dermat. et syph., *28:*167, 1972 (French)

Nasal cavity, schwannoma of (Iwamura *et al*). Arch. Otolaryng., *96:*176, 1972

Nose, glioma of (Aptenko *et al*). Arkh. Patol., *34:*72, 1972 (Russian)

Electrocoagulation in treatment of skin cancers of nose, ear and eye areas (Whelan). Bull. Soc. Internat. Chir., *31:*557, 1972

Carcinoma, nasal premaxillary complex (Briant *et al*). Can. J. Otolaryngol., *1:*30, 1972

Esthesioneuroepithelioma: report of two cases and discussion of management (Blokmanis). Can. J. Otolaryngol., *1:*43, 1972

Nose, basal cell carcinoma: with report of two atypical cases (Toppozada *et al*). J. Laryng. & Otol., *86:*933, 1972

Neoplasms, congenital, of nose (Macomber) (Follow-Up Clinic). PRS, *50:*77, 1972

Intranasal schwannoma (Wolfowitz *et al*). S. Afr. Med. J., *46:*55, 1972

Nose Neoplasms – Cont.

laringol., *2*:49, 1974

Nose tip, *mycosis fungoides* on (Uzel, Yormuk), PRS, *57*:114, 1976. Acta Oncol. Turcica, *8*:26, 1975

Giant keratoacanthoma of the nose (Rapaport). Arch. Dermat., *111*:73, 1975

Olfactory neuroblastoma. Management and prognosis (Bailey *et al*). Arch. Otolaryng., *101*:1, 1975

Nasal glomus (Enfores, Herngren), PRS, *57*:670, 1976. J. Laryng. & Otol., *89*:863, 1975

Inverted Schneiderian papilloma: a clinical and pathological study (Vrabec). Laryngoscope, *85*:186, 1975

Nasal reconstruction (Walter). Laryngoscope, *85*:1227, 1975

Dermatofibroma of the nose (Zakrzewski *et al*). Otolaryngol. Pol., *29*:617, 1975 (Polish)

Syndrome, Gardner's, extra-abdominal manifestations of (Neale, Pickrell, Quinn). PRS, *56*:92, 1975

Papillomas of the nasal and paranasal cavities (Claimont *et al*). South. Med. J., *68*:41, 1975

Cylindromas of the nose and paranasal sinuses (Volkov *et al*). Vestn. Otorinolaringol., *1*:55, 1975 (Russian)

Neurilemmoma of the nose and accessory sinuses (Volkov *et al*). Vestn. Otorinolaringol., *3*:34, 1975 (Russian)

Cancer of the skin of the nose. Treatment by total skin excision and three-quarter thickness skin graft (Goepfert *et al*). Arch. Otolaryng., *102*:90, 1976

Fresh tissue chemosurgery for tumors of the nose (Stegman *et al*). Eye Ear Nose Throat Mon., *55*:26, 1976

Gliomas, frontonasal tumors, diagnosis and management (Griffith). PRS, *57*:692, 1976

Nose, Sinuses of: See *Paranasal Sinus Neoplasms*

Nose, Surgery of (See also *Rhinoplasty*)

Nasal bones, giant-cell tumor of (Sgouras, Georgiades). PRS, *48*:184, 1971

Bilobed flap in nasal repair (Tardy *et al*). Arch. Otolaryng., *95*:1, 1972

Effective haemostasis with local anaesthesia in nasal surgery (Hirshowitz *et al*). Brit. J. Plast. Surg., *25*:335, 1972

Nose, lateral, subperiosteal osteotomy using rhinotome (Olivari), PRS, *52*:205, 1973. Chir. Plast., *1*:261, 1972

Nose, anatomically weak and aging, surgery of (Patterson). N. C. Med. J., *33*:692, 1972

Nose, Surgery of – Cont.

Nose, small defects of, use of complete transverse nasal flap in repair (Lipshutz, Penrod). PRS, *49*:629, 1972

Chondromucosal flap in nasal vestibule, versatility of (Millard). PRS, *50*:580, 1972

Nasal tip lesions, surgical treatment of (Pitanguy, Casancao, Garcia), PRS, *51*:701, 1973. Rev. brasil. cir., *61*:77, 1972

Nose tip surgery by hook flap technique (Psillakis, Albano), PRS, *52*:594, 1973. Rev. brasil. clin. terapeut., *1*:587, 1972

Nose, repair of prominent nasal tip (Spina, Kamakura, Psillakis), PRS, *53*:104, 1974. Rev. Soc. Med. Chir. San Jose, *5*:5, 1972

Nasal obstruction, judicious turbinectomy for (Fry), PRS, *52*:205, 1973. Australian & New Zealand J. Surg., *42*:291, 1973

Nose, half, reconstruction (Garcia-Velazco), PRS, *54*:234, 1974. Brit. J. Plast. Surg., *26*:412, 1973

Nostrils, modification in technique of closure (Gadre). J. Laryng. & Otol., *58*:903, 1973

Flap, dorsal nasal (Rigg). PRS, *52*:361, 1973

Nose, superior osteotomy: adjunct to osteoplastic nasal surgery (Graham, Royster), PRS, *53*:240, 1974. Rev. Latino Am. cir. plast., *17*:33, 1973

Making intranasal operations easier (Klusener). Z. Laryngol. Rhinol. Otol., *52*:93, 1973 (German)

Nose, dorsum of, reconstruction by osteoperiosteal grafts (Ditroi), PRS, *55*:634, 1975. Acta chir. plast., *16*:171, 1974

Extramucous rhinoplasty (Aytemiz *et al*), PRS, *57*:114, 1976. Bull. Milit. M. Acad., *16*:299, 1974

Cutaneous plastic surgery of the nose. Rieger's flap (Mazauric *et al*). J. Fr. Otorhinolaryngol., *23*:513, 1974 (French)

Operative management of the nose and associated tissues of the face (Walter). Laryngol. Rhinol. Otol. (Stuttg.), *53*:548, 1974 (German)

Reconstructive flaps in otolaryngology (McFarland). Laryngoscope, *84*:1267, 1974

Flap, dorsal nasal (Avakoff) (Letter to the Editor). PRS, *53*:671, 1974

Nose reconstruction with large forehead flap (Daver, Antia). PRS, *55*:360, 1975

Septum and columella, loss from unusual form of child abuse (Orton). PRS, *56*:345, 1975

Nose, free skin flap from retroauricular region to (Fujino, Harashina, Nakajima). PRS, *57*:338, 1976

Nasal alae, absent, of Johanson-Blizzard syndrome, surgical correction of (Fox, Golden, Edgerton). PRS, *57*:484, 1976

NOSTI, J. C., AND DAVIS, J. W.: Treatment of hypospadias by Byars technique. PRS, 52:128, 1973

NOTEA, E. et al: Lyophilized amnion in burns and skin loss. Harefuah, 88:265, 1975 (Hebrew)

NOTERMAN, J.: Interfascicular dissection of peripheral nerve with surgical microscope, PRS, 56:466, 1975. Acta chir. belg., 74:192, 1975

NOTERMAN, J.: Surgical pathology of the peripheral nerve. Introduction. Acta. chir. belg. (Suppl.), 1:9, 1975 (French)

NOTES, B.: Letter: Terminology. J.A.M.A., 234:1321, 1975

NOVAK, J.: Cervicoaural fistula. Cesk. Otolaryngol., 21:86, 1972 (Czechoslovakian)

NOVAK, J.: Bilateral occurrence of supernumerary deciduous and permanent canine tooth, PRS, 54:630, 1974. Czas. Stomatol., 2:148, 1974

NOVAK, J. et al: Fire hazards of clothing, especially of synthetic fibers. Orv. Hetil., 112:2095, 1971 (Hungarian)

NOVAK, J. et al: Primary homotransplantation (biological dressing) without excision in the treatment of burns. Orv. Hetil., 112:3078, 1971 (Hungarian)

NOVAK, R., AND DAVIS, J.: Effects of low-pass filtering on rate of learning and retrieval from memory of speech-like stimuli, PRS, 57:683, 1976. J. Speech & Hearing Res., 17:279, 1974

NOVELLI, G. P., MARSILI, M., AND PIERACEIOLI, E.: Anti-shock action of steroids other than cortisone, PRS, 53:375, 1974. Europ. Surg. Res., 5:169, 1973

NOVER, A. et al: Diseases of anterior segment of eye. Diagnosis and therapy. Fortschr. Med., 92:233, 1974 (German)

NOVICH, M. M.: What really happens in boxing? PRS, 54:370, 1974. Phys. & Sports Med., 2:28, 1974

NOWINSKI, J.: Advantages of vestibular approach in plastic operations of the nose. Otolaryngol. Pol., 26:59, 1972 (Polish)

NOYEK, A. M. et al: Osteoma of maxillary sinus – its occurrence following surgery. Can. J. Otolaryngol., 3:90, 1974

NUMMI, J. et al: Post-traumatic tenolysis in the hand. Handchirurgie, 3:11, 1971 (German)

NUNEZ, F. D.: Relationship of hematocrit levels to skin flap survival in the dog (with Earle, Fratianne). PRS, 54:341, 1974

NUNIS, E. M.: Plastic and reconstructive surgery and surgical nursing. Berita Jururawat., 12:65, 1972

NUNN, D. B. et al: Trachea – innominate artery fistula following tracheostomy. Successful repair using an innominate vein graft. Ann. Thorac. Surg., 20:698, 1975

Nursing

Nursing Care of the Plastic Surgery Patient. Ed. by Donald Wood-Smith and Pauline C. Porowski. C. V. Mosby Co., St. Louis, 1967.

Nursing device for use in cleft palate care (Shirley, Cocke). PRS, 48:83, 1971

Plastic and reconstructive surgery and surgical nursing (Nunis). Berita Jururawat., 12:65, 1972

Nursing the plastic surgery patient (Gill). A. O. R. N., 18:505, 1973

Caring for patients with facial or intraoral reconstruction (Trowbridge). Am. J. Nurs., 73:1930, 1973

Field of activity of pediatric nurse in mouth, jaw and plastic surgery as illustrated in West German jaw hospital (Kreidler). Dtsch. Krankenpflegez, 26:127, 1973 (German)

Nurse's functions in office of cosmetic department (Stepanova). Med. Sestra., 32:41, 1973 (Russian)

Eating with a tracheostomy (Weber), PRS, 56:355, 1975. Am. J. Nursing, 74:1439, 1974

Nursing, bedside. Attendance of aged, blind, mute patient – understanding needs of patient with pharyngeal cancer following tracheotomy (Okamatsu). Jap. J. Nurs., 38:63, 1974 (Japanese)

Nurses' reactions to transsexual surgery (Lark), PRS, 57:767, 1976. A.O.R.N., 22:743, 1975

NUSEIBEH, I. M.: Split skin graft and treatment of pressure sores, PRS, 56:114, 1975. Paraplegia, 12:1, 1974

Nutrition

Intravenous nutrition, total, adjunct to management of infants with ruptured omphalocele (Filler et al), PRS, 48:612, 1971. Am. J. Surg., 121:454, 1971

Venous cannulation, prolonged central, morbid and mortal complications. Awareness, recognition, and prevention (Henzel, DeWeese), PRS, 49:477, 1972. Am. J. Surg., 121:600, 1971

Parenteral nutrition utilizing common facial vein, catheter placement in infants needing total (Zumbro, Mullin, Nelson), PRS, 48:92, 1971. Arch. Surg., 102:71, 1971

Subclavian vein, right, anatomic relationships (Land), PRS, 48:197, 1971. Arch. Surg., 102:178, 1971

Nutritive solutions given parenterally,

Nutrition — Cont.

growth of *Candida albicans* in (Brennan *et al*), PRS, *50:*312, 1972. Arch. Surg., *103:*705, 1971

Trauma, major, intracellular cation alterations following: effect of supranormal caloric intake (Curreri *et al*), PRS, *49:*476, 1972. J. Trauma, *11:*390, 1971

Hypophosphatemia in hyperalimentation (Ruberg *et al*), PRS, *49:*670, 1972. Surg. Forum, *22:*87, 1971

Catheters, intravenous, bacteriologic nature and prevention of contamination to (Crenshaw *et al*), PRS, *50:*424, 1972. Am. J. Surg., *123:*264, 1972

Infants and children, high caloric parenteral therapy in (Asch, Huxtable, Hays), PRS, *50:*638, 1972. Arch. Surg., *104:*434, 1972

Intravenous hyperalimentation (Vogel, Kingsbury, Baue), PRS, *51:*610, 1973. Arch. Surg., *105:*414, 1972

Fluid therapy for infants and children on a plastic surgical service, brief guide to (Pickrell, Mladick). PRS, *49:*404, 1972

Hyperalimentation, central venous catheter placement using common facial vein (Zumbra, Mullin, Nelson), PRS, *52:*603, 1973. Am. J. Surg., *125:*654, 1973

Veins, cephalic and basilic, used for introduction of central venous catheters (Webre, Arens), PRS, *53:*250, 1974. Anesthesiology, *38:*389, 1973

Subclavian vein catheterization, complications of (Glaser, Radoman, Canonne), PRS, *53:*606, 1974. Ann. Chir., *27:*911, 1973

Aphagia following traumatic coma. Attempts at physiopathogenic interpretation. Treatment (Lallemant *et al*). Ann. Otolaryngol. Chir. Cervicofac., *90:*329, 1973

Parenteral nutrition in thermally injured patients, 10% intravenous fat emulsion for (Wilmore *et al*), PRS, *53:*686, 1974. Ann. Surg., *178:*503, 1973

Osteomyelitis of clavicle following subclavian vein catheterization (Manny, Haruzi, Yosipovitch), PRS, *52:*454, 1973. Arch. Surg., *106:*342, 1973

Soybean oil, total intravenous nutrition (Yeo *et al*), PRS, *53:*376, 1974. Arch. Surg., *106:*792, 1973

Catheters, silicone rubber for long-term hyperalimentation, new method of fixation (Filler), PRS, *53:*247, 1974. J. Pediat. Surg., *8:*395, 1973

Infants, long-term intravenous feeding using peripheral veins (Coran), PRS, *54:*697, 1974. J. Pediat. Surg., *8:*801, 1973

Central venous catheter thrombosis, hazard of medical progress (Warden, Wilmore,

Nutrition — Cont.

Pruitt), PRS, *53:*489, 1974. J. Trauma, *13:*620, 1973

Nutrition, parenteral, of burned child (Popp, Law, MacMillan), PRS, *54:*378, 1974. Ann. Surg., *179:*219, 1974

Weight loss after operation, oral and intravenous nutrition (Daly *et al*), PRS, *55:*645, 1975. Ann. Surg., *180:*709, 1974

Infants, seriously ill, complications of intravenous alimentation (Dimmick *et al*), PRS, *55:*120, 1975. Canad. J. Surg., *17:*186, 1974

Subclavian vein, infraclavicular percutaneous catheterization of (Wang, Ho), PRS, *54:*692, 1974. Chinese M.J., *5:*80, 1974

Subclavian venipuncture and catheterization by supraclavicular approach (Shanghai Chung Shan Hospital), PRS, *54:*692, 1974. Chinese M.J., *5:*81, 1974

Candida osteomyelitis and arthritis from hyperalimentation therapy (Noble, Lyne), PRS, *55:*259, 1975. J. Bone & Joint Surg., *56A:*825, 1974

Feeding techniques for dysphagic patients (Gaffney, Campbell), PRS, *56:*114, 1975. Am. J. Nursing, *74:*2194, 1975

Nutrition, surgical problems managed by elemental diet (Rivard, LaPoint), PRS, *56:*116, 1975. Canad. J. Surg., *18:*90, 1975

Nutrition, total parenteral, in pediatrics (Winters), PRS, *57:*268, 1976. Pediatrics, *56:*17, 1975

NWAKO, F.: Combined one stage urethroplasty in treatment of hypospadias, PRS, *55:*638, 1975. J. Pediat. Surg., *4:*467, 1974

NWOKU, A. L.: Problems and results of free mucosa transplantation in the oral cavity. Z. W. R., *81:*586, 1972 (German)

NWOKU, A. L.: Results of surgical correction of open bite using Schuchardt's method. Fortschr. Kiefer. Gesichtschir., *18:*209, 1974 (German)

NWOKU, A. L. *et al*: Problems of correction of asymmetric mandibular prognathism. Int. J. Oral Surg., *3:*229, 1974

NWOKU, A. L. *et al*: Technic and results in tear duct reconstruction in facial injuries. Fortschr. Kiefer. Gesichtschir., *19:*148, 1975 (German)

NWOKUS, A. L.: Recurrence of oral cancer in patients with radio-osteomyelitis of jaw, PRS, *53:*682, 1974. J. Maxillo-facial Surg., *1:*157, 1973

NWOKUS, A. L., AND KOCH, H.: Effect of radiation injury on growing face, PRS, *56:*459, 1975. J. Maxillo-facial Surg., *3:*28, 1975

NWOKUS, A. L. N., AND KOCH, H.: Temporomandibular joint — rare localization for bone tumors, PRS, *55:*379, 1975. J. Maxillo-facial Surg., *2:*113, 1974

NYBROE, L., FEJERSKOV, O., AND PHILIPSEN, H. P.: The histology of autologous skin grafts in the human oral cavity. Acta Odontol. Scand., *30:*643, 1972

NYHAN, W. L.: Malformation syndromes in human genetic disease. PRS, *52:*237, 1973

NYLEN, B.: Plastic surgery in a developing country. Nord. Med., *86:*1220, 1971 (Swedish)

NYLEN, B.: Plastic surgery – a rapidly developing specialty. Nord. Med., *86:*1223, 1971 (Swedish)

NYLEN, B.: Bone grafting of skull defects (with Körlof, Rietz). PRS, *52:*378, 1973

NYLEN, B.: Open fractures: new fixation method in cross-leg cases (arm-leg) (Follow-Up Clinic). PRS, *54:*604, 1974

NYLEN, B. *et al*: Observations from a Saigon hospital for reconstructive pediatric surgery. Lakartidningen, *69:*1125, 1972 (Swedish)

NYLEN, B. *et al*: Primary, early bone grafting in complete clefts of lip and palate, PRS, *56:*683, 1975. Scand. J. Plast. Reconstr. Surg., *8:*79, 1974

O

OARA, Y. *et al*: Decompression incision in finger burns – chemical burn of the finger. Orthop. Surg. (Tokyo), *22:*881, 1971 (Japanese)

OATA, N: Clinical and cinefluorographic studies on postoperative dysphagia after mandibulectomy for malignant tumors. J. Jap. Stomatol. Soc., *39:*611, 1972 (Japanese)

OATIS, G. W. *et al*: Dermoid cyst of floor of mouth, PRS, *56:*597, 1975. J. Oral Surg., *39:*192, 1975

OATIS, G. W. *et al*: Cleidocranial dysostosis with mandibular cyst, case report. Oral Surg., *40:*62, 1975

OBER, K. G. *et al*: Reconstructive and plastic surgery in gynecology. Dtsch. Med. J., *23:*565, 1972 (German)

OBERFIELD, R. A., CADY, B., AND BOOTH, J. C.: Regional arterial chemotherapy for advanced carcinoma of head and neck, PRS, *54:*235, 1974. Cancer, *32:*82, 1973

OBERHOLZER, D.: Priorities in the treatment of acute hand injuries. Proc. Mine. Med. Off. Assoc., *53:*2, 1973

OBERNIEDERMAYR, A.: Harelip and cleft palate, current status of therapy and problems of postoperative care. Dtsch. Med. J., *21:*107, 1970 (German)

Obesity (See also *Abdominoplasty; Lipodystrophy; Mammaplasty*)

Plastic operations for pendulous abdomen in obese subjects (Szczawinski *et al*). Pol.

Obesity – Cont.

Przegl. Chir., *43:*1317, 1971 (Polish)

Metabolic disorders, acute, after intestinal short circuit operations because of massive obesity (Bunte, Husemann), PRS, *53:*365, 1974. Bull. Soc. Internat. Chir., *32:*415, 1973

Intestinal short circuit operations for massive obesity, acute metabolic disorders after (Bunte, Husemann), PRS, *53:*365, 1974. Internat. Chir., *32:*415, 1973

Psychoneurosis and obesity – the hen and egg dilemma (Valsrub). J.A.M.A., *230:*591, 1974

Diet, latest fad – lockjaw, PRS, *55:*647, 1975. Med. World News, Feb. 8, 1974

Obesity, current status of jejuno-ileal bypass for, PRS, *56:*678, 1975. Nutrition Rev., *32:*333, 1974

Weight reduction, massive, surgical reduction after (McCraw). PRS, *53:*349, 1974

Obesity: personal reaction to weight loss (Pescatore), PRS, *56:*116, 1975. Am. J. Nursing, *74:*2227, 1975

Massive weight loss patient (Zook). Clin. Plast. Surg., *2:*457, 1975

Editorial: surgery for obesity (Friedell). Int. Surg., *60:*70, 1975

Surgical treatment of severe obesity (Montorsi). Minerva Med., *66:*2629, 1975 (Italian)

Plastic surgical treatment of obesity (Sanders). Proc. Roy. Soc. Med., *68:*664, 1975

OBI, L. J., AND BAYLES, D. E.: New instrument for treatment of rhinophyma. PRS, *50:*414, 1972

Obituaries (See also *Classic Reprints; History of Plastic Surgery*)

In memoriam Assistant Professor Teobald Adamczak, M.D. (Peskova). Acta chir. plast. (Praha), *16:*256, 1974

Bales, Harold W., Jr., M.D., PRS, *54:*703, 1974

Beatty, Hugh G., M.D., PRS, *50:*640, 1972

Bransfield, John W., M.D., PRS, *52:*690, 1973

Brown, James Barrett, M.D., PRS, *48:*101, 1971

Browne, Harold R., M.D., PRS, *48:*406, 1971

Burt, Glen B., M.D., PRS, *52:*690, 1973

Caltagirone, Joseph V., M.D., PRS, *56:*685, 1975

Carlin, Gene A., M.D., PRS, *56:*685, 1975

Coffey, Richard J., M.D., PRS, *52:*690, 1973

Cowan, James A., Jr., M.D., PRS, *52:*690, 1973

De Cholnoky, Tibor, M.D., PRS, *56:*685, 1975

Obituaries – Cont.

DeStefano, George A., M.D., PRS, *50:*640, 1972

Douglas, Beverly, M.D., PRS, *56:*685, 1975; PRS, *57:*408, 1976

Finley, Marcus L., M.D., PRS, *56:*685, 1975

Haynes, Leigh K., M.D., PRS, *50:*640, 1972

Hill, John Robert, M.D., PRS, *52:*690, 1973

Howard, Lot Duncan, M.D., PRS, *54:*632, 703, 1974

Hyslop, Volney B., M.D., PRS, *54:*703, 1974

Ivy, Robert H., M.D., PRS, *54:*704, 1974, PRS, *55:*122, 1975. Cleft Palate J., *11:*508, 1974. Rozhl. Chir., *54:*661, 1975

Kazanjian, Varaztad H., M.D., PRS, *55:*524, 1975; PRS, *56:*686, 1975. New England J. Med., *292:*806, 1975. Trans. Am. Acad. Ophthalmol. Otolaryngol., *80:*267, 1975

Kitlowski, Edward A., M.D., PRS, *48:*615, 1971

LaDage, Leo H., M.D., PRS, *52:*691, 1973

Limberg, Alexander A., M.D., PRS, *56:*239, 686, 1975

Lipshutz, Herbert, M.D., PRS, *54:*704, 1974

McNichol, J. Wallace, M.D., PRS, *56:*686, 1975

McWhirt, Joseph R., M.D., PRS, *54:*704, 1974

Mills, James Theodore, M.D., PRS, *54:*251, 704, 1974

Morley, George Henry, M.D., Brit. J. Plast. Surg., *24:*419, 1971

Moran, Robert E., M.D., PRS, *50:*641, 1972; (Obituary by Letterman), PRS, *51:*493, 1973

Neumann, Charles G., M.D., PRS, *52:*691, 1973

O'Connor, Gerald Brown, M.D., PRS, *51:*612, 1973; PRS, *52:*691, 1973

O'Malley, Joseph E., M.D., PRS, *52:*691, 1973

Potter, Leo Edward, M.D., PRS, *52:*691, 1973

Sanvenero-Rosselli, Gustavo, M.D., PRS, *54:*513, 704, 1974. Brit. J. Plast. Surg., *27:*297, 1974. Acta chir. plast. (Praha), *16:*199, 1974. Minerva Med., *65:*4380, 1974 (Italian)

Straatsma, Clarence Ralph, M.D., PRS, *55:*648, 1975; *56:*686, 1975

Tamerin, Joseph A., M.D. (Obituary by Crikelair). PRS, *56:*480, 686, 1975

Trusler, Harold M., M.D., PRS, *51:*713, 1973; PRS, *52:*691, 1973

Vincent, Richard W., PRS, *49:*590, 1972; PRS, *50:*641, 1972

Walker, John C., Jr., M.D., PRS, *56:*686, 1975

Wallace, Alexander B., J. R. Coll. Surg. Edinb., *20:*142, 1975. Lancet, *1:*52, 1975. Rozhl. Chir., *54:*420, 1975 (Czechoslovakian)

Obituaries – Cont.

Wallace, Alister B., F.R.C.S., PRS, *56:*686, 1975; PRS, *57:*269, 1976

Webster, Jerome Pierce, M.D., PRS, *50:*510, 1972. PRS, *55:*728, 1975. PRS, *56:*686, 1975. J. Hist. Med., *30:*67, 1975

OBLAK, P.: Trigonometric method of analysis of upper part of mouth cavity, PRS, *57:*258, 1976. J. Maxillo-facial Surg., *3:*88, 1975

OBLAK, P.: New concept of morphogenesis of clefts in lip, alveolus, and palate, PRS, *57:*675, 1976. J. Maxillo-facial Surg., *3:*182, 1975

OBLAK, P.: New guiding principles in the treatment of clefts. J. Maxillo-facial Surg., *3:*231, 1975

OBREJA, S. *et al*: Advantages of free skin autografts in the treatment of rhinophyma. Otorinolaringologie, *16:*297, 1971 (Rumanian)

OBREJA, S. *et al*: On a case of total branchial fistula. Otorinolaringologie, *16:*345, 1971 (Rumanian)

OBREJA, S. *et al*: Critical study of the surgical approach to the maxillary sinus, using an osteoplastic flap. Rev. Chir. (Otorinolaringol.), *19:*335, 1974 (Rumanian)

O'BRIEN, B. M., AND SHANMUGAN, N.: Experimental transfer of composite free flaps with microvascular anastomoses, PRS, *54:*117, 1974. Australian & New Zealand J. Surg., *43:*285, 1973

O'BRIEN, B. M., AND MILLER, G. D. H.: Digital reattachment and revascularization, PRS, *53:*244, 1974. J. Bone & Joint Surg., *55A:*714, 1973

O'BRIEN, B. M. *et al*: Saving the amputated digit and hand. M. J. Australia, *1:*558, 1973

O'BRIEN, B. M. *et al*: Successful transfer of large island flap from groin to foot by microvascular anastomoses. PRS, *52:*271, 1973

O'BRIEN, B. M. *et al*: Clinical replantation of digits. PRS, *52:*490, 1973

O'BRIEN, B. M., AND HAYHURST, J. W.: Metallized microsutures and new micro needle holder. PRS, *52:*673, 1973

O'BRIEN, B. M., AND MACLEOD, A. M.: Replantation surgery in upper limb, PRS, *52:*680, 1973. Proc. Roy. Australasian Coll. Surg., *46:*427, 1973

O'BRIEN, B. M. *et al*: Free flap transfers with microvascular anastomoses, PRS, *56:*683, 1975. Brit. J. Plast. Surg., *27:*220, 1974

O'BRIEN, B. M. *et al*: Major replantation surgery in upper limb, PRS, *56:*228, 1975. Hand, *6:*217, 1974

OBSTBAUM, S., AND PODOS, S.: Ocular compression and non-corticosteroidal anti-inflammatory agents, PRS, *57:*113, 1976. Am. J. Ophth., *79:*1008, 1975

OBWEGESER, H.: Correction of jaw position in an adult cleft patient. Dtsch. Zahnaerztl. Z., *28:*688, 1973 (German)

OBWEGESER, H. L.: Late reconstruction of large maxillary defects after tumor-resection. J. Maxillo-facial Surg., *1:*19, 1973

OBWEGESER, H. L.: Maxillofacial surgeon's responsibility in middle face surgery. Arch. Otorhinolaryngol. (N.Y.), *207:*229, 1974 (German)

OBWEGESER, H. L.: Correction of skeletal anomalies of otomandibular dysostosis, PRS, *55:*378, 1975. J. Maxillo-facial Surg., *2:*73, 1974

OBWEGESER, H. L., FREIHOFER, H. P. M., AND HOREGS, J.: Variations of fibrous dysplasia in jaws, PRS, *53:*603, 1974. J. Maxillo-facial Surg., *1:*161, 1973

OBWEGESER, H. L. *et al*: Another way of treatment of fractures of atrophic edentulous mandible. J. Maxillo-facial Surg., *1:*213, 1973

OCANA LOSA, J. M., AND MARTINEZ CARO, A.: Duplication of urethra with epispadias, PRS, *53:*107, 1974. Rev. med. Hosp. Gen. Asturias, *5:*131, 1970

OCHSNER, S. F., AND COLLINS, V. P.: Interstitial radiotherapy for intraoral carcinoma, PRS, *55:*642, 1975. South. M.J., *67:*1150, 1974

O'CONNOR, G. B. *et al*: Advancement of soft tissues to correct mild midfacial retrusion. PRS, *52:*42, 1973

O'CONNOR, R. L.: Digital nerve compression secondary to palmar aneurysm. Clin. Orthop., *83:*149, 1972

O'CONOR, C. M.: Carcinoma of lips – reparative plasties, PRS, *48:*194, 1971. Bull. Acad. Argent. Cir., *54:*542, 1970

O'CONOR, C. M.: Progressive facial hemiatrophy, PRS, *52:*688, 1973. Bol. y trab. Acad. argent. cir., *56:*543, 1972

O'CONOR, C. M. *et al*: Reparative plasty in large defects of palate, PRS, *51:*346, 1973. Prensa med. argent., *59:*992, 1972

Ocular: See *Eye*

Ocular Hypertelorism: See *Hypertelorism*

Ocular Hypotelorism: See *Hypotelorism*

ODASSO, M. *et al*: Anatomical and clinical features of mesenchymal tumors of the jaws. Minerva Stomatol., *22:*269, 1973 (Italian)

O'DELL, A. J.: Objectives and standards in care of patient with radical neck dissection. Nurs. Clin. North Am., *8:*159, 1973

O'DONNELL, J. P., KRISCHER, J. P., AND SHIERE, F. R.: Analysis of presurgical orthopedics in treatment of unilateral cleft lip and palate, PRS, *56:*108, 1975. Cleft Palate J., *11:*374, 1974

O'DONNELL, T. F., JR.: Minor infections of hand in Marine recruits: analysis of 100 consecutive cases, PRS, *48:*93, 1971. Mil. Med., *136:*30, 1971

O'DONOGHUE, M. N., AND ZAREM, H. A.: Stimulation of neovascularization – comparative efficacy of fresh and preserved skin grafts. PRS, *48:*474, 1971

Odontogenic Cysts (See also *Jaw Cysts*)

Cyst, odontogenic, calcifying (Herd). Aust. Dent. J., *17:*421, 1972

Keratocysts, odontogenic, radiological features of (McIvor). Brit. J. Oral Surg., *10:*116, 1972

Jaws, keratocysts of (Klammt). Dtsch. Stomatol., *22:*501, 1972 (German)

Therapy of tooth eruption disorders caused by cysts (Hotz *et al*). Fortschr. Kieferorthop., *33:*19, 1972

Maxilla, odontogenic keratocyst of (Kotton). J. Laryng. & Otol., *86:*1169, 1972

Odontogenic cysts in man, metaplasia and degeneration in (Browne). J. Oral. Pathol., *1:*145, 1972

Jaws, keratocysts of (Donoff *et al*). J. Oral Surg., *30:*880, 1972

Jaws, keratocysts of, note on origin (Stoelinga *et al*). Int. J. Oral Surg., *2:*37, 1973

Odontogenic keratocysts, use of exfoliative cytology and protein estimations in preoperative diagnosis of (Kramer *et al*). Int. J. Oral Surg., *2:*143, 1973

Odontodysplasia, regional, with associated midline mandibular cyst, case report (Burch *et al*). J. Oral Surg., *31:*44, 1973

Odontogenic cysts, surgical treatment (De la Mata Pages). Rev. Esp. Estomatol., *21:*413, 1973 (Spanish)

Adenomatoid odontogenic tumor. Periodontal aspects on diagnosis and treatment, (Berghagen). Sven. Tandlak. Tidskr., *66:*467, 1973

Retrograde root-filling in oral surgery (Ross). Trans. Int. Conf. Oral Surg., *4:*98, 1973

Various problems in the treatment of odontogenic cysts (Penev). Cesk. Stomatol., *74:*153, 1974 (Czechoslovakian)

Odontogenic keratocyst – an approach to treatment (Bramley). Int. J. Oral Surg., *3:*337, 1974

Odontogenic cysts, irradiated allogeneic bone grafts in treatment of (Spengos). J. Oral Surg., *32:*674, 1974

Dentinal dysplasia: report of a family (McFarlane *et al*). J. Oral Surg., *32:*867, 1974

Odontogenic keratocyst, case report (Sher *et al*). Oral Surg., *37:*518, 1974

Analysis of the recurrence of odontogenic

Odontogenic Cysts — Cont.
keratocysts (Forssell *et al*). Proc. Finn. Dent. Soc., *70:*135, 1974

Dental cyst, review of recent experimental work on (Harris), PRS, *56:*225, 1975. Proc. Roy. Soc. Med., *67:*1259, 1974

Study of odontogenic cysts with special reference to comparisons between keratinizing and nonkeratinizing cysts (Borg *et al*). Sven. Tandlak. Tidskr., *67:*311, 1974

Keratinizing squamous epithelial cysts (keratocysts) in the jaws (Stiebitz *et al*). Wien. Klin. Wochenschr., *86:*643, 1974 (German)

Factor XIII concentrate in osteotomies and cystectomies with heterologous bone implantation (Mannheim). Z. W. R., *83:*323, 1974 (German)

Odontogenic cysts bulging into maxillary sinuses, analysis and therapeutic results in (Lewandowski). Czas. Stomatol., *28:*649, 1975 (Polish)

Lateral periodontal cyst: report of a case (Lederman). J. Oral Med., *30:*62, 1975

Ultrastructure of the keratinizing and calcifying odontogenic cyst (Chen *et al*). Oral Surg., *39:*769, 1975

Calcifying odontogenic cyst (Anneroth *et al*). Oral Surg., *39:*794, 1975

Calcifying odontogenic cyst. A review and analysis of seventy cases (Freedman *et al*). Oral Surg., *40:*93, 1975

Odontogenic keratocysts (Richter *et al*). Schweiz. Monatsschr. Zahnheilkd., *85:*487, 1975 (French)

OELSNITZ, G. V. D.: Results of funnel chest operation in pediatric surgical clinic in Bremen, PRS, *55:*108, 1975. Ztschr. Kinderchir., *15:*25, 1974

OESER, R. *et al*: Significance of acral oscillography in functional circulation disorders caused by work with compressed-air tools. Dtsch. Gesundheitsw., *27:*942, 1972 (German)

O'FALLON, W. M.: Enzyme analysis as test of skin viability (with Georgiade, King). PRS, *53:*67, 1974

OGANESIAN, O. Z.: Conduction anesthesia in surgery of the hand. Vestn. Khir., *111:*111, 1973 (Russian)

OGAWA, T. K. *et al*: Air-fluid levels in the sphenoid sinus in epistaxis and nasal packing. Radiology, *118:*351, 1976

OGBUOKIRI, C. G., LOW, E. J., AND MACMILLAN, B. G.: Superior mesenteric artery syndrome in burned children, PRS, *51:*234, 1973. Am. J. Surg., *124:*75, 1972

OGG, M. J.: Patients' refusal of surgery after Innovar premedication (with Briggs). PRS, *51:*158, 1973

OGINO, Y. *et al*: Experience in external nasal reconstruction and discussion on various problems. Jap. J. Plast. Reconstr. Surg., *14:*456, 1971 (Japanese)

OGO, K.: Treatment of micrognathia in neonatal period; report of 65 cases (with Monroe). PRS, *50:*317, 1972

OGO, K. *et al*: Ten-year survey of macrostomia, PRS, *54:*106, 1974. Jap. J. Plast. Reconstr. Surg., *16:*431, 1973

OGURA, J., BILLER, H. F., AND WETTE, R.: Elective neck dissection for pharyngeal and laryngeal cancers: evaluation, PRS, *50:*309, 1972. Ann. Otol. Rhin. & Laryng., *80:*646, 1971

OGURA, J. H.: Plastic surgery research in otolaryngology. Laryngoscope, *81:*1985, 1971

OGURA, J. H.: Conservation surgery of the larynx and pharynx. Tex. Med., *68:*106, 1972

OGURA, J. H.: Selection of patients for conservation surgery of larynx and pharynx. Trans. Am. Acad. Ophthalmol. Otolaryngol., *76:*741, 1972

OGURA, J. H. *et al*: Use of regional flaps in reconstructive surgery of head and neck. Can. J. Otolaryngol., *1:*290, 1972

OGURA, J. H. *et al*: Cancer of the head and neck. Hypopharynx and larynx. Surgical management. J.A.M.A., *221:*77, 1972

OGURA, J. H. *et al*: Conservation surgery of larynx and hypopharynx — selection of patients and results. Can. J. Otolaryngol., *2:*11, 1973

OGURA, J. H. *et al*: Surgical results of orbital decompression for malignant exophthalmos. Laryngoscope, *84:*637, 1974

OGURA, J. H. *et al*: Long term therapeutic results — cancer of the larynx and hypopharynx. Preliminary report. Laryngoscope, *85:*1746, 1975

OGURA, J. H. *et al*: Conservation surgery for epidermoid carcinoma of the marginal area (aryepiglottic fold extension). Laryngoscope, *85:*1801, 1975

OGURA, J. H. *et al*: Conservation surgery for epidermoid carcinoma of the supraglottic larynx. Laryngoscope, *85:*1808, 1975

OH, S. J., AND KIM, K. W.: Thrombophlebitis-induced median neuropathy, PRS, *55:*510, 1975. South. M.J., *67:*1041, 1974

O'HARA, A. E. *et al*: Sialography in unusual case of subcutaneous emphysema of neck. Arch. Otolaryng., *98:*354, 1973

O'HARA, J. P., III *et al*: Angiography in the diagnosis of osteoid-osteoma of the hand. J. Bone & Joint Surg. (Am.), *57:*163, 1975

O'HARA, K. *et al*: Prediction of survival time of rats in severe heat, PRS, *57:*127, 1976. J. Appl. Physiol., *38:*724, 1975

OHARA, Y.: Incision for reduction of tension in burned hands. Shujutsu, 26:48, 1972 (Japanese)

OHBA, T. et al: Mandibular metastasis of osteogenic sarcoma, case report. Oral Surg., 39:821, 1975

OHHATA, N.: Clinical and cinefluorographic studies on postoperative dysphagia after mandibulectomy for malignant tumors. J. Jap. Stomatol. Soc., 39:611, 1972 (Japanese)

OHLSÉN, L.: Growth of cartilage from free perichondrial graft placed across defect in rabbit's trachea (with Sohn). PRS, 53:55, 1974

OHMORI, K.: Successful clinical transfer of ten free flaps by microvascular anastomoses (with Harii, Ohmori), PRS, 53:259, 1974. Discussion by Goldwyn, PRS, 53:469, 1974

OHMORI, K.: Hair transplantation with free scalp flaps (with Harii, Ohmori). PRS, 53:410, 1974

OHMORI, K.: Free groin flaps in children (with Harii). PRS, 55:588, 1975

OHMORI, K.: Free gracilis muscle transplantation with microneurovascular anastomoses for treatment of facial paralysis (with Harii, Torii). PRS, 57:133, 1976

OHMORI, K.: Free musculocutaneous flap (with Harii, Sekiguchi), PRS, 57:294, 1976. Discussion by Cannon, PRS, 57:511, 1976

OHMORI, S.: Use of gastroepiploic vessels as recipient or donor vessels in free transfer of composite flaps by microvascular anastomoses (with Harii). PRS, 52:541, 1973

OHMORI, S.: Successful clinical transfer of ten free flaps by microvascular anastomoses (with Harii, Ohmori), PRS, 53:259, 1974. Discussion by Goldwyn, PRS, 53:469, 1974

OHMORI, S.: Hair transplantation with free scalp flaps (with Harii, Ohmori). PRS, 53:410, 1974

OHMORI, S.: Recent progress in plastic surgery, especially on craniofacial surgery. Neurol. Surg. (Tokyo), 3:277, 1975 (Japanese)

OHMORI, S., AND MATSUMOTO, K.: Treatment of cryptotia using Teflon string. PRS, 49:33, 1972

OHMORI, S., MATSUMOTO, K., AND NAKAI, H.: Reconstruction of microtic ear by use of silicone rubber frame, PRS, 56:352, 1975. Jap. J. Plast. Reconstr. Surg., 17:484, 1974

OHMORI, S., MATSUMOTO, K., AND NAKAI, H.: Follow-up study on reconstruction of microtia using silicone framework, PRS, 53:555, 1974

OHTSUKA, H. et al: Clinical application of cryosurgery in plastic and reconstructive surgery, PRS, 55:384, 1975. Jap. J. Plast. Reconstr. Surg., 17:371, 1974

OHYAMA, H., AND HASHIMOTO, K.: Collagenolytic activity in malignant melanoma: physi-

ochemical studies, PRS, 54:116, 1974. Cancer Res., 33:2507, 1973

OIKARINEN, V. J. et al: Laboratory screening tests prior to outpatient oral surgery. Proc. Finn. Dent. Soc., 69:110, 1973

OIKAWA, K. et al: Effect of lymphadenectomy on neoplasm immunity. Hokkaido J. Med. Sci., 50:84, 1975 (Japanese)

OJAJARVI, J.: An evaluation of antiseptics used for hand disinfection in wards. J. Hyg. (Camb.), 76:75, 1976

OJEDA, F. X.: Tendon graft: evaluation of flexor profundus of fingers, PRS, 53:606, 1974. Rev. Latino Am. cir. plast., 17:57, 1973

OJEDA, F. X. et al: Midline cleft of lower lip and mandible, PRS, 57:263, 1976. Cir. Plast. Ibero-Latino Am., 1:51, 1975

OKA, M. et al: Respiratory management in Pierre Robin syndrome – with special reference to acidbase equilibrium. Jap. J. Anesthesiol., 21:1352, 1972 (Japanese)

OKAMATSU, T.: Bedside nursing. Attendance of aged, blind, mute patient – understanding needs of patient with pharyngeal cancer following tracheotomy. Jap. J. Nurs., 38:63, 1974 (Japanese)

O'KEEFFE, P. J.: Trephining sebaceous cysts. Brit. J. Plast. Surg., 25:411, 1972

OKSALA, A.: Blow-out fracture of orbit. Duodecim, 90:171, 1974 (Finnish)

OKSENBERG, J.: et al: Anatomical and clinicosurgical aspects of malar region. Odontol. Chil., 20:15, 1972 (Spanish)

OKUN, M. R.: On skin pigmentation (Letter to the Editor). PRS, 57:738, 1976

OKUN, M. R. et al: Malignant melanoma developing from intradermal nevi, PRS, 57:264, 1976. Arch. Dermat., 110:599, 1974

OLAH, Z.: Experiences with movable bulbar implant of hydrophile gel methylacrylate Hydron, following enucleation. Cesk. Oftalmol., 31:180, 1975 (Slovakian)

OLBOURNE, N. A.: Congenital urethral fistula. PRS, 57:237, 1976

OLBOURNE, N. A. et al: Malignant melanoma in childhood. Brit. J. Plast. Surg., 27:305, 1974

OLBOURNE, N. A., SAAD, M. N., AND CLEMENT, R.: Benign osteoblastoma of metacarpal bone, PRS, 56:229, 1975. Hand, 6:198, 1974

OLBOURNE, N. A. et al: Rotation flap for distal nasal defects. Brit. J. Plast. Surg., 28:64, 1975

OLDER, J. J., AND ALLANSMITH, M. R.: Penetrating keratoplasty in patient with 75% third degree burns, PRS, 56:223, 1975. Ann. Ophth., 7:309, 1975

OLDER, J. J. et al: Surgical removal of basal cell carcinoma of the eyelids utilizing frozen section control. Trans. Am. Acad. Ophthalmol.

Otolaryngol., *79:*658, 1975

OLDHOFF, J. *et al:* Melanotic neuroectodermal tumour of infancy. Trans. Int. Conf. Oral Surg., *4:*55, 1973

OLESHKO, N. A. *et al:* Remote results of treatment of perilunar dislocations of the hand and dislocations of the wrist semilunar bone. Ortop. Travmatol. Protez., *32:*27, 1971 (Russian)

OLEWINSKI, T. *et al:* Emergency treatment of penile skin defect by means of skin transplantation using a transplant of medium thickness. Pol. Przegl. Chir., *44:*863, 1972 (Polish)

OLIN, R.: Arterial occlusion caused by jobs that are hard on the hands. Med. Times. *99:*178, 1971

OLIVARI, A., PRADIER, R., AND ROJAS, F.: Immunologic study of 100 patients with head and neck neoplasias, PRS, *57:*679, 1976. Bol. y trab. Acad. argent cir., *59:*308, 1975

OLIVARI, N.: Lateral, subperiosteal osteotomy using rhinotome, PRS, *52:*205, 1973. Chir. Plast., *1:*261, 1972

OLIVARI, N.: One-stage reconstruction of whole lower lip. Brit. J. Plast. Surg., *26:*66, 1973

OLIVARI, N.: Selective early excision of burns and its significance for the prophylaxis of burn complications. In *Plastische und Wiederherstellungs-Chirurgie*, ed. by Hohler; pp. 227–36. Schattauer, Stuttgart, 1975 (German)

OLIVARI, N., SCHRUDDE, J., AND WAHLE, H.: Surgical treatment of bedsores in paraplegics. PRS, *50:*477, 1972

OLIVARI, N., REISMANN, B., AND BAYER, H. W.: Operative treatment of infected pilonidal cysts by sliding graft, PRS, *52:*602, 1973. Bruns' Beitr. klin. Chir., *220:*306, 1973

OLIVARI, N. *et al:* Treatment of hemangioma in childhood, surgical therapy. Z. Allgemeinmed., *49:*60, 1973 (German)

OLIVARI, N. *et al:* Discussion comment on paper of Olivari and Schrudde: Treatment of hemangioma in childhood, surgical therapy. Z. Allgemeinmed., *49:*895, 1973 (German)

OLIVARI, N. *et al:* X-ray injury of the skin and its treatment. In *Plastische und Wiederherstellungs-Chirurgie*, ed. by Hohler; pp. 341–51. Schattauer, Stuttgart, 1975 (German)

OLIVER, L. P.: Aneurysmal bone cyst, case report. Oral Surg., *35:*67, 1973

OLIVER, R. F.: Fate of cutaneously and subcutaneously implanted trypsin purified dermal collagen in pig. Brit. J. Exp. Pathol., *53:*540, 1972

OLIVERAS MORENO, J. M.: Fractures of lateral component of middle third of face. An. Esp. Odontoestomatol., *34:*199, 1975 (Spanish)

OLLEY, P. C.: Aspects of plastic surgery. Psychiatric aspects of referral. Brit. Med. J., *3:*248, 1974

OLLEY, P. C.: Aspects of plastic surgery. Social and psychological sequelae. Brit. Med. J., *3:*322, 1974

OLLSON, C. A.: Pedicle patch urethroplasty for cure of urethral stricture (with Anastasi). PRS, *51:*1, 1973

OLLSTEIN, R. N. *et al:* Alternate case study of topical sulfamylon and silver sulfadiazine in burns. PRS, *48:*311, 1971

OLOFSSON, J. *et al:* Growth and spread of laryngeal and hypopharyngeal carcinoma with reflections on effect of preoperative irradiation. One hundred and thirty-nine cases studied by whole organ serial sectioning. Acta Otolaryngol. (Suppl.) (Stockh.), *308:*1, 1973

OLOW-NORDENRAM, M. *et al:* Partial tongue excision in treatment of apertognathia. Oral Surg., *35:*152, 1973

OLSEN, J. A. *et al:* Occasional occurrence of serious renal complications after methoxyflurane (Penthrane) anesthesia. PRS, *52:*160, 1973

OLSEN, R. F. *et al:* Orthosurgical teamwork. J. Am. Dent. Assoc., *90:*998, 1975

OLSHANSKY, K.: *Extensor indicis proprius* syndrome, clinical test (with Spinner). PRS, *51:*134, 1973

OLSON, N. R., AND MILES, W. K.: Treatment of acute blunt laryngeal injuries, PRS, *50:*305, 1972. Ann. Otol. Rhin. & Laryng., *80:*704, 1971

OLSON, P. S.: Thrombus formation in arterial and venous circulation in hypofibrinogenemic dogs, PRS, *55:*512, 1975. Europ. Surg. Res., *6:*176, 1974

OLSON, R. E.: Vitamin E and its relation to heart disease, PRS, *54:*119, 1974. Circulation, *48:*179, 1973

OLSSON, C. A. *et al:* True hermaphroditism, PRS, *48:*514, 1971. J. Urol., *105:*586, 1971

OLSZEWSKI, W. *et al:* Primary lymphatic edema of lower limbs. 1. Lymphographic and histologic examination of vessels and lymph nodes in primary lymphedema. Pol. Przegl. Chir., *44:*657, 1972 (Polish)

OLUMIDE, A. A. *et al:* Osteoma of the ethmofrontal sinus. Case report. J. Neurosurg., *42:*343, 1975

OLUMIDE, F.: Thyroglossal cyst presenting with severe laryngeal obstruction. Niger. Med. J., *3:*52, 1973

OLUWASANMI, J. O.: Keloids in the African. Clin. Plast. Surg., *1:*179, 1974

OLUWASANMI, J. O., LAGUNDOYE, S. B., AND AKINYEMI, O. O.: Ankylosis of mandible from *cancrum oris. PRS,* *57:*342, 1976

OMER, G. E.: Sensibility of hand as opposed to sensation in hand, PRS, 53:108, 1974. Ann. Chir., 27:479, 1973

OMER, G. E. et al: Neurovascular cutaneous island pedicles for deficient median nerve sensibility, PRS, 49:104, 1972. J. Bone & Joint Surg., 52A:1181, 1970

OMER, G. E., JR. et al: Evaluation of ice application with postoperative dressings. Clin. Orthop., 81:117, 1971

OMER, G. E., JR. et al: Initial management of severe open injuries and traumatic amputations of foot. Arch. Surg., 105:696, 1972

OMER, G. E., JR., AND THOMAS, S. R.: Management of chronic pain syndromes in upper extremity, PRS, 56:679, 1975. Clin. Orthop., 104:37, 1974

OMORI, K. et al: Free groin flaps: their vascular basis. Brit. J. Plast. Surg., 28:238, 1975

OMORI, S.: The 39th Congress of the American Society of Plastic Surgery. Jap. J. Plast. Reconstr. Surg., 14:189, 1971 (Japanese)

OMORI, S.: Current trends observed at the International Confederation of Plastic and Reconstructive Surgery. Jap. J. Plast. Reconstr. Surg., 15:24, 1972 (Japanese)

OMORI, S.: Reparative surgery of the nose and ear. Surg. Ther. (Osaka), 26:548, 1972 (Japanese)

OMORI, S.: Congenital deformities of the auricle. Clin. Plast. Surg., 1:3, 1974

OMORI, S. et al: Thermal injuries of the hand and their sequelae observed at the Department of Plastic Surgery, Tokyo Keisatsu Byoin. Orthop. Surg. (Tokyo), 21:930, 1970 (Japanese)

ONEAL, R. M.: Areolar sharing to reconstruct absent nipple (with Wexler). PRS, 51:176, 1973

ONEAL, R. M., GREER, D. M., JR., AND NOBEL, G. L.: Secondary correction of bilateral cleft lip deformities with Millard's midline muscular closure. PRS, 54:45, 1974

O'NEILL, J. A., JR.: Comparison of xenograft and prosthesis for burn wound care, PRS, 54:506, 1974. J. Pediat. Surg., 5:705, 1973

O'NEILL, J. A., JR.: Evaluation and treatment of burned child, PRS, 57:121, 1976. Pediat. Clin. N. Am., 22:407, 1975

O'NEILL, J. A. et al: Patterns of injury in battered child syndrome, PRS, 53:691, 1974. J. Trauma, 13:332, 1973

O'NEILL, J. V. et al: Cryosurgery of the supraglottic cavernous hemangioma. Arch. Otolaryng., 102:55, 1976

ONG, T. H., AND SOLOMON, J. R.: Fat necrosis of scrotum, PRS, 54:377, 1974. J. Pediat. Surg., 8:919, 1973

ONISHI, M. et al: Calcifying epithelial odonto-genic tumor of the mandible of an 11-year-old child. Report of a case. J. Jpn. Stomatol. Soc., 41:286, 1974 (Japanese)

ONIZUKA, T.: Review of rhinoplasty. Jap. J. Plast. Reconstr. Surg., 14:465, 1971 (Japanese)

ONIZUKA, T.: Thiersch graft. Shujutsu, 25:1271, 1971 (Japanese)

ONIZUKA, T.: Repair of columella base deformity in unilateral cleft lip. Brit. J. Plast. Surg., 25:33, 1972

ONIZUKA, T.: Progress in the technic of facial skin flap. Surg. Ther. (Osaka), 26:519, 1972 (Japanese)

ONIZUKA, T.: Planning the repair of cleft lip deformities. Brit. J. Plast. Surg., 26:181, 1973

ONIZUKA, T.: Philtrum formation in secondary cleft lip repair. PRS, 56:522, 1975

ONIZUKA, T.: Surgical correction of lobster claw feet. PRS, 57:98, 1976

ONIZUKA, T., TAI, Y., AND KONDO, S.: New method of columella reconstruction using cross lip flap, PRS, 50:305, 1972. Jap. J. Plast. Reconstr. Surg., 14:373, 1971

ONIZUKA, T. et al: Reconstruction of the prominence of the columellar sill of the nose. Jap. J. Plast. Reconstr. Surg., 15:175, 1972 (Japanese)

ONIZUKA, T., AND TAI, Y.: Supernumerary nostril. PRS, 50:403, 1972.

ONIZUKA, T. et al: Development of the palatal arch in relation to unilateral cleft lip and palate surgery: a comparison of the effects of different surgical approaches. Cleft Palate J., 12:444, 1975

ONLAND, J. M. et al: Surgical treatment of mandibular prognathism. Ned. Tijdschr. Tandheelkd., 79:174, 1972 (Dutch)

ONO, Y. et al: Method of treatment of vascular tumor, head and neck region. J. Otolaryngol. Japan, 75:1091, 1972 (Japanese)

OOI, B. S. et al: Lymphocytotoxins in aging, PRS, 56:366, 1975. Transplantation, 18:190, 1974

OOSTERHUIS, J. W., VERSCHUEREN, R. C. J., AND OLDHOFF, J.: Experimental surgery on Cloudman S91 melanoma with carbon-dioxide laser, PRS, 57:680, 1976. Acta chir. belg., 74:422, 1975

OOSTERLINCK, W., AND RENDERS, G.: Treatment of Peyronie's disease with procarbazine, PRS, 57:120, 1976. Brit. J. Urol., 47:219, 1975

OPANASHCHENKO, G. A. et al: Diagnosis and treatment of cylindromas of otorhinolaryngologic organs. Zh. Ushn. Nos. Gorl. Bolexn., 33:104, 1973 (Russian)

OPOLSKI, M. et al: Plastic surgery of a large

defect of skull soft tissue following burn wound due to electric current. Wiad. Lek., *25*:383, 1972 (Polish)

OPPENHEIMER, R. P.: Airway—instantly. J. A. M. A., *230*:76, 1974

OPPENHEIMER, R. P.: Treatment of comminuted fractures of the anterior sinus wall. Trans. Am. Acad. Ophthalmol. Otolaryngol., *80*:507, 1975

OPPERBECK, J.: Submucous cleft palate as a cause of rhinolalia aperta after tonsillectomy. Z. Laryngol. Rhinol. Otol., *49*:805, 1970 (German)

Oral Surgery (See also *Vestibuloplasty*)

Practical Oral Surgery. 3rd ed. By Henry B. Clark, Jr. Lea & Febiger, Philadelphia, 1965

Textbook of Oral Surgery. Ed. by Walter C. Guralnick. Little, Brown & Co., Boston, 1968

Oral Surgery. 5th edition. Ed. by Kurt H. Thoma. C. V. Mosby Co., St. Louis, 1969

An Outline in Oral Surgery, Part II. By H. C. Killey, G. R. Seward, and L. W. Kay. John Wright & Sons, Ltd., Bristol, 1971. PRS, *51*:209, 1973

Fundamentals of Oral Surgery. By Emmett R. Costich and Raymond P. White, Jr. W. B. Saunders Co., Philadelphia, 1971

Minor Oral Surgery. By Geoffrey L. Howe. Williams & Wilkins Co., Baltimore, 1971. PRS, *50*:180, 1972

Preprosthetic surgery from the viewpoint of the prosthodontist (Miller). J. Oral Surg., *29*:760, 1971

Preprosthetic surgery with dentures. Clinical viewpoints on management of carrying out follow-up studies (Sigurdson). Sven. Tandlak. Tidskr., *64*:383, 1971 (Swedish)

Atlas of Oral Surgery. By Benjamin J. Gans. C. V. Mosby Co., St. Louis, 1972

Textbook of Practical Oral Surgery. Ed. by Daniel E. Waite. Lea & Febiger, Philadelphia, 1972

Dentistry out of surgery—birth of specialty (Fickling). Aust. Dent. J., *17*:178, 1972

Grafts: some intraoral uses (McKee). J. Contra Costa Dent. Soc., *16*:16, 1972

Diastema, maxillary midline, closure of, with frenectomy and corticotomy (Massey). J. Ga. Dent. Assoc., *46*:26, 1972

Oral surgery, clinical expermentation of DA 2370 (Zepelin) in (D'Angelo). Minerva Stomatol., *21*:270, 1972 (Italian)

Oral cavity, retention cysts, surgery in treatment of (Rocha). Rev. Gaucha. Odontol., *20*:258, 1972 (Portuguese)

Oral and maxillofacial surgery coming of age

Oral Surgery—Cont.

in Puerto Rico (Valls). Rev. Odontol. P. R., *10*:31, 1972

Tooth buds, transplanted, behavior and fate of (Sharav, Metzger, Weinrele), PRS, *51*: 611, 1973. Transplantation, *13*: 360, 1972

Oral surgery, development and advances in (Kole). Wien. Med. Wochenschr., *122*: 687, 1972 (German)

Fasciitis, fatal necrotizing, after tooth extraction (Crowson), PRS, *53*:602, 1974. Am. Surgeon, *39*:525, 1973

Dental surgery in children, outpatient, ketamine for (Bamber, Ratcliffe, McEwan), PRS, *53*:373, 1974. Anesthesia, *28*:446, 1973

Some dental problems, and the surgeon (Hopkins). Ann. R. Coll. Surg. Engl., *53*:95, 1973

Syndrome, Hunter's, two cases—anesthetic and operative difficulties in oral surgery (Hopkins *et al*). Brit. J. Oral Surg., *10*:286, 1973

Dental surgeon and oral surgeon, life and work of, in Peoples Republic of China (Kerr). Brit. J. Oral Surg., *11*:36, 1973

Oral surgery, ambulatory, therapy recommendations (Editorial). Dtsch. Stomatol., *23*:360, 1973 (German)

Periodontics, therapy recommendations for (Editorial). Dtsch. Stomatol., *23*:884, 1973

Anchor oral endosteal implant (Cranin *et al*). J. Biomed. Mater. Res., *7*:235, 1973

Tooth implant, self supportive polymer (Hodosh, Povar, Shklar), PRS, *53*:372, 1974. J. Biomed. Mater. Res., *7*:205, 1973

Tooth vitality after alveolar segmental osteotomy (Pepersack), PRS, *53*:251, 1974. J. Maxillo-facial Surg., *1*:85, 1973

Osteotomy, alveolar segmental, tooth vitality after (Pepersack), PRS, *53*:251, 1974. J. Maxillo-facial Surg., *1*:85, 1973

Viral hepatitis: hazard to oral surgeons (Glazer *et al*). J. Oral Surg., *31*:504, 1973

Mandibular vestibuloplasty with free graft of mucoperiosteal layer from hard palate (Morgan, Gallegos, Frileck), PRS, *51*:359, 1973

Oral and plastic surgeon, pioneer: Simon P. Hullihen (Goldwyn), PRS, *52*:250, 1973

Oral surgery, outpatient, laboratory screening tests prior to (Oikarinen *et al*). Proc. Finn. Dent. Soc., *69*:110, 1973

Oral surgery, use of biocompatible interface for combining tissues and prostheses in (Hinds, Homsy, Kent). Trans. Congr. Int. Assoc. Oral Surg., *4*:210, 1973

Current Advances in Oral Surgery, Vol. 1. By William B. Irby. C. V. Mosby Co., St.

Oral Surgery — Cont.
Louis, 1974
Textbook of Oral Surgery. 4th edition. Ed. by Gustav O. Kruger. C. V. Mosby Co., St., Louis, 1974
Periodontal ligament, donor, evidence of alloimmunogenic potential of (Robinson *et al*). Am. J. Pathol., *75:*503, 1974
Oral surgery, some economic aspects of (Lowry). Brit. J. Oral Surg., *11:*249, 1974
Dentistry, allergic reactions to metals used in (Fisher), PRS, *56:*116, 1975. Cutis, *14:*797, 1974
Tooth, supernumerary deciduous and permanent canine, bilateral (Novak), PRS, *54:*630, 1974. Czas. Stomatol., *2:*148, 1974
Maxillary implants, subperiosteal (Ricciardi). Dent. Surv., *50:*24, 1974
Tooth vitality following mobilization of the alveolar process (Pepersack). Fortschr. Kiefer. Gesichtschir., *18:*280, 1974 (German)
Oral surgeon's experience with interosseous blade implant (Rakower). Int. J. Oral Surg., *3:*282, 1974
Maxillary permanent incisor, unerupted, surgical and orthodontic management (Gatoff *et al*). J. Am. Dent. Assoc., *89:*897, 1974
Hospital Committees, participation on (Devlin). J. Oral Surg., *32:*487, 1974
Oral and Maxillofacial Surgery, Department of, Jacksonville Hospitals Educational Program, University of Florida Affiliate (Editorial). J. Oral Surg., *32:*541, 1974
Use of steroids in the prevention of some complications after traumatic oral surgery (Hooley *et al*). J. Oral Surg., *32:*864, 1974
Frenum, hypertrophic, submucosal frenotomy (Maloney), PRS, *55:*507, 1975. J. Oral Surg., *38:*23, 1974
Lateral trepanation of lower third molars (Summers). L. Aust. Dent. J., *19:*149, 1974
Dental treatment, incidence of bacteremia following, on pediatric patients (De Leo *et al*), PRS, *55:*120, 1975. Oral Surg., *37:*37, 1974
Oral surgical procedures, custom cast splints for (Brudvik), PRS, *55:*506, 1975. Oral Surg., *38:*15, 1974
Transplantation of third molar into edentulous site (Conklin). Oral Surg., *38:*193, 1974
Functional compensation of muscles after postoperative rehabilitation in reference to electromyographic analysis (Grosfeld). Oral Surg., *38:*829, 1974
Tooth reimplantation and transplantation problems in one of our own cases (Bagi).

Oral Surgery — Cont.
Orv. Hetil., *115:*1110, 1974 (Hungarian)
Epulis tumor, congenital (Bowe), PRS, *53:*227, 1974
Teeth, six imperfectly erupted permanent, surgical, orthodontic and prosthetic treatment of (Posti *et al*). Proc. Finn. Dent. Soc., *70:*75, 1974 (Finnish)
Treatment of bone pockets (Singer). Z. W. R., *83:*207, 1974 (German)
Oral & Maxillofacial Surgery. 5th edition. By W. Harry Archer. W. B. Saunders Co., Philadelphia, 1975
Oral surgery, therapeutic cosmetic effects of (Wehner), PRS, *57:*259, 1976. AORN, *22:*52, 1975
A variation in subperiosteal implant design. A case report (L'Estrange *et al*). Brit. Dent. J., *138:*141, 1975
Jaundice following oral surgery: Gilbert's syndrome (Quinn *et al*). Brit. J. Oral Surg., *12:*285, 1975
Cryosurgery and its application to oral surgery (Leopard). Brit. J. Oral Surg., *13:*128, 1975
Oral surgery, resins in (Mastrocola, Ziter), PRS, *57:*266, 1976. Dent. Clin. N. Am., *19:*407, 1975
Globulomaxillary cyst treated by marsupialization (Litwiller). Dent. Radiogr. Photogr., *48:*42, 1975
Periodontal defects, comparison of iliac marrow and biodegradable ceramic in (Levin *et al*), PRS, *57:*114, 1976. J. Bio-Med. Mater., *9:*183, 1975
Preprosthetic surgery (Fisher). J. Can. Dent. Assoc., *41:*297, 1975
Corticalosteotomy, segmental alveolar movement after experimental animal research (Duker), PRS, *57:*395, 1976. J. Maxillo-facial Surg., *3:*81, 1975
Treatment of maxillary alveolar hyperplasia by total maxillary alveolar osteotomy (Hall *et al*). J. Oral Surg., *33:*180, 1975
Letter: Frustrations of oral surgery (Wallace). J. Oral Surg., *33:*247, 1975
Letter: The status of oral surgery. J. Oral Surg., *33:*487, 1975
Teeth, dislocated and disrupted (Tolmeijer), PRS, *57:*115, 1976. Nederl. tijdschr. geneesk., *119:*949, 1975
Effect of postmortem tissue fixation on tooth mobility and pocket depth in human beings (Gillette). Oral Surg., *39:*130, 1975

ORANDI, A.: One-stage urethroplasty: four-year follow-up, PRS, *51:*604, 1973. J. Urol., *107:*977, 1972

Orbit—Cont.

122:Suppl 5:3, 1972 (German)

Motility disorders of the eye in injuries of the osseous orbit (x-ray report) (Ellegast). Wien. Med. Wochenschr., 122:Suppl 5:7, 1972 (German)

Motility disorders of the eye in injuries of the osseous orbit (ophthalmologic report) (Friemel). Wien. Med. Wochenschr., 122: Suppl 5:10, 1972 (German)

Orbital reconstruction after radical resection (Habal et al). Ann. chir. plast., 18:183, 1973

Reconstruction of conjunctival cavity: holding in place of prosthetic form by transorbitary pin (Souyris et al). Ann. chir. plast., 18:315, 1973 (French)

Orbit, giant conjunctival cyst of (Allison et al). Ann. Ophth., 5:199, 1973

Ophthalmic surgery, orbit (Trokel), PRS, 52:451, 1973. Arch. Ophth., 89:152, 1973

Intraorbital implants, insertion of secondary (Soll). Arch. Ophth., 89:214, 1973

Orbital injury, differential diagnosis (Smith, Wiggs), PRS, 53:240, 1974. Arch. Ophth., 89:484, 1973

Orbital reconstruction after radical resection (Habal, Murray), PRS, 52:205, 1973. Arch. Surg., 106:353, 1973

Orbital reconstructive surgery, indications and contraindications for (La Ruffa), PRS, 53:601, 1974. Bol. y. trab. Soc. argent. cir., 34:294, 1973

Fronto-orbital epidermoid cyst (Ravault et al). Bull. Soc. Ophtalmol. Fr., 73:793, 1973 (French)

Orbital fissure, superior, operative and rehabilitative treatment of syndrome (Ostachowicz et al). Czas. Stomatol., 26:727, 1973 (Polish)

Csapody's orbitoplasty by means of Meller's epithelial graft. Klin. Oczna, 43:49, 1973 (Polish)

Orbital roof repair by duplication of frontal bone flap (Marchac et al). Nouv. Presse Med., 2:2413, 1973 (French)

Indication of infraorbital nerve decompression (Pfaltz). O. R. L., 35:214, 1973

Orbital cyst, microphthalmos and (Kok-van Alphen et al). Ophthalmologica, 167:389, 1973

Orbital floor repair with nasal septal cartilage (Wiesenbaugh et al). Trans. Int. Conf. Oral Surg., 4:308, 1973

Orbital corrections with the use of alloplastic material (Borghouts et al). Trans. Int. Conf. Oral Surg., 4:321, 1973

Transplantation of homologous dura in reconstruction of the orbital floor. The re-

Orbit—Cont.

sults of five years experience (Luhr et al). Trans. Int. Conf. Oral Surg., 4:340, 1973

Orbital spatula—light guide (Brovkina et al). Vestn. Oftalmol., 1:79, 1973 (Russian)

Orbital deformities, correction of posttraumatic enophthalmos (Spira, Gerow, Hardy), PRS, 55:632, 1975. Acta chir. plast., 16:107, 1974

Orbit concavities, modification of Csapody's method of conjunctival sac reconstruction (Morozov, Grechischlina), PRS, 56:351, 1975. Acta chir. plast., 16:209, 1974

Orbit, severe lesion repaired by repositioning or osteotomy and bone grafting (Marchac et al), PRS, 55:375, 1975. Ann. chir. plast., 19:41, 1974

Orbital sepum, surgical anatomy of (Putterman, Urist), PRS, 54:686, 1974. Ann. Ophth., 6:290, 1974

Orbit, the (Trokel). Arch. Ophth., 91:233, 1974

Orbital cavity, neurosurgeon in (Schurmann). Arch. Otorhinolaryngol. (NY), 207:253, 1974 (German)

Orbit, rhino-surgical tasks in (Mennig). Arch. Otorhinolaryngol. (NY), 207:285, 1974

Orbital meningoencephalocele communicating with lacrimal sac, case report (Chohan et al). Clin. Pediatr. (Phila.), 13:330, 1974

Craniofacial surgery (Converse et al). Clin. Plast. Surg., 1:499, 1974

Maxillary resection prosthesis with magnetic connection to the eye epithesis (Ariely et al). Dtsch. Zahnaerztl. Z., 29:819, 1974 (German)

Surgical correction of the skeleton in the area of the orbit and maxilla (Schmid). Fortschr. Kiefer. Gesichtschir., 18:28, 1974 (German)

Cranial approach in the surgical repositioning of displaced orbital contents (Reichert). Fortschr. Kiefer. Gesichtschir., 18:34, 1974 (German)

Surgical decompression of the orbit for endocrine exophthalmos (Spira et al). Fortschr. Kiefer. Gesichtschir., 18:35, 1974

Decompression of the retrobulbar space and the optic nerve (Chuden). HNO, 22:320, 1974 (German)

Orbital cellulitis (Amies). J. Laryng. & Otol., 88:559, 1974

Flap, nasal wall, rotated to reconstruct defect of orbital floor (Niederdellmann, Munker, Lange), PRS, 55:375, 1975. J. Maxillo-facial Surg., 2:153, 1974

Orbital contents, ultrasonic display of (Dadd, Kossoff, Hughes), PRS, 54:618, 1974. M. J.

Orbit—Cont.

Australia, *1:*580, 1974

Progress in the field of eyelid and orbit surgery (Walser). Med. Klin., *69:*1720, 1974 (German)

Orbital correction by means of alloplastic materials (Borghouts *et al*). Ned. tijdschr. geneeskd., *118:*521, 1974 (Dutch)

Orbit, removal of glass fragment from (Posazhennikov). Oftalmol. Zh., *28:*302, 1974 (Russian)

Orbitocranial foreign body, case report (Dujovny *et al*). Ophthalmologica, *168:*261, 1974

Developing field of craniofacial surgery (Whitaker *et al*). Pediatrics, *54:*571, 1974

Use of temporal aponeurosis for closing of periorbital tears during certain cases of diplopia (Hosxe *et al*). Rev. Stomatol. Chir. Maxillofac., *74:*393, 1974

Destructive injuries of the craniofacial sphere. Value of primary overall repair (Stricker *et al*). Rev. Stomatol. Chir. Maxillofac., *75:*274, 1974 (French)

Orbital hemorrhage from retrobulbar injection, central retinal artery closure during (Kraufhar, Seelenfreund, Froelich), PRS, *54:*382, 1974. Tr. Am. Acad. Ophth., *78:*65, 1974

Transplantation of homologous dura in reconstruction of the orbital floor. The results of five years experience (Luhr *et al*). Trans. Int. Conf. Oral Surg., *4:*340, 1974

Transantral orbital decompression in dysthyroid eye disease (Taylor). Trans. Opthalmol. Soc. N.Z., *26:*51, 1974

Diagnosis and surgical tactics in rhinogenic intraocular complications (Mlechin *et al*). Vestn. Otorinolaringol., *2:*32, 1974 (Russian)

Correction of fronto-orbital defects (Schlondorff). Z. Laryngol. Rhinol. Otol., *53:*104, 1974 (German)

Proceedings. 2nd International Symposium on Orbital Disorders, Amsterdam, 1973. Ed. by G. M. Bleeker. Albert J. Phiebig, White Plains, N. Y., 1975

Cyst, aneurysmal bone, of orbit (Powell, Glaser), PRS, *56:*591, 1975. Arch. Ophth., *93:*340, 1975

Nodular fasciitis causing unilateral proptosis (Perry *et al*). Brit. J. Ophthalmol., *59:*404, 1975

Various bone materials for the reconstruction of defects of the orbital floor (Schmelzle). Fortschr. Kiefer. Gesichtschir., *19:*191, 1975 (German)

Topographical anatomy of the total osteotomy of the midface (Matras *et al*). J. Max-

Orbit—Cont.

illo-facial Surg., *3:*260, 1975

Proceedings: endocrine exophthalmos treated by orbital decompression (Clarke). J. Neurol. Neurosurg. Psychiatry, *38:*822, 1975

Transcranial orbital decompression in severe cases of unilateral exophthalmos (Palva *et al*). J. Laryng. & Otol., *89:*1123, 1975

Orbital surgery, advances in (Chwirot). Klin. Oczna., *45:*575, 1975 (Polish)

Recent progress in plastic surgery, especially on craniofacial surgery (Ohmori). Neurol. Surg. (Tokyo), *3:*277, 1975 (Japanese)

Paget's disease of bone. Report of a case (Akin *et al*). Oral Surg., *39:*707, 1975

Surgical treatment of exophthalmos. A review (Lanier). PRS, *55:*56, 1975

Orbitotomy performed with use of ultrasonic instruments (Brovkina *et al*). Vestn. Oftalmol., *2:*46, 1975

Problems of face and neck surgery near the orbital base of the skull (Mennig). Z. Aerztl. Fortbild. (Jena), *69:*949, 1975 (German)

Ectoprosthesis after exenteration of the orbit (Bernhoft). Nor. Tannlageforen Tid., *86:*57, 1976 (Norwegian)

Chrome cobalt and gold implant for the reconstruction of a traumatized orbital floor (Kummoona). Oral Surg., *41:*293, 1976

Orbit, Fracture (See also *Craniofacial Injuries, Facial Injuries, Zygoma*)

Orbital cavity floor and malar bone, treatment of comminuted fractures using a hydropneumatic method of immobilization (Carvalhal Franca), PRS, *48:*510, 1971. Rev. Latino Am. cir. plast., *13:*106, 1969

Fractures of the Orbit. Ed. by G. M. Bleeker and T. Keith Lyle. Williams & Wilkins Co., Baltimore, 1970. PRS, *48:*589, 1971

Orbit, blowout fracture concomitant with rupture of globe (Dodick, Gallin, Kwitko), PRS, *48:*293, 1971. Arch. Ophth., *84:*707, 1970

Blowout fractures of the orbit (Singer *et al*). Nebr. Med. J., *55:*352, 1970

Orbital floor fractures and ocular complications (Fradkin). Am. J. Ophth., *72:*699, 1971

Analysis and results of 34 orbit base fractures (Schlondorff *et al*). Arch. Klin. Exp. Ohren Nasen Kehlkopfheilkd., *199:*647, 1971 (German)

Visual loss complicating repair of orbital floor fractures (Nicholson, Guzak), PRS, *49:*356, 1972. Arch. Ophth., *86:*369, 1971

Unrecognized forms of orbital floor fractures and their treatment (Woillez *et al*).

Orbit, Fracture – Cont.

nert). Fortschr. Kiefer. Gesichtschir., *19:*185, 1975 (German)

Studies for the treatment planning in orbital fractures (Schule *et al*). Fortschr. Kiefer. Gesichtschir., *19:*188, 1975 (German)

Orbital fracture treated by internal indirect fixation with hooks (Mektubjian), PRS, *57:*394, 1976. J. Maxillo-facial Surg., *3:*132, 1975

Orbital fractures, treatment by infraorbital-transantral approach (Livingston *et al*). J. Oral Surg., *33:*586, 1975

Primary bone grafting in management of facial fractures (Bonanno *et al*). N. Y. State J. Med., *75:*710, 1975

Treatment of enophthalmic narrow palpebral fissure after blow-out fracture (Putterman *et al*). Ophthalmic Surg., *6:*45, 1975

Orbitonasal surgery, xeroradiography examination in (Maillard, Otto, Clodius), PRS, *55:*664, 1975

Coronal incision for exposure in initial treatment of facial fractures (Shaw, Parsons), PRS, *56:*254, 1975

Fractures, orbital, ocular injuries in (Jabaley, Lerman, Sanders), PRS, *56:*410, 1975

Orbit, Neoplasms of

Frozen sections, application to diagnosis of orbital tumors (Howard), PRS, *48:*509, 1971. Am. J. Ophth., *71:*221, 1971

Orbit, exenterated in children due to retinoblastomas, reconstruction of (Murillo), PRS, *51:*346, 1973. Cir. cir. Mexico, *40:*76, 1972

Orbit, malignant melanoma primary in, case report (Henderson *et al*). Trans. Am. Acad. Ophthalmol., Otolaryngol., *76:*1487, 1972

Orbital Tumors. By J. W. Henderson. W. B. Saunders Co., Philadelphia, 1973

Tumors, orbital, reconstruction after radical resection (Habal, Murray), PRS, *52:*205, 1973. Arch. Surg., *106:*353, 1973

Craniofacial resection, combined, for tumor involving orbital walls (Wilson, Westbury), PRS, *54:*685, 1974. Brit. J. Plast. Surg., *26:*44, 1973

Head and neck rhabdomyosarcoma in children (Donaldson *et al*), PRS, *52:*214, 1973. Cancer, *31:*26, 1973

Tumor, recurrent mixed of lacrimal gland, cranio-orbital resection and neck dissection for (Habal, Murray), PRS, *51:*689, 1973

Orbital region, malignant disease of, treatment (Vickers). Proc. Roy. Soc. Med., *66:*689, 1973

Indications and technique of hemimaxillectomy for treatment of advanced malig-

Orbit, Neoplasms of – Cont.

nancy of the maxilla (Sammis). Trans. Int. Conf. Oral Surg., *4:*154, 1973

Orbit, exenteration of, sliding bridge graft in (Carbajal). Trans. Ophthalmol. Soc., N. Z., *25:*136, 1973

Orbital melanoma, primary (Jakobiec *et al*). Am. J. Ophth., *78:*24, 1974

Astrocytoma of the optic nerve and chiasm associated with microphthalmos and orbital cyst (Bonner *et al*). Brit. J. Ophthalmol., *58:*828, 1974

Orbit exenteration. Practical note (Taglioni *et al*). Bull. Soc. Ophtalmol. Fr., *74:*341, 1974 (French)

Orbital hemangioma – clinical analysis of 79 cases (Shanghai First Medical College), PRS, *55:*633, 1975. Chinese M. J., *9:*162, 1974

Rhabdomyosarcoma of orbit (Aviles), PRS, *55:*245, 1975. Internat. Surg., *59:*297, 1974

Ultrasonic display of orbital contents (Dadd, Kossoff, Hughes), PRS, *54:*618, 1974. M. J. Australia, *1:*580, 1974

Extended subfrontal approach to tumors of the orbit (Cophignon *et al*). Neurochirurgie, *20:*161, 1974 (French)

Orbit invaded by morpheic basal cell carcinoma (Gilkes, Borrie), PRS, *55:*385, 1975. Proc. Roy. Soc. Med., *67:*437, 1974

Tumor of orbit, benign fibrous (Case, LaPiana), PRS, *57:*256, 1976. Ann. Ophth., *7:*813, 1975

Orbit, primary malignant melanoma of, in Negro (Drews), PRS, *56:*591, 1975. Arch. Ophth., *93:*335, 1075

Orbit, aneurysmal bone cyst of (Powell, Glaser), PRS, *56:*591, 1975. Arch. Ophth., *93:*340, 1975

Orbital tumors, metastatic: case of orbital metastasis in malignant melanoma of skin (Hotz). Klin. Monatsbl. Augenheilkd., *166:*176, 1975 (German)

Flap, temporal muscle, for reconstruction after orbito-maxillary resections for cancer (Bakamjian, Souther), PRS, *56:*171, 1975

ORD, R., AND MATZ, G.: Tuberculous cervical lymphadenitis, PRS, *54:*687, 1974. Arch. Otolaryng., *99:*327, 1974

O'REILLY, K.: Treatment by nylon setons of lymphedema of the arm following radical mastectomy. M. J. Australia, *1:*1269, 1972

O'REILLY, R. J., AND BLATT, G.: High pressure injection injury: potential hazard of "enhanced recovery," PRS, *57:*534, 1976. J.A.M.A., *233:*533, 1975

O'REILLY, R. J. *et al*: Accidental high-pressure injection-gun injuries of the hand; the role of the emergency radiologic examination. J. Trauma, *15:*24, 1975

ORENTREICH, N.: Hair transplantation. N. Y. State J. Med., *72:*578, 1972

ORENTREICH, N. *et al*: Cosmetic improvement of factitial defects. Med. Trial Tech. Q., *172:*80, 1971

ORENTREICH, N. *et al*: Autograft repigmentation of leukoderma. Arch. Dermat., *105:*734, 1972

ORENTREICH, N., AND DURR, N. P.: Mammogenesis in transsexuals, PRS, *55:*512, 1975. J. Invest. Dermat., *63:*142, 1974

ORGEL, M. G. *et al*: Electrical burns of mouth in children: method for assessing results. J. Trauma, *15:*285, 1975

O'RIAIN, S.: New and simple test of nerve function in hand, PRS, *53:*489, 1974. Brit. M. J., *3:*615, 1973

O'RIAIN, S. *et al*: Speech results in cleft palate surgery. A survey of 249 patients. Brit. J. Plast. Surg., *25:*380, 1972

ORIBE, J. A. *et al*: Temporomandibular condylectomies in comparative anatomy. Rev. Asoc. Odontol. Argent., *62:*22, 1973 (Spanish)

O'RIORDAN, B. C.: Oral submucous fibrosis, PRS, *55:*723, 1975. Proc. Roy. Soc. Med., *67:*877, 1974

ORKIN, M. *et al*: Cerebriform intradermal nevus. A cause of cutis verticis gyrata. Arch. Dermat., *110:*575, 1974

ORLANDO, J. C., SMITH, J. W. AND GOULIAN, D.: Dupuytren's contracture, PRS, *56:*680, 1975. Brit. J. Plast. Surg., *27:*211, 1974

ORLANDO, J. C. *et al*: Superomedial dermal pedicle for nipple transposition. Brit. J. Plast. Surg., *28:*42, 1975

ORLIAN, A. I.: Benign hemangiopericytoma of tongue. J. Oral Surg., *31:*936, 1973

ORLIAN, A. I.: Sialolithiasis of submaxillary duct. N.Y. State Dent. J., *39:*548, 1973

ORLICH, C., AND GURDIAN-MORALES, M.: Trauma and repair of external genital organs in men, PRS, *50:*307, 1972. Rev. Latino Am. cir. plast., *15:*45, 1972

ORLOV, A. N. *et al*: Early surgical treatment of deep chemical burns. Voen. Med. Zh., *8:*33, 1971 (Russian)

ORLOV, A. N. *et al*: Surgical treatment of some dermatoses. Vestn. Dermatol. Venerol., *0:*65, 1974 (Russian)

ORLOV, A. N. *et al*: Present-time problems of the treatment of burns. Vestn. Khir., *114:*69, 1975 (Russian)

Oroantral Fistula

Surgical treatment of oro-antral fistula (a report on 362 cases of oro-antral fistula treated by the buccal flap operation (Kil-

Oroantral Fistula – Cont.

ley). Minerva Stomatol., *20:*166, 1971

Oroantral fistulae, treatment of (Wowern). Arch. Otolaryng., *96:*99, 1972

Antro-alveolary fistulae, established, treatment (Goodman *et al*). Can. J. Otolaryngol., *1:*97, 1972

Clinical and radiographic findings after surgical closure of mouth-antrum connection in combination with radical surgery in maxillary antrum (Rink). Dtsch. Stomatol., *22:*251, 1972 (German)

Observations based on the surgical closure of 362 oro-antral fistulas (Killey *et al*). Int. Surg., *57:*545, 1972

Combined buccal and reverse palatal flap for closure of oral-antral fistula (Ziemba). J. Oral Surg., *30:*727, 1972

Maxillary sinus, complications resulting from dento-surgical operations in area of. Surgical closure combined with radical operation in maxillary sinus. (With changes of mucosa of maxillary sinus.) (Stellmach *et al*). Quintessence Int., *3:*11, 1972

Maxillary sinus, complications resulting from dento-surgical operations in area of. Plastic closure in connection with tooth extraction (Stellmach *et al*). Quintessence Int., *3:*17, 1972

Maxillary sinus, complications resulting from dento-surgical operations in area of. Plastic closure of suction cup perforation of hard palate (Stellmach, Frenkel). Quintessence Int., *3:*21, 1972

Maxillary sinus, complications resulting from dento-surgical operations in area of. Surgical closure with double flap repair (Stellmach, Frenkel). Quintessence Int., *3:*23, 1972

Closure of perforations of the floor of the maxillary sinus (Babaev). Stomatologiia (Mosk.), *51:*61, 1972 (Russian)

Oroantral fistula (Ishrat-Husain). Int. Surg., *58:*58, 1973

Oroantral fistula, correlation between the development of and size of corresponding bony defect (Wowern). J. Oral Surg., *31:*98, 1973

Oroantral fistula, gold foil closure (Meyerhoff *et al*). Laryngoscope, *83:*940, 1973

Oroantral fistulas, surgical closure of (Da Reis *et al*). Rev. Bras. Odontol., *30:*134, 1973 (Portuguese)

Oroantral fistulas following dental extraction (Dos Reis). Rev. Port. Estomatol. Cir. Maxilofac., *14:*79, 1973 (Portuguese)

Various methods for the closure of bucconasal communications (Landais). Rev. Stomatol. Chir. Maxillofac., *74:*642, 1973

Oroantral Fistula — Cont.
(French)

Closure of oroantral fistula using lyophilized dura (Stoehr). Stomatol. D.D.R., *23:*481, 1973 (German)

Acquired defects of the antrum (Hjorting-Hansen *et al*). Trans. Int. Conf. Oral Surg., *4:*19, 1973

An original procedure for closing large oroantral openings where conventional procedures have failed (Moose). Trans. Int. Conf. Oral Surg., *4:*175, 1973

Mucosal and cutaneous fistulas of dental and salivary origin (Llado Olivar). An. Esp. Odontoestomatol., *33:*385, 1974 (Spanish)

Bucco-sinusal communications (Freche *et al*). Ann. Chir., *28:*781, 1974 (French)

Palatal island flap in the closure of oro-antral fistulae (Henderson). Brit. J. Oral Surg., *12:*141, 1974

Radiological appearance of maxillary sinuses prior to treatment of oroantral fistula and during late control examinations (Dobaczewski). Czas. Stomatol., *27:*1043, 1974 (Polish)

Follow-up studies on hospitalized patients with sinus perforation (Ivankievicz *et al*). Fogorv. Sz., *67:*207, 1974

Oroantral communication, treatment of (Haanaes *et al*). Int. J. Oral Surg., *3:*124, 1974

Results of apicoectomy of maxillary canines, premolars and molars with special reference to oroantral communication as a prognostic factor (Ericson *et al*). Int. J. Oral Surg., *3:*386, 1974

Radiographic and clinical follow-up study of 150 oroantral communications (Haanaes). Int. J. Oral Surg., *3:*412, 1974

Oroantral fistulas, modified palatal flap technique for closure (Choukas). J. Oral Surg., *32:*112, 1974

Gold foil technique to close oroantral fistula (Mainous, Hammer), PRS, *55:*375, 1975. J. Oral Surg., *32:*528, 1974

Fistula, oral-antral, after antral packing (Cheesman), PRS, *55:*634, 1975. Proc. Roy. Soc. Med., *67:*716, 1974

Our experience with 107 buccosinusal communications without failure of closure (Landais). Rev. Stomatol. Chir. Maxillofac., *75:*186, 1974 (French)

Use of a tubular flap for replacement of extensive losses of palatine tissue (Slesinger). Rev. Stomatol. Chir. Maxillofac., *75:*188, 1974 (French)

Case of large bucco-sinusal communication, following partial resection of the maxilla, repaired by tubular flap and bone graft

Oroantral Fistula — Cont.

(Rossi *et al*). Rev. Stomatol. Chir. Maxillofac., *75:*192, 1974 (French)

Skin grafts in the closure of bucconasal and buccosinusal communications (Souyris *et al*). Rev. Stomatol. Chir. Maxillofac., *75:*195, 1974 (French)

Closure of buccosinusal communications with double pedicle flaps (Merlini *et al*). Rev. Stomatol. Chir. Maxillofac., *75:*199, 1974 (French)

Application of several principles of surgery of congenital abnormalities to buccosinusonasal communications (Vailiant *et al*). Rev. Stomatol. Chir. Maxillofac., *75:*203, 1974 (French)

Treatment of perforations of the roof of the mouth. Alveolar buccosinusal communications (Lachard *et al*). Rev. Stomatol. Chir. Maxillofac., *75:*208, 1974 (French)

Closing orosinusal communication with double flap (Merlini *et al*). Riv. Ital. Stomatol., *29:*73, 1974

Long-term study after treatment of oroantral fistulae (Dobaczewski). Czas. Stomatol., *28:*707, 1975 (Polish)

Oral antrostomy (Haanaes *et al*). Int. J. Oral Surg., *4:*55, 1975

Sinusitis, maxillary, sequela following closure of curative oro-antral fistula (Baumann, Pajarola), PRS, *57:*672, 1976. J. Maxillo-facial Surg., *3:*164, 1975

Oronasal fistula following anterior maxillary osteotomy (Granite). J. Oral Surg., *33:*129, 1975

ORTICOCHEA, M.: Results of dynamic muscle sphincter operation in cleft palates, PRS, *48:*197, 1971. Brit. J. Plast. Surg., *23:*108, 1970

ORTICOCHEA, M.: Use of intact side of face for reconstruction of injured side, PRS, *48:*399, 1971. Brit. J. Plast. Surg., *23:*235, 1970

ORTICOCHEA, M.: Reconstruction of the thumb using two flaps from the same hand. Brit. J. Plast. Surg., *24:*345, 1971

ORTICOCHEA, M.: Eye socket reconstruction with composite grafts, PRS, *48:*343, 1971

ORTICOCHEA, M.: Musculocutaneous flap method, immediate and heroic substitute for method of delay, PRS, *52:*105, 1973. Brit. J. Plast. Surg., *25:*106, 1972

ORTICOCHEA, M.: New method of total reconstruction of penis. Brit. J. Plast. Surg., *25:*347, 1972

ORTICOCHEA, M.: Use of buttock to reconstruct breast. Brit. J. Plast. Surg., *26:*304, 1973

ORTICOCHEA, M.: Indications and convenient surgical moment of dynamic muscle sphincter of pharynx, PRS, *54:*619, 1974. Ann. chir. plast., *19:*5, 1974

ORTICOCHEA, M.: Reconstruction of the short columella in bilateral cleft lip patients using the nasal septum. Brit. J. Plast. Surg., *28:*97, 1975

ORTIZ, J. M.: Internal wire splint for adduction contracture of thumb (with Araico, Valdes), PRS, *48:*339, 1971

ORTIZ, M. A., AND KRAUSHAR, M. F.: Lacrimal drainage following repair of inferior canaliculus, PRS, *57:*113, 1976. Ann. Ophth., *7:*739, 1975

ORTIZ-MONASTERIO, FERNANDO: Taliacottii's *De Curtorum Chirurgia per Insitionem.* Libreria Manuel Porrua, S. A., Mexico D. F., Mexico, 1973. PRS, *53:*466, 1974

ORTIZ-MONASTERIO, F.: Surgical management of bilateral cleft lip (with Viale-Gonzalez, Barreto), PRS, *51:*530, 1973

ORTIZ-MONASTERIO, F.: Primary simultaneous correction of lip and nose in unilateral cleft lip (with Velazquez), PRS, *54:*558, 1974

ORTIZ-MONASTERIO, F.: Mobile unit for detection and care of craniofacial anomalies PRS, *55:*186, 1975

ORTIZ-MONASTERIO, F. *et al*: Congenital absence of vagina, long-term follow-up in 21 patients treated with skin grafts, PRS, *49:*165, 1972

ORTIZ-MONASTERIO, F., AND TRIGOS, I.: Management of patients with complications from injection of foreign materials into breasts, PRS, *50:*42, 1972

ORTIZ-MONASTERIO, F., ARAICO, J., AND TRIGOS, I.: Record card for burn patient, PRS, *52:*325, 1973. Rev. Latino Am. cir. plast., *16:*25, 1972

ORTIZ-MONASTERIO, F., LOPEZ-MAS, J., AND ARAICO, J.: Rhinoplasty in thick-skinned nose, PRS, *56:*593, 1975. Brit. J. Plast. Surg., *27:*19, 1974

ORTIZ-MONASTERIO, F., AND JAIME, C.: Simple disimpacting device for chisels, PRS, *53:*233, 1974

ORTIZ-MONASTERIO, F. *et al*: Integration and training of a multidisciplinary team for craniofacial surgery. Prensa Med. Mex., *39:*183, 1974 (Spanish)

ORTIZ-MONASTERIO, F. *et al*: Final results from delayed treatment of patients with clefts of lip and palate, PRS, *56:*468, 1975. Scand. J. Plast. Reconstr. Surg., *8:*109, 1974

ORTIZ-MONASTERIO, F. *et al*: Craniofacial surgery, PRS, *57:*116, 1976. Bol. Med. Hosp. Infant., *32:*587, 1975

ORTON, C. I.: Loss of columella and septum from unusual form of child abuse, PRS, *56:*345, 1975

ORTON, H. S.: Treatment of class II facial deformity. Orthodontic considerations. Brit. J. Oral Surg., *10:*243, 1973

OSBON, D. B.: Intermediate and reconstructive care of maxillofacial missile wounds. J. Oral Surg., *31:*429, 1973

OSBORNE, A., DOREY, L. R., AND HARVEY, J. P.: Volkmann's contracture associated with prolonged external pressure on forearm, PRS, *51:*348, 1973. Arch. Surg., *104:*794, 1972

OSCHATZ, R. *et al*: Congenital arteriovenous fistula of the hand. Zentralbl. Chir., *98:*1783, 1973 (German)

OSHMIANSKAIA, A. I.: Combined therapy for malignant tumors of neck. Med. Radiol. (Mosk.), *17:*78, 1972 (Russian)

OSHMIANSKAIA, A. I. *et al*: Diagnosis and treatment of lymphangiosarcoma in the presence of lymphostasis of the upper extremity following mastectomy. Khirurgiia (Mosk.), *2:*23, 1975 (Russian)

OSTACHOWICZ, M. *et al*: Operative and rehabilitative treatment of syndrome of superior orbital fissure. Czas. Stomatol., *26:*727, 1973 (Polish)

Osteomyelitis (See also *Jaw, Infection of*)

Osteomyelitis, traumatic chronic, malignant transformation of a rare complication (Triantafyllou, Tutuntzakis, Avramidis), PRS, *48:*397, 1971. Trans. 1st Panhellenic Cong. Orthop. Surg. & Traum., *1:*277, 1969

Antibiotic penetration of experimental bone hematomas (Wilson *et al*), PRS, *50:*310, 1972. J. Bone & Joint Surg., *53:*1622, 1971

Bone defects, infected, surgical treatment of (Burri, Henkemeyer, Rüedi), PRS, *49:*588, 1972. Langenbeck's Arch. Chir., *330:*54, 1971

Primary skin-grafting in the treatment of chronic osteomyelitis (Naylor *et al*). Brit. J. Surg., *59:*117, 1972

Fistulae of osteomyelitic origin, myoplastic closure of (Popkirov), PRS, *51:*610, 1973. Bruns' Beitr. klin. Chir., *219:*658, 1972

Osteomyelitis in long bones, surgical treatment (Overton, Tully), PRS, *54:*117, 1974. Am. J. Surg., *126:*736, 1973

Vein catheterization, subclavian, osteomyelitis of clavicle following (Manny, Haruzi, Yosipovitch), PRS, *52:*454, 1973. Arch. Surg., *106:*342, 1973

Osteomyelitis treated by excision and graft at open operations (Roy-Camille *et al*), PRS, *55:*253, 1975. Chirurgie, *100:*480, 1974

Antibiotic concentrations in human bone (Kolczun *et al*), PRS, *54:*507, 1974. J. Bone & Joint Surg., *56A:*305, 1974

Osteomyelitis — Cont.

Osteomyelitis of mandible, intraoral partial resection and reconstruction (Sailer), PRS, *55:*716, 1975. J. Maxillo-facial Surg., *2:*173, 1974

Osteomyelitis of mandible, chronic, surgical treatment (Glahn), PRS, *55:*717, 1975. J. Maxillo-facial Surg., *2:*238, 1974

Osteogenesis, experimental, with decalcified allogenic bone matrix in palatal defects (Narang, Wells), PRS, *55:*118, 1975. Oral Surg., *37:*153, 1974

Osteomyelitis of mandible, suppurative, secondary to fracture (Limongelli *et al*), PRS, *56:*353, 1975. Oral Surg., *38:*850, 1974

Retropharyngeal infection with disc space involvement and osteomyelitis, following pharyngeal flap operation (Tucker, Hubbard). PRS, *53:*477, 1974

Osteomyelitis, current concepts in treatment (Medoff), PRS, *57:*405, 1976. Postgrad. Med., *58:*157, 1975

OSTERWALD, G.: Microsurgery of rhinobasis in injuries. Arch. Klin. Exp. Ohren Nasen Kehlkopfheilkd., *205:*213, 1973 (German)

OSTRANDER, R. B. *et al*: Pigmented neuroectodermal tumor of infancy: report of two cases. J. Oral Surg., *32:*626, 1974

OSTROVSKIL, G. G.: Some complications of tracheostomy in children. Zh. Ushn. Nos. Gorl. Bolezn., *3:*100, 1974 (Russian)

ÖSTRUP, L. T., AND FREDRICKSON, J. M.: Distant transfer of free, living bone graft by microvascular anastomoses. PRS, *54:*274, 1974

ÖSTRUP, L. T., AND FREDRICKSON, J. M.: Reconstruction of mandibular defects after radiation, using free, living bone graft transferred by microvascular anastomoses. PRS, *55:*563, 1975

ÖSTRUP, L. T. *et al*: Bone formation in a free, living bone graft transferred by microvascular anastomoses. A quantitative microscopic study using fluorochrome markers. Scand. J. Plast. Reconstr. Surg., *9:*101, 1975

OTSUKA, M.: Clinical epidemiological studies on harelip and cleft palate. J. Otolaryngol. Jpn., *78:*345, 1975 (Japanese)

OTANI, Y. *et al*: 2 cases of hand injury by a roller. Orthop. Surg. (Tokyo), *22:*995, 1971 (Japanese)

Otoplasty (See also *Ear Deformities, Acquired; Ear Deformities, Congenital; Ear, Reconstruction of*)

Simple surgical technic for external ear correction (Wieland). Arch. Klin. Exp. Ohren Nasen Kehlkopfheilkd., *199:*514, 1971

Otoplasty — Cont.

(German)

Otoplasty, experimental, using rabbit's ear (Pischke, Bortnick), PRS, *49:*469, 1972. Arch. Otolaryng., *94:*220, 1971

Results of plastic surgery of the ear using the McEvitt, Joseph and Converse methods (Kleinfeldt *et al*). Dtsch. Gesundheitsw., *26:*1840, 1971 (German)

Late results following surgical correction of prominent ears (Birke *et al*). Dtsch. Gesundheitsw., *26:*2370, 1971 (German)

When your patient asks about plastic surgery (Meijer). Med. Times. *99:*117, 1971

Ear, cupped, surgical correction of (Kislov). PRS, *48:*121, 1971

Sculptured ear (Klein). South. Med. J., *64:*1150, 1971

Otoplasty (Zohar). Arch. Otolaryng., *96:*187, 1972

Otoplasty: plastic surgery of protruding ear (Correia, Melega, Carvalho), PRS, *53:*680, 1974. Ars. Curandi, *5:*148, 1972

Correction of prominent ears (Tolhurst). Brit. J. Plast. Surg., *25:*261, 1972

Ears, protruding, simple and physiologic method to correct (Muhlbauer), PRS, *51:*229, 1973. Chir. Plastica, *1:*126, 1972

Ears, prominent, surgical methods and results in 240 corrections (Tempel). Deutsche Stomatol., *22:*773, 1972 (German)

Ears, protruding (Rebattu). J. Med. Lyon, *53:*1633, 1972 (French)

Otoplasty, new knife for (Jakubik). PRS, *53:*601, 1974. Acta chir. plast., *15:*55, 1973

Ears, protruding, relative place of operation on osseous planes and cartilaginous structures in treatment of (Ampe *et al*). Acta Otorhinolaryngol. Belg., *27:*10, 1973 (French)

Mustardé's technique, correction of protruding ears with (Roucher). Ann. chir. plast., *18:*74, 1973 (French)

Ears, protruding, technique of anterior cartilaginous striation in correction of (Batisse *et al*). Ann. Otolaryngol. Chir. Cervicofac., *90:*389, 1973 (French)

Ears, protruding, conchal hypertrophy and correction of (Schneider, Clodius). PRS, *55:*105, 1975. Brit. J. Plast. Surg., *26:*115, 1973

Otoplasty, mattress suture: histopathologic study (Bohsali). Eye, Ear, Nose & Throat Month., *52:*57, 1973

Otoplasty: cryptotia: pathology and repair (Washio). PRS, *52:*648, 1973

Otoplasty, new marking instrument for (Brusis). Ztschr. Laryng. Rhin. Otol., *52:*51, 1973 (German)

Otoplasty—Cont.

Ears, prominent, method for correction of (Bowen). Brit. J. Plast. Surg., *27:*92, 1974

Otoplasty (Mallen). Can. J. Otolaryngol., *3:*74, 1974

Notes on esthetic surgery in the Indonesian (Wiratmadja). Clin. Plast. Surg., *1:*173, 1974

Ears, bat, simple operation for (Wieland). Laryngol. Rhinol. Otol. (Stuttg.), *53:*556, 1974 (German)

Otoplasty as procedure for outpatient clinic (Philipszoon). O.R.L., *36:*58, 1974

Otoplasty, revision techniques in, evaluation and management (Feuerstein). Otolaryngol. Clin. North Am., *7:*133, 1974

Ears, lop, surgery for (Abramczyk). Otolaryngol. Pol., *28:*307, 1974 (Polish)

Concha-mastoid suture for correcting prominent ears (Pandeya, Furnas) (Letter to the Editor), PRS, *53:*670, 1974

Lop ear, congenital, simplified technique for correction (Kaye, Lotuaco). PRS, *54:*667, 1974

Surgery of anomalies of position and shape of the pinna (Haas). Z. Laryngol. Rhinol. Otol., *53:*93, 1974 (German)

Ears, protruding, use of dermal flaps in treatment of (Elsahy), PRS, *57:*755, 1976. Acta chir. plast., *17:*71, 1975

Method of prominent ear correction (Schetrumpf). Brit. J. Plast. Surg., *28:*292, 1975

Keloidal cicatrices encountered during surgery for protruding ears (Millard *et al*). Ann. Otolaryngol. Chir. Cervicofac., *92:*432, 1975 (French)

Medial conchal excision in otoplasty (Smith *et al*). Laryngoscope, *85:*738, 1975

Prevention of meatal stenosis in conchal setback otoplasty (Small). Laryngoscope, *85:*1782, 1975

Ear, lop (Tanzer). PRS, *55:*406, 1975

Mattress suture otoplasty: histopathologic study (Bohsali). Eye, Ear, Nose & Throat Month., *52:*57, 1976

OTRADOVEC, J. AND BOROVANSKY, V.: Hydraulic orbital fractures (blowout fractures), their diagnosis and treatment. Cesk. Oftalmol., *29:*16, 1973 (Czechoslovakian)

OTT, G.: Skin prostheses. Ergeb. Chir. Orthop., *54:*45, 1970 (German)

OTT, J.: Eyes' dual function—part III. Eye Ear Nose Throat Mon., *53:*465, 1974

OTTE, M. J.: Correcting inverted nipples, aid to breast feeding, PRS, *56:*605, 1975. Am. J. Nursing, *75:*454, 1975

OTTO, A. J. *et al*: Secondary correction of posttraumatic changes in orbit with alloplastic material. Ophthalmologica, *165:*519, 1972

OTTO, R.: Xeroradiography examinations in orbitonasal surgery (with Maillard, Clodius). PRS, *55:*664, 1975

OTTOLENGHI, C. E.: Massive osteo and osteoarticular bone grafts, technic and results of 62 cases. Clin. Orthop., *87:*156, 1972

OTTOLENGHI, F.: Simple method to facilitate free skin grafts. G. Ital. Dermatol., *47:*4, 1972 (Italian)

OULIE, J.: Use of areolo-mammary flap with internal pedicle in reduction mammoplasty. Ann. chir. plast., *20:*251, 1975 (French)

OURA, T.: Wound healing and plastic surgery in ulcer. Surg. Ther. (Osaka), *26:*498, 1972 (Japanese)

OURA, T. *et al*: Experience and problems in nasal reconstruction. Jap. J. Plast. Reconstr. Surg., *15:*165, 1972 (Japanese)

OVCHINNIKOV, V. A. *et al*: Median cysts and fistulas of the neck and their treatment. Vestn. Khir., *112:*23, 1974 (Russian)

OVERBECK, W. *et al*: Primary tumors and injuries of lymphatic system. Chirurg., *44:*107, 1973 (German)

OVERTON, J. H. *et al*: Aspects of management of burned child. Anaesth. Intensive Care, *1:*535, 1973

OVERTON, L., AND TULLY, W.: Surgical treatment of chronic osteomyelitis in long bones, PRS, *54:*117, 1974. Am. J. Surg., *126:*736, 1973

OWENS, D. E. *et al*: Retropharyngeal hematoma, complication of therapy with anticoagulants, PRS, *57:*765, 1976. Arch. Otolaryng., *101:*565, 1975

OWEN-SMITH, M. S.: Congenital constriction band of the thigh, PRS, *54:*503, 1974. Australian & New Zealand J. Surg., *44:*57, 1974

OWSLEY, J. Q.: Cinefluorographic analysis and treatment of cleft palate speech (Follow-Up Clinic). PRS, *49:*335, 1972

OWSLEY, J. Q., CREECH, B. J., AND DEDO, H. H.: Poor speech following pharyngeal flap operation; etiology and treatment, PRS, *52:*325, 1973. Cleft Palate J., *9:*312, 1972

OWSLEY, J. Q., JR.: Camouflage and augmentation mammaplasty, PRS, *54:*374, 1974. West. J. Med., *120:*101, 1974

OWSLEY, J. Q., JR.: Some current trends in ethics of medical practice (Editorial). PRS, *56:*567, 1975

OWSLEY, J. Q., JR., AND HINMAN, F., JR.: One-stage reconstruction of external genitalia in female with exstrophy of bladder. PRS, *50:*227, 1972

OWSLEY, J. Q., JR., LAWSON, L. I., AND CHIERICI, G. J.: Re-do pharyngeal flap. PRS, *57:*180, 1976

OZENBERGER, J. M. *et al*: Cryosurgery in allergic rhinitis. Minerva Med., *65:*3714, 1974

OZINKOVSKII, V. V. *et al*: Case of giant osteochondroma of upper jaw. Zh. Ushn. Nos. Gorl. Bolezn., *31:*108, 1971 (Russian)

OZINKOVSKII, V. V. *et al*: Fistula of the soft palate after opening of a peritonsillar abscess. Zh. Ushn. Nos. Gorl. Bolezn., *6:*95, 1974 (Russian)

OZSAHINOGLU, C. *et al*: Comparison of methods of extra temporal facial nerve repair. J. Laryng. & Otol., *89:*1095, 1975

P

PAARLBERG, D. *et al*: Lipomas of the hand. Including a case of lipoblastomatosis in a child. Mayo Clin. Proc., *47:*121, 1972

PACKER, K. J.: Methoxyflurane analgesia for burns dressings. Postgrad. Med. J., *48:*128, 1972

PADDISON, G. M., AND HANKS, G. E.: Chondrosarcoma of maxilla, PRS, *49:*474, 1972. Cancer, *28:*616, 1971

PADGETT, A. M. *et al*: Enlarged styloid processes as complication in mandibular prognathism surgery, case report. Va. Dent. J., *51:*26, 1974

PADOVAN, I. F.: Combination of extranasal and intranasal approach in surgery of the nasal pyramid and nasal septum (decortication). Can. J. Otolaryngol., *4:*522, 1975

PADOVAN, I. F. *et al*: Pathogenesis of mediastinal emphysema and pneumothorax following tracheotomy. Chest, *66:*553, 1974

PAEGLE, R. D., AYRES, S., AND DAVIS, S.: Rapid tracheal injury by cuffed airways and healing with loss of ciliated epithelium, PRS, *52:*462, 1973. Arch. Surg., *106:*31, 1973

PAEZ, P. *et al*: Stridor as the presenting symptom of lingual thyroglossal duct cyst in an infant. Clin. Pediatr. (Phila.), *13:*1077, 1974

PAFF, GEORGE H.: *Anatomy of the Head and Neck*. W. B. Saunders Co., Philadelphia, 1973. PRS, *53:*468, 1974

PAGE, C. P. *et al*: Thyroid carcinomas arising in thyroglossal ducts. PRS, *55:*636, 1975. Arch. Surg., *180:*799, 1974

PAGE, D. L.: Cutaneous melanoma: 20-year retrospective study with clinicopathologic correlation (with Franklin, Reynolds). PRS, *56:*277, 1975

PAGE, R. E.: Hand injuries at work, PRS, *57:*261, 1976. Hand, *7:*51, 1975

PAGLIA, M. A., KNAPPER, W. H., AND FORTNER, J. G.: Regional node dissection in treatment of malignant melanoma, PRS, *50:*98, 1972. Clin. Bull. Memorial Sloan-Kettering Cancer Center, *1:*136, 1971

PAGLIA, M. A. *et al*: Peutz-Jeghers syndrome. Surgical challenge. NY State J. Med., *75:*402, 1975

PAJAROLA, G. F.: Giant cell epulis in edentulous jaw. Schweiz. Monatsschr. Zahnheilkd., *83:*1261, 1973 (German)

PAJIC, D.: Torticollis myogenes in children. Med. Pregl., *27:*209, 1974 (Serbian)

PAKHOMOV, S. P.: Surgery in cicatricial contractures of the hand and fingers after burns in children. Ortop. Travmatol. Protez., *31:*30, 1970 (Russian)

PAKHOMOV, S. P.: Active surgical treatment in extensive deep burns. Ortop. Travmatol. Protez., *34:*13, 1973 (Russian)

PAKHOMOV, S. P. *et al*: Local antibacterial therapy during preparation of burn wounds for autodermoplasty. Khirurgiia (Mosk.), *9:*37, 1974 (Russian)

PAKHOMOV, S. P. *et al*: Prevention and treatment of postburn deformations of the breasts. Vestn. Khir., *115:*124, 1975 (Russian)

PAKHOMOVA, A. I.: Technics of tenorrhaphy of levator muscle in correction of ptosis of upper eyelid. Oftalmol. Zh., *29:*452, 1974 (Russian)

PAKKANEN, M. *et al*: Use of mesh graft in skin autotransplantation. Duodecim, *89:*955, 1973 (Finnish)

PALANDE, D. D. *et al*: Opponensplasty in intrinsic-muscle paralysis of thumb in leprosy, PRS, *57:*674, 1976. J. Bone & Joint Surg., *57A:*489, 1975

PALANT, D. I. *et al*: Unusual facies, cleft palate, mental retardation, and limb abnormalities in siblings—a new syndrome. J. Pediatr., *78:*686, 1971

Palatal Neoplasms (See also *Jaw, Neoplasms; Mouth, Neoplasms*)

Palatal neoplasms of salivary origin, 10 cases (Carlier *et al*). Acta Stomatol. Belg., *69:*257, 1972 (French)

Cylindroma therapy, results of (Schettler). Fortschr. Kiefer. Gesichtschir., *15:*84, 1972 (German)

Myxoma of hard palate (Pradhan, Varma, Pradhan), PRS, *51:*234, 1973. Internat. Surg., *57:*341, 1972

Carcinoma of hard palate and its relation to reverse smoking (Ramulu, Reddy), PRS, *51:*484, 1973. J. Internat. Surg., *57:*8, 1972

Chondrosarcoma of the hard palate (Gregoriades). J. Laryng. & Otol., *86:*513, 1972

Palate, primary reconstruction after radical maxillectomy for cancer (Bakamjian) (Follow-Up Clinic). PRS, *49:*335, 1972

Palate, benign chondroma of, case report (Snyder *et al*). J. Oral Surg., *31:*873, 1973

Anatomical and clinical features of mesen-

Palatal Neoplasms—Cont.

chymal tumors of the jaws (Odasso *et al*). Minerva Stomatol., *22:*269, 1973 (Italian)

Renal carcinoma presenting as metastasis to uvula (Lansigan *et al*). Urology, *2:*449, 1973

Place of surgery in the treatment of carcinomas of the oral cavity (Mendes da Costa *et al*). Acta chir. belg., *73:*529, 1974 (French)

Cervical node metastasis from epidermoid carcinoma of the oral cavity and oropharynx. A critical assessment of current staging (Spiro *et al*). Am. J. Surg., *128:*562, 1974

Management of the palatal pleomorphic adenoma (Worthington). Brit. J. Oral Surg., *12:*132, 1974

Palate, low-grade papillary adenocarcinoma of (Allen *et al*). Cancer, *33:*153, 1974

Tumors, benign, of hard palate (Ramulu *et al*), PRS, *55:*246, 1975. Indian J. Surg., *36:*113, 1974

Ectopic localization of mixed tumors of the salivary glands (Udovcki). J. Med. Pregl., *27:*313, 1974 (Serbian)

Mucoepidermoid tumors of minor salivary glands. Clinical note (D'Angelo *et al*). Minerva Stomatol., *23:*116, 1974 (Italian)

Preliminary study of histological effects of three different types of electrosurgical currents (Friedman *et al*). N.Y. State Dent. J., *40:*349, 1974

Fibrolipoma of the palate: report of two cases (Steward *et al*). N.Y. State Dent. J., *40:*603, 1974

Angiomyoma of the oral cavity (Gutmann *et al*). Oral Surg., *38:*269, 1974

Effectiveness of combined and radiotherapy of malignant tumors of the minor salivary glands of the maxilla (Vorob'ev). Stomatologiia (Mosk.), *53:*20, 1974 (Russian)

End results of surgical treatment of 622 cases of tumors of the salivary glands (Catania *et al*). Tumori, *60:*307, 1974 (Italian)

Intraoral complete resection of the upper jaw (Shinbirev). Zdravookhr. Ross. Fed., *5:*106, 1974 (Russian)

Immediate reconstruction of the hard palate following maxillectomy for carcinoma (Lissaois). Int. Surg., *60:*477, 1975

Clinical-pathological conference: Case 10, part 2. Neurofibrosarcoma (Carpenter *et al*). J. Oral Surg., *33:*38, 1975

Intraoral junctional nevus: review of the literature and report of case (Grossman *et al*). J. Oral Surg., *33:*275, 1975

Emotional aspects of new prostheses for previously treated maxillofacial patients (Davidson *et al*). J. Prosthet. Dent., *34:*55,

Palatal Neoplasms—Cont.

1975

Palatal reconstruction utilizing retrieved forehead flap (Chambers *et al*). J. Surg. Oncol., *7:*191, 1975

Leiomyosarcoma of the head and neck: a review of the literature and report of two cases (Mindell *et al*). Laryngoscope, *85:*904, 1975

Tumor, mixed, of velum palatinum, case report (Penha, Ribeiro), PRS, *57:*671, 1976. Med. Universal, *18:*8, 1975

Palate, glandular tumors of (Coates *et al*), PRS, *56:*462, 1975. Surg. Gynec. & Obst., *140:*589, 1975

Tumors of minor salivary gland origin (Antalik *et al*). Trans. Pa. Acad. Ophthalmol. Otolaryngol., *28:*42, 1975

Palate (See also Cleft Palate)

Tensor palati, functional anatomy (Ross), PRS, *48:*609, 1971. Arch. Otolaryng., *93:*1, 1970

Palatal defect, gross, surgical repair of (Beare), PRS, *48:*515, 1971. Proc. Roy. Soc. Med., *64:*71, 1971

Palate, primary, and nose in man, development of (Azzolini, Mangiante), PRS, *49:*359, 1972. Rev. Ital. chir. plast., *3:*1, 1971

Double, overlapping hinge flap to close palatal fistula (Rintala). Scand. J. Plast. Reconstr. Surg., *5:*91, 1971

Experience in the use of protective plates in resection of the maxilla (Iroshnikova). Stomatologiia (Mosk.), *50:*96, 1971 (Russian)

Palate, studies on variability of maxilla (Michalek), PRS, *52:*321, 1973. Acta chir. plast., *14:*73, 1972

Palatal fistulae, secondary, closure with intraoral tissue and bone grafting (Jackson), PRS, *52:*100, 1973. Brit. J. Plast. Surg., *25:*93, 1972

Palate, normal and cleft primary and secondary, vascular patterns (Frederiks), PRS, *52:*209, 1973. Brit. J. Plast. Surg., *25:*207, 1972

Palate, hard, myxoma of (Pradhan, Varma, Pradhan), PRS, *51:*234, 1973. Internat. Surg., *57:*341, 1972

Median palatal cyst: report of case (Thornton *et al*). J. Oral Surg., *30:*661, 1972

Palate, reparative plasty in large defects of (O'Conor *et al*), PRS, *51:*346, 1973. Prensa med. argent., *59:*992, 1972

Palate, secondary, role of mitotic activity in formation of (Jelinek, Dostal), PRS, *54:*628, 1974. Acta chir. plast., *15:*216, 1973

Hard palate, invasive pleomorphic adenoma

Palate — Cont.

of (Joachims *et al*). J. Laryng. & Otol., *87:*1147, 1973

Various methods for the closure of bucconasal communications (Landais). Rev. Stomatol. Chir. Maxillofac., *74:*642, 1973 (French)

Palate, secondary, development studies, rapid technique for contrasting embryonic tissues in (Dostal, Behounkova), PRS, *56:*367, 1975. Acta chir. plast., *16:*243, 1974

Reconstructive experience with the medially-based deltopectoral flap (Park *et al*). Am. J. Surg., *128:*548, 1974

Closure of a palatal fistula using a mucoperiosteal island flap (Herbert). Brit. J. Plast. Surg., *27:*332, 1974

Palate, soft, electrical stimulation of (Peterson), PRS, *55:*382, 1975. Cleft Palate J., *11:*72, 1974

Palatal processes, effect of Vitamin A on fusion *in vivo* and *in vitro* in rats (Nanda), PRS, *55:*383, 1975. Cleft Palate J., *11:*123, 1974

Palate, bony, of pig, growth consequent to transpositioning oral and nasal mucoperiosteum (Atherton, Lovius, Maisels), PRS, *56:*110, 1975. Cleft Palate J., *11:*429, 1974

Surgery of the pterygoid fossa (Harpman). Eye Ear Nose Throat Mon., *53:*354, 1974

Palatoplasty, effect on facial and dental relations (Bishara), PRS, *55:*513, 1975. Internat. J. Oral Surg., *3:*65, 1974

Bilateral fibrous hyperplasia of the palate (Killey). Internat. J. Oral Surg., *3:*302, 1974

Palate in Golden Syrian hamster, light microscopic and histochemical observations on development of (Ravindra, Chaudhry), PRS, *55:*259, 1975. J. Anat., *117:*1, 1974

Crossbite correction with a therapeutic pacifier (Rutrick). J. Dent. Child., *41:*442, 1974

Use of steroids in the prevention of some complications after traumatic oral surgery (Hooley *et al*). J. Oral Surg., *32:*864, 1974

Prosthetic management of surgically induced defects of the palate (Guerra). Mo. Med., *71:*690, 1974

Palatal defects, experimental osteogenesis with decalcified allogenic bone matrix in (Narang, Wells), PRS, *55:*118, 1975. Oral Surg., *37:*153, 1974

Palatal abnormalities in syndrome of gonadal dysgenesis and its variants and in Noonan's syndrome (Horowitz, Morishima), PRS, *56:*358, 1975. Oral Surg., *38:*839, 1974

Palate, soft, pathologic changes in lepromatous leprosy (Reichart), PRS, *56:*593, 1975.

Palate — Cont.

Oral Surg., *38:*898, 1974

Palate, primitive, and cleft cyst of upper maxilla, embryogenesis of (Fortunato), PRS, *57:*401, 1976. Riv. ital. chir. plast., *6:*53, 1974

Palate, hard, timing of repair (Robertson, Jolleys), PRS, *56:*468, 1975. Scand. J. Plast. Reconstr. Surg., *8:*49, 1974

Fistula of the soft palate after opening of a peritonsillar abscess (Ozinkovskil *et al*). Zh. Ushn. Nos. Gorl. Bolezn., *6:*95, 1974 (Russian)

Palatal mucosal grafts, fenestrated, for vestibuloplasty (Shepherd, Maloney, Doku), PRS, *56:*467, 1975. J. Oral Surg., *33:*34, 1975

Combined anterior and posterior maxillary ostectomy: a new technique (Wolford *et al*). J. Oral Surg., *33:*842, 1975

Use of a free connective tissue graft to increase the width of attached gingiva (Edel). Oral Surg., *39:*341, 1975

Palate, double (Gupta), PRS, *57:*537, 1976. Oral Surg., *40:*53, 1975

Maxillary exostoses. Surgical management of an unusual case (Blakemore *et al*). Oral Surg., *40:*200, 1975

Le Fort III osteotomy to correct dish-face deformity resulting from facial trauma (Lewis *et al*). S. Afr. Med. J., *49:*1915, 1975

PALETTA, F. X.: Hidradenitis suppurativa: pathologic study and use of skin flaps (Follow-Up Clinic). PRS, *49:*334, 1972

PALETTA, F. X.: Further concepts in gustatory sweating (with McGibbon). PRS, *49:*639, 1972

PALETTA, F. X.: Lower eyelid reconstruction. PRS, *51:*653, 1973

PALETTA, F. X., AND RYBKA, F. J.: Treatment of hamartomas of median nerve, PRS, *51:*705, 1973. Ann. Surg., *176:*217, 1972

PALETTA, F. X., WALKER, J., AND KING, J.: Hemangioma-thrombocytopenia syndrome (Follow-Up Clinic). PRS, *50:*183, 1972

PALFER-SOLLIER, M. *et al*: Osteosynthesis with steel wire. The "eversant" point in mandibular osteosynthesis. Rev. Stomatol. Chir. Maxillofac., *74:*214, 1973 (French)

PALKOSKA, F.: Homoplastic skin transplantation after chemical sterilization and preservation. 1. Method: bacteriological, histological and histochemical studies. 2. Clinical testing and evaluation. Z. Exp. Chir., *4:*62, 1971 (German)

PALMER, B.: Sympathetic denervation and reinnervation of cutaneous blood vessels following surgery. Experimental study on rats by histochemical fluorescence method, PRS, *49:*472, 1972. Scand. J. Plast. Reconstr. Surg., *4:*93, 1970

PALMER, B.: The influence of stress on survival of experimental skin flaps. A study on rats. Scand. J. Plast. Reconstr. Surg., *6:*110, 1972

PALMER, J. D.: Treatment of malignant melanomas of the skin. Laval. Med., *42:*926, 1971

PALMIERI, T. J.: High pressure injection injuries of the hand; treatment by early mobilization. Bull. Hosp. Joint Dis., *35:*18, 1974

PALOMO, F. *et al*: Forty-four-month evaluation of patient treated by surgical orthodontics, case report. Oral Surg., *38:*520, 1974

PALUBIS, J. E.: Cleft lip and palate with delayed eruption and congenital absence of teeth. Birth Defects, *7:*265, 1971

PALUBIS, J. E. *et al*: Lip pits with cleft lip and palate. Birth Defects, *7:*245, 1971

PALVA, A., JOKINEN, K., AND NIEMELA, T.: Tracheostomy in children, PRS, *57:*532, 1976. Arch. Otolaryng., *101:*536, 1975

PALVA, A. *et al*: Tumors of parotid region. J. Laryng. & Otol., *89:*419, 1975

PALVA, T. *et al*: Transcranial orbital decompression in severe cases of unilateral exophthalmos. J. Laryng. & Otol., *89:*1123, 1975

PAMURZIN, L. G. *et al*: Use of inorganic reducing agents to neutralize the toxic effect of "chronic alkalis" in thermochemical burns. Farmakol. Toksikol., *35:*498, 1972 (Russian)

PANDEY, S. *et al*: An unusual arrow injury. Int. Surg., *57:*589, 1972

PANDEYA, N. K. *et al*: Letter: Further risk with bleomycin. J. Am. Osteopath. Assoc., *74:*260, 1974

PANDEYA, N. K., AND FURNAS, D. W.: Correcting prominent ears (Letter to the Editor). PRS, *53:*670, 1974

PANDYA, N. H. *et al*: One-stage technique for constructing female external genitalia in male transsexuals. Brit. J. Plast. Surg., *26:*277, 1973

PANDYA, N. J.: Experimental production of "cauliflower ear" in rabbits. PRS, *52:*534, 1973

PANDYA, N. J.: Skin, dartos, and nerve biopsies as aids to diagnosis in leprosy, PRS, *54:*70, 1974. Discussion by Brand, PRS, *54:*218, 1974

PANDYA, N. J., AND STUTEVILLE, O. H.: Vertical wedge ostectomy in mandibular rami for correction of prognathism. PRS, *48:*140, 1971

PANDYA, N. J., AND STUTEVILLE, O. H.: Treatment of ameloblastoma. PRS, *50:*242, 1972

PANDYA, N. J., AND ZAREM, H. A.: Absence of vascularization in porcine skin grafts on mice. PRS, *53:*211, 1974

PANDYA, M. P. *et al*: Mammography – prelimi-

nary experience with 50 cases, PRS, *55:*247, 1975. Indian J. Surg., *36:*102, 1974

PANET-RAYMOND, G., AND JOHNSON, W. C.: Adenocarcinoma of eccrine sweat gland, PRS, *52:*685, 1973. Arch. Dermat., *107:*94, 1973

PANEVA-HOLEVITCH, E.: New technique to correct thumb opposition in thenar muscle paralysis, PRS, *53:*106, 1974. Acta Orthop. Belg., *38:*308, 1972

PANEVA-KHOLEVICH, E.: Osteosynthesis of the tubular bones of the hand with metal plate. Ortop. Travmatol. Protez., *35:*59, 1974 (Russian)

PANKIN, V. I., AND CHIRKOVA, A. M.: Comparative evaluation of transplantation of heterologous cartilage stored frozen and in 70° alcohol, PRS, *54:*510, 1974. Acta chir. plast., *15:*155, 1973

PANNBACKER, M.: Survey of publications for parents of cleft palate children: a preliminary report. Cleft Palate J., *13:*57, 1976

PANNIKE, A. *et al*: Experiences and rehabilitation results in single and repeated plastic surgery of flexor tendons. Monatsschr. Unfallheilk., *74:*211, 1971 (German)

PANTAZOPOULOS, P. *et al*: Current views on treatment of cancer of maxillary sinus. Stomatologia (Athenai), *31:*27, 1974 (Greek)

PANZONI, E.: Changes in tooth sensitivity following Caldwell-Luc radical surgery of maxillary sinus. Riv. Ital. Stomatol., *28:*59, 1973 (Italian)

PAP, G. S.: Management of neck contractures resulting from burn injuries, PRS, *51:*351, 1973. Internat. Surg., *57:*413, 1972

PAP, G. S.: Comparison of three methods of eyelid reconstruction. PRS, *49:*513, 1972

PAP, G. S.: First branchial cleft sinus and pouch. PRS, *52:*583, 1973

PAP, G. S.: Dermoid cysts of face – recommendation for early excision. Eye, Ear, Nose, Throat Mon., *53:*239, 1974

PAPADOPOULOS, C.: Corrective operation for laterognathism. Odontostomatol. Proodos., *27:*161, 1973 (Greek)

PAPAIOANNOU, A. N., AND CRITSELIS, A. N.: Xanthogranuloma of thigh, PRS, *47:*308, 1971. Acta chir. Hellenica, *2:*203, 1970

PAPAIOANNOU, A. N., CRITSELIS, A. N., AND GIAMALAKIS, C. S.: Comparison of operative repairs of oral floor cancer, PRS, *49:*474, 1972. Acta chir. Hellenica, *18:*376, 1971

PAPAIOANNOU, A., CRITSELIS, A., AND YAMALAKIS, C.: Radical groin lymph node dissection, PRS, *56:*473, 1975. Tr. 8th Panhellenic Cong. Surg. Soc., *A:* 276, 1973

PAPAKONSTANTINOU, A. *et al*: Special method of arthroplasty of the temporomandibular joint. Stomatologia (Athenai), *32:*145, 1975 (Greek)

PAPANGELOU, L.: Correction of the nasal septum deviation: a new conservative technique. J. Laryng. & Otol., *86:*83, 1972

PAPARELLA, MICHAEL M., AND SHUMRICK, DONALD A.: *Otolaryngology, Volume III. Head and Neck.* W. B. Saunders Co., Philadelphia, 1973. PRS, *53:*218, 1974

PAPE, H. D.: Indications for multiple wire osteosynthesis in mid-facial fractures. Fortschr. Kiefer. Gesichtschir., *19:*151, 1975 (German)

PAPILLON, J.: Value of mammography in cosmetic surgery of breasts (with Perras). PRS, *52:*132, 1973

PAPILLON, J. *et al*: Cutaneous radio-cancer of both hands. J. Radiol. Electrol. Med. Nucl., *50:*750, 1969 (French)

PAPOUTSAKIS, S. *et al*: Therapeutic problem of pilonidal cyst disease: comparison of operative methods and conclusions on 1147 personal cases, PRS, *50:*100, 1972. Trans. 7th Panhellenic Cong. Surg. Soc., *2:*384, 1971

PAPPAS, J. C.: Repair of nostril defect with contralateral nasolabial flap (with Santos). PRS, *57:*704, 1976

PAQUIN, M. *et al*: Functional prostheses for the mutilated hand. Acta Orthop. Belg., *39:*1188, 1973 (French)

PARADIS, R. *et al*: Flotation pad therapy for decubitus ulcers, PRS, *56:*111, 1975. Arch. Phys. Med. & Rehab., *56:*40, 1975

PARADISE, J. L.: Middle ear problems associated with cleft palate. An internationally-oriented review. Cleft Palate J., *12:*17, 1975

Paranasal Sinus Neoplasms

Paranasal sinus exenteration or laryngectomy, hyposmia after (Hoye, Ketcham, Henkin), PRS, *48:*391, 1971. Am. J. Surg., *120:*485, 1970

Paranasal sinuses, metastatic tumors of oral cavity, pharynx and (Jortay), PRS, *50:*635, 1972. Acta chir. belg., *70:*715, 1971

Maxillary sinus carcinoma, diagnosis and TNM classification (Sakai *et al*). Acta Otolaryngol. (Stockh.), *74:*123, 1972

Peripheral nerve tumors involving paranasal sinuses: a case report and review of the literature (Robitaille *et al*). Cancer, *35:*1254, 1972

Maxillary sinus, rhabdomyosarcoma of (Bailey *et al*). Trans. Am. Acad. Ophthalmol. Otolaryngol., *76:*1375, 1972

Ossifying cementoma (cementifying fibroma) (Montgomery). Trans. Am. Acad. Ophthalmol. Otolaryngol., *76:*1380, 1972

Ethmoid sinuses: re-evaluation of surgical resection (Ketcham *et al*). Am. J. Surg., *126:*469, 1973

Paranasal Sinus Neoplasms – Cont.

Maxillary sinus cancers, radio-surgical treatment (Torre *et al*). Ann. Otolaryngol. Chir. Cervicofac., *90:*353, 1973 (French)

Cancer, ethmoid sinuses, combined intracranial and facial approach for excision and repair of (Millar *et al*). Aust. N.Z. J. Surg., *43:*179, 1973

Maxillary sinus, tumors of. Study of 53 cases treated with radiotherapy and surgery combined or isolated radiotherapy (Pourquier *et al*). J. Radiol. Electrol. Med. Nucl., *54:*27, 1973 (French)

Maxillary sinus cancer therapy contribution of curietherapy (Robillard *et al*). J. Radio. Electrol. Med. Nucl., *54:*153, 1973 (French)

Paranasal sinuses, radiorecurrent cancer of, pseudomonas meningitis complicating radical resection for: report of two patients successfully treated with intrathecal polymyxin (Geelhoed *et al*). J. Surg. Oncol., *5:*365, 1973

Paranasal sinuses, leiomyoangioma of, case report (Schwartzman *et al*). Laryngoscope, *83:*1856, 1973

Roentgenologic appearances of sphenoethmoidal mucocele (Takahashi *et al*). Neuroradiology, *6:*45, 1973

Cancer, frontal sinus, primary (Rusanova). Vopr. Onkol., *19:*95, 1973 (Russian)

Combined radiological and surgical therapy of cancer of the ethmoid. (Elner *et al*). Acta Otolaryngol., *78:*270, 1974

Ameloblastoma of the maxillary sinus (De Gandt *et al*). Acta Otorhinolaryngol. Belg., *28:*365, 1974 (French)

Sinuses, ethmoid and sphenoid, problems in tumors of (Lapayowker, Ronis), PRS, *56:*677, 1975. Adv. Oto-rhino-laryngol., *21:*19, 1974

Adenoid cystic carcinoma of salivary origin. A clinicopathologic study of 242 cases (Spiro *et al*). Am. J. Surg., *128:*512, 1974

Pseudosarcomatous changes in antrochoanal polyps (Smith, Echevarria, McLelland), PRS, *54:*699, 1974. Arch. Otolaryng., *99:*228, 1974

Neurilemmoma of the sphenoid sinus (Calcaterra *et al*). Arch. Otolaryng., *100:*383, 1974

Fibrous histiocytomas of the nose and paranasal sinuses (Rice *et al*). Arch. Otolaryng., *100:*398, 1974

Benign bone tumors of the nose and paranasal sinuses in childhood. Review of cases in the Hospital Infantilede Mexico (Shubich *et al*). Bol. Med. Hosp. Infant. Mex., *31:*831, 1974 (Spanish)

Maxillary sinus, osteoma of–its occurrence

Paranasal Sinus Neoplasms—Cont.

following surgery (Noyek *et al*). Can. J. Otolaryngol., *3:*90, 1974

Juvenile fibroma of antral origin (Ramanjaneyulu). Int. Surg., *59:*423, 1974

Carcinoma of maxillary sinus following thorotrast instillation (Rankow, Conley, Fodor), PRS, *55:*386, 1975. J. Maxillo-facial Surg., *2:*119, 1974

Maxillary antrum, carcinoma of, in 8-year-old child. Clinical-Pathological Conference (Caldwell *et al*). J. Oral Surg., *32:*367, 1974

Cancer, maxillary sinus, management of (Sako). J. Surg. Oncol., *6:*325, 1974

Tumors of the paranasal sinuses involving the orbit (Reichert). Laryngol. Rhinol. Otol. (Stuttg.), *53:*443, 1974 (German)

Maxillary antrum, carcinoma of: role of preoperative irradiation (Pearlman *et al*). Laryngoscope, *84:*400, 1974

Paranasal sinus neoplasm, proptosis caused by (Miglets). Ohio State Med. J., *70:*171, 1974

Maxillary sinus, cancer of, current views of treatment (Pantazopoulos *et al*). Stomatologia (Athenai), *31:*27, 1974 (Greek)

Paranasal sinuses and adjacent areas, polytomography of (Saunders *et al*). Trans. Am. Acad. Ophthalmol. Otolaryngol., *78:*168, 1974

Atypical fibroxanthoma of ethmoid sinus (Lesica *et al*). Arch. Otolaryng., *101:*506, 1975

Maxillary sinus sarcomas. Case report and literature review (Prasanna *et al*). Can. J. Otolaryngol., *4:*704, 1975

Osteoma of the ethmofrontal sinus. Case report (Olumide *et al*). J. Neurosurg., *42:*343, 1975

Complex odontoma of the maxillary sinus: report of case (Curreri *et al*). J. Oral Surg., *33:*45, 1975

Frontal sinus disease. III. Experimental and clinical factors in failure of the frontal osteoplastic operation (Schenck). Laryngoscope, *85:*76, 1975

Mucosal melanomas of the head and neck (Barton). Laryngoscope, *85:*93, 1975

Inverted Schneiderian papilloma: a clinical and pathological study (Vrabec). Laryngoscope, *85:*186, 1975

Alveolar rhabdomyosarcoma of the ethmoid sinus (Makishima *et al*). Laryngoscope, *85:*400, 1975

Adenoma, benign pleomorphic, of hard palate, radiologic features of (Pinto *et al*). Oral Surg., *39:*976, 1975

Papillomas of the nasal and paranasal cavities (Claimont *et al*). South. Med. J., *68:*41,

Paranasal Sinus Neoplasms—Cont.

1975

Cylindromas of the nose and paranasal sinuses (Volkov *et al*). Vestn. Otorinolaringol., *1:*55, 1975 (Russian)

Neurilemmoma of the nose and accessory sinuses (Volkov *et al*). Vestn. Otorinolaringol., *3:*34, 1975 (Russian)

Late Flavobacterium species meningitis after craniofacial exenteration (Bagely *et al*). Arch. Intern. Med., *136:*229, 1976

Adenocarcinoma of the para-nasal sinuses (Saunders *et al*). J. Laryngl. Otol., *90:* 157, 1976

PARANT, M.: Parotid fistulas, therapeutic result. Rev. Fr. Odontostomatol., *19:*244, 1972

PARANT, M. *et al*: Technic for partial segment osteotomy of the upper maxillary. Orthod. Fr., *41:*325, 1970 (French)

PARANT, M. M.: Parotidean fistulae: therapeutic result. Actual Odontostomatol. (Paris), *26:*281, 1972 (French)

Paraplegia and Quadriplegia (See also *Pressure Sores*)

Ischial tuberosity, pressure sores over, method of treatment (Sundarason), PRS, *48:*298, 1971. Singapore M. J., *11:*34, 1970

Paraplegics, surgical management of pressure sores in (Ganguli, Roy), PRS, *50:*636, 1972. Indian J. Surg., *33:*273, 1971

Paraplegia, electromicturition in: implication of spinal neuro-prosthesis (Nashold *et al*), PRS, *50:*419, 1972. Arch. Surg., *104:*195, 1972

Paralytic upper extremities, control systems for function in traumatic quadriplegia (Stauffer, Nickel), PRS, *52:*452, 1973. Paraplegia, *10:*3, 1972

Paraplegia, sexual function in (Tarabulcy), PRS, *52:*453, 1973. Paraplegia, *10:*201, 1972

Decubitus ulcers, massive, an alternative to total-thigh flap for coverage of (Burkhardt). PRS, *49:*433, 1972

Paraplegics, surgical treatment of bedsores in (Olivari, Schrudde, Wahle). PRS, *50:*477, 1972

Bladder, urinary, plastic operation in neurogenic disorders of micturition (Savchenko, Mokhort), PRS, *54:*504, 1974. Acta chir. plast., *15:*223, 1973

Paraplegic bladder, chronic electrical stimulation (Grimes, Nashold, Currie), PRS, *52:*596, 1973. J. Urol., *109:*242, 1973

Water bed, use of, for prevention of pressure sores (Siegel, Vistnes, Laub). PRS, *51:*31, 1973

Paraplegics, elevated bathtubs for, PRS,

Paraplegia and Quadriplegia – Cont.

55:260, 1975. Am. J. Physical Med., 53:208, 1974

Blood volume and capacitance vessel compliance in quadriplegic patient (Desmond, Laws), PRS, 55:110, 1975. Canad. Anaesth. Soc. J., 21:421, 1974

Sphincterotomy, external: rationale for procedure and experiences with 150 patients (Schellhammer, Hackler, Bunts), PRS, 56:106, 1975. Paraplegia, 12:5, 1974

Paraplegic patients, beds to prevent ischemia in, comparison of four (Carpendale), PRS, 56:115, 1975. Paraplegia, 12:21, 1974

Paraplegic, value of sinography in management of decubitus ulcers (Lopez, Aranha). PRS, 53:208, 1974

Ulcer, sacral decubitus, repaired by turnover flap of *gluteus maximus* muscle (Stallings, Delgado, Converse). PRS, 54:52, 1974

Paraplegics, young, use of long island flap to bring sensation to the sacral area (Dibbell). PRS, 54:220, 1974

Penis necrosis with decubitus ulcer: debridement and closure with scrotal flap (Lanier, Neale). PRS, 54:609, 1974

Vascular status and function in paraplegics and tetraplegics (Faubel, Flach), PRS, 54:239, 1974. Ztschr. Orthop., 112:111, 1974

Paraplegics and pressure sores, an operant conditioning approach to prevention (Malament, Dunn, Davis), PRS, 56:470, 1975. Arch. Phys. Med. & Rehab., 56:161, 1975

Paraplegic, Cloran telescoping oral orthotic device for (Materson, Lotz), PRS, 57:543, 1976. Arch. Phys. Med. Rehabil., 56:409, 1975

Transplantation of the musculocutaneous nerve on the median nerve in an attempt at improving the function of the hand of a tetraplegic (Kiwerski). Chir. Narzadow. Ruchu Ortop. Pol., 40:173, 1975 (Polish)

Sometimes deleterious influence of the brachioradialis radial extensors and finger flexors on residual hand function in spastic tetraplegics (Treanor *et al*). Paraplegia, 13:12, 1975

Tendon transfers to improve grasp in patients with cervical spinal cord injury (Freehaver). Paraplegia, 13:15, 1975

Ulcers, preventing recurrent tissue breakdowns after pressure "sore" closures (Rogers, Wilson), PRS, 56:419, 1975. Discussion by Brand, PRS, 56:573, 1975

PARDINA, A. J., AND FRONTERA VACA, J. L.: Leporine nose, PRS, 48:394, 1971. Bull. Plast. Reconstr. Surg. Argent., 1:12, 1970

PARDOE, R.: Effect of commonly used antisep-

tics on wound healing (with Gruber, Vistnes). PRS, 55:472, 1975

PARDUE, A. M.: Repair of torn earlobe with preservation of the perforation for an earring. PRS, 51:472, 1973

PARK, J. S. *et al*: Reconstructive experience with the medially based deltopectoral flap. Am. J. Surg., 128:548, 1974

PARKASH, A., PANDIT, P., AND SHARMA, L.: Studies in wound healing in experimental diabetes, PRS, 54:242, 1974. Internat. Surg., 59:25, 1974

PARKER, M.: Avoiding bone resorption under plastic chin implants, PRS, 53:250, 1974. Arch. Otolaryng., 98:100, 1973

PARKER, R.: Case of juvenile angiofibroma, PRS, 53:248, 1974. Arch. Otolaryng., 98:129, 1973

PARKER, R., AND WILKINSON, T.: Prevention of adhesions in injury of extensor mechanism of fingers, PRS, 55:109, 1975. South. M. J., 67:796, 1974

PARKES, A.: "Lumbrical plus" finger. J. Bone & Joint Surg. (Br.), 53:236, 1971

PARKES, A.: Ischemic effects of external and internal pressure on upper limb, PRS, 54:236, 1974. Hand, 5:105, 1973

PARKES, A.: Paralytic claw fingers – a graft tenodesis operation. Hand, 5:192, 1973

PARKES, A.: Some thoughts on examination of the hand. Hand, 7:104, 1975

PARKES, M.: Avoiding bone resorption under plastic chin implants. Arch. Otolaryng., 98:100, 1973

PARKES, M. *et al*: Pinch technique for repair of cosmetic eyelid deformities. Arch. Ophth., 89:324, 1973

PARKES, M. L. *et al*: Rhinoplastic dressings. Eye, Ear, Nose, Throat Mon., 52:166, 1973

PARKES, M. L., AND BRENNAN, H. G.: Familial choanal atresia in rhinoplasty candidate, case report, PRS, 53:240, 1974. Eye, Ear, Nose & Throat Month., 52:222, 1973

PARKES, M. L., AND KAMER, F. M.: The mature nose. Laryngoscope, 83:157, 1973

PARKS, B. J. *et al*: Electric burns of the hand. J. Occup. Med., 15:967, 1973

PARKS, B. J. *et al*: Bites of the hand. Rocky Mt. Med. J., 71:85, 1974

PARMER, D. E. *et al*: Arthroplasty for bilateral temporomandibular joint ankylosis, case report. J. Oral Surg., 30:816, 1972

PARNES, E. I. *et al*: Necrosis of the anterior maxilla following osteotomy. Oral Surg., 33:326, 1972

Parotid Gland

Resection of tympanic plexus in Frei's syndrome and recurrent parotiditis (Bouche *et*

Parotid Gland—Cont.

al). Ann. Otolaryngol. Chir. Cervicofac., *88:*449, 1971 (French)

Tonsillectomy blade for superficial parotidectomy (Smith). Arch. Otolaryng., *94:*364, 1971

Sialography, role in extraparotid disease (Mandel, Baurmash), PRS, *48:*195, 1971. Oral Surg., *31:*164, 1971

Leriche's operation for the treatment of parotid gland fistula (Uchikoshi *et al*). Otolaryngology (Tokyo), *43:*919, 1971 (Japanese)

Parotid duct transplantation for correction of drooling in patients with cancer of head and neck (Cohen, Holmes, Edgerton), PRS, *49:*361, 1972. Surg. Gynec. & Obst., *133:*663, 1971

Parotidean fistulae: therapeutic result (Parant). Actual Odontostomatol. (Paris), *26:*281, 1972 (French)

Parotid disease, historical and pathological curiosities of (Maynard). Guys Hosp. Rep., *121:*45, 1972

Stensen's duct, external parotid fistulae by section of (Pena, Gruart), PRS, *51:*702, 1973. Orientacion Med. Argent., *21:*844, 1972

Parotid fistulas, therapeutic result (Parant). Rev. Fr. Odontostomatol., *19:*244, 1972

Parotidectomy for inflammatory lesions (Lachard *et al*). Rev. Stomatol. Chir. Maxillofac., *73:*235, 1972 (French)

Parotid niche, unusual air cavity of (Poncet). Ann. Otolaryngol. Chir. Cervicofac., *90:*376, 1973 (French)

Chronic recurrent parotitis in children (Wagenaar). Arch. chir. neerl., *25:*13, 1973

Salivary symptoms in Parkinson's disease (Patson, Gibberd, Wilson), PRS, *53:*365, 1974. Arch. Neurol., *29:*274, 1973

Correction of extreme dilatation of Stensen's duct resulting from chronic partial obstruction (Christensen, Mashberg, Turk). J. Oral Surg., *31:*136, 1973

Parotid fistula: a complication of mandibular osteotomy (Goldberg, Marco, Google). J. Oral Surg., *31:*207, 1973

Parotid surgery, identification of facial nerve in (Maran). J. R. Coll. Surg. Edinb., *18:*58, 1973

Parotid duct injuries, treatment of (Abramson). Laryngoscope, *83:*1764, 1973

Sialorrhea in mentally retarded patients managed by trans-tympanic neurectomy (Townsend, Morimoto, Kraleman), PRS, *54:*105, 1974. Mayo Clin. Proc., *48:*776, 1973

Parotid surery, current status (Wehmer).

Parotid Gland—Cont.

Med. Klin., *68:*410, 1973 (German)

Parotid duct calculus (Thomson), PRS, *53:*681, 1974. Proc. Roy. Soc. Med., *66:*352, 1973

Parotid surgery with special care of facial nerve (Birnmeyer). Z. Laryngol. Rhinol. Otol., *52:*813, 1973 (German)

Parotidectomy in patient with family history of hyperthermia (Wadhwa *et al*). Anesthesiology, *40:*191, 1974

Syndrome, Sjögren's, nasal and mucous membrane biopsy (Powell, Larson, Hankin), PRS, *55:*246, 1975. Ann. Int. Med., *81:*25, 1974

Syndrome, Sjögren's, in systemic *lupus erythematosus* (Alarcon-Segovia, Velazquez-Forero, Gonzalez-Jimenez), PRS, *56:*237, 1975. Ann. Int. Med., *81:*577, 1974

Hydatid cysts in children (Saled *et al*). Chirurgie, *100:*294, 1974 (French)

Interpretation of the 99mTcO-4-salivary gland scans (Breunsbach *et al*). Fortschr. Geb. Roentgenstr. Nuklearmed., *121:*500, 1974 (German)

Dribbling of saliva in children with cerebral palsy and its management (Makhani). Indian J. Pediatr., *41:*272, 1974

Oral surgical approach to the treatment of Sjögren's syndrome (Berenyi). Int. J. Oral Surg., *3:*309, 1974

Parotitis, recurrent, in childhood (Garvar, Kringstein), PRS, *55:*246, 1975. J. Oral Surg., *32:*373, 1974

Parotid, diagnosis and treatment of diseases of (Ungerecht). Munch. Med. Wochenschr., *116:*439, 1974 (German)

Transparotid approach in mandibular ameloblastoma recurrences (Gouiric *et al*). Rev. Stomatol. Chir. Maxillofac., *75:*58, 1974 (French)

Anesthesia for operations on the parotid gland (Klementov *et al*). Stomatologiia (Mosk.), *53:*97, 1974 (Russian)

Juxtaoral organ: the importance of knowledge of this organ in oral pathology and surgery (Krammer *et al*). Wien. Klin. Wochenschr., *86:*639, 1974 (German)

Postmaxillectomy rhinorrhea: corrected by transposition of parotid duct opening (Clark *et al*). Arch. Otolaryng., *101:*492, 1975

Parotid area swelling caused by prominent transverse process of atlas (Emistein, Katz), PRS, *57:*395, 1976. Arch. Otolaryng., *101:*558, 1975

Parotid surgery, identification of facial nerve in (Heeneman). Can. J. Otolaryngol., *4:*145, 1975

Parotid Gland—Cont.

Surgical method for exteriorizing the orifice of Stensen's duct for long-term collection of parotid saliva (Tamarin *et al*). J. Dent. Res., *54:*458, 1975

Parotid gland cysts. Review and report of two unusual cases (Shaheen *et al*). J. Laryng. Otol., *89:*435, 1975

Parotid gland, unusual lesions of (Katz). J. Surg. Oncol., *7:*219, 1975

Syndrome, Sjögren's (Akin, Kreller, Walters), PRS, *56:*462, 1975. Oral Surg., *33:*27, 1975

Morphological aspects of xerophthalmia after transplantation of Stensen's duct into the conjunctival cavity (Kurbanaeva *et al*). Vestn. Oftalmol., *2:*43, 1975 (Russian)

Parotid Neoplasms (See also *Salivary Gland Neoplasms*)

Frey's syndrome, Jacobson's neurectomy for (Smith *et al*), PRS, *48:*604, 1971. Am. J. Surg., *120:*478, 1970

Parotid gland tumors (Toraya *et al*), PRS, *49:*238, 1972. Am. J. Surg., *120:*629, 1970

Diagnosis and therapy of parotid neoplasms (Werner). Dtsch. Gesundheitsw., *25:*358, 1970 (German)

Articulotemporal syndrome. Report of 4 cases (Meyer). Monatsschr. Ohrenheilkd. Laryngorhinol., *104:*413, 1970 (German)

Prevention of complications after parotidectomy (Timosca). Rev. Stomatol. Chir. Maxillofac., *71:*673, 1970 (French)

Parotid gland cystadenolymphoma (Warthin's tumor) (Storgard Jensen, Husted), PRS, *48:*92, 1971. Scand. J. Plast. Reconstr. Surg., *4:*114, 1970

Malignant oncocytoma of the parotid gland (Whittam *et al*). Brit. J. Surg., *58:*851, 1971

Parotid gland, submandibular gland and palate region, salivary gland tumors in (Eneroth), PRS, *49:*237, 1972. Cancer, *27:*1415, 1971

Parotid gland, sebaceous lymphoma of (Wasan), PRS, *49:*475, 1972. Cancer, *28:*1019, 1971

Parotid tumors, giant (Bhargava, Elhence), PRS, *48:*604, 1971. Internat. Surg., *55:*448, 1971

Clinical and histological experiences in 54 malignant parotid tumors (Ronay *et al*). Langenbecks Arch. Chir., *330:*45, 1971 (German)

Parotid gland tumor, mixed of enormous dimensions (Bobic). Med. Arh., *25:*75, 1971 (Serbian)

Parotid Neoplasms—Cont.

Parotid gland tumors (Lambert), PRS, *48:*518, 1971. Mil. Med., *136:*484, 1971

Parotid gland neoplasms, experiences in treatment of (Catania). Minerva Chir., *26:*1422, 1971 (Italian)

Swelling of the parotid region, its surgical treatment. Report of 56 cases (Pazat *et al*). Rev. Stomatol. Chir. Maxillofac., *72:*725, 1971 (French)

Total parotidectomy with conservation of the facial nerve (Bortot *et al*). Riv. Ital. Stomatol., *26:*446, 1971 (Italian)

Surgical treatment of benign tumors of the parotid gland (Sointsev *et al*). Stomatologiia (Mosk.), *50:*34, 1971 (Russian)

Children, vascular tumors of the parotid region in (Martinez-Mora, Boix-Ochoa, Tressera), PRS, *50:*96, 1972. Surg. Gynec. & Obst., *133:*973, 1971

Adenocarcinoma in 12-year-old girl, superficial parotidectomy for (Garas *et al*), PRS, *51:*483, 1973. Acta chir. Hellenica, *44:*586, 1972

Parotid gland surgery, management of facial nerve in (Beahrs, Chong), PRS, *51:*349, 1973. Am. J. Surg., *124:*473, 1972

Syndrome, Frey's (Clabaugh *et al*). Arch. Dermat., *106:*597, 1972

Reinnervation after resection of the facial nerve (Trojaborg *et al*). Arch. Neurol., *26:*17, 1972

Parotid gland, branchiogenic cysts within (Sisson *et al*). Arch. Otolaryng., *96:*165, 1972

Parotidectomy, amputation neuroma of great auricular nerve after (Hobsley). Brit. J. Surg., *59:*735, 1972

Parotid clear-cell adenoma of possible myoepithelial origin (Saksela *et al*). Cancer, *30:*742, 1972

Parotid gland, congenital hemangioma of, in six-month-old child (Chaves, Oliveira), PRS, *53:*111, 1974. Folha Med. Brazil, *65:*385, 1972

Parotid gland tumors, mixed, malignant degeneration of (Lentrodt). Fortschr. Kiefer. Gesichtschir., *15:*101, 1972 (German)

Parotidectomy, conservative, results in, in pleomorphous adenomas—report of 110 cases (Rehrmann *et al*). Fortschr. Kiefer. Gesichtschir., *15:*106, 1972 (German)

Extensive postoperative surgical emphysema with pneumomediastinum and pneumothorax (Mehdiratta *et al*). Int. Surg., *57:*666, 1972

Parotid gland, mass in, management of (Rosenfeld *et al*). J. Tenn. Med. Assoc., *65:*1007, 1972.

Parotid Neoplasms—Cont.

Malignant papillary cystadenoma lymphomatosum (Dobrossy, Ronay, Moinar). Oncology, *26:*457, 1972

Therapeutic methods in angiotenic tumor of the head and neck (Koike *et al*). Otolaryngology (Tokyo), *44:*93, 1972 (Japanese)

Gustatory sweating, further concepts in (McGibbon, Paletta). PRS, *49:*639, 1972

Parotid tumor, benign, ipsilateral, spontaneous facial nerve paralysis associated with (Cimorra, Ferreira, Martinez-Tello). PRS, *50:*523, 1972

Parotid gland neoplasms, surgery of benign and mixed (Kosokovic *et al*). Rad. Med. Fak. Zagrebu., *20:*239, 1972 (Croatian)

Parotid angioma, case (Crepy *et al*). Rev. Stomatol. Chir. Maxillofac., *73:*213, 1972 (French)

Parotidectomy, anterior traction of mandible during (Gaillard). Rev. Stomatol. Chir. Maxillofac., *73:*579, 1972 (French)

Auto-transplantation of motor nerves after surgery of parotid neoplasms with involvement of the facial nerve (Burlibasa *et al*). Stomotologia (Bucur.), *19:*81, 1972 (Rumanian)

Primary myoplasty in removal of the parotid gland together with branches of the facial nerve (Naumov *et al*). Stomatologiia (Mosk.), *51:*30, 1972 (Russian)

Parotid gland tumor, clinical and histological findings in 220 cases of (Ronay *et al*). Zentralbl. Chir., *97:*1082, 1972

Significance and treatment of lymph node metastases of malignant mucous and salivary gland tumors (Rafla). Am. J. Roentgenol. Radium Ther. Nucl. Med., *117:*595, 1973

Parotid tumor, mixed, with tyrosine crystals (Micheau). Ann. Anat. Pathol. (Paris), *18:*469, 1973 (French)

Syndrome, Gardner's. Apropos of two familial cases (Leroux—Robert *et al*). Ann. Otolaryngol. Chir. Cervicofac., *90:*161, 1973

Papillary cystadenolymphoma of parotid gland associated with cervical lymph node tuberculosis (Lallemant *et al*). Ann. Otolaryngol. Chir. Cervicofac., *90:*224, 1973 (French)

Parotid tumor, giant mixed (Cachin *et al*). Ann. Otolaryngol. Chir. Cervicofac., *90:*363, 1973 (French)

Parotid gland, benign tumors of (Coevorden, Horree), PRS, *54:*106, 1974. Arch. chir. neerl., *25:*435, 1973

Parotid gland, malignant epithelial tumors of. Classification, staging and treatment (Langezaal *et al*). Arch. chir. neerl.,

Parotid Neoplasms—Cont.

*25:*441, 1973

Malignant tumours in the ENR-region. IV. Tumours of the parotid gland (Lange *et al*). Arch. Geschwulstforsch., *42:*358, 1973 (German)

Parotid gland, sebaceous gland carcinoma of (Zechner *et al*). Arch. Klin. Exp. Ohren Nasen Kehlkopfheilkd., *205:*119, 1973 (German)

Parotid tumors of deep lobe (Sheridan *et al*). Aust. N. Z. J. Surg., *43:*129, 1973

Parotid tumors (Vargas *et al*), PRS, *55:*376, 1975. Bol. Soc. Venezuelana Cir., *27:*133, 1973

Tumors of pharyngeal prolongation of parotid (Yoel), PRS, *54:*107, 1974. Bol. y trab. Acad. argent. cir., *57:*250, 1973

Carcinoma, parotid and radiotherapy (Patey). Brit. Med. J., *1:*236, 1973

Parotid glands, oncocytoma of. Case presentation and review of literature (Hernandez *et al*). Del. Med. J., *45:*219, 1973

Parotid gland, neoplasms of. Review of 185 operated cases (Garas *et al*). Int. Surg., *58:*178, 1973

Parotid tumor, mixed, histologically benign, with hepatic metastasis (Young *et al*). J. Pathol., *109:*171, 1973

Parotid gland, mixed tumors of, diagnosis and treatment of 153 (Verhaeghe *et al*). Lille Med., *18:*385, 1973 (French)

Lymphangioma, parotid: congenital tumor (Kornblut *et al*). O. R. L., *35:*303, 1973

Tumors, major salivary gland, surgical decisions in treatment of (Rankow). PRS, *51:*514, 1973

Parotid gland swelling: neurilemmoma of facial nerve (Conley, Janecka). PRS, *52:*55, 1973

Carcinoma, adenoid cystic, of head and neck (Newton *et al*), PRS, *52:*600, 1973. Proc. Roy. Australasian Coll. Surgeons, *46:*720, 1973

Tumors of deep lobe of parotid gland (Sheridan, Newton), PRS, *52:*600, 1973. Proc. Roy. Australasian Coll. Surg., *46:*744, 1973

Parotid, malignant cystadenolymphoma. Histological and ultrastructural study (Cernea *et al*). Rev. Stomatol. Chir. Maxillofac., *74:*141, 1973 (French)

Parotid region, tumors of (Dupuis). Rev. Stomatol. Chir. Maxillofac., *74:*493, 1973 (French)

Parotid, successive bilateral cylindroma of (Arsac *et al*). Sem. Hop. Paris, *49:*2031, 1973 (French)

Parotid gland, tumors of, management (Hugo *et al*). Surg. Clin. North Am.,

Parotid Neoplasms — Cont.
123:49, 1975
Parotid gland tumors. Clinicopathologic study (Sinha *et al*). Am. J. Surg., 129:75, 1975
Parotid gland tumors, clinicopathologic study (Sinha, Buntine), PRS, 57:672, 1976. Am. J. Surg., 129:675, 1975
Prognosis of malignant tumors of the parotid gland with facial paralysis (Conley *et al*). Arch. Otolaryng., 101:39, 1975
Benign lymphoepithelial lesions of the salivary glands (Kelly *et al*). Arch. Otolaryng., 101:71, 1975
Process of atlas, prominent, causing parotid area swelling (Emistein, Katz), PRS, 57:395, 1976. Arch. Otolaryng., 101:558, 1975
Acinic cell carcinoma (Levin, Robinson, Lin), PRS, 55:724, 1975. Arch. Surg., 110:64, 1975
Neurilemmoma of facial nerve, intraparotid (Aston, Sparks), PRS, 57:116, 1976. Arch. Surg., 110:757, 1975
Injury of the facial nerve during surgery of the parotid gland (Ward). Brit. J. Surg., 62:401, 1975
Pericardial effusion secondary to mucoepidermoid carcinoma of the parotid gland. A report of an unusual case (Becker *et al*). Cancer, 36:1080, 1975
Parotid region, tumors of (Palva *et al*). J. Laryng. & Otol., 89:419, 1975
Parotidectomy, conservative, in infancy and childhood (Scheunemann), PRS, 56:462, 1975. J. Maxillo-facial Surg., 3:37, 1975
Parotid gland, mixed tumors of, conservative surgical treatment (Stea), PRS, 57:258, 1976. J. Maxillo-facial Surg., 3:135, 1975
Parotid biopsy, technique for (Kraaijenhagen). J. Oral Surg., 33:328, 1975
Pleomorphic adenoma of the parotid gland. A review of results of treatment (Haw). J. R. Coll. Surg. Edinb., 20:25, 1975
Unusual lesions of the parotid gland (Katz). J. Surg. Oncol., 7:219, 1975
Free dermis fat transplantation as adjunct in the surgery of the parotid gland (Walter). Laryngol. Rhinol. Otol. (Stuttg.), 54:435, 1975 (German)
Identification of facial nerve at secondary surgery (Janecka). Laryngoscope, 85:896, 1975
Parotid gland tumors in infants and children, management of (Chong *et al*). Mayo Clin. Proc., 50:279, 1975
Papillary cystadenoma lymphomatosum (Warthin's tumor). Analysis of 14 operated cases (Garas *et al*). Minerva Med., 66:1683,

Parotid Neoplasms — Cont.
1975 (Italian)
Synchronous malignant mucoepidermoid tumor of parotid gland and Warthin's tumor in adjacent lymph node (Lumerman *et al*). Oral Surg., 39:953, 1975
Papillary cystadenoma lymphomatosum (Warthin's tumour). Review of 14 operated cases (Garas *et al*). Panminerva Med., 17:78, 1975
Tumors of salivary glands (Richardson *et al*). PRS, 55:131, 1975
Tumor, "benign mixed," of parotid, rare, inexorable, lethal (McDowell) (Editorial). PRS, 55:214, 1975
Tumor, benign teratoid, of parotid (Shadid, Engeron, Glass). PRS, 55:363, 1975
Parotid gland, hemangiomas of, in children (Williams). PRS, 56:29, 1975
Tumor, parotid, rare, inexorable, lethal "benign mixed" (Conley) (Letter to the Editor). PRS, 56:205, 1975
Therapy of parotid gland tumors (Cancura). Wien. Med. Wochenschr., Suppl 31:3, 1975 (German)
Parotidectomy (Smith). Am. J. Nurs., 76:422, 1976
Recurrent benign mixed tumor and the facial nerve (Work *et al*). Arch. Otolaryng., 102:15, 1976
A bump under the ear (Zwaveling). Ned. tijdschr. geneeskd., 120:409, 1976 (Dutch)
Technique for the rapid performance of parotidectomy with minimal risk (Woods *et al*). Surg. Gynec. & Obst., 142:87, 1976

PARRISH, H. M. *et al*: Hospital management of pit viper venenations. Clin. Toxicol., 3:501, 1970
PARRY, C. B.: *Rehabilitation of the Hand.* 3rd edition. Butterworth & Co., Ltd., London and Toronto, 1974
PARRY, C. B.: Problems in rehabilitation of the burnt hand. Hand, 2:140, 1970
PARRY, C. B.: Restoration of hand function. Rehabilitation of the injured hand. Trans. Med. Soc. Lond., 90:101, 1974
PARRY, C. B. *et al*: New types of lively splints for peripheral nerve lesions affecting the hand. Hand, 2:31, 1970
PARRY, C. B. W.: Management of injuries of brachial plexus, PRS, 55:719, 1975. Proc. Roy. Soc. Med., 67:488, 1974
PARRY, R. G.: Laryngeal chondroplasty for appearance (with Wolfort). PRS, 56:371, 1975
PARRY, R. G., WOLFORT, F. G., AND COCHRAN, T. C.: Simple method for producing graph or text lecture slides. PRS, 57:751, 1976
PARSONS, R. W.: Heterotopic cervical salivary

gland, case report with sialogram. PRS, *49:*464, 1972

PARSONS, R. W.: Exposure through coronal incision for initial treatment of facial fractures (with Shaw). PRS, *56:*254, 1975

PARSONS, R. W.: Editorial: Military plastic surgery and esthetic surgery. Mil. Med., *141:*117, 1976

PARSONS, R. W. *et al:* An approach to reconstruction of complex lower face injuries. Brit. J. Plast. Surg., *25:*23, 1972

PARSONS, R. W., BECKWITH, M. M., AND THERING, H. R.: Surgical rehabilitation after extensive losses in the lower face from war injuries. PRS, *49:*633, 1972

PARSONS, R. W., BURTON, F. C., AND SHAW, R. C.: Versatile mammaplasty pattern of Wise. PRS, *55:*1, 1975

PARSONS, R. W., AND KNIESER, M. R.: "De-epithelization" of the dermal pedicle in reduction mammaplasty. PRS, *57:*619, 1976

PARTYKA, W. *et al:* Neurilemmomas of the face and oral cavity. Czas. Stomatol., *29:*147, 1976 (Polish)

PARUI, R.: Results of various operations for sacrococcygeal pilonidal disease (with Sood, Green). PRS, *56:*559, 1975

PARULEKAR, S. S.: Open injuries to the neck front. J. Laryng. & Otol., *88:*1195, 1974

PASCUAL-CASTROVIEJO, I.: Aerodysostosis. An. Esp. Pediatr., *7:*342, 1974 (Spanish)

PASHA, N. I.: Experience with mesh grafting. J. Med. Liban., *24:*143, 1971

PASHAYAN, H. *et al:* Nostril asymmetry not a microform of cleft lip. Cleft Palate J., *8:*185, 1971

PASHAYAN, H. *et al:* Bilateral aplasia of the tibia, polydactyly and absent thumb in father and daughter. J. Bone & Joint Surg. (Br.). *53:*495, 1971

PASLIN, D. A.: Psoriasis on scars, PRS, *54:*379, 1974. Arch. Dermat., *108:*665, 1973

PASLIN, D. A.: Effects of biopsy on incidence of metastases in hamsters bearing malignant melanoma. J. Invest. Dermatol., *61:*33, 1973

PASNIKOWSKI, T.: Plastic surgery in cases of defects of pharynx and upper esophagus following laryngectomy and pharyngectomy. Otolaryngol. Pol., *26:*439, 1972 (Polish)

PASNIKOWSKI, T.: Role of plastic surgery in complex treatment of malignant neoplasms of head and neck. Pol. Tyg. Lek., *28:*1743, 1973 (Polish)

PASNIKOWSKI, T. *et al:* Juvenile fibromas. Otolaryngol. Pol., *28:*245, 1974 (Polish)

PASTORIZA, J. *et al:* Cranioplasties of skull dome. Ann. chir. plast., *18:*261, 1973 (French)

PASZENKO, Z. *et al:* Experimental evaluation of

some methods of plastic operations on the common carotid artery. Neurol. Neurochir. Pol., *6:*447, 1972 (Polish)

PATAKY, P. E., GRAHAM, W. P., III, AND MUNGER, B. L.: Terminal neuromas treated with triamcinolone acetonide, PRS, *53:*607, 1974. J. Surg. Res., *14:*36, 1973

PATEL, M. R.: *Flexor digitorum sublimis* transfer for multiple extensor tendon ruptures in rheumatoid arthritis (with Nalebuff). PRS, *52:*530, 1973

PATERSON, H. H. *et al:* Posterior pharyngeal tension pneumatocele. Can. Med. Assoc. J., *111:*243, 1974

PATERSON, W. D.: Pseudosarcoma (atypical fibroxanthoma). Brit. J. Dermatol., *90:*359, 1974

PATEY, D.: Tumors of salivary glands. Brit. Med. J., *4:*492, 1972

PATEY, D.: Radiotherapy and carcinoma of parotid. Brit. Med. J., *1:*236, 1973

PATHAK, I. C. *et al:* Anterior abdominal wall defects. Indian. Pediatr., *11:*781, 1974

PATKIN, M. *et al:* Gelfoam dressing for donor sites. M. J. Australia, *2:*750, 1973

PATMAN, R. D., AND THOMPSON, J. E.: Fasciotomy in peripheral vascular surgery, PRS, *49:*359, 1972. Arch. Surg., *101:*663, 1970

PATSON, M. C., GIBBERD, F. B., AND WILSON, R. S. E.: Salivary symptoms in Parkinson's disease, PRS, *53:*365, 1974. Arch. Neurol., *29:*274, 1973

PATTBERG, B.: Report on congenital cutis verticis gyrata (fibroepithelioma) in two infants. Klin. Paediatr., *185:*495, 1973 (German)

PATTERSON, C. N.: Surgery of anatomically weak and aging nose. N. C. Med. J., *33:*692, 1972

PATTERSON, C. N. *et al:* Facial analysis in patient evaluation for physiologic and cosmetic surgery. Laryngoscope, *84:*1004, 1974

PATTERSON, R. P. *et al:* Proportionally controlled externally powered hand splint. Arch. Phys. Med. Rehabil., *52:*434, 1971

PATTERSON, T. J. S.: "Mr. Lucas" and the "B. L." letter (Letter to the Editor). PRS, *48:*68, 1971

PATTERSON, T. J. S., BERRY, R. J., AND WIERNIK, G.: The effect of X-radiation on survival of skin flaps in pig, PRS, *52:*216, 1973. Brit. J. Plast. Surg., *25:*17, 1972

PAUL, U.: Paralysis of accessory nerve after minor surgery on the triangle of neck side. Zentralbl. Chir., *95:*1298, 1970 (German)

PAULSHICK, B. Z.: Letter: Breast reconstruction. Am. Fam. Physician, *12:*30, 1975

PAVEK, V.: Foreign objects in the lip. Cesk. Stomatol., *72:*41, 1972 (Czech)

PAVEL, A. *et al*: Prophylactic antibiotics in clean orthopedic surgery, PRS, *55:*388, 1975. J. Bone & Joint Surg., *56A:*777, 1974

PAVKOVA, L. *et al*: Problem of infection in patients with burns, PRS, *54:*623, 1974. Rozhl. chir., *53:*195, 1974

PAVLIN, E. G. *et al*: Difficulty in removal of tracheostomy tubes. Anesthesiology, *44:*69, 1976

PAVLOV, B. L.: Surface osteosynthesis in osteoplasty of the mandible. Stomatologiia (Mosk.), *50:*86, 1971 (Russian)

PAVLOV, B. L.: Delayed results of osteoplasty of the mandible. Vestn. Khir., *107:*86, 1971 (Russian)

PAVLOV, B. L.: Classification of mandibular defects. Stomatologiia (Mosk.), *53:*43, 1974 (Russian)

PAVLOVSKII, V. M.: Post-traumatic nasal hemorrhage requiring unilateral ligation of external and internal carotid arteries. Zh. Ushn. Nos. Gorl. Bolezn., *2:*105, 1974 (Russian)

PAVLOVSKY, P.: Occurrence and development of psychopathologic phenomena in burned persons and their relation to severity of burns, age, and premorbid personality, PRS, *52:*327, 1973. Acta chir. plast., *4:*112, 1972

PAXTON, B. R., DAVIDORF, F. H., AND MAKLEY, T. A., JR.: Carcinoma of lacrimal canaliculi and lacrimal sac, PRS, *48:*293, 1971. Arch. Ophth., *84:*749, 1970

PAZAT, P. *et al*: Swelling of the parotid region, its surgical treatment. Report of 56 cases. Rev. Stomatol. Chir. Maxillofac., *72:*725, 1971 (French)

PEACOCK, E., JR.: Biologic frontiers in control of healing, PRS, *54:*114, 1974. Am. J. Surg., *126:*708, 1973

PEACOCK, E. E.: Full-time plastic surgical research, and sour grapes (Letter to the Editor). PRS, *51:*440, 1973

PEACOCK, E. E., JR.: Influence of modern connective tissue biology upon surgery of the hand. Surg. Annu., *3:*249, 1971

PEACOCK, E. E., JR.: Biological basis for management of benign disease of the breast; case against subcutaneous mastectomy, PRS, *55:*14, 1975. Discussion by Watson, PRS, *55:*225, 1975

PEACOCK, E. E., JR., MADDEN, J. W., AND TRIER, W. C.: Biologic basis for the treatment of keloids and hypertrophic scars, PRS, *51:*709, 1973. South. M. J., *63:*755, 1970

PEACOCK, E. E., JR., MADDEN, J. W., AND TRIER, W. C.: Postoperative recovery of flexor tendon function, PRS, *50:*538, 1972. Am. J. Surg., *122:*686, 1971

PEACOCK, ERLE E., AND VAN WINKLE, WALTON, JR.: *Surgery and Biology of Wound Repair*. W. B. Saunders Co., Philadelphia, 1970. PRS, *48:*371, 1971

PEARL, R. M., AND KAPLAN, E. N.: Cephalometric study of facial growth in children after combined pushback and pharyngeal flap operations. PRS, *57:*480, 1976

PEARLMAN, A. W. *et al*: Carcinoma of maxillary antrum: role of preoperative irradiation. Laryngoscope, *84:*400, 1974

PEARLMAN, B. A.: An oral contraceptive drug and gingival enlargement; the relationship between local and systemic factors. J. Clin. Periodontol., *1:*47, 1974

PEARLMAN, C. K.: Reconstruction following iatrogenic burn of the penis. J. Pediatr. Surg., *11:*121, 1976

PEARMAN, R. O.: Insertion of Silastic penile prosthesis for treatment of organic sexual impotence, PRS, *50:*632, 1972. J. Urol., *107:*802, 1972

PEARN, J. H.: Survival after snake-bite with prolonged neurotoxic envenomation. M. J. Australia, *2:*259, 1971

PEARSON, B. W.: Epistaxis, PRS, *57:*257, 1976. Postgrad. Med., *57:*116, 1975

PEARSON, B. W. *et al*: S.M.R., septoplasty, and surgical relief of nasal obstruction. Can. J. Otolaryngol., *2:*238, 1973

PEARSON, D.: Radiotherapy in malignant melanoma. Proc. Roy. Soc. Med., *67:*96, 1974

PEARSON, F. G. *et al*: Detection and management of tracheal stenosis following cuffed tube tracheostomy. Ann. Thorac. Surg., *12:*359, 1971

PEARSON, F. G. *et al*: Adenoid cystic carcinoma of trachea. Experience with 16 patients managed by tracheal resection. Ann. Thorac. Surg., *18:*16, 1974

PEASE, G. L. *et al*: Surgical management of osteogenic sarcoma of the mandible. Arch. Otolaryng., *101:*761, 1975

PECH, A. CANNONI, M., AND LISBONNIS, J. M.: Technic of conservative cervical lymphadenectomy. Ann. chir. plast., *18:*37, 1973 (French)

PECH, A. *et al*: Combination of two products with antidepressive and tranquilizing actions. Their interest in an O.R.L. and facial surgery department. J. Fr. Otorhinolaryngol., *23:*267, 1974 (French)

PECHATNIKOVA, E. A. *et al*: Medical disability evaluation of patients with thermal burns. Khirurgiia (Mosk.), *48:*46, 1972 (Russian)

PECK, D., AND LOWMAN, R. M.: Mammography appraisal, PRS, *54:*373, 1974. Conn. Med., *38:*103, 1974

PECK, G. C.: Discussion of "Tripod resection for 'Pinocchio' nose deformity," by Fredricks. PRS, *53:*674, 1974

Pectoralis Muscle, Absence of (See also *Syndactylism)*

Congenital absence of *pectoralis* muscle (Ramirez, Marti), PRS, *53:*604, 1974. An. med. y cir., *53:*293, 1973

Syndrome, Poland's (Glicenstein, Pennecot, Duhamel), PRS, *54:*630, 1974. Ann. chir. plast., *19:*41, 1974

Syndrome, Poland's (Martinez Sahuquillo, Morales Lupianes), PRS, *54:*630, 1974. Rev. españ. cir. plast., *7:*1, 1974

PEDERSEN, B.: Moistening of the inspired air in nasally intubated and tracheostomy patients. Ugeskr. Laeger, *136:*2238, 1974 (Danish)

PEDERSEN, G. W.: Horizontal osteotomy for correction of maxillary retrusion: report of case. J. Oral Surg., *30:*581, 1972

PEDERSEN, G. W.: Central giant-cell lesion of maxilla: enucleation and immediate reconstruction. Oral Surg., *36:*790, 1973

PEDERSON, G. W., AND BLATTO, D. M.: Total maxillary osteotomy for cleft palate rehabilitation, PRS, *57:*121, 1976. Oral Surg., *39:*669, 1975

PEDERSEN, G. W. *et al:* Correction of mandibular dentoalveolar retrusion by anterior segmental advancement. Oral Surg., *41:*281, 1976

PEDERSEN, K. N. *et al:* Oral tumors with localization at the openings of the major salivary glands. Nor. Tannlaegeforen Tid., *85:*7, 1975 (Norwegian)

PEER, G. *et al:* Use of Gosset's operation on the spastic hand. Beitr. Orthop. Traumatol., *18:*74, 1971 (German)

PEER, L. A.: Does growth occur in young rabbit ear cartilage grafts transplanted in young rabbits? (Follow-Up Clinic). PRS, *49:*208, 1972

PEGG, S. P.: Adult burns. A three-year survey with assessment of sulfamylon. M. J. Australia, *1:*350, 1972

PEICHOCKI, M. *et al:* Analysis of 3046 cases of maxillofacial fractures treated at Department of Dental Surgery, Institute of Stomatology in Gdansk in years 1946–1971. Czas. Stomatol., *26:*997, 1973 (Polish)

PEIKO, M. A.: Primary closure of cleft palate using palatal mucosal flap: attempt to prevent growth impairment, PRS, *54:*622, 1974. J. Maxillo-facial Surg., *2:*40, 1974

PEKING ANESTHESIA COORDINATING GROUP: Clinical application of ketamine anesthesia,

PRS, *55:*646, 1975. Chinese M. J., *7:*121, 1974

PEKING CHISCHUEITAN HOSPITAL: Replantation of severed limbs – analysis of 40 cases, PRS, *55:*254, 1975. Chinese M. J., *6:*67, 1973

PEKING HOSPITAL OF WORKERS: Microcirculatory disturbances in septic shock – clinical analyses of 263 cases, PRS, *57:*763, 1976. Chinese M. J., *1:*174, 1975

PELED, I., KAPLAN, I., AND STEPHENSON, M.: Surgical uses of carbon dioxide laser, PRS, *57:*123, 1976. Folha Med., Brazil, *70:*5, 1975

PELERIN, J.: Embryonal remnant with parotid symptomatology. Rev. Laryngol. Otol. Rhinol. (Bord.), *92:*851, 1971 (French)

PELFRENE, A. F.: Letter: Malignant melanoma during treatment with levodopa. Nouv. Presse Med., *4:*1365, 1975 (French)

PELLERIN, D. *et al:* Ureterocolonic implantation in the treatment of bladder exstrophy: 42 cases out of 68 bladder exstrophies from 1945 to 1969. Ann. Chir. Infant., *12:*400, 1971 (French)

PELLERIN, D. *et al:* Transintestinal cutaneous ureterostomy for bladder exstrophy: 17 cases of which 13 use an ileal intraperitoneal loop and 4 a sigmoid loop. Ann. Chir. Infant., *12:*447, 1971 (French)

PELZER, R. H.: Reconstruction of female escutcheon in exstrophy of bladder (with Ship). PRS, *49:*643, 1972

PEMBERTON, L. B.: Comprehensive view of tracheostomy. Am. Surg., *38:*251, 1972

PENA, A. *et al:* Oral neoplastic lesions and their prevention. Rev. Port. Estomatol. Chir. Maxilofac., *14:*5, 1973 (Portuguese)

PENA, C. A., AND GRUART, J. F.: External parotid fistulae by section of Stensen's duct, PRS, *51:*702, 1973. Orientacion Med. Argent., *21:*844, 1972

PENDERGRAST, W. J., JR.: Marjolin's ulcer: an immunologically privileged tumor? (with Bostwick, Vasconez). PRS, *57:*66, 1976

PENDERGRAST, W. J., JR. *et al:* Regional lymphadenectomy and tumor immunity. Surg. Gynec. & Obst., *142:*385, 1976

PENEV, P. D.: Various problems in the treatment of odontogenic cysts. Cesk. Stomatol., *74:*153, 1974 (Czechoslovakian)

PENHA, R., AND RIBEIRO, V.: Velum palatinum mixed tumor, report of a case, PRS, *57:*671, 1976. Med. Universal, *18:*8, 1975

PENHOLZ, H.: Treatment of peripheral nerve injuries with homologous nerve grafts, PRS, *53:*250, 1974. Langenbecks Arch. Chir., *333:*1, 1973

PENICHE, J.: Metastasis of carcinoma of pancreas to skin, PRS, *49:*108, 1972. Dermat. Rev. Mexicana, *431:*14, 1970

PENICHE, J., AND ALBORES, J.: Topical chemotherapy of skin tumors with 5-FU, PRS, *48*:92, 1971. Dermat. Rev. Mexicana, *14*:189, 1970

Penis (See also *Epispadias; Hypospadias; Transsexualism; Urethra*)

Balanitis xerotica obliterans (Rheinschild, Olsen), PRS, *48*:295, 1971. J. Urol., *104*:860, 1970

Penis, basal cell carcinoma of (Fegen, Beebe, Persky), PRS, *49*:235, 1972. J. Urol., *104*:864, 1970

Penis, hemangio-endothelial sarcoma of: report of case and review of literature (Hodgins, Hancock), PRS, *49*:235, 1972. J. Urol., *104*:867, 1970

Incomplete testicular feminization (Blizzard). Birth Defects, 7:310, 1971

Rapid method for constructing a functional sensitive penis (Kaplan). Brit. J. Plast. Surg., *24*:342, 1971

Procedure for lengthening the phallus in boys with exstrophy of the bladder (Kelley *et al*). J. Pediatr. Surg., *6*:645, 1971

Penis and scrotum, transposition in twin brothers (Datta *et al*), PRS, *48*:607, 1971. J. Urol., *105*:739, 1971

Microphallus, surgical management (Hinman), PRS, *49*:585, 1972. J. Urol., *105*:901, 1971

Prepubertal phallus, local application of testosterone cream to (Immergut *et al*), PRS, *49*:585, 1972. J. Urol., *105*:905, 1971

Penile urethra, recurrent fistula of (Malament), PRS, *50*:200, 1972. J. Urol., *106*:704, 1971

Fractures of penis: rationale of surgical treatment (Gross, Arnold, Waterhouse), PRS, *50*:95, 1972. J. Urol., *106*:708, 1971

Corpora cavernosa, iatrogenic dislocation of (Kish, Srivastova), PRS, *50*:200, 1972. J. Urol., *106*:711, 1971

Glans penis, successful replantation of traumatically amputated (Tuerk, Weir). PRS, *48*:499, 1971

Penis and scrotum, avulsion of skin (Sanchez Galindo, Almendral), PRS, *48*:608, 1971. Rev. españ. cir. plast., *4*:27, 1971

Remote results of alloplasty of the penis in impotence (Vainberg *et al*). Urol. Nefrol. (Mosk.), *36*:44, 1971 (Russian)

Free dermatoplasty in lacerated wounds of the skin of the genital organs (Stepakov *et al*). Urol. Nefrol. (Mosk.), *36*:60, 1971 (Russian)

Plastic surgery in traumatic amputation of the penis (Pozdniakova). Vestn. Khir., *107*:59, 1971 (Russian)

Penis and scrotum, traumatic scalpation,

Penis – Cont.

late sequelae (Kipikasa *et al*), PRS, *52*:680, 1973. Acta chir. plast., *14*:255, 1972

Priapism: treatment by corpus cavernosum-saphenous vein anastomosis (Lee *et al*). Ann. Surg., *175*:279, 1972

Penis, new method of total reconstruction (Orticochea). Brit. J. Plast. Surg., *25*:347, 1972

Circumcision, complications of (Gallagher). Brit. J. Urol., *44*:720, 1972

Penis, keratoacanthoma, unusual case report (Brown, Leuy), PRS, *52*:327, 1973. Cutis, *8*:585, 1972

Impotence, implantable fluid transfer system for treatment of (Kothari *et al*). J. Biomech., *5*:567, 1972

Penis, congenital absence of (Farah, Reno), PRS, *50*:539, 1972. J. Urol., *107*:154, 1972

Penis, surgical management of squamous cell carcinoma of (Skinner, Leadbetter, Kelley), PRS, *50*:542, 1972. J. Urol., *107*:273, 1972

Penis, webbed, without chordee (Perlmutter, Chamberlain), PRS, *50*:632, 1972. J. Urol., *107*:320, 1972

Peyronie's disease (Poutasse), PRS, *51*:604, 1973. J. Urol., *107*:419, 1972

Priapism, atypical case with unusual sequelae (Rheinschild *et al*), PRS, *51*:604, 1973. J. Urol., *107*:423, 1972

Microphallus, characteristics and choice of treatment (Hinman), PRS, *51*:604, 1973. J. Urol., *107*:499, 1972

Silastic penile prosthesis, insertion for organic sexual impotence (Pearman), PRS, *50*:632, 1972. J. Urol., *107*:802, 1972

Cavernospongiosum shunt in treatment of priapism (Sacher *et al*), PRS, *51*:233, 1973. J. Urol., *108*:97, 1972

Spongiocavernosum shunt in surgical treatment of idiopathic persistent priapism (Falk, Loos), PRS, *51*:233, 1973. J. Urol., *108*:101, 1972

Heparin induced priapism and surgical treatment (Klein, Hall, Smith), PRS, *51*:233, 1973. J. Urol., *108*:104, 1972

Diphallia: report of case (Aleem), PRS, *51*:232, 1973. J. Urol., *108*:357, 1972

Carcinoma of penis, analysis of therapy in 100 consecutive cases (Hardner *et al*), PRS, *51*:349, 1973. J. Urol., *108*:428, 1972

Penile gangrene, accidental (Markland, Merrill), PRS, *51*:348, 1973. J. Urol., *108*:494, 1972

Penile agenesis (Soderdahl, Brosman, Goodwin), PRS, *51*:348, 1973. J. Urol., *108*:496, 1972

Microphallus, surgical treatment for (Har-

Penis—Cont.

Isolated lesions of penis in children (Blanco Lopez *et al*). An. Esp. Peadiatr., 7:319, 1974 (Spanish)

Erythroplasia of Queyrat treated with topically administered fluorouracil (Goete), PRS, *56*:680, 1975. Arch. Dermat., *110*:271, 1974

Incomplete urethral duplication and urinary retention (Fellows *et al*). Brit. J. Urol., *46*:449, 1974

Rare combination of duplication of genitourinary tract, hindgut, vertebral column and other associated anomalies (Dutta *et al*). Brit. J. Urol., *46*:577, 1974

Lengthening of the congenital or acquired short penis (Johnston). Brit. J. Urol., *46*:685, 1974

Femoro-pudendal by-pass, internal iliac thromboendarterectomy and direct arterial anastomosis to the cavernous body in the treatment of erectile impotence (Michal *et al*). Bull. Soc. Int. Chir., *33*:343, 1974

Developmental defects of the prepuce (Svab *et al*). Cas. Lek. Cesk., *113*:298, 1974 (Czech)

Surgical construction of the male external genitalia (Engel). Clin. Plast. Surg., *1*:229, 1974

Long-term psychologic follow-up of intersexed patients (Money). Clin. Plast. Surg., *1*:271, 1974

Surgical treatment of impotence (Tudoriu). Helv. Chir. Acta, *41*:451, 1974 (German)

Penis, neural and vascular development (Dail, Evan), PRS, *55*:250, 1975. Invest. Urol., *11*:427, 1974

Priapism as a surgical emergency (Kondo *et al*). Jap. J. Urol., *65*:189, 1974 (Japanese)

Penis and scrotum, chronic lymphedema of (Keeler *et al*). J. Med. Soc. N. J., *71*:575, 1974

Impotence, surgical treatment with penile prosthesis and psychiatric evaluation (Gee *et al*), PRS, *54*:505, 1974. J. Urol., *111*:41, 1974

Peyronie's disease, surgical treatment with dermal graft (Devine, Horton), PRS, *54*:504, 1974. J. Urol., *111*:44, 1974

Penis, melanoma of (Bracken, Diokno), PRS, *54*:621, 1974. J. Urol., *111*:198, 1974

Penis: repair of genital defects associated with persistent cloaca (Ambrose), PRS, *54*:504, 1974. J. Urol., *111*:256, 1974

Penis, webbed (Mashih *et al*). J. Urol., *111*:690, 1974

Erythroplasia of Queyrat (Rege, Evans), PRS, *57*:536, 1976. J. Urol., *111*:784, 1974

Congenital curvature of the penis (Gavrell).

Penis—Cont.

J. Urol., *112*:489, 1974

Penis, congenital curvature of (Pond, Brannan), PRS, *57*:536, 1976. J. Urol., *112*:491, 1974

Comparison between cavernosaphenous and cavernospongiosum shunting in the treatment of idiopathic priapism: a report of 5 operations (Dahl *et al*). J. Urol., *112*:614, 1974

Penis, recurrent flail, unusual complication of penile prosthesis (Jacobs, McCullough), PRS, *57*:536, 1976. J. Urol., *112*:768, 1974

Surgery of male impotence; intracavernous prosthesis of the penis (Subrini *et al*). J. Urol. Nephrol. (Paris), *80*:269, 1974 (French)

Penis for female-to-male transsexual, surgical construction (Noe, Birdsell, Laub). PRS, *53*:511, 1974

Scrotal flap for necrosis of penis with decubitus ulcer (Lanier, Neale). PRS, *54*:609, 1974

Priapism, new operation for (Ebbehoj), PRS, *56*:357, 1975. Scand. J. Plast. Reconstr. Surg., *8*:241, 1974

Failure of chemotherapy in treatment of giant condyloma acuminata (Buschke-Loewenstein tumor) (Redman *et al*). South. Med. J., *67*:742, 1974

Penile and scrotal skin, avulsion of (Thomsen *et al*). Ugeskr. Laeger, *136*:255, 1974 (Danish)

Lipogranulomatosis of external genitalia (Engelman *et al*). Urology, *3*:358, 1974

Penile implant, Pearson, fracture (Albert *et al*). Urology, *3*:502, 1974

Penis, seborrheic keratosis of (Cheng). Urology, *3*:595, 1974

Preputial skin-bridging. Complication of circumcision (Klauber *et al*). Urology, *3*:722, 1974

Male urinary incontinence. Correction with ischiocavernous muscles collaring method (Chen). Urology, *4*:348, 1974

Injection technique to induce penile erection (Gittes *et al*). Urology, *4*:473, 1974

High bilateral funiculo-orchiectomy: secondary to avulsion injury (McGinnis *et al*). Urology, *4*:596, 1974

Duplication of penis (Johnson *et al*). Urology, *4*:722, 1974

Subcutaneous splinting of the penis with two lateral polyethylene prostheses as a method of treatment of impotence (Krasulin *et al*). Urol. Nefrol. (Mosk.), *39*:42, 1974 (Russian)

Complications in phallo- and urethroplasty (Mendel'). Vestn. Khir., *113*:124, 1974

Penis – Cont.

(Russian)

Penis, exceptionally large epidermoid cyst of, in newborn (Rupp, Knothe), PRS, *55:*250, 1975. Ztschr. Kinderchir., *15:*236, 1974

Rupture of the corpus cavernosum of the penis (Hudson). Brit. J. Clin. Pract., *29:*191, 1975

Peyronie's disease (Chesney), PRS, *57:*262, 1976. Brit. J. Urol., *47:*209, 1975

Peyronie's disease treated with procarbazine (Oosterlinck, Renders), PRS, *57:*120, 1976. Brit. J. Urol., *47:*219, 1975

Leiomyosarcoma of penis (Hamal), PRS, *57:*120, 1976. Brit. J. Urol., *47:*319, 1975

Peyronie's disease, epitheloid sarcoma masquerading as (Moore *et al*). Cancer, *35:*1706, 1975

Anomalies of penis, congenital and acquired (Lopez-Engelking), PRS, *55:*638, 1975. Cir. Cir., *42:*169, 1975

Reconstruction of the penoscrotal skin after avulsion (Sangmit). Int. Surg., *60:*563, 1975

Three cases of congenital torsion of the penis (Sugiura *et al*). Jpn. J. Urol., *66:*160, 1975 (Japanese)

Treatment of organic erectile impotence. Experience with the Scott procedure (Ambrose). J. Med. Soc. N. J., *72:*805, 1975

Diphallus, probable, with complete duplication of urethra (Redman, Bissada), PRS, *56:*230, 1975. J. Pediat. Surg., *10:*135, 1975

Chordee corrected by dermal graft (Devine, Horton), PRS, *57:*675, 1976. J. Urol., *113:*56, 1975

Penile and scrotal lymphedema, surgical management of (Vaught, Litvok, McRoberts), PRS, *57:*761, 1976. J. Urol., *113:*204, 1975

Scrotal skin recession phalloplasty (Malkin *et al*). J. Urol., *113:*343, 1975

Congenital micropenile skin sleeve (Shiraki *et al*). J. Urol., *114:*469, 1975

External shunt in the treatment of idiopathic priapism (Cate *et al*). J. Urol., *114:*726, 1975

Balanitis xerotica obliterans in children (McKay *et al*). J. Urol., *114:*773, 1975

Four cases of peno-scrotal avulsions (Michaud *et al*). J. Urol. Nephrol. (Paris), *81:*558, 1975 (French)

Skin replacement on the penis (Anderl). Langenbecks Arch. Chir., *339:*433, 1975 (German)

Penis, secondary closures of skin incisions of (Horton, Devine). PRS, *55:*630, 1975

Four V-flap repair of preputial stenosis, al-

Penis – Cont.

ternative to circumcision (Emmett). PRS, *55:*687, 1975

Transposition of scrotum and penis, congenital (Griffin, Hayes). PRS, *55:*710, 1975

Cavernospongiosum shunt in the treatment of priapism (Srougi *et al*). Rev. Hosp. Clin. Fac. Med. Sao Paulo, *30:*397, 1975 (Portuguese)

Priapism – pathogenesis and therapy (Tscholl). Schweiz. Med. Wochenschr., *105:*517, 1975 (German)

Injuries to the skin of the male external genitalia in Southern Africa (Malherbe). S. Afr. Med. J., *49:*147, 1975

Reconstruction of the male external genitalia (Boxer). Surg. Gynec. & Obst., *141:*939, 1975

Implantable penile prostheses in impotent males (Bias *et al*). Urology, *5:*224, 1975

Penile prosthesis, Small-Carrion. New implant for management of impotence (Small *et al*). Urology, *5:*479, 1975

Penis, lateral curvature, surgical correction of (Redman *et al*). Urology, *5:*508, 1975

Penile dressing, ideal (Chiu *et al*). Urology, *5:*670, 1975

Reanastomosis of completely transected penis in canine. Review of current concepts (Raney *et al*). Urology, *6:*735, 1975

Operative treatment of male pseudohermaphroditism (Carl *et al*). Urologe (A.), *14:*178, 1975 (German)

Penile prosthesis, silicone, to treat organic impotence (Shishito, Shirai, Matsuda), PRS, *56:*466, 1975. Urol. int., *30:*211, 1975

Sapheno-cavernous anastomosis as a method of treatment of priapism (Nikol'skii *et al*). Urol. Nefrol. (Mosk.), *1:*58, 1975 (Russian)

Reconstruction following iatrogenic burn of the penis (Pearlman). J. Pediatr. Surg., *11:*121, 1976

Penis, congenital urethral fistula (Olbourne). PRS, *57:*237, 1976

Penis, silicone granuloma of (Lighterman). PRS, *57:*517, 1976

Penis and scrotum, syphilitic elephantiasis of (Elsahy). PRS, *57:*601, 1976

PENKAVA, J.: Correction of nasal saddle deformity using lateral part of tip cartilage, PRS, *50:*94, 1972. Acta chir. plast., *13:*25, 1971

PENKAVA, J.: Complicated reconstruction after mutilating operation of lip and bilateral cleft of primary and secondary palate, PRS, *54:*623, 1974. Acta chir. plast., *16:*8, 1974

PENKAVA, J.: Median cleft of upper lip and jaw,

PRS, *56:*358, 1975. Acta chir. plast., *16:*201, 1974

PENKAVA, J.: Middle cleft of upper lip and jaw, PRS, *54:*506, 1974. Cesk. Stomatol., *2:*142, 1974

PENKAVA, J. *et al:* Oblique facial clefts. Cesk. Stomatol., *74:*277, 1974

PENN, I.: Immunosuppression and cancer. Importance in head and neck surgery. Arch. Otolaryng., *101:*667, 1975

PENN, I. *et al:* De novo malignant tumors in organ transplant recipients. Transplant Proc., *3:*773, 1971

PENN, I., AND STARZL, T. E.: Malignant tumors arising *de novo* in immunosuppressed organ transplant recipients, PRS, *51:*483, 1973. Transplantation, *14:*407, 1972

PENN, JACK: *The Right to Look Human.* McGraw-Hill Book Co., Johannesburg, New York, 1974. PRS, *56:*664, 1975

PENN, J.: Kiel-bone implants to chin and nose (Follow-Up Clinic). PRS, *52:*432, 1973

PENN, J. G.: Zigzag pectoro-subaxillary flap (with Penn). PRS, *51:*27, 1973

PENNEC, J.: Current treatment of leprosy in the Malta pavilion of the Hopital Saint-Louis. Ann. Med. Interne (Paris), *125:*561, 1974 (French)

PENNISI, V. R. *et al:* Facial burns. Med. Trial Tech. Q., *18:*361, 1972

PENNISI, V. R., AND CAPOZZI, A.: Transposition of fat in cervicofacial rhytidectomy. PRS, *49:*423, 1972

PENNISI, V. R. *et al:* Marlex 50 as replacement for mandibular condyle (Follow-Up Clinic). PRS, *49:*565, 1972

PENNISI, V. R., CAPOZZI, A., AND FRIEDMAN, G.: Travase, effective enzyme for burn debridement. PRS, *51:*371, 1973

PENNISI, V. R., AND CAPOZZI, A.: Treatment of chronic cystic disease of breast by subcutaneous mastectomy. PRS, *52:*520, 1973

PENNISI, V. R., AND CAPOZZI, A.: Incidence of carcinoma in subcutaneous mastectomy, PRS, *56:*9, 1975. Discussion by Snyderman, PRS, *56:*208, 1975

PENOFF, J. H.: Screw syringe for injecting steroids into scars. PRS, *53:*484, 1974

PENROD, D. S.: Use of complete transverse nasal flap in repair of small defects of the nose (with Lipshutz). PRS, *49:*629, 1972

PEPERSACK, W.: Tooth vitality following mobilization of the alveolar process. Fortschr. Kiefer. Gesichtschir., *18:*280, 1974 (German)

PEPERSACK, W.: Remote results of the correction of mandibular protrusion by sagittal osteotomy of the mandibular rami. Rev. Stomatol. Chir. Maxillofac., *75:*142, 1974 (French)

PEPERSACK, W. J.: Tooth vitality after alveolar segmental osteotomy, PRS, *53:*251, 1974. J. Maxillo-facial Surg., *1:*85, 1973

PERA ERRO, E.: Grafting palmar areas of hand with plantar skin of feet, PRS, *53:*248, 1974. Rev. españ. cir. plast., *5:*175, 1972

PERCY, E. C.: Tendon lacerations of the hands. Can. Med. Assoc. J., *105:*635, 1971

PERCZYNSKA-PARTYKA, W.: Modern views on treatment of clefts of upper lip, alveolar process and palate. Czas. Stomatol., *26:*547, 1973 (Polish)

PERDIKIS, P.: Lid-load operation in facial palsy. S. Afr. J. Surg., *11:*197, 1973

PEREIRA, L. G.: Glossectomy in mandibular prognathism. Rev. Asoc. Paul. Cir. Dent., *27:*349, 1973 (Portuguese)

PEREIRA, L. G. *et al:* Anomalies of maxillofacial region. Incisivo, *2:*14, 1973 (Portuguese)

PEREIRA, L. G. *et al:* Plastic surgery for maxillary prognathism. Incisivo, *2:*18, 1973 (Portuguese)

PEREZ, C. A. *et al:* Regional lymphadenectomy and tumor curability. Experimental observations in a murine lymphosarcoma. Am. J. Roentgenol. Radium Ther. Nucl. Med., *123:*621, 1975

PEREZ, L. *et al:* Surgical treatment of funnel chest and of pigeon breast in children. Bol. Med. Hosp. Infant Mex., *31:*1171, 1974 (Spanish)

PEREZ FERNANDEZ, A.: Syndrome of dysfunction of temporomandibular joint, PRS, *53:*242, 1974. Rev. españ. cir. plast., *4:*13, 1971

PEREZ FERNANDEZ, A., AND QUETGLAS, J.: Oro-digito-facial syndrome, PRS, *53:*116, 1974. Rev. españ. cir. plast., *5:*153, 1972

PERI, G. *et al:* Mandibular external cortex osteosynthesis using intraoral approach. Ann. chir. plast., *17:*184, 1972 (French)

PERI, G. *et al:* Recent injuries of cranio-facial middle third (therapeutic attitudes). Ann. chir. plast., *17:*260, 1972 (French)

PERI, G. *et al:* Problems raised by fistula of low parotid region (originating from first branchial pocket). Ann. chir. plast., *18:*83, 1973 (French)

PERI, G. *et al:* Holes especially for reconstruction of certain segments of facial bones. Ann. chir. plast., *18:*169, 1973 (French)

PERICOTS AYATS, J. AND PERICOT, J. A., JR.: Facial deformity – surgical treatment. Trans. Congr. Int. Assoc. Oral Surg., *4:*345, 1973

PERINETTI, P. W., MANFREDI, A., AND ANCHEL-ERGUEZ, R.: Importance of lymphatic drainage in edema following reimplantation of an amputated limb, PRS, *54:*111, 1974. Bol. y trab. Soc. argent. cir., *34:*465, 1973

Periodontal Cyst (See also *Jaw Cysts; Odontogenic Cysts; Oral Surgery*)

Lateral periodontal cyst: report of a case (Lederman). J. Oral Med., *30:*62, 1975

PERKASH, I.: Intermittent catheterization: urologist's point of view, PRS, *54:*504, 1974. J. Urol., *111:*356, 1974

PERKO, M.: Surgical therapy of jaw deformities caused by cleft lip and cleft palate. Indications and late results. Osterr. Z. Stomatol., *67:*287, 1970 (German)

PERKO, M.: Contribution to problem of velopharyngeal incompetence, PRS, *53:*246, 1974. J. Maxillo-facial Surg., *1:*96, 1973

PERKO, M.: Indications and contraindications for surgical management of temporomandibular joint. Schweiz. Monatsschr. Zahnheilkd., *83:*73, 1973 (German)

PERKO, M.: Behavior of the maxillary sinuses after orthopedic jaw operations. Fortschr. Kiefer. Gesichtschir., *18:*213, 1974 (German)

PERKO, M.: Advantages and disadvantages of various mucosal incisions. Schweiz. Monatsschr. Zahnheilkd., *85:*167, 1975 (German)

PERKO, M. *et al*: Primary treatment of cleft lip and cleft palate. Minerva Stomatol., *20:*193, 1971 (Italian)

PERKO, M. *et al*: Late results of osteosynthesis treatments in juvenile jaw fractures. Fortschr. Kiefer. Gesichtschir., *19:*206, 1975 (German)

PERKO, M. A.: Primary closure of the cleft palate using a palatal mucosal flap: an attempt to prevent growth impairment. J. Maxillofacial Surg., *2:*40, 1974

PERL, T. Z.: Segmental sagittal splitting of the mandible in the surgical treatment of carcinoma of the floor of the mouth. J. Oral Surg., *30:*656, 1972

PERLMAN, G. S. *et al*: Basal cell carcinoma of the eyelids: review of patients treated by surgical excision. Surg. Forum, *26:*540, 1975

PERLMAN, R. *et al*: Histoplasmosis of the common palmar tendon sheath. J. Bone & Joint Surg. (Am.), *54:*676, 1972

PERLMUTTER, A. D., AND CHAMBERLAIN, J. W.: Webbed penis without chordee, PRS, *50:*632, 1972. J. Urol., *107:*320, 1972

PERLMUTTER, A. D. *et al*: Meatal advancement for distal hypospadias without chordee. J. Urol., *113:*850, 1975

PERLMUTTER, S. *et al*: Metastasis to gingiva, PRS, *56:*364, 1975. Oral Surg., *38:*749, 1974

PERMUY RODRIGUEZ, J. *et al*: Facial paralysis

with or without surgical treatment. Pre and postoperative neurophysiological control. Idiopathic facial paralysis. Electrophysiological patterns. Rev. Esp. Otoneurooftalmol. Neurocir., *31:*333, 1973 (Spanish)

PERNA, A. M. *et al*: Fatal respiratory distress syndrome after prolonged mechanical ventilation; its pathogenesis and prevention, PRS, *51:*353, 1973. J. Surg. Res., *11:*584, 1972

PERNET, A., AND PISTELLI, J. L.: Indications and therapy in congenital anomalies of hand, PRS, *50:*538, 1972. Rev. Latino Am. cir. plast., *14:*17, 1970

PERNOT, C. *et al*: Holt-Oram syndrome and hand malformations associated with congenital heart disease. Arch. Mal. Coeur, *63:*1428, 1970 (French)

PERRAS, C., AND PAPILLON, J.: Value of mammography in cosmetic surgery of the breasts, PRS, *52:*132, 1973

PERRIMAN, A. AND UTHMAN, A.: Periostitis ossificans. Brit. J. Oral Surg., *10:*211, 1972

PERRIN, C.: Filling of traumatic notch at base of nose using eyebrow incision. J. Fr. Otorhinolaryngol., *22:*242, 1973 (French)

PERRIN, C. *et al*: Conservative curettage of neck. Practical management. J. Fr. Otorhinolaryngol., *22:*229, 1973 (French)

PERRIN, E. R.: Use of soluble steroids within inflatable breast prostheses. PRS, *57:*163, 1976

PERRY, C. B. W.: *Rehabilitation of the Hand.* 3rd Ed. Butterworth, London, 1974

PERRY, J. F.: Use of a surgical glove in treatment of edema in the hand. Phys. Ther., *54:*498, 1974

PERRY, J. F. *et al*: Protective sensation in hand and its co-relation to Ninhydrin sweat test following nerve laceration, PRS, *55:*248, 1975. Am. J. Phys. Med., *53:*113, 1974

PERRY, J. F. *et al*: Evaluation procedures for patients with hand injuries. Phys. Ther., *54:*593, 1974

PERRY, R. H. *et al*: Nodular fasciitis causing unilateral proptosis. Brit. J. Ophthalmol., *59:*404, 1975

PERS, M.: Operation for correction of snub-nose deformity, PRS, *53:*602, 1974. Scand. J. Plast. Reconstr. Surg., *7:*64, 1973

PERS, M., AND BRETTEVILLE-JENSEN, G.: Reduction mammaplasty based on vertical bipedicle and "tennis ball" assembly, PRS, *51:*103, 1973. Scand. J. Plast. Reconstr. Surg., *6:*61, 1972

PERS, M. *et al*: Pedicle muscle flaps and their applications in the surgery of repair. Brit. J. Plast. Surg., *26:*313, 1973

PERSKY, L. AND OWENS, R.: Genitourinary tract abnormalities in Turner's syndrome (gonadal dysgenesis), PRS, *48:*514, 1971. J. Urol., *105:*309, 1971

PERSON, E. *et al*: Transsexual syndrome in males. II. Secondary transsexualism. Am. J. Psychother., *28:*174, 1974

PERSSON, G.: Remarkable recurrence of keratocyst in bone graft. Int. J. Oral Surg., *2:*69, 1973

PESCATORE, E. A.: Personal reaction to weight loss, PRS, *56:*116, 1975. Am. J. Nursing, *74:*2227, 1975

PESKOVA, H.: In memoriam of Prof. Gustavo Sanvenero-Rosselli. Acta chir. plast. (Praha), *16:*199, 1974

PESKOVA, H.: In memoriam Assistant Professor Teobald Adamczak, M.D. Acta chir. plast. (Praha), *16:*256, 1974

PESKOVA, H.: 70th birthday of Prof. V. Karfik, D.Sc. Cas. Lek. Cesk, *113:*288, 1974 (Czech)

PESKOVA, H.: Seventieth birthday of Prof. Dr. V. Karfik M.D., D.Sc., Rozhl. Chir., *53:*145, 1974 (Czechoslovakian)

PETER, J. P., AND CHINSKY, R. R.: Sociological aspects of cleft palate adults. I. Marriage, PRS, *55:*514, 1975. Cleft Palate J., *11:*295, 1974. II. Education, PRS, *56:*109, 1975. Cleft Palate J., *11:*443, 1974

PETERS, C.: Construction of perineal body in female (with Pickrell, Neale). PRS, *55:*529, 1975

PETERS, C.: Transposition of lips for correction of facial paralysis (with Pickrell, Puckett), PRS, *57:*427, 1976

PETERS, C. R. *et al*: Office and emergency room care of the injured hand. South. Med. J., *69:*53, 1975

PETERS, P. E. *et al*: Current status of endolymphatic therapy with radionuclides. Lymphology, *7:*49, 1974

PETERS, R. A. *et al*: Snowmobile injuries and oral surgeon: survey of snowmobile injuries in central Wisconsin, PRS, *51:*700, 1973. J. Oral Surg., *30:*794, 1972

PETERS, R. A. *et al*: Technique for open reduction of subcondylar fractures. Oral Surg., *41:*273, 1976

PETERSEN, N. C.: Cosmetic surgery. Ugeskr. Laeger, *133:*2441, 1971 (Danish)

PETERSEN, N. C.: Malignant melanoma of the skin. Ugeskr. Laeger, *134:*214, 1972 (Danish)

PETERSEN, N. C.: Unknown lip-flap procedures by Stein, PRS, *54:*499, 1974. Scand. J. Plast. Reconstr. Surg., *7:*82, 1973

PETERSEN, N. C.: Commentary on "Lip repair (cheiloplasty) performed by a new method," by Stein (Classic Reprint). PRS, *53:*332, 1974

PETERSEN, N. C., AND BITTMAN, S.: Epidemiology of pressure sores, PRS, *48:*614, 1971.

Scand. J. Plast. Reconstr. Surg., *5:*62, 1971

PETERSON, A.: Electrosurgical correction of maxillary double lip. Dent. Dig., *78:*182, 1972

PETERSON, H. D.: Treatment of eyelid deformities due to burns (with Silverstein). PRS, *51:*38, 1973

PETERSON, H. D., AND BURT, G. B.: Role of steroids in prevention of circumferential capsular scarring in augmentation mammaplasty. PRS, *54:*28, 1974

PETERSON, L. J.: Immediate surgical closure of multiple maxillary diastemas. J. Oral Surg., *31:*522, 1973

PETERSON, L. J. *et al*: Preoperative interview and psychological evaluation of orthognathic surgery patient. J. Oral Surg., *32:*583, 1974

PETERSON, L. J. *et al*: Psychological considerations in corrective maxillary and midfacial surgery. J. Oral Surg., *34:*157, 1976

PETERSON, S. J.: Electrical stimulation of soft palate, PRS, *55:*382, 1975. Cleft Palate J., *11:*72, 1974

PETERSON, S. J., AND PRUZANSKY, S.: Palatal anomalies in syndromes of Apert and Crouzon, PRS, *56:*109, 1975. Cleft Palate J., *11:*394, 1974

PETIT, P.: Ureterocolonic transplantations. Palliative treatment of bladder exstrophy. Ann. Chir. Infant., *12:*394, 1971 (French)

PETKOV, I., AND ANDREEV, V. C.: Unusual localization of dermatofibrosarcoma protuberans. Hautarzt, *23:*508, 1972 (German)

PETRANYI, G. *et al*: Inhibition of skin allograft rejection by antilymphocytic serum pretreatment of the donor. Immunological preparation of the graft. Acta Med. Acad. Sci. Hung., *28:*155, 1971

PETRES, J.: Experiences with plastic surgery in the therapy of skin neoplasms. Arch. Derm. Forsch., *244:*156, 1972 (German)

PETRES, J.: Plastic surgery following the excision of skin tumors. Hautarzt, *23:*271, 1972

PETRES, J. *et al*: Possibilities of dermatosurgery in neoplasms in the hand region. Fortschr. Med., *92:*1054, 1974 (German)

PETRES, J. *et al*: Surgical therapy of extended skin tumors of the torso. Hautarzt, *25:*566, 1974 (German)

PETRIE, P. W. R., AND LAMB, D. W.: Severe hand problems in drug addicts, PRS, *54:*236, 1974. Hand, *5:*130, 1973

PETRIELLA, V. M. *et al*: Gigantic ameloblastoma of mandible, case report. J. Oral Surg., *32:*44, 1974

PETROLATI, M. *et al*: Immediate treatment of complex injuries of the face. Minerva Chir., *26:*842, 1971 (Italian)

PETROLATI, M., GNUCCI, M. L., AND DELL'ANTONIO, A.: Morphological and functional results of burn scar treatment, PRS, 56:361, 1975. Riv. ital. chir. plast., 5:345, 1973

PETROLATI, M., AND DIARA, A.: Posttraumatic injuries of peripheral nerves, PRS, 57:675, 1976. Riv. ital. chir. plast., 6:185, 1974

PETROV, M. A.: Transplantations of nerves and roots of spinal cord. Reconstr. Surg. Traumatol., 12:250, 1971

PETROV, V. I.: Diagnosis and treatment of skin cancer from ulcers and osteomyelitic fistulas. Vopr. Onkol., 18:72, 1972 (Russian)

PETROV, V. I. et al: Osteosynthesis of fragments of the mandible by homologous grafting of sections and ultrasonic coagulation. Stomatologiia (Mosk.), 54:29, 1975 (Russian)

PETROVIC, S.: Our experience with secondary osteoplasty in the treatment of cleft palate. Dtsch. Zahn. Mund. Kieferheilkd., 57:230, 1971 (German)

PETROVIC, S.: Surgical therapy of irreparable paresis of facial nerve. Combination of static and dynamic hinges. Cesk. stomatol., 72:410, 1972 (Slovakian)

PETROVIC, S.: Surgical treatment of vertically open bite, PRS, 53:682, 1974. Acta chir. plast., 15:39, 1973

PETROVIC, S.: Treatment of mandibular prognathism. Triple osteotomy of body of mandible. Cesk. Stomatol., 73:107, 1973 (Slovakian)

PETROVIC, S.: Surgical arrangement of deformations of facial region. Mobilization of facial bones. Cesk. Stomatol., 73:232, 1973 (Slovakian)

PETROVIC, S.: Reconstruction of the defect of alveolar process of the maxilla using bone graft as a pre-prosthetic arrangement in adult patients with cleft palate. Cesk. Stomatol., 75:131, 1975 (Slovakian)

PETROVIC, S. et al: Surgical treatment of anomalies of prognathic character. Cesk. Stomatol., 71:294, 1971 (Czechoslovakian)

PETROVIC, S. et al: Traumatic aneurysm of the radial artery in a 10-year-old child. Med. Pregl., 24:517, 1971 (Serbian)

PETROVSKII, B. V.: Organization and prospects for the development of the surgical service in the USSR; a report to the 29th All-Union Congress of Surgeons. Khirurgiia (Mosk.), 10:3, 1974 (Russian)

PETTAVEL, J.: Place of surgery in treatment of malignant melanoma. Schweiz. Med. Wochenschr., 103:1424, 1973 (French)

PETTAVEL, J. et al: Treatment of advanced or recurrent malignant melanoma. Schweiz. Med. Wochenschr., 100:988, 1970 (French)

PETTY, C. T., THEOGARAJ, S. D., AND COHEN, I.

K.: Secondary reconstruction of cervical esophagus, PRS, 56:70, 1975

PETZ, R.: Complex fractures of zygoma and mandibular ramus. Dtsch. Stomatol., 21:619, 1971 (German)

PETZ, R.: New method of fixation in mandibular fractures. Dtsch. Stomatol., 21:653, 1971 (German)

PETZ, R.: Evaluation of surgery of fractures in the temporomandibular joint region. Dtsch. Stomatol., 22:411, 1972 (German)

PETZ, R.: Tissue tolerance and biomechanical questions of monomandibular wire fixation. Zentralbl. Chir., 97:1008, 1972 (German)

PETZOID, D.: Excision of freckles. Munch. Med. Wochenschr., 114:932, 1972 (German)

Peutz-Jeghers Syndrome

Peutz-Jeghers disease, surgical treatment of case (Altunkov et al). Khirurgiia (Sofiia), 26:260, 1973 (Bulgarian)

Syndrome, Peutz-Jeghers (Szklanny et al). Pol. Przegl. Chir., 45:1095, 1973 (Polish)

Syndrome, Peutz-Jeghers (Schott et al). Dtsch. Med. Wochenschr., 99:1525, 1974 (German)

Syndrome, Peutz-Jeghers (Bugaj). Pol. Przegl. Chir., 46:1153, 1974 (Polish)

Peutz-Jeghers-Touraine syndrome (Jonderko et al). Pol. Tyg. Lek., 29:1669, 1974 (Polish)

Syndrome, Peutz-Jeghers, comments on, (observations of three personal cases) (Gaspar Fuentes et al). Rev. Esp. Enferm. Apar. Dig., 43:261, 1974 (Spanish)

Syndrome, Peutz-Jeghers. Surgical challenge (Paglia et al). NY State J. Med., 75:402, 1975

PEYCHL, L.: Demonstration of parasites in toxoplasmatic lymphadenitis. Cesk. Patol., 10:86, 1974 (Czechoslovakian)

PEYCHL, L. et al: Histopathology of lymph node toxoplasmosis. Cas. Lek. Cesk., 113:392, 1974

PEYTRAL, C. et al: Facial nerve neuromas, PRS, 56:353, 1975. Ann. Otolaryng., 10:555, 1974

PFALTZ, C. R.: Indication of infraorbital nerve decompression. O. R. L., 35:214, 1973

PFALTZ, C. R. et al: Indication for infraorbital nerve decompression following maxillofacial injuries. H. N. O., 20:302, 1972 (German)

PFEIFER, G.: Indications, technic and results of block and segmental osteotomies on the maxilla and mandible in dysgnathias. Fortschr. Kiefer. Gesichtschir., 18:248, 1974 (German)

PFEIFER, G. et al: Etiology of cleft lip and cleft palate in humans and in animal experiments. Experientia, 29:225, 1973 (German)

PFEIFER, G., SCHLOTE, H. H., AND VAN KREY-

BIG, T.: Clefts of face in animal experiments, PRS, *55:*721, 1975. J. Maxillo-facial Surg., *2:*230, 1974

PFEIFER, G. *et al*: Course and effect of the changes in therapy in maxillofacial fractures. Fortschr. Kiefer. Gesichtschir., *19:*62, 1975 (German)

PFEIFFER, K. M.: Sprains and dislocations of fingers, PRS, *50;*306, 1972. Ther. Umsch., *28:*815, 1971

PFEIFFER, K. M.: Open reduction and screw fixation of fresh fractures of scaphoid bone of hand, PRS, *51:*479, 1973. Helvet. chir. acta, *39:*471, 1972

PFEIFFER, K. M.: Position of osteosynthesis in the management of hand fractures. Ther. Umsch., *29:*679, 1972 (German)

PFEIFLE, K. *et al*: Pain syndromes as late sequelae of neck dissection. Dtsch. Zahnaerztl. Z., *28:*968, 1973 (German)

PFEIFLE, K. *et al*: Pseudotumors of clavicle following neck dissection, PRS, *54:*502, 1974. J. Maxillo-facial Surg., *2:*14, 1974

PFITZER, P., AND PAPE, H. D.: Investigation of DNA content of leukoplakia cells of oral mucosa, PRS, *57:*115, 1976. J. Maxillo-facial Surg., *3:*119, 1975

PFLUG, J.: Physiopathology and treatment of lymphedema. Phlebologie, *27:*393, 1974 (French)

PFRETZSCHNER, C. *et al*: Complications of tracheotomy. Z. Laryngol. Rhinol. Otol., *52:*616, 1973

PHALEN, G. S., KENDRICK, J. I., AND RODRIQUEZ, J. M.: Lipomas of upper extremity, PRS, *48:*512, 1971. Am. J. Surg., *121:*298, 1971

Pharyngeal Neoplasms (See also *Larynx; Pharyngectomy*)

Hypopharynx, carcinoma of, at early age (Rao *et al*). J. Laryng. & Otol., *88:*1069, 1962

Pharyngoesophageal tract, new method of plastic operation in case of extensive laryngectomy due to cancer (Lukovskyi, Tytar), PRS, *48:*511, 1971. Acta chir. plast., *12:*157, 1970

Carcinomas, squamous cell, in oropharynx and laryngopharynx, combination of radiation and surgery in (Fletcher *et al*). Aktuel Probl. Chir., *14:*347, 1970

Indications, methods and results of conservative surgery in the treatment of cancer of the sinus piriformis (Andre *et al*). Arch. Ital. Otol., *81:*247, 1970 (French)

Surgery of the mandible and transmandibular surgery of the bucco-pharyngeal cavity

Pharyngeal Neoplasms — Cont.
tumors (Richard). Cancro, *23:*301, 1970 (French)

Pharynx, paranasal sinuses, oral cavity and, metastatic tumors of (Jortay), PRS, *50:*635, 1972. Acta chir. belg., *70:*715, 1971

Carcinoma of the posterior pharyngeal wall (Wilkins). Am. J. Surg., *122:*477, 1971

Methods of repair after surgery for cancer of the pharyngeal wall, postcricoid area, and cervical esophagus (Ballantyne). Am. J. Surg., *122:*482, 1971

Difficult repair of 2 pharyngostomas with modified crosswise flaps (Abbes *et al*). Ann. chir. plast., *16:*247, 1971 (French)

Major cervico-facial surgery and geriatrics (Andre *et al*). Ann. Otolaryngol. Chir. Cervicofac., *88:*295, 1971 (French)

What must we think of the staged transmaxillary buccopharyngectomy (Richard *et al*). Ann. Otolaryngol. Chir. Cervicofac., *88:*663, 1971 (French)

Pharyngeal and laryngeal cancers, elective neck dissection for; an evaluation (Ogura, Biller, Wette), PRS, *50:*309, 1972. Ann. Otol. Rhin. & Laryng., *80:*646, 1971

Surgery of cancer of the throat (Goonatilake). Ceylon Med. J., *17:*69, 1971

Pharynx and mouth, epidermoid carcinoma of, 1960–1964 (Farr, Arthur), PRS, *50:*97, 1972. Clin. Bull. Memorial Sloan-Kettering Cancer Ctr., *1:*130, 1971

Cigarette smoking and cancer of mouth, larynx, and pharynx (Moore), PRS, *49:*473, 1972. J.A.M.A., *218:*553, 1971

Surgical pathology of hypopharyngeal neoplasms (Harrison). J. Laryng. & Otol., *85:*1215, 1971

Visceral replacement after laryngo-pharyngectomy (Ranger). J. Laryng. & Otol., *85:*1218, 1971

Conventional surgical management of carcinoma of the hypopharynx (Bryce). J. Laryng. & Otol., *85:*1221, 1971

Integrated radiation and operation in the treatment of carcinoma of the head and neck: experience in 101 patients (Rush *et al*). J. Surg. Oncol., *3:*151, 1971

Pattern of lymphatic spread in pharyngeal cancer (Silva *et al*). J. Surg. Oncol., *3:*415, 1971

Delayed contralateral cervical metastases with laryngeal and laryngopharyngeal cancers (Biller *et al*). Laryngoscope, *81:*1499, 1971

Bakamjian's method for reconstruction of the hypopharynx (Van den Broek *et al*). Ned. tijdschr. geneeskd., *115:*1675, 1971 (Dutch)

Pharyngeal Neoplasms – Cont.

Medially based chest flap for treatment of cancer of the hypopharynx (Van den Broek *et al*). Pract. Otorhinolaryngol. (Basel), *33*:339, 1971

Prophylactic removal of lymph nodes and cellular tissue of the neck in patients with laryngeal and laryngopharyngeal cancer (Baradulina *et al*). Vestn. Otorinolaringol., *33*:55, 1971 (Russian)

Functional rehabilitation of the pharynx in surgically treated neoplasms (Zehm *et al*). Z. Laryngol. Rhinol. Otol., *50*:776, 1971 (German)

Planned preoperative irradiation and surgery for advanced cancer of the oral cavity, pharynx and larynx (Roswit *et al*). Am. J. Roentgenol. Radium Ther. Nucl. Med., *114*:59, 1972

Pharynx and mouth, epidermoid carcinoma, prognostic significance of histologic grade (Arthur, Farr), PRS, *52*:102, 1973. Am. J. Surg., *124*:489, 1972

Nasopharynx carcinoma, review of 146 patients with emphasis on radiation dose and time factors (Moench, Phillips), PRS, *52*:102, 1973. Am. J. Surg., *124*:515, 1972

Cancers, pharyngolaryngeal, treated with bleomycin. Histopathological assessment (Renault *et al*). Ann. Otolaryngol. Chir. Cervicofac., *89*:229, 1972 (French)

Epitheliomas of glosso-epiglottal sulcus. Apropos of 122 cases treated at the Gustave-Roussy Institute between 1960 and 1967 (Vandenbrouck *et al*). Ann. Otolaryngol. Chir. Cervicofac., *89*:517, 1972 (French)

Role of surgery in the management of postcricoid and cervical esophageal neoplasms (Harrison). Ann. Otol. Rhin. & Laryng., *81*:465, 1972

Pharynx and neck, teratoma of (Hawkins *et al*). Ann. Otol. Rhin. & Laryng., *81*:848, 1972

Carcinoma in a pharyngeal pouch: five-year survival after resection (Kune). Aust. N. Z. J. Surg., *41*:249, 1972

Cancer, hypopharyngeal, conventional pharyngolaryngectomy in surgical management of (Bryce). Can. J. Otolaryngol., *231*, 1972

Airway obstruction, upper, in newborn secondary to hemangiopericytoma (Baden *et al*). Can. Med. Assoc. J., *107*:1202, 1972

Problem of laryngopharyngeal and pharyngeal carcinomas (Chiadek). Cesk. Otolaryngol., *21*:102, 1972 (Czechoslovakian)

Pharyngeal Neoplasms – Cont.

Resection of the mandible in oral tumours (Rosemann). H. N. O., *20*:166, 1972 (German)

Cancer of the head and neck. Hypopharynx and larynx. Surgical management (Ogura *et al*). J.A.M.A., *221*:77, 1972

Palliative surgery (Gaisford). J.A.M.A., *221*:83, 1972

Reconstruction (Edgerton). J.A.M.A., *221*:1258, 1972

Neurilemmoma of the pharynx (Iliades *et al*). Laryngoscope, *82*:430, 1972

Pharyngolarynx: new aspects of the use of the larynx for reconstruction in hypopharyngeal carcinoma (Siirala *et al*). Laryngoscope, *82*:504, 1972

Carcinoma, larynx and laryngopharynx, high dosage preoperative radiation and surgery for. Fourteen-year program (Goldman *et al*). Laryngoscope, *82*:1306, 1972

Carcinoma, laryngopharynx, hypothyroidism following combined therapy in (Murken *et al*). Laryngoscope, *82*:1306, 1972

Surgery in cancer of head and neck. Use of posterior cervical flap (Lenczyk *et al*). N. Y. State J. Med., *72*:239, 1972

Radiological appearance of lower pharynx following laryngectomy and management of tissue defect by modified method of Messerklinger (Wazny. Czerwonka). Otolaryngol. Pol., *26*:681, 1972 (Polish)

Primary reconstructive surgery of head and neck tumors with pedicle flaps. II. Application of a pedicle flap of the anterior chest wall to partially pharyngectomized cases (Murakami *et al*). Otolaryngology (Tokyo), *44*:289, 1972 (Japanese)

Cancer surgery, oropharyngeal, massive, catastrophic breakdown after, management of (Mladick *et al*), PRS, *49*:316, 1972

Cancers, piriform sinus, conservative surgery in treatment of, indications, technics and results of (Andre *et al*). Probl. Actuels Otorhinolaryngol. *201*:24, 1972 (French)

Laryngeal reconstruction after hemi-laryngopharyngectomy (Andre *et al*). Rev. Laryngol. Otol. Rhinol. (Bord.), *93*:88, 1972 (French)

Hemi-pharyngolaryngectomy with monoblock lymph node dissection and reconstruction (Portmann *et al*). Rev. Laryngol. Otol. Rhinol. (Bord.), *93*:94, 1972 (French)

Parapharyngeal neurilemmoma with intracranial extension (Smith *et al*). South. Med. J., *65*:1171, 1972

Combined hydroxyurea and radiotherapy: a

Pharyngeal Neoplasms—Cont.

new dosage schedule (Hussey *et al*). South. Med. J., *65:*137, 1972

Conservation surgery of the larynx and pharynx (Ogura). Tex. Med., *68:*106, 1972

Cancers, hypopharynx, results of surgical treatment. Experience at Institut Gustave-Roussy, Villejuif, 1960–1970 (Cachin *et al*). Acta Otorhinolaryngol. Belg., *27:*1010, 1973 (French)

Cancers, hypopharynx, results of surgical treatment of 253 cases (Piquet *et al*). Acta Otorhinolaryngol. Belg. *27:*1029, 1973 (French)

Cancer, larynx and hypopharynx, treatment of lymphatic involvement in (Agazzi). Acta Otorhinolaryngol. Belg., *27:*1041, 1973 (French)

Epithelioma of hypopharynx (round table discussion). Acta Otorhinolaryngol. Belg., *27:*1063, 1973 (French)

Our experience with surgery of cancer of the pharynx with suture of the pharynx to the cricoid cartilage (Ramirez Mohedano *et al*). Acta Otorinolaryngol. Iber. Am., *24:*91, 1973 (Spanish)

Laryngeal and hypopharyngeal carcinoma, growth and spread of, with reflections on effect of preoperative irradiation. One hundred and thirty nine cases studied by whole organ serial sectioning (Olofsson *et al*). Acta Otolaryngol. (Suppl.) (Stockh.), *308:*1, 1973

Carcinoma, tonsil and nasopharynx; 20-year results (Mater). Am. J. Roent. Radium Ther., *117:*517, 1973

Cancers, larynx and hypopharynx, importance of combined radiotherapy and surgery in treatment of (Piquet *et al*). Ann. Otolaryngol. Chir. Cervicofac., *90:*633, 1973

Verrucous carcinoma of pyriform sinus (Thomas *et al*). Arch. Otolaryng., *97:*488, 1973

Comparison of preoperative and primary radiotherapy in treatment of carcinoma of hypopharynx (Lord). Brit. J. Radiol., *46:*175, 1973

Hypopharynx, carcinoma of, preoperative radiotherapy in (Morrison). Brit. J. Radiol., *46:*646, 1973

Carcinoma, hypopharynx (Briant *et al*). Can. J. Otolaryngol., *2:*4, 1973

Carcinoma of hypopharynx, treatment of (Inoue, Shigematsu, Sato), PRS, *52:*460, 1973. Cancer, *31:*649, 1973

Lipoma of pharynx (report of four cases) (Toppozada *et al*). J. Laryng. & Otol., *87:*787, 1973

Pharyngeal Neoplasms—Cont.

Hypopharynx, cancer of (Stell). J. R. Coll. Surg. Edinb., *18:*20, 1973

Hypopharynx and larynx, conservation surgery of (Schechter, McLarey), PRS, *53:*683, 1974. Mil. Med., *138:*639, 1973

Pharyngeal reconstruction using the deltopectoral flap (Stell). O. R. L., *35:*317, 1973

Pharynx, middle, case of neurofibroma of (Sekula *et al*). Otolaryngol. Pol., *27:*527, 1973 (Polish)

Pharynx, atypical fibroxanthoma in (Berschadsky *et al*). PRS, *52:*443, 1973

Temporal island flap for replacement of oral and pharyngeal mucosa (McKee). South Med. J., *66:*534, 1973

Radiotherapy of epipharyngeal neoplasms (Gauwerky *et al*). Strahlentherapie, *146:*125, 1973 (German)

Cancers, nonfixed of glottic region, surgical management of irradiation failures of (Ballantyne *et al*). Am. J. Roentgenol. Radium Ther. Nucl. Med., *120:*164, 1974

Hypopharynx, carcinoma of (Raven). Am. J. Roentgenol. Radium Ther. Nucl. Med., *120:*173, 1974

Triple drug intra-arterial infusion combined with X-ray therapy and surgery for head and neck cancer (Cruz *et al*). Am. J. Surg., *128:*573, 1974

Results of high dose radiation and surgery in the treatment of advanced cancer of the head and neck (Carifi *et al*). Am. J. Surg., *128:*580, 1974

Hypopharynx, total reconstruction of, with tongue flap and dermal graft (Lore). Ann. Otol. Rhin. & Laryng., *83:*476, 1974

Carcinoma, posterior pharyngeal wall, surgery for (Seda *et al*). Arch. Otolaryng., *99:*297, 1974

Selection of treatment for in situ and early invasive carcinoma of the glottis (DeSanto). Can. J. Otolaryngol., *3:*552, 1974

Resection of the mandibular angle with plastic occlusion of the pharynx in monoblock surgery of tonsillar cancer (Tichy). Cesk. Otolaryngol., *23:*349, 1974 (Czech)

Hamartoma of the hypopharynx (Wey *et al*). H. N. O., *22:*217, 1974 (German)

Greater omentum in repair of complication following surgery and radiotherapy for certain cancers (Abbes *et al*). Int. Surg., *59:*81, 1974

Retropharyngeal lipoma (Kenefick). J. Laryng. & Otol., *88:*805, 1974

Role of radiotherapy in the treatment of oral cancer (Vermund *et al*). J. Oral Surg., *32:*690, 1974

Prevention of complications of composite re-

Pharyngeal Neoplasms—Cont.

section after high dose preoperative radiotherapy (Tucker *et al*). Laryngoscope, *84:*933, 1974

A study of tumors of the parapharyngeal space (Work *et al*). Laryngoscope, *84:*1748, 1974

Carcinoma, laryngeal and hypopharyngeal, recurrent, radical neck dissection (Bleuler). O.R.L., *36:*7, 1974 (German)

Pharyngeal carcinoma, lower, treated surgically, case (Kamieniec *et al*). Otolaryngol. Pol., *28:*237, 1974 (Polish)

Repair of a large pharyngostome in irradiated tissues. 7-year cure (Stricker *et al*). Rev. Stomatol. Chir. Maxillofac., *75:*227, 1974 (French)

Development of closure procedures in pharyngostomes and orostomes in irradiated tissues (Soussaline *et al*). Rev. Stomatol. Chir. Maxillofac., *75:*229, 1974 (French)

Indications, limits and results of functional latero-cervical lymph node excision (Pignataro). Tumori, *60:*585, 1974 (Italian)

Pharynx, reticuloplasmacytoma of (Betkowski *et al*). Wiad. Lek., *27:*751, 1974 (Polish)

Control by irradiation alone of nonfixed clinically positive lymph nodes from squamous cell carcinoma of the oral cavity, oropharynx, supraglottic larynx, and hypopharynx (Schneider *et al*). Am. J. Roentgenol. Radium Ther. Nucl. Med., *123:*42, 1975

Comparison of long-term carcinologic results between radical and conservative cervical surgery (Andre *et al*). Ann. Otolaryngol. Chir. Cervicofac., *92:*113, 1975 (French)

Pyriform sinus cancer: a clinical and laboratory study (Kirchner). Ann. Otol. Rhin. & Laryng., *84:*793, 1975

Head and neck rhabdomyoma, parapharyngeal (Shapiro *et al*), PRS, *57:*117, 1976. Arch. Otol., *101:*323, 1975

Stomal recurrence following laryngectomy (Bonneau *et al*). Arch. Otolaryng., *101:*408, 1975

Evaluation of total pharyngolaryngectomy for hypopharyngeal cancer (Iwai *et al*). Arch. Otorhinolaryngol. (N.Y.), *209:*223, 1975

Subtotal pharyngolaryngectomy conservation surgery for carcinoma of sinus pyriformis extending toward the larynx (Iwai *et al*). Arch. Otorhinolaryngol. (N.Y.), *209:*271, 1975

Use of a tongue flap for the repair of defects following radical surgery of the head and neck (Robertson). Aust. N. Z. J. Surg., *45:*395, 1975

Pharyngeal Neoplasms—Cont.

Combined pre-operative irradiation and surgery for advanced cancer of the larynx and laryngopharynx (a 14 year correlative statistical and histopathological study) (Goldman *et al*). Can. J. Otolaryngol., *4:*251, 1975

Prolonged depression of cellular immunity in cured laryngopharyngeal cancer patients treated with radiation therapy (Tarpley *et al*). Cancer, *35:*638, 1975

Efficacy of combining radiation therapy with a surgical procedure in patients with cervical metastasis from squamous cancer of the oropharynx and hypopharynx (Jesse *et al*). Cancer, *35:*1163, 1975

Combination of radiotherapy and surgery in the treatment of head and neck cancers (Cachin *et al*). Cancer Treat. Rev., *2:*177, 1975

Temporo-frontal flap. Its value in post-irradiation buccal-pharyngeal surgery (Junien-Lavillauroy *et al*). J. Fr. Otorhinolaryngol., *24:*763, 1975 (French)

One stage reconstruction of hypopharynx following total laryngopharyngectomy (Draf). Laryngol. Rhinol. Otol. (Stuttg.), *54:*572, 1975 (German)

Long term therapeutic results—cancer of the larynx and hypopharynx. Preliminary report (Ogura *et al*). Laryngoscope, *85:*1746, 1975

Cancer, head and neck, fiberoptic endoscopy in (Dellon, Hall, Chretien). PRS, *55:*466, 1975

Management of oral and pharyngeal cancer: a multi-disciplinary approach (El-Domeiri *et al*). Surg. Clin. North Am., *55:*107, 1975

Carcinoma of the oropharynx. Results of megavoltage radiation therapy in 305 patients (Weller *et al*). Am. J. Roentgenol., *126:*236, 1976

Pharyngectomy (See also *Larynx; Pharyngeal Neoplasms*)

Esophagoplasty, secondary, after pharyngolaryngectomy, using modified deltopectoral flap (Jackson, Lang). PRS, *48:*155, 1971

Laryngectomy and subtotal esophagectomy, cervical esophageal reconstruction after (Armstrong, Peters). PRS, *48:*382, 1971

Primary reconstructive surgery of head and neck tumors with pedicle flaps. I. Application of a pedicle flap of the anterior chest wall to partially pharyngectomized cases (Murakami *et al*). Otolaryngology (Tokyo), *44:*289, 1972 (Japanese)

Pharyngectomy—Cont.

Primary reconstructive surgery of head and neck tumors with pedicle flaps. II. Application of a pedicle flap of the anterior chest wall to partially pharyngectomized cases (Murakami *et al*). Otolaryngology (Tokyo), *44:*289, 1972 (Japanese)

Selective compressor for pharyngostomas (Martinez Andres). Acta Otorinolaryngol. Iber. Am., *24:*87, 1973 (Polish)

Pharyngostome, reconstruction with fibroscopic study of interior luman (La Ruffa), PRS, *53:*683, 1974. Bol. y trab. Soc. argent. cir., *34:*263, 1973

Pharyngoesophageal reconstruction, cervical, prefabrication techniques in (Bakamjian, Holbrook), PRS, *55:*107, 1975. Brit. J. Plast. Surg., *26:*214, 1973

Pharyngo-esophagostomy (Harcourt). Eye, Ear, Nose, Throat, Mon., *52:*26, 1973

Fistulae, cervical, use of prefolded flap to provide lining and cover in repair of (Shapiro, Fleury). PRS, *51:*319, 1973

Oropharyngeal defect, massive, total flap reconstruction for (Griffin *et al*), PRS, *51:*457, 1973. Discussion by Edgerton, PRS, *51:*582, 1973

Oral and pharyngeal mucosa, temporal island flap for replacement of (McKee). South. Med. J., *66:*534, 1973

Epithelized skin flap in plastic surgery for gaping defects of pharyngeal walls and jugular portion of esophagus (Chudakov). Vestn. Khir., *111:*83, 1973 (Russian)

Combined closure of open defects of pharynx and cervical portion of esophagus by local tissues and Filatov's tube (Babaiants). Vestn. Otorinolaringol., *35:*96, 1973 (Russian)

Use of split thickness grafts in the repair of excisions of the oropharynx, base of the tongue, and larynx (Ruch *et al*). Am. J. Surg., *128:*553, 1974

Pharyngoesophageal defects, everting closure of (Sobol, Tucker, Tucker), PRS, *55:*107, 1975. Arch. Otolaryng., *100:*148, 1974

Anterior pharyngeal pouch (Maguire *et al*). Can. J. Otolaryngol., *3:*225, 1974

Defects, oropharyngeal surgical, reconstruction with triangular cervical flap (Poisson, Franchebois), PRS, *54:*500, 1974. Canad. J. Surg., *17:*167, 1974

Clinical conference: Failure in understanding needs of patient following total pharyngectomy. Jap. J. Nurs., *38:*548, 1974 (Japanese)

Pretherapy speech intelligibility of a glossectomee (Riviere *et al*). J. Commun. Disord.,

Pharyngectomy—Cont.

*7:*357,1974

Management of fistulae of the head and neck after radical surgery (Stell *et al*). J. Laryng. & Otol., *88:*819, 1974

Pharyngoesophagostoma, management of (Aviles). Laryngoscope, *84:*317, 1974

Pharyngeal fistulas, postoperative (Francesconi *et al*), PRS, *57:*397, 1976. Riv. ital. chir. plast., *6:*81, 1974

Pharyngostome repairs (Guthrie *et al*). Surg. Clin. North Am., *54:*767, 1974

Device for irrigation of the margins of pharyngostomas stimulating healing of the preparations (Mostovoi *et al*). Zh. Ushn. Nos. Gorl. Bolezn., *6:*97, 1974 (Russian)

Our procedure for pharyngoplasty in transmandibular pharyngectomies (Andre *et al*). Ann. Otolaryngol. Chir. Cervicofac., *92:*149, 1975 (French)

Esophageal reconstruction, cervical, secondary (Petty, Theogaraj, Cohen. PRS, *56:*70, 1975

Fistula, pharyngoesophageal, repaired by microvascular transfer of free skin flap (Fujino, Saito). PRS, *56:*549, 1975

New principle of production of obturating apparatus in gaping defects of the esophagus and pharynx (Balon *et al*). Vestn. Khir., *115:*108, 1975 (Russian)

Laryngopharyngectomy, new suction obturator to control saliva after (Javor). PRS, *57:*106, 1976

Pharynx

Pharyngostomas, plastic repair (Vieta *et al*), PRS, *48:*295, 1971. Bull. Soc. Plast. Surg. Cordoba, *1:*1, 1970

Pharyngeal constrictor muscle, superior, innervation of (Smith, Dedo), PRS, *48:*196, 1971. Ann. Otol. Rhin. & Laryng., *80:*92, 1971

Cricopharyngeal myotomy in dysphagia (Stevens *et al*). Laryngoscope, *81:*1616, 1971

Can we rehabilitate children exposed to prolonged intubation? (Krivosic-Horber, Tempe, Gauthier-Lafaye). Anesth. Analg. (Paris), *29:*411, 1972 (French)

Management of pharyngocutaneous fistula (Myers). Arch. Otolaryng., *95:*10, 1972

Penetrating injuries of parapharyngeal space (Shanon *et al*). Arch. Otolaryng., *96:*256, 1972

Zenker's diverticulum: importance of pharyngo-esophageal sphincter (Ribet *et al*). J. Chir. (Paris), *104:*37, 1972 (French)

Pharyngoesophageal diverticulum. Analysis of clinical patterns, surgical management, and results of treatment (Sugahara *et al*).

Pharynx—Cont.

Rev. Paul. Med., *82:*117, 1973 (Portuguese)

Pharyngoplasty using transplantation of skeletal muscle as free autograft (Thompson), PRS, *56:*355, 1975. Riv. ital. chir. plast., *5:*495, 1973

Present status of one-stage pharyngo-esophageal diverticulectomy (Welsh *et al*). Surg. Clin. North Am., *53:*935, 1973

Pharyngostomy, cervical. Safe alternative for gastrointestinal decompression (Lyons). Am. J. Surg., *127:*387, 1974

Cricopharyngeal achalasia (Helsper *et al*). Am. J. Surg., *128:*521, 1974

Late assessment of results of cricopharyngeal myotomy for cervical dysphagia (Akl *et al*). Am. J. Surg., *128:*818, 1974

Functional restitution of denervated gullet (Zehm). Arch. Otolaryng., *99:*279, 1974

Posterior pharyngeal tension pneumatocele (Paterson *et al*). Can. Med. Assoc. J., *111:*243, 1974

Changes of resonance during-speech after surgical interventions in the meso- and epipharynx (Krahulec *et al*). Cesk. Otolaryngol, *23:*363, 1974 (Slovakian)

Pharyngotomy for colonic anastomosis during total esophagoplasty (Laccourreye *et al*). J. Chir. (Paris), *107:*83, 1974 (French)

Cricopharyngeal myotomy for paralytic dysphagia (Hirano). J. Fr. Otorhinolaryngol., *23:*732, 1974

Laceration of hypopharynx (Vogel *et al*). J. Pediatr. Surg., *9:*557, 1974

Letter: Cricopharyngeus (Barclay). N. Z. Med. J., *80:*314, 1974

Letter: Ambulatory enteral nutrition. A new method (Choubrac *et al*). Nouv. Presse Med., *3:*1959, 1974 (French)

Hypopharynx, endotracheal tube perforation of (Hawkins *et al*), PRS, *54:*373, 1974. West. J. Med., *120:*282, 1974

Anticoagulants, therapy with, retropharyngeal hematoma complication (Owens *et al*), PRS, *57:*765, 1976. Arch. Otolaryng., *101:*565, 1975

Dysphagia secondary to cricopharyngeal muscle dysfunction, surgical management (Calcaterra *et al*). Arch. Otolaryng., *101:*726, 1975

Significance of myotomy of cricopharyngeal muscle and the surface fibers of the esophagus in pharyngo-esophageal dyskinesia. Apropos of 7 cases (Desaulty *et al*). J. Fr. Otorhinolaryngol., *24:*527, 1975 (French)

Pharyngoplasty through cross palatopharyngeal flaps (Heller), PRS, *57:*117, 1976. J. Maxillo-facial Surg., *3:*94, 1975

Atelectasis, further experiences with the ary-

Pharynx—Cont.

tenoid-epiglottic flap for chronic aspiration pneumonia (Vecchione, Habal, Murray). PRS, *55:*318, 1975

Cricopharyngeal myotomy for dysphagia in oculopharyngeal muscular dystrophy. Report of a case (Dayal *et al*). Arch. Otolaryng., *102:*115, 1976

PHELPS, M. D., JR.: Stasis ulcers, PRS, *53:*373, 1974. Lahey Clin. Bull., *22:*54, 1973

PHILIPSZOON, A. J.: Otoplasty as procedure for outpatient clinic. O. R. L., *36:*58, 1974

PHILLIPS, C. W., LUTTERBECK, E. F., AND WILKOLM, L.: Xeroradiography of breast, PRS, *55:*379, 1975. Internat. Surg., *58:*607, 1973

PHILLIPS, J. *et al*: Clostridial myonecrosis of abdominal wall. Management after extensive resection. Am. J. Surg., *128:*436, 1974

PHILLIPS, J. A., III: *Aeromonas hydrophila* wound infection (with Rosenthal, Bernhardt). PRS, *53:*77, 1974

PHILLIPS, S. J., AND VICK, J. A.: Pretreatment of E. coli endotoxin shock with WR 2823: new alphadrenergic blocking agent, PRS, *48:*299, 1971. Surgery, *69:*510, 1971

Photography

Plastic surgery, value of photography in (Talamas), PRS, *49:*478, 1972. Tribuna Med. Mexico, *20:*3; 1971

Strobe light unit explosion (Graham) (Letter to the Editor). PRS, *49:*331, 1972

Photodrawer (Weisman). PRS, *50:*627, 1972

Medical Photography. By H. L. Gibson. Eastman Kodak Co., Rochester, N. Y., 1973. PRS, *54:*602, 1974

Photography of operative field—a simple device (Adhia, Adhia), PRS, *54:*119, 1974. Indian J. Surg., *35:*593, 1973

Photogrammetry—a planning tool in facial reconstruction (Wright *et al*) In *Biostereometrics 74,* ed. Herron; Falls Church, Va., Am. Soc. Photogrammetry, 1974 pp. 154–60

Preoperative photography as an aid in orthopedic jaw surgery (Selle). Fortschr. Kiefer. Gesichtschir., *18:*106, 1974 (German)

Photographs shown preoperatively to patients (Goin) (Letter to the Editor). PRS, *54:*90, 1974

Photographs of results in other patients, views of several prominent attorneys on the preoperative showing of (DeMere) (Letter to the Editor), PRS, *54:*91, 1974

Photographs, black and white, how to make from good color transparencies (Schneider). PRS, *56:*218, 1975

Slides, lecture, graph or text, simple method for producing (Parry, Wolfort, Cochran).

Photography—Cont.
PRS, *57:*751, 1976

Physical Therapy

Physical therapy, analysis of results in 681 burned patients (Dobbs, Curreri), PRS, *52:*101, 1973. J. Trauma, *12:*242, 1972

PICAUD, A. J.: Ablation of sebaceous cysts of the face. Presse Med., *79:*2237, 1971 (French)

PICAUD, A. J. *et al*: Is it permissible to reconstruct a breast with prosthesis after mastectomy for cancer? When and how? Ann. chir. plast., *17:*278, 1972 (French)

PICHIMAIER, H. *et al*: Surgical therapy of thyroid malignoma. Med. Klin., *70:*158, 1975 (German)

PICKARD, B. H. *et al*: Fractures of the ethmoid involving the orbit. Trans. Ophthalmol. Soc. U.K., *91:*515, 1971

PICKENS, R. L., AND LATTIMER, J. K.: Disseminated intravascular coagulation, diagnosis and treatment of hemorrhagic diathesis after prostatectomy, PRS, *52:*98, 1973. J. Urol., *108:*951, 1972

PICKRELL, K. L.: Xeroderma pigmentosa (Follow-Up Clinic). PRS, *49:*83, 1972

PICKRELL, K. L.: Results of pushback operations in treatment of submucous cleft palate (with Massengill, Robinson). PRS, *51:*432, 1973

PICKRELL, K. L.: Appearance and attire of medical students (Editorial). PRS, *51:*438, 1973

PICKRELL, K. L.: Reply to "Evaluation of submucous cleft palate surgery," by Dellon, Hoopes (Letter to the Editor). PRS, *53:*339, 1974

PICKRELL, K. L.: Intralesional BCG, intravenous immune lymphocytes, and immunization with neuraminidase-treated tumor cells to manage melanoma (with Seigler, Shingleton). PRS, *55:*294, 1975

PICKRELL, K. L.: Dynamic correction of unilateral paralysis of lower lip (with Puckett, Neale). PRS, *55:*397, 1975

PICKRELL, K. L. *et al*: Study of 100 operated cleft lip-palate patients operated upon 22 to 27 years ago by one surgeon. PRS, *49:*149, 1972

PICKRELL, K. L., AND MLADICK, R.: Brief guide to fluid therapy for infants and children on plastic surgical service. PRS, *49:*404, 1972

PICKRELL, K. L., PETERS, C., AND NEALE, H.: Construction of perineal body in female. PRS, *55:*529, 1975

PICKRELL, K. L., PUCKETT, C., AND PETERS, C.: Transposition of lips for correction of facial paralysis. PRS, *57:*427, 1976

PICO, G.: Modified technique of external dacry-ocystorhinostomy. Am. J. Ophth., *72:*679, 1971

PIERCE, H. E.: Cryosurgery for hypertrophic scars and keloids. Preliminary report. J. Natl. Med. Assoc. *66:*174, 1974

PIERCE, J. M., JR.: Urethroplasty for anterior urethral stricture, PRS, *52:*596, 1973. J. Urol., *109:*422, 1973

PIERCE, R. E., AND TENEYCK, F. D.: Hereditary hyperpigmentation anomalies in blacks, PRS, *57:*542, 1976. J. Heredity, *65:*157, 1974

PIERCELL, M. P., WAITE, D. E., AND NELSON, R.: Prevention of self-inflicted trauma in semicomatose patients, PRS, *56:*353, 1975. J. Oral Surg., *32:*903, 1974

PIERCELL, M. P. *et al*: Central hemangioma of the mandible: intraoral resection and reconstruction. J. Oral Surg., *33:*225, 1975

PIERRE, M. L., AND JOUGLARD, J. P.: Treatment of unilateral congenital hypoplasia or absence of breast. PRS, *56:*146, 1975

Pierre Robin Syndrome (See also *Cleft Palate; Micrognathia*)

Glossoptotic hypoxia and micrognathia—the Pierre Robin syndrome reviewed. Early recognition and prompt surgical treatment is important for survival (Farnsworth *et al*). Clin. Pediatr. (Phila.), *10:*600, 1971

Pierre Robin syndrome—case report and statistical study (Kubo *et al*). Iryo, *25:*311, 1971 (Japanese)

Pierre-Robin syndrome. New personal surgical-orthopaedical treatment (Sossi). Minerva Stomatol., *20:*179, 1971

Pierre Robin syndrome in association with combined congenital lengthening and shortening of long bones (Walden, Logosso, Brennan). PRS, *48:*80, 1971

Management of Pierre Robin syndrome in infancy by prolonged nasoesophageal intubation (Stern *et al*). Am. J. Dis. Child, *124:*78, 1972

Tracheotomy in pediatrics (Tucker *et al*). Ann. Otol. Rhin. & Laryng., *81:*818, 1972

Pierre Robin syndrome: unusual associated developmental defects (Holthusen). Ann. Radiol. (Paris), *15:*253, 1972 (Multi-language)

Problems and results of Eschler's dorsal masseter transposition for the treatment of Robin's syndrome (Harle *et al*). Dtsch. Zahnaerztl. Z., *27:*47, 1972 (German)

Respiratory management in Pierre Robin syndrome—with special reference to acid-base equilibrium (Oka *et al*). Jap. J. Anesthesiol., *21:*1352, 1972

Glossopharyngeal airway obstruction, late development in mandibular hypoplasia

Pierre Robin Syndrome—Cont.
(Cosman, Crikelair). PRS, *50:*573, 1972

Long-term evolution of some cases of Robin's syndrome of the newborn (Michelet *et al*). Rev. Stomatol. Chir. Maxillofac., *73:*77, 1972 (French)

Syndrome, Pierre Robin, management of (Davies). Dev. Med. Child. Neurol., *15:*359, 1973

Emergency situation following surgery for cleft palate in children with Robin syndrome and its therapy (Harle *et al*). Osterr. Z. Stomatol., *70:*131, 1973 (German)

Syndrome, Pierre Robin, treatment of, by Duhamel's method (Gross *et al*). Pediatr. Pol., *45:*1215, 1973 (Polish)

Pierre Robin syndrome, Duhamel procedure for treatment of (Minervini) (Letter to the Editor). PRS, *51:*686, 1973

Micrognathia, treatment of respiratory obstruction in, by use of nasogastric tube (McEvitt), PRS, *52:*138, 1973. Discussions by Lindsay, McDowell, Randall, PRS, *52:*306, 1973

Syndrome, Pierre Robin, eye abnormalities and skeletal deformities in (Cosman, Keyser), PRS, *56:*109, 1975. Cleft Palate J., *11:*404, 1974

Micrognathia and glossoptosis in the newborn. Surgical tacking of the tongue in small jaw syndromes (Hawkins *et al*). Clin. Pediatr. (Phila.), *13:*1066, 1974

Pre- intra- and post-operative problems in a new therapeutic trend in the Pierre Robin syndrome (Mocavero *et al*). Minerva Anestesiol., *41:*294, 1975 (Italian)

Airway obstruction in Pierre Robin syndrome relieved by fastening base of tongue forward to hyoid (Lapidot, Ben-Hur). PRS, *56:*89, 1975

Obstruction, respiration, in micrognathia, relief by use of large nasogastric tube (Benfield) (Letter to the Editor). PRS, *56:*570, 1975

PIESSENS, W. F.: Evidence for human cancer immunity, PRS, *48:*93, 1971. Cancer, *26:*1212, 1970

PIETRUSCHKA, G. *et al*: Incidence, therapy and prognosis of chemical eye burns. Z. Aerztl. Fortbild. (Jena), *65:*835, 1971 (German)

PIETRUSKI, J.: Topodiagnosis of intratemporal facial nerve palsy. Otolaryngol. Pol., *26:*619, 1972 (Polish)

PIETRUSKI, J.: Electrogustometry in diagnosis of facial nerve palsy. Otolaryngol. Pol., *27:*125, 1973 (Polish)

PIETRUSKI, J.: Results of surgical and conservative treatment of peripheral facial nerve pa-

ralysis using our computational methods. A comparative study. Otolaryngol. Pol., *29:*531, 1975 (Polish)

PIETRUSKI, J. *et al*: Salivation test in diagnosis and prognosis in Bell's palsy. Otolaryngol. Pol., *27:*253, 1973 (Polish)

PIETRUSKI, J. *et al*: Complex treatment of large osteoma of frontal sinus. Otolaryngol. Pol., *28:*103, 1974 (Polish)

PIGGOT, T. A., AND BLACK, M. J. M.: Importance of not damaging the volar digital arteries when using zig-zag incision on a finger (Letter to the Editor). PRS, *53:*80, 1974

PIGNATARO, O.: Indications, limits and results of functional latero-cervical lymph node excision. Tumori, *60:*585, 1974 (Italian)

PIGOSSI, N.: Glycerin preserved dura implants, PRS, *49:*362, 1972. Rev. Latino Am. plast. surg., *14:*29, 1970

PIGOTT, R. W.: Results of nasopharyngoscopic assessment of pharyngoplasty, PRS, *56:*354, 1975. Scand. J. Plast. Reconstr. Surg., *8:*148, 1974

PIHRT, J.: Surgery of medial cysts and fistulas from cosmetic point of view. Cesk. Otolaryngol., *22:*246, 1973 (Czechoslovakian)

PIKE, D.: Studies of tendon healing in the rat. Remodeling of distal stump after severance (with Greenlee). PRS, *48:*260, 1971

PIKE, R. L. *et al*: Composite autogenous marrow and surface-decalcified implants in mandibular defects. J. Oral Surg., *31:*905, 1973

PIKE, R. L., AND BOYNE, P. J.: Use of surface-decalcified allogenic bone and autogenous marrow in extensive mandibular defects, PRS, *55:*119, 1975. J. Oral Surg., *32:*177, 1974

PILAR-SVOBODA, B.: Unilateral hypertrophy of the facial bones. Chir. Maxillofac. Plast., *8:*3, 1971 (Croatian)

PILGER, T. W.: Craniofacial hereditary syndrome of Crouzon. Int. J. Orthod., *12:*25, 1974

PILGRIM, M. C. *et al*: Reconstructive nasal surgery. Am. J. Nurs., *73:*451, 1973

PILHEU, F. R.: Melanoma, clinical experience in 77 patients, PRS, *56:*112, 1975. Bol. y Trab. Acad. argent. cir., *58:*392, 1974

PILHEU, F. R. *et al*: Current status of mouth cancer treatment. Prensa med. argent., *58:*1812, 1971 (Spanish)

PILHEU, R. F.: Clinical experience with 77 patients with melanoma, PRS, *57:*124, 1976. Prensa med. argent., *62:*97, 1975

PILLERON, J. P.: Malignant melanoma. Laval. Med., *42:*933, 1971 (French)

Pilonidal Cysts

Pilonidal cyst disease, comparison of operative methods and conclusions on 1147 per-

Pilonidal Cysts—Cont.

sonal cases (Papoutsakis *et al*), PRS, *50:*100, 1972. Trans. 7th Panhellenic Cong. Surg. Soc., *2:*384, 1971

Pilonidal sinus, postnatal, treatment of 48 cases by modified Patey, Lord, and Millar technique (Evangelou *et al*), PRS, *51:*487, 1973. Acta chir. Hellenica, *44:*684, 1972

Pilonidal sinus, ambulant treatment of (Swierstra), PRS, *51:*110, 1973. Arch. chir. neerl., *24:*1, 1972

Pilonidal cysts, operative treatment by sliding graft (Olivari, Reismann, Bayer), PRS, *52:*602, 1973. Bruns' Beitr. klin. Chir., *220:*306, 1973

Pilonidal sinus, large, treatment of (Berger, Millesi, Simma), PRS, *53:*249, 1974. Chir. Praxis, *17:*285, 1973

Pilonidal sinus, treatment by block excision and primary suture (Verbeek, Bender), PRS, *55:*722, 1975. Arch. chir. neerl., *26:*311, 1974

Treatment of pilonidal sinus by "Z" plasty (Lodha). J. Indian Med. Assoc., *62:*307, 1974

Sacrococcygeal pilonidal disease, results of various operations for (Sood, Green, Parui). PRS, *56:*559, 1975

PIMENIDIS, M. Z. *et al*: Effect of early postnatal condylectomy on the growth of the mandible. Am. J. Orthod., *62:*42, 1972

PINDBORG, J. J.: *Atlas of Diseases of Oral Mucosa*. 2nd Ed. W. B. Saunders Co., Philadelphia, 1973

PINEL, J. *et al*: Plasmocytoma of nasal fossae with multifocal bone involvement. Case followed 13 years. Ann. Otolaryngol. Chir. Cervicofac., *90:*462, 1973 (French)

PINEL, J. *et al*: Vascular sarcomas of the ethmoid sinus (hemangioendothelioma). Ann. Otolaryngol. Chir. Cervicofac., *92:*557, 1975 (French)

PINKERT, R.: Histological studies of rabbit jaw on tissue reaction following Kallocryl-K implantation. Stomatol. D.D.R., *24:*342, 1974 (German)

PINKERTON, J. A., JR. *et al*: Digital ischemia: hypothenar hammer syndrome J. Kans. Med. Soc., *76:*125, 1975

PINKUS, N. B.: Dangers of oral feeding in presence of cuffed tracheostomy tubes. M. J. Australia, *1:*1238, 1973

PINSKY, L.: Community of human malformation syndromes that shares ectodermal dysplasia and deformities of the hands and feet. Teratology, *11:*227, 1975

PINTO, C. T. *et al*: Adenomeloblastoma, PRS, *53:*110, 1974. Gazeta sanit., *3:*127, 1972

PINTO, E. B. S.: Esthetic solution for *pectus excavatum* in female patients, PRS, *56:*678, 1975. Rev. brasil. cir., *64:*136, 1974

PINTO, R. S. *et al*: Radiologic features of benign pleomorphic adenoma of hard palate. Oral Surg., *39:*976, 1975

PIONER, L.: Plastic surgery for aged. Zahnaerztl. Prax., *22:*1, 1971 (German)

PIOTTI, F.: Causes of failure in esthetic surgery: mammaplasty, PRS, *57:*759, 1976 (Italian). Riv. ital. chir. plast., *7:*447, 1975

PIOTTI, F., MASCETTI, M., AND GAMBARO, G.: Reconstructive plastic surgery of skin cancer of face, PRS, *57:*670, 1976. Riv. ital. chir. plast., *6:*203, 1974

PIPKIN, GARRET, AND BUHLER, VICTOR: *The Illness of Trauma*. Charles C Thomas, Springfield, Ill., 1971. PRS, *50:*519, 1972

PIQUET, J. J. *et al*: Results of surgical treatment of cancers of hypopharynx, 253 cases. Acta Otorhinolaryngol. Belg., *27:*1029, 1973 (French)

PIQUET, J. J. *et al*: Importance of combined radiotherapy and surgery in treatment of cancers of larynx and hypopharynx. Ann. Otolaryngol. Chir. Cervicofac., *90:*633, 1973

PIQUET, J. J. *et al*: Subtotal reconstructive surgery in the treatment of laryngeal cancers. Ann. Otolaryngol. Chir. Cervicofac., *91:*311, 1974 (French)

PIRAGINE, F.: Direct cervical microlymphography as method of checking patients after unilateral radical neck dissection. Ateneo. Parmense (Acta Biomed.), *1:*3, 1972 (Italian)

PIRES, E. D.: Initial surgery of war wounds of hand, PRS, *48:*94, 1971. Rev. port. Mil. Med., *18:*2, 1970

PIROTTA, T.: Hairgrafting. Australas. J. Dermatol., *14:*121, 1973

PIRSIG, W.: Acute nasal trauma in children. Z. Laryngol. Rhinol. Otol., *52:*265, 1973 (German)

PIRSIG, W.: Regeneration of septal cartilage in children after septoplasty. A histological study. Acta Otolaryngol. (Stockh.), *79:*451, 1975 (German)

PIRSIG, W. *et al*: Rhinoplasty in children: follow-up study in 92 cases. Laryngol. Rhinol. Otol. (Stuttg.), *53:*250, 1974 (German)

PISCEVIC, A. *et al*: Correction of jaw deformities by surgical procedures on alveolar process. Stomatol. Glas. Srb., *205:*12, 1972 (Croatian)

PISCEVIC, A. *et al*: Maxillary alveolar protrusions. Rev. Stomatol. Chir. Maxillofac., *75:*128, 1974 (French)

PISCEVIC, A. *et al*: Late results in the surgical treatment of progenia in the area of the mandibular ramus. Med. Pregl., *28:*461, 1975 (Serbian)

PISCEVIC, S. *et al*: Closed injury of common carotid. Vojnosanit. Pregl., *31:*119, 1974 (Serbian)

PISCHKE, F. J., AND BORTNICK, E.: Experimental otoplasty using rabbit ear, PRS, *49:*469, 1972. Arch. Otolaryng., *94:*220, 1971

PITANGUY, I.: Facial hemiatrophy, PRS, *48:*292, 1971. Cir. Plast. Uruguay, *11:*7, 1970

PITANGUY, I.: Dermolipectomies crurales. Ann. chir. Plast., *17:*40, 1972 (French)

PITANGUY, I.: Abdominal lipectomy. Clin. Plast. Surg., *2:*401, 1975

PITANGUY, I.: Correction of lipodystrophy of the lateral thoracic aspect and inner side of the arm and elbow dermosenescence. Clin. Plast. Surg., *2:*477, 1975

PITANGUY, I., AND CANSANCAO, A.: Nipple reduction, PRS, *49:*582, 1972. Rev. brasil. cir., *61:*73, 1971

PITANGUY, I., CANSANCAO, A., AND GARCIA, L. C.: Surgical treatment of nasal tip lesions, PRS, *51:*701, 1973. Rev. brasil. cir., *61:*77, 1972

PITANGUY, I., AND CANSANCAO, A.: Hypermentonism, PRS, *50:*94, 1972. Rev. brasil. cir., *61:*119, 1971

PITANGUY, I., CANSANCAO, A., AND GARCIA, L. C.: Rhytidectomy, PRS, *52:*320, 1973. Rev. brasil. cir., *61:*173, 1971

PITANGUY, I. *et al*: Reconstruction of ear lobe: technical contribution by employing preauricular flap, PRS, *51:*602, 1973. Rev. brasil. cir., *62:*51, 1972

PITANGUY, I. *et al*: Our scheme for rhinoplasty, PRS, *51:*602, 1973. Rev. brasil. cir., *62:*63, 1972

PITANGUY, I., RAMOS, H., AND GARCIA, L. C.: Philosophy, technique, and complications of rhytidectomies through observation and analysis of 2600 personal cases, PRS, *53:*239, 1974. Rev. brasil. cir., *62:*277, 1972

PITANGUY, I. *et al*: Pitanguy-Costa maxillofacial splint, PRS, *51:*711, 1973. Rev. brasil cir., *62:*1212, 1972

PITANGUY, I., DAHER, J. C., AND SOUZA MOTTA, E. F.: Negroid tip of nose; personal contribution to treatment, PRS, *53:*364, 1974. Rev. brasil cir., *63:*52, 1973

PITANGUY, I. *et al*: Rhytidoplasty in men, PRS, *54:*105, 1974. Rev. brasil. cir., *63:*109, 1973

PITANGUY, I. *et al*: Hypoplastic senile chin associated with submandibular adiposity, PRS, *54:*233, 1974. Rev. brasil. cir., *63:*217, 1973

PITANGUY, I., CARREIRAO, S. E., AND GARCIA, L. C.: Transareolar incision for augmentation mammaplasty, PRS, *54:*501, 1974. Rev. brasil. cir., *63:*301, 1973

PITANGUY, I., LESSA, S. F., AND GARCIA, L. C.: Acquired fissures of lip and palate, PRS, *54:*687, 1974. Rev. brasil. cir., *63:*317, 1973

PITANGUY, I. *et al*: Inverted nipple, PRS, *57:*673, 1976. Rev. brasil. cir., *64:*199, 1974

PITANGUY, I. *et al*: Functional alterations in breast hypertrophy, PRS, *57:*673, 1976. Rev. brasil. cir., *64:*209, 1974

PITTMAN, M. R. *et al*: Mesenchymal chondrosarcoma, case report. J. Oral surg., *32:*443, 1974

PITTMAN, M. R. *et al*: Experimental study of autoclaved autogenous mandible in combination with cancellous bone and marrow. J. Oral Surg., *33:*171, 1975

PIZER, M. E. *et al*: Mouth cancer – concepts of treatment. Va. Med. Mon., *99:*148, 1972

PLAGMANN, H. C. *et al*: Experimental studies on epithelial regeneration in heterotopic connective tissue transplantations. Dtsch. Zahnaerztl. Z., *29:*497, 1974 (German)

PLAKHOTNIUK, V. IA. *et al*: Device for dissection of necrotic skin (necrotome). Ortop. Travmatol. Protez., *33:*71, 1972 (Russian)

PLANAS, J.: Introduction of breast implants through the abdominal route. PRS, *57:*434, 1976

PLANAS, J. *et al*: Capsular retraction in mammary prostheses, PRS, *56:*594, 1975. Rev. españ. cir. plast., *7:*206, 1974

PLANQ, V.: Ear aplasia and forked hand. An association of these 2 congenital abnormalities. Ann. chir. plast., *15:*229, 1970 (French)

PLANE, C. *et al:* Section of the optic nerve due to orbital injury. Electrophysiologic examination. Rev. Otoneuroophthalmol., *41:*73, 1969

Plantar Warts (See also *Calluses; Warts*)

Can radiotherapy of plantar warts still be justified? (Sauerbrey). Z. Allgemeinmed., *47:*1584, 1971 (German)

Plantar warts, treatment by blunt dissection (Pringle, Helms), PRS, *54:*376, 1974. Arch. Dermat., *108:*79, 1973

Warts, plantar, plantar calluses, and such (McDowell) (Editorial). PRS, *51:*196, 1973

Keratosis *palmaris et plantaris* (Kisner, Hendrix). PRS, *51:*424, 1973

Keratosis *palmaris et plantaris* – some prospective thoughts (Climo, Kisner) (Letters to the Editor). PRS, *52:*568, 1973

Ultrasound and plantar warts: double blind study (Braatz, McAlistar, Broaddus). PRS, *54:*699, 1974. Mil. Med., *139:*199, 1974

Lichen planus, plantar, treatment by excision and skin grafting (King, Karkowski, Miller). PRS, *56:*668, 1975

Plasma Scalpel

Some technical problems in plasma scalpel hepatectomies (Hishimoto *et al*). ACEMB, *22:*24, 1969

Plasma Scalpel — Cont.

Surgical application of the plasma jet — plasma scalpel surgery (Hishimoto, Goldman). Asian M.J., *15:*264, 1972

Development and evaluation of plasma scalpel: tool for bloodless surgery (Link, Incropera, Glover). HTGDL-9, School of Mechanical Engineering, Purdue Univ., 1973

Laser excision of acute third-degree burns followed by immediate autograft replacement: an experimental study in pigs (Stellar *et al*). J. Trauma, *13:*45, 1973

Wound healing of mouse skin incised with plasma scalpel (Link *et al*). J. Surg. Res., *14:*505, 1973

Thermal response of tissue subjected to plasma scalpel heating (Link, Incropera, Glover). 73-WA/Bio-32, ASME Winter Annual Mtg, Detroit, Mich., 1973

Scalpel, plasma, use of carbon dioxide laser for debridement of third degree burns (Levine *et al*). Ann. Surg., *172:*246, 1974

Carbon dioxide laser excision of acute burns with immediate autografting (Fidler *et al*). J. Surg. Res., *17:*1, 1974

Gas transport resulting from plasma scalpel surgery (Henderson *et al*). Med. Biol. Eng., *12:*208, 1974

Scalpel, plasma, to excise burns (Link, Zook, Glover). PRS, *55:*657, 1975

Laser, scalpel, electrosurgical, and tangential excisions of third degree burns (Levine *et al*). PRS, *56:*286, 1975

Plastic Surgery

Primary Repair of Soft Tissue Injuries. By R. V. S. Thompson. Melbourne (Australia) University Press, 1969. PRS, *48:*276, 1971

Atlas of Surgical Techniques. By Philip Thorek. J. B. Lippincott and Co., Philadelphia and Toronto, 1970. PRS, *55:*356, 1975

Plastic and Reconstructive Surgery. Third Edition. By Hans May. F. A. Davis Co., Philadelphia, 1971. PRS, *48:*589, 1971

Plastic Surgery in Infancy and Childhood. Ed. by John Clarke Mustardé. E. & S. Livingstone, Edinburgh, 1971. PRS, *49:* 451, 1972

Reconstruction Surgery and Traumatology, Volume 12. Ed. by G. Chapchal. Albert J. Phiebig, White Plains, N. Y., 1971.

Can round table discussions be changed? (Vilain). Ann. chir. plast., *16:*191, 1971 (French)

Problems of cutaneous closing (Ducourtioux). Bull. Mem. Soc. Chir. Paris, *61:*310, 1971 (French)

False primary truths, false friends in facial plastic surgery (Jost). Cah. Med., *12:*1275, 1971

Plastic Surgery — Cont.

Should a plastic surgeon take part in treatment of patients with multiple injuries? (Chytilova *et al*). Cas. Lek. Cesk., *110:*673, 1971 (Czechoslovakian)

Soft-tissue lesions, urgent surgery of (Wilflingseder). Langenbeck's Arch. Chir., *329:*88, 1971

Plastic surgery research in otolaryngology (Ogura). Laryngoscope, *81:*1985, 1971

Plastic surgery, reconstructive, post-graduate training in, in East Africa (Rees, Wood). PRS, *48:*5, 1971

JCAH, ill-fated, or who is going to inspect hospitals? (McDowell) (Editorial). PRS, *48:*65, 1971

Plastic surgery, forces and directions in the future of (Lindsay). PRS, *48:*303, 1971

Army, plastic surgery in, short historical account (Jennings). PRS, *48:*413, 1971

Reconstructive and plastic surgery of the face (Neuner). Schweiz. Monatsschr. Zahnheilkd., *81:*947, 1971 (German)

Blood loss and hemostasis in plastic surgery of the skin (Tychinkina *et al.)*. Vestn. Khir., *107:*94, 1971 (Russian)

Clinical use of POR 8 in plastic and reconstructive surgery (Bruck). Wien. Med. Wochenschr., *121:*691, 1971 (German)

Plastic surgery for aged (Pioner). Zahnaerztl. Prax., *22:*1, 1971 (German)

Beyond Plastic Surgery. By Charles Beaver Edwards. Wayne State University Press, Detroit, 1972. PRS, *51:*329, 1973

Early Care of the Injured Patient. By the Committee on Trauma, American College of Surgeons. W. B. Saunders Co., Philadelphia, 1972. PRS, *55:*615, 1975

Fundamental Techniques of Plastic Surgery and their Surgical Applications. 5th Edition. By Ian A. McGregor. Williams & Wilkins Co., Baltimore, 1972. PRS, *53:*342, 1974

Manual of Surgical Therapeutics, Second Edition. Ed. by Robert E. Condon and Lloyd M. Nyhus. Little, Brown & Co., Boston, 1972. PRS, *52:*82, 1973

Plastic and Reconstructive Surgery of the Face and Neck. Ed. by John Conley and John T. Dickinson. Grune & Stratton, New York; Georg Thieme Verlag, Stuttgart, 1972. PRS, *53:*86, 1974

Supportive Care of the Surgical Patient. By William H. Stahl. Grune & Stratton, New York, 1972. PRS, *52:*661, 1973

The Unfavorable Result in Plastic Surgery: Avoidance and Treatment. By Robert M. Goldwyn. Little, Brown & Co., Boston, 1972. PRS, *52:*186, 1973

Plastic surgery, dermatologic. Medico-social

Plastic Surgery—Cont.

Trans. Stud. Coll. Physicians Phila., *41:*124, 1973

Plastic surgery, current possibilities of (Kohnlein). Z. Allgemeinmed., *49:*45, 1973 (German)

The Accident Man. Ed. by D. Mollowitz. Joh. Ambrosius Barth, Frankfurt, 1974. PRS, *56:*333, 1975

Diagnosis and Early Management of Trauma Emergencies: A Manual for the Emergency Service. By Robert J. Touloukian and Thomas J. Krizek. Charles C Thomas, Springfield, Ill., 1974. PRS, *56:*206, 1975

Indication for Operation. Ed. by G. Heberer and G. Hegemann. Springer-Verlag, New York, 1974. PRS, *56:*445, 1975

Is it Moral to Modify Man? Ed. by Claude A. Frazier. Charles C Thomas, Springfield, Ill., 1974. PRS, *55:*356, 1975

Principles of Surgery, 2nd Ed. Ed. by Seymour I. Schwartz *et al.* McGraw-Hill, N. Y., 1974. PRS, *56:*207, 1975

Reconstructive Surgery and Traumatology, Vol. 14. By G. Chapchal. Albert J. Phiebig, White Plains, N. Y., 1974.

Textbook of Surgery: The Biological Basis of Modern Surgical Practice. Ed. by David Sabiston. W. B. Saunders Co., Philadelphia, 1974. PRS, *56:*81, 1975

The Year Book of Plastic and Reconstructive Surgery. Ed. by Kathryn Lyle Stephenson. Year Book Medical Publishers, Inc., Chicago, 1974. PRS, *55:*355, 1975

Knife blades—changing after skin incisions (Jacobs), PRS, *54:*241, 1974. Ann. Surg., *179:*102, 1974

Surgical manpower. Symposium (Chase *et al*). Arch. Surg., *108:*637, 1974

Sequelae, surgical treatment of (Feijo), PRS, *55:*722, 1975. Ars Curandi, *7:*54, 1974

Records, clinical, for plastic surgery, computer storage (Lister), PRS, *56:*684, 1975. Brit. J. Plast. Surg., *27:*47, 1974

United States, production and distribution of surgeons in (Wangensteen, Moore, Waldhausen), PRS, *55:*258, 1975. Bull. Am. Coll. Surgeons, *59:*17, 1974

Surgical and esthetic aspects of the facial profile (D'ottaviano *et al*). Int. J. Oral Surg., *3:*243, 1974

Letter: Who treats facial fractures? (Dupuis *et al*). J. Trauma, *14:*990, 1974

Letter: Who treats facial fractures? (Guralnick). J. Trauma, *14:*990, 1974

Letter: Survey of surgical privileges: a study in futility (Laskin). J. Trauma, *14:*990, 1974

Plastic Surgery—Cont.

Organization and prospects for the development of the surgical service in the USSR; a report to the 29th All-Union Congress of Surgeons (Petrovskii). Khirurgiia (Mosk.), *10:*3, 1974 (Russian)

Editorial: Cosmetic surgery. M. J. Australia, *2:*763, 1974

Progress in American medicine. Current successes, current problems (Schweisheimer). Med. Klin., *69:*711, 1974 (German)

V-Y-S-plasty for closure of round defect (Argamaso). PRS, *53:*99, 1974

Medical service, out-of-country, residency participation in (Henjyoji, Laub). PRS, *53:*660, 1974

Symmetry, natural facial, as preoperative and postoperative consideration (Gorney, Harries). PRS, *54:*187, 1974

Vitamin A-treated mice, enhanced resistance to certain infections in (Cohen, Elin). PRS, *54:*192, 1974

Plastic surgery, role in academic medicine (Edgerton). PRS, *54:*523, 1974

Editorial: Esthetic surgery (Verdan). Rev. Med. Suisse Romande., *94:*8957, 1974 (French)

Surgery in 21st century (Dunphy), PRS, *54:*511, 1974. Surgery, *75:*332, 1974

Consultation with a Plastic Surgeon. By R. L. Dicker and V. R. Syracuse. Nelson-Hall Publishers, Chicago, 1975. PRS, *57:*741, 1976

· *Fundamental Techniques of Plastic Surgery.* 6th edition. By Ian A. McGregor. Longman, Inc., New York, 1975

Plastic Surgery. By Tord Skoog. W. B. Saunders Co., Philadelphia, 1975

Practice of Surgery. Current Review Volume II. By Walter F. Ballinger and Theodore Drapanas. C. V. Mosby Co., St. Louis, 1975. PRS, *57:*374, 1976

Proceedings. (Reconstruction Surgery and Traumatology Series, Vol. 15.) Ed. by G. Chapchal. Albert J. Phiebig, White Plains, N. Y., 1975.

Year Book of Plastic and Reconstructive Surgery. Ed. by Frederick J. McCoy *et al.* Year Book Medical Pub., Inc., Chicago, 1975

Accepting disfigurement when death is the alternative (Tierney). Am. J. Nurs., *75:*2149, 1975

Truncus, plastic surgery of, study of dermal elastic fibers during (Mitz, Elbaz, Vilde), PRS, *56:*233, 1975. Ann. chir. plast., *20:*31, 1975

Medicine and surgery of the profile (Vilain). Ann. chir. plast., *20:*113, 1975 (French)

Three-pronged plasty (Glicenstein *et al*).

Plastic Surgery—Cont.

Ann. chir. plast., *20:*257, 1975 (French)

Aspects of cutaneous plastic surgery in the tropics (Bourrel *et al*). Ann. chir. plast., *20:*375, 1975 (French)

Surgical experiences in Nepal (Melsom). Ann. R. Coll. Surg. Engl., *57:*268, 1975

Regional plastic surgery (Conley). Arch. Otolaryng., *101:*205, 1975

Diagnostic coding in a plastic surgery unit (Crockett). Brit. J. Plast. Surg., *28:*286, 1975

Present and future role of plastic surgery in Africa. A viewpoint (Ejide). East Afr. Med. J., *52:*599, 1975

Problems of plastic and reconstructive surgery in the face (Buschmann). Fortschr. Med., *93:*1691, 1975 (German)

Present status of plastic surgery (Stephenson). J.A.M.A., *234:*929, 1975

Letter: Terminology (Notes). J.A.M.A., *234:*1321, 1975

Memory, interference with, in aging (Smith), PRS, *57:*267, 1976. J. Gerontol., *30:*319, 1975

Letter: Frustrations of oral surgery (Wallace). J. Oral Surg., *33:*247, 1975

Correcting facial deformity (Tempest). Nurs. Times, *71:*1163, 1975

Children, suture removal facilitated in (Johnson). PRS, *55:*97, 1975

Plastic surgery in rural Ethiopia (Finseth), PRS, *55:*545, 1975

Ink, Bonney's blue marking (Johnson). PRS, *56:*155, 1975

Plastic surgery, world of, increasing complexities in (Harding). PRS, *56:*609, 1975

Pigmentation, skin, current concepts and relevance to plastic surgery (Morgan, Gilchrest, Goldwyn), PRS, *56:*617, 1975

Letter: Regional plastic surgeons (Smith). Postgrad. Med., *57:*27, 1975

Molds, metallic facial, direct wax method for fabrication (Zini), PRS, *56:*115, 1975. Prosth. Dent., *33:*95, 1975

Health and disease in rural Ethiopia (Finseth *et al*). Yale J. Biol. Med., *48:*105, 1975

Dog-ears: "crown" excision of facial skin lesions (Robbins), PRS, *57:*251, 1976

Staged operations for better results, "piecemeal principle" (Weisman), PRS, *57:*570, 1976

Lecture slides, graph or text, simple method for producing (Parry, Wolfort, Cochran), PRS, *57:*751, 1976

Plastic Surgery Articles, Reviews of

Plastic surgery—a rapidly developing speciality (Nylen). Nord. Med., *86:*1223, 1971

Plastic Surgery Articles, Reviews of—Cont.
(Swedish)

What is new in plastic surgery? (Strömbeck). Lakartidningen, *69:*2187, 1972 (Swedish)

Recent advances in plastic surgery (Jackson). Scott. Med. J., *17:*153, 1972

Reviews in Plastic Surgery and General Plastic and Reconstructive Surgery. Ed. by Magdy N. Saad and Peter Lechtveld. Excerpta Medica, Amsterdam. American Elsevier Publishing Co., Inc. New York, 1974. PRS, *57:*91, 1976

Recent Advances in Plastic Surgery, Number One. Ed. by James Calnan. Longman, Inc., New York, 1976

Plastic Surgery Books: See *Books*

Plastic Surgery History: See *History of Plastic Surgery*

Plastic Surgery, Medicolegal Aspects: See *Legal Aspects*

Plastic Surgery, Military: See *War Injuries*

Plastic Surgery, Office

Outpatient surgery, comfortable mattress for (McKinney, Monn). PRS, *52:*446, 1973

Plastic surgery in office surgical unit (Williams). PRS, *52:*513, 1973

Office surgery: plastic surgery operatory unit (Dingman, Pickens). PRS, *56:*673, 1973

Office surgery and pursuit of excellence (Davis) (Editorial). PRS, *54:*345, 1974

Office plastic surgery (Tipton). PRS, *54:*660, 1974

Costs and charges for use of office operating room (Barker). PRS, *57:*7, 1976

Plastic Surgery, Psychology of (See also *Factitious Lesions*)

Errors in indications for plastic operations (Coerdt). Langenbecks Arch. Chir., *327:*652, 1970 (German)

Psychiatric complications, long-term incidence in severely burned adults (Andreasen, Norris, Hartford), PRS, *49:*666, 1972. Ann. Surg., *174:*785, 1971

Psychological response to trauma, management and study (Titchener), PRS, *48:*95, 1971. J. Trauma, *10:*974, 1971

Somatic delusions, problem in patients seeking cosmetic surgery (Druss, Symonds, Crikelair). PRS, *48:*246, 1971

Motivational patterns of patients seeking cosmetic (esthetic) surgery (Edgerton, Knorr). PRS, *48:*551, 1971

Psychopathologic phenomena in burned persons (Pavlovsky), PRS, *52:*327, 1973. Acta

Plastic Surgery, Psychology of—Cont.

chir. plast., *4:*112, 1972

Emotional reactions, management in seriously burned adults (Andreasen *et al*), PRS, *51:*107, 1973. New England J. Med., *286:*65, 1972

Adulthood of 98 cleft lip-palate children, psychological findings (Clifford, Crocker, Pope). PRS, *50:*234, 1972

Operating for the aging face (Goldwyn). Psychiatry Med., *3:*187, 1972

Psychological Aspects of the "Cleft Palate Problem," Vol. I. By D. C. Spriestersbach. Vol. II. By D. C. Spriestersbach, Gene R. Powers, *et al.* University of Iowa Press, Iowa City, 1973. PRS, *54:*215, 1974

Rehabilitation of the Facially Disfigured. Prevention of Irreversible Psychic Trauma by Early Reconstruction. By J. J. Longacre. Charles C Thomas Co., Springfield, Ill., 1973. PRS, *54:*93, 1974

Otolaryngology, psychological problems in (Lucente). Laryngoscope, *83:*1684, 1973

Plastic surgery in prison. An apparently negative result (Lehman *et al*). Ohio State Med. J., *69:*893, 1973

Deformed delinquent adolescents, is plastic surgery effective in the rehabilitation of? (Meyer *et al*). PRS, *51:*53, 1973

Psychological disturbances: suicide attempts related to congenital facial deformities (Berger). PRS, *51:*323, 1973

Psychological aspects of esthetic plastic surgery of face (Edson-Sperli), PRS, *53:*239, 1974. Rev. Latino Am. cir. plast., *17:*15, 1973

Disease and Social Behavior—An Interdisciplinary Perspective. By Horacio Fabrega, Jr. M. I. T. Press, Cambridge, Mass., 1974. PRS, *55:*699, 1975

The Right to Look Human. By Jack Penn, McGraw-Hill Book Co., Johannesburg, New York, 1974. PRS, *56:*664, 1975

Plastic surgery, aspects. Psychiatric aspects of referral (Olley). Brit. Med. J., *3:*248, 1974

Aspects of plastic surgery. Social and psychological sequelae (Olley). Brit. Med. J., *3:*322, 1974

Psychological aspects of hand injury (Cone, Hueston), PRS, *54:*236, 1974. M. J. Australia, *1:*104, 1974

Psychosexual dynamics of patients undergoing mammary augmentation (Baker, Kolin, Bartlett). PRS, *53:*652, 1974

Sex reassignment: gender dysphoria syndromes: position statement on so-called "transsexualism" (Meyer, Hoopes). PRS, *54:*444, 1974

Plastic Surgery, Psychology of—Cont.

Special psychological aspect of the relation between client and surgeon in cosmetic surgery (Janvier *et al*). Rev. Med. Suisse Romande., *94:*963, 1974 (French)

Psychiatry of aging. An outline for plastic surgery (Bochnik). In *Plastische und Wiederherstellungs-Chirurgie,* ed. by Hohler; pp. 3-12. Schattauer, Stuttgart, 1975 (German)

Weight loss, personal reaction to (Pescatore), PRS, *56:*116, 1975. Am. J. Nursing, *74:*2227, 1975

Accepting disfigurement when death is the alternative (Tierney). Am. J. Nurs., *75:*2149, 1975

Psychological implications of cosmetic surgery (Lejour, Lecocq), PRS, *56:*603, 1975. Acta chir. belg., *74:*5, 1975

Psychology and plastic surgery: service rendered to patients (Grignon), PRS, *57:*681, 1976. Ann. chir. plast., *20:*95, 1975

Happiness, mood as indicant of (Cameron), PRS, *57:*267, 1976. J. Gerontol., *30:*216, 1975

Elderly medical-surgical patients, unrecognized psychiatric illness in (Schuckit, Miller, Hahlbohm), PRS, *57:*683, 1976. J. Gerontol., *30:*655, 1975

Children, psychological preparation for surgery, stress responses and adjustments (Visintainer, Wolfer), PRS, *57:*544, 1976. Pediatrics, *56:*187, 1975

Motivation: factors influencing patient satisfaction with results of esthetic plastic surgery (Reich). PRS, *55:*5, 1975

Emotionally disturbed patient, plastic surgeon's obligations to (Edgerton) (Editorial). PRS, *55:*81, 1975

Neurosis, obsessive, loss of columella and septum from unusual form of child abuse (Orton). PRS, *56:*345, 1975

Operate, decision to, a socioeconomic perspective in urban state (Scott, Mackie), PRS, *57:*768, 1976. Surgery, *77:*311, 1975

Maladjustment, use of behavior modification therapy in recalcitrant burned child (Zide, Pardoe). PRS, *57:*378, 1976

PLATH, P. *et al*: Tracheotomy or long-time intubation? H. N. O., *20:*29, 1972 (German)

PLAUE, R.: Operative treatment of decubitus ulcers. Arch. Orthop. Unfallchir., *77:*223, 1973 (German)

PLAZA CARRANZA, F.: Recurrences of ameloblastomas of the jaws. Rev. Stomatol. Chir. Maxillofac., *75:*53, 1974 (French)

PLENK, H. JR. *et al*: Microscopic observations on the course of muscles and the construction of the upper lip of man. Verh. Anat. Ges., 65:341, 1971 (German)

PLESS, J.: Laminate-plasty reconstruction of partial auricular defects, PRS, 57:394, 1976. Scand. J. Plast. Reconstr. Surg., 9:40, 1975

PLESS, J.: Replantation of severed ear parts (with Larsen), PRS, 57:176, 1976. Discussion by Mladick, PRS, 57:375, 1976

PLESS, J., AND SONDERGAARD, W.: Effect of halothane on tissue necrosis in pedicle skin flaps in pigs, PRS, 51:109, 1973. Scand. J. Plast. Reconstr. Surg., 6:13, 1972

PLETCHER, J. D. et al: Preoperative embolization of juvenile angiofibromas of the nasopharynx. Ann. Otol. Rhin. & Laryng., 84:740, 1975

PLEWIG, G.: Dermabrasion for nodular cutaneous elastosis with cysts and comedones. Arch. Dermat., 105:294, 1972

PLINER, M. A. et al: A case of combined lesions of the cervical lymph nodes from actinomycosis and tuberculosis. Probl. Tuberk., 49:78, 1971 (Russian)

PLOTNIKOV, N. A.: Problem of osteoplasty of lower jaw. Stomatologiia (Mosk.), 52:43, 1973 (Russian)

PLOTNIKOV, N. A. et al: Roentgenological assessment of reconstruction of articular end of lyophilized jaw transplanted into defect of lower jaw following its resection with exarticulation. Stomatologiia (Mosk.), 52:35, 1973 (Russian)

POATE, W. J.: Subcutaneous mastectomy with immediate reconstruction of the breast. Aust. N. Z. J. Surg., 45:383, 1975

POCTA, J. et al: Ketalar in burns. Rozhl. Chir., 51:7, 1972 (Czechoslovakian)

PODDUBNYI, V. P.: Neurilemmoma of the parotid region. Vestn. Otorinolaringol., 4:64, 1974 (Russian)

PODLESCH, I.: Technic of anesthesia in ankylosis of the temporomandibular joints. Fortschr. Kiefer. Gesichtschir., 18:121, 1974 (German)

PODLEWSKI, J. et al: Skin carcinoma in contused head injury treated surgically. Wiad. Lek., 27:557, 1974 (Polish)

PODLUZHNIY, G. A.: Single-stage correction of chordee and urethral plasty in penile forms of hypospadias. Acta Chir. Plast. (Praha), 15:190, 1973

PODOSHIN, L. et al: Use of the foley balloon catheter in zygomatic-arch fractures. Brit. J. Oral Surg., 12:246, 1974

PODOSHIN, L. et al: Unusual presentation of a frontal mucocoele. Eye Ear Nose Throat Mon., 54:69, 1975

PODOSWA, G., AND TALAVERA, S.: Osteoma cutis, PRS, 48:198, 1971. Dermat. Rev. Mexicana, 14:163, 1970

PODOSWA, G., LAGUNA, O., AND ARMENDARES, S.: Congenital universal alopecia, PRS, 57:267, 1976. Dermat. Ibero Lat. Am., 13:223, 1971

POGASIAN, L. R.: Treatment of poisonous snake bites. Khirurgiia (Mosk.), 48:129, 1972 (Russian)

POHL, A. L., LARSON, D. L., AND LEWIS, S. R.: Thumb reconstruction in severely burned hand. PRS, 57:320, 1976

POHL, G.: Time for surgery – urgency and delayed operation. Beitr. Orthop. Traumatol., 21:21, 1974 (German)

POIRIER, R. A., AND STANSEL, H. C., JR.: Arterial aneurysms of hand, PRS, 51:230, 1973. Am. J. Surg., 124:72, 1972

POISSON, R., AND FRANCHEBOIS, P.: Triangular cervical flap for primary reconstruction of oropharyngeal surgical defects, PRS, 54:500, 1974. Canad. J. Surg., 17:167, 1974

POISSON R. et al: Triangular cervical flap in primary reconstruction of buccopharyngeal cavity. Union Med. Can., 103:1420, 1974 (French)

POKROVSKII, A. V. et al: Indications and technic of creating a lympho-venous anastomosis in lymphedema of the extremities. Klin. Khir., 9:11, 1971 (Russian)

POKROVSKLI, A. V. et al: Pathogenesis and surgical treatment of post-thrombophlebitic and varicose leg ulcers. Khirurgiia (Mosk.), 11:73, 1974 (Russian)

POLIAKOVA, A. M. et al: Sutureless fixation of free skin transplants during removal of cicatricial deformities of the eyelids. Vestn. Oftalmol., 3:56, 1971 (Russian)

POLK, H. C., JR.: Modern trends in care of burn patient. D. M., 1:39, 1973

POLK, HIRMAN C., JR., AND STONE, H. HARLAN: Contemporary Burn Management. Little, Brown & Co., Boston, 1971.

POLK, H. C., JR., AND LINN, B. S.: Selective regional lymphadenectomy for melanoma, a mathematical aid to clinical judgment, PRS, 50:97, 1972. Ann. Surg., 174:402, 1971

POLK, H. C., JR. et al.: "Prophylactic" regional lymph node dissection. Ann. Surg., 180:257, 1974

POLLACK, R. S.: Carotid body tumors – idiosyncracies. Oncology, 27:81, 1973

POLLAN, L. D. et al: Osseous cryosurgery and its effect on adjacent pulpal tissues. Oral Surg., 38:668, 1974

POLLET, J.: Views of plastic surgeon concerning nasal obstructions. Probl. Actuels Otorhinolaryngol., 203:22, 1971 (French)

POLLET, J.: Skin resection for Corbin's beaked nose. Ann. chir. plast., 17:15, 1972 (French)

POLLET, J.: Use of osteo-cartilaginous fragments removed during rhinoseptoplasty. Ann. chir. plast., *17:*90, 1972 (French)

POLLET, J.: Three autogenous struts for nasal tip support. PRS, *49:*527, 1972

POLLET, J.: Crow's feet. Ann. chir. plast., *18:*191, 1973 (French)

POLLET, J.: Breast augmentation prostheses. Critical study of results. Ann. chir. plast., *18:*301, 1973 (French)

POLLET, J. *et al*: Cutaneous resections for correction of so-called "crow's beak" deformity after rhinoplasty. Ann. Otolaryngol. Chir. Cervicofac., *90:*481, 1973 (French)

POLLOCK, W. J., VIRNELLI, F. R., AND RYAN, R. F.: Axillary hidradenitis suppurativa, simple, effective surgical technique. PRS, *49:*22, 1972

POLLOCK, W. J., COLON, G. A., AND RYAN, R. F.: Reconstruction of lower eyelid by different lid-splitting operation. PRS, *50:*184, 1972

POLLOCK, W. J., BITSEFF, E. L., AND RYAN, R. F.: Rapid transfer of thoracoacromial flaps to face and neck. PRS, *50:*433, 1972

Polychondritis

E. N. T. changes of atrophic polychondritis: report of a case (Iglesias Cendon). Acta Otorinolaryngol. Iber. Am., *22:*351, 1971 (Spanish)

Polychondritis, relapsing (Jones). PRS, *51:*331, 1973

POMERANCE, H. H.: Congenital prolabial-maxillary scar: a possible minor expression of cleft lip. J. Pediatr., *78:*868, 1971

POMOSOV, D. V. *et al*: Catheterization of the bronchial tree via tracheocentesis. Voen. Med. Zh., *9:*71, 1975 (Russian)

POMPINO, H. J.: Reply to the article by W. Schmitt and coworkers: "Surgery of bladder exstrophy using ureterosigmoideostomy and cystectomy" in: Zschr. Urol., *64:*509, 1971. Z. Urol. Nephrol., *65:*289, 1972 (German)

POMPINO, H. J.: Possibilities of operative treatment of children with exstrophy of bladder. Munch. Med. Wochenschr., *116:*1187, 1974 (German)

POMPNER, K.: Foreign body injuries of hands. Zentralbl. Chir., *98:*1438, 1973 (German)

PONCET, E. *et al*: Restoration of the external ear in aplasias using skin grafts in the canal. Ann. Otolaryngol. Chir. Cervicofac., *91:*526, 1974 (French)

PONCET, E., *et al*: Severe emergency epistaxis. Ann. Otolaryngol. Chir. Cervicofac., *92:*145, 1975 (French)

PONCET, P.: Operations on residual or recurrent cervical adenopathies following curative doses of cobalt therapy. Ann. Otolaryngol. Chir. Cervicofac., *89:*405, 1972 (French)

PONCET, P.: Salvage laryngectomy and pharyngolaryngectomy after cancericidal cobalt therapy. Acta Otorhinolaryngol. Belg., *27:*1005, 1973 (French)

PONCE, P.: Unusual air cavity of parotid niche. Ann. Otolaryngol. Chir. Cervicofac., *90:*376, 1973 (French)

POND, H. S., AND BRANNAN, W.: Correction of congenital curvature of penis, PRS, *57:*536, 1976. J. Urol., *112:*491, 1974

PONIECKI, A. *et al*: Romberg-type hemiatrophy in a case of severe rheumatoid arthritis. Wiad. Lek., *24:*1313, 1971 (Polish)

PONS, J. *et al*: Facial injuries caused by shot wounds. Rev. Stomatol. Chir. Maxillofac., *72:*743, 1971 (French)

PONS, J. *et al*: Prosthetic reconstruction of a therapeutic destruction of the facial massif (technical considerations). Rev. Stomatol. Chir. Maxillofac., *72:*821, 1971 (French)

PONS, J. *et al*: Injuries of medial vertical third of face. Rev. Fr. Odontostomatol., *19:*27, 1972 (French)

PONS, J. *et al*: Trans-buccal subtotal mandibular resection with immediate reconstruction. Ann. chir. plast., *18:*155, 1973 (French)

PONS, J. *et al*: Rare variant of odontogenic tumor. Rev. Stomatol. Chir. Maxillofac., *74:*506, 1973 (French)

PONTEN, B.: Follow-up study of skin transplantation in leg ulcer. Nord. Med., *88:*1221, 1971 (Swedish)

PONTEN, B.: Plastic surgery treatment of chronic venous ulcers of the leg. Scand. J. Plast. Reconstr. Surg., *6:*74, 1972

PONTEN, B. *et al*: New observations on tissue changes along pathway of current in electrical injury. Case report, PRS, *49:*472, 1972. Scand. J. Plast. Reconstr. Surg., *4:*75, 1970

PONTES, R.: Technique of reduction mammaplasty. Brit. J. Plast. Surg., *26:*365, 1973

PONTES, R.: Single stage reconstruction of missing breast. Brit. J. Plast. Surg., *26:*377, 1973

POPA, D. P. *et al*: Possibilities of ensuring lacrimal drainage by permeabilization of the obstructed nasolacrimal duct. Rev. Chir. (Oftalmol.), *19:*307, 1975 (Rumanian)

POPE, B. A.: Psychological findings in adulthood of 98 cleft lip-palate children (with Clifford, Crocker). PRS, *50:*234, 1972

POPELKA, S.: Surgical treatment of the rheumatic hand. Handchirurgie, *1:*223, 1969 (German)

POPELKA, S.: Technic of plastic surgery of metacarpophalangeal joints in patients with chronic arthritis. Acta Chir. Orthop. Traumatol. Cech., *39:*147, 1972 (Czechoslovakian)

POPESCU, V.: Temporomandibular arthroplasty by interposition of full-thickness skin graft, PRS, *49:*103, 1972. Rev. port. maxillofacial surg., *2:*223, 1970

POPESCU, V. *et al*: Surgical treatment of severe dento-maxillary irregularities. Int. Dent. J., *21:*346, 1971

POPESCU, V. *et al*: Plastic reconstitution of functional rehabilitation after great surgical ablations in maxillofacial tumors. J. Med. Lyon, *53:*303, 1972 (French)

POPESCU, V. *et al*: Reduction of bleeding by vasoconstrictive drug infiltration in the surgery cleft lip and cleft palate. Stomatologia (Bucur.), *19:*51, 1972 (Rumanian)

POPESCU, V. *et al*: Corrective osteotomies in the sequelae of operations for congenital labio-maxillo-palatine malformations. Rev. Stomatol. Chir. Maxillofac., *75:*86, 1974

POPESCU, V. *et al*: Vertical osteotomy of ascending rami mandibular retrognathism. J. Maxillo-facial Surg., *3:*65, 1975

POPESCU, V. *et al*: Plombage with osseous homotransplants in some mandibular tumors. Rev. Chir. (Stomatol.), *22:*209, 1975 (Rumanian)

POPESCU, V. *et al*: Results obtained with bone homograft in cystic tumors of the jaw. Rev. Odontostomatol. (Paris), *4:*51, 1975 (French)

POPESCU, V. C.: Advancement of middle third of face without bone grafting in Crouzon's disease, PRS, *55:*716, 1975. J. Maxillo-facial Surg., *2:*219, 1974

POPESCU, V. D.: Vertical osteotomy of ascending rami in mandibular retrognathism, PRS, *57:*530, 1976. J. Maxillo-facial Surg., *3:*65, 1975

POPKIROV, S.: Diagnosis and therapy of bone infections of the hand. Hefte Unfallheilkd., *107:*225, 1970 (German)

POPKIROV, S.: Myoplastic closure of fistulae of osteomyelitic origin, PRS, *51:*610, 1973. Bruns' Beitr. klin. Chir., *219:*658, 1972

POPOVIC, D. *et al*: Current war injuries of extremities. Vojnosanit. Pregl., *32:*546, 1975 (Serbian)

POPOVIC, V. *et al*: Reconstructive plastic surgery of the nose. Med. Glas., *25:*72, 1971 (Croatian)

POPP, M. B., LAW, E. J., AND MACMILLAN, B. G.: Parenteral nutrition in burned child: study of 26 patients, PRS, *54:*378, 1974. Ann. Surg., *179:*219, 1974

POPPERS, P. J. *et al*: Evaluation of Etidocaine, new local anesthetic agent with modified bilateral ulnar nerve block technique, PRS, *54:*248, 1974. J. Anesth., *40:*13, 1974

POPSTEFANOW, A. *et al*: Topographic-anatomic tables for the graphical demonstration of di-

agnosis of open and covered hand injuries. Beitr. Orthop. Traumatol., *19:*167, 1972 (German)

PORADOVSKA, W., JAWORSKA, M., AND HANC, I.: Donohue's syndrome (leprechaunism) in female infant, PRS, *51:*233, 1973. Acta chir. plast., *14:*4, 1972

PORADOWSKA, W. *et al*: Diagnosis and treatment of anterior encephalocele, PRS, *54:*630, 1974. Acta chir. plast., *15:*137, 1973

PORLSEN, C. O., AND JACOBSEN, G. K.: Chemotherapy of human malignant melanoma transplanted in nude mouse, PRS, *57:*678, 1976. Cancer Res., *35:*2990, 1975

PORTER, B. B. *et al*: Limb and joint transplantation. Review of research and clinical experience. Clin. Orthop., *104:*249, 1974

PORTER, J. M. *et al*: Diagnosis and treatment of Raynaud's phenomenon, PRS, *56:*107, 1975. Surgery, *77:*11, 1975

PORTERFIELD, J. D.: Director of JCAH replies (Letter to the Editor). PRS, *48:*584, 1971

PORTMANN, G. *et al*: Hemi-pharyngolaryngectomy with monoblock lymph node dissection and reconstruction. Rev. Laryngol. Otol. Rhinol. (Bord.), *93:*94, 1972 (French)

PORTUGALOVA, V. V.: Histochemical data on human skin melanoma in relation to treatment. Vopr. Onkol., *20:*3, 1974 (Russian)

Port-Wine Stains: See *Hemangioma*

PORWOLIK, E. *et al*: Tracheotomy tube with tightening balloon. Pol. Przegl. Chir., *46:*781, 1974 (Polish)

POSAZHENNIKOV, A. P.: Removal of glass fragment from the orbit. Oftalmol. Zh., *28:*302, 1974 (Russian)

POSCH, J. L.: Use of cross-finger flap for treatment of congenital broad constricting bands of fingers (with Artz). PRS, *52:*645, 1973

POSNER, D. M.: Ehlers-Danlos syndrome, coexisting with a Martin-Gruber anastomosis. A case report. Ohio State Med. J., *69:*453, 1973

POSNER, M. A. *et al*: Advancement pedicle flap for thumb injuries. J. Bone & Joint Surg. (Am.), *53:*1618, 1971

POST, B.: Clinical picture and histology of metastasizing spinalioma, treated with bleomycin. Z. Hautkr., *48:*1019, 1973 (German)

POSTHUMUS MYEJES, F. E.: Acute peripheral facial nerve paralysis, prognostic criteria and value of surgical decompression. Ned. tijdschr. geneeskd., *116:*319, 1972 (Dutch)

POSTI, J. J. *et al*: Surgical orthodontic and prosthetic treatment of six imperfectly erupted permanent teeth. Proc. Finn. Dent. Soc., *70:*75, 1974

POSTLETHWAIT, R. W., WILLIGAN, D. A., AND ULIN, A. W.: Human tissue reaction to sutures, PRS, *56:*233, 1975. Ann. Surg., *181:*144, 1975

Poswillo, D.: Otomandibular deformity: pathogenesis as guide to reconstruction. PRS, *55:*378, 1975. J. Maxillo-facial Surg., *2:*64, 1974

Poswillo, D.: Surgery of temporomandibular joint. Oral Sci. Rev., *6:*87, 1974

Poswillo, D.: Pathogenesis of submucous cleft palate, PRS, *56:*359, 1975. Scand. J. Plast. Reconstr. Surg., *8:*34, 1974

Poswillo, D.: Pathogenesis of Treacher Collins syndrome (mandibulofacial dysostosis), PRS, *57:*528, 1976, Brit. J. Oral Surg., *13:*1, 1975

Poswillo, D.: Evaluation, surveillance and treatment of panoral leukoplakia. J. Maxillofacial Surg., *3:*205, 1975

Poswillo, D. E.: Cryosurgery and electrosurgery compared in the treatment of experimentally induced oral carcinoma. Brit. Dent. J., *131:*347, 1971

Poswillo, D. E.: Late effects of mandibular condylectomy. Oral Surg., *33:*500, 1972

Poswillo, D. E.: Orofacial malformations, PRS, *55:*375, 1975. Proc. Roy. Soc. Med., *67:*343, 1974

Poswillo, D. E.: Cryosurgery of the oral mucous membranes. Proc. Roy. Soc. Med., *68:*608, 1975

Potapov, I. I. *et al*: Local cryotherapy in treatment of benign and malignant tumors of otorhinolaryngeal organs. Vestn. Otorinolaringol., *35:*8, 1973 (Russian)

Potdar, G. G. *et al*: Mixed salivary tumors. Indian J. Cancer, *10:*217, 1973

Potenza, A. D.: Flexor tendon injuries. Orthop. Clin. North Am., *1:*355, 1970

Potenza, A. D.: Technique for arthrodesis of finger joints, PRS, *54:*108, 1974. J. Bone & Joint Surg., *55A:*1534, 1973

Potgieter, M. G.: Some aspects of facial nerve paralysis. I. Introduction, etiology, applied anatomy and topognosis, and degree of paralysis. South African M. J., *47:*27, 1973

Potgieter, M. G.: Some aspects of facial nerve paralysis. 3. Complications, prognosis and management. South African M. J., *47:*100, 1973

Potsic, W. P. *et al*: Reimplantation of amputated pinna. Arch. Otolaryng., *100:*73, 1974

Potter, Guy D.: *Sectional Anatomy and Tomography of the Head*. Grune and Stratton, New York, 1971. PRS, *51:*84, 1973

Poulton, D. R.: Treatment planning in maxillary prognathism. Am. J. Orthod., *65:*430, 1974

Poulton, D. R.: Case report (chin). Angle Orthod., *44:*167, 1974

Poulton, D. R. and Ware, W. H.: Surgical-orthodontic treatment of severe mandibular retrusion. Am. J. Orthod., *63:*237, 1973

Pourquier, H. *et al*: Tumors of maxillary sinus. Study of 53 cases treated with radiotherapy and surgery combined or isolated radiotherapy. J. Radiol. Electrol. Med. Nucl., *54:*27, 1973 (French)

Pous, J. G.: Ileal bladder controlled by the anal sphincter. Ann. Chir. Infant., *12:*443, 1971 (French)

Pous, J. G. *et al*: Aneurisms of the hand and fingers in children. Ann. Chir., *29:*1005, 1975 (French)

Poutasse, E. F.: Peyronie's disease, PRS, *51:*604, 1973. J. Urol., *107:*419, 1972

Povstianof, N. E. *et al*: Post-burn defects of the hand. Khirurgiia (Mosk.), *4:*36, 1975 (Russian)

Powell, J., and Glaser, J.: Aneurysmal bone cyst of orbit, PRS, *56:*591, 1975. Arch. Ophth., *93:*340, 1975

Powell, R. O., Larson, A. L., and Hankin, R. I.: Nasal and mucous membrane biopsy, Sjögren's syndrome, PRS, *55:*246, 1975. Ann. Int. Med., *81:*25, 1974

Powers, G. L., and Starr, C. D.: Effect of muscle exercise on velopharyngeal gap and nasality, PRS, *55:*251, 1975. Cleft Palate J., *11:*28, 1974

Powers, Gene R.: *Cleft Palate*. Bobbs-Merrill Co., Inc., Indianapolis, Ind., 1973

Powley, Philip: *Trauma Surgery Excepting Bones and Joints*. 1st Edition. John Wright and Sons, Ltd., Bristol, England, 1973. PRS, *53:*585, 1974

Poyzer, K. G. *et al*: Pseudorecidivism of irradiated basal cell carcinoma. Australas. J. Dermatol., *15:*77, 1974

Pozatek, Z. W., Kaban, L. B., and Guralnick, W. C.: Fractures of zygomatic complex: evaluation of surgical management with special emphasis on eyebrow approach. J. Oral Surg., *31:*141, 1973

Pozdniakova, T. N.: Plastic surgery in traumatic amputation of the penis. Vestn. Khir., *107:*59, 1971 (Russian)

Poznanski, A. K. *et al*: New family with the hand-foot-genital syndrome—a wider spectrum of the hand-foot-uterus syndrome. Birth Defects, *11:*127, 1975

Pradhan, A. C., Varma, R. K., and Pradhan, S.: Myxoma of hard palate, PRS, *51:*234, 1973. Internat. Surg., *57:*341, 1972

Pradier, R. *et al*: Deltopectoral flap in reconstruction for resection of head and neck cancer, PRS, *54:*626, 1974. Rev. argent. cir., *26:*32, 1974

Pradier, R. N. *et al*: Deltopectoral flap in surgery of head and neck cancer, PRS *51:*485,

Pressure Scores — Cont.

Spinal injuries, bactericidal effect of air-fluidized bed (Sharbaugh, Gargest, Wright), PRS, *52:*602, 1973. Am. Surgeon, *39:*253, 1973

Ischiectomy associated with muscular plasty, in treatment of ischiatic bedsores (Dupuis, Debray, Vilain). Ann. chir. plast., *18:*27, 1973 (French)

Decubitus ulcers, operative treatment of (Plaue). Arch. Orthop. Unfallchir., *77:*223, 1973 (German)

Flaps, delaying of, useful adjunct (in treatment of decubitus ulcer) (Williams). Brit. J. Plast. Surg., *26:*61, 1973

Decubitus ulcers, severe, treatment using Beaufort-Winchester water bed (Grahame *et al*). Brit. J. Plast. Surg., *26:*75, 1973

Decubitus ulcers, chronic, in paraplegics with stationary neurological lesions, surgical treatment (Riebelova). Cas. Lek. Cesk., *112:*25, 1973 (Czechoslovakian)

Decubitus ulcers, principles in treatment of (Sundell *et al*). Duodecim, *89:*1234, 1973 (Finnish)

Decubitus ulcers: prevention and treatment (Guthrie *et al*). Geriatrics, *28:*67, 1973

Decubitus ulcer and its incidence in rehabilitation of neurological patients (Chantraine *et al*). J. Belge Rhumatol. Med. Phys., *28:*386, 1973 (French)

Pressure sores, use of water bed for prevention of (Siegel, Vistnes, Laub), PRS, *51:*31, 1973

Decubitus ulcers in paraplegic. II. Surgical treatment (Fissette *et al*). Rev. Med. Liege, *28:*475, 1973 (French)

Trophic ulcers, Clofazimine ointment in treatment (Ellis, Taube). South African M. J., *47:*378, 1973

Surgical treatment of bedsores (Brodeur *et al*). Union Med. Can., *102:*1921, 1973

Debridement of decubitus ulcers with carbon dioxide laser (Stellar *et al*), PRS, *54:*242, 1974. Ann. Surg., *179:*230, 1974

Decubitus ulcer, surgical treatment in adult patients with spinal cord injuries (Remus *et al*). Arch. Orthop. Unfallchir., *79:*119, 1974 (German)

Wheelchair cushions to reduce pressure under bony prominences (Souther, Carr, Vistnes), PRS, *55:*519, 1975. Arch. Phys. Med., *55:*460, 1974

Enzyme spray to heal decubitus ulcers (Yucel, Basmajian), PRS, *55:*640, 1975. Arch. Phys. Med. & Rehab., *55:*517, 1974

Surgical treatment of pressure sores — study of results (Glaumann *et al*). Lakartidningen, *71:*493, 1974 (Swedish)

Pressure Scores — Cont.

Ascorbic acid supplementation in treatment of pressure sores (Taylor *et al*), PRS, *55:*254, 1975. Lancet, *2:*544, 1974

Decubitus ulcer, particular type (Sanders *et al*). Ned. tijdschr. geneeskd., *118:*233, 1974 (Dutch)

Pressure sores, split-skin graft and treatment of (Nuseibeh), PRS, *56:*114, 1975. Paraplegia, *12:*1, 1974

Beds to prevent tissue ischemia in paraplegic patients, comparison of four (Carpendale), PRS, *56:*115, 1975. Paraplegia, *12:*21, 1974

Decubitus ulcers, value of sinography in the management of (Lopez, Aranha), PRS, *53:*208, 1974

Pressure necrosis: knee-to-knee syndrome (Carlin), PRS, *53:*353, 1974

Pressure, tissue ischemia, and operating table pads (Souther, Vistnes) (Letter to the Editor), PRS, *53:*465, 1974

Decubitus ulcer, sacral, repaired by turnover island flap of gluteus maximus muscle (Stallings, Delgado, Converse), PRS, *54:*52, 1974

Decubitus ulcer, use of a long island flap to bring sensation to the sacral area in young paraplegics (Dibbell), PRS, *54:*220, 1974

Ulcer, decubitus, with necrosis of penis: debridement and closure with scrotal flap (Lanier, Neale), PRS, *54:*609, 1974

Myelomeningocele, reconstructive surgical procedures (Curtin), PRS, *54:*505, 1974. South. M. J., *67:*406, 1974

Bacteroides bacteremia from decubitus ulcers (Rissing *et al*), PRS, *55:*646, 1975. South, M. J., *67:*1179, 1974

Decubitus ulcers, flotation pad therapy for (Paradis), PRS, *56:*111, 1975. Arch. Phys. Med. & Rehab., *56:*40, 1975

Pressure sores, operant conditioning approach to prevention (Malament, Dunn, Davis), PRS, *56:*470, 1975. Arch. Phys. Med. & Rehab., *56:*161, 1975

Pressure sores, treatment in handicapped children (Lang), PRS, *57:*683, 1976. Cutis, *16:*158, 1975

Hydrotherapy and topical collagenase for decubitus ulcers (Vetra *et al*). Geriatrics, *30:*53, 1975

Early dermoplasty of decubitus ulcer in spine and spinal cord injuries (Bazilevskaia). Khirurgiia (Mosk.), *11:*128, 1975 (Russian)

Treatment of decubitus ulcers (Berecek). Nurs. Clin. North Am., *10:*171, 1975

Pressure "sore" closures, preventing recurrent tissue breakdowns after (Rogers, Wilson), PRS, *56:*419, 1975. Discussion by Brand, PRS, *56:*573, 1975

Pressure Scores—Cont.

Advances in the surgical treatment of pressure sores (Landa *et al*). Rev. Surg., *33:*1, 1976

PREUS, M. *et al*: Lobster claw defect with ectodermal defects, cleft lip-palate, tear duct anomaly and renal anomalies. Clin. Genet., *4:*369, 1973

PRÉVOST, Y.: Simplifying Le Fort I type of maxillary osteotomy (with Dupont, Ciaburro), PRS, *54:*142, 1974

PRÉVOST-THIÉRIOT, G. *et al*: Pathological and clinical study of 15 keloid scars, PRS, *51:*608, 1973. Ann. dermat. & syph., *99:*269, 1972

PREVOT, J: Apropos of Bricker's operation. Ann. Chir. Infant., *12:*462, 1971 (French)

PRICE, E. *et al*: Solitary keratoacanthoma in child. Am. J. Dis. Child., *128:*110, 1974

PRICE, E. W.: Nodular subepidermal fibrosis in non-filarial endemic elephantiasis of legs. Brit. J. Dermatol., *89:*451, 1973

PRICE, E. W.: Management of endemic (non-filarial) elephantiasis of lower legs. Trop. Doct., *5:*70, 1975

PRICE, R. I. M.: Failure of steroid instillation to prevent capsular contracture after augmentation mammaplasty (Letter to the Editor), PRS, *57:*371, 1976

PRICE, R. I. M., AND ECKER, M. L.: Z-plasty skin closure after lengthening Achilles tendon, PRS, *52:*309, 1973. Discussion by Goldwyn, PRS, *52:*431, 1973

PRICHARD, J. F.: Critical study of autogeneic bone transplants. Actual Odontostomatol. (Paris), *27:*341, 1973 (French)

PRIEBE, C. J., JR.: Defense of tracheostomy in children. J.A.M.A., *232:*1009, 1975

PRIEST, N.D.: Effects of hydrocortisone on mandibular condylar cartilage of rat, PRS, *56:*225, 1975. Proc. Roy. Soc. Med., *68:*128, 1975

PRIMIANO, G. A., AND REEP, T. C.: Disruption of proximal carpal arch of hand, PRS *54:*503, 1974. J. Bone & Joint Surg., *56A:*328, 1974

PRINGLE, R. G.: Amputations of thumb, PRS, *51:*703, 1973. Injury, *3:*211, 1972

PRINGLE, W. M., AND HELMS, D. C.: Treatment of plantar warts by blunt dissection, PRS, *54:*376, 1974. Arch. Dermat., *108:*79, 1973

PROBERT, J. C., PARKER, B. R., AND KAPLAN, H. S.: Growth retardation in children after megavoltage radiation of spine, PRS, *54:*699, 1974. Cancer, *32:*634, 1973

PROBST, C. E., JR. *et al*: A digastric flexor digitorum superficialis: case report. Bull. Hosp. Joint Dis., *36:*52, 1975

PROBST, J.: Evaluation of hand infections. Hefte Unfallheilkd., *107:*236, 1970 (German)

PROCHAZKOVA, L. *et al*: Melanoblastoma of the mucous membrane of the oral cavity. Cesk. Stomatol., *72:*289, 1972 (Czechoslovakian)

PROCTOR, D. S.: Treatment of burns: a comparative trial of antibiotic dressings. S. Afr. Med. J., *45:*231, 1971

PROFETA, G. *et al*: Diagnosis and therapy of unilateral exophthalmos. Acta Neurol. (Napoli), *28:*85, 1973 (Italian)

PROFFIT, W. R. *et al*: Combined orthodontic and surgical management of maxillary protrusion in adults. Am. J. Orthod., *64:*368, 1973

Prognathism

Surgical treatment of upper prognathism (Dautrey *et al*). Acta Stomatol. Belg., *68:*335, 1971 (French)

Surgical treatment of mandibular prognathism (Mayer). Acta Stomatol. Belg., *68:*383, 1971 (French)

One-stage mandibular-maxillary reconstruction in the treatment of gross disproportion of the jaws (Winstock). Brit. J. Oral Surg., *9:*115, 1971

Hapsburg jaw (Hart), PRS, *48:*292, 1971. Canad. M. A. J., *104:*601, 1971

Surgical treatment of anomalies of prognathic character (Petrovic *et al*). Cesk. Stomatol., *71:*294, 1971 (Czechoslovakian)

Surgery or orthodontics—a philosophy of approach (Walker *et al*). Dent. Clin. North Am., *15:*771, 1971

Surgical treatment of severe dento-maxillary irregularities (Popescu *et al*). Int. Dent. J., *21:*346, 1971

Mandibular prognathism, surgical correction of, by sagittal osteotomy of ascending ramus (Takahashi *et al*). Jap. J. Oral Surg., *17:*528, 1971) (Japanese)

New system for integrated three dimensional craniofacial mapping (Baumrind *et al*). J. Dent. Res., *50:*1496, 1971

Study of facial height changes after mandibular osteotomy in 46 patients (White *et al*). J. Oral Surg., *29:*858, 1971

Mandibular prognathism, calculation of degrees of (Dachateau, Carteau). Orthod. Fr., *42:*566, 1971 (French)

Prognathism, correction of, vertical wedge ostectomy in mandibular rami for (Pandya, Stuteville), PRS, *48:*140, 1971

Prognathism, correction of, associated with maxillary retrusion (Rusconi, Brusati), PRS, *48:*558, 1971

Mandibular prognathism (Arienza). Rev. Asoc. Odontol. Argent., *59:*12, 1971 (Spanish)

Can the turning of the upper fragment in

Prognathism — Cont.
operations for progeny by Kostecka technic be prevented? (Muska). Sb. Ved. Pr. Lek. Fak. Karlovy. Univ., *14:*337, 1971 (Czech)

Modified fixation of bone fragments in the treatment of prognathism (Mushka). Stomatologiia (Mosk.), *50:*78, 1971 (Russian)

Mandibular protrusion, changes in facial topography by stereometric method after surgical treatment (Wictorin *et al*). Sven. Tandlak. Tidskr., *64:*373, 1971

Soft tissue profile change produced by reduction of mandibular prognathism (Robinson *et al*). Angle Orthod., *42:*227, 1972

Prognathism, current directions in surgical treatment of (Rusconi). Ann. Stomatol. (Roma), *21:*115, 1972 (Italian)

Prognathism, surgical treatment by means of splitting mandibular ramus (Cwioro). Czas. Stomatol., *25:*833, 1972 (Polish)

Prognathism, evaluation of therapeutic methods in (Malinowski). Czas. Stomatol., *25:*1227, 1972 (Polish)

Prognathism, maxillary, surgical and prosthetic treatment, case (Cataloglu). Dentoral (Istanbul), *4:*180, 1972 (Turkish)

Mandibular prognathism, surgical treatment of (Brotsos). Hell. Stomatol. Chron., *16:*171, 1972 (Greek)

Cephalometric examinations in prognathism, presurgical and postsurgical (Borcbakan, Uner), PRS, *57:*117, 1976. J. Fac. M. Univ. Ankara, *25:*1464, 1972

Prognathism, sagittal osteotomy of ascending branch of mandible by endobuccal approach to correct (Dumas, Freidel), PRS, *50:*418, 1972. J. Fr. Otorhinolaryng., *21:*317, 1972

Prognathism and right displacement with open bite of mandible, L-shaped osteotomy performed for (Min *et al*). J. Korean Dent. Assoc., *10:*373, 1972 (Korean)

Midline splitting of the maxilla for correction of malocclusion (Steinhauser). J. Oral Surg., *30:*413, 1972

Complications of sagittal osteotomy of the mandibular ramus (Behrman). J. Oral Surg., *30:*554, 1972

Total maxillary osteotomy and repositioning of the maxilla: report of case (Cruickshank *et al*). J. Oral Surg., *30:*586, 1972

Sagittal osteotomy, short lingual cut in (Simpson). J. Oral Surg., *30:*811, 1972

Syndrome, Mendelson's, case in patient with rigid intermaxillary block after Obwegeser-Dal Pont intervention for correction of prognathism (Antognini *et al*). Mondo Odontostomatol., *14:*933, 1972 (Italian)

Surgical correction of deformities of the facial

Prognathism — Cont.
skeleton (Lovely). N. S. Med. Bull., *51:*55, 1972

Surgical treatment of mandibular prognathism (Onland *et al*). Ned. tijdschr. tandheelkd., *79:*174, 1972 (Dutch)

Surgical treatment of mandibular prognathism (Onland *et al*). Ned. tijdschr. tandheelkd., *79:*233, 1972 (Dutch)

Dental aspects of surgical orthodontics (Gibbs). N. Y. State J. Med., *72:*233, 1972

Mandibular prognathism, surgical treatment of case (Walsh, Donaldson, Harding). New Zealand Dent. J., *68:*14, 1972

Surgical and orthodontic management of Class 3 malocclusion (Demetriades *et al*). Odontostomatol. Proodos., *26:*183, 1972 (Greek)

The Obwegeser osteotomy (Simpson). Orthodontist, *4:*48, 1972

Prognathism, preventive retention after mandibular surgery for (Monti *et al*). Ortodoncia, *36:*151, 1972

Prognathic profiles of face (Quetglas, Perez, Escribano), PRS, *54:*104, 1974. Rev. españ. cir. plast., *5:*235, 1972

Prognathism, early surgical correction, case (Rabe). Tandlakartidningen, *64:*620, 1972 (Swedish)

Mandibular prognathism, correcting (Crooks). A.O.R.N., *17:*66, 1973

Surgical-orthodontic correction of mandibular prognathism (Bell, Creekmore). Am. J. Orthodontics, *63:*256, 1973

Prognathism, larynx, incompetence in: unusual postoperative complication (Banks). Brit. J. Oral Surg., *11:*94, 1973

Mandibular prognathism, treatment of. Triple osteotomy of body of mandible (Petrovic). Cesk. Stomatol., *73:*107, 1973 (Slovakian)

Prognathism, critical evaluation of surgical results in 101 cases of, with special reference to Obwegeser-Dal Pont's method (Grimm *et al*). Dtsch. Zahn. Mund. Kieferheilkd., *61:*295, 1973 (German)

Prognathism, maxillary, plastic surgery for (Pereira *et al*). Incisivo, *2:*18, 1973 (Portuguese)

Open subcondylar osteotomy in the treatment of mandibular deformities (Berenyl). Int. J. Oral Surg., *2:*81, 1973

Oblique sliding osteotomy of the mandibular rami in 55 patients with mandibular prognathism (Astrand *et al*). Int. J. Oral Surg., *2:*89, 1973

Maxillo-mandibular surgery for correction of dentofacial deformities. 2. Mandibular prognathism (Weinberg *et al*). J. Can.

Prognathism — Cont.

Fortschr. Kiefer. Gesichtschir., *18:*143, 1974 (German)

Osteosynthesis in sagittal osteotomy using the Obwegeser-Dal Pont method (Spiessl). Fortschr. Kiefer. Gesichtschir., *18:*145, 1974 (German)

Intraoral Redon drainage in osteotomy of the ascending ramus of the mandible (Schmelzle *et al*). Fortschr. Kiefer. Gesichtschir., *18:*148, 1974 (German)

Sensitivity of the lower lip after protection or resection of the inferior alveolar nerve in progenia operations (Koblin *et al*). Fortschr. Kiefer. Gesichtschir., *18:*151, 1974 (German)

End results of the lateral oblique osteotomy for mandibular prognathism (Rankow *et al*). Fortschr. Kiefer. Gesichtschir., *18:*155, 1974 (German)

Results of prognathism operations in the Westdeutsche Kieferklinik (West German Jaw Clinic). Differential analysis of treatment in 98 cases (Biermann *et al*). Fortschr. Kiefer. Gesichtschir., *18:*159, 1974 (German)

Median osteotomy for reduction of the mandible in dysgnathia (Spiessl). Fortschr. Kiefer. Gesichtschir., *18:*163, 1974 (German)

Neurologic disorders following surgical correction of progenia and microgenia (Niederdellmann *et al*). Fortschr. Kiefer. Gesichtschir., *18:*186, 1974 (German)

Single-step surgical treatment of pronounced prognathia (Wunderer). Fortschr. Kiefer. Gesichtschir., *18:*195, 1974 (German)

Treatment of the gnathic open bite (Steinhardt *et al*). Fortschr. Kiefer. Gesichtschir., *18:*199, 1974 (German)

Single-step correction of mandibular prognathism and habitual jaw luxation (Koberg). Fortschr. Kiefer. Gesichtschir., *18:*234, 1974 (German)

Osteotomy of mandibular rami, oblique sliding (Arand, Ericson), PRS, *55:*508, 1975. Internat. J. Oral Surg., *3:*49, 1974

Problems of correction of asymmetric mandibular prognathism (Nwoku *et al*). Int. J. Oral Surg., *3:*229, 1974

Surgical orthodontic treatment of facial asymmetry using direct bonding plastic brackets (Kawamura *et al*). Int. J. Oral Surg., *3:*252, 1974

Mandibular asymmetry (Erickson *et al*). J. Am. Dent. Assoc., *89:*1369, 1974

A method of intermaxillary fixation for repair of mandibular prognathism with resin postcrowns (Matsuo *et al*). J. Jpn. Stomatol. Soc., *41:*151, 1974 (Japanese)

Prognathism — Cont.

Ramus "C" osteotomy with body sagittal split (Byrne *et al*). J. Oral Surg., *32:*259, 1974

Simplified sigmoid notch retractor for extraoral osteotomies (Zallen *et al*). J. Oral Surg., *32:*386, 1974

Sagittal split osteotomy of mandibular ramus, radioisotope study of vascular response to (Grammer *et al*). J. Oral Surg., *32:*578, 1974

Intraoral oblique osteotomy of the mandibular ramus (Massey *et al*). J. Oral Surg., *32:*755, 1974

Use of a new instrument in the osteotomy of the ascending mandibular ramus (Tamas). Magy. Traumatol. Orthop., *17:*223, 1974 (Hungarian)

Multiple osteotomy at a single stage (Curioni *et al*). Minerva Stomatol., *23:*106, 1974 (Italian)

Segmental alveolar osteotomy in the correction of maxillofacial malformations (Torrielli *et al*). Minerva Stomatol., *22:*218, 1974 (Italian)

Prognathism, patients with, neurotic or pseudoneurotic character development in (Stamen *et al*). Ned. tijdschr. geneeskd., *118:*778, 1974 (Dutch)

Prognathism, orthodontic treatment during intermaxillary immobilization period following surgical correction of (Elias *et al*). Oral Surg., *37:*526, 1974

Prognathism surgery, effect on speech (Goodstein, Cooper, Wallace), PRS, *56:*354, 1975. Oral Surg., *37:*846, 1974

Evaluation of the surgical procedure of sagittal split osteotomy of the mandibular ramus (Wang *et al*). Oral Surg., *38:*167, 1974

Medical correction of maxillary and mandibular prognathism (Van Put). Rev. Belge Med. Dent., *29:*465, 1974 (Dutch)

Intermaxillary and internal wiring fixation. Review of techniques and report of cases (Barakat). Rev. Dent. Libn., *24:*39, 1974

Experiences and results in the treatment of malformations of the jaws by segmental osteotomies (Torrielli *et al*). Rev. Stomatol. Chir. Maxillofac., *75:*125, 1974 (French)

Remote results of the correction of mandibular protrusion by sagittal osteotomy of the mandibular rami (Pepersack). Rev. Stomatol. Chir. Maxillofac., *75:*142, 1974 (French)

Eight cases of sagittal osteotomies of the mandibular rami (Daieff *et al*). Rev. Stomatol. Chir. Maxillofac., *75:*145, 1974 (French)

Maxillofacial orthopedic surgery. New methods (Meyer). Rev. Stomatol. Chir. Maxillo-

Prognathism—Cont.

fac., *75:*153, 1974 (French)

Radiography of the temporomandibular joint after oblique sliding osteotomy of the mandibular rami (Hollender *et al*). Scand. J. Dent. Res., *82:*466, 1974

Osteotomy, mandibular, to correct prognathism (Hoffman), PRS, *56:*105, 1975. South. M. J., *67:*1427, 1974

Surgical management of mandibular prognathism by intraoral operation of the ascending ramus (Chrysafes). Stomatologia (Athenai), *31:*231, 1974 (Greek)

Prognathism, mandibular, surgery, enlarged styloid processes as complication in (Padgett *et al*). Va. Dent. J., *51:*26, 1974

Prognathism: surgical treatment (Gigurere). Can. J. Otolaryngol., *4:*679, 1975 (French)

Surgical treatment of progenia and associated open occlusion using technic of vertical osteotomy of ramus mandibulae (Halmos). Cesk. Stomatol., *75:*83, 1975

Mandibular prognathism, surgery of (Ribeiro Soares, Ribeiro Soares), PRS, *57:*757, 1976. Cir. Plast. Ibero-Latino Am., *1:*13, 1975

Analysis of morphological and functional conditions of the temporomandibular joints prior to and following treatment of prognathism (Baranczak *et al*). Czas. Stomatol., *28:*159, 1975 (Polish)

Surgical orthognathics. Redefined role based upon etiologic factors (Zambito). Dent. Clin. North Am., *19:*515, 1975

General anesthesia in surgical correction of prognathism (Beres *et al*). Fogorv. Sz., *68:*289, 1975 (Hungarian)

Correction of pseudoprognathism in adults (Bogi *et al*). Fogorv. Sz., *68:*344, 1975 (Hungarian)

Integumental profile changes caused by surgical treatment of mandibular protrusion (Wisth). Int. J. Oral Surg., *4:*32, 1975

Late results after advancing the mandible by sagittal splitting of the rami (Freihofer *et al*). J. Maxillo-facial Surg., *3:*230, 1975

Simplified technique to reduce perioral edema in intraoral sagittal split osteotomies (Weinberg *et al*). J. Oral Surg., *33:*61, 1975

Lap joint mandibular ostectomy (Whinery). J. Oral Surg., *33:*223, 1975

Prognathism, minimal, treatment of by midline mandibular ostectomy (MacDonald *et al*). J. Oral Surg., *33:*386, 1975

Middle-third facial osteotomies: their use in the correction of acquired and developmental dentofacial and craniofacial deformities (Epker *et al*). J. Oral Surg., *33:*491, 1975

Prognathism—Cont.

Osteotomies of mandibular ramus, comparison of vertical and sagittal split (Wang, Waite), PRS, *57:*672, 1976. J. Oral Surg., *33:*596, 1975

An appliance that permits early mobilization after correction of mandibular prognathism (Ryan *et al*). J. Oral Surg., *33:*875, 1975

Mandibular prognathism (Wang-Norderud *et al*). J. Oslo City Hospital, *25:*57, 1975

Late results in the surgical treatment of progenia in the area of the mandibular ramus (Piscevic *et al*). Med. Pregl., *28:*461, 1975) (Serbian)

Surgical correction of jaw abnormalities causing severe facial deformities (Berenyi *et al*). Orv. Hetil., *116:*1767, 1975 (Hungarian)

Surgical treatment of prognathism (Malinowski *et al*). Otolaryngol. Pol., *29:*481, 1975 (Polish)

Surgical correction of mandibular prognathism (Semenchenko *et al*). Stomatologiia (Mosk.), *54:*54, 1975 (Russian)

Orthognathic surgery. Review of mandibular body procedures (Keller *et al*). Mayo Clin. Proc., *51:*117, 1976

Patient motivation and response to surgical correction of prognathism (Laufer *et al*). Oral Surg., *41:*309, 1976

Prognathism in patient with Hand-Schuller-Christian's disease (Corwin, Greer), PRS, *57:*513, 1976

PROKOPYSHIN, M. V.: Surgical treatment of superficial varicose veins of the lower limbs. Klin. Khir., *1:*5, 1975 (Russian)

PROSNAK, M: External gel-filled prosthesis of the breast. Pol. Przegl. Chir., *48:*81, 1976

Prostheses (See also *Hands, Prosthetic; Implants; Silicones*)

Intraosseous anchorage of dental prostheses. I. Experimental studies (Branemark *et al*), PRS, *48:*97, 1971. II. Review of clinical approaches (Adell *et al*), PRS, *49:*102, 1972. Scand. J. Plast. Reconstr. Surg., *3:*81, 1969; Part II, *4:*19, 1970

Prostheses, mammary, personal experience and critical study of (Vrebos), PRS, *50:*199, 1972. Acta chir. belg., *70:*300, 1971

Tissue reactions after subcutaneous implantation of Hydrom sponge (Smahel *et al*). Acta chir. plast. (Praha), *13:*193, 1971

Silicone-Dacron reinforced gliding prosthesis prior to tendon grafting, two stage procedure in flexor tendon reconstruction in severely damaged hands (Hunter, Salis-

Prostheses — Cont.

prostheses after autoclaving (Talcott) (Letter to the Editor), PRS, *55:*216, 1975

Mammary prosthesis, prevention of postoperative shifting (Zackin, Goulian), PRS, *55:*713, 1975

Polyurethane covers of some breast prostheses, foreign body reactions to (Cocke, Leathers, Lynch), PRS, *56:*527, 1975

Prosthesis, silicone penile, to treat organic impotence (Shishito, Shirai, Matsuda), PRS, *56:*466, 1975. Urol. int., *30:*211, 1975

Breast prostheses, inflatable, use of soluble steroids within (Perrin), PRS, *57:*163, 1976

PROTOPOPOV, A. A. *et al*: Treatment of cancer of lower lip in initial stages. Vopr. Onkol., *20:*96, 1974 (Russian)

PROTOPOPOV, A. A. *et al*: Recurrences and metastases of cancer of the lower lip. Vopr. Onkol., *21:*83, 1975 (Russian)

PROUZA, Z., MOSEROVA, J., AND JANECEK, J.: Subcutaneous temperature measurements in a non-contact burn, PRS, *52:*684, 1973. Acta chir. plast., *14:*168, 1972

PROWLER, J. R.: Anterior Z-plasty ridge extension. Oral Surg., *33:*172, 1972

PROWLER, J. R.: Simple method for avoidance of relapse in mandibular osteotomy. Trans. Congr. Int. Assoc. Oral Surg., *4:*242, 1973

PRPIC, I.: Surgery of the rheumatoid arthritis of the hand. Reumatizam, *21:*167, 1974 (Croatian)

PRPIC, I. *et al:* Lyophilized corium grafts for repair of abdominal wall defects, PRS, *54:*700, 1974. Brit. J. Plast. Surg., *26:*35, 1973

PRPIC, I. *et al*: Use of xenograft corium for reconstruction of abdominal wall defects, PRS, *56:*678, 1975. Brit. J. Plast. Surg., *27:*125, 1974

PRUITT, B. A., JR.: Complications of thermal injury. Clin. Plast. Surg., *1:*667, 1974

PRUITT, B. A., JR.: Discussion of "Open and closed treatment of burns with povidone-iodine," by Georgiade. PRS, *53:*82, 1974

PRUITT, B. A., JR., FOLEY, F. D., AND MONCRIEF, J. A.: Curling's ulcer: a clinical-pathology study of 323 cases, PRS, *48:*90, 1971. Ann. Surg., *172:*523, 1970

PRUITT, B. A., AND CURRERI, W. P.: Burn wound and its care, PRS, *49:*667, 1972. Arch. Surg., *103:*461, 1971

PRUITT, B. A., JR., MASON, A. D., JR., AND MONCRIEF, J. A.: Hemodynamic changes in early postburn patient: influence of fluid administration and of vasodilator (hydralazine), PRS, *49:*587, 1972. J. Trauma, *11:*36, 1971

PRUITT, B. A., JR., AND FOLEY, F. D.: Use of biopsies in burn patient care, PRS, *52:*683, 1973. Surgery, *73:*887, 1973

PRUITT, B. S., JR., AND MOYLAN, J. A., JR.: Current management of thermal burns. Adv. Surg., *6:*237, 1972

PRUSAK, M. *et al*: Studies in management of contaminated wound. IX. Quantitation of Evans blue dye content of open and primarily closed surgical wounds, PRS, *52:*601, 1973. Am. J. Surg., *125:*585, 1973

PRUSKI, J.: Diagnosis and planned surgical treatment of mandibular prognathism. Czas. Stomatol., *27:*173, 1974 (Polish)

PRUSZEWICZ, A. *et al*: Electromyographic studies on palatal, pharyngeal and lip muscles during phonation and deglutition in patients with cleft palate. HNO, *19:*77, 1971 (German)

PRUZANSKY, S.: Challenge and opportunity in craniofacial anomalies. Cleft Palate J., *8:*239, 1971

PRUZANSKY, S.: Longitudinal study of growth in bilateral cleft lip and palate, from infancy to adolescence (with Friede). PRS, *49:*392, 1972

PRUZANSKY, S. *et al*: Two sisters with unoperated bilateral cleft lip and palate, age 6 and 4 years. Brit. J. Plast. Surg., *28:*251, 1975

PRUZANSKY, S. *et al*: Letter: for parents of newborn babies with cleft lip/palate — pamphlet. Cleft Palate J., *13:*76, 1976

PRYDSO, U. *et al*: Bone formation in palatal clefts subsequent to palato-vomer plasty, PRS, *56:*359, 1975. Scand. J. Plast. Reconstr. Surg., *8:*73, 1974

PRZYWARA, S. *et al*: Cryosurgical treatment of postradiotherapy recurrences of skin carcinoma. Wiad. Lek., *26:*1173, 1973 (Polish)

PSAUME, J.: Early bone deformities in monolateral facial clefts, PRS, *57:*762, 1976 (French). Ann. chir. plast., *20:*299, 1975

PSILLAKIS, J.: New method for correction of prominent nasal tip (with Spina, Kamakura). PRS, *51:*416, 1973

PSILLAKIS, J. M.: Total reconstruction of the ear in congenital microtia (with Spina, Kamakura). PRS, *48:*349, 1971

PSILLAKIS, J. M. *et al*: Skin allograft contemporaneous with heart transplant, PRS, *52:*603, 1973. Rev. paulista med., *78:*63, 1971

PSILLAKIS, J. M. *et al*: Deformities of the middle 3rd of the face: nasomaxillary hypoplasia. Rev. Asoc. Med. Bras., *18:*185, 1972 (Portuguese)

PSILLAKIS, J. M., AND ALBANO, A. M.: Rhinoplasty: surgery of tip of nose by hood flap technique, PRS, *52:*594, 1973. Rev. brasil. clin. terapeut., *1:*587, 1972

PSILLAKIS, J. M., AND ERHART, E. A.: Reinnervation of skin grafts: experimental study, PRS, *52:*324, 1973. Rev. bras. clin. terap., *1:*607, 1972

PSILLAKIS, J. M., LAPA, F., AND SPINA, V.: Surgical correction of midfacial retrusion (nasomaxillary hypoplasia) in the presence of normal dental occlusion. PRS, *51:*67, 1973

PSILLAKIS, J. M., PEREIRA, W. C., AND ISHIDA, J.: Ocular hypertelorism: analysis of twenty cases, PRS, *52:*451, 1973. Rev. bras. clin. terap., *2:*55, 1973

PSILLAKIS, J. M. *et al*: Surgical treatment of hypertelorism. I. Facial osteotomy. Rev. Paul. Med., *82:*151, 1973 (Portuguese)

PSILLAKIS, J. M. *et al*: Fluid silicone gel of Japanese origin, PRS, *56:*684, 1975. Rev. Asoc. med. Brasil, *19:*191, 1974

PSILLAKIS, J. M., KAMAKURA, L., AND SPINA, V.: Reconstruction of labial philtrum with auricular composite grafts, PRS, *56:*676, 1975. Rev. Asoc. med. Brasil, *20:*297, 1974

PSILLAKIS, J. M. *et al*: Surgical treatment of hypertelorism. II. Craniofacial osteotomy. Rev. Paul. Med., *83:*129, 1974 (Portuguese)

Psychology: See *Plastic Surgery, Psychology of*

Ptosis: See *Blepharoptosis; Breasts, Ptosis*

PUCKETT, C.: Transposition of lips for correction of facial paralysis (with Pickrell, Peters).PRS, *57:*427, 1976

PUCKETT, C. L., NEALE, H. W., AND PICKRELL, K. L.: Dynamic correction of unilateral paralysis of the lower lip. PRS, *55:*397, 1975

PUK, E.: Use of mucosal-periosteal flaps from the vomer in the treatment of asymmetrical palatal clefts. Czas. Stomatol., *27:*1037, 1974 (Polish)

PULATOV, A. T.: Development of reconstructive surgery in the Tadzhik S.S.R. Vestn. Khir., *108:*6, 1972 (Russian)

PULEC, J. L.: Bell's palsy: diagnosis, management and results of treatment. Laryngoscope, *84:*2119, 1974

PULVERTAFT, R. G.: Reconstruction of the severely mutilated hand. Rheumatol. Phys. Med., *11:*90, 1971

PULVERTAFT, R. G.: Twenty-five years of hand surgery. Personal reflections. J. Bone & Joint Surg. (Br.), *55:*32, 1973

PULVERTAFT, R. G.: Psychological aspects of hand injuries. Hand, *7:*93, 1975

PURANIK, R. S., MENCIA, L. F., AND GILBERT, M. G.: Artificial testicles in children: new Silastic gel testicular prosthesis, PRS, *52:*595, 1973. J. Urol., *109:*735, 1973

PURI, P.: Webbed penis without chordee. J.

Pediatr. Surg., *11:*125, 1976

PURITA, F.: Hair transplants in accidental baldness. Hospital (Rio de J.), *77:*1303, 1970 (Portuguese)

PUTNIK, M. *et al*: Clinical features and results of surgical treatment of malignant melanomas of skin. Vojnosanit. Pregl., *29:*401, 1972 (Croatian)

PUTTERMAN, A. M.: Clamp for strengthening Muller's muscle in the treatment of ptosis. Modification, theory, and clamp for the Fasanella-Servat ptosis operation. Arch. Ophth., *87:*665, 1972

PUTTERMAN, A. M.: Jaw-winking blepharoptosis treated by Fasanella-Servat procedure. Am. J. Ophth., *75:*1016, 1973

PUTTERMAN, A. M.: Fixation of Pyrex tubes in conjunctivodacryocystorhinostomy. Am. J. Ophth., *78:*1026, 1974

PUTTERMAN, A. M.: Temporary blindness after cosmetic blepharoplasty. Am. J. Ophth., *80:*1081, 1975

PUTTERMAN, A. M., AND URIST, M.: Surgical treatment of upper eyelid retraction, PRS, *50:*417, 1972. Arch. Ophth., *87:*401, 1972

PUTTERMAN, A. M., AND URIST, M. J.: Baggy eyelids—true hernia, PRS, *54:*686, 1974. Ann. Ophth., *5:*1029, 1973

PUTTERMAN, A. M. *et al*: Simplified levator recession in treatment of overcorrected blepharoptosis. Surg. Forum, *24:*504, 1973

PUTTERMAN, A. M. *et al*: Transconjunctival isolation and transcutaneous resection of levator palpebrae superioris muscle. Am. J. Ophth., *77:*90, 1974

PUTTERMAN, A. M., STEVENS, T., AND URIST, M. J.: Non-surgical management of blow-out fractures of orbital floor, PRS, *55:*508, 1975. Am. J. Ophth., *77:*232, 1974

PUTTERMAN, A. M. *et al*: Simplified levator palpebrae superioris muscle recession to treat over-corrected blepharoptosis. Am. J. Ophth., *77:*358, 1974

PUTTERMAN, A. M., AND URIST, M. J.: Surgical anatomy of orbital septum, PRS, *54:*686, 1974. Ann. Ophth., *6:*290, 1974

PUTTERMAN, A. M. *et al*: Müller muscle-conjunctiva resection. Technique for treatment of blepharoptosis. Arch. Ophth., *93:*619, 1975

PUTTERMAN, A. M. *et al*: Treatment of enophthalmic narrow palpebral fissure after blow-out fracture. Ophthalmic Surg., *6:*45, 1975

PYBUS, P. K.: New method for a Le Fort type 3 fracture of the maxilla. S. Afr. Med. J., *45:*991, 1971

PYBUS, P. K.: Le Fort type 3 fracture of the maxilla. S. Afr. Med. J., *46:*40, 1972

PYKE, R. *et al*: Local anaesthesia combined

with diazepam for nasal surgery. J. Laryng. & Otol., *87:*1243, 1973

Q

QUANTE, M. *et al:* Middle ear exudates as regular finding in cleft lip, jaw and palate. Arch. Klin. Exp. Ohren Nasen Kehlkopfheilkd., *199:*483, 1971 (German)

QUARNER, V. *et al:* Surgical research with mucous grafts, PRS, *50:*99, 1972. Tribuna Med. Mexico, *21:*3, 1972

QUETGLAS, J.: Dupuytren's disease, comments on 80 cases operated, PRS, *52:*679, 1973. Acta chir. plast., *14:*244, 1972

QUETGLAS, J.: Delayed closure of hand injuries, PRS, *51:*232, 1973. Rev. español. cir. plast., *2:*193, 1972

QUETGLAS, J., PEREZ, A., AND ESCRIBANO, F.: Prognathic profiles of face, PRS, *54:*104, 1974. Rev. español. cir. plast., *5:*235, 1972

QUETGLAS, J. *et al:* Fibrous dysplasia of mandible, PRS, *57:*532, 1976. Cir. Plast. Ibero-Latino Am., *1:*25, 1975

QUINBY, S. V. *et al:* How children live after disfiguring burns. Psychiatry Med., *2:*146, 1971

QUINBY, W. C., JR.: Restrictive effects of thoracic burns in children. J. Trauma, *12:*646, 1972

QUINLIVAN, J. K.: Elastin fibers in scar tissue (with Bhangoo, Connelly). PRS, *57:*308, 1976

QUINN, G. W. *et al:* Treatment of mandibular prognathism in cleft palate patients. Am. J. Orthod., *59:*76, 1971

QUINN, J. H. *et al:* Trigeminal neuralgia: treatment by repetitive peripheral neurectomy. Supplemental report. J. Oral Surg., *33:*591, 1975

QUINN, N. W. *et al:* Jaundice following oral surgery: Gilbert's syndrome. Brit. J. Oral. Surg., *12:*285, 1975

QUINTARELLI, G.: Lymphoscintigraphy in lymph node metastases from oral cancer. Minerva Stomatol. *23:*147, 1974 (Italian)

R

RABE, T.: Case of early surgical correction of prognathism. Tandlakartidningen, *64:*620, 1972 (Swedish)

RABISCHONG, P.: Basic problems in the restoration of prehension. Ann. Chir., *25:*927, 1971 (French)

RABKIN, I. KH. *et al:* X-ray diagnosis of post-tracheostomic stenoses. Grudn. Khir., *5:*83, 1974 (Russian)

RABUZZI, D. D.: Midfacial fractures. N. Y. State J. Med., *71:*2412, 1971

RABUZZI, D. D.: Revision surgery of malaligned midfacial fractures. Otolaryngol. Clin. North Am., *7:*107, 1974

RACHMAN, R.: Soft tissue injury by mercury from broken thermometer, PRS, *54:*249, 1974. Am. J. Clin. Path., *61:*296, 1974

Radial Nerve: See *Nerve, Radial*

Radiation Injuries

Acute accidental radiodermatitis (Mestdagh *et al*). Arch. Belg. Dermatol. Syphilligr., *24:*73, 1968 (French)

Radionecrosis of jaws: its prophylaxis (Camillo), PRS, *48:*603, 1971. Rev. port. Oral Surg., *2:*207, 1970

Free skin grafts on the parietal pleura: report of a case (Butters *et al*). Brit. J. Plast. Surg., *24:*412, 1971

Treatment of osteoradionecrosis by bone removal and grafting (Dupuis *et al*). Rev. Stomatol. Chir. Maxillofac., *73:*410, 1972

Radiation injury, local, and its surgical treatment. Report of 170 cases (Holmström, Johanson). Scand. J. Plast. Reconstr. Surg., *6:*156, 1972

Experience in surgical treatment of late radiation injuries (Bogatskii). Stomatologiia (Mosk.), *51:*33, 1972 (Russian)

Omental lengthening, surgical technique based on arterial anatomy (Alday, Goldsmith), PRS, *51:*354, 1973. Surg. Gynec. & Obst., *135:*103, 1972

Plastic surgical treatment of radiation scars after plantar warts (Krogh). Ugeskr. Laeger, *134:*2155, 1972 (Danish)

Mandibular osteoradionecrosis, therapeutic aspects of (De Coninck *et al*). Acta Stomatol. Belg., *70:*387, 1973 (French)

Radiation-induced ulcer, surgical therapy of (Gerhard). Allgemeinmed., *49:*1699, 1973 (German)

Mandibular osteoradionecrosis, one stage surgical repair with jaw preservation (Nickell *et al*), PRS, *53:*682, 1974. Am. J. Surg., *126:*502, 1973

Radionecrosis of flexor folds, axilla, groin, neck, treatment of, using the great omentum supporting dermo-epidermal free flaps (Kiricuta). Ann. chir. plast., *18:*65, 1973 (French)

Hand, radiodermatitis of, series of 104 operated cases of (179 hands) (Lagrot *et al*). Ann. chir. plast., *18:*233, 1973 (French)

Radionecrosis, jugomandibular complex. Therapeutic problems (Lallemant *et al*). Ann. Otolaryngol. Chir. Cervicofac.,

Radiation Treatment of Benign Conditions—Cont.

*88:*215, 1970

Can radiotherapy of plantar warts still be justified? (Sauerbrey). Z. Allgemeinmed., *47:*1584, 1971 (German)

Radiation to infant breast, mammary hypoplasia following (Skalkeas, Gogas, Pavlatos), PRS, *52:*679, 1973. Acta chir. plast., *14:*240, 1972

Radiation Treatment of Cancer

Radiotherapy and surgery combined, trend toward, in management of cancer of oral cavity (Leonard, Hass), PRS, *48:*398, 1971. Am. J. Surg., *120:*514, 1970

Radiation and surgery to treat squamous cell cancer of supraglottic larynx (Flynn, Jesse, Lindberg), PRS, *52:*102, 1973. Am. J. Surg., *124:*477, 1972

Radiotherapy, treatment of squamous cell carcinoma of oral cavity (Fayos, Lampe), PRS, *52:*102, 1973. Am. J. Surg., *124:*493, 1972

Radiation dose and time factors in carcinoma of nasopharynx, review of 146 patients (Moench, Phillips), PRS, *52:*102, 1973. Am. J. Surg., *124:*515, 1972

Radiation, management of problems of teeth and jaw in patients undergoing (Daly, Drane, MacComb), PRS, *52:*213, 1973. Am. J. Surg., *124:*539, 1972

Radiotherapy, endolymphatic, in malignant melanoma of lower extremities (Kalkoff, Baumeister, Gehring). Arch. Derm. Forsch., *244:*250, 1972 (German)

Salivary gland function, effect of fractionated radiotherapy on (Eneroth, Henrikson, Jakobsson), PRS, *51:*476, 1973. Cancer, *30:*1147, 1972

Peripheral nerve regeneration after effect of ionizing radiation (Miehlke). O. R. L., *34:*88, 1972 (German)

Radiotherapy for postoperative recurrent squamous cell carcinoma in head and neck (Deutsch *et al*), PRS, *54:*108, 1974. Arch. Otolaryng., *98:*316, 1973

Radiotherapy and carcinoma of parotid (Patey). Brit. Med. J., *1:*236, 1973

Tumor therapy, interstitial, use of iridium-192 in (Stella *et al*), PRS, *53:*375, 1974. Cancer, *32:*665, 1973

Radiotherapy, role of dentist in (Santiago), PRS, *53:*604, 1974. J. Prosth. Dent., *39:*196, 1973

Radiotherapy for retinoblastoma, osteogenic sarcoma developing after (Shah, Arlen, Miller), PRS, *55:*255, 1975. Am. Surgeon, *40:*485, 1974

Radiation Treatment of Cancer—Cont.

Radiation, microwave, to cure cancer—preliminary hypothesis (Holt), PRS, *55:*116, 1975. Australasian Radiol., *18:*15, 1974

Radiotherapy to cure metastatic hemangiopericytoma (Dube, Paulson), PRS, *55:*388, 1975. J. Bone & Joint Surg., *56A:*833, 1974

Radiotherapy of next decade (Fowler), PRS, *55:*644, 1975. Proc. Roy. Soc. Med., *67:*743, 1974

Radiotherapy, interstitial, for intraoral carcinoma (Ochsner, Collins), PRS, *55:*642, 1975. South. M.J., *67:*1150, 1974

Radiosensitivity of lymph node metastases (Henk), PRS, *56:*231, 1975. Proc. Roy. Soc. Med., *68:*85, 1975

Radiation Treatment of Keloids

Radiation therapy of keloids (Asakura *et al*), PRS, *54:*118, 1974. Jap. J. Plast: Reconstr. Surg., *16:*496, 1973

X-rays and keloids (Editorial). Brit. Med. J., *3:*592, 1974

Radical Neck Dissection: See *Neck Dissections*

Radicular Cyst: See *Jaw Cysts*

Radioactive Isotopes

Gallium 76 for localization of septic lesions (Littenberg *et al*), PRS, *54:*512, 1974. Ann. Int. Med., *77:*403, 1973

Thorotrast-induced hepatoma presenting as hyperparathyroidism (Kiely, Titus, Orivs), PRS, *54:*235, 1974. Cancer, *31:*1312, 1973

Iridium-192 used in interstitial tumor therapy (Stella *et al*), PRS, *53:*375, 1974. Cancer, *32:*665, 1973

Radioactive isotopes to localize deep abscesses (Allen *et al*), PRS, *56:*367, 1975. Henry Ford Hosp. M.J., *21:*111, 1973

Radionuclides in renal transplants, techniques (De Murphy, Tovar Zamora), PRS, *56:*357, 1975. Prensa Med. Mex., *39:*247, 1974

Radon seed implants. Residual radioactivity after 33 years (Goldstein). Arch. Dermat., *111:*757, 1975

RADLOWSKA, Z. *et al*: Treatment of skin defects by dermo-epidermal homografts in children. Pol. Tyg. Lek., *26:*1820, 1971 (Polish)

RADNOT, M.: "Fingerprint" inclusions in orbicular muscle of eye. Ophthalmologica, *168:*282, 1974 (German)

RADNOT, M. *et al*: Ultrastructural changes in senile atrophy of orbicularis oculi muscle. Am. J. Ophth., *78:*689, 1974

RAFATY, F. M.: Browlift operation, PRS, 57:393, 1976. Arch. Otolaryng., 101:467, 1975

RAFF, M., et al: Treatment of burns with reference to hypertrophic scars. Wien Med. Wochenschr., 115:395, 1973

RAFFI, A. et al: Acute disseminated lupus erythematosus with gangrene of the fingers of the hand. Pediatrie, 23:358, 1968 (French)

RAFLA, S.: Significance and treatment of lymph node metastases of malignant mucous and salivary gland tumors. Am. J. Roentgenol. Radium Ther. Nucl. Med., 117:595, 1973

RAFLA, S. et al: Aggressive management of advanced head and neck tumors. Am. J. Roentgenol. Radium Ther. Nucl. Med., 120:608, 1974

RAGAB, R. R. et al: Eosinophilic granuloma with bilateral involvement of both jaws. Int. J. Oral Surg., 4:73, 1975

RAGNHILDSTVEIT, E. et al: Gas producing infection caused by Bacteroides. Tidsskr. Nor. Laegeforen, 96:240, 1976 (Norwegian)

RAGNI, M. V. et al: Primary malignant melanoma of vagina and vulva. Obstet. Gynecol., 43:658, 1974

RAHMAT, A., NORMAN, J. N., AND SMITH, G.: Effect of zinc deficiency on wound healing, PRS, 54:698, 1974. Brit. J. Surg., 61:271, 1974

RAHMEL, R.: Angiography of the upper extremity. Handchirurgie, 2:91, 1970 (German)

RAHMEL, R.: Disastrous results in infected minor hand injuries. Hefte Unfallheilkd., 107:251, 1970 (German)

RAHN, B. et al: Biomechanics of osteosynthesis in the mandible. Fortschr. Kiefer. Gesichtschir., 19:37, 1975 (German)

RAICK, A. N.: Cell differentiation and tumor-promoting action in skin carcinogenesis, PRS, 55:517, 1975. Cancer Res., 34:2915, 1974

RAIE, R. E.: Reconstructive surgery in impaired opposition of the thumb. Vestn. Khir., 105:102, 1970 (Russian)

RAINE, A. C.: Office conjunctivorhinostomy. Ann. Ophth., 3:1097, 1971

RAINER, W. G. et al: Effects of graded compression on nerve conduction velocity, PRS, 53:684, 1974. Arch. Surg., 107:719, 1973

RAITHEL, D., MÜHE, E., AND DECKER, D.: Therapy of stress ulcers, PRS, 51:110, 1973. Chirurg., 43:328, 1972

RAJU, S. et al: Unreliability of visual inspection to monitor skin graft survival times in AG-B-incompatible rat strains. Transplantation, 17:325, 1974

RAKOFSKY, S. I.: Adequacy of surgical excision of basal cell carcinoma. Ann. Ophth., 5:596, 1973

RAKOWER, W.: Oral surgeon's experience with interosseous blade implant. Int. J. Oral

Surg., 3:282, 1974

RAKSIN, S. Z. et al: Submandibular duct sialolith of unusual size and shape. J. Oral Surg., 33:142, 1975

RAM, S.: Reconstruction of mammary hypoplasia associated with chest wall deformities (with Hawtof, Alani). PRS, 57:172, 1976

RAMA, G. et al: Arion's sutures in blepharoptosis correction. Am. J. Ophth., 76:276, 1973

RAMAKRISHNAN, K. M., THOMAS, K. P., AND SUNDARARAJAN, M. S.: Study of 1,000 patients with keloids in South India. PRS, 53:276, 1974

RAMANATHAN, K.: Burkitt's lymphoma in West Malaysia, PRS, 52:103, 1973. Southeast Asian J. Trop. Med., 3:249, 1972

RAMANATHAN, K. et al: Frequency of oral precancerous conditions in 407 Malaysians — with correlation to oral habits, PRS, 52:458, 1973. Med. J. Malaya, 27:173, 1973

RAMANATHAN, K., AND LAKSHIMI, S.: Oral carinoma in Chinese female, PRS, 55:245, 1975. M. J. Malaysia, 28:84, 1973

RAMANATHAN, K., AND LAKSHIMI, S.: Oral carcinoma in Chinese male, PRS, 54:246, 1974. Asian J. Med., 10:3, 1974

RAMANATHAN, K., AND LAKSHIMI, S.: Oral carcinoma in Malay female, PRS, 55:642, 1975. Asian J. Med., 10:129, 1974

RAMANJANEYULU, P.: Juvenile fibroma of antral origin. Int. Surg., 59:423, 1974

RAMIRES, A. T.: Study of surgical infection among burn patients, PRS, 51:706, 1973. Asian J. Med., 8:512, 1972

RAMIREZ, A. et al: Functional recuperation of replanted extremities, PRS, 55:121, 1975. Antioquia Med., 21:575, 1971

RAMIREZ, A., AND MARTI, V.: Congenital absence of pectoralis muscle, PRS, 53:604, 1974. An. med. cir., 53:293, 1973

RAMIREZ, M.: Treatment of facial paralysis by static suspension with dermal flaps (with Guerrero-Santos, Espaillat). PRS, 48:325, 1971

RAMIREZ-BARRIA, R.: Phoniatric-surgical management in cleft palate cases, PRS, 50:420, 1972. Rev. Latino Am. cir. Plast., 15:41, 1972

RAMIREZ-GOMEZ, A. et al: Osteosynthesis of the long bones of the hand using the AO technic. Acta Orthop. Belg., 39:973, 1973 (French)

RAMIREZ MOHEDANO, M. A. et al: Our experience with surgery of cancer of the pharynx with suture of the pharynx to the cricoid cartilage. Acta Otorinolaryngol. Iber. Am., 24:91, 1973 (Spanish)

RAMIREZ YUSTI, N.: Skeletal traction in hand burns, PRS, 55:515, 1975. Rev. Latino Am. cir. plast., 17:25, 1973

RAMSDEN, D. et al: Adenoid cystic carcinoma of

head and neck: report of 30 cases. Aust. N.Z.J. Surg., *43:*102, 1973

RAMSDEN, R. T., AND MARAN, A. C. D.: Protection of facial nerve in radical neck dissection, PRS, *54:*618, 1974. Brit. J. Surg., *61:*297, 1974

RAMSTAD, T.: Post-orthodontic retention and postprosthodontic occlusion in adult complete unilateral and bilateral cleft subjects. Cleft Palate J., *10:*34, 1973

RAMSTAD, T.: Cleft lip and cleft palate. Prosthetic treatment. 7. Tidsskr. Nor. Laegeforen, *93:*2487, 1973 (Norwegian)

RAMULU, C., AND REDDY, C. R. R. M.: Carcinoma of hard palate and relation to reverse smoking, PRS, *51:*484, 1973. J. Internat. Surg., *57:*8, 1972

RAMULU, C. *et al*: Benign tumors of hard palate, PRS, *55:*246, 1975. Indian J. Surg., *36:*113, 1974

RANCHOD, M.: Metastatic melanoma with balloon cell changes, PRS, *51:*351, 1973. Cancer, *30:*1006, 1972

RANDALL, P.: Lip adhesion operation in cleft lip surgery (Follow-Up Clinic). PRS, *50:*182, 1972

RANDALL, P.: Discussion of "Treatment of respiratory obstruction in micrognathia by use of a nasogastric tube," by McEvitt. PRS, *52:*306, 1973

RANDALL, P.: Direct approach to "hanging columella." PRS, *53:*544, 1974

RANDALL, P.: Cleft lip. Clin. Plast. Surg., *2:*215, 1975

RANDALL, P.: Preservation of a posterior pharyngeal flap during maxillary advancement (with Ruberg, Whitaker). PRS, *57:*335, 1976

RANDALL, P., AND PADGETT, E. C.: Endotracheal tube holder and bite block. PRS, *50:*412, 1972

RANDALL, P., WHITAKER, L. A., AND LaROSSA, D.: Importance of muscle reconstruction in primary and secondary cleft lip repair. PRS, *54:*316, 1974

RANDELL, J.: Transvestism and trans-sexualism. Brit. J. Psychiatry, spec. no. *9:*201, 1975

RANEY, A. M. *et al*: Reanastomosis of completely transected penis in canine. Review of current concepts. Urology, *6:*735, 1975

RANGER, D.: Visceral replacement after laryngopharyngectomy. J. Laryng. & Otol., *85:*1218, 1971

RANK, B. K.: President's address to the Fifth International Congress of Plastic Surgery. PRS, *48:*207, 1971

RANK, B. K.: Surgery and skin cancer. Ann. R. Coll. Surg. Engl., *52:*148, 1973

RANK, B. K., WAKEFIELD, A. R., AND HUESTON, J. T.: *Surgery of Repair as Applied to Hand Injuries.* 4th Edition. Williams & Wil-

kins Co., Baltimore, 1973. PRS, *53:*672, 1974

RANKOW, R. M.: Surgical decisions in treatment of major salivary gland tumors. PRS, *51:*514, 1973

RANKOW, R. M. *et al*: End results of the lateral oblique osteotomy for mandibular prognathism. Fortschr. Kiefer. Gesichtschir., *18:*155, 1974 (German)

RANKOW, R. M., CONLEY, J., AND FODOR, P.: Carcinoma of maxillary sinus following thorotrast instillation, PRS, *55:*386, 1975. J. Maxillo-facial Surg., *2:*119, 1974

RANKOW, R. M., AND POLAYES, I. M.: *Diseases of the Salivary Glands.* W. B. Saunders Co., Philadelphia, 1975

RANKOW, R. M. *et al*: Surgery of orbital floor fractures. Fortschr. Kiefer. Gesichtschir., *19:*169, 1975

RANNEY, D. A.: Hand in leprosy. Hand, *5:*1, 1973

RANNEY, D. A.: Reconstruction of the transverse metacarpal arch in ulnar palsy by transfer of the *extensor digiti minimi.* PRS, *52:*406, 1973

RANNEY, D. A.: Mechanism of arch reversal in the surgically corrected claw hand. Hand, *6:*266, 1974

RANNEY, D. A.: Role of punch grafting in eyebrow replacement. Lepr. Rev., *45:*153, 1974

RANNEY, D. A., AND FURNESS, M. A.: Results of *temporalis* transfer in lagophthalmos due to leprosy. PRS, *51:*301, 1973

RANSFORD, A. O., AND PROVAN, J. L.: Anterior tibial compartment syndrome complicating femoral embolectomy, PRS, *48:*393, 1971. Canad. J. Surg., *14:*231, 1971

RANTA, R.: Asymmetric formation in permanent dentition of cleft-affected children, PRS, *54:*694, 1974. Scand. J. Plast. Reconstr. Surg., *7:*59, 1973

RANTA, R. *et al*: Effect of periosteal flap technique on cleft width and formation of alveolar ridge in relation to bite level in surgery for cleft lip and palate, PRS, *56:*682, 1975. Scand. J. Plast. Reconstr. Surg., *8:*62, 1974

Ranula

Operative treatment of retention cysts by the method of coagulation (Khiterer). Stomatologiia (Mosk.), *50:*84, 1971 (Russian)

Ranula, plunging—case report (Rayne). Brit. J. Oral Surg., *11:*139, 1973

Ranulas, plunging, mucous extravasation theory as cause of (Roediger *et al*). Brit. J. Surg., *60:*720, 1973

Plunging ranula (Khafif *et al*). J. Oral Surg., *33:*537, 1975

Letter: Treatment of plunging ranula (Swank). J. Oral Surg., *33:*823, 1975

Ranula – Cont.
  Gland, sublingual, sarcoidosis and ranula of (Narang, Dixon), PRS, *57:*258, 1976. J. Oral Surg., *39:*376, 1975

Rao, B. D. *et al*: Intranasal meningoencephalocele. Int. Surg., *59:*421, 1974

Rao, P. B. *et al*: Carcinoma of hypopharynx at early age. J. Laryng. & Otol., *88:*1069, 1972

Rao, P. M. *et al*: Cylindroma – recurrence in postoperative fibrosis (a case report). J. Postgrad. Med., *21:*161, 1975

Rapaport, F. T. *et al*: Pulmonary microembolization in severe thermal injury. Proc. Soc. Exp. Biol. Med., *139:*1013, 1972

Rapaport, Felix T., and Dausset, Jean: *Tissue Typing Today: Proceedings of an International Symposium on the Role of Histocompatibility Typing in Clinical Organ Transplantation.* Grune & Stratton, N. Y. and London, 1971. PRS, *50:*518, 1972

Rapaport, Felix T., and Merrill, John P.: *Artificial Organs and Cardiopulmonary Support Systems.* Grune & Stratton, New York, 1972. PRS, *51:*85, 1973

Rapaport, Felix T., Balner, Hans, and Kountz, Samuel L.: *Transplantation Today.* (Proceedings of the 4th Int. Cong. of the Transplantation Society, San Francisco, Sept. 1972) Grune & Stratton, New York, 1973. PRS, *53:*218, 1974

Rapaport, J.: Giant keratoacanthoma of the nose. Arch. Dermat., *111:*73, 1975

Rapoport, A. *et al*: Neurogenic sarcoma (neurofibrosarcoma) of tongue, PRS, *54:*234, 1974. Internat. Surg., *58:*738, 1973

Rappaport, I., and Yim, D.: Congenital arteriovenous fistulas of head and neck, PRS, *52:*454, 1973. Arch. Otolaryng., *97:*350, 1973

Rapperport, A. S.: Simple and inexpensive dermabrader. PRS, *48:*386, 1971

Raque, C. J. *et al*: Snuff dippers keratosis (snuff-induced leukoplakia). South. Med. J., *68:*565, 1975

Rasi, H. B.: Fate of preserved human cartilage (Follow-Up Clinic). PRS, *49:*83, 1972

Raskin, M. B.: Agenesis of the vagina: report of case. J. Am. Osteopath. Assoc., *75:*206, 1975

Rasmussen, J. E.: Syndrome of trichoepitheliomas, milia, and cylindromas. Arch. Dermat., *111:*610, 1975

Rasmussen, T., Mathieson, G., and Le Blanc, F.: Surgical therapy of typical and forme fruste variety of Sturge-Weber syndrome. Schweiz. Arch. Neurol. u. Psychiat., *111:*393, 1972

Ratliff, A. H.: Deformities of the thumb in rheumatoid arthritis. Hand, *3:*138, 1971

Ratliff, A. H. *et al*: An extension to an operating table for hand surgery. Hand, *3:*112, 1971

Ravault, M. P. *et al*: Fronto-orbital epidermoid cyst. Bull. Soc. Ophtalmol. Fr., *73:*793, 1973 (French)

Raven, R. W.: British Association of Surgical Oncology. Ann. R. Coll. Surg. Engl., *53:*305, 1973

Raven, R. W.: Carcinoma of hypopharynx. Am. J. Roentgenol. Radium Ther. Nucl. Med., *120:*173, 1974

Raven, R. W.: Combination therapy in certain cancerous disease of head and neck. Am. J. Roentgenol. Radium Ther. Nucl. Med., *120:*178, 1974

Ravindra, M. S., and Chaudhry, A. P.: Light microscopic and histochemical observations on development of palate in Golden Syrian hamster, PRS, *55:*259, 1975. J. Anat., *117:*1, 1974

Ravisse, P. *et al*: Odontogenic calcifying epithelial tumor (Pindborg's tumor), case report. Ann. Anat. Pathol. (Paris), *18:*463, 1973 (French)

Ravon, R. W.: Progress in surgical oncology, PRS, *55:*725, 1975. Proc. Roy. Soc. Med., *67:*737, 1974

Rawat, S. S. *et al*: Congenital double columella. Brit. J. Plast. Surg., *28:*153, 1975

Rawat, S. S. *et al*: One-stage repair of full-thickness alar defects. Brit. J. Plast. Surg., *28:*317, 1975

Rawis, H. C., III, *et al*: Surgical correction of permanently dislocated mandible. J. Oral Surg., *31:*385, 1973

Rayne, J.: Plunging ranula – case report. Brit. J. Oral Surg., *11:*139, 1973

Rayner, C. R. W.: Disseminated candidiasis in severely burned patient. PRS, *51:*461, 1973

Rayner, C. R. W.: Repair of full-thickness defects in abdominal wall in rats avoiding visceral adhesions, PRS, *56:*678, 1975. Brit. J. Plast. Surg., *27:*130, 1974

Razvozova, E. P.: Use of ultrasonics for prevention of contractures after burns. Ortop. Travmatol. Protez., *34:*13, 1974 (Russian)

Reagan, B., and Folse, R.: Lower limb-venous dynamics in normal persons and children of patients with varicose veins, PRS, *48:*92, 1971. Surg. Gynec. & Obst., *132:*15, 1971

Rebattu, J. P.: Reflections on the laryngo-tracheal sequelae of assisted respiration with intubation or tracheotomy. From functional disorders to lesions. J. Fr. Otorhinolaryngol., *24:*67, 1975 (French)

Rebattu, J. P. *et al*: Protruding ears. J. Med. Lyon, *53:*1633, 1972 (French)

Rebattu, J. P. *et al*: Functional surgery and esthetic surgery of nose. Lyon Med., *228:*805, 1972 (French)

RECHNAGEL, K.: Arthrodesis of wrist joint, follow-up of 60 cases, PRS, *49:*583, 1972. Scand. J. Plast. Reconstr. Surg., *5:*120, 1971

RECKLER, J. M.: Superior mesenteric artery syndrome as consequence of burn injury, PRS, *53:*493, 1974. J. Trauma, *12:*979, 1973

RECKLING, F. W. *et al:* Severe electrical burns with impending renal failure. J. Kans. Med. Soc., *72:*410, 1971

RECKLING, F. W., HERMRECK, A. S., AND PELTIER, L. F.: Trauma conference: method of teaching management of injured patient, PRS, *57:*541, 1976. J. Trauma, *14:*841, 1974

Rectum

Anorectal malformations (Beltran-Brown, Nasrallah), PRS, *51:*481, 1973. Cir. y cir. Mexico, *40:*57, 1972

Rectum, duplication of (Ruiz-Moreno), PRS, *50:*420, 1972. El Medico, *21:*58, 1972

Rectum, transplantation of small bowel mucosa to (Brody) (Follow-Up Clinic). PRS, *50:*183, 1972

Lymphogranuloma, surgically treated local, case (Szabo *et al*). Fogorv. Sz., *66:*172, 1973

Lymphogranuloma venereum, radical perineal resection for far-advanced (Hirschberg, Horton). PRS, *51:*217, 1973

Fistulectomies, surgery for incontinence after (Garriz *et al*), PRS, *53:*107, 1974. Prensa Med. Argent., *60:*492, 1973

Incontinence, fecal, electromyographic and electromanometric studies after *gracilis* transplantations for (Holschneider, Lahoda), PRS, *54:*631, 1974. Ztschr. Kinderchir., *14:*288, 1974

From anal atresia to continent organ (Scharli). Arch. chir. neerl., *27:*179, 1975 (German)

Gracilis plastic surgery using Pickrell's technic (Blessing *et al*). Helv. Chir. Acta, *42:*231, 1975 (German)

Perineal body, construction in female (Pickrell, Peters, Neale). PRS, *55:*529, 1975

REDDICK, L. P., AND MYERS, R. T.: Neurilemmoma of cervical portion of vagus nerve, PRS, *53:*111, 1974. Am. J. Surg., *125:*744, 1973

REDDY, L. N.: One-stage repair of hypospadias. Urology, *5:*475, 1975

REDING, R.: Results in the treatment of burns. Zentralbl. Chir., *96:*1032, 1971 (German)

REDMAN, J., AND BISSADA, N.: Complete duplication of urethra with probable diphallus, PRS, *56:*230, 1975. J. Pediat. Surg., *10:*135, 1975

REDMAN, J. C.: Suspected early primary malignant melanoma. Rocky Mt. Med. J., *71:*161, 1974

REDMAN, J. C.: Suspected early primary malignant melanoma, PRS, *56:*113, 1975. Cutis, *15:*98, 1975

REDMAN, J. F.: Noonan's syndrome and cryptorchidism, PRS, *52:*596, 1973. J. Urol., *109:*909, 1973

REDMAN, J. F.: Technique to preserve preputial blood supply, PRS, *53:*110, 1974. J. Urol., *109:*1019, 1973

REDMAN, J. F. *et al:* Failure of chemotherapy in treatment of giant condyloma acuminata (Buschke-Loewenstein tumor). South. Med. J., *67:*742, 1974

REDMAN, J. F. *et al:* Surgical dressing for hypospadias repair. Urology, *4:*739, 1974

REDMAN, J. F. *et al:* Perineal corporeal compression: techniques to evaluate chordee. Urology, *5:*351, 1975

REDMAN, J. F. *et al:* Surgical correction of lateral curvature of penis. Urology, *5:*508, 1975

REDPATH, T. H.: Mandibular reconstruction in Nigeria. Brit. J. Oral Surg., *9:*85, 1971

REEF, T. C. *et al:* Extensor digitorum brevis manus and its clinical significance. J. Bone & Joint Surg. (Am.), *57:*704, 1975

REEH, M. J.: Blepharoptosis. Mil. Med., *136:*760, 1971

REEMTSMA, K., AND MALONEY, J. V., JR.: Economics of instant medical news, PRS, *56:*236, 1975. New England J. Med., *290:*439, 1974

REES, B. I. *et al:* Delayed exposed skin grafting in surgery for breast cancer and melanoma. Clin. Oncol., *1:*131, 1975

REES, T. D.: Transfer of free composite grafts of skin and fat (Follow-Up Clinic). PRS, *49:*84, 1972

REES, T. D.: Correction of ectropion resulting from blepharoplasty. PRS, *50:*1, 1972

REES, T. D.: Discussion of "Bone deformation beneath alloplastic implants," by Jobe *et al.* PRS, *51:*174, 1973

REES, T. D.: Discussion of "Acute retrobulbar hemorrhage during elective blepharoplasty," by Hartley *et al*, PRS, *52:*12, 1973. Erratum, PRS, *52:*470, 1973

REES, T. D.: Mammary asymmetry. Clin. Plast. Surg., *2:*371, 1975

REES, T. D.: Reconstruction of breast areola by intradermal tattooing and transfer. PRS, *55:*620, 1975

REES, T. D.: Effect of hematoma on thickness of pseudosheaths around silicone implants (with Williams, Aston). PRS, *56:*194, 1975

REES, T. D.: Dry eye complication after blepharoplasty. PRS, *56:*375, 1975

REES, T. D., AND WOOD, A. M.: Post-graduate training in reconstructive plastic surgery in East Africa. PRS, *48:*5, 1971

REES, T. D. *et al*: Breast reduction: is it an aid to cancer detection? Brit. J. Plast. Surg., *25:*144, 1972

REES, T. D., AND CASSON, P. R.: Indications for cutaneous dermal overgrafting (Follow-Up Clinic). PRS, *49:*566, 1972

REES, T. D., LEE, Y. C., AND COBURN, R. J.: Expanding hematoma after rhytidectomy, retrospective study. PRS, *51:*149, 1973

REES, T. D., ASHLEY, F. L., AND DELGADO, J. P.: Silicone fluid injections for facial atrophy. PRS, *52:*118, 1973

REES, T. D., AND COBURN, R. J.: Silicone treatment of partial lipodystrophy, PRS, *55:*505, 1975. J.A.M.A., *230:*868, 1974

REES, T. D., GUY, C. L., AND COBURN, R. J.: Use of inflatable breast implants, PRS, *52:*609, 1973. Addendum, PRS, *54:*213, 1974

REES, THOMAS D., AND WOOD-SMITH, DONALD: *Cosmetic Facial Surgery.* W. B. Saunders Co., Philadelphia, 1973. PRS, *52:*427, 1973

REGE, P. R., AND EVANS, A. T.: Erythroplasia of Queyrat, PRS, *57:*536, 1976. J. Urol., *111:*784, 1974

REGE, S. R. *et al*: Combined approach for massive nasopharyngeal fibroma. J. Laryng. & Otol., *89:*1219, 1975

REGENSBURGER, D. *et al*: Errors of indication in funnel chest operations. Langenbecks Arch. Chir., *327:*570, 1970 (German)

REGNAULT, P.: Complete face and forehead lifting with double traction on "crow's-feet." PRS, *49:*123, 1972

REGNAULT, P.: Reduction mammaplasty by "B" technique. PRS, *53:*19, 1974

REGNAULT, P.: Nipple hypertrophy. Physiologic reduction by circumcision. Clin. Plast. Surg., *2:*391, 1975

REGNAULT, P.: Abdominal dermolipectomies. Clin. Plast. Surg., *2:*411, 1975

REGNAULT, P.: Abdominoplasty by W technique. PRS, *55:*265, 1975

REGNAULT, P., AND STEPHENSON, K. L.: Dr. Suzanne Noël, first woman to do esthetic surgery. PRS, *48:*133, 1971

REGNAULT, P. *et al*: Clinical trial and evaluation of proposed new inflatable mammary prosthesis. PRS, *50:*220, 1972

REGNIER, R.: Usefulness of radiotherapy in the treatment of cutaneous melanoma. Acta Chir. Belg., *73:*237, 1974 (French)

Rehabilitation

Rehabilitation of cancer patient. 2. Paraplegia, amputations and head and neck surgery (Downie). Nurs. Mirror, *135:*36, 1972

Rehabilitation even for disfigured persons (Ehring *et al*). Oeff. Gesundheitswes., *34:*529, 1972 (German)

Rehabilitation – Cont.

Rehabilitation, primary, after total glossectomy and laryngectomy with mandibulectomy for advanced cancer of mouth (Terz, King, Lawrence). Surg. Gynec. & Obst., *136:*276, 1973

REHAK, G. *et al*: Experience with orthodontic treatment before surgical correction of unilateral and bilateral cleft lip and palate in infants. Orv. Hetil., *115:*2672, 1974 (Hungarian)

REHDER, H. *et al*: XX-male-syndrome. Pathogenesis and aspects of diagnostic pitfalls. Urologe. (A), *14:*182, 1975 (German)

REHN, J.: Treatment of skin defects on extremities and on trunk. Langenbecks Arch. Chir., *334:*609, 1973 (German)

REHRMANN, A.: Effect of early bone grafting on the growth of upper jaw in cleft lip and palate children. A computer evaluation. Minerva Chir., *26:*874, 1971

REHRMANN, A.: Creation of alveolar ridge after bone transplantation to mandible (Follow-Up Clinic). PRS, *48:*368, 1971

REHRMANN, A.: Two stage surgery of mandibular cystic adamantinomas. Fortschr. Kiefer. Gesichtschir., *15:*195, 1972 (German)

REHRMANN, A.: Construction of upper lip, columella, and *orbicularis* muscle in bilateral clefts, PRS, *56:*468, 1975. J. Maxillo-facial Surg., *3:*2, 1975

REHRMANN, A. *et al*: Fractures of central facial bones in their relation to skull base. Langenbecks Arch. Chir., *329:*548, 1971 (German)

REHRMANN, A. *et al*: Results in conservative parotidectomy in pleomorphous adenomas – report of 110 cases. Fortschr. Kiefer. Gesichtschir., *15:*106, 1972 (German)

REHRMANN, A., AND KREIDLER, J.: Late results after arthroereisis of temporomandibular joint by autoplastic bone graft, PRS, *53:*241, 1974. J. Maxillo-facial Surg., *1:*99, 1973

REHRMANN, A., BLESSING, M. H., AND REIL, B.: Clinical and histological late findings on pedicle skin flaps in oral cavity, PRS, *57:*540, 1976. J. Maxillo-facial Surg., *3:*155, 1975

REICH, H.: Hemangiopericytoma of child. Monatsschr. Kinderheilkd., *120:*430, 1972 (German)

REICH, J.: Esthetic plastic surgery, development and place in medical practice, PRS, *51:*712, 1973. M. J. Australia, *1:*1152, 1972

REICH, J.: Surgical improvement in appearance of female body, PRS, *56:*236, 1975. M. J. Australia, *2:*767, 1974

REICH, J.: Factors influencing patient satisfaction with results of esthetic plastic surgery. PRS, *55:*5, 1975

REICH, M. P., AND EISEMAN, B.: Tissue oxygenation following resuscitation with crystalloid solution following experimental acute blood loss, PRS, *48:*519, 1971. Surgery, *69:*928, 1971

REICHART, P.: Pathologic changes in soft palate in lepromatous leprosy, PRS, *56:*593, 1975. Oral Surg., *38:*898, 1974

REICHENBACH, E.: Karl Schuchardt and the development of jaw and face surgery (on his 70th birthday, 24 December 1971). Dtsch. Zahn. Mund. Kieferheilkd., *57:*266, 1971 (German)

REICHERT, H.: Cranial approach in the surgical repositioning of displaced orbital contents. Fortschr. Kiefer. Gesichtschir., *18:*34, 1974 (German)

REICHERT, H.: Lateral velopharyngoplasty: new method for correction of open nasality, PRS, *55:*381, 1975. J. Maxillo-facial Surg., *2:*95, 1974

REICHERT, R.: Tumors of the paranasal sinuses involving the orbit. Laryngol. Rhinol. Otol. (Stuttg.), *53:*443, 1974

REICHMANN, J.: Burn scar carcinoma, avoidable sequelae of burns? Z. Aerztl. Fortbild. (Jena), *65:*1197, 1971 (German)

REICHMANN, W.: Late results of radical surgery for extensive racemose lymphangioma of the arm. Handchirurgie, *3:*41, 1971 (German)

REICHMANN, W.: Late results following extirpation of melanosarcoma of the hand by superficial lymphangiectomy and lymphadenectomy. Handchirurgie, *3:*42, 1971 (German)

REICHMANN, W.: Proceedings: Acute suppurating infections of hands and fingers and their treatment. Langenbecks Arch. Chir., *334:*499, 1973 (German)

REID, D. A.: An unusual mutilating injury of the hand. Brit. J. Plast. Surg., *25:*53, 1972

REID, D. A.: Corrective osteotomy in the hand. Hand, *6:*50, 1974

REID, D. A.: Post-operative complications in hand surgery. Hand, *7:*115, 1975

REID, D. A. C.: Escalator injuries of hand, PRS, *54:*376, 1974. Injury, *5:*47, 1973

REID, D. A. C.: Hand injuries requiring skin replacement and restoration of tendon function, PRS, *56:*679, 1975. Brit. J. Plast. Surg., *27:*5, 1974

REID, H. A.: Principles of snakebite treatment. Clin. Toxicol., *3:*473, 1970

REID, R. L. *et al*: Acute necrosis of the second interosseous compartment of the hand. J. Bone & Joint Surg. (Am.), *55:*1095, 1973

REID, S. P. *et al*: Essential blepharospasm. J. Ir. Med. Assoc., *67:*64, 1974

REID, W. H.: Care of burned hand, PRS, *54:*690, 1974. Hand, *6:*163, 1974

REIL, B. *et al*: Diagnostic and therapeutic regime for reducing mortality after resection of tumors in head and neck. J. Maxillo-facial Surg., *3:*54, 1975

REILL, P.: Severe hand injuries in old age. Hefte Unfallheilkd., *121:*137, 1975 (German)

REIN, J. M., AND COSMAN, B.: Bacteroides necrotizing fasciitis of upper extremity. PRS, *48:*592, 1971

REINHARDT, K.: Calcification of fatty tissue transplants in the mamma. Roentgenblaetter, *27:*418, 1974 (German)

REINISCH, J., AND MYERS, B.: Effect of local anesthesia with epinephrine on skin flap survival. PRS, *54:*324, 1974

REINISCH, J. F.: Pathophysiology of skin flap circulation. PRS, *54:*585, 1974

REINISCH, J. F.: Reply to "Is arteriovenous shunting the correct explanation of flap delay phenomenon?" by Freshwater (Letter to the Editor). PRS, *55:*698, 1975

REIS, N. D.: Gillies "cocked hat" reconstruction for total loss of ulnar four fingers. Hand, *5:*229, 1973

REIS, N. D.: Screw fixation in Zancolli capsuloplasty, PRS, *56:*229, 1975. Hand, *6:*150, 1974

REISIN, J. H., GUTHRIE, R. H., AND GOULIAN, D., JR.: Timing of pedicled flap delays by measurements of flap oxygen and carbon dioxide, PRS, *56:*365, 1975. J. Surg. Oncol., *6:*79, 1974

REITZIK, M.: Surgically corrected mandibular prognathism. Cephalometric analysis of 50 cases. Am. J. Orthod., *66:*82, 1974

REMAGEN, W. *et al*: Benign osteoblastoma. Oral Surg., *39:*279, 1975

REMARK, F. L.: Airless paint gun injury of the hand. A surgical emergency. Mo. Med., *69:*196, 1972

REMARK, F. L. *et al*: Management of the acutely injured hand. Mo. Med., *68:*767, 1971

REMARK, F. L. *et al*: Management of major nasal defects. South. Med. J., *65:*623, 1972

REMENSNYDER, J. P.: Topography of tissue oxygen tension changes in acute burn edema, PRS, *51:*606, 1973. Arch. Surg., *105:*477, 1972

REMENSNYDER, J. P.: Burn contractures of the neck: natural history and surgical treatment. In *Plastische und Wiederherstellungs-Chirurgie,* ed. by Hohler; pp. 259-66. Schattauer, Stuttgart, 1975

REMUS, W. *et al*: Surgical treatment in adult patients with spinal cord injuries. Arch. Orthop. Unfallchir., *79:*119, 1974 (German)

RENARD, A., AND MORGAN, B. L.: Nasolabial cyst, PRS, *57:*240, 1976

RENAUD, Y. *et al*: Cylindroma of oral cavity. Rev. Stomatol. Chir. Maxillofac., *74:*1, 1973 (French)

RENAULT, P. *et al*: Pharyngolaryngeal cancers treated with bleomycin. Histopathological assessment. Ann. Otolaryngol. Chir. Cervicofac., *89:*229, 1972

RENK, H.: Use of Kiel bone graft in restorative surgery in ENT fields. H. N. O., *21:*114, 1973 (German)

RENKIELSKI, J.: Treatment of urinary bladder exstrophy. Pol. Przegl. Chir., *45:*1201, 1973 (Polish)

RENNEFARTH, I.: Cervicofacial actinomycosis. Z. Aerztl. Fortbild. (Jena), *64:*395, 1970 (German)

RENNER, A. *et al*: Arthroplasty of the hand with silicone rubber prosthesis. Magy. Traumatol. Orthop., *15:*44, 1972 (Hungarian)

RENY, A. *et al*: Surgical treatment of epithelioma of the external and internal canthal regions. Bull. Soc. Ophtalmol. Fr., *74:*1037, 1974 (French)

RENY, M. A.: Full thickness graft from eyelid to eyelid. Bull. Soc. Ophtalmol. Fr., *74:*637, 1974 (French)

Replantation

Successful replantation of severed extremities (Nasseri *et al*). Langenbecks Arch. Chir., *327:*771, 1970 (German)

Replantation of amputated extremities, functional recuperation (Ramirez *et al*), PRS, *55:*121, 1975. Antioquia Med., *21:*575, 1971

Replantation of an almost totally amputated limb (Coppilino *et al*). Minerva Med., *62:*4732, 1971 (Italian)

Pocket principle, new technique for reattachment of severed ear part (Mladick *et al*). PRS, *48:*219, 1971

Ear half, severed, successful replantation of (McDowell). PRS, *48:*281, 1971

New technic for the reimplantation of a completely severed auricle (Baudet *et al*). Ann. chir. plast., *17:*67, 1972 (French)

Replantation of the mutilated external ear. New method (Baudet). Nouv. Presse Med., *1:*344, 1972 (French)

Amputated tissues of the head and neck, fate of, following replacement (Grabb, Dingman). PRS, *49:*28, 1972

Ear, replantation of severed part (Gifford) (Letter to the Editor). PRS, *49:*202, 1972

Ear, amputated, salvage of (Conroy) (Letter to the Editor). PRS, *49:*564, 1972

Thumb, totally severed, successful replantation (Snyder, Stevenson, Browne). PRS, *50:*553, 1972

Limb replantation, experimental study (Maquieira *et al*), PRS, *51:*354, 1973. Rev. argent. cir., *22:*66, 1972

Replantation – Cont.

Ear, mutilated, reimplantation of pinna (Baudet *et al*). Rev. Laryngol. Otol. Rhinol. (Bord.), *93:*241, 1972 (French)

Ear lobe, reimplantation of, after quasi-total section (Vergon *et al*). Ann. Otolaryngol. Chir. Cervicofac., *90:*711, 1973 (French)

Reattachment of totally amputated auricle (Clemons *et al*). Arch. Otolaryng., *97:*269, 1973

Vascular problems in replantation of limbs (Danese, Cree, Singer), PRS, *53:*606, 1974. Arch. Surg., *107:*715, 1973

Replantation of amputated finger (Lendvay), PRS, *53:*685, 1974. Asian J. Med., *9:*249, 1973

Amputations of upper limb, traumatic, microvascular repair in (Miller), PRS, *53:*367, 1974. Australian & New Zealand J. Surg., *43:*19, 1973

Amputated limb, importance of lymphatic drainage in edema following replantation (Perinetti, Manfredi, Anchelerguez), PRS, *54:*111, 1974. Bol. y trab. Soc. argent. cir., *34:*465, 1973

Reattachment of severed limbs. Brit. Med. J., *1:*564, 1973

Replantation of severed limbs and fingers (Shanghai Sixth Peoples Hospital), PRS, *51:*703, 1973. Chinese M.J., *1:*1, 1973

Replantation of severed limbs, analysis of 40 cases (Peking Chischueit'an Hospital), PRS, *55:*254, 1975. Chinese M.J., *6:*67, 1973

Replantation of severed fingers (Chung Shan Medical College, Kwangchow), PRS, *55:*248, 1975. Chinese M.J., *6:*71, 1973

Limb replantation after resection of neoplastic segment—report of 8 cases (Shanghai Sixth People's Hospital), PRS, *55:*255, 1975. Chinese M.J., *6:*72, 1973

Reimplantation of limbs after resection of neoplastic segment, report of 8 cases. Chinese Med. J. *6:*338, 1973 (Chinese)

Experiments in transplantation of severed limbs. Chinese Med. J., *6:*348, 1973 (Chinese)

Regeneration of veins and lymphatics after limb reimplantation in dogs. Chinese Med. J., *6:*353, 1973 (Chinese)

Replantation of severed index finger to replace amputated thumb (Limb Replantation Research Group), PRS, *53:*487, 1974. Chinese M.J., *8:*110, 1973

Replantation of severed limbs, complications and management (Shanghai First Peoples Hospital), PRS, *53:*494, 1974. Chinese M.J., *9:*122, 1973

Ear replantation, successful, of subtotally

Replantation — Cont.

separated ear using local hypothermia (Mühlbauer). Chirurg., *44:*85, 1973 (German)

Digital reattachment and revascularization (O'Brien, Miller), PRS, *53:*244, 1974. J. Bone & Joint Surg., *55A:*714, 1973

Reanastomosis of amputated penis (Schulman), PRS, *52:*596, 1973. J. Urol., *109:*432, 1973

Saving the amputated digit and hand (O'Brien *et al*). M. J. Australia, *1:*558, 1973

Ear fragment, large severed, successful replantation of (Baudet) (Letter to the Editor). PRS, *51:*82, 1973

Replantation of avulsed anterior teeth in patients with jaw fractures (Lu). PRS, *51:*377, 1973

Otoplasty: ear reattachment by modified pocket principle (Mladick, Carraway). PRS, *51:*584, 1973

Nasal tip replantation (Cort). PRS, *52:*194, 1973

Replantation surgery in China (American Replantation Mission). PRS, *52:*476, 1973

Replantation of digits, clinical (O'Brien *et al*). PRS, *52:*490, 1973

Amputation of fingers or extremities: get in there and replant! (McDowell) (Editorial). PRS, *52:*562, 1973

Replantation of completely amputated distal thumb without venous anastomosis (Serafin, Kutz, Kleinert), PRS, *52:*579, 1973. Commentary by Buncke, PRS, *52:*581, 1973

Micro needle holder, new, and metallized microsutures (O'Brien, Hayhurst), PRS, *52:*673, 1973

Replantation surgery in upper limb (O'Brien, MacLeod), PRS, *52:*680, 1973. Proc. Roy. Australasian Coll. Surg., *46:*427, 1973

Replantation of amputated extremities. Necessity for re-evaluation (Balas). Vasc. Surg., *7:*1, 1973

Replantation of severed fingers (Corry, Russell), PRS, *54:*502, 1974. Ann. Surg., *179:*225, 1974

Reimplantation of amputated pinna (Potsic *et al*). Arch. Otolaryng., *100:*73, 1974

Replantation of little finger in 20-month-old child (Tamai *et al*), PRS, *56:*679, 1975. Brit. J. Plast. Surg., *27:*1, 1974

Replantation, limb, experimental study of effect of ilex pubescens on vessels of isolated organs, with report on clinical use (Chung Shan Medical College, Kwangchow), PRS, *55:*250, 1975. Chinese M.J., *2:*28, 1974

Replantation of upper limb in 43-year-old

Replantation — Cont.

woman (Harvey *et al*), PRS, *56:*356, 1975. Clin. Orthop., *102:*167, 1974

Tooth replantation (Massler), PRS, *55:*506, 1975. Dent. Clin. N. Am., *18:*2, 1974

Fingers replanted after prolonged cooling, experimental (Hayhurst *et al*), PRS, *56:*227, 1975. Hand, *6:*134, 1974

Replantation surgery, major, in upper limb (O'Brien *et al*), PRS, *56:*228, 1975. Hand, *6:*217, 1974

Prognostic value of thermography in operations of transplantation for saving a limb (Baudet *et al*). J. Radiol. Electrol. Med. Nucl., *55:*239, 1974 (French)

Replantation of a hand severed through the palm (Kolos *et al*). M. J. Australia, *2:*559, 1974

Replantation of portions of 4 fingers in one hand (Chunprapaph), PRS, *55:*248, 1975. New England J. Med., *291:*460, 1974

Replantation, improved patency rates in microvascular surgery when using magnesium sulfate and silicone rubber vascular cuff (Nomoto, Buncke, Chater), PRS, *54:*157, 1974

Reimplantations in arts (Tosatti), PRS, *54:*511, 1974. Surgery, *75:*389, 1974

Future of constructive surgery. (Russell). Transplant Proc., *6:*147, 1974

Structure and properties of the aldolase in the muscles of a replanted extremity in dogs (Lisova *et al*). Ukr. Biokhim. Zh., *46:*418, 1974 (Ukrainian)

Long term nerve function in replantation surgery of the hand and digits (Morrison *et al*). Ann. Chir., *29:*1041, 1975 (French) (English)

Replantation of severed limbs, hyperbaric oxygen therapy in (Shanghai Sixth People's Hospital), PRS, *57:*763, 1976. Canad. J. Surg., *18:*403, 1975

Limbs, severed, hyperbaric oxygen therapy in replantation (Shanghai Sixth People's Hospital), PRS, *57:*763, 1976. Chinese M.J., *1:*197, 1975

Replantation of severed limbs (Editorial). Analysis of 40 cases. Chinese Med. J., *1:*265, 1975

Surgery in China: part 1. (Critchley). M. J. Australia, *1:*693, 1975

Replantation of amputated extremities. Report of five cases (Jaffe *et al*). Ohio State Med. J., *71:*381, 1975

Reimplantation of teeth in monkeys, storage before (Nasjleti, Castelli), PRS, *57:*115, 1976. Oral Surg., *39:*20, 1975

Replantation of limb and certain principles of

Replantation–Cont.

restoration of blood and lymph circulation (Kirpatovskii *et al*). Ortop. Travmatol. Protez., *4:*58, 1975

Magnesium sulfate or heparin, experimental effects on patency of microvascular anastomoses (Engrav *et al*). PRS, *55:*618, 1975

Replantation and transplantation, microvascular, study of washout solutions for (Harashina, Buncke). PRS, *56:*542, 1975

Replantation, hand, experience with 8 cases (Ferreira *et al*), PRS, *57:*533, 1976. Rev. Assoc. med. bras., *21:*149, 1975

Replantation of severed ear parts (Larsen, Pless), PRS, *57:*176, 1976. Discussion by Mladick. PRS, *57:*357, 1976

Hand: cross-hand digital transfer (Edgerton). PRS, *57:*281, 1976

RESL, M.: Postmortem bacteriological findings in trachea of tracheotomized and nontracheotomized subjects. Sb. Ved. Pr. Lek. Fak. Karlovy Univ. (Suppl.), *15:*395, 1972 (Czechoslovakian)

RETHI, A.: Surgery of the cleft-lip profile. Laryngol. Rhinol. Otol. (Stuttg.), *54:*132, 1975 (German)

Retrognathism (See also *Micrognathia*)

One-stage mandibular-maxillary reconstruction in the treatment of gross disproportion of the jaws (Winstock). Brit. J. Oral Surg., *9:*115, 1971

Surgical treatment of severe dento-maxillary irregularities (Popescu *et al*). Int. Dent. J., *21:*346, 1971

Sectional osteotomies of the jaws. Their value in the correction of profile abnormalities (Merville *et al*). Rev. Fr. Odontostomatol., *18:*1094, 1971 (French)

Horizontal osteotomy for correction of maxillary retrusion: report of case (Pedersen). J. Oral Surg., *30:*581, 1972

Surgical correction of retrognathism by forward movement of a part of the maxilla with simultaneous bone transplantation (Zisser). Osterr. Z. Stomatol., *69:*143, 1972 (German)

Surgical-orthodontic treatment of severe mandibular retrusion (Poulton, Ware). Am. J. Orthodontics, *63:*237, 1973

Retrognathism, mandibular, treatment of, using retrocondylar cartilage graft (Trauner procedure) (Lachard, Vitton). Ann. chir. plast., *18:*50, 1973 (French)

Maxillo-mandibular surgery for correction of dentofacial deformities. 5. Mandibular retrusion (Weinberg *et al*). J. Can. Dent. Assoc., *39:*544, 1973

Retrognathism – Cont.

Retrognathia, correction of, by modified "C" osteotomy of ramus and sagittal osteotomy of mandibular body (Hayes). J. Oral Surg., *31:*682, 1973

Trauner's operation in the treatment of retrognathia (Vitton *et al*). Rev. Stomatol. Chir. Maxillofac., *74:*632, 1973 (French)

Bilateral vertical osteotomy with notching for a butt joint of a retrognathic mandible (Smylski). Trans. Int. Conf. Oral Surg., *4:*41, 1973

Bilateral vertical osteotomy with notching for a butt joint of a retrognathic mandible (Smylski). Trans. Int. Conf. Oral Surg., *4:*237, 1973

Surgical treatment of maxillary protrusion and retrognathism (Kole). Fortschr. Kiefer. Gesichtschir., *18:*46, 1974 (German)

Treatment of childhood retrognathism through transposition of the masseter muscle (Spiessl *et al*). Fortschr. Kiefer. Gesichtschir., *18:*176, 1974 (German)

Standard method for the correction of symmetrical "bird-face" (Chausse). Fortschr. Kiefer. Gesichtschir., *18:*182, 1974 (German)

Indications, technic and results of block and segmental osteotomies on the maxilla and mandible in dysgnathias (Pfeifer). Fortschr. Kiefer. Gesichtschir., *18:*248, 1974

Mandibular retrusion surgically corrected by bilateral subcondylar ramus osteotomy and bone transplantation (Nordenram *et al*). Nor. Tannlaegeforen Tid., *84:*52, 1974 (Norwegian)

Evaluation of the surgical procedure of sagittal split osteotomy of the mandibular ramus (Wang *et al*). Oral Surg., *38:*167, 1974

Le Fort I type of maxillary osteotomy, simplifying (Dupont, Ciaburro, Prévost). PRS, *54:*142, 1974

Retrognathia and bird face, surgical treatment of (Kruger). Quintessenz, *25:*25, 1974 (German)

Discussion of indications for alveolar segmental osteotomy of the jaws (Cros *et al*). Rev. Stomatol. Chir. Maxillofac., *75:*107, 1974 (French)

Multiple osteotomies in a single surgical stage (Curioni). Rev. Stomatol. Chir. Maxillofac., *75:*116, 1974 (French)

Eight cases of sagittal osteotomies of the mandibular rami (Daieff *et al*). Rev. Stomatol. Chir. Maxillofac., *75:*145, 1974 (French)

Use of a Le Fort I osteotomy as a surgical approach (Hopkins *et al*). Brit. J. Oral

Retrognathism—Cont.
Surg., *13:*27, 1975
Mandibular retrusion, surgical correction of, in combination with mandibular alveolar protrusion (Steinhauser *et al*). J. Am. Dent. Assoc., *91:*132, 1975
Teamwork approach to correct a severe prosthodontic problem (Belinfante *et al*). J. Am. Dent. Assoc., *91:*357, 1975
Mandibular retrognathism, vertical osteotomy of ascending rami in (Popescu), PRS, *57:*530, 1976. J. Maxillo-facial Surg., *3:*65, 1975
Late results after advancing the mandible by sagittal splitting of the rami (Freihofer *et al*). J. Maxillo-facial Surg., *3:*230, 1975
Treatment of exophthalmia and retrognathia (van der Meulen *et al*). Ned. tijdschr. geneeskd., *119:*1757, 1975 (Dutch)
Surgical correction of jaw abnormalities causing severe facial deformities (Berenyi *et al*). Orv. Hetil., *116:*1767, 1975
Maxillary advancements: anesthetic management of and intraoperative care of patients undergoing major facial osteotomies (Davies, Munro). PRS, *55:*50, 1975
Mandibular retrognathia: a review of the literature and selected cases (Fox *et al*). J. Oral Surg., *34:*53, 1976
Interdental osteotomy for immediate repositioning of dental-osseous elements (Merrill *et al*). J. Oral Surg., *34:*118, 1976
Modification of the sagittal ramus-split osteotomy for retrognathia (Gallo *et al*). J. Oral Surg., *34:*178, 1976
Retrognathic mandible—surgical correction (Hull *et al*). Oral Surg., *41:*2, 1976
Correction of mandibular dentoalveolar retrusion by anterior segmental advancement (Pedersen *et al*). Oral Surg., *41:*281, 1976

RETTIG, H., AND OEST, O.: On disease pattern of morbus Dupuytren, PRS, *54:*247, 1974. Ztschr. Orthop., *112:*187, 1974
REUTER, G.: Treatment with lemon juice in prevention of recurrences of keloid. Zentralbl. Chir., *98:*604, 1973 (German)
REUTER, G.: Exomphalos-macroglossia-gigantism syndrome from surgical viewpoint (EMG syndrome). Zentralbl. Chir., *99:*668, 1974 (German)
REUTER, S. H.: Bivalve teflon nasal septal splint. Trans. Am. Acad. Ophthalmol. Otolaryngol., *77:*1146, 1973
REUTHER, J. *et al*: Primary and secondary treatment in chin defect fractures. Fortschr. Kiefer. Gesichtschir., *19:*215, 1975 (German)
REVENKO, T. A. *et al*: Dermatoglyphic data in

congenital hand deformities. Ortop. Travmatol. Protez., *10:*65, 1974 (Russian)
REVZIN, M. E.: Corrective procedures to repair inadequately treated fractured mandibles and maxillae. Trans. Int. Conf. Oral Surg., *4:*299, 1973
REYCHLER, A. *et al*: Frontal cross bite. Acta Stomatol. Belg., *71:*91, 1974 (Dutch)
REYES-GUERRA, A., JR.: Intraoral use of Kirschner pins. J. Oral Surg., *33:*304, 1975
REYMANN, F.: Follow-up study of treatment of basal cell carcinoma with 5-fluorouracil ointment. Dermatologica, *144:*205, 1972
REYMANN, F.: Treatment of basal cell carcinoma of skin with curettage, PRS, *53:*612, 1974. Arch. Dermat., *108:*528, 1973
REYMANN, F.: Multiple basal cell carcinoma treated with currettage. Ugeskr. Laeger, *136:*2523, 1974 (Danish)
REYMANN, F.: Multiple basal cell carcinomas of the skin, PRS, *57:*679, 1976. Arch. Dermat., *111:*877, 1975
REYNAUD, J.: Possibilities and indications of functional and restorative surgery for a leprous nose. Ann. chir. plast., *17:*137, 1972 (French)
REYNOLDS, B., WRAY, R. C., AND WEEKS, P. M.: Should an incompletely severed tendon be sutured? PRS, *57:*36, 1976. Discussion by Kleinert, PRS, *57:*236, 1976
REYNOLDS, V. H.: Cutaneous melanoma: 20-year retrospective study with clinicopathologic correlation (with Franklin, Page), PRS, *56:*277, 1975
RHEINSCHILD, G. W., AND OLSEN, B. S.: Balanitis xerotica obliterans, PRS, *48:*295, 1971. J. Urol., *104:*860, 1970
RHEINSCHILD, G. W. *et al*: Atypical case of priapism with unusual sequelae, PRS, *51:*604, 1973. J. Urol., *107:*423, 1972

Rhinolalia: See *Cleft Palate; Cleft Palate, Velopharyngeal Incompetence*

Rhinophyma

Rhinophyma patients, experiences with 8 operated (Fara), PRS, *51:*475, 1973, Acta chir. plast., *13:*254, 1971
Advantages of free skin autografts in the treatment of rhinophyma (Obreja *et al*). Otorinolaringologie, *16:*297, 1971 (Rumanian)
Rhinophyma skin grafts (Crikelair), PRS, *49:*98, 1972
Rhinophyma, new instrument for treatment (Obi, Bayles), PRS, *50:*414, 1972
Surgical treatment of rosaceà (Domeneci Llavallol). Acta otorinolaryngol. Iber. Am., *24:*94, 1973 (Spanish)

Rhinophyma – Cont.

Rhinophyma, severe (Chadfield). Brit. J. Dermatol., *88:*517, 1973

Rhinophyma and intranasal carcinoma (Kornblut). J. Laryng. & Otol., *87:*1137, 1973

Rhinophyma, cryosurgical treatment of (Nolan), PRS, *52:*437, 1973

Rhinophyma – cold knife paring and contour dermabrasion (Kirschner *et al*). Eye Ear Nose Throat Mon., *53:*421, 1974

Rhinophymous masses of acne conglobata, surgical treatment (Stellmach), PRS, *56:*471, 1975. J. Maxillo-facial Surg., *3:*58, 1975

Rhinoplasty (See also *Nose*)

False primary truths, false friends in facial plastic surgery (Jost). Cah. Med., *12:*1275, 1971 (French)

Experience in external nasal reconstruction and discussion on various problems (Ogino *et al*). Jap. J. Plast. Reconstr. Surg., *14:*456, 1971 (Japanese)

Surgery of alae nasi (Cvejic). Med. Glas., *25:*75, 1971 (Croatian)

Esthetic considerations of patient and surgeon: the nose-chin relationship (Grignon). Actual Odontostomatol. (Paris), *26:*455, 1972

Use of osteo-cartilaginous fragments removed during rhinoseptoplasty (Pollet). Ann. chir. plast., *17:*90, 1972 (French)

Rhinoplasty, craft of (Caplan). Can. J. Otolaryngol., *1:*102, 1972

Variables in rhinoplasties in identical twins (Goodwin). Eye Ear Nose Throat Mon., *51:*109, 1972

Rhinoplasty using Converse method (Fabre, Castelnau). J. Fr. Otorhinolaryngol., *21:*938, 1972 (French)

Rhinoplasty, cosmetic – the prerogative of plastic surgeon or rhinologist (Bridger). J. Otolaryngol. Soc. Aust., *3:*428, 1972

Nose, esthetic anatomy (Bernstein). Laryngoscope, *82:*2000, 1972

Rhinoplasty, reflections on corrective or modeling (Muntenescu *et al*). Otorinolaringologie, *17:*419, 1972 (Rumanian)

Advantages of vestibular approach in plastic operations of the nose (Nowinski). Otolaryngol. Pol., *26:*59, 1972 (Polish)

Rhinoplasty, new method to correct nasolabial angle (Caronni), PRS, *50:*338, 1972

Rhinoplasty, our scheme for (Pitanguy *et al*), PRS, *51:*602, 1973. Rev. brasil. cir., *62:*63, 1972

Rhinoplasty, controlled extra-mucosal, with preoperative measurement of profile modi-

Rhinoplasty–Cont.

fication (Robin). Ann. chir. plast., *18:*119, 1973 (French)

Nose, lateral cartilages of, study of junction between (Jost *et al*). Ann. chir. plast., *18:*175, 1973 (French)

Rhinoplasty, use of scissors in (Jost). Ann. chir. plast., *18:*279, 1973 (French)

Rhinoplasty, esthetic (Serson Neto). Ann. chir. plast., *18:*307, 1973 (French)

Rhinoplasty (Kataye). Ann. Otolaryngol. Chir. Cervicofac., *90:*123, 1973 (French)

Corrective rhinoplasty. Study of 5,000 personal cases (Bruck). Arch. Otolaryng., *97:*441, 1973

Rhinoplasty, external approach (Goodman). Can. J. Otolaryngol., *2:*207, 1973

Rhinoplasty training, videotaped and real-time color television in (Conway *et al*). Can. J. Otolaryngol., *2:*282, 1973

Rhinoplasty, corrective (Chabrier). Inf. Dent., *55:*45, 1973 (French)

Rhinoplasty and plastic facial repair (Stein). J. Am. Osteopath. Assoc., *72:*827, 1973

Nose, external, and profile plasty (Walter). Z. Laryngol. Rhinol. Otol., *52:*409, 1973 (German)

Sex change: secondary surgery in transsexuals (Bellinger, Goulian). PRS, *51:*628, 1973

Columellar-lip angle, cosmetic repair of acute (Guerrero-Santos), PRS, *52:*246, 1973

Rhinoplasty. Cosmetic surgery. 2. (Talamas). Postgrad. Med., *54:*129, 1973

Nose, plastic surgery of (Gervais). Rev. Infirm., *23:*715, 1973

Rhinoplasty, superior osteotomy: adjunct to osteoplastic nasal surgery (Graham, Royster), PRS, *53:*240, 1974. Rev. Latino Am. cir. plast., *17:*33, 1973

Nose, plastic surgery of (Geine). Vestn. Otorinolaringol., *35:*3, 1973 (Russian)

Corrective osteotomy in region of apertura piriformis to widen nostril (Werner). Z. Laryngol. Rhinol. Otol., *52:*89, 1973 (German)

Rhinoplasty, general points (Haas). Z. Laryngol. Rhinol. Otol., *52:*405, 1973 (German)

Nasal bones, correction of deformities; special care to avoid technical errors (Haas). Z. Laryngol. Rhinol. Otol., *52:*590, 1973 (German)

Nasal cartilage deformities, correction of, with special attention to sources of error (Haas). Z. Laryngol. Rhinol. Otol., *52:*699, 1973 (German)

Fractures in rhinoplasty (Mir y Mir), PRS, *54:*499, 1974. Acta chir. plast., *16:*48, 1974

Rhinoplasty–Cont.

Rhinorrheography in nose morphology and septorhinoplasties (Riu). Ann. chir. plast., *19:*181, 1974 (French)

Musculus depressor septi nasi. Study of its action and the role played in its resection during the postoperative course of cosmetic rhinoplasties (Mahe *et al*). Ann. chir. plast., *19:*257, 1974 (French)

Rhinoplasty, corrective, applied anatomy in (Bernstein). Arch. Otolaryng., *99:*67, 1974

Osteotomy and infraction in rhinoplasty (Smith). Arch. Otolaryng., *100:*266, 1974

Nasal surgery in childhood, clinical evaluation through 43 cases (Avila Lozada *et al*). Bol. Med. Hosp. Infant. Mex., *31:*799, 1974 (Spanish)

Assessment and management of bony deformities of the middle and lower face (Henderson). Brit. J. Plast. Surg., *27:*287, 1974

Nasal xeroradiography (McKinney *et al*). Brit. J. Plast. Surg., *27:*352, 1974

Cosmetic surgery (Horton *et al*). Brit. Med. J., *3:*566, 1974

Rhinoplasty, extramucous (Aytemiz *et al*), PRS, *57:*114, 1976. Bull. Milit. M. Acad., *16:*299, 1974

Surgical treatment of male transsexuals (Edgerton). Clin. Plast. Surg., *1:*285, 1974

Role of physical anthropology in plastic surgery today (Rogers). Clin. Plast. Surg., *1:*439, 1974

Rhinoplasty, corrective, new aspects in (Meyer *et al*). H. N. O., *22:*154, 1974 (German)

Surgical and esthetic aspects of the facial profile (D'ottaviano *et al*). Int. J. Oral Surg., *3:*243, 1974

Surgery of the nasal septum and pyramid (Gilchrist). J. Laryng. & Otol., *88:*759, 1974

Rhinoplasty in children: follow-up study in 92 cases (Pirsig *et al*). Laryngol. Rhinol. Otol. (Stuttg.), *53:*250, 1974 (German)

External approach to rhinoplasty (Goodman *et al*). Laryngoscope, *84:*2195, 1974

Otorhinolaryngology. Rhinology (Fleischer *et al*). Munch. Med. Wochenschr., *116:*1791, 1974 (German)

Allergic patient and rhinoplasty procedures (Soss). Otolaryngol. Clin. North Am., *7:*845, 1974

"Hanging columella," direct approach to (Randall), PRS, *53:*544, 1974

Rhinoplasty, asymptomatic rhinolith in (Mahler, Kaufman), PRS, *54:*490, 1974

Rhinoplasty and maxillary osteotomies (Aiach). Rev. Stomatol. Chir. Maxillofac.,

Rhinoplasty – Cont.

*75:*159, 1974 (French)

Modifications of the upper lip after rhinoplasty (Aiach). Rev. Stomatol. Chir. Maxillofac., *75:*1119, 1974 (French)

Internal fixation of grafts during rhinoplasty (Soubiran). Rev. Stomatol. Chir. Maxillofac., *75:*1125, 1974 (French)

Rhinoplasty (Kitsera *et al*). Vestn. Otorinolaringol., *4:*31, 1974 (Russian)

Anomalies in the development of the nasal cavity in children and their treatment (Shevrygin *et al*). Zh. Ushn. Nos. Gorl. Bolezn., *6:*30, 1974 (Russian)

Role of endo-oral incision during lateral osteotomies (Senechal *et al*). Ann. chir. plast., *20:*233, 1975 (French)

Resection of the depressor muscle of the tip in esthetic rhinoplasties (Mahe *et al*). Ann. Otolaryngol. Chir. Cervicofac., *92:*381, 1975 (French)

Combination of extranasal and intranasal approach in surgery of the nasal pyramid and nasal septum (decortication) (Padovan). Can. J. Otolaryngol., *4:*522, 1975

Negroid nose (Acosta da Almeida *et al*). Int. Surg., *60:*554, 1975

Long-term experience with poly (glycolmonomethacrylate) gel in plastic operations of the nose (Voldrich *et al*). J. Biomed. Mater. Res., *9:*675, 1975

Clinical rhinomanometry and septo-rhinoplasty (Willemot). J. Fr. Otorhinolaryngol., *24:*681, 685, 691, 1975 (French)

Conservative management of the Negro nose (Kamer *et al*). Laryngoscope, *85:*551, 1975

Sequential septo-rhinoplasty (Smithdeal). Laryngoscope, *85:*1216, 1975

Combined correction of the nasal pyramid and septum (Firica *et al*). Rev. Chir. (Otorinolaryngol.), *20:*101, 1975 (Rumanian)

Rhinoplasty and additional techniques of profiloplasty (Hinderer), PRS, *57:*756, 1975. Rev. Iber. Latinoamericana Cir. Plast., *1:*245, 1975

Undermining and redraping in rhinoplasty (Felt). Trans. Am. Acad. Ophthalmol. Otolaryngol., *80:*540, 1975

Technique for the non-caucasian nose (Stucker). Trans. Pa. Acad. Ophthalmol. Otolaryngol., *28:*48, 1975

Use of a correcting negative mask in cosmetic operations on the external nose (Bystrenin *et al*). Vestn. Otorinolaringol., *1:*43, 1975 (Russian)

Rhinoplasty, Anesthesia for

Nasal surgery, local anaesthesia combined with diazepam for (Pyke *et al*). J. Laryng.

Rhinoplasty, Anesthesia for — Cont.

& Otol., *87*:1243, 1973

Anesthesia, ketamine, and intranasal or intraoral operations (Bryant), PRS, *51*:562, 1973

Rhinoplasty, use of cocaine as topical anesthetic in (Feehan, Mancusi-Ungaro), PRS, *57*:62, 1975

Rhinoplasty, Augmentation

Saddle nose (Senechal). Probl. Actuels Otorhinolaryngol., *187*:99, 1970 (French)

Correcture of the saddle nose (Nagel). Z. Laryngol. Rhinol. Otol., *49*:250, 1970 (German)

Nasal saddle nose deformity, correction of, using lateral part of nasal tip cartilage (Penkava), PRS, *50*:94, 1972. Acta chir. plast., *13*:25, 1971

Long-term behaviour of preserved homologous rib cartilage in the correction of saddle nose deformity (Muhlbauer *et al*). Brit. J. Plast. Surg., *24*:325, 1971

Reconstruction of a saddle nose (Sabiek). Med. Glas., *25*:81, 1971 (Croatian)

Nose, middle third, correction of post-traumatic saddle of (Arbour). Can. J. Otolaryngol., *1*:304, 1972

Airway obstruction due to prolapse of the lower lateral cartilages in saddle deformity (Stallings *et al*). Laryngoscope, *82*:515, 1972

Saddle nose deformity, correction (Sessions *et al*). Laryngoscope, *82*:2000, 1972

Bone and cartilage grafts: current concepts (Goode). Otolaryngol. Clin. North Am., *5*:447, 1972

Nasal hump implant, homologous (Bernstein). Arch. Otolaryng. *98*:385, 1973

Saddle nose: its correction after extensive septal cartilage removal (Soss). Arch. Otolaryng., *98*:391, 1973

Saddle nose (Smith). Arch. Otolaryng., *98*:435, 1973

Saddle nose, relapsing polychondritis (Jones), PRS, *51*:331, 1973

Rhinoplasty for snub nose (Pers), PRS, *53*:602, 1974. Scand. J. Plast. Reconstr. Surg., *7*:64, 1973

Saddle nose, problems particular to correction of bony or bony-chondral (Haas). Z. Laryngol. Rhinol. Otol., *52*:866, 1973 (German)

Nasal actinomycosis following heterograft. A case report (Thomas *et al*). Arch. Otolaryng., *100*:377, 1974

Oriental rhinoplasty (Furukawa). Clin. Plast. Surg., *1*:129, 1974

Notes on esthetic surgery in the Indonesian

Rhinoplasty, Augmentation — Cont.

(Wiratmadja). Clin. Plast. Surg., *1*:173, 1974

Saddle nose deformity, operative method for (Aoyagi *et al*), PRS, *56*:461, 1975. Jap. J. Plast. Reconstr. Surg., *17*:531, 1974

Experience with prefabricated silicone implants for reconstruction in facially deformed patients (Habal *et al*). J. Prosthet. Dent., *32*:292, 1974

Rhinoplasty, augmentation, with polyamide: saddle nose deformity, etiology, prevention, and treatment (Beekhuis). Laryngoscope, *84*:2, 1974

Saddle depression of the nose (Tunstall). Nurs. Times, *70*:1774, 1974

Saddle nose deformity, correction with upper-lateral turnover procedure (Woolf) (Follow-Up Clinic), PRS, *54*:482, 1974

Augmentation, nasal, by the intraoral route (Flowers), PRS, *54*:570, 1974

Plastic surgery of the face in leprosy (Maillard *et al*). Rev. Med. Suisse Romande., *94*:729, 1974 (French)

Tolerance of the cortical bone to silicone materials (Bruchet *et al*). Ann. chir. plast., *20*:227, 1975 (French)

Complications of augmentation rhinoplasty in orientals (Mutou). Brit. J. Plast. Surg., *28*:160, 1975

Surgical correction of saddle nose deformity (Beekhuis). Trans. Am. Acad. Ophthalmol. Otolaryngol., *80*:596, 1975

Rhinoplasty, Complications

Rhinoplasty, some errors and difficulties (Leoni). Acta Otorinolaryngol. Iber. Am., *22*:139, 1971 (Italian)

Massive bleeding due to primary fibrinolysis following rhinoplasty (Seligsohn *et al*). Harefuah, *82*:219, 1972 (Hebrew)

Rhinoplasty, esthetic, new anatomical concept of postoperative complications in (Safian), PRS, *51*:162, 1973

Hypersomnia caused by upper airway obstructions: a new syndrome in otolaryngology (Simmons *et al*). Ann. Otol. Rhin. & Laryng., *83*:670, 1974

Staphylococcal endocarditis following septorhinoplasty (Coursey). Arch. Otolaryng., *99*:454, 1974

Nose, thick-skinned, rhinoplasty in (Ortiz-Monasterio, Lopez-Mas, Araico), PRS, *56*:593, 1975. Brit. J. Plast. Surg., *27*:19, 1974

Rhinoplasty, central nervous system histoplasmosis after (Gilden *et al*). Neurology (Minneap.), *24*:874, 1974

Rhinoplasty, secondary (Sheen), PRS,

Rhinoplasty, Complications — Cont.
56:137, 1975
Nose, postoperative asymmetry of (Jost, Vergnon, Hadjean), PRS, 57:257, 1976. Ann. chir. plast., 20:123, 1975
Rhinoplasty, valvular obstruction of nasal airway (DesPrez, Kiehn), PRS, 56:307, 1975
Carotid-cavernous sinus fistula occurring after a rhinoplasty (Song, Bromberg), PRS, 55:92, 1975

Rhinoplasty, Deviated Nose

Importance of corrective plastic surgery of the septum in the treatment of cartilaginous deviated nose (Muller). Z. Aerztl. Fortbild. (Jena), 64:349, 1970 (German)
Method of repairing defects and deformities of the nasal septum with free grafts of the concha auriculae (Balon). Vestn. Khir., 107:80, 1971 (Russian)
Rhinoplasty, combined, surgery of nasal pyramid and septum in one stage (Barletta), PRS, 50:418, 1972. Prensa méd. argent., 59:112, 1972
Straightening the crooked nose (Anderson). Trans. Am. Acad. Ophthalmol. Otolaryngol., 76:938, 1972
Rhinoplasty, judicious turbinectomy for nasal obstruction (Fry), PRS, 52:205, 1973. Australian & New Zealand J. Surg., 42:291, 1973
Problem of cartilage bending in nose surgery, experimental and clinical aspects (Hellmich). H. N. O., 21:223, 1973 (German)
Nasal septum, treatment of deflection of anterocaudal portion of (Francesconi, Fenili), PRS, 51:542, 1973
Submucosal septal resection followed by immediate reconstruction by bone grafting (Compte, Lisbonne), PRS, 54:618, 1974. Ann. chir. plast., 19:55, 1974
One stage repair of the twisted nose (Kean). Eye Ear Nose Throat Mon., 52:502, 1974
Diagnosis, clinical aspects and surgical treatment of traumatic curvature of the nose in the residual period of the injury (Martinkenas). Vestn. Otorinolaringol., 2:49, 1975 (Russian)

Rhinoplasty, Function in

Repositioning of the nasal septum without mucosal dissection (Neveu). Ann. chir. plast., 16:231, 1971 (French)
Initial experiences with Cottle's nasal septus reconstruction (Salus *et al*). H.N.O., 19:311, 1971 (German)
Septoplasty or reposition of the nasal septum, basic element of rhinoplasty (its func-

Rhinoplasty, Function in — Cont.
tional and esthetic value) (Cajgfinger *et al*). J. Med. Lyon, 52:1513, 1971 (French)
Results with Cottle's method of septum surgery (Kleinfeldt). Dtsch. Gesundheitsw., 27:362, 1972 (German)
Functional surgery and esthetic surgery of nose (Rebattu *et al*). Lyon Med., 228:805, 1972
Rhinoplasty, treatment of resistant forms of vasomotor allergic rhinitis as preliminary stage to (Demidov *et al*). Vestn. Otorinolaringol., 34:56, 1972 (Russian)
Rhinoplasty and septal perforations (Senechal *et al*). Ann. Otolaryngol. Chir. Cervicofac., 90:659, 1973 (French)
Septorhinoplasty surgery in children (Crysdale). Can. J. Otolaryngol., 2:211, 1973
S. M. R., septoplasty, and surgical relief of nasal obstruction (Pearson *et al*). Can. J. Otolaryngol., 2:238, 1973
Nose, functional plastic surgery of (Wille). Schweiz. Med. Wochenschr., 103:452, 1973 (German)
Rhinoplasties, esthetic, functional and anatomic viewpoint in (Haas). Z. Laryngol. Rhinol. Otol., 52:235, 1973 (German)
Rhinoplasty and nasal function (Kastenbauer). Munch. Med. Wochenschr., 116:399, 1974 (German)
Resection of the nasal septum with reimplantation of autocartilage (Kostyshin). Vestn. Otorinolaringol., 3:93, 1975 (Russian)

Rhinoplasty, History (See also *History of Plastic Surgery*)

Rhinoplasty from its beginning to the 19th century (Galanti *et al*). Clin. Otorinolaringoiatr., 22:339, 1970 (Italian)
Rhinoplasty. Its development and present day usages (Sokol *et al*). Ohio State Med. J., 68:556, 1972
History of rhinoplasty in Russia (Mirskii). Vestn. Khir., 108:132, 1972 (Russian)

Rhinoplasty, Implants in

Silicone nasal implants, fate of (Milward), PRS, 52:217, 1973. Brit. J. Plast. Surg., 25:276, 1972
Nose, chip implants in, preoperative assessment of risk factors (Hellmich). H.N.O., 20:218, 1972 (German)
Operative technique of rhinoplastic implants (Hellmich). Z. Laryngol. Rhinol. Otol., 51:298, 1972 (German)
Nasal implants, prefabricated silicone (Antia *et al*), PRS, 52:264, 1973
Nose chip implants, synthetic, late results in (Gerth). Z. Aerztl. Fortbild. (Jena), 67:880,

Rhinoplasty, Implants in – Cont.

1973 (German)

Nasal augmentation by intraoral route (Flowers), PRS, *54:*570, 1974

Rhinoplasty, Instruments for

Rhinotome used in lateral, subperiosteal osteotomy (Olivari), PRS, *52:*205, 1973. Chir. Plast., *1:*261, 1972

New osteoclast (Marechal). Ann. Otolaryngol. Chir. Cervicofac., *91:*537, 1974 (French)

Rhinoplasty, cutting forceps for lateral osteotomy in (Goumain), PRS, *53:*358, 1974

Rhinoplasty, Postoperative Care

Rhinoplasty, corrective, reducing eyelid edema and ecchymosis following (Shehadi). PRS, *49:*508, 1972

Rhinoplasty, employment of carica papaya endopeptidase associated with benzidamine (Lopez), PRS, *52:*104, 1973. Tribuna Med. Argent., *15:*611, 1972

Need of mini-cast for nose (Daieff). Ann. chir. plast., *18:*189, 1973

Rhinoplasty, suture technics in, using the extramucosal technic (Jost). Ann. chir. plast., *18:*271, 1973 (French)

Rhinoplastic dressings (Parkes *et al*). Eye, Ear, Nose, Throat, Mon., *52:*166, 1973

Rhinoplasty, suitability of tissue adhesive histoacryl in (Kastenbauer). Z. Laryngol. Rhinol. Otol., *52:*240, 1973 (German)

Post-rhinoplasty edema, prevention of (Stucker). Laryngoscope, *84:*536, 1974

Nasal surgery, care after (Ventura). Nursing (Jenkintown), *4:*87, 1974

An absorbent, non-adherent nasal pack (Kamer *et al*). Laryngoscope, *85:*384, 1975

External immobilizing plaster cast (Zakrzewski *et al*). Otolaryngol. Pol., *29:*505, 1975 (Polish)

Rhinoplasty, Psychology of (See also *Plastic Surgery, Psychology of*)

When your patient asks about plastic surgery (Meijer). Med. Times, *99:*117, 1971

Feminine loss of identity in rhinoplasty (Knorr). Arch. Otolaryng., *96:*11, 1972

Rhinoplasty, preoperative selection and counseling of patients (Thomson), PRS, *50:*174, 1972

Aspects of plastic surgery. Social and psychological sequelae (Olley). Brit. Med. J., *3:*322, 1974

A psychological study of patients undergoing cosmetic surgery (Wright *et al*). Arch. Otolaryng., *101:*145, 1975

Rhinoplasty, Psychology of – Cont.

Incidence of schizophrenia and severe psychological disorders in patients 10 years after cosmetic rhinoplasty (Gipson *et al*). Brit. J. Plast. Surg., *28:*155, 1975

Rhinoplasty in transsexuals, psychological considerations (Trop, Golden), PRS, *55:*593, 1975

Rhinoplasty, Reconstructive

Rhinoplasties, total (Blanchart), PRS, *48:* 89, 1971. Rev. españ. cir. plast., *2:*21, 1969

Nasal reconstruction of losses due to oncological surgery: 15 years' experience (Barrera, Serrano-Rebeil, Ortiz-Monasterio), PRS, *48:*89, 1971. Mem. V Cong. Mexicano Dermat., *5:*541, 1970

Successful late management of a severed nose tip (Moritsch). Monatsschr. Ohrenheilkd. Laryngorhinol., *104:*365, 1970 (German)

Method of primary reconstruction of nose and upper lip (Zehm). Arch. Klin. Exp. Ohren Nasen Kehlkopfheilkd., *199:*638, 1971 (German)

Use of pedunculated frontal flaps for rhinoplasty (Bardach). Dtsch. Stomatol., *21:*625, 1971 (German)

Nasal reconstructions after resection of cutaneous tumors (Garcia-Velazco), PRS, *50:*536, 1972. Invest. Clin. Mexico, *10:*229, 1971

Total reconstruction of the external nose, particularly on the method using a tubed pedicle flap (Takahashi *et al*). Jap. J. Plast. Reconstr. Surg., *14:*447, 1971 (Japanese)

Rhinoplasty by using a forehead flap (Soeda). Jap. J. Plast. Reconstr. Surg., *14:*475, 1971 (Japanese)

Experience in total reconstruction of the external nose with Millard's method (Sugimoto *et al*). Jap. J. Plast. Reconstr. Surg., *14:*482, 1971 (Japanese)

Total reconstruction of the external nose, with special reference to rhinoplasty for the syphilitic saddle nose (Uchida *et al*). Jap. J. Plast. Reconstr. Surg., *14:*495, 1971 (Japanese)

Reconstructive plastic surgery of the nose (Popovic *et al*). Med. Glas., *25:*72, 1971 (Croatian)

Composite ear grafts for construction of columella (Meade) (Follow-Up Clinic). PRS, *48:*73, 1971

Use of free transplantation of previously cooled auricles of the external ear and local

Rhinoplasty, Reconstructive – Cont.

plastic surgery to replace defects in the nasal dorsum, apex, alae and septum (Balon). Vestn. Khir., *106:*63, 1971 (Russian)

Remote results of rhinoplasty using Filatov's graft with decalcified bone (Vasil'eva). Vestn. Khir., *106:*102, 1971 (Russian)

Reconstruction of the cutaneocartilaginous part of the nasal septum by grafting an auricular transplant (Kostylev). Vestn. Khir., *107:*84, 1971 (Russian)

Possibilities and indications of functional and restorative surgery for a leprous nose (Reynaud). Ann. chir. plast., *17:*137, 1972 (French)

Reconstruction of the columella (Kaplan). Brit. J. Plast. Surg., *25:*37, 1972

Chondro-mucosal grafts (Bleracque *et al*). Bull. Soc. Ophtalmol. Fr., *72:*1125, 1972 (French)

Nasal skin defects, one stage reconstruction with local flaps (Lejour), PRS, *52:*205, 1973. Chir. Plast., *1:*254, 1972

Experience and problems in nasal reconstruction (Oura *et al*). Jap. J. Plast. Reconstr. Surg., *15:*165, 1972 (Japanese)

Nasolabial flap in reconstruction of the nose (Burnam). J. Fla. Med. Assoc., *59:*32, 1972

Reconstruction of columella of nasal septum (Meyer). O. R. L., *34:*170, 1972 (French)

Nasal reconstruction using pedicle skin flaps (Gunter). Otolaryngol. Clin. North Am., *5:*457, 1972

Nasal reconstructions, midline forehead flap, in patients with low browlines (Richardson, Hanna, Gaisford). PRS, *49:*130, 1972

Nasal flap, use of complete transverse, in repair of small defects of nose (Lipshutz, Penrod). PRS, *49:*629, 1972

Nasolabial fold, reconstruction (Clodius). PRS, *50:*467, 1972

Auricular composite graft and forehead flap with periosteum, reconstructive rhinoplasty with (Fujino). PRS, *50:*526, 1972

Nasal vestibule, versatility of chondromucosal flap in (Millard). PRS, *50:*580, 1972

Columellar losses, surgical treatment of (Ferreira *et al*). Rev. Paul. Med., *79:*127, 1972 (Portuguese)

Management of major nasal defects (Remark *et al*). South. Med. J., *65:*623, 1972

Reparative surgery of the nose and ear (Omori). Surg. Ther. (Osaka), *26:*548, 1972 (Japanese)

Nasal surgery, reconstructive (Pilgrim *et al*). Am. J. Nurs., *73:*451, 1973

Columella, reconstruction after tumor resection at nose entrance (Schaupp *et al*). Arch.

Rhinoplasty, Reconstructive – Cont.

Klin. Exp. Ohren Nasen Kehlkopfheilkd., *205:*332, 1973 (German)

Rhinoplasty, half (Garcia-Velazco), PRS, *54:*234, 1974. Brit. J. Plast. Surg., *26:*412, 1973

Nasal reconstruction, total: further application of delto-pectoral flap (Song *et al*). Brit. J. Plast. Surg., *26:*414, 1973

Nasal reconstruction, pedicle flap: design and execution (Tardy). Can. J. Otolaryngol., *2:*342, 1973

Nose wing, reconstruction of, using a fronto-temporal flap (Schaupp). H. N. O., *21:*187, 1973 (German)

Nasal reconstruction, auricular composite graft in: report of 3 cases (Kawai *et al*). Jap. J. Oral Surg., *19:*95, 1973 (Japanese)

Nasal pyramid, repair of partial loss of skin substance from (Mazauric *et al*). J. Fr. Otorhinolaryngol., *22:*815, 1973 (French)

Nasolabial flaps, reconstructions of nose and upper lip with (Cameron, Latham, Dowling). PRS, *52:*145, 1973

Columellar reconstruction, one-stage (Snow) (Follow-Up Clinic). PRS, *52:*299, 1973

Nose, partial loss of substance of, treatment of (Montandon). Rev. Med. Suisse Romande., *93:*769, 1973 (French)

Nasal defects, development of method for reconstruction of, using Filatov's graft (Khitrov). Stomatologiia (Mosk.), *52:*36, 1973 (Russian)

Nose, correction of cicatricial deformations and defects of, after deep facial burns (Kabakov *et al*). Vestn. Khir., *111:*91, 1973

Nasal ala, reconstruction of (Kastenbauer). Z. Laryngol. Rhinol. Otol., *52:*83, 1973 (German)

Local flaps in the repair of nasal skin defects (Verheecke *et al*). Ann. chir. plast., *19:*193, 1974 (French)

Plastic surgery, Italian, of nose and face, experiences with (Denecke). Laryngol. Rhinol. Otol. (Stuttg.), *53:*248, 1974 (German)

Plastic management of nasal defects with special consideration of composite grafts (Feldmann). Laryngol. Rhinol. Otol. (Stuttg.), *53:*384, 1974 (German)

Reconstruction of nasal defects (Haas). Laryngol. Rhinol. Otol. (Stuttg.), *53:*530, 1974 (German)

Reconstruction of nasal defects (Haas). Laryngol. Rhinol. Otol. (Stuttg.), *53:*548, 1974 (German)

Operative management of the nose and associated tissues of the face (Walter). Laryngol. Rhinol. Otol. (Stuttg.), *53:*548, 1974

Rhinoplasty Reconstructive—Cont.
(German)
Reconstructive flaps in otolaryngology (McFarland). Laryngoscope, *84:*1267, 1974
Rhinoplasty, reconstructive, for lower half of nose (Millard). PRS, *53:*133, 1974
Cheek flap for subtotal nose reconstruction (Fryer). PRS, *53:*436, 1974
Nasal defects, small, off-midline forehead flap for repair of (Dhawan, Aggarwal, Hariharan). PRS, *53:*537, 1974
Regional flaps in head and neck surgery (Komorn). Tex. Med., *70:*70, 1974
Reconstruction of soft tissues of the nasal dorsum (Iarchuk). Vestn. Khir., *113:*80, 1974 (Russian)
Rhinoplasty, reconstruction after trauma (Jacobs, Walter), PRS, *57:*114, 1976. Actuel. Chir., *10:*157, 1975
Nasal defects, distal rotation flap for (Olbourne *et al*). Brit. J. Plast. Surg., *28:*64, 1975
Congenital double columella (Rawat *et al*). Brit. J. Plast. Surg., *28:*153, 1975
One-stage repair of full-thickness alar defects (Rawat *et al*). Brit. J. Plast. Surg., *28:*317, 1975
Modern methods of partial nasal reconstruction (Krisch). Laryngol. Rhinol. Otol. (Stuttg.), *54:*424, 1975 (German)
Nasal reconstruction (Walter). Laryngoscope, *85:*1227, 1975
Reconstruction of nose tip with a cylindrical flap (Preferansow *et al*). Otolaryngol. Pol., *29:*71, 1975 (Polish)
Rhinoplasty, large Indian forehead (Daver, Antia), PRS, *55:*360, 1975
Filatov's flap in otorhinolaryngology (on the centenary of the birth of Academician V. P. Filatov) (Kurilin *et al*). Zh. Ushn. Nos. Gorl. Bolezn., *2:*4, 1975 (Russian)
Nasolabial flap, contralateral, to repair nostril defect (Santos, Pappas), PRS, *57:*704, 1976
Rhinoplasty, reconstructive, for lower two-thirds of nose (Millard), PRS, *57:*722, 1976

Rhinoplasty Reduction

Simple procedure for correction of the hump nose (Neuner). Brit. J. Plast. Surg., *24:*375, 1971
Reduction rhinoplasty, five most important points in (Tamerin), PRS, *48:*214, 1971
Skin resection for Corbin's beaked nose (Pollet). Ann. chir. plast., *17:*15, 1972 (French)
Osteotomy, lateral, subperiosteal, using rhinotome (Olivari), PRS, *52:*205, 1973. Chir. Plast., *1:*261, 1972
Rhinoplasties, reduction, planning (Cardoso

Rhinoplasty, Reduction—Cont.
et al). Rev. Asoc. Med. Bras., *18:*401, 1972 (Portuguese)
Transfixion, high septal (Brennan, Parkes), PRS, *54:*234, 1974. Internat. Surg., *58:*732, 1973
Rhinoplasty, reduction, skin excisions in (Webster), PRS, *51:*289, 1973
Rhinoplasty in thick-skinned nose (Ortiz-Monasterio, Lopez-Mas, Araico), PRS, *56:*593, 1975. Brit. J. Plast. Surg., *27:*19, 1974
Nose, "Pinocchio" deformity, tripod resection for (Fredricks), PRS, *53:*531, 1974. Discussion by Peck, PRS, *53:*674, 1974
Rhinoplasty: direct approach to "hanging columella" (Randall), PRS, *53:*544, 1974
Rhinoplasty, corrective, for enlargement of nose due to acromegaly (Hirshowitz, Mayblum, Kanter), PRS, *56:*665, 1975
Nose hump, more accurate removal in rhinoplasty (Snow), PRS, *57:*253, 1976

Rhinoplasty, Reviews of (See also *Plastic Surgery Articles, Reviews of*)

Review of rhinoplasty (Onizuka). Jap. J. Plast. Reconstr. Surg., *14:*465, 1971 (Japanese)
Review of rhinoplasty (Tani). Jap. J. Plast. Reconstr. Surg., *14:*489, 1971 (Japanese)
Rhinoplasty today (Meyer). Rev. Med. Suisse Romande., *94:*971, 1974 (French)

Rhinoplasty, Secondary

Re-operations in nasal hypoplasia (Firica *et al*). Otorinolaringologie, *16:*339, 1971 (Rumanian)
Rhinoplasty, so-called "crow's beak" deformity after, cutaneous resections for correction of (Pollet *et al*). Ann. Otolaryngol. Chir. Cervicofac., *90:*481, 1973 (French)
Rhinoplasty, unsuccessful, revision in (Kerth *et al*). Otolaryngol. Clin. North Am., *7:*65, 1974
Rhinoplasty, revision (Stucker). Trans. Pa. Acad. Ophthalmol. Otolaryngol., *27:*42, 1974
Secondary rhinoplasty (Sheen), PRS, *56:*137, 1975
Secondary nasal revisions after rhinoplasties (Walter). Trans. Am. Acad. Ophthalmol. Otolaryngol., *80:*519, 1975

Rhinoplasty, Tip Corrections

Nasal tip, studies on support of (Janeke, Wright), PRS, *49:*102, 1972. Arch. Otolaryng., *93:*5, 1971
Problems of a corrective technic for the lower

Rhinoplasty, Tip Corrections – Cont.
cartilaginous arch of the nasal pyramid (Fruttero). Minerva Otorinolaringol., *21*:211, 1971 (Italian)

Nasal tip retrusion, congenital, and three little composite ear grafts (Millard), PRS, *48*:501, 1971

Corbin's beaked nose (Jost *et al*). Ann. chir. plast., *17*:5, 1972 (French)

Correction of projection defect of tip of nose (Jost). Ann. chir. plast., *17*:245, 1972

Nasal tip projection (Beekhuis). Eye Ear Nose Throat Mon., *51*:92, 1972

Nasal tip support, three autogenous struts for (Pollet), PRS, *49*:527, 1972

Nasal tip reconstruction, use of ear cartilage grafts for (Falces, Gorney), PRS, *50*:147, 1972

Rhinoplasty: surgery of tip of nose by hook flap technique (Psillakis, Albano), PRS, *52*:594, 1973. Rev. brasil. clin. terapeut., *1*:587, 1972

Rhinoplasty, repair of prominent nasal tip (Spina, Kamakura, Psillakis), PRS, *53*:104, 1974. Rev. Soc. Med. San Jose, *5*:5, 1972

Nasal tip surgery, thoughtful (Smith). Arch. Otolaryng., *97*:244, 1973

Rhinoplasty tip ptosis: etiology and prevention (Tardy). Laryngoscope, *83*:923, 1973

Columellar advancement for nasal tip elevation (Goode *et al*). Laryngoscope, *83*:1123, 1973

Rhinoplasty: new method for correction of prominent nasal tip (Spina, Kamakura, Psillakis), PRS, *51*:416, 1973

Nasal tip correction in rhinoplasty (Webster, White, Courtiss), PRS, *51*:384, 1973

Nasal tip deformity: crossed alar wing procedure for correction of late deformity in unilateral cleft lip nose (Whitlow, Constable), PRS, *52*:38, 1973

Negroid tip of nose, treatment (Pitanguy, Daher, Souza Motta), PRS, *53*:364, 1974. Rev. brasil cir., *63*:52, 1973

Evaluation of surgical techniques on nasal tip projection (Bortnick). Laryngoscope, *84*:1316, 1974

Rhinoplasty: tripod resection for "Pinocchio" nose deformity (Fredricks), PRS, *53*:531, 1974. Discussion by Peck, PRS, *53*:674, 1974

Columella, hanging, direct approach to (Randall), PRS, *53*:544, 1974

Alar base resection for wide-flaring nostrils (Ship). Brit. J. Plast. Surg., *28*:77, 1975

Nose: achieving more nasal tip projection by use of small autogenous vomer or septal cartilage graft (Sheen), PRS, *56*:35, 1975.

Rhinoplasty, Tip Corrections – Cont.
Discussion by Horton, PRS, *56*:211, 1975

Graft, bone, small, absorption of, in nasal tip (Sheen) (Letter to the Editor), PRS, *56*:332, 1975

Alar cartilages, surgical treatment (Martins). Rev. Asoc. Med. Bras., *21*:55, 1975 (Portuguese)

Rhinoplasty: nasal tip projection (Lamont) (Letter to the Editor), PRS, *57*:228, 1976

RHOADS, J. E., JR. *et al*: Use of tissue-matched meshed homografts in treatment of massive burns. Rev. Surg., *30*:451, 1973

RHODE, C. M., AND JENNINGS, W. D., JR.: Operative treatment of stiff proximal interphalangeal joint, PRS, *48*:94, 1971. Am. Surgeon, *37*:44, 1971

RHODE, C. M. *et al*: Pacinian corpuscle neuroma of digital nerves. South. Med. J., *68*:86, 1975

RHODES, G. A.: Cutaneous and subcutaneous necrosis as complication of coumarin-congener therapy (with Kahn, Stern), PRS, *48*:160, 1971

Rhytidectomy

Face-Lift Operation. By John Conley. Charles C Thomas, Springfield, Ill., 1968

Ptoses, facial skin, corrective surgery of (Jost). Probl. Actuels Otorhinolaryngol., *201*:10, 1970 (French)

Surgical correction of facial skin sagging (Vrebos). Brux. Med., *51*:569, 1971 (French)

Rhytidectomy, sectional (Gonzalez-Ulloa, Stevens-Flores), PRS, *50*:198, 1972. Internat. Surg., *56*:266, 1971

Surgery in aging of soft tissue of the face (Frishberg). Khirurgiia (Mosk.)., *47*:43, 1971 (Russian)

Submental lipectomy, simplified technique in (Weisman), PRS, *48*:443, 1971

Rhytidectomy (Pitanguy, Cansançao, Garcia), PRS, *52*:320, 1973. Rev. brasil. cir., *61*:173, 1971

Wrinkles. Etiopathogenetic theory (Abreu). Rev. Paul. Med., *78*:93, 1971

Age changes in the forehead area and a surgical method of treating them (Mirov). Vestn. Dermatol. Venerol., *45*:74, 1971 (Russian)

Aged, plastic surgery for (Pioner). Zahnaerztl. Prax., *22*:1, 1971 (German)

Facelift patients (Hurwitz). A. N. A. Clin. Sess., p. 185, 1972

Wrinkles of face (Malbec, Quaife, Arce Gonzalez), PRS, *50*:198, 1972. El Dia Medico Argent., *44*:15, 1972

Rhytidectomy — Cont.

tion of (Barker), PRS, *54:*651, 1974

Wrinkles of frontal region, surgical treatment of, (Spina *et al*), PRS, *55:*244, 1975. Rev. Hosp. clin., *29:*76, 1974

Refining aspects of rhytidoplasty (Tabari). In *Plastiche und Wiederherstellungs-Chirurgie,* ed. by Hohler; pp. 27–33. Schattauer, Stuttgart, 1975 (German)

Facelifting and blepharoplasty. Surgical and suture techniques (Hohler). In *Plastische und Wiederherstellungs-Chirurgie,* ed. by Hohler; pp. 35–47. Schattauer, Stuttgart, 1975 (German)

Hairbearing preauricular rotation flap and additional corrections in the treatment of the aging face (Hinderer). In *Plastische und Wiederherstellungs-Chirurgie,* ed. by Hohler; pp. 49–66. Schattauer, Stuttgart, 1975

Extra adipose tissue resection with the facelift (Zischinsky). In *Plastiche und Wiederherstellungs-Chirurgie,* ed. by Hohler; pp. 67–8. Schattauer, Stuttgart, 1975 (German)

Error in facial stretching (Schmidt-Tintemann). In *Plastische und Wiederherstellungs-Chirurgie,* ed. by Hohler; pp. 69–73. Schattauer, Stuttgart, 1975 (German)

Hair loss: a rare complication of facelift (Kratochwil). In *Plastische und Wiederherstellungs-Chirurgie,* ed. by Hohler; pp. 321–2. Schattauer, Stuttgart, 1975 (German)

Granuloma after subcutaneous injection of facial wrinkles with Teflon paste (Lemperle *et al*). In *Plastische und Wiederherstellungs-Chirurgie,* ed. by Hohler; pp. 335–9. Schattauer, Stuttgart, 1975 (German)

The tuck-up operation. A new technique of secondary rhytidectomy (Anderson). Arch. Otolaryng., *101:*739, 1975

Plication: should subcutaneous tissue be plicated in face lift? (Gurdin) (Letter to the Editor), PRS, *55:*84, 1975

Face-lift incision, modification in, to facilitate suturing around the earlobe (Hirshowitz), PRS, *55:*368, 1975

Rhytidectomy, factors in production of inconspicuous scars (Wray, Holtmann, Weeks), PRS, *56:*86, 1975

Rhytidectomy, estrogen therapy after, ancillary effects of (Gonzalez-Ulloa) (Letter to the Editor), PRS, *56:*203, 1975

Rhytidectomy, segmental approach to (Lewis), PRS, *56:*297, 1975

Flaccidity of cheeks: cutaneous resection with quadrangular preauricular incision (Spadafora, Durand, de los Rios), PRS,

Rhytidectomy — Cont.

*57:*670, 1976, Prensa Univ. Arg., *6:*8361, 1975

Two-stage concept of rhytidectomy (Kamer *et al*). Trans. Am. Acad. Ophthalmol. Otolaryngol., *80:*546, 1975

Rhytidectomy, repair of submental depression occurring after (Wilkinson), PRS, *57:*33, 1976

Rhytidectomy, male, sideburn relationship (Sturman), PRS, *57:*248, 1976

Rhytidectomy, reconstruction of sideburn for alopecia after (Juri, Juri, de Antueno), PRS, *57:*304, 1976

Hypertension, postoperative, as etiological factor in hematoma after rhytidectomy, prevention with chlorpromazine (Berner, Morain, Noe), PRS, *57:*314, 1976

Rhytidoplasty, forehead, and brow lifting (Viñas, Caviglia, Cortinas), PRS, *57:*445, 1976

RIABINA, V. P. *et al*: Cylindroma of ear. Vestn. Otorinolaringol., *35:*93, 1973 (Russian)

RIBEIRO, L.: New technique for reduction mammaplasty, PRS, *55:*330, 1975

RIBEIRO, L., AND BACKER, E.: Mastoplasty with safety pedicle, PRS, *53:*486, 1974. Rev. españ. cir. plast., *6:*223, 1973

RIBEIRO SOARES, V., AND RIBEIRO SOARES, V.: Surgery of mandibular prognathism, PRS, *57:*757, 1976. Cir. Plast. Ibero-Latino Am., *1:*13, 1975

RIBET, M. *et al*: Zenker's diverticulum: importance of pharyngo-esophageal sphincter. J. Chir. (Paris), *104:*37, 1972 (French)

Rib Grafts: See Bone Grafts, Various Categories; Cranioplasty; Jaw, Bone Grafts to

RIBOLDI, A. *et al*: Occupational diseases of the milker's hand. Berufsdermatosen, *20:*166, 1972 (German)

RICBOURG, B., MITZ, V., AND LASSAU, J. P.: Superficial temporal artery, PRS, *57:*262, 1976. Ann. chir. plast., *20:*197, 1975

RICCABONA, A.: Lateral pharyngotomy in treatment of carcinoma of root of tongue. Wien. Klin. Wochenschr., *85:*333, 1973 (German)

RICCIARDI, A.: Maxillary subperiosteal implants. Dent. Surv., *50:*24, 1974

RICE, C. O.: Adenomammectomy: technique and advantages. Northwest. Med., *71:*375, 1972

RICE, D. H. *et al*: Fibrous histiocytomas of the nose and paranasal sinuses. Arch. Otolaryng., *100:*398, 1974

RICH, A. M.: Four years' experience with Morel-Fatio palpebral spring (with Morgan),

PRS, *53:*404, 1974

RICH, A. M.: Surgical management of paralyzed orbicularis oculi. Trans. Am. Acad. Ophthalmol. Otolaryngol., *78:*622, 1974

RICH, N. M. *et al*: Repair of lower extremity venous trauma: more aggressive approach required, PRS, *57:*535, 1976. J. Trauma, *14:*639, 1974

RICHARD, J.: Surgery of the mandible and transmandibular surgery of the bucco-pharyngeal cavity tumors. Cancro, *23:*301, 1970 (French)

RICHARD, J. *et al*: What must we think of the staged transmaxillary buccopharyngectomy. Ann. Otolaryngol. Chir. Cervicofac., *88:*663, 1971 (French)

RICHARD, J. *et al*: Indications for surgery in pelvigingival cancers. J. Radiol. Electrol. Med. Nucl., *53:*475, 1972 (French)

RICHARDS, A. T., STRICKE, L., AND SPITZ, L.: Sacrococcygeal chordomas in children, PRS, *54:*381, 1974. J. Pediat. Surg., *8:*911, 1973

RICHARDS, G. J., JR., AND CHAMBERS, R. G.: Hydroxyurea in treatment of neoplasms of head and neck, PRS, *53:*688, 1974. Am. J. Surg., *126:*513, 1973

RICHARDS, K. E., AND FELLER, I.: Grid escharotomy for debriding burns, PRS, *53:*685, 1974. Surg. Gynec. & Obst., *137:*843, 1973

RICHARDS, M. T.: Breast surgery – as office procedure. Can. Med. Assoc. J., *109:*305, 1973

RICHARDSON, G. S., HANNA, D. C., AND GAISFORD, J. C.: Midline forehead flap nasal reconstructions in patients with low browlines, PRS, *49:*130, 1972

RICHARDSON, G. S. *et al*: Tumors of salivary glands, PRS, *55:*131, 1975

RICHARDSON, J. E. *et al*: Thyroid cancer in young patients in Great Britain. Brit. J. Surg., *61:*85, 1974

RICHARDSON, J. R., LINTON, P. C., AND LEADBETTER, G. W., JR.: New concept in treatment of stomal stenosis, PRS, *51:*236, 1973. J. Urol., *108:*159, 1972

RICHIE, J. P.: Intestinal loop urinary diversion in children. J. Urol., *111:*687, 1974

RICHMAN, L. C.: Behavior and achievement of cleft palate children. Cleft Palate J., *13:*4, 1976

RICHMOND, D. A.: Uncommon causes of nerve compression with hand symptoms, PRS, *54:*374, 1974. Hand, *5:*209, 1973

RICHTER, K. J. *et al*: Central giant cell lesion in angle of mandible: review of literature and report of case. J. Oral Surg., *31:*26, 1973

RICHTER, K. J. *et al*: Chondrosarcoma of temporomandibular joint, case report. J. Oral Surg., *32:*777, 1974

RICHTER, M. *et al*: Vestibuloplasty with and without suture fixation. Deutsch. Zahnaertzl. Z., *28:*206, 1973

RICHTER, M. *et al*: Odontogenic keratocysts. Schweiz. Monatsschr. Zahnheilkd., *85:*487, 1975 (French)

RICHTER, S. *et al*: Mixed tumors of the parotid gland in the eyelid. Klin. Monatsbl. Augenheilkd., *166:*201, 1975 (German)

RICKER, J. H.: Efficacy of local steroid injection in treatment of stenosing tenovaginits (with Clark, MacCollum), PRS, *51:*179, 1973

RICKETSON, G.: Obituary of Beverly Douglas, M.D., PRS, *57:*408, 1976

RICKHAM, P. O.: Cervical teratoma. Helv. Pediatr. Acta, *27:*549, 1972 (German)

RIEBELOVA, V.: Surgical treatment of chronic decubitus ulcers in paraplegics with stationary neurological lesions. Cas. Lek. Cesk., *112:*25, 1973 (Czechoslovakian)

RIEDLER, L. *et al*: Clinic and therapy of thyroglossal and branchial cysts and fistulas. Langenbecks Arch. Chir., *336:*247, 1974 (German)

RIEGER, H. J.: Fee entitlement in failed cosmetic surgery. Dtsch. Med. Wochenschr., *99:*2068, 1974 (German)

RIETZ, K. A.: Bone grafting of skull defects (with Korlof, Nylén), PRS, *52:*378, 1973

RIGG, B. M.: Dorsal nasal flap, PRS, *52:*361, 1973

RIGG, B. M.: Method for intraoperative selection of best size for mammary prosthesis, PRS, *52:*589, 1973

RIGG, B. M.: Surgical management of familial benign chronic pemphigus, PRS, *54:*364, 1974

RIGG, B. M.: Transfer of free groin flap to heel by microvascular anastomosis, PRS, *55:*36, 1975

RIGG, B. M.: Microirrigator, PRS, *56:*349, 1975

RIGG, B. M., AND MARTYN, J. W.: Unusual congenital dermal sinus of buttock, PRS, *56:*581, 1975

RIGHTOR, M.: Augmentation of wound strength by pretreatment with epinephrine (with Myers), PRS, *54:*201, 1974. Discussion by Weeks, PRS, *54:*351, 1974

RIGOPOULOS, C., AND CONSTANDINIDIS, E.: Compound fractures with immediate internal fixation, PRS, *48:*399, 1971. Trans. 1st Panhellenic Cong. Orthop. Surg. & Traum., *1:*80, 1969

RILEY, C.: Surgical stents for vestibuloplasty and alveolar ridge skin grafts. J. Prosthet. Dent., *26:*511, 1971

RILEY, F. C.: Surgical management of ophthalmopathy in Graves' disease. Transfrontal orbital decompression. Mayo Clin. Proc., *47:*986, 1972

RINALDI, E.: "Swan-neck" deformity of the fingers in the rheumatoid hand: surgical correction. Reumatismo, 24:175, 1972 (Italian)

RINALDI, I.: Value of preoperative angiography in the surgical management of cervical hourglass neurofibroma. Case report. J. Neurosurg., 36:97, 1972

RINK, B.: Clinical and radiographic findings after surgical closure of mouth-antrum connection in combination with radical surgery in maxillary antrum. Dtsch. Stomatol., 22:251, 1972 (German)

RINK, B.: Treatment of bite wounds in maxillofacial region. Stomatol. D.D.R., 24:461, 1974 (German)

RINSKY, L. A. et al: Freeman-Sheldon ("whistling face") syndrome. J. Bone & Joint Surg. (Am.), 58:148, 1976

RINTALA, A.: Surgical therapy of basal cell carcinoma. Correlation of the macroscopic and microscopic control of excision with recurrence. Scand. J. Plast. Reconstr. Surg., 5:87, 1971

RINTALA, A.: Double, overlapping hinge flap to close palatal fistula. Scand. J. Plast. Reconstr. Surg., 5:91, 1971

RINTALA, A.: Surgical treatment of cleft lip and palate. Suom. Hammaslaak. Toim., 68:35, 1972 (Finnish)

RINTALA, A. et al: Carcinoma arising in a postburn scar. Duodecim, 88:639, 1972 (Finnish)

RINTALA, A. et al: Separate epignathi of the mandible and the nasopharynx with cleft palate: a case report. Brit. J. Plast. Surg., 27:103, 1974

RINTALA, A. et al: Cheilitis granulomatosa, Melkersson-Rosenthal syndrome, PRS, 54:687, 1974. Scand. J. Plast. Reconstr. Surg., 7:130, 1974

RINTALA, A. et al: Bone forming capacity of periosteal flap in surgery for cleft lip and palate, PRS, 56:681, 1975. Scand. J. Plast. Reconstr. Surg., 8:58, 1974

RINTALA, A. E.: How a patient experienced cleft lip operation in 1763. PRS, 57:158, 1976

RINTALA, A. E., AND SVINHUFVUD, U.: Effect of augmentation mammaplasty on mammography and thermography. PRS, 54:390, 1974

RIORDAN, D. C.: Fowler procedure for correction of paralytic claw hand (with Enna). PRS, 52:352, 1973

RIORDAN, D. C.: Functional anatomy of the hand and forearm. Orthop. Clin. North Am., 5:199, 1974

RIORDAN, D. C.: Rehabilitation and re-education in tendon transfers. Orthop. Clin. North Am., 5:445, 1974

RIORDAN, D. C. et al: Synovitis of the extensors of the fingers associated with extensor digitorum brevis manus muscle. A case report.

Clin. Orthop., 95:278, 1973

RIOS, A. et al: Active specific immunotherapy of minimal residual tumors: excision plus neuraminidase-treated tumor cells. Int. J. Cancer, 13:71, 1974

RISSANEN, P. M.: End results of treatment in cancer of the tongue. Ann. Chir. Gynaecol. Fenn., 61:112, 1972

RISSING, J. P. et al: Bacteroides bacteremia from decubitus ulcers, PRS, 55:646, 1975. South. M.J., 67:1179, 1974

RISTIC, J. et al: Reticulosarcoma of the maxilla. Med. Pregl., 28:541, 1975 (Serbian)

RISTOW, B. v. B., O'GRADY, W., AND FARR, H.: Resection of large skin carcinoma of neck; coverage with deltopectoral flap. PRS, 49:570, 1972

RISTOW, W. et al: Unilateral cerebral circulation decrease following unilateral neck dissection. Arch. Klin. Exp. Ohren Nasen Kehlkopfheilkd., 202:523, 1972 (German)

RITA, L. et al: Ketamine hydrochloride for pediatric premedication. I. Comparison with pentazocine, PRS, 54:627, 1974. Anesth. & Analg., 53:375, 1974

RITA, L., AND SELENY, F. L.: Ketamine hydrochloride for pediatric premedication. II. Prevention of postanesthetic excitement, PRS, 54:627, 1974. Anesth. & Analg., 53:375, 380, 1974

RITLAND, D., AND BUTTERFIELD, W.: Extremity complications of drug abuse, PRS, 54:109, 1974. Am. J. Surg., 126:639, 1973

RITSILA, V. et al: Use of free periosteum for bone formation in congenital clefts of the maxilla. A preliminary report. Scand. J. Plast. Reconstr. Surg., 6:57, 1972

RITSILA, V. et al: Role of zygomatic arch in growth of skull in rabbits. Proc. Finn. Dent. Soc., 69:164, 1973

RITSILA, V., AND ALHOPURO, S.: Reconstruction of experimental tracheal cartilage defects with free periosteum, PRS, 54:689, 1974. Scand. J. Plast. Reconstr. Surg., 7:116, 1973

RITTER, K.: Chemodectomas in otorhinolaryngology. H. N. O., 22:6, 1974

RITTER, M. A.: Anatomy and function of the palmar fascia. Hand, 5:263, 1973

RITTMANN, W. W., AND PERREN, S. M.: Cortical Bone Healing after Internal Fixation and Infection. Springer-Verlag, New York, 1974. PRS, 57:91, 1976

RITZAU, M.: Weight changes in patients with intermaxillary immobilization after jaw fractures. Int. J. Oral Surg., 2:122, 1973

RITZE, H.: Pre- and post-surgical prosthesis. Dent. Labor ⬩(Munch.), 21:235, 1973 (German)

RIU, R.: Rhinorrheography in nose morphology

and septorhinoplasties. Ann. chir. plast., 19:181, 1974 (French)

RIVAL, J. M. et al: Binder's maxillo-nasal dysostosis. Apropos of 10 cases. J. Genet. Hum., 22:263, 1974 (French)

RIVARD, J., AND LAPOINT, R.: Clinical experience in using elemental diet in management of various surgical nutritional problems, PRS, 56:116, 1975. Canad. J. Surg., 18:90, 1975

RIVAS RODERO, S. et al: Case of primary malignant melanoma of mouth. An. Esp. Odontoestomatol., 31:389, 1972 (Spanish)

RIVAS, J. et al: Ventral hernia. Importance of its effects on respiration, PRS, 53:605, 1974. Chir. Mem. Acad., 99:547, 1973

RIVES, J. et al: Dacron prosthesis in treatment of adult inguinal hernia (183 cases), PRS, 53:605, 1974. Chir. Mem. Acad., 99:564, 1973

RIVIERE, C. L. et al: Pretherapy speech intelligibility of a glossectomee. J. Commun. Disord., 7:357, 1974

RIX, R. R.: Combined nerve and tendon injury in the palm. J.A.M.A., 217:480, 1971

ROA-ROA, T. T.: Some considerations concerning application of liquid silicone in mammarian hypotrophies, PRS, 50:419, 1972. Rev. Latino Am. Cir. Plast., 15:17, 1972

ROB, C., AND SMITH, R.: Pulvertaft's Hand. J. B. Lippincott Co., Philadelphia, 1970.

ROBACK, H. et al: Gender identification and the female impersonator. South. Med. J., 68:459, 1975

ROBBETT, W. F.: Self-retaining midfacial retractor. Trans. Am. Acad. Ophthalmol. Otolaryngol., 77:1149, 1973

ROBBINS, T. H.: "Crown" excision of facial skin lesions, PRS, 57:251, 1976

ROBBINS, T. H.: Use of fascio-muscle flaps to repair defects in leg, PRS, 57:460, 1976

ROBERSON, G. H. et al: Presurgical internal maxillary artery embolization in juvenile angiofibroma. Laryngoscope, 82:1524, 1972

ROBERT, J. et al: Topographic diagnosis of nevocarcinomas and their metastases, using labelled bleomycin. Bull. Soc. Fr. Dermatol. Syphiligr., 79:166, 1972 (French)

ROBERTS, G. D. D., WRIGHT, C. J., AND SHAMIA, R. I.: Operative management of ankylosis of jaw, PRS, 55:655, 1975. Trop. Doctor, 4:121, 1974

ROBERTS, G. J.: Growth of cartilages of cranial base: preliminary studies on Rattus norvegicus, PRS, 56:225, 1975. Proc. Roy. Soc. Med., 68:130, 1975

ROBERTSO, P. A.: Respiratory care in local anesthesia, PRS, 56:470, 1975. AORN, 21:797, 1975

ROBERTSON, D. C.: The technique of inferior

flap mammaplasty (Follow-Up Clinic), PRS, 52:433, 1973

ROBERTSON, M. S.: Use of a tongue flap for the repair of defects following radical surgery of the head and neck. Aust. N. Z. J. Surg., 45:395, 1975

ROBERTSON, N. R.: Recent trends in early treatment of cleft lip and palate. Dent. Pract. Dent. Rec., 21:326, 1971

ROBERTSON, N. R. et al: Some observations on rapid expansion followed by bone grafting in cleft lip and palate. Cleft Palate J., 9:236, 1972

ROBERTSON, N. R. E., AND JOLLEYS, A.: Timing of hard palate repair, PRS, 56:468, 1975. Scand. J. Plast. Reconstr. Surg., 8:49, 1974

ROBICSEK, F. et al: Technical considerations in the surgical management of pectus excavatum and carinatum. Ann. Thorac. Surg., 18:549, 1974

ROBILLARD, J. et al: Maxillary sinus cancer therapy contribution of curietherapy. J. Radiol. Electrol. Med. Nucl., 54:153, 1973 (French)

ROBIN, J. L.: Controlled extra-mucosal rhinoplasty with pre-operative measurement of profile modification. Ann. chir. plast., 18:119, 1973 (French)

ROBINOW, M. et al: Acrodysostosis. A syndrome of peripheral dysostosis, nasal hypoplasia, and mental retardation. Am. J. Dis. Child., 121:195, 1971

ROBINS, P., AND MENN, H.: Chemosurgery in treatment of skin cancer, PRS, 52:599, 1973. Hosp. Practice, 5:40, 1970

ROBINS, P. et al: Basal cell carcinoma: treatment by the Mohs technique. Laryngoscope, 82:965, 1972

ROBINS, R. E. et al: Analysis of mortality and morbidity in 100 composite resections for oral carcinoma. Am. J. Surg., 130:178, 1975

ROBINSON, D. C. et al: The prevalence and natural history of cleft lip and palate in Uganda. Dev. Med. Child. Neurol., 12:636, 1970

ROBINSON, D. W.: K. U. M. C. Burn Center. First six months. J. Kans. Med. Soc., 75:233, 1974

ROBINSON, D. W.: What's new in surgery? (plastic surgery), PRS, 55:723, 1975. Contemp. Surg., 6:21, 1975

ROBINSON, D. W.: Surgical problems in excision and repair of radiated tissue, PRS, 55:41, 1975

ROBINSON, D. W.: Plastic surgery and burns. Surg. Gynec. & Obst., 140:208, 1975

ROBINSON, H. et al: Role of erythropoietin in anemia of thermal injury, PRS, 53:608, 1974. Ann. Surg., 178:565, 1973

ROBINSON, H. S. et al: Functional results of

excisional arthroplasty for rheumatoid hand, PRS, *52:*688, 1973. Canad. M. A. J., *108:*1495, 1973

ROBINSON, J. L., AND DAVIES, N. J.: Bipolar diathermy, PRS, *56:*116, 1975. Canad. J. Surg., *17:*287, 1974

ROBINSON, M.: Bone resorption under plastic chin implants. Follow-up of a preliminary report. Arch. Otolaryng., *95:*30, 1972

ROBINSON, M.: Results of pushback operations in treatment of submucous cleft palate (with Massengill, Pickrell), PRS, *51:*432, 1973

ROBINSON, M. J.: Familial melanomas. J.A.M.A., *220:*277, 1972

ROBINSON, P. J. *et al*: Evidence of alloimmunogenic potential of donor periodontal ligament. Am. J. Pathol., *75:*503, 1974

ROBINSON, S. W. *et al*: Soft tissue profile change produced by reduction of mandibular prognathism. Angle Orthod., *42:*227, 1972

ROBINSON, T. J. *et al*: Alterations in pulmonary ventilation and blood gases in acute burns, PRS, *52:*209, 1973. Brit. J. Plast. Surg., *25:*250, 1972

ROBITAILLE, A. *et al*: Correction of keloids and finger contractures in burn patients, PRS, *54:*113, 1974. Arch. Phys. Med., *54:*515, 1973

ROBITAILLE, Y. *et al*: Peripheral nerve tumors involving paranasal sinuses: a case report and review of the literature. Cancer, *35:*1254, 1972

ROBSON, M. C.: Potential pitfalls in use of deltopectoral flap (with Krizek). PRS, *50:*326, 1972

ROBSON, M. C.: Current use of prophylactic antibiotics in plastic and reconstructive surgery (with Krizek, Koss). PRS, *55:*21, 1975

ROBSON, M. C.: Scalping injury (with Koss, Krizek). PRS, *55:*439, 1975

ROBSON, M. C.: Resection and immediate reconstruction for patients with "inoperable" recurrent head and neck cancer. Surg. Clin. North Am., *56:*111, 1976

ROBSON, M. C. *et al*: Quantitative comparison of biological dressings. Surg. Forum, *23:*503, 1972

ROBSON, M. C., DUKE, W. F., AND KRIZEK, T. J.: Rapid bacterial screening in treatment of civilian wounds, PRS, *53:*687, 1974. J. Surg. Res., *14:*426, 1973

ROBSON, M. C., SAMBURG, J. L., AND KRIZEK, T. J.: Quantitative comparison of biological dressings, PRS, *51:*706, 1973. Surg. Forum, *23:*504, 1972; PRS, *53:*689, 1974. J. Surg. Res., *14:*431, 1973

ROBSON, M. C., AND KRIZEK, T. J.: Predicting skin graft survival, PRS, *52:*330, 1973. J. Trauma, *13:*213, 1973

ROBSON, M. C. *et al*: Amniotic membranes as temporary wound dressing, PRS, *52:*601,

1973. Surg. Gynec. & Obst., *136:*904, 1973

ROBSON, M. C. *et al*: Efficacy of systemic antibiotics in treatment of granulating wounds, PRS, *54:*695, 1974. J. Surg. Res., *16:*299, 1974

ROBSON, M. C., SCHAERF, R. H. M., AND KRIZEK, T. J.: Evaluation of topical povidone-iodine ointment in experimental burn wound sepsis, PRS, *54:*328, 1974

ROCA, P. D.: Painful ophthalmoplegia: the Tolosa-Hunt syndrome, PRS, *57:*256, 1976. Ann. Ophth., *7:*828, 1875

ROCCHIO, M. A., DICOLA, V., AND RANDALL, H. T.: Role of electrolyte solutions in treatment of hemorrhagic shock, PRS, *53:*109, 1974. Am. J. Surg., *125:*488, 1973

ROCHA, E.: Surgery in treatment of retention cysts in oral cavity. Rev. Gaucha. Odontol., *20:*258, 1972 (Portuguese)

ROCHET, Y. *et al*: Personal operative technic for the treatment of congenital absence of the vagina with functional uterus. Bull. Fed. Soc. Gynecol. Obstet. Lang. Fr., *23:*467, 1971 (French)

ROCHET, Y. *et al*: Surgical treatment of congenital absence of the vagina with functional uterus (2 cases operated on successfully by a personal technic). Lyon Chir., *67:*265, 1971 (French)

ROCHET, Y. *et al*: Treatment of vaginal aplasia using a cleavage operation with two surgical teams, two cases. Chirurgie, *99:*838, 1973 (French)

ROCHET, Y., AND GAGNAIRE, J. C.: Study of different surgical techniques and results in 57 cases of vaginal aplasia, PRS, *56:*466, 1975. J. Gynec. Obst. Biol. Reprod., *3:*223, 1975

ROCKWOOD, CHARLES A., AND GREEN, DAVID P.: *Fractures*. J. B. Lippincott Co., Philadelphia, 1975. PRS, *57:*740, 1976

RODEHEAVER, G. T. *et al*: Wound cleansing by high pressure irrigation, PRS, *57:*402, 1976. Surg. Gynec. & Obst., *141:*357, 1975

RODIER, D. *et al*: Immediate massive bone graft after block surgery of cancers of the buccal cavity. Chirurgie, *97:*785, 1972 (French)

RODING, H., AND JAEGER, A.: Epidemiology of thermal trauma in DDR (East Germany), PRS, *52:*685, 1973. Zentralbl. Chir., *98:*289, 1973

RODRIGUES, M. M., LUBOWITZ, R. M., AND SHANNON, G. M.: Mucinous (adenocystic) carcinoma of eyelid, PRS, *53:*601, 1974. Arch. Ophth., *89:*493, 1973

RODRIGUES, R. J., AND WOLFF, W. J.: Fungal septicemia in surgical patients, PRS, *55:*645, 1975. Ann. Surg., *180:*741, 1974

RODRIGUEZ, J. H. *et al*: Paradental maxillary cyst. Rev. Circ. Argent. Odontol., *35:*50, 1972

(Spanish)

RODRIGUEZ, J. M. et al: Lipomas in the hand and wrist: diagnosis and treatment. Clev. Clin. Q., 32:201, 1970

RODRIGUEZ DE LIMA, A.: Secondary effects following use of inner implants, PRS, 50:543, 1972. Rev. Latino Am. cir. plast., 14:73, 1970

RODRIGUEZ-FORNOS, S., AND NARBONA ARNAU, B.: Branchial cysts and fistulas, PRS, 54:111, 1974. Cir. Españ., 27:339, 1973

ROE, E. et al: Effects of topical chemoprophylaxis on transferable antibiotic resistance in burns. Lancet, 2:109, 1972

ROEDIGER, W. E. et al: Mucous extravasation theory as cause of plunging ranulas. Brit. J. Surg., 60:720, 1973

ROED-PETERSEN, B.: Absorbable synthetic suture material for internal fixation of fractures of mandible. Int. J. Oral Surg., 3:133, 1974

ROED-PETERSEN, B. et al: Study of Danish snuff-induced oral leukoplakias. J. Oral Pathol., 2:301, 1973

ROENIGK, H. et al: Immunotherapy of malignant melanoma with vaccinia virus, PRS, 55:115, 1975. Arch. Dermat., 109:668, 1974

ROETTINGER, W. et al: Role of inoculation site as a determinant of infection in soft tissue wounds, PRS, 53:687, 1974. Am. J. Surg., 126:354, 1973

ROGERS, B. O.: Chronologic history of cosmetic surgery, PRS, 48:400, 1971. Bull. N. Y. Acad. Med., 47:265, 1971

ROGERS, B. O.: Surgery in the Revolutionary War, contributions of John Jones, M.D., PRS, 49:1, 1972

ROGERS, B. O.: Role of physical anthropology in plastic surgery today. Clin. Plast. Surg., 1:439, 1974

ROGERS, B. O.: Obituary on Gustavo Sanvenero-Rosselli, M.D., PRS, 54:513, 1974

ROGERS, J., AND WILSON, L. F.: Preventing recurrent tissue breakdowns after pressure "sore" closures, PRS, 56:419, 1975. Discussion by Brand, PRS, 56:573, 1975

ROGERS, P. A., AND NARDI, W.: Fracture of orbital floor: case report with serious delayed sequelae, PRS, 52:205, 1973. M. J. Australia, 1:175, 1973

ROGGE, C. W. O.: Ambroise Paré (1510–1590) and evolution of surgical instrumentarium, PRS, 57:126, 1976. Arch. chir. neerl., 27:1, 1975

ROGGENDORF, E.: Symetroplast and its use in face and neck surgery. Dtsch. Stomatol., 22:845, 1972 (German)

ROHDE, B. et al: Steotocystoma multiplex. Hautarzt, 25:29, 1974

ROHENER, T. J., JR., AND BLANCHARD, T. W.:

Management of urethral injuries in war casualties, PRS, 48:91, 1971. Mil. Med., 135:748, 1970

ROHRT, T. et al: Transmaxillary reconstruction in orbital floor fractures. J. Oslo City Hosp., 24:3, 1974

ROLAND, C. G.: Thoughts about medical writing, PRS, 57:682, 1976. Anesth. Analg., Cleve., 54:366, 1975

ROLANDER, T. et al: Fibrous xanthoma of larynx. Arch. Otolaryng., 96:168, 1972

ROLES, N. C., AND MAUDSLEY, R. H.: Radial tunnel syndrome, PRS, 52:679, 1973. J. Bone & Joint Surg., 54B:499, 1972

ROLFFS, J.: Results of primary orbital reconstructions in mid-facial fractures. Fortschr. Kiefer. Gesichtschir., 19:184, 1975 (German)

ROLFFS, J. et al: Maxillary cementoblastoma, case report. Dtsch. Zahnaerztl. Z., 29:713, 1974 (German)

ROLING, U. et al: Cytological studies after autotransplantation in the oral cavity. Dtsch. Zahnaerztl. Z., 29:875, 1974 (German)

ROLLER, N. W. et al: Lidocaine topical film strip for oral mucosal biopsies. J. Oral Med., 30:55, 1975

ROMANIUK, K. et al: Two cases of aneurysmal bone cysts of jaws. Int. J. Oral Surg., 1:48, 1972

ROMBOUTS, J. J., AND NOEL, H.: Parosteal osteogenic sarcoma of skeleton of hand, PRS, 56:465, 1975. Rev. chir. orthop., 61:71, 1975

ROMBOUTS, J. J. et al: Juxtacortical osteogenic sarcoma localized in the hand. Presentation of 2 cases. Rev. Chir. Orthop., 61:75, 1975 (French)

ROMIEU, C.: Congress of the French Chapter of the International College of Surgeons, organized by the Reims University Surgical Clinic, June 7, 8,and 9, 1974. Breast cancer, current problems. Conclusion. Ann. Chir., 29:877, 1975 (French)

ROMIEU, C. et al: Malignant melanomas of the face. J. Fr. Otorhinolaryngol., 20:1121, 1971 (French)

ROMIEU, C., AND SERROU, B.: Present aspects of immunology of cancer, PRS, 55:516, 1975. J. Internat. Surg., 59:393, 1974

ROMODANOV, A. P. AND LIASHCHENKO, D. S.: Craniofacial dysostosis. Zh. Nevropatol. Psikhiatr., 72:1487, 1972 (Russian)

ROMUALDI, P.: Surgery in bladder exstrophy. Minerva Pediatr., 24:1168, 1972

RONAY, P. et al: Clinical and histological experiences in 54 malignant parotid tumors. Langenbecks Arch. Chir., 330:45, 1971 (German)

RONAY, P. et al: Clinical and histological findings in 220 cases of parotid gland tumor. Zentralbl. Chir., 97:1082, 1972

RONCHESE, E.: Occupation marks. Practitioner, 210:507, 1973

RONDEAU, Y. et al: Prolonged intubation or tracheotomy in neonatal and pediatric resuscitation. Union Med. Can., 99:1662, 1970 (French)

RONNING, O. et al: Changes in dentition of guinea-pig following partial section of inferior alveolar nerve. Arch. Oral Biol., 18:1059, 1973

RONTAL, E. et al: Lateral alveolo-maxillary osteotomies. Revascularization studies. Arch. Otolaryng., 95:18, 1972

RONTAL, E. et al: Transoral reduction of mandibular fractures. Arch. Otolaryng., 97:279, 1973

RONTAL, E. et al: External fixation of facial fractures. Arch. Otolaryng., 98:393, 1973

RONTAL, E. et al: Biphase external fixation: technique and application. Laryngscope, 84:1404, 1974

ROPER, A. L.: Homograft reconstruction of nasal septum. Arch. Otolaryng., 97:235, 1973

ROSE, E. H., KSANDER, G. A., AND VISTNES, L. M.: Skin tension lines in the domestic pig. PRS, 57:729, 1976

ROSEMANN, G.: Resection of the mandible in oral tumours. H. N. O., 20:166, 1972 (German)

ROSEMANN, G. et al: Treatment of hemispasmus facialis by scarification of nerve. Arch. Klin. Exp. Ohren Nasen Kehlkopfheilkd., 205:205, 1973 (German)

ROSEN, A. D.: Innervation of the hand: an electromyographic study. Electromyogr. Clin. Neurophysiol., 13:175, 1973

ROSEN, G.: Facial nerve surgery. Harefuah, 88:416, 1975 (Hebrew)

ROSEN, Y. et al: Eccrine sweat gland tumor of clear cell origin involving the eyelids. Cancer, 36:1034, 1975

ROSENBAUM, R. W., HAYES, M. F., AND MATSUMOTO, T.: Efficacy of steroids in treatment of septic and cardiogenic shock, PRS, 52;461, 1973. Surg. Gynec. & Obst., 136:914, 1973

ROSENBERG, H.: Anesthesia orientation for medical student, PRS, 57:267, 1976. Anesth. & Analg. Cleve., 54:328, 1975

ROSENBERG, V. I.: Some fiber-optic retractors for use in plastic surgery. PRS, 48:286, 1971

ROSENBERG, V. I.: New bipolar forceps for electrocoagulation. PRS, 48:390, 1971

ROSENBERG, V. I.: Fiber-optic nasal septal retractors. PRS, 49:468, 1972

ROSENBERG, V. I.: New fingertip-controlled bipolar forceps for electrocoagulation. PRS, 54:228, 1974

ROSENFELD, L. et al: Management of mass in parotid gland. J. Tenn. Med. Assoc., 65:1007, 1972

ROSENGARTEN, D. S.: Regimen designed to abolish postoperative venous thrombosis, PRS, 52:687, 1973. Proc. Roy. Australasian Coll. Surg., 46:737, 1973

ROSENGREN, B.: On lacrimal drainage. Ophthalmologica, 164:409, 1972

ROSENHOUSE, L.: President Cleveland's secret surgery, PRS, 55:387, 1975. Private Practice, 6:43, 1974

ROSENQUIST, J.: Preprosthetic surgery in the front region of the mandible. Int. J. Oral Surg., 4:18, 1975

ROSENSTEIN, S.: Orthodontic and bone grafting procedures in a cleft lip and palate series: an interim cephalometric evaluation. Angle Orthod., 45:227, 1975

ROSENSTEIN, S. W.: An orthodontist's view of surgical orthodontics. J. Oral. Surg., 31:177, 1973

ROSENSTEIN, S. W. et al: A series of cleft lip and palate children five years after undergoing orthopedic and bone grafting procedures. Angle Orthod., 42:1, 1972

ROSENTHAL, A. M. et al: Hyperbaric treatment of pressure sores. Arch. Phys. Med. Rehabil., 52:413, 1971

ROSENTHAL, S. G.: Glabellar rhytidoplasty, new approach. PRS, 50:361, 1972

ROSENTHAL, S. G., BERNHARDT, H. W., AND PHILLIPS, J. A., III: Aeromonas hydrophila wound infection. PRS, 53:77, 1974

ROSENTHAL, S. R., HAWLEY, P. L., AND HAKIM, A. A.: Purified burn toxic factor and its competitin, PRS, 50:421, 1972. Surgery, 71:527, 1972

ROSS, D. E. et al: En bloc ethmoidectomy for cancer. (A progress report.) Laryngoscope, 82:682, 1972

ROSS, J. W.: Retrograde root-filling in oral surgery. Trans. Int. Conf. Oral Surg., 4:98, 1973

ROSS, J. W.: Mandibular ostectomy in acromegalic. Int. J. Oral Surg., 3:256, 1974

ROSS, M. B.: Functional anatomy of the tensor palati, PRS, 48:609, 1971. Arch. Otolaryng., 93:1, 1970

ROSS, R. B.: Management of dental arch deformity in cleft lip and palate. Clin. Plast. Surg., 2:325, 1975

ROSS, R. B., AND JOHNSTON, M. C.: Cleft Lip and Palate. Williams & Wilkins Co., Baltimore, 1972. PRS, 51:444, 1973

ROSSELLI, D. et al: Preliminary observations on 105 cases of hare lip operated on with Skoog's periosteal flap. Ann. chir. plast., 17:106, 1972 (French)

ROSSELLI, D. et al: Postoperative development of maxillary bone and incisor in rabbit operated when few days old, PRS, 57:395, 1976.

Riv. ital. chir. plast., *6:*227, 1974

ROSSETTI, M.: Surgical technic of cervical esophageal diverticula. Helv. Chir. Acta, *38:*237, 1971 (German)

ROSSI, G. *et al*: Case of large bucco-sinusal communication, following partial resection of the maxilla, repaired by tubular flap and bone graft. Rev. Stomatol. Chir. Maxillofac., *75:*192, 1974 (French)

ROSSMAN, K.: Combined radiation therapy and surgery in the treatment of advanced head and neck cancer. Ariz. Med., *32:*869, 1975

ROSWIT, B. *et al*: Planned preoperative irradiation and surgery for advanced cancer of the oral cavity, pharynx and larynx. Am. J. Roentgenol. Radium Ther. Nucl. Med., *114:*59, 1972

ROTH, H.: Partially successful reimplantation of the hand. Helv. Chir. Acta, *37:*234, 1970 (German)

ROTHMAN, D.: Use of peritoneum in construction of vagina. Obstet. Gynecol., *40:*835, 1972

ROTHMAN, D. *et al*: Giant pilomantrixoma (Malherbe calcifying epithelioma). Arch. Surg., *111:*86, 1976

ROTHMANN, M., VAKILZADEH, F., AND RUPEC, M.: Hydrotherapy in cauterization wounds, PRS, *56:*599, 1975. Arch. Dermat. Forsch., *251:*281, 1975

ROTHNER, A. D.: Aberrant salivary fistulas, PRS, *54:*378, 1974. J. Pediat. Surg., *8:*931, 1973

ROUCHER, F.: Can burn patients be treated in a general surgery unit? Cah. Med., *12:*1137, 1970 (French)

ROUCHER, F.: What is the practical value of intravenous locoregional anesthesia in surgery of the hand? Presse Med., *79:*2330, 1971 (French)

ROUCHER, F.: Correction of protruding ears with Mustardé's technique. Ann. chir. plast., *18:*74, 1973 (French)

ROUCHER, F.: Chronic ulcer of leg of venous origin, PRS, *57:*119, 1976. Lyon chir., *70:*388, 1974

ROUCHER, F., MALLARD, G., AND LATREILLE, R.: Cutaneous degloving of lower limbs run over by vehicle, PRS, *55:*511, 1975. Lyon chir., *70:*312, 1974

ROUCHON, C. *et al*: Indication of different flaps in orostome closure. Rev. Stomatol. Chir. Maxillofac., *75:*219, 1974 (French)

ROUCHON, C. *et al*: Osseous desmoid fibroma of the mandible, apropos of 1 case: Rev. Stomatol. Chir. Maxillofac., *76:*527, 1975 (French)

ROUGERIE, J. *et al*: Craniostenosis and craniofacial dysmorphism. Principles of new method of treatment and its results. Neurochirurgie, *18:*429, 1972 (French)

ROUGIER, J.: Surgical treatment of blepharophimosis. Ann. chir. plast., *18:*141, 1973 (French)

ROULAUD, J. P. *et al*: Problems posed during surgical repair of a gunshot wound in the mandible. Rev. Stomatol. Chir. Maxillofac., *76:*493, 1975 (French)

ROULLET, J.: Surgery of tenosynovitis of the extensors during chronic rheumatoid polyarthritis. Rev. Chir. Orthop., *58:*407, 1972 (French)

ROULLET, J. *et al*: Pollicization. Lyon Chir., *67:*114, 1971 (French)

ROUSSO, M.: Metacarpophalangeal arthroplasties with silicone implants. Ann. Chir., *25:*951, 1971 (French)

ROUSSO, M.: Severe burns of the dorsum of the hand. Reconstruction of the web space. A five-flap technique. Part 1. The first web space. Ann. Chir., *29:*475, 1975 (French)

ROUSSO, M.: Severe burns of the dorsum of the hand. Part 2. Reconstruction of the 2nd, 3rd and 4th web space areas. The modified five-flap technique. Ann. Chir., *29:*1015, 1975 (French)

ROUSSOS, J.: Total eversion of upper lids. Ann. Ophth., *6:*633, 1974

ROUTLEDGE, R. T.: Treatment using chemotherapy-surgery combination, PRS, *49:*238, 1972. Proc. Roy. Soc. Med., *64:*737, 1971

ROUTSAW, P. D.: Infiltrating malignant melanoma of heel: case report. J. Am. Podiatry Assoc., *63:*319, 1973

ROUX, J. P. *et al*: The management of paediatric hermaphroditism. S. Afr. Med. J., *48:*2088, 1974

ROWE, M. I., AND ARANGO, A.: Choice of intravenous fluid in shock resuscitation, PRS, *57:*122, 1976. Pediat. Clin. N. Am., *22:*269, 1975

ROWE, N. L.: Surgery of temporomandibular joint, PRS, *50:*537, 1972. Proc. Roy. Soc. Med., *65:*383, 1972

ROWE, N. L.: Fractures of the orbital floor. Trans. Int. Conf. Oral Surg., *4:*302, 1973

ROWE, W.: Genetic factors in natural history of marine leukemia virus infection, PRS, *54:*242, 1974. Cancer Res., *33:*3061, 1973

ROWINSKA, J. *et al*: Diagnostic difficulties in mandibular tumors in primary hyperparathyroidism. Czas. Stomatol., *27:*19, 1974 (Czechoslovakian)

ROWLAND, M. D.: Surgery for sex reassignment, PRS, *57:*769, 1976. AORN, *22:*735, 1975

ROWLAND, S. A.: Prosthetic replacement for irreparable hands. Tex. Med., *68:*121, 1972

ROWLAND, S. A.: Palmar incision for release of the carpal tunnel. Clin. Orthop., *103:*89, 1974

ROY-CAMILLE, R. *et al*: Treatment of osteitis by excision and graft at open operations by Papineau's method, PRS, *55*:253, 1975. Chirurgie, *100*:480, 1974

ROYDHOUSE, R. H., AND HORAN, J. D.: Temporomandibular and mandibular dysfunction, PRS, *49*:470, 1972. Canad. M. A. J., *105*:1320, 1971

ROYSTER, H. P.: Autotransfusion for blood loss in some major esthetic operations (with Noone, Graham). PRS, *51*:559, 1973

ROYSTER, H. P.: Conjunctival approach for exploration of orbital floor (with Lynch, Lamp). PRS, *54*:153, 1974

ROZENBLIT, J. *et al*: Klippel-Fell syndrome associated with multiple developmental anomalies. Pol. Tyg. Lek., *28*:833, 1973 (Polish)

ROZNOVAN, V. K.: Condition of oxidation-reduction processes in patients with chronic osteomyelitis of the jaw and phlegmons of the maxillofacial area in connection with surgical intervention and anesthesia. Stomatologiia (Mosk.), *54*:33, 1975 (Russian)

ROZOVSKY, L. F.: Sex and single hospital. Can. Hosp., *50*:29, 1973

ROZOWSKAJA, T. P. *et al*: Restoration of work capacity in combined lesions of flexor tendons and nerves of the fingers. Chir. Narzadow. Ruchu Ortop. Pol., *37*:375, 1972 (Polish)

RUBERG, R. L. *et al*: Hypophosphatemia with hypophosphaturia in hyperalimentation, PRS, *49*:670, 1972. Surg. Forum, *22*:87, 1971

RUBERG, R. L., RANDALL, P., AND WHITAKER, L. A.: Preservation of a posterior pharyngeal flap during maxillary advancement, PRS, *57*:335, 1976

RUBIN, G., AND GEARHART, D. F.: Cosmetic hand cover for hook, PRS, *53*:366, 1974. Bull. Prosthetics Res., *17*:83, 1973

RUBIN, L. R.: Anatomy of a smile; its importance in treatment of facial paralysis. PRS, *53*:384, 1974

RUBIN, L. R.: Burned female breast. N.Y. State J. Med., *75*:865, 1975

RUBIN, L. R.: Cushioned augmentation repair after a subcutaneous mastectomy. PRS, *57*:23, 1976

RUBIN, L. R., AND BONGIOVI, J., JR.: Human skin – antibacterial *in vitro*? PRS, *49*:472, 1972. J. Surg. Res., *11*:321, 1971

RUBIN, L. R., BROMBERG, B. E., AND WALDEN, R. H.: Long-term human reaction to synthetic plastics, PRS, *49*:110, 1972. Surg. Gynec. & Obst., *132*:603, 1971

RUBIN, L. R., AND MARSHALL, J. H.: Oral airway for use around edematous lip adhesions. PRS, *49*:354, 1972

RUBIN, L. R. *et al*: Total ear reconstruction by composite grafts (Follow-Up Clinic). PRS, *49*:454, 1972

RUBIN, R. J., AND COREY, L.: Preventing rabies in humans, PRS, *56*:115, 1975. South. M. J., *67*:1472, 1974

RUBIN, R. L. *et al*: Squamous cell carcinoma of floor of mouth with extensive mandibular involvement, PRS, *56*:600, 1975. J. Oral Surg., *39*:184, 1975

RUBINCHIK, L. Z.: Remote results of tunnel implants of phtoroplast into the orbital cavity after enucleation. Oftalmol. Zh., *29*:288, 1974 (Russian)

RUCH, M. *et al*: Giant frontal mucocele. Plastic surgery with acrylic resin. Ann. Otolaryngol. Chir. Cervicofac., *88*:403, 1971 (French)

RUDAKOV, B. IA.: Use of hyperbaric oxygen in experimental burns. Eksp. Khir. Anesteziol., *16*:82, 1971 (Russian)

RUDERT, H.: Wire suture osteosynthesis in facial and skull traumatology. Z. Laryngol. Rhinol. Otol., *50*:640, 1971 (German)

RUDERT, H.: Principles of orbital fracture management. Arch. Klin. Exp. Ohren Nasen Kehlkopfeilkd., *205*:282, 1973 (German)

RUDGE, P.: Tourniquet paralysis with prolonged conduction block. An electro-physiological study. J. Bone & Joint Surg. (Br.), *56-B*:716, 1974

RUDIGER, R. A. *et al*: Severe developmental failure with coarse facial features, distal limb hypoplasia, thickened palmar creases, bifid uvula, and ureteral stenosis: a previously unidentified familial disorder with lethal outcome. J. Pediatr., *79*:977, 1971

RUDIN, *et al*: Histologic analysis of extrophied bladder after anatomical closure. J. Urol., *108*:802, 1972

RUDOLPH, R. *et al*: Isotopic measurement of collagen turnover in skin grafts. Surg. Forum, *22*:489, 1971

RUDOLPH, R., AND KLEIN, L.: Inhibition of mature ^{3}H-collagen destruction by triamcinolone, PRS, *53*:692, 1974. J. Surg. Res., *14*:435, 1973

RUDOLPH, R., AND KLEIN, L.: Healing processes in skin grafts, PRS, *53*:498, 1974. Surg. Gynec. & Obst., *136*:641, 1973

RUDOLPH, R., AND KLEIN, L.: Pathways of radioactive collagen loss from skin grafts, PRS, *55*:114, 1975. Surg. Gynec. & Obst., *138*:55, 1974

RUDOLPH, R. *et al*: Fournier's syndrome: synergistic gangrene of scrotum. Am. J. Surg., *129*:591, 1975

RUDOLPH, R. I., AND WOOD, M. G.: Giant pigmented nevus, PRS, *55*:641, 1975. Cutis, *14*:223, 1974

RUDOWSKI, W.: Present and future trends in research on burns and treatment of thermal injuries. Pol. Przegl. Chir., *46:*73, 1974 (Polish)

RUDOWSKI, W. *et al*: Bacteriological and clinical studies on sulfamylon in the treatment of burns. Brit. J. Plast. Surg., *25:*135, 1972

RUEDI, T. *et al*: Experience with stable osteosynthesis in metacarpal fractures. Langenbecks Arch. Chir., *328:*285, 1971 (German)

RÜEDI, T. P., BURRI, C., AND PFEIFFER, K. M.: Stable internal fixation of fractures of hand, PRS, *49:*584, 1972. J. Trauma, *11:*381, 1971

RUIZ-MORENO, F.: Duplication of rectum, PRS, *50:*420, 1972. El Medico, *21:*58, 1972

RUKAVINA, K.: Operative treatment of Dupuytren's contracture, PRS, *51:*478, 1973. Bruns' Beitr. klin. Chir., *219:*551, 1972

RULLI, M. A.: Wound healing granulation tissue of sialoadenectomized rats. Rev. Fac. Odontol. Aracatuba, *2:*171, 1973 (Portuguese)

RUMELT, M. B. *et al*: Isolated blowout fractures of the medial orbital wall with medial rectus muscle entrapment. Am. J. Ophth., *73:*451, 1972

RUMPF, G. *et al*: Indirect injuries of the orbital floor (blow out fractures). Dtsch. Gesundheitsw., *27:*222, 1972 (German)

RUPP, J. P., AND KNOTHE, W.: Exceptionally large epidermoid cyst of penis in newborn, PRS, *55:*250, 1975. Ztschr. Kinderchir., *15:*236, 1974

RUPRECHT, A. *et al*: Simple bone cyst, report of two cases. Oral Surg., *39:*826, 1975

RUSAKOV, A. B. *et al*: Results of prognosis of outcome of auto-dermoplasty in burned patients. Ortop. Travmatol. Protez., *34:*56, 1973 (Russian)

RUSAKOV, A. B. *et al*: Prognostic value of cytological characteristics of burn wound prior to autodermoplasty. Ortop. Travmatol. Protez., *2:*62, 1975 (Russian)

RUSANOVA, N. I.: Primary cancer of frontal sinus. Vopr. Onkol., *19:*95, 1973 (Russian)

RUSCONI, L.: Current directions in surgical treatment of prognathism. Ann. Stomatol. (Roma), *21:*115, 1972 (Italian)

RUSCONI, L., AND BRUSATI, R.: Correction of prognathism associated with maxillary retrusion. PRS, *48:*558, 1971

RUSCONI, L. *et al*: Restricted opening of mouth from symmetrical bilateral hyperplasia of coronoid processes. J. Oral Surg., *32:*452, 1974

RUSENAS, I.: Changes in primate pacinian corpuscles following volar pad excision and skin grafting (with Miller). PRS, *57:*627, 1976

RUSINIAK, K.: Effect of tissue on electrical properties of chromium-cobalt implants in dogs. Protet. Stomatol., *24:*183, 1974 (Polish)

RUSH, B. F., JR. *et al*: Transoral and transverse incision for excision of the maxillary sinus. J. Surg. Oncol., *3:*53, 1971

RUSH, B. F., JR. *et al*: Integrated radiation and operation in the treatment of carcinoma of the head and neck: experience in 101 patients. J. Surg. Oncol., *3:*151, 1971

RUSH, B. F., JR. *et al*: Use of split thickness grafts in the repair of excisions of the oropharynx, base of the tongue, and larynx. Am. J. Surg., *128:*553, 1974

RUSSELL, A. S. *et al*: Deforming arthropathy in systemic lupus erythematosus. Ann. Rheum. Dis., *33:*204, 1974

RUSSELL, D. J., AND BEASON, E. S.: Maxillary recession for bucktooth deformity. PRS, *51:*220, 1973

RUSSELL, J. D., AND WITT, W. S.: Cell size and growth characteristics of cultured fibroblasts isolated from normal and keloid tissue. PRS, *57:*207, 1976

RUSSELL, P. S.: The future of constructive surgery. Transplant Proc., *6:*147, 1974

RUTRICK, R. E.: Crossbite correction with a therapeutic pacifier. J. Dent. Child., *41:*442, 1974

RUTRICK, R. E. *et al*: Multidisciplinary responsibilities in orthopedic-occlusal rehabilitation. Am. J. Orthod., *64:*491, 1973

RUTSTEIN, DAVID D.: *Blueprint for Medical Care*. M. I. T. Press, Cambridge, Mass., 1974. PRS, *55:*486, 1975

RUZIN, G. P. *et al*: Brephroplasty in treatment of jaw cysts in children. Stomatologiia (Mosk.), *53:*44, 1974 (Russian)

RUZIN, G. P. *et al*: Bone brephroplasty in cleft palate. Stomatologiia (Mosk.), *54:*38, 1975 (Russian)

RYAN, D. E. *et al*: An appliance that permits early mobilization after correction of mandibular prognathism. J. Oral Surg., *33:*875, 1975

RYAN, J. F., AND KERR, W. S., JR.: Malignant hyperthermia, catastrophic complication, PRS, *52:*602, 1973. J. Urol., *109:*879, 1973

RYAN, J. J., HOOPES, J. E., AND JABALEY, M. E.: Drug injection injuries of hands and forearms in addicts. PRS, *53:*445, 1974

RYAN, J. J., AND HOOPES, J. E.: Needle aspiration of flexor digital sheath as aid in diagnosing tenosynovitis. PRS, *56:*152, 1975

RYAN, M. D. *et al.*: Primary fibrosarcoma of the tongue: report of case. J. Oral Surg., *30:*135, 1972

RYAN, R. F.: Axillary hidradenitis suppurativa (with Pollock, Virnelli). PRS, *49:*22, 1972

RYAN, R. F.: Obituary on Richard W. Vincent. PRS, *49:*590, 1972

RYAN, R. F.: Rapid transfer of thoracoacromial flaps to face and neck (with Pollock, Bitseff). PRS, *50:*433, 1972

RYAN, R. F.: Topical therapy of burns. Postgrad. Med., *52:*105, 1972

RYAN, R. F.: Standardization of measurements in medicine by conversion to metric system (with Buren). PRS, *54:*459, 1974

RYAN, R. F. *et al*: Basal cell carcinoma as seen by plastic surgeon. J. La. State Med. Soc., *124:*361, 1972

RYAN, R. F., AND COLEMAN, W. P., III: Use of student-written programmed texts for teaching "core" knowledge in surgery. PRS, *53:*429, 1974

RYAN, T. J.: Diseases of skin. Management of varicose ulcers and eczema. Brit. Med. J. *1:*192, 1974

RYDOSZ, J.: Buried continuous suture in plastic surgery in the oral vestibule. Czas. Stomatol., *27:*1205, 1974 (Polish)

RYGARD, J. *et al*: Lip cancer. Ugeskr. Laeger, *135:*1866, 1973 (Danish)

RYKALIN, I. K. *et al*: Treatment of suppurative diseases of the hand. Khirurgiia (Mosk.), *48:*94, 1972 (Russian)

S

SAAD, MAGDY N., AND LECHTVELD, PETER: *Reviews in Plastic Surgery and General Plastic and Reconstructive Surgery*. Excerpta Medica, Amsterdam. American Elsevier Publishing Co., Inc., New York, 1974. PRS, *57:*91, 1976

SAAD, M. N. *et al*: Further applications of the rotation advancement technique. Brit. J. Plast. Surg., *25:*116, 1972

SAAD, M. N., AND MAISELS, D. O.: Facial incisions and approaches, PRS, *54:*697, 1974. Brit. J. Surg., *61:*566, 1974

SAADI, M. H.: Accessory exstrophic bladder. Brit. J. Clin. Pract., *29:*275, 1975

SAALFELD, J. *et al*: Congenital curvature of penis. Successful results with variations in corporoplasty. J. Urol., *109:*64, 1973

SAAVEDRA GONZALES, M. *et al*: Tumors of cutaneous glomus. Rozhl. Chir., *52:*822, 1973 (Czechoslovakian)

SABAS, A. A., MANGIONE, S., AND SIMONI, E.: Graft of *dura mater* in trachea, PRS, *57:*758, 1976. Rev. argent. cir., *28:*32, 1975

SABERMAN, M. N. *et al*: Clostridial infection of paranasal sinuses. Trans. Am. Acad. Ophthalmol. Otolaryngol., *76:*1356, 1972

SABIEK, T.: Reconstruction of a saddle nose. Med. Glas., *25:*81, 1971 (Croatian)

SABISTON, DAVID: *Textbook of Surgery: The Biological Basis of Modern Surgical Practice*. W. B. Saunders Co., Philadelphia, 1974. PRS, *56:*81, 1975

SABISTON, D. W.: Management of fractures of orbit. Trans. Aust. Coll. Ophthalmol., *3:*147, 1971

SABISTON, W. R.: Letter: seven come eleven. J.A.M.A., *234:*1222, 1975

SACHER, E. C. *et al*: Cavernospongiosum shunt in treatment of priapism, PRS, *51:*233, 1973. J. Urol., *108:*97, 1972

SACKER, M. A. *et al*: Pathogenesis and prevention of tracheo-bronchial damage with suction procedures, PRS, *53:*610, 1974. Chest, *64:*285, 1973

Sacrococcygeal Chordoma

Sacrococcygeal teratoma, giant, in newborn (Salaymeh), PRS, *49:*107, 1972. Internat. Surg., *56:*56, 1971

Sacrococcygeal chordomas in children (Richards, Stricke, Spitz), PRS, *54:*381, 1974. J. Pediat. Surg., *8:* 911, 1973

SADE, J.: Facial nerve reconstruction and its prognosis. Ann. Otol. Rhin. & Laryng., *84:*695, 1975

SADLOWSKI, R. W. *et al*: Further experience with one-stage hypospadias repair. J. Urol., *112:*677, 1974

SADOYAMA, J. A.: Muscle and fascial grafts in carotid artery protection. Laryngoscope, *85:*841, 1975

SAEBOE-LARSSEN, J.: Hand injuries. Tidsskr. nor. laegeforen, *91:*1886, 1971 (Norwegian)

SAEKI, K. *et al*: Inhibition of granulation tissue growth by histamine, PRS, *57:*268, 1976. J. Pharmacol. & Exper. Therap., *193:*910, 1975

SAFFRON, M. H.: Jerome Pierce Webster, 1888–1974. J. Hist. Med., *30:*67, 1975

SAFIAN, J.: Late report on early operation for "baggy eyelids." PRS, *48:*347, 1971

SAFIAN, J.: New anatomical concept of postoperative complications in esthetic rhinoplasty. PRS, *51:*162, 1973

SAFMAN, B. L.: Bilateral pathology in Bell's palsy, PRS, *51:*704, 1973. Arch. Otolaryng., *93:*55, 1971

SAFRA, M., AND OAKLEY, G., JR.: Association between cleft lip with or without cleft palate and prenatal exposure to diazepam, PRS, *57:*676, 1976. Lancet, *2:*478, 1975

SAGE, M. *et al*: Ketamine anaesthesia for burns surgery. Postgrad. Med. J., *48:*156, 1972

SAGEBIEL, R. W.: Histologic artifacts of benign pigmented nevi, PRS, *51:*483, 1973. Arch. Dermat., *106:*691, 1972

SAHATCHIEV, A. *et al*: Results of radical treatment of cancer of anterior two-thirds of tongue. Cancer, *30:*703, 1972

SAHYOUN, I.: Extensive radicular cyst of maxilla, case report. Rev. Dent. Liban., *23:*83, 1973

SAIJO, M., MUNRO, I. R., AND MANCER, K.: Lymphedema, clinical review and follow-up study. PRS, 56:513, 1975

SAIJO, M., MUNRO, I. R., AND MANCER, K.: Lymphangioma, long-term follow-up study. PRS, 56:642, 1975

SAIK, R. P., WALZ, C. A., AND RHOADS, J. E.: Evaluation of bacitracin-neomycin surgical skin preparation, PRS, 51:611, 1973. Am. J. Surg., 121:557, 1971

SAIKIA, N. K.: Pemphigus and malignancy. Brit. J. Dermatol., 88:407, 1973

SAILER, H. F.: Perimandibular cavernous hemangioma. Schweiz. Monatsschr. Zahnheilkd., 83:1267, 1973 (German)

SAILER, H. F.: Experiences with intraoral partial resection and simultaneous reconstruction of mandible in preoperatively non-infected cases, PRS, 55:716, 1975. J. Maxillofacial Surg., 2:173, 1974

SAILER, R., AND STAUCH, G.: Experimental investigations on prophylaxis of adhesions in peritonitis caused by enterococci with chondroitin-sulfates, PRS, 53:366, 1974. Bruns' Beitr. klin. Chir., 220:637, 1973

SAILER, R. et al: Therapy of gas gangrene. Comparison of results of the standard and hyperbaric oxygen therapy. Med. Klin., 69:1620, 1974 (German)

SAITO, H. et al: Management of orbital fat herniation by facial injury. Shujutsu, 25:1197, 1971 (Japanese)

SAITO, J. et al: Temporal bone findings in trisomy D, PRS, 55:717, 1975. Arch. Otolaryng., 100:386, 1974

SAITO, S.: Repair of pharyngoesophageal fistula by microvascular transfer of free skin flap (with Fujino). PRS, 56:549, 1975

SAITOH, H. et al: External fixation with resin in mandibular fracture, PRS, 55:378, 1975. Jap. J. Plast. Reconstr. Surg., 17:225, 1974

SAKABE, T. et al: Effects of lidocaine on canine cerebral metabolism and circulation related to electroencephalogram, PRS, 54:693, 1974. Anesthesiology, 40:433, 1974

SAKAGUCHI, S. et al: Thompson's operation on lymphedema of extremity, PRS, 56:467, 1975. Operation, 29:211, 1975

SAKAI, S. et al: Diagnosis and TNM classification of maxillary sinus carcinoma. Acta Otolaryngol. (Stockh.), 74:123, 1972

SAKAI, T.: Development in the Japan Society of Cancer Research of the Head and Neck Region in the last few years. J. Otolaryngol. Jap., 74:550, 1971 (Japanese)

SAKATA, S.: Scanning electron microscopic study on 3-dimensional ultrastructure of normal skin and scarred skin (atrophic scar, hypertrophic scar and keloid), PRS, 53:610,

1974. Jap. J. Plast. Reconstr. Surg., 16:412, 1973

SAKAUE, M.: New technique for nerve suture, epineurium anchoring funicular suture (with Tsuge, Ikuta). PRS, 56:496, 1975

SAKELLARIDES, H. T.: Dupuytren's contracture of hand and surgical correction by limited fasciectomy, PRS, 54:109, 1974. Acta orthop. belg., 38:190, 1972

SAKELLARIDES, H. T. et al: Reinnervation of the denervated muscles by nerve transplantation. Clin. Orthop., 83:195, 1972

SAKO, K.: Management of cancer of maxillary sinus. J. Surg. Oncol., 6:325, 1974

SAKO, K., MARCHETTA, F. C., AND HAYES, R. L.: Cryotherapy of intraoral leukoplakia, PRS, 52:102, 1973. Am. J. Surg., 124:482, 1972

SAKO, K. et al: Speech and vocational rehabilitation of laryngectomized patient, PRS, 57:532, 1976. J. Surg. Oncol., 6:197, 1974

SAKSELA, E. et al: Parotid clear-cell adenoma of possible myoepithelial origin. Cancer, 30:742, 1972

SAKUDA, M. et al: Changes of cheek pressure during swallowing following expansion of the maxillary dental arch in repaired cleft palates. J. Oral Rehabil., 2:145, 1975

SAKURAI, S. et al: Reconstruction of the skull defect using dimethyl polysiloxan (DMPS) following surgery of bone tumor in the frontal sinus. Otolaryngology (Tokyo), 43:607, 1971 (Japanese)

SALA, O. et al: Radiotherapy of maxillary tumors. Monatsschr. Ohrenheilkd. Laryngorhinol., 106:396, 1972 (German)

SALACZ, T. et al: Role of arteriography in the reconstruction of severe hand injuries. Magy. Traumatol. Orthop., 17:88, 1974 (Hungarian)

SALAM, A. A.: Brachial plexus paralysis: unusual complication of anticoagulant therapy, PRS, 51:350, 1973. Am. Surgeon, 38:454, 1972

SALAMA, R., AND WEISSMAN, S. L.: Congenital bilateral anomalous band between flexor and extensor pollicis longus tendons, PRS, 57:260, 1976. Hand, 7:25, 1975

SALASIN, R. I., AND BRIGGS, R. M.: Closure of large myelomeningocele. PRS, 51:464, 1973

SALAYMEH, M. T.: Giant sacrococcygeal teratoma in newborn, PRS, 49:107, 1972. Internat. Surg., 56:56, 1971

SALAZKIN, M. A. et al: Early plastic surgery of facial nerve. Vopr. Neurokhir., 36:30, 1972 (Russian)

SALED, H. et al: Hydatid cysts in children. Chirurgie, 100:294, 1974 (French)

SALEM, J. E. et al: In vivo fabrication of a temporary prosthesis for maxillofacial avulsion wounds: a clinical trial in Vietnam. J.

Trauma, *12:*501, 1972

SALEM, L. E., AND TRAVEZAN, R.: Malignant melanoma of head and neck, PRS, *54:*115, 1974. Internat. Surg., *58:*790, 1973

SALIBA, M. J., DEMPSEY, W. C., AND KRUGGEL, J. L.: Large burns in humans: treatment with heparin, PRS, *53:*246, 1974. J. A. M. A., *25:*261, 1973

SALISBURY, R. E.: Evaluation of Orenzyme in the prevention of swelling after hand surgery. Rev. Surg., *28:*455, 1971

SALISBURY, R. E.: Effect of early surgical excision and homografting on survival of burned rats and of intraperitoneally-infected burned rats (with Levine, Mason). PRS, *56:*423, 1975

SALISBURY, R. E., AND HUNTER, J. M.: Evaluation of oral trypsin-chymotrypsin for prevention of swelling after hand surgery. PRS, *49:*171, 1972

SALISBURY, R. E. *et al*: Biological dressings for skin graft donor sites, PRS, *52:*456, 1973. Arch. Surg., *106:*705, 1973

SALISBURY, R. E., AND PALM, L.: Dynamic splinting for dorsal burns of hand. PRS, *51:*226, 1973

SALISBURY, R. E. *et al*: Management of electrical burns of upper extremity. PRS, *51:*648, 1973

SALISBURY, R. E. *et al*: Ischemic necrosis of the intrinsic muscles of the hand after thermal injuries. J. Bone & Joint ˙Surg. (Am.), *56A:*1701, 1974

SALISBURY, R. E., SILVERSTEIN, P., AND GOODWIN, M. N., JR.: Upper extremity fungal invasions secondary to large burns. PRS, *54:*654, 1974

SALISBURY, ROGER E.: *Burns of the Upper Extremity.* W. B. Saunders Co., Philadelphia, 1976

Salivary Duct Calculi

Wharton duct problem (Lyons). J. La. State Med. Soc., *123:*348, 1971

Diagnosis and surgical treatment of salivary gland diseases (Bochenek). Otolaryngol. Pol., *25:*597, 1971 (Polish)

Sialolithotomy (Kruger). Am. Fam. Physician, *5:*116, 1972

Parotid calculus (Jackson). J. R. Nav. Med. Serv., *58:*59, 1972

Giant calculi of submandibular gland, case (Brocheriou *et al*). Rev. Stomatol. Chir. Maxillofac., *73:*517, 1972 (French)

Salivary calculi (diagnosis and treatment) (Beetke). Zentralbl. Chir., *97:*1073, 1972 (German)

Child, submandibular sialolithiasis in (Longhurst). Brit. Dent. J., *135:*291, 1973

Salivary Duct Calculi—Cont.

Submandibular gland, large calculus of, case report (Brusati *et al*). J. Oral Surg., *31:*710, 1973

Sialothithiasis of submaxillary duct (Orlian). N.Y. State Dent. J., *39:*548, 1973

Salivary gland, lingual, aberrant, lithiasis of (Dos Reis). Rev. Port. Estomatol. Cir. Maxilofac., *14:*191, 1973 (Portuguese)

Sialoliths in efferent duct of submandibular gland, surgical management (Vermeeren), PRS, *55:*507, 1975. Arch. chir. neerl., *26:*189, 1974

Salivary calculus of sublingual gland (Bozzay). Forgorv. Sz., *67:*134, 1974 (Hungarian)

Transoral surgical removal of a sialolith in the submandibular gland (Moose). Int. J. Oral Surg., *3:*318, 1974

Oral surgical care in the Rostock District—a pilot study (Andra *et al*). Stomatol. DDR, *24:*582, 1974 (German)

Significance of the anatomical structure of the submandibular salivary gland in calculi (Lesovaia). Stomatologiia (Mosk.), *53:*25, 1974 (Russian)

Salivary calculi in the minor salivary glands (Lomov-Oppokov *et al*). Stomatologiia (Mosk.), *53:*91, 1974 (Russian)

Anesthesia for operations on the parotid gland (Klementov *et al*). Stomatologiia (Mosk.), *53:*97, 1974 (Russian)

Surgical excision of the submandibular salivary glands in diabetic retinitis (Motta *et al*). Surv. Ophthalmol., *19:*63, 1974

Submandibular gland calculus with canalization—case report (Shteyer *et al*). Brit. J. Oral Surg., *12:*302, 1975

Emergency sialography (Fordham, Schatz), PRS, *56:*593, 1975. Emergency Med., *7:*101, 1975

Submandibular duct sialolith of unusual size and shape (Raksin *et al*). J. Oral Surg., *33:*142, 1975

Salivary gland disorders, some aspects of (Kenefick), PRS, *57:*395, 1976. Proc. Roy. Soc. Med., *68:*283, 1975

Case of large calculus of the submandibular gland (Koumoura). Stomatologia (Athenai), *32:*157, 1975 (Greek)

Surgical treatment method of sialolithiasis of the parotid gland (Solov'ev *et al*). Stomatologiia (Mosk.), *54:*46, 1975 (Russian)

Salivary Gland

Parotidean fistulae: therapeutic result (Parant). Actual Odontostomatol. (Paris), *26:*281, 1972 (French)

Salivary Gland — Cont.

Sublingual gland, submental herniation of, case report (Schneider *et al*). J. Oral Surg., *30:*824, 1972

Heterotopic cervical salivary gland (Parsons). PRS, *49:*464, 1972

Sjögren's disease with widespread lymphoid deposits (Grundy). Proc. Roy. Soc. Med., *65:*167, 1972

Salivary gland, Fibrir. foam as filling material for defects in surgery of. Animal experiments and clinical results (Jung *et al*). Arch. Klin. Exp. Ohren Nasen Kehlkopfheilkd., *204:*105, 1973 (German)

Sialography in unusual case of subcutaneous emphysema of neck (O'Hara *et al*). Arch. Otolaryng., *98:*354, 1973

Salivary fistulas, aberrant (Rothner), PRS, *54:*378, 1974. J. Pediat. Surg., *8:*931, 1973

Salivation, uncontrolled, parasympathectomy, surgical treatment for (Sartawi *et al*). Surg. Neurol., *1:*291, 1973

Salivary gland disorders. I. Recognition, diagnosis, treatment (Schwartz, Friedman). New York J. Med., *73:*297, 1973

Salivary obstruction, submandibular, new approach to, chorda tympani neurectomy (Zalin *et al*). Brit. J. Surg., *61:*392, 1974

Salivary gland counterbalance (Samuels *et al*). Oral Surg., *38:*535, 1974

Diseases of the Salivary Glands. By R. M. Rankow and I. M. Polayes. W. B. Saunders Co., Philadelphia, 1975

Gland, salivary, disorders of (Kenefick), PRS, *57:*395, 1976. Proc. Roy. Soc. Med., *68:*283, 1975

Salivary Gland Neoplasms (See also *Parotid Neoplasms*)

Salivary glands, treatment of malignant tumors of, at Gustave-Roussy institute (Lacour *et al*). Aktuel Probl. Chir., *14:*389, 1970

Mucoepidermoid tumors of major salivary glands (Tharvaldsson *et al*), PRS, *48:*199, 1971. Am. J. Surg., *120:*432, 1970

Submaxillary gland excision (Frable), PRS, *48:*294, 1971. Surg. Gynec. & Obst., *131:*1155, 1970

Adenoid cystic carcinoma of major and minor salivary glands (Leafstedt *et al*), PRS, *51:*608, 1973. Am. J. Surg., *122:*756, 1971

Salivary gland tumors in parotid gland, submandibular gland, and palate region (Eneroth), PRS, *49:*237, 1972. Cancer, *27:*1415, 1971

Leriche's operation for the treatment of parotid gland fistula (Uchikoshi *et al*). Oto-

Salivary Gland Neoplasms — Cont.

laryngology (Tokyo), *43:*919, 1971 (Japanese)

Examinations catalogued, results of 41 cylindroma cases (Spiessl, Schuchardt), PRS, *51:*707, 1973. Adv. Jaw & Face Surg., Year Book, 1972

Mucoepidermoid carcinoma of salivary gland (Connell, Evans), PRS, *52:*213, 1973. Am. J. Surg., *124:*519, 1972

Salivary gland tumor, mixed, of palate of child (Buehrie *et al*). Arch. Otolaryng., *96:*163, 1972

Salivary gland tumors (Editorial). Brit. Med. J., *4:*252, 1972

Salivary gland tumors (Patey). Brit. Med. J., *4:*492, 1972

Tumors of major salivary glands in children (Castro *et al*), PRS, *50:*97, 1972. Cancer, *29:*312, 1972

Treatment of minor salivary gland malignancies of upper food and air passage epithelium. A review of 87 cases (Kadish *et al*). Cancer, *29:*1021, 1972

Carcinoma, small cell (oat cell), of minor salivary gland origin (Koss *et al*). Cancer, *30:*737, 1972

Salivary gland tumors, mixed, diagnosis and therapy (Cendelin). Dtsch. Stomatol., *22:*509, 1972 (German)

Salivary glands, epithelial tumors of (Seifert). Fortschr. Kiefer, Gesichtschir., *15:*2, 1972

Mixed tumors of salivary glands, 184 cases, at Northwest German Dental Clinic from 1946–1967 (Schuchardt *et al*). Fortschr. Kiefer. Gesichtschir., *15:*28, 1972 (German)

Salivary gland tissue, aberrant, tumors of (Zehm). Forschr. Kiefer. Gesichtschir., *15:*43, 1972 (German)

Mixed tumors of soft tissues of mouth (Milde *et al*). Fortschr. Kiefer. Gesichtschir., *15:*56, 1972 (German)

Cylindromas of maxillofacial region (Stiebitz). Fortschr. Kiefer. Gesichtschir., *15:*60, 1972 (German)

Salivary gland tumors of palate, clinical and therapeutic aspects of (Schule). Fortschr. Kiefer. Gesichtchir., *15:*65, 1972 (German)

Cylindromas, radical treatment of (Wannemacher). Fortschr. Kiefer. Gesichtschir., *15:*81, 1972 (German)

Cylindroma therapy, results of (Schettler). Fortschr. Kiefer. Gesichtschir., *15:*84, 1972 (German)

Salivary gland tumor, differential diagnosis and therapy of (Andreevski). God. Zb.

Salivary Gland Neoplasms — Cont.

Med. Fak. Skopje., *18:*207, 1972 (Croatian)

Historical mixed tumor of soft palate? (Or mixed tumor of pharyngeal extension of parotid gland.) (Mazauric *et al*). J. Fr. Otorhinolaryngol., *21:*515, 1972 (French)

Salivary gland tumours (Butler). J. Laryng., & Otol., *86:*775, 1972

Mucoepidermoid carcinoma of minor salivary glands: report of 17 cases with follow-up (Eversole *et al*). J. Oral Surg., *30:*107, 1972

Submandibular gland swelling, unilateral, after induction of general anesthesia, case report (Smith *et al*). J. Oral Surg., *30:*911, 1972

Mixed tumors of submandibular glands (Udovicki *et al*). Med. Pregl., *25:*335, 1972 (Serbian)

Salivary glands, mixed tumors of, histopathological and prognostic considerations in 14 (Gianni). Minerva Stomatol., *21:*173, 1972 (Italian)

Salivary gland neoplasms in records of Slovak Institute of Oncology in years 1960 to 1969 (Knotek *et al*). Nowotwory, *22:*245, 1972 (Polish)

Salivary gland tumors, diagnostic possibilities of sialography in, on basis of 100 cases confirmed surgically (Benendo-Kapuscinska *et al*). Pol. Przegl. Radiol., *36:*721, 1972 (Polish)

Salivary gland tumors, X-ray treatment of postoperative recurrences of malignant (Borejko). Pol. Przegl. Radiol., *36:*795, 1972 (Polish)

Salivary gland, minor vestibular, muco-epidermoid cancer of (Crepy *et al*). Rev. Stomatol. Chir. Maxillofac., *73:*223, 1972 (French)

Salivary glands, mixed tumors (Lanier *et al*). South. Med. J., *65:*1485, 1972

Neoplasms of minor and lesser major salivary glands (Batsakis), PRS, *51:*351, 1973. Surg. Gynec. & Obst., *135:*289, 1972

Lymph node metastases of mucous and salivary gland tumors. Am. J. Roent. Radium Ther., *117:*595, 1973

Submaxillary gland tumors, malignant (Byers *et al*), PRS, *53:*682, 1974. Am. J. Surg., *126:*458, 1973

Salivary glands, carcinoma in pleomorphic adenomas of (Boles *et al*). Ann. Otol. Rhin. & Laryng., *82:*684, 1973

Salivary gland tumors, serous acinocellular (Galil-Ogly *et al*). Arkh. Patol., *35:*47, 1973 (Russian)

Salivary gland, mixed tumor, submandibu-

Salivary Gland Neoplasms — Cont.

lar duct lithiasis associated with (Hinder *et al*). Brit. J. Surg:, *60:*246, 1973

Tumors of minor salivary glands (Spiro *et al*), PRS, *52:*214, 1973. Cancer, *31:*117, 1973

Cylindroma, jaw and face, current aspects of therapy based on long-term observations (Schettler *et al*). Chirurg., *44:*370, 1973 (German)

Salivary glands, removal (Kowalik). Czas. Stomatol. *26:*1069, 1973 (Polish)

Salivary tumors, mixed (Potdar *et al*). Indian J. Cancer, *10:*217, 1973

Salivary glands, intraoral minor, mucoepidermoid tumors of, clinicopathologic study of 54 cases (Melrose *et al*). J. Oral Pathol., *2:*314, 1973

Cylindroma of head and neck, analysis of (Steinhoff *et al*). J. Surg. Oncol., *5:*17, 1973

Salivary gland tumors (Borcbakan *et al*), PRS, *57:*116, 1976. Kanser, *3:*38, 1973

Salivary glands, oncocytic and oncocytoid tumors of (Johns *et al*). Laryngoscope, *83:*1940, 1973

Salivary tumors. Salivary gland disorders. II. (Schwartz, Friedman). N. Y. State J. Med., *73:*439, 1973

Salivary gland tumors, major, surgical decisions in treatment of (Rankow). PRS, *51:*514, 1973

Head and neck, adenoid cystic carcinoma of (Newton *et al*), PRS, *52:*600, 1973. Proc. Roy. Australasian Coll. Surgeons, *46:*720, 1973

Cylindroma of oral cavity (Renaud *et al*). Rev. Stomatol. Chir. Maxillofac., *74:*1, 1973 (French)

Salivary gland tumors (Berdal). Tidsskr. Nor. Laegeforen, *93:*1899, 1973 (Norwegian)

Salivary glands, tumors of (Marlowe *et al*). Trans. Pa. Acad. Ophthalmol. Otolaryngol., *26:*36, 1973

Salivary gland tumors — synopsis of 692 cases (Glaser). Z. Aertl. Fortbild. (Jena), *67:*915, 1973 (German)

Malignancy in pleomorphic adenoma. Clinical and microspectrophotometric study (Eneroth *et al*). Acta Otolaryngol. (Stockh.), *77:*426, 1974

Adenoid cystic carcinoma of salivary origin. A clinicopathologic study of 242 cases (Spiro *et al*). Am. J. Surg., *128:*512, 1974

Salivary duct carcinoma (Fayemi, Toker), PRS, *55:*116, 1975. Arch. Otolaryng., *99:*366, 1974

Head and neck, adenoid cystic carcinoma in (cylindroma) (Conley, Dingman), PRS,

Salivary Gland Neoplasms—Cont.
lar). South. Med. J., *68:*347, 1975
Tumors of minor salivary gland origin (Antalik *et al*). Trans Pa. Acad. Ophthalmol. Otolaryngol., *28:*42, 1975

SALMAN, L. *et al*: Decompression of a median mandibular cyst: report of case. J. Oral Surg., *30:*503, 1972

SALMON, L. F. W.: Tracheostomy, PRS, *57:*260, 1976. Proc. Roy. Soc. Med., *68:*347, 1975

SALOMON, J. *et al*: Tracheal stenosis following tracheostomy. Int. Surg., *57:*498, 1972

SALTER, M. I.: Sensory re-education of the hand. Prog. Phys. Ther., *1:*264, 1970

SALTMACHER, F.: Reflections on classification and first aid of burned victims in diasters. Z. Aerztl. Fortbild. (Jena), *64:*1282, 1970 (German)

SALUS, W. G. *et al*: Initial experiences with Cottle's nasal septus reconstruction. H.N.O., *19:*311, 1971 (German)

SALVI, V.: Indications and possibilities of surgery for "rheumatic hand." Reumatismo, *21:*57, 1969 (Italian)

SALVI, V.: Methods in the surgical treatment of chronic arthropathies of the hand. Reumatismo, *22:*208, 1970 (Italian)

SALVI, V.: Delayed primary suture in flexor tendon division. Hand, *3:*181, 1971

SALVI, V.: Personal experience with McCash's "open palm" technique for Dupuytren's contracture, PRS, *54:*376, 1974. Hand, *5:*161, 1973

SALYER, K. E.: Vascularization of porcine skin heterografts (with Toranto, Myers), PRS, *54:*195, 1974. Discussion by Ben-Hur, PRS, *54:*352, 1974

SALYER, K. E., AND NICKELL, W. B.: Newer concepts of reconstructive surgery in patients with cancer of head and neck, PRS, *51:*485, 1973. South. M. J., *65:*1364, 1972

SALYER, K. E. *et al*: Survival of vascular pedicle island flaps. Surg. Forum, *23:*505, 1972

SALYER, K. E. *et al*: Interrelated role of maxillofacial prosthetics and reconstructive surgery, PRS, *53:*692, 1974. Am. J. Surg., *126:*496, 1973

SALYER, K. E., AND KYGER, E. R., III: Study in rats of survival of composite homotransplants of skin and subcutaneous tissue, with microvascular anastomoses. PRS, *51:*672, 1973

SALYER, K. E., AND NICKELL, W. B.: Surgical correction of facial paralysis, PRS, *55:*634, 1975. South. M.J., *67:*1166, 1974

SALYER, K. E. *et al*: Difficulties and problems to be solved in the approach to craniofacial malformations. Birth Defects, *11:*315, 1975

SALZMANN, J. A.: An appraisal of surgical orthodontics. Am. J. Orthod., *61:*105, 1972

SAMANT, H. C. *et al*: Congenital midline fistula of tongue, PRS, *56:*597, 1975. Oral Surg., *39:*34, 1975

SAMENGO, L. A.: Advanced maxillofacial tumors, PRS, *48:*517, 1971. Rev. argent. cir., *19:*89, 1970

SAMENGO, L. A.: Parotidectomy: personal technique for investigation of facial trunk, PRS, *54:*618, 1974. Prensa med. Argent., *50:*41, 1974

SAMII, M.: Operative surgical restitution of injured nerves, PRS, *51:*480, 1973. Langenbecks Arch. Chir., *332:*255, 1972

SAMII, M.: Restoring sensation to cut inferior alveolar nerve by direct anastomosis or by free autologous nerve grafting (with Hausamen, Schmidseder). PRS, *53:*83, 1974

SAMIIAN, M. R.: Advantages of the bilobed flap for closure of small defects of the face (with Morgan). PRS, *52:*35, 1973

SAMITZ, M. H.: Prevention of occupational skin diseases from exposure to chromic acid and chromates: use of ascorbic acid, PRS, *54:*371, 1974. Cutis, *13:*569, 1974

SAMMIS, F. C., JR.: Indications and technique of hemimaxillectomy for treatment of advanced malignancy of the maxilla. Trans. Int. Conf. Oral Surg., *4:*154, 1973

SAMOKHVALOV, V. V. *et al*: Comparative pathomorphological characteristics of methods of accelerated fixation of free skin grafts. Ortop. Travmatol. Protez., *32:*81, 1971 (Russian)

SAMUELS, H. S. *et al*: Salivary gland counterbalance. Oral Surg., *38:*535, 1974

SAMUELS, P. B., KATZ, D. J., AND DARROW, A. K.: Mechanized skin suturing, PRS, *55:*640, 1975. Arch. Surg., *109:*838, 1974

SAMUELS, P. B. *et al*: Skin closure using a new skin clip. Am. J. Surg., *129:*345, 1975

SANCHEZ GALINDO, J., AND ALMENDRAL, J.: Avulsion of skin of penis and scrotum, PRS, *48:*608, 1971. Rev. españ. cir. plast., *4:*27, 1971

SANCHEZ TORRES, J. *et al*: Central mandibular hemangioma, case report. Oral Surg., *37:*509, 1974

SANCHO, A. M.: New method of digital reconstruction by neurosensitive tubular flap, PRS, *57:*760, 1976. Rev. port. med. mil., *22:*212, 1974

SANCHO RODRIGUEZ-FORNOS, S., AND NARBONA ARNAU, B.: Branchial cysts and fistulas, PRS, *54:*111, 1974. Cir. Españ., *27:*339, 1973

SANDERS, B. *et al*: Management of wound breakdown after primary repair of facial laceration. J. Oral Surg., *32:*531, 1974

SANDERS, B. *et al*: Modified technique for palatal mucosal grafts in mandibular labial vestibuloplasty. J. Oral Surg., *33:*950, 1975

SANDERS, D. W. *et al*: Ameloblastic fibro-odontoma: case report. J. Oral Surg., *32:*281, 1974

SANDERS, G. B.: Complete axillary node dissection with preservation of the pectoralis major muscle. Arch. Surg., *103:*518, 1971

SANDERS, H. J.: Ocular injuries in orbital fractures, review of 119 cases (with Jabaley, Lerman). PRS, *56:*410, 1975

SANDERS, R.: Tourniquet, instrument or weapon? PRS, *54:*236, 1974. Hand, *5:*119, 1973

SANDERS, R.: Plastic surgical treatment of obesity. Proc. Roy. Soc. Med., *68:*664, 1975

SANDERS, R. J. *et al*: A particular type of decubitus (ulcer). Ned. tijdschr. geneeskd., *118:*233, 1974 (Dutch)

SANDNER, O.: Conservative and surgical treatment of condylar fractures of temporomandibular joint. Int. J. Oral Surg., *3:*218, 1974

SANDZEN, S. C.: Management of acute fingertip injury in child, PRS, *56:*228, 1975. Hand, *6:*190, 1974

SANDZEN, S. C., JR.: Treating acute fingertip injuries. Am. Fam. Physician, *5:*68, 1972

SANDZEN, S. C., JR.: Crush injuries of the hand and fingers. 1. Med. Trial Tech. Q., *19:*144, 1972

SANDZEN, S. C., JR.: Crush injuries of the hand and fingers. 2. Med. Trial Tech. Q., *19:*282, 1973

SANDZEN, S. C. JR.: Crush injuries of the hand and fingers. 3. Med. Trial Tech. Q., *19:*418, 1973

SANDZEN, S. C., JR.: Treating acute hand and finger injuries. 1. Am. Fam. Physician, *9:*74, 1974

SANDZEN, S. C., JR.: Treating acute hand and finger injuries. Am. Fam. Physician, *9:*100, 1974

SANDZEN, S. C., JR., AND STEEL, H. H.: Thumb repositioning in 4-digit hand. PRS, *53:*91, 1974

SANFELIPPO, P. M., BEAHRS, O. H., AND HAYLES, A. B.: Indications for thyroidectomy in pediatric patient, PRS, *51:*702, 1973. Am. J. Surg., *122:*472, 1971

SANGMIT, S.: Reconstruction of the penoscrotal skin after avulsion. Int. Surg., *60:*563, 1975

SANNER, J. *et al*: Salivary retention phenomenon following surgical lowering of floor of mouth. J. Oral Surg., *32:*377, 1974

SANO, K. *et al*: Surgically treated case of brachydactylia of the metacarpal bone. Orthop. Surg. (Tokyo), *22:*146, 1971 (Japanese)

SANTHA, E. *et al*: Arthrodesis of the fingers. Magy. Traumatol. Orthop., *15:*161, 1972 (Hungarian)

SANTIAGO, A.: Role of the dentist in radiotherapy, PRS, *53:*604, 1974. J. Prosth. Dent., *39:*196, 1973

SANTLER, R. AND FREILINGER, G.: Surgery of neoplasms in dermatology. Arch. Derm. Forsch., *244:*418, 1972 (German)

SANTONI-RUGIU, P. *et al*: Restoration of maxillary cleft using periosteum flaps in the case of complete labio-palatine cleft. Ann. chir. plast., *16:*326, 1971 (French)

SANTOS, O. A., AND PAPPAS, J. C.: Repair of nostril defect with contralateral nasolabial flap. PRS, *57:*704, 1976

SANTOS, V. B. *et al*: Bilateral pseudocysts of auricle in female. Ann. Otol. Rhin. & Laryng., *83:*9, 1974

SANTOS, V. B. *et al*: Role of surgery in head and neck cancer with fixed nodes. Arch. Otolaryng., *101:*645, 1975

SANVENERO-ROSSELLI, D. G.: Restoration of severe injuries in the frontal, nasal and ethmodal region. Dtsch. Zahn. Mund. Kieferheilkd., *57:*285, 1971 (Italian)

SANY, J.: Prosthesis and rehabilitation of the hand in chronic rheumatoid arthritis. Rev. Rhum. Mal. Osteoartic., *40:*216, 1973 (French)

SAPELLI, P. L.: Depressed fractures of the upper part of the face. Rev. Stomatol. Chir. Maxillofac., *75:*259, 1974 (French)

SAPONE, J. *et al*: Traumatic bone cyst of jaws: diagnosis, treatment and prognosis. Oral Surg., *32:*127, 1974

SARDAK, G. A. *et al*: Free autodermoplasty in esophageal surgery. Klin. Khir., *3:*16, 1974 (Russian)

SARKIN, T. L.: Surgery of the hand in infants with cerebral palsy. S. Afr. Med. J., *45:*655, 1972

SARKISOV, M. A. *et al*: Amputation and prosthesis after electric trauma of the upper limbs. Vestn. Khir., *113:*103, 1974 (Russian)

SARNAT, B. G. *et al*: Facial skeletal changes after mandibular condylectomy in growing and adult monkeys. Am. J. Orthod., *62:*428, 1972

SARNQUIST, F., AND LARSON, P. C.: Drug induced heat stroke, PRS, *53:*610, 1974. Anesthesiology, *39:*348, 1973

SARRAT, R.: Evolutive and embryological development of facial region, PRS, *57:*753, 1976. Cir. Plast. Ibero-Latino Am., *1:*7, 1975

SARTAN, V. A.: Industrial injuries of the fingers and hands. Ortop. Travmatol. Protez., *32:*65, 1971 (Russian)

SARTAN, V. A.: Primary blind suture in open combined injuries of the fingers and hand. Ortop. Travmatol. Protez., *34:*59, 1973 (Russian)

SARTAN, V. A.: Case of primary combined plastic surgery in severe open complicated hand injury. Ortop. Travmatol. Protez., *3:*58, 1975 (Russian)

SARTAWI, M. *et al*: Parasympathectomy: surgical treatment for uncontrolled salivation. Surg. Neurol., *1:*291, 1973

SARWAR, M.: Orbital orbicularis sling operation for ptosis. Ann. Ophth., *4:*250, 1972

SASHIKOVA, V. G.: Use of "catgut ligatures" in treatment of trophic ulcers of the lower limbs. Vestn. Khir., *115:*57, 1975 (Russian)

SATAVA, R. M., JR. *et al*: Success rate of cervical exploration for hyperparathyroidism. Arch. Surg., *110:*625, 1975

SATERNUS, K. S.: Fatal complications of tracheotomy. H.N.O., *20:*274, 1972 (German)

SATKO, I.: Main principles in treatment of facial bone fractures. Cesk. Stomatol., *74:*46, 1974 (Slovakian)

SATO, F. *et al*: Clinical observation of neck swelling—metastatic cancer of the neck without detectable primary site. Jap. J. Cancer Clin., *18:*274, 1972 (Japanese)

SATO, Y.: Treatment of malignant tumor of head and neck region through team work with radiology department. J. Otolaryngol. Jap., *76:*1301, 1973 (Japanese)

SATTEL, W. *et al*: Bone tumors of the hand. Handchirurgie, *3:*103, 1971

SAUBIER, E. C. *et al*: Problem of thoracic wall reconstruction after removal of large tumor mass, PRS, *51:*103, 1973. Lyon chir., *68:*256, 1972

SAUCIER, J. L.: Psychological repercussions of genital operations. Union Med. Can., *103:*1233, 1974 (French)

SAUER, H. *et al*: Orthopedic jaw operations on the tuberculum articulare. Fortschr. Kiefer. Gesichtschir., *18:*238, 1974 (German)

SAUERBREY, W.: Can radiotherapy of plantar warts still be justified? Z. Allgemeinmed., *47:*1584, 1971 (German)

SAUNDERS, S. H. *et al*: Adenocarcinoma of the paranasal sinus. J. Laryng. & Otol., *90:*157, 1976

SAUNDERS, W. H.: Otorhinolaryngology. Surg. Gynec. & Obst., *138:*209, 1974

SAUNDERS, W. H. *et al*: Polytomography of paranasal sinuses and adjacent areas. Trans. Am. Acad. Ophthalmol. Otolaryngol., *78:*168, 1974

SAUNDERS, W. H. *et al*: Rehabilitation of the shoulder after radical neck dissection. Ann. Otol. Rhin. & Laryng., *84:*812, 1975

SAVAGE, J.: Aluminum hydroxide granuloma, PRS, *54:*118, 1974. Proc. Roy. Soc. Med., *66:*984, 1973

SAVAGE, T. M. *et al*: Cardiorespiratory effects of Althesin and ketamine, PRS, *53:*373, 1974. Anaesthesia, *28:*391, 1973

SAVANI, A., SAVOIA, A., AND TAIDELLI, G.: Our experience with ½% silver nitrate in treatment of burns, PRS, *50:*308, 1972. Acta chir. plast., *13:*87, 1971

SAVANI, A. *et al*: Reparative surgery of genitoperineal region. Minerva Chir., *26:*1474, 1971 (Italian)

SAVCHENKO, N. E. *et al*: On the necessity and possibility of unification in the treatment of hypospadias. Urol. Nefrol. (Mosk.), *37:*69, 1972 (Russian)

SAVCHENKO, N. Y., AND MOKHORT, V. A.: Plastic operation on urinary bladder in neurogenic disorders of micturition, PRS, *54:*504, 1974. Acta chir. plast., *15:*223, 1973

SAVELIEV, V. I. *et al*: Preparation and gas sterilization of mandibular homografts. Stomatologiia (Mosk.), *53:*34, 1975 (Russian)

SAVELYEV, V. I.: Methods of preparation and conservation of tissue grafts without aseptic technique, PRS, *50:*542, 1972. Acta chir. plast., *13:*121, 1971

SAVIN, R. C.: Hair transplants in burn scars and other alopecias. Conn. Med., *37:*501, 1973

SAWHNEY, C. P.: Combined autograft and homograft cover in extensive deep burns. Brit. J. Plast. Surg., *25:*141, 1972

SAWHNEY, C. P.: Geometry of single cleft lip repair. PRS, *49:*518, 1972

SAWHNEY, C. P.: Evaluation of Thompson's buried dermal flap operation for lymphedema of limbs, PRS, *56:*680, 1975. Brit. J. Plast. Surg., *27:*278, 1974

SAWHNEY, C. P.: Considerations in management of contractures of neck, PRS, *55:*384, 1975. Indian J. Plast. Surg., *7:*6, 1974

SAWHNEY, K. K. *et al*: Liposarcoma of the hand. Am. Surg., *41:*117, 1975

SAWHNEY, K. L. *et al*: Hemangioma of maxilla. Ann. Otol. Rhin. & Laryng., *82:*254, 1973

SAWHNEY, O. P.: Free composite lip grafts (with Walker). PRS, *50:*142, 1972

SAXENA, R. C.: Canaliculo-dacryocysto-rhinostomy. A simple technique. J. All India Ophthalmol. Soc., *18:*173, 1970

SAXENA, R. C.: Few observations on dacryocystorhinostomy in lacrimal fistula. Indian J. Ophthalmol., *20:*133, 1972

SAXENA, R. C. *et al*: Severe epistaxis after dacryocystorhinostomy. Indian J. Ophthalmol., *20:*136, 1972

SAXENA, V. S.: Cancer of tongue: study of regional lymph node spread, PRS, *48:*199, 1971. Cancer, *27:*38, 1971

SAXMAN, J. H.: A call for new directions in cleft palate speech research. Cleft Palate J., *9:*274, 1972

SAYOC, B. T.: Surgery of the Oriental eyelid. Clin. Plast. Surg., *1*:157, 1974

SAZIMA, H., SCOTT, W., AND MOORE, D.: Maxillofacial rehabilitation in South Vietnam, PRS, *54*:235, 1974. Mil. Med., *138*:824, 1973

SAZIMA, H. J.: Diagnosis and treatment of fractures of malar eminence. Mil. Med., *136*:888, 1971

SBAITI, A.: Ocular changes in case of ectodermal dysplasia. Klin. Monatsbl. Augenheilkd., *164*:267, 1974 (German)

SBOKOS, C. G. *et al*: Surgical correction of pectus excavatum using a retrosternal bar. Thorax, *30*:40, 1975

Scalp (See also *Hair*)

Hair transplants in accidental baldness (Purita). Hospital (Rio de J.), *77*:1303, 1970 (Portuguese)

Treatment of scalping (Laube *et al*). Zentralbl. Chir., *95*:994, 1970 (German)

Surgical possibilities in the treatment of baldness (Fevrier). Bord. Med., *4*:3255, 1971 (French)

Split-thickness scalp flap for resurfacing full thickness forehead and temporal scalp defects (Ship *et al*). Brit. J. Plast. Surg., *24*:351, 1971

Scalp and skull, major resection for cancer with immediate complete reconstruction in 14 cases (Gaisford, Hanna, Susen) (Follow-Up Clinic). PRS, *48*:369, 1971

Scalp vein sites of needle insertion during intravenous therapy, prevention of infection (Crenshaw *et al*), PRS, *51*:354, 1973. Am. J. Surg., *124*:43, 1972

Pilonidal cyst of the scalp (Moyer). Arch. Dermat., *105*:578, 1972

Use of scalp flaps following resection of oral cancer (Dhawan *et al*). Aust. N.Z. J. Surg., *41*:363, 1972

Experience of reconstruction of the head with a giant jump flap (Fukuda). Jap. J. Plast. Reconstr. Surg., *15*:203, 1972 (Japanese)

Scalp, hair-covered, therapy of large defects of (Mehler *et al*). Langenbecks Arch. Chir., *331*:265, 1972 (German)

Hair transplantation (Orentreich). N.Y. State J. Med., *72*:578, 1972

Scalp defect, large, autotransplant of omentum with microsurgical revascularization (McLean, Buncke). PRS, *49*:268, 1972

Brain development, fetal, scalp hair patterning as clue to (Smith, Gong), PRS, *54*:370, 1974. J. Pediat., *83*:374, 1973

Scalp and skull defect in patient with systemic form of scleroderma, coverage of

Scalp – Cont.

(Losken, Davies, Gordon). PRS, *51*:212, 1973

Arteriovenous malformation, congenital defect of the skull and scalp due to (Vasconez). PRS, *51*:692, 1973

Scalp, extensive turban tumor of, treatment (single observation) (Kupchik *et al*). Vopr. Onkol., *19*:77, 1973 (Russian)

Scalp cyst, taping of, method to facilitate removal of (Witkowski *et al*). Acta Physiol. Scand., *91*:226, 1974

Taping of a cyst: a method to facilitate removal of a scalp cyst (Witkowski *et al*). Atherosclerosis, *20*:226, 1974

Clinical success of distant transfer of free skin flap in head and neck regions by microvascular anastomoses (Fujino *et al*). Keio J. Med., *23*:47, 1974

Scalp and skull, electrical burn of (Luce, Hoopes), PRS, *54*:359, 1974

Flaps, free scalp, hair transplantation with (Harii, Ohmori, Ohmori), PRS, *53*:410, 1974

Scalp lesion, nevus sebaceous of Jadassohn (Baker), PRS, *57*:403, 1976. Arch. Otolaryng., *101*:515, 1975

Scalp defects, surgical closure (Widmaier), PRS, *57*:527, 1976. J. Maxillo-facial Surg., *3*:149, 1975

Scalp defects, congenital, in 4 generations (Weippl, Ader), PRS, *56*:460, 1975. Klin. Paediatr., *187*:84, 1975

Fundamental technique of microvascular surgery (Harii). Neurol. Surg. (Tokyo), *3*:889, 1975 (Japanese)

Scalping injury (Koss, Robson, Krizek), PRS, *55*:439, 1975

Scalp, large denudation covered by autotransplant of omentum (Ikuta), PRS, *55*:490, 1975

Free skin flap transfer (Harii *et al*). Clin. Plast. Surg., *3*:111, 1976

Scalp Avulsions

Avulsion of scalp and its reconstruction (Jeremiah), PRS, *48*:604, 1971. Internat. Surg., *55*:265, 1971

Avulsion laceration of the scalp, treatment with primary punch grafts and an overlay sheet of split-skin graft (Hight, Anderton), PRS, *52*:663, 1973

Avulsion, scalp (Koss, Robson, Krizek), PRS, *55*:439, 1975

Scalpel, Plasma: See *Plasma Scalpel*

SCARAMELLA, L. F. *et al*: Facial nerve anastomosis. Laryngoscope, *83*:1834, 1973

Scars (See also *Burn Scars; Collagen; Keloids; Scars, Hypertrophic; Wound Healing*)

Scars, linear, Z- and W-plasty in revisions (Borges), PRS, *49:*241, 1972. Internat. Surg., *56:*182, 1971

Skin incisions, strength development in young and old rats (Holm-Pedersen, Zederfeldt), PRS, *48:*610, 1971. Scand. J. Plast. Reconstr. Surg., *5:*7, 1971

Scar Tissue, its Use and Abuse: The Surgical Correction of Deformation Due to Hypertrophic Scar and the Prevention of its Formation. By J. J. Longacre. Charles C Thomas, Springfield, Ill., 1972. PRS, *52:*187, 1973

Value of an enzyme inhibitor in cicatrization (animal experimentation; application to hand surgery) (Comtet *et al*). Ann. chir. plast., *17:*145, 1972 (French)

Scar formation, inhibition by proline analog cis-hydroxyproline (Lane *et al*), PRS, *52:*104, 1973. J. Surg. Res., *13:*135, 1972

Scars, skin grafts, and flaps, growth in young minipigs (Baran, Horton). PRS, *50:*487, 1972

Elective Incisions and Scar Revision. By Albert F. Borges. Little, Brown & Co., Boston, 1973. PRS, *54:*216, 1974

Scar tissue, huge midline hernias in, repair (Chaimoff, Dintsman), PRS, *53:*110, 1974. Am. J. Surg., *125:*767, 1973

Scar tissue, biologic frontiers in control of healing (Peacock), PRS, *54:*114, 1974. Am. J. Surg., *126:*708, 1973

Scars, psoriasis on (Paslin), PRS, *54:*379, 1974. Arch. Dermat., *108:*665, 1973

Scarring, severe, secondary to chickenpox (Smith *et al*). Brit. J. Plast. Surg., *26:*344, 1973

Scars, vaccination, in deltoid area, pitfall of surgical excision of (Musgrave) (Letter to the Editor). PRS, *51:*198, 1973

Lymph outflow, facial scars and (Clodius). Praxis, *62:*336, 1973 (German)

Vitamin E, influence in anomalous scar (Gras Artero), PRS, *56:*363, 1975. Riv. ital. chir. plast., *5:*309, 1973

Scars and scar revision (Eskeland). Tidsskr. Nor. Laegeforen, *93:*1067, 1973 (Norwegian)

Peritoneum, method of restoring (Mansberger, Kang), PRS, *54:*247, 1974. Am. Surgeon, *40:*117, 1974

Scars. Aspects of plastic surgery (Crockett). Brit. Med. J., *2:*648, 1974

Control and prevention of hypertrophic scarring and contracture (Noordhoff). Clin. Plast. Surg., *1:*49, 1974

Scars — Cont.

Scars, smallpox-induced: treatment by dermabrasion (Vukas). Dermatologica, *148:*175, 1974

Scars, suture techniques and, and their correction (Haas). Laryngol. Rhinol. Otol. (Stuttg.), *53:*234, 1974 (German)

Scar revision. (Mathog). Minn. Med., *57:*31, 1974

Scars, head and neck, revision (Gunter). Otolaryngol. Clin. North Am., *7:*119, 1974

Scars, hypertrophic, and keloids (Ketchum, Cohen, Masters). PRS, *53:*140, 1974

Scars, inconspicuous, factors in production of (Wray, Holtmann, Weeks). PRS, *56:*86, 1975

Pregnancy estrogens, presumptive evidence of effect on keloid growth (Moustafa, Abdel-Fattah). PRS, *56:*450, 1975

Z-plasty, subcutaneous (Vecchione, Pickering). PRS, *56:*579, 1975

Scars, skin pigmentation, current concepts and relevance to plastic surgery (Morgan, Gilchrest, Goldwyn). PRS, *56:*617, 1975

Action of corticosteroids on cutaneous cicatrization. Use in maxillofacial surgery (Grellet *et al*). Rev. Stomatol. Chir. Maxillofac., *76:*379, 1975 (French)

Tissue growth, cell size and growth characteristics of cultured fibroblasts isolated from normal and keloid tissue (Russell, Witt). PRS, *57:*207, 1976

Scar tissue, elastin fibers in (Bhangoo, Quinlivan, Connelly). PRS, *57:*308, 1976

Scars, healed, disruption of, in scurvy — result of disequilibrium in collagen metabolism (Cohen, Keiser), PRS, *57:*213, 1976. Discussion by Chvapil, PRS, *57:*376, 1976

Tension lines, skin, in domestic pig (Rose, Ksander, Vistnes). PRS, *57:*729, 1976

Scars, Burn: See *Burn Scars*

Scars, Hypertrophic (See also *Burn Scars; Collagen; Keloid; Wound Healing*)

Keloids, hypertrophic scars and, treatment by corticoid intralesional injections with dermo-jet (Henel, Pinto), PRS, *48:*519, 1971. A Folha Med., *61:*337, 1970

Hypertrophic scars and keloids, biologic basis for treatment (Peacock, Madden, Trier), PRS, *51:*709, 1973. South. M.J., *63:*755, 1970

Hypertrophic scars and keloids, follow-up on treatment with triamcinolone (Ketchum, Robinson, Masters). PRS, *48:*256, 1971

Collagen synthesis in human keloid and hypertrophic scar (Cohen, Keiser,

Scars, Hypertrophic — Cont.

Sjoerdsma), PRS, *50:*205, 1972. Surg. Forum, *22:*488, 1971

Scars and keloids, treatment of (Sugimoto), PRS, *51:*610, 1973. Jap. J. Plast. Reconstr. Surg., *15:*157, 1972

Cis-hydroxyproline for inhibition of scar formation (Lane *et al*), PRS, *52:*104, 1973. J. Surg. Res., *13:*135, 1972

Collagen and histamine synthesis in keloid and hypertrophic scar (Cohen *et al*), PRS, *51:*709, 1973. Surg. Forum, *23:*509, 1972

Scars and keloids in children, Kenacort A in treatment of (Jaworski), PRS, *54:*624, 1974. Acta chir. plast., *15:*206, 1973

Scars, keloid (Garcez, Saraiva, Braga), PRS, *53:*248, 1974. Folha Med. Brazil, *66:*57, 1973

Scars, atrophic, hypertrophic, ʼand keloid, electron microscopic study on 3-dimensional ultrastructure of normal and scarred skin (Sakata), PRS, *53:*610, 1974. Jap. J. Plast. Reconstr. Surg., *16:*412, 1973

Scar, hypertrophic, origin of (Linares *et al*), PRS, *53:*495, 1974. J. Trauma, *13:*70, 1973

Osteitis: coverage of scalp and skull defect in patient with systemic form of scleroderma (Losken, Davies, Gordon), PRS, *51:*212, 1973

Hypertrophic scars, and keloids, intralesional injection with Dermo-Jet (Vallis) (Follow-Up Clinic), PRS, *52:*434, 1973

Scars, hypertrophic, modifying evolution of (Linares), PRS, *55:*517, 1975. Rev. Latino Am. cir. plast., *17:*51, 1973

Control and prevention of hypertrophic scarring and contracture (Noordhoff). Clin. Plast. Surg., *1:*49, 1974

Hypertrophic scar: *dermatofibrosarcoma protuberans* or keloid — a warning (Manalan, Cohen, Theogaraj). PRS, *53:*96, 1974

Hypertrophic scars and keloids (Ketchum, Cohen, Masters), PRS, *53:*140, 1974

Scars, hypertrophic burn, reappraisal of shaving and skin grafting for (Moustafa, Abdel-Fattah). PRS, *57:*463, 1976

SCARTASCINI, J. F. *et al*: Surgical correction of tooth malposition. Trib. Odontol. (B. Aires), *57:*40, 1973 (Spanish)

SCHAAF, N. G.: Materials in maxillofacial prosthetics, PRS, *57:*266, 1976. Dent. Clin. N. Am., *19:*347, 1975

SCHAAF, N. G.: Prosthesis after maxillectomy. Otolaryngol. Clin. North Am., *9:*301, 1976

SCHAAF, N. G. *et al*: Prosthetic rehabilitation of head and neck cancer patient. J. Surg. Oncol., *6:*311, 1974

SCHABERG, S. J. *et al*: Blood loss and hypotensive anesthesia in oral-facial corrective surgery. J. Oral Surg., *34:*147, 1976

SCHADE, G. J.: Epidemiological aspects of cleft lip and cleft palate. Ned. Tijdschr. Trandheelkd., *78:*300, 1971 (Dutch)

SCHADE, G. J.: Induction of cleft palate by amniotic sac puncture. Acta Morphol. Neerl. Scand., *13:*104, 1975

SCHADE, K.: Clinical experiences in 2000 facial soft-tissue injuries. Zentralbl. Chir., *96:*1389, 1971 (German)

SCHADE, K.: Surgical therapy of lateral middle face fractures. Dtsch. Stomatol., *22:*769, 1972 (German)

SCHADE, K.: Critical evaluation of Nasteff-Rosenthal's surgical method in cystic tumors of jaw region. Dtsch. Stomatol., *23:*40, 1973 (German)

SCHAERF, R. H. M.: Evaluation of topical povidone-iodine ointment in experimental burn wound sepsis (with Robson, Krizek). PRS, *54:*328, 1974

SCHANEWEDE, H. VON: Prosthetic treatment after surgical removal of tumors in the jaw region. Dtsch. Stomatol., *21:*765, 1971 (German)

SCHANTZ, A., AND CASTLEMAN, B.: Parathyroid carcinoma, PRS, *52:*458, 1973. Cancer, *31:*600, 1973

SCHARF, F. *et al*: Report on results of the treatment of mandibular fractures with osteosynthesis plates. Fortschr. Kiefer. Gesichtschir., *19:*82, 1975 (German)

SCHARGUS, G. *et al*: Experimental and histological studies in fracture healing on osteotomized rabbit mandibles after immobilization of the fragments by wire sutures and osteosynthesis plates. Fortschr. Kiefer. Gesichtschir., *19:*21, 1975 (German)

SCHARGUS, G. *et al*: Cryosurgical devitalization of bone and its regeneration, PRS, *57:*405, 1976. J. Maxillofacial Surg., *3:*128, 1975

SCHARLI, A. F.: From anal atresia to continent organ. Arch chir. neerl., *27:*179, 1975 (German)

SCHARLZER, E.: Acute closed hand injuries. Dtsch. Med. J., *21:*1327, 1970 (German)

SCHARLZER, E.: Anatomy of the arterial pattern of the palmar arch of the hand. Handchirurgie, *2:*122, 1970 (German)

SCHARLZER, E.: Rehabilitation — conservative measures following surgical treatment of tendon injuries of the hand. Handchirurgie, *3:*99, 1971 (German)

SCHATTEN, W. E.: Cervicofacial actinomycosis (with Hartley), PRS, *51:*44, 1973

SCHATTEN, W. E.: Acute retrobulbar hemorrhage during elective blepharoplasty (with Hartley, Lester), PRS, *52:*8, 1973. Discussions by Lemoine, Rees, Newell, PRS, *52:*12, 1973

SCHATTEN, W. E.: Subcutaneous mastectomy; excess skin problem (with Hartley, Griffin), PRS, *56:*5, 1975

SCHATTEN, W. E., HARTLEY, J. H., JR., AND HAMM, W. G.: Reduction mammaplasty by Dufourmentel-Mouly method, PRS, *48:*306, 1971

SCHATTEN, W. E. *et al:* Effect of dextran on metastasis of V2 carcinoma in rabbits (Follow-Up Clinic), PRS, *50:*78, 1972

SCHATTEN, W. E. *et al:* Further experience with lateral wedge resection mammaplasties. Brit. J. Plast. Surg., *28:*37, 1975

SCHAUERHAMER, R. A. *et al:* Studies in management of contaminated wound. VII. Susceptibility of surgical wounds to postoperative surface contamination, PRS, *49:*668, 1972. Am. J. Surg., *122:*74, 1971

SCHAUPP, H.: Reconstruction of nose wing using a frontotemporal flap. H.N.O., *21:*187, 1973 (German)

SCHAUPP, H. *et al:* Reconstruction of columella after tumor resection at nose entrance. Arch. Klin. Exp. Ohren Nasen Kehlkopfheilkd., *205:*332, 1973 (German)

SCHAUPP, H. *et al:* Treatment of skin cancer in head and neck region. Z. Laryngol. Rhinol. Otol., *52:*245, 1973 (German)

SCHAUPP, H. *et al:* Covering of defects in the lateral head and neck regions with shoulder flaps. H.N.O., *23:*160, 1975 (German)

SCHECHTER, G. L., AND McLAREY, D.: Conservation surgery of larynx and hypopharynx, PRS, *53:*683, 1974. Mil. Med., *138:*639, 1973

SCHECHTER, I. *et al:* Prolonged retention of glutaraldehyde-treated skin homografts in humans. Brit. J. Plast. Surg., *28:*198, 1975

SCHEGG, H. K.: Excision of mucosa. Schweiz. Monatsschr. Zahnheilkd., *83:*1295, 1973 (German)

SCHEGG, H. K.: Preparation, aftercare and definitive management in large preprosthetic interventions. Schweiz. Monatsschr. Zahnheilkd., *83:*1483, 1973

SCHEGG, H. K.: Case of traumatic mandibular fracture related to radicular cyst. Schweiz. Monatsschr. Zahnheilkd., *84:*291, 1974 (German)

SCHELLANDER, F. *et al:* Basal cell hamartoma and cellular naevus: unusual combined malformation. Brit. J. Dermatol., *90:*413, 1974

SCHELLHAMMER, P. AND DONNELLY, J.: Mode of treatment for incarceration of penis. J. Trauma, *13:*171, 1973

SCHELLHAMMER, P. F., HACKLER, R. H., AND BUNTS, R. C.: External sphincterotomy: rationale for procedure and experiences with 150 patients, PRS, *56:*106, 1975. Paraplegia, *12:*5, 1974

SCHENCK, N. L.: Frontal sinus disease. III. Experimental and clinical factors in failure of the frontal osteoplastic operation. Laryngoscope, *85:*76, 1975

SCHENKE, H.: Surgical suture materials and suture techniques in oto-rhino-laryngology. H.N.O., *22:*356, 1974 (German)

SCHENKEIN, I. *et al:* Increased nerve-growth stimulating activity in disseminated neurofibromatosis, PRS, *54:*377, 1974. New England J. Med., *290:*613, 1974

SCHER, C. *et al:* High-pressure paint gun injuries of the hand: a report of two cases. Brit. J. Plast. Surg., *26:*167, 1973

SCHERER, E. *et al:* New radiological-surgical concepts in primary treatment of malignant melanomas. Fortschr. Geb. Roentgenstr. Nuklearmed., *118:*174, 1973 (German)

SCHERR, D. D. *et al:* Tissue-viability assessment with the Doppler ultrasonic flowmeter in acute injuries of extremities. J. Bone & Joint Surg. (Am)., *55:*157, 1973

SCHERZ, W., AND DOHLMAN, C.: Is the lacrimal gland dispensable: keratoconjunctivitis sicca after lacrimal gland removal, PRS, *56:*460, 1975. Arch. Ophth., *93:* 281, 1975

SCHETRUMPF, J.: Cortico-medullary peg for interphalangeal joint fusion, PRS, *56:*596, 1975. Hand, 7:81, 1975

SCHETRUMPF, J. R.: Method of prominent ear correction. Brit. J. Plast. Surg., *28:*292, 1975

SCHETTLER, D.: Results of cylindroma therapy. Fortschr. Kiefer. Gesichtschir., *15:*84, 1972 (German)

SCHETTLER, D.: Intra- and postoperative complications in surgical repair of clefts in infancy. J. Maxillo-facial Surg., *1:*40, 1973

SCHETTLER, D. *et al:* Cylindroma of jaw and face, current aspects of therapy based on long-term observations. Chirurg., *44:*370, 1973 (German)

SCHETTLER, D. *et al:* Growing jaw during and after orthopedic-surgical extension in children with congenital microgenia. Fortschr. Kiefer. Gesichtschir., *18:*166, 1974 (German)

SCHETTLER, D., AND REHRMANN, A.: Long-term results of functional treatment of condylar fractures with long bridle according to A. Rehrmann, PRS, *56:*463, 1975. J. Maxillo-facial Surg., *3:*14, 1975

SCHEUNEMANN, H.: Pull-through surgery in mouth floor-tongue neoplasms. Acta Stomatol. Belg., *72:*229, 1975

SCHEUNEMANN, H.: Conservative parotidectomy in infancy and childhood, PRS, *56:*462, 1975. J. Maxillo-facial Surg., *3:*37, 1975

SCHEUNEMANN, H.: Surgical procedures in cleft-palate patients, with reference to phonetic function: primary and secondary methods. Langenbecks Arch. Chir., *339:*355, 1975 (German)

SCHEUNEMANN, H. *et al*: Surgical mobilization of a clamped jaw following radiotherapy. Fortschr. Kiefer. Gesichtschir., *18:*244, 1974 (German)

SCHIELE, H. P. *et al*: Radiographic changes in burns of the upper extremity. Radiology, *104:*13, 1972

SCHIERHORN, H.: Technics and hazards of intragluteal injections. Dtsch. Gesundheitsw., *26:*2360, 1971 (German)

SCHILLI, W. *et al*: Functionally stable osteosynthesis in mandible. Int. J. Oral Surg., *3:*349, 1974

SCHILLI, W. *et al*: Time plan for the treatment of cheilognatho-uranoschisis. Z. Allgemelomed., *51:*1312, 1975 (German)

SCHILLING, F.: Psychological examinations of the diagnostic valency of manual dexterity in childhood. Monatsschr. Kinderheilkd., *122:*763, 1974 (German)

SCHINDEL, J. *et al*: Cherubism, PRS, *54:*689, 1974. Internat., Surg., *59:*225, 1974

SCHINDLER, R. *et al*: Carcinoma of lacrimal sac. Can. J. Ophthalmol., *8:*161, 1973

SCHINK, W.: Treatment of malignant tumors in the region of the hand. Handchirurgie, *1:*154, 1969 (German)

SCHINK, W.: Pyogenic infections of the hand. Chirurg., *42:*356, 1971 (German)

SCHINK, W.: Tendon injuries of the hand, PRS, *51:*603, 1973. Langenbecks Arch. Chir., *332:*495, 1972

SCHINK, W.: Management of facial injuries in general hospital. Initial treatment by general surgeon. Langenbecks Arch. Chir., *334:*407, 1973 (German)

SCHLEGEL, D.: Management of tumors of oral cavity. Zahnaerztl. Prax., *22:*76, 1971 (German)

SCHLEGEL, D.: Technic and results of intraoral prognathism operations. Fortschr. Kiefer. Gesichtschir., *18:*135, 1974 (German)

SCHLENKER, J. D. *et al*: Calcinosis circumscripta of the hand in scleroderma. J. Bone & Joint Surg. (Am.), *55:*1051, 1973

SCHLIESSER, H.: Hearing acuity before and after pharyngeal flap procedure (with LeWorthy), PRS, *56:*49, 1975

SCHLIETER, F.: Conservative therapy of malignant melanoma of conjunctiva originating from melanotic preblastomatosis Dubreuilh. Klin. Monatsbl. Augenheilkd., *16:*416, 1972 (German)

SCHLIETER, F.: Therapy of malignant melanoma of the conjunctiva. Ber. Dtsch. Ophthalmol. Ges., *73:*391, 1975 (German)

SCHLONDORFF, G.: Surgical correction of hypertelorism. Laryngol. Rhinol. Otol. (Stuttg.), *53:*98, 1974 (German)

SCHLONDORFF, G.: Correction of fronto-orbital defects. Laryngol. Rhinol. Otol. (Stuttg.), *53:*104, 1974 (German)

SCHLONDORFF, G. *et al*: Analysis and results of 34 orbit base fractures. Arch. Klin. Exp. Ohren Nasen Kehlkopfheilkd., *199:*647, 1971 (German)

SCHLOSS, M. D.: Laryngeal and tracheal complications following prolonged intubation and tracheostomy. Can. J. Otolaryngol., *1:*135, 1972

SCHLOSSHAUER, B.: Prevention and management of tracheal and laryngeal stenosis in children. H.N.O., *23:*342, 1975 (German)

SCHLOTE, H. H. *et al*: Technic and results of the treatment of orbital floor defect fractures with lyophilized dura. Fortschr. Kiefer. Gesichtschir., *19:*169, 1975 (German)

SCHLUMS, D.: Location relationship of N. facialis to parotid and N. auriculotemporalis. Dtsch. Zahnaerztl. Z., *27:*917, 1972 (German)

SCHMAUSS, A. K.: Gas gangrene following intramuscular injections. Z. Aerztl. Fortbild. (Jena), *68:*41, 1974 (German)

SCHMAUS, A. K. *et al*: "Spontaneous" and "posttraumatic" hand pressure edema, a model of typical but seldom timely recognized artifact. Z. Aerztl. Fortbild. (Jena), *65:*141, 1971 (German)

SCHMAUSS, A. K. *et al*: Classification, diagnosis and treatment of gas gangrene. Bruns Beitr. Klin. Chir., *221:*134, 1974 (German)

SCHMELZLE, R.: Various bone materials for the reconstruction of defects of the orbital floor. Fortschr. Kiefer. Gesichtschir., *19:*191, 1975 (German)

SCHMELZLE, R. *et al*: Intraoral Redon drainage in osteotomy of the ascending ramus of the mandible. Fortschr. Kiefer. Gesichtschir., *18:*148, 1974 (German)

SCHMELZLE, R., AND SCHMIDT, U.: Results of animal experiments on transplantability of Cialite-preserved human dura, PRS, *54:*626, 1972. J. Maxillo-facial Surg., *2:*49, 1974

SCHMELZLE, R. *et al*: Effect of trimethaphan-camphorsulfonate on blood pressure during neuroleptoanalgesia in surgery of jaw and face. Med. Welt., *25:*521, 1974 (German)

SCHMID, E.: Secondary plastic surgery of lid injuries. Klin. Monatsbl. Augenheilkd., *160:*581, 1972 (German)

SCHMID, E.: Surgical correction of the skeleton in the area of the orbit and maxilla. Fortschr. Kiefer. Gesichtschir., *18:*28, 1974 (German)

SCHMID, E.: Reconstitution of lip, tongue and glottis function. Acta Stomatol. Belg., *72:*301, 1975 (German)

SCHMID, E. *et al*: Development of cleft upper jaw following primary osteoplasty and orthodontic treatment, PRS, *55:*381, 1975. J. Maxillo-facial Surg., *2:*92, 1974

SCHMID, E. *et al*: On mucoepidermoid tumors with rare locations in laryngological areas. Laryngol. Rhinol. Otol. (Stuttg.), *54:*290, 1975 (German)

SCHMID, F.: Neuroanatomy, pathogenesis and therapy of temporomandibular pain. Dtsch. Zahnaerztl. Z., *28:*976, 1973 (German)

SCHMID, F.: Surgical and social pediatric viewpoints in treatment of cleft lip and palate, PRS, *55:*111, 1975. Ztschr. Kinderchir., *15:*9, 1974

SCHMIDSEDER, R.: Restoring sensation to cut inferior alveolar nerve by direct anastomosis or by free autologous nerve grafting (with Hausamen, Samii), PRS, *53:*83, 1974

SCHMIDSEDER, R. *et al*: Familial congenital occurrence of multiple odontomas. Dtsch. Zahnaerztl. Z., *28:*628, 1973 (German)

SCHMIDSEDER, R. *et al*: Multiple odontogenic tumors and other anomalies. An autosomal dominantly inherited syndrome. Oral Surg., *39:*249, 1975

SCHMIDT, A.: Tumors in the region of the hand. Zentralbl. Chir., *96:*1113, 1971 (German)

SCHMIDT, A. *et al*: Therapy of recent burns of the hands. Zentralbl. Chir., *97:*609, 1972 (German)

SCHMIDT, B., AND RASTAN, H.: Cardiac alterations in case of Klippel-Trenaunay syndrome, PRS, *51:*478, 1973. Ztschr. Kinderchir., *11:*468, 1972

SCHMIDT, G. B. *et al*: Death precipitated by tracheostomy in a child. J.A.M.A., *231:*277, 1975

SCHMIDT, H.: The flat vestibulum. Problems, indications for surgery, modification of vestibuloplasty and evaluation of success. Stomatol. DDR, *25:*612, 1975 (German)

SCHMIDT, H. W. *et al*: Three cases of primary multiple malignant melanoma of skin. Arch. Dermatol. Forsch., *248:*391, 1974 (German)

SCHMIDT, J.: Potential complications of nasal and sinus therapy. J. Med. Trial Tech. Q., *20:*75, 1973

SCHMIDT, J. G. *et al*: Orbito-craniobasal impaling injuries. Klin. Monatsbl. Augenheilkd., *159:*624, 1971 (German)

SCHMIDT, P. H. *et al*: Intranasal meningoencephalocele. Arch. Otolaryng., *99:*402, 1974

SCHMIDT-MARTENS, F. *et al*: Surgical repair of disrupted lacrimal duct by means of tapered pigtail probe and soft polyethylene tube. Klin. Monatsbl. Augenheilkd., *162:*531, 1973 (German)

SCHMIDT-TINTEMANN, U.: Treatment and prevention of scars following burns. Munch. Med. Wochenschr., *115:*718, 1973 (German)

SCHMIDT-TINTEMANN, U.: Error in facial stretching. In *Plastische und Wiederherstellungs-Chirurgie,* ed. by Hohler; pp. 69-73, Schattauer, Stuttgart, 1975 (German)

SCHMITT, W. *et al*: Surgery of bladder exstrophy with ureterosigmoidostomy and cystectomy. Z. Urol. Nephrol., *64:*509, 1971 (German)

SCHMITZ, R. *et al*: Chemically induced abnormalities of the masticatory skull in experimental animals. I. Effect of cyclophosphamide and 6-mercaptopurine on embryonic and fetal development of the rat. Dtsch. Zahn. Mund. Kieferheilkd., *59:*385, 1972 (German)

SCHMITZ, R. *et al*: Indication, technic and clinical results of compression osteosynthesis in mandibular fractures (5-year experience). Fortschr. Kiefer. Gesichtschir., *19:*74, 1975 (German)

SCHMOKER, R. *et al*: Excentric-dynamic compression plate. Experimental study as contribution to a functionally stable osteosynthesis in mandibular fractures. Schweiz. Monatsschr. Zahnheilkd., *83:*1496, 1973 (German)

SCHMOKER, R. *et al*: Results of surgical management of zygomatic fractures with special reference to fracture classification. Fortschr. Kiefer. Gesichtschir., *19:*154, 1975 (German)

SCHMOKER, R. *et al*: Functionally stable osteosynthesis of the mandible by means of an excentric dynamic compression plate. Results of a follow-up of 25 cases. Schweiz. Monatsschr. Zahnheilkd., *86:*167, 1976 (German)

SCHNEEWIND, J. H.: Surgical emergencies of the hand. Surg. Clin. North Am., *52:*203, 1972

SCHNEIDER, H. R. *et al*: Effect of hemimandibulectomy on the remaining temporo-mandibular joint. Pract. Otorhinolaryngol. (Basel), *33:*1, 1971 (German)

SCHNEIDER, H. R., WEY, W., AND ROSLI, A.: Effect of hemimandibulectomy on remaining temporomandibular joint. Schweiz. Monatsschr. Zahnheilkd., *83:*82, 1973 (German)

SCHNEIDER, J. J. *et al*: Control by irradiation alone of nonfixed clinically positive lymph nodes from squamous cell carcinoma of the oral cavity, oropharynx, supraglottic larynx, and hypopharynx. Am. J. Roentgenol. Radium Ther. Nucl. Med., *123:*42, 1975

SCHNEIDER, K.: Facial injuries. Praxis, *60:*1228, 1971 (German)

SCHNEIDER, K.: Abdominal-thoracic round pedicle graft. Helv. Chir. Acta, *39:*335, 1972 (German)

SCHNEIDER, K., AND CLODIUS, L.: Conchal hypertrophy and correction of protruding ears,

experiences with bone plate osteosynthesis in fractures of the edentulous mandible-V. Z. W. R., *83:*1042, 1974 (German)

SCHROLL, K.: Indications for transcutaneous and surgical treatment of zygomatic fractures. Fortschr. Kiefer. Gesichtschir., *19:*159, 1975 (German)

SCHRUDDE, J.: Influence of primary osteoplasty on the treatment of patients with clefts of the lip, palate and jaw. Brit. J. Plast. Surg., *24:*189, 1971

SCHRUDDE, J.: On problem of reconstruction after burns. Panminerva Med., *14:*241, 1972

SCHRUDDE, J.: Surgical treatment of bedsores in paraplegics (with Olivari, Wahle), PRS, *50:*477, 1972

SCHRUDDE, J.: Injuries to face caused by shatterproof glass. Langenbecks Arch. Chir., *334:*421, 1973 (German)

SCHUBERT, J. *et al*: Treatment of hypospadias. Z. Urol. Nephrol., *68:*579, 1975 (German)

SCHUCHARDT, K. *et al*: 184 cases of mixed tumors of salivary glands at Northwest German Dental Clinic from 1946–1967. Fortschr. Kiefer. Gesichtschir., *15:*28, 1972 (German)

SCHUCKIT, M. A., MILLER, P. L., AND HAHLBOHM, D.: Unrecognized psychiatric illness in elderly medical-surgical patients, PRS, *57:*683, 1976. J. Gerontol., *30:*655, 1975

SCHUHR, E. U.: Surgical procedure in unusual injury of lower leg. Zentralbl. Chir., *98:*1708, 1973 (German)

SCHULE, H.: Studies on evaluation of conservative and surgical measurements in temporomandibular joint disfunction. Dtsch. Zahnaerztl. Z., *27:*826, 1972 (German)

SCHULE, H.: Clinical and therapeutic aspects of salivary gland tumors of palate. Fortschr. Kiefer. Gesichtchir., *15:*65, 1972 (German)

SCHULE, H.: Progress in cosmetic surgery of bony facial profile. Zahnaerztl. Prax., *24:*371, 1973 (German)

SCHULE, H.: Esthetic aspects in the planning of chin operations. Fortschr. Kiefer. Gesichtchir., *18:*114, 1974 (German)

SCHULE, H. *et al*: Studies for the treatment planning in orbital fractures. Fortschr. Kiefer. Gesichtchir., *19:*188, 1975 (German)

SCHULER, F. A., III, GRAHAM, J. K., AND HORTON, C. E.: Benign symmetrical lipomatosis (Madelung's disease), PRS, *57:*663, 1976

SCHULITZ, K. P.: Synovectomy and articular cartilage, PRS, *54:*247, 1974. Ztschr. Orthop., *112:*118, 1974

SCHULITZ, K. P. *et al*: Skeletal growth disorders following radiotherapy and their treatment. Ztschr. Orthop., *111:*249, 1973 (German)

SCHULMAN, M. L.: Reanastomosis of amputated penis, PRS, *52:*596, 1973. J. Urol., *109:*432, 1973

SCHULSTAD, I.: Madelung's deformity with extensor tendon rupture, PRS, *49:*583, 1972. Scand. J. Plast. Reconstr. Surg., *5:*153, 1971

SCHULTZ, L., BULL, B. S., AND BRAUNWALD, N. S.: Use of tissue culture techniques to evaluate new material developed to serve as artificial heart linings, PRS, *48:*299, 1971. Surgery, *69:*510, 1971

SCHULTZ, R. C.: Changing character and management of soft tissue windshield injuries, PRS, *52:*106, 1973. J. Trauma, *12:*24, 1972

SCHULTZ, R. C.: Management of common facial fractures. Surg. Clin. North Am., *53:*3, 1973

SCHULTZ, R. C.: "Dry eye" following blepharoplasty (with Swartz, Seaton), PRS, *54:*644, 1974

SCHULTZ, R. C.: Maxillofacial injuries from vehicular accidents. Foreword. Clin. Plast. Surg., *2:*1, 1975

SCHULTZ, R. C.: Frontal sinus and supraorbital fractures from vehicle accidents. Clin. Plast. Surg., *2:*93, 1975

SCHULTZ, R. C., AND McMASTER, W. C.: Treatment of dog bite injuries, especially those of the face, PRS, *49:*494, 1972

SCHULTZ, R. C. *et al*: Midfacial fractures from vehicular accidents. Clin. Plast. Surg., *2:*173, 1975

SCHULTZ, R. J.: Traumatic entrapment of *extensor digiti minimi proprius* in progressive restriction of motion of metacarpophalangeal joint of little finger, PRS, *54:*621, 1974. J. Bone & Joint Surg., *56A:*428, 1974

SCHULTZ, R. J. *et al*: Anomalous median nerve and an anomalous muscle belly of the first lumbrical associated with carpal-tunnel syndrome. J. Bone & Joint Surg. (Am.), *55:*1744, 1973

SCHULZ, P. *et al*: Results in therapy of odontogenic jaw tumors. Z. W. R., *83:*432, 1974 (German)

SCHULZ, R. *et al*: Pharyngeal flap surgery and voice quality—factors related to success and failure. Cleft Palate J., *10:*166, 1973

SCHULZE, F. Differential diagnosis of the blowout fractures of the orbit. Dtsch. Gesundheitsw., *26:*1737, 1971 (German)

SCHULZE-BERGMANN, G.: Limits of conservative and surgical treatment of varicose symptom complex. Z. Hautkr., *50:*147, 1975 (German)

SCHUMACHER, G. H. *et al*: Vestibuloplasty, an intervention in muscular system of stomoschisis. Dtsch. Stomatol., *22:*734, 1972 (German)

SCHUMACHER, G. H. *et al*: Vestibuloplasty and intervention into the musculatory system of mouth. Dtsch. Stomatol., *22:*889, 1972 (German)

SCHUMACHER, H. R., JR.: Joint involvement in

progressive systemic sclerosis (scleroderma): light and electron microscopic study of synovial membrane and fluid, PRS, *53:*693, 1974. Am. J. Clin. Path., *60:*593, 1973

SCHURMANN, K.: Neurosurgeon in orbital cavity. Arch. Otorhinolaryngol. (NY), *207:*253, 1974 (German)

SCHURTER, M.: Inframammary-based dermofat flaps in mammary reconstruction following subcutaneous mastectomy (with Letterman), PRS, *55:*156, 1975

SCHURTER, M. *et al*: Breast deformities and their surgical repair. J. Invest. Dermatol., *63:*138, 1974

SCHURTER, M., AND LETTERMAN, G.: Suggested anatomical nomenclature for nose, PRS, *57:*490, 1976

SCHURTER, M. A.: Surgical correction of massive gynecomastia (with Letterman), PRS, *49:*259, 1972

SCHURTER, M. A.: Surgical correction of exophthalmos; history, technique, and long-term follow-up (with Moran, Letterman), PRS, *49:*595, 1972

SCHURTER, M. A.: Will Durston's "mammaplasty" (with Letterman), PRS, *53:*48, 1974

SCHWAGER, R. G. *et al*: Inversion of human female nipple, with simple method of treatment, PRS, *54:*564, 1974

SCHWAGER, R. G., SMITH, J. W., AND GOULIAN, D., JR.: Small, deep forearm lacerations; differential diagnosis of muscle and nerve injuries, PRS, *55:*190, 1975

SCHWAGER, R. G., AND IMBER, G.: Inflatable splint to immobilize extremities after skin grafting, PRS, *57:*523, 1976

SCHWAIGER, M: Modern trends in surgical treatment of cancer of breast, PRS, *53:*365, 1974. Langenbecks Arch. Chir., *332:*619, 1972

SCHWARTZ, A. E. *et al*: Labial flap for reconstruction of the anterior oral cavity. Surg. Gynec. & Obst., *135:*276, 1972

SCHWARTZ, A. E., SCHWARTZ, J. S., AND FRIEDMAN, E. W.: Cytotoxic effect of viruses on Harding-Passey melanoma in tissue culture, PRS, *53:*496, 1974. J. Surg. Res., *14:*16, 1973

SCHWARTZ, A. E., AND FRIEDMAN, E. W.: Salivary gland disorders. I. Recognition, diagnosis, treatment. New York J. Med., *73:*297, 1973

SCHWARTZ, A. E., AND FRIEDMAN, E. W.: Salivary gland disorders. II. Salivary tumors. N. Y. State J. Med., *73:*439, 1973

SCHWARTZ, A. W.: Median rhomboid glossitis, PRS, *52:*91, 1973

SCHWARTZ, A. W.: Technique for excision of abdominal fat. Brit. J. Plast. Surg., *27:*44, 1974

SCHWARTZ, D. L. *et al*: Diaphragmatic hernia,

three legs, two penises, and imperforate anus: complete salvage problem in newborn. J. Pediatr. Surg., *9:*525, 1974

SCHWARTZ, HARRY: *The Case for American Medicine: A Realistic Look at our Health Care System.* David McKay Co., New York, 1972. PRS, *53:*85, 1974

SCHWARTZ, H.: American medicine after Watergate, PRS, *54:*248, 1974. Bull. Am. Coll. Surgeons, *59:*7, 1974

SCHWARTZ, M. F.: Developing a direct, objective measure of velopharyngeal inadequacy. Clin. Plast. Surg., *2:*305, 1975

SCHWARTZ, M. L. *et al*: Local anti-coagulation of prosthetic heart valves, PRS, *53:*501, 1974. Circulation, suppl. #3, *47, 48:*85, 1973

SCHWARTZ, SEYMOUR I. *et al: Principles of Surgery*, 2nd Ed. McGraw-Hill, N. Y., 1974. PRS, *56:*207, 1975

SCHWARTZMAN, J. *et al*: Leiomyoangioma of paranasal sinuses: case report. Laryngoscope, *83:*1856, 1973

SCHWARZ, G.: Neurovascular free flaps (with Daniel, Terzis), PRS, *56:*13, 1975

SCHWARZ, G.: Dorsal dislocation of index MP joint (with Cunningham), PRS, *56:*654, 1975

SCHWARZWALD, M.: Skin carcinoma and its treatment. Lijec. Vjesn., *96:*589, 1974 (Croatian)

SCHWEISHEIMER, W.: Progress in American medicine. Current successes, current problems. Med. Klin., *69:*711, 1974 (German)

SCHWEITZER, H. C.: Occlusion effect in bilateral mandibulectomy patient. J. Speech, Hear. Disord., *39:*360, 1974

SCHWEITZER, R. J.: Protection of femoral vessels after groin dissection, PRS, *49:*109, 1972, Am. J. Surg., *122:*23, 1971

SCHWENZER, N.: Surgical improvement of alveolar ridge in cases of atrophy of alveolar process. Acta Odontol. Venez., *9:*213, 1971 (Spanish)

SCHWENZER, N.: Complications in the surgical fixation of the mid-facial region. Dtsch. Stomatol., *21:*592, 1971 (German)

SCHWENZER, N.: Free skin transplantation in oral cavity. Z. W. R., *80:*523, 1971 (German)

SCHWENZER, N.: Surgical possibilites and limits of surgery of the deep bite. Dtsch. Zahnaerztl. Z., *27:*549, 1972 (German)

SCHWENZER, N.: Change in management of facial skull injuries after second world war. Dtsch. Zahn. Mund. Kieferheilkd., *60:*361, 1973 (German)

SCHWENZER, N.: Correction of noses associated with clefts of lip and palate, PRS, *53:*240, 1974. J. Maxillo-facial Surg., *1:*91, 1973

SCHWENZER, N.: Possible applications of stepwise osteotomy of the ascending ramus.

Fortschr. Kiefer. Gesichtschir., *18:*138, 1974 (German)

SCHWENZER, N.: Rare clefts of face, PRS, *55:*720, 1975. J. Maxillo-facial Surg., *2:*224, 1974

SCHWENZER, N.: Carcinoma of the mouth floor. Possibilities and limitations of surgical treatment. Acta Stomatol. Belg., *72:*277, 1975 (French)

SCHWENZER, N.: Problem of metal damage and stability in wire osteosynthesis in the midfacial region. Fortschr. Kiefer. Gesichtschir., *19:*145, 1975 (German)

SCHWENZER, N.: Findings in the maxillary sinus following mid-facial fractures. Fortschr. Kiefer. Gesichtschir., *19:*167, 1975 (German)

SCHWENZER, N. *et al*: Study of fractures in general. 6. Reproduction of form and function. Zahnaerztl. Prax., *24:*518, 1973 (German)

SCHWENZER, N. *et al*: Study of fractures in general. 9. Surgical therapy. Zahnaerztl. Prax., *24:*628, 1973 (German)

SCHWENZER, N. *et al*: Special study of fractures. 3. Surgical treatment of mandibular fractures. Zahnaerztl. Prax., *25:*139, 1974

SCHWERDTNER, U.: Case report on lipomatosis dolorosa (dercum). Z. Gesamte Inn. Med., *29:*726, 1974 (German)

SCHWOPE, A. D. *et al*: Development of a synthetic burn covering. Trans. Am. Soc. Artif. Inter. Organs, *20A:*103, 1974

SCHWORER, J. *et al*: Mediastinal emphysema following fracture in the region of the paranasal sinuses. Fortschr. Geb. Roentgenstr. Nuklearmed., *115:*684, 1971 (German)

Scleroderma

Coup de sabre, a linear form of scleroderma, repair of (Zamick, Weiss), PRS, *50:*520, 1972

Dimethyl sulfoxide in the treatment of scleroderma (Engel), PRS, *52:*332, 1973. South M. J., *65:*71, 1972

Scleroderma, joint involvement in, light and electron microscopic study of synovial membrane and fluid (Schumacher), PRS, *53:*693, 1974. Am. J. Clin. Path., *60:*593, 1973

Syndrome, Werner's. Familial ulcerous scleroderma with cataracts and diabetes (Vandaele). Arch. Belg. Dermatol., *29:*251, 1973 (French)

Skull, and scalp defect in patient with systemic form of scleroderma, coverage of (Losken, Davies, Gordon), PRS, *51:*212, 1973

SCOFIELD, H. H., WERNING, J. T., AND SHUKES, R. C.: Solitary intraoral keratoacanthoma, PRS, *55:*106, 1975. Oral Surg., *37:*889, 1974

SCOPPA, J. *et al*: Non-chromaffin paraganglioma of the nasopharynx. J. Laryng. & Otol., *89:*653, 1975

SCOTT, A. A.: Pressure monitoring device for low pressure cuffs on tracheostomy tubes. Can. Anesth. Soc. J., *21:*120, 1974

SCOTT, D. L.: Hypnoanalgesia for major surgery. A psychodynamic process. Am. J. Clin. Hypn., *16:*84, 1973

SCOTT, D. L.: Hypnosis in plastic surgery. Am. J. Clin. Hypn., *18:*98, 1975

SCOTT, F. B. *et al*: Management of erectile impotence. Use of implantable inflatable prosthesis. Urology, *2:*80, 1973

SCOTT, H. D., AND MACKIE, A.: Decisions to hospitalize and operate, a socioeconomic perspective in urban state, PRS, *57:*768, 1976. Surgery, *77:*311, 1975

SCOVILLE, W. B.: Proceedings: Surgery for motor tics of the face and neck. J. Neurol. Neurosurg. Psychiatry, *38:*408, 1975

Scrotum (See also *Hypospadias; Transsexual Surgery*)

Management of peno-scrotal skin avulsions (Buzelin *et al*). Ann. Urol. (Paris), *5:*263, 1971

Perineal masses in male subjects (Gray, Gillenwater, Mulholland), PRS, *50:*200, 1972. J. Urol., *106:*236, 1971

Carcinoma of scrotum, radical excision and repair using ox fascia: case report (El-Domeiri, Paglia), PRS, *50:*94, 1972. J. Urol., *106:*575, 1971

Doughnut scrotum (Datta, Rheinschild), PRS, *48:*608, 1971. J. Urol., *105:*692, 1971

Scrotum and penis, transposition in twin brothers (Datta *et al*), PRS, *48:*607, 1971. J. Urol., *105:*739, 1971

Scrotal wall hemangioma in an infant (Mininberg, Harley), PRS, *50:*94, 1972. J. Urol., *106:*789, 1971

Scrotum, enormous elephantiasis of (Holubec), PRS, *52:*681, 1973. Acta chir. plast., *14:*191, 1972

Scrotum and penis, traumatic scalpation, late sequelae (Kipikasa *et al*), PRS, *52:*680, 1973. Acta chir. plast., *14:*255, 1972

Fertility disorders, male, surgical correction (Kaufmann). Dtsch. Med. Wochenschr., *97:*1510, 1972 (German)

Paget's disease of scrotum: case report with local lymph node invasion (Vermillion, Page), PRS, *50:*539, 1972. J. Urol., *107:*281, 1972

Scrotum — Cont.

Fournier's gangrene (Burpee, Edwards), PRS, *50:*633, 1972. J. Urol., *107:*812, 1972

Scrotum, lymphedema as complication of testicular prosthesis (Elsahy), PRS, *52:*207, 1973. J. Urol., *108:*595, 1972

Scrotal testicular ectopia, bilateral (Mininberg, Richman), PRS, *52:*324, 1973. J. Urol., *108:*652, 1972

Fournier's disease. Apropos of 3 cases (Doremieux, Rezieiner, Kohler). J. Urol. Nephrol. (Paris), *78:*696, 1972 (French)

Fournier's disease, presentation of case of, with favorable course, with cutaneous plasty (Guillemin, Parietti). J. Urol. Nephrol. (Paris), *78:*703, 1972 (French)

Skin avulsion of penis and scrotum (Huffstadt). Ned. tijdschr. geneeskd., *116:*57, 1972 (Dutch)

Dermatome grafting of totally denuded testes (Campbell) (Follow-Up Clinic), PRS, *50:*280, 1972

Traumatic scalping of penile and scrotal skin (Brygman). Pol. Przegl. Chir., *44:* (Suppl):1157, 1972 (Polish)

Testicular torsion in utero (Schneider *et al*). Am. J. Obstet. Gynecol., *117:*1126, 1973

Fat necrosis of scrotum (Ong, Solomon), PRS, *54:*377, 1974. J. Pediat. Surg., *8:*919, 1973

Scrotum, two-stage reconstruction of, for tropical elephantiasis (Hasham). J. Urol., *109:*659, 1973

Penile gangrene successfully treated by debridement and scrotal skin bridge, case report (Myers, Kelalis), PRS, *52:*596, 1973. J. Urol., *109:*733, 1973

Perineal resection, radical, for far-advanced lymphogranuloma venereum (Hirschberg, Horton), PRS, *51:*217, 1973

Surgical construction of the male external genitalia (Engel). Clin. Plast. Surg., *1:*229, 1974

Hemangioma of the scrotum: a case report review and comparison with varicocele (Cooper *et al*). J. Urol., *112:*623, 1974

Traumatic amputation of the penis (Englman *et al*). J. Urol., *112:*774, 1974

Accessory scrotum: a case report (Takayasu *et al*). J. Urol., *112:*826, 1974

Scrotal dressing, useful (Straffon). M. J. Australia, *1:*320, 1974

Flap, scrotal, for necrosis of penis with decubitus ulcer: debridement and closure with (Lanier, Neale), PRS, *54:*609, 1974

"Thumb" urethroplasty. A modification and comparative study (Kishev). Urology, *4:*320, 1974

Hidradenitis suppurativa of scrotum and per-

Scrotum — Cont.

ineum (Ward *et al*). Urology, *4:*463, 1974

Syndrome, Fournier's: synergistic gangrene of scrotum (Rudolph *et al*). Am J. Surg., *129:*591, 1975

Reconstruction of the penoscrotal skin after avulsion (Sangmit). Int. Surg., *60:*563, 1975

Scrotal and penile lymphedema, surgical management of (Vaught, Litvok, McRoberts), PRS, *57:*761, 1976. J. Urol., *113:*204, 1975

Operative management of chronic hidradenitis suppurativa of the scrotum and perineum (Vickers). J. Urol., *114:*414, 1975

Four cases of peno-scrotal avulsions (Michaud *et al*). J. Urol. Nephrol. (Paris), *81:*558, 1975 (French)

Scrotum and penis, congenital transposition of (Griffin, Hayes), PRS, *55:*710, 1975

Reconstruction of the male external genitalia (Boxer). Surg. Gynec. & Obst., *141:*939, 1975

Scrotum, trauma of (Culp), PRS, *56:*106, 1975. Tribuna Med., *28:*15, 1975

Two-stage urethroplasty. Improved method for treating bulbomembranous strictures (Fernandes *et al*). Urology, *6:*568, 1975

Treatment of hypospadias (Schubert *et al*). Z. Urol. Nephrol., *68:*579, 1975 (German)

Webbed penis without chordee (Puri). J. Pediatr. Surg., *11:*125, 1976

Syphilis, elephantiasis of penis and scrotum (Elsahy), PRS, *57:*601, 1976

Scrub, Surgical

Skin preparation, surgical, evaluation of bacitracin-neomycin (Saik, Walz, Rhoads), PRS, *51:*611, 1973. Am. J. Surg., *11:*557, 1971

pHisoHex and Betadine surgical scrub solutions, an assessment of effectiveness in management of contaminated wound, Study V (Custer *et al*), PRS, *49:*587, 1972. Am. J. Surg., *121:*572, 1971

Scrubbing, gentle, therapeutic value in prolonging limited period of effectiveness of antibiotics in contaminated wounds. Study V (Edlich *et al*), PRS, *49:*668, 1972. Am. J. Surg., *121:*668, 1971

Skin disinfection and skin bacteria (Selwyn, Ellis), PRS, *51:*109, 1973. Brit. M. J., *1:*136, 1972

pHisoHex and Betadine, evaluation as antiseptic agents in surgical preparation of hands (Gross *et al*), PRS, *53:*114, 1974. Am. J. Surg., *126:*49, 1973

Scrubbing, preoperative hand, evaluation of (McBride, Duncan, Knox), PRS, *53:*615,

Scrub, Surgical — Cont.

1974. Surg. Gynec. & Obst., *137:*934, 1973

Skin disinfection with ethanol, without and with additives (Kuiper), PRS, *54:*511, 1974. Arch. chir. neerl., *24:*15, 1974

Hexachlorophene in mice (Stenback), PRS, *56:*115, 1975. Arch. Environmental Health, *30:*32, 1975

Skin necrosis due to cetrimide application (August), PRS, *57:*127, 1976. Brit. M. J., *1:*70, 1975

SCRUGGS, H. J. *et al*: Use of thermography to evaluate the optimum time for surgery after preoperative radiation. Laryngoscope, *85:*726, 1975

SCUDERI, G. *et al*: Conjunctival melanoma in anophthalmic orbit. Ophthalmologica, *166:*172, 1973

SEABAUGH, D. R. *et al*: Disseminated intravascular coagulation and urologist, PRS, *50:*540, 1972. J. Urol., *106:*267, 1971

SEALY, R. *et al*: Treatment of head and neck cancer with intra-arterial cytotoxic drugs and radiotherapy. Cancer, *30:*187, 1972

SEAR, A. J.: Intra-oral condylectomy applied to unilateral condylar hyperplasia. Brit. J. Oral Surg., *10:*143, 1972

SEASHORE, J. H., MacNAUGHTON, R. J., AND TALBERT, J. L.: Treatment of gastroschisis and omphalocele with biological dressings, PRS, *56:*226, 1975. J. Pediat. Surg., *10:*9, 1975

SEATON, J. R., JR.: "Dry eye" following blepharoplasty (with Swartz, Schultz). PRS, *54:*644, 1974

SEATON, J. R., JR.: Soft tissue facial injuries related to vehicular accidents. Clin. Plast. Surg., *2:*79, 1975

Sebaceous Cysts

Ablation of sebaceous cysts of the face (Picaud). Presse Med., *79:*2237, 1971 (French)

Minimal incision for removing sebaceous cysts (Vivakananthan). Brit. J. Plast. Surg., *25:*60, 1972

Sebaceous cysts, trephining (O'Keeffe). Brit. J. Plast. Surg., *25:*411, 1972

Carbon dioxide laser in head and neck surgery (Kaplan *et al*). Am. J. Surg., *128:*543, 1974

Taping of a cyst: a method to facilitate removal of a scalp cyst (Witkowski *et al*). Atherosclerosis, *20:*226, 1974

Steotocystoma multiplex (Rohde *et al*). Hautarzt, *25:*29, 1974

Carcinoma sebaceum (adenoma sebaceum malignum) (Wojnerowicz *et al*). Przegl. Dermatol., *61:*865, 1974 (Polish)

Staphylococcal septicemia following removal

Sebaceous Cysts — Cont.

of sebaceous cysts (Itarut *et al*). Rocky Mt. Med. J., *71:*576, 1974

Sebaceous cyst extraction through mini-incisions (Moore *et al*). Brit. J. Plast. Surg., *28:*307, 1975

Sebaceous Gland Neoplasms

Sebaceous gland adenoma, intraoral (Epker, Henny), PRS, *48:*609, 1971. Cancer, *27:*987, 1971

Sebaceous lymphangioma of parotid gland (Wasan), PRS, *49:*475, 1972. Cancer, *28:*1019, 1971

SEBASTIAN, G. *et al*: Analysis of therapy of recurrent basaliomas. Dermatol. Monatsschr., *159:*216, 1973 (German)

SEBEK, V.: Neoplasty of female urethra. Rozhl. Chir., *53:*47, 1974 (Czechoslovakian)

SEDA, H. J. *et al*: Surgery for carcinoma of posterior pharyngeal wall. Arch. Otolaryng., *99:*297, 1974

SEDDON, SIR HERBERT: *Surgical Disorders of the Peripheral Nerve*. Williams & Wilkins Co., Baltimore, 1972. PRS, *52:*82, 1973

SEDEE, G. *et al*: Submucosal resection of nasal septum: its current status. Acta Otorhinolaryngol. Belg., *27:*539, 1973 (French)

SEDGWICK, C. E.: Embryology and developmental abnormalities. Major Probl. Clin. Surg., *15:*5, 1974

SEDGWICK, C. E.: Surgical technique. Major Probl. Clin. Surg., *15:*170, 1974

SEDIN, N. S.: Surgical treatment of deformities of the forearm and hand in patients with infantile cerebral palsy. Ortop. Travmatol. Protez., *33:53:* 1972 (Russian)

SEEBACHER, J., NOZIK, D., AND MATHIEU, A.: Inadvertent intracranial introduction of a nasogastric tube, complication of severe maxillofacial trauma, PRS, *56:*238, 1975. Anesthesiology, *42:*100, 1975

SEEBERT, C. T.: Halothane anesthesia in burn patient: nine consecutive anesthetics in one having 30 percent second-and third-degree burns. South. Med. J., *66:*1057, 1973

SEEMAYER, T. A. *et al*: Epithelioid sarcoma. Can. J. Surg., *17:*37, 1974

SEERY, G. *et al*: Prevention of burns. S. Afr. Med. J., *46:*550, 1972

SEGAL, E. *et al*: Isolation of Candida tropicalis from orbital infection as complication of maxillary osteomyelitis. Infection, *2:*111, 1974

SEGARRA, J. A., AND BENNETT, J. E.: Distal necrosis of dorsal pedicle flaps in rat: immediate versus delayed terminal inset, PRS, *51:*710, 1973. Surg. Forum, *23:*521, 1972

SEGMULLER, G.: Diagnosis of hand tumors.

Helv. Chir. Acta, *40:*241, 1973 (German)

SEGMULLER, G. *et al*: Problems of fracture fixation in growing hand bones. Handchirurgie, *3:*109, 1971 (German)

SEGMULLER, GOTTFRIED: *Operative Stabilization of the Hand Skeleton.* Verlag Hans Huber, Bern, Stuttgart, Wien, 1973. PRS, *55:*357, 1975

SEGURA, J. W. *et al*: Long-term results of ureterosigmoidostomy in children with bladder exstrophy. J. Urol., *114:*138, 1975

SEHDEV, M. K. *et al*: Ameloblastoma of maxilla and mandible, PRS, *56:*225, 1975. Cancer, *33:*324, 1974

SEHGAL, V. N.: Vitamin E, melanotoxic agent, PRS, *53:*502, 1974. Dermatologica, *145:*56, 1972

SEIFERT, G.: Epithelial tumors of salivary glands. Fortschr Kiefer. Gesichtschir., *15:*2, 1972 (German)

SEIFERT, G.: Surgery for prognathism. Zahnaerztl. Prax., *24:*290, 1973 (German)

SEIFETDINOV, E. A.: Clinical picture and diagnosis of traumatic epidermal cysts of the hand. Vestn. Khir., *108:*111, 1972 (Russian)

SEIFFERT, K. E.: Tendon transplantation and tendon replacement. Langenbecks Arch. Chir., *327:*1106, 1970 (German)

SEIGLER, H. F. *et al*: Non-specific and specific immunotherapy in patients with melanoma. Surgery, 72:162, 1972

SEIGLER, H. F., SHINGLETON, W. W., AND PICKRELL, K. L.: Intralesional BCG, intravenous immune lymphocytes, and immunization with neuraminidase-treated tumor cells to manage melanoma. PRS, *55:*294, 1975

SEIJI, M., AND OHSUMI, T.: Statistical study on melanoma in Japan (1961–1970), PRS, *53:*111, 1974. Asian M. J., *16:*101, 1973

SEITCHICK, M. W.: Anterior ethmoid nerve block for treatment of nasal fractures. PRS, *48:*187, 1971

SEKIGUCHI, J.: Free musculocutaneous flap (with Harii, Ohmori), PRS, *57:*294, 1976. Discussion by Cannon, PRS, *57:*511, 1976

SEKIGUCHI, T. *et al*: Management of facial burns. Shujutsu, *25:*1127, 1971 (Japanese)

SEKIYAMA, S. *et al*: Postoperative management of radical neck dissection with continuous suction drainage. Jap. J. Oral Surg., *19:*276, 1973 (Japanese)

SEKULA, J. *et al*: Case of neurofibroma of middle pharynx. Otolaryngol. Pol., *27:*527, 1973 (Polish)

SELDIN, E. B.: Percutaneous drilling technique for upper border wiring of fractures of angle of mandible. J. Oral Surg., *31:*720, 1973

SELIGMAN, M.: Use of Morris splint in mandibular fractures. Trans. Int. Conf. Oral Surg., *4:*333, 1973

SELIGMAN, R.: Psychiatric classification system for burned children. Am. J. Psychiatry, *131:*41, 1974

SELIGSOHN, U. *et al*: Massive bleeding due to primary fibrinolysis following rhinoplasty. Harefuah, *82:*219, 1972 (Hebrew)

SELIM, M. M. E., AND KANDIL, E.: Rifampicin in treatment of cutaneous leishmaniasis, PRS, *53:*502, 1974. J. Kuwait M. A., *6:*159, 1972

SELING, A.: Simplified corrective surgery of funnel chest (Letter). Dtsch. Med. Wochenschr., *99:*479, 1974 (German)

SELLARS, S. L.: Neurofibroma of facial nerve. S. Afr. Med. J., *46:*1332, 1972

SELLE, G.: Pathogenesis, clinical aspects and therapy of habitual jaw luxation. Dtsch. Zahnaerztl. Z., *27:*831, 1972 (German)

SELLE, G.: Preoperative photography as an aid in orthopedic jaw surgery. Fortschr. Kiefer. Gesichtschir., *18:*106, 1974 (German)

SELMANOWITZ, V. J., LERER, W. N., AND ORENTREICH, N.: Multiple noduli cutanei and urinary tract abnormalities, PRS, *48:*295, 1971. Cancer, *26:*1256, 1970

SELVAPANDIAN, A. J.: Reconstructive surgery in leprosy deformities. Int. J. Lepr., *39:*660, 1971

SELWYN, S., AND ELLIS, H.: Skin bacteria and skin disinfection reconsidered, PRS, *51:*109, 1973. Brit. Med. J., *1:*136, 1972

SEMENCHENKO, G. I.: Substantiation of the optimal terms of surgical reconstruction of the upper lip and palate in congenital clefts. Stomatologiia (Mosk.), *49:*68, 1970 (Russian)

SEMENCHENKO, G. I. *et al*: Surgical correction of mandibular prognathism. Stomatologiia (Mosk.), *54:*54, 1975 (Russian)

SEMENIUK, V. M. *et al*: Method of removing mandible from cadaver with forensic stomatological expertise and replacing it with prosthesis. Sud. Med. Ekspert, *16:*55, 1973 (Russian)

SEN, D. K.: Temporalis transplantation procedure for paralytic lagophthalmos, PRS, *50:*304, 1972. Internat. Surg., *56:*410, 1971

SEN, R.: Hemangiopericytoma of hand. PRS, *57:*746, 1976

SENECHAL, G.: Saddle nose. Probl. Actuels Otorhinolaryngol., *187:*99, 1970 (French)

SENECHAL, G.: Perforations of nasal septum. Probl. Actuels Otorhinolaryngol., 335, 1972 (French)

SENECHAL, G. *et al*: Means of fixing traction bands during palliative surgery of facial paralysis. Ann. Otolaryngol. Chir. Cervicofac., *90:*585, 1973 (French)

SENECHAL, G. *et al*: Septal perforations and rhinoplasty. Ann. Otolaryngol. Chir. Cervicofac., *90:*659, 1973 (French)

SENECHAL, G. *et al*: Role of endo-oral incision during lateral osteotomies. Ann. chir. plast., *20:*233, 1975 (French)

SEPULVEDA, A. O.: Surgical exploration of facial nerve, PRS, *48:*391, 1971. Rev. Latino Am. cir. plast., *14:*57, 1970

SERAFIN, D., KUTZ, J. E., AND KLEINERT, H. E.: Replantation of completely amputated distal thumb without venous anastomosis, PRS, *52:*579, 1973. Commentary by Buncke, PRS, *52:*581, 1973

SERAFIN, D., VILLARREAL RIOS, A., AND GEORGIADE, N.: Fourteen free groin flap transfers. PRS, *57:*707, 1976

SERALS, J. C., AND BIGGS, D. R.: Surgically induced maxillary growth inhibition in rats, PRS, *55:*247, 1975. Cleft Palate J., *11:*1, 1974

SERENA, A.: 65 autotransplants in burned patients. G. Ital. Dermatol., *46:*546, 1971 (Italian)

SERENKOVA, M. G.: Free skin transplantation using "SITO" graft in treatment of faulty stumps of lower limb, PRS, *54:*626, 1974. Acta chir. plast., *16:*16, 1974

SERGEEVA, P. A. *et al*: Modification of operation of congenital ptosis in children. Oftalmol. Zh., *29:*146, 1974 (Russian)

SERJEANT, G. R.: Leg ulceration in sickle cell anemia, PRS, *54:*503, 1974. Arch. Intern. Med., *133:*681, 1974

SERJEANT, G. R.: Leg ulceration in sickle cell anemia. Arch. Intern. Med., *133:*690, 1974

SERJEANT, G. R. *et al*: Shortening of the digits in sickle cell anaemia: a sequela of the hand-foot syndrome. Trop. Geogr. Med., *23:*341, 1971

SEROPIAN, R., AND REYNOLDS, B. W.: Wound infections after preoperative depilatory versus razor preparation, PRS, *48:*518, 1971. Am. J. Surg., *121:*251, 1971

SERRA, M.: Actinic chronic cheilitis and its relations to epitheliomas of the lower lip. G. Ital. Dermatol., *46:*397, 1971 (Italian)

SERRES, P. *et al*: Karate and cheek fracture. Rev. Stomatol. Chir. Maxillofac., *74:*177, 1973 (French)

SERROU, B. *et al*: Current aspects of treatment of maxillary sinus. J. Fr. Otorhinolaryngol., *22:*435, 1973 (French)

SERSON, D.: Geometrical planning for abdominal dermolipectomy, PRS, *48:*605, 1971. Rev. españ. cir. plast., *4:*37, 1971

SERSON NETO, D., AND MARTINS, L. C.: Surgical treatment for facial palsy, PRS, *48:*88, 1971. Ars. Curandi, *3:*62, 1970

SERSON NETO, D., AND MARTINS, L. C.: Chemical peeling of face, PRS, *49:*477, 1972. Ars. Curandi, *2:*52, 1971

SERSON NETO, D.: Esthetic rhinoplasty. Ann. chir. plast., *18:*307, 1973 (French)

SERVANT, J. M., IKUTA, Y., AND HARADA, Y.: Scanning electron microscope study of microvascular anastomoses, PRS, *57:*329, 1976

SESIA, G.: Two cases of bladder exstrophy treated by cystosigmoidostomy. Follow-up of 15 years. Minerva Urol., *25:*143, 1973 (Italian)

SESSIONS, D. G. *et al*: Correction of saddle nose deformity. Laryngoscope, *82:*2000, 1972

SESSIONS, D. G. AND PORUBSKY, E. S.: Temporomandibular arthroplasty for chronic dislocation of mandible. Laryngoscope, *82:*2273, 1972

SESSIONS, D. G. *et al*: Total glossectomy for advanced carcinoma of base of tongue. Laryngoscope, *83:*39, 1973

SESSIONS, D. G., DEDO, D. D., AND OGURA, J. H.: Tongue flap reconstruction in cancer of oral cavity, PRS, *57:*395, 1976. Arch. Otolaryng., *101:*166, 1975

SETHI, P. K. *et al*: Mycetoma of the hand. A report of three cases. Indian J. Med. Sci., *26:*656, 1972

SETHI, S. M. *et al*: Osteoarthropathy associated with solitary pulmonary metastasis from melanoma. Can. J. Surg., *17:*221, 1974

SEVELYEV, V. E., AND SISOLYATIN, P. G.: Brepho- and homo-bone plasty with sterilized transplants in maxillofacial surgery, PRS, *53:*499, 1974. Acta chir. plast., *15:*65, 1973

SEVEREID, L. R.: Longitudinal study of the efficacy of adenoidectomy in children with cleft palate and secretory otitis media. Trans. Am. Acad. Ophthalmol. Otolaryngol., *76:*1319, 1972

SEVERINOV, A. V.: Surgical therapy of median cysts and neck fistulas. Vestn. Otorinolaringol., *33:*64, 1971 (Russian)

SEVITT, S.: *Reactions to Injury and Burns and their Clinical Importance*. J. B. Lippincott Co., Philadelphia, 1975. PRS, *56:*444, 1975

SEWARD, G.: Replacement of anterior part of mandible by bone grafts, PRS, *55:*717, 1975. J. Maxillofacial Surg., *2:*168, 1974

SEWARD, G. R.: Treatment of class II facial deformity. Maxillary operations. Brit. J. Oral Surg., *10:*254, 1973

SEWELL, R. L.: Excessive axillary sweating. Tex. Med., *70:*67, 1974

SEYDEL, H. G. *et al*: Carcinoma of soft palate and uvula. Am. J. Roentgenol. Radium Ther. Nucl. Med., *120:*603, 1974

SEYFRIED: Characteristics of dynamic data of fingers in the healthy and rheumatoid hand. Z. Gesamte. Hyg., *18:*59, 1972 (German)

SEYMOUR, R. L., FUNKE, F. W., AND IRBY, W. B.: Adenoameloblastoma, PRS, *56:*235, 1975. Oral Surg., *38:*860, 1974

SEYMOUR, R. L. *et al*: Temporomandibular ankylosis secondary to rheumatoid arthritis.

Report of a case. Oral Surg., *40:*584, 1975

SEYMOUR, R. L. *et al*: Dislocation of the condyle into the middle cranial fossa. J. Oral Surg., *34:*180, 1976

SGOURAS, N., AND GEORGIADES, D.: Giant-cell tumor of nasal bones. PRS, *48:*184, 1971

SHAABAN, I.: New surgical method for removal of lower lip cancer. Syria Dent. J., *9:*7, 1973 (Arabic)

SHADID, E. A.: Examination and care of the acutely injured hand. J. Okla. State Med. Assoc., *66:*139, 1973

SHADID, E. A., ENGERON, O., AND GLASS, R. T.: Benign teratoid tumor of parotid. PRS, *55:*363, 1975

SHAFER, W. G.: Initial mismanagement and delay in diagnosis of oral cancer. J. Am. Dent. Assoc., *90:*1262, 1975

SHAFRIR, A. *et al*: Electroencephalogram in hyperhidrosis palmo-plantaris. Harefuah, *86:*238, 1974 (Hebrew)

SHAH, I., ARLEN, M., AND MILLER, T.: Osteogenic sarcoma developing after radiotherapy for retinoblastoma, PRS, *55:*255, 1975. Am. Surgeon, *40:*485, 1974

SHAH, J. H. *et al*: Treatment of burns in children using 0.5 per cent silver nitrate spray locally. A preliminary report. J. Postgrad. Med., *18:*74, 1972

SHAH, J. P.: Amelanotic melanoma. Prog. Clin. Cancer, *6:*195, 1975

SHAH, J. P., AND GOLDSMIGHT, H. S.: Malignant melanoma in North American Negro, PRS, *49:*668, 1972. Surg. Gynec. & Obst., *133:*437, 1971

SHAH, J. P., AND GOLDSMITH, H. S.: Prognosis of malignant melanoma in relation to clinical presentation, PRS, *50:*309, 1972. Am. J. Surg., *123:*286, 1972

SHAH, J. P. *et al*: Epidermoid carcinoma of the supraglottic larynx. Role of neck dissection in initial surgical treatment. Am. J. Surg., *128:*494, 1974

SHAH, J. T. *et al*: Partial or total closure of nostrils in atrophic rhinitis. Arch. Otolaryng., *100:*196, 1974

SHAHEEN, N. A. *et al*: Cysts of parotid gland. Review and report of two unusual cases. J. Laryng. & Otol., *89:*435, 1975

SHAHEEN, O. H.: Arterial epistaxis. J. Laryng. & Otol., *89:*17, 1975

SHAKIR-ALIEV, R. IA.: Urethroplasty in hypospadias. Urol. Nefrol. (Mosk.), *36:*47, 1971 (Russian)

SHALIMOV, A. A. *et al*: Appraisal of prognostic significance of various factors in results of autotransplantation of skin in burned patients, PRS, *57:*762, 1976. Acta chir. plast., *17:*42, 1975

SHANDALOVA, L. B.: Contour plastic surgery with adipose tissue. Vestn. Khir., *108:*62, 1972 (Russian)

SHANGHAI ACUPUNCTURE ANESTHESIA COORDINATING GROUP: Acupuncture anesthesia, PRS, *56:*602, 1975. Chinese M. J., *1:*13, 1975

SHANGHAI CHUNG SHAN HOSPITAL: Subclavian venipuncture and catheterization by supraclavicular approach, PRS, *54:*692, 1974. Chinese M. J., *5:*81, 1974

SHANGHAI FIRST MEDICAL COLLEGE: Small vessel anastomosis—effect of anticoagulant therapy on patency rate, PRS, *54:*239, 1974. Chinese M. J., *1:*6, 1974

SHANGHAI FIRST MEDICAL COLLEGE: Orbital hemangioma—clinical analysis of 79 cases, PRS, *55:*633, 1975. Chinese M. J., *9:*162, 1974

SHANGHAI FIRST PEOPLES HOSPITAL: Complications in replantation of severed limbs and management, PRS, *53:*494, 1974. Chinese M. J., *9:*122, 1973

SHANGHAI SIXTH PEOPLES HOSPITAL: Replantation of severed limbs and fingers, PRS, *51:*703, 1973. Chinese M. J., *1:*1, 1973

SHANGHAI SIXTH PEOPLE'S HOSPITAL: Replantation of limbs after resection of neoplastic segment—report of 8 cases, PRS, *55:*255, 1975. Chinese M. J., *6:*72, 1973

SHANGHAI SIXTH PEOPLE'S HOSPITAL: Hyperbaric oxygen therapy in replantation of severed limbs—report of 21 cases, PRS, *57:*763, 1976. Chinese M. J., *1:*197, 1975

SHANNON, G. M.: Treatment of carcinoma of lids and orbit. J. Med. Soc. N. J., *70:*914, 1973

SHANNON, J. P. *et al*: Improved method for repair of pectus chest deformities. Ann. Thorac. Surg., *16:*629, 1973

SHANON, E. *et al*: Penetrating injuries of parapharyngeal space. Arch. Otolaryng., *96:*256, 1972

SHAPIRA, E., GILADI, A., AND NEUMAN, Z.: Use of water-soluble papain (WIP) for debridement of burn eschar and necrotic tissue. PRS, *52:*279, 1973

SHAPIRO, C. S., AND FLEURY, A. F.: Use of prefolded flap to provide lining and cover in repair of cervical fistulae. PRS, *51:*319, 1973

SHAPIRO, L., JUHLIN, E. A., AND BROWNSTEIN, M. H.: Rudimentary polydactyly, PRS, *54:*376, 1974. Arch. Dermat., *108:*223, 1973

SHAPIRO, R. S. *et al*: Parapharyngeal rhabdomyoma, PRS, *57:*117, 1976. Arch. Otol., *101:*323, 1975

SHAPIRO, S. L.: On management of intractable epistaxis. Eye, Ear, Nose, Throat Mon., *53:*153, 1974

SHARAV, Y., METZGER, Z., AND WEINRELE, M. M.: Behavior and fate of transplanted tooth buds, PRS, *51:*611, 1973. Transplantation,

*13:*360, 1972

SHARBAUGH, R. J., GARGEST, T. S., AND WRIGHT, F. A.: Further studies on bactericidal effect of air-fluidized bed, PRS, *52:*602, 1973. Am. Surgeon, *39:*253, 1973

SHARMA, L. K.: Median cleft of upper lip, PRS, *53:*155, 1974

SHARMA, L. K., KOSHAL, A., AND PRAKASH, A.: Degloving injury of penis, PRS, *54:*238, 1974. Internat. Surg., *58:*9, 1973

SHARMA, L. K. *et al:* Hand injuries in childhood – a survey of fifty patients. J. Ir. Med. Assoc., *66:*598, 1973

SHARMA, R. N. *et al:* Whitlow trephine. J. Indian Med. Assoc., *57:*209, 1971

SHARP, P. M. *et al:* Case of mixed anaerobic infection of jaw. J. Oral Surg., *32:*457, 1974

SHARPE, C.: Tissue cover for thumb web: a review, PRS, *51:*231, 1973. Arch. Surg., *104:*21, 1972

SHARRARD, W. J.: Lumbar and sacral ulceration in older paraplegic children with special reference to progressive kyphosis. Proc. Roy. Soc. Med., *64:*1145, 1971

SHAW, D. T. *et al:* Interdigital butterfly flap in the hand (the double-opposing Z-plasty). J. Bone & Joint Surg. (Am.), *55:*1677, 1973

SHAW, E. B.: Endotracheal intubation and tracheostomy, clinical concepts. D. M., 1–35, 1974

SHAW, H. J.: Repair of laryngo-pharynx and cervical esophagus after radiation, PRS, *49:*238, 1972. Proc. Roy. Soc. Med., *64:*734, 1971

SHAW, H. J.: Operability of metastatic neck cancer. Brit. J. Clin. Pract., *26:*187, 1972

SHAW, H. J. *et al:* Elective tracheostomy in head and neck tumor surgery. J. Leg. Med., *88:*599, 1974

SHAW, M. H.: Serious complication of operation for axillary hyperhidrosis. Brit. J. Plast. Surg., *27:*196, 1974

SHAW, R. C.: Versatile mammaplasty pattern of Wise (with Parsons, Burton). PRS, *55:*1, 1975

SHAW, R. C., AND PARSONS, R. W.: Exposure through coronal incision for initial treatment of facial fractures. PRS, *56:*254, 1975

SHCHECHKIN, V. N.: Hemangioendothelioma of the nose and accessory sinuses. Vestn. Otorinolaringol., *4:*56, 1974 (Russian)

SHCHEGOLEVA, V. D.: Comparative study of late postoperative results following plastic surgery of the palate. Stomatologiia (Mosk.), *53:*39, 1974 (Russian)

SHCHERBATIUK, D. I.: Local use of corticosteroids in surgical interventions in maxillofacial region. Stomatologiia (Mosk.), *54:*37, 1975 (Russian)

SHCHERBTIUK, D. I. Change in function of adrenal cortex after operations in connection with malignant neoplasms in maxillofacial region. Stomatologiia (Mosk.), *52:*97, 1973 (Russian)

SHCHIPACHEVA, V. I.: Plastic treatment of scar contractures of neck with Filatov pedicled flap in children, PRS, *57:*766, 1976. Acta chir. plast., *17:*49, 1975

SHCHUR, V. V. *et al:* Use of a quantum generator (Laser) in the treatment of wounds. Vestn. Khir., *108:*85, 1972 (Russian)

SHEA, P. C., JR.: Comments on current burn therapy. J. Med. Assoc. Ga., *60:*373, 1971

SHEAR, M. *et al:* Morphological changes in lymph node deposits of oral squamous carcinoma. Int. J. Oral Surg., *2:*1, 1973

SHEDBALKAR, A. R., AND JONES, F. R.: Periareolar incision for augmentation mammaplasty (Letter to the Editor). PRS, *53:*217, 1974

SHEDD, D. *et al:* Reed-fistula method of speech rehabilitation after laryngectomy, PRS, *52:*107, 1973. Am. J. Surg., *124:*510, 1972

SHEDD, D. P.: Rehabilitation problems of head and neck cancer patients. J. Surg. Oncol., *8:*11, 1976

SHEDD, D. P., AND GAETA, J. F.: *In vivo* staining of pharyngeal and laryngeal cancer, PRS, *49:*108, 1972. Arch. Surg., *102:*442, 1971

SHEEHY, E.: Primary excision: innovation in pediatric burn care. R. N., *37:*21, 1974

SHEEN, J. H.: Supratarsal fixation in upper blepharoplasty. PRS, *54:*424, 1974

SHEEN, J. H.: Secondary rhinoplasty. PRS, *56:*137, 1975

SHEEN, J. H.: Achieving more nasal tip projection by use of small autogenous vomer or septal cartilage graft, PRS, *56:*35, 1975. Discussion by Horton, PRS, *56:*211, 1975

SHEEN, J. H.: Absorption of small bone graft in nasal tip (Letter to the Editor). PRS, *56:*332, 1975

SHEHADI, S. I.: Reducing eyelid edema and ecchymosis after corrective rhinoplasty. PRS, *49:*508, 1972

SHEIL, A. G. R.: Organ transplantation: balance sheet to date, PRS, *54:*117, 1975. Australian & New Zealand J. Surg., *43:*209, 1973

SHENTAL, V. V. *et al:* Plastic closure of extensive defects of the maxillofacial area following extensive surgical operations for cancer. Stomatologiia (Mosk.), *54:*36, 1975 (Russian)

SHEPARD, G. H.: Healing of wounds after delayed primary closure. Experimental study. PRS, *48:*358, 1971

SHEPARD, G. H.: Storage of split-skin grafts on their donor sites. Clinical and experimental study, PRS, *49:*115, 1972; Letter to the Editor, PRS, *50:*178, 1972

SHEPHARD, G. H., AND RICH, N. M.: Treatment of soft tissue war wounds by American military surgeon, PRS, *51:*711, 1973. Mil. Med., *137:*264, 1972

SHEPARD, G. H., MELVIN, M., AND KLEINERT, H. E.: Complications of moustache or traumatic hair lip. PRS, *49:*346, 1972

SHEPHERD, N. *et al*: Expanded split-thickness mucosal grafts. J. Oral Surg., *31:*687, 1973

SHEPHERD, N. S., MALONEY, P. L., AND DOKU, H. C.: Fenestrated palatal mucosal grafts for vestibuloplasty, PRS, *56:*467, 1975. J. Oral Surg., *33:*34, 1975

SHER, M. R. *et al*: Treatment of facial asymmetry with Silastic implant. J. Oral Surg., *32:*460, 1974

SHER, M. R. *et al*: Odontogenic keratocyst, case report. Oral Surg., *37:*518, 1974

SHERIDAN, B. F. *et al*: Tumors of deep lobe of parotid. Aust. N. Z. J. Surg., *43:*129, 1973

SHERIDAN, B. F., AND NEWTON, N. C.: Tumors of deep lobe of parotid gland, PRS, *52:*600, 1973. Proc. Roy. Australasian Coll. Surg., *46:*744, 1973

SHERLOCK, E. C.: Examination of the hand. Am. Surg., *37:*661, 1971

SHESTERNIA, N. A.: 11-Oxycorticosteroids in peripheral blood of patients with thermic burns, PRS, *48:*396, 1971. Acta chir. plast., *12:*209, 1970

SHETTY, D. K. *et al*: Clinical aspects and therapy of macrostomia. Zahn. Mund. Kieferheilkd., *62:*745, 1974 (German)

SHEVCHENKO, I. T. *et al*: Analysis of the survival of patients with pigmented neoplasms. Klin. Khir., *1:*36, 1972

SHEVKUNOV, V. A.: Treatment of suppurative diseases of the fingers and hand. Khirurgiia (Mosk.), *49:*19, 1973 (Russian)

SHEVRYGIN, B. V. *et al*: Anomalies in the development of the nasal cavity in children and their treatment. Zh. Ushn. Nos. Gorl. Bolezn., *6:*30, 1974 (Russian)

SHIBATA, S. *et al*: Case of von Recklinghausen's disease with unilateral pulsating exophthalmos. Clin. Neurol., *14:*512, 1974 (Japanese)

SHIELDS, C. *et al*: Hand infections secondary to human bites. J. Trauma, *15:*235, 1975

SHIELDS, J., AND FONT, R.: Meibomian gland carcinoma presenting as lacrimal gland tumor, PRS, *55:*641, 1975. Arch. Ophth., *92:*304, 1974

SHIELDS, M. B., AND REED, J. W.: Aniridia and congenital ptosis, PRS, *56:*223, 1975. Ann. Ophth., *7:*203, 1975

SHIFFMAN, N. J.: Squamous cell carcinomas of skin of pinna, PRS, *57:*403, 1976. Canad. J. Surg., *18:*279, 1975

SHIMAZAKI, S. *et al*: Problems of sulfamylon treatment for burns. Surg. Ther. (Osaka), *26:*589, 1972

SHIMIZU, M.: Experience in indwelling aspiration by a tube drain following surgery of cervical metastases of malignant oral cancer. J. Jap. Stomatol. Soc., *38:*574, 1971 (Japanese)

SHIMIZU, M.: Suture method of abdominal area after collecting skin flap for mobilization of jaw joint—application of "U" plasty. J. Jap. Stomatol. Soc., *40:*169, 1973 (Japanese)

SHIMKIN, M. B.: Upon man and beast: adventures in cancer epidemiology, PRS, *55:*116, 1975. Cancer Res., *34:*1525, 1974

SHIMO, G.: Middle ear problems associated with cleft palate. Can. J. Otolaryngol., *1:*9, 1972

SHINBIREV, N. A.: Intraoral complete resection of upper jaw. Zdravookhr. Ross. Fed., *5:*106, 1974 (Russian)

SHINBIREV, N. A. *et al*: Use of split skin graft in formation of fronto-nasal anastomosis. Vestn. Otorinolaringol., *35:*13, 1973 (Russian)

SHINDARSKI, B. *et al*: Surgical treatment of deep thermal burns in children by means of free autologous and homologous skin transplantations. Khirurgiia (Sofiia), *25:*267, 1972 (Bulgarian)

SHINDLE, R. D. AND LEONE, C. R., JR.: Cicatricial ectropion associated with lamellar ichthyosis. Arch. Ophth., *89:*62, 1973

SHINGLETON, W. W.: Intralesional BCG, immune lymphocytes, and immunization with neuraminidase-treated tumor cells to manage melanoma (with Seigler, Pickrell). PRS, *55:*294, 1975

SHINODA, T.: Manual myotomy for congenital muscular torticollis in infants. Orthop. Surg. (Tokyo), *22:*1099, 1971 (Japanese)

SHINTANI, A. *et al*: Rapid microvascular repair using plastic adhesive. Stroke, *3:*34, 1972

SHIP, A. G.: Permanent cutaneous cystostomy by interposition of abdominal skin-lined, tubed flap (Follow-Up Clinic). PRS, *52:*298, 1973

SHIP, A. G.: Alar base resection for wide-flaring nostrils. Brit. J. Plast. Surg., *28:*77, 1975

SHIP, A. G. *et al*: Split-thickness scalp flap for resurfacing full thickness forehead and temporal scalp defects. Brit. J. Plast. Surg., *24:*351, 1971

SHIP, A. G., AND PELZER, R. H.: Reconstruction of female escutcheon in exstrophy of bladder. PRS, *49:*643, 1972

SHIPACHEVA, V. I.: Repair with Filatov's flap in defects and deformations of the oral region. Vestn. Khir., *113:*65, 1974 (Russian)

SHIRAKI, I. W. *et al*: Congenital micropenile

skin sleeve. J. Urol., *114:*469, 1975

SHIRCLIFFE, A. C. *et al*: Technique for obtaining porcine heterografts for use on burned patients. J. Trauma, *14:*168, 1974

SHIRLEY, W. L., AND COCKE, W. L.: Nursing device for use in cleft palate care. PRS, *48:*83, 1971

SHISHITO, S., AND SHIRAI, M.: Repair of hypospadias by 4 layer sutures, PRS, *53:*368, 1974. Operation, *27:*559, 1973

SHISHITO, S. *et al*: Surgical repair for hypospadias. Urethroplasty by quadruple layer sutures. Urol. int., *29:*382, 1974

SHISHITO, S., SHIRAI, M., AND MATSUDA, S.: Treatment of organic impotence by implantation of silicone penile prosthesis, PRS, *56:*466, 1975. Urol. int., *30:*211, 1975

Shock (See also *Burn Shock*)

Hypoxemia immediately after operation (Thompson, Eason), PRS, *49:*361, 1972. Am. J. Surg., *120:*649, 1970

Coma, hyperosmolar, surgical significance (Flanigan *et al*), PRS, *48:*202, 1971. Am. J. Surg., *120:*652, 1970

Autotransfusion, intraoperative, early clinical experience with disposable unit for (Klebanoff), PRS, *48:*202, 1971. Am. J. Surg., *120:*718, 1970

Shock, recovery patterns and lethal manifestations of live *E. coli* organism (Hinshaw *et al*), PRS, *48:*201, 1971. J. Trauma, *10:*787, 1970

Pulmonary changes following treatment for hemorrhagic shock: saline *versus* colloid infusion (Siegel *et al*), PRS, *48:*201, 1971. Surg. Forum, *21:*17, 1970

Pluronic F-68, beneficial effect on microcirculation in experimental hemorrhagic shock (Grover, Newman, Paton), PRS, *48:*96, 1971. Surg. Forum, *21:*30, 1970

Surgical procedure, extensive, total circulating albumin deficits occurring with (Hoye, Paulson, Ketcham), PRS, *48:*202, 1971. Surg. Gynec. & Obst., *131:*943, 1970

Shock, infusion of Ringer's lactate solution during (Canizaro, Prager, Shires), PRS, *51:*710, 1973. Am. J. Surg., *122:*494, 1971

Shock, clinical, hemodynamic changes, treatment, and prognosis (Wilson, Sarver, Rizzo), PRS, *49:*241, 1972. Arch. Surg., *102:*21, 1971

Industrial surfactant, pluronic F-68, influence in treatment of hemorrhagic shock (Hymes, Safavian, Gunther), PRS, *48:*612, 1971. J. Surg. Res., *11:*191, 1971

WR 2823, pretreatment of *E. coli* endotoxin shock with new alphadrenergic blocking

Shock—Cont

agent (Phillips, Vick), PRS, *48:*299, 1971. Surgery, *69:*510, 1971

Tissue oxygenation following resuscitation with crystalloid solution following experimental acute blood loss (Reich, Eiseman), PRS, *48:*519, 1971. Surgery, *69:*928, 1971

Shock, traumatic and non-traumatic, effect on allograft survival (Markley, Thornton, Smallman), PRS, *49:*362, 1972. Surgery, *70:*667, 1971

Physiologic management of septicemic shock in man (Sugerman *et al*), PRS, *49:*476, 1972. Surg. Forum, *22:*3, 1971

Lipid, availability for energy metabolism during hypovolemia (Farago *et al*), PRS, *49:*476, 1972. Surg. Forum, *22:*7, 1971

Post-injury state, clinical significance of functional residual capacity in (Monaco *et al*), PRS, *49:*588, 1972. Surg. Forum, *22:*42, 1971

Shock, dilemma of vasopressors and vasodilators in therapy of (Shoemaker, Brown), PRS, *48:*400, 1971. Surg. Gynec. & Obst., *132:*51, 1971

Shock, problem of acute severe trauma and (Hardaway), PRS, *49:*669, 1972. Surg. Gynec. & Obst., *133:*799, 1971

Physiology ad physiopathology of low pressure venous system (Schneider), PRS, *51:*605, 1973. Ann dermat. & syph., *99:*393, 1972

Coagulation changes of hemorrhagic shock in baboons (Herman, Moquin, Horwitz), PRS, *50:*311, 1972. Ann. Surg., *175:*197, 1972

Mesenteric circulatory responses to hemorrhagic shock in baboon (Barton, Reynolds, Swan), PRS, *50:*311, 1972. Ann. Surg., *175:*204, 1972

Insulin release, pancreatic, decline during hemorrhagic shock in baboon (Moss *et al*), PRS, *50:*423, 1972. Ann. Surg., *175:*210, 1972

Hemorrhage, regulation of ventilation, alterations in response to CO_2 (Baue, Nara), PRS, *51:*710, 1973. Ann. Surg., *176:*80, 1972

Lymph lysosomal enzyme acid phosphatase in hemorrhagic shock (Clermont, Williams), PRS, *51:*710, 1973. Ann. Surg., *176:*90, 1972

Glucose, hypertonic, effect in hypovolemic shock in man (McNamara *et al*), PRS, *51:*710, 1973. Ann. Surg., *176:*247, 1972

Infants and children on plastic surgical service, brief guide to fluid therapy (Pickrell, Mladick). PRS, *49:*404, 1972

Bile salts producing stress ulcers during ex-

Shock — Cont.

perimental shock (Hamza, DenBesten), PRS, *50:*100, 1972. Surgery, *71:*161, 1972

Dextran 70 and dextran 40, comparative effects in experimental animals (Litwin), PRS, *50:*100, 1972. Surgery, *71:*295, 1972

Shock, septic, in burn illness (Matejicek *et al*), PRS, *54:*507, 1974. Acta chir. plast., *15:*263, 1973

Electrolyte solutions, role in treatment of hemorrhagic shock (Rocchio, DiCola, Randal), PRS, *53:*109, 1974. Am. J. Surg., *125:*488, 1973

Blood pressure and diuresis, effect in rats of intravenous injection of rabbit anti-rat lymphocyte globulin on (Dalton, Davison), PRS, *53:*614, 1974. Europ. Surg. Res., *5:*116, 1973

Steroids other than cortisone, anti-shock action of (Novelli, Marsili, Pieraceioli), PRS, *53:*375, 1974. Europ. Surg. Res., *5:*169, 1973

Blood volume changes in surgical treatment of oral-facial deformities: preliminary report (Kelly, Terry). J. Oral Surg., *31:*90, 1973

Phenoxybenzamine and methylprednisolone on precapillary and postcapillary resistance in endotoxin-shocked dogs (Motsay *et al*), PRS, *53:*609, 1974. J. Surg. Res., *14:*406, 1973

Trauma, patients with multiple, adverse effects of salt and water retention on pulmonary function of (Abrams, Deane, Davis), PRS, *53:*500, 1974. J. Trauma, *13:*788, 1973

Hemorrhagic shock treated with new vasodilator (Vick *et al*), PRS, *53:*109, 1974. Mil. Med., *138:*490, 1973

Steroids in treatment of septic and cardiogenic shock, efficacy of (Rosenbaum, Hayes, Matsumoto), PRS, *52:*461, 1973. Surg. Gynec. & Obst., *136:*914, 1973

Cardiovascular effects of carbon dioxide in man (Cullen, Eger), PRS, *55:*727, 1975. Anesthesiology *41:*345, 1974

Shock treatment, experimental, new pharmocodynamic approach — use of solution of glucose, insulin, and potassium in (Alvarez-Cordero *et al*), PRS, *56:*362, 1975. Cir. Cir., *42:*49, 1974

Pulmonary changes due to hemorrhagic shock; resuscitation with isotonic and hypertonic saline (Fulton, Fisher), PRS, *54:*624, 1974. Surgery, *75:*881, 1974

Shock, septic, microcirculatory disturbances in (Peking Hospital of Workers), PRS, *57:*763, 1976. Chinese M. J., *1:*174, 1975

Intravenous therapy, trouble in long run (Munster), PRS, *56:*597, 1975. Emergency Med., *7:*230, 1975

Shock — Cont.

Resuscitation following trauma, selection of plasma volume expanders for (Mandelson), PRS, *57:*676, 1976. Mil. Med., *140:*258, 1975

Shock resuscitation, choice of intravenous fluid in (Rowe, Arango), PRS, *57:*122, 1976. Pediat. Clin. N. Am., *22:*269, 1975

Blood volume relationship to hematocrit, CVP, pulmonary wedge pressure, and cardiorespiratory changes (Back *et al*), PRS, *57:*407, 1976. Surgery, *78:*304, 1975

Glucose, cellular, used during hemorrhagic shock in pig (Wright, Henderson), PRS, *57:*676, 1976. Surgery, *78:*322, 1975

Pulmonary surfactant system, normal electron histochemistry and effect of hemorrhagic shock on (Moss, Newson, Das Gupta), PRS, *56:*469, 1975. Surg. Gynec. & Obst., *140:*53, 1975

SHOEMAKER, W. C., AND BROWN, R. S.: Dilemma of vasopressors and vasodilators in therapy of shock, PRS, *48:*400, 1971. Surg. Gynec. & Obst., *132:*51, 1971

SHOEMAKER, W. C. *et al*: Burn pathophysiology in man. I. Sequential hemodynamic alterations, PRS, *53:*493, 1974. J. Surg. Res., *14:*64, 1973

SHONS, A. R. *et al*: Cervical-pectoral flaps in the treatment of advanced oral cancer. J. Surg. Oncol., *7:*213, 1975

SHORT, S. G., AND OGLE, R. G.: Extractions in hemophilia — use of EACA (epsilon aminocarpoic acid), PRS, *54:*247, 1974. Minnesota Med., *57:*77, 1974

SHPRINTZEN, R. J. *et al*: Three dimensional cinefluoroscopic analysis of velopharyngeal closure during speech and non-speech activities in normals, PRS, *56:*114, 1975. Cleft Palate J., *11:*412, 1974

SHREWSBURY, M. M., JOHNSON, R. K., AND OUSTERHOUT, D. K.: Palmaris brevis — reconsideration of anatomy and possible function, PRS, *50:*307, 1972. J. Bone & Joint Surg., *54:*344, 1972

SHTEYER, A. *et al*: Submandibular gland calculus with canalization — case report. Brit. J. Oral Surg., *12:*302, 1975

SHTIL, A. A.: Repeated surgery in malignant tumors of the accessory sinuses of the nose. Vestn. Otorinolaringol., *34:*92, 1972 (Russian)

SHTIL, A. A.: Evaluation of results of combined treatment of malignant neoplasms of nose and accessory sinuses. Vestn. Otorinolaringol., *2:*49, 1974 (Russian)

SHUANGSHOTI, S., NETSKY, M. G., AND FITZHUGH, G. S.: Parapharyngeal meningioma with special reference to cell of origin, PRS,

49:237, 1972. Ann. Otol. Rhin. & Laryng., 80:464, 1971

SHUANGSHOTI, S. et al: Ectopic meningiomas. Arch. Otolaryng., 98:102, 1973

SHUBICH, I. et al: Benign bone tumors of the nose and paranasal sinuses in childhood. Review of cases in the Hospital Infantilede Mexico. Bol. Med. Hosp. Infant. Mex., 31:831, 1974 (Spanish)

SHUBICH, NEIMAN I. et al: Kartagener's syndrome in childhood. Report of 2 cases. Bol. Med. Hosp. Infant. Mex., 32:493, 1975 (Spanish)

SHUCK, J. M.: Burn treatment with Sulfamylon cream and Sulfamylon solution: coordinated techniques, PRS, 54:112, 1974. Rev. Latino Am. cir. plast., 17:75, 1973

SHUCK, J. M.: Current practices in burn management. Am. Surg., 40:145, 1974

SHUCK, J. M.: Preparing and closing burn wound. Clin. Plast. Surg., 1:577, 1974

SHUCK, J. M., BEDEAU, G. W., AND THOMAS, P. R. S.: Homograft skin for early management of difficult wounds, PRS, 52:105, 1973. J. Trauma, 12:215, 1972

SHUCK, J. M., EINFELDT, L. E., AND TRAINOR, M. P.: Sulfamylon solution dressings in management of burn wounds: preliminary clinical report, PRS, 53:492, 1974. J. Trauma, 12:999, 1972

SHUCK, J. M. et al: Mafenide acetate solution dressings: an adjunct in burn wound care. J. Trauma, 15:595, 1975

SHUERT, G. T. et al: Guillain-Barre syndrome after mandibular surgery, case report. J. Oral Surg., 30:913, 1972

SHUL'GA, A. O. et al: Surgical treatment of patients with malignant tumors of nose and paranasal sinuses. Zh. Ushn. Nos. Gorl. Bolezn., 32:66, 1972 (Russian)

SHULMAN, J. A. et al: Colonization with gentamicin-resistant Pseudomonas aeruginosa, pyocine type 5, in a burn unit. J. Infect. Dis., 124:18, 1971

SHUMAKHER, G. KH. et al: Anatomical principles of plastic operations in the vestibule of the oral cavity. Stomatologiia (Mosk.), 53:83, 1974 (Russian)

SHUMRICK, D. A.: Carotid artery rupture. Laryngoscope, 83:1051, 1973

SHURMAN, J.: Bilateral hypertrophy of coronoid processes, PRS, 57:117, 1976. Anesthesiology, 42:491, 1975

SHUSTER, M. M.: Internal nasal mold, made of silicone rubber, for grafts or flaps inside the nose, PRS, 52:203, 1973

SHVARTS, F. G.: Treatment of burn trauma under the conditions of a garrison hospital. Voen. Med. Zh., 1:40, 1974 (Russian)

SHVYKROV, M. B.: Topical diagnosis of maxillary fractures. Stomatologiia (Mosk.), 53:40, 1974 (Russian)

SIBILLY, A. et al: Frontal sinus fractures and injuries of the facial bones. Rev. Stomatol. Chir. Maxillofac., 72:495, 1971 (French)

SIBULKIN, D., AND HEALEY, W. V.: Invisible glomus tumor, PRS, 55:115, 1975. Arch. Surg., 109:111, 1974

SIDHU, S. S. et al: Reconstruction by maxillofacial prosthesis following extensive cancer surgery. Newsl. Int. Coll. Dent. (India), 10:1, 1973

SIDORENKO, L. N. et al: Pathogenetic therapy of dyshormonal hyperplasia of male breast. Vopr. Onkol., 18:27, 1972 (Russian)

SIEDSCHLAG, W. D. et al: Treatment of transorbital brain injuries caused by foreign bodies. Zentralbl. Neurochir., 32:95, 1973 (German)

SIEGEL, D. C. et al: Pulmonary changes following treatment for hemorrhagic shock: saline versus colloid infusion, PRS, 48:201, 1971. Surg. Forum, 21:17, 1970

SIEGEL, M. I.: Mechanisms of early maxillary growth — implications for surgery. J. Oral Surg., 34:106, 1976

SIEGEL, R. J.: Correction of enophthalmos in anophthalmic orbit (with Iverson, Vistnes). PRS, 51:545, 1973

SIEGEL, R. J., AND VISTNES, L. M.: Epinephrine requirements for effective hemostasis in local anesthetics, PRS, 51:711, 1973. Surg. Forum., 23:515, 1972

SIEGEL, R. J., VISTNES, L. M., AND LAUB, D. R.: Use of water bed for prevention of pressure sores. PRS, 51:31, 1973

SIEGEL, R. J., VISTNES, L. M., AND IVERSON, R. E.: Effective hemostasis with less epinephrine, experimental and clinical study. PRS, 51:129, 1973

SIEGLER, H. F. et al: Non-specific and specific immunotherapy in patients with melanoma, PRS, 50:636, 1972. Surgery, 72:162, 1972

SIEGLER, J.: Place of septal replacement operation in treatment of nasal obstruction. J. Laryng. & Otol., 87:153, 1973

SIEMSSEN, S. O. et al: Use of deltopectoral flap in radical cancer surgery in head and neck region. Ugeskr. Laeger, 134:2137, 1972 (Danish)

SIENKIEWICZ, H. et al: Case of melanoma of the posterior pharyngeal wall. Otolaryngol. Pol., 26:89, 1972 (Polish)

SIERRA, E. B.: Functional levels for finger amputation, PRS, 51:702, 1973. Rev. Latino Am. cir. plast., 14:45, 1970

SIERRA, J. G.: Surgical treatment of gingival melanosis. Rev. Fed. Odontol. Colomb., 22:51, 1973 (Spanish)

SIFFERT, R. S.: Experimental and clinical experiences in epiphyseal transplantation (with Hoffman, Simon), PRS, *50:*58, 1972

SIGEL, B. *et al*: Diagnosis of lower limb venous thrombosis by Doppler ultrasound technique. Arch. Surg., *104:*174, 1972

SIGURDSON, A.: Preprosthetic surgery with dentures. Clinical viewpoints on management of carrying out follow-up studies. Sven. Tandlak. Tidskr., *64:*383, 1971 (Swedish)

SIIRALA, U. *et al*: Pharyngolarynx: new aspects of the use of the larynx for reconstruction in hypopharyngeal carcinoma. Laryngoscope, *82:*504, 1972

SIIRALA, U. *et al*: The problem of advanced supraglottic carcinoma. Laryngoscope, *85:*1633, 1975

SILBER, S. J., AND CRUDOP, J.: Kidney transplantation in inbred rats, PRS, *52:*681, 1973. Am. J. Surg., *125:*551, 1973

SILBERMANN, M. *et al*: Skeletal open bite associated with bimaxillary dento-alveolar protrusion, evaluation and treatment. Brit. J. Oral Surg., *10:*223, 1972

SILBERMANN, M. *et al*: Sponteneous healing of large osteomyelitic defect in mandible, case report. J. Oral Surg., *30:*821, 1972

SILBERMANN, M. *et al*: Mandibular osteomyelitis in patient with chronic alcoholism: etiology, management, and statistical correlation. Oral Surg., *38:*530, 1974

SILBERMANN, M. *et al*: Mandibular actinomycosis: report of case. J. Am. Dent. Assoc., *90:*162, 1975

Silicones (See also *Implants; Prostheses*)

Silicone polymers, low molecular, chemicobiological properties of, and employment in conserving homologous tissues of mesenchymal origin (Nikitin), PRS, *50:*206, 1972. Acta chir. plast., *13:*61, 1971

Complications of silastic implants. Experience with 137 consecutive cases (Davis *et al*). Brit. J. Plast. Surg., *24:*405, 1971

Silicoma, case of (Bisaggio), PRS, *50:*635, 1972. Folia med. Brazil, *63:*59, 1971

Tumor, malignant foreign body granuloma of breast incident to (Yamazaki *et al*), PRS, *50:*305, 1972. Geka Surg. Ther. Osaka, *33:*1283, 1971

Dimethylpolysiloxane fluid in soft tissue augmentation, experience with (Blocksma). PRS, *48:*564, 1971

Experiences with silastic in plastic surgery of the face (Haas). Z. Laryngol. Rhinol. Otol., *50:*751, 1971 (German)

Silicone mesh sheet as suspension material (Arai, Fukuda, Akiyama), PRS, *52:*463, 1973. Jap. J. Plast. Reconstr. Surg., *15:*447,

Silicones — Cont.

1972

Silicone ear framework, our experiences with; report of 17 ears in 15 patients (Monroe), PRS, *49:*428, 1972

Foreign materials into breasts, management of patients with complications from injection of (Ortiz-Monasterio, Trigos), PRS, *50:*42, 1972

Silicone spheres, treatment of facial hemangioma by intravascular embolization with (Longacre, Benton, Unterthiner), PRS, *50:*618, 1972

Silicone, liquid, in mammarian hypotrophies, some considerations concerning application of (Roa-Roa), PRS, *50:*419, 1972. Rev. Latino Am. Cir. Plast., *15:*17, 1972

Forehead reconstruction with silicone elastomer sponge (Calcaterra *et al*). Arch. Otolaryng., *98:*389, 1973

Otorhinolaryngology, synthetic implants in (Cote *et al*). Can. J. Otolaryngol., *2:*263, 1973 (French)

Silicone granuloma of penis (Datta, Kern), PRS, *52:*596, 1973. J. Urol., *109:*840, 1973

Silicone granulomatous disease of breast simulating cancer (Kuiper), PRS, *52:*452, 1973. Mich. Med., *72:*215, 1973

Silicone fluid, augmentation of surface contour by subcutaneous injections of (Ashley, Thompson, Henderson), PRS, *51:*8, 1973

Silicone gel pillows, retropharyngeal implantation of, for velopharyngeal incompetence (Brauer), PRS, *51:*254, 1973

Plastic surgery, use of silicones in, retrospective view (Braley), PRS, *51:*280, 1973

Silicone-bone compound implants for mandibular reconstruction (Swanson *et al*), PRS, *51:*402, 1973

Silicone gel breast implants, treatment of bilateral breast carcinomas in patient with (Benavent), PRS, *51:*588, 1973

Silicone implants, fate of pseudosheath pocket around (Thomson), PRS, *51:*667, 1973

Silicone fluid injections for facial atrophy (Rees, Ashley, Delgado), PRS, *52:*118, 1973

Silicone rubber, internal nasal mold made of, for grafts or flaps inside nose (Shuster), PRS, *52:*203, 1973

Silicone implants, prefabricated nasal (Antia *et al*), PRS, *52:*264, 1973

Silastic, permanent fixation of, to temporal bone, reconstruction of temporomandibular joint by (Stratigos). Trans. Congr. Int. Assoc. Oral Surg., *4:*284, 1973

Silicone injection to correct form of face and body (Lisbonne, Comte), PRS, *54:*631, 1974. Ann. chir. plast., *19:*31, 1974

Silicones — Cont.

Silicone granuloma, mammary (Delage, Shane, Johnson), PRS, *54:*373, 1974. Arch. Dermat., *108:*105, 1973

Facial furrows, silicone for (Goin). J.A.M.A., *229:*1581, 1974

Silicone treatment of partial lipodystrophy (Rees, Coburn), PRS, *55:*505, 1975. J.A.M.A., *230:*868, 1974

Silicones for medical application (Evans), PRS, *56:*474, 1975. J. Polym. Med., *4:*135, 1974

Mammaplasty: new soft, round silicone gel breast implant (Wiener, Aiache, Silver), PRS, *53:*174, 1974

Silicone gel inflatable mammary prosthesis (Dahl, Baccari, Arfai), PRS, *53:*234, 1974

Prosthesis, silicone rubber, after mandibular condylectomy (Hartwell, Hall), PRS, *53:*440, 1974

Silicone framework, reconstruction of microtia with, follow-up study (Ohmori, Matsumoto, Nakai), PRS, *53:*555, 1974

Silicone elastomer: fibrous capsule formation after subcutaneous implantation of synthetic materials in experimental animals (Imber *et al*), PRS, *54:*183, 1974

Silicone: nasal augmentation by intraoral route (Flowers), PRS, *54:*570, 1974

Silicone gel, fluid, of Japanese origin (Psillakis *et al*), PRS, *56:*684, 1975. Rev. Asoc. med. Brasil, *19:*191, 1974

Catastrophic results after silicone injections (Jenny). In *Plastische und Wiederherstellungs-Chirurgie*, ed. by Hohler; pp. 331–4. Schattauer, Stuttgart, 1975

Corns, treatment by injectable silicone (Balkin), PRS, *57:*543, 1976. Arch. Dermat., *111:*1143, 1975

Silicone injections used for facial defects (Berger), PRS, *57:*393, 1976. Arch. Otolaryng., *101:*525, 1975

Silicone elastomer implant, repair of concavity of thoracic wall with (Baker, Mara, Douglas), PRS, *56:*212, 1975

Silicone granuloma of penis (Lighterman), PRS, *57:*517, 1976

Capsule formation, long-term study of reactions to various silicone breast implants in rabbits (Lilla, Vistnes), PRS, *57:*637, 1976

Silla, M: Immediate reconstruction in primary tumors of lower lip, PRS, *57:*671, 1976. Riv. ital. chir. plast., *6:*257, 1974

Silsby, J. J.: Nipple reconstruction, PRS, *57:*667, 1976

Silva, N. *et al*: Pattern of lymphatic spread in pharyngeal cancer. J. Surg. Oncol., *3:*415, 1971

Silva, P. F. *et al*: Importance of preservation of vascular pedicles in esophagoplasties. Results observed in 60 patients with caustic stenosis of esophagus operated on consecutively. Rev. Asoc. Med. Bras., *20:*219, 1974 (Portuguese)

Silver, C. M.: An adjustable device to increase mouth opening. J. Bone & Joint Surg. (Am.), *53:*1217, 1971

Silver, C. M., Simon, S. D., and Litchman, H. M.: Surgical treatment of arthritic temporomandibular joint, PRS, *52:*206, 1973. Surg. Gynec. & Obst., *136:*251, 1973

Silver, D. *et al*: Surgical treatment of the refractory postphlebitic ulcer, PRS, *49:*584, 1972. Arch. Surg., *103:*554, 1971

Silver, H. L.: Treating complications of augmentation mammaplasty, PRS, *49:*637, 1972

Silver, L.: Preservation of traumatically amputated fingertips (with Weiner, Aiache), PRS, *49:*609, 1972

Silver, L.: New soft, round, silicone gel breast implant (with Weiner, Aiache), PRS, *53:*174, 1974

Silverman, F. N. *et al*: Acroosteolysis (Hajdu-Cheney syndrome). Birth Defects, *10:*106, 1974

Silverstein, F. *et al*: Myoelectric hand splint. Am. J. Occup. Ther., *28:*99, 1974

Silverstein, M. L. *et al*: Malignant melanoma metastatic to bladder. Regression following intratumor injection of BCG vaccine. J.A.M.A., *229:*688, 1974

Silverstein, P.: Upper extremity fungal invasions secondary to large burns (with Salisbury, Goodwin), PRS, *54:*654, 1974

Silverstein, P. *et al*: Evaluation of formalin-fixed skin as temporary dressing for granulating wounds, PRS, *49:*668, 1972. Surg. Forum, *22:*60, 1971

Silverstein, P. *et al*: Subcutaneous tissue infiltration as an adjunct to split-thickness skin grafting. Am. J. Surg., *123:*624, 1972

Silverstein, P. *et al*: Laboratory evaluation of enzymatic burn wound debridement *in vitro* and *in vivo*, PRS, *52:*212, 1973. Surg. Forum, *23:*31, 1972

Silverstein, P., and Peterson, H. D.: Treatment of eyelid deformities due to burns, PRS, *51:*38, 1973

Silverstein, P. *et al*: In vitro evaluation of enzymatic debridement of burn wound eschar. Surgery, *73:*15, 1973

Simaga, D. *et al*: Indications for conservative surgery in the treatment of phagedenic ulcer, cancerous or noncancerous. Bull. Soc. Med. Afr. Noire Lang. Fr., *15:*267, 1970 (French)

Simes, R. J. *et al*: Ultrastructure of an odontogenic myxoma. Oral Surg., *39:*640, 1975

SIMMONS, F. B. *et al*: Hypersomnia caused by upper airway obstructions: a new syndrome in otolaryngology. Ann. Otol. Rhin. & Laryng., *83*:670, 1974

SIMON, B. E.: Experimental and clinical experiences in epiphyseal transplantation (with Hoffman, Siffert), PRS, *50*:58, 1972

SIMON, B. E.: Experiences with Pitanguy method of correction of trochanteric lipodystrophy (with Hoffman), PRS, *55*:551, 1975

SIMON, B. E.: Mondor's disease, unusual complication of mammaplasty (with Fischl, Kahn), PRS, *56*:319, 1975

SIMON, B. E., HOFFMAN, S., AND KAHN, S.: Classification and surgical correction of gynecomastia, PRS, *51*:48, 1973

SIMON, H.: Regional neck lymph nodes and primary tumors. 1. Neck lymph node metastases. Laryngol. Rhinol. Otol. (Stuttg.), *54*:997, 1975 (German)

SIMONETTA, C.: Use of "A. O." plates in the hand. Hand, *2*:43, 1970

SIMONS, F. E. R., AND SCHALLER, J. G.: Benign rheumatoid nodules, PRS, *57*:123, 1976. Pediatrics, *56*:29, 1975

SIMONS, J. N.: Malignant melanoma of head and neck, PRS, *52*:102, 1973. Am. J. Surg., *124*:485, 1972

SIMONS, R. L. *et al*: Prolongation of skin allografts in man using anti-lymphoblast globulin, PRS, *53*:112, 1974. ALG Therapy & Stand. Workshop, Behringwerke Ag. Marburg, *51*:149, 1972

SIMONS, R. L., AND LAWSON, W.: Chin reduction in profileplasty, PRS, *57*:528, 1976. Arch. Otolaryng., *101*:207, 1975

SIMPSON, D. C.: Gripping surfaces for artificial hands. Hand, *3*:12, 1971

SIMPSON, D. C.: External powered prostheses. Hand, *3*:211, 1971

SIMPSON, H. E.: Basal-cell carcinoma and peripheral ameloblastoma. Oral Surg., *38*:233, 1974

SIMPSON, W.: The Obwegeser osteotomy. Orthodontist, *4*:48, 1972

SIMPSON, W.: Results of surgery for mandibular prognathism. Brit. J. Oral Surg., *12*:166, 1974

SIMPSON, W. J.: Short lingual cut in sagittal osteotomy. J. Oral Surg., *30*:811, 1972

SIMUN, L. *et al*: Injuries of the extensors of the hand and fingers (analysis of 1000 cases). Acta Chir. Orthop. Traumatol. Cech., *38*:298, 1972 (Slovakian)

SIMUN, L. *et al*: Treatment of the hand damaged by burns and pressure. Acta Chir. Orthop. Traumatol. Cech., *40*:264, 1973 (Slovakian)

SINCLAIR, S., BECKMAN, E., AND ELLMAN, L.:

Biopsy of enlarged superficial lymph nodes, PRS, *54*:694, 1974. J.A.M.A., *228*:602, 1974

SINGER, B.: Treatment of bone pockets. Z.W.R., *83*:207, 1974 (German)

SINGER, C. F., JR., GIENGER, G. L., AND KULLBOM, T. L.: Solitary intraosseous neurofibroma involving mandibular canal: case report. J. Oral Surg., *31*:127, 1973

SINGER, J. A. *et al*: Blowout fractures of the orbit. Nebr. Med. J., *55*:352, 1970

SINGER, J. B.: Addition of adhesive backing to nasal splints, PRS, *48*:505, 1971

SINGH, D. S., AND GARG, R. S.: Polyethylene intubation of nasolacrimal duct in chronic dacryocystitis. Review of 40 cases with one-year follow-up. Brit. J. Ophth., *56*:914, 1972

SINGH, J. P. *et al*: Neonatal cervical teratoma, case report. Indian Pediatr., *9*:229, 1972

SINGH, S., BABOO, M. L., AND PATHAK, I. C.: Cystic lymphangioma in children, report of 32 cases, PRS, *48*:517, 1971. Surgery, *69*:947, 1971

SINGHA, S. S. *et al*: Cicatricial ectropion of lower lid. Indian J. Opththalmol., *21*:82, 1973

SINGLETON, E. B. *et al*: Peripheral dysostosis. Birth Defects, *10*:510, 1974

SINGLETON, M. A., AND GROSS, C. W.: Management of keloids by surgical excision and local injections of steroid, PRS, *52*:331, 1973. South. M. J., *64*:1377, 1971

SINHA, B. K., AND BUNTINE, D. W.: Prognosis of cutaneous malignant melanoma, clinicopathological study, PRS, *56*:113, 1975. Canad. J. Surg., *17*:328, 1974

SINHA, B. H., AND BUNTINE, D. W.: Parotid gland tumors, clinicopathologic study, PRS, *57*:672, 1976. Am. J. Surg., *129*:675, 1975

SINHA, R. N.: Burns in tropical countries. Clin. Plast. Surg., *1*:121, 1974

SINILO, M. I. *et al*: Free skin grafts on weight-bearing and functionally active limb surfaces. Vestn. Khir., *113*:70, 1974 (Russian)

SIN'KEVICH, V. P.: Treatment of varicose ulcers and their preparation for skin plastic surgery using bacteriostatic hemopaste. Vestn. Khir., *106*:37, 1971 (Russian)

SIRBAN, I. *et al*: On fractures of the upper jaw. Otorinolaringologie, *17*:17, 1972 (Rumanian)

SIRSAT, M. V., SAMPAT, M. B., AND SHRIKHANDE, S. S.: Primary intra-alveolar squamous cell carcinoma of mandible. Report of a case. Oral Surg., *35*:366, 1973

SISIRUCA, H., AND GONZALES, A.: Experience with physiological amputation and immediate prosthesis at University Hospital in Caracas, PRS, *50*:538, 1972. Bol. Soc. Ven. Cir., *25*:1091, 1971

SISLER, H. A.: Wound closure after lacrimal sac surgery. Ann. Ophth., *3*:1357, 1971

SISSON, G. A. *et al*: Branchiogenic cysts within the parotid gland, case report. Arch. Otolaryng., *96:*165, 1972

SISSON, G. A. *et al*: Transsternal radical neck dissection. Postoperative complications and management. Arch. Otolaryng., *101:*46, 1975

SISSON, G. A. *et al*: Voice rehabilitation after laryngectomy—results with hypopharyngeal prosthesis, PRS, *57:*396, 1976. Arch. Otolaryng., *101:*178, 1975

SITKOVSKII, M. B. *et al*: Reconstructive operative interventions in rectovaginal fistulae in girls. Pediatr. Akush. Ginekol., *4:*58, 1972 (Ukrainian)

SIVALOGANATHAN, V.: Surgical management of patients with advanced buccal pouch cancer, PRS, *51:*108, 1973. M. J. Malaya, *26:*116, 1971

SIVALOGANATHAN, V.: Cleft lips in Malaysians, PRS, *49:*176, 1972

SIVALOGANATHAN, V. *et al*: Plastic surgery on elephantiasis of legs: case report. Southeast Asian J. Trop. Med. Public Health, *4:*279, 1973

SIVULA, A., AND SOMER, T.: Mondor's disease, observations on 14 patients and survey of literature, PRS, *54:*117, 1974. Ann. chir. et gynaec. Fenniae, *62:*361, 1973

SIXTH PEOPLE'S HOSPITAL, SHANGHAI: Understanding and progress of replantation of severed limbs and digits, PRS, *51:*703, 1973. Chinese M.J., *1:*1, 1973

SIZER, J. S. *et al*: Digital amputations in diabetic patients. Surgery, *72:*980, 1972

SKALKEAS, G., GOGAS, J., AND PAVLATOS, F.: Mammary hypoplasia following radiation to infant breast, PRS, *52:*679, 1973. Acta chir. plast., *14:*240, 1972

SKALOUD, F. *et al*: Experimental homotransplantation in mandibular defects. Fogorv. Sz., *64:*305, 1971 (Hungarian)

SKAROPOULOS, G. *et al*: Results of surgical treatment of 26 cases of craniostenosis. Rev. Otoneuroophtalmol., *46:*453, 1974 (French)

SKELLY, M. *et al*: Changes in phonatory aspects of glossectomee intelligibility through vocal parameter manipulation. J. Speech Hear. Disord., *37:*379, 1972

SKERIK, S. K. *et al*: Functional evaluation of congenital hand anomalies. Am. J. Occup. Ther., *25:*98, 1971

Skin

Studies made by Russian scientists on skin transplantation (Mirskif). Horm. Metab. Res., *1:*67, 1969 (Russian)

Experimental studies on the blood supply of autologous, free full-skin transplants in the postoperative phase in man (Gloor *et al*). Med. Welt., *21:*967, 1970 (German)

Skin—Cont.

Blood vessels, cutaneous, sympathetic denervation and reinnervation of following surgery. Experimental study on rats by means of histochemical fluorescence method (Palmer), PRS, *49:*472, 1972. Scand. J. Plast. Reconstr. Surg., *4:*93, 1970

Depilatory, preoperative, versus razor preparation, wound infections after (Seropian, Reynolds), PRS, *48:*518, 1971. Am. J. Surg., *121:*251, 1971

Congenital universal alopecia (Podoswa, Laguna, Armendares), PRS, *57:*267, 1976. Dermat. Ibero Lat. Am., *13:*223, 1971

Treatment of wounds with avulsed skin (Tani *et al*). Jap. J. Plast. Reconstr. Surg., *14:*145, 1971 (Japanese)

Skin, human—antibacterial *in vitro*? (Rubin, Bongiovi), PRS, *49:*472, 1972. J. Surg. Res., *11:*321, 1971

Skin, normal and burnt, evaporative water loss from (Lamke), PRS, *49:*665, 1972. Thesis, Dept. Surg., Linkoping Univ., Sweden, 1971

Blood loss and hemostasis in plastic surgery of the skin (Tychinkina *et al*). Vestn. Khir., *107:*94, 1971 (Russian)

Free full skin transplantation by the Corachan method (Anke *et al*). Zentralbl. Chir., *96:*799, 1971 (German)

Skin temperature, thermographic study of wound healing (Viitanen, Viljanto), PRS, *52:*105, 1973. Ann. chir. et gynaec. Fenniae, *60:*101, 1972

Anticoagulant therapy, complication, hemorrhagic necrosis of skin (Von Empel, Smeenk), PRS, *52:*99, 1973. Arch. chir. neerl., *24:*353, 1972

Skin lesions, necrotizing, in heroin addicts (Dunne, Johnson), PRS, *50:*538, 1972. Arch. Dermat., *105:*544, 1972

Tissue adhesives in cutaneous surgery (Wilkinson). Arch. Dermat., *106:*834, 1972

Skin, quantitative histochemical investigations on DNA content of facultatives and obligatory precanceroses of (Ehlers, Stephan), PRS, *51:*107, 1973. Arch. Derm. Forsch., *243:*114, 1972

Stratified squamous skin (Gibson). Brit. J. Plast. Surg., *25:*1, 1972

Closure of rhomboid skin defects: the flaps of Limberg and Dufourmentel (Lester *et al*). Brit. J. Plast. Surg., *25:*300, 1972

Skin trauma in patients receiving systemic corticosteroid therapy (David), PRS, *50:*637, 1972. Brit. M.J., *2:*614, 1972

Skin characteristics of importance to surgeon (Whitaker). Int. Surg., *57:*877, 1972

Lipid of skin, waterholding: ethyl linoleate,

Skin – Cont.

A. The evidence, studies in burns (Jalenko, Wheeler, Scott), PRS, *52:*210, 1973. J. Trauma, *12:*968, 1972

Friction blister (Akers, Sulzberger), PRS, *50:*98, 1972. Mil. Med., *137:*1, 1972

Skin infections in Vietnam (Allen *et al*), PRS, *52:*103, 1973. Mil. Med., *137:*295, 1972

Reticulosis, systemic, of surface of skin, experiences in methodical aphoresis (Mian, Francesconi, Crudeli), PRS, *53:*692, 1974. Minerva dermat., *47:*8, 1972

Experimental studies on tensile strength of healing wound of fascia and muscle (Tukallo *et al*). Pol. Med. J., *11:*939, 1972

Autoradiographic investigations of connective tissue wounds of skin (Helpap, Cremer), PRS, *51:*484, 1973. Res. Exper. Med., *157:*289, 1972

Nonsuture immobilization of skin, studies in (Wilkinson, Rybka, Paletta), PRS, *51:*709, 1973. South. M.J., *65:*25, 1972

The Integument: A Textbook of Skin Biology. By R. I. C. Spearman. Cambridge Univ. Press, London, 1973.

High-power nendymium-YAG laser surgery (Goldman *et al*). Acta Derm. Venereol. (Stockh.), *53:*45, 1973

Skin, normal and scarred, microscopic study of (Sakata), PRS, *53:*610, 1974. Jap. J. Plast. Reconstr. Surg., *16:*412, 1973

Skin, human, as elastic membrane (Danielson), PRS, *53:*375, 1974. J. Bio-Mechanics, *6:*539, 1973

Granuloma, swimming pool, *Mycobacterium marinum* infection of hand (Cortez, Panpey), PRS, *52:*322, 1973. J. Bone & Joint Surg., *55A:*363, 1973

Skin defects, management of. Closure of skin defect by free transplants. Basic principles of application and technique (Bruck). Langenbecks Arch. Chir., *334:*567, 1973 (German)

Skin defects, extremities and trunk, treatment of (Rehn). Lagenbecks Arch. Chir., *334:*609, 1973 (German)

Sunscreen, more effective – PABA (Garcia, Davis), PRS, *53:*114, 1974. Mil. Med., *138:*331, 1973

Skin, histological and histochemical examinations of, after irradiation by ruby laser (Boxduganov *et al*). Radiobiol. Radiother. (Berl.), *14:*703, 1973 (German)

Amino acid composition of normal and pathologic skin (Micali, Scuderi), PRS, *56:*367, 1975. Riv. ital. chir. plast., *5:*573, 1973

Oscillometry, photoelectric, physiological and technical study factors in measurement of skin circulation (Medgyesi), PRS,

Skin – Cont.

*53:*501, 1974. Scand. J. Plast. Reconstr. Surg., *7:*29, 1973

Skin defects, repair of, with autologous skin homogenisate and wound contraction (Gloor *et al*). Z. Hautkr., *48:*755, 1973

Skin strips, use of, in orthopedics (Bezouglis *et al*). Z. Orthop., *111:*617, 1973 (German)

Skin, mechanical properties of (Arion), PRS, *54:*628, 1974. Ann. chir. plast., *19:*37, 1974

Skin, normal human, surface microtopography of (Tring, Murgatroyd), PRS, *54:*382, 1974. Arch. Dermat., *109:*223, 1974

Prostaglandin E_1 effects in epidermal cell growth *in vitro* (Bem, Greaves), PRS, *56:*474, 1975. Arch. Dermat. Forsch., *251:*35, 1974

Chromic acid and chromates, prevention of occupational skin disease by use of ascorbic acid (Samitz), PRS, *54:*371, 1974. Cutis, *13:*569, 1974

Aging skin (AMA Committee on Cutaneous Health and Cosmetics), PRS, *54:*383, 1974. Hospital Med., *10:*72, 1974

Skin viability determination during trauma of limbs (Winninger), PRS, *54:*624, 1974. J. chir., *107:*205, 1974

Ectodermal dysplasia, ocular changes in, case of (Sbaiti). Klin. Monatsbl. Augenheilkd., *164:*267, 1974 (German)

Skin blood pressure, simple method for approximate measurement of (Chavatzas, Jamieson), PRS, *55:*119, 1975. Lancet, *1:*711, 1974

Skin wrinkling in cystic fibrosis (Moynahan), PRS, *56:*356, 1975. Lancet, *2:*907, 1974

Enzyme analysis as test of skin viability (Georgiade, King, O'Fallon), PRS, *53:*67, 1974

Face peeling, chemical, long-term histological study of skin after (Baker *et al*), PRS, *53:*522,1974

Skin tension, new theory regarding lines of (Bulacio Nuñez), PRS, *53:*663, 1974

Face peeling, chemical, histological changes following (Bhangoo) (Letter to the Editor), PRS, *54:*599, 1974

Skin Signs of Systemic Disease. By Irwin M. Braverman. W. B. Saunders, Philadelphia, London, Toronto, 1975. PRS, *57:*657, 1976

Dermis, elastic fibers of, study during plastic surgery of truncus (Mitz, Elbaz, Vilde), PRS, *56:*233, 1975. Ann. chir. plast., *20:*31, 1975

Immunosuppressive and cytotoxic drugs in dermatology (Dantzig), PRS, *57:*768, 1976. Arch. Dermat., *110:*393, 1975

Skin – Cont.

Skin, normal, effect of topical fluorouracil on (Zelickson, Mottaz, Weiss), PRS, *57:*543, 1976. Arch. Dermat., *111:*1301, 1975

Dyes, hair, percutaneous penetration following use of (Maibach, Leaffer, Skinner), PRS, *57:*681, 1976. Arch. Dermat., *111:*1444, 1975

Phenol, decontamination of skin exposed to (Brown), PRS, *56:*114, 1975. Arch. Environmental Health., *30:*1, 1975

Necrosis of skin from cetrimide application (August), PRS, *57:*127, 1976. Brit. M.J., *1:*70, 1975

Allergy to cosmetics, what goes on under make-up (Taub), PRS, *57:*681, 1976. Eye, Ear, Nose, & Throat Month., *54:*278, 1975

Skin temperature measurement, correction factors in (Jirak *et al*), PRS, *57:*127, 1976. J. Appl. Physiol., *38:*752, 1975

Dermatitis, contact, from methylmethacrylate bone cement (Fries *et al*), PRS, *57:*406, 1976. J. Bone & Joint Surg., *57A:*547, 1975

Tissues mechanics (Kenedi *et al*). Phys. Med. Biol., *20:*699, 1975

Estrogen therapy after rhytidectomy, ancillary effects of (Gonzalez-Ulloa) (Letter to the Editor), PRS, *56:*203, 1975

Itch, pharmacology and physiology of (Greaves), PRS, *57:*682, 1976. Proc. Roy. Soc. Med., *68:*529, 1975

Skin cycle, lack of effect of, on survival of experimental skin flaps in rats (Myers, Donovan, Falterman), PRS, *57:*650, 1976

Skin, Congenital Absence of

Cutis, congenital aplasia of, in 3 successive generations (Fisher, Schneider), PRS, *57:*267, 1976. Arch. Dermat., *108:*252, 1973

Congenital absence of skin (aplasia cutis congenita) (Croce, Purohit, Janovski), PRS, *53:*376, 1974. Arch. Surg., *106:*732, 1973

Aplasia cutis congenita (Wright *et al*), PRS, *54:*702, 1974. J. Pediat. Surg., *9:*415, 1974

Skin Diseases

A note on infantile and juvenile leucodermata and their palliative cosmetic treatment (Castellani). Arch. Ital. Sci. Med. Trop. Parassitol., *51:*49, 1970

Noduli cutanei, multiple, and urinary tract anomalies (Selmanowitz, Lerer, Orentreich), PRS, *48:*295, 1971. Cancer, *26:*1256, 1970

Venereal and skin diseases. Literature review 1970–1971. Dtsch. Med. J., *23:* June 10, 1972 (German)

Rifampicin in treatment of cutaneous leish-

Skin Diseases – Cont.

maniasis (Selim, Kandil), PRS, *53:*502, 1974. J. Kuwait M.A., *6:*159, 1972

Dermatophytosis, skin infections in Vietnam (Allen *et al*), PRS, *52:*103, 1973. Mil. Med., *137:*295, 1972

Xeroderma pigmentosa (Pickrell) (Follow-Up Clinic), PRS, *49:*83, 1972

Fibrinolytic activity in lesions of hereditary hemorrhagic telangiectasia (Kwaan, Silverman), PRS, *52:*597, 1973. Arch. Dermat., *107:*571, 1973

Psoriasis on scars (Paslin), PRS, *54:*379, 1974. Arch. Dermat., *108:*665, 1973

Skin, congenital absence of (aplasia cutis congenita) (Croce, Purohit, Janovski), PRS, *53:*376, 1974. Arch. Surg., *106:*732, 1973

Vitiligo, treatment with autologous thin Thiersch's grafts (Behl *et al*). Int. J. Dermatol., *12:*329, 1973

Ascorbic acid to prevent occupational skin diseases from exposure to chromic acid and chromates (Samitz), PRS, *54:*371, 1974. Cutis, *13:*569, 1974

Chromomycosis simulating basal cell carcinoma (Baumal, Hanson, Jeerapaet), PRS, *55:*640, 1975. Cutis, *14:*227, 1974

Lupus erythematosus, systemic, hand in (Bleifeld, Inglis), PRS, *55:*510, 1975. J. Bone & Joint Surg., *56A:*1207, 1974

Axilla: surgical management of familial benign chronic pemphigus (Rigg), PRS, *54:*364, 1974

Usefulness of surgical treatment in some skin diseases (Szmczykowa *et al*). Przegl. Dermatol., *61:*825, 1974 (Polish)

Nodules, benign rheumatoid (Simons, Schaller), PRS, *57:*123,1976. Pediatrics, *56:*29, 1975

Skin Disinfection: See *Scrub, Surgical*

Skin Flaps (See also *Composite Flap; Cross-Arm Flap; Cross-Finger Flap; Cross-Leg Flap; Cross-Lip Flap; Cross-Thigh Flap; Free Flaps; etc.*)

Bipedicled island flaps (Holevich, Paneva-Holevich), PRS, *50:*307, 1972. Acta chir. plast., *13:*106, 1971

Difficult repair of 2 pharyngostomas with modified crosswise flaps (Abbes *et al*). Ann. chir. plast., *16:*247, 1971 (French)

Infrared thermometry in surgical flaps (Karl *et al*). Dtsch. Stomatol., *21:*657, 1971 (German)

Skin flaps in plastic surgery (Bisaggio), PRS, *51:*109, 1973. Folha Med. Brazil, *63:*59, 1971

Skin Flaps — Cont.

50:433, 1972

Flaps, skin grafts and scars, growth in young minipigs (Baran, Horton), PRS, *50:*487, 1972

Compound fractures of tibia: soft tissue defect (Brown). Proc. Roy. Soc. Med., *65:*625, 1972

Preauricular flap to reconstruct earlobe (Pitanguy *et al*), PRS, *51:*602, 1973. Rev. brasil. cir., *62:*51, 1972

Flap, Mustardé, to reconstruct lower limb (Milke), PRS, *53:*368, 1974. Rev. Soc. Med. Cir. San Jose, *5:*83, 1972

Halothane, effect on tissue necrosis in pedicled skin flaps in pigs (Pless, Sondergaard), PRS, *51:*109, 1973. Scand. J. Plast. Reconstr. Surg., *6:*13, 1972

Hernias, large incisional, repair with skin flaps (Medgyesi), PRS, *51:*486, 1973. Scand. J. Plast. Reconstr. Surg., *6:*69, 1972

Flaps, skin influence of stress on survival of experimental. A study on rats. Scand. J. Plast. Reconstr. Surg., *6:*110, 1972

Circulation adequacy, tissue gas levels as index: relation between ischemia and development of collateral circulation (delay phenomenon) (Myers, Cherry, Milton), PRS, *50:*101, 1972. Surgery, *71:*15, 1972

Skin flaps rotated into delayed or primary recipient sites, wound healing of (Hentz *et al*), PRS, *52:*329, 1973. Surg. Forum, *23:*34, 1972

Flaps, arterial experimental (Daniel *et al*). Surg. Forum, *23:*507, 1972

Sickle cell anemia, exchange transfusion for flap surgery in (Ashbell), PRS, *51:*705, 1973. Surg. Forum, *23:*517, 1972

Flaps in rat, distal necrosis of: immediate *vs.* delayed terminal inset (Segarra, Bennett), PRS, *51:*710, 1973. Surg. Forum, *23:*521, 1972

Oral cavity defects, use of tubed flaps in reconstructing (Trichilis), PRS, *52:*450, 1973. Acta chir. Hellenica, *45:*99, 1973

Flap, double Filatov, for large tissue defects in one or both legs and feet (Kenerman), PRS, *53:*689, 1974. Acta chir. plast., *15:*120, 1973

Flap, split, in head and neck reconstruction (Krizek, Robson), PRS, *53:*613, 1974. Am. J. Surg., *126:*488, 1973

Flaps, pectoral skin, cutaneous vascular anatomy of (Calcaterra, Cherney, Saffouri), PRS, *53:*613, 1974. Ann. Otol. Rhin. & Laryng., *82:*691, 1973

Flaps, skin, to reconstruct head and neck region (Lichtfeld, Snow), PRS, *54:*117, 1974. Arch. chir. neerl., *25:*379, 1973

Skin Flaps — Cont.

Forehead flap. Technique and complications (Biller *et al*). Arch. Otolaryng., *97:*316, 1973

Skin flap avulsion of leg due to minor trauma after renal transplantation (Marshall), PRS, *54:*116, 1974. Australian & New Zealand J. Surg., *43:*223, 1973

Flaps, axial pattern, vascular basis of (Smith), PRS, *55:*117, 1975. Brit. J. Plast. Surg., *26:*150, 1973

Flaps, single pedicled, axial and random patterned (McGregor, Morgan), PRS, *55:*118, 1975. Brit. J. Plast. Surg., *26:*202, 1973

Blood supply in flaps, control and measurement (Köhnlein, Ilg), PRS, *52:*597, 1973. Bruns' Beitr. klin. Chir., *220:*313, 1973

Abdominal area, suture method of, after collecting skin flap for mobilization of jaw joint — application of "U" plasty (Shimizu). J. Jap. Stomatol. Soc., *40:*169, 1973 (Japanese)

Our experience with the intermediary flap plastic of Blair-Kettesy (Molnar). Klin. Monatsbl. Augenheilkd., *163:*590, 1973 (Polish)

Graft, sliding, from adjacent skin, fundamentals of utilization and technique of, in covering defects (Willebrand). Langenbecks Arch. Chir., *334:*575, 1973 (German)

Flap circulation, new visual aid: cholesteric liquid crystals (Hoehn, Binkert), PRS, *48:*209, 1973

Pectoro-subaxillary zigzag flap (Penn, Penn), PRS, *51:*27, 1973

Flap, experimental pedicle, studies on the action of dimethyl sulfoxide on (Adamson) (Follow-Up Clinic), PRS, *51:*88, 1973

Flap viability, bromphenol blue in assay of rheomacrodex effects in (Goulian) (Follow-Up Clinic), PRS, *51:*206, 1973

Flap, will a wider have a greater viable length? (McDowell) (Editorial), PRS, *52:*76, 1973

Reverse dermal-fat flap: alternative cross-leg flap (Clodius, Smahel), PRS, *52:*85, 1973

Thermography, infrared, viability prediction in pedicle flaps by (Bloomenstein) (Follow-Up Clinic), PRS, *52:*185, 1973

Plantar flap to repair lesions of heel (Mir y Mir), PRS, *53:*498, 1974. Rev. españ. cir. plast., *6:*89, 1973

Skin flaps, pedicled, improving circulation in (Coiffman), PRS, *55:*518, 1975. Rev. Latino Am. cir. plast., *17:*21, 1973

Skin flaps, local and regional, in head and neck surgery (Jarrett *et al*). Rocky Mt. Med. J., *70:*51, 1973

Flap, skin, photoplethysmography of (Cher-

Skin Flaps – Cont.

geshtav). Stomatologiia, 52:20, 1973

Reconstructive experience with the medially based deltopectoral flap (Park et al). Am. J. Surg., 128:548, 1974

Thermography, value in assessment of skin grafts and flaps (Abbes, Demard, Aubanel), PRS, 55:642, 1975. Ann. chir. plast., 19:325, 1974

Flap, large rotational, for neck dissection and facial skin replacement (Smith et al). Arch. Otolaryng., 99:122, 1974

Flaps, local arterial, to reconstruct lip defects (Karapandzic), PRS, 56:676, 1975. Brit. J. Plast. Surg., 27:93, 1974

Flaps, leg, local delayed (Bowen, Meares), PRS, 56:683, 1975. Brit. J. Plast. Surg., 27:167, 1974

Flap, triangular cervical, for primary reconstruction of oropharyngeal surgical defects (Poisson, Franchebois), PRS, 54:500, 1974. Canad. J. Surg., 17:167, 1974

Trauma, determination of skin viability after (Winninger), PRS, 54:624, 1974. J. chir., 107:205, 1974

Flap delays, pedicled, timing by measurements of flap oxygen and carbon dioxide (Reisin, Guthrie, Goulian), PRS, 56:365, 1975. J. Surg. Oncol., 6:79, 1974

Healing of lined and unlined parasitic and nonparasitic flaps (Whitaker et al). J. Surg. Oncol., 6:511, 1974

Otolaryngology, reconstructive flaps in (McFarland). Laryngoscope, 84:1267, 1974

Cancer, breast, transverse abdominal flap for reconstruction after radical operations (Tai, Hasegawa), PRS, 53:52, 1974

Flap, rotational: V-Y-S-plasty for closure of round defect (Argamaso), PRS, 53:99, 1974

Skin flap viability, intravenous fluorescein test as measure of (Thorvaldsson, Grabb), PRS, 53:576, 1974

Flap rotation, repair for small defects of helix of ear (Elsahy), PRS, 53:598,1974

Flaps, local triangular, for closure of axillary hidradenitis defects (Lipshutz), PRS, 53:677, 1974

Pulp, fingertip, restoration of sensation with dorsolateral island flap after injury (Joshi), PRS, 54:175, 1974

Vascularization: augmentation of wound strength by pretreatment with epinephrine (Myers, Rightor), PRS, 54:201, 1974. Discussion by Weeks, PRS, 54:351, 1974

Skin flap survival, effect of local anesthesia with epinephrine on (Reinisch, Myers), PRS, 54:324, 1974

Limberg and Dufourmental flaps, further application of (Jervis et al), PRS, 54:335, 1974

Skin Flaps – Cont.

Skin flap survival in the dog, relationship of hematocrit levels to (Earle, Fratianne, Nunez), PRS, 54:341, 1974

Flaps: tissue transfers for functional reconstruction in thoracic surgery (Cervino, Bales, Emerson), PRS, 54:437, 1974

Skin flap circulation, pathophysiology of (Reinisch), PRS, 54:585, 1974

Arm flap repair of extensive thoracic wall defect (Farina), PRS, 54:680, 1974

Flaps, skin, influence of varying pressure and duration of treatment with hyperbaric oxygen on survival (Jurell, Kaijser), PRS, 54:701, 1974. Scand. J. Plast. Reconstr. Surg., 7:25, 1974

Flaps, vomer, skin graft to, in cleft palate cases (Stenström, Thilander), PRS, 56:682, 1975. Scand. J. Plast. Reconstr. Surg., 8:67, 1974

Repair with Filatov's flap in defects and deformations of the oral region (Shipacheva). Vestn. Khir., 113:65, 1974 (Russian)

Flaps, dermal, used to treat protruding ears (Elsahy), PRS, 57:755, 1976. Acta chir. plast., 17:71, 1975

Flaps, abdominal, dermo-dermal uniting (Lalardrie et al), PRS, 57:258, 1976. Ann. chir. plast., 20:183, 1975

Use of the Doppler ultrasonic flowmeter for pedicle flaps (Davis et al). Ann. Otol. Rhin. & Laryng., 84:213, 1975

Silicone elastomer sheeting in development of pedicled flaps (Guthrie et al), PRS, 57:404, 1976. Arch. Otolaryng., 101:89, 1975

Flap, tongue, to reconstruct after cancer of oral cavity (Sessions, Dedo, Ogura), PRS, 57:395, 1976. Arch. Otolaryng., 101:166, 1975

Blood flow measurements in skin flaps (Nathanson, Jackson), PRS, 57:265, 1976. Arch. Otolaryng., 101:354, 1975

The viability of triangular skin flaps (Stell et al). Brit. J. Plast. Surg., 28:247, 1975

Temperature measurement, skin, correction factors in (Jirak et al), PRS, 57:127, 1976. J. Appl. Physiol., 38:752, 1975

Flaps, pedicled skin, in oral cavity, clinical and histological late findings (Rehrmann, Blessing, Reil), PRS, 57:540, 1976. J. Maxillo-facial Surg., 3:155, 1975

Defatting the pendulous flap, one stage correction (Kiehn et al), PRS, 55:33, 1975

Arteriovenous axis flap to protect femoral vessels (D'Hooghe, Hendrickx), PRS, 55:87, 1975

Dorsalis pedis arterialized flap (McGraw, Furlow), PRS, 55:177, 1975

Skin Flaps—Cont.

Cutaneous circulation: deltopectoral flap: anatomical and hemodynamic approach (Daniel, Cunningham, Taylor), PRS, *55:*276, 1975

Transverse abdominal flaps and the deep epigastric arcade (Brown, Vasconez, Jurkiewicz), PRS, *55:*416, 1975

Arteriovenous shunting, is it the correct explanation of flap delay phenomenon? (Freshwater) (Letter to the Editor), PRS, *55:*697, 1975

Flap, deltoscapular (Doldan, Shatkin), PRS, *55:*708, 1975

Flaps, skin, toward anatomical and hemodynamic classification of (Daniel) (Letter to the Editor), PRS, *56:*330, 1975

Flap: goodbye to the term "length-to-width ratio" (Grabb) (Letter to the Editor), PRS, *56:*330, 1975

Defect, large chest wall, one-stage coverage with giant bipedicled flap (LeWinn, Guthrie, Kovachev), PRS, *56:*336, 1975

Flap, cross-foot (Taylor, Hopson), PRS, *55:*677, 1975. Discussion by Cannon, PRS, *56:*83, 1975

Flap, chin, to reconstruct lower lip (Tomasoni), PRS, *57:*756, 1976 (Italian). Riv. ital. chir. plast., *7:*403, 1975

Skin Flaps. By William C. Grabb and M. Bert Myers. Little, Brown & Co., Boston, 1976

Flaps, local, rotated to repair forehead defects (Worthen), PRS, *57:*204, 1976

Groin flap for coverage of foot and ankle defects in children (Furnas), PRS, *57:*246, 1976

Flap, auriculo-mastoid, earlobe construction with (Brent), PRS, *57:*389, 1976

Limb, lower, use of fascio-muscle flaps to repair defects of (Robbins), PRS, *57:*460, 1976

Skin flaps in rats, experimental, lack of effect of skin cycle on survival of (Myers, Donovan, Falterman), PRS, *57:*650, 1976

Skin tension lines in domestic pig (Rose, Ksander, Vistnes), PRS, *57:*729, 1976

Skin Flaps, Compound: See *Composite Flap*

Skin Flaps, Deltopectoral

Deltopectoral flap, modified used in secondary esophagoplasty after pharyngolaryngectomy (Jackson, Lang), PRS, *48:*155, 1971

Reconstruction surgery of the esophagus with deltopectoral flap (Lammli *et al*).

Skin Flaps, Deltopectoral—Cont.

Pract. Otorhinolaryngol. (Basel), *33:*11, 1971 (German)

Bipedicled deltopectoral flap and Ticonium prosthesis in reconstruction of lower jaw area (Wurlitzer, Ballantyne), PRS, *49:*220, 1972

Deltopectoral flap, complications with the (Gingrass *et al*), PRS, *49:*501, 1972

Deltopectoral flap, potential pitfalls in the use of (Krizek, Robson), PRS, *50:*326, 1972

Head and neck cancer, radiated, deltopectoral flap for reconstruction (Krizek, Robson), PRS, *52:*105, 1973. Surg. Gynec. & Obst., *135:*787, 1972

Reconstructive experience with the medially based deltopectoral flap (Park *et al*). Am. J. Surg., *128:*548, 1974

Head and neck cancer, deltopectoral flap for reconstruction in (Pradier *et al*), PRS, *54:*626, 1974. Rev. argent. cir., *26:*32, 1974

Deltopectoral flap: anatomical and hemodynamic approach (Daniel, Cunningham, Taylor), PRS, *55:*276, 1975

Deltopectoral dermal-fat flap, free, microvascular transfer of (Fujino, Tanino, Sugimoto), PRS, *55:*428, 1975

Neck: deltoscapular flap (Doldan, Shatkin), PRS, *55:*708, 1975

Deltopectoral flap: secondary reconstruction of cervical esophagus (Petty, Theogaraj, Cohen), PRS, *56:*70, 1975

Skin Flaps to Face

Bipedicled V-Y flap technique for primary repair of lower lip defects (Hollmann), PRS, *48:*391, 1971. Acta chir. plast. *12:*223, 1970

Cutler-Beard bridge flap, an upside-down (Hecht), PRS, *48:*293, 1971. Arch Ophth., *84:*760, 1970

Deltopectoral flap (Lore, Zingapan), PRS, *49:*477, 1972. Arch. Otolaryng., *94:*13, 1971

Flaps, subcutaneous, in facial surgery (Albertengo, Abriata), PRS, *51:*710, 1973. An. cir., *37:*20, 1972

Nose, skin defects, one stage reconstruction with local flaps (Lejour), PRS, *52:*205, 1973. Chir. Plast., *1:*254, 1972

Flap, retroauricular temporal, further experience with (Washio), PRS, *50:*160, 1972

Neck to cheek rotation flaps (Stark, Kaplan), PRS, *50:*230, 1972

Face and neck, rapid transfer of thoracoacromial flaps (Pollock, Bitseff, Ryan), PRS, *50:*433, 1972

Deltopectoral flap for reconstruction of radiated cancer of head and neck (Krizek,

Skin Flaps to Hand — Cont.

Nakamura), PRS, *54:*286, 1974

Flap for soft tissue replacement on distal segment of thumb, rotation-transposition method (Argamaso), PRS, *54:*366, 1974

Flap, groin, resurfacing hand injuries with (Nickell), PRS, *54:*690, 1974. South. M.J., *67:*567, 1974

Flap, abdominal, in surgery of hand (Baudet, Lemaire), PRS, *57:*265, 1976. Ann. chir. plast., *20:*215, 1975

Flaps, vascular, in secondary surgery after hand trauma (Vilain, Mitz), PRS, *56:*596, 1975. Hand, *7:*56, 1975

Flap, pendulous, one stage correction (Kiehn *et al*), PRS, *55:*33, 1975

Flaps, adjacent, from opposing body surfaces, hand sandwich (Smith, Furnas), PRS, *57:*351, 1976

Skin Flaps, Homoplastic (Parabiosis)

Homotransplantation of skin flaps in dogs by microvascular technique, rejection phenomena after (Harashina *et al*), PRS, *52:*390, 1973

Skin Flaps, Island

Island pedicles, neurovascular cutaneous, for deficient median nerve sensibility (Omer *et al*), PRS, *49:*104, 1972. J. Bone & Joint Surg., *52A:*1181, 1970

Island flaps, bipedicled (Holevich, Paneva-Holevich), PRS, *50:*307, 1972. Acta chir. plast., *13:*106, 1971

Island flaps, neurovascular (Lievano), PRS, *49:*471, 1972. Rev. Latino Am. cir. plast., *15:*33, 1971

Flaps, island, vascular pedicle, survival of (Salyer *et al*). Surg. Forum, *23:*505, 1972

Island pedicle flap in thumb and index finger injuries (Sullivan) (Follow-Up Clinic), PRS, *51:*208, 1973

Flap, island, extended neurovascular, in thumb reconstruction (Storvik), PRS, *54:*503, 1974. Scand. J. Plast. Reconstr. Surg., *7:*147, 1973

Flap, large island, to reconstruct skin defects of cheek (Lejour), PRS, *56:*473, 1975. Acta chir. belg., *74:*183, 1975

Skin Flaps, Jump

Experience of reconstruction of the head with a giant jump flap (Fukuda). Jap. J. Plast. Reconstr. Surg., *15:*203, 1972 (Japanese)

Flaps, open jump, in repair of massive soft tissue defects (Morgan, Zbylski), PRS, *50:*265, 1972

Flap, abdominal, for orbital recostruction

Skin Flaps, Jump — Cont.

after radical resection (Habal, Murray), PRS, *52:*205, 1973. Arch. Surg., *106:*353, 1973

Skin Flaps, Subcutaneous Pedicle

De-epithelized flap, buried, 20-year follow-up of a patient with hemifacial atrophy treated by (Converse, Betson), PRS, *48:*278, 1971

Dermal flaps, treatment of facial paralysis by static suspension with (Guerrero-Santos, Ramirez, Espaillat), PRS, *48:*325, 1971

Facial surgery, subcutaneous pedicle flaps in (Albertengo, Abriata), PRS, *51:*710, 1973. An. cir., *37:*20, 1972

Dermal flaps, use of, for attachment of rhytidoplasty flaps (Cameron *et al*), PRS, *51:*596, 1973

Nasolabial subcutaneous flap (Grate, Hicks), PRS, *53:*613, 1974. South. M.J., *66:*1234, 1973

Face, flaps on, subcutaneous pedicled (Spira, Gerow, Hardy), PRS, *56:*676, 1975. Brit. J. Plast. Surg., *27:*258, 1974

Flap, buried dermal, for lymphedema of limbs (Sawhney), PRS, *56:*680, 1975. Brit. J. Plast. Surg., *27:*278, 1974

Flap, de-epithelialized hypogastric, to protect femoral vessels (D'Hooghe, Hendrickx), PRS, *55:*87, 1975

Skin Flaps, Tubed

Skin tube constructor, hand (Arai, Fukuda), PRS, *49:*240, 1972. Jap. J. Plast. Reconstr. Surg., *14:*330, 1971

Vascularization of tubed pedicle, experimental study on (Yano), PRS, *50:*310, 1972. Otorhinolaryng. Tokyo, *14:*471, 1971

Tubed flap in palate repair (Evans), PRS, *48:*395, 1971. Proc. Roy. Soc. Med., *64:*73, 1971

Flap, tubed abdominal, primary application of one-stage (Li *et al*), PRS, *51:*232, 1973. Hand, *4:*184, 1972

Abdominal-thoracic round pedicle graft (Schneider). Helv. Chir. Acta, *39:*335, 1972 (German)

Tubed flap, small, for cylindrical defects in leg; "cork" procedure (Hagstrom, Brown, Landa), PRS, *49:*224, 1972

Tissue respiration of Filatov's pedicled graft at various stages of plastic operations (Neupokoev). Stomatologiia (Mosk.), *51:*11, 1972 (Russian)

Flaps, tubed, in reconstructing defects of oral cavity (Trichilis), PRS, *52:*450, 1973. Acta chir. Hellenica, *45:*99, 1973

Skin Flaps, Tubed — Cont.

Legs and feet, large tissue defects in one or both, use of double Filatov flap for (Kenerman), PRS, *53:*689, 1974. Acta chir. plast., *15:*120, 1973

Tubed flaps, on lack of any effect of gravity on survival of (Myers, Cherry, Bombet), PRS, *51:*428, 1973

Flap, tubed, abdominal skin-lined, permanent cutaneous cystostomy by interposition of a (Ship) (Follow-Up Clinic), PRS, *52:*298, 1973

Pedicles, tubed, review of 196 (Stranc *et al*). Brit. J. Plast. Surg., *28:*54, 1975

Skin Grafts

Skin transplantation and skin substitutes (Kohnlein). Langenbecks Arch. Chir., *327:*1090, 1970 (German)

Die Freien Hauttransplantationen. By Fritz Andina. Springer Verlag, Berlin, Heidelberg, New York, 1970. PRS, *48:*176, 1971

Re-vascularisation of a free skin autograft (Lily). Acta Chir. Acad. Sci. Hung., *12:*181, 1971

Covering of old and infected losses of the skin surface (Bazant *et al*). Acta Chir. Orthop. Traumatol. Cech., *38:*230, 1971 (Czechoslovakian)

Head and neck surgery, delayed skin grafting in (Jackson), PRS, *50:*99, 1972. Acta chir. plast., *13:*16, 1971

Clinical and ultrastructural study of fragmented skin grafts (Colson *et al*). Ann. chir. plast., *16:*299, 1971 (French)

Epidermal grafting (Falabella), PRS, *50:*100, 1972. Arch. Dermat., *104:*592, 1971

Free skin grafts on the parietal pleura: report of a case (Butters *et al*). Brit. J. Plast. Surg., *24:*412, 1971

Skin cover in hand injuries (Bailey), PRS, *48:*606, 1971. Injury, *2:*294, 1971

Open skin grafting for granulation wounds (Fukuda *et al*). Jap. J. Plast. Reconstr. Surg., *14:*183, 1971 (Japanese)

Skin grafting of burns: a centennial. A tribute to George David Pollock (Freshwater *et al*). J. Trauma, *11:*862, 1971

Enzyme therapy as a method of preparing trophic ulcers and protractedly nonhealing wounds for dermato-autoplasty (Grigorian *et al*). Klin. Khir., *9:*1, 1971 (Russian)

pH measurement in transplantation of skin autografts (Glinz), PRS, *48:*518, 1971. Med. & Hygiene, *955:*437, 1971

Effects of 5-fluorouracil on skin-graft survival (Kerry *et al*). Ohio State Med. J., *67:*1093, 1971

Treatment of chronic osteomyelitis by sau-

Skin Grafts — Cont.

cerization and skin grafting (Evans). Proc. Roy. Soc. Med., *64:*1204, 1971

Isotopic measurement of collagen turnover in skin grafts (Rudolph *et al*). Surg. Forum, *22:*489, 1971

Facial plastic surgery with a rotation fatcutaneous graft (Mukhin). Vestn. Khir., *107:*46, 1971 (Russian)

Subcutaneous tissue infiltration as an adjunct to split-thickness skin grafting (Silverstein *et al*). Am. J. Surg., *123:*624, 1972

Epidermoid cyst after a total skin graft for eventration (Nini *et al*). Chirurgie, *98:*50, 1972 (French)

Simple method to facilitate free skin grafts (Ottolenghi). G. Ital. Dermatol., *47:*4, 1972 (Italian)

Versatile skin-grafting technique. Geriatrics, *27:*68, 1972

Free skin graft, primary, in head and neck surgery. Practical course of regional, plastic and constructive surgery. Basic considerations, technique and indication (Nagel). H.N.O., *20:*319, 1972 (German)

Free skin transplantation with local use of glucocorticoids (Vasil'ev *et al*). Khirurgiia (Mosk.), *49:*13, 1972 (Russian)

Skin plastic surgery in scar contractures of the neck following burns (Dmitriev *et al*). Ortop. Travmatol. Protez., *33:*7, 1972 (Russian)

Skin transplantation under ambulatory conditions (Klassen *et al*). Ortop. Travmatol. Protez., *33:*15, 1972 (Russian)

Epithelial cells, living, implanted into the subcutis, fate of (Ben Hur) (Follow-Up Clinic), PRS, *49:*455, 1972

Testes, totally denuded, dermatome grafting (Campbell) (Follow-Up Clinic), PRS, *50:*280, 1972

Steroids, skin grafting in systemic lupus erythematosus patients who are on (Tuerk), PRS, *50:*382, 1972

Doughnut skin graft for orbital lining (Hébert) (Follow-Up Clinic), PRS, *50:*402, 1972

Palmar areas of hand grafted with plantar skin of feet (Pera Erro), PRS, *53:*248, 1974. Rev. españ. cir. plast., *5:*175, 1972

Skin grafts, ^{3}H-collagen turnover in (Klein, Rudolph), PRS, *51:*352, 1973. Surg. Gynec. & Obst., *135:*49, 1972

Specificity of free skin graft of the face (Ito). Surg. Ther. (Osaka), *26:*515, 1972 (Japanese)

Skin grafting in ulcerating "cancer en cuirasse" — case report (Gruner). Acta Chir. Scand., *139:*492, 1973

Neck, burned, devices for preventing con-

Skin Grafts—Cont.

tractures after secondary repair (Colin, Janvier), PRS, *54:*113, 1974. Ann. chir. plast., *18:*15, 1973

Skin grafts, recipient areas for, studies of metabolic activity after tangential excision of burns (Lawrence, Carney), PRS, *54:*695, 1974. Brit. J. Plast. Surg., *26:*93, 1973

Skin cover, protection of damaged tissue by (Lawrence, Stone), PRS, *54:*696, 1974. Brit. J. Plast. Surg., *26:*101, 1973

Skin grafts, cutting without anesthesia: case of familial dysautonomia (Goldin *et al*). Brit. J. Plast. Surg., *26:*184, 1973

Graft conditioning with non-specific ribonucleic acid (Lerf), PRS, *52:*463, 1973. Bruns' Beitr. klin. Chir., *220:*206, 1973

Autologous skin homogenizate to treat chronic and acute skin defects (Klein, Kohler), PRS, *52:*461, 1973. Bruns' Beitr. klin. Chir., *220:*214, 1973

Psoriasis in autologous grafts (Haneke). Dermatol. Monatsschr., *159:*227, 1973 (German)

Revascularization of skin autografts (Lessa *et al*), PRS, *53:*112, 1974. Folha Med. Brazil, *66:*17, 1973

Skin, free transplants, selection of transplantation thickness in (Ganzoni *et al*). Helv. Chir. Acta, *40:*267, 1973 (German)

Graft, tension releasing, to extensive burn scar on face (Matsumoto *et al*), PRS, *53:*607, 1974. J. Jap. Accident Med. Assoc., *21:*329, 1973

Skin graft survival, predicting (Robson, Krizek), PRS, *52:*330, 1973. J. Trauma, *13:*213, 1973

Skin grafting of exposed arterial vein grafts: clinical and experimental study (Gingrass, Cunningham, Paletta), PRS, *53:*689, 1974. J. Trauma, *13:*951, 1973

Dermatoplasty (Khristich *et al*). Khirurgiia (Mosk.), *49:*122, 1973 (Russian)

Grafts or flaps, inside nose, internal nasal mold, made of silicone rubber, for (Shuster), PRS, *52:*203, 1973

Hypothenar region as donor area for lesions of fingertip volar surface (Badim *et al*), PRS, *53:*498, 1974. Rev. brasil. cir., *62:*163, 1973

Grafting, partial-thickness, for fingertip injuries (Nelson), PRS, *55:*510, 1975. Rev. Latino Am. cir. plast., *17:*47, 1973

Skin grafts, healing processes in (Rudolph, Klein), PRS, *53:*498, 1974. Surg. Gynec. & Obst., *136:*641, 1973

Skin graft, split, use of in formation of frontonasal anastomosis (Shinbirev *et al*). Vestn. Otorinolaringol., *35:*13, 1973 (Russian)

Skin Grafts—Cont.

Skin, reparative regeneration of, derivative neoformation in (Khanin *et al*). Zh. Eksp. Klin. Med., *13:*8, 1973 (Russian)

Graft, "SITO," in treatment of faulty stumps of lower limb (Serenkova), PRS, *54:*626, 1974. Acta chir. plast., *16:*16, 1974

Revascularization of free skin grafts in dependence on recipient bed (Brozman), PRS, *55:*643, 1975. Acta chir. plast., *16:*136, 1974

Topical refrigeration analgesia for skin transplantation in patients with burns (Magierski). Anaesth. Resusc. Intensive Ther., *2:*77, 1974

Grafts and flaps, skin, value of thermography in assessment (Abbes, Demard, Aubanel), PRS, *55:*642, 1975. Ann. chir. plast., *19:*325, 1974

Autografts, new method for covering large surface area wounds. I. *In vitro* multiplication of rabbitskin epithelial cells (Freeman *et al*), PRS, *55:*114, 1975. II. Surgical application of tissue culture expanded rabbitskin autografts (Igel *et al*), PRS, *55:*114, 1975. Arch. Surg., *108:*721, 724, 1974

Skin grafting (Zani), PRS, *55:*725, 1975. Ars Curandi, *7:*49, 1974

Finger resurfacing by multiple subcutaneous pedicle or louvre flaps (Emmett), PRS, *56:*683, 1975. Brit. J. Plast. Surg., *27:*370, 1974

Head and neck surgery, delayed skin grafting in (Beekhuis), PRS, *54:*625, 1974. J. Maxillo-facial Surg., *2:*3, 1974

Free total transplantation in lid surgery (Neubauer). Klin. Monatsbl. Augenheilkd., *165:*86, 1974 (German)

Principles of reconstructive operations on the face using flaps and free grafts (Haas). Laryngol. Rhinol. Otol. (Stuttg.), *53:*371, 1974 (German)

Use of skin grafts. M. J. Australia, *1:*121, 1974

Granulating wound, method of "transfers" in free skin transplantation on (Kovinskii *et al*). Ortop. Travmatol. Protez., *35:*85, 1974 (Russian)

Skin grafting and muscle transposition to cover exposed bone (Vasconez, Bostwick, McCraw), PRS, *53:*526, 1974

Skin grafts, effect of various methods of postoperative procedures aiming at healing (Kobus). Pol. Przegl. Chir., *46:*723, 1974 (Polish)

Grafting, primary and delayed split-skin, effect on wound contraction (Stone, Madden), PRS, *57:*765, 1976. Surg. Forum, *25:*41, 1974

Collagen loss, radioactive, from skin grafts

Skin Grafts—Cont.

(Rudolph, Klein), PRS, *55:*114, 1975. Surg. Gynec. & Obst., *138:*55, 1974

Future of constructive surgery (Russell). Transplant Proc., *6:*147, 1974

Simplified method of skin transplantation (D'Hooghe, Hendrickx), PRS, *57:*766, 1976. Acta chir. belg., *5:*500, 1975

Skin autotransplantation in burned patients, appraisal of prognostic significance of various factors (Shalimov *et al*), PRS, *57:*762, 1976. Acta chir. plast., *17:*42, 1975

Laryngotracheal stenosis, repair of extended (Friedman, Billar, Som), PRS, *57:*759, 1976. Arch. Otolaryng., *101:*152, 1975

Skin graft, free, relay transplantation, new method of expanding (Smahel *et al*). Brit. J. Plast. Surg., *28:*49, 1975

Aspergillus infection in skin transplantation and its therapy (Bauer *et al*). Chirurg., *46:*279, 1975 (German)

Skin grafting: contemporary concepts and applications (Leis *et al*). J. Am. Osteopath. Assoc., *74:*631, 1975

Grafting, free skin (Huffstadt), PRS, *57:*125, 1976. Nederl. tijdschr. geneesk., *119:*589, 1975

Skin graft survival on avascular defects (Gingrass, Grabb, Gingrass), PRS, *55:*65, 1975

Graft, functional, of heel (Mir y Mir) (Follow-Up Clinic), PRS, *55:*702, 1975

Feet, plantar lichen planus, treatment by excision and skin grafting (King, Karkowski, Miller), PRS, *56:*668, 1975

Skin Grafts, Accordion or *Sieve:* See *Skin Grafts, Meshed*

Skin Grafts, Delayed

Skin grafting, delayed, in head and neck surgery (Jackson), PRS, *50:*99, 1972. Acta chir. plast., *13:*16, 1971

Skin grafting, delayed, in head and neck surgery (Beekhuis), PRS, *54:*625, 1974. J. Maxillo-facial Surg., *2:*3, 1974

Delayed exposed skin grafting in surgery for breast cancer and melanoma (Rees *et al*). Clin. Oncol., *1:*131, 1975

Skin grafts, delayed, method to keep dressing moist prior to (Jackson), PRS, *56:*347, 1975

Skin Grafts, Donor Sites

Donor site treatment, controlled trial with Fucidin gauze (Johansen, Sorensen), PRS, *51:*109, 1973. Scand. J. Plast. Reconstr. Surg., *6:*47, 1972

Skin graft donor sites, biological dressings

Skin Grafts, Donor Sites—Cont.

for (Salisbury *et al*), PRS, *52:*456, 1973. Arch. Surg., *106:*705, 1973

Hemostatic agent as definitive dressing in management of donor sites in partial thickness skin grafting (Hagstrom) (Follow-Up Clinic), PRS, *51:*89, 1973

Skin graft donor site as model for evaluation of hemostatic agents (Wilkinson, Tenery, Zufi), PRS, *51:*541, 1973

Silastic sheet dressings, effect of, on healing split-skin graft donor sites (Harris, Filarski, Hector), PRS, *52:*189, 1973

Donor sites, painless (Koonin, Melmed), PRS, *54:*697, 1974. South African M. J., *47:*2241, 1973

Forearm as donor site for split-skin grafts (Xavier, Lamb), PRS, *56:*465, 1975. Hand, *6:*243, 1974

Skin of healed superficial burns used as donor site for split-skin grafts (Mariani), PRS, *57:*191, 1976

Skin Grafts, Dressings for

Comparative pathomorphological characteristics of methods of accelerated fixation of free skin grafts (Samokhvalov *et al*). Ortop. Travmatol. Protez., *32:*81, 1971 (Russian)

Significance of the duration of pressure bandage for the result of autologous, free, full-skin transplantation. Experimental studies in guinea pigs (Gloor *et al*). Dermatol. Monatsschr., *158:*190, 1972 (German)

Tissue adhesive spray in skin grafting (Matsumoto, De Laurentis, Morello), PRS, *53:*113, 1974. Internat. Surg., *57:*978, 1972

Skin grafts on small animals, internal stent for securing (Bryant), PRS, *52:*106, 1973. J. Surg. Res., *13:*241, 1972

Our experience of fixing free skin grafts by overlap with cyacrin (Andruson *et al*). Ortop. Travmatol. Protez., *33:*58, 1972 (Russian)

Sutureless fixation of grafts in free skin plastic surgery (literature review) (Andruson *et al*). Ortop. Travmatol. Protez., *33:*78, 1972 (Russian)

Immobilization of extremities after skin grafting with inflatable splint (Schwager, Imber), PRS, *57:*523, 1976

Skin Grafts, Full-Thickness

Naso-labial full thickness graft (Beare *et al*). Brit. J. Plast. Surg., *25:*315, 1972

Skin grafts, free, full thickness, revascularization of (Gloor *et al*). Arch. Dermatol. Forsch., *246:*211, 1973

Skin grafts, full-thickness, for closure of de-

Skin Grafts, Full-Thickness—Cont.
fects in radiation-damaged skin (Andra), PRS, *54:*625, 1974. J. Maxillo-facial Surg., *2:*9, 1974

Full-thickness skin graft, innervated, to restore sensibility to fingertips and heels (Maquieira), PRS 53:568, 1974

Skin Grafts, Growth of
Growth potential of grafts, flaps, and tubes (Baran *et al*). Surg. Forum, *22:*481, 1971

Skin grafts, flaps, and scars, growth of, in young minipigs (Baran, Horton), PRS, *50:*487, 1972

Grafts, free skin, growth of (Iso), PRS, *53:*371, 1974. Jap. J. Plast. Reconstr. Surg., *16:*265, 1973

Skin Grafts, Homografts and Heterografts
Skin grafts and rejection phenomenon (Aguirre), PRS, *52:*329, 1973. Rev. Latino Am. cir. plast., *14:*17, 1970

Skin allografts in rats with extensive skin loss (Holta, Ballantyne, Converse), PRS, *49:*478, 1972. Scand. J. Plast. Reconstr. Surg., *4:*89, 1970

Homograft rejection, effect on wound healing (Kim *et al*), PRS, *48:*202, 1971. Surg. Gynec. & Obst., *131:*495, 1970

Inhibition of skin allograft rejection by anti-lymphocytic serum pretreatment of the donor. Immunological preparation of the graft (Petranyi *et al*). Acta Med. Acad. Sci. Hung., *28:*155, 1971

Use of cutaneous homografts in severely burned patients (Faguer *et al*). Ann. Chir., *25:*919, 1971 (French)

Cell-mediated and humoral mechanisms in allograft and xenograft skin rejection (Hamilton *et al*). Brit. J. Surg., *58:*858, 1971

Skin graft, successful, on renal allograft (Wu, Gault, MacLean), PRS, *48:*97, 1971. Canad. J. Surg., *14:*80, 1971

Supplement to the cutaneous homograft case report presented in 1950 (Caby). Chirurgie, *97:*722, 1971 (French)

Wide use of skin allografts (Giladi *et al*). Harefuah, *80:*594, 1971 (Hebrew)

Skin allografts in leprosy, prolonged survival of (Hans, Weiser, Kau), PRS, *51:*611, 1973. Internat. J. Leprosy, *39:*1, 1971

Rejection of allografts prevented by use of "Trasicor" (Ageeb *et al*), PRS, *52:*463, 1973. Kasr el Fini J. Surg., *12:*10, 1971

Evaluation of homotransplantation of skin preserved by lyophilization and freezing (Donetskii *et al*). Khirurgiia (Mosk.), *47:*22, 1971 (Russian)

Experience in the use of ALS and ALG for

Skin Grafts, Homografts and Heterografts—Cont.
prolonging the viability of skin grafts in burn patients (Spasokukotskii *et al*). Klin. Khir., *10:*31, 1971

Xenotransplantation as biologic dressing in severe burns (Bohmert *et al*), PRS, *48:*516, 1971. Med. & Hygiene, *955:*438, 1971

Treatment of skin defects by dermo-epidermal homografts in children (Radlowska *et al*). Pol. Tyg. Lek., *26:*1820, 1971 (Polish)

Homografts, cadaver (Hackett), PRS, *50:*202, 1972. Proc. Roy. Soc. Med., *64:*1291, 1971

Skin grafts, role in organ grafting (Lagrot, Micheau, Costagliola), PRS, *48:*613, 1971. Rev. españ. cir. plast., *4:*57, 1971

Skin homografts in epidermolysis bullosa (Castro Fariña), PRS, *48:*611, 1071. Rev. españ. cir. plast., *4:*109, 1971

Skin allograft contemporaneous with heart transplant (Psillakis *et al*), PRS, *52:*603, 1973. Rev. paulista med., *78:*63, 1971

Corticosteroids applied topically as pretreatment of rabbit skin allografts (Klaue, Jolley), PRS, *49:*362, 1972. Surgery, *70:*718, 1971

Cyclophosphamide-induced immunologic tolerance to skin homografts (Nirmul *et al*). Surg. Forum, *22:*287, 1971

Platelet activity in allograft rejection (Coburn *et al*). Surg. Forum, *22:*476, 1971

Skin allografts, inhibiting collagen cross-linking on survival of (Weiner, Happel, Madden), PRS, *50:*99, 1972. Surg. Forum, *22:*486, 1971

Skin homografts in man prolonged by use of anti-lymphoblast globulin (Simons *et al*), PRS, *53:*112, 1974. ALG Therapy & Stand. Workshop, Behringwerke Ag. Marburg, *51:*149, 1972

Porcine zenograft burn dressings (German *et al*), PRS, *50:*634, 1972. Arch. Surg., *104:*806, 1972

Porcine skin grafts (Capozzi). Calif. Med., *116:*56, 1972

Vitamin C deficient guinea pigs, prolonged skin allograft survival in (Kalden, Buthy), PRS, *51:*484, 1973. Europ. Surg. Res., *4:*114, 1972

Homograft skin for early management of difficult wounds (Shuck, Bedeau, Thomas), PRS, *52:*105, 1973. J. Trauma, *12:*215, 1972

Skin grafts, brephoplastic (Wallace) (Follow-Up Clinic), PRS, *50:*183, 1972

Homografting, autograft rejection induced by (Cramer) (Follow-Up Clinic), PRS, *50:*401, 1972

Inhibitory effect of alpha-globulin on the second set allograft reaction (Glaser *et al*).

Skin Grafts, Homografts and Heterografts —
Cont.

Proc. Soc. Exper. Biol. Med., *140:*996, 1972

Heterografts as first surgical dressing for burns (Sturla *et al*), PRS, *52:*598, 1973. Rev. argent. cir., *23:*49, 1972

Wound dressing, radiation-sterilized split skin, new type of biological. Preliminary report (Körlof *et al*). Scand. J. Plast. Reconstr. Surg., *6:*126, 1972

Cross species immunosuppressive effects of antilymphocyte serum in mice and rats (Motoji *et al*). Transplantation, *14:*536, 1972

Comparison of skin allograft rejection and cytotoxic antibody production in two lines of mice genetically selected for "high" and "low" antibody synthesis (Liacopoulos-Briot *et al*). Transplantation, *14:*590, 1972

Evidence for adaptation of skin grafts in enhanced irradiated mice (McKenzie *et al*). Transplantation, *14:*661, 1972

Rabbit anti-rat lymphocyte serum: in vitro antimacrophage activity of different types of antisera and relationship to immunosuppression (Jakobsen). Acta Pathol. Microbiol. Scand., *81:*353, 1973

Graft, porcine, to treat close-range shotgun wounds to extremities with vascular injury (Ledgerwood, Lucas), PRS, *53:*249, 1974. Am. J. Surg., *125:*690, 1973

Increased homograft survival. Internal thoracic duct-esophageal shunt (Flintoff *et al*). Arch. Otolaryng., *97:*251, 1973

Porcine skin grafting of exposed arterial vein grafts in massive thigh injuries with vascular disruption (Ledgerwood, Lucas), PRS, *53:*368, 1974. Arch. Surg., *107:*201, 1973

Heterografts, lyophilized pigskin, for donor site cover (Chang, Gomez, Edelstein), PRS, *55:*118, 1975. Brit. J. Plast. Surg., *26:*147, 1973

Antigenicity, graft conditioning with nonspecific ribonucleic acid (Lerf), PRS, *52:*463, 1973. Bruns' Beitr. klin. Chir., *220:*206, 1973

Homografts in extensive third degree burns (Chinese PLA Burns Unit), PRS, *54:*241, 1974. Chinese M. J., *11:*148, 1973

Evaluation of antilymphocyte serum: comparison of skin allograft survival and rosette inhibition (Kissling *et al*). Experientia, *29:*105, 1973

Skin grafts in weak histocompatibility systems, variation in time taken for rejection of, analysis of relative contributions by donor and recipient to (Matousek *et al*). Folia Biol. (Praha), *19:*402, 1973

Skin Grafts, Homografts and Heterografts —
Cont.

Homografts, skin, study of lymphocyte depletion and hypogamma-globulinemia on survival (Lahoti, Sharma), PRS, *53:*497, 1974. Indian J. Surg., *35:*375, 1973

Grafts, skin, experimental studies of resurfacing effects of autograft, homograft, heterograft, fibrin membrane, and P.V.F. for large skin defect in rats (Namba, Uchida, Date), PRS, *54:*382, 1974. Jap. J. Plast. Reconstr. Surg., *16:*375, 1973

Transplantation and cutaneous genetics (Billingham *et al*) J. Invest. Dermatol., *60:*509, 1973

Heterografts, porcine, for burn wound care compared with prosthesis (O'Neill), PRS, *54:*506, 1974. J. Pediat. Surg., *5:*705, 1973

Skin, homograft and heterograft, clinical evaluation of Epigard as substitute for (Alexander *et al*), PRS, *53:*500, 1974. J. Trauma, *13:*374, 1973

Cellular immune response of humans to pigskin (McCabe *et al*), PRS, *51:*181, 1973

Antigenic properties of skin: study in rats of survival of composite homotransplants of skin and subcutaneous tissue, with microvascular anastomoses (Salyer, Kyger), PRS, *51:*672, 1973

Antilymphocyte serum, preparation of, by transplantation of lymphoid heterografts to the anterior chamber of the rabbit eye (White), PRS, *52:*66, 1973

Grafts, commercial porcine skin, for wound dressing (Elliott, Hoehn), PRS, *52:*401, 1973

Homografts, use in deep dermal burns (Zdrawic), PRS, *53:*686, 1974. Riv. ital. chir. plast., *4:*19, 1973

Homografts, heart and skin, in inbred rats, factors responsible for differential survival of (Warren, Lofgreen, Steinmuller), PRS, *53:*689, 1974. Transplantation, *16:*458, 1973

Tissues, preserved, immunological properties of (Artsimovich), PRS, *55:*646, 1975. Acta chir. plast., *16:*96, 1974

Neomycin toxicity from porcine skin heterografts (Sugarbaker, Sabath, Morgan), PRS, *54:*240, 1974. Ann. Surg., *179:*183, 1974

Active enhancement of mouse skin allografts: effect of Bordetella pertussis and regional lymphadenectomy (Clark *et al*). Brit. J. Surg., *61:*325, 1974

Triamcinolone acetonide used in successful pretreatment of rabbit-skin homotransplants (Klaue), PRS, *55:*117, 1975. Bruns' Beitr. klin. Chir., *221:*313, 1974

Homograft rejection, cryo-biological tissue

Skin Grafts, Meshed

Technic and indications of net grafts. Outcome of the cicatrices (Baux *et al*). Ann. chir. plast., *16:*237, 1971 (French)

Dermatome, simplified mesh (Kojima, Onizuka), PRS, *49:*239, 1972. Jap. J. Plast. Reconstr. Surg., *14:*269, 1971

Experience with mesh grafting (Pasha). J. Med. Liban., *24:*143, 1971

Mesh grafts, experiments with (Smahel, Ganzoni), PRS, *52:*330, 1973. Acta chir. plast., *14:*90, 1972

Graft, the "relay" (Smahel). Brit. J. Plast. Surg., *25:*432, 1972

Skin grafts, wide-mesh net for immobilization (Freeman) (Follow-up Clinic), PRS, *49:*207, 1972

Skin grafts, meshed, split thickness, useful and inexpensive carrier for (Myers *et al*). Am. Surg., *39:*238, 1973

Graft, mesh, use of in skin autotransplantation (Pakkanen *et al*). Duodecim, *89:*955, 1973 (Finnish)

Dermatome for mesh skin grafts, follow-up (Morotomi *et al*), PRS, *53:*371, 1974. Jap. J. Plast. Reconstr. Surg., *16:*258, 1973

Graft, mesh, nonexpanded, use of (Neale). J. Trauma, *14:*247, 1974

Mesh skin grafting, new biological indication for (Mir y Mir), PRS, *54:*246, 1974. Rev. españ. cir. plast., *7:*25, 1974

Surgical mesh technic for covering large skin defects (Konz). Hautarzt, *26:*277, 1975 (German)

Meshed skin grafting, aid to (Lehv), PRS, *56:*584, 1975

Skin graft, mesh, studies on degree of taking (Zietkiewicz *et al*). Pol. Tyg. Lek., *30:*853, 1975 (Polish)

Grafts, split-skin, simple apparatus for expanding (D'Hooghe), PRS, *57:*387, 1976

Skin Grafts to Mouth

Skin grafts, thin, use of in therapy of some buccal mucosa lesions (Kuffer, Soubiran). Bull. Soc. franc. dermat. et syph., *78:*632, 1971 (French)

Dermal-epidermal free grafts in preprosthetic surgery (Brusati *et al*). Riv. Ital. Stomatol., *26:*731, 1971 (Italian)

Oral cavity, human, histology of autologous skin grafts in (Nybore, Fejerskov, Philipsen). Acta Odontol. Scand., *30:*643, 1972

Skin grafts, autogenous, free, to alveolar ridge in humans, histologic follow-up study of (Moller *et al*). Int. J. Oral Surg., *1:*283, 1972

Skin graft, autologous, study of in muco-

Skin Grafts to Mouth – Cont.

membranous floor by microspectrophotometry (Harada, Kurozumi). J. Otolaryngol. Jap., *75:*1072, 1972 (Japanese)

Skin graft, intraoral, occurrence of verruca vulgaris on. Unique growth with significant implications (Hertz). Oral Surg., *34:*934, 1972

Use of split thickness grafts in the repair of excisions of the oropharynx, base of the tongue, and larynx (Rush *et al*). Am. J. Surg., *128:*553, 1974

Skin grafts, intraoral, stabilized by "parachute" stent (Goshgarian, Miller), PRS, *57:*530, 1976. Am. J. Surg., *130:*370, 1975

Skin Grafts, Nerve Regeneration in

Re-innervation of a free skin autograft (Lily). Acta Chir. Acad. Sci. Hung., *12:*237, 1971

Skin grafts in head and neck surgery (Goldstein). Otolaryngol. Clin. North Am., *5:*513, 1972

Skin grafts, reinnervation of (Psillakis, Erhart), PRS, *52:*324, 1973. Rev. bras. clin. Therap., *1:*607, 1972

Sensation revival in transplantations and cutaneous grafts of hand (Celli, Caroli), PRS, *51:*104, 1973. Riv. Chir. della Mano, *8:*23, 1972

Sensation in grafted skin, and factors which influence long-term result (Namba), PRS, *53:*612, 1974. Jap. J. Plast. Reconstr. Surg., *16:*338, 1973

Graft, innervated full-thickness skin, to restore sensibility to fingertips and heels (Maquieira), PRS, *53:*568, 1974

Skin grafting, extensive head and neck, elective postoperative I.O.P.V. for (Delilkan *et al*). Anaesth. Intensive Care., *3:*68, 1975

Skin Grafts, Pigmentation of

Facial plastic surgery with a rotation fat-cutaneous graft (Mukhin). Vestn. Khir., *107:*46, 1971 (Russian)

Autograft repigmentation of leukoderma (Orentreich *et al*). Arch. Dermat., *105:*734, 1972

Skin graft pigmentation, new approach to prevention (Lopez-Mas *et al*), PRS, *49:*18, 1972

Melanin and melanocytes in human skin autografts (Tsukada), PRS, *53:*200, 1974

Grafts, skin pigmentation, current concepts and relevance to plastic surgery (Morgan, Gilchrest, Goldwyn), PRS, *56:*617, 1975

Skin Grafts, Pinch (Reverdin)

Pinch grafts for cutaneous ulcers (Smith *et al*). South. Med. J., *64:*1166, 1971

Skin Grafts, Preservation of

Skin grafts stored at +4°C, histological examination of (Běhounková), PRS, *50:*543, 1972. Acta chir. plast., *13:*128, 1971

Skin bank and viable frozen human skin, clinical experience (Bondoc, Burke), PRS, *50:*99, 1972. Ann. Surg., *174:*371, 1971

Skin grafts, fresh and preserved, comparative efficacy of, in stimulation of neovascularization (O'Donoghue, Zarem), PRS, *48:*474, 1971

Formalin fixed skin, evaluation as temporary dressing for granulating wounds (Silverstein *et al*), PRS, *49:*668, 1972. Surg. Forum, *22:*60, 1971

Skin grafts, split, storage on their donor sites; clinical and experimental study (Shepard), PRS, *49:*115, 1972

Healing of split-skin autografts after storage in deuterated medium (Wandall), PRS, *51:*110, 1973. Scand. J. Plast. Reconstr. Surg., *6:*36, 1972

Skin, human, preserved in cialit, use in plastic surgery (Morel-Fatio *et al*). Ann. chir. plast., *18:*101, 1973 (French)

Viability of skin grafts stored in various media (Hurst, Lindsay, Lee), PRS, *52:*687, 1973. Canad. J. Surg., *16:*206, 1973

Skin, rat, effect of cryostorage on oxygen uptake and autograft viability of (Lessler *et al*). Cryobiology, *10:*185, 1973

Grafts, split-skin, from pigs following incubation on autologous blood or serum for various periods, viability of (Creech, DeVito, Eade), PRS, *51:*572, 1973

Freeze drying of skin, *in vitro* studies of vitality (Sørensen, Jemec), PRS, *53:*502, 1974. Scand. J. Plast. Reconstr. Surg., *7:*35, 1973

Immunological properties of preserved tissues (Artsimovich), PRS, *55:*646, 1975. Acta chir. plast., *16:*96, 1974

Skin grafts, inexpensive method for cooling (Lepaw), PRS, *55:*518, 1975. Cutis, *14:*595, 1974

Skin preservation, comparative evaluation of certain methods of (Margolin). Ortop. Travmatol. Protez., *35:*26, 1974 (Russian)

Preserved cadaver skin for the coverage of large-scale third-degree burns (Zellner). Zentralbl. Chir., *99:*1105, 1974 (German)

Skin Grafts, Split (Thiersch)

Clinical evaluation of "reinforced" split-skin grafts (Monty). Brit. J. Surg., *58:*917, 1971

Dermatomes, drum-type, skin cleaning fluids for use with (Hawtof) (Letter to the Editor), PRS, *48:*171, 1971

Thiersch graft (Onizuka). Shujutsu, *25:*1271, 1971 (Japanese)

Skin Grafts, Split (Thiersch)—Cont.

Endogenous eczema in a split-thickness skin graft (Harnack *et al*). Dermatol. Monatsschr., *158:*28, 1972 (German)

Models for improvement of split skin transplantation (Meyer). Dtsch. Zahn. Mund. Kieferheilkd., *58:*328, 1972 (German)

Skin donor sites, use of heterogenous peritoneum for treating (Madykenov *et al*). Khirurgiia (Mosk.), *49:*28, 1972 (Russian)

Split-skin grafts, storage on their donor sites (Ashbell, Shepard) (Letter to the Editor), PRS, *50:*178, 1972

Split skin autografts, healing after storage in deuterated medium (Wandall), PRS, *51:*110, 1973. Scand. J. Plast. Reconstr. Surg., *6:*36, 1972

Skin, split, radiation-sterilized: new type of biological wound dressing. Preliminary report (Körlof *et al*). Scand. J. Plast. Reconstr. Surg., *6:*126, 1972

Skin, partial thickness, and wound granulations, nature of bond between (Burleson, Eiseman), PRS, *51:*353, 1973. Surgery, *72:*315, 1972

Grafts, split-skin, two from same donor area (Malherbe, Van der Walt), PRS, *53:*113, 1974. Arch. chir. neerl., *25:*81, 1973

Skin graft donor sites, biological dressings for (Salisbury *et al*). Arch. Surg., *106:*705, 1973

Skin grafting: effective safety devices for Padgett dermatome (Brent), PRS, *51:*467, 1973

Split-skin grafts from pigs following incubation on autologous blood or serum for various periods, viability of (Creech, DeVito, Eade), PRS, *51:*572, 1973

Graft, split-skin donor sites, effect of Silastic sheet dressings on healing of (Harris, Filarski, Hector), PRS, *52:*189, 1973

Keratinization of human split skin autografts. Light and electron microscopic study (Eriksson). Scand. J. Plast. Reconstr. Surg., *7:*15, 1973

Grafts, painless donor sites (Koonin, Melmed), PRS, *54:*697, 1974. South African M. J., *47:*2241, 1973

Rapid production of fresh granulation tissue suitable for transplantation following acquired chronic skin defects. Z. Haut. Geschlechtskr., *48:*153, 1973 (German)

Skin graft donor sites, improved management of (Lloyd). Arch. Surg., *108:*561, 1974

Grafts, split-skin, technique for obtaining uniform (Vecchione), PRS, *55:*640, 1975. Arch. Surg., *109:*837, 1974

Grafts, split-skin, forearm as donor site (Xavier, Lamb), PRS, *56:*465, 1975. Hand, *6:*243, 1974

Skin Grafts, Split (Thiersch) – Cont.

Donor sites, split-skin graft, deleterious effect of split-skin homograft coverage on (Miller), PRS, *53:*316, 1974.

Clinical and histological results after extensive split skin transplantation (Kunert *et al*). In *Plastische und Wiederherstellungs-Chirurgie,* ed. by Hohler, pp. 251–7. Schattauer, Stuttgart, 1975 (German)

Donor sites: effect of commonly used antiseptics on wound healing (Gruber, Vistnes, Pardoe), PRS, *55:*472, 1975

Donor site of healed superficial burns used for split-skin grafts (Mariani), PRS, *57:*191, 1976

Skin Grafts to Vagina: See Vagina

Skin Neoplasms (See also *Cancer, Basal Cell; Hemangioma; Melanoma; Nevi; etc.*)

Intraepidermic epithelioma of Borst and Jadassohn (Nicolis, Capetanakis, Panas), PRS, *49:*473, 1972. Ann. Dermat. et Syph., *98:*161, 1971

Sweat gland carcinoma: clinico-pathological study of 83 patients (El-Domeiri *et al*), PRS, *48:*93, 1971. Ann. Surg., *173:*270, 1971

Skin and subcutaneous metastases from gastrointestinal carcinoid tumors (Norman, Cunningham, Cleveland), PRS, *50:*421, 1972. Arch. Surg., *103:*767, 1971

Multiple self-healing squamous epithelioma (Ferguson-Smith *et al*). Birth Defects, *7:*157, 1971

Turban tumors (cylindromatosis) (Harper). Birth Defects, *7:*338, 1971

Sweat gland carcinomas, multiple primary (Futrell *et al*), PRS, *49:*473, 1972. Cancer, *28:*686, 1971

Cryosurgery for cancer of the skin (Zacarian). Cancro, *24:*349, 1971

Possibilities and limits in the serial excision of pigmented nevi (Sholz et al). Dermatol. Monatsschr., *157:*412, 1971 (German)

Skin and mucous membranes, benign lesions of, cryosurgical therapy of (Hansen), PRS, *50:*424, 1972. Internat. Surg., *56:*403, 1971

Cutaneous tumors, nasal reconstructions after resections of (Garcia-Velazco), PRS, *50:*536, 1972. Invest. Clin. Mexico, *10:*229, 1971

Primary malignant tumors of the hand (Kendall *et al*). J. Kans. Med. Soc., *72:*376, 1971

Chemosurgery for the microscopically controlled excision of skin cancer (Mohs). J. Surg. Oncol., *3:*257, 1971

Plastic surgical treatment of facial skin can-

Skin Neoplasms – Cont.

cer (Murray *et al*). J. Surg. Oncol., *3:*269, 1971

Curettage and electrodesiccation as a method of treatment for epitheliomas of the skin (Crissey). J. Surg. Oncol., *3:*287, 1971

Hidradenoma, clear cell, with metastasis, case report with review of literature (Chung, Heffernan), PRS, *48:*177, 1971

Our experiences in the treatment of skin hemangiomas (Arneri *et al*). Vojnosanit. Pregl., *28:*561, 1971 (Croatian)

Leiomyosarcoma in skin. Case report (Chaves *et al*). Acta Derm. Venereol. (Stockh.), *52:*288, 1972

Carcinoma of sweat glands in adolescents (Futrell *et al*), PRS, *51:*708, 1973. Am. J. Surg., *123:*594, 1972

Histochemical investigations, quantitative, on DNA content of facultatives and obligatory precanceroses of skin (Ehlers, Stephan), PRS, *51:*107, 1973. Arch. Derm. Forsch., *243:*114, 1972

Skin neoplasms, experiences with plastic surgery in therapy (Petres). Arch. Derm. Forsch., *244:*156, 1972 (German)

Dermatology, surgery of neoplasms in (Santler, Freilinger). Arch. Derm. Forsch., *244:*418, 1972 (German)

Lymphangiography and surgery in lymphangioma of the skin (Edwards *et al*). Brit. J. Surg., *59:*36, 1972

Primary skin-grafting in the treatment of chronic osteomyelitis (Naylor *et al*). Brit. J. Surg., *59:*117, 1972

Skin cancers, electrocoagulation in treatment of nose, ear and eye areas (Whelan). Bull. Soc. Internat. Chir., *31:*557, 1972

Adenoacanthoma: review of 20 cases, compared with literature (Carapeto *et al*). Dermatologica, *145:*269, 1972

Skin cancer: statistical approach of 482 primary skin neoplasms (Lissaios *et al*), PRS, *52:*457, 1973. Galenus, *14:*731, 1972

Plastic surgery following the excision of skin tumors (Petres). Hautarzt, *23:*271, 1972 (German)

Trichoepithelioma, solitary (Steigleder). Hautarzt, *23:*323, 1972 (German)

Chemosurgery (Mohs' technique) in the treatment of epitheliomas (Tolman). Med. Clin. North Am., *56:*739, 1972

Epitheliomas, cutaneous, in patients less than 40 years old (Marchac). Nouvelle Presse Med., *1:*3035, 1972 (French)

Carcinoma, large skin, of neck; coverage with a deltopectoral flap (Ristow, O'Grady, Farr), PRS, *49:*570, 1972

Skin Neoplasms — Cont.

Jadassohn, premalignant nature of sebaceous nevus of (Constant, Davis), PRS, *50:*257, 1972

Poroma, eccrine, of hand (Mamoun *et al*), PRS, *50:*295, 1972

Cancer, skin, current management (Menn). Postgrad. Med., *52:*161, 1972

Surgical treatment of skin cancer (Apton). Proc. Rudolph Virchow Med. Soc. City N.Y., *29:*111, 1972-73

Tumor transplants in alymphatic skin islands (Ziegler *et al*). Surg. Forum, *23:*127, 1972

Epithelioma, cutaneous, review of 445 recurrences of, after surgery and radiotherapy (Basso Ricci *et al*). Tumori, *58:*361, 1972 (Italian)

Skin cancer (Jensen *et al*). Ugeskr. Laeger, *134:*107, 1972 (Danish)

Cancer, skin, from ulcers and osteomyelitic fistulas, diagnosis and treatment (Petrov). Vopr. Onkol., *18:*72, 1972 (Russian)

Skin cancer relapses, results of treating (Dryzhak). Vopr. Onkol., *18:*73, 1972 (Russian)

Use of optical quantum generators (lasers) in oncology (Moskalik *et al*). Vopr. Onkol., *18:*97, 1972 (Russian)

Carcinoma, skin, treatment of 443 cases of, with curettage and soft roentgen rays by Ebbehoj method (Jensen *et al*). Acta Radiol. (Ther.) (Stockh.), *12:*369, 1973

Carcinoma, skin, basal cell and squamous (Clabaugh). Am. Fam. Physician, *7:*78, 1973

Epithelioma, remote results of surgery and critical study of carcinologic results, apropos of 330 cases (Vandenbussche *et al*). Ann. chir. plast., *18:*44, 1973 (French)

Epithelioma, skin, treatment of, by chemosurgery: Mohs' technic (Tapernoux *et al*). Ann. Dermatol. Syphiligr. (Paris), *100:*169, 1973 (French)

Skin cancer and surgery (Rank). Ann. R. Coll. Surg. Engl., *52:*148, 1973

Woringer-Kolopp disease, epidermotropic cutaneous reticulosis, "Pagetoid reticulosis" (Grosshans *et al*). Arch. Belg. Dermatol., *29:*195, 1973 (French)

Skin fibrosarcoma, recurrent, preceded by inflammation (Welvaart, Polano), PRS, *52:*459, 1973. Arch. chir. neerl., *25:*35, 1973

Skin, spread of tumors to (Brownstein, Helwig), PRS, *52:*460, 1973. Arch. Dermat., *107:*80, 1973

Eccrine sweat gland, adenocarcinoma of (Panet-Raymond, Johnson), PRS, *52:*685,

Skin Neoplasms — Cont.

1973. Arch. Dermat., *107:*94, 1973

Skin cancer, recurrent (Freeman, Duncan), PRS, *52:*685, 1973. Arch. Dermat., *107:*395, 1973

Trichoepitheliomas (Brownstein, Shapiro), PRS, *57:*264, 1976. Arch. Dermat., *107:*866, 1973

Carcinomas, squamous cell, multiple cutaneous, during immunosuppresive therapy (Westburg *et al*). Arch. Dermat., *107:*893, 1973

Eccrine hidrocystoma (Wolf *et al*). Arch. Dermat., *108:*50, 1973

Curettage to treat basal cell carcinoma of skin (Reymann), PRS, *53:*612, 1974. Arch. Dermat., *108:*528, 1973

Epithelioma, calcifying (pilomatrixoma) (Moehlenbeck), PRS, *53:*687, 1974. Arch. Dermat., *108:*532, 1973

Skin, squamous cell carcinoma of, treatment of (Honeycutt, Jansen), PRS, *54:*380, 1974. Arch. Dermat., *108:*670, 1973

Tumors, skin, in immunosuppressed patients (Marshall), PRS, *54:*115, 1974. Australian & New Zealand J. Surg., *43:*214, 1973

Fluorouracil-5, clinical trial in treatment of some cutaneous malignancies (Littlewood, Murray), PRS, *55:*116, 1975. Brit. J. Plast. Surg., *26:*140, 1973

Skin cancer, chemotherapy of (Klein, Case, Burgess), PRS, *53:*250, 1974. Cancer, *23:*228, 1973

Cancer of skin of face, nose, eyelids, and ears (Whelan, Deckers), PRS, *52:*214, 1973. Cancer, *31:*159, 1973

Fibroxanthoma of skin, atypical (Fretzin, Helwig), PRS, *54:*243, 1974. Cancer, *31:*1541, 1973

Tumor, skin, spontaneously resolving, immunological reaction in keratoacanthoma (Brown, Tan), PRS, *53:*496, 1974. Cancer Res., *33:*2030, 1973

Skin cancer, treatment (Cuccia). Del. Med. J., *45:*323, 1973

Skin tumors, use of lasers for treatment (Lazarev *et al*). Klin. Khir., *11:*36, 1973 (Russian)

Cutis verticis gyrata (fibroepithelioma), congenital, in two infants, report on (Pattberg). Klin. Paediatr., *185:*495, 1973 (German)

Skin lesions, clinical application of 5-Fluorouracil in treatment of (Snyderman) (Follow-Up Clinic), PRS, *52:*298, 1973

Skin tumors, cryosurgery in treatment of (Adamus *et al*). Pol. Tyg. Lek., *28:*440, 1973 (Polish)

Skin Neoplasms—Cont.

ground of ulcers, osteomyelitic fistulas and scars (Dryzhak). Klin. Khir., *10:*78, 1975 (Russian)

Treatment of skin cancer by cryosurgery (Woolridge *et al*). Mo. Med., *72:*28, 1975

Tumor, nevus of Ota (Yeschua, Wexler, Neuman), PRS, *55:*229, 1975

Malignant transformation in tropical ulcers (Ariyan, Krizek), PRS, *55:*324, 1975

Skin cancer, immunobiology of (Dellon *et al*), PRS, *55:*341, 1975

Cancer: cutaneous melanoma, 20-year retrospective study with clinicopathologic correlation (Franklin, Reynolds, Page), PRS, *56:*277, 1975

Perineum, multicentric pigmented Bowen's disease of (Emmerson), PRS, *57:*399, 1976. Proc. Roy. Soc. Med., *68:*345, 1975

Cryosurgery for facial skin lesions (Leopard). Proc. Roy. Soc. Med., *68:*606, 1975

Malignant oncology of integuments, plastic surgery and (Micheli-Pellegrini, Francesconi, Fenili), PRS, *57:*766, 1976 (Italian). Riv. ital. chir. plast., 7:197, 1975

Review of the treatment of malignant skin neoplasms during the past 10 years at the clinical Center for Plastic Surgery in Kosice (Kipikasa *et al*). Rozhl. Chir., *54:*416, 1975 (Slovakian)

Surgery or irradiation of skin neoplasms? (Krenar *et al*). Rozhl. Chir., *54:*421, 1975 (Czechoslovakian)

Cryosurgery in dermatologic office practice: special reference to dermatofibroma and mucous cyst of the lip (Spiller *et al*). South. Med. J., *68:*157, 1975

Editorial: A philosophy of approach to treatment of hemangiomas (Green). South. Med. J., *68:*383, 1975

Epithelioma, painful Malherbe and Chenantais calcifying, case (Jonecko *et al*). Wiad. Lek., *28:*673, 1975 (Polish)

Exophytic bowenoid squamous cell carcinoma (Goertz). Z. Hautkr., *50:*798, 1975 (German)

Giant pilomatrixoma (Malherbe calcifying epithelioma) (Rothman *et al*). Arch. Surg., *111:*86, 1976

Cancer, skin: increasing incidence of melanoma (Cosman, Heddle, Crikelair), PRS, *57:*50, 1976

Skin Pigmentation

Skin lightener, butylated hydroxytoluene as (Bentley-Phillips, Bayles), PRS, *54:*382, 1974. Arch. Dermat., *109:*216, 1974

Pigmentary irregularities in blacks (Pierce,

Skin Pigmentation—Cont.

Teneyck), PRS, *57:*542, 1976. J. Heredity, *65:*157, 1974

Skin pigmentation, current concepts and relevance to plastic surgery (Morgan, Gilchrest, Goldwyn), PRS, *56:*617, 1975

Skin pigmentation (Okun) (Letter to the Editor), PRS, *57:*738, 1976

SKINNER, D. G.: Management of extensive, localized neoplasms of lower abdominal wall. Pubectomy and scrotal skin transfer technique. Urology, *3:*34, 1974

SKINNER, D. G., LEADBETTER, W. F., AND KELLEY, S. B.: Surgical management of squamous cell carcinoma of penis, PRS, *50:*542, 1972. J. Urol., *107:*273, 1972

SKINSNES, O. K. *et al:* Pathogenesis of extremity deformity in leprosy. A pathologic study on large sections of amputated extremities in relation to radiological appearance. Int. J. Lepr., *40:*375, 1972

SKIPPER, H. E.: Combination therapy: some concepts and results. Cancer Chemother. Rep. (Suppl.), *4:*137, 1974

SKIVOLOCKI, W., HARRIS, B. H., AND BOLES, E. T., JR.: New method for skin grafting burned patient who has *epidermolysis bullosa*, PRS, *53:*355, 1974

SKOBLIN, A. P. *et al:* Conduction anesthesia in hand and finger injuries. Vestn. Khir., *106:*96, 1971 (Russian)

SKOKIJEV, A. *et al:* Fractures of the zygomatic maxillary complex. Vojnosanit. Pregl., *32:*536, 1975 (Serbian)

SKOLNIC, M. L., AND McCALL, G. N.: Radiographic technique for demonstrating causes of persistent nasality in patients with pharyngeal flaps, PRS, *54:*689, 1974. Brit. J. Plast. Surg., *26:*12, 1973

SKOLNICK, M. L.: Velopharyngeal function in cleft palate. Clin. Plast. Surg., *2:*285, 1975

SKOLNICK, M. L. *et al:* Radiological evaluation of velopharyngeal closure. J.A.M.A., *218:*96, 1971

SKOLNICK, M. L. *et al:* Velopharyngeal competence and incompetence following pharyngeal flap surgery: video-fluoroscopic study in multiple projections. Cleft Palate J., *9:*1, 1972

SKOLNICK, M. L. *et al:* Patterns of velopharyngeal closure in subjects with repaired cleft palate and normal speech: a multi-view videofluoroscopic analysis. Cleft Palate J., *12:*369, 1975

SKOLNIK, E. M. *et al:* Dermoid cysts of the nose. Laryngoscope, *81:*1632, 1971

SKOLNICK, E. M. *et al:* Posterior triangle in

radical neck surgery. Arch. Otolaryng., *102:*1, 1976

SKONIECZNY, J. *et al:* Carcinoma of the external ear. Otolaryngol. Pol., *29:*61, 1975 (Polish)

SKOOG, TORD: *Plastic Surgery.* W. B. Saunders Co., Philadelphia, 1975.

SKOOG, T.: Repair of unilateral cleft lip deformity: maxilla, nose and lip, PRS, *48:*295, 1971. Scand. J. Plast. Reconstr. Surg., *3:*109, 1969

SKOOG, T.: Modern surgical approach to treatment of Dupuytren's contracture, PRS, *49:*358, 1972. Woman Phys., *25:*769, 1970

SKOOG, T., AND JOHANSSON, S. H.: Formation of articular cartilage from free perichondrial grafts. PRS, *57:*1, 1976

SKORNICK, W. A., AND DRESSLER, D. P.: Topical antisepsis studies in burned rat, PRS, *49:*666, 1972. Arch. Surg., *103:*469, 1971

SKORNICK, W. A., AND DRESSLER, D. P.: Evaluation of 5% Sulfamylon cream in control of experimental burn wound sepsis, PRS, *53:*492, 1974. Surgery, *74:*540, 1973

SKROBACKI, A.: Unhappy love affair of Johann Friedrich Dieffenbach. Wiad. Lek., *27:*1121, 1974 (Polish)

SKUDE, G., AND ROTHMAN, U.: Amylase isoenzymes in serum after maxillofacial surgery, PRS, *55:*120, 1975. Scand. J. Plast. Reconstr. Surg., *7:*105, 1974

SLADCZYK, E.: Treatment of hypospadias. Z. Urol. Nephrol., *64:*823, 1971 (German)

SLATER, R. M. *et al:* Simplified method of treating burns of the hands. Brit. J. Plast. Surg., *24:*296, 1971

SLAVIK, M.: Unusual indication for interthoracoscapular amputation. Acta Chir. Orthop. Traumatol. Cech., *39:*164, 1972 (Czechoslovakian)

SLAVKIN, D. M. *et al:* Bilateral granular cell myoblastoma of lip: report of case. J. Oral Surg., *31:*848, 1973

SLESINGER, M: Use of a tubular flap for replacement of extensive losses of palatine tissue. Rev. Stomatol. Chir. Maxillofac., *75:*188, 1974 (French)

SLESINGER, M. J.: Treatment of hemoangioma of the face. Acta Stomatol. Belg., *72:*495, 1975 (French)

SLIM, M. S. *et al:* Carotid neurifobroma in a child. Am. J. Surg., *123:*343, 1972

SLOCUM, D. B. *et al:* Late reconstruction of ligamentous injuries of medial compartment of knee. Clin. Orthop., *100:*23, 1974

SLOGOFF, S. *et al:* Tracheoesophageal fistula following prolonged tracheal intubation. Anesthesiology, *39:*453, 1973

SLOGOFF, S. *et al:* Clinical experience with sub-anesthetic ketamine, PRS, *54:*628, 1974. Anesth. & Analg., *53:*354, 1974

SLONIUM, L. *et al:* Folded breast prosthesis: new clinical and radiological entity. Australas. Radiol., *16:*159, 1972

SLOTH, M. *et al:* Late complications after septum surgery. Ugeskr. Laeger, *138:*88, 1976 (Danish)

SLOVIN, A. J.: Arterial below knee bypass grafts. Experience with modified bovine heterograft. Am. J. Surg., *128:*58, 1974

SLY, R. E. *et al:* Objective assessment of digital clubbing in caucasian, Negro, and oriental subjects, PRS, *54:*503, 1974. Chest, *64:*689, 1973

SMAHEL, J.: The "relay" graft. Brit. J. Plast. Surg., *25:*432, 1972

SMAHEL, J. *et al:* Tissue reactions after subcutaneous implantation of Hydrom sponge. Acta chir. plast. (Praha), *13:*193, 1971

SMAHEL, J., AND GANZONI, N.: Experiments with mesh grafts, PRS, *52:*330, 1973. Acta chir. plast., *14:*90, 1972

SMAHEL, J. *et al:* Relay transplantation: new method of expanding free skin graft. Brit. J. Plast. Surg., *28:*49, 1975

SMAHEL, Z.: Anthropology in genetic counseling, PRS, *54:*629, 1974. Rozhl. chir., *53:*159, 1974

SMALL, A.: Prevention of meatal stenosis in conchal setback otoplasty. Laryngoscope, *85:*1782, 1975

SMALL, D. F.: Letter: Handlebar palsy. New England J. Med., *292:*322, 1975

SMALL, E. W.: Inside-out and bottom-up: management of maxillofacial trauma patients. Mil. Med., *136:*553, 1971

SMALL, E. W.: Acute alcoholism and craniofacial trauma: problem of differential diagnosis, PRS, *54:*372, 1974. J. Oral Surg., *32:*275, 1974

SMALL, E. W.: Correlation of psychological findings and treatment results in temporomandibular joint pain-dysfunction syndrome, PRS, *56:*105, 1975. J. Oral Surg., *32:*589, 1974

SMALL, E. W.: Lingual splinting and interosseous fixation for early mobilization of mandibular symphysis/condyle fractures. Fortschr. Kiefer. Gesichtschir., *19:*96, 1975 (German)

SMALL, G. S. *et al:* A "true giant cell tumor" in the mandible? J. Oral Surg., *33:*296, 1975

SMALL, I. A.: Chalmers J. Lyons memorial lecture: Metal implants and the mandibular staple bone plate. J. Oral Surg., *33:*571, 1975

SMALL, I. A. AND GOODMAN, P. A.: Giant cemento-ossifying fibroma of maxilla: report of case and discussion. J. Oral Surg., *31:*113, 1973

SMALL, I. A. *et al:* Mandibular staple implant for the atrophic mandible. J. Biomed. Mater. Res., *8:*365, 1974

SMALL, M. P. *et al:* Small-Carrion penile prosthesis. New implant for management of impotence. Urology, *5:*479, 1975

SMALLEY, J. J., AND CUNNINGHAM, M. P.: Forehead flap rotation to protect carotid artery, PRS, *49:*96, 1972

SMART, C. R. *et al:* Cancer of head and neck in Utah, PRS, *57:*540, 1976. Am. J. Surg., *128:*463, 1974

SMATT, V.: Immediate prosthetic replacement after completion of maxillary surgery. J. Med. Liban., *26:*73, 1973 (French)

SMATT, V.: Outer mandibular plate osteosynthesis by endoral approach. Rev. Dent. Liban., *23:*38, 1973

SMIGIEL, M. R. *et al:* Exophthalmos. More commonly encountered neurosurgical lesions. Mayo Clin. Proc., *50:*345, 1975

SMILEY, G. R.: Possible genesis for cleft palate formation, PRS, *50:*390, 1972

SMILEY, K., AND PERRY, M. O.: Balloon catheter tamponade of major vascular wounds, PRS, *48:*515, 1971. Am. J. Surg., *121:*326, 1971

SMIRNITSKII, V. V.: Neurofibromatosis of cervico-occipital region. Vestn. Khir., *110:*124, 1973 (Russian)

SMITH, A. D.: Aging and interference with memory, PRS, *57:*267, 1976. J. Gerontol., *30:*319, 1975

SMITH, A. J.: Perphenazine side effects presenting in oral surgical practice. Brit. J. Oral Surg., *10:*349, 1973

SMITH, B.: Late bilateral naso-orbital fracture and dacryostenosis. Trans. Am. Acad. Ophthalmol. Otolaryngol., *76:*1378, 1972

SMITH, B.: Anesthesia for lacrimal surgery. Trans. Ophthalmol. Soc. U.K., *93:*619, 1973

SMITH, B., AND WIGGS, E. O.: Differential diagnosis in orbital injury, PRS, *53:*240, 1974. Arch. Ophth., *89:*484, 1973

SMITH, B. *et al:* Severe scarring secondary to chickenpox, case report. Brit. J. Plast. Surg., *26:*344, 1973

SMITH, B. C. *et al:* Complications of orbital fractures. N. Y. State J. Med., *71:*2407, 1971

SMITH, B. E.: Teratology in anesthesia, PRS, *55:*639, 1975. Clin. Obst. Gynec., *17:*145, 1974

SMITH, BYRON, AND CHERUBINI, THOMAS D.: *Oculo-Plastic Surgery. A Compendium of Principles and Techniques.* C. V. Mosby Co., St. Louis, 1970. PRS, *49:*80, 1972

SMITH, C., ECHEVARRIA, R., AND MCLELLAND,

C.: Pseudosarcomatous changes in antrochoanal polyps, PRS, *54:*699, 1974. Arch. Otolaryng., *99:*228, 1974

SMITH, D.: De-epithelialized overflap technique in repair of hypospadias, PRS, *55:*110, 1975. Brit. J. Plast. Surg., *26:*106, 1973

SMITH, D. E. *et al:* Treatment of burns in a non-urban community hospital. Northwest. Med., *71:*103, 1972

SMITH, D. M.: Rhabdomyosarcoma of the head and neck. Can. J. Otolaryngol., *3:*618, 1974

SMITH, D. W., AND GONG, B. T.: Scalp hair patterning as clue to early fetal brain development, PRS, *54:*370, 1974. J. Pediat., *83:*374, 1973

SMITH, E.: Hypospadias repair–elimination of fistulae, PRS, *52:*681, 1973. Proc. Roy. Australasian Coll. Surg., *46:*370, 1973

SMITH, E. B. *et al:* Stasis ulcer and "fibrinogen Baltimore." Arch. Dermat., *104:*221, 1971

SMITH, G. L. *et al:* Unilateral submandibular gland swelling after induction of general anesthesia, case report. J. Oral Surg., *30:*911, 1972

SMITH, H. G. *et al:* Eradication of microscopic lymph node metastases after injection of living BCG adjacent to the primary tumor. J. Natl. Cancer Inst., *55:*1345, 1975

SMITH, H. W.: Saddle nose. Arch. Otolaryng., *98:*435, 1973

SMITH, H. W.: Symposium on maxillofacial trauma. IV. Pitfalls in treatment of mid-facial trauma. Laryngoscope, *83:*547, 1973

SMITH, H. W. *et al:* Congenital choanal atresia – a technique for surgical correction. Trans. Am. Acad. Ophthalmol. Otolaryngol., *80:*527, 1975

SMITH, H. W. *et al:* Nasopharyngeal pushback in treatment of velopharyngeal insufficiency. Arch. Otolaryng., *102:*83, 1976

SMITH, I.: Fractures of middle third of facial skeleton – new method of treatment, PRS, *55:*384, 1975. J. Maxillo-facial Surg., *2:*128, 1974

SMITH, J., AND ABRAMSON, M: Membranous *vs* endochondral bone autografts, PRS, *54:*701, 1974. Arch. Otolaryng., *99:*203, 1974

SMITH, J. D. *et al:* Pinch grafts for cutaneous ulcers. South. Med. J., *64:*1166, 1971

SMITH, J. F. *et al:* Snuff-dipper's lesion, PRS, *49:*361, 1972, Arch. Otolaryng., *92:*450, 1970

SMITH, J. R.: Lymphatic cannulation of head and neck (Follow-Up Clinic), PRS, *49:*545, 1972

SMITH, J. W.: Substitution of skin grafts for pedicled tissues in hand reconstruction (Follow-Up Clinic), PRS, *48:*173, 1971

SMITH, J. W.: Advances in facial nerve repair.

Surg. Clin. North Am., *52:*1287, 1972

SMITH, J. W.: Small, deep forearm lacerations; differential diagnosis of muscle and nerve injuries (with Schwager, Goulian), PRS, *55:*190, 1975

SMITH, J. W., AND CONWAY, H.: Selection of appropriate surgical procedures in lymphedema (Follow-Up Clinic), PRS, *49:*334, 1972

SMITH, JAMES W., AND BAKER, SAMM SINCLAIR: *"Doctor, Make Me Beautiful!"* David McKay Co., New York, 1973. PRS, *53:*219, 1974

SMITH, M. L.: Parotidectomy. Am. J. Nurs., *76:*422, 1976

SMITH, N.: Suture of the palate (Classic Reprint), PRS, *48:*61, 1971

SMITH, P. J.: Vascular basis of axial pattern flaps, PRS, *55:*117, 1975. Brit. J. Plast. Surg., *26:*150, 1973

SMITH, P. J. et al: Anatomical basis of groin flap, PRS, *49:*41, 1972

SMITH, R.: Tonsillectomy blade for superficial parotidectomy. Arch. Otolaryng., *94:*364, 1971

SMITH, R.: Managing epistaxis. Postgrad. Med., *55:*143, 1974

SMITH, R. et al: Large rotational flap for neck dissection and facial skin replacement. Arch. Otolaryng., *99:*122, 1974

SMITH, R. et al: Blood supply to levator scapulae muscle relative to carotid artery protection. Trans. Am. Acad. Ophthalmol. Otolaryngol., *78:*1128, 1974

SMITH, R. et al: Medial conchal excision in otoplasty. Laryngoscope, *85:*738, 1975

SMITH, R. B.: Reason for taking iliac bone grafts from left side in young patients (Letter to the Editor), PRS, *52:*425, 1973

SMITH, R. B.: Pharyngitis as source of postoperative infection around breast implant (Letter to the Editor), PRS, *54:*347, 1974

SMITH, R. B. et al: Technic for tracheostomy tube change. Anesth. Analg. (Cleve.), *53:*627, 1974

SMITH, R. C., AND FURNAS, D. W.: Hand sandwich: adjacent flaps from opposing body surfaces, PRS, *57:*351, 1976

SMITH, R. F., AND BETTGE, C. L.: Comparative characteristics of human and porcine staphylococci and their differentiation in burn xenografting procedures. Appl. Microbiol., *24:*929, 1972

SMITH, R. F. et al: Autograft rejection in acutely burned patients; relation to colonization by Streptococcus agalactiae. Appl. Microbiol., *25:*493, 1973

SMITH, R. F. et al: Colonization of burns by Streptococcus faecalis related to contami-

nated porcine xenografts. Tex. Rep. Biol. Med., *31:*47, 1973

SMITH, R. F. et al: Bacteremia and postmortem microbiology in burned children, PRS, *56:*469, 1975. Am. J. Clin. Path., *63:*502, 1975

SMITH, R. J.: Anomalous muscle belly of the flexor digitorum superficialis causing carpal-tunnel syndrome. Report of a case. J. Bone & Joint Surg. (Am.), *53:*1215, 1971

SMITH, R. J.: Non-ischemic contractures of intrinsic muscles of hand, PRS, *49:*665, 1972. J. Bone & Joint Surg., *53A:*1313, 1971

SMITH, R. J. et al: Treatment of the one-digit hand. J. Bone & Joint Surg. (Am.), *55:*113, 1973

SMITH, R. O., JR. et al: Jacobson's neurectomy for Frey's syndrome, PRS, *48:*604, 1971. Am. J. Surg., *120:*478, 1970

SMITH, R. O., JR. et al: Parapharyngeal neurilemmoma with intracranial extension. South. Med. J., *65:*1171, 1972

SMITH, R. R., AND DEDO, H. H.: Innervation of superior pharyngeal constrictor muscle, PRS, *48:*196, 1971. Ann. Otol. Rhin. & Laryng., *80:*92, 1971

SMITH, R. T., AND TS'AO, C. H.: Fibrin degradation products in postoperative period, PRS, *53:*693, 1974. Am. J. Clin. Path., *60:*644, 1973

SMITH, R. V., AND FISHER, R. G.: Struthers' ligament: source of median nerve compression above elbow, PRS, *53:*366, 1974. J. Neurosurg., *38:*778, 1973

SMITH, S. M.: Subjective experiences during 32-year period after resurfacing of hands for severe and acute radiation burns, PRS, *51:*23, 1973

SMITH, T. W.: Hair transplant. Arch. Otolaryng., *96:*227, 1972

SMITH, T. W.: Thoughtful nasal tip surgery. Arch. Otolaryng., *97:*244, 1973

SMITH, T. W.: Osteotomy and infraction in rhinoplasty. Arch. Otolaryng., *100:*266, 1974

SMITH, T. W.: Letter: Regional plastic surgeons. Postgrad. Med., *57:*27, 1975

SMITH, T. W.: Letter: Peer review of cosmetic surgeons. Eye Ear Nose Throat Mon., *55:*17, 1976

SMITH, V. H.: Medial decompression of orbit for endocrine exophthalmos. Trans. Ophthalmol. Soc. U.K., *92:*485, 1972

SMITHDEAL, C. D.: Sequential septo-rhinoplasty. Laryngoscope, *85:*1216, 1975

SMITHDEAL, C. D., CORSO, P. F., AND STRONG, E. W.: Dermis grafts for carotid artery protection: yes or no? PRS, *57:*536, 1976. Am. J. Surg., *128:*484, 1974

SMYLSKI, P. T.: Bilateral vertical osteotomy with notching for a butt joint of retrognathic mandible. Trans. Congr. Int. Assoc. Oral Surg., *4:*237, 1973

Snake Bite: See *Bites and Stings*

SNEDDON, J.: Sepsis in hand injuries. Hand, 2:58, 1970

SNEDDON, JOAN: *The Care of Hand Infection.* Williams & Wilkins Co., Baltimore, 1970

SNELL, G. E.: History of rhinoplasty. Can. J. Otolaryngol., *2:*224, 1973

SNELL, J. A.: Internal fixation of certain fractures of mandible with bone plating (Follow-Up Clinic), PRS, *57:*512, 1976

SNEZHKO, L. A.: Combinations of skin cancer and malignant tumors of other localities. Vopr. Onkol., *17:*8, 1971 (Russian)

SNIDER, R. L., AND PORTER, J. M.: Treatment of experimental frostbite with intra-arterial sympathetic blocking drugs, PRS, *57:*403, 1976. Surgery, 77:557, 1975

SNOW, G. B.: Incisions for neck dissection and laryngectomy. O.R.L., *36:*61, 1974

SNOW, G. B., AND SINDRAM, P. J.: Intra-arterial infusion chemotherapy in head and neck cancer, PRS, *54:*246, 1974. Arch. chir. neerl., 25:363, 1973

SNOW, J. C. *et al:* Broken disposable needle during axillary approach to block brachial plexus, PRS, *54:*249, 1974. Anesth. Analg. (Cleve.), 53:89, 1974

SNOW, J. C. *et al:* Fire hazard during CO_2 laser microsurgery on the larynx and trachea. Anesth. Analg. (Cleve.), *55:*146, 1976

SNOW, J. W.: Use of retrograde tendon flap in repairing severed extensor in PIP joint area, PRS, *51:*555, 1973

SNOW, J. W.: One-stage columellar reconstruction (Follow-Up Clinic), PRS, *52:*299, 1973

SNOW, J. W.: Use of volar flap for repair of fingertip amputations (Follow-Up Clinic), PRS, *52:*299, 1973

SNOW, J. W.: More accurate removal of the hump in rhinoplasty, PRS, *57:*253, 1976

SNOW, J. W.: Method for reconstruction of central slip of extensor tendon of finger, PRS, *57:*455, 1976

SNOW, J. W., AND FINK, G. H.: Use of transverse carpal ligament window for pulley in tendon transfers for median nerve palsy, PRS, *48:*238, 1971

SNOW, J. W. *et al:* New method for permanent preservation of anatomical specimens, PRS, *48:*387, 1971

SNOW, J. W., AND JOHNSON, H. C.: One-stage reconstruction of lacrimal apparatus, PRS, *48:*453, 1971

SNOW, J. W. *et al:* Flexion contractures of the hand. J. Fla. Med. Assoc., *62:*19, 1975

SNOW, J. W., AND SWITZER, H.: Method of

studying relationships between finger joints and flexor and extensor mechanisms, PRS, *55:*242, 1975

SNOW, R. S.: Constructing improved splint for mallet finger deformity, PRS, *52:*586, 1973

SNYDER, C. C.: Carpal tunnel syndrome caused by hand injuries (with Browne), PRS, *56:*41, 1975

SNYDER, C. C., LEVINE, G. A., AND DINGMAN, D. L.: Trial of sternoclavicular whole joint graft as substitute for temporomandibular joint, PRS, *48:*447, 1971

SNYDER, C. C., STRAIGHT, R., AND GLENN, J.: Snakebitten hand, PRS, *49:*275, 1972

SNYDER, C. C. *et al:* Successful replantation of totally severed thumb, PRS, *50:*553, 1972

SNYDER, C. C. *et al:* Mandibular lengthening by gradual distraction, PRS, *51:*506, 1973

SNYDER, C. C. *et al:* Bridging the gap between premedical and medical education (Editorial), PRS, *53:*214, 1974

SNYDER, G. B.: Use of homografts in keloids. Brit. J. Plast. Surg., 26:32, 1973

SNYDER, G. B.: Button compression for keloids of lobule. Brit. J. Plast. Surg., 27:186, 1974

SNYDER, G. B.: Planning an augmentation mammaplasty, PRS, *54:*132, 1974

SNYDER, G. B.: Cervico-mentoplasty with rhytidectomy, PRS, *54:*404, 1974

SNYDER, G. B.: Treatment of exposed breast implant by reimplantation behind posterior wall of capsule, PRS, *56:*97, 1975

SNYDER, G. B. *et al:* Mandibular ankylosis: surgical-orthodontic treatment. J. Fla. Med. Assoc., 61:569, 1974

SNYDER, S. R. *et al:* Eosinophilic granuloma of bone: case report. J. Oral Surg., 31:712, 1973

SNYDERMAN, REUVEN K.: *Symposium on Neoplastic & Reconstructive Problems of the Female Breast.* Vol. 7. C. V. Mosby Co., St. Louis, 1973

SNYDERMAN, R. K.: Discussion of "Subcutaneous mastectomy for central tumors of breast, with immediate reconstruction," by Freeman, PRS, *51:*445, 1973

SNYDERMAN, R. K.: "Subcutaneous mastectomy with immediate prosthetic reconstruction" – operation in search of patients (Letter to the Editor), PRS, *53:*582, 1974

SNYDERMAN, R. K.: Discussion of "Incidence of obscure carcinoma in subcutaneous mastectomy. Results of national survey," by Pennisi, Capozzi, PRS, *56:*208, 1975

SNYDERMAN, R. K.: Letter: Breast prostheses. Lancet, *1:*494, 1976

SNYDERMAN, R. K.: Breast reconstruction after mastectomy for cancer (Editorial), PRS, *57:*224, 1976

SNYDERMAN, R. K., AND STARZYNSKI, T. E.:

Clinical application of 5-fluorouracil in treatment of skin lesions (Follow-Up Clinic), PRS, *52:*298, 1973

SOARES, V. R. *et al*: Plastic surgery in basalioma of the nose. Rev. Bras. Med. *28:*269, 1971 (Portuguese)

SOBANSKI, J. *et al*: Decreased mortality of patients with intranuclear malignant melanoma after enucleation of eyeball followed by orbit X-ray irradiation. Pol. Med. J., *11:*1512, 1972

SOBCZAK, O. M.: Use of ketamine in pediatric dentistry, PRS, *56:*604, 1975. Anesth. Analg., Cleve., *54:*248, 1975

SOBOL, S., TUCKER, W., AND TUCKER, H.: Everting closure of pharyngoesophageal defects, PRS, *55:*107, 1975. Arch. Otolaryng., *100:*148, 1974

SOBOTKOWSKA, K.: Gestational tumor of oral cavity. Czas. Stomatol., *27:*895, 1974 (Polish)

Societies, Associations, and Congresses of Plastic Surgery

All the National Societies of Plastic Surgery, PRS, *48:*402, 1971; *49:*479, 1972; *50:*425, 1972; *51:*489, 1973; *52:*465, 1973; *53:*503, 1974; *54:*516, 1974; *55:*520, 1975; *56:*476, 1975; *57:*545, 1976

Argentine Society of Esthetic Surgery, PRS, *49:*243, 1972; *53:*121, 1974

Argentine Society of Plastic Surgery, PRS, *53:*253, 1974; *56:*483, 1975

Argentine: Mar del Plata Society of Plastic, Oral, and Maxillofacial Surgery, PRS, *50:*430, 1972

Asian Pacific Section of the International Confederation for Plastic and Reconstructive Surgery, PRS, *56:*483, 1975

Royal Australasian College of Surgeons, PRS, *49:*484, 1972; *50:*544, 1972; *56:*483, 1975

Austrian Society for Plastic Surgery, PRS, *49:*243, 1972; *52:*334, 1973

Belgian Society of Plastic Surgery, PRS, *49:*365, 1972

Brazilian Society of Plastic Surgery, PRS, *50:*315, 1972; *54:*255, 635, 1974

British Association of Plastic Surgeons, PRS, *49:*594, 1972; *51:*716, 1973; *52:*607, 1973; *53:*617, 1974, *55:*732, 1975

Bulgarian Society of Plastic Surgery, PRS, *51:*614, 1973

Canadian Society of Plastic Surgeons, PRS, *49:*364, 1972; *54:*384, 1974; *57:*412, 1976

Colombian Association for Plastic Surgery and Surgery of the Hand, PRS, *48:*106, 1971; *52:*607, 1973

Chilean Society of Plastic and Reconstructive Surgery, PRS, *51:*496, 1973; *57:*272, 1976

Societies, Associations and Congresses of Plastic Surgery – Cont.

Costa Rica Plastic and Reconstructive Surgery Society, PRS, *56:*607, 1975

Czechoslovak Society of Plastic Surgery, PRS, *49:*113, 1972; *54:*125, 1974

Danish Society of Plastic and Reconstructive Surgery, PRS, *49:*593, 1972; *53:*120, 1974; *57:*412, 1976

Ecuadorian Society of Plastic Surgery, PRS, *51:*717, 1973; *55:*732, 1975

European Association for Maxillofacial Surgery, PRS, *50:*104, 1972; *52:*334, 1973; *56:*485, 1975; *57:*551, 1976

Finnish Society of Plastic Surgeons, PRS, *51:*718, 1973

French Society of Plastic and Reconstructive Surgery, PRS, *48:*105, 301, 1971; *49:*365, 1972; *51:*716, 1973; *52:*218, 1973; *53:*509, 1974; *54:*520, 1974; *57:*685, 1976; joint meeting with British Association of Plastic Surgeons, *49:*113, 1972

French Association of Maxillofacial Surgeons, meeting of, PRS, *56:*242, 1975

Association of German Plastic Surgeons, PRS, *50:*105, 1972; *51:*614, 1973; *52:*218, 1973; *53:*617, 1974; *55:*394, 1975

German Society for Plastic and Reconstructive Surgery, PRS, *55:*395, 1975; *56:*119, 1975

German Society of Maxillofacial Surgeons, PRS, *51:*615, 1973

Greece: Hellenic Society of Plastic and Reconstructive Surgery, PRS, *48:*204, 1971; *50:*430, 1972; *54:*705, 1974

Hungarian Society of Plastic Surgery, PRS, *52:*218, 1973

Ibero Latin-American Federation for Plastic and Reconstructive Surgery, PRS, *54:*634, 1974

International Confederation for Plastic and Reconstructive Surgery, European Section of, PRS, *50:*208, 1972

International Society of Aesthetic Plastic Surgery, PRS, *48:*617, 1971; *52:*606, 1973; *55:*651, 1975; *57:*551, 1976

International Association for Maxillofacial Surgery, PRS, *48:*106, 1971; *53:*618, 1974; *56:*120, 1975; *57:*412, 1976

International Society of Clinical Plastic Surgeons, PRS, *57:*131, 1976

Iranian Society for Plastic Surgery, PRS, *54:*124, 1974; *57:*131, 1976

Israel Association of Plastic Surgeons, PRS, *49:*113, 1972; *54:*705, 1974; *56:*687, 1975

Italian Society of Plastic Surgery, PRS, *49:*483, 594, 1972; *52:*110, 1973; *53:*617, 1974; *55:*394, 1975

Japan Society of Plastic and Reconstructive Surgery, PRS, *49:*593, 1972; *51:*113, 1973;

Societies of Surgery, National – Cont.
  55:263, 1975; 57:130, 1976
  Southern Medical Association, PRS, 49:594, 1972; 51:716, 1973; 53:616, 1974
  Teratology Society, PRS, 51:496, 1973; 53:618, 1974; 57:552, 1976
  Transplantation Society, PRS, 53:380, 1974; 57:412, 1976
  Twelfth International Congress of Orthopaedic Surgery and Traumatology, PRS, 50:105, 1972
  Western Surgical Association, PRS, 50:554, 1972; 54:634, 1974; 56:607, 1975
  World Microsurgery Congress, PRS, 57:552, 1976

Societies of Plastic Surgery, State and Regional, etc.

  Regional Societies of Plastic and Reconstructive Surgery, PRS, 48:99, 1971; 49:111, 1972; 50:102, 1972; 51:111, 1973; 52:108, 1973; 54:120, 1974; 55:126, 1975; 56:117, 1975; 57:128, 1976
  Alabama Society of Plastic and Reconstructive Surgeons, PRS, 55:262, 1975
  Buffalo Plastic Surgical Society, PRS, 53:252, 1974
  California Society of Plastic Surgeons, PRS, 48:410, 1971; 50:546, 1972; 57:130, 1976
  Chicago Society of Plastic Surgery, PRS, 54:255, 1974; 56:484, 1975
  District of Columbia Metropolitan Area Society of Plastic and Reconstructive Surgeons, PRS, 49:365, 1972; 51:357, 1973; 53:509, 1974; 55:527, 1975
  Florida Society of Plastic and Reconstructive Surgeons, PRS, 48:410, 1971; 50:546, 1972; 53:252, 1974; 54:521, 635, 1974; 57:411, 1976
  Plastic and Maxillofacial Surgical Society of Northeast Florida, PRS, 51:496, 1973; 52:335, 1973
  Georgia Society for Plastic Surgery, PRS, 50:104, 1972; 53:695, 1974; 56:119, 1975
  Houston Society of Plastic Surgery, PRS, 50:431, 1972
  Kentucky Society for Plastic and Reconstructive Surgery, PRS, 49:673, 1972
  Massachusetts Society of Plastic Surgeons, PRS, 52:607, 1973; 54:385, 1974
  Greater Miami Society of Plastic and Reconstructive Surgeons, PRS, 56:688, 1975; 57:412, 1976
  Midwestern Association of Plastic Surgeons, PRS, 49:114, 1972; 50:544, 1972; 53:120, 1974
  Association of Military Plastic Surgeons, PRS, 51:716, 1973
  Mississippi Society of Plastic and Reconstructive Surgeons, PRS, 56:485, 1975
  New England Society of Plastic and Recon-

Societies of Plastic Surgery, State and Regional, etc. – Cont.
  structive Surgeons, PRS, 52:469, 1973; 55:651, 1975; 56:608, 1975
  New Jersey Society of Plastic and Reconstructive Surgeons, PRS, 49:114, 1972; 53:616, 1974; 57:272, 1976
  New York Regional Society of Plastic and Reconstructive Surgery, PRS, 50:643, 1972; 51:717, 1973; 57:552, 1976
  Northwest Society of Plastic Surgeons, PRS, 50:544, 1972
  Ohio Valley Society for Plastic and Reconstructive Surgery, PRS, 48:410, 1971; 50:314, 1972; 52:469, 1973
  Ivy Society of Plastic Surgery (Pennsylvania): PRS, 49:243, 1972; 50:315, 546, 1972; 52:692, 1973
  Quebec Society of Plastic and Reconstructive Surgery, PRS, 50:314, 1972; 52:110, 1973; 55:129, 1975
  Rocky Mountain Association of Plastic and Reconstructive Surgeons, PRS, 50:545, 1972
  Skoog, Tord, Society of Plastic Surgeons, PRS, 50:314, 1972
  Southeastern Society of Plastic and Reconstructive Surgeons, PRS, 49:114, 1972; 50:544, 1972, 52:469, 1973, 54:520, 1974
  Tennessee Society of Plastic and Reconstructive Surgeons, PRS, 48:301, 1971
  Texas Society of Plastic Surgeons, PRS, 55:395, 1975; 57:130, 1976
  Virginia Society of Plastic and Reconstructive Surgery, PRS, 52:470, 1973; 57:770, 1976
  Wisconsin Society of Plastic and Reconstructive Surgery, PRS, 54:521, 1974

SODERDAHL, D. W., BROSMAN, S. A., AND GOODWIN, W. E.: Penile agenesis, PRS, 51:348, 1973. J. Urol., 108:496, 1972
SOEDA, S.: Theory and practice of free composite graft. Jap. J. Plast. Reconstr. Surg., 14:97, 1971 (Japanese)
SOEDA, S.: Rhinoplasty by using a forehead flap. Jap. J. Plast. Reconstr. Surg., 14:475, 1971 (Japanese)
SOEHREN, S. E. *et al*: Clinical and histologic studies of donor tissues utilized for free grafts of masticatory mucosa. J. Periodontol., 44:727, 1973
SOHN, S. A., AND OHLSEN, L.: Growth of cartilage from free perichondrial graft placed across defect in rabbit's trachea, PRS, 53:55, 1974
SOIN, K.: Some unusual osteoarticular injuries of hand, PRS, 53:106, 1974. Proc. Roy. Australasian Coll. Surg., 46:270, 1973
SOINTSEV, A. M. *et al*: Surgical treatment of

benign tumors of the parotid gland. Stomatologiia (Mosk.), *50:*34, 1971 (Russian)

SOKOL, A. B. *et al*: Rhinoplasty. Its development and present day usages. Ohio State Med. J., *68:*556, 1972

SOKOL, A. B., AND BERGGREN, R. B.: Thermograms after repair of nerve injuries in hand, PRS, *51:*449, 1973

SOKOLOV, E. F.: Treatment of burn wounds with the skin of the convalescents. Khirurgiia (Mosk.), *4:*21, 1975 (Russian)

SOKOLOV, N. N.: Use of decalcified heterologous bone in plastic facial surgery. Vestn. Khir., *106:*100, 1971 (Russian)

SOKOLOVA, L. A.: Free adipodermal grafts in surgical treatment of progressive lipodystrophy, PRS, *52:*686, 1973. Acta chir. plast., *14:*157, 1972

SOLL, D. B.: Insertion of secondary intraorbital implants. Arch. Ophth., *89:*214, 1973

SOLNIT, A. J. *et al*: Psychological reactions to facial and hand burns in young men. Can I see myself through your eyes? Psychoanal. Study Child., *30:*549, 1975

SOLOGUB, V. K. *et al*: Burns in light of A.V. Vishnevskii's school of thought. Khirurgiia (Mosk.), *9:*21, 1974 (Russian)

SOLOMENNYI, S. M.: Comparative study of results of autologous grafting of postoperative defects of mandibular canal using minced muscle tissue and coagulated blood. Stomatologiia (Mosk.), *53:*82, 1974 (Russian)

SOLOMON, A. A.: Testicular prosthesis: new insertion operation, PRS, *51:*348, 1973. J. Urol., *108:*435, 1972

SOLOMON, L. M. *et al*: Epidermal and other congenital organoid nevi. Curr. Probl. Pediatr., *6:*1, 1975

SOLOMON, M. P. *et al*: Intraoral submucosal pseudosarcomatous fibromatosis. Oral Surg., *38:*264, 1974

SOLONEN, K. A.: Experiences of a hand-surgeon in intravenous regional anesthesia. Handchirurgie, *1:*132, 1969 (German)

SOLOWAY, M. S. *et al*: Effect of regional lymphadenectomy on development of concomitant immunity. Surg. Forum, *23:*101, 1972

SOLOV'EV, A. E.: Epispadias of the double urethra. Vestn. Khir., *107:*90, 1971 (Russian)

SOLOV'EV, M. M. *et al*: Myxoma of the jaw: clinical picture, diagnosis and treatment. Stomatologiia (Mosk.), *54:*37, 1975 (Russian)

SOLOV'EV, M. M. *et al*: Surgical treatment method of sialolithiasis of the parotid gland. Stomatologiia (Mosk.), *54:*46, 1975 (Russian)

SOLOVKO, A. Iu.: Bone development in angioma. Vestn. Khir., *107:*123, 1971 (Russian)

SOLOWAY, H. B.: Drug-induced bleeding, PRS, *54:*622, 1974. Am. J. Clin. Path., *61:*622, 1974

SOLOWAY, H. B., AND ROBINSON, E. F.: Coagulation mechanism in experimental pulmonary fat embolism, PRS, *52:*325, 1973. J. Trauma, *12:*630, 1972

SOLTAN, M.: Surgical treatment of lower lip carcinoma with simultaneous plastic reconstruction of tissue defect. Czas. Stomatol., *28:*1089, 1975 (Polish)

SOLVIO, A. I. *et al*: Cleft lip and palate treatment and organization of the patient care in Finland. Suom. Hammaslaak. Toim., *68:*32, 1972 (Finnish)

SOM, M. L.: Elective neck dissection for carcinoma of tongue and floor of mouth. Trans. Am. Acad. Ophthalmol. Otolaryngol., *77:*182, 1973

SOM, M. L.: Laryngotracheal autograft for postcricoid carcinoma, reevaluation. Ann. Otol. Rhin. & Laryng., *83:*481, 1974

SOM, M. L.: Surgical management of carcinoma of maxilla. Arch. Otolaryng., *99:*270, 1974

SOM, M. L.: Surgery in premalignant lesions. Can. J. Otolaryngol., *3:*551, 1974

SOM, M. L. *et al*: Surgical management of recurrent head and neck cancer. Otolaryngol. Clin. North Am., *7:*163, 1974

SOMAN, C. S., AND SIRSAT, M. V.: Primary malignant melanoma of oral cavity in Indians, PRS, *56:*224, 1975. Oral Surg., *38:*426, 1974

SOMERS, G.: One-stage reconstruction for exstrophy of bladder in girls (with Furnas, Haq), PRS, *56:*61, 1975. Discussion by Devine, PRS, *56:*209, 1975

SOMMERLAD, B. C.: A long-term follow-up of hypospadias patients. Brit. J. Plast. Surg., *28:*324, 1975

SOMOGYI, J. *et al*: Development of mortality from malignant melanoma in Slovakia compared with Bohemia and some selected countries. Neoplasma, *18:*649, 1971

SONG, I. C.: Split-rib mandibular reconstruction (with Bromberg, Craig), PRS, *50:*357, 1972

SONG, I. C.: Evaluation of mammaplasty techniques in municipal teaching hospital (with Bromberg, Norwitz), PRS, *53:*33, 1974

SONG, I. C. *et al*: Total nasal reconstruction: further application of delto-pectoral flap. Brit. J. Plast. Surg., *26:*414, 1973

SONG, I. C., CRAMER, M. S., AND BROMBERG, B. E.: Primary vaginal reconstruction after pelvic exenteration, PRS, *51:*509, 1973

SONG, I. C., AND BROMBERG, B. E.: Pharyngopalatoplasty with free transplantation of *palmaris longus*, PRS, *56:*677, 1975. Brit. J. Plast. Surg., *27:*337, 1974

SONG, I. C., AND BROMBERG, B. E.: Carotid-cavernous sinus fistula occurring after rhinoplasty, PRS, *55:*92, 1975

SONNELAND, J.: "Inoperable" breast carcinoma. Successful result using zinc chloride fixative, PRS, *51:*347, 1973. Am. J. Surg., *124:*391, 1972

SONNENBURG, M.: Surgical treatment of mandibular fractures. Stomatol. DDR, *25:*673, 1975

SOOD, G. C. *et al*: Modified dacryocystorhinostomy. Indian J. Ophthalmol., *20:*127, 1972

SOOD, J. C., SEN, D. K., AND SETA, L. D.: Human bone as buried implant after enucleation, PRS, *48:*88, 1971. Internat. Surg., *54:*1, 1970

SOOD, S. C., GREEN, J. R., AND PARUI, R.: Results of various operations for sacrococcygeal pilonidal disease, PRS, *56:*559, 1975

SOOD, V. P. *et al*: Desmoplastic fibroma of maxilla. J. Laryng. & Otol., *89:*329, 1975

SOONG, T. T., AND HUANG, W. N.: Stochastic model for biological tissue elasticity in simple elongation, PRS, *53:*375, 1974. J. Bio-Mechanics, *6:*451, 1973

SOPEK, A. *et al*: Juvenile fibroma with atypical course. Wiad. Lek., *27:*915, 1974 (Polish)

SØRENSEN, B.: Medical education, epidemiology and surgery. Int. J. Epidemiol., *2:*387, 1973

SØRENSEN, B., AND HALL, K. V.: Mortality and causes of death in burned patients treated by exposure method, PRS, *51:*59, 1973

SØRENSEN, B., AND JEMEC, B.: Freeze drying of skin; *in vitro* studies of vitality, PRS, *53:*502, 1974. Scand. J. Plast. Reconstr. Surg., *7:*35, 1973

SORRELLS, R. B.: Examination of the injured hand. J. Arkansas Med. Soc., *71:*403, 407, 1975

SOSATH, G.: Burns and hyperbaric oxygenation. Med. Klin., *67:*1638, 1972 (German)

SOSS, T. L.: Saddle nose: its correction after extensive septal cartilage removal. Arch. Otolaryng., *98:*391, 1973

SOSS, T. L.: Allergic patient and rhinoplasty procedures. Otolaryngol. Clin. North Am., *7:*845, 1974

SOSSI, G.: Pierre-Robin syndrome. New personal surgical-orthopaedical treatment. Minerva Stomatol., *20:*179, 1971

SOTIROPOULOS, A. *et al*: Duplication of external genitalia in men. Urology, *4:*688, 1974

SOTO, D.: Parosteal sarcoma, PRS, *49:*474, 1972. Rev. Latino Am. cir. plast., *15:*45, 1971

SOUBIRAN, J. M.: Vermilionectomy. Actual Odontostomatol. (Paris), *26:*501, 1972

SOUBIRAN, J. M.: Internal fixation of grafts during rhinoplasty. Rev. Stomatol. Chir. Maxillofac., *75:*1125, 1974 (French)

SOUBIRAN, J. M. *et al*: Use of heterologous bone in surgical treatment of fractures of zygoma (25 cases). Ann. chir. plast., *17:*296, 1972

SOUBIRAN, J. M. *et al*: Indications for skin grafts in chronic diseases of the mouth. Rev. Stomatol. Chir. Maxillofac., *75:*103, 1974 (French)

SOUDIJN, E. R. *et al*: Cleft palates and middle ear effusions in babies. Cleft Palate J., *12:*229, 1975

SOUGARD, J.: Hand injuries caused by high pressure syringes. Ugeskr. Laeger, *136:*909, 1974 (Danish)

SOUQUET, R. *et al*: Value of bipedicled flap in covering lesions of the back of the hand. Ann. chir. plast., *18:*56, 1973 (French)

SOUSA-LENNOX, J.: Congenital anomalies, PRS, *54:*629, 1974. Semana med. Mexico, *79:*243, 1974

SOUSSALINE, M.: Trial of a new technic in the surgical treatment of tattoos. Ann. chir. plast., *19:*193, 251, 1974 (French)

SOUSSALINE, M. *et al*: Development of closure procedures in pharyngostomes and orostomes in irradiated tissues. Rev. Stomatol. Chir. Maxillofac., *75:*229, 1974 (French)

SOUTER, W. A.: Splintage in the rheumatoid hand. Hand, *3:*144, 1971

SOUTER, W. A.: Problem of boutonniere deformity. Clin. Orthop., *104:*116, 1974

SOUTHER, S. G.: Use of temporal muscle flap for reconstruction after orbito-maxillary resections for cancer (with Bakamjian), PRS, *56:*171, 1975

SOUTHER, S. G., CARR, S. D., AND VISTNES, L. M.: Wheelchair cushions to reduce pressure under bony prominences, PRS, *55:*519, 1975. Arch. Phys. Med., *55:*460, 1974

SOUTHER, S. G., CORBOY, J. M., AND THOMPSON, J. B.: Fasanella-Servat operation for ptosis of upper eyelid, PRS, *53:*123, 1974

SOUTHER, S. G., AND VISTNES, L. M.: Pressure, tissue ischemia, and operating table pads (Letter to the Editor), PRS, *53:*465, 1974

SOUTHMAYD, W. W. *et al*: Rupture of flexor tendons of index finger after Colles' fracture, PRS, *57:*398, 1976. J. Bone & Joint Surg., *57A:*562, 1975

SOUTHWICK, H. W.: Cancer of tongue. Surg. Clin. North Am., *53:*147, 1973

SOUTHWICK, H. W.: Malignant melanoma. Role of node dissection reappraised. Cancer, *37:*202, 1976

SOUYRIS, F. *et al*: Maxillase 3000 in plastic and reparative surgery of face. Rev. Odontostomatol. Midi Fr., *30:*57, 1972 (French)

SOUYRIS, F. *et al*: Segmental osteotomies of the upper jaw. Rev. Stomatol. Chir. Maxillofac., *73:*43, 1972 (French)

SOUYRIS, F. *et al*: Reconstruction of conjunctival cavity: holding in place of prosthetic form by transorbitary pin. Ann. chir. plast., *18:*315, 1973 (French)

SOUYRIS, F. *et al*: Osteosynthesis using screws and plates in maxillofacial and craniofacial surgery. Ann. chir. plast., *19:*131, 1974 (French)

SOUYRIS, F. *et al*: Segmental osteotomies of the jaws in orthodontic disorders. Rev. Stomatol. Chir. Maxillofac., *75:*122, 1974 (French)

SOUYRIS, F. *et al*: Skin grafts in the closure of bucconasal and buccosinusal communications. Rev. Stomatol. Chir. Maxillofac., *75:*195, 1974 (French)

SOUYRIS, F. *et al*: Phonetic results of velopharyngoplasties. Apropos of 67 cases. Rev. Stomatol. Chir. Maxillofac., *76:*423, 1975 (French)

SOUZA, W. N.: Hydration of burned patients in first postburn 48 hours, PRS, *55:*722, 1975. Ars Curandi, 7:34, 1974

SPADAFORA, A., TOLEDO RIOS, R., AND DE LOS RIOS, E.: Inguinocrural cutaneous flaccidity, PRS, *49:*233, 1972. Prensa med. argent., *58:*1393, 1971

SPADAFORA, A., DE LOS RIOS, E., AND TOLEDO RIOS, R.: Flat cheekbones (platyzygion), PRS, *49:*581, 1972. Prensa med. argent., *58:*1946, 1971

SPADAFORA, A., AND DE LOS RIOS, E. R.: Tuberous hemangioma of cheek skin, PRS, *49:*475, 1972. Prensa Univ. Arg., *5:*6825, 1971

SPADAFORA, A., AND DURAND, A. S.: Pendulous abdomen: reconstruction of umbilicus in anterolateral low dermolipectomy, PRS, *55:*509, 1975. Proc. Second Argent. Cong. Aesth. Surg., 66, 1974

SPADAFORA, A., DURAND, A. S., AND DE LOS RIOS, E.: Flaccidity of cheeks: cutaneous resection with quadrangular preauricular incision, PRS, *57:*670, 1976. Prensa Univ. Arg., *6:*8361, 1975

SPAETH, E. B.: Analysis of causes, types, and factors important to correction of congenital blepharoptosis, PRS, *48:*509, 1971. Am. J. Ophth., *71:*696, 1971

SPAETH, E. B.: Shrunken socket and related orbital hypoplasia. Surgical correction. Int. Ophthalmol. Clin., *10:*879, 1971

SPAETH, E. B.: Review of early history of ophthalmic plastic surgery. Trans. Pa. Acad. Ophthalmol. Otolaryngol., *26:*95, 1973

SPAETH, P. G.: Superior sulcus deformity and ptosis. Surgical correction. Int. Ophthalmol. Clin., *10:*791, 1971

SPANOS, B. *et al*: Hydroxyproline of urine after thermal injury in burns, PRS, *56:*469, 1975. Tr. 8th Panhellenic Cong. Surg. Soc., A:314, 1973

SPANOS, P. K., AND McQUARRIE, D. G.: Early

total ischiectomy with primary closure for decubitus ulcer, PRS, *53:*247, 1974. Am. J. Surg., *126:*98, 1973

SPASOKUKOTSKII, IU. A. *et al*: Experience in the use of ALS and ALG for prolonging the viability of skin grafts in burn patients. Klin. Khir., *10:*31, 1971 (Russian)

SPEARMAN, R. I. C.: *The Integument: A Textbook of Skin Biology.* Cambridge Univ. Press, London, 1973

SPECTOR, G. J. *et al*: Craniofacial dysjunction: otolaryngological point of view. Laryngoscope, *84:*1297, 1974

Speech Defects (See also *Cleft Palate; Cleft Palate, Velopharyngeal Incompetence*)

Reed-fistula method of speech rehabilitation after laryngectomy (Shedd *et al*), PRS, *52:*107, 1973. Am. J. Surg., *124:*510, 1972

Voice tunnels in laryngectomies, observations on (Kothary, Potdar, De Souza), PRS, *52:*97, 1973. Am. J. Surg., *124:*535, 1972

Speech defects in children, aged 7: national study (Butler, Peckham, Sheridan), PRS, *52:*455, 1973. Brit. M.J., *1:*253, 1973

Speech and vocational rehabilitation of laryngectomized patient (Sako *et al*), PRS, *57:*532, 1976. J. Surg. Oncol., *6:*197, 1974

Speech, effect of surgery for prognathism on (Goodstein, Cooper, Wallace), PRS, *56:*354, 1975. Oral Surg., *37:*846, 1974

SPENCE, H. M.: Surgical correction of hypospadias. Tex. Med., *68:*47, 1972

SPENCE, H. M. *et al*: Genital reconstruction in female with adrenogenital syndrome. Brit. J. Urol., *45:*126, 1973

SPENCE, H. M. *et al*: Exstrophy of the bladder. I. Long-term results in a series of 37 cases treated by ureterosigmoidostomy. J. Urol., *114:*133, 1975

SPENCE, V. A. *et al*: Current status of thermography in peripheral vascular disease. J. Cardiovasc. Surg. (Torino), *16:*572, 1975

SPENGOS, M. N.: Irradiated allogeneic bone grafts in treatment of odontogenic cysts. J. Oral Surg., *32:*674, 1974

SPERLI, A. E.: Cosmetic reduction of nipple with functional preservation. Brit. J. Plast. Surg., *27:*42, 1974

SPERLING, R. L., AND KRIMMER, B. M.: Malignant mixed tumors of lacrimal gland, PRS, *50:*81, 1972

SPERLING, R. L., AND GOLD, J. J.: Use of antiestrogen after reduction mammaplasty to prevent recurrence of virginal hypertrophy of breasts, PRS, *52:*439, 1973

SPIER, W.: Management of fresh hand injuries.

Ther. Ggw., *110:*1428, 1971 (German)
SPIER, W.: Reconstructive surgery on the hand. Ther. Ggw., *111:*684, 1972 (German)
SPIESSL, B.: Rigid internal fixation of fractures of lower jaw, PRS, *51:*476, 1973. Traum. Reconstr. Surg., *13:*124, 1972
SPIESSL, B.: Osteosynthesis in sagittal osteotomy using the Obwegeser-Dal Pont method. Fortschr. Kiefer. Gesichtschir., *18:*145, 1974 (German)
SPIESSL, B.: Median osteotomy for reduction of the mandible in dysgnathia. Fortschr. Kiefer. Gesichtschir., *18:*163, 1974 (German)
SPIESSL, B.: Functionally stable osteosynthesis in mandibular fractures—problems and technic. Fortschr. Kiefer. Gesichtschir., *19:*68, 1975 (German)
SPIESSL, B. *et al*: Routine exploration of the maxillary sinus in median facial fractures. D.D.Z., *23:*407, 1969 (German)
SPIESSL, B. *et al*: Planning pre- and postoperative treatment in orthodontic surgical procedures. Dtsch. Stomatol., *21:*734, 1971 (German)
SPIESSL, B. *et al*: Occlusion problems in functionally stable osteosynthesis of the mandible with teeth. Dtsch. Zahn. Mund. Kieferheilkd., *57:*293, 1971 (German)
SPIESSL, B., AND PREIN, J.: Late complications after fractures of zygoma, PRS, *50:*94, 1972. Ther. Umsch., *28:*811, 1971
SPIESSL, B., AND SCHUCHARDT, K.: Results of catalogued examinations of 41 cylindroma cases, PRS, *51:*707, 1973. Adv. Jaw & Face Surg., Year Book, 1972
SPIESSL, B., AND PREIN, J.: Morphology and malignancy of adamantinomas, PRS, *51:*708, 1973. Adv. Jaw & Face Surg., Year Book, 1972
SPIESSL, B. *et al*: Diagnosis and treatment of tumors of facial bones. Ther. Umsch., *29:*664, 1972 (German)
SPIESSL, B., AND PREIN, J.: Treatment of ankylosis of TMJ. Schweiz. Monatsschr. Zahnheilkd., *83:*89, 1973 (German)
SPIESSL, B. *et al*: Treatment of childhood retrognathism through transposition of the masseter muscle. Fortschr. Kiefer. Gesichtschir., *18:*176, 1974 (German)
SPILLER, W. F.: Cryosurgery in dermatologic office practice with special reference to basal cell carcinoma. Tex. Med., *68:*84, 1972
SPILLER, W. F. *et al*: Cryosurgery in dermatologic office practice: special reference to dermatofibroma and mucous cyst of the lip. South. Med. J., *68:*157, 1975
SPILLNER, G. *et al*: Treatment of soft part deficiencies and tendon injuries of the hand. Z. Allgemeinmed., *49:*68, 1973 (German)
SPINA, V.: Proposed modification for the classi-

fication of cleft lip and cleft palate. Cleft Palate J., *10:*251, 1973
SPINA, V.: Surgical correction of midfacial retrusion (nasomaxillary hypoplasia) in presence of normal dental occlusion (with Psillakis, Lapa), PRS, *51:*67, 1973
SPINA, V., AND HARO HERNANDES, J.: Surgical management of perforations of nasal septum, PRS, *48:*510, 1971; *52:*321, 1973. Rev. Latino Am. cir. plast., *13:*54, 1969
SPINA, V., KAMAKURA, L., AND PSILLAKIS, J. M.: Total reconstruction of ear in congenital microtia, PRS, *48:*349, 1971
SPINA, V. *et al*: Classification of cleft lip and cleft palate. Suggested changes. Rev. Hosp. Clin. Fac. Med. Sao Paulo, *27:*5, 1972 (Portuguese)
SPINA, V., FERREIRA, M. C., AND PSILLAKIS, J. M.: Dermafat grafts in repair of facial deformities, PRS, *52:*330, 1973. Rev. paulista med., *80:*19, 1972
SPINA, V., KAMAKURA, L., AND PSILLAKIS, J. M.: Prominent nasal tip, its repair, PRS, *53:*104, 1974. Rev. Soc. Med. Chir. San Jose, *5:*5, 1972
SPINA, V., KAMAKURA, L., AND PSILLAKIS, J.: New method for correction of prominent nasal tip, PRS, *51:*416, 1973
SPINA, V. *et al*: Surgical treatment of wrinkles of frontal region, PRS, *55:*244, 1975. Rev. Hosp. clin., *29:*76, 1974
SPINA, V., PSILLAKIS, J. M., AND FERREIRA, M. C.: Hemangiomas of face, PRS, *55:*723, 1975. Rev. paulista med., *83:*115, 1974
SPINK, M. S., AND LEWIS, G.: *Albucassis on Surgery and Instruments.* University of California Press, Berkeley, 1973
SPINNER, MORTON: *Injuries of the Major Branches of Peripheral Nerves of the Forearm.* W. B. Saunders Co., Philadelphia, 1972. PRS, *50:*611, 1972
SPINNER, M. *et al*: Impending ischemic contracture of hand, early diagnosis and management, PRS, *50:*341, 1972
SPINNER, M., AND OLSHANSKY, K.: *Extensor indicis proprius* syndrome, clinical test, PRS, *51:*134, 1973
SPINNER, M., AND SPENCER, P. S.: Nerve compression lesions of upper extremity, PRS, *56:*679, 1975. Clin. Orthop., *104:*46, 1974
SPIRA, M.: Discussion of "Bone deformation beneath alloplastic implants," by Jobe *et al*, PRS, *51:*174, 1973
SPIRA, M.: Silicone bag treatment of burned hands (Follow-Up Clinic), PRS, *52:*80, 1973
SPIRA, M.: Simplified design for reduction mammaplasty (with Gerow, Hardy), PRS, *53:*271, 1974
SPIRA, M.: What is maxillofacial surgery and who are maxillofacial surgeons? (Editorial),

PRS, *56:*438, 1975

SPIRA, M. *et al*: A comparison of chemical peeling, dermabrasion, and 5-fluourouracil in cancer prophylaxis. J. Surg. Oncol., *3:*367, 1971

SPIRA, M. *et al*: Maxims in maxillofacial management. South. Med. J., *65:*1136, 1972

SPIRA, M., GEROW, F. J., AND HARDY, S. B.: Modified Bonnacolto dacryocystorhinostomy, PRS, *52:*511, 1973

SPIRA, M., GEROW, F. J., AND HARDY, S. B.: Correction of posttraumatic enophthalmos, PRS, *55:*632, 1975. Acta chir. plast., *16:*107, 1974

SPIRA, M., GEROW, F. J., AND HARDY, S. B.: Subcutaneous pedicle flaps on face, PRS, *56:*676, 1975. Brit. J. Plast. Surg., *27:*258, 1974

SPIRA, M. *et al*: Surgical decompression of the orbit for endocrine exophthalmos. Fortschr. Kiefer. Gesichtschir., *18:*35, 1974

SPIRA, M., GEROW, F. J., AND HARDY, S. B.: Complications of chemical face peeling, PRS, *54:*397, 1974

SPIRO, R. H., AND STRONG, E. W.: Epidermoid carcinoma of mobile tongue, treatment by partial glossectomy alone, PRS, *51:*607, 1973. Am. J. Surg., *122:*707, 1971

SPIRO, R. H., AND STRONG, E. W.: Discontinuous partial glossectomy and radical neck dissection in selected patients with epidermoid carcinoma of mobile tongue, PRS, *53:*602, 1974. Am. J. Surg., *126:*544, 1973

SPIRO, R. H. *et al*: Epidermoid carcinoma of oral cavity and oropharynx. Elective vs. therapeutic radical neck dissection as treatment. Arch. Surg., *107:*382, 1973

SPIRO, R. H. *et al*: Tumors of minor salivary glands, PRS, *52:*214, 1973. Cancer, *31:*117, 1973

SPIRO, R. H. *et al*: Adenoid cystic carcinoma of salivary origin. A clinicopathologic study of 242 cases. Am. J. Surg., *128:*512, 1974

SPIRO, R. H. *et al*: Cervical node metastasis from epidermoid carcinoma of the oral cavity and oropharynx. A critical assessment of current staging. Am. J. Surg., *128:*562, 1974

SPIRO, R. H., AND STRONG, E. W.: Surgical treatment of cancer of tongue, PRS, *55:*516, 1975. Surg. Clin. N. Am., *54:*759, 1974

SPIVACK, J.: Reconstruction of rheumatoid hands. J. Med. Soc. N.J., *69:*547, 1972

SPLER, W.: Hand injuries in patients with multiple injuries. Med. Welt., *5:*169, 1971 (German)

Splints, Finger: See *Fingers, Splints for*

Splints, Hand: See *Hands, Splints*

Splints, Jaw

Splint for mandibular fixation, Morris biphasic external (Baumgarten, DesPrez), PRS, *50:*66, 1972

Pitanguy-Costa maxillofacial splint (Pitanguy *et al*), PRS, *51:*711, 1973. Rev. brasil. Cir., *62:*1212, 1972

Splints, custom cast, for oral surgical procedures (Brudvik), PRS, *55:*506, 1975. Oral Surg., *38:*15, 1974

Headcap, Orthoplast, for external fixation of facial fractures (Greer, Moore, Coleman), PRS, *54:*614, 1974

SPOHN, W. G.: Cranial-orbital defects. Prosthetic correction. Int. Ophthalmol. Clin., *10:*897, 1971

SPONHOLZ, H. *et al*: Value and significance of mouth vestibulum deepening under special consideration of cicatricial contracture. Dtsch. Stomatol., *22:*40, 1972 (German)

SPONHOLZ, H. *et al*: Experience with surgical deepening of the oral vestibulum in the mandible. Stomatol. DDR, *25:*607, 1975 (German)

SPREKELSEN, GASSO C. *et al*: Current surgical treatment of the intratemporal facial palsy. Rev. Esp. Otoneurooftalmol. Neurocir., *32:*149, 1974 (Spanish)

SPRETER, VON KREUDENSTEIN: Alloplastic reconstruction of chin in bird face by intraosseous anchorage of plastic implants. Zahnaerztl. Prax., *22:*37, 1971 (German)

SPRIESTERSBACH, D. C., POWERS, GENE R. *et al*: *Psychological Aspects of the "Cleft Palate Problem,"* Vols. I & II. University of Iowa Press, Iowa City, 1973. PRS, *54:*215, 1974

SPRIESTERSBACH, D. C. *et al*: Clinical research in cleft lip and cleft palate: the state of the art. Cleft Palate J., *10:*113, 1973

SPRINGER, H. A., AND WHITEHOUSE, J. S.: Launois-Bensaude adenolipomatosis, PRS, *50:*291, 1972

SRINIVASAN, H.: Extensor diversion graft operation for correction of intrinsic minus fingers in leprosy. J. Bone & Joint Surg. (Br.), *55:*58, 1973

SRINIVASAN, H.: Simple and direct method for simultaneously measuring angles of adjacent finger joints, PRS, *57:*524, 1976

SRIVASTAVA, K. P. *et al*: Congenital constriction bands of lower extremity. Indian. J. Pediatr., *38:*76, 1971

SRIVASTAVA, V. K., AND BHARGAVA, K. S.: Dermatofibrosarcoma protuberans. Indian J. Cancer, *9:*257, 1972

SRIVASTAVA, Y. C.: Oral leukoplakia, PRS, *56:*224, 1975. Internat. Surg., *58:*614, 1975

SRIVASTVA, K. N. *et al*: Stenson duct "implantation" in xerophthalmia—a surgical technique. Two case studies. Eye Ear Nose Throat Mon., *49:*522, 1970

SROUGI, M. *et al*: Cavernospongiosum shunt in the treatment of priapism. Rev. Hosp. Clin. Fac. Med. Sao Paulo, *30:*397, 1975 (Portuguese)

SROUR, R. K. *et al*: Neurotrophism in relation to muscle and nerve grafts in rats. Surg. Forum, *25:*508, 1974

SRSEN, S. *et al*: Hereditary gingival fibromatosis. Acta Univ. Carol. (Med. Monogr.), (Praha), *56:*141, 1973

SRUGI, S., AND ADAMSON, J. E.: Comparative study of tendon suture materials in dogs, PRS, *50:*31, 1972

STACK, G.: Tension in the lumbrical muscle. Hand, 2:166, 1970

STACK, H. B.: *Palmar Fascia.* Longman, London, 1974

STACK, H. G.: Button hole deformity. Hand, *3:*152, 1971

STACK, H. G. *et al*: Zig-zag deformity in the rheumatoid hand. Hand, *3:*62, 1971

STACK, R. E.: Carpal tunnel syndrome, PRS, *53:*367, 1974. Fam. Phys., *8:*88, 1973

STADAAS, J. *et al*: Burn problems illustrated by a case. J. Oslo City Hosp., *21:*97, 1971

STADAAS, J. *et al*: Problems with burns illustrated by a case. Tidsskr. nor. laegeforen, *91:*2007, 1971 (Norwegian)

STADAAS, J. O.: Chondritis of ear in burns. Tidsskr. nor. laegeforen, *93:*678, 1973 (Norwegian)

STADELMANN, W.: Lingua fixata. Surgical correction of shortened lingual frenum. Quintessenz, *24:*107, 1973 (German)

STADEN, D. A. VAN: An approach to the extensively injured hand. S. Afr. Med. J., *47:*380, 1973

STADNICKI, G. *et al*: The association of cleft palate with the Klippel-Feil syndrome. Oral Surg., *33:*335, 1972

STÄDTLER, K. *et al*: Research on burn toxins, PRS, *50:*308, 1972. Ther. Umsch., *28:*847, 1971

STÄDTLER, K. *et al*: Formation of specific "burn toxin" in mouse skin by thermal injuries, PRS, *51:*482, 1973. Europ. Surg. Res., *4:*198, 1972

STAEMMLER, H. J.: Gynecological remarks on the problem of the artificial vagina. Langenbecks Arch. Chir., *339:*417, 1975 (German)

STAFFILENO, H.: Significant differences and advantages between the full thickness and split thickness flaps. J. Periodontol., *45:*421, 1974

STAHL, WILLIAM H.: *Supportive Care of the Surgical Patient.* Grune & Stratton, New York, 1972. PRS, *52:*661, 1973

STAHNKE, H. L.: Arizona's lethal scorpion. Ariz. Med., *29:*490, 1972

STAGE, A. H.: Severe burns in pregnant patient, PRS, *54:*240, 1974. Obst. & Gynec., *42:*259, 1973

STAINES, N. A. *et al*: Passive enhancement of mouse skin allografts. Specificity of antiserum for major histocompatibility. Transplantation, *18:*192, 1974

STALEY, C. J. *et al*: Elective neck dissection in carcinoma of the larynx. Otolaryngol. Clin. North Am., *3:*543, 1970

STALLARD, H. B.: Evolution of lateral orbitotomy (Presidential Address). Trans. Ophthalmol. Soc. U. K., *93:*3, 1973

STALLARD, M. C., AND SAAD, M. N.: Aglossia-adactylia syndrome, PRS, *57:*92, 1976

STALLINGS, J. O.: Triple flap attack on the double cleft. Laryngoscope, *82:*141, 1972

STALLINGS, J. O.: Subcutaneous mastectomy with reconstruction. Am. Fam. Physician, *10:*184, 1974

STALLINGS, J. O. *et al*: Reverse dermis graft: a versatile technic, PRS, *49:*669, 1972. Am. Surgeon, *37:*539, 1971

STALLINGS, J. O. *et al*: Congenital microtia, PRS, *49:*233, 1972. Arch. Otolaryng., *94:*176, 1971

STALLINGS, J. O. *et al*: Reverse dermis graft—a choice not a flap. J. Iowa Med. Soc., *61:*606, 1971

STALLINGS, J. O. *et al*: Autografting of small second degree thermal burns. Am. Surg., *38:*136, 1972

STALLINGS, J. O. *et al*: Triple flap attack on the double cleft. Laryngoscope, *82:*141, 1972

STALLINGS, J. O. *et al*: Airway obstruction due to prolapse of the lower lateral cartilages in saddle deformity. Laryngoscope, *82:*515, 1972

STALLINGS, J. O., PAKIAM, A.I., AND CORY, C. C.: Late treatment of enophthalmos, PRS, *54:*686, 1974. Brit. J. Plast. Surg., *26:*57, 1973

STALLINGS, J. O., DELGADO, J. P., AND CONVERSE, J. M.: Turnover island flap of *gluteus maximus* muscle for repair of sacral decubitus ulcer, PRS, *54:*52, 1974

STALLWORTH, J. M. *et al*: Chronically swollen painful extremity, detailed study for possible etiological factors, PRS, *54:*690, 1974. J.A.M.A., *228:*1656, 1974

STAMATIN, S. I. *et al*: Bone plasty in the treatment of benign bone neoplasms and certain precancerous conditions. Ortop. Travmatol. Protez., *10:*25, 1974 (Russian)

STAMEN, F. C. *et al*: Neurotic or pseudoneurotic character development in patients with prognathism. Ned. tijdschr. geneeskd., *118:*778,

1974 (Dutch)

STANDFORD, J. R., KILMAN, J. W., AND ZEIGER, J. P.: Use of nitroblue tetrazolium (NBT) dye test as indicator of infection in surgical patients, PRS, 57:767, 1976. Am. J. Surg., 128:668, 1974

STANISAVLJEVIC, B.: Rare case of accidental maxillary injury. Srp. Arh. Celok. Lek., 101:383, 1973 (Serbian)

STANKO, V.: Errors in treatment of injuries of middle part of face. Cesk. Stomatol., 75:175, 1975 (Slovakian)

STANTON, S. L.: Gynecologic complications of epispadias and bladder exstrophy. Am. J. Obstet. Gynecol., 119:749, 1974

STANTON-HICKS, M. et al: Effects of peridural block, PRS, 57:768, 1976. Anesthesiology, 42:398, 1975

STARCHENKO, M. E.: Functional state of restored skin cover in persons who have suffered burn disease. Vestn. Khir., 110:82, 1973 (Russian)

STARK, C. R. et al: Temporal-spatial clustering of oral-cleft births in Michigan and Montana. Cleft Palate J., 7:826, 1970

STARK, D. B.: Nasal lining in cleft palate repair (Follow-Up Clinic), PRS, 49:333, 1972

STARK, E. W., AND BORTON, T. E.: Klippel-Feil syndrome and associated hearing loss, PRS, 52:682, 1973. Arch. Otolaryng., 97:415, 1973

STARK, N.: Implantation of small lacrimal tube for improved drainage of aqueous humor into subconjunctival space. Ber. Dtsch. Ophthalmol. Ges., 71:647, 1972 (German)

STARK, R. B.: Oral cancer: reconstruction and rehabilitation, PRS, 52:327, 1973. Ca-A Cancer J. Clin., 22:303, 1972

STARK, R. B.: Deliberate hypotension for blepharoplasty and rhytidectomy (Follow-Up Clinic), PRS, 49:453, 1972

STARK, R. B.: Development of face, PRS, 53:600, 1974. Surg. Gynec. & Obst., 137:403, 1973

STARK, R. B.: Commentary on "Building out the malar prominences as an addition to rhytidectomy," by Gonzalez-Ulloa, PRS, 53:469, 1974

STARK, R. B.: Unusual cleft lip deformity (Letter to the Editor), PRS, 54:346, 1974

STARK, R. B.: Variation in rhytidectomy incision at front of ear, PRS, 54:369, 1974

STARK, R. B.: Parable of 3 doyens, PRS, 56:487, 1975

STARK, R. B., AND KAPLAN, J. M.: Cross-leg flaps in patients over fifty years of age, PRS, 52:207, 1973. Brit. J. Plast. Surg., 25:20, 1972

STARK, R. B., AND KAPLAN, J. M.: Rotation flaps, neck to cheek, PRS, 50:230, 1972

STARK, R. B., AND KAPLAN, J. M.: Manage-

ment of cleft lip and palate, PRS, 50:540, 1972. Tribuna Med. Mexico, 21:11, 1972

STARK, R. B., AND KAPLAN, J. M.: Development of cleft lip nose, PRS, 51:413, 1973

STARR, C. D. et al: Nasality and cleft uvula. Cleft Palate J. 8:189, 1971

STARZYNSKI, S.: Mixed tumor of parotid intraductal gland. Patol. Pol., 25:169, 1974 (Polish)

STASINOPOULOS, E. et al: Surgical reconstruction of the alveolar ridges. Current modification of technic. Stoma. (Thessalonike), 2:122, 1970 (Greek)

STATE, D. et al: Clinical use of porcine xenografts in conditions other than burns. Surg. Gynec. & Obst., 138:13, 1974

Statistics

Statistics for clinical research (McCrum), PRS, 56:367, 1975. Henry Ford Hosp. M. J., 21:117, 1973

Statistical applications in physical medicine (Daniel, Coogler), PRS, 56:604, 1975. Part I: Am. J. Phys. Med., 53:271, 1974; Part II: 54:25, 1975

STAUFFER, E. S., AND NICKEL, V. L.: Control systems for upper extremity function in traumatic quadriplegia, PRS, 52:452, 1973. Paraplegia, 10:3, 1972

STAVEM, P.: Bleeding time from incisions standardized by protruding skin fold method. Brit. J. Haematol., 26:153, 1974

STEA, G.: Surgical treatment of cheilognathopalatoschisis. Mondo Odontostomatol., 14:101, 1971 (Italian)

STEA, G.: Treatment of ameloblastoma of the mandible: resection via the intraoral route and simultaneous reconstruction by means of autogenous bone transplant. Riv. Ital. Stomatol., 26:395, 1971

STEA, G.: Our experience with mandibular resection by endobuccal approach and immediate transplantation of autologous bone. Rev. Stomatol. Chir. Maxillofac., 75:55, 1974 (French)

STEA, G.: Conservative surgical treatment of mixed tumors of parotid gland, PRS, 57:258, 1976. J. Maxillo-facial Surg., 3:135, 1975

STECHMILLER, G. M., AND SEIGLER, H. F.: Characterization of chimpanzee anti-human melanoma antiserum, PRS, 57:403, 1976. Cancer Res., 35:2132, 1975

STECKLER, R. M. et al: Craniofacial injuries due to impalement on an auto gearshift lever. J. Trauma, 12:161, 1972

STECKLER, R. M. et al: "Andy Gump." Am. J. Surg., 128:545, 1974

STECKLER, R. M. et al: The philosophy of head

and neck cancer surgery. J. Prosthet. Dent., *32:*307, 1974

STEDMAN, THOMAS L.: *Stedman's Medical Dictionary,* 22nd Edition. Williams & Wilkins Co., Baltimore, 1972. PRS, *50:*612, 1972. 23rd Edition, 1976

STEENBERGHE, D. *et al*: Midfacial necrosis: apropos of 2 cases and review of the literature. Rev. Stomatol. Chir. Maxillofac., *76:*509, 1975 (French)

STEFANI, F. H. *et al*: Progressive lethal ulceration of the nose (Kraus-Chatellier). Klin. Monatsbl. Augenheilkd., *167:*110, 1975 (German)

STEFANOVIC, B. *et al*: Rare vascular tumor of the neck: cystic hygroma of the neck. Srp. Arh. Celok. Lek., *98:*1065, 1970 (Serbian)

STEFFANOFF, D. N.: Late development of squamous cell carcinoma in split-skin graft lining vagina, PRS, *51:*454, 1973

STEFFENSEN, W. H., AND RHOADS, H. T., JR.: Obituary on Clarence R. Straatsma, M.D., PRS, *55:*648, 1975

STEGMAN, S. J. *et al*: Fresh tissue chemosurgery for tumors of the nose. Eye Ear Nose Throat Mon., *55:*26, 1976

STEHLIN, J. S. *et al*: Results of hyperthermic perfusion for melanoma of the extremities. Surg. Gynec. & Obst., *140:*339, 1975

STEICHEN, F. M.: Clinical experience with autosuture instruments, PRS, *48:*300, 1971. Surgery, *69:*609, 1971

STEIDL, L. *et al*: Five year experience and results obtained in surgical treatment of ischemic lesions of 7th nerve. Cas. Lek. Cesk., *111:*802, 1972 (Czechoslovakian)

STEIDL, L. *et al*: Proceedings: Unusual reinnervation after resection of the facial nerve. Electroencephalogr. Clin. Neurophysiol., *39:*547, 1975

STEIGLEDER, G. K.: Solitary trichoepithelioma. Hautarzt, *23:*323, 1972 (German)

STEIN, F.: Method for rapid and good thumb reconstruction (with Morgan), PRS, *50:*131, 1972

STEIN, G.: Malignant melanoma of the skin. Z. Haut. Geschlechtskr., *46:*409, 1971 (German)

STEIN, H. I.: Rhinoplasty and plastic facial repair. J. Am. Osteopath. Assoc., *72:*827, 1973

STEIN, J. J.: Osteogenic sarcoma (osteosarcoma): results of therapy. Am. J. Roentgenol. Radium Ther. Nucl. Med., *123:*607, 1975

STEIN, J. M., AND PRUITT, B. A.: Suppurative thrombophlebitis—lethal iatrogenic disease, PRS, *49:*236, 1972. New England J. Med., *282:*1452, 1970

STEIN, S. A. V.: Lip repair (cheiloplasty) performed by a new method (Classic Reprint), PRS, *53:*332, 1974

STEINER, A. K. *et al*: Localized leukocyte mobilization in patients with solid malignant tumors, PRS, *51:*484, 1973. Schweiz. med. Wchnschr., *102:*1165, 1972

STEINER, B. W. *et al*: Gender identity project. Organization of multidisciplinary study. Can. Psychiatr. Assoc. J., *19:*7, 1974

STEINHARDT, G. *et al*: Treatment of the gnathic open bite. Fortschr. Kiefer. Gesichtschir., *18:*199, 1974 (German)

STEINHAUSER, E. *et al*: Correction of speech in patients with cleft lip and palate by surgical positioning of the maxilla. Dtsch. Zahnaerztl. Z., *27:*203, 1972 (German)

STEINHAUSER, E. W.: Vestibuloplasty—skin grafts. J. Oral Surg., *29:*777, 1971

STEINHAUSER, E. W.: Midline splitting of the maxilla for correction of malocclusion. J. Oral Surg., *30:*413, 1972

STEINHAUSER, E. W.: Treatment of ankylosis in children. Int. J. Oral Surg., *2:*129, 1973

STEINHAUSER, E. W.: Advancement of mandible by sagittal ramus split and suprahyoid myotomy. J. Oral Surg., *31:*516, 1973

STEINHAUSER, E. W.: Changes in the soft tissues after corrective osteotomies in the jaw region. Dtsch. Zahnaerztl. Z., *29:*1065, 1974 (German)

STEINHAUSER, E. W. *et al*: Surgical correction of mandibular retrusion in combination with mandibular alveolar protrusion. J. Am. Dent. Assoc., *91:*132, 1975

STEINHAUSER, E. W. *et al*: Correction of severe open-bite associated with muscular disease. Report of a case. Oral Surg., *39:*509, 1975

STEINHILBER, W.: Correction of dysgnathias by means of osteotomy of alveolar process. Dtsch. Zahnaerztl. Z., *29:*755, 1974 (German)

STEINHILBER, W.: Indications, technic and results of unilateral osteotomy on the body of the mandible for the correction of prognathism. Fortschr. Kiefer. Gesichtschir., *18:*131, 1974 (German)

STEINHOFF, N. G. *et al*: Analysis of cylindroma of head and neck. J. Surg. Oncol., *5:*17, 1973

STEINHUSER, E. W.: Mid-line splitting of the maxilla for correction of dental-facial disharmonies. Fortschr. Kiefer. Gesichtschir., *18:*189, 1974

STEINMETZ, E.: Emergency tracheotomy via a cannula. Ugeskr. Laeger, *136:*2244, 1974

STEINMETZ, L. *et al*: Complete scalping of penis. Pol. Przegl. Chir., *45:*275, 1973 (Polish)

STEINMULLER, D.: Reinnervation after orthotopic grafting of peripheral nerve segments in inbred rats (with Bucko), PRS, *53:*326, 1974

STEINMULLER, D. *et al*: Differential survival of skin and heart allografts in radiation chimaeras provides further evidence for skin histocompatibility antigen. Nature, 248:796, 1974

STELINSKA, A. et al: Lipomas of oral cavity. Czas. Stomatol., 25:931, 1972 (Polish)

STELL, P. M.: First laryngectomy for carcinoma. Arch. Otolaryng., 98:293, 1973

STELL, P. M.: Cancer of hypopharynx. J. R. Coll. Surg. Edinb., 18:20, 1973

STELL, P. M.: Pharyngeal reconstruction using the delto-pectoral flap. O.R.L., 35:317, 1973

STELL, P. M.: Limitations of surgery in the treatment of head and neck cancer. Can. J. Otolaryngol., 4:408, 1975

STELL, P. M.: Management of cervical lymph nodes in head and neck cancer, PRS, 56:226, 1975. Proc. Roy. Soc. Med., 68:83, 1975

STELL, P. M., AND MARAN, A. G. D.: Head and Neck Surgery. J. B. Lippincott Co., Philadelphia, 1972. PRS, 52:295, 1973

STELL, P. M. et al: Skin flaps in head and neck surgery. J. Laryng. & Otol., 86:419, 1972

STELL, P. M. et al: Management of fistulae of the head and neck after radical surgery. J. Laryng. & Otol., 88:819, 1974

STELL, P. M. et al: The viability of triangular skin flaps. Brit. J. Plast. Surg., 28:247, 1975

STELLA, J. G. et al: Use of iridium-192 in interstitial tumor therapy, PRS, 53:375, 1974. Cancer, 32:665, 1973

STELLAR, S. et al: Laser excision of acute third degree burns followed by immediate autograft replacement: experimental study in pig, PRS, 53:685, 1974. J. Trauma, 13:45, 1973

STELLAR, S. et al: Carbon dioxide laser debridement of decubitus ulcers, followed by immediate rotation flap or skin graft closure, PRS, 54:242, 1974. Ann Surg., 179:230, 1974

STELLBRINK, G.: Synovectomy in the upper limbs. Indications and results. Beitr. Orthop. Traumatol., 18:117, 1971 (German)

STELLBRINK, G.: Trigger finger syndrome in rheumatoid arthritis not caused by flexor tendon nodules. Hand, 3:76, 1971

STELLBRINK, G.: Compression of the palmar branch of the median nerve by the atypical palmaris longus muscle. Handchirurgie, 4:155, 1972 (German)

STELLBRINK, G.: Injured hand. Munch. Med. Wochenschr., 115:1959, 1973 (German)

STELLBRINK, G. et al: Ganglioplastic tumors of the hand. Handchirurgie, 2:152, 1970 (German)

STELLMACH, R.: Surgical consequences in cylindroma of submandibular gland with invasion of common carotid artery. Fortschr. Kiefer. Gesichtschir., 15:97, 1972 (German)

STELLMACH, R.: Surgical procedures for im-

provement of lip esthetics. Zahnaerztl. Prax., 24:237, 1973 (German)

STELLMACH, R.: Possibilities of surgical treatment of unilateral mandibular dysostosis in adults. Fortschr. Kiefer. Gesichtschir., 18:49, 1974 (German)

STELLMACH, R.: Surgical treatment of acne conglobata of face, PRS, 56:471, 1975. J. Maxillofacial Surg., 3:58, 1975

STELLMACH, R.: Reconstruction and rehabilitation of the mandible in unilateral agenesis of the articular process. Z.W.R., 85:74, 1976 (German)

STELLMACH, R., REHRMANN, A., AND KOCH, H.: Malignant degeneration of basal cell carcinoma of face: basal-squamous carcinoma, PRS, 48:471, 1971

STELLMACH, R. et al: Complications resulting from dento-surgical operations in area of maxillary sinus. Surgical closure combined with radical operation in maxillary sinus. (With changes of mucosa of maxillary sinus.) Quintessence Int., 3:11, 1972

STELLMACH, R. et al: Complications resulting from dento-surgical operations in area of maxillary sinus. Plastic closure in connection with tooth extraction. Quintessence Int., 3:17, 1972

STELLMACH, R., AND FRENKEL, G.: Complications resulting from dento-surgical operations in area of maxillary sinus. Plastic closure of suction cup perforation of hard palate. Quintessence Int., 3:21, 1972

STELLMACH, R., AND FRENKEL, G.: Complications resulting from dento-surgical operations in area of maxillary sinus. Surgical closure with double flap repair. Quintessence Int., 3:23, 1972

STELLMACH, R. et al: Oral surgery procedures II. Dysostosis mandibularis. Dent. Dienst., 25:45, 1973 (German)

STELLMACH, R. K.: Biographical sketch and commentary on Karl Schoenborn (Classic Reprint), PRS, 49:561, 1972

STENBACK, F.: Hexachlorophene in mice, PRS, 56:115, 1975. Arch. Environmental Health, 30:32, 1975

STENHOUSE, D.: Intraoral actinomycosis. Report of five cases. Oral Surg., 39:547, 1975

STENHOUSE, D., AND MacDONALD, D. G.: Low grade osteomyelitis of jaws with actinomycosis, PRS, 55:508, 1975. Internat. J. Oral Surg., 3:64, 1974

STENSTROM, S.: Alar cartilage and nasal deformity in unilateral cleft lip (Follow-Up Clinic), PRS, 55:359, 1975

STENSTRÖM, S. et al: Wound healing with ordinary adhesive tape. A clinical and experimental study. Scand. J. Plast. Reconstr.

Surg., *6:*40, 1972

STENSTRÖM, S., AND THILANDER, B.: Management of cleft palate cases using modified Dunn procedure with skin graft to vomer flaps, PRS, *56:*682, 1975. Scand. J. Plast. Reconstr. Surg., *8:*67, 1974

STENSTRÖM, S. J., AND THILANDER, B. L.: Healing of surgically created defects in the septal cartilages of young guinea pigs, PRS, *49:*194, 1972

STENSTRÖM, S. J., AND THILANDER, B. L.: Bone grafting in secondary cases of cleft lip and palate (Follow-Up Clinic), PRS, *49:*333, 1972

Stent (See also Skin Grafts, Inlay; Skin Grafts, Dressings for)

Stent, internal, for securing large skin grafts on small animals (Bryant), PRS, *52:*106, 1973. J. Surg. Res., *13:*241, 1972

Stent: internal nasal mold, made of silicone rubber, for grafts or flaps inside the nose (Shuster). PRS, *52:*203, 1973

Stent, "parachute" (Goshgarian, Miller), PRS, *57:*530, 1976. Am. J. Surg., *130:*370, 1975

STEPAKOV, A. I. *et al*: Free dermatoplasty in lacerated wounds of the skin of the genital organs. Urol. Nefrol. (Mosk.), *36:*60, 1971 (Russian)

STEPANIK, J.: Diaphanoscopy in Toti's dacryocystorhinostomy. Klin. Monatsbl. Augenheilkd., *164:*270, 1974

STEPANOVA, R. A.: Nurse's functions in office of cosmetic department. Med. Sestra., *32:*41, 1973 (Russian)

STEPHENS, F. O.: Place of chemotherapy in treatment of advanced squamous carcinoma of head and neck and in other situations, PRS, *55:*386, 1975. M. J. Australia, *2:*587, 1974

STEPHENS, F. O. *et al*: Effect of cortisone and vitamin A on wound infection, PRS, *51:*609, 1973. Am. J. Surg., *121:*569, 1971

STEPHENS, F. O., HUNT, T. K., AND DUNPHY, J. E.: Study of traditional methods of care on the tensile strength of skin wounds in rats, PRS, *49:*587, 1972. Am. J. Surg., *122:*78, 1971

STEPHENS, F. O., DUNPHY, J. E., AND HUNT, T. K.: Effect of delayed administration of corticosteroids on wound contracture, PRS, *48:*96, 1971. Ann. Surg., *173:*214, 1971

STEPHENS, F. O. *et al*: Use of an automatic stapling device for closure of surgical wounds. Aust. N. Z. J. Surg., *44:*398, 1974

STEPHENS, R., HANSEN, H., AND MUGGIA, F.: Hypercalcemia in epidermoid tumors of head, neck, and esophagus, PRS, *54:*108, 1974. Cancer, *31:*1487, 1973

STEPHENSON, A. L.: Reduction mammaplasty – experience with lateral approach of Dufourmentel and Mouly, PRS, *52:*678, 1973. Proc. Roy. Australasian Coll. Surg., *46:*441, 1973

STEPHENSON, HUGH JR.: *Immediate Care of the Acutely Ill and Injured*, C. V. Mosby Co., St. Louis, 1974. PRS, *57:*509, 1976

STEPHENSON, H. E., JR. *et al*: Immunologic factors in human melanoma "metastatic" to products of gestation (with exchange-transfusion in infant to mother), PRS, *48:*297, 1971. Surgery, *69:*515, 1971

STEPHENSON, K. L.: Dr. Suzanne Noël, first woman to do esthetic surgery (with Regnault). PRS, *48:*133, 1971

STEPHENSON, K. L.: Present status of plastic surgery. J.A.M.A., *234:*929, 1975

STEPHENSON, KATHRYN LYLE: *The Year Book of Plastic and Reconstructive Surgery*. Year Book Medical Publishers, Inc., Chicago, 1974. PRS, *55:*355, 1975

STERN, H. D.: Cutaneous and subcutaneous necrosis as a complication of coumarin-congener therapy (with Kahn, Rhodes). PRS, *48:*160, 1971

STERN, L. M. *et al*: Management of Pierre Robin syndrome in infancy by prolonged nasoesophageal intubation. Am. J. Dis. Child, *124:*78, 1972

STERN, O. S.: New fixation device for cross-leg flaps. PRS, *50:*194, 1972

STERNLICHT, H. C.: Contiguous mucosal graft. J. Periodontol., *46:*221, 1975

STERNSCHEIN, M. J. *et al*: Causalgia, PRS, *56:*107, 1975. Arch. Phys. Med. & Rehab., *56:*58, 1975

Sternum

Sternum, congenital cleft, repair of (Vilar-Sancho, Bermudez-Piernagorda), PRS, *48:*605, 1971. Rev. españ. cir. plast., *4:*87, 1971

Sternum, stabilization after funnel chest operation (Gross), PRS, *57:*398, 1976. Ztschr. Kinderchir., *17:*67, 1975

Congenital bifid sternum (Lambrecht), PRS, *57:*760, 1976. Ztschr. Kinderchir., *17:*128, 1975

STEVENS, A. H.: Staphyloraphe, or palate suture, successfully performed (Classic Reprint). PRS, *48:*61, 1971

STEVENS, D. M.: Liabilities engendered in emergency department practice, PRS, *54:*383, 1974. J. Legal Med., *2:*17, 1974

STEVENS, K. M. *et al*: Cricopharyngeal myotomy in dysphagia. Laryngoscope, *81:*1616, 1971

STEVENSON, R. M.: Successful transplantation

of totally severed thumb (with Snyder, Browne). PRS, *50:*553, 1972

STEWARD, D. J.: Experiences with outpatient anesthesia service for children, PRS, *53:*693, 1974. Anesth. Analg., Cleve., *52:*877, 1973

STEWART, J. M. *et al*: Familial hand abnormality and sensori-neural deafness: a new syndrome. J. Pediatr., *78:*102, 1971

STEWART, S. *et al*: Large sublingual dermoid cyst. J. Oral Surg., *31:*620, 1973

STEWART, S. *et al*: Large bilateral traumatic bone cysts of mandible, case report. J. Oral Surg., *31:*685, 1973

STEWART, S. *et al*: Lymphoepithelial (branchial) cyst of parotid gland. J. Oral Surg., *32:*100, 1974

STEWART, S. *et al*: Fibrolipoma of the palate: report of two cases. N. Y. State Dent. J., *40:*603, 1974

STEWART, S. S. *et al*: Myxoma of lower jaw. Oral Surg., *36:*800, 1973

STIEBITZ, R.: Cylindromas of maxillofacial region. Fortschr. Kiefer. Gesichtschir., *15:*60, 1972 (German)

STIEBITZ, R. *et al*: Keratinizing squamous epithelial cysts (keratocysts) in the jaws. Wien. Klin. Wochenschr., *86:*643, 1974 (German)

STIEGLITZ, L. N. *et al*: Blepharochalasis. Am. J. Ophth., *77:*100, 1974

STIEGLITZ, R. *et al*: Burns caused by electric arc. Z. Aerztl. Fortbild. (Jena), *66:*364, 1972 (German)

STIEN, R. *et al*: Acute peripheral facial palsy. Indications for surgical treatment. Arch. Otolaryng., *98:*187, 1973

STILL, J. M., JR., AND GEORGIADE, N.: Burn wound therapy. Am. Surgeon, *39:*82, 1973

STILL, J. M., JR., AND KLEINERT, H. E.: Anomalous muscles and nerve entrapment in the wrist and hand. PRS, *52:*394, 1973

STIMMEL, B.: Crisis in medical education, PRS *54:*511, 1974. Ann. Int. Med., *79:*119, 1973

Stings: See *Bites and Stings*

STINSON,V.: Porcine skin dressings for burns. Am. J. Nurs., *74:*111, 1974

STIVERS, F. E., STEFFEK, A. J., AND YARINGTON, C. T., JR.: Effect of lathyrogens on developing midfacial structures in rat, PRS, *49:*586, 1972. J. Surg. Res., *11:*415, 1971

STOCK, A.: Importance of the skin in primary treatment of injured hands. Zentralbl. Chir., *99:*1010, 1974 (German)

STCEHR, K.: Closure of oroantral fistula using lyophilized dura. Stomatol. DDR, *23:*481, 1973 (German)

STOELINGA, P. J.: Recurrences and multiplicity of cysts. Trans. Int. Conf. Oral Surg., *4:*77, 1973

STOELINGA, P. J. *et al*: Note on origin of keratocysts of jaws. Int. J. Oral Surg., *2:*37, 1973

STOELINGA, P. J. *et al*: Combined correction of the upper jaw and nose in patients with schisis. Ned. tijdschr. geneeskd., *117:*1604, 1973 (Dutch)

STOELTING, R. K., AND PETERSON, C.: Methoxyflurane anesthesia in pediatric patients, PRS, *57:*681, 1976. Anesthesiology, *42:*16, 1975

STOKER, N. C., AND EPKER, B. N.: Posterior maxillary ostectomy: retrospective study of treatment results, PRS, *55:*717, 1975. Internat. J. Oral Surg., *3:*153, 1974

STOKSTED, P. *et al*: Nasal fractures, their diagnoses, complications and treatment. H. N. O., *21:*304, 1973 (German)

STOLL, A. M. *et al*: Heat transfer through fabrics as related to thermal injury. Trans. N. Y. Acad. Sci., *33:*649, 1971

STOLLER, R. J.: Male transsexualism: uneasiness. Am. J. Psychiatry, *130:*536, 1973

STOLP, A.: Surgical-plastic treatment of facial skin neoplasms. Dermatol. Monatsschr., *160:*387, 1974 (German)

STONE, E. J. *et al*: Lymphedema. Surg. Gynec. & Obst., *135:*625, 1972

STONE, H. H.: Stress ulcers in patients with major burns. Am. Surg., *38:*107, 1972

STONE, H. H., AND KOLK, L. D.: The evolution and spread of gentamicin-resistant *Pseudomonas*, PRS, *49:*106, 1972. J. Trauma, *7:*586, 1971

STONE, H. H. *et al*: Periurethral abscess in patients with major burns. Am. Surg., *38:*318, 1972

STONE, H. H. *et al*: *Candida* sepsis: pathogenesis and principles of treatment, PRS, *54:*702, 1974. Ann. Surg., *179:*697, 1974

STONE, J. W.: Comprehensive care of bilateral maxillary fractures. Laryngoscope, *83:*179, 1973

STONE, J. W. *et al*: Methods of bone grafting the mandible. South. Med. J., *65:*815, 1972

STONE, P. A.: Hand burns caused by electric fires, PRS, *53:*370, 1974. Injury, *4:*240, 1973

STONE, P. A., AND LAWRENCE, J. C.: Healing of tangentially excised and grafted burns in man, PRS, *54:*696, 1974. Brit. J. Plast. Surg., *26:*20, 1973

STONE, P. A., AND MADDEN, J. W.: Effect of primary and delayed split-skin grafting on wound contraction, PRS, *57:*765, 1976. Surg. Forum, *25:*41, 1974

STONER, D. L., AND COOKE, J. P.: Intratracheal cuffs and aeromedical evacuation, PRS, *55:*643, 1975. Anesthesiology, *41:*302, 1974

STOPPA, R. *et al*: Original plastic procedure for inguinal hernia, PRS, *52:*463, 1973. Chirurgie, *99:*119, 1973

STORCK, H.: Clinical aspects and therapy of malignant melanoma. Hautarzt, *21:*187, 1970 (German)

STORGARD JENSEN, P., AND HUSTED, E.: Cystadenolymphoma (Warthin's tumor) of parotid gland, PRS, *48:*92, 1971. Scand. J. Plast. Reconstr. Surg., *4:*114, 1970

STORRS, J.: Bilateral eosinophilic granuloma of the mandible. Oral Surg., *41:*93, 1976

STORTENBEEK, W.: Modern concepts of surgical shock. Arch. chir. neerl., *25:*215, 1973

STORVIK, H. M.: Extended neurovascular island flap in thumb reconstruction, PRS, *54:*503, 1974. Scand. J. Plast. Reconstr. Surg., *7:*147, 1973

STOUGH, B.: Current trends in hair transplantation, PRS, *54:*104, 1974. Arch. Otolaryng., *98:*370, 1973

STOUGH, D. B.: Corrective surgical office procedures of face. Am. Fam. Physician, *7:*68, 1973

STOUGH, D. B., III *et al:* Chemical peel for facial wrinkles. Am. Fam. Physician, *10:*106, 1974

STRAATSMA, B. R.: Discussion of "Successful early relief of blindness occurring after blepharoplasty" by Hueston, Heinze (with Hepler, Sugimura). PRS, *57:*233, 1976

STRAFFON, W. G.: Useful scrotal dressing. M. J. Australia, *1:*320, 1974

STRAHAN, R. W. *et al:* Current concepts in management of keloids. Otolaryngol. Clin. North Am., *5:*521, 1972

STRAIGHT, R.: Snakebitten hand (with Snyder, Glenn). PRS, *49:*275, 1972

STRAIT, J.: Transsexual patient after surgery. Am. J. Nurs., *73:*462, 1973

STRAKA, J. A.: Problems complicating tracheotomy. Trans. Pa. Acad. Ophthalmol. Otolaryngol., *28:*60, 1975

STRANC, M. F.: Severe degloving injury of upper limb. Hand, *5:*76, 1973

STRANC, M. F., AND BUNCE, A. H.: Dacryocystography in midfacial fractures, PRS, *52:*96, 1973. Brit. J. Plast. Surg., *25:*269, 1972

STRANC, M. F. *et al:* Review of 196 tubed pedicles. Brit. J. Plast. Surg., *28:*54, 1975

STRANDNESS, D. E., JR. *et al:* Ultrasonic velocity detector in the diagnosis of thrombophlebitis. Arch. Surg., *104:*180, 1972

STRATIGOS, G. T.: Reconstruction of temporomandibular joint by permanent fixation of Silastic to temporal bone. Trans. Congr. Int. Assoc. Oral Surg., *4:*284, 1973

STRAUCH, B.: Dorsal thumb flap for release of adduction contracture of the first web space. Bull. Hosp. Joint Dis., *36:*34, 1975

STRAUCH, B. *et al:* Experimental approach to mandibular replacement: island vascular composite rib grafts. Brit. J. Plast. Surg.,

*24:*334, 1971

STRAULI, P.: Barrier function of lymph nodes. Review of experimental studies and their implications for cancer surgery. Aktuel Probl. Chir., *14:*161, 1970

STRAUSS, P.: Reconstruction of the posterior canal wall with homograft septal cartilage − first results. Z. Laryngol. Rhinol. Otol., *53:*24, 1974 (German)

STRAUSS, S. A.: Official re-registration of a female transsexual following medical treatment. Forensic Sci., *3:*19, 1974

STRELI, R.: Treatment of the cleft hand through syndactylization, a new simple method. Handchirurgie, *1:*104, 1969 (German)

STRELIS, A. K. *et al:* Microtracheostomy in treatment of patients with destructive tuberculosis complicated by bronchitis. Probl. Tuberk., *51:*30, 1973 (Russian)

STREMMEL, W.: Importance of blood glycogen following stress-induced disturbances of metabolism, PRS, *52:*602, 1973. Bruns' Beitr. klin. Chir., *220:*297, 1973

Stress

Injury, reaction of body as whole (Gelin), PRS, *48:*96, 1971. J. Trauma, *10:*932, 1971

Diuresis under stress, the polyuria of sepsis (Hermreck, Berg, Ruhlen), PRS, *52:*330, 1973. Surg. Forum, *23:*53, 1972

Glycogen, blood, importance following stress-induced disturbances of metabolism (Stremmel), PRS, *52:*602, 1973. Bruns' Beitr. klin. Chir., *220:*297, 1973

Plasma citrate levels, hypocitricemic effect of surgical stress (Costello, Balkissoon, Stacey), PRS, *54:*119, 1974. J. Surg. Res., *15:*182, 1973

Stress responses and adjustments of surgical pediatric patients (Visintainer, Wolfer), PRS, *57:*544, 1976. Pediatrics, *56:*187, 1975

STRICKER, M.: Reconstruction of peripheral part of facial nerve. J. Maxillo-facial Surg., *1:*142, 1973

STRICKER, M.: The periorbit. Its role in the genesis of static and dynamic sequelae of orbital fractures. Ann. chir. plast., *20:*157, 1975 (French)

STRICKER, M. *et al:* Value of composite grafts in reconstruction of the eyelids. Bull. Soc. Ophtalmol. Fr., *70:*925, 1970 (French)

STRICKER, M. *et al:* Vascular tumors of the face. Ann. chir. plast., *16:*220, 1971 (French)

STRICKER, M. *et al:* Restoration of the lacrimal apparatus. Value of venous grafts. Ann. chir. plast., *16:*314, 1971 (French)

STRICKER, M. *et al:* Cranio-orbito-facial osteotomies in severe malformations. Minerva Stomatol., *20:*161, 1971

STRICKER, M. *et al*: Osteotomy of skull and face. Ann. chir. plast., *17:*233, 1972 (French)

STRICKER, M. *et al*: Palatal gaps: problems posed by their repair. Ann. chir. plast., *17:*267, 1972 (French)

STRICKER, M. *et al*: Orbitary, orbito-facial, orbito-cranio-facial osteotomies. Rev. Otoneuroophtalmol., *44:*441, 1972 (French)

STRICKER, M. *et al*: Facial actinomycosis. Rev. Stomatol. Chir. Maxillofac., *73:*495, 1972 (French)

STRICKER, M. *et al*: Correction of paralyzed face: muscle transposition. Ann. chir. plast., *18:*213, 1973 (French)

STRICKER, M. *et al*: Trimethoprim-sulfamethoxazole combination (Eusaprim T. M.) in maxillofacial surgery. J. Fr. Otorhinolaryngol., *22:*657, 1973 (French)

STRICKER, M. *et al*: Repair of vault of skull: value of cranioplasty, PRS, *56:*103, 1975. Ann. chir. plast., *19:*289, 1974

STRICKER, M. *et al*: Internasal vestibular flap in cheilorhinoplasty for sequelae of cleft. Rev. Stomatol. Chir. Maxillofac., *75:*71, 1974 (French)

STRICKER, M. *et al*: Repair of a large pharyngostome in irradiated tissues, 7-year cure. Rev. Stomatol. Chir. Maxillofac., *75:*227, 1974 (French)

STRICKER, M. *et al*: Destructive injuries of the craniofacial sphere. Value of primary overall repair. Rev. Stomatol. Chir. Maxillofac., *75:*274, 1974 (French)

STRICKER, M. *et al*: Heavy injuries of craniofacial border area, importance of primary overall repair, PRS, *57:*758, 1976. (French) Ann. chir. plast., *20:*285, 1975

STRICKLAND, D. M.: New mastopexy operation for mild or moderate breast ptosis (with Bartels, Douglas). PRS, *57:*687, 1976

STRICKLAND, J. W.: Bone, nerve, and tendon injuries of hand in children, PRS, *57:*261, 1976. Pediat. Clin. N. Am., *22:*451, 1975

STROHMENGER, P.: Rectal bladder as a treatment for bladder exstrophy. Acta Urol. Belg., *41:*25, 1973

STROHMENGER, P. *et al*: Urinary diversion through isolated bowel segments. Langenbecks Arch. Chir., *340:*91, 1975 (German)

STROMBECK, J. O.: What is new in plastic surgery? Lakartidningen, *69:*2187, 1972 (Swedish)

STROMBECK, J. O.: Reconstruction surgery of the breast. Arch. Gynaekol., *219:*121, 1975 (German)

STROME, M.: Cryosurgery: complications in head and neck. Trans. Am. Acad. Ophthalmol. Otolaryngol., *77:*1372, 1973

STROME, M. *et al*: Multiple postintubation complications. Ann. Otol. Rhin. & Laryng., *83:*432, 1974

STRONG, M. L., JR.: Chondromas of the tendon sheath of the hand. Report of a case and review of the literature. J. Bone & Joint Surg. (Am.), *57:*1164, 1975

STRONG, M. S. *et al*: Laser surgery in aerodigestive tract, PRS, *53:*486, 1974. Am. J. Surg., *126:*529, 1973

STRONG, M. S. *et al*: Head and neck cancer manpower study. Am. J. Surg., *129:*273, 1975

STRUPLER, W.: Diagnosis and treatment of isolated blow-out fractures of the orbital floor. Arch. Klin. Exp. Ohren Nasen Kehlkopfheilkd., *201:*57, 1972 (German)

STRUPLOVA, V. *et al*: Surgery of lacrimal duct injuries. Cesk. Oftalmol., *28:*237, 1972 (Czech)

STRUVE-CHRISTENSEN, E. *et al*: Fistula formation in temporary elective tracheostomy. Ugeskr. Laeger, *136:*2241, 1974 (Danish)

STRYCHALSKI, J.: Basal cell adenoma of intraoral minor salivary gland origin. J. Oral Surg., *32:*595, 1974

STRZYZEWSKI, H.: Surgical management of neglected cases of multiple flexor tendon and nerve injuries above the wrist. Chir. Narzadow. Ruchu Ortop. Pol., *37:*455, 1972 (Polish)

STRZYZEWSKI, H. *et al*: Value of compression arthrodesis of finger joints. Chir. Narzadow. Ruchu Ortop. Pol., *36:*741, 1971 (Polish)

STRZYZEWSKI, H. *et al*: Functional efficiency of the hand following surgical treatment in severe ulnar deviation of fingers in rheumatoid arthritis. Chir. Narzadow. Ruchu Ortop. Pol., *37:*49, 1972 (Polish)

STRZYZEWSKI, H. *et al*: Hand function following tendon synovectomy at the wrist. Chir. Narzadow. Ruchu Ortop. Pol., *37:*381, 1972 (Polish)

STUCKER, F. J.: Prevention of post-rhinoplasty edema. Laryngoscope, *84:*536, 1974

STUCKER, F. J.: Revision rhinoplasty. Trans. Pa. Acad. Ophthalmol. Otolaryngol., *27:*42, 1974

STUCKER, F. J.: Technique for non-caucasian nose. Trans. Pa. Acad. Ophthalmol. Otolaryngol., *28:*48, 1975

STUCKEY, J. G.: Avulsive injuries to the heel. South. Med. J., *64:*1472, 1971

STUEBER, K. *et al*: Carotid artery replacement with saphenous vein graft for other than arteriosclerotic obstructive disease. Med. Ann. D.C., *43:*237, 1974

STUPPLER, S. A. *et al*: Incarceration of penis by foreign body. Urology, *2:*308, 1973

STURIM H. S.: Treatment of electrical injuries. J. Trauma, *11:*959, 1971

STURIM, H. S.: Bleeding complications with pharyngeal flap construction in humans following Teflon pharyngoplasty, PRS, *55:*514, 1975. Cleft Palate J., *11:*292, 1974

STURIM, H. S., AND JACOB, C. T., JR.: Teflon pharyngoplasty. PRS, *49:*180, 1972

STURLA, F. *et al*: Employment of heterografts as first surgical dressing for burns, PRS, *52:*598, 1973. Rev. argent. cir., *23:*49, 1972

STURM, J. T. *et al*: Milroy's disease, thrombocytosis, and strokes. Minn. Med., *57:*689, 1974

STURMAN, M. J.: Sideburn relationship in the male face-lift. PRS, *57:*248, 1976

STURUP, G. K.: Treatment of sex offender. Castration: total treatment. Int. Psychiatry Clin., *8:*175, 1971

STURUP, G. K.: Male transsexuals: a long-term follow-up after sex reassignment operations. Acta Psychiatr. Scand., *53:*51, 1976

STUTEVILLE, O. H.: Vertical wedge ostectomy in mandibular rami for correction of prognathism (with Pandya). PRS, *48:*140, 1971

STUTEVILLE, O. H.: Treatment of ameloblastoma (with Pandya). PRS, *50:*242, 1972

Stuteville, Orion H., Society of Plastic Surgery. PRS, *51:*241, 1973

STUTSMAN, A. C. *et al*: Ultraconservative management of superficially invasive epidermoid carcinoma of the true vocal cord. Ann. Otol. Rhin. & Laryng., *80:*507, 1971

SUAREZ NUNEZ, J.: Vascular area of temporomandibular joint, PRS, *51:*229, 1973. Rev. Esp. Estomatologia, *17:*367, 1972

SUBHEDAR, V. Y.: A new surgical procedure for correction of ulnar deviation of fingers in rheumatoid arthritis. Rheumatol. Phys. Med., *12:*89, 1973

SUBRINI, L.: Surgical treatment of virile impotence: intracavernous intubation. J. Urol. Nephrol. (Paris), *79:*647, 1973 (French)

SUBRINI, L. *et al*: Surgery of male impotence, intracavernous prosthesis of the penis. J. Urol. Nephrol. (Paris), *80:*269, 1974 (French)

SUBRTOVA, I. *et al*: Reversed occlusions in frontal region of teeth treated by corticotomy. Cesk. Stomatol., *74:*206, 1974 (Czechoslovakian)

SUBTELNY, J. D. *et al*: Ratings and measures of cleft palate speech. Cleft Palate J., *9:*18, 1972

SUCKLING, R. D.: Treatment of cancer of the lid edge. Trans. Ophthalmol. Soc. N. Z., *27:*69, 1975

SUGA, F. *et al*: Cryosurgery of the tongue and tonsil. J. Otolaryngol. Jap., *74:*514, 1971

SUGAHARA, M. *et al*: Pharyngoesophageal diverticulum. Analysis of clinical patterns, surgical management and results of treatment. Rev. Paul. Med., *82:*117, 1973 (Portuguese)

SUGAR, H. S.: Deep lamellar resection of intra- and extraocular epithelial implantation cyst. Am. J. Ophth., *76:*451, 1973

SUGAR, O.: Comments on Crouzon's disease and diagnosis of arteriovenous fistula. J. Neurosurg., *38:*127, 1973

SUGARBAKER, E. V. *et al*: Survival and regional disease control after isolation-perfusion for invasive stage I melanoma of the extremities. Cancer, *37:*188, 1976.

SUGARBAKER, P. H., SABATH, L. D., AND MORGAN, A. P.: Neomycin toxicity from porcine skin xenografts, PRS, *54:*240, 1974. Ann. Surg., *179:*183, 1974

SUGARMAN, G. I. *et al*: The facial-digital-genital (Aarskog) syndrome. Am. J. Dis. Child., 126:248, 1973

SUGERMAN, H. J. *et al*: Physiologic management of septicemic shock in man, PRS, *49:*476, 1972. Surg. Forum, *22:*3, 1971

SUGIMOTO, C.: Treatment of scars and keloids, PRS, *51:*610, 1973. Jap. J. Plast. Reconstr. Surg., *15:*157, 1972

SUGIMOTO, C.: Microvascular transfer of free deltopectoral dermal-fat flap (with Fujino, Tanino), PRS, *55:*428, 1975

SUGIMOTO, C. *et al*: Experience in total reconstruction of the external nose with Millard's method. Jap. J. Plast. Reconstr. Surg., *14:*482, 1971 (Japanese)

SUGIMURA, G. I.: Discussion of "Successful early relief of blindness occurring after blepharoplasty" by Hueston, Heinze (with Hepler, Straatsma), PRS, *57:*233, 1976

SUGIMURA, M. *et al*: Case of neurilemmoma in mandible. Int. J. Oral. Surg., *3:*194, 1974

SUGIURA, H. *et al*: Three cases of congenital torsion of the penis. Jpn. J. Urol., *66:*160, 1975. (Japanese)

SUH, K. W. *et al*: Bleeding as initial sign of carcinoma of tonsil, PRS, *56:*355, 1975. Oral Surg., *38:*695, 1974

SUHLER, A. *et al*: Healthy pregnancy 24 years after ureterosigmoidostomy for bladder exstrophy, in spite of prolonged treatment with chloraminophen and corticosteroids for chronic rheumatoid arthritis. J. Urol. Nephrol. (Paris), *79:*599, 1973 (French)

SUIT, H., RUSSELL, W., AND MARTIN, R.: Management of patients with sarcoma of soft tissue in an extremity, PRS, *54:*244, 1974. Cancer, *31:*1247, 1973

SUKACHEV, V. A. *et al*: Combination of 2 methods of restoration of the brows. Stomatologiia (Mosk.), *51:*79, 1972 (Russian)

SUKHORUKOV, IU. A.: Splint for treating fractures of the metacarpals and digital phalanges. Ortop. Travmatol. Protez., *32:*76, 1971 (Russian)

SULLIVAN, D. E.: Role of orthopedic hospital in Shriners burns program, PRS, *51*:293, 1973

SULLIVAN, G. L.: Caveat chirurgicus. Trans. Am. Ophthalmol. Soc., *70*:328, 1972

SULLIVAN, J.: Bilateral pharyngoplasty as aid to velopharyngeal closure (Follow-Up Clinic), PRS, *48*:587, 1971

SULLIVAN, J. G.: Primary application of an island pedicle flap in thumb and index finger injuries (Follow-Up Clinic), PRS, *51*:208, 1973

SULTANOV, M. I.: Cosmetic aspect of external dacryocystorhinostomy. Oftal. zhur., *27*:302, 1972 (Russian)

SULTANOV, M. I.: Comparative evaluation of effectiveness of three modifications of external dacryocystorhinostomy. Vestn. Oftalmol., *3*:77, 1975 (Russian)

SULTANOV, M. IU.: Comparative evaluation of hammerless methods of forming openings in the bone. Vestn. Oftalmol., *3*:83, 1971 (Russian)

SULTANOV, M. IU.: Operation for activization of the lower lacrimal canal. Oftalmol. Zh., *29*:624, 1974 (Russian)

SULTANOV, M. IU. *et al*: Results of surgery activating the upper lacrimal duct by P. A. Erlyshev's method in reflex lacrimation. Oftalmol. Zh., *26*:391, 1971 (Russian)

SUMMERS, G. W.: Physiologic problems following ablative surgery of head and neck. Otolaryngol. Clin. North Am., *7*:217, 1974

SUMMERS, J. L., WILKERSON, J. E., AND WEGRYN, J. F.: Conservative therapy for Kaposi's sarcoma of external genitalia, PRS, *51*:704, 1973. J. Urol., *108*:287, 1972

SUMMERS, L.: Lateral trepanation of lower third molars. Aust. Dent. J., *19*:149, 1974

SUMMERS, L. *et al*: Intraoral condyloma acuminatum. Oral Surg., *38*:273, 1974

SUMMERS, L. *et al*: Temporo-mandibular joint ankylosis and oro-nasal fistula as complications of facial trauma. Aust. N.Z. J. Surg., *45*:94, 1975

SUMNER, D. S. *et al*: Prediction of tissue loss in human frostbite with Xenon-133, PRS, *48*:515, 1971. Surgery, *69*:899, 1971

SUMNER, D. S., CRIBLEZ, T. L., AND DOOLITTLE, W. H.: Host factors in human frostbite, PRS, *54*:691, 1974. Mil. Med., *141*:454, 1974

SUMRALL, A.: Clinical diagnosis and biological behavior of cutaneous malignant melanoma. J. Natl. Med. Assoc., *64*:359, 1972

SUNDARARAJAN, M. S.: Study of 1,000 patients with keloids in South India (with Ramakrishnan, Thomas), PRS, *53*:276, 1974

SUNDARASON, R., AND RATNAM, S. S.: Surgery of male transsexual, PRS, *52*:680, 1973. Proc. Roy. Australasian Coll. Surg., *46*:445, 1973

SUNDELL, B.: Evaluation of fluid resuscitation in the burned patient. Ann. Chir. Gynaecol. Fenn., *60*:192, 1971

SUNDELL, B.: Thermal burns. Retrospective study on 240 patients. I. Distribution of material and admission factors. Ann. Chir. Gynaecol. Fenn., *62*:339, 1973

SUNDELL, B.: Thermal burns. Retrospective study on 192 fresh burns. II. Care of burn wound and mortality. Ann. Chir. Gynaecol. Fenn., *62*:344, 1973

SUNDELL, B. *et al*: Principles in treatment of decubitus ulcers. Duodecim, *89*:1234, 1973 (Finnish)

SUNDERLAND, S.: Internal anatomy of nerve trunks in relation to neural lesions of leprosy. Observations on pathology, symptomatology and treatment. Brain, *96*:865, 1973

SUNDERLAND, S.: Restoration of median nerve function after destructive lesions which preclude end-to-end repair, PRS, *57*:537, 1976. Brain, *97*:1, 1974

SUNDMARK, E.: Zygomatic fractures. Nord. Med., *86*:1189, 1971 (Swedish)

SUNG, W. H.: New one-stage technique for repair of penoscrotal hypospadias, PRS, *52*:681, 1973. Proc. Roy. Australasian Coll. Surg., *46*:386, 1973

SUNKAT, R. *et al*: Treatment of arterial circulation disorders. Clinical results after lumbar sympathectomy. Fortschr. Med., *92*:694, 1974 (German)

SUSSMAN, L. N.: Clotting time – an enigma, PRS, *53*:694, 1974. Am. J. Clin. Path., *60*:651, 1973

SUSTER, M. *et al*: Hydraulic fractures of orbit and possibilities of their surgical reconstruction. Cesk. Otolaryngol., *23*:138, 1974 (Slovakian)

SUTCLIFFE, B. *et al*: Polythene and Plastazote hand-resting splint. Physiotherapy, *58*:138, 1972

SUTHERLAND, S.: Addendum to "Free vascularized nerve graft," by Taylor, Ham, PRS, *57*:425, 1976

Sutures (See also *Tissue Adhesives*)

Polyglycolic acid polymer as new absorbable synthetic suture, clinical use of (Dardik, Dardik, Laufman), PRS, *49*:477, 1972. Am. J. Surg., *121*:656, 1971

Suture materials, surgical tensile strength and knot security (Hermann), PRS, *49*:110, 1972. Am. Surgeon, *37*:209, 1971

Autosuture instruments, clinical experience with (Steichen), PRS, *48*:300, 1971. Surgery, *69*:609, 1971

Suture material, ideal (Ulin), PRS, *51*:237, 1973. Surg. Gynec. & Obst., *133*:475, 1971

Sutures—Cont.

Sutures, iodized gut, reduction of experimental wound infection with (Ludewig, Rudolf, Wangensteen), PRS, *49:*670, 1972. Surg. Gynec. & Obst., *133:*946, 1971

Thermographic studies on healing of differently tied fascial sutures (Tauber *et al*), PRS, *51:*609, 1973. Bruns' Beitr. klin. Chir., *219:*667, 1972

Polyglycolic acid, clinical trial of new absorbable suture material (Turner *et al*), PRS, *51:*486, 1973. Canad. J. Surg., *15:*389, 1972

Suture, ideal, search for (Nathan), PRS *50:*637, 1972. Internat. Surg., *57:*26, 1972

Dexon absorbable suture material used in general surgery (Anscombe), PRS, *53:*251, 1974. Internat. Surg., *57:*887, 1972

Skin, studies in nonsuture immobilization of (Wilkinson, Rybka, Paletta), PRS, *51:*709, 1973. South M.J., *65:*25, 1972

Dexon—a new suture material: its use in plastic surgery (Cocke). South. Med. J., *65:*629, 1972

Suture material, considerations in choice for various tissues (Van Winkle, Hastings), PRS, *51:*353, 1973. Surg. Gynec. & Obst., *135:*113, 1972

Skin closure, sterile, "use-once" clip applicator for (Annis). Brit. J. Surg., *60:*686, 1973

Sterilization of catgut by conventional methods and by radiation, tissue reaction after implantation in parenchymatous organs (Helpap *et al*), PRS, *53:*114, 1974. Bruns' Beitr. klin. Chir., *220:*323, 1973

Sutures, history of (Mackenzie), PRS, *53:*502, 1974. Med. Hist., *17:*158, 1973

Sutures: studies of urethral healing in dogs (Everingham, Horton, Devine), PRS, *51:*312, 1973

Suture, buried—new, self-adapting intracutaneous suture (Wahl). Zentralbl. Chir., *98:*1720, 1973 (German)

Vicryl, synthetic absorbable sutures (Horton *et al*), PRS, *56:*363, 1975. Am. Surgeon, *40:*729, 1974

Skin suturing, mechanized (Samuels, Katz, Darrow), PRS, *55:*640, 1975. Arch. Surg., *109:*838, 1974

Use of an automatic stapling device for closure of surgical wounds (Stephens *et al*). Aust. N. Z. J. Surg., *44:*398, 1974

Knot properties of surgical suture materials (Holmlund), PRS, *56:*366, 1975. Europ. Surg. Res., *6:*65, 1974

Wound closure, stitchless, surgical experiences with (Kugler). Fortschr. Med., *92:*621, 1974 (German)

Sutures, small bowel, different types, vascular regeneration after (Juvara, Necula,

Sutures—Cont.

Murgu), PRS, *54:*238, 1974. Lyon chir., *70:*52, 1974

Sutures, painless removal (Bialostozky). Surgery, *76:*356, 1974

Sutures, human tissue reaction to (Postlethwait, Willigan, Ulin), PRS, *56:*233, 1975. Ann. Surg., *181:*144, 1975

Suture, polyglycolic acid, in strabismus surgery (Blau *et al*), PRS, *57:*394, 1976. Arch. Ophth., *93:*538, 1975

Suture removal in children facilitated (Johnson), PRS, *55:*97, 1975

Suturing, interrupted, in microvascular anastomoses, method of successive (Fujino, Aoyagi), PRS, *55:*240, 1975

Sutures, factors in production of inconspicuous scars (Wray, Holtmann, Weeks), PRS, *56:*86, 1975

Vascular surgery, use of monofilament suture in (Dean, Pinkerton, Foster), PRS, *57:*407, 1976. Surgery, *78:*165, 1975

Suture materials, effect on healing skin wounds (Van Winkle *et al*), PRS, *56:*599, 1975. Surg. Gynec. & Obst., *140:*7, 1975

New technique for skin closure (Tejani *et al*). Surg. Gynec. & Obst., *142:*406, 1976

SUWANWELA, C., INDARAKOSES, A., AND AKSARANUGRAHA, S.: Posterior interosseous nerve paralysis, PRS, *52:*206, 1973. J. M. A. Thailand, *55:*610, 1972

SUZUKI, K.: Flexor tendon injury of the hand—reconstructive surgery and evaluation. J. Jap. Orthop. Assoc., *45:*651, 1971

SUZUKI, K.: Reconstruction of post-traumatic boutonniere deformity, PRS, *54:*375, 1974. Hand, *5:*145, 1973

SUZUKI, K. *et al*: Injuries of the flexor tendon of the hand—free tendon graft following pedicle flap transfer. Othop. Surg. (Tokyo), *22:*870, 1971 (Japanese)

SUZUKI, M.: Study of biological chemistry on nature of jaw cysts, PRS, *57:*116, 1976. J. Maxillo-facial Surg., *3:*106, 1975

SVAB, J. *et al*: Developmental defects of the prepuce. Cas. Lek. Cesk., *113:*298, 1974 (Czech)

SVEEN, K.: Foreign bodies in maxillary sinus. Nor. Tannlaegeforen Tid., *84:*152, 1974 (Norwegian)

SVEEN, K. *et al*: Myxomas in jaw. Case of bilateral maxillary myxomas. Nor. Tannlaegeforen Tid., *85:*230, 1975

SVEND-HANSEN, H.: Late results of operative correction of funnel chest. Ugeskr. Laeger, *136:*2302, 1974 (Danish)

SVINHUFVUD, U.: Effect of augmentation mammaplasty on mammography and thermography (with Rintala), PRS, *54:*390, 1974

SVISTUNOV, I. A.: Causes of recurrences of lip cancer and their treatment. Med. Radiol. (Mosk.), *19:*67, 1974 (Russian)

SVISTUNOVA, T. M. *et al*: Late results of low-voltage roentgen therapy and spontaneous regression of cutaneous hemangiomas in children. Vopr. Onkol., *17:*99, 1971 (Russian)

SVOBODA, O.: Filling of postoperative cavities in bones. Cesk. Stomatol., *72:*264, 1972 (Czechoslovakian)

SWAIN, R. *et al*: Experimental analysis of causative factors and protective methods in carotid artery rupture, PRS, *55:*110, 1975. Arch. Otolaryng., *99:*235, 1974

SWAIN, R. E. *et al*: Fibrosarcoma of head and neck: clinical analysis of forty cases. Ann. Otol. Rhin. & Laryng., *83:*439, 1974

SWANK, R. L., II: Letter: Treatment of plunging ranula. J. Oral Surg., *33:*823, 1975

SWANK, R. L., II: *et al*: Cervical esophageal atresia. J. Pediatr. Surg., *10:*795, 1975

SWANSON, A. B.: Surgery of established rheumatoid deformities in hand, PRS, *52:*322, 1973. Rev. Latino. Am. cir. plast., *15:*37, 1971

SWANSON, A. B.: Flexible implant resection arthroplasty. Hand, *4:*119, 1972

SWANSON, A. B.: Flexible implant arthroplasty for arthritic finger joints, PRS, *51:*105, 1973. J. Bone & Joint Surg., *54A:*435, 1972

SWANSON, A. B.: Disabling arthritis of base of thumb, PRS, *51:*104, 1973. J. Bone & Joint Surg., *54A:*456, 1972

SWANSON, A. B.: Treatment of war wounds of the hand. Clin. Plast. Surg., *2:*615, 1975

SWANSON, A. B. *et al*: Pathogenesis and pathomechanics of rheumatoid deformities in the hand and wrist. Orthop. Clin. North Am., *4:*1039, 1973

SWANSON, ALFRED B.: *Flexible Implant Resection Arthroplasty in the Hand and Extremities.* C. V. Mosby Co., St. Louis, 1973. PRS, *54:*350, 1974

SWANSON, A. E.: Sagittal osteotomy for correction of maxillo-mandibular deformities. J. Can. Dent. Assoc., *39:*785, 1973

SWANSON, L.: Congenital absence of the nose and anterior nasopharynx; report of two cases (with Gifford, MacCollum), PRS, *50:*5, 1972

SWANSON, L. T. *et al*: Compound silicone-bone implants for mandibular reconstruction, PRS, *51:*402, 1973

SWANSON, L.. T. *et al*: Midface correction for craniofacial dysostosis. Birth Defects, *10:*189, 1974

SWARTZ, E. M.: Will it happen again? Arch. Surg., *104:*19, 1972

SWARTZ, R. M., SCHULTZ, R. C., AND SEATON,

J. R., JR.: "Dry eye" following blepharoplasty, PRS, *54:*644, 1974

SWARTZ, W. M., RUECKERT, F., AND BROWN, F. E.: Panniculectomy specimens as a convenient and inexpensive source of homograft skin, PRS, *55:*628, 1975

Sweat Glands (See also *Hidradenitis; Hyperhidrosis; Skin Neoplasms*)

Sweating, gustatory, further concepts in (McGibbon, Paletta), PRS, *49:*639, 1972

Eccrine poroma of the hand (Mamoun *et al*), PRS, *50:*295, 1972

Sweat gland carcinoma with regional lymph node metastasis (Meijer *et al*). Arch. chir. neerl., *27:*77, 1975

Eccrine sweat gland tumor of clear cell origin involving the eyelids (Rosen *et al*). Cancer, *36:*1034, 1975

SWEENEY, N. V.: Composite grafts of skin and fat, PRS, *54:*700, 1974. Brit. J. Plast. Surg., *26:*72, 1973

SWEENY, P. R. *et al*: Metaplasia of adult oral mucous membrane. J. Surg. Res., *19:*303, 1975

SWEET, R. A. *et al*: Study of incidence of hypospadias in Rochester, Minn. 1940–1970; case control comparison of possible etiologic factors, PRS, *54:*238, 1974. Mayo Clin. Proc. Staff Meet., *49:*52, 1974

SWENSON, S. A., JR. *et al*: Surgical treatment of familial plantar hyperkeratosis. Nebr. Med. J., *57:*377, 1972

SWEZEY, R. L. *et al*: Inappropriate intrinsic muscle action in the rheumatoid hand. Ann. Rheum. Dis., *30:*619, 1971

SWEZEY, R. L. *et al*: Resorptive arthropathy and the opera-glass hand syndrome. Semin. Arthritis Rheum., *2:*191, 1972–73

SWEZEY, R. L. *et al*: Nerve conduction studies in resorptive arthropathies: opera-glass hand. J. Bone & Joint Surg. (Am.), *55:*1680, 1973

SWIERSTRA, J. C. C.: Ambulant treatment of pilonidal sinus, PRS, *51:*110, 1973. Arch. chir. neerl., *24:*1, 1972

SYKES, P. J.: Pre-auricular sinus: clinical features and the problems of recurrence. Brit. J. Plast. Surg., *25:*175, 1972

SYKES, P. J.: Unusual penetrating injury of cheek: case report. Injury, *4:*347, 1973

SYKES, P. J.: Composite reconstruction of the mandible and the temporomandibular joint, following hemimandibulectomy (with Ho, Bailey), PRS, *53:*414, 1974

SYKES, P. J., AND HO, L. C. Y.: Hypospadias, report on 193 treated cases, PRS, *50:*452, 1972

SYKORA, G. F.: Use of angiography in outlining

solitary solid tumors of the head and neck (with Mandel, Kiehn), PRS, *52:*61, 1973

SYLLA, S. *et al:* Anatomical landmarks useful in locating the facial nerve. Bull. Soc. Med. Afr. Noire Lang. Fr., *19:*333, 1974 (French)

SYLWANOWICZ, L.: Difficulties encountered during the removal of tracheal cannulas in infants and children. Wiad. Lek., *26:*2161, 1973 (Polish)

SYLWANOWICZ, L. *et al:* Lymphangioma cavernosum palati molli et uvulae. Otolaryngol. Pol., *26:*467, 1972 (Polish)

SYMONDS, F. C.: Problem of somatic delusions in patients seeking cosmetic surgery (with Druss, Crikelair), PRS, *48:*246, 1971

SYMONDS, F. C. *et al:* Pitfalls in management of penetrating injuries of forearm, PRS, *49:*582, 1972. J. Trauma, *11:*47, 1971

Symposia, Seminars, etc.

Symposium on Esthetic Surgery, PRS, *48:*302, 1971

Sumner L. Koch seminar in hand surgery, PRS, *48:*520, 1971

Symposium on Problems of the Female Breast, PRS, *48:*520, 1971

Symposium on Esthetic Plastic Surgery in Mexico, PRS, *49:*594, 1972; *51:*242, 1973; *52:*220, 1973; *54:*125, 1974; *56:*120, 1975

Symposium on Head and Neck malignancy, PRS, *49:*592, 1972

Symposium on Orofacial Anomalies at Duke, PRS, *50:*316, 1972; *54:*522, 1974

International Symposium on Biomaterials, PRS, *50:*644, 1972; *52:*336, 1973; *54:*706, 1974; *56:*486, 1975

Symposium on Cleft Lip and Palate Patient, PRS, *51:*241, 1973

Symposium on Hand Surgery, Tape Recordings, PRS, *51:*242, 1973; *53:*695, 1974

Symposium at Kings County Hospital, Downstate Medical Center, PRS, *51:*242, 1973

Rehabilitation Seminar in Louisiana, PRS, *51:*357, 1973

Symposium on Esthetic Surgery in Spain, PRS, *51:*358, 1973

Symposium on Cancer of the Head and Neck, PRS, *51:*614, 1973

Symposium on Orofacial Anomalies, PRS, *52:*220, 1973

Symposium on the Treatment of Burns, PRS, *52:*334, 607, 1973

Symposium on Injured Human Face, PRS, *52:*336, 1973

Symposium on Plastic Surgery of the Orbital Region, PRS, *52:*692, 1973

Symposium on the Nose, PRS, *52:*692, 1973

International Symposium on Wound Heal-

Symposia, Seminars, etc.—Cont.

ing, PRS, *53:*253, 1974

Seminar on Hand Disability, PRS, *53:*509, 1974

Symposium on Progress in Hand Surgery, PRS, *53:*617, 1974

Symposium on Evaluation of Recent Advances in Craniofacial Surgery, PRS, *53:*695, 1974

Symposium on Reconstructions In and About the Orbit, PRS, *54:*255, 1974

Symposium on Corrective Rhinoplasty, PRS, *54:*520, 1974

Symposium on Mammaplasty and Lipectomy, PRS, *54:*521, 1974

Symposium and Workshop on Microsurgery, PRS, *54:*521, 1974

Symposium on Skin Tumors, PRS, *54:*521, 1974

Fourth International Conference on Gender Identity (Harry Benjamin), PRS, *54:*705, 1974

Symposium on Cosmetic Surgery, PRS, *54:*706, 1974

Symposium on Military Plastic Surgery, PRS, *54:*706, 1974

Symposium on Esthetic Plastic Surgery, PRS, *55:*129, 1975

Symposium on Esthetic Surgery at Straith Memorial Hospital, PRS, *55:*395, 1975

Session on Hand Surgery, PRS, *56:*120, 1975

International Symposium on Pre-Prosthetic Surgery, PRS, *56:*370, 1975

Symposium of Military Plastic Surgery, PRS, *56:*486, 1975

Symposium on Velopharyngeal Insufficiency, PRS, *56:*687, 1975

Syndactylism (See also *Fingers, Deformities; Pectoralis Muscle, Absence of*)

Isolated acrosyndactyly: avoiding post-operative contracture (Thomson). Brit. J. Plast. Surg., *24:*357, 1971

Pseudo-syndactyly, surgical treatment in case of epidermolysis bullosa dystrophica (Anderl, Weiser), PRS, *53:*115, 1974. Chir. Plast., *1:*145, 1972

Syndactylism, anatomy and surgical treatment (Losch, Duncker), PRS, *50:*167, 1972

Art of incisions for recurrent syndactyly (Blauth *et al*). Arch. Orthop. Unfallchir., *77:*97, 1973

Syndactyly, surgical, after wedge resection for macrodactyly of foot (Diamond, Gould), PRS, *54:*691, 1974. South. M.J., *67:*645, 1974

Syndactyly in burned hands (Huang, Larson, Lewis), PRS, *56:*21, 1975. Discussion by Bennett, PRS, *56:*442, 1975

Syndactylism — Cont.

Syndactyly, burn, lateral-volar finger flap in treatment (MacDougal, Wray, Weeks), PRS, *57:*167, 1976

SYNDER, B. S.: Mandibular and maxillofacial fractures. J. Am. Osteopath. Assoc., *72:*637, 1973

SYNDER, S. R. *et al*: Benign chondroma of palate, case report. J. Oral Surg., *31:*873, 1973

SYSOLIATIN, P. G.: Replacement of defects of the mandible by preserved allogenic bone in children. Stomatologiia (Mosk.), *55:*67, 1976 (Russian)

SYSOLIATIN, P. G. *et al*: Bone homoplasty in treatment of ununited fractures of lower jaw complicated by chronic osteomyelitis. (Vestn. Khir., *111:*108, 1973 (Russian)

SYSOLIATIN, P. G. *et al*: Homologous bone embryonic graft in oral surgery. Stomatologiia (Mosk.), *53:*92, 1974 (Russian)

SZABO, G. *et al*: Benign symmetrical lipomatosis. Orv. Hetil., *113:*2652, 1972 (Hungarian)

SZABO, G. *et al*: Case of surgically treated local lymphogranuloma. Fogorv. Sz., *66:*172, 1973

SZADOK, D. AND DRZYZGA, F.: Surgical treatment of ankylosed temporomandibular joints using the Kelikian method in ankylosing spondylitis. Wiad. Lek., *26:*169, 1973 (Polish)

SZAL, G. J., AND MILLER, T.: Surgical repair of facial nerve branches, PRS, *57:*395, 1976. Arch. Otolaryng., *101:*160, 1975

SZCZAWINSKI, A. *et al*: Plastic operations for pendulous abdomen in obese subjects. Pol. Przegl. Chir., *43:*1317, 1971 (Polish)

SZCZAWINSKI, A. *et al*: Plastic operations for pendulous abdomen in obese subjects. Pol. Med. J., *11:*922, 1972

SZEKELY, O. *et al*: Hyperbaric oxygen therapy in injured subjects. Injury, *4:*294, 1973

SZKLANNY, J. *et al*: Peutz-Jeghers syndrome. Pol. Przegl. Chir., *45:*1095, 1973 (Polish)

SZLAZAK, L. *et al*: Nasopharyngeal hemangioma. Otolaryngol. Pol., *28:*329, 1974 (Polish)

SZMEJA, Z. *et al*: Ganglioneuroma of the auricle. Case report. Otolaryngol. Pol., *28:*687, 1974 (Polish)

SZTABA, R. *et al*: Supracystic urinary drainage in children. Pol. Przegl. Chir., *46:*1453, 1974 (Polish)

SZYFELBEIN, S. K., AND RYAN, J. F.: Use of controlled hypotension for primary surgical excision in extensively burned child, PRS, *55:*515, 1975. Anesthesiology, *41:*501, 1974

SZYMANKIEWICZ, S.: Results of conservative and surgical treatment of chemical and thermal eye burns based on clinical research between 1957 and 1966. Klin. Oczna., *41:*559,

1971 (Polish)

SZYMCZYKOWA, B. *et al*: Usefulness of surgical treatment in some skin diseases. Przegl. Dermatol., *61:*825, 1974 (Polish)

T

TABARI, K.: Refining aspects of rhytidoplasty. In *Plastische und Wiederherstellungs-Chirurgie* ed. by Hohler; pp. 27–33. Schattauer, Stuttgart, 1975 (German)

TABOR, G. L.: Benign lymphocytic lymphoma of upper eyelid and left plica semilunaris. Ann. Ophth., *5:*964, 1973

TAEN, A. *et al*: Reconstruction of mental region by Millard's method in case of ameloblastoma of mandible. Jap. J. Oral Surg., *19:*150, 1973 (Japanese)

TAGLIONI, M. *et al*: Orbit exenteration. Practical note. Bull. Soc. Ophtalmol. Fr., *74:*341, 1974 (French)

TAHARA, I. *et al*: Respiratory insufficiency in patients with severe burn, PRS, *49:*237, 1972. Operation, *25:*765, 1971

TAI, Y., AND HASEGAWA, H.: Transverse abdominal flap for reconstruction after radical operations for recurrent breast cancer, PRS, *53:*52, 1974

TAIARA, C. *et al*: Correction of enophthalmos and deep supratarsal sulcus by posterior subperiosteal glass bead implantation. Brit. J. Ophthalmol., *57:*741, 1973

TAIARA, C., SARGENT, R. A., AND SMITH, B.: Dacryocystorhinostomy: Kasper operation, PRS, *56:*104, 1975. Ann. Ophth., *6:*1333, 1974

TAIDELLI, G., SAVANI, A., AND GRISOTTI, A.: Vaccination against Pseudomonas infection in burned patients: aspects and problems, PRS, *50:*308, 1972. Acta chir. Plast., *13:*94, 1971

TAILLENS, J. P.: Intercarotid glomus and its glomic tumor. J. Fr. Otorhinolaryngol., *22:*595, 1973 (French)

TAINMONT, J.: Medical and surgical aspects of severe cyclic epistaxis. Acta Otorhinolaryngol. Belg., *28:*187, 1974 (French)

TAJIMA, S.: Handling of open wounds and granulation wounds. Jap. J. Plast. Reconstr. Surg., *14:*135, 1971 (Japanese)

TAJIMA, S.: Early diagnosis of facial fracture — methods of early diagnosis and emergency treatment. Surg. Ther. (Osaka), *26:*563, 1972 (Japanese)

TAJIMA, S.: Longitudinal study on electrical pulp testing following Le Fort type osteotomy and Le Fort type fracture, PRS, *57:*259, 1976. J. Maxillo-facial Surg., *3:*74, 1975

TAJIMA, S. *et al*: Surgical treatment of malunited fracture of zygoma with diplopia and with comments on blowout fracture, PRS, 55:716, 1975. J. Maxillo-facial Surg., 2: 201, 1974

TAJIMA, T.: Treatment of open crushing type of industrial injuries of the hand and forearm: degloving, open circumferential, heat-press, and nail-bed injuries. J. Trauma, 14:995, 1974

TAJIMA, Y. et al: Plastic surgery for total lid defect due to resection of the cancer. Folia Ophthalmol. Jap., 22:949, 1971 (Japanese)

TAJIMA, Y., MARUYAMA, N., AND IKEGAMI, M: Endoscopic observations on internal surface of lacrimal sac following dacryocystorhinostomy. Acta Soc. Ophthalmol. Japan, 76:1242, 1972 (Japanese)

TAJIMA, Y., AND IKEGAMI, M: Endoscopic observation of lacrimal sac following dacryocystorhinostomy, PRS, 54:118, 1974. Jap. J. Ophth., 17:175, 1973

TAKACSI-NAGY, L.: Role of telecobalt therapy in the treatment of inoperable ameloblastomas. Radiobiol. Radiother. (Berl.), 15:453, 1974 (German)

TAKACSI-NAGY, L.: Mesenchymal tumors of the mouth. Dtsch. Zahnaerztl. Z., 30:827, 1975 (German)

TAKACSI-NAGY, L. et al: Role of radiotherapy in the treatment of primary tumours of the frontal sinuses. J. Laryng. & Otol., 90:211, 1976

TAKAGI, M. et al: Autopsy case of leiomyosarcoma of maxilla. J. Oral Pathol., 1:125, 1972

TAKAGI, M. et al: Fibrous tumor of infancy—report of case originating in oral cavity. J. Oral Pathol., 2:293, 1973

TAKAGISHI, N. et al: Measures for prevention of hand injuries and their results in industry. Orthop. Surg. (Tokyo), 21:932, 1970 (Japanese)

TAKAHASHI, M. et al: Roentgenologic appearances of sphenoethmoidal mucocele. Neuroradiology, 6:45, 1973

TAKAHASHI, R.: Surgery of frontal cranial base. J. Otolaryngol. Jap., 76:1231, 1973 (Japanese)

TAKAHASHI, R. et al: Total reconstruction of the external nose, particularly on the method using a tubed pedicle flap. Jap. J. Plast. Reconstr. Surg., 14:447, 1971 (Japanese)

TAKAHASHI, S. et al: Surgical correction of mandibular prognathism by sagittal osteotomy of ascending ramus. Jap. J. Oral Surg., 17:528, 1971 (Japanese)

TAKAKU, S.: Indications for meniscectomy of temporomandibular joint. Jap. J. Oral Surg., 19:400, 1973 (Japanese)

TAKASAKI, K.: Clinical and histopathological study on chemotherapy of maxillary cancer with special reference to bleomycin. J. Oto-

laryngol. Jap., 74:1129, 1971 (Japanese)

TAKATS, G.: Sympathectomy revisited: dodo or phoenix? Surgery, 78:644, 1975

TAKAYAMA, I. et al: Therapy of malignant tumor of the head and neck region. J. Otolaryngol. Jap., 74:422, 1971 (Japanese)

TAKAYAMA, T. et al: Three cases of dacryocytorhinostomy. Otolaryngology (Tokyo), 43:673, 1971 (Japanese)

TAKAYASU, H. et al: Accessory scrotum: a case report. J. Urol., 112:826, 1974

TAKEDA, C. et al: Reconstructive surgery of head and neck cancer. J. Otolaryngol. Jap., 75:1085, 1972 (Japanese)

TAKIGAWA, K.: Chondroma of the bones of the hand. A review of 110 cases. J. Bone & Joint Surg., (AM.), 53:1591, 1971

TAL, Y. et al: Frequency of cleft lip and palate in northern Israel. Isr. J. Med. Sci., 10:515, 1974

TALAAT, S. M. et al: Prevention of early histopathological changes in liver in extensive burns, PRS, 55:112, 1975. Brit. J. Plast. Surg., 26:132, 1973

TALAMAS, I.: Value of photography in plastic surgery, PRS, 49:478, 1972. Tribuna Med. Mexico, 20:3, 1971

TALAMAS, I.: Cosmetic surgery. The face-lift. Postgrad. Med., 53:120, 1973

TALAMAS, I.: Cosmetic surgery. 2. Rhinoplasty. Postgrad. Med., 54:129, 1973

TALARA, C. et al: Palpebral dacryoadenectomy. Am. J. Ophth., 75:461, 1973

TALBOT, I. C., et al: Fibrous dysplasia of craniofacial bones. Clinico-pathological survey of seven cases. J. Laryng. & Otol., 88:429, 1974

TALBOT, W. R.: Soft tissue glass impaction. Oral Surg., 32:161, 1974

TALCOTT, T. D.: Strength of gel-bag prostheses after autoclaving (Letter to the Editor), PRS, 55:216, 1975

TALEISNIK, J.: Palmar cutaneous branch of median nerve and approach to carpal tunnel, PRS, 53:684, 1974. J. Bone & Joint Surg., 55:1212, 1973

TALMANT, J. C. et al: New data on the embryology of congenital labiopalatine defects. Rev. Stomatol. Chir. Maxillofac., 73:257, 1972 (French)

TAMAI, S. et al: Microvascular surgery in orthopedics and traumatology, PRS, 51:705, 1973. J. Bone & Joint Surg., 54B:637, 1972

TAMAI, S. et al: Little finger replantation in 20-month-old child, PRS, 56:679, 1975. Brit. J. Plast. Surg., 27:1, 1974

TAMARIN, A. et al: Surgical method for exteriorizing the orifice of Stensen's duct for long-term collection of parotid saliva. J. Dent. Res., 54:458, 1975

TAMAS, F.: Use of a new instrument in the osteotomy of the ascending mandibular ramus. Magy. Traumatol. Orthop., *17:*223, 1974 (Hungarian)

TAMAS, F. *et al*: Severe deep bite corrected by surgery and prosthodontics. Orv. Hetil., *114:*2911, 1973 (Hungarian)

TAMERIN, J. A.: Five most important points in reduction rhinoplasty, PRS, *48:*214, 1971

TAMIR, D. *et al*: Treatment of hypospadias: ten year follow-up study. Harefuah, *81:*370, 1971 (Hebrew)

TAN, K. L. *et al*: Congenital lip pits with cleft lip or palate. J. Singapore Paediatr. Soc., *13:*75, 1971

TANAKA, Y. *et al*: Six cases of male pseudohermaphroditism treated by feminization surgery with special reference to their classification and prognosis. Clin. Endocrinol. (Tokyo), *19:*467, 1971 (Japanese)

TANDON, S. N. *et al*: Pretibial lacerations. Brit. J. Plast. Surg., *26:*172, 1973

TANGE, I.: Evaluation of primary cleft lip repair, PRS, *52:*455, 1973. Jap. J. Plast. Reconstr. Surg., *15:*412, 1972

TANGEN, I. G.: Ankylosis of temporomandibular joint. Nor. Tannlaegeforen Tid., *83:*322, 1973 (Norwegian)

TANGEN, I. G.: Ameloblastoma. Nor. Tannlaegeforen Tid., *84:*308, 1974 (Norwegian)

TANI, T.: Review of rhinoplasty. Jap. J. Plast. Reconstr. Surg., *14:*489, 1971 (Japanese)

TANI, T.: Follow-up study of circumoral reconstruction of old facial palsy, PRS, *52:*462, 1973. Jap. J. Plast. Reconstr. Surg., *15:*486, 1972

TANI, T. *et al*: Treatment of wounds with avulsed skin. Jap. J. Plast. Reconstr. Surg., *14:*145, 1971 (Japanese)

TANINO, R.: Microvascular transfer of free deltopectoral dermal-fat flap (with Fujino, Sugimoto), PRS, *55:*428, 1975

TANZER, R. C.: "Know thyself" (Presidential Address), PRS, *50:*549, 1972

TANZER, R. C.: Constricted (cup and lop) ear, PRS, *55:*406, 1975

TANZER, R. C.: Obituary of Jerome Pierce Webster, M.D., PRS, *55:*728, 1975

TANZER, R. C., AND CHAISSON, R.: Protective guard for use during reconstruction of the auricle, PRS, *53:*236, 1974

TANZER, RADFORD C., AND EDGERTON, MILTON T.: *Symposium on the Reconstruction of the Auricle.* C. V. Mosby Co., St. Louis, 1974. PRS, *56:*571, 1975

TAPERNOUX, B.: Chemosurgical treatment of skin tumors using Mohs' technic. Praxis, *62:*1393, 1973 (French)

TAPERNOUX, B. *et al*: Treatment of skin epithe-lioma by chemosurgery: Mohs' technic. Ann. Dermatol. Syphiligr. (Paris), *100:*169, 1973 (French)

TAPLEY, N. DU V. *et al*: Applications of electron beam in management of lymphatics of neck in head and neck cancers. Am. J. Roentgenol. Radium Ther. Nucl. Med., *117:*575, 1973

TARABULCY, E.: Sexual function in normal and in paraplegia, PRS, *52:*453, 1973. Paraplegia, *10:*201, 1972

TARAPON, I. G. *et al*: Surgical tactics in crural varicose ulcers. Klin. Khir., *12:*49, 1973 (Russian)

TARAPON, IU. G. *et al*: Treatment of microtrauma of the hand and fingers and prevention of their suppurative complications. Ortop. Travmatol. Protez., *3:*62, 1975 (Russian)

TARDY, M. E., JR.: Regional flaps. Principles and application. Otolaryngol. Clin. North Am., *5:*551, 1972

TARDY, M. E., JR.: Pedicle flap nasal reconstruction: design and execution. Can. J. Otolaryngol., *2:*342, 1973

TARDY, M. E., JR.: Rhinoplasty tip ptosis: etiology and prevention. Laryngoscope, *83:*923, 1973

TARDY, M. E., JR. *et al*: Bilobed flap in nasal repair. Arch. Otolaryng., *95:*1, 1972

TARPLEY, J. L. *et al*: Prolonged depression of cellular immunity in cured laryngopharyngeal cancer patients treated with radiation therapy. Cancer, *35:*638, 1975

TARSITANO, J. J. *et al*: Correction of maxillary protrusion with severe vertical dysplasia—multidisciplinary approach. J. Oral Surg., *31:*675, 1973

TASANEN, A. *et al*: Closed condylotomy in the treatment of idiopathic and traumatic pain-dysfunction syndrome of the temporomandibular joint. Int. J. Oral Surg., *2:*102, 1973

TASANEN, A. *et al*: Osteochondromatosis of the temporomandibular joint. Report of a case. Oral Surg., *38:*845, 1974

TASANEN, A. *et al*: External skeletal fixation in maxillofacial surgery. Proc. Finn. Dent. Soc., *70:*229, 1974

TASANEN, A. *et al*: A methodological analysis and follow-up of vestibular plasty and skin grafting. Proc. Finn. Dent. Soc., *71:*176, 1975

TASCHE, C., ANGELATS, J., AND JAYARAM, B.: Surgical treatment of hidradenitis suppurativa of the axilla, PRS, *55:*559, 1975

TASH, E. L. *et al*: Training voluntary pharyngeal wall movements in children with normal and inadequate velopharyngeal closure. Cleft Palate J., *8:*277, 1971

TASHIMA, C. K.: Association of malignant melanoma and malignant lymphoma. Lancet,

*1:*266, 1973

TASIC, D.: First aid in mass treatment of burns. Srp. Arh. Celok. Lek., *99:*51, 1971 (Serbian)

TATE, R. J.: Facial injuries associated with the battered child syndrome. Brit. J. Oral Surg., *9:*41, 1971

TATO, J. M.: Adipose tissue graft in otorhinology. Arch. Otolaryng., *100:*467, 1974

TATRAI, J.: Clinical experience with mandibular osteosynthesis by compression plates. Forgorv. Sz., *68:*241, 1975 (Hungarian)

Tattoos, Commercial

Treatment of skin wound surfaces with a collagen film after elimination of tattooing with a dermatome (Ezrokhin *et al*). Sov. Med., *34:*149, 1971 (Russian)

Reliable regional anaesthesia of the upper limb: augmented axillary block allowing the shaving and overgrafting of multiple forearm tattoos (Harrison *et al*). Brit. J. Plast. Surg., *25:*195, 1972

Tattoos, dermal, removal (Gupta) (Follow-Up Clinic), PRS, *50:*401, 1972

Tattoo removal, analysis of results of treatment of skin surface wounds after, according to data of Moscow Research Institute for Cosmetology for 1964–1970 (Ezrokhin). Vestn. Dermatol. Venerol., *46:*61, 1972 (Russian)

Tattoo removal. New simple technique (Manchester). California Med., *118:*10, 1973

Tattoos, salabrasion for (Editorial). M. J. Australia, *2:*352, 1973

Tattoos, removal, experimental use of optic quantum generators (lasers) for (Alborova *et al*). Vestn. Dermatol. Venerol., *47:*35, 1973 (Russian)

Trial of a new technic in the surgical treatment of tattoos (Soussaline). Ann. chir. plast., *19:*193, 1974 (French)

Tattoos, trial of new technic in surgical treatment of (Soussaline). Ann. chir. plast., *19:*251, 1974 (French)

Tattoos (Morgan). Brit. Med. J., *2:*34, 1974

Abrasion with table salt, removal of commercial tattoos by (Manchester), PRS, *53:*517, 1974

Tattoo erasing (McDowell) (Editorial), PRS, *53:*580, 1974

Tattoo removal by superficial dermabrasion (Clabaugh), PRS, *55:*401, 1975

Tattoos, Dirt

Care of the traumatic tattoo (Zook). Med. Times, *102:*90, 1974

TAURAS, A. P.: Periareolar incision for aug-

mentation mammaplasty (with Jones), PRS, *51:*641, 1973

TAURAS, S. P. *et al*: Temporomandibular joint ankylosis corrected with a gold prosthesis. J. Oral Surg., *30:*767, 1972

TAUB, S., AND SPIRO, R. H.: Vocal rehabilitation of laryngectomees. Preliminary report of new technic, PRS, *51:*236, 1973. Am. J. Surg., *124:*87, 1972

TAUB, S., AND BERGNER, L. H.: Air bypass voice prosthesis for vocal rehabilitation of laryngectomees, PRS, *53:*114, 1974. Am. J. Surg., *125:*748, 1973

TAUB, S. J.: What goes on under your make-up if you are allergic to cosmetics, PRS, *57:*681, 1976. Eye, Ear, Nose & Throat Month., *54:*278, 1975

TAUB, S. J.: Some aspects of nasal allergy: a review, PRS, *57:*671, 1976. Eye, Ear, Nose & Throat Month., *54:*326, 1975

TAUBER, R. *et al*: Thermographic studies on healing of differently tied fascial sutures, PRS, *51:*609, 1973. Bruns' Beitr. klin. Chir., *219:*667, 1972

TAUTIN, F. S., AND SCHAAF, N. G.: Superiorly based obturator, PRS, *56:*105, 1975. Prosth. Dent., *33:*96, 1975

TAWASHY, K.: Adenocarcinoma of nasal septum. Can. J. Otolaryngol., *3:*93, 1974

TAYLER, W. B., AND WILKING, J. W., JR.: Nevoid basal cell carcinoma of palm, PRS, *49:*361, 1972. Arch. Dermat., *102:*654, 1970

TAYLOR, G. A. *et al*: Ten years' experience in surgical treatment of basal cell carcinoma. Study of factors associated with recurrence. Brit. J. Surg., *60:*522, 1973

TAYLOR, G. A., AND HOPSON, W. L. G.: Cross-foot flap, PRS, *55:*677, 1975. Discussion by Cannon, PRS, *56:*83, 1975

TAYLOR, G. I.: Distant transfer of island flap by microvascular anastomoses (with Daniel), PRS, *52:*111, 1973

TAYLOR, G. I.: Deltopectoral flap: anatomical and hemodynamic approach (with Daniel, Cunningham), PRS, *55:*276, 1975

TAYLOR, G. I., AND DANIEL, R. K.: Free flap; composite tissue transfer by vascular anastomosis, PRS, *55:*642, 1975. Australian & New Zealand J. Surg., *43:*1, 1973

TAYLOR, G. I., MILLER, G. D. H., AND HAM, F. J.: Free vascularized bone graft, clinical extension of microvascular techniques, PRS, *55:*533, 1975

TAYLOR, G. I., AND DANIEL, R. K.: Anatomy of several free flap donor sites, PRS, *56:*243, 1975

TAYLOR, G. I., AND HAM, F. J.: Free vascularized nerve graft, PRS, *57:*413, 1976

TAYLOR, N. *et al*: Evaluation of hand function

in children. Arch. Phys. Med. Rehabil., *54:*378, 1973

TAYLOR, P. H. *et al*: Use of angiography in case of recurrent epistaxis after multiple arterial ligation. Brit. J. Surg., *61:*721, 1974

TAYLOR, T. V. *et al*: Ascorbic acid supplementation in treatment of pressure sores, PRS, *55:*254, 1975. Lancet, *2:*544, 1974

TAYLOR, W.: Transantral orbital decompression in dysthyroid eye disease. Trans. Ophthalmol. Soc. N. Z., *26:*51, 1974

TAYLOR, W. O. A.: Car seat belts and the eye, PRS, *55:*727, 1975. Injury, *6:*3, 1974

TAZUEV, A. SH.: Clinical assessment of final results in the treatment of metastases of cancer of the lower lip. Stomatologiia (Mosk.), *54:*40, 1975 (Russian)

TEARSTON, G. M. *et al*: Body sculpturing. Surg. Clin. North Am., *55:*151, 1975

TEGTMEIER, R. E.: Self-retaining retractors for hand surgery, PRS, *53:*485, 1974

TEICH-ALASIA, S.: "Open-air" treatment of lesions from burns, PRS, *53:*491, 1974. Riv. ital. chir. plast., *4:*1, 1973

TEICH-ALASIA, S.: Modern orientations in surgical treatment of burns, PRS, *57:*676, 1976. Riv. ital. chir. plast., *6:*279, 1974

TEICH-ALASIA, S. *et al*: Recovery of sensation in pedicle and skin grafts of the hand. Minerva. Chir., *26:*1397, 1971 (Italian)

TEICH-ALASIA, S., AND BARBERIS, M. L.: Value of "cross-arm" flap in reconstructive surgery of hand, PRS, *53:*113, 1974. Chir. Plast., *1:*134, 1972

TEICHMANN, K. D. *et al*: Semicircular probe for threading of the lacrimal ducts. Klin. Monatsbl. Augenheilkd., *165:*678, 1974 (German)

TEICHMANN, W. *et al*: Therapy of severe tetanus. Zentralbl. Chir., *100:*1450, 1975 (German)

TEIXEIRA, A. C.: Correction of facial profile of leprous patients, PRS, *57:*113, 1976. Rev. Asoc. med. Bras., *21:*124, 1975

TEIXEIRA, C. P. *et al*: True hermaphroditism. Report of case and review of literature. Rev. Asoc. Med. Bras., *19:*231, 1973 (Portuguese)

TEJANI, F. *et al*: New technique for skin closure. Surg. Gynec. & Obst., *142:*406, 1976

TELES, J. C. B., CARDOSO, A. S., AND GONCALVES, A. R.: Blue nevus of oral mucosa, PRS, *56:*234, 1975. Oral Surg., *38:*905, 1974

TELESYNSKI, M. *et al*: Morton's neuroma. Chir. Narzadow. Ruchu Ortop. Pol., *39:*199, 1974 (Polish)

TEMPEL, V.: Surgical methods and results in 240 corrections of prominent ears. Deutsche Stomatol., *22:*773, 1972 (German)

TEMPERO, K. F.: Use of diazepam in treatment of tetanus. Am. J. Med. Sci., *266:*4, 1973

TEMPEST, M.: Correcting facial deformity. Nurs. Times, *71:*1163, 1975

TEMPEST, M. N.: Cancrum oris, PRS, *50:*535, 1972. Trop. Doctor, *1:*164, 1972

TEMPEST, M. N.: Comment on "Simple method for emergency orotracheal intubation" (Letter to the Editor), PRS, *51:*82, 1973

TEMPEST, M. N.: Urea treatment of skin malignancies. Lancet, *1:*266, 1974

TEMPLE, W. J. *et al*: Effect of nutrition, diet and suture material on long term wound healing. Ann. Surg., *182:*93, 1975

Temporomandibular Joint (See also *Jaw, Ankylosis; Jaw, Dislocations; Mandibular Condyle; Temporomandibular Joint Syndrome*)

Critical study of Ward's technic in the treatment of temporo-mandibular ankylosis. Analysis of a homogeneous series of 15 cases (Freidel *et al*). Ann. chir. plast., *16:*334, 1971 (French)

Surgical treatment of mandibular joint disorders (James). Ann. R. Coll. Surg. Engl., *49:*310, 1971

Sada's treatment for temporomandibular ankylosis (Yoel), PRS, *49:*581, 1972. Bol. y trab. Acad. argent cir., *55:*375, 1971

Surgical correction of recurrent bony ankylosis of the temporomandibular joint (Martinez-Garcia). Brit. J. Oral Surg., *9:*110, 1971

Temporomandibular and mandibular dysfunction (Roydhouse, Horan), PRS, *49:*470, 1972. Canad. M. A. J., *105:*1320, 1971

Surgery of the temporomandibular joint (Trauner). Dtsch. Zahn. Mund. Kieferheilkd., *57:*327, 1971 (German)

An adjustable device to increase mouth-opening (Silver). J. Bone Joint Surg. (Am.), *53:*1217, 1971

Changes in the temporomandibular joint after surgical treatment. A radiologic follow-up study (Agerberg *et al*). Oral Surg., *32:*865, 1971

Sternoclavicular whole joint graft as substitute for temporomandibular joint, trial of (Snyder, Levine, Dingman), PRS, *48:*447, 1971

Unilateral mandibular resection-disarticulation by an intraoral method and immediate reconstruction by bone auto-graft (Bortot *et al*). Riv. Ital. Stomatol., *26:*605, 1971 (Italian)

Surgery in bilateral ankylosis of the temporomandibular joint and microgenia (Titova). Vestn. Khir., *106:*58, 1971 (Russian)

Hyperplasia, condylar, unilateral, intra-oral condylectomy applied to (Sear). Brit. J.

Temporomandibular Joint — Cont.

Schweiz. Monatsschr. Zahnheilkd., *83:*23, 1973 (French)

Temporomandibular joint, indications and contraindications for surgical management of (Perko). Schweiz. Monatsschr. Zahnheilkd., *83:*73, 1973 (German)

Hemimandibulectomy, effect of, on remaining temporomandibular joint (Schneider, Wey, Rosli). Schweiz. Monatsschr. Zahnheilkd., *83:*82, 1973 (German)

Temporomandibular joint, treatment of ankylosis of (Spiessl, Prein). Schweiz. Monatsschr. Zahnheilkd., *83:*89, 1973 (German)

Restriction of jaw movement due to abnormalities of the coronoid process (Findlay). Trans. Int. Conf. Oral Surg., *4:*269, 1973

Arthroplasty of ankylosed temporomandibular joint (Walker). Trans. Congr. Int. Assoc. Oral Surg., *4:*279, 1973

Reconstruction of the temporomandibular joint by permanent fixation of Silastic to the temporal bone (Stratigos). Trans. Int. Conf. Oral Surg., *4:*284, 1973

Facial deformity — surgical treatment (Ayats *et al*). Trans. Int. Conf. Oral Surg., *4:*345, 1973

Kelikian method in ankylosing spondylitis, surgical treatment of ankylosed temporomandibular joints using (Szadok, Drzyzga). Wiad. Lek., *26:*169, 1973 (Polish)

Temporomandibular joint (articulatio temporomandibularis), topographic and applied anatomy of, of various domestic animals with special reference to resection possibilities of discus articularis. 4. Swine (Sus srofa domesticus) (Meister *et al*). Z. Exp. Chir., *6:*437, 1973 (German)

Experimental results of mandibular nearthrosis (Domarus *et al*). Zahnaerztl. Prax., *24:*147, 1973 (German)

Nasotracheal intubation in maxillofacial surgery using bronchofibroscopy (Gille *et al*). Anesth. Analg. (Paris), *31:*551, 1974 (French)

Temporomandibular joint ankylosis, bilateral with associated micrognathia, case report (Fieldhouse). Brit. J. Oral Surg., *11:*213, 1974

Tomography of temporomandibular joint (Coin), PRS, *55:*377, 1975. Dent Radiogr. Photogr., *47:*23, 1974

Technic of anesthesia in ankylosis of the temporomandibular joints (Podlesch). Fortschr. Kiefer. Gesichtschir., *18:*121, 1974 (German)

Orthopedic jaw operations on the tuberculum articulare (Sauer *et al*). Fortschr. Kiefer

Temporomandibular Joint — Cont.

Gesichtschir., *18:*238, 1974 (German)

Conservative and surgical treatment of condylar fractures of the temporomandibular joint (Sandner). Int. J. Oral Surg., *3:*218, 1974

Bone tumors, rare, in temporomandibular joint (Nwokus, Koch), PRS, *55:*379, 1975. J. Maxillo-facial Surg., *2:*113, 1974

Temporomandibular joint, surgical treatment of ankylosis of (El-Mofty), PRS, *55:*106, 1975. J. Oral Surg., *32:*202, 1974

Chondrosarcoma of the temporomandibular joint: report of case (Richter *et al*). J. Oral Surg., *32:*777, 1974

Temporomandibular joint, load of, physical calculations and analyses (Hekneby), PRS, *54:*372, 1974. J. Prosth. Dent., *31:*303, 1974

Surgery of the temporomandibular joint (Poswillo). Oral Sci. Rev., *6:*87, 1974

Joint surgery, temporomandibular, use of biocompatible interface for binding tissues and prostheses (Hinds, Honsy, Kent), PRS, *56:*105, 1975. Oral Surg., *28:*512, 1974

Osteochondromatosis of the temporomandibular joint. Report of a case (Tasanen *et al*). Oral Surg., *38:*845, 1974

Temporomandibular joint replacement, total, new procedure for (Kiehn, DesPrez, Converse), PRS, *53:*221, 1974

Temporomandibular joint and mandible, composite reconstruction of, following hemimandibulectomy (Ho, Bailey, Sykes), PRS, *53:*414, 1974

Temporomandibular joint, condylectomy with silicone rubber replacement (Hartwell, Hall), PRS, *53:*440, 1974

Cases of bilateral temporomandibular ankylosis (Beauvais *et al*). Rev. Stomatol. Chir. Maxillofac., *75:*851, 1974 (French)

Statistics of temporomandibular joint disorders from the viewpoint of maxillofacial surgery (Birke *et al*). Stomatol. DDR, *24:*683, 1974 (German)

New surgical treatment method for temporomandibular ankyloses. Conservation of the meniscus in attempt at reconstruction of an equvalent structure and mobilization in propulsion (Delaire). Actual Odontostomatol. (Paris), *110:*173, 1975 (French)

Temporomandibular joint ankylosis and oronasal fistula as complications of facial trauma (Summers *et al*). Aust. N. Z. J. Surg., *45:*94, 1975

Discotemporal plastic treatment of hypermobile jaw joint (Bilder *et al*). Cesk. Stomatol., *75:*190, 1975 (Czechoslovakian)

Examination of the structure and surface of articular disc in surgically treated arthro-

Temporomandibular Joint Syndrome—Cont.
joints (Michelet *et al*). Rev. Stomatol. Chir. Maxillofac., *74:*647, 1973 (French)

Temporomandibular joint luxation and subluxation, habitual, author's own therapeutic method for (Neuner). Schweiz. Monatsschr. Zahnheilkd., *83:*61, 1973 (German)

Temporomandibular joint, arthritic, surgical treatment (Silver, Simon, Litchman), PRS, *52:*206, 1973. Surg. Gynec. & Obst., *136:*251, 1973

Use of biocompatible interface for combining tissues and prostheses in oral surgery (Hinds *et al*). Trans. Int. Conf. Oral Surg., *4:*210, 1973

Arthroplasty of the ankylosed temporomandibular joint (Walker). Trans. Int. Conf. Oral Surg., *4:*279, 1973

Reconstruction of the temporomandibular joint by permanent fixation of Silastic to the temporal bone (Stratigos). Trans. Int. Conf. Oral Surg., *4:*284, 1973

Temporomandibular capsular rearrangement (Toller). Brit. J. Oral Surg., *11:*207, 1974

Joint, temporomandibular, tomography of (Coin), PRS, *55:*377, 1975. Dent. Radiogr. Photogr., *47:*23, 1974

Arthrography, opaque, of temporomandibular joint (Toller), PRS, *55:*717, 1975. Int. J. Oral Surg., *3:*17, 1974

Joint, temporomandibular, pain-dysfunction syndrome, correlation of psychological findings and treatment results (Small), PRS, *56:*105, 1975. J. Oral Surg., *32:*589, 1974

Head and neck pain: T-M joint syndrome (Norris *et al*). Laryngoscope, *84:*1466, 1974

Surgery of the temporomandibular joint (Poswillo). Oral Sci. Rev., *6:*87, 1974

Functional compensation of muscles after postoperative rehabilitation in reference to electromyographic analysis (Grosfeld). Oral Surg., *38:*829, 1974

Temporomandibular arthropathy (Toller), PRS, *54:*372, 1974. Proc. Roy. Soc. Med., *67:*153, 1974

Statistics of temporomandibular joint disorders from the viewpoint of maxillofacial surgery (Birke *et al*). Stomatol. DDR, *24:*683, 1974 (German)

Discotemporal plastic treatment of hypermobile jaw joint (Bilder *et al*). Cesk. Stomatol., *75:*190, 1975 (Czechoslovakian)

Correlation of clinical, surgical and histopathological findings in temporomandibular arthropathies (Hornova *et al*). Cesk. Stomatol., *75:*196, 1975 (Czechoslovakian)

Temporomandibular Joint Syndrome—Cont.
Temporomandibular joint pain dysfunction syndrome, treatment of patients with (Zarb *et al*). J. Can. Dent. Assoc., *41:*410, 1975

Condyle: surgical correction of lesions of the temporomandibular joints (Dingman, Dingman, Lawrence), PRS, *55:*335, 1975. Discussion by Kiehn, PRS, *55:*484, 1975

Hydrocortisone, effects on mandibular condylar cartilage of rat (Priest), PRS, *56:*225, 1975. Proc. Roy. Soc. Med., *68:*128, 1975

Special method of arthroplasty of the temporomandibular joint (Papakonstantinou *et al*). Stomatologia (Athenai), *32:*145, 1975 (Greek)

TEMTAMY, S. A. *et al:* Coffin-Lowry syndrome: an inherited faciodigital mental retardation syndrome. J. Pediatr. *86:*724, 1975

Tendon

Dislocation, traumatic, of long-finger extensor tendon (Kettelkamp, Flatt, Moulds), PRS, *49:*664, 1972. J. Bone & Joint Surg., *53:*229, 1971

Tendon healing in rat, remodeling of distal stump after severance (Greenlee, Pike), PRS, *48:*260, 1971

Prenatal development of tendon sheaths in hands of human embryos (Zauner, Negel), PRS, *49:*664, 1972. Surg. Forum, *22:*430, 1971

Tendons, collagen metabolism in iso- and homografts of (Tobias, Seiffert), PRS, *52:*105, 1973. Brit. J. Plast. Surg., *25:*83, 1972

Tendon grafts, homologous, preserved in cialit, surgical use (Iselin) (Follow-Up Clinic), PRS, *49:*208, 1972

Tendons, long flexor, avulsion injury (Chang, Thoms, White), PRS, *50:*260, 1972

Tendons, surface phenomenon on (Wilson, Hueston), PRS, *54:*375, 1974. Hand, *5:*155, 1973

Tendon sheath formed around silicone rod in chickens (Farkas *et al*), PRS, *53:*614, 1974. J. Bone & Joint Surg., *55:*1149, 1973

Tenolysis, results of, controlled evaluation in chickens (Hurst, McCain, Lindsay), PRS, *52:*171, 1973

Z-plasty skin closure after lengthening the Achilles tendon (Price, Ecker), PRS, *52:*309, 1973. Discussion by Goldwyn, PRS, *52:*431, 1973

Tendon transfer, pedicled, with silicone rod (Van der Meulen) (Letter to the Editor), PRS, *51:*328, 1973

Tendon injury: dynamic tenodesis of distal

Tendon – Cont.

interphalangeal joint, for use after severance of *profundus* alone (Kahn), PRS, *51:*536, 1973

Tendon prosthesis (Tkachenko, Dedushkin, Belousov), PRS, *55:*643, 1975. Acta chir. plast., *16:*185, 1974

Tendon, *flexor digitorum superficialis* in fingers of human hand (Kuczynski), PRS, *56:*227, 1975. Hand, *6:*121, 1974

Tendon, flexor, reconstruction of digital pulleys (Wray, Weeks), PRS, *53:*534, 1974

Chicken toe, some practical notes on anatomy of, for surgeon investigators (Farkas, Thomson, Martin), PRS, *54:*452, 1974

Tendon, rabbit, microcirculation in (Lundborg), PRS, *57:*261, 1976. Hand, *7:*1, 1975

Tendons, flexor and *extensor pollicis longus*, congenital bilateral anomalous band between (Salama, Weissman), PRS, *57:*260, 1976. Hand, *7:*25, 1975

Tendon, *superficialis*, dilemma of intact (Nichols), PRS, *56:*596, 1975. Hand, *7:*85, 1975

Tendon healing, role of tendon tissues in (Furlow), PRS, *57:*39, 1976

Tendon Injuries (See also *Hands, Tendon Injuries*)

Tendon, flexor, atraumatic retrieval (Kilgore *et al*), PRS, *49:*358, 1972. Am. J. Surg., *122:*430, 1971

Flexor tendon function, postoperative recovery of (Peacock, Madden, Trier), PRS, *50:*538, 1972. Am. J. Surg., *122:*686, 1971

Flexor tendon repair, recent advances in (Van Der Meulen), PRS, *49:*358, 1972. Arch. chir. neerl., *23:*129, 1971

Flexor tendon lesions of hand, treatment of (Schokkenbroek), PRS, *49:*358, 1972. Thesis, Univ. Utrecht, 1971

Tendon injuries of hand (Schink), PRS, *51:*603, 1973. Langenbecks Arch. Chir., *332:*495, 1972

Tendon insertion, profundus, avulsion in football players (Wenger), PRS, *52:*452, 1973. Arch. Surg., *106:*145, 1973

Tendon, extensor, injuries of hand (McFarlane, Hampole), PRS, *53:*488, 1974. Canad. J. Surg., *16:*366, 1973

Flexor pollicis longus tendon laceration, delayed repair by advancement, free graft, or direct suture (Urbaniak, Goldner), PRS, *53:*684, 1974. J. Bone & Joint Surg., *55:*1123, 1973

Tendon suture, primary, in thumb and fingers (Jensen, Weilby), PRS, *56:*356, 1975. Hand, *6:*297, 1974

Tendons, digital flexor, repair potential of (Matthews, Richards), PRS, *56:*679, 1975.

Tendon Injuries – Cont.

J. Bone & Joint Surg., *56:*618, 1974

Tendon, flexor, repairs in no-man's-land (Green, Niebauer), PRS, *55:*509, 1975. J. Bone & Joint Surg., *56A:*1216, 1974

Flexor tendon lacerations in "some-man's land," purposeful delay of primary repair (Arons), PRS, *53:*638, 1974. Discussion by Hartrampf, PRS, *54:*95, 1974

Tendon, flexor, repair reaction within digital sheath (Matthews, Richards), PRS, *57:*261, 1976. Hand, *7:*27, 1975

Tendon, incompletely severed, should it be sutured? (Reynolds, Wray, Weeks), PRS, *57:*36, 1976. Discussion by Kleinert, PRS, *57:*236, 1976

Tendon, Reconstructive Surgery (See also *Hands, Reconstructive Surgery*)

Flexor tendon reconstruction in severely damaged hands (Hunter, Salisbury), PRS, *50:*632, 1972. J. Bone & Joint Surg., *53:*829, 1971

Tendon repairs with nylon and modified pull-out technique (Mangus *et al*), PRS, *48:*32, 1971

Flexor profundus tendons, reconstruction with tendon grafts (Gonzalez, Ojeda), PRS, *49:*582, 1972. Semana méd. Mexico, *69:*147, 1971

Tendon plasty of hand and finger flexor tendons, homologous (Kovalenko, Demichev), PRS, *51:*603, 1973. Acta chir. plast., *14:*60, 1972

Collagen metabolism in iso- and homografts of tendons (Tobias, Seiffert), PRS, *52:*105, 1973. Brit. J. Plast. Surg., *25:*83, 1972

Tendon material, homologous preserved, possibility of using (Vooerhoeve), PRS, *50:*423, 1972. Chir. Praxis, *16:*1, 1972

Flexor tendon surgery, half century of, current status and changing philosophies (Verdan), PRS, *51:*105, 1973. J. Bone & Joint Surg., *54A:*472, 1972

Tendon suture materials, comparative study in dogs (Srugi, Adamson), PRS, *50:*31, 1972

Silicone rod to form tendon sheath in chickens (Farkas *et al*), PRS, *53:*614, 1974. J. Bone & Joint Surg., *55:*1149, 1973

Achilles tendon, Z-plasty skin closure after lengthening (Price, Ecker), PRS, *52:*309, 1973. Discussion by Goldwyn, PRS, *52:*431, 1973

Tendon function restored after hand injuries (Reid), PRS, *56:*679, 1975. Brit. J. Plast. Surg., *27:*5, 1974

Flexor tendon repairs in no-man's-land (Green, Niebauer), PRS, *55:*509, 1975. J. Bone & Joint Surg., *56A:*1216, 1974

Tendon, Reconstructive Surgery — Cont.

Compression, median nerve, complicating tendon graft prosthesis (DeLuca *et al*), PRS, *57:*398, 1976. J. Bone & Joint Surg., *57A:*553, 1975

Tendon Rupture (See also *Fingers, Baseball Injuries; Hands, Rheumatoid Disease of; Hands Tendon Ruptures in*)

Madelung's deformity with extensor tendon rupture (Schulstad), PRS, *49:*583, 1972. Scand. J. Plast. Reconstr. Surg., *5:*153, 1971

Flexor tendons, ruptures in hands of non-rheumatoid patients (Folmar, Nelson, Phalen), PRS, *51:*106, 1973. J. Bone & Joint Surg., *54A:*579, 1972

Profundus tendon insertion, avulsion in football players (Wenger), PRS, *52:*452, 1973. Arch. Surg., *106:*145, 1973

Tendon transfer, *flexor digitorum sublimis,* for multiple extensor tendon ruptures in rheumatoid arthritis (Nalebuff, Patel), PRS, *52:*530, 1973

Tendons, flexor, of index finger ruptured after Colles' fracture (Southmayd *et al*), PRS, *57:*398, 1976. J. Bone & Joint Surg., *57A:*562, 1975

Tendon Transplantation

Flexor tendon grafts in fingers and thumb. Study of factors influencing results in 1000 cases (Boyes, Stark), PRS, *50:*630, 1972. J. Bone & Joint Surg., *53:*1332, 1971

Tendon, long flexor of index finger, transfer to proximal phalanx of long finger during index-ray amputation (Eversmann, Burkhalter, Dunn), PRS, *49:*664, 1972. J. Bone & Joint Surg., *53:*1343, 1971

Tendon transfers for median nerve palsy, use of transverse carpal ligament window for pulley in (Snow, Fink), PRS, *48:*238, 1971

Tendon grafts, reconstruction of *flexor profundus* tendons with (Gonzalez, Ojeda), PRS, *49:*582, 1972. Semana méd. Mexico, *69:*147, 1971

Homografts and isografts of tendons, collagen metabolism in (Tobias, Seiffert), PRS, *52:*105, 1973. Brit. J. Plast. Surg., *25:*83, 1972

Tendon, pedicled, transfer with silicone rod in complicated secondary flexor tendon repairs (Kessler), PRS, *49:*439, 1972

Tendon graft function (Colville), PRS, *54:*375, 1974. Hand, *5:*152, 1973.

Strain test on tendons, surface phenomenon (Wilson, Hueston), PRS, *54:*375, 1974. Hand, *5:*155, 1973

Tendon Transplantation — Cont.

Tendon laceration, *flexor pollicis longus,* delayed repair by advancement, free graft, or direct suture (Urbaniak, Goldner), PRS, *53:*684, 1974. J. Bone & Joint Surg., *55:*1123, 1973

Tendon transfer for treatment of chronic, painful metatarsal callus (Kiehn, Earle, DesPrez), PRS, *51:*154, 1973

Tenodesis: *flexor pollicis longus* tendon transfer for restoration of opposition of thumb (Mangus), PRS, *52:*155, 1973

Transfer, *flexor digitorum sublimis,* for multiple extensor tendon ruptures in rheumatoid arthritis (Nalebuff, Patel), PRS, *52:*530, 1973

Graft, tendon, evaluation of *flexor profundus* (Ojeda), PRS, *53:*606, 1974. Rev. Latino Am. cir. plast., *17:*57, 1973

Grafts, tendon, experimental tendon sheath formation out of vasal tissue (Biro, Horvath, Herber), PRS, *55:*119, 1975. Bruns' Beitr. klin. Chir., *221:*319, 1974

Arthritis, rheumatoid, tendon transfer for radial rotation of wrist in (Clayton, Ferlic), PRS, *55:*637, 1975. Clin. Orthop., *100:*176, 1974

Grafts, flexor tendon, postoperative care (Tubiana), PRS, *56:*230, 1975. Hand, *6:*152, 1974

Tendon surgery: some practical notes on anatomy of chicken toe for surgeon investigators (Farkas, Thomson, Martin), PRS, *54:*452, 1974

Tendon transfer for congenital aplasia or hypoplasia of finger extensors (Tsuge), PRS, *57:*398, 1976. Hand, *7:*15, 1975

Tendon, *extensor pollicis longus,* used as distal extension for *opponens* transfer (Kaplan, Dinner, Chait), PRS, *57:*186, 1976

Tendon, Tumors of

Tendons and aponeurosis, clear cell sarcoma of (Berumen-Cervantes, Calderon-Lopez, Villarreal-Cantu), PRS, *55:*515, 1975. Sem. Med. Mexico, *81:*165, 1974

TENERY, J. H.: Skin graft donor site as a model for evaluation of hemostatic agents (with Wilkinson, Zufi), PRS, *51:*541, 1973

Tenosynovitis, Stenosing

Tuberculous tenosynovitis, chronic recurrent, of finger flexors (Anderl, Semenitz), PRS, *52:*206, 1973. Handsurg., *4:*3, 1972

Tendovaginitis, stenosing, of radial, dorsal, and volar compartments of hand (Fara, Hrivnakova, Dobias), PRS, *53:*606, 1974.

Tenosynovitis, Stenosing — Cont.
Acta chir. plast., *15:*93, 1973
Tenovaginitis, stenosing, efficacy of local steroid injection in treatment of (Clark, Ricker, MacCollum), PRS, *51:*179, 1973
Tenosynovitis, aid in diagnosing, needle aspiration of flexor digital sheath (Ryan, Hoopes), PRS, *56:*152, 1975

TENZEL, R.: Reconstruction of central one-half of eyelid, PRS, *56:*223, 1975. Arch. Ophth., *93:*125, 1975

TENZEL, R. R.: Periosteal elevator for orbital surgery. Am. J. Ophth., *74:*1211, 1972

TENZEL, R. R.: Complications of orbital fractures, their prevention and treatment, PRS, *57:*670, 1976. Eye, Ear, Nose & Throat Month., *54:*305, 1975

TENZEL, R. R.: Surgical judgment in ptosis repair. Trans. Am. Acad. Ophthalmol. Otolaryngol., *79:*679, 1975

TENZER, J. A.: Partial glossectomy in preprosthetic surgery. Oral Surg., *35:*616, 1973

TEODOROVICH, E. *et al*: Early complications following tracheotomy in surgical patients. Eksp. Khir. Anesteziol., *16:*86, 1971 (Russian)

TEPMONGKOL, P.: Mitomycin-C in treatment of advanced malignant tumors, PRS, *52:*213, 1973. Siriraj Hosp. Gaz., *24:*1265, 1972

TERAHATA, K.: Malpractice and new legal decisions. II. Treatment of blepharoptosis following plastic surgery of eyelids. Iryo, *26:*264, 1972 (Japanese)

TER-ANDRIASOV, E. L.: Classification of postburn cicatricial deformations of the eyelids. Voen. Med. Zh., *8:*20, 1973 (Russian)

TER-ASATUROV, G. P. *et al*: Rehabilitation time in patients following restoration of the continuity of the fractured mandible. Stomatologiia (Mosk.), *53:*50, 1974 (Russian)

TERBIZAN, A.: Experiences with myo-electrical and reciprocal ortheses. Handchirurgie, *4:*81, 1972 (German)

TERRAHE, K. *et al*: Hazards and complications of transmaxillary ethmoid-sphenoid cavity scraping. Arch. Klin. Exp. Ohren Nasen Kehikopfheilkd., *205:*284, 1973

TERRILL, R. E.: Denervated Meissner corpuscle, sequential histological study after nerve division in rhesus monkey (With Dellon, Witebsky), PRS, *56:*182, 1975

TERRY, B. C. *et al*: Alveolar ridge augmentation in edentulous maxilla with use of autogenous ribs. J. Oral Surg., *32:*429, 1974

TERSHAKOWEC, M. G.: Variation of Biesenberger technique of reduction mammaplasty (with Carlsen), PRS, *55:*653, 1975

TERZ, J. J., KING, R. E., AND LAWRENCE, W., JR.: Primary rehabilitation after total glossectomy and laryngectomy with mandibulectomy for advanced cancer of mouth. Surg., Gynec. & Obst., *136:*276, 1973

TERZ, J. J. *et al*: Primary oropharyngeal cancer and hypercalcemia. Cancer, *33:*334, 1974

TERZ, J. J. *et al*: Primary reconstruction of mandible with wire mesh prosthesis. Surg. Gynec. & Obst., *139:*198, 1974

TERZIS, J.: Neurovascular free flap (with Daniel, Schwarz), PRS, *56:*13, 1975

TERZIS, J.: Restoration of sensation to an anesthetic hand by free neurovascular flap from foot (with Daniel, Midgley), PRS, *57:*275, 1976

TERZIS, J.: Single fascicular recordings: intraoperative diagnostic tool for management of peripheral nerve lesions (with Williams), PRS, *57:*562, 1976. Discussion by Collins, PRS, *57:*744, 1976

TERZIS, J., FAIBISOFF, B., AND WILLIAMS, H. B.: Diamond knife for microsurgical repair of peripheral nerves, PRS, *54:*102, 1974

TERZIS, J., FAIBISOFF, B. A., AND WILLIAMS, H. B.: Polyethylene bag background in microsurgical repair of peripheral nerves, PRS, *53:*596, 1974

TERZIS, J., FAIBISOFF, B., AND WILLIAMS, H. B.: Nerve gap: suture under tension *vs.* graft. PRS, *56:*166, 1975

TESNIER, D.: Etiology and treatment of glossodynias. Rev. Stomatol. Chir. Maxillofac., *76:*417, 1975 (French)

TESSIER, P.: Treatment of facial dysmorphias in craniofacial dysostosis, Crouzon's and Apert's diseases. Total osteotomy and sagittal displacement of the facial massive. Faciostenosis, sequelae of Le Fort 3 fracture. Dtsch. Zahn. Mund. Kieferheilkd., *57:*302, 1971 (French)

TESSIER, P.: Orbito-cranial surgery. Minerva Chir., *26:*878, 1971 (French)

TESSIER, P.: Treatment of facial dysmorphisms in craniofacial dysostosis (DCF). Crouzon and Apert diseases. Total osteotomy of the facial massif. Sagittal displacement of the facial massif. Neurochirurgie, *17:*295, 1971 (French)

TESSIER, P.: Relationship of craniostenoses to crainofacial dystostoses, and to faciostenoses, study with therapeutic implications. PRS, *48:*224, 1971

TESSIER, P.: Definitive plastic surgical treatment of the severe facial deformities of cranial dysostosis, Crouzon's and Apert's diseases. PRS, *48:*419, 1971

TESSIER, P.: Total osteotomy of the middle third of the face for faciostenosis or for sequelae of Le Fort III fractures. PRS, *48:*533, 1971

Tessier, P.: Commentary on Le Fort (Classic Reprint), PRS, *50:*605, 1972

Tessier, P.: Biographical sketch of Le Fort (Classic Reprint), PRS, *50:*606, 1972

Tessier, P.: Conjunctival approach to orbital floor and maxilla in congenital malformation and trauma, PRS, *53:*247, 1974. J. Maxillo-facial Surg., *1:*3, 1973

Tessier, P.: Orbital hypertelorism. Fortschr. Kiefer. Gesichtschir., *18:*14, 1974

Tessier, P.: Experiences in treatment of orbital hypertelorism. PRS, *53:*1, 1974

Tessier, P. *et al*: Orbital hypertelorism. II. Definite treatment of orbital hypertelorism (OR. H.) by extracranial osteotomies. Scand. J. Plast. Surg., *7:*39, 1973

Tetanus

Immunization, active, against smallpox and tetanus, peripheral nerve and root disturbance following (Deliyannakis), PRS, *48:*608, 1971. Mil. Med., *136:*458, 1971

Tetanus, use of diazepam in treatment of (Tempero). Am. J. Med. Sci., *266:*4, 1973

Toxoid, tetanus, injection causing aluminum hydroxide granuloma (Savage), PRS, *54:*118, 1974. Proc. Roy. Soc. Med., *66:*984, 1973

Tetanus in patients three years of age and up. A personal series of 230 consecutive patients (Garnier). Am. J. Surg., *129:*459, 1975

Tetanus following minor burn (Larkin *et al*). J. Trauma, *15:*546, 1975

Therapy of severe tetanus (Teichmann *et al*). Zentralbl. Chir., *100:*1450, 1975 (German)

Tetsch, P.: Development of raised temperature after osteotomies, PRS, *55:*387, 1975. J. Maxillo-facial Surg., *2:*141, 1974

Texier, M. *et al*: Treatment of thoracic radio-dermatitis with pediculated autoplasty of large mesentery followed by skin graft, PRS, *53:*243, 1974. Chirurg., *99:*262, 1973

Thane, D. *et al*: Experimental facial nerve paralysis, influence of decompression, PRS, *57:*530, 1976. Ann. Otol. Rhin. & Laryng., *83:*582, 1974

Thangaraj, R. H.: Intravenous regional analgesia for hand surgery in leprosy. Lepr. Rev., *42:*266, 1971

Thawley, S. E.: Air in the neck. Laryngoscope, *84:*1445, 1974

Thawley, S. E. *et al*: Basal cell adenoma of the salivary glands. Laryngoscope, *84:*1756, 1974

Thawley, S. E., and Ogura, J. H.: Granular cell myoblastoma of head and neck, PRS, *55:*515, 1975. South M. J., *67:*1020, 1974

Theogaraj, S. D.: Selection of procedure in unilateral cleft lip repair. Indian. Pediatr., *8:*774, 1971

Theogaraj, S. D.: On management of intersexual anomalies. PRS, *51:*632, 1973

Theogaraj, S. D.: Secondary reconstruction of cervical esophagus (with Petty, Cohen), PRS, *56:*70, 1975

Thering, H. R.: Surgical rehabilitation after extensive losses in lower face from war injuries (with Parsons, Beckwith), PRS, *49:*533, 1972

Thevenin, R.: Indications and technic of osteosynthesis using a flexible screw. Acta Orthop. Belg., *39:*980, 1973 (French)

Thevenin, R., and Iselin, F.: Treatment of fractures of metacarpals and phalanges, PRS, *50:*419, 1972. J. Chir. Paris, *103:*251, 1972

Thiers, H. *et al*: Malignant melanoma of the palate. Bull. Soc. Fr. Dermatol. Syphiligr., *78:*174, 1971 (French)

Thilander, B., and Stenström, S.: Maxillary growth after implantation of Surgicel in clefts of maxilla, PRS, *56:*681, 1975. Scand. J. Plast. Reconstr. Surg., *8:*52, 1974

Thilander, B. L.: Healing of surgically created defects in the septal cartilages of young guinea pigs (with Stenström). PRS, *49:*194, 1972

Thio, R. T.: False aneurysm of ulnar artery after surgery employing tourniquet, PRS, *50:*540, 1972. Am. J. Surg., *123:*356, 1972

Thoma, Kurt H.: *Oral Surgery*. 5th edition. C. V. Mosby Co., St. Louis, 1969

Thomas, A. N.: Management of tracheoesophageal fistula caused by cuffed tracheal tubes, PRS, *51:*230, 1973. Am. J. Surg., *124:*181, 1972

Thomas, C. *et al*: Dacryorhinostomy operation: some technical procedures. Bull. Soc. Ophtalmol. Fr., *71:*468, 1971 (French)

Thomas, C. Y. *et al*: Hyperbaric oxygen therapy for pyoderma gangrenosum, PRS, *57:*405, 1976. Arch. Dermat., *110:*445, 1975

Thomas, E. H. *et al*: Surgical treatment of a pseudoarthrosis of the mandible. Rev. Stomatol. Chir. Maxillofac., *76:*489, 1975 (French)

Thomas, G. G. *et al*: Nasal actinomycosis following heterograft. A case report. Arch. Otolaryng., *100:*377, 1974

Thomas, G. K. *et al*: Subglottic enlargement using cartilage-mucosa autograft. A preliminary study. Arch. Otolaryng., *101:*689, 1975

Thomas, J. A. B.: Some aspects of dysphagia, PRS, *55:*718, 1975. Proc. Roy. Soc. Med., *67:*477, 1974

Thomas, J. R. *et al*: Verrucous carcinoma of pyriform sinus. Arch. Otolaryng., *97:*488,

1973

THOMAS, K. P.: Study of 1,000 patients with keloids in South India (with Ramakrishnan, Sundararajan), PRS, 53:276, 1974

THOMAS, M. L.: Phlebography. Arch. Surg., 104:145, 1972

THOMAS, M. L. et al: Angiography in venous dysplasias of the limbs. Am. J. Roentgenol. Radium Ther. Nucl. Med., 113:722, 1971

THOMAS, T. et al: Disordered blood coagulation in burned children receiving high molecular weight dextran. J. Clin. Pathol., 25:473, 1972

THOMPSON, D. P.: Augmentation of surface contour by subcutaneous injections of silicone fluid (with Ashley, Henderson), PRS, 51:8, 1973

THOMPSON, D. S., AND EASON, C. N.: Hypoxemia immediately after operation, PRS, 49:361, 1972. Am. J. Surg., 120:649, 1970

THOMPSON, G. E. et al: Experiences with outpatient anesthesia, PRS, 53:693, 1974. Anesth. Analg., Cleve., 52:881, 1973

THOMPSON, I. M. et al: Rectal flap urethroplasty. J. Urol., 107:667, 1972

THOMPSON, J. B.: Fasanella-Servat operation for ptosis of the upper eyelid (with Souther, Corboy), PRS, 53:123, 1974

THOMPSON, L. W., GOSLING, C. C., AND HAYES, J. E.: Facial moulage technique for plastic surgeon. PRS, 49:190, 1972

THOMPSON, L. W. et al: Simplified art course for plastic surgeon. PRS, 49:408, 1972

THOMPSON, M. et al: Synovectomy of the metacarpophalangeal joints in rheumatoid arthritis. Proc. Roy. Soc. Med., 66:197, 1973

THOMPSON, N.: Autogenous free grafts of skeletal muscle, preliminary experimental study. PRS, 48:11, 1971

THOMPSON, N.: Investigation of autogenous skeletal muscle free grafts in dog. With report on successful free graft of skeletal muscle in man, PRS, 50:423, 1972. Transplantation, 12:353, 1971

THOMPSON, N.: New pharyngoplasty using transplantation of skeletal muscle as free autograft, PRS, 56:355, 1975. Riv. ital. chir. plast., 5:495, 1973

THOMPSON, N., AND ELL, P. J.: Dermal overgrafting in treatment of venous stasis ulcers. Substitute for skin flap repairs in some injuries of extremities. PRS, 54:290, 1974

THOMPSON, R. V. S.: Primary Repair of Soft Tissue Injuries. Melbourne (Australia) University Press, 1969. PRS, 48:276, 1971

THOMPSON, V.: Transamygdaline method and neck lymphatics, PRS, 56:466, 1975. Prensa med. argent., 62:21, 1975

THOMS, O. J.: Avulsion injury of long flexor tendons (with Chang, White), PRS, 50:260,

1972

THOMSEN, K. et al: Glomus jugulare tumours (A series of 21 cases). J. Laryng. & Otol., 89:1113, 1975

THOMSEN, K. A.: Surgical treatment of juvenile nasopharyngeal angiofibroma. Arch. Otolaryng., 94:191, 1971

THOMSEN, M.: Hydrofluoric acid burns. Ugeskr. Laeger, 135:1183, 1973 (Danish)

THOMSEN, M.: Burns. Zentralbl. Chir., 99:1098, 1974 (German)

THOMSEN, M. et al: Avulsion of penile and scrotal skin. Ugeskr. Laeger, 136:255, 1974 (Danish)

THOMSON, H. G.: Isolated acrosyndactyly: avoiding post-operative contracture. Brit. J. Plast. Surg., 24:357, 1971

THOMSON, H. G.: Home-made dynamic finger splint. PRS, 50:302, 1972

THOMSON, H. G.: Fate of the pseudosheath pocket around silicone implants. PRS, 51:667, 1973

THOMSON, H. G.: Some practical notes on anatomy of chicken toe for surgeon investigators (with Farkas, Martin), PRS, 54:452, 1974

THOMSON, H. G., AND SHORE, B.: Bathtub burn – pediatric disaster, PRS, 49:472, 1972. Canad. J. Surg., 14:399, 1971

THOMSON, H. G., AND WRIGHT, A. M.: Surgical tattooing of the port-wine stain. PRS, 48:113, 1971

THOMSON, H. G., AND HARWOOD-NASH, D.: Fate of infractured hamuli. PRS, 50:354, 1972

THOMSON, H. G., AND SVITEK, V.: Small animal bites, role of primary closure, PRS, 52:687, 1973. J. Trauma, 13:20, 1973

THOMSON, H. G., AND HOFFMAN, H. J.: Intracranial use of breast prosthesis to temporarily stablize reduction cranioplasty. PRS, 55:704, 1975

THOMSON, H. S.: Aids in preoperative selection and counseling of patients for rhinoplasty (Editorial), PRS, 50:174, 1972

THOMSON, J. P. S.: Parotid duct calculus, PRS, 53:681, 1974. Proc. Roy. Soc. Med., 66:352, 1973

THOREK, PHILIP: Atlas of Surgical Techniques. J. B. Lippincott and Co., Philadelphia and Toronto, 1970. PRS, 55:356, 1975

THORMANN, T.: Benign juvenile melanoma (Spitz), Paediatr. Grenzgeb., 13:91, 1974 (German)

THORMANN, T.: Therapy of capillary hemangiomas. Paediatr. Grenzgeb., 13:109, 1974 (German)

THORNE, F. L.: Pocket photoplethysmograph; aid in determining the viability of pedicle flaps (with Creech), PRS, 49:380, 1972

THORNTON, W. F. et al: Median palatal cyst:

report of case. J. Oral Surg., *30:*661, 1972

THORTON, S. P. *et al*: Dacryocystorhinostomy with nasolacrimal duct prosthesis. Ophthalmic Surg., *6:*50, 1975

THORVALDSSON, S. E., AND GRABB, W. C.: Intravenous fluorescein test as measure of skin flap viability. PRS, *53:*576, 1974

Thumb (See also *Fingers, Various Categories*)

Thumb, rupture of ulnar collateral ligament of (gamekeeper's thumb), correction by dynamic repair (Neviaser, Wilson, Lievano), PRS, *50:*306, 1972. J. Bone & Joint Surg., *53:*1357, 1971

Thumb, adduction contracture of, internal wire splint for (Araico, Valdes, Ortiz), PRS, *48:*339, 1971

Thumb, surgical treatment of osteoarthritis of carpometacarpal joint (Weilby), PRS, *49:*583, 1972. Scand. J. Plast. Reconstr. Surg., *5:*136, 1971

Several operations for restoring thumb opposition (Briantseva). Vestn. Khir., *106:*68, 1971 (Russian)

Thumb opposition in cases of thenar muscle paralysis, new technique to correct (Paneva-Holevitch), PRS, *53:*106, 1974. Acta Orthop. Belg., *38:*308, 1972

Thumb web, tissue cover for (Sharpe), PRS, *51:*231, 1973. Arch. Surg., *104:*21, 1972

Amputations of thumb (Pringle), PRS, *51:*703, 1973. Injury, *3:*211, 1972

Modified technique for stabilising the spastic thumb (Lam). J. Bone & Joint Surg. (Br.), *54:*522, 1972

Arthritis, disabling, of base of thumb (Swanson), PRS, *51:*104, 1973. J. Bone & Joint Surg., *54A:*456, 1972

Thumb, reconstruction of metacarpophalangeal joint in rheumatoid arthritis (Inglis *et al*), PRS, *51:*105, 1973. J. Bone & Joint Surg., *54A:*704, 1972

Bowler's thumb, diagnosis and treatment (Dobyns *et al*), PRS, *51:*347, 1973. J. Bone & Joint Surg., *54A:*751, 1972

Replantation, successful, of totally severed thumb (Snyder, Stevenson, Browne), PRS, *50:*553, 1972

Arthritis, rheumatoid, etiology and management of adduction contracture of thumb (Kessler), PRS, *54:*376, 1974. Hand, *5:*170, 1973

Thumb reconstruction using radial innervated cross-finger pedicled graft (Miura), PRS, *52:*595, 1973. J. Bone & Joint Surg., *55A:*563, 1973

Thumb, extensor indicis proprius opponensplasty (Burkhalter, Christensen, Brown),

Thumb – Cont.

PRS, *53:*243, 1974. J. Bone & Joint Surg., *55A:*825, 1973

Palliative treatment of paralytic deformities of the thumb (Tubiana). Orthop. Clin. North Am., *4:*1141, 1973

Thumb, degenerative arthritis of carpometacarpal joint (Lee), PRS, *53:*106, 1974. Orthop. Rev., *2:*45, 1973

Flexor pollicis longus tendon transfer for restoration of opposition of thumb (Mangus), PRS, *52:*155, 1973

Thumb, flag flap (Iselin), PRS, *52:*374, 1973

Thumb, injured, sensory rehabilitation of (Adamson) (Follow-Up Clinic), PRS, *52:*432, 1973

Thumb, clinical replantation of digits (O'Brien *et al*), PRS, *52:*490, 1973

Thumb tip injuries, delayed volar advancement for (Millender, Albin, Nalebuff), PRS, *52:*635, 1973

Thumb, congenital camptodactyly of (Borras, Azcoytia, Dargallo), PRS, *56:*229, 1975. Barcelona Quirurgica, *18:*233, 1974

Thumb, locking metacarpophalangeal joint of (Tsuge, Watari), PRS, *56:*227, 1975. Hand, *6:*255, 1974

Thumb and fingers, primary tendon suture in (Jensen, Weilby), PRS, *56:*356, 1975. Hand, *6:*297, 1974

Thumb, human, carpometacarpal joint of (Kuczynski), PRS, *56:*229, 1975. J. Anat., *118:*119, 1974

Thumb repositioning in 4-digit hand (Sandźen, Steel), PRS, *53:*91, 1974

Thumb, bifid, construction of one good thumb from both parts (Hartrampf, Vasconez, Mathes), PRS, *54:*148, 1974

Thumb, distal segment, rotation-transposition method for soft tissue replacement on (Argamaso), PRS, *54:*366, 1974

Anomalies of thumb, congenital, pollicization in (Montanana, Codina, Rodes), PRS, *54:*621, 1974. Rev. españ. cir. plast., *7:*63, 1974

Thumb, post-traumatic stiffening in adduction (Monet, Gosset), PRS, *57:*674, 1976. Chirurgie, *101:*402, 1975

Thumb in leprosy, opponensplasty in intrinsic muscle paralysis of (Palande *et al*), PRS, *57:*674, 1976. J. Bone & Joint Surg., *57A:*489, 1975

Thumb: acute monomyelocytic leukemia presenting as felon (Chang, Whitaker, LaRossa), PRS, *55:*623, 1975

Thumb opposition, use of *extensor pollicis longus* tendon as distal extension for *opponens* transfer (Kaplan, Dinner, Chait), PRS, *57:*186, 1976

Thumb, Reconstruction (See also *Fingers, Transplantation; Toe to Finger [or Thumb] Transplants*)

Pollicization of the index finger in children (Malek *et al*). Ann. Chir. Plast., *16:*198, 1971 (French)

Reconstruction of the thumb using two flaps from the same hand (Orticochea). Brit. J. Plast. Surg., *24:*345, 1971

Pollicization in children (Harrison). Hand, *3:*204, 1971

Pollicization of index finger, method and results in aplasia and hypoplasia of thumb (Buck-Gramcko), PRS, *50:*306, 1972. J. Bone & Joint Surg., *53:*1605, 1971

Advancement pedicle flap for thumb injuries (Posner *et al*). J. Bone & Joint Surg. (Am.), *53:*1618, 1971

Pollicization (Roullet *et al*). Lyon Chir., *67:*114, 1971 (French)

Skin plastic surgery in phalangization of the 1st metacarpal bone (Titov). Ortop. Travmatol. Protez., *32:*50, 1971 (Russian)

Thumb amputations (Pringle), PRS, *51:*703, 1973. Injury, *3:*211, 1972

Thumb reconstruction, method for rapid and good (Morgan, Stein), PRS, *50:*131, 1972

Thumb reconstruction by radial nerve innervated cross finger flap (Wilkinson), PRS, *51:*476, 1973. South. M. J., *65:*992, 1972

Thumb reconstruction using ring finger (Garcia-Velazco), PRS, *54:*109, 1974. Brit. J. Plast. Surg., *26:*406, 1973

Thumb, amputated, autotransplantation of severed index finger (Limb Replantation Research Group), PRS, *53:*487, 1974. Chinese M. J., *8:*110, 1973

Thumb reconstruction by transfer of toe (Millesi), PRS, *53:*107, 1974. Chir. Plast., *1:*347, 1973

Phalangization of thumb (Minkow, Stein), PRS, *54:*375, 1974. J. Trauma, *13:*649, 1973

Thumb, completely amputated, replantation without venous anastomosis (Serafin, Kutz, Kleinert), PRS, *52:*579, 1973. Commentary by Buncke, PRS, *52:*581, 1973

Pollicization for congenital deformities of hand (Harrison), PRS, *53:*683, 1974. Proc. Roy. Soc. Med., *66:*634, 1973

Thumb reconstruction, extended neurovascular island flap in (Storvik), PRS, *54:*503, 1974. Scand. J. Plast. Reconstr. Surg., *7:*147, 1973

Thumbs, missing, reconstruction with improved "cocked hat" operation (Lanchow General Hospital), PRS, *55:*637, 1975. Chinese M. J., *10:*177, 1974

Thumb reconstruction, reverse pollicization

Thumb, Reconstruction — Cont.

for (Elsahy), PRS, *56:*357, 1975. Hand, *6:*233, 1974

Hand, 4-digit, thumb repositioning in (Sandźen, Steel), PRS, *53:*91, 1974

Polydactylia, construction of one good thumb from both parts of a congenitally bifid thumb (Hartrampf, Vasconez, Mathes), PRS, *54:*148, 1974

Pollicization in congenital anomalies of thumb (Montanana, Codina, Rodes), PRS, *54:*621, 1974. Rev. espan. cir. plast., *7:*63, 1974

Thumb reconstruction using amputated phalanges (De Macedo, Baroudi, Tozzi Netto), PRS, *57:*534, 1976. Cir. Plast. Ibero-Latino Am., *1:*97, 1975

Thumb reconstruction (De Macedo, Baroudi, Tozzi-Netto), PRS, *57:*674, 1976. Rev. Iber. Latinoamericana Cir. Plast., *1:*293, 1975

Pollicization of thumb in severely burned hand (Pohl, Larson, Lewis), PRS, *57:*320, 1976

THURSTON, J. B. *et al*: Scanning electron microscopy study of micro-arterial damage and repair. PRS, *57:*197, 1976

Thyroglossal Cysts and Fistulas

Median cervical cysts and fistulae, their surgical correction with partial resection of the hyoid bone (Bohme *et al*). Bruns Beitr. Klin. Chir., *218:*617, 1971 (German)

Surgical therapy of median cysts and neck fistulas (Severinov). Vestn. Otorinolaringol., *33:*64, 1971 (Russian)

Thyroglossal tract cyst, tumoral process developed in cicatrix of (Leroux-Robert *et al*). J. Fr. Otorhinolaryngol., *21:*617, 1972 (French)

Thyroglossal duct remnants in infants and children (Guimaraes *et al*). Mayo Clin. Proc., *47:*117, 1972

Thyroglossal tract, fistulas of (Bodea *et al*). Otorinolaringologie, *17:*425, 1972 (Rumanian)

Midline cysts and fistulas of the neck (Kulczynski). Otolaryngol. Pol., *26:*49, 1972 (Polish)

Congenital fistulas and cysts of the neck in our clinical material (Jarzebski). Wiad. Lek., *25:*767, 1972 (Polish)

Thyroglossal cyst presenting with severe laryngeal obstruction (Olumide). Niger. Med. J., *3:*52, 1973

Carcinoma, squamous cell, arising in thyroglossal duct cyst (Mobini *et al*). Am. Surg., *40:*290, 1974

Thyroglossal Cysts and Fistulas – Cont.

Thyroid carcinomas arising in thyroglossal ducts (Page *et al*), PRS, *55:*636, 1975. Arch. Surg., *180:*799, 1974

Carcinoma arising in median ectopic thyroid (including thyroglossal duct tissue) (Li-Volsi *et al*). Cancer, *34:*1303, 1974

Stridor as the presenting symptom of lingual thyroglossal duct cyst in an infant (Paez *et al*). Clin. Pediatr. (Phila.), *13:*1077, 1974

Thyroglossal cysts and fistulae (MacDonald). Int. J. Oral Surg., *3:*342, 1974

Clinic and therapy of thyroglossal and branchial cysts and fistulas (Riedler *et al*). Langenbecks Arch. Chir., *336:*247, 1974 (German)

Lingual and subhyoid thyroid glands, undescended, management of (Wertz). Laryngoscope, *84:*507, 1974

Embryology and developmental abnormalities (Sedgwick). Major Probl. Clin. Surg., *15:*5, 1974

Cut-throat surgery (Wade), PRS, *57:*397, 1976. Proc. Roy. Soc. Med., *68:*357, 1975

TICHY, S.: Resection of the mandibular angle with plastic occlusion of the pharynx in monoblock surgery of tonsillar cancer. Cesk. Otolaryngol., *23:*349, 1974 (Czech)

TIDEMAN, H.: Technique of vestibular plasty using free mucosal graft from cheek. Int. J. Oral Surg., *1:*76, 1972

TIDEMAN, H.: Preprosthetic surgery. 7. Indications and discussion of various patients. Ned. Tijdschr. Tandheelkd., *79:*262, 1972 (Dutch)

TIEDEMANN, R. *et al*: Specialized, plastic and reconstructive surgery. Cooperative care of mid-facial injuries. H.N.O., *22:*24, 1974 (German)

TIERNEY, E. A.: Accepting disfigurement when death is the alternative. Am. J. Nurs., *75:*2149, 1975

TILLEY, A. R. *et al*: Staged treatment of lymphedema praecox. Can. Med. Assoc. J., *110:*309, 1974

TILLMAN, K.: Rheumatic hand and its surgical treatment. Orthopedic additional report. Handchirurgie, *1:*197, 1969 (German)

TILNEY, N. L., GRIFFITH, H. J. G., AND EDWARDS, E. A.: Natural history of major venous thrombosis of upper extremity, PRS, *48:*92, 1971. Arch. Surg., *101:*792, 1970

TIMAR, T. *et al*: Benign mesenchymoma of epiglottis in infant. Orv. Hetil., *115:*873, 1974 (Hungarian)

TIMAR, T. *et al*: Long-term intratracheal intubation. Orv. Hetil., *115:*1035, 1974 (Hungarian)

TIMMIS, H. H.: Tracheostomy: overview of implications, management and morbidity. Adv. Surg., *7:*199, 1973

TIMOSCA, G.: Morphofunctional reconstitution of the mandible after extirpation of benign tumors or tumors with a local clinical malignancy. J. Med. Lyon, *53:*353, 1972 (French)

TIMOSCA, G.: Radical therapy, without recurrence, of ameloblastic tumors of the jaws. Rev. Stomatol. Chir. Maxillofac., *75:*47, 1974 (French)

TIMOSCA, G. *et al*: Cheiloplasty after surgical excision of cancer of lower lip. Rev. Med. Chir. Soc. Med. Nat. Iasi., *75:*909, 1971 (Rumanian)

TINDALL, J. P., AND HARRISON, C. M.: Pasteurella multocida infections following animal injuries, especially cat bites, PRS, *51:*485, 1973. Arch. Dermat., *105:*412, 1972

TINDER, L. E.: Relationship of mid-face fractures to mandibular fractures in various forms of trauma, PRS, *53:*603, 1974. Mil. Med., *138:*672, 1973

TIPTON, J. B.: Should incisions in orbital septum be sutured in blepharoplasty? PRS, *49:*613, 1972

TIPTON, J. B.: Should subcutaneous tissue be plicated in a face lift? PRS, *54:*1, 1974

TIPTON, J. B.: Office plastic surgery. PRS, *54:*160, 1974

Tissue Adhesives

Tissue adhesives, assessment for repair of contaminated tissue. Part VII of studies in management of contaminated wound (Edlich *et al*), PRS, *49:*361, 1972. Am. J. Surg., *122:*394, 1971

Acrylate and bakelite adhesive in surgery, application of (Köhnlein, Brehmer), PRS, *50:*422, 1972. Brun's Beitr. klin. Chir., *219:*159, 1972

Tissue glueing, technique and results (Heiss), PRS, *52:*216, 1973. Bull. Soc. Internat. Chir., *6:*549, 1972

Adhesives for primary closure of skin incisions (Fischl) (Follow Up Clinic), PRS, *49:*333, 1972

Wound closure of skin incisions using tissue adhesives (Lindorf). Dtsch. Zahnaerztl. Z., *28:*1131, 1973 (German)

Wound closure, surgical tape: disenchantment (Ellenberg) (Follow-Up Clinic), PRS, *52:*80, 1973

Otorhinolaryngology, usefulness of cyanoacrylic glues in (Czarnecki *et al*). Otolaryngol. Pol., *28:*141, 1974 (Polish)

Tissue Survival

Elasticity, biological tissue, in simple elongation, stochastic model for (Soong, Huang),

Tissue Survival — Cont.
   PRS, *53:*375, 1974. J. Bio-Mechanics, *6:*451, 1973

TITCHENER, J. L.: Management and study of psychological response to trauma, PRS, *48:*95, 1971. J. Trauma, *10:*974, 1971

TITOV, V. E.: Skin plastic surgery in phalangization of the 1st metacarpal bone. Ortop. Travmatol. Protez., *32:*50, 1971 (Russian)

TITOVA, A. T.: Surgery in bilateral ankylosis of the temporo-mandibular joint and microgenia. Vestn. Khir., *106:*58, 1971 (Russian)

TITZE, A.: Indications and limitations of conservative management of bone fractures in the area of the hand. Zentralbl. Chir., *97:*1723, 1972 (German)

TIWARI, R. M.: Hodgkins disease of maxilla. J. Laryng & Otol., *87:*85, 1973

TKACHENKO, A. M.: Clinico-roentgenological characteristics of arthroplasty by lyophilized bone homograft in ankylosis of the temporomandibular joint. Stomatologiia (Mosk.), *51:*84, 1972 (Russian)

TKACHENKO, S. S. *et al*: Treatment of injuries to the flexor tendons of the fingers at the level of the fibro-osseous canals. Vestn. Khir., *107:*80, 1971 (Russian)

TKACHENKO, S. S. *et al*: Intraosseous administration of olemorphocycline in the primary surgical treatment of open fractures of the hand and foot. Vestn. Khir., *111:*103, 1973 (Russian)

TKACHENKO, S. S., DEDUSHKIN, V. S., AND BELOUSOV, A. Y.: Tendon prosthesis, PRS, *55:*643, 1975. Acta chir. plast., *16:*185, 1974

TOBIAS, M., AND SEIFFERT, K. E.: Collagen metabolism in iso- and homografts of tendons, PRS, *52:*105, 1973. Brit. J. Plast. Surg., *25:*83, 1972

TOBIN, H. A.: Conservation in head and neck surgery. J. Maine Med. Assoc., *63:*137, 1972

TOBIN, H. A.: Increased cerebrospinal fluid pressure following unilateral radical neck dissection. Laryngoscope, *82:*817, 1972

TOBIN, H. A.: New instrument for application of wires in maxillofacial surgery. Trans. Am. Ophthalmol. Otolaryngol., *80:*261, 1975

Toe-to-Finger (or Thumb) Transplants

   Thumb replacement: great toe transplantation by microvascular anastomosis (Buncke *et al*), PRS, *55:*109, 1975. Brit. J. Plast. Surg., *26:*194, 1973

   Toe transplantation to reconstruct thumb (Millesi), PRS, *53:*107, 1974. Chir. Plast., *1:*347, 1973

TOFIELD, J. J.: Somersault flap for reconstruc-

tion of helix. Brit. J. Plast. Surg., *28:*71, 1975

TOGAWA, K. *et al*: Surgery of extra-temporal facial nerve paralysis, PRS, *49:*233, 1972. J. Otol. Japan, *74:*122, 1971

TOLAROVA, M.: Empirical recurrence risk figures for genetic counseling of clefts, PRS, *52:*683, 1973. Acta chir. plast., *14:*234, 1972

TOLAROVA, M.: Theory and practice of genetic counseling of inborn and developmental defects, PRS, *54:*629, 1974. Rozhl. chir., *53:*151, 1974

TOLHURST, D. E.: Correction of prominent ears. Brit. J. Plast. Surg., *25:*261, 1972

TOLHURST, D. E.: Myxoma of the palm. Hand, *5:*260, 1973

TOLHURST, D. E.: Modification of Foley catheter for use in perineal urethrostomy. PRS, *55:*503, 1975

TOLIN, S.: Long survival in metastatic melanoma. Arch. Surg., *107:*492, 1973

TOLLEFSEN, H. R., AND SPIRO, R. H.: Median labiomandibular glossotomy, PRS, *48:*297, 1971. Ann. Surg., *173:*415, 1971

TOLLER, P. A.: Immunological factors in cysts of jaws, PRS, *49:*470, 1972. Proc. Roy. Soc. Med., *64:*555, 1971

TOLLER, P. A.: Temporomandibular capsular rearrangement. Brit. J. Oral Surg., *11:*207, 1974

TOLLER, P. A.: Opaque arthrography of temporomandibular joint, PRS, *55:*717, 1975. Int. J. Oral Surg., *3:*17, 1974

TOLLER, P. A.: Temporomandibular arthropathy, PRS, *54:*372, 1974. Proc. Roy. Soc. Med., *67:*153, 1974

TOLMAN, E. L.: Chemosurgery (Mohs' technique) in the treatment of epitheliomas. Med. Clin. North Am., *56:*739, 1972

TOLMEIJER, J. A.: Dislocated and disrupted teeth, PRS, *57:*115, 1976. Nederl. tijdschr. geneesk., *119:*949, 1975

TOLSDORFF, P. *et al*: Technic and application of retroauricular insular flap. Laryngol. Rhinol. Otol. (Stuttg.), *53:*887, 1974 (German)

TOMAN, J.: Problems of laterognathism. Cesk. Stomatol., *72:*377, 1972

TOMAN, J.: Surgery of laterognathism of articular origin. Rev. Stomatol. Chir. Maxillofac., *75:*148, 1974 (French)

TOMAN, J.: Mandibular deformities caused by benign tumors. Acta Stomatol. Belg., *72:*311, 1974 (German)

TOMANEK, R. J., AND LUND, D. D.: Degeneration of different types of skeletal muscle fibres, PRS, *55:*258, 1975. J. Anat., *116:*395, 1973

TOMASEO, I. *et al*: Gardner's syndrome as a surgical problem. Lijec. Vjesn. *96:*610, 1974

(Croatian)

TOMASONI, S.: Reconstruction of lower lip through chin flap, PRS, *57:*756, 1976 (Italian). Riv. ital. chir. plast., *7:*403, 1975

TOMI, M. *et al:* Contracture of the adduction muscles of the thumb in cerebral palsy. Orthop. Surg. (Tokyo), *21:*950, 1970 (Japanese)

TOMICH, C. E. *et al:* Adenoid squamous cell carcinoma of the lip: report of cases. J. Oral Surg., *30:*592, 1972

TOMILOV, I. I. *et al:* Removal of sewing needle from soft tissues of neck. Zh. Ushn. Nos. Gorl. Bolexn., *33:*108, 1973 (Russian)

TOMILOVA, L. I., AND CZECHOVA, S. P.: Some plastic operations in ophthalmology with use of sterilized homologous tissues, PRS, *51:*486, 1973. Acta chir. plast., *13:*235, 1971

TOMLINSON, F. B., AND HOVEY, L. M.: Transconjunctival lower lid blepharoplasty for removal of fat. PRS, *56:*314, 1975

Tongue

Glossotomy, median labiomandibular (Tollefsen, Spiro), PRS, *48:*297, 1971. Ann. Surg., *173:*415, 1971

Glossopharyngeal nerve block (Barton, Williams), PRS, *49:*105, 1972. Arch. Otolaryng., *93:*2, 1971

Dorsum of tongue pedicle flap replacing the epiglottis: an experimental study (Lapidot *et al*). Arch. Otolaryng., *94:*197, 1971

Cryosurgery of the tongue and tonsil (Suga *et al*). J. Otolaryngol. Jap., *74:*514, 1971 (Japanese)

Tongue, growth anomaly of, its relation to jaw anomalies and its surgical treatment (Gasparini *et al*). Riv. Ital. Stomatol., *26:*160, 1971 (Italian)

Tongue flap, closure of secondary palatal fistulae with intraoral tissue and bone grafting (Jackson), PRS, *52:*100, 1973. Brit. J. Plast. Surg., *25:*93, 1972

Tongue flaps, use to resurface lip defects and close palatal fistulae in children (Jackson), PRS, *49:*537, 1972

Corticotomy and wedge-shaped tongue excision as supporting therapy in late orthodontic cases (Machtens, Karwetzky, Meisel). Z. W. R., *81:*1070, 1972 (German)

Tongue flaps, vascularization, morphology and use (Cadenat *et al*). Ann. Chir. Plast., *18:*223, 1973 (French)

Tongue necrosis attributed to ergotamine in temporal arteritis (Wolpaw, Brotten, Martin), PRS, *53:*241, 1974. J.A.M.A., *225:*514, 1973

Tongue, protrusive, effect on, force of detachment of genioglossus muscle (McWilliams *et al*). J. Am. Dent. Assoc., *86:*1310, 1973

Tongue—Cont.

Tongue-skin flap, indications for, in reconstruction of oral tissue loss (Gosserez *et al*). J. Fr. Otorhinolaryngol., *22:*921, 1973 (French)

Lingual thyroid, alternative management: excision with implantation (Danis), PRS, *54:*371, 1974. J. Pediat. Surg., *6:*869, 1973

Innervated partial hemi-tongue pseudoepiglottis: experimental study. Laryngoscope, *83:*1841, 1973

Unusual cause of hypothyroidism (following excision of lingual thyroid) in Chinese boy (Cheah *et al*). Med. J. Malaysia, *27:*217, 1973

Tongue, partial excision in treatment of apertognathia (Olow-Nordenram *et al*). Oral Surg., *35:*152, 1973

Partial glossectomy in preprosthetic surgery (Tenzer). Oral Surg., *35:*616, 1973

Tongue flap, median transit (Calamel), PRS, *51:*315, 1973

Tongue: use of pterygoid muscle sling to provide glossomimic function after total glossectomy (Washio), PRS, *51:*497, 1973

Lingual frenum, surgical correction of shortened (lingua fixata) (Stadelmann). Quintessenz, *24:*107, 1973 (German)

Tongue, reconstruction of (DeFries). Ann. Otol. Rhin. & Laryng., *83:*471, 1974

Influence of tongue asymmetries on the development of jaws and the position of teeth (Austermann *et al*). Int. J. Oral Surg., *3:*261, 1974

Ankyloglossia with psychological implications (Ketty *et al*). J. Dent. Child., *41:*43, 1974

Tongue trauma, prevention in semicomatose patients (Piercell, Wait, Nelson), PRS, *56:*353, 1975. J. Oral Surg., *32:*903, 1974

Tongue flap for reconstruction of lips in electrical burns (Zarem, Greer), PRS, *53:*310, 1974

Anomalies, congenital (Sousa-Lennox), PRS, *54:*629, 1974. Semana med. Mexico, *79:*243, 1974

Reconstitution of lip, tongue and glottis function (Schmid). Acta Stomatol. Belg., *72:*301, 1975 (German)

Tongue, partial necrosis of, caused by endotracheal tube, report (Bagenyi *et al*). Anaesthesist, *24:*136, 1975 (German)

Lingual thyroid, case report and review of literature (Fahey, Monroe), PRS, *57:*672, 1976. Arch. Otolaryng., *101:*574, 1975

Mandibular osteotomy and lingual flaps. Use in patients with cancer of the tonsil area and tongue base (De Santo *et al*). Arch. Otolaryng., *101:*652, 1975

Tongue — Cont.

Use of a tongue flap for the repair of defects following radical surgery of the head and neck (Robertson). Aust. N. Z. J. Surg., *45:*395, 1975

Ankyloglossia (Lessa, Carreirao), PRS, *57:*258, 1976. Folha Med. Brazil, *70:*295, 1975

Tongue, congenital midline fistula of (Samant *et al*), PRS, *56:*597, 1975. Oral Surg., *39:*34, 1975

Note on lingual mutilations and their possible surgical repair (Lebourg). Rev. Stomatol. Chir. Maxillofac., *76:*311, 1975 (French)

Case of post-traumatic ischemic necrosis of the tongue (Brami). Rev. Stomatol. Chir. Maxillofac., *76:*455, 1975 (French)

Aglossia-adactylia syndrome (Stallard, Saad), PRS, *57:*92, 1976

Tongue, Diseases (See also *Tongue, Glossodynia*)

Lingual thyroid and lingual thryoglossal tract remnants. Clinical and histopathologic study with review of literature (Baughman). Oral Surg., *34:*781, 1972

Glossitis, median rhomboid (Schwartz), PRS, *52:*91, 1973

Lingual cysticercosis (Navarrete *et al*). Bol. Med. Hosp. Infant. Mex., *31:*101, 1974 (Spanish)

Tongue and floor of mouth, dermoid, epidermoid and teratomatous cysts of (Gold *et al*). J. Oral Surg., *32:*107, 1974

Tongue, epidermoid cyst of, case report (Akerson *et al*). J. Oral Surg., *32:*117, 1974

Tongue, gastric mucosal cyst of (Harris, Courtemanche), PRS, *54:*612, 1974

Anesthesia and resuscitation in operations for diseases and injuries of the tongue, and the floor of the mouth (Aleksandrov *et al*). Vestn. Khir., *112:*88, 1974 (Russian)

Psychosomatic disorders of the mouth and face (Harris). Practitioner, *214:*372, 1975

Tongue, Glossodynia

Glossodynia and its treatment (Georgieva). Vutr. Boles, *10:*63, 1971 (Bulgarian)

Tongue, "burning," differential diagnosis of (Jung). Fortschr. Med., *90:*1043, 1972

Treatment of glossodynia with Ambosex (Joob-Fancsaly). Forgorv. Sz., *66:*185, 1973 (Hungarian)

Glossodynia, diagnosis of (Hary *et al*). Stomatologiia (Bucur.), *20:*355, 1973 (Rumanian)

Etiopathogenesis and treatment of glossalgia (Bendik). Stomatologiia (Mosk.), *52:*76,

Tongue, Glossodynia — Cont.

1973 (Russian)

Etiology and pathogenesis of the glossalgia syndrome (Evdokimov *et al*). Stomatologiia (Mosk.), *53:*12, 1974 (Russian)

Psychosomatic disorders of mouth and face (Harris). Practitioner, *214:*372, 1975

Etiology and treatment of glossodynias (Tesnier). Rev. Stomatol. Chir. Maxillofac., *76:*417, 1975 (French)

Tongue Neoplasms

Carcinoma, epidermoid, of mobile tongue (Spiro, Strong), PRS, *51:*607, 1973. Am. J. Surg., *122:*707, 1971

Cancer of the tongue: review of thirteen-year experience — 1955–1968 (Maddox *et al*). Am. Surg., *37:*624, 1971

Subglottic cancer, pathology and management (Harrison), PRS, *48:*200, 1971. Ann. Otol. Rhin. & Laryng., *80:*6, 1971

Lipoma of the tongue (De Vleeschouwer *et al*). Arch. Belg. Dermatol. Syphiligr., *27:*123, 1971 (Dutch)

Cancer of tongue: study of regional lymph node spread (Saxena), PRS, *48:*199, 1971. Cancer, *27:*38, 1971

Review of the treatment of cancer of the mobile portion of the tongue (Frazell). Cancer, *28:*1178, 1971

Tongue, base of, cervical lymph node metastases in squamous cell carcinoma (Barkley *et al*), PRS, *52:*103, 1973. Am. J. Surg., *124:*462, 1972

End results of treatment in cancer of the tongue (Rissanen). Ann. Chir. Gynaecol. Fenn., *61:*112, 1972

Carcinoma, tongue, postoperative complications after combined treatment for (Backstrom *et al*). Arch. Klin. Exp. Ohren Nasen Kehlkopfheilkd., *201:*273, 1972

Pre-irradiation tattooing (Baluyot *et al*). Arch. Otolaryng., *96:*151, 1972

Carcinoma of tongue (Hughes). Brit. Med. J., *2:*768, 1972

Lymph node invasion in cancers of mobile portion of tongue (Moyse *et al*). Bull. Cancer (Paris), *59:*161, 1972 (French)

Cancer, tongue, anterior two-thirds, results of radical treatment (Sahatchiev *et al*). Cancer, *30:*703, 1972

Functional disorders following resection of the tongue and floor of the mouth (Kowalik). Czas. Stomatol., *25:*369, 1972 (Polish)

Primary fibrosarcoma of the tongue: report of case (Ryan *et al*). J. Oral Surg., *30:*135, 1972

Cancer, tongue, surgical results in (Matsumura, Kubo, Ono). J. Otolaryngol. Jap.,

Tongue Neoplasms — Cont.

75:1086, 1972 (Japanese)

Carcinoma, lingual, glossectomy rehabilitation by mandibular tongue prosthesis (Moore), PRS, *52:*332, 1973. J. Prosth. Dent., *28:*429, 1972

Carcinoma, oral tongue, occult regional metastasis (Lee *et al*). Laryngoscope, *82:*1273, 1972

Carcinoma, squamous cell, base of tongue, surgical treatment (Whicker *et al*). Laryngoscope, *82:*1853, 1972

Role of total glossectomy in the management of cancer of the oral cavity (Meyers). Otolaryngol. Clin. North Am., *5:*343, 1972

Cancer of tongue; results of treatment in 258 consecutive cases (Whitaker, Lehr, Askovitz), PRS, *50:*363, 1972

Tongue cancer. Current results of treatment. Postgrad. Med., *51:*247, 1972

Treatment of cancer of the vestibule of the larynx and of the root of the tongue (Elinek). Vestn. Otorinolaringol., *34:*89, 1972 (Russian)

Tongue, carcinoma of. Incidence and management of regional lymph node metastasis (Elbrond *et al*). Acta Otolaryngol. (Stockh.), *75:*310, 1973

Tongue, cancer of (Jeppsson *et al*). Acta Otolaryngol. (Stockh.), *75:*314, 1973

Tongue, carcinoma of, combined radiotherapy and surgery in treatment (Jakobsson *et al*). Acta Otolaryngol. (Stockh.), *75:*321, 1973

Carcinoma linguae. Series of 96 patients (Elbrond *et al*). Acta Radiol. (Ther.) (Stockh.), *12:*465, 1973

Carcinoma, epidermoid, of tongue, partial glossectomy and neck dissection for (Spiro, Strong), PRS, *53:*602, 1974. Am. J. Surg., *126:*544, 1973

Rhabdomyosarcoma of tongue in infant: results of combined radiation and chemotherapy (Leibert, Stool), PRS, *53:*681, 1974. Ann. Surg., *178:*621, 1973

Cancer of tongue, role of radiotherapy in treatment (Vermund, Gollin), PRS, *54:*106, 1974. Cancer, *32:*333, 1973

Tongue, fibrosarcoma of (Nagy). Int. J. Oral Surg., *2:*303, 1973

Sarcoma, neurogenic (neurofibrosarcoma) of tongue (Rapoport *et al*), PRS. *54:*234, 1974. Internat. Surg., *58:*738, 1973

Tongue cancers, surgical treatment of (Coudry *et al*). J. Fr. Otorhinolaryngol., *22:*869, 1973 (French)

Cancer, tongue, mobile part. Therapeutic indications (Horiot). J. Fr. Otorhinolaryngol., *22:*875, 1973 (French)

Tongue Neoplasms — Cont.

Indications, technic and results of total subglossolaryngectomy (Andre). J. Fr. Otorhinolaryngol., *22:*881, 1973 (French)

Tongue, mucoepidermoid carcinoma of (Heidelberger *et al*). J. Laryng. & Otol., *87:*1239, 1973

Tongue, benign hemangiopericytoma of (Orlian). J. Oral Surg., *31:*936, 1973

Carcinoma, base of tongue, total glossectomy for advanced (Sessions *et al*). Laryngoscope, *83:*39, 1973

Tongue, neurofibroma (Ukleja *et al*). Otolaryngol. Pol., *27:*121, 1973 (Polish)

Lingual tumors, benign, in children, late results of surgical treatment (Bozek *et al*). Pediatr. Pol., *45:*1193, 1973 (Polish)

Carcinoma, squamous cell, of faucial arch, tonsillar fossa and base of tongue, incidence and causes of local failure of irradiation in (Gelinas *et al*). Radiology, *108:*383, 1973

Carcinoma, tongue, mobile (Grellet). Rev. Stomatol. Chir. Maxillofac., *74:*111, 1973

Local and lymph node treatment of epitheliomas of the mobile part of the tongue (Moyse *et al*). Rev. Stomatol. Chir. Maxillofac., *74:*574, 1973 (French)

Tongue, cancer of (Southwick). Surg. Clin. North Am., *53:*147, 1973

Tongue, carcinoma of root of, lateral pharyngotomy in treatment of (Riccabona). Wien. Klin. Wochenschr., *85:*333, 1973 (German)

Place of surgery in the treatment of carcinomas of the oral cavity (Mendes da Costa *et al*). Acta Chir. Belg., *73:*529, 1974 (French)

Carbon dioxide laser in head and neck surgery (Kaplan *et al*). Am. J. Surg., *128:*543, 1974

Use of split thickness grafts in the repair of excisions of the oropharynx, base of the tongue, and larynx (Rush *et al*). Am. J. Surg., *128:*553, 1974

Rhabdomyosarcoma of the head and neck (Smith). Can. J. Otolaryngol., *3:*618, 1974

Radical neck dissection in advanced tumors of the head and neck. Considerations on 52 cases (Caldarola *et al*). Cancro, *27:*187, 1974 (Italian)

Evaluation and rehabilitation of glossectomy speech behavior (Amerman *et al*). J. Commun. Disord., *7:*365, 1974

Synovial sarcoma of the tongue, report of a case (Moussavi *et al*). J. Laryng. & Otol., *88:*795, 1974

Cryosurgery in otolaryngology (Editorial). J. Otolaryngol. Jpn., *77:*799, 1974 (Japanese)

Cryosurgical treatment of recurrent head and neck malignancies — a comparative

Tongue Neoplasms — Cont.

study (Goode *et al*). Laryngoscope, *84:*1950, 1974

Tongue, carcinoma of, in child. Case report and review of literature (Turner *et al*). Oral Surg., *37:*663, 1974

Cyst, gastric mucosal, of the tongue (Harris, Courtemanche), PRS, *54:*612, 1974

Indications for skin grafts in chronic diseases of the mouth (Soubiran *et al*). Rev. Stomatol. Chir. Maxillofac., *75:*103, 1974 (French)

Head and neck myoblastoma (Thawley, Ogura), PRS, *55:*515, 1975. South. M. J., *67:*1020, 1974

Cancer of tongue, surgical treatment of (Spiro, Strong), PRS, *55:*516, 1975. Surg. Clin. N. Am., *54:*759, 1974

Indications, limits and results of functional laterocervical lymph node excision (Pignataro). Tumori, *60:*585, 1974 (Italian)

Anesthesia and resuscitation in operations for diseases and injuries of the tongue, and the floor of the mouth (Aleksandrov *et al*). Vestn. Khir., *112:*88, 1974 (Russian)

Postoperative bronchopulmonary complications in malignant neoplasms of maxillofacial localization (Dunaevskii *et al*). Vestn. Khir., *113:*69, 1974 (Russian)

Surgical technic in combined treatment of cancer of the tongue and mouth floor (Becker). Acta Stomatol. Belg., *72:*247, 1975 (German)

Technical possibilities of destruction and reconstruction in surgery of cancer of the tongue and mouth floor (Torielli *et al*). Acta Stomatol. Belg., *72:*259, 1975 (French)

Treatment of neoplasms of the mobile part of the tongue (Tuglimana *et al*). Acta Stomatol. Belg., *72:*291, 1975 (French)

Preoperative cytostasis of extensive flat epithelial cancer of the tongue and floor of the mouth (Gruneberg). Acta Stomatol. Belg., *72:*437, 1975 (German)

Analysis of mortality and morbidity in 100 composite resections for oral carcinoma (Robins *et al*). Am. J. Surg., *130:*178, 1975

Combined chemotherapy and cryosurgery for oral cancer (Benson). Am. J. Surg., *130:*596, 1975

Tongue flap reconstruction in cancer of oral cavity (Sessions, Dedo, Ogura), PRS, *57:*395, 1976. Arch. Otolaryng., *101:*166, 1975

Mandibular osteotomy and lingual flaps. Use in patients with cancer of the tonsil area and tongue base (DeSanto *et al*). Arch. Otolaryng., *101:*652, 1975

Tongue Neoplasms — Cont.

Efficacy of combining radiation therapy with a surgical procedure in patients with cervical metastasis from squamous cancer of the oropharynx and hypopharynx (Jesse *et al*). Cancer, *35:*1163, 1975

Heteroptic gastric mucosa in the tongue (Giarelli *et al*). Dtsch. Zahnaerztl. Z., *30:*823, 1975 (German)

Mesenchymal tumors of the mouth(Takacsi-Nagy). Dtsch. Zahnaerztl. Z., *30:*827, 1975 (German)

Neurilemmoma of the tongue (Mosadomi). J. Oral Med., *30:*44, 1975

Sclerosing hemangioma of the tongue: report of case (Friedlander *et al*). J. Oral Surg., *33:*212, 1975

Cervical-pectoral flaps in the treatment of advanced oral cancer (Shons *et al*). J. Surg. Oncol., *7:*213, 1975

Leiomyosarcoma of head and neck: review of literature and report of two cases (Mindell *et al*). Laryngoscope, *85:*904, 1975

Tongue, lymphangioma of, associated with cervical cystic hygroma and anterior open bite (Mendex *et al*), PRS, *57:*757, 1976. O Medico, *79:*199, 1975

Lingual osseous choristoma (McClendon), PRS, *56:*593, 1975. Oral Surg., *39:*39, 1975

Swallowing and speech after radical total glossectomy with tongue prosthesis (De Souza *et al*). Oral Surg., *39:*356, 1975

Carcinoma, squamous cell, tongue and floor of mouth, management of, after excisional biopsy (Ange *et al*). Radiology, *116:*143, 1975

Daily practice: appreciation of the oncologic risk of oral lichen planus (Castermans-Elias *et al*). Rev. Belge. Med. Dent., *30:*33, 1975 (French)

Management of oral and pharyngeal cancer: a multi-disciplinary approach (El-Domeiri *et al*). Surg. Clin. North Am., *55:*107, 1975

Oncocytoma of tongue in a child (Das *et al*). J. Pediatr. Surg., *11:*113, 1976

Resection and immediate reconstruction for patients with "inoperable" recurrent head and neck cancer (Robson). Surg. Clin. North Am., *56:*111, 1976

TOPAZIAN, R. G.: Rehabilitation of the atrophic edentulous maxilla by bone grafting. J. Am. Dent. Assoc., *90:*625, 1975

TOPAZIAN, R. G. *et al*: Use of ceramics in augmentation and replacement of portions of the mandible. J. Biomed. Mater. Res., *6:*311, 1972

TOPPOZADA, H. H. *et al*: Basal cell carcinoma of nose: with report of two atypical cases. J.

Laryng. & Otol., *86:*933, 1972

TOPPOZADA, H. H. *et al*: Lipoma of pharynx (report of four cases). J. Laryng. & Otol., *87:*787, 1973

TORANTO I. R., SALYER, K. E., AND MYERS, M. B: Vascularization of porcine skin heterografts, PRS, *54:*195, 1974. Discussion by Ben-Hur, PRS, *54:*352, 1974

TORII, S.: Free *gracilis* muscle transplantation with microneurovascular anastomoses for the treatment of facial paralysis (with Harii, Ohmori), PRS, *57:*133, 1976

TORRE, P. *et al*: Radio-surgical treatment of cancers of maxillary sinus. Ann. Otolaryngol. Chir. Cervicofac., *90:*353, 1973 (French)

TORRES-BALDO, S.: Wrist and hand pathology related to sports, PRS, *52:*323, 1973. Rev. Latino Am. cir. plast., *15:*17, 1971

TORRIELLI, F.: Immediate intra-oral mandibular bone transplants. Minerva Stomatol., *20:*110, 1971 (Italian)

TORRIELLI, F. *et al*: Osteotomy of ramus of mandible with particular reference to stepped management. Minerva Stomatol., *22:*41, 1973 (Italian)

TORRIELLI, F. *et al*: Segmental alveolar osteotomy in the correction of maxillofacial malformations. Minerva Stomatol., *22:*218, 1973 (Italian)

TORRIELLI, F. *et al*: Experiences and results in the treatment of malformations of the jaws by segmental osteotomies. Rev. Stomatol. Chir. Maxillofac., *75:*125, 1974 (French)

TORRIELLI, F. *et al*: Technical possibilities of destruction and reconstruction in surgery of cancer of the tongue and mouth floor. Acta Stomatol. Belg., *72:*259, 1975 (French)

Torticollis

Manual myotomy for congenital muscular torticollis in infants (Shinoda). Orthop. Surg. (Tokyo), *22:*1099, 1971 (Japanese)

Experience of manual myotomy for muscular torticollis in infants (Kasai). Orthop. Surg. (Tokyo), *22:*1107, 1971 (Japanese)

Prognosis in muscular torticollis (Kawamura *et al*. Orthop. Surg. (Tokyo), *23:*44, 1972 (Japanese)

Torticollis, analysis of 271 cases (Armstrong) (Follow-Up Clinic), PRS, *49:*565, 1972

Wry-neck, operative treatment. Follow-up study over period of 27 years (Bosch). Wien. Klin. Wochenschr., *84:*688, 1972 (German)

Anesthetic problems in surgery for varying levels of respiratory obstruction in infants and children (Wilson *et al*). Anesth. Analg. (Cleve.), *53:*878, 1974

Surgical treatment and after care in muscu-

Torticollis—Cont.

lar torticollis (Manitz). Beitr. Orthop. Traumatol., *21:*376, 1974 (German)

Torticollis myogenes in children (Pajic). Med. Pregl., *27:*209, 1974 (Serbian)

Torticollis, so-called bilateral muscular (Dol'nitskii *et al*). Ortop. Travmatol. Protez., *35:*69, 1974

TOSATTI, B.: Transplantation and reimplantation in arts, PRS, *54:*511, 1974. Surgery, *75:*389, 1974

TOSATTI, E.: Unsolved problem of peripheral lymphedema (Editorial). Lymphology, *6:*167, 1973

TOSOVSKY, V. *et al*: Local therapy of burns in children. Cesk. Pediatr., *27:*404, 1972 (Czechoslovakian)

TOSOVSKY, V., STRYKAL, F., AND KOLIKOVA, E.: Bone changes in meningomyelocele, PRS, *51:*234, 1973. Kinderchir., *11:*254, 1972

TOTH, B. B. *et al*: Central adenocarcinoma of the mandible. Oral Surg., *39:*436, 1975

TOTH, B. B. *et al*: Central pacinian neurofibroma of the maxilla. Oral Surg., *39:*630, 1975

TOTSUKA, G. *et al*: Selective facial nerve branch blocking. Arch. Otolaryng., *95:*360, 1972

TOULOUKIAN, ROBERT J., AND KRIZEK, THOMAS J.: *Diagnosis and Early Management of Trauma Emergencies: A Manual for the Emergency Service.* Charles C Thomas, Springfield, Ill., 1974. PRS, *56:*206, 1975

TOUMIEUX, B. *et al*: Tracheal resections for stenosis caused by respiratory resuscitation. Ann. Chir. Thorac. Cardiovasc., *11:*395, 1972 (French)

TOUSSI, T. *et al*: Metastatic melanoma treated in a pregnant woman: pre- and postnatal implications. Union Med. Can., *103:*1968, 1974 (French)

TOWERS, J. F.: Secondary tumours of the maxilla. Trans. Int. Conf. Oral Surg., *4:*138, 1973

TOWERS, J. F. *et al*: Simple reconstruction of mandible following resection. Proc. Roy. Soc. Med., *67:*607, 1974

TOWERS, J. F., AND MCANDREWS, P. G.: Maxillary sinusitis mimicking malignant disease, PRS, *57:*126, 1976. J. Oral Surg., *39:*718, 1975

TOWNES, P. L. *et al*: Hereditary syndrome of imperforate anus with hand, foot, and ear anomalies. J. Pediatr., *81:*321, 1972

TOWNS, T. M.: Chronic sclerosing osteomyelitis of maxilla and mandible: review of literature and case report. J. Oral Surg., *30:*903, 1972

TOWNSEND, G. L., MORIMOTO, A. M., AND KRALEMANN, H.: Management of sialorrhea in mentally retarded patients by trans-tympanic neurectomy, PRS, *54:*105, 1974. Mayo

Clin. Proc., *48:*776, 1973

TOWNSEND, P. L.: Silicone rubber casts of the distal urethra in studying fistula formation and other hypospadias problems. Brit. J. Plast. Surg., *28:*320, 1975

TOWNSEND, P. L. G.: Nipple sensation following breast reduction and free nipple transplantation, PRS, *56:*678, 1975. Brit. J. Plast. Surg., *27:*308, 1974

Trachea (See also *Anesthesia; Tracheotomy*)

Tracheal injury, incidence and pathogenesis following cuffed tube tracheostomy with assisted ventilation (Andrews, Pierson), PRS, *49:*233, 1972. Ann. Surg., *173:*249, 1971

Wounds, penetrating, of larynx and cervical trachea (LeMay), PRS, *49:*670, 1972. Arch. Otolaryng., *94:*558, 1971

Trachea, experimental plastic elongation: preliminary report (Uhlschmid), PRS, *48:*510, 1971. Helvet. chir. acta, *1:*207, 1971

Tracheal injury from cuffed tracheostomy tubes, reappraisal of (Bryant, Trinkle, Dubilier), PRS, *48:*392, 1971. J.A.M.A., *215:*625, 1971

Tracheostomy balloon cuffs, new concept in (Hinshaw *et al*), PRS, *49:*669, 1972. Surg. Forum, *22:*194, 1971

Tracheoesophageal fistula caused by cuffed tracheal tubes, management of (Thomas), PRS, *51:*230, 1973. Am. J. Surg., *124:*181, 1972

Trachea, thoracic, experimental elongation of (Uhlschmid), PRS, *51:*603, 1973. Langenbecks Arch. Chir., *331:*255, 1972

Orotracheal intubation, emergency, simple method for (Manchester, Mani, Masters), PRS, *49:*312, 1972

Tracheal reconstruction with autogeneous mucochondrial graft (Krizek, Kirchner), PRS, *50:*123, 1972

Tracheal defects in dog, replacement by preformed composite graft; a later report (Farkas *et al*), PRS, *50:*238, 1972

Comments on paper by P. Wilflingseder: Reconstruction of trachea using segment transplant from nasal septum. Wien. Klin. Wschr., *84:*226, 1972. (Brucke *et al*). Wien. Klin. Wochenschr., *84:*797, 1972 (German)

Tracheostomy, indications, technics, and tubes—reappraisal (Hardy), PRS, *53:*105, 1974. Am. J. Surg., *126:*300, 1973

Tracheal complications after long-term ventilation, amelioration of—new method of cuff inflation (Wolff *et al*), PRS, *57:*541, 1976. Anaesthetist, *22:*317, 1973

Trachea, composite nasal septal autografts of (Furstoss *et al*). Ann. Otol. Rhin. & Lar-

Trachea—Cont.

yng., *82:*831, 1973

Tracheal injury, rapid, by cuffed airways and healing with loss of ciliated epithelium (Paegle, Ayres, Davis), PRS, *52:*462, 1973. Arch. Surg., *106:* 31, 1973

Trachea and bronchus, damage by suction procedures (Sacker *et al*), PRS, *53:*610, 1974. Chest, *64:*285, 1973

Tracheal cartilage defects, experimental, reconstruction with free periosteum (Ritsila, Alhopuro), PRS, *54:*689, 1974. Scand. J. Plast. Reconstr. Surg., *7:*116, 1973

Tracheostomies, aspiration in patients with (Cameron, Reynolds, Zuidema), PRS, *52:*206, 1973. Surg. Gynec. & Obst., *126:*68, 1973

Trachea, adenoid cystic carcinoma of. Experience with 16 patients managed by tracheal resection (Pearson *et al*). Ann. Thorac. Surg., *18:*16, 1974

Trachea, focal muscular hyperplasia of (Benisch *et al*), PRS, *54:*690, 1974. Arch. Otolaryng., *99:*226, 1974

Tracheal injury by cuffed tracheostomy tubes, determinants of (Dunn, Dunn, Moser), PRS, *54:*501, 1974. Chest, *65:*128, 1974

Tracheal defect, growth of cartilage from free perichondrial graft placed across defect in rabbit's trachea (Sohn, Ohlsen), PRS, *53:*55, 1974

Trachea, free periosteal transplants in reconstruction of (Kugan, Pasila), PRS, *55:*718. 1975. Ztschr. Kinderchir., *15:*371, 1974

Tracheostomy (Salmon), PRS, *57:*260, 1976. Proc. Roy. Soc. Med., *68:*347, 1975

Graft of *dura mater* in trachea (Sabas, Mangione, Simone), PRS, *57:*758, 1976. Rev. argent. cir., *28:*32, 1975

Tracheotomy

Tracheotomy or long-term intubation in acute respiratory insufficiency? (Mantel *et al*). Langenbecks Arch. Chir., *327:*906, 1970 (German)

Avoidance of tracheotomy damage through a changed surgical technic (Berger *et al*). Langenbecks Arch. Chir., *327:*922, 1970 (German)

Tracheotomy or intubation, prolonged, in neonatal and pediatric resuscitation (Rondeau *et al*). Union Med. Can., *99:*1662, 1970 (French)

Tracheostomy cuff designed to prevent suffocation (Myerowitz *et al*). Am. J. Surg., *122:*835, 1971

Detection and management of tracheal stenosis following cuffed tube tracheostomy

Tracheotomy—Cont.

(Pearson *et al*). Ann. Thorac. Surg., *12:*359, 1971

Reflections of difficult decannulation (Wind). Arch. Otolaryng., *94:*426, 1971

Skin-lined tube as a complication of tracheostomy (Hughes *et al*). Arch. Otolaryng., *94:*568, 1971

Incidence and pathogenesis of tracheal injury following tracheostomy with cuffed tube and assisted ventilation. Analysis of a 3-year prospective study (Andrews). Brit. J. Surg., *58:*749, 1971

Tracheotomy in the multi-injured (Lehmann *et al*). Cah. Anesthesiol., *19:*335, 1971 (French)

Harare staff clinical conference. Tracheostomy versus naso-tracheal intubation (Duthie). Cent. Afr. J. Med., *17:*222, 1971

Early complications following tracheotomy in surgical patients (Teodorovich *et al*). Eksp. Khir. Anesteziol., *16:*86, 1971 (Russian)

Tracheostomy and prolonged intubation in the management of trauma (Austin). Injury, *2:*191, 1971

Management of tracheal stenosis secondary to prolonged ventilation utilizing a cuffed tracheostomy tube—a case report (Chaney *et al*). J. Indiana State Med. Assoc., *64:*1196, 1971

Acquired laryngotracheal stenosis in children (Louhimo *et al*). J. Pediatr. Surg., *6:*730, 1971

The contribution of cuff volume and pressure in tracheostomy tube damage (Ching *et al*). J. Thorac. Cardiovasc. Surg., *62:*402, 1971

Low-pressure cuff for tracheostomy tubes to minimize tracheal injury. A comparative clinical trial (Grillo *et al*). J. Thorac. Cardiovasc. Surg., *62:*898, 1971

Respiration monitor for infants with tracheostomy (Harris). Lancet, *2:*583, 1971

Tracheotomy and tracheostomy in plastic surgery (Fittipaldi). Minerva Chir., *26:*1454, 1971 (Italian)

Divided tracheotomy tube for registering respiration, introducing gas mixtures and connection to an artifical respiration apparatus (Mitagvariia *et al*). Patol. Fiziol. Eksp. Ter., *15:*86, 1971 (Russian)

Emergency tracheotomy. A new technical variant (Koatz). Prensa Med. Argent., *58:*1666, 1971 (Spanish)

Critical considerations on tracheotomy (Ibarra-Perez *et al*). Prensa Med. Mex., *36:*465, 1971 (Spanish)

Automatic intermittent insufflation of the tracheotomy tube cuff (Franzen). Rev.

Tracheotomy—Cont.

Bras. Anestesiol., *21:*103, 1971 (Portuguese)

The cuff: a mixed blessing (Barton). Surgery, *70:*800, 1971

Balloon cuffs, tracheostomy, new concept in (Hinshaw *et al*), PRS, *49:*669, 1971. Surg. Forum, *22:*194, 1971

Unavoidable adverse sequelae of tracheostomy and possible ways of lessening them (Isakov). Vestn. Khir., *107:*130, 1971 (Russian)

Contemporary viewpoints on tracheotomy (Aslamazova). Vestn. Otorinolaringol., *33:*68, 1971 (Russian)

Problems of tracheotomy in the surgical routine (Borchert *et al*). Zentralbl. Chir., *96:*1005, 1971 (German)

Tracheostomy in adult, technic of (Giradet). Am. J. Surg., *125:*327, 1972

Comprehensive view of tracheostomy (Pemberton). Am. Surg., *38:*251, 1972

Tracheal resections for stenosis caused by respiratory resuscitation (Toumieux *et al*). Ann. Chir. Thorac. Cardiovasc., *11:*395, 1972 (French)

Tracheotomy, late cataclysmic tracheal hemorrhage following: new surgical success and over-all results of 10 operations (Couraud *et al*). Ann. Chir. Thorac. Cardiovasc., *11:*401, 1972 (French)

Decannulation problems in infants (Baker *et al*). Ann. Otol. Rhin. & Laryng., *81:*555, 1972

Tracheotomy in pediatrics (Tucker *et al*). Ann. Otol. Rhin. & Laryng., *81:*818, 1972

Tracheostomy closure and scar revisions (Kulber *et al*). Arch. Otolaryng., *96:*22, 1972

Inspired oxygen concentrations using a humidifier-tracheostomy T-piece system (Nakamura *et al*). Brit. J. Anaesth., *44:*61, 1972

Tracheostomy tubes, pre-stretched cuffs on (Wandless *et al*). Brit. J. Anaesth., *44:*1222, 1972

Speaking valve for attachment to tracheostomy tube (Emery). Brit. Med. J., *2:*466, 1972

Respiratory problems, tracheostomy in management of, in developing country: study at Lagos University Teaching Hospital (Ffoulkes-Crabbe, Emma). Can. Anaesth. Soc. J., *19:*478, 1972

Tracheostomy and prolonged intubation, laryngeal and tracheal complications following (Schloss). Can. J. Otolaryngol., *1:*135, 1972

Subglottic stenosis in infants and children: clinical problem and experimental surgical

Tracheotomy — Cont.

correction (Fearon *et al*). Can. J. Otolaryngol., *1:*281, 1972

Tracheostomy dependence in children. Review of ten cases (Ayim). East Afr. Med. J., *49:*830, 1972

Tracheotomy or long-time intubation? (Plath *et al*). H. N. O., *20:*29, 1972 (German)

Tracheotomy, fatal complications of (Saternus). H. N. O., *20:*274, 1972 (German)

Tracheal stenosis following tracheotomy (Middendorp). Helv. Chir. Acta, *39:*555, 1972 (German)

Tracheostomy: surgical problems and complications (Greenway). Int. Anesthesiol. Clin., *10:*151, 1972

Tracheal stenosis following tracheostomy (Salomon *et al*). Int. Surg., *57:*498, 1972

Prolonged endotracheal intubation versus tracheostomy in infants and children (Guinee). J. Arkansas Med. Soc., *68:*259, 1972

Tracheostomy, fatal hemorrhage following. Case report (Kantawala *et al*). J. Postgrad. Med., *18:*156, 1972

Use of a one-way valve to aid in tracheostomy decannulation (Ashcraft *et al*). J. Thorac. Cardiovasc. Surg., *64:*161, 1972

Clinical and experimental evaluation of controlled-pressure intratracheal cuff (Magovern *et al*). J. Thorac. Cardiovasc. Surg., *64:*747, 1972

An aseptic tracheostomy suction catheter (Morrell *et al*). Lancet, *1:*76, 1972

Prevention of ulceration during use of cuffed tracheostomy tube (Gilston). Lancet, *1:*1074, 1972

Tracheotomy in neonates (Gibson *et al*). Laryngoscope, *82:*643, 1972

Arytenoids, use of an epiglottic flap to, in surgical treatment of life-endangering chronic aspiration pneumonia (Habal, Murray), PRS, *49:*305, 1972

Tracheostomy: its management and alternatives (McClelland). Proc. Roy. Soc. Med. *65:*401, 1972

Trachea of tracheotomized and nontracheotomized subjects, postmortem bacteriological findings in (Resl). Sb. Ved. Pr. Lek. Fak. Karlovy Univ. (Suppl.), *15:*395, 1972 (Czechoslovakian)

Ventilatory work, influence of tracheotomy or intubation cannulas on (Atlan *et al*). Sem. Hop. Paris, *48:*2979, 1972 (French)

Tracheal stenosis and sterilization of tracheotomy cannulas with ethylene oxide (Mantz *et al*). Sem. Hop. Paris, *48:*3367, 1972 (French)

Tracheotomy tubes, flow resistance in (Cavo *et al*). Surg. Forum, *23:*490, 1972

Tracheotomy — Cont.

Neck, enlarged, tracheotomy tube for management of (Abramson). Trans. Am. Acad. Ophthalmol. Otolaryngol., *76:*1010, 1972

Tracheotomy, advantages and disadvantages of. Follow up results (Knoch *et al*). Z. Aerztl. Forbild. (Jena), *66:*675, 1972 (German)

Tracheostomy: overview of implications, management and morbidity (Timmis). Adv. Surg., *7:*199, 1973

Airway, tracheostomy — indications, techniques, and tubes (Hardy), PRS, *53:*105, 1974. Am. J. Surg., *126:*300, 1973

Tracheoesophageal fistula following prolonged tracheal intubation (Slogoff *et al*). Anesthesiology, *39:*453, 1973

Evaporation — optimal physiological principle for artificial climatization of inspired air (Wallis *et al*). Arch. Klin. Exp. Ohren Nasen Kehlkopfheilkd., *205:*363, 1973 (German)

Tracheal stenoses, benign, resection of, following tracheostomy and longtime intubation (Brucke *et al*). Bruns Beitr. Klin. Chir., *220:*387, 1973 (German)

Tracheal tube cuff designs, evaluation of (Carroll). Crit. Care Med., *1:*45, 1973

Proper use of large diameter, large residual volume cuffs (Carroll *et al*). Crit. Care Med., *1:*153, 1973

Recommended performance specifications for cuffed endotracheal and tracheostomy tubes: joint statement of investigators, inventors and manufacturers (Carroll *et al*). Crit. Care Med., *1:*155, 1973

Tracheostomy and endotracheal cuffs, pressure dynamics of. 1. Use of tracheal model to evaluate performance (Wu *et al*). Crit. Care Med., *1:*197, 1973

Tracheotomy or long-term intubation? (Fritsche). H. N. O., *21:*297, 1973 (German)

Tracheostomy, hemorrhage following (Brantigan), PRS, *53:*604, 1974. J. Trauma, *13:*235, 1973

Tracheostomy tubes, fenestrated (Freeman). Lancet, *1:*259, 1973

Tracheostomy tubes, fenestrated (Lange). Lancet, *2:*444, 1973

Tracheostomy tubes, fenestrated (Battersby *et al*). Lancet, *2:*963, 1973

Tracheostomy tubes, cuffed, dangers of oral feeding in presence of (Pinkus). M. J. Australia., *1:*1238, 1973

Tracheostomy in infants and children, an improved technique for (White, Haller). Med. Times, *101:*120, 1973

Tracheostomy, treatment of subostial stenosis secondary to (Turitto *et al*). Minerva

Tracheotomy – Cont.

Anestesiol., *39:*105, 1973 (Italian)

Tracheotomy in resuscitation (Gianasi *et al*). Minerva Anestesiol., *39:*194, 1973 (Italian)

Tracheostomy, postponed (Coluccio). Minerva chir., *28:*148, 1973 (Italian)

Tracheostomy and prolonged tracheal intubation in young children, aspects of controversy concerning. Current status of problem (Ciurea *et al*). Otorinolaringologie, *18:*107, 1973 (Rumanian)

Microtracheostomy in treatment of patients with destructive tuberculosis complicated by bronchitis (Strelis *et al*). Probl. Tuberk., *51:*30, 1973 (Russian)

Tracheal cuffs, recent developments in (Cross). Resuscitation, *2:*77, 1973

Tracheotomy or tracheal intubation, prolonged, obstructive complications of assisted ventilation using. Prevention and supervision using systematic laryngoscopy, 185 cases (Gautier *et al*). Sem. Hop. Paris, *49:*2779, 1973 (French)

Aspiration in patients with tracheostomies (Cameron, Reynolds, Zuidema), PRS, *52:*266, 1973. Surg. Gynec. & Obst., *126:*68, 1973

Tracheotomy material (Lind). Tidsskr. Nor. Laegeforen, *93:*2380, 1973 (Norwegian)

Tracheostomy and intubation, fusion of vocal cords following (Kirchner *et al*). Trans. Am. Acad. Ophthalmol. Otolaryngol., 77:188, 1973

Tracheostomy in system of resuscitation and anesthesiological measures in maxillofacial surgery (Dunaevskii *et al*). Tsitologiia, *15:*74, 1973 (Russian)

Tracheal cannulas in infants and children, difficultues encountered during the removal of (Sylwanowicz). Wiad Lek., *26:*2161, 1973 (Polish)

Tracheotomy, complications of (Pfretzschner *et al*). Z. Laryngol. Rhinol. Otol., *52:*616, 1973

Tracheotomy, modern concepts of indications for (Liande). Zh. Ushn. Nos. Gorl. Bolezn., *33:*69, 1973 (Russian)

Tracheotomy tube (foreign body) in bronchus, long-term symptomless presence (Vendelovskii *et al*). Zh. Ushn. Nos. Gorl. Bolezn., *33:*76, 1973 (Russian)

Tracheotomy tube, combined (Gapanovich *et al*). Zh. Ushn. Nos. Gorl. Bolezn. *33:*113, 1973 (Russian)

Improved tracheotomy tube obdurator (Emerson). Am. Fam. Physician, *10:*155, 1974

Tracheostomy, eating with (Weber), PRS, *56:*355, 1975. Am. J. Nursing, *74:*1439,

Tracheotomy – Cont.

1974

Tracheostomy complicating massive burn injury. Plea for conservatism (Eckhauser *et al*). Am. J. Surg., *127:*418, 1974

Tracheostomy tube change, technic for (Smith). Anesth. Analg. (Cleve.), *53:*627, 1974

Tissue reaction to cuffed tube materials (Lam *et al*). Anaesth. Intensive Care, *2:*260, 1974

Tracheal resection, extensive, for post-tracheotomy stenosis or tumor. Postoperative radiological and functional study (Arnaud *et al*). Ann. Chir. Thorac. Cardiovasc., *13:*73, 1974 (French)

Tracheal T-tube, silicone (Montgomery). Ann. Otol. Rhin. & Laryng., *83:*71, 1974

Tracheotomy decannulation, bilateral pneumothorax five days after (Lehmann). Ann. Otol. Rhin. & Laryng., *83:*128, 1974

Multiple postintubation complications (Strome *et al*). Ann. Otol. Rhin. & Laryng., *83:*432, 1974

Tracheostome maintenance by obturator for prolonged or future needs (Friedberg *et al*). Ann. Otol. Rhin. & Laryng., *83:*520, 1974

Hypersomnia caused by upper airway obstructions: a new syndrome in otolaryngology (Simmons *et al*). Ann. Otol. Rhin. & Laryng., *83:*670, 1974

Tracheostomies, prevention of aspiration in patients with. Aspiration pneumonia (Bone *et al*). Ann. Thorac. Surg., *18:*30, 1974

Acceptability of swivel connectors (Holdcroft *et al*). Brit. J. Anaesth., *46:*298, 1974

Tracheostomy tubes, pressure monitoring device for low pressure cuffs on (Scott). Can. Anesth. Soc. J., *21:*120, 1974

Tracheotomy, pediatric (Friedberg *et al*). Can. J. Otolaryngol., *3:*147, 1974

Delayed decannulation – investigation and management (Crysdale). Can. J. Otolaryngol., *3:*156, 1974

Transtracheal catheter ventilation: clinical experiences in 36 patients (Jacobs *et al*). Chest, *65:*36, 1974

Letter: Cuff pressure measurements (Ching *et al*). Chest, *66:*604, 1974

Pathogenesis of mediastinal emphysema and pneumothorax following tracheotomy (Padovan *et al*). Chest, *66:*553, 1974

Technique for changing tracheostomy tubes in the early postoperative patient (Widmann). Crit. Care Med., *2:*277, 1974

Tracheostomy and endotracheal intubation, clinical concepts (Shaw). D. M., 1–35, 1974

X-ray diagnosis of posttracheostomic stenoses (Rabkin *et al*). Grudn. Khir., *0:*83,

Tracheotomy—Cont.

1974 (Russian)

Airway-instantly (Oppenheimer). J.A.M.A., *230:*76, 1974

Tracheostomy, delayed massive hemorrhage from (Comer), PRS, *55:*508, 1975. J. Cardiovasc. Surg., *15:*389, 1974

Elective tracheostomy in head and neck tumour surgery (Shaw *et al*). J. Laryng. & Otol., *88:*599, 1974

Laryngo-tracheoplasty (Evans *et al*). J. Leg. Med., *88:*589, 1974

Problem stoma (Helsper). J. Surg. Oncol., *6:*151, 1974

Bilateral stress pneumothorax during tracheostomy (Chistikhin). Khirurgiia (Mosk.), *0:*138, 1974 (Russian)

Clinical experience with new low-pressure high-volume tracheostomy cuffs. Importance of limiting intracuff pressure (Ching *et al*). N. Y. State J. Med., *74:*2379, 1974

Tracheal stenoses. Development and latest state of experimental surgery (Flemming *et al*). O. R. L., *36:*179, 1974

Long-term intratracheal intubation (Timar *et al*). Orv. Hetil., *115:*1035, 1974 (Hungarian)

Tracheotomy tube with tightening balloon (Porwolik *et al*). Pol. Przegl. Chir., *46:*781, 1974 (Polish)

Surgery of cervical trachea (Weerda *et al*). Prax. Pneumol., (Suppl) *28:* 1007, 1974 (German)

Artificial airways in children (Aberdeen *et al*). Surg. Clin. North Am., *54:* 1155, 1974

Tracheal healing following tracheostomy (Bardin *et al*). Surg. Forum, *25:*210, 1974

Tracheal stenosis after intubation, tracheostomy and respiratory therapy (Andersen *et al*). Ugeskr. Laeger, *136:*2235, 1974 (Danish)

Moistening of the inspired air in nasally intubated and tracheostomy patients (Pedersen). Ugeskr. Laeger, *136:*2238, 1974 (Danish)

Fistula formation in temporary elective tracheostomy (Struve-Christensen *et al*). Ugeskr. Laeger, *136:*2241, 1974 (Danish)

Emergency tracheotomy via a cannula (Steinmetz). Ugeskr. Laeger, *136:*2244, 1974 (Danish)

Editorial: Complications after tracheostomy (Kristensen). Ugeskr. Laeger, *136:*2255, 1974 (Danish)

Postoperative bronchopulmonary complications in malignant neoplasms of maxillofacial localization (Dunaevskii *et al*). Vestn. Khir., *113:*69, 1974 (Russian)

Tracheostomy, inspired air humidifier in

Tracheotomy—Cont.

(Marshin *et al*). Voen. Med. Zh., *4:*80, 1974 (Russian)

Tracheotomy in intensive therapy (Kroesen *et al*). Z. Allgemeinmed., *50:*285, 1974 (German)

Some complications of tracheostomy in children (Ostrovskil). Zh. Ushn. Nos. Gorl. Bolezn., *3:*100, 1974 (Russian)

Retractor for tracheotomy (Ioffe). Zh. Ushn. Nos. Gorl. Bolezn., *3:*107, 1974 (Russian)

Tracheostomy and long-term intubation, complications to, follow-up study (Aass). Acta Anaesthesiol. Scand., *19:*127, 1975

Reconstitution of lip, tongue and glottis function (Schmid). Acta Stomatol. Belg., *72:*301, 1975 (German)

Letter: Safe alternative to tracheostomy in acute epiglottis (Coker *et al*). Am. J. Dis. Child., *129:*136, 1975

Helping patients with endotracheal and tracheostomy tubes communicate (Lawless). Am. J. Nurs., *75:*2151, 1975

Vocalization via a cuffed tracheostomy tube. A new principle (Hansen *et al*). Anaesthesia, *30:*878, 1975

Decannulation of tracheostomised children (Manzano *et al*). An. Esp. Pediatr., *8:*297, 1975 (Spanish)

Tracheal incision as a contributing factor to tracheal stenosis. An experimental study (Lulenski *et al*). Ann. Otol. Rhin. & Laryng., *84:*781, 1975

Stomal recurrence following laryngectomy (Bonneau *et al*). Arch. Otolaryng., *101:*408, 1975

Trachea—innominate artery fistula following tracheostomy. Successful repair using an innominate vein graft (Nunn *et al*). Ann. Thorac. Surg., *20:*698, 1975

Tracheostomy in children (Palva, Jokinen, Niemela), PRS, *57:*532, 1976. Arch. Otolaryng., *101:*536, 1975

Surgery to prevent aspiration (Montgomery). Arch. Otolaryng., *101:*679, 1975

Subglottic enlargement using cartilage-mucosa autograft. A preliminary experimental study (Thomas *et al*). Arch. Otolaryng., *101:*689, 1975

Tracheostomy: emergency or élective? (Johnson). Ariz. Med., *32:*411, 1975

Injuries to tracheal cartilage produced during 3 different technics for fixation of the trachea during tracheotomy (Vivar-Mejia *et al*). Bol. Med. Hosp. Infant. Mex., *32:*97, 1975 (Spanish)

Letter: swivel connections (Holdcroft *et al*). Brit. J. Anaesth., *48:*642, 1975

Picture of tracheotomy in children (Hybasek

Tracheotomy – Cont.

et al). Cesk. Otolaryngol., *24:*351, 1975 (Czechoslovakian)

Prospective study of complications after tracheostomy for assisted ventilation (Dane *et al*). Chest, *67:*398, 1975

Recurrent problems in emergency room management of maxillofacial injuries (Baker *et al*). Clin. Plast. Surg., *2:*65, 1975

Twenty-five years experience with glottis widening surgery in our clinic (Horbst *et al*). H. N. O., *23:*147, 1975 (German)

Prevention and management of tracheal and laryngeal stenosis in children (Schlosshauer). H. N. O., *23:*342, 1975 (German)

Laryngostomy instead of tracheostomy (Kneafsey *et al*). Ir. Med. J., *68:*279, 1975

Death precipitated by tracheostomy in a child (Schmidt *et al*). J.A.M.A., *231:*277, 1975

Letter: Airway – instantly. J.A.M.A., *231:*347, 1975

Tracheostomy in children, defense of (Priebe). J. A. M. A., *232:*1009, 1975

Tracheostomy or not? (Greene). J.A.M.A., *234:*1150, 1975

Letter: seven come eleven (Sabiston). J.A.M.A., *234:*1222, 1975

Reflections on the laryngo-tracheal sequellae of assisted respiration with intubation or tracheotomy. From functional disorders to lesions (Rebattu). J. Fr. Otorhinolaryngol., *24:*67, 1975 (French)

Laryngeal and tracheal stenosis: an adapted speaking aid tracheostomy tube (Cowan). J. Laryng. & Otol., *89:*531, 1975

Fatal hemorrhage from the innominate artery complicating tracheostomy (Gnanapragasam). J. Laryng. & Otol., *89:*853, 1975

Analysis of bacteriological cultures in tracheostomized patients (Guduric *et al*). Med. Pregl., *28:*385, 1975 (Serbian)

Arytenoid-epiglottic flap for chronic aspiration pneumonia, further experiences with (Vecchione, Habal, Murray), PRS, *55:*318, 1975.

Scar, tracheostomy, subcutaneous Z-plasty for (Vecchione, Pickering), PRS, *56:*579, 1975

Care and complications of tracheotomy (Manzano *et al*). Rev. Esp. Anestesiol. Reanim., *22:*490, 1975 (Spanish)

Tracheal size following tracheostomy with cuffed tracheostomy tubes: an experimental study (Leverment *et al*). Thorax, *30:*271, 1975

Problems complicating tracheotomy (Straka). Trans. Pa. Acad. Ophthalmol.

Tracheotomy – Cont.

Otolaryngol., *28:*60, 1975

Safe replacement of tracheostomy tubes (McQuarrie). Surg. Gynec. & Obst., *140:*769, 1975

Catheterization of the bronchial tree via tracheocentesis (Pomosov *et al*. Voen. Med. Zh., *9:*71, 1975 (Russian)

Difficulty in removal of tracheostomy tubes (Pavlin *et al*). Anesthesiology, *44:*69, 1976

Cricothyroidotomy: elective use in respiratory problems requiring tracheotomy (Brantigan *et al*). J. Thorac. Cardiovasc. Surg., *71:*72, 1976

TRAIL, M. L. *et al*: Anomalies of the first branchial cleft. South. Med. J., *65:*716, 1972

TRAIL, M. L. *et al*: Tumors of submandibular gland. Laryngoscope, *84:*1225, 1974

TRAIL, M. O. *et al*: Congenital choanal atresia. South. Med. J., *66:*460, 1973

TRAN-NGOC-NINH, *et al*: Cystic hygroma in children: report of 126 cases. J. Pediatr. Surg., *9:*191, 1974

Transplantation (See also *Bone Grafts, Various Categories; Cartilage Grafts; Skin Grafts; etc.*)

Human Organ Support and Replacement. Transplantation and Artificial Prostheses. Ed. by James D. Hardy, Charles C Thomas, Springfield, Ill., 1971. PRS, *49:*81, 1972

Immunobiology of Transplantation. By Rupert Billingham and Willys Silvers. Prentice-Hall, Inc., Englewood Cliffs, N. J., 1971. PRS, *50:*399, 1972

Tissue Typing Today: Proceedings of an International Symposium on the Role of Histocompatibility Typing in Clinical Organ Transplantation. Ed. by Felix T. Rapaport and Jean Dausset. Grune & Stratton, N. Y. and London, 1971. PRS, *50:*518, 1972

Transplantation Reviews. Vol. 7. By Goran Moller. *Immunological Surveillance Against Neoplasia.* Williams & Wilkins Co., Baltimore, 1971. PRS, *51:*86, 1973

Transplantation Today, Third Congress. Ed. by Hans Balner, D. W. van Bekkum, and Felix T. Rapaport. Grune & Stratton, New York, 1971. PRS, *49:*205, 1972

Tissue grafts, methods of preparation and conservation, without aseptic technique (Savelyev), PRS, *50:*542, 1972. Acta chir. plast., *13:*121, 1971

Renal allograft, successful skin graft on (Wu, Gault, McLean), PRS, *48:*97, 1971. Canad. J. Surg., *14:*80, 1971

Metacarpophalangeal joint, autogenous

TRAYCOFF, R. B. *et al*: Thermographic demonstration of tenosynovitis. A case report. Ohio State Med. J., *70:*632, 1974

TREANOR, W. J. *et al*: Sometimes deleterious influence of the brachioradialis radial extensors and finger flexors on residual hand function in spastic tetraplegics. Paraplegia, *13:*12, 1975

TREISTER, G. *et al*: Metastatic gangrene of lid in *Pseudomonas* septicemia, PRS, *57:*113, 1976. Ann. Ophth., *7:*639, 1975

TRELFORD, J. D. *et al*: Amniotic membrane as living surgical dressing in human patients. Oncology, *28:*358, 1973

TRELFORD, J. D. *et al*: Amnion autografts, permanent structure. J. Med., *6:*243, 1975

TRESLEY, I. J. *et al*: Augmentation mentoplasty, reflections. Laryngoscope, *82:*2092, 1972

TRESSERRA LLAURADO, L.: Congenital labiopalatine fissures. An. Esp. Odontoestomatol., *30:*407, 1971 (Spanish)

TRESSERRA LLAURADO, L.: Congenital labiopalatine fissures. An. Esp. Odontoestomatol., *30:*483, 1971 (Spanish)

TRET'IAK, D. N.: Malignant melanomas of the maxillary sinus. Zh. Ushn. Nos. Gorl. Bolezn., *30:*98, 1970 (Russian)

TREUHAFT, P. S. *et al*: Rapid method for evaluating the structure and function of the rheumatoid hand. Arthritis Rheum., *14:*75, 1971

TRICHILIS, E.: Urgent surgical management of zygomatic arch and orbital fractures, PRS, *52:*594, 1973. Trans. 7th Panhel. Cong. Surg., *1:*274, 1971

TRICHILIS, E.: Use of tube flaps in reconstructing defects of oral cavity, PRS, *52:*450, 1973. Acta chir. Hellenica, *45:*99, 1973

TRIEDMAN, L. J. *et al*: Principles and techniques of autogenous bone grafting to mandible. R. I. Med. J., *55:*305, 1972

TRIGOS, I.: Management of patients with complications from injections of foreign materials into the breasts (with Ortiz-Monasterio), PRS, *50:*42, 1972

TRING, F. C., AND MURGATROYD, L. B.: Surface microtopography of normal human skin, PRS, *54:*382, 1974. Arch. Dermat., *109:*223, 1974

TRISHKIN, V. A.: Lymphography for determining the radicality of regional lymph node removal in malignant neoplasms of the skin of the extremities. Vopr. Onkol., *17:*3, 1971 (Russian)

TRIVEDI, L. K. *et al*: Conjunctive-rhinostomy. J. All India. Ophthalmol. Soc., *18:*170, 1970

TRNKA, J.: 5-fluorouracil and Bucky rays in the treatment of superficial basaliomas. Cesk. Dermatol., *47:*80, 1972 (Czechoslovakian)

TRODAHL, J. N.: Acinic cell adenocarcinoma of minor salivary gland origin. Mil. Med., *137:*234, 1972

TROIANO, M. F., AND CHRIST, T.: Postmortem recovery of mandibular osseous grafts with cellulose acetate filter, PRS, *57:*541, 1976. J. Maxillo-facial Surg., *3:*200, 1975

TROJABORG, W. *et al*: Reinnervation after resection of the facial nerve. Arch. Neurol., *26:*17, 1972

TROKEL, S. L.: The orbit, PRS, *52:*451, 1973. Arch. Ophth., *89:*152, 1973

TROKEL, S. L.: The orbit. Arch. Ophth., *91:*233, 1974

TROMOVITCH, T., AND STEGEMAN, S.: Microscopically controlled excision of skin tumors, PRS, *55:*255, 1975. Arch. Dermat., *110:*231, 1974

TRONCZYNSKA, J.: Electrorhinopneumography as an objective method of assessment of velopharyngeal insufficiency in cleft-palate patients. Folia Phoniatr. (Basel), *24:*371, 1972

TROP, J. L., AND GOLDEN, J. S.: Rhinoplasty in transsexuals; psychological considerations. PRS, *55:*593, 1975

TROQUES, R.: Implantation of mammary prosthesis by axillary incision. Nouv. Presse Med., *1:*2409, 1972

TROQUES, R.: Fractures of the metacarpals and phalanges. Their treatment by screws. Nouv. Presse Med., *3:*1367, 1974 (French)

TROSHEV, K.: Frantisek Burian Academy – 1st steps in plastic surgery. Khirurgiia (Sofiia), *23:*178, 1970 (Bulgarian)

TROSHEV, K.: Frantisek Burian in Balkan Wars, PRS, *55:*647, 1975. Acta chir. plast., *16:*193, 1974

TROSHKOV, A. A. *et al*: Prevention and treatment of keloid scars after cutiplastic operations in children. Vestn. Khir., *113:*73, 1974 (Russian)

TROWBRIDGE, J. E.: Caring for patients with facial or intraoral reconstruction. Am. J. Nurs., *73:*1930, 1973

TROZAK, D. J. *et al*: Metastatic malignant melanoma in prepubertal children. Pediatrics, *55:*191, 1975

Trunk

Trunk, congenital ring-constriction of (Evans). Brit. J. Plast. Surg., *26:*340, 1973
Diaphragm, defects of, function of pedicled muscle flaps (Brandesky), PRS, *54:*620, 1974. Ztschr. Kinderchir., *14:*260, 1974

TRUNKEY, D. D.: Doctor George Goodfellow, the first civilian trauma surgeon. Surg. Gynec. & Obst., *141:*97, 1975

TRUSHKEVICH, I. N. *et al*: Technic and direct

results of cryosurgery of lip cancer. Stomatologiia (Mosk.) 55:37, 1976 (Russian)

TRUSHKEVICH. L. I. et al: Cryosurgery of lip
neoplasms. Klin. Khir., 10:54, 1974 (Russian)

TSAI, T. M.: Experimental and clinical application of microvascular surgery, PRS, 56:605,
1975. Ann. Surg., 181:169, 1975

TSCHIRKOV, F. et al: Surgery of leg ulcers due to
disordered venous and arterial hemodynamics in lower extremities. Z. Haut. Geschlechtskr., 47:911, 1972 (German)

TSCHOLL, R.: Priapism — pathogenesis and therapy. Schweiz. Med. Wochenschr., 105:517,
1975 (German)

TSCHOPP, H. M.: Acute postoperative streptococcus gangrene of face, PRS, 52:204, 1973.
Chir. Plast., 1:244, 1972

TSCHOPP, H. M.: Plastic-surgical principles in
the rehabilitation of severe mid-facial injuries. Fortschr. Kiefer. Gesichtschir., 19:137,
1975 (German)

TSCHOPP, H. M.: Principles in restoration of soft
tissue damage of face. Helv. Chir. Acta,
42:165, 1975 (German)

TSCHOPP, H. M.: Small artery anastomosis using cuff of dura mater and tissue adhesive,
PRS, 55:606, 1975

TSUGE, K.: Congenital aplasia or hypoplasia of
finger extensors, PRS, 57:398, 1976. Hand,
7:15, 1975

TSUGE, K.: Treatment of established Volkmann's contracture. J. Bone & Joint Surg.
(Am.), 57:925, 1975

TSUGE, K.: Free muscle transplantation in dogs
by microneurovascular anastomoses (with
Kubo, Ikuta). PRS, 57:495, 1976

TSUGE, K., AND WATARI, S.: Locking metacarpophalangeal joint of thumb, PRS, 56:227,
1975. Hand, 6:255, 1974

TSUGE, K. et al: Intra-tendinous tendon suture
in the hand—a new technique. Hand, 7:250,
1975

TSUGE, K., IKUTA, Y., AND SAKAUE, M.: New
technique for nerve suture, anchoring funicular suture. PRS, 56:496, 1975

TSUKADA, S.: Melanocytes and melanin in human skin autografts. PRS, 53:200, 1974

TSUKAMOTO, K.: Experimental observation on
nerve regeneration after reconstructive surgery of the facial nerve. J. Otolaryngol. Jap.,
74:1340, 1971 (Japanese)

TSUKAMOTO, S. et al: Electromyographic activities of jaw muscles before and after condylectomy. Brit. J. Oral Surg., 10:78, 1972

TSUKANOV, V. A.: Experience with surgical
treatment of tropical ulcers. Klin. Khir.,
4:77, 1974 (Russian)

TSUTSUI, H. et al: Case of gigantic ameloblastoma developing to size of infant's head. To-

kushima J. Exp. Med., 21:69, 1974

TSUTSUMI, M. et al: Results of vidian neurectomy. J. Otolaryngol. Japan, 75:1207, 1972
(Japanese)

TUBIANA, R.: Palliative treatment of paralysis
of intrinsic muscles of the thumb with tendon
transfer. Ann. Chir., 25:971, 1971 (French)

TUBIANA, R.: On the rheumatoid hand. Introduction. Rev. Chir. Orthop., 58:399, 1971
(French)

TUBIANA, R.: Therapeutic indications in the
rheumatoid hand. Rev. Chir. Orthop.,
58:464, 1972 (French)

TUBIANA, R.: Positions for immobilization of
the hand. Ann. Chir., 27:459, 1973 (French)

TUBIANA, R.: Palmar island skin flaps, PRS,
53:249, 1974. Ann. Chir., 27:503, 1973

TUBIANA, R.: Results and complications of
flexor tendon grafting. Orthop. Clin. North
Am., 4:877, 1973

TUBIANA, R.: Palliative treatment of paralytic
deformities of the thumb. Orthop. Clin.
North Am., 4:1141, 1973

TUBIANA, R.: Use of tourniquet on limbs. Dangers and their prevention. Rev. Chir. Orthop., 59:239, 1973 (French)

TUBIANA, R.: Postoperative care following
flexor tendon grafts, PRS, 56:230, 1975.
Hand, 6:152, 1974

TUBIANA, R.: Hand reconstruction. Acta Orthop. Scand., 46:446, 1975

TUBIANA, R.: Planning of surgical treatment.
Hand, 7:223, 1975

TUBIANA, R., HUESTON, J. T. et al: Maladie de
Dupuytren. Second Edition. L'Expansion,
Paris, 1972. PRS, 51:210, 1973

TUBIANA, R. et al: 5th metacarpal phalanx formation. Chirurgie, 98:68, 1972 (French)

TUBIANA, R. et al: Lyell's syndrome treated in
specialized burn unit, PRS, 52:456, 1973. Chirurgie, 99:40, 1973

TUBIANA, R. et al: Phalangization of the first
and fifth metacarpals. Indications, operative
technique, and results. J. Bone & Joint Surg.
(Am.), 56:447, 1974

TUCKER, A. L.: Plea for primary closure of
naso-alveolar openings during cleft palate repairs, (Letter to the Editor), PRS, 55:614,
1975

TUCKER, A. L., AND HUBBARD, J. G.: Retropharyngeal infection with disc space involvement and osteomyelitis, following pharyngeal flap operation. PRS, 53:477, 1974

TUCKER, H. M. et al: Surgical management of
premaxillary malignancy. Report of three
cases. Arch. Otolaryng., 95:42, 1972

TUCKER, H. M. et al: Massive surgery for palliation in malignancy of head and neck. Laryngoscope, 83:1635, 1973

TUCKER, H. M. *et al*: Prevention of complications of composite resection after high dose preoperative radiotherapy. Laryngoscope, *84:*933, 1974

TUCKER, J. A. *et al*: Tracheotomy in pediatrics. Ann. Otol. Rhin. & Laryng., *81:*818, 1972

TUCKER, K. *et al*: Tower of London bomb explosion. Brit. Med. J., *3:*287, 1975

TUDORIU, T.: Surgical treatment of impotence. Helv. Chir. Acta, *41:*451, 1974 (German)

TUERK D.: Surgical treatment of Moebius syndrome by platysma and *temporalis* muscle transfers (with Edgerton, Fisher), PRS, *55:*305, 1975

TUERK, D., AND EDGERTON, M. T.: Surgical treatment of congenital webbing (pterygium) of popliteal area. PRS, *56:*339, 1975

TUERK M.: New material for dermabrasion. PRS, *49:*661, 1972

TUERK M.: Skin grafting in systemic lupus erythematosus patients who are on steroids. PRS, *50:*382, 1972

TUERK M.: Possible dangers of using Fabricut as a dermabrasive (Letter to the Editor), PRS, *51:*441, 1973

TUERK, M., AND WEIR, W. H., JR.: Successful replantation of a traumatically amputated glans penis. PRS, *48:*499, 1971

TUGILIMANA, M. *et al*: Treatment of neoplasms of the mobile part of the tongue. Acta Stomatol. Belg., *72:*291, 1975 (French)

TUKALLO, K. *et al*: Experimental studies on tensile strength of healing wound of fascia and muscle. Pol. Med. J., *11:*939, 1972

TULLEY, W. J.: Management of cleft lip and palate. Introduction. Ann. R. Coll. Surg. Engl., *48:*30, 1971

TULLI, A., RUSCIANI, L., AND FABRI, G.: Surgical reconstruction in case of amputation of fingertip, PRS, *56:*595, 1975. Chron. Dermat., *5:*2, 1974

TUNBRIDGE, R.: Mobility for disabled, PRS, *55:*725, 1975. Proc. Roy. Soc. Med., *67:*399, 1974

TUNCER, M. *et al*: Bilateral choanal atresia in newborn. Two case reports. Turk. J. Pediatr., *13:*147, 1971

TUNNELL, W. P.: Role of pediatric surgery in general surgical education. J. Pediatr. Surg., *9:*743, 1974

TUNSTALL, M. N.: Saddle depression of the nose. Nurs. Times, *70:*1774, 1974

TURBEY, W. J., BUNTAIN, W. L., AND DUDGEON, D. L.: Surgical management of pediatric breast masses, PRS, *57:*674, 1976. Pediatrics, *56:*736, 1975

TURBOW, M. E.: Abdominal compression following circumferential burn: cardiovascular responses, PRS, *53:*608, 1974. J. Trauma, *13:*535, 1973

TURITTO, P. *et al*: Treatment of subostial stenosis secondary to tracheostomy. Minerva Anestesiol., *39:*105, 1973 (Italian)

TURNBULL, A., SHAH, J., AND FORTNER, J.: Recurrent melanoma of extremity treated by major amputation, PRS, *52:*599, 1973. Arch. Surg., *106:*496, 1973

TURNBULL, A. *et al*: Cystosarcoma phylloides. J. R. Coll. Surg. Edinb., *19:*104, 1974

TURNER, F. W. *et al*: Clinical trial of new absorbable synthetic suture material: polyglycolic acid, PRS, *51:*486, 1973. Canad. J. Surg., *15:*389, 1972

TURNER, H. *et al*: Carcinoma of tongue in child. Case report and review of literature. Oral Surg., *37:*663, 1974

TURNER-WARWICK, R.: Use of pedicle grafts in repair of urinary tract fistulae, PRS, *52:*324, 1973. Brit. J. Urol., *44:*644, 1972

TURUT, P.: Arion's thread in ptosis surgery. Bull. Soc. Ophtalmol. Fr., *75:*347, 1975 (French)

TURVEY, T. A. *et al*: Soft tissue procedures adjunctive to orthognathic surgery for improvement of facial balance. J. Oral Surg., *32:*572, 1974

TUSON, K. W.: Epignathus: basicranial teratoma. A case report and review of the literature. Brit. J. Surg., *58:*935, 1971

TWEED, W. A., MINUCK, M., AND MYMIN, D.: Circulatory responses to Ketamine anesthesia, PRS, *51:*605, 1973. Anesthesiology, *37:*613, 1972

TYCHINKINA, A. K. *et al*: Blood loss and hemostasis in plastic surgery of the skin. Vestn. Khir., *107:*94, 1971 (Russian)

TYLDESLEY, W. R.: Tobacco chewing in English coal miners. A preliminary report. Brit. J. Oral Surg., *9:*21, 1971

TYLDESLEY, W. R. *et al*: Haemangioma of the maxilla: a case report. Brit. J. Oral Surg., *13:*56, 1975

TYRER, E.: Another knife injury. Radiography, *38:*307, 1972

TYRONE, N.O., WYKER, A. W., AND GILLENWATER, J. Y.: Anterior urethral transposition, modification of technique, PRS, *48:*608, 1971. J. Urol., *105:*729, 1971

TYSZIEWICZ, S. *et al*: Multifocal form of fibromatosis palmaris. Chir. Narzadow. Ruchu Ortop. Pol., *40:*89, 1975 (Polish)

TYSZKA, E.: Motivational mechanisms behind the wish for plastic surgery in persons with minor facial disfigurements. Psychiatr. Pol., *7:*621, 1973 (Polish)

TYTAR, G. M. *et al*: Means of indirect evaluation of palatopharyngeal closure. Zh. Ushn. Nos. Gorl. Bolezn., *31:*85, 1971 (Russian)

U

UBIGLIA, G., SANTONI RUGIU, P., AND MASSEI, A.: Our experience in hypospadias treatment, PRS, 56:358, 1975. Riv. ital. chir. plast., 5:527, 1973

UCHIDA, A. et al: Innovation of attachment for urinary tract for easier urination for patients following penile amputation. Jap. J. Nurs., 37:1156, 1973 (Japanese)

UCHIDA, J.: New technic for repairing the nostril deformity in cleft lip. Jap. J. Plast. Reconstr. Surg., 14:405, 1971 (Japanese)

UCHIDA, Y.: Management of wounds, particularly granulation wounds. Jap. J. Plast. Reconstr. Surg., 14:174, 1971 (Japanese)

UCHIDA, Y. et al: Total reconstruction of the external nose, with special reference to rhinoplasty for the syphilitic saddle nose. Jap. J. Plast. Reconstr. Surg., 14:495, 1971 (Japanese)

UCHIKOSHI, S. et al: Leriche's operation for the treatment of parotid gland fistula. Otolaryngology (Tokyo), 43:919, 1971 (Japanese)

UCHINISHI, K. et al: Neurovascular island flap in functional reconstruction of the thumb. Orthop. Surg. (Tokyo), 22:955, 1971 (Japanese)

UDOVICKI, J.: Ectopic localization of mixed tumors of the salivary glands. J. Med. Pregl., 27:313, 1974 (Serbian)

UDOVICKI, J. et al: Mixed tumors of submandibular glands. Med. Pregl., 25:335, 1972 (Serbian)

UEBA, Y.: Lengthening short fourth toe with silicone block prosthesis, PRS, 55:380, 1975. Jap. J. Plast. Reconstr. Surg., 17:296, 1974

UHLER, I. V. et al: Actinomycosis of the tongue. Oral Surg., 34:199, 1972

UHLSCHMID, G.: Experimental plastic elongation of trachea, PRS, 48:510, 1971. Helvet. chir. acta, 1:207, 1971

UHLSCHMID, G.: Experimental elongation of thoracic trachea, PRS, 51:603, 1973. Langenbecks Arch. Chir., 331:255, 1972

UKLEJA, Z. et al: Lingual neurofibroma. Otolaryngol. Pol., 27:121, 1973 (Polish)

ULASOVETS, A. F.: Detachment of mucosa and perichondrium of nasal septum with subsequent ligation of terminal branch of anterior ethmoids artery for stopping nasal hemorrhaging. Zh. Ushn. Nos. Gorl. Bolezn., 104, Mar–Apr., 1974

Ulcers (See also *Curling's Ulcer; Leg Ulcer; Pressure Sores*)

Treatment of phagedenic ulcers (Grigorian *et al*). Vestn. Khir., 106:42, 1971 (Russian)
Application of a combined flat pedicled graft

Ulcers – Cont.

for plastic surgery of trophic ulcers of the leg and foot (Bondar'). Vestn. Khir., 107:116, 1971 (Russian)

Physical therapy of chronic ulcers and torpidly granulating wounds (Kaliko *et al*). Vopr. Kurortol. Fizioter. Lech. Fiz. Kult., 36:458, 1971 (Russian)

Buruli disease and patients' activities (Barker *et al*). East Afr. Med. J., 49:260, 1972

Wound healing and plastic surgery in ulcer (Oura). Surg. Ther. (Osaka), 26:498, 1972 (Japanese)

Ulcers, tropical, experience with surgical treatment of (Tsukanov). Klin. Khir., 4:77, 1974 (Russian)

Tropical ulcers (Ariyan, Krizek), PRS, 55:324, 1975

ULIN, A. W.: Ideal suture material, PRS, 51:237, 1973. Surg. Gynec. & Obst., 133:475, 1971

ULITSKYI, G. I., AND MALYGIN, G. D.: Roentgenological dynamics of reparative regeneration lengthening of metacarpals by distraction method, PRS, 53:487, 1974. Acta chir. plast., 15:82, 1973

ULMER, E.: Bilateral free-end denture with consideration for simplified supplementation of anterior dentition (patient requested that natural mandibular anterior teeth be retained). Quintessence Int., 5:35, 1974

UNGERECHT, K.: Diagnosis and treatment of diseases of parotid. Munch. Med. Wochenschr., 116:439, 1974 (German)

UNSWORTH, I. P.: Gas gangrene in New South Wales. M. J. Australia, 1:1077, 1973

URBANIAK, J. R.: Prosthetic arthroplasty of hand, PRS, 56:679, 1975. Clin. Orthop., 104:9, 1974

URBANIAK, J. R., AND GOLDNER, J. L.: Laceration of *flexor pollicis longus* tendon: delayed repair by advancement, free graft, or direct suture, PRS, 53:684, 1974. J. Bone & Joint Surg., 55:1123, 1973

URBANIAK, J. R. et al: Vascularization and the gliding mechanism of free flexor-tendon grafts inserted by the silicone-rod method. J. Bone & Joint Surg. (Am.), 56:473, 1974

Urethra (See also *Epispadias; Hypospadias; Penis*)

Urethra, female, malignant melanoma, report of case with 5-year survival and review of literature (Block, Hotchkiss), PRS, 48:518, 1971. J. Urol., 105:251, 1971

Triamcinolone, transurethral injection in treatment of urethral stricture (Hebert), PRS, 51:603, 1973. J. Urol., 105:403, 1971

Urethra – Cont.

Urinary diversion by anterior transposition of urethra (Dorsey), PRS, *48:*607, 1971. J. Urol., *105:*725, 1971

Urethral transposition, anterior: modification of technique (Tyrone, Wyker, Gillenwater), PRS, *48:*608, 1971. J. Urol., *105:*729, 1971

Urethra, penile, repair of recurrent fistula of (Malament), PRS, *50:*200, 1972. J. Urol., *106:*704, 1971

Urinary tract fistulae, use of pedicle grafts in repair (Turner-Warwick), PRS, *52:*324, 1973. Brit. J. Urol., *44:*644, 1972

Urethroplasty (Williams *et al*). Brit. J. Urol., *44:*719, 1972

Urethral construction, functional, in female epispadias (Harrold, Champion, Ford), PRS, *50:*539, 1972. J. Urol., *107:*144, 1972

Urethroplasty, one-stage, 4-year follow-up (Orandi), PRS, *51:*604, 1973. J. Urol., *107:*977, 1972

Fenestration, interurethral, for case of double urethra with hypospadias (Durrani, Shah, Kakalia), PRS, *52:*98, 1973. J. Urol., *108:*586, 1972

Incontinence, male, crucification operation for (Wallace). Proc. Roy. Soc. Med., *65:*303, 1972

Congenital shortness of urethra (Almendral Lucas, Martin Laborda), PRS, *53:*244, 1974. Rev. espan. cir. plast., *5:*201, 1972

Urethrostomy, perineal, use of Foley catheter in (Elsahy), PRS, *53:*488, 1974. Acta chir. plast., *15:*131, 1973

Urethral strictures, anterior, experience with free graft urethroplasty (Brannon, Ochsner, Fuselier), PRS, *52:*680, 1973. J. Urol., *109:*265, 1973

Incontinence, congenital urethral perineal fistulas (Gehring, Vitenson, Woodhead), PRS, *53:*245, 1974. J. Urol., *109:*419, 1973

Urethral stricture, urethroplasty for (Pierce), PRS, *52:*596, 1973. J. Urol., *109:*422, 1973

Urethroplasty, new spiral-flap (Gellman, Bellingham, Malament), PRS, *54:*110, 1974. J. Urol., *110:*546, 1973

Infants and children, scrotal flap urethroplasty for strictures of the deep urethra (McGuire, Weiss), PRS, *54:*110, 1974. J. Urol., *110:*599, 1973

Urethra, meatal and parameatal tumors in young men (Huvos, Grabstald), PRS, *54:*110, 1974. J. Urol., *110:*688, 1973

Urethritis after urethral extrusion of penile prosthesis (Jepson, Silber), PRS, *53:*244, 1974. J. Urol., *109:*838, 1973

Urethroplasty, pedicle patch, for cure of ure-

Urethra – Cont.

thral stricture (Anastasi, Ollson), PRS, *51:*1, 1973

Urethral healing; studies of, in dogs (Everingham, Horton, Devine), PRS, *51:*312, 1973

Urethrostomy, perineal: treatment of hypospadias by Byars technique (Nosti, Davis), PRS, *52:*128, 1973

Cystostomy, permanent cutaneous, by interposition of an abdominal skin-lined tubed flap (Ship) (Follow-Up Clinic), PRS, *52:*298, 1973

Continence: technique for epispadias repair (Khanna), PRS, *52:*365, 1973

Incontinence, surgery of (Garriz *et al*), PRS, *53:*107, 1974. Prensa méd. argent., *60:*492, 1973

Urethra reconstruction (Zenteno Alanis), PRS, *54:*621, 1974. Rev. espan. cir. plast., *6:*255, 1973

Urethral stricture, treatment of, by free full-thickness skin graft (Devine) urethroplasty (Abrahams *et al*). Urology, *1:*93, 1973

Urethra, congenital polyps, in children (Mildenberger, Schweizer), PRS, *53:*368, 1974. Ztschr. Kinderchir., *13:*240, 1973

Urethroplasties, scrotal inlay, personal experience with 37 Turner-Warwick (Ashken). Brit. J. Urol., *46:*313, 1974

Urethra, melanoma of (Bracken, Diokno), PRS, *54:*621, 1974. J. Urol., *111:*198, 1974

Bladder function: intermittent catheterization (Perkash), PRS, *54:*504, 1974. J. Urol., *111:*356, 1974

Urethral catheters, indwelling (Degroot, Kunin), PRS, *56:*596, 1975. Am. J. Nursing, *75:*448, 1975

Urethroplasty, one-stage island patch, technique and results (Blandy *et al*). Brit. J. Urol., *47:*83, 1975

Urethra, complete duplication, with probable diphallus (Redman, Bissada), PRS, *56:*230, 1975. J. Pediat. Surg., *10:*135, 1975

Urethral fistula, congenital, with chordee (Goldstein), PRS, *57:*761, 1976. J. Urol., *113:*138, 1975

Urethrostomy, perineal, modification of Foley catheter for use in (Tolhurst), PRS, *55:*503, 1975

Current Operative Urology. Ed. by E. D. Whitehead. Harper & Row, Hagerstown, Md., 1975. PRS, *57:*232, 1976

Congenital urethral fistula (Olbourne), PRS, *57:*237, 1976

URMOSI, J. *et al*: Malignant melanoma in retroperitoneum 15 years following removal of primary eye tumor. Orv. Hetil., *115:*1353, 1974 (Hungarian)

URTILA, E.: An original method of plastic surgery after treatment of cancer of the lower lip by resection. Rev. Stomatol. Chir. Maxillofac., *76:*579, 1975 (French)

URVOY, M. *et al:* Role of sarcoidosis in etiology of unilateral exophathalmos. Bull. Soc. Ophtalmol. Fr., *73:*581, 1973 (French)

USTOL'TSEVA, E. V.: Giant cell tumors of the tendon sheaths of the hand. Ortop. Travmatol. Protez., *32:*18, 1971 (Russian)

UTHMAN Z. Z. *et al:* Myxoma of mandible. Case report. Brit. J. Oral Surg., *9:*151, 1971

UZEL, S., AND YORMUK, E.: Case of *mycosis fungoides* with rare localization – preliminary report, PRS, *57:*114, 1976. Acta Oncol. Turcica, *8:*26, 1975

UZHUMETSKENE I. I.: Correction of anomalies of dento-maxillofacial system as method of treatment of arthropathies in adults. Stomatologia (Mosk.), *52:*51, 1973 (Russian)

V

VAAGE, J., DOROSHOW, J. H., AND DUBOIS, T. T.: Radiation induced changes in established tumor immunity, PRS, *54:*244, 1974. Cancer Res., *34:*129, 1974

Vagina (See also *Genitalia; Transsexual Surgery*)

Vagina, artifical, reinnervation of mucous membrane (Giliazumdinova *et al*). Akush. Ginekol. (Mosk.), *47:*49, 1971 (Russian)

Personal operative technic for the treatment of congenital absence of the vagina with functional uterus (Rochet *et al*). Bull. Fed. Soc. Gynecol. Obstet. Lang. Fr., *23:*467, 1971 (French)

Vagina construction by intestinal mucosa-muscularis graft (Wilflingseder), PRS, *51:*704, 1973. Chir. Plast., *1:*15, 1971

Surgical treatment of congenital absence of the vagina with functional uterus (2 cases operated on successfully by a personal technic (Rochet *et al*). Lyon Chir., *67:*265, 1971 (French)

Anatomical study of the possibilities of using the sigmoid colon in the surgical treatment of congenital absence of the vagina (Vuillard *et al*). Lyon Chir., *67:*311, 1971 (French)

Vaginal agenesis, clinical and therapeutic consideration on (Micali *et al*). Minerva Chir., *26:*1480, 1971 (Italian)

Aplasia vaginae et uteri associated with dystopic solitary kidney – colpoplasty, using sigmoid colon (Zeffer *et al*). Orv. Hetil.,

Vagina – Cont.

*112:*1710, 1971 (Hungarian)

Morphologic changes and cytologically determined hormonal effects in the artificial vagina constructed from large intestine (Gyory *et al*). Zentralbl. Gynekol., *93:*1121, 1971 (German)

Vagina reconstruction by thick skin graft (Fara, Vesely, Kafka), PRS, *52:*324, 1973. Acta chir. plast., *14:*127, 1972

Free dermatoplasty in correction of vagina defects (Kozlov). Akush. Ginekol. (Mosk.), *48:*57, 1972 (Russian)

Intestinal mucosa-muscularis grafts in vagina, subsequent behavior (Wilflingseder, Dapunt, Fodisch), PRS, *52:*207, 1973. Chir. Plast., *1:*281, 1972

Gynecology, reconstructive and plastic surgery in (Ober *et al*). Dtsch. Med. J., *23:*565, 1972 (German)

Reconstruction of the vagina with a graft composed of intestinal mucosa (Wilflingseder). Nouv. Presse Med., *1:*1794, 1972 (French)

Vagina reconstruction after extensive perineal resection. A case report (Lucas *et al*). Obstet. Gynecol., *39:*73, 1972

Creation of a neovagina. A simplified technic (Capraro *et al*). Obstet. Gynecol., *39:*545, 1972

Squamous cell carcinoma developing in an artificial vagina (Duckler). Obstet. Gynecol., *40:*35, 1972

Vagina, use of peritoneum in construction (Rothman). Obstet. Gynecol., *40:*835, 1972

Rectovaginal fistulae in girls, reconstructive operative interventions in (Sitkovskii *et al*). Pediatr. Akush. Ginekol., *4:*58, 1972 (Ukrainian)

Skin grafts for congenital absence of vagina; long-term follow-up in 21 patients (Ortiz-Monasterio *et al*), PRS, *49:*165, 1972

Vaginal reconstruction following pelvic exenteration: surgical and psychological considerations (Morley *et al*). Am. J. Obstet. Gynecol., *116:*996, 1973

Vagina, congenital absence of, with uterine aplasia, treatment of, using peritoneal colpoplasty (Muller). Chirurgie, *99:*830, 1973 (French)

Vaginal aplasia, treatment using a cleavage operation with two surgical teams, two cases (Rochet *et al*). Chirurgie, *99:*838, 1973 (French)

Vaginal agenesis, simple operation for correction (Ariyamitr *et al*). J. Med. Assoc. Thai., *56:*680, 1973

Venereum, lymphogranuloma, radical perineal resection for far-advanced (Hirsch-

Vagina – Cont.

berg, Horton), PRS, *51:*217, 1973

Vagina, late development of squamous cell carcinoma in split-skin graft lining a (Steffanoff), PRS, *51:*454, 1973

Pelvic exenteration, primary vaginal reconstruction after (Song, Cramer, Bromberg), PRS, *51:*509, 1973

Vagina, squamous carcinoma in a split-skin graft lining (Crow) (Letter to the Editor), PRS, *52:*293, 1973

Vagina formation from peritoneum of Douglas' pouch (Davydov, Zhvitiashvli), PRS, *54:*622, 1974. Acta chir. plast., *16:*35, 1974

Vaginal function, re-establishment of, through the creation of neo-vagina. Description of simple and reasonable method (Centaro *et al*). Ann. Ostet. Ginecol. Med. Perinat., *94:*79, 1974 (Italian)

Rare combination of duplication of genitourinary tract, hindgut, vertebral column and other associated anomalies (Dutta *et al*). Brit. J. Urol., *46:*577, 1974

Letter: Congenital absence of vagina (Beazley). Brit. Med. J., *3:*344, 1974

Psychosomatic development of women with artificial vagina (Doka *et al*). Cesk. Gynekol., *39:*187, 1974 (Slovakian)

Surgical construction of female genitalia (Jones). Clin. Plast. Surg., *1:*255, 1974

Surgical treatment of male transsexuals (Edgerton). Clin. Plast. Surg., *1:*285, 1974

Vagina aplasia (Kirchhoff). Fortschr. Med., *92:*495, 1974 (German)

Vaginal construction using cecal and sigmoid bowel segments in transsexual patients (Markland, Hastings), PRS, *54:*622, 1974. J. Urol., *111:*217, 1974

Surgical management of female congenital adrenal hyperplasia (adrenogenital syndrome) (Fay *et al*). J. Urol., *112:*813, 1974

Construction of the vagina with transposition of the sigmoid colon (Zangl). Langenbacks Arch. Chir., *339:*413, 1974 (German)

Vagina, artificial, squamous carcinoma arising in (Dellon) (Letter to the Editor), PRS, *53:*584, 1974

Vagina, artificial, construction of (Castanares)(Follow-Up Clinic), PRS, *54:*605, 1974

Unusual case of congenital abnormality of the urogenital apparatus associated with exstrophy of the bladder in a female patient (Lodovici *et al*). Rev. Asoc. Med. Bras., *20:*374, 1974 (Portuguese)

Vaginoplasty in intersexual status (Lodovici). Rev. Asoc. Med. Bras., *20:*405, 1974 (Portuguese)

Adenocarcinoma of vagina – reconstruction after radical surgery (Bivens, Zimmer-

Vagina – Cont.

man), PRS, *55:*511, 1975. Rocky Mountain M. J., *71:*512, 1974

Vaginoplasty at the Chelsea hospital for women: a comparison of two techniques (Feroze *et al*). Brit. J. Obstet. Gynaecol., *82:*536, 1975

Agenesis of the vagina: report of case (Raskin). J. Am. Osteopath. Assoc., *75:*206, 1975

Vaginal aplasia, surgical techniques and results in 57 cases (Rochet, Gagnaire), PRS, *56:*466, 1975. J. Gynec. Obst. Biol. Reprod., *3:*223, 1975

Construction of the vagina by means of split-skin or mucosal grafts (Wilflingseder). Langenbecks Arch. Chir., *339:*403, 1975 (German)

Gynecological remarks on the problem of the artificial vagina (Staemmler). Langenbecks Arch. Chir., *339:*417, 1975 (German)

Rectovaginal reconstruction in female (Pickrell, Peters, Neale), PRS, *55:*529, 1975

Fistulas, rectovaginal and urethrovaginal, operative correction of recurrent (Holschneider, Hecker), PRS, *57:*761, 1976. Ztschr. Kinderchir., *17:*227, 1975

Vaginal agenesis (Capraro *et al*). Am. J. Obstet. Gynecol., *124:*98, 1976

VAGNER, R. I. *et al*: Ilio-inguinal lymphadenectomy in the treatment of regional metastases of cutaneous melanoblastomas of the lower extremities. Vestn. Khir., *107:*55, 1971 (Russian)

VAGNER, R. I. *et al*: Indications for regional lymphadenectomy in melanoblastoma of the skin of the extremities. Vopr. Onkol., *20:*33, 1974 (Russian)

VAHLENSIECK, W.: Hypospadias repair with histoacrylic tissue adhesive and without indwelling catheter drainage. Urol. Res., *1:*2, 1973

VAILLANT, J. M. *et al*: Symmetrical adenolipomatosis. Two cases. Rev. Stomatol. Chir. Maxillofac., *74:*125, 1973 (French)

VAILLANT, J. M. *et al*: Current attitudes towards fractures of the dentate portion of the mandible. 350 cases. Rev. Stomatol. Chir. Maxillofac. *74:*216, 1973 (Czech)

VAILLANT, J. M. *et al*: Case of massive maxillary fibromyxoma. Rev. Stomatol. Chir. Maxillofac., *74:*473, 1973 (French)

VAILLANT, J. M. *et al*: Application of several principles of surgery of congenital abnormalities to buccosinusonasal communications. Rev. Stomatol. Chir. Maxillofac., *75:*203, 1974 (French)

VAILLANT J. M. *et al*: A parotid tumor ulcerating the skin. Rev. Stomatol. Chir. Maxillofac., *75:*873, 1974 (French)

VAILLANT, J. M. *et al*: Value of grafts and microplates in mandibular graft resections. Rev. Stomatol. Chir. Maxillofac., *75:*1013, 1974 (French)

VAINBERG, Z. S. *et al*: Remote results of alloplasty of the penis in impotence. Urol. Nefrol. (Mosk.), *36:*44, 1971 (Russian)

VAINIO, K.: Surgery of the rheumatoid hand. Mod. Trends Orthop., *5:*219, 1972

VAINIO, K.: Synovectomy of the hand. Rev. Rhum. Mal. Osteoartic., *40:*205, 1973 (French)

VAINSHTEIN, E. A.: Surgical treatment of ankylosis of the temporomandibular joint. Stomatologiia (Mosk.), *55:*42, 1976 (Russian)

VALDES, J. L.: Internal wire splint for adduction contracture of the thumb (with Araico, Ortiz), PRS, *48:*339, 1971

VALDINA, E. A. *et al*: Cancer from remnants of thyrolingual duct. Vopr. Onkol., *21:*16, 1975 (Russian)

VALENTIN, P.: Mechanism of finger deformities in the rheumatoid hand. Rev. Chir. Orthop., *58:*445, 1972 (French)

VALLIS, C. P.: Intralesional injection of keloids and hypertrophic scars with the Dermo-Jet (Follow-Up Clinic), PRS, *52:*434, 1973

VALLIS, C. P.: Hair transplantation to upper lip to create moustache, PRS, *54:*606, 1974

VALLS, C. F.: Oral and maxillo facial surgery coming of age in Puerto Rico. Rev. Odontol. P. R., *10:*31, 1972

VALSRUB, S.: Psychoneurosis and obesity—the hen and egg dilemma (Editorial). J. A. M. A., *230:*591, 1974

VANCE, J. P. *et al*: Incidence and aetiology of post-operative nausea and vomiting in plastic surgical unit. Brit. J. Plast. Surg., *26:*336, 1973

VAN CLOOSTER, R. *et al*: Reconstruction of eye socket for prosthesis. Acta Stomatol. Belg., *69:*331, 1972 (Dutch)

VANDAELE, R.: Werner's syndrome. Familial ulcerous scleroderma with cataracts and diabetes. Arch. Belg. Dermatol., *29:*251, 1973 (French)

VAN DE LANDE, J. L. *et al*: Hypoplasia of the breast, a psychosocial disease. Ned. tijdschr. geneeskd., *116:*428, 1972 (Dutch)

VAN DEMARK, D. R.: Some results of speech therapy for children with cleft palate, PRS, *55:*251, 1975. Cleft Palate J., *11:*41, 1974

VAN DEMARK, D. R.: Assessment of articulation for children with cleft palate, PRS, *55:*383, 1975. Cleft Palate J., *11:*200, 1974

VAN DEMARK, D. R.: Assessment of velopharyngeal competency for children with cleft

palates, PRS, *55:*514, 1975. Cleft Palate J., *11:*310, 1974

VAN DEMARK, D. R.: Comparison of articulation abilities in velopharyngeal competency between Danish and Iowa children with cleft palates, PRS, *56:*109, 1975. Cleft Palate J., *11:*463, 1974

VAN DEMARK, R. F.: The all-ulnar hand. S. D. J. Med., *26:*21, 1973

VAN DEN BROEK, P. *et al*: Bakamjian's method for reconstruction of the hypopharynx. Ned. tijdschr. geneeskd., *115:*1675, 1971 (Dutch)

VAN DEN BROEK, P. *et al*: Medially based chest-flap for treatment of cancer of the hypopharynx. Pract. Otorhinolaryngol. (Basel), *33:*330, 1971

VANDENBROUCK, C.: Mandibular osteoradionecrosis. J. Radiol. Electrol. Med. Nucl., *53:*477, 1972 (French)

VANDENBROUCK, C. *et al*: Epitheliomas of glosso-epiglottal sulcus. Apropos of 122 cases treated at the Gustave-Roussy Institute between 1960 and 1967. Ann. Otolaryngol. Chir. Cervicofac., *89:*517, 1972 (French)

VANDENBUSSCHE, F. *et al*: Partial eyelid autoplasty with one-stage mucosal or chondromucosal graft. Ann. Chir. Plast., *16:*322, 1971 (French)

VANDENBUSSCHE, F. *et al*: Dubreuilh's melanosis: therapeutic paradox. Ann. chir. plast., *17:*289, 1972 (French)

VANDENBUSSCHE, F. *et al*: Keratoacanthomas: diagnostic pitfall in skin tumor pathology. Rational therapeutic attitude. Ann. chir. plast., *17:*289, 1972 (French)

VANDENBUSSCHE, F. *et al*: Remote results of epithelioma surgery and critical study of carcinologic results, apropos of 330 cases. Ann. chir. plast., *18:*44, 1973 (French)

VANDENBUSSCHE, F. *et al*: Malignant melanomas of Lille, 1967–1972: comparison between "histoprognosis" and actual outcome, PRS, *57:*680, 1976. Acta chir. belg., *74:*406, 1975

VANDERLINDEN, E.: Ten free flap transfers: use of intra-arterial dye injection to outline a flap exactly (with Boeckx, de Coninck), PRS, *57:*716, 1976

VAN DER MEULEN, J. C.: Recent advances in flexor tendon repair, PRS, *49:*358, 1972. Arch. chir. neerl., *23:*129, 1971

VAN DER MEULEN, J. C.: Canthopexy, new approach, PRS, *50:*474, 1972

VAN DER MEULEN, J. C.: Pedicled tendon transfer with a silicone rod (Letter to the Editor), PRS, *51:*328, 1973

VAN DER MEULEN, J. C.: Hypertelorism. Ned. tijdschr. geneeskd., *118:*451, 1974 (Dutch)

VAN DER MEULEN, J. C., RAMSELAAR, J. M., AND BLOEM, J. J. A. M.: Primary treatment of naso-orbital fractures, PRS, *55:*107, 1975. Nederl. tijdschr. geneesk., *118:*841, 1974

VAN DER MEULEN, J. C. *et al*: Treatment of exophthalmia and retrognathia. Ned. tijdschr. geneeskd., *119:*1757, 1975 (Dutch)

VAN DER PLOEZ, E., AND KOOPS, H. S.: Modified technique of groin dissection, PRS, *51:*479, 1973. Arch. chir. neerl., *24:*31, 1972

VAN DER WAAL, I. *et al*: Case of gigantiform cementoma. Int. J. Oral Surg., *3:*440, 1974

VAN DE WATER, J.: Safeguards in the repair of pharyngoesophageal diverticulum. Surg. Gynec. & Obst., *133:*851, 1971

VAN DE WATER, J. M. *et al*: Prevention of post-operative pulmonary complications, PRS, *51:*355, 1973. Surg. Gynec. & Obst., *135:*229, 1972

VAN DONGEN, J. A., AND LICHTVELD, P.: Breast reconstruction after mastectomy: indications, PRS, *57:*397, 1976. Nederl. tijdschr. geneesk., *119:*997, 1975

VAN DOORN, M. E.: Enucleation and primary closure of jaw cysts. Int. J. Oral Surg., *1:*17, 1972

VAN DROOGENBROECK, J. B.: Eyebrow transplantation. Int. J. Lepr., *39:*629, 1971

VAN GELDER, L.: Open nasal speech following adenoidectomy and tonsillectomy. J. Commun. Disord., *7:*263, 1974

VANGELISTA, D. *et al*: Immediate management of open hand injuries. Possible technical errors. Fracastoro, *62:*177, 1969 (Italian)

VANGGAARD, L.: Frostbite (with Holm), PRS, *54:*544, 1974

VAN MIEROP, L. H.: Poisonous snakebite: a review. 2. Symptomatology and treatment. J. Fla. Med. Assoc., *63:*201, 1976

VAN OOST, A.: Surgical treatment of case of axillary hyperhidrosis. Arch. Belg. Dermatol. Syphiligr., *28:*421, 1972 (French)

VAN PUT, E.: Medical correction of maxillary and mandibular prognathism. Rev. Belge. Med. Dent., *29:*465, 1974 (Dutch)

VAN RECK, J.: Adams' cranial suspension method. Acta Stomatol. Belg., *71:*125, 1974 (French)

VANTTINEN, E. *et al*: Femoropopliteal and femorotibial arterial reconstructive surgery. Special reference to the autogenous venous bypass procedure using unreversed vein after eversion valvectomy. Acta Chir. Scand., *141:*341, 1975

VAN WETTER, P.: Fractures and dislocations of the hand. General conclusions. Acta Orthop. Belg., *39:*1129, 1973 (French)

VANWIJCK, R. *et al*: Preliminary results of immunosurgical treatment of primary melanoma, PRS, *57:*403, 1976. Acta chir. belg., *74:*430, 1975

VANWINKLE, W., JR., AND HASKINGS, J. C.: Considerations in choice of suture material for various tissues, PRS, *51:*353, 1973. Surg. Gynec. & Obst., *135:*113, 1972

VAN WINKLE, W. *et al*: Effects of suture materials on healing skin wounds, PRS, *56:*599, 1975. Surg. Gynec. & Obst., *140:*7, 1975

VAN ZYL, J. A. *et al*: Use of double transverse incision with radical block dissection of the neck. S. Afr. J. Surg., *13:*43, 1975 (Afrikaans)

VAN ZYL, J. J.: Gas gangrene, modern therapeutic approach. S. Afr. J. Surg., *11:*181, 1973 (Afrikaans)

VARAVVA, L. A.: Modified apparatus for intraosseous infusions and irrigation of burns. Vestn. Khir., *106:*107, 1971 (Russian)

VARAVVA, L. A.: Plastic surgery of skin in treatment of bone fractures of extremities with traumatic skin defects. Vestn. Khir., *111:*97, 1973 (Russian)

VARELA-IRIJOA, F. *et al*: Giant hemangioma. Angiologia, *27:*234, 1975 (Spanish)

VARGAS, G. P. E. *et al*: Parotid tumors, PRS, *55:*376, 1975. Bol. Soc. Venezuelana Cir., *27:*133, 1973

VARGAS-CORTES, F., WINKELMANN, R. K., AND SOULE, E. H.: Atypical fibroxanthomas of skin. Further observations with 19 additional cases. Proc. Staff Meet. Mayo Clin., *48:*211, 1973

VARIAN, J. P.: Ridged plaster volar slab. Hand, *7:*78, 1975

Varicose Ulcer: See Leg Ulcer

VARMA, S. K. *et al*: Conservative management of congenital lower limb amputee, PRS, *55:*249, 1975. Indian J. Surg., *36:*193, 1974

VARNER, E. A. *et al*: History of rotational method of plastic surgery of skin (priority of Dr. E. B. Eshe). Khirurgiia (Mosk.), *50:*136, 1974 (Russian)

VASCONEZ, L. O.: Congenital defect of skull and scalp due to arteriovenous malformation, PRS, *51:*692, 1973

VASCONEZ, L. O.: Treatment of macromastia in actively enlarging breast (with Mayl, Jurkiewicz), PRS, *54:*6, 1974

VASCONEZ, L. O.: Construction of one good thumb from both parts of a congenitally bifid thumb (With Hartrampf, Mathes), PRS, *54:*148, 1974

VASCONEZ, L. O.: Transverse abdominal flaps and deep epigastric arcade (with Brown, Jurkiewicz), PRS, *55:*416, 1975

VASCONEZ, L. O.: Basal cell carcinoma of medial canthal area (with Bostwick, Jurkiewicz), PRS, *55:*667, 1975

VASCONEZ, L. O.: Marjolin's ulcer: immunologically privileged tumor? (with Bostwick, Pendergrast), PRS, *57:*66, 1976

VASCONEZ, L. O., JURKIEWICZ, M. J., AND TYRAS, D.: Helpful maneuver for excision of intraoral malignant tumors, PRS, *52:*601, 1973. Surg. Gynec. & Obst., *136:*985, 1973

VASCONEZ, L. O., BOSTWICK, J., III, AND MC-CRAW, J.: Coverage of exposed bone by muscle transposition and skin grafting, PRS, *53:*526, 1974

VASIL'EV, S. F.: Clinical classification of the open combined injuries of the hand and fingers. Ortop. Travmatol. Protez., *35:*57, 1974 (Russian)

VASIL'EV, V. B. *et al*: Free skin transplantation with local use of glucocorticoids. Khirurgiia (Mosk.), *49:*13, 1972 (Russian)

VASIL'EVA, N. G.: Remote results of rhinoplasty using Filatov's graft with decalcified bone. Vestn. Khir., *106:*102, 1971 (Russian)

VAUGHT, S. K., LITVOK, A. S., AND MC-ROBERTS, J. W.: Surgical management of scrotal and penile lymphedema, PRS, *57:*761, 1976. J. Urol., *113:*204, 1975

VECCHIONE, T. R.: Technique for obtaining uniform split-skin grafts, PRS, *55:*640, 1975. Arch. Surg., *109:*837, 1974

VECCHIONE, T. R.: Method for recontouring domed nipple, PRS, *57:*30, 1976

VECCHIONE, T. R., HABAL, M. B., AND MURRAY, J. E.: Further experiences with arytenoid-epiglottic flap for chronic aspiration pneumonia, PRS, *55:*318, 1975

VECCHIONE, T. R., AND PICKERING, P. P.: Subcutaneous Z-plasty, PRS, *56:*579, 1975

VELAZQUEZ, J. M., AND ORTIZ-MONASTERIO, F.: Primary simultaneous correction of lip and nose in unilateral cleft lip, PRS, *54:*558, 1974

VELEZ-GUTIERREZ, J. A.: Amputation or reconstruction, PRS, *55:*258, 1975. Rev. el Medico, *24:*19, 1974

VELIKOV, K., PAPUROV, G., AND MARKOV, D.: Tissue reaction after implantation of various polymers to thymectomized and non-thymectomized rats, PRS, *53:*614, 1974. Acta chir. plast., *15:*29, 1973

VELLER, D. G. *et al*: Surgeons' injuries during operations. Klin. Khir., *0:*43, 1974 (Russian)

Velopharyngeal Incompetence: See *Cleft Palate, Velopharyngeal Incompetence*

VENDELOVSKII, I. I. *et al*: Long-term symptomless presence of foreign body (tracheotomy tube) in bronchus. Zh. Ushn. Nos. Gorl. Bolezn., *33:*76, 1973 (Russian)

VENNE, J. P.: Chondrosternal malformations. Union Med. Can., *102:*1352, 1973 (French)

VENTURA, M. R.: Care after nasal surgery. Nursing (Jenkintown), *4:*87, 1974

VERA, C. L. *et al*: Central functional changes

after facial-spinal-accessory anastomosis in man and facial-hypoglossal anastomosis in the cat. J. Neurosurg., *43:*181, 1975

VERBECK, C. *et al*: Prevention of recurrence in surgery for ankylosis. Fortsch. Kiefer. Gesichtschir., *18:*241, 1974 (German)

VERBEEK, H. O. F., AND BENDER, J.: Results of treatment of pilonidal sinus by block excision and primary suture, PRS, *55:*722, 1975. Arch. chir. neerl., *26:*311, 1974

VERDAN, C.: Some difficult situations in restorative surgery of the mutilated hand. Chirurgie, *98:*295, 1972 (French)

VERDAN, C.: Functional reconstruction of a congenital lobster-claw hand. Handchirurgie, *5:*93, 1973 (German)

VERDAN, C.: Editorial: Esthetic surgery. Rev. Med. Suisse Romande., *94:*8957, 1974 (French)

VERDAN, C. *et al*: Esthetics in surgery of the hand. Rev. Med. Suisse Romande., *94:*989, 1974 (French)

VERDAN, C. *et al*: Anatomic and functional relations between the tendons of the long palmar muscle and the long flexor muscle of the thumb at their crossing in the carpus. Ann. chir. plast., *20:*191, 1975 (French)

VERDAN, C. E.: Half century of flexor tendon surgery. Current status and changing philosophies, PRS, *51:*105, 1973. J. Bone & Joint Surg., *54A:*472, 1972

VERDAN, C. E.: Proceedings: Surgical reconstructive possibilities in severely mutilated hands. Hefte Unfallheilkd., *114:*157, 1973 (German)

VERDICH, M.: Dacrocystorhinostomy. Ugeskr. Laeger, *136:*1196, 1974 (Danish)

VERGNON, L. *et al*: Nostril stenosis and atresia. Dilator tube. Ann. Otolaryngol. Chir. Cervicofac., *88:*675, 1971 (French)

VERGON, L. *et al*: Reimplantation of ear lobe after quasi-total section. Ann. Otolaryngol. Chir. Cervicofac., *90:*711, 1973 (French)

VERHAEGHE, M. *et al*: Diagnosis and treatment of 153 mixed tumors of parotid gland. Lille Med., *18:*385, 1973 (French)

VERHEECKE, G. *et al*: Local flaps in the repair of nasal skin defects. Ann. chir. plast., *19:*193, 1974 (French)

VERIN *et al*: Plastic restoration of major losses of palpebral substance: technic and indications. Bull. Soc. Ophtalmol. Fr., *70:*827, 1970

VERMEEREN, J. I. J. F.: Surgical management of sialoliths in efferent duct of submandibular gland, PRS, *55:*507, 1975. Arch. chir. neerl., *26:*189, 1974

VERMILLION, C. D., AND PAGE, D. L.: Paget's disease of scrotum: case report with local lymph node invasion, PRS, *50:*539, 1972. J.

Urol., *107:*281, 1972

VERMUND, H., AND GOLLIN, F.: Role of radiotherapy in treatment of cancer of tongue, PRS, *54:*106, 1974. Cancer, *32:*333, 1973

VERMUND, H. *et al*: Role of radiotherapy in the treatment of oral cancer. J. Oral Surg., *32:*690, 1974

VERNE, D.: Surgical treatment of common abnormalities in relation to oral prosthesis. J. Oral Surg., *29:*768, 1971

VERONESI, U. *et al*: Therapeutic planning and prognosis in cutaneous malignant melanoma. Arch. Ital. Chir., *95:*607, 1969 (Italian)

VERRAZ, R.: Traumatic exophthalmos. Nosographic considerations and clinical case report. Arch. Sci. Med. (Torino), *127:*383, 1970 (Italian)

VERSCHUEREN, R. C. J., KOUDSTAAL, J., AND OLDHOFF, J.: Carbon dioxide laser, some possibilities in surgery, PRS, *56:*362, 1975. Acta chir. belg., *73:*197, 1974

VERSTREKEN, J.: New approach to the excision of Dupuytren contractures in the hand. Acta Orthop. Belg., *37:*290, 1971

VESELY, D. G.: Sculpture of the hand. A dramatization of anatomy. Clin. Orthop., *89:*94, 1972

VESELY, K.: Risk of gynaecologists participating in operations of transsexualism. Cesk. Gynekol., *40:*720, 1975 (Czechoslovakian)

VESSE, M. *et al*: Treatment of an old temporomandibular joint luxation. Rev. Stomatol. Chir. Maxillofac., *76:*443, 1975 (French)

Vestibuloplasty (See also *Oral Surgery*)

Surgical improvement of alveolar ridge in cases of atrophy of alveolar process (Schwenzer). Acta Odontol. Venez., *9:*213, 1971 (Spanish)

Mediastinal emphysema following fracture in the region of the paranasal sinuses (Schworer *et al*). Fortschr. Geb. Roentgenstr. Nuklearmed., *115:*684, 1971 (German)

Preprosthetic surgery from the viewpoint of the prosthodontist (Miller). J. Oral Surg., *29:*760, 1971

Surgical treatment of common abnormalities in relation to oral prosthesis (Verne). J. Oral Surg., *29:*768, 1971

Vestibuloplasty—skin grafts (Steinhauser). J. Oral Surg., *29:*777, 1971

Vestibuloplasty, mucosal grafts (palatal and buccal) (Hall). J. Oral Surg., *29:*786, 1971

Surgical stents for vestibuloplasty and alveolar ridge skin grafts (Riley). J. Prosthet. Dent., *26:*511, 1971

Mandible, bone transplantation to, creation of alveolar ridge after (Rehrmann) (Fol-

Vestibuloplasty—Cont.

low-Up Clinic), PRS, *48:*368, 1971

An experimental investigation into the relapse problem in vestibuloplasties with secondary epithelialization (Egyedi). Aust. Dent. J., *17:*67, 1972

Fibromatosis gingivae (Bartosova). Cesk. Stomatol., *72:*435, 1972 (Czechslovakian)

Value and significance of mouth vestibulum deepening under special consideration of cicatricial contracture (Sponholz *et al*). Dtsch. Stomatol., *22:*40, 1972 (German)

Vestibuloplasty, an intervention in muscular system of stomoschisis (Schumacher *et al*). Dtsch. Stomatol., *22:*734, 1972 (German)

Vestibuloplasty and intervention into musculatory system of mouth (Schumacher *et al*). Dtsch. Stomatol., *22:*889, 1972 (German)

Studies on the width of the gingiva proper after vestibuloplasty with and without periostal fenestration (Diedrich *et al*). Dtsch. Zahnaerztl. Z., *27:*346, 1972 (German)

Technique of vestibular plasty using free mucosal graft from cheek (Tideman). Int. J. Oral Surg., *1:*76, 1972

Free buccal mucosal grafts for vestibuloplasty (Maloney *et al*). J. Oral Surg., *30:*716, 1972

Microbuccal fold extension for implant and other surgical procedures (Weber). J. Prosthet. Dent., *27:*423, 1972

Preprosthetic surgery. 7. Indications and discussion of various patients (Tideman). Ned. Tijdschr. Tandheelkd., *79:*262, 1972 (Dutch)

Vestibuloplasty, involving lingual side of mandible, healing of mylohyoid musculature after ("lowering floor of mouth") (Courage *et al*). Oral Surg., *34:*581, 1972

Vestibuloplasty and plastic surgery, experiences with, on floor of mouth in edentulous mandibles (Immertreu). Quintessenz, *23:*15, 1972 (German)

Vestibular extension in periodontal surgery. Edjan and Mejchar technic (Cattoni). Rev. Dent. (St. Domingo), *18:*5, 1972 (Spanish)

Problems of prosthetic treatment of the edentulous mandible, especially before and after total plastic surgery of the floor of the mouth and the vestibulum by means of free skin flaps (Geering). Schweiz. Monatsschr. Zahnheilkd., *82:*263, 1972 (German)

Sulcus-extension surgery as preprosthetic treatment in front region of lower jaw. Clinical roentgenographic evaluation (Berthold *et al*). Sven. Tandlak. Tidskr., *65:*255, 1972

Fibromatosis, gingival, hereditary (Srsen *et*

Vestibuloplasty — Cont.

al). Acta Univ. Carol. (Med. Monogr.), (Praha), *56:*141, 1973

Mouth, edentulous, and vestibule of mouth, Obwegeser's method of plastic surgery of (Andrie *et al*). Cesk. Stomatol., *83:*122, 1973 (Czechoslovakian)

Results of treatment of certain periodontal conditions by increasing depth of vestibule and widening gingival area (Kaczmarczyk-Stachowska *et al*). Czas. Stomatol., *26:*783, 1973 (Polish)

Therapy recommendations for periodontics (Editorial). Dtsch. Stomatol., *23:*884, 1973

Vestibuloplasty, with and without suture fixation (Richter). Deutsch. Zahnaertzl. Z., *28:*206, 1973

Vestibuloplasty, electron microscopic studies in (Flores de Jacoby *et al*). Dtsch. Zahnaerztl. Z., *28:*1230, 1973 (German)

Current technics in preprosthetic surgery (Vialatel *et al*). Inf. Dent., *55:*23, 1973 (French)

Surgical approach to problem lower denture (Montano). J. Conn. State Dent. Assoc., *47:*95, 1973

Mandibular vestibuloplasty (Morrow *et al*). J. Ky. Dent. Assoc., *25:*13, 1973

Dentures, vestibular preparation for (Glogoff *et al*). J. Mercer. Dent. Soc., *27:*14, 1973

Vestibuloplasty — skin and palatal mucosal grafts, case report (Brown). J. Mich. State. Dent. Assoc., *55:*70, 1973

Jaw anomalies, preprosthetic surgery of (Martes *et al*). Odontiatrike, 213-8, 1973 (Greek)

Mandible, edentulous, reconstruction of floor of mouth and vestibule of (Immertreu). Quintessence Int., *4:*9, 1973

Vestibuloplasty, mandibular, with free graft of mucoperiosteal layer from hard palate (Morgan, Gallegos, Frileck), PRS, *51:*359, 1973

Reconstruction of maxillary vestibular sulcus. Pre and retropyromidal sulcus (Gallardo). Rev. Esp. Estomatol., *21:*30, 1973 (Spanish)

Fibromatosis gingivae, excision of mucosa (Schegg). Schweiz. Monatsschr. Zahnheilkd., *83:*1295, 1973 (German)

Fibromatosis gingivae, new pathways in surgical treatment of (Neuner *et al*). Schweiz. Monatsschr. Zahnheilkd., *83:*1327, 1973 (German)

Preparation, aftercare and definitive management in large preprosthetic interventions (Schegg). Schweiz. Monatsschr. Zahnheilkd., *83:*1483, 1973

Pre-prosthetic surgery — a new technique in

Vestibuloplasty — Cont.

the edentulous lower jaw (Edlan). Trans. Int. Conf. Oral Surg., *4:*191, 1973

Twelve years of free skin vestibuloplasty (Coffin). Trans. Int. Conf. Oral Surg., *4:*195, 1973

Free mucosal grafts in major reconstructive oral surgery (Guernsey). Trans. Int. Conf. Oral Surg., *4:*198, 1973

Mandibular alveolar atrophy, transoral rib grafting for, a progress report (Davis *et al*). Trans. Congr. Int. Assoc. Oral Surg., *4:*206, 1973

Experience of pre-prosthetic surgery on the atrophic endentulous mandible (Hopkins *et al*). Brit. Dent. J., *137:*341, 1974

Buried continuous suture in plastic surgery in the oral vestibule (Rydosz). Czas. Stomatol., *27:*1205, 1974 (Polish)

Cytological studies after autotransplantation in the oral cavity (Roling *et al*). Dtsch. Zahnaerztl. Z., *29:*875, 1974 (German)

Edentulous ridges, deficient, restoration of, by bone grafting and use of subperiosteal metal implants (Boyne). Int. J. Oral Surg., *3:*278, 1974

Mandible, atrophic, mandibular staple implant for (Small *et al*). J. Biomed. Mater. Res., *8:*365, 1974

Vestibuloplasty and floor of mouth revision with application of split-thickness skin graft (Bell). J. N.C. Dent. Soc., *57:*14, 1974

Vestibuloplasty, immediate, with free mucosal grafts (Maloney, Shepherd, Doku), PRS, *55:*246, 1975. J. Oral Surg., *32:*343, 1974

Mouth, floor of, surgical lowering, salivary retention phenomenon following (Sanner *et al*). J. Oral Surg., *32:*377, 1974

Alveolar ridge augmentation in edentulous maxilla with use of autogenous ribs (Terry *et al*). J. Oral Surg., *32:*429, 1974

Use of steroids in the prevention of some complications after traumatic oral surgery (Hooley *et al*). J. Oral Surg., *32:*864, 1974

Gingivectomy, blood volume lost during, using two different anesthetic techniques (Hecht *et al*). J. Periodontol., *45:*9, 1974

Degenerative denture ridge — care and treatment (Wendt). J. Prosthet. Dent., *32:*477, 1974

Mandibular staple implant for an atrophic mandibular ridge: solving retention difficulties of a denture (Metz). J. Prosthet. Dent., *32:*572, 1974

Maxillary denture stabilization, intramucosal insert, simplified technique for (Fagan). Oral Implantol., *4:*504, 1974

Vestibuloplasty, asutural maxillary (Malo-

Vestibuloplasty — Cont.
  ney *et al*). Oral Surg., *37:*858, 1974
  Fibrosis, oral submucous (O'Riordan), PRS, *55:*723, 1975. Proc. Roy. Soc. Med., *67:*877, 1974
  Closure of buccosinusal communications with double pedicle flaps (Merlini *et al*). Rev. Stomatol. Chir. Maxillofac., *75:*199, 1974 (French)
  Treatment of perforations of the roof of the mouth. Alveolar buccosinusal communications (Lachard *et al*). Rev. Stomatol. Chir. Maxillofac., *75:*208, 1974 (French)
  Preliminary results of deepening of the vestibulum by means of Edlan's and Mejchar's methods (Kleber *et al*). Stomatol. DDR, *24:*670, 1974 (German)
  Anatomical principles of plastic operations in the vestibule of the oral cavity (Shumakher *et al*). Stomatologiia (Mosk.), *53:*83, 1974 (Russian)
  Preprosthetic surgery (Kruger). Z. W. R., *83:*8, 1974
  Vestibuloplasty, open, using lyophilized dura in (Krekeler). Z. W. R., *83:*639, 1974 (German)
  Preprosthetic surgery in relation to oral anomalies (Faraco Munuera). An. Esp. Odontoestomatol., *34:*435, 1975 (Spanish)
  Clinical results with Edlan and Mejchar's vestibuloplasty (De Jacoby *et al*). Dtsch. Zahnaerztl. Z., *30:*581, 1975 (German)
  Current views on periodontal surgery. I. Surgery of periodontal soft tissues (Gera). Fogorv. Sz., *68:*225, 1975 (Hungarian)
  Preprosthetic surgery in the front region of the mandible (Rosenquist). Int. J. Oral Surg., *4:*18, 1975
  Vestibuloplasty, oral, tattoo marking for registration of relapse after (Hillerup). Int. J. Oral Surg., *4:*65, 1975
  Rehabilitation of the atrophic edentulous maxilla by bone grafting (Topazian). J. Am. Dent. Assoc., *90:*625, 1975
  Denture tolerance before and after mandibular vestibuloplasty with skin grafting, patient survey (Landesman *et al*). J. Am. Dent. Assoc., *90:*806, 1975
  Long-term ridge augmentation with rib graft (Davis *et al*). J. Maxillofac. Surg., *3:*103, 1975
  Vestibuloplasty, fenestrated palatal mucosal grafts for (Shepherd, Maloney, Doku), PRS, *56:*467, 1975. J. Oral Surg., *33:*34, 1975
  Letter: The status of oral surgery. J. Oral Surg., *33:*487, 1975
  Maxillary "pocket inlay" vestibuloplasty (Boudreau *et al*). J. Oral Surg., *33:*601,

Vestibuloplasty — Cont.
  1975
  Modified technique for palatal mucosal grafts in mandibular labial vestibuloplasty (Sanders *et al*). J. Oral Surg., *33:*950, 1975
  Role of the prosthodontist in preprosthetic surgery (Wilkie). J. Prosthet. Dent., *33:*386, 1975
  A methodological analysis and follow-up of vestibular plasty and skin grafting (Tasanen *et al*). Proc. Finn. Dent. Soc., *71:*176, 1975
  Experience with surgical deepening of the oral vestibulum in the mandible (Sponholz *et al*). Stomatol. DDR, *25:*607, 1975 (German)
  The flat vestibulum. Problems, indications for surgery, modification of vestibuloplasty and evaluation of success (Schmidt). Stomatol. DDR, *25:*612, 1975 (German)
  Vestibuloplasty with skin grafting (Yrastorza). J. Oral Surg., *34:*29, 1976
  Partial vestibuloplasty with secondary epithelization (Baumann). Schweiz. Monatsschr. Zahnheilkd., *86:*17, 1976 (German)

VETRA, H. *et al*: Hydrotherapy and topical collagenase for decubitus ulcers. Geriatrics, *30:*53, 1975

VEVERKA, K. *et al*: Unusual injuries of soft tissues of the lower lip during work. Cesk. Stomatol., *72:*46, 1972 (Czechoslovakian)

VIALATEL, C. *et al*: Current technics in preprosthetic surgery. Inf. Dent., *55:*23, 1973 (French)

VIALE-GONZALEZ, M., BARRETO, F., AND ORTIZ-MONASTERIO, F.: Surgical management of bilateral cleft lip, PRS, *51:*530, 1973

VIBILD, O. *et al*: Flexion contracture in the interphalangeal joints following splinting for simple metacarpal fractures. Ugeskr. Laeger, *136:*1439, 1974 (Danish)

VIC-DUPONT, V. *et al*: Gas gangrene. Apropos of 32 cases. Ann. Med. Interne (Paris), *125:*469, 1974 (French)

VICHARE, N. A.: Anomalous muscle belly of the flexor digitorum superficialis. Report of a case. J. Bone & Joint Surg. (Br.), *52:*757, 1970

VICK, J. A. *et al*: Treatment of hemorrhagic shock with new vasodilator, PRS, *53:*109, 1974. Mil. Med., *138:*490, 1973

VICKERS, H. R.: Treatment of malignant disease of orbital region. Proc. Roy. Soc. Med., *66:*689, 1973

VICKERS, M. A.: Operative management of chronic hidradenitis suppurativa of scrotum and perineum. J. Urol., *114:*414, 1975

VICKERY, I. M.: Hemifacial atrophy. Brit. J. Oral Surg., 9:102, 1971

VICTOR, D. I., BRESNAN, M. J., AND KELLER, R. B.: Brain abscess complicating use of halo traction, PRS, 52:602, 1973. J. Bone & Joint Surg., 55A:635, 1973

VIEHWEGER, G. et al: Comparative angiographic investigations of the upper limb under local, regional and general anesthesia. Fortschr. Geb. Roentgenstr. Nuklearmed., 121:303, 1974 (German)

VIGONI, M.: Ulcers and hypodermitis. Phlebologie, 25:353, 1972 (French)

VIITANEN, S. M., AND VILJANTO, J.: Wound healing, thermographic study, PRS, 52:105, 1973. Ann. chir. et gynaec. Fenniae, 60:101, 1972

VIJAYARAGHAVAN, K. et al: Post-operative relapse following sagittal split osteotomy. Brit. J. Oral Surg., 12:63, 1974

VIJAYARAGHAVEN, K. et al: An unusual case of "haemorrhagic" bone cyst. Brit. J. Oral Surg., 13:64, 1975

VIKTOROV, L. A. et al: External carotid artery ligation in epistaxis. Vestn. Otorinolaringol., 34:115, 1972 (Russian)

VILAIN, R.: Infection and superinfection of burn patients. Is the burn center a septic ghetto? Anesth. Analg. (Paris), 28:761, 1971 (French)

VILAIN, R.: Can round table discussions be changed? Ann. chir. plast., 16:191, 1971 (French)

VILAIN, R.: Breast esthetics and carcinology, PRS, 54:620, 1974. Ann. chir. plast., 19:1, 1974

VILAIN, R.: Medicine and surgery of the profile. Ann. chir. plast., 20:113, 1975 (French)

VILAIN, R.: Treatment of steatomery in the female: theory and practice. Ann. chir. plast., 20:135, 1975 (French)

VILAIN, R.: Note of surgical technic. The technic called in a setting sun in abdominal dermodystrophies. Ann. chir. plast., 20:239, 1975 (French)

VILAIN, R.: Some considerations in surgical alteration of the feminine silhouette. Clin. Plast. Surg., 2:449, 1975

VILAIN, R.: Surgical correction of steatomeries. Clin. Plast. Surg., 2:467, 1975

VILAIN, R. et al: Use of flag-shaped flap in palmar defects. Ann. Chir., 25:1031, 1971 (French)

VILAIN, R., AND MICHON, J.: Infections de la Main Chez l'Enfant et l'Adulte. Masson & Cie, Paris, 1972. PRS, 52:661, 1973

VILAIN, R., AND Dupuis, J. F.: Use of flag flap for coverage of small area on finger or palm, PRS, 51:397, 1973

VILAIN, R., AND MITZ, V.: Vascular flaps in secondary surgery after hand trauma, PRS, 56:596, 1975. Hand, 7:56, 1975

VILAIN, RAYMOND et al: Osteo-Articular Injuries of the Hand. Expansion Scientifique Francaise, Paris, 1971. PRS, 49:656, 1972

VILARDELL, E.: Gynecomastia, PRS, 51:230, 1973. Med. Clinica, 48:344, 1972

VILAR-SANCHO, B., AND BERMUDEZ-PIERNAGORDA, M.: Repair of congenital cleft of sternum, PRS, 48:605, 1971. Rev. españ. cir. plast., 4:87, 1971

VILASCO, J. et al: 7 cases of ameloblastoma recurrence. Rev. Stomatol. Chir. Maxillofac., 75:42, 1974 (French)

VILJANTO, J. et al: Stimulation of granulation tissue growth in burns. Ann. Chir. Gynaec. Fenn., 62:18, 1973

VILLA, C. et al: Surgical treatment of the postphlebitis syndrome. I. Minerva Chir., 30:16, 1975 (Italian)

VILLA, C. et al: Surgical treatment of the postphlebitis syndrome. II. Minerva Chir., 30:21, 1975 (Italian)

VILLANO, J. B.: Follow-up of bone grafts to the nose (with Farina), PRS, 48:251, 1971

VILLANUEVA, R.: Rehabilitation needs of the cancer patient. South. Med. J., 68:169, 1975

VILLARREAL RIOS, A.: Fourteen free groin flap transfers (with Serafin, Georgiade), PRS, 57:707, 1976

VINAGERAS GUARNEROS, E. et al: Correction of a nostril deformity secondary to cleft lip and palate. Bol. Med. Hosp. Infant. Mex., 31:771, 1974 (Spanish)

VINAGERAS GUARNEROS, E. et al: Modification of the muscular flap in the rotation technic and Millard's advancement technic in cleft-lip closure. Bol. Med. Hosp. Infant. Mex., 32:457, 1975 (Spanish)

VIÑAS, J. C.: Ischemic face lift (Letter to the Editor), PRS, 52:293, 1973

VIÑAS, J. C. et al: Surgical treatment of double chin, PRS, 50:119, 1972

VIÑAS, J. C., CAVIGLIA, C., AND CORTINAS, J. L.: Forehead rhytidoplasty and brow lifting, PRS, 57:445, 1976

VINOGRADOVA, O. I. et al: Use of plastubol for the treatment of burns. Khirurgiia (Mosk.), 4:30, 1975 (Russian)

VIRET, J.: Limitations of the role of social insurance, especially disability insurance, in cases of esthetic damage. Rev. Med. Suisse Romande., 94:1005, 1974 (French)

VIRNELLI, F. R.: Axillary hidradenitis suppurativa (with Pollock, Ryan), PRS, 49:22, 1972

VISENTINI, P., MAZZOLENI, F., AND LINDA, G.: Lipomatosis at prevailing cervical localization, PRS, 56:363, 1975. Riv. ital. chir. plast., 5:483, 1973

VISHNEVSKII, A. A. *et al*: Prognosis of autograft for burns using the table methods. Fksp. Khir. Anesteziol., *16*:3, 1971 (Russian)

VISHNEVSKII, A. A. *et al*: Pathogenesis and clinical picture of burn sepsis. Klin. Med. (Mosk.), *50*:7, 1972 (Russian)

VISHNEVSKII, A. A. *et al*: The past and present of the Soviet military-field surgery. Sov. Med., *5*:3, 1975 (Russian)

VISINTAINER, M. A., AND WOLFER, J. A.: Psychological preparation for surgical pediatric patients: effect on children's and parents' stress responses and adjustment, PRS, *57*:544, 1976. Pediatrics, *56*:187, 1975

VISSAIN, L., AND VAILLAUD, J. C.: Oro-facial-digital syndrome, 11th case in same family, PRS, *51*:605, 1973. Ann. dermat. & syph., *99*:5, 1972

VISTNES, L.: Effect of commonly used antiseptics on wound healing (with Gruber, Pardoe), PRS, *55*:472, 1975

VISTNES, L. M.: Skin coverage in common hand injuries. Postgrad. Med., *51*:180, 1972

VISTNES, L. M.: Use of water bed for prevention of pressure sores (with Siegel, Laub), PRS, *51*:31, 1973

VISTNES, L. M.: Effective hemostasis with less epinephrine, experimental and clinical study (with Siegel, Iverson), PRS, *51*:129, 1973

VISTNES, L.: Bone deformation beneath alloplastic implants (with Jobe, Iverson), PRS, *51*:169, 1973. Discussions by Rees, Spira, PRS, *51*:174, 1973

VISTNES, L. M.: Correction of enophthalmos in the anophthalmic orbit (with Iverson, Siegel), PRS, *51*:545, 1973

VISTNES, L. M.: Effect of hydrotherapy on clinical course and pH of experimental cutaneous chemical burns (with Gruber, Laub), PRS, *55*:200, 1975

VISTNES, L. M.: Long-term study of reactions to various silicone breast implants in rabbits (with Lilla), PRS, *57*:637, 1976

VISTNES, L. M.: Skin tension lines in domestic pig (with Rose, Ksander), PRS, *57*:729, 1976

VISTNES, L. M., AND HOGG, G. R.: Burn eschar, histopathological study, PRS, *48*:56, 1971

VISTNES, L. M., AND KERNAHAN, D.A.: Melkersson-Rosenthal syndrome, PRS, *48*:126, 1971

VISTNES, L. M., IVERSON, R. E., AND LAUB, D. R.: Anophthalmic orbit, surgical correction of lower eyelid ptosis, PRS, *52*:346, 1973

VISTNES, L. M., LILLA, J. A., AND SIEGEL, R. J.: Heterotopic transplantation of ureter as free graft, PRS, *56*:231, 1975. Invest. Urol., *12*:8, 1974

VISTNES, L. M., AND IVERSON, R. E.: Surgical treatment of contracted socket, PRS, *53*:563, 1974

VISTNES, L. M., HARRIS, D. R., AND FAJARDO, L. F.: Evaluation of cryosurgery for basal cell carcinoma, PRS, *55*:71, 1975

VISUTHIKOSOL, V., AND BURI, P.: Treatment of thermal burns by amniotic membranes, PRS, *56*:232, 1975. Asian J. Mod. Med., *11*:17, 1975

VITIELLO, F.: Surgical technics for correction of nasal septum deviation. Minerva Stomatol., *23*:180, 1974 (Italian)

VITIELLO, F.: Reconstructive surgical treatment of neoplasms of nasal pyramid. Minerva Stomatol., *23*:188, 1974 (Italian)

VITTON, J.: Experimental study on the role of the condyle in mandibular growth. Rev. Stomatol. Chir. Maxillofac., *75*:1001, 1974 (French)

VITTON, J. *et al*: Trauner's operation in the treatment of retrognathia. Rev. Stomatol. Chir. Maxillofac., *74*:632, 1973 (French)

VITURIN, B. M. *et al*: Indications for surgical treatment of cervical chemodectomas. Vestn. Khir., *108*:3, 1972 (Russian)

VIVAKANANTHAN, C.: Minimal incision for removing sebaceous cysts. Brit. J. Plast. Surg., *25*:60, 1972

VIVAR-MEJIA, G. *et al*: Injuries to tracheal cartilage produced during 3 different technics for fixation of the trachea during tracheotomy. Bol. Med. Hosp. Infant. Mex., *32*:97, 1975 (Spanish)

VLACH, O. *et al*: On the problem of operation treatment of spastic hand. Acta Chir. Orthop. Traumatol. Cech., *41*:40, 1974 (Czechoslovakian)

VLADECK, B. C. *et al*: Burn pathophysiology in man. II. Sequential oxygen transport and acid base alterations, PRS, *53*:609, 1974. J. Surg. Res., *14*:74, 1973

VLADOVIC-RELJA, T., MONTANI, D., AND ZECEVIC, D.: Mortality in burn injury over a period of ten years, PRS, *54*:623, 1974. Acta chir. plast., *15*:231, 1973

VODIANOV, N. M.: Treatment of patients with isolated injuries of tendons of the flexor digitorum profundus. Ortop. Travmatol. Protez., *34*:8, 1973 (Russian)

VODIANOV, N. M. *et al*: Primary reconstructive surgery on the hand following severe frostbite. Vestn. Khir., *107*:97, 1972 (Russian)

VODOLATSKII, M. P.: Use of self-hardening plastic material Protacryl for bone preservation. Stomatologiia (Mosk.), *53*:38, 1974 (Russian)

VODOVOZOV, A. M.: Surgery for spastic ectropion. Oftalmol. Zh., *27*:390, 1972 (Russian)

VOENA, G. *et al*: Clinical remarks and considerations on preservation of the mandible in the Commando operation. Minerva Otorinolaringol., *21*:186, 1971 (Italian)

VOGEL, C. M., KINGSBURY, R. J., AND BAUE, A. E.: Intravenous hyperalimentation: review of 2¹/₂ years' experience, PRS, 51:610, 1973. Arch. Surg., 105:414, 1972

VOGEL, T. T. et al: Laceration of hypopharynx. J. Pediatr. Surg., 9:557, 1974

VOGELGESANG, G. W.: Hunt's syndrome; case report. J. Am. Osteopath. Assoc., 73:762, 1974

VOITOVICH, V. V.: Method of investigation of the function of the hand and fingers. Ortop. Travmatol. Protez., 34:65,1973 (Russian)

VOLDER, J. G. R., AND OOSTERWIJK, W. M.: Surgical treatment of venous leg ulcers, PRS, 51:704, 1973. Arch. chir. neerl., 24:245, 1972

VOLDRICH, Z. et al: Long-term experience with poly (glycolmonomethacrylate) gel in plastic operations of the nose. J. Biomed. Mater. Res., 9:675, 1975

VOLKAN, V. D. et al: Dreams of transsexuals awaiting surgery. Compr. Psychiatry, 14:269, 1973

VOLKOV, I. et al: Our experience with the joining of tissues using cyacrin. Vestn. Otorinolaringol., 2:81, 1975 (Russian)

VOLKOV, IU. N. et al: Cylindromas of the nose and paranasal sinuses. Vestn. Otorinolaringol., 1:55, 1975 (Russian)

VOLKOV, IU. N. et al: Neurilemmoma of the nose and accessory sinuses. Vestn. Otorinolaringol., 3:34, 1975 (Russian)

VOLKOV, L. A.: Diagnostic errors in lip neoplasms. Sov. Med., 35:142, 1972 (Russian)

VOLKOV, L. F. et al: Classification of burns of the lower limbs. Khirurgiia (Mosk.), 48:28, 1972 (Russian)

VOLKOV, V. V. et al: Size and localization of bone aperture in external dacrocystorhinostomy. Oftalmol. Zh., 30:179, 1975 (Russian)

VOLOGODSKALA, M. E. et al: Cranioplasty with roentgenocontrast acrylic plates. Vestn. Khir., 110:118, 1973 (Russian)

VOLOIR, P.: Post-traumatic algo-dystrophies. Bull. Mem. Soc. Chir. Paris, 60:293, 1970 (French)

VON BARSEWISCH, B.: Reconstruction of lacrimal apparatus. Laryngol. Rhinol. Otol. (Stuttg.), 53:482, 1974 (German)

VON DAMARUS, H.: Pains in face and jaws, due to Wegener's granuloma. Z. Laryngol. Rhinol. Otol., 52:901, 1973 (German)

VON EMPEL, C. H., AND SMEENK, G.: Hemorrhagic necrosis of skin as complication of anticoagulant therapy, PRS, 52:99, 1973. Arch. chir. neerl., 24:353, 1972

VON KOPPENFELS, R. et al: Clinical aspects and therapy of eosinophilic granuloma in facial skull. Dtsch. Zahnaerztl. Z., 28:514, 1973

VON LEDEN, H.: Cryosurgery of head and neck. Acta Otorinolaryngol. Iber. Am., 22:275, 1971 (Spanish)

VON LEDEN, H.: New horizons in laryngology. Acta Otolaryngol. (Stockh.), 74:332, 1972

VON LEDEN, H.: Cryosurgery of the head and neck. Tex. Med., 68:108, 1972

VON LEDEN, H.: Cryogenic surgery in head and neck tumors. Arch. Klin. Exp. Ohren Nasen Kehlkopfheilkd., 205:84, 1973 (German)

VON LUTZKI, A. et al: Esthetic-surgical breast enlargement, exchange mastectomy, and breast reconstruction following mamma amputation. New clinical and radiographic findings. Med. Welt., 26:381, 1975 (German)

VON PRINCE, K. M. et al: Application of fingernail hooks in splinting of burned hands. Am. J. Occup. Ther., 24:556, 1970

VON PRINCE, K. M. P., AND YAEKEL, M.: The Splinting of Burn Patients. Charles C Thomas, Springfield, Ill., 1974. PRS, 56:664, 1975

VOORHOEVE, A.: Possibility to use homologous preserved tendon material, PRS, 50:423, 1972. Chir. Praxis, 16:1, 1972

VORLOVA, Z.: Testing new materials for blood clotting properties by in vitro method, PRS, 56:475, 1975. J. Polym. Med., 4:119, 1974

VOROB'EV, IU I.: Effectiveness of combined and radiotherapy of malignant tumors of the minor salivary glands of the maxilla. Stomatologiia (Mosk.), 53:20, 1974 (Russian)

VOROB'EVA, R. G. et al: Endotracheal anesthesia in children during operations in the maxillofacial region. Stomatologiia (Mosk.), 50:83, 1971 (Russian)

VOURC'H, G.: Various considerations on use of ketamine. Anesth. Analg. (Paris), 30:1043, 1973 (French)

VOZDVIZHENSKII, S. I. et al: Experience with work of children's units for treatment of burns and norms for their demand. Ortop. Travmatol. Protez., 34:69, 1973 (Russian)

VRABEC, D. P.: Inverted Schneiderian papilloma: a clinical and pathological study. Laryngoscope, 85:186, 1975

VRABEC, R.: Therapy of burns in Egypt. Rozhl. chir., 50:652, 1971 (Czechoslovakian)

VRABEC, R.: Importance of allografts and xenografts in surgical treatment of skin losses, PRS, 54:626, 1974. Rozhl. chir., 53:187, 1974

VRABEC, R., KOLAŘ, J., AND DRUGOVA, B.: Curling's ulcer, PRS, 50:541, 1972. Acta chir. plast., 13:176, 1971

VRABEC, R. et al: Basic Problems in Burns: Proceedings. Symposium, Prague, September 1973. Springer-Verlag, New York, 1975

VRABEC, R. et al: Clinical experience with enzymatic debridement of burned skin with the use of collagenase. J. Hyg. Epidemiol. Microbiol. Immunol. (Praha), *18:*496, 1974

VRACHNOS, T., PARASKEVAS, P., AND STYLO-GIANNIS, S.: Surgical management of advanced cancer of head and neck, PRS, *56:*473, 1975. Tr. 8th Panhellenic Cong. Surg. Soc., *A:*190, 1973

VREBOS, J.: Personal experience and critical study of mammary prostheses, PRS, *50:*199, 1972. Acta chir. belg., *70:*300, 1971

VREBOS, J.: Surgical correction of facial skin sagging. Brux. Med., *51:*569, 1971 (French)

VREBOS, J.: Personal and clinical experience with mammary prosthesis implantations. Ann. chir. plast., *17:*114, 1972 (French)

VREBOS, J.: Ring constriction of extremities, PRS, *56:*602, 1975. Brux. Med., *54:*693, 1974

VUILLARD, P. *et al*: Anatomical study of the possibilities of using the sigmoid colon in the surgical treatment of congenital absence of the vagina. Lyon Chir., *67:*311, 1971 (French)

VUKAS, A.: Smallpox-induced scars: treatment by dermabrasion. Dermatologica, *148:*175, 1974

VUKAS, A. *et al*: Regenerative properties of tissues involved in chronic pathological processes. Preliminary report of experimental study. Gerontologia, *20:*9, 1974

VULCAN, P., AND GEORGESCU, C.: Proliferating epidermoid cyst, PRS, *57:*255, 1976. Dermat. Vener., *18:*47, 1973

Vulva (See also *Vagina*)

Vulvectomy, extensive superficial, with primary skin grafting for premalignant lesions (Marchac), PRS, *54:*691, 1974. Brit. J. Plast. Surg., *26:*40, 1973

Clitoroplasty: experience during 19-year period. (Kumar *et al*). J. Urol., *111:*81, 1974

Elephantiasis, vulvar (Cardinal), PRS, *54:*377, 1974. Rev. Medico, *24:*43, 1974

Labia minora graft for nipple reconstruction (Silsby), PRS, *57:*667, 1976

VYTRISHCHAK, V. IA.: Use of standard V. S. Vasiliev dental band bars in mandibular fractures. Stomatologiia (Mosk.), *50:*89, 1971 (Russian)

W

WACHSMUTH, W., AND WILHELM, A.: *Allgemeine und Spezielle Chirurgische Operationslehre: Die Operationen an der Hand.* Springer-Verlag, Berlin, 1972. PRS, *51:*580, 1973

WADA, T. *et al*: Growth and changes in maxillary arch form in complete unilateral cleft lip and cleft palate children. Cleft Palate J., *12:*115, 1975

WADE, J. S. H.: Cut-throat surgery, PRS, *57:*397, 1976. Proc. Roy. Soc. Med., *68:*357, 1975

WADHWA, R. K. *et al*: Parotidectomy in patient with family history of hyperthermia. Anesthesiology, *40:*191, 1974

WADSWORTH, T. G.: Traction hand splint. Hand, *5:*268, 1973

WAGENAAR, J.: Chronic recurrent parotitis in children. Arch. chir. neerl., *25:*13, 1973

WAGENKNECHT, L. V., AND ANVERT, J.: Substitute of human ureter by synthetic material, PRS, *51:*106, 1973. Chirurg, *43:*334, 1972

WAGENKNECHT, L. V. *et al*: Derivation of the upper urinary ways in bladder exstrophy. Z. Urol. Nephrol., *67:*589, 1974 (German)

WAGH, P., AND READ, R.: Defective collagen synthesis in inguinal herniation, PRS, *52:*103, 1973. Am. J. Surg., *124:*819, 1972

WAGNER, D., AND SCHWARTZ, G.: Electrical burns of mouth, PRS, *56:*232, 1975. Emerg. Med., *7:*275, 1975

WAGNER, D. F. *et al*: A new approach to radical retroperitoneal iliac and femoral node dissection. Arch. Surg., *103:*681, 1971

WAGNER, R. I. *et al*: Laser therapy of human benign and malignant neoplasms of the skin. Acta Radiol. (Ther.) (Stockh.), *14:*417, 1975

WAHL, D.: Buried suture – new, self-adapting intracutaneous suture. Zentralbl. Chir., *98:*1720, 1973 (German)

WAHLE, H.: Surgical treatment of bedsores in paraplegics (with Olivari, Schrudde), PRS, *50:*477, 1972

WAHLE, H. *et al*: Conservative and surgical therapy of decubital ulcers in paraplegics. Fortschr. Neurol. Psychiatr., *39:*653, 1971 (German)

WAISBREN, B. A., STEIN, M., AND COLLENTINE, G. E.: Methods of burn treatment: comparison by probit analysis, PRS, *56·*232, 1975. J.A.M.A., *231:*255, 1974

WAITE, DANIEL E.: *Textbook of Practical Oral Surgery.* Lea & Febiger, Philadelphia, 1972

WAITE, D. E.: Mandibular asymmetry. Trans. Congr. Int. Assoc. Oral Surg., *4:*246, 1973

WAKASUGI, B.: Facial nerve block in the treatment of facial spasm. Arch. Otolaryng., *95:*356, 1972

WAKELIN, D. *et al*: Pedunculated malignant melanoma of conjunctiva – the sequel. Can. J. Ophthalmol., *10:*90, 1975

WALCHER, K.: Hand injuries in skiing. Munch. Med. Wochenschr., *113:*1573, 1971 (German)

WALCHER, K., AND STURZ, H.: Further observations on capacity for regeneration in hyaline cartilage, PRS, *51:*109, 1973. Langenbecks Arch. Chir., *331:*1, 1972

WALDEN, R. *et al*: Upper thoracic sympathectomy for palmar hyperhydrosis. Harefuah, *85:*357, 1973 (Hebrew)

WALDEN, R. H., LOGOSSO, R. D., AND BRENNAN, L.: Pierre Robin syndrome in association with combined congenital lengthening and shortening of the long bones, PRS, *48:*80, 1971

WALDHART, F.: Surgical correction of bilateral hypertrophy of masseter muscle and mandibular angle. Osterr. Z. Stomatol., *68:*462, 1971 (German)

WALDHART, F.: Statistical report on 150 zygoma fractures. Osterr. Z. Stomatol., *69:*136, 1972 (German)

WALDHART, E.: Experiences with vertical osteotomy of the ascending ramus of the mandible in the treatment of prognathism. Fortschr. Kiefer. Gesichtschir., *18:*143, 1974 (German)

WALDHART, E., AND LYNCH, J. B.: Benign hypertrophy of masseter muscles and mandibular angles, PRS, *48:*294, 1971. Arch. Surg., *102:*115, 1971

WALDRON, C. A. *et al*: Benign fibro-osseous lesions of jaws: clinical-radiologic-histologic review of 65 cases. Oral Surg., *35:*190, 1973

WALIKE, J. W., AND BAILEY, B. J.: Head and neck hemangiopericytoma, PRS, *48:*298, 1971. Arch. Otolaryng., *93:*345, 1971

WALKER, J. C., JR., AND SAWHNEY, O.P.: Free composite lip grafts, PRS, *50:*142, 1972

WALKER, R. V.: Arthroplasty of the ankylosed temporomandibular joint. Trans. Int. Conf. Oral Surg., *4:*279, 1973

WALKER, R. V. *et al*: Surgery or orthodontics – a philosophy of approach. Dent. Clin. North Am., *15:*771, 1971

WALKER, W. W.: Surgical enigma of gynecomastia. J. Natl. Med. Assoc., *63:*385, 1971

WALL, N. R., CAMERON, R. R., AND LATHAM, W. D.: Restoring overhang of upper lip in repairs of oral commissure, PRS, *49:*626, 1972

WALLACE, A. B.: Grant of arms. Brit. J. Plast. Surg., *25:*266, 1972

WALLACE, A. F.: Brephoplastic skin grafts (Follow-Up Clinic), PRS, *50:*183, 1972

WALLACE, D. C., EXTON, L. A., AND McLEOD, G. R. C.: Genetic factor in malignant melanoma, PRS, *48:*609, 1971. Cancer, *27:*1262, 1971

WALLACE, D. C., BEARDMORE, G. L., AND EXTON, L. A.: Familial malignant melanoma, PRS, *52:*215, 1973. Ann. Surg., *177:*15, 1973

WALLACE, D. M.: Crucifaction operation for male incontinence. Proc. Roy. Soc. Med., *65:*303, 1972

WALLACE, J., AND MacDONALD, G. D.: Calcifying epithelial odontogenic tumor (Pindborg tumor), PRS, *56:*683, 1975. Brit. J. Plast. Surg., *27:*23, 1974

WALLACE, J. R.: Letter: Frustrations of oral surgery. J. Oral Surg., *33:*247, 1975

WALLACE, L. *et al*: Bilateral ankylosis of mandible in open position. Review of literature and report of case. Oral Surg., *37:*179, 1974

WALLACE, R. M. *et al*: Use of hair plugs from skin excised during face lifting. Arch. Dermat., *109:*96, 1974

WALLACE, W. A.: Damaged digital nerve, PRS, *57:*760, 1976. Hand, *7:*139, 1975

WALLER, L. C.: Electronic auscultation of metallic foreign bodies, PRS, *51:*610, 1973. Am. J. Surg., *123:*626, 1972

WALLER, R. R.: Management of myogenic (myopathic) ptosis. Trans. Am. Acad. Ophthalmol. Otolaryngol., *79:*697, 1975

WALLIS, W. *et al*: Evaporation – optimal physiological principle for artificial climatization of inspired air. Arch. Klin. Exp. Ohren Nasen Kehlkopfheilkd., *205:*363, 1973 (German)

WALSER, F.: Simple ptosis operation with modified tarsectomy. Klin. Monatsbl. Augenheilkd., *160:*589, 1972 (German)

WALSER, F.: Progress in the field of eyelid and orbit surgery. Med. Klin., *69:*1720, 1974 (German)

WALSH, J. P., DONALDSON, K. I., AND HARDING, J. F.: Surgical treatment of case of mandibular prognathism. New Zealand Dent. J., *68:*14, 1972

WALTER, C.: Reconstruction of auricle, PRS, *50:*418, 1972. Arch. Klin. Exp. Ohren Nasen Kehlkopfheilkd., *202:*252, 1972

WALTER, C.: Survey of use of composite grafts in head and neck region. Otolaryngol. Clin. North Am., *5:*571, 1972

WALTER, C.: Problems of facial soft tissue injury. H. N. O., *21:*182, 1973 (German)

WALTER, C.: External nose and profile plasty. Z. Laryngol. Rhinol. Otol., *52:*409, 1973 (German)

WALTER, C.: Should free dermis-fat transplantation still be considered for use in face? H. N. O., *22:*110, 1974 (German)

WALTER, C.: Operative management of the nose and associated tissues of the face. Laryngol. Rhinol. Otol. (Stuttg.), *53:*548, 1974 (German)

WALTER, C.: Free dermis fat transplantation as adjunct in the surgery of the parotid gland. Laryngol. Rhinol. Otol. (Stuttg.), *54:*435, 1975 (German)

WALTER, C.: Nasal reconstruction. Laryngoscope, *85:*1227, 1975

WALTER, C. D.: Secondary nasal revisions after rhinoplasties. Trans. Am. Acad. Ophthalmol. Otolaryngol., *80:*519, 1975

WALTER, W. L.: Early surgical repair of blow-out fracture of orbital floor by using transantral approach. South. Med. J., *65:*1229, 1972

WALTHER, H.: Therapy of the ulcus cruris. Munch. Med. Wochenschr., *114:*1069, 1972 (German)

WALTON, S.: Injection gun injury of the hand with anticorrosive paint and paint solvent. A case report. Clin. Orthop., *74:*141, 1971

WAN, S. H. *et al*: Effect of route of administration and effusion on methotrexate pharmacokinetics, PRS, *55:*516, 1975. Cancer Res., *34:*3487, 1974

WANDALL, J. H.: Healing of split skin autografts after storage in deuterated medium, PRS, *51:*110, 1973. Scand. J. Plast. Reconstr. Surg., *6:*36, 1972

WANDLESS, J. G. *et al*: Pre-stretched cuffs on tracheostomy tubes. Brit. J. Anaesth., *44:*1222, 1972

WANDSCHNEIDER, G.: Rotation plasty in the surgical treatment of acquired penile urethral fistulas and abnormalities. Z. Urol. Nephrol., *68:*727, 1975 (German)

WANEBO, H. J. *et al*: Reappraisal of surgical management of sarcoma of buttock, PRS, *52:*460, 1973. Cancer, *31:*97, 1973

WANEBO, H. J. *et al*: Treatment of minimal breast cancer. Cancer, *33:*349, 1974

WANEBO, H. J. *et al*: Malignant melanoma of the extremities: a clinicopathologic study using levels of invasion (microstage). Cancer, *35:*666, 1975

WANG, C. C., SCHULTZ, M. D., AND MILLER, D.: Combined radiation therapy and surgery for carcinoma of supraglottis and pyriform sinus, PRS, *52:*213, 1973. Am. J. Surg., *124:*551, 1972

WANG, J. H. *et al*: Evaluation of surgical procedure of sagittal split osteotomy of mandibular ramus. Oral Surg., *38:*167, 1974

WANG, J. H., AND WAITE, D. E.: Comparison of vertical and sagittal split osteotomies of mandibular ramus, PRS, *57:*672, 1976. J. Oral Surg., *33:*596, 1975

WANG J. K.: Acupuncture in China, PRS, *54:*249, 1974. Anesth. & Analg., *53:*111, 1974

WANG, K. H.: Lateral anastomosis of the lacrimal apparatus and lacrimal ductules. Chinese Med. J. (Engl.), *6:*424, 1975 (Chinese)

WANG, S., AND HO, J.: Infraclavicular percutaneous catheterization of subclavian vein, PRS, *54:*692, 1974. Chinese M. J., *5:*80, 1974

WANG, Y., AND LI, C.: Metal-plastic jaw implant in repair of major mandibular defect ameloblastoma resection, PRS, *54:*701, 1974. Chinese M. J., *5:*84, 1974

WANGENSTEEN, S. L., MOORE, F. D., AND

WALDHAUSEN, J. A.: Production and distribution of surgeons in United States, PRS, *55:*258, 1975. Bull. Am. Coll. Surgeons, *59:*17, 1974

WANG-NORDERUD, R. *et al*: Mandibular prognathism. J. Oslo City Hospital, *25:*57, 1975

WANG-NORDERUD, R., AND RAGAB, R. R.: Osteocartilaginous exostosis of mandibular condyle, PRS, *57:*672, 1976. Scand. J. Plast. Reconstr. Surg., *9:*165, 1975

WANNEMACHER, M. F.: Radical treatment of cylindromas. Fortschr. Kiefer. Gesichtschir., *15:*81, 1972 (German)

War Injuries (See also *Blast Injuries; Gunshot Wounds*)

War surgery in forward surgical hospital in Vietnam, continuing report (Byerly, Pendse), PRS, *48:*612, 1971. Mil. Med., *136:*221, 1971

Pulsating water jet devices in debridement of combat wounds (Bhaskar *et al*), PRS, *48:*612, 1971. Mil. Med., *136:*264, 1971

Casualties from napalm in Vietnam (Zhukov). Voen. Med. Zh., *8:*85, 1971 (Russian)

Current status of the problem of treatment of maxillofacial wounds in field conditions (Kabakov). Voen. Med. Zh., *11:*16, 1971 (Russian)

Combat casualties, clinical fat embolism in (McNamara *et al*), PRS, *51:*711, 1973. Ann. Surg., *176:*54, 1972

War casualties, ketamine as anesthetic agent (Austin, Tamlyn), PRS, *53:*615, 1974. J. Roy. Army M. Corps, *18:*15, 1972

American military surgeon, treatment of soft tissue war wounds by (Shephard, Rich), PRS, *51:*711, 1973. Mil. Med., *137:*264, 1972

Vietnam, skin infections in (Allen *et al*), PRS, *52:*103, 1973. Mil. Med., *137:*295, 1972

War injuries, surgical rehabilitation after extensive losses in lower face (Parsons, Beckwith, Thering), PRS, *49:*533, 1972

Exostosis following grenade injury to hand (Lagundoye, Oluwasanmi), PRS, *54:*375, 1974. Hand, *5:*149, 1973

Vietnam, snakebites in, treatment (Berlinger, Flowers), PRS, *52:*601, 1973. Mil. Med., *138:*139, 1973

Facial fractures in combat, midface and mandibular (Linder), PRS, *53:*105, 1974. Mil. Med., *138:*487, 1973

Vietnam, South, maxillofacial rehabilitation in (Sazima, Scott, Moore), PRS, *54:*235, 1974. Mil. Med., *138:*824, 1973

Review of the treatment of facial injuries in the Nigerian Civil War (Awty *et al*). Trans. Int. Conf. Oral Surg., *4:*291, 1973

War injuries of upper extremity (Brara,

War Injuries—Cont.
  Kathpalia, Char), PRS, *56:*228, 1975. Indian J. Surg., *36:*379, 1974
  War, maxillofacial injuries in (Acharyya), PRS, *56:*225, 1975. Indian J. Surg., *36:*392, 1974
  Methods of treatment of after-effects of battle injuries in war invalids (Grigor'ev). Ortop. Travmatol. Protez., *34:*1, 1974 (Russian)
  CMRI hospital in Saigon, report on (Barsky) (Letter to the Editor), PRS, *53:*464, 1974
  Paralysis, facial, produced by combat wounds, treatment of (Morgan, Cramer), PRS, *53:*647, 1974
  Israel war, recent, initial burn experience in (Levin, Bornstein), PRS, *54:*432, 1974
  Maxillo-facial injuries from the war in Cambodia (Hor). Rev. Stomatol. Chir. Maxillofac., *75:*1021, 1974 (French)
  Vietnam conflict, incidence of postoperative wound infections during (Latina), PRS, *57:*677, 1976. Mil. Med., *140:*354, 1975
  Vietnam, Barsky Unit, end of chapter, end of story? (Mills) (Letter to the Editor), PRS, *57:*654, 1976

WARD, C. M.: Injury of the facial nerve during surgery of the parotid gland. Brit. J. Surg., *62:*401, 1975
WARD, J. N. *et al*: Hidradenitis suppurativa of scrotum and perineum. Urology, *4:*463, 1974
WARD, P. H. *et al*: Serious cosmetic complications of osteoplastic frontal bone. Arch. Otolaryng., *98:*389, 1973
WARD, P. H. *et al*: Juvenile angiofibroma: a more rational therapeutic approach based upon clinical and experimental evidence. Laryngoscope, *84:*2181, 1974
WARD, V. J.: Clinical assessment of use of free gingival graft for correcting localized recession associated with frenal pull. J. Periodontal., *45:*78, 1974
WARDA, F. *et al*: Tumors and tumor-like lesions of the hand. Chir. Narzadow. Ruchu Ortop. Pol., *39:*773, 1974 (Polish)
WARDEN, G. D. *et al*: Hypernatremic state in hypermetabolic burn patients, PRS, *52:*598, 1973. Arch. Surg., *106:*420, 1973
WARDEN, G. D., WILMORE, D. W., AND PRUITT, B. A.: Central venous thrombosis: hazard of medical progress, PRS, *53:*489, 1974. J. Trauma, *13:*620, 1973
WARDEN, G. D. *et al*: Suppression of leukocyte chemotaxis *in vitro* by chemotherapeutic agents used in management of thermal injuries, PRS, *57:*263, 1976. Ann. Surg., *181:*363, 1975
WARKANY, JOSEPH: *Congenital Malformations: Notes and Comments.* Year Book Medical Publishers, Chicago, 1971. PRS, *52:*570, 1973

WARREN, D. W.: The determination of velopharyngeal incompetence by aerodynamic and acoustical techniques. Clin. Plast. Surg., *2:*229, 1975
WARREN, D. W., TRIER, W. C., AND BEVIN, A. G.: Effect of restorative procedures on nasopharyngeal airway in cleft palate, PRS, *56:*108, 1975. Cleft Palate J., *11:*367, 1974
WARREN, J. M.: Operations for fissure of hard and soft palate (Classic Reprint), PRS, *48:*271, 1971
WARREN, K. S.: Marked prolongation of skin homograft survival with niridazole (with Mandel, Mahmoud), PRS, *55:*76, 1975
WARREN, R. F. *et al*: Prolonged traumatic dislocation of mandible. J. Oral Surg., *32:*555, 1974
WARREN, R. P., LOFGREEN, J. S., AND STEINMULLER, D.: Factors responsible for differential survival of heart and skin allografts in inbred rats, PRS, *53:*689, 1974. Transplantation, *16:*458, 1973
WARTHAN, T. L., RUDOLPH, R. I., AND GROSS, P. R.: Isolated plantar fibromatosis, PRS, *54:*379, 1974. Arch. Dermat., *108:*823, 1973

Warts

  Warts, periungual, causing bone destruction of distal phalanx (Gardner, Acker), PRS, *52:*452, 1973. Arch. Dermat., *107:*275, 1973

Warts, Plantar: See *Plantar Warts*

WASAN, S. M.: Sebaceous lymphadenoma of parotid gland, PRS, *49:*475, 1972. Cancer, *28:*1019, 1971
WASHIO, H.: Intestinal conduit for free transplantation of other tissues, PRS, *48:*48, 1971
WASHIO, H.: Further experiences with retroauricular flap, PRS, *50:*160, 1972
WASHIO, H.: Use of pterygoid muscle sling to provide glossomimic function after total glossectomy, PRS, *51:*497, 1973
WASHIO, H.: Cryptotia: pathology and repair, PRS, *52:*648, 1973
WASIK, F. *et al*: Fibroxanthoma resembling hemangioma of group of solitary blue rubber bleb nevus. Dermatol. Monatsschr., *160:*35, 1974 (German)
WASSERMAN, B. S.: Development of an oral cancer detection program in a hospital. N. Y. State Dent. J., *41:*77, 1975
WATANABE, Y. *et al*: Bleomycin therapy of oral cancer. Trans. Int. Conf. Oral Surg., *4:*147, 1973
WATERHOUSE, C.: Gamma globulin production and light-chain metabolism in patients with metastatic cancer, PRS, *56:*472, 1975. Cancer Res., *35:*987, 1975

WATERS, W. R.: Branchio-skeleto-genital syndrome, new hereditary syndrome (with Elsahy), PRS, *48:*542, 1971

WATSON, A. C.: Innervated muco-muscular flap for correction of defects of vermilion border of lip. Brit. J. Plast. Surg., *26:*355, 1973

WATSON, A. C. *et al*: Thermography in plastic surgery. J. R. Coll. Surg. Edinb., *17:*247, 1972

WATSON, H. K. *et al*: Post-traumatic interosseus-lumbrical adhesions. A cause of pain and disability in the hand. J. Bone & Joint Surg., (Am.), *56:*79, 1974

WATSON, J.: Soft tissue aspects of facial fractures. Proc. Roy. Soc. Med., *65:*918, 1972

WATSON, T. A.: Discussion of "Biological basis for management of benign disease of the breast: case against subcutaneous mastectomy," by Peacock, PRS, *55:*225, 1975

WATTS, G. T.: Letter: Breast prostheses. Lancet, *2:*280, 1975

WATTS, G. T.: Letter: Breast prostheses. Lancet, *1:*145, 1976

WAZNY, M. AND CZERWONKA, R.: Radiological appearance of lower pharynx following laryngectomy and management of tissue defect by modified method of Messerklinger. Otolaryngol. Pol., *26:*681, 1972 (Polish)

WEATHERALL, J. A. C.: Detection of incidence of congenital malformations in community, PRS, *48:*91, 1971. Proc. Roy. Soc. Med., *63:*1251, 1970

WEATHERLEY-WHITE, R. C. A. *et al*: Submucous cleft palate, incidence, natural history, indications for treatment, PRS, *49:*297, 1972

WEAVER, A. W. *et al*: Management of penetrating wounds of neck, PRS, *49:*241, 1972. Surg. Gynec. & Obst., *133:*49, 1971

WEAVER, A. W., AND SMITH, D. B.: Frozen autogenous mandibular stent-graft for immediate reconstruction in oral cancer surgery, PRS, *53:*499, 1974. Am. J. Surg., *126:*505, 1973

WEAVER, A. W., AND SMITH, D. B.: Cryosurgery for head and neck cancer, PRS, *57:*540, 1976. Am. J. Surg., *128:*466, 1974

WEAVER, P. C., AND COPEMAN, P. W. M.: Simple surgery for axillary hyperhidrosis, PRS, *48:*606, 1971. Proc. Roy. Soc. Med., *64:*607, 1971

WEAVER, P. C. *et al*: Salvage procedures for locally advanced malignant melanoma of the lower limb (with special reference to the role of isolated limb perfusion and radical lymphadenectomy). Clin. Oncol., *1:*45, 1975

WEBB, F. W. S.: Calcinosis, PRS, *55:*719, 1975. Proc. Roy. Soc. Med., *67:*466, 1974

WEBB, P. J.: Hand table. Hand, *7:*187, 1975

WEBBER, W. B.: Finger-flexion device for flexor tendon injuries, PRS, *48:*284, 1971

WEBBER, W. B.: Proximal interphalangeal joint flexion contracture secondary to injury of anomalous ulnar lumbrical muscle insertion, PRS, *55:*226, 1975

WEBER, B.: Eating with a trach, PRS, *56:*355, 1975. Am. J. Nursing, *74:*1439, 1974

WEBER, G. *et al*: Combined cytostatic and surgical treatment of extensive basal cell epitheliomata. Brit. J. Dermatol., *86:*408, 1972

WEBER, J., JR. *et al*: Restrictive pharyngeal flap. Brit. J. Plast. Surg., *23:*347, 1970

WEBER, S. P.: Microbuccal fold extension for implant and other surgical procedures. J. Prosthet. Dent., *27:*423, 1972

WEBRE, D. R., AND ARENS, J. F.: Use of cephalic and basilic veins for introduction of central venous catheters, PRS, *53:*250, 1974. Anesthesiology, *38:*389, 1973

WEBSTER, G. V.: Ischemic face-lift, PRS, *50:*560, 1972

WEBSTER, G. V.: Skin excisions in reduction rhinoplasty, PRS, *51:*289, 1973

WEBSTER, R. C.: Use of double W-plasty in upper blepharoplasty (with Courtiss, White), PRS, *53:*25, 1974

WEBSTER, R. C.: Selection of alternatives in augmentation mammaplasty (with Courtiss, White), PRS, *54:*552, 1974

WEBSTER, R. C., WHITE, M. F., AND COURTISS, E. H.: Nasal tip correction in rhinoplasty, PRS, *51:*384, 1973

WECKESSER, ELDEN, C.: *Treatment of Hand Injuries. Preservation and Restoration of Function.* Year Book Medical Publishers, Chicago, 1974. PRS, *55:*700, 1975

WEED, J. C. *et al*: Vulvoplasty in cases of exstrophy of bladder. Obstet. Gynecol., *43:*512, 1974

WEEKS, P. M.: Discussion of "Fibrotic arch around the deep branch of the ulnar nerve in the hand," by Lotem *et al*, PRS, *52:*556, 1973

WEEKS, P. M.: Reconstruction of digital pulleys (with Wray), PRS, *53:*534, 1974

WEEKS, P. M.: Discussion of "Augmentation of wound strength by pretreatment with epinephrine," by Myers, Rightor, PRS, *54:*351, 1974

WEEKS, P. M.: Plastic surgery and burns. Surg. Gynec. & Obst., *138:*212, 1974

WEEKS, P. M.: Factors in production of inconspicuous scars (with Wray, Holtmann), PRS, *56:*86, 1975

WEEKS, P. M.: Should an incompletely severed tendon be sutured? (with Reynolds, Wray), PRS, *57:*36, 1976. Discussion by Kleinert, PRS, *57:*236, 1976

WEEKS, P. M.: Lateral-volar finger flap for treatment of burn syndactyly (with Mac-

Dougal, Wray), PRS, *57:*167, 1976

WEEKS, P. M.: Spontaneous regression of primary lesion of metastatic malignant melanoma (with MacDougal, Wray), PRS, *57:*355, 1976

WEEKS, PAUL M., AND WRAY, R. CHRISTIE: *Management of Acute Hand Injuries. A Biological Approach.* C. V. Mosby Co., St. Louis, 1973. PRS, *54:*216, 1974

WEERDA, H.: Prosthetic cover in carcinomas of jaw and face. Z. Laryngol. Rhinol. Otol., *52:*445, 1973 (German)

WEERDA, H. *et al*: Surgery of cervical trachea. Prax. Pneumol., *Suppl 28:*1007, 1974 (German)

WEHBY, V., AND SALTI, I.: Significance of gynecomastia, PRS, *56:*677, 1975. Lebanese M. J., *27:*719, 1974

WEHMER, W.: Current status of parotid surgery. Med. Klin., *68:*410, 1973 (German)

WEHNER, R. J.: Therapeutic, cosmetic effects of oral surgery, PRS, *57:*259, 1976. AORN, *22:*52, 1975

WEHNERT, J.: Correlation between hypospadias and other congenital anomalies, PRS, *56:*466, 1975. Ztschr. Urol., *67:*857, 1975

WEHNERT, J. *et al*: Value of supplementary measures for improvement of results in the hypospadias surgery. Z. Urol. Nephrol., *67:*595, 1974 (German)

WEIDNER, F.: Prognosis in malignant melanoma. Med. Klin., *68:*419, 1973 (German)

WEIDNER, F. AND HORNSTEIN, O. P.: Regional lymph node metastasis in malignant melanoma. Arch. Derm. Forsch., *245:*50, 1972 (German)

WEIGERT, M. *et al*: Silicone rubber-implants in hand surgery. Arch. Orthop. Unfallchir., *73:*189, 1972 (German)

WEIJERMAN, J. E. *et al*: Perforation in a case of submucous cleft palate due to an aphthous ulcer. Brit. J. Oral Surg., *10:*217, 1972

WEIL, P. H., AND STEICHEN, F. M.: Treatment of penetrating injuries of neck, PRS, *49:*110, 1972. J. Trauma, *11:*590, 1971

WIELAND, H.: Simple operation for bat ears. Laryngol. Rhinol. Otol. (Stuttg.), *53:*556, 1974 (German)

WEILBY, A.: Surgical treatment of osteoarthritis of carpometacarpal joint of thumb, PRS, *49:*583, 1972. Scand. J. Plast. Reconstr. Surg., *5:*136, 1971

WEINBERG, B. *et al*: Relationship between three oral breath pressure ratios and ratings of severity of nasality for talkers with cleft palate. Cleft Palate J., *8:*251, 1971

WEINBERG, F. B.: External physiognomic prostheses as adjunct to surgery. Trans. Pa. Acad. Ophthalmol. Otolaryngol., *26:*107,

1973

WEINBERG, S. *et al*: Maxillo-mandibular surgery for correction of dentofacial formities. 1. Preoperative evaluation. J. Can. Dent. Assoc., *39:*263, 1973

WEINBERG, S. *et al*: Maxillo-mandibular surgery for correction of dentofacial deformities. 2. Mandibular prognathism. J. Can. Dent. Assoc., *39:*342, 1973

WEINBERG, S. *et al*: Maxillo-mandibular surgery for correction of dentofacial deformities. 3. Maxillary protrusion. J. Can. Dent. Assoc., *39:*416, 1973

WEINBERG, S. *et al*: Maxillo-mandibular surgery for correction of dentofacial deformities. 4. Maxillary retrusion. (Mandibular pseudoprognathism.) J. Can. Dent. Assoc., *39:*465, 1973

WEINBERG, S. *et al*: Maxillo-mandibular surgery for correction of dentofacial deformities. 5. Mandibular retrusion (retrognathia). J. Can. Dent. Assoc., *39:*544, 1973

WEINBERG, S. *et al*: Maxillo-mandibular surgery for correction of dentofacial deformities. 6. Apertognathia (open bite). J. Can. Dent. Assoc., *39:*623, 1973

WEINBERG, S., *et al*: Simplified technique to reduce perioral edema in intraoral sagittal split osteotomies. J. Oral Surg., *33:*61, 1975

WEINER, D. L.: On subcutaneous mastectomy (Editorial), PRS, *49:*654, 1972

WEINER, D. L., SILVER, L., AND AIACHE, A.: Preservation of traumatically amputated fingertips, PRS, *49:*609, 1972

WEINER, D. L. *et al*: Single dermal pedicle for nipple transposition in subcutaneous mastectomy, reduction mammaplasty, or mastopexy, PRS, *51:*115, 1973

WEINER, D. L. AIACHE, A. E., AND SILVER, L.: New soft, round silicone gel breast implant, PRS, *53:*174, 1974

WEINER, D. L. *et al*: Breast augmentation with improved implant material. R. N., *37:*12, 1974

WEINER, L. J. *et al*: Biologic principles affecting repair of flexor tendons. Adv. Surg., *5:*145, 1971

WEINER, L. J., HAPPEL, T. J., AND MADDEN, J. W.: Inhibiting collagen cross-linking on survival of skin allografts, PRS, *50:*99, 1972. Surg. Forum, *22:*486, 1971

WEINERT, C. R., JR. *et al*: Immune response to sarcomas, PRS, *56:*364, 1975. Clin. Orthop., *102:*207, 1974

WEINGARTEN, C. A.: Simultaneous bilateral radical neck dissection. Preservation of external jugular vein. Arch. Otolaryng., *97:*309, 1973

WEINSTEIN, G. D.: Epithelial neoplasms. Clin.

Pharmacol. Ther., *16:*922, 1974

WEINSTEIN, I. R.: Surgical treatment of mandibular asymmetry: report of a case. J. Oral Surg., *30:*303, 1972

WEINSTEIN, L. *et al:* Gas gangrene. New England J. Med., *289:*1129, 1973

WEINSTOCK, F. J.: Only an eye opener, PRS, *56:*104, 1975. Emerg. Med., *7:*123, 1975

WEINTRAUB, W. H. *et al:* Chickenpox epidemic in pediatric burn unit. Surgery, *76:*490, 1974

WEIPPL, G., AND ADER, H.: Congenital scalp defects in 4 generations, PRS, *56:*460, 1975. Klin. Paediatr., *187:*84, 1975

WEIR, N. F.: Theodore Billroth: first laryngectomy for cancer. J. Laryng. & Otol., *87:*1161, 1973

WEISFELD M.: Illustrated technique for the complete removal of nail matrix and hyponychium without skin incisions (Suppan nail technique no. 2). J. Am. Podiatry Assoc., *65:*481, 1975

WEISMAN, P. A.: Simplified technique in submental lipectomy, PRS, *48:*443, 1971

WEISMAN, P. A.: Indications for pharyngeal flap in primary repair of cleft palate, PRS, *48:*568, 1971

WEISMAN, P. A.: Photodrawer, PRS, *50:*627, 1972

WEISMAN, P. A.: "Piecemeal principle," staged operations for better results, PRS, *57:*570, 1976

WEISS, C. E.: Significance of Passavant's pad in post-obturator patients. Folia Phoniatr. (Basel), *24:*51, 1972

WEISS, C. E.: Speech pathologist's role in dealing with obturator-wearing school children, PRS, *56:*110, 1975. J. Speech & Hearing Disorders, *39:*153, 1974

WEISS, H. W.: Physiology of human penile erection, PRS, *50:*633, 1972. Ann. Int. Med., *76:*793, 1972

WEISS, I. S.: Complications following use of cheek flap rotation to reconstruct the lower lid. Ophthalmic Surg., *6:*42, 1975

WEISS, M. W. *et al:* Pilot study of 198 normal children's pinch strength and hand size in the growing hand. Am. J. Occup. Ther., *25:*10, 1971

WEISSMAN, S. L., AND PLASCHKES, Y.: Surgical correction of lobster-claw feet, PRS, *49:*89, 1972

WEISZ, G. M., RANG, M., AND SALTER, R. B.: Posttraumatic fat embolism in children: review of literature and experience in Hospital for Sick Children, PRS, *53:*500, 1974. J. Trauma, *13:*529, 1973

WEITZNER, S.: Subcutaneous liposarcoma. Int. J. Dermatol., *12:*283, 1973

WEITZNER, S.: Adenoid squamous-cell carcinoma of vermilion mucosa of lower lip. Oral Surg., *37:*589, 1974

WEITZNER, S.: Basal-cell carcinoma of the vermillion mucosa and skin of the lip. Oral Surg., *39:*634, 1975

WELCH, G. S. *et al:* Frostbite of the hands. Hand, *6:*33, 1974

WELHAM, R. A.: Canalicular obstruction and Lester-Jones tube—what to do when all else fails. Trans. Ophthalmol. Soc. U. K., *93:*623, 1973

WELHAM, R. A. *et al:* Results of dacryocystorhinostomy—analysis of causes for failure. Trans. Ophthalmol. Soc. U. K., *93:*601, 1973

WELLER, R. M.: Anaesthesia for cystic hygroma in a neonate. Anaesthesia, *29:*588, 1974

WELLER S. A. *et al:* Carcinoma of the oropharynx. Results of megavoltage radiation therapy in 305 patients. Am. J. Roentgenol., *26:*236, 1976

WELLING, R. E., AND TAGGART, J. P.: Carcinoid tumor metastatic to neck, PRS, *55:*724, 1975. Arch. Surg., *110:*111, 1975

WELLMANN, K. F.: Finger mutilation and polydactylia on prehistoric rock pictures in North America. Dtsch. Med. Wochenschr., *97:*527, 1972 (German)

WELLS, S. A. *et al:* Transplantation of parathyroid glands in man; clinical indications and results, PRS, *57:*404, 1976. Surgery, *78:*34, 1975

WELMAN, A. J.: Paralysis or disorders of body coordination. Ned. tijdschr. geneeskd., *116:*1029, 1972 (Dutch)

WELSH, B. E.: Non-endotracheal airway for surgery of head in outpatients. Anesthesiology, *40:*298, 1974

WELSH, G. F. *et al:* Present status of one-stage pharyngo-esophageal diverticulectomy. Surg. Clin. North Am., *53:*935, 1973

WELSH, N. H.: Mucous membrane grafting. Arch. Ophth., *92:*362, 1974

WELTY, M. J. *et al:* Patient with maxillofacial cancer. 1. Surgical treatment and nursing care. Nurs. Clin. North Am., *8:*137, 1973

WELVAART, K., AND POLANO, M. K.: Recurrent fibrosarcoma of skin preceded by inflammation, PRS, *52:*459, 1973. Arch. chir. neerl., *25:*35, 1973

WENDT, D. C.: Degenerative denture ridge—care and treatment. J. Prosthet. Dent., *32:*477, 1974

WENDT, H.: Combination of plastic operations by Meyer-Burgdorff, and Chocholka methods in one-stage surgical treatment of hypospadias. Z. Urol. Nephrol., *67:*861, 1974 (German)

WENGER, D. R.: Avulsion of profundus tendon insertion in football players, PRS, *52:*452,

1973. Arch. Surg., *106:*145, 1973

WENTGES, R. T.: Surgical anatomy of the pterygopalatine fossa. J. Laryng. & Otol., *89:*35, 1975

WENZEL, R. *et al*: Treatment of hand burns in general practice. Z. Allgemeinmed., *48:*1452, 1972 (German)

WEPNER, F., AND HOLLMANN, K.: Midface anthropometry on cephalometric radiograph in cleft lip and palate cases, PRS, *57:*537, 1976. J. Maxillo-facial Surg., *3:*188, 1975

WERB, A.: Aspects of treatment. Surgery of lacrimal sac. Ann. R. Coll. Surg. Engl., *54:*236, 1974

WERELDS, R. J. *et al*: Frenectomy in dental practice. Acta Stomatol. Belg., *68:*475, 1971 (Dutch)

WERNER, A.: Acceleration-deceleration neck trauma, remarks by a neurosurgeon. Praxis, *63:*1535, 1974 (French)

WERNER, R.: Plastic surgery of leishmaniasis of the face. Z. Laryngol. Rhinol. Otol., *51:*197, 1972 (German)

WERNER, R.: Leprosy in mouth, jaw, and facial region. Dtsch. Zahnaerztl. Z., *28:*64, 1973 (German)

WERNER, R.: Corrective osteotomy in region of apertura piriformis to widen nostril. Z. Laryngol. Rhinol. Otol., *52:*89, 1973 (German)

WERNER, U.: Diagnosis and therapy of parotid neoplasms. Dtsch. Gesundheitsw., *25:*358, 1970 (German)

WERNER-BRZEZINSKA, H., DABSKA, M., AND ADAMUS, J.: Fibrosarcoma of skin. Polski tygodnik lek., *28:*102, 1973 (Polish)

WERTZ, M. L.: Management of undescended lingual and subhyoid thyroid glands. Laryngoscope, *84:*507, 1974

WESLEY, R. K. *et al*: Primary malignant hemangioendothelioma of the gingiva. Report of a case and review of the literature. Oral Surg., *39:*103, 1975

WESSELS, J. V. *et al*: Effect of nitrous oxide on ketamine anesthesia. Anesthesiology, *39:*382, 1973

WESSER, D. R.: Repair of cryptotic ear with trefoil flap, PRS, *50:*192, 1972

WESSINGHAGE, D.: Principles of reconstructive surgery of the rheumatic hand. Langenbecks Arch. Chir., *339:*395, 1975 (German)

WEST, R. A. *et al*: Posterior maxillary surgery, its place in the treatment of dentofacial deformities. J. Oral Surg., *30:*562, 1972

WEST, R. A. *et al*: Maxillary ostectomies for preprosthetic surgery. J. Oral Surg., *32:*13, 1974

WEST, R. A. *et al*: Maxillary alveolar hyperplasia, diagnosis and treatment planning. J. Maxillo-facial Surg., *3:*239, 1975

WESTBROOK, K. C. *et al*: Chemodectomas of neck, selective management, PRS, *52:*102, 1973. Am. J. Surg., *124:*760, 1972

WESTBURG, S. P. *et al*: Multiple cutaneous squamous cell carcinomas during immunosuppressive therapy. Arch. Dermat., *107:*893, 1973

WESTON, E. G., AND KUKRAL, A. J.: Clostridia, PRS, *53:*691, 1974. Rocky Mountain M. J., *70:*43, 1973

WESTWOOD, R. M., AND TILSON, H. B.: Complications of maxillary osteotomies, PRS, *57:*116, 1976. J. Oral Surg., *33:*104, 1975

WETTE, R.: Probability model for survival in radical neck surgery and the estimation of expected survival in elective neck surgery. Ann. Otol. Rhin. & Laryng., *80:*651, 1971

WETTLAUGER, J. N.: Cutaneous chordee, fact or fancy. Urology, *4:*293, 1974

WEXLER, M. R.: Nasal septum: experimental and clinical correlation of surgery or injury. Laryngoscope, *81:*1409, 1971

WEXLER, M. R., AND NEUMAN, Z.: Use of foam rubber sponge in tie-over dressings for skin grafting, PRS, *50:*301, 1972

WEXLER, M. R. *et al*: Demonstrating the Z-plasty. Brit. J. Plast. Surg., *26:*417, 1973

WEXLER, M. R., AND ONEAL, R. M.: Areolar sharing to reconstruct the absent nipple, PRS, *51:*176, 1973

WEXLER, M. R. *et al*: Tendon grafts for isolated injuries of the flexor digitorum profundus tendon. Isr. J. Med. Sci., *10:*1448, 1974

WEXLER, M. R., AND NOVARK, B. W.: Hanhart's syndrome, PRS, *54:*99, 1974

WEXLER, M. R., YESCHUA, R., AND NEUMAN, Z.: Early treatment of burns of dorsum of hand by tangential excision and skin grafting, PRS, *54:*268, 1974

WEXLER, M. R. *et al*: Cross-hand, cross-finger neurovascular flap: a preliminary report. Brit. J. Plast. Surg., *28:*216, 1975

WEXLER, M. R. *et al*: Reconstruction of breast in cases of macromastia and ptosis. Harefuah, *88:*213, 1975 (Hebrew)

WEY, W. *et al*: Hamartoma of the hypopharynx. H. N. O., *22:*217, 1974 (German)

WHEELER, E. S., AND MILLER, T. A.: Blister and the second degree burn in guinea pigs: effect of exposure, PRS, *57:*74, 1976

WHELAN, C. S.: Electrocoagulation in treatment of skin cancers of nose, ear and eye areas. Bull. Soc. Internat. Chir., *31:*557, 1972

WHELAN, C. S., AND DECKERS, P. J.: Electrocoagulation and curettage for carcinoma involving skin of face, nose, eyelids, and ears, PRS, *52:*214, 1973. Cancer, *31:*159, 1973

WHICKER, J. H. *et al*: Hemilateral rhinotomy in treatment of hereditary hemorrhagic telangiectasis. Arch. Otolaryng., *96:*319, 1972

WHICKER, J. H. *et al*: Surgical treatment of squamous cell carcinoma of base of tongue. Laryngoscope, *82:*1853, 1972

WHICKER, J. H. *et al*: Wilfred Batten Lewis Trotter, 1872 to 1939. His legacy to pharyngeal surgeons. Arch. Otolaryng., *97:*423, 1973

WHICKER J. H. *et al*: Surgical treatment of squamous cell carcinoma of tonsil. Laryngoscope, *84:*90, 1974

WHINERY, J. G.: Lap joint mandibular ostectomy. J. Oral Surg., *33:*223, 1975

WHITAKER, L. *et al*: Prospective and randomized series comparing superior and inferior based posterior pharyngeal flaps, PRS, *52:*100, 1973. Cleft Palate J., *9:*304, 1972

WHITAKER, L. A.: Characteristics of skin of importance to surgeon. Int. Surg., *57:*877, 1972

WHITAKER, L. A.: Importance of muscle reconstruction in primary and secondary cleft lip repair (with Randall, LaRossa), PRS, *54:*316, 1974

WHITAKER, L. A.: Structural goals in craniofacial surgery. Cleft Palate J., *12:*23, 1975

WHITAKER, L. A.: Preservation of a posterior pharyngeal flap during maxillary advancement (with Ruberg, Randall, PRS, *57:*335, 1976

WHITAKER, L. A. *et al*: Retaining articular cartilage in finger joint amputations, PRS, *49:*542, 1972

WHITAKER, L. A., LEHR, H. B., AND ASKOVITZ, S. I.: Cancer of the tongue. Results of treatment in 258 consecutive cases, PRS, *50:*363, 1972

WHITAKER, L. A., AND GRAHAM, W. P., III: Management of hand infections in the narcotic addict, PRS, *52:*384, 1973

WHITAKER, L. A., KANTOWITZ, J. A., AND RANDALL, P.: Nasolacrimal apparatus in congenital facial anomalies, PRS, *55:*381, 1975. J. Maxillo-facial Surg., *2:*59, 1974

WHITAKER, L. A. *et al*: Healing of lined and unlined parasitic and nonparasitic flaps. J. Surg. Oncol., *6:*511, 1974

WHITAKER, L. A. *et al*: Developing field of craniofacial surgery. Pediatrics, *54:*571, 1974

WHITE, A. A., III: Disappearing bone disease with arthropathy and severe scarring of the skin. A report of four cases seen in South Vietnam. J. Bone & Joint Surg. (Br.), *53:*303, 1971

WHITE, A. A., III *et al*: Management of the foot in leprosy. Clin. Orthop., *85:*115, 1972

WHITE, C. E.: Preparation of antilymphocyte serum by transplantation of lymphoid heterografts to anterior chamber of rabbit eye, PRS, *52:*66, 1973

WHITE, D. K. *et al*: Median mandibular cyst: review of literature and report of two cases. J. Oral Surg., *33:*372, 1975

WHITE, D. K. *et al*: Odontogenic myxoma. Clinical and ultrastructural study. Oral Surg., *39:*901, 1975

WHITE, J. A., III *et al*: Facial fractures in small children. South. Med. J., *64:*1207, 1971

WHITE, J. H.: Tycron for canalicular repair. Am. J. Ophth., *75:*731, 1973

WHITE, J. J., AND HALLER, J. A., JR.: An improved technique for tracheostomy in infants and children. Med. Times, *101:*120, 1973

WHITE, J. S., AND WEXLER, H. R.: Baby with tail, PRS, *54:*382, 1974. J. Pediat. Surg., *8:*833, 1973

WHITE, M. F.: Nasal tip correction in rhinoplasty (with Webster, Courtiss), PRS, *51:*384, 1973

WHITE, M. F.: Use of double W-plasty in upper blepharoplasty (with Courtiss, Webster), PRS, *53:*25, 1974

WHITE, M. F.: Selection of alternatives in augmentation mammaplasty (with Courtiss, Webster), PRS, *54:*552, 1974

WHITE, P. F., AND JOHNSTON, R. R.: Interaction of ketamine and halothane in rats, PRS, *57:*267, 1976. Anesthesiology, *42:*179, 1975

WHITE, R. H., JR. *et al*: Polyglycolic acid sutures in ophthalmic surgery. Trans. Am. Acad. Ophthalmol. Otolaryngol., *78:*632, 1974

WHITE, R. P., JR. *et al*: Study of facial height changes after mandibular osteotomy in 46 patients. J. Oral Surg., *29:*858, 1971

WHITE, W. F.: Flexor muscle slide in the spastic hand: the Max Page operation. J. Bone & Joint Surg. (Br.), *54:*453, 1972

WHITE, W. L.: Healing of second degree burns; comparison of effects of early application of homografts and coverage with tape (with Miller), PRS, *49:*552, 1972

WHITE, W. L.: Avulsion injury of long flexor tendons (with Chang, Thoms), PRS, *50:*260, 1972

WHITE, W. L.: Plastic surgery and burns. Surg. Gynec. & Obst., *134:*274, 1972

WHITEHEAD, E.: Atrophic rhinitis: proplast as an implant material in surgical treatment. Can. J. Otolaryngol., *4:*505, 1975

WHITEHEAD, F. D.: *Current Operative Urology.* Harper & Row, Hagerstown, Md., 1975. PRS, *57:*232, 1976

WHITLOW, D. R.: Our present technique for rhytidectomy (with Baker, Gordon), PRS, *52:*232, 1973

WHITLOW, D. R., AND CONSTABLE, J. D.: Crossed alar wing procedure for correction of late deformity in unilateral cleft lip nose,

PRS, *52:*38, 1973

WHITNEY, C. R., ANDERSON, R. P., AND ALLANSMITH, M. R.: Preoperatively administered antibiotics, PRS, *50:*93, 1972. Arch. Ophth., *87:*155, 1972

WHITSON, T. C., AND ALLEN, B. D.: Management of burned hand, PRS, *49:*106, 1972. J. Trauma, *11:*606, 1971

WHITTAM, D. E. *et al*: Malignant oncocytoma of the parotid gland. Brit. J. Surg., *58:*851, 1971

WICTORIN, L. *et al*: Changes in facial topography by stereometric method after surgical treatment of mandibular protrusion. Sven. Tandlak. Tidskr., *64:*373, 1971

WIDMAIER, W.: Intraoral closure of subcutaneous clefts of lip, PRS, *57:*121, 1976. J. Maxillo-facial Surg., *3:*84, 1975

WIDMAIER, W.: Surgical closure of exposed skull, PRS, *57:*527, 1976. J. Maxillo-facial Surg., *3:*149, 1975

WIDMANN, W. D.: Technique for changing tracheostomy tubes in the early postoperative patient. Crit. Care Med., *2:*277, 1974

WIEDEMAN, M. P. *et al*: Effects of cooling in the microvasculature after thermal injury. Microvasc. Res., *3:*154, 1971

WIEDEMANN, H. R. *et al*: Left-side idiopathic gynecomastia in twenty-eight-month-old boy. Helv. Paediatr. Acta, *28:*413, 1973 (German)

WIELAND, H.: Simple surgical technic for external ear correction. Arch. Klin. Exp. Ohren Nasen Kehlkopfheilkd., *199:*514, 1971 (German)

WIESENBAUGH, J. M., JR. *et al*: Orbital floor repair with nasal septal cartilage. Trans. Int. Conf. Oral Surg., *4:*308, 1973

WIGGERS, I. M.: USAF plastic surgeons and dentists aid disfigured and spread good will. Dent. Dig., *78:*13, 1972

WIGGINS, H. E., JR. *et al*: Free palatal mucosa grafts. Evaluation in 26 cases. Oral Surg., *35:*35, 1973

WIGGINS, H. E., JR. *et al*: Cementoblastoma of the maxilla: report of case. J. Oral Surg., *33:*302, 1975

WIKKELING, O. M. *et al*: In vitro studies on lines of osteotomy in pterygoid region. J. Maxillo-facial Surg., *1:*209, 1973

WILCOX, J. W. *et al*: Osteogenic sarcoma of mandible: review of literature and report of case. J. Oral Surg., *31:*49, 1973

WILD, H.: Surgical methods and results in congenital ptosis. Z. Aerztl. Fortbild. (Jena), *65:*976, 1971 (German)

WILDING, K. *et al*: Actinomycosis of bone. Aust. N. Z. J. Surg., *45:*61, 1975

WILFERT, H. *et al*: Experimental bases for administration of the Kiel bone chip as bone substitute in jaw surgery. Dtsch. Zahnaerztl Z., *27:*405, 1972 (German)

WILFLINGSEDER, P.: Construction of vagina by an intestinal mucosa-muscularis graft, PRS, *51:*704, 1973. Chir. Plast., *1:*15, 1971

WILFLINGSEDER, P., *et al*: Urgent plastic surgery of large soft-tissue lesions. Langenbeck's Arch. Chir., *329:*88, 1971

WILFLINGSEDER, P.: Reconstruction of the vagina with a graft composed of intestinal mucosa. Nouv. Presse Med., *1:*1794, 1972 (French)

WILFLINGSEDER, P.: Advances in the surgical treatment of skin tumors. Wien. Med. Wochenschr., *124:*593, 1974 (German)

WILFLINGSEDER, P.: Ten years experience with alloplastics in facial paresis. In *Plastische und Wiederherstellungs-Chirurgie*, ed. by Hohler; pp. 107–9. Schattauer, Stuttgart, 1975 (German)

WILFLINGSEDER, P.: Construction of the vagina by means of split-skin or mucosal grafts. Langenbecks Arch. Chir., *339:*403, 1975 (German)

WILFLINGSEDER, P., DAPUNT, O., AND FODISCH, H.: Subsequent behavior of small bowel composite grafts in vagina, PRS, *52:*207, 1973. Chir. Plast., *1:*281, 1972

WILGIS, E. F.: Tourniquet in reconstructive surgery of the hand. Handchirurgie, *4:*99, 1972

WILGIS, E. F. S.: Observations on the effects of tourniquet ischemia, PRS, *49:*664, 1972. J. Bone & Joint Surg., *53:*1343, 1971

WILGIS, E. F. S. *et al*: Evaluation of small-vessel flow, study of dynamic non-invasive techniques, PRS, *55:*509, 1975. J. Bone & Joint Surg., *56A:*1199, 1974

WILHELM, A.: Tendon sutures, tendon transplantations and tendon transfer on the hand. Chirurg., *46:*301, 1975 (German)

WILHELM, K.: Stable osteosynthesis in fractures of the hand bone. Arch. Orthop. Unfallchir., *70:*275, 1971 (German)

WILHELM, K.: Stable AO-osteosynthesis in open hand fractures. Arch. Orthop. Unfallchir., *71:*6, 1971 (German)

WILHELM, K.: Post-traumatic carpal tunnel syndrome. Arch. Orthop. Unfallchir., *72:*87, 1972 (German)

WILHELM, K.: Bridling of nerve defects using lyophilized homologous grafts. Handchirurgie, *4:*25, 1972 (German)

WILHELM, K.: Proceedings: Conservative or surgical treatment of hand fractures. Munch. Med. Wochenschr., *117:*364, 1975 (German)

WILHELM, K. *et al*: Indications for the AO treatment of fractures of the bones of the hand. Munch. Med. Wochenschr., *115:*371, 1973

(German)

WILKE, A.: Excision or radiation of basaliomas of the lids. Klin. Monatsbl. Augenheilkd., *165:*676, 1974 (German)

WILKERSON, D. C.: Gastrointestinal bleeding as manifestation of von Recklinghausen's disease of the skin, PRS, *49:*108, 1972. Am. Surgeon, *37:*298, 1971

WILKIE, N. D.: Role of the prosthodontist in preprosthetic surgery. J. Prosthet. Dent., *33:*386, 1975

WILKINS, S. A., JR.: Carcinoma of the posterior pharyngeal wall. Am. J. Surg., *122:*477, 1971

WILKINSON, F. J. *et al:* Probability in lymph node sectioning. Cancer, *33:*1269, 1974

WILKINSON, T. S.: Tissue adhesives in cutaneous surgery. Arch. Dermat., *106:*834, 1972

WILKINSON, T.S.: Reconstruction of thumb by radial nerve innervated cross finger flap, PRS, *51:*476, 1973. South. M. J., *65:*992, 1972

WILKINSON, T. S.: Repair of a submental depression occurring after rhytidectomy, PRS, *57:*33, 1976

WILKINSON, T. S., RYBKA, F. J., AND PALETTA, F. X.: Studies in nonsuture immobilization of skin, PRS, *51:*709, 1973. South. M. J., *65:*25, 1972

WILKINSON, T. S., TENERY, J. H., AND ZUFI, D.: Skin graft donor site as model for evaluation of hemostatic agents, PRS, *51:*541, 1973

WILKINSON, T. S., AND IGLESIAS, J.: Tissue adhesive as adjunct in hair transplantation, PRS, *56:*103, 1975. South. M. J., *67:*1408, 1974

WILKINSON, T. S. *et al:* Room temperature vulcanizing Silastic in facial contour reconstruction. J. Trauma, *15:*479, 1975

WILLE, H. P.: Functional plastic surgery of nose. Schweiz. Med. Wochenschr., *103:*452, 1973 (German)

WILLEBRAND, H.: Fundamentals of utilization and technique of sliding graft from adjacent skin in covering defects. Langenbecks Arch. Chir., *334:*575, 1973 (German)

WILLEBRAND, H. *et al:* Primary surgical treatment of extensive soft tissue defects of the hand. Handchirurgie, *2:*34, 1970 (German)

WILLEMOT, J.: Clinical rhinomanometry and septorhinoplasty. J. Fr. Otorhinolaryngol., *24:*681, 685, 691, 1975 (French)

WILLEN, R. *et al:* Squamous cell carcinoma of gingiva. Histological classification and grading of malignancy. Acta Otolaryngol. (Stockh.), *79:*146, 1975

WILLIAMS, B.: Some surgeons and their hand injuries. Practitioner, *213:*717, 1974

WILLIAMS, C., ASTON, S., AND REES, T. D.: Effect of hematoma on thickness of pseudosheaths around silicone implants, PRS,

*56:*194, 1975

WILLIAMS, C. S.: Initial treatment of acute hand injuries. J. La. State Med. Soc., *124:*205, 1972

WILLIAMS, C. S. *et al:* Mycobacterium marinum (atypical acid-fast bacillus) infections of the hand. J. Bone & Joint Surg. (Am.), *55:*1042, 1973

WILLIAMS, C. S., AND RIORDAN, D.: High velocity injection injuries of hand, PRS, *54:*502, 1974. South. M. J., *67:*295, 1974

WILLIAMS, C. W.: Delaying of flaps. Useful adjunct. Brit. J. Plast. Surg., *26:*61, 1973

WILLIAMS, C. W.: Hypospadias, critical assessment of management (with Dickie), PRS, *54:*579, 1974

WILLIAMS, C. W. *et al:* Silastic sheeting in hand surgery. Hand, *4:*273, 1972

WILLIAMS, D. C.: Factors in tumor dissemination, PRS, *55:*723, 1975. Proc. Roy. Soc. Med., *67:*847, 1974

WILLIAMS, D. F., AND ROAF, ROBERT: *Implants in Surgery.* W. B. Saunders Co., London, Philadelphia, Toronto, 1973. PRS, *54:*480, 1974

WILLIAMS, D. I., *et al:* Further progress with reconstruction of the exstrophied bladder. Brit. J. Surg., *60:*203, 1973

WILLIAMS, E. O. *et al:* Mandibular replacements – a review of embedded implants. J. Prosthet. Dent., *35:*207, 1976

WILLIAMS, H. B.: Free transfer of skin flaps by microvascular anastomoses (with Daniel), PRS, *52:*16, 1973

WILLIAMS, H. B.: Hemangiomas of parotid gland in children, PRS, *56:*29, 1975

WILLIAMS, H. B.: Nerve gap: suture under tension *vs.* graft (with Terzis, Faibisoff), PRS, *56:*166, 1975

WILLIAMS, H. B., AND TERZIS, J.: Single fascicular recordings: intraoperative diagnostic tool for management of peripheral nerve lesions, PRS, *57:*562, 1976. Discussion by Collins, PRS, *57:*744, 1976

WILLIAMS, J. E.: Experiences with large series of Silastic breast implants, PRS, *49:*253, 1972

WILLIAMS, J. E.: Plastic surgery in an office surgical unit, PRS, *52:*513, 1973

WILLIAMS, J. L. *et al:* Urethroplasty. Brit. J. Urol., *44:*719, 1972

WILLIAMS, J. L. *et al:* Fibrous dysplastic lesions of jaws in Nigerians. Brit. J. Oral Surg., *11:*118, 1973

WILLIAMS, R. G.: Management of cancer of mouth. Ann. Roy. Coll. Surgeons England, *52:*49, 1973

WILLIAMS, R. G: Recurrent head and neck cancer: results of treatment, PRS, *57:*124, 1976. Brit. J. Surg., *61:*691, 1974

WIND, J.: Reflections of difficult decannulation. Arch. Otolaryng., *94:*426, 1971

WINE, W. M. *et al*: Marsupialization of a dentigerous cyst of the mandible: report of case. J. Oral Surg., *29:*742, 1971

WINE, W. M. *et al*: Iliac bone graft for restoration of avulsion defects of mandible. Case report. W. Va. Dent. J., *47:*7, 1973

WINEGAR, L., AND GRIFFIN, W.: Occult primary tumor, PRS, *54:*501, 1974. Arch. Otolaryng., *98:*159, 1973

WINKELMAN, N. Z. *et al*: Variant high sensory branch of the median nerve to the third web space. Bull. Hosp. Joint Dis., *34:*161, 1973

WINKLER, E.: Basic rules and problems with reduction mammaplasty in light of personal experience, PRS, *51:*230, 1973. Chir. Plast. *1:*85, 1972

WINNIE, A. P. *et al*: Interscalene cervical plexus block: single-injection technic, PRS, *57:*543, 1976. Anesth. Analg., Cleve., *54:*370, 1975

WINNINGER, A. L.: Anterior approach for fractures of the diaphyse and base of the first metacarpal. Nouv. Presse Med., *1:*1997, 1972 (French)

WINNINGER, A. L.: Determination of skin viability during trauma of limbs, PRS, *54:*624, 1974. J. chir., *107:*205, 1974

WINNINGER, A. L.: Simple technic for anesthesia of the hand and fingers. Nouv. Presse Med., *3:*1303, 1974 (French)

WINSLOW, R. B.: Altering the dimensions of canine face by induction of new bone formation (with Calabrese, Latham), PRS, *54:*467, 1974

WINSLOW, R. B. *et al*: Treatment of velopharyngeal incompetency by bilateral island sandwich flap combined with superiorly based pharyngeal flap, PRS, *55:*513, 1975. Cleft Palate J., *11:*272, 1974

WINSLOW, R. B. *et al*: Initial care for lacerations of flexor tendons of the hand. N. C. Med. J., *35:*38, 1974

WINSTOCK, D.: One-stage mandibular-maxillary reconstruction in the treatment of gross disproportion of the jaws. Brit. J. Oral Surg., *9:*115, 1971

WINSTON, M. F.: Results of treatment of injuries to the flexor tendons. Hand, *4:*45, 1972

WINSTON, P.: Traumatic nasal deformities, PRS, *55:*375, 1975. Proc. Roy. Soc. Med., *67:*713, 1974

WINTER, G. D.: Epidermal wound healing under new polyurethane foam dressing. (Lyofoam), PRS, *56:*531, 1975

WINTERS, R. W.: Total parenteral nutrition in pediatrics, PRS, *57:*268, 1976. Pediatrics, *56:*17, 1975

WINTHER, S. *et al*: Idiopathic gingival fibromatosis. Survey of literature and report of five cases. Tandlaegebladet, *77:*313, 1973 (Danish)

WINTSCH, K.: Skin neoplasms. Chirurg., *45:*313, 1974 (German)

WIRATMADJA, R. M.: Notes on esthetic surgery in the Indonesian. Clin. Plast. Surg., *1:*173, 1974

WISE, K. S.: Anatomy of the metacarpo-phalangeal joints, with observations of the aetiology of ulnar drift. J. Bone & Joint Surg. (Br.), *57:*485, 1975

WISE, L., MARGRAF, H. W., AND BALLINGER, W. F.: Adrenal cortical function in severe burns, PRS, *51:*606, 1973. Arch. Surg., *105:*213, 1972

WISE, L., MARGRAF, H. W., AND BALLINGER, W. F.: Effect of surgical trauma on conjugation pattern of 17-hydroxycorticosteroids, PRS, *52:*217, 1973. Surgery, *73:*163, 1973

WISE, R. J.: New inflatable implant for breast augmentation, PRS, *53:*360, 1974

WISKEMANN, A.: Nevi and nevus-similar syndrome, PRS, *53:*111, 1974. Chir. Praxis, *16:*629, 1972

WISSINGER, H. A.: Resection of hook of hamate, its place in treatment of median and ulnar nerve entrapment in hand, PRS, *56:*501, 1975

WISTH, P. J.: Integumental profile changes caused by surgical treatment of mandibular protrustion. Int. J. Oral Surg., *4:*32, 1975

WITEBSKY, F. G.: Denervated Meissner corpuscle, sequential histological study after nerve division in rhesus monkey (with Dellon, Terrill), PRS, *56:*182, 1975

WITEK, R.: Surgical treatment of crural varicose ulcers by Babcock-Linton method. Pol. Przegl. Chir., *45:*1209, 1973 (Polish)

WITKOWSKI, J. A. *et al*: Taping of cyst: method to facilitate removal of scalp cyst. Acta Physiol. Scand., *91:*226, 1974

WITKOWSKI, J. A. *et al*: Taping of a cyst: a method to facilitate removal of a scalp cyst. Atherosclerosis, *20:*226, 1974

WITSCHEL, H.: Mixed tumor of lacrimal gland with adenoid-cystic carcinoma. Klin. Monatsbl. Augenheilkd., *164:*206, 1974 (German)

WITT, W. S.: Cell size and growth characteristics of cultured fibroblasts isolated from normal and keloid tissue (with Russell), PRS, *57:*207, 1976

WITTELS, W.: Antibiotics and corticosteroids in the corticosteroid treatment of burns. Wien. Klin. Wochenschr., *83:*936, 1971 (German)

WITTELS, W.: Burns and their treatment. Z. Haut. Geschlechtskr., *46:*761, 1971 (German)

WITWICKA, Z. *et al*: Reconstruction of pharynx and cervical part of esophagus following

thermal burns. Am. J. Surg., *124:*720, 1972

Wood, P. B.: Wound infection in undressed sutured wounds of the hand. Brit. J. Surg., *58:*543, 1971

Wood, T.: Eye complications with blepharoplasty or other eyelid surgery (with DeMere, Austin), PRS, *53:*634, 1974

Wood, V. F.: Treatment of central polydactyly. Clin. Orthop., *74:*196, 1971

Woods, J. E.: Influence of immunologic responsiveness on head and neck cancer; therapeutic implications (Editorial), PRS, *56:*77, 1975

Woods, J. E. *et al*: Technique for the rapid performance of parotidectomy with minimal risk. Surg. Gynec. & Obst., *142:*87, 1976

Wood-Smith, D.: Report on 50 craniofacial operations (with Converse, McCarthy), PRS, *55:*283, 1975

Wood-Smith, D.: Orbital hypotelorism (with Converse, McCarthy), PRS, *56:*389, 1975

Wood-Smith, D. *et al*: Australian experience in craniofacial osteotomy for facial deformity. Aust. N. Z. J. Surg., *44:*382, 1974

Woodward, A. H. *et al*: Lymphangiosarcoma arising in chronic lymphedematous extremities. Cancer, *30:*562, 1972

Woolf, R. M.: Bilateral cleft lip repairs; review of 160 cases and description of present management (with Broadbent), PRS, *50:*36, 1972

Woolf, R. M.: Correction of saddle nose deformity with the upper-lateral turnover procedure (Follow-Up Clinic), PRS, *54:*482, 1974

Woolf, R. M., and Broadbent, T. R.: Four-flap Z-plasty, PRS, *49:*48, 1972

Woolridge, W. E. *et al*: Treatment of skin cancer by cryosurgery. Mon. Med., *72:*28, 1975

Work, W. P. *et al*: A study of tumors of the parapharyngeal space. Laryngoscope, *84:*1748, 1974

Work, W. P. *et al*: Recurrent benign mixed tumor and the facial nerve. Arch. Otolaryng., *102:*15, 1976

Worle, M. *et al*: Reposition and retention of lateral mid-facial fractures by means of a balloon catheter. Fortschr. Kiefer. Gesichtschir., *19:*178, 1975 (German)

Worley, R. *et al*: Treatment of continuity defect of mandible. J. Oral Surg., *31:*942, 1973

Worley, R. D.: Experimental use of poly (methyl methacrylate) implants in mandibular defects. J. Oral Surg., *31:*170, 1973

Worms, F. W. *et al*: Surgical orthodontic treatment planning: profile analysis and mandibular surgery. Angle Orthod., *46:*1, 1976

Worst, J.: Remarks on surgery of lacrimal apparatus in children. Annee Ther. Clin. Ophtalmol., *22:*187, 1971 (French)

Worst, P. K. M., Valentine, E. A., and Fu-

senig, N. E.: Formation of epidermis after reimplantation of pure primary epidermal cell cultures from perinatal mouse skin, PRS, *55:*518, 1975. J. Natl. Cancer Inst., *53:*1061, 1974

Worthen, E. F.: Regeneration of skull following deep electrical burn, PRS, *48:*1, 1971

Worthen, E. F.: Palmar split skin graft. Brit. J. Plast. Surg., *26:*408, 1973

Worthen, E. F.: Repair of forehead defects by rotation of local flaps, PRS, *57:*204, 1976

Worthington, P.: Management of the palatal pleomorphic adenoma. Brit. J. Oral Surg., *12:*132, 1974

Wound Healing

Wound infections after preoperative depilatory *versus* razor preparation (Seropian, Reynolds), PRS, *48:*518, 1971. Am. J. Surg., *121:*251, 1971

Vitamin A and cortisone, effect on wound infection (Stephens *et al*), PRS, *51:*609, 1973. Am. J. Surg., *121:*569, 1971

Wound, contaminated, studies in management, V. Assessment of effectiveness of pHisoHex and Betadine surgical scrub solutions (Custer *et al*), PRS, *49:*587, 1972. Am. J. Surg., *121:*572, 1971

Wound fluid zinc levels during tissue repair. Sequential determination by surgically implanted Teflon cylinders (Lichti *et al*), PRS, *49:*588, 1972. Am. J. Surg., *121:*665, 1971

Wound, contaminated, studies in management, VI. Therapeutic value of gentle scrubbing in prolonging limited period of effectiveness of antibiotics in contaminated wounds (Edlich *et al*), PRS, *49:*668, 1972. Am. J. Surg., *121:*668, 1971. VIII. Assessment of tissue adhesives for repair of contaminated tissue, PRS, *49:*361, 1972. Am. J. Surg., *122:*394, 1971

Wounds, surgical, susceptibility to postoperative surface contamination. Part VII. Studies in management of contaminated wound. (Schauerhamer *et al*), PRS, *49:*668, 1971. Am. J. Surg., *122:*74, 1971

Skin wounds in rats, study of traditional methods of care on tensile strength of (Stephens, Hunt, Dunphy), PRS, *49:*587, 1972. Am. J. Surg., *122:*78, 1971

Wound contracture, effect of delayed administration of corticosteroids (Stephens, Dunphy, Hunt), PRS, *48:*96, 1971. Ann. Surg., *173:*214, 1971

Wound healing, studies on biology of collagen during. III. Dynamic metabolism of scar collagen and remodeling of dermal wounds (Madden, Peacock), PRS, *51:*235,

Wound Healing—Cont.

1973. Ann. Surg., *174:*511, 1971

Blood supply of healing wounds: functional and angiographic (Myers, Cherry), PRS, *48:*299, 1971; *51:*708, 1973. Arch. Surg., *102:*49, 1971

Healing incisions in animals, simple standardized method for studying tensile strength of (Nagy, Zingg), PRS, *48:*202, 1971. Canad. J. Surg., *14:*136, 1971

Wound healing, effect of germ-free state (Donati *et al*), PRS, *48:*610, 1971. J. Surg. Res., *11:*163, 1971

Wound healing, studies of effects of diapulse treatment of various aspects in experimental animals (Constable, Scapicchio, Opitz), PRS, *48:*610, 1971. J. Surg. Res., *11:*254, 1971

Wounds, infected, effect of antibiotics and chemical adhesives on (Beasley *et al*), PRS, *49:*588, 1972. Mil. Med., *136:*566, 1971

Wounds, contaminated, effect of vancomycin, streptomycin and tetracycline pulsating jet lavage on (Cutright *et al*), PRS, *50:*98 1972. Mil. Med., *136:*810, 1971

Triamcinolone, follow-up on treatment of hypertrophic scars and keloids with (Ketchum, Robinson, Masters), PRS, *48:*256, 1971

Wound healing after delayed primary closure. Experimental study (Shepard), PRS, *48:*358, 1971

Strength development of skin incisions in young and old rats (Holm-Pedersen, Zederfeldt), PRS, *48:*610, 1971. Scand. J. Plast. Reconstr. Surg., *5:*13, 1971

Tissue culture techniques, use to evaluate new material developed to serve as artificial heart linings (Schultz, Bull, Braunwald), PRS, *48:*299, 1971. Surgery, *69:*510, 1971

Abscesses, deep soft tissue, secondary to nonpenetrating trauma (Heeb), PRS, *48:*298, 1971. Surgery, *69:*550, 1971

Wound healing, effect of iron deficiency anemia (Macon, Pories), PRS, *48:*399, 1971. Surgery, *69:*792, 1971

Wounds, granulating, evaluation of formalin-fixed skin as a temporary dressing (Silverstein *et al*), PRS, *49:*668, 1972. Surg. Forum, *22:*60, 1971

Wound infection, experimental, reduction with iodized gut sutures (Ludewig, Rudolf, Wangensteen), PRS, *49:*670, 1972. Surg. Gynec. & Obst., *133:*946, 1971

Wound healing, effect of laser radiation on (Mester *et al*). Z. Exp. Chir., *4:*307, 1971 (German)

Epidermal Wound Healing. Ed. by H. I.

Wound Healing—Cont.

Maibach and D. T. Rovee. Year Book Medical Publishers, Chicago, 1972. PRS, *52:*429, 1973

Wound healing, stimulation of, by laser rays (Mester *et al*). Acta Chir. Acad. Sci. Hung., *13:*315, 1972

Oxygen supply in healing tissue (Niinikoski, Hunt, Dunphy), PRS, *50:*422, 1972. Am. J. Surg., *123:*247, 1972

Wound fluid and plasma zinc levels in rats during tissue repair (Lichti, Schilling, Shurley), PRS, *50:*422, 1972. Am. J. Surg., *123:*253, 1972

Wounds, contaminated crushed, effectiveness of pulsating water jet lavage in treatment of (Gross, Cutright, Bhaskar), PRS, *51:*352, 1973. Am. J. Surg., *124:*373, 1972

Edema and healing rate of stasis ulcers of legs, relationship between (Myers, Rightor, Cherry), PRS, *51:*605, 1973. Am. J. Surg., *124:*666, 1972

Wound healing, thermographic study (Viitanen, Viljanto), PRS, *52:*105, 1973. Ann. chir. et gynaec. Fenniae, *60:*101, 1972

Vitamin E, inhibitory effects on collagen synthesis and wound repair (Ehrlich, Tarver, Hunt), PRS, *50:*421, 1972. Ann. Surg., *175:*235, 972

Wounds and burns, appraisal of allografts and xenografts as biological dressings for (Artz, Rittenburg, Yarbrough), PRS, *51:*236, 1973. Ann. Surg., *175:*934, 1972

Wound sepsis in plastic surgery unit (Morrison *et al*). Brit. J. Plast. Surg., *25:*435, 1972

Wound closure, technique and results of tissue glueing (Heiss), PRS, *52:*216, 1973. Bull. Soc. Internat. Chir., *6:*549, 1972

Cartilage extract, saline, for healing experimental long bone defects (Herold, Hurvitz, Tadmor), PRS, *51:*487, 1973. Internat. Surg., *57:*246, 1972

Wound healing, enzyme activity in regenerating epithelium. I. Acid phosphatase (Im, Hoopes, Sohn), PRS, *52:*103, 1973; II β-glucuronidase, PRS, *52:*104, 1973; III. β-galactosidase and β-glucosidase, PRS, *52:*104, 1973. J. Surg. Res., *12:*402, and 406, 1972. IV. Amino transferases and NADP-dependent enzymes, PRS, *53:*611, 1974. J. Surg. Res., *15:*262, 1973

Wounds, difficult, homograft skin for early management (Shuck, Bedeau, Thomas), PRS, *52:*105, 1973. J. Trauma, *12:*215, 1972

Cartilage, hyaline, further observations on capacity for regeneration (Walcher, Sturz), PRS, *51:*109, 1973. Langenbecks Arch. Chir., *331:*1, 1972

Wound healing complications following open

Wound Healing — Cont.

hand injuries (Geldmacher), PRS, *53:*367, 1974. Langenbecks Arch. Chir., *332:*479, 1972

Antiseptic agents and pulsating jet lavage on contaminated wounds, effects of (Gross *et al*), PRS, *50:*542, 1972. Mil. Med., *137:*145, 1972

Overgrafting, cutaneous dermal, indications for (Rees) (Follow-Up Clinic), PRS, *49:*566, 1972

Wounds of skin, autoradiographic investigations of connective tissue proliferation in (Helpap, Cremer), PRS, *51:*484, 1973. Res. Exper. Med., *157:*289, 1972

Tensile properties and morphology of healing wounds in young and old rats (Holm-Pedersen, Viidik), PRS, *51:*108, 1973. Scand. J. Plast. Reconstr. Surg., *6:*24, 1972

Wound oxygen, measurement with implanted Silastic tube (Niinikoski, Hunt), PRS, *50:*98, 1972. Surgery, *71:*22, 1972

Oxygen tension and wound healing (Chase), PRS, *50:*98, 1972. Surgery, *71:*150, 1972

Wounds, metabolic and circulatory contributions to oxygen gradients in (Ehrlich, Grislis, Hunt), PRS, *51:*352, 1973. Surgery, *72:*578, 1972

Wound healing, byssal thread formation: collagen-glycosaminoglycan interaction (Keiter, Bakowski, Weeks), PRS, *52:*328, 1973. Surg. Forum, *23:*27, 1972

Wound healing of skin flaps rotated into delayed or primary recipient sites (Hentz *et al*), PRS, *52:*329, 1973. Surg. Forum, *23:*34, 1972

Wound healing, influence of pure virus infection on (Bruckner *et al*), PRS, *52:*329, 1973. Surg. Forum, *23:*41, 1972

Wound contraction, effect of local smooth muscle antagonist (Morton, Madden, Peacock), PRS, *51:*709, 1973. Surg. Forum, *23:*511, 1972

Wound healing, stimulation of, by means of laser rays. (Clinical and electron microscopical study.) (Mester *et al*). Acta Chir. Acad. Sci. Hung., *14:*347, 1973

Ultrasound to strengthen sutured skin wounds in animals (Drastichova, Samohyl, Slavetinska), PRS, *53:*611, 1974. Acta chir. plast., *15:*114, 1973

Regeneration of limb after lengthening by distraction epiphysiolysis (Eydelshteyn, Udalova, Bochkarev), PRS, *54:*511, 1974. Acta chir. plast., *15:*149, 1973

Wounds, surgical, open and primarily closed, Evans blue dye content of (Prusak *et al*), PRS, *52:*601, 1973. Am. J. Surg., *125:*585, 1973

Wound Healing — Cont.

Wounds, contaminated, skin dressings in the treatment of (Allen *et al*), PRS, *53:*110, 1974. Am. J. Surg., *126:*45, 1973

Inoculation site, role as determinant of infection in soft tissue wounds (Roettinger *et al*), PRS, *53:*687, 1974. Am. J. Surg., *126:*354, 1973

Wound, surgical, resistance to antimicrobial prophylaxis and mechanism of development (Edlich, Smith, Edgerton), PRS, *54:*114, 1974. Am. J. Surg., *126:*583, 1973

Healing, biologic frontiers in control of (Peacock), PRS, *54:*114, 1974. Am. J. Surg., *126:*708, 1973

Acidification of wounds, chemical, adjuvant to healing and unfavorable action of alkalinity and ammonia (Leveen *et al*), PRS, *54:*114, 1974. Ann. Surg., *178:*745, 1973

Granulomas, starch (Leonard), PRS, *52:*603, 1973. Arch. Dermat., *107:*101, 1973

Wound infection, surgical, prospective study of 20,822 operations of incidence (Davis, Cohen, Rao), PRS, *53:*371, 1974. Australian & New Zealand J. Surg., *43:*75, 1973

Skin wound, chronic. New method for treatment (Klein). Hefte Unfallheilkd., *114:*162, 1973 (German)

Bacterial screening in treatment of civilian wounds (Robson, Duke, Krizek), PRS, *53:*687, 1974. J. Surg. Res., *14:*426, 1973

Wound healing of mouse skin incised with plasma scalpel (Link *et al*), PRS, *54:*113, 1974. J. Surg. Res., *14:*505, 1973

Zinc and wound healing in normal and chronically ill rats (Elias, Chvapil), PRS, *53:*495, 1974. J. Surg. Res., *15:*59, 1973

Amino transferases and NADP-dependent enzymes (Im, Hoopes), PRS, *53:*611, 1974. J. Surg. Res., *15:*262, 1973

Donor sites, split-skin graft, effect of Silastic sheet dressings on the healing of (Harris, Filarski, Hector), PRS, *52:*189, 1973

Fibroblast, contractile, relevance in plastic surgery (Montandon *et al*), PRS, *52:*286, 1973

Fibroblast, on the contractile (Madden) (Editorial), PRS, *52:*291, 1973

Wound healing, use of commercial porcine skin for wound dressings (Elliott, Hoehn), PRS, *52:*401, 1973

Wound healing: exudation, inflammatory cell migration and granulation tissue formation in preformed cavities (Lundgren, Lindhe), PRS, *54:*698, 1974. Scand. J. Plast. Reconstr. Surg., *7:*1, 1973

Estrogen and progesterone, influence on exudation, inflammatory cell migration, and granulation tissue formation in preformed

Wound Healing—Cont.

cavities (Lundgren), PRS, *54:*697, 1974. Scand. J. Plast. Reconstr. Surg., 7:20, 1973

Estrogen and progesterone, influence on vascularization of granulation tissue in preformed cavities (Lundgren), PRS, *54:*698, 1974. Scand. J. Plast. Reconstr. Surg., 7:85, 1973

Blood flow and respiratory gas tensions in wounds in young and old rats (Holm-Pedersen, Zederfeldt), PRS, *54:*508, 1974. Scand. J. Plast. Reconstr. Surg., 7:91, 1973

Wound healing research, standards for (Hunt), PRS, *52:*216, 1973. Surgery, 73:153, 1973

Corticosteroid metabolites, effect of surgical trauma on conjugation pattern (Wise, Margraf, Ballinger), PRS, *52:*217, 1973. Surgery, 73:163, 1973

Healing processes in skin grafts (Rudolph, Klein), PRS, *53:*498, 1974. Surg. Gynec. & Obst., *136:*641, 1973

Skin wounds in rats, effect of skin dressing and topical antibiotics on healing (Burleson, Eiseman), PRS, *52:*461, 1973. Surg. Gynec. & Obst., *136:*958, 1973

Wound healing, effect of Travase on (Harris *et al*). Tex. Rep. Biol. Med., *31:*771, 1973

Vitamin C, influence on healing of wounds and bones and on prognosis of polytrauma (Bellmann *et al*), PRS, *52:*686, 1973. Zentralbl. Chir., 98:510, 1973

Wound Healing. By J. E. Dunphy. Med. Com., New York, 1974

Tissue conservation theory, static, questions of (Feygelman), PRS, *55:*725, 1975. Acta chir. plast., *16:*113, 1974

Infection in surgical patients, use of nitroblue tetrazolium (NBT) dye test as indicator of (Standford, Kilman, Zeiger), PRS, *57:*767, 1976. Am. J. Surg., *128:*668, 1974

Wound, healing, vascularization of (Myers, Wolf), PRS, *56:*471, 1975. Am. Surgeon, *12:*716, 1974

Wound healing, effect of anemia on (Heughan, Grislis, Hunt), PRS, *54:*379, 1974. Ann. Surg., *179:*163, 1974

Zinc deficiency, effect on wound healing (Rahmat, Norman, Smith), PRS, *54:*698, 1974. Brit. J. Surg., *61:*271, 1974

Endothelium, fibroblastic, experiments for developing on synthetic preparations (Götz *et al*), PRS, *54:*247, 1974. Bruns' Beitr. klin. Chir., *221:*142, 1974

Wound infection, local use of antibiotics to prevent (Bingham *et al*), PRS, *56:*362, 1975. Clin. Orthop., *99:*194, 1974

Wounds of hand, soft tissue, spontaneous healing and wound contraction of (Con-

Wound Healing—Cont.

olly), PRS, *54:*690, 1974. Hand, 6:26, 1974

Wound healing, effects of estrogen on—experimental study (Murthy *et al*), PRS, *55:*254, 1975. Indian J. Surg., *36:*1, 1974

Wound healing in experimental diabetes (Parkash, Pandit, Sharma), PRS, *54:*242, 1974. Internat. Surg., *59:*25, 1974

Wound healing, formation of epidermis after implantation of epidermal cell cultures from perinatal mouse skin (Worst, Valentine, Fusenig), PRS, *55:*518, 1975. J. Natl. Cancer Inst., *53:*1061, 1974

Wound healing, epidermal, glycogen metabolism in (Hoopes, Im), PRS, *56:*471, 1975. J. Surg. Oncol., *6:*408, 1974

Wounds, granulating, efficacy of systemic antibiotics in treatment of (Robson *et al*), PRS, *54:*695, 1974. J. Surg. Res., *16:*299, 1974

Bowel, small, sutures, vascular regeneration after different types (Juvara, Necula, Murgu), PRS, *54:*238, 1974. Lyon chir., *70:*52, 1974

Aeromonas hydrophila wound infection (Rosenthal, Bernhardt, Phillips), PRS, *53:*77, 1974

Hypertrophic scars and keloids (Ketchum, Cohen, Masters), PRS, *53:*140, 1974

Wound healing, clinical aspects, teaching exercises for medical students (Graham), PRS, *53:*433, 1974

Histological study of skin after chemical face peeling, long-term (Baker *et al*), PRS, *53:*522, 1974

Tension, skin, new theory regarding lines of (Bulacio Nuñez), PRS, *53:*663, 1974

Wound healing: augmentation of wound strength by pretreatment with epinephrine (Myers, Rightor), PRS, *54:*201, 1974. Discussion by Weeks, PRS, *54:*351, 1974

Gas tensions in healing tissues of traumatized patients (Heppenstall *et al*), PRS, *54:*625, 1974. Surgery, 75:874, 1974

Wound contraction, effect of primary and delayed split-skin grafting on (Stone, Madden), PRS, *57:*765, 1976. Surg. Forum, *25:*41, 1974

Wound healing, role of infection (DeHaan, Ellis, Wilks), PRS, *54:*698, 1974. Surg. Gynec. & Obst., *138:*693, 1974

Wound healing, surface hydrogen ion concentration to determine timing of closure (Lipton *et al*), PRS, *55:*114, 1975. Surg. Gynec. & Obst., *139:*189, 1974

Plastubol spray in management of extensive surgical wounds (Kabza, Pasz), PRS, *56:*471, 1975. Wiad. Lek., *27:*1275, 1974

Latest studies on the effect of laser beams on

Wound Healing – Cont.

wound healing (clinical and electronoptic experiences) (Mester *et al*). Z. Exp. Chir., 7:9, 1974 (German)

Infection, body's response to (Meakins), PRS, 57:264, 1976. AORN, 22:37, 1975

Skin closure using a new skin clip (Samuels *et al*). Am. J. Surg., 129:345, 1975

Dermo-dermal uniting, an experimental study (Lalardrie *et al*), PRS, 57:268, 1976. Ann. chir. plast., 20:183, 1975

Wound infections, effect of differing ambient oxygen tensions on (Hunt *et al*), PRS, 56:599, 1975. Ann. Surg., 181:35, 1975

Wound contracture and epithelialization in rabbits, effects of cortisone acetate, methylprednisolone and medroxyprogesterone on (Lenco, McKnight, MacDonald), PRS, 56:470, 1975. Ann. Surg., 181:67, 1975

Effect of nutrition, diet and suture material on long term wound healing (Temple *et al*). Ann. Surg., 182:93, 1975

Acid wounds, hydrotherapy in (Rothmann, Vakilzadeh, Rupec), PRS, 56:599, 1975. Arch. Dermat. Forsch., 251:281, 1975

Botulism, wound (Cherington, Ginsburg), PRS, 56:596, 1975. Arch. Surg., 110:436, 1975

Clinicosurgical treatment of synergistic necrotizing cellulitis (Corrao, Beveraggi, Pietravello), PRS, 57:764, 1976. Bol. y trab. soc. argent. cir., 36:271, 1975

Wound healing research (Heughan, Hunt), PRS, 56:470, 1975. Canad. J. Surg., 18:118, 1975

Wound infection, prophylactic antibiotic therapy in surgery (MacLean), PRS, 57:405, 1976. Canad. J. Surg., 18:243, 1975

Wound healing: what's new in surgery (Robinson), PRS, 55:723, 1975. Contemp. Surg., 6:21, 1975

Healing of surgical defects in bone (Horton *et al*), PRS, 57:257, 1976. J. Oral Surg., 39:536, 1975

Granulomas, inhibition of growth by histamine (Saeki *et al*), PRS, 57:268, 1976. J. Pharmacol. & Exper. Therap., 193:910, 1975

Wound infections, postoperative, incidence during Vietnam conflict (Latina), PRS, 57:677, 1976. Mil. Med., 140:354, 1975

Wound infection: current use of prophylactic antibiotics in plastic and reconstructive surgery (Krizek, Koss, Robson), PRS, 55:21, 1975

Wound healing, surgical problems in excision and repair of radiated tissue (Robinson), PRS, 55:41, 1975

Wound healing, effect of commonly used an-

Wound Healing – Cont.

tiseptics on (Gruber, Vistnes, Pardoe), PRS, 55:472, 1975

Wound dehiscence, secondary closures of penile skin incisions (Horton, Devine), PRS, 55:630, 1975

Meissner corpuscle, denervated, sequential histological study after nerve division in rhesus monkey (Dellon, Witebsky, Terrill), PRS, 56:182, 1975

Tissue breakdowns after pressure "sore" closures, preventing recurrent (Rogers, Wilson), PRS, 56:419, 1975. Discussion by Brand, PRS, 56:573, 1975

Wound healing, epidermal, under new polyurethane foam dressing (Lyofoam) (Winter), PRS, 56: 531, 1975

Wound healing, effects of suture materials on (Van Winkle *et al*), PRS, 56:599, 1975. Surg. Gynec. & Obst., 140:7, 1975

Tendon tissues, role of, in tendon healing (Furlow), PRS, 57:39, 1976

Fibroblasts, cultured, isolated from normal and keloid tissue, cell size and growth characteristics (Russell, Witt), PRS, 57:207, 1976

Wound healing, disruption of healed scars in scurvy – result of disequilibrium in collagen metabolism (Cohen, Keiser), PRS, 57:213, 1976. Discussion by Chvapil, PRS, 57:376, 1976

Wound healing: elastin fibers in scar tissue (Bhangoo, Quinlivan, Connelly), PRS, 57:308, 1976

Wound healing in bats, elastogenesis in (Bhangoo, Church), PRS, 57:468, 1976

Lines, skin tension, in domestic pig (Rose Ksander, Vistnes), PRS, 57:729, 1976

Wowern, N. von: Treatment of oroantral fistulae. Arch. Otolaryng., 96:99, 1972

Wowern, N. von: Correlation between the development of an oroantral fistula and the size of corresponding bony defect. J. Oral Surg., 31:98, 1973

Wray, J. B.: Principles of early management in massive injuries of the hand. J. Indiana State Med. Assoc., 64:1277, 1971

Wray, R. C., Jr.: Should an incompletely severed tendon be sutured? (with Reynolds, Weeks), PRS, 57:36, 1976. Discussion by Kleinert, PRS, 57:236, 1976

Wray, R. C., Jr.: Lateral-volar finger flap for treatment of burn syndactyly (with MacDougal, Weeks), PRS, 57:167, 1976

Wray, R. C., Jr.: Spontaneous regression of primary lesion of metastatic malignant melanoma (with MacDougal, Weeks), PRS, 57:355, 1976

WRAY, R. C., JR. *et al*: Silastic frameworks in total reconstruction of auricle. Brit. J. Plast. Surg., *26:*296, 1973

WRAY, R. C., JR., AND WEEKS, P. M.: Reconstruction of digital pulleys, PRS, *53:*534, 1974

WRAY, R. C., HOOPES, J. E., AND DAVIS, G. M.: Correction of extreme gynecomastia, PRS, *56:*677, 1975. Brit. J. Plast. Surg., *27:*39, 1974

WRAY, R. C., JR., MOORE, D. L., AND WEEKS, P. M.: Use of silicone chin implants in plastic surgery: method of chin augmentation, PRS, *54:*510, 1974. South. M. J., *67:*456, 1974

WRAY, R. C., JR., HOLTMANN, B., AND WEEKS, P. M.: Factors in production of inconspicuous scars, PRS, *56:*86, 1975

WRIGHT, A. M.: Surgical tattooing of the portwine stain (with Thomson), PRS, *48:*113, 1971

WRIGHT, A. M. *et al*: Photogrammetry—a planning tool in facial reconstruction. In *Biostereometrics 74*, ed. by Herron; pp. 154-60. Falls Church, Va.; Am. Soc. Photogrammetry, 1974

WRIGHT, J. A. *et al*: Fibrosarcoma of mandible, case report. Oral Surg., *36:*16, 1973

WRIGHT, J. E. *et al*: Continuous monitoring of visually evoked response during intraorbital surgery. Trans. Ophthalmol. Soc. U. K., *93:*311, 1973

WRIGHT, J. E. *et al*: *Aplasia cutis congenita*, PRS, *54:*702, 1974. J. Pediat. Surg., *9:*415, 1974

WRIGHT, M. R. *et al*: A psychological study of patients undergoing cosmetic surgery. Arch. Otolaryng., *101:*145, 1975

WRIGHT, P., AND HENDERSON, K.: Cellular glucose utilization during hemorrhagic shock in pig, PRS, *57:*676, 1976. Surgery, *78:*322, 1975

WRIGHT, R. C. *et al*: Scleromyxedema. Arch. Dermat., *112:*63, 1976

Wringer Injuries

Two cases of hand injury by a roller. (Otani *et al*). Orthop. Surg. (Tokyo), *22:*995, 1971 (Japanese)

Wringer and crush injuries of hand (Buck-Gramcko), PRS, *51:*476, 1973. Langenbecks Arch. Chir., *332:*465, 1972

Current treatment of wringer injuries (Golden *et al*). Va. Med. Mon., *99:*1073, 1972

Wringer injuries, household (McCullock, Boswick, Jonas), PRS, *52:*679, 1973. J. Trauma, *13:*1, 1973

Primary closure of fresh injuries of the hand caught in rollers (Gershkovich). Ortop. Travmatol. Protez., *7:*54, 1974 (Russian)

Treating wringer injuries (Graham *et al*). Pa. Med., *78:*67, 1975

WRONSKI, J. *et al*: Cerebral complications following injury to the orbit with a pencil. Neurol. Neurochir. Pol., *5:*597, 1971 (Polish)

WU, K. T., GAULT, M. H., AND MACLEAN, L. D.: Successful skin graft on renal allograft, PRS, *48:*97, 1971. Canad. J. Surg., *14:*80, 1971

WU, K. T., JORDAN, F. R., AND ECKERT, C.: Lipoma, cause of paralysis of deep radial (posterior interosseous) nerve: report of case and review of literature, PRS, *54:*508, 1974. Surgery, *75:*790, 1974

WU, P. T. *et al*: Total resection of temporal bone for carcinoma of middle ear and temporal bone, PRS, *55:*635, 1975. Chinese M. J., *2:*23, 1974

WU, W. H. *et al*: Pressure dynamics of endotracheal and tracheostomy cuffs. 1. Use of tracheal model to evaluate performance. Crit. Care Med., *1:*197, 1973

WUESTER, W. O.: Surgical approach to the treatment of melanoma. J. Med. Soc. N. J., *69:*235, 1972

WULLSTEIN, H. L.: Position on development of regional plastic and rehabilitation surgery. H. N. O., *21:*22, 1973 (German)

WUNDERER, S.: Experiences with vertical osteotomy in the maxilla. Dtsch. Zahn. Mund. Kieferheilkd., *59:*5, 1972 (German)

WUNDERER, S.: Indication for surgical orthodontic interventions—results and failures. Osterr. Z. Stomatol., *70:*382, 1973 (German)

WUNDERER, S.: Single-step surgical treatment of pronounced prognathia. Fortschr. Kiefer. Gesichtschir., *18:*195, 1974 (German)

WUNDERER, S.: Comparative scintigraphic studies following osteosynthesis. Fortschr. Kiefer. Gesichtschir., *19:*24, 1975 (German)

WURLITZER, F., AND BALLANTYNE, A. J.: Reconstruction of lower jaw area with bipedicled deltopectoral flap and Ticonium prosthesis, PRS, *49:*220, 1972

WYNDER, E. L., AND CHAN, P. C.: Possible role of riboflavin deficiency in epithelial neoplasia. II. Effect on skin tumor development, PRS, *48:*93, 1971. Cancer, *26:*1221, 1970

WYNN, S. K.: Primary nostril reconstruction in complete cleft lips, the round nostril technique, PRS, *49:*56, 1972

WYNN, S. K.: On the article "reconstruction of a traumatic subtotal ear loss with two skin tubes" (Letter to the Editor), PRS, *49:*332, 1972

WYNN, S. K.: Immediate composite graft to loss of nasal ala from dog-bite, PRS, *50:*188, 1972

WYNN, S. K. *et al*: Speech status of post-adolescents following bone flap palatal surgery. Cleft Palate J., *8:*196, 1971

WYNNE-DAVIES, R.: Genetics and malformations of the hand. Hand, *3:*184, 1971

WYNNE-DAVIES, R.: Genetics and congenital malformation of the hand. J. Ir. Med. Assoc., *66:*596, 1973

WYSOCKI, J. P. *et al*: Role of wounds in epidemiology of nosocomial infections due to *Pseudomonas aeruginosa*, PRS, *55:*258, 1975. Invest. Urol., *11:*370, 1974

WYSS, T.: Rehabilitation of leprosy patient by correction of nasal deformities. New ways in correction of the saddle-nose. Praxis, *62:*1305, 1973 (German)

X

Xanthomas

Face, atypical fibroxanthoma of skin of (Fretzin, Helwig), PRS, *54:*243, 1974. Cancer, *31:*1541, 1973

Xanthelasma, new method for surgery of (Fuchs). Klin. Monatsbl. Augenheilkd., *163:*324, 1973 (German)

Fibroxanthoma, atypical, with ganglial metastases (Jaimovich, Abulafia), PRS, *57:*264, 1976. Med. Cut., *2:*15, 1973

Fibroxanthoma, atypical, in the pharynx (Berschadsky *et al*), PRS, *52:*443, 1973

XAVIER, T. S., AND LAMB, D. W.: Forearm as donor site for split-skin grafts, PRS, *56:*465, 1975. Hand, *6:*243, 1974

Y

YABLON, I. G., FRAZBLAU, C., AND LEACH, R. E.: Response of transplanted articular cartilage to growth hormone, PRS, *54:*510, 1974. J. Bone & Joint Surg., *56A:*322, 1974

YACAMOTTI, J. D.: Enzymatic debridement of facial burns, PRS, *53:*491, 1974. Prensa med. argent., *60:*1055, 1973

YADEV, S. S.: Limb deformities in leprosy. Indian J. Med. Sci., *28:*542, 1974

YAGHNAM, F. C.: Management of cutaneous hemangioma in children, PRS, *56:*683, 1975. Jordan M. J., *9:*128, 1974

YAMADA, S. *et al*: En bloc subtotal temporal bone resection for cancer of external ear. J. Neurosurg., *39:*370, 1973

YAMAMOTO, Y. *et al*: Methods of therapeutic evaluation in peripheral nerve injuries of the hand and its significance. Orthop. Surg. (Tokyo), *21:*969, 1970 (Japanese)

YAMANISHI, Y. *et al*: Collagenolytic activity in malignant melanoma: physiochemical studies, PRS, *54:*115, 1974. Cancer Res., *33:*2507, 1973

YAMAZAKI, Z. *et al*: Foreign body granuloma of breast: incidence of malignant tumor, PRS, *50:*305, 1972. Geka Surg. Ther. Osaka, *33:*1283, 1971

YANAGIHARA, N. *et al*: Denervation in Bell's palsy. Evoked electromyographic study. O. R. L., *36:*361, 1974

YANAGISAWA, E.: Symposium on maxillofacial trauma. 3. Pitfalls in management of zygomatic fractures. Laryngoscope, *83:*527, 1973

YANO, K.: Experimental study on vascularization of the tubed pedicle, PRS, *50:*310, 1972. Otorhinolaryng. Tokyo, *14:*471, 1971

YAO, S. T. *et al*: Gunshot wounds of face, PRS, *52:*107, 1973. J. Trauma, *12:*523, 1972

YAO, S. T. *et al*: Method for assessing ischemia of hand and fingers, PRS, *51:*348, 1973. Surg. Gynec. & Obst., *135:*373, 1972

YAO, S. T. *et al*: Limb blood flow in congenital arteriovenous fistula, PRS, *52:*208, 1973. Surgery, *73:*80, 1973

YARCHUK, N. I., AND TERTISIONAS, P. V.: Reconstruction of eyebrows with free skin grafts, PRS, *52:*205, 1973. Acta chir. plast., *14:*82, 1972

YARINGTON, C. T., JR.: Single-stage repair of bilateral cleft lip. Arch. Otolaryng., *97:*263, 1973

YARNINGTON, C. T., JR. *et al*: Radical neck dissection. Mortality and morbidity. Arch. Otolaryng., *97:*306, 1973

YASSIN, J. G. *et al*: Entropion of lower lid: repair by double triangle tarsectomy. Ophthalmic Surg., *5:*65, 1974

YAWALKAR, S. J.: *Leprosy for Practitioners*. Popular Prakashan, Ltd., Bombay, India, 1974. PRS, *55:*616, 1975

YELLIN, A. E., AND SHORE, E. H.: Surgical management of arterial occlusion following percutaneous femoral angiography, PRS, *52:*453, 1973. Surgery, *73:*772, 1973

YELLIN, H.: Muscle cross-reinnervation. Nature, *249:*596, 1974

YEO, M. T. *et al*: Total intravenous nutrition, PRS, *53:*376, 1974. Arch. Surg., *106:*792, 1973

YESCHUA, R.: Early treatment of burns of dorsum of hand by tangential excision and skin grafting (with Wexler, Neuman), PRS, *54:*268, 1974

YESCHUA, R., WEXLER, M. R., AND NEUMAN, Z.: Nevus of Ota, PRS, *55:*229, 1975

YIM, D. *et al*: Carotid artery and dermal graft, PRS, *54:*692, 1974. Arch. Otolaryng., *99:*242, 1974

YIP, W. K., *et al*: Benign osteoblastoma of the maxilla. Oral Surg., *38:*259, 1974

YOEL, J.: Sada's treatment for temporomandibular ankylosis, PRS, *49:*581, 1972. Bol. y trab. Acad. argent. cir., *55:*375, 1971

YOEL, J.: Tumors of pharyngeal prolongation of parotid, PRS, *54:*107, 1974. Bol. y trab. Acad. argent. cir., *57:*250, 1973

YOEL, JOSE: *Pathology and Surgery of the Salivary Glands.* Charles C Thomas, Springfield, Ill., 1975. PRS, *57:*230, 1976

YONEMOTO, R. H. *et al:* Composite operation in cancer of head and neck (commando procedure), PRS, *51:*235, 1973. Arch. Surg., *104:*809, 1972

YONGCHIYUD, U. *et al:* Maduromycosis of hand due to *Phialophora jeanselme,* PRS, *52:*97, 1973. Southeast Asian J. Trop. Med., *3:*138, 1972

YONKERS, A. J. *et al:* Early management of facial trauma. Am. Fam. Physician, *6:*68, 1972

YONKERS, A. J. *et al:* Cancer of the lip. Laryngoscope, *82:*625, 1972

YOSIPOVITCH, Z. *et al:* Subcutaneous Achilles tenotomy in the treatment of perforating ulcer of the foot in leprosy. Int. J. Lepr., *39:*631, 1971

YOUNG, G. R. *et al:* Histologically benign mixed parotid tumor with hepatic metastasis. J. Pathol., *109:*171, 1973

YOUNG, H. HERMAN: *Year Book of Orthopedics and Traumatic Surgery.* Year Book Medical Publishers, Chicago, 1974. PRS, *56:*81, 1975

YOUNG, I. M. *et al:* Hearing impairment following radical neck dissection. Trans. Pa. Acad. Ophthalmol. Otolaryngol., *28:*155, 1975

YOUNG, L. W. *et al:* New syndrome manifested by mandibular hypoplasia, acroosteolysis, stiff joints and cutaneous atrophy (mandibuloacral dysplasia) in two unrelated boys. Birth Defects, *7:*291, 1971

YOUNG, R. A. *et al:* Anterior maxillary osteotomy: a retrospective evaluation of sinus health, patient acceptance and relapses. J. Oral Surg., *30:*69, 1972

YRASTORZA, J. A.: Vestibuloplasty with skin grafting. J. Oral Surg., *34:*29, 1976

YU, S. W.: Mixed tumor of the nasal septum. Can. J. Otolaryngol., *3:*630, 1974

YU, W. *et al:* Flexor digitorum sublimis to profundus tendon transfer for flexion deformities in spastic paralysis. Can. J. Surg., *17:*225, 1974

YUCEL, V. E., AND BASMAJIAN, J. V.: Decubitus ulcers: healing effect of enzymatic spray, PRS, *55:*640, 1975. Arch. Phys. Med. & Rehab., *55:*517, 1974

YULES, RICHARD B.: *Atlas for Surgical Repair of Cleft Lip, Cleft Palate, and Noncleft Velopharyngeal Incompetence.* Charles C Thomas, Springfield, Ill., 1971. PRS, *50:*399,

1972

YULES, R. B.: Current concepts of treatment of ear disease in cleft palate children and adults. Cleft Palate J., *12:*315, 1975

YUSUPOV, I. A.: Joining of lymph routes and autotransplantation of lymph nodes in experiments, PRS, *48:*394, 1971. Acta chir. Plast., *12:*235, 1970

YVROUD, M.: Role of the dermis in differentiation of the nasolacrimal duct in Discoglossus pictus (anourous amphibian). C. R. Acad. Sci. (D.) (Paris), *279:*81, 1974 (French)

Z

Z-Plasty

Z-plasty and W-plasty in revision of linear scars, historical review (Borges), PRS, *49:*241, 1972. Internat. Surg., *56:*182, 1971

Z-plasty, four-flap (Woolf, Broadbent), PRS, *49:*48, 1972

Z-plasty, four-flap (Mir-y-Mir) (Letter to the Editor), PRS, *50:*509, 1972

Z-plasty, demonstrating the (Wexler *et al*). Brit. J. Plast. Surg., *26:*417, 1973

Tendon, achilles, Z-plasty skin closure after lengthening the (Price, Ecker), PRS, *52:*309, 1973. Discussion by Goldwyn, PRS, *52:*431, 1973

Six-flap Z-plasty (Mir-y-Mir), PRS, *52:*625, 1973

Z-plasty, earlobe, in Borneo (Abrahams), PRS, *53:*548, 1974

Z-plasties, 5 single (Borges), PRS, *55:*387, 1975. Virginia M. Month., *101:*618, 1974

Letter: Z-plasty (Wolfe). New England J. Med., *292:*319, 1975

Z-plasty operation for sacrococcygeal pilonidal disease (Sood, Green, Parui), PRS, *56:*559, 1975

Neck, subcutaneous Z-plasty (Vecchione, Pickering), PRS, *56:*579, 1975

ZABOLOSKIL, A. T. *et al:* Preservation and autotransplantation of skin in elephantiasis of extremities. Klin. Khir., *3:*45, 1974 (Russian)

ZABOLOTSKIL, A. T.: Surgical treatment of elephantiasis of the upper extremities. Vestn. Khir., *115:*67, 1975 (Russian)

ZABRODSKY, S. *et al:* High attachment of lower lip frenum. Its consequence and therapy. Cesk. Stomatol., *72:*86, 1972

ZACARIAN, S. A.: Cryosurgery for cancer of the skin. Cancro, *24:*349, 1971

ZACARIAN, S. A.: Cancer of the eyelid—a cryosurgical approach. Ann. Ophth., *4:*473, 1972

ZACARIAN, SETRAG A.: *Review of Cryosurgery of Tumors of the Skin and Oral Cavity.*

Charles C Thomas, Springfield, Ill., 1973. PRS, *55:*486, 1975

ZACHARIAE, L.: Dupuytren's contracture, etiological role of trauma, PRS, *49:*583, 1972. Scand. J. Plast. Reconstr. Surg., *5:*116, 1971

ZACKIN, H., AND GOULIAN, D., JR.: Prevention of postoperative shifting of mammary prostheses, PRS, *55:*713, 1975

ZAFFIRI, O.: Hypnosis in anesthesia. Minerva Med., *66:*3894, 1975 (Italian)

ZAGUBELIUK, N. K.: Plastic repair of postoperative cavities of the jaw. Stomatologiia (Mosk.), *50:*39, 1971 (Russian)

ZAHORSKY, C. L.: New approach to the elusive dynamic pharyngeal flap, preliminary report (with McCoy), PRS, *49:*160, 1972

ZAIDENBERG, M. A. *et al*: Changes of hexosamines and sialic acids in blood serum in burns. Klin. Med. (Mosk.), *51:*86, 1973 (Russian)

ZAIKOVA, M. V. *et al*: Outcome of primary plastic surgery in tumors of eyelids. Oftalmol. Zh., *28:*485, 1973 (Russian)

ZAJAC, S. *et al*: Dorsal intertendinous fascia of the hand. Folia Morphol. (Warsz.), *33:*121, 1974

ZAJDELA, Z.: Celesnik procedure in the surgical treatment of bilateral complete clefts. J. Maxillo-facial Surg., *1:*137, 1973

ZAKHAROV, IU. S. *et al*: Use of preserved homologous embryonic bone in the reconstruction or restoration of defects following excision of cysts and benign tumors of the jaws. Stomatologiia (Mosk.), *53:*90, 1974 (Russian)

ZAKHAROV, IU. S. *et al*: Compression osteosynthesis by spikes with supports in fractures of the mental portion of the mandible. Stomatologiia (Mosk.), *54:*71, 1975 (Russian)

ZAKHAROV, V. A.: Lacoorostomy with permanent intubation. Oftal. zhur., *27:*297, 1972 (Russian)

ZAKRZEWSKI, A. *et al*: Dermatofibroma of the nose. Otolaryngol. Pol., *29:*617, 1975 (Polish)

ZAKRZEWSKI, J. *et al*: External immobilizing plaster cast. Otolaryngol. Pol., *29:*505, 1975 (Polish)

ZALESIN, H. M. *et al*: Central cavernous hemangioma of the mandible treated by an intraoral approach. J. Oral Surg., *33:*877, 1975

ZALIN, H. *et al*: Chorda tympani neurectomy — new approach to submandibular salivary obstruction. Brit. J. Surg., *61:*392, 1974

ZALLEN, R. D.: Congenital lip sinuses of the lower lip: report of case. J. Oral Surg., *29:*732, 1971

ZALLEN, R. D. *et al*: Simplified sigmoid notch retractor for extraoral osteotomies. J. Oral Surg., *32:*386, 1974

ZAMBITO, R. F.: Surgical orthognathics. Rede-

fined role based upon etiologic factors. Dent. Clin. North Am., *19:*515, 1975

ZAMICK, P. *et al*: Deep dermal burns treated by excision, skin grafts, and tri-iodothyronine. Surg. Forum, *22:*491, 1971

ZAMICK, P., AND WEISS, R. M.: Repair of *coup de sabre,* linear form of scleroderma, PRS, *50:*520, 1972

ZAMICK, P., AND MEHREGAN, A. H.: Effect of 1-tri-iodothyronine on marginal scars of skin grafted burns in rats, PRS, *51:*71, 1973

ZAMPAKOS, I. *et al*: Immediate reconstruction of major defects following surgery for oral cancer based on arterial skin flaps. Stomatologia (Athenai), *29:*347, 1972 (Greek)

ZANCOLLI, E.: Surgery for the quadriplegic hand with active, strong wrist extension preserved. A study of 97 cases. Clin. Orthop., *112:*101, 1975

ZANCOLLI, E., AND MITRE, H.: *Latissimus dorsi* transfer to restore elbow flexion, PRS, *53:*684, 1974. J. Bone & Joint Surg., *55:*1265, 1973

ZANGL, A.: Construction of the vagina with transposition of the sigmoid colon. Langenbecks Arch. Chir., *339:*413, 1975 (German)

ZANI, R.: Masseter muscle rotation in the treatment of inferior facial paralysis (with Correia), PRS, *52:*370, 1973

ZANI, R.: Surgical anatomy of the facial nerve as related to ancillary operations in rhytidoplasty (with Correia), PRS, *52:*549, 1973

ZANI, R.: Skin grafting, PRS, *55:*725, 1975. Ars Curandi, *7:*49, 1974

ZAPATER, R. C. *et al*: Hand onychomycosis. Arch. Argent. Dermatol., *19:*183, 1969 (Spanish)

ZARB, G. A. *et al*: Treatment of patients with temporomandibular joint pain dysfunction syndrome. J. Can. Dent. Assoc., *41:*410, 1975

ZAREM, H. A.: Stimulation of neovascularization — comparative efficacy of fresh and preserved skin grafts (with O'Donoghue), PRS, *48:*474, 1971

ZAREM, H. A.: Induced resolution of cavernous hemangiomas following prednisolone therapy (Follow-Up Clinic), PRS, *51:*207, 1973

ZAREM, H. A.: Management of complications in head and neck surgery. Surg. Clin. North Am., *53:*191, 1973

ZAREM, H. A.: Absence of vascularization in porcine skin grafts on mice (with Pandya), PRS, *53:*211, 1974

ZAREM, H. A., RATTENBORG, C., AND HARMEL, M.: Carbon monoxide toxicity in human fire victims, PRS, *54:*112, 1974. Arch. Surg., *107:*1, 1973

ZAREM, H. A. *et al*: Surgical management of hand deformities in recessive dystrophic epidermolysis bullosa. Brit. J. Plast. Surg., 27:176, 1974

ZAREM, H. A., AND GREER, D. M., JR.: Tongue flap for reconstruction of lips in electrical burns, PRS, 53:310, 1974

ZARINS, C. K., AND SKINNER, D. B.: Circulation in profound hypothermia, PRS, 53:115, 1974. J. Surg. Res., 14:97, 1973

ZARIVCHATSKII, M. F.: Plastic surgery of skin with A. K. Tychinkina's modification in treatment of persistently unhealing wounds and ulcers of foot and shin. Vestn. Khir., 111:80, 1973 (Russian)

ZAUNER, J. C., AND NAGEL, D.: Prenatal development of tendon sheaths in hands of human embryos, PRS, 49:664, 1972. Surg. Forum, 22:430, 1971

ZAUSAEV, V. I.: Objective analysis of persistent deformities of the palate following surgical interventions and assessment of the results of uranostaphyloplasty. Stomatologiia (Mosk.), 51:51, 1972 (Russian)

ZAWACKI, B. E.: Reversal of capillary stasis and prevention of necrosis in burns, PRS, 55:113, 1975. Ann. Surg., 180:98, 1974

ZAWACKI, B. E.: Treatment of extensive burns. New England J. Med., 290:862, 1974

ZAWACKI, B. E.: Effect of Travase on heat-injured skin, PRS, 56:111, 1975. Surgery, 77:132, 1975

ZAWACKI, B. E., AND ASCH, M.: Technique for autografting large burns from limited donor sites, PRS, 53:498, 1974. Surgery, 74:774, 1973

ZAWISTOWSKA, J. et al: Difficulties and modifications of intubation technique in infants with labial, alveolar, and palatal clefts. Anaesth. Resusc. Intensive Ther., 1:211, 1973

ZBYLSKI, J. R.: Repair of massive soft tissue defects by open jump flaps (with Morgan), PRS, 50:265, 1972

ZBRODOWSKI, A.: Vascularization of flexor tendons within the carpal tunnel and the hand. Chir. Narzadow. Ruchu Ortop. Pol., 38:589, 1973 (Polish)

ZBRODOWSKI, A.: Anatomical model of the mesotenon of the flexor tendons in the carpal tunnel. Chir. Narzadow. Ruchu Ortop. Pol., 39:57, 1974 (Polish)

ZBRODOWSKI, A. et al: Anatomic model of the ligamentous apparatus of the tendons of the extensor digitorum muscle of the hand in man. Folia Morphol. (Warsz.), 32:381, 1973

ZDRAWIC, F.: Use of homografts in deep dermal burns, PRS, 53:686, 1974. Riv. ital. chir. plast., 4:19, 1973

ZDRAVIC, F.: Initial treatment of burns and burn scars, PRS, 56:361, 1975. Riv. ital. chir. plast., 5:305, 1973

ZECHNER, G. et al: Sebaceous gland carcinoma of parotid gland. Arch. Klin. Exp. Ohren Nasen Kehlkopfheilkd., 205:119, 1973 (German)

ZEFFER, J. et al: Aplasia vaginae et uteri associated with dystopic solitary kidney—colpoplasty, using sigmoid colon. Orv. Hetil., 112:1710, 1971 (Hungarian)

ZEGARELLI, D. J. et al: Large dental granuloma (? inflammatory pseudotumor) with unusual features, case report. J. Am. Dent. Assoc., 89:891, 1974

ZEHM, S.: Method of primary reconstruction of nose and upper lip. Arch . Klin. Exp. Ohren Nasen Kehlkopfheilkd., 199:638, 1971 (German)

ZEHM, S.: Surgery of retromaxillary space. Monatsschr. Ohrenheilkd. Laryngorhinol., 105:147, 1971 (German)

ZEHM, S.: Tumors of aberrant salivary gland tissue. Fortschr. Kiefer. Gesichtschir., 15:43, 1972 (German)

ZEHM, S.: Plastic surgery of frontal bone defect with special reference to tantalum. H. N. O., 21:79, 1973 (German)

ZEHM, S.: Functional restitution of denervated gullet. Arch. Otolaryng., 99:279, 1974

ZEHM, S. et al: Functional rehabilitation of the pharynx in surgically treated neoplasms. Z. Laryngol. Rhinol. Otol., 50:776, 1971 (German)

ZEHNDER, P. R. et al: Chondrosarcoma of maxilla: surgery and reconstruction. J. La. State Med. Soc., 126:243, 1974

ZEITZ, J. et al: Split skin transplantation after grinding off hypertrophic burn scars. In Plastische und Wiederherstellungs-Chirurgie, ed. by Hohler; pp. 327-9. Schattauer, Stuttgart, 1975 (German)

ZELENIN, R. P. et al: Experience with the treatment of angiomas and angiomatosis. Klin. Khir., 11:75, 1974 (Russian)

ZELICKSON, A. S., MOTTAZ, J., AND WEISS, L. W.: Effects of topical fluorouracil on normal skin, PRS, 57:543, 1976. Arch. Dermat., 111:1301, 1975

ZELLNER, P. R.: Local treatment of recent burns, PRS, 50:201, 1972. Langenbecks Arch. Chir., 329:889, 1971

ZELLNER, P. R.: Current treatment methods in burn injuries. Krankenpflege, 26:47, 1972 (German)

ZELLNER, P. R.: Heat-induced injuries of hand, PRS, 51:476, 1973. Langenbecks Arch. Chir., 332:485, 1972

ZELLNER, P. R.: Therapy of burn injuries. Med. Klin., 67:657, 1972 (German)

ZELLNER, P. R.: Preserved cadaver skin for the coverage of large-scale third-degree burns. Zentralbl. Chir., 99:1105, 1974 (German)

ZELLNER, P. R.: Skin substitution in neck and facial burns. Magy. Traumatol. Orthop., *18*:265, 1975 (Hungarian)

ZELLNER, P. R. *et al*: Transplantation and preservation of tissue-typed skin in burns. Chirurg., *46*:319, 1975 (German)

ZEMLOWA, J.: Jaw cysts in children. Czas. Stomatol., *25*:759, 1972 (Polish)

ZENTENO, A. S.: Fracture of the penis, PRS, *52*:669, 1973

ZENTENO, A. S.: New instrument for mammary surgery. Brit. J. Plast. Surg., *28*:164, 1975

ZENTENO, S.: Elongation of cleft lip, PRS, *54*:240, 1974. Rev. españ. cir. plast., *7*:13, 1974

ZENTENO ALANIS, S.: Reconstruction of urethra, PRS, *54*:621, 1974. Rev. españ. cir. plast., *6*:255, 1973

ZERBINATI, A. *et al*: Apropos of case of microinvasive carcinoma of oral cavity. Minerva Stomatol., *23*:211, 1974 (Italian)

ZEROMSKA, B.: Immunological aspects of maxillary sinusitis, PRS, *55*:726, 1975. J. Maxillofacial Surg., *2*:242, 1974

ZEYLAND-MALAWKA, E.: Function of the hand following injuries of the flexor and extensor tendons. Chir. Narzadow. Ruchu Ortop. Pol., *36*:33, 1971 (Polish)

ZHILLIS, B. G. *et al*: Anesthesia in burns. Khirurgiia (Mosk.) *4*:33, 1975 (Russian)

ZHUKOV, G. A.: Casualties from napalm in Vietnam. Voen. Med. Zh., *8*:85, 1971 (Russian)

ZIDE, B., AND PARDOE, R.: Use of behavior modification therapy in a recalcitrant burned child, PRS, *57*:378, 1976

ZIEGLER, M. M. *et al*: Tumor transplants in alymphatic skin islands. Surg. Forum, *23*:127, 1972

ZIEGLER, M. M. *et al*: Regional lymphadenectomy and varied tumor antigenicity. Surg. Forum, *26*:170, 1975

ZIELINSKI, T.: Reconstructive surgery in treatment of skin neoplasms and keratoacanthoma. Przegl. Dermatol., *60*:543, 1973 (Polish)

ZIELINSKI, W. *et al*: Malherbe's calcifying epithelioma in children. Pediatr. Pol., *49*:75, 1974 (Polish)

ZIEMBA, R. B.: Combined buccal and reverse palatal flap for closure of oral-antral fistula. J. Oral Surg., *30*:727, 1972

ZIEROTT, G.: Classification, diagnosis and therapy of gas gangrene. Bruns Beitr. Klin. Chir., *221*:140, 1974 (German)

ZIEROTT, G. *et al*: Changes in evaluation and therapy of gas edema through administration of hyperbaric oxygenation. Clinical comparative study of 31 cases of gas edema. Bruns

Beitr. Klin. Chir., *220*:292, 1973 (German)

ZIEROTT, G., AND VON MEISSNER, F.: Candidiasis in cases of postoperative intensive care, PRS, *53*:691, 1974. Chirurg., *44*:509, 1973

ZIETKIEWICZ, W. *et al*: Effect of the pH of solutions used topically on the bacterial flora of burn wounds. Pol. Tyg. Lek., *27*:949, 1972 (Polish)

ZIETKIEWICZ, W. *et al*: Studies on degree of taking mesh skin graft. Pol. Tyg. Lek., *30*:853, 1975 (Polish)

ZIKRIA, B. A. *et al*: What is clinical smoke poisoning, PRS, *56*:598, 1975. Ann. Surg., *181*:151, 1975

ZINI, I. *et al*: Direct wax method for fabrication of metallic facial molds, PRS, *56*:115, 1975. Prosth. Dent., *33*:95, 1975

ZIPP, P., AND KOUNTZ, S. L.: Analysis of immunosuppressive and oncogenic effects of heterologous antilymphocyte serum, PRS, *49*:109, 1972. Am. J. Surg., *122*:204, 1971

ZIRKLE, T. J., AND SEIDENSTRICKER, E. L.: Adjustable double clamp for use in microvascular surgery, PRS, *51*:340, 1973

ZIRKLE, T. J., AND THOMPSON, R. J.: Deltopectoral flaps, PRS, *54*:690, 1974. Arch. Surg., *108*:770, 1974

ZOOK, E. G.: Care of the traumatic tattoo. Med. Times, *102*:90, 1974

ZOOK, E. G.: Reinforced tongue blade for Dingman mouth gag, PRS, *54*:682, 1974

ZOOK, E. G.: Massive weight loss patient. Clin. Plast. Surg., *2*:457, 1975

ZOOK, E. G.: Plasma scalpel excision of burns (with Link, Glover), PRS, *55*:657, 1975

ZOOK, E. G. *et al*: Ketamine anesthesia in pediatric plastic surgery, PRS, *48*:241, 1971

ZRUBECKY, G.: Operative and conservative restoration of grip in the flaccid hand-paralysis due to cervical cord injuries. Handchirurgie, *4*:71, 1972 (German)

ZRUBECKY, G.: Surgical reconstruction of prehensile function in tetraplegics. Paraplegia, *11*:144, 1973

ZUBASHICH, V. F. *et al*: Cryosurgical device with adjustable cooling capacity. Med. Tekh., *3*:44, 1973 (Russian)

ZUBASHICH, V. F. *et al*: Cryosurgical device with adjustable cold output. Biomed. Eng. (N. Y.), *7*:175, 1974

ZUBENKO, A. P.: Effect of exercise therapy on rheographic values in patients with burns. Vrach. Delo., *4*:131, 1972 (Russian)

ZUBIRI, J. S.: Breast-halving incision for subcutaneous mastectomy (with Corso), PRS, *56*:1, 1975

ZUFI, D.: Skin graft donor site as model for evaluation of hemostatic agents (with Wilkinson, Tenery), PRS, *51*:541, 1973

ZUHLKE, D.: Proceedings: Surgical therapy of salivary gland tumors. H. N. O., *22*:381, 1974 (German)

ZUHLKE, V. *et al*: Surgical therapy of esophageal erosions and their consequences. Bruns Beitr. Klin. Chir., *220*:792, 1973

ZUMBRA, G. L., JR., MULLIN, M. J., AND NELSON, T. G.: Central venous catheter placement utilizing common facial vein, technique useful in hyperalimentation and venous pressure monitoring, PRS, *52*:603, 1973. Am. J. Surg., *125*:654, 1973

ZUMBRO, G., MULLIN, M. J., AND NELSON, T. G.: Catheter placement in infants needing total parenteral nutrition, using common facial vein, PRS, *48*:92, 1971. Arch. Surg., *102*:71, 1971

ZUPPINGER, A. *et al*: Therapy of oral neoplasms. Schweiz. Med. Wochenschr., *102*:657, 1972 (German)

ZURMAEV, I. A.: Open combined injuries of the hand and fingers and their treatment. Ortop. Travmatol. Protez., *3*:59, 1975 (Russian)

ZWAVELING, A.: A bump under the ear. Ned. tijdschr. geneeskd., *120*:409, 1976 (Dutch)

ZWEIG, J. *et al*: Transfer of the extensor digiti quinti to restore pinch in ulnar palsy of the hand. J. Bone & Joint Surg. (Am.), *54*:51, 1972

ZWILLICH, C., AND PIERSON, D. J.: Nasal necrosis; complication of nasotracheal intubation, PRS, *53*:681, 1974. Chest, *64*:376, 1973

Zygoma (See also *Facial Injuries; Orbit, Fracture*)

Fractures of the zygomatic complex (Hopkins). Ann. R. Coll. Surg. Engl., *49*:403, 1971

Fractures, orbital floor, visual loss complicating repair of (Nicholson, Guzak), PRS, *49*:356, 1972. Arch. Ophth., *86*:369, 1971

Therapy of fractures of the zygomatic arch (Berenyi). Dtsch. Stomatol., *21*:599, 1971 (German)

Therapy of zygomatic fractures (Grimm). Dtsch. Stomatol., *21*:605, 1971 (German)

Complex fractures of zygoma and mandibular ramus (Petz). Dtsch. Stomatol., *21*:619, 1971 (German)

Diagnosis and treatment of fractures of malar eminence (Sazima). Mil. Med., *136*:888, 1971

Midfacial fractures (Rabuzzi). N. Y. State J. Med., *71*:2412, 1971

Zygomatic fractures (Sundmark). Nord. Med., *86*:1189, 1971 (Swedish)

Platyzygion – flat cheek-bones (Spadafora, De Los Rios, Toledo Rios), PRS, *49*:581,

Zygoma – Cont.

1972. Prensa med. argent., *58*:1946, 1971

Contention in fractures of the zygomatic bone (Delaire *et al*). Rev. Stomatol. Chir. Maxillofac., *72*:623, 1971 (French)

Management of fractures of the zygoma, orbital floor and maxilla (Makino). Shujutsu, *25*:1187, 1971 (Japanese)

Fractures of zygoma, late complications after (Spiessl, Prein), PRS, *50*:94, 1972. Ther. Umsch., *28*:811, 1971

Fractures of zygomatic arch and orbit, urgent surgical management (Trichilis), PRS, *52*:594, 1973. Trans. 7th Panhellenic Cong. Surg., *1*:274, 1971

Fractures of orbital floor, current concepts in diagnosis and management of (Miller, Morris), PRS, *50*:629, 1972. Am. J. Surg., *123*:560, 1972

Zygoma, fractures of, use of heterologous bone in surgical treatment (Soubiran *et al*). Ann. chir. plast., *17*:296, 1972

Metastatic basal cell epithelioma discovered by chemosurgery (Mikhail *et al*). Arch. Dermat., *105*:103, 1972

Fractures of zygoma (Fung), PRS, *50*:630, 1972. Asian J. Med., *8*:202, 1972

Pneumocephalus as a rare complication of mid-facial fractures (Mikulickova *et al*). Cesk. Stomatol., *72*:285, 1972 (Czechoslovakian)

Zygoma and arch fractures, new reduction apparatus for (Fujino), PRS, *51*:610, 1973. Jap. J. Plast. Reconstr. Surg., *15*:209, 1972

Repair of trauma about the orbit (Fryer *et al*). J. Trauma, *12*:290, 1972

Anatomical and clinico-surgical aspects of malar region (Oksenberg *et al*). Odontol. Chil., *20*:15, 1972 (Spanish)

Statistical report on 150 zygoma fractures (Waldhart). Osterr. Z. Stomatol., *69*:136, 1972 (German)

Zygomatic arch, treatment of fractures of, by means of metallic osteosynthesis (Arlotta *et al*). Rass. Int. Stomatol. Prat., *23*:189, 1972 (Italian)

Zygomatic-malar complex, fractures of (Melmed). S. Afr. Med. J., *46*:569, 1972

Zygomatic fractures, alternate method of treatment (Elsahy, Vistnes), PRS, *53*:603, 1974. Acta chir. plast., *15*:51, 1973

Fractures of malar bone (apropos of 149 cases) (Bourguet *et al*). Ann. Otolaryngol. Chir. Cervicofac., *90*:55, 1973 (French)

Fracture, blowout, differential diagnosis in orbital injury (Smith, Wiggs), PRS, *53*:240, 1974. Arch. Ophth., *89*:484, 1973

Use of the Status-X-Panorama roentgen apparatus for diagnosis of zygoma and zygo-

Zygoma – Cont.

matic arch fractures (Wiltschke). Dtsch. Stomatol., *23:*673, 1973 (German)

Zygomatic complex, fractures of, evaluation of surgical management with special emphasis on eyebrow approach (Pozatek, Kaban, Guralnick). J. Oral Surg., *31:*141, 1973

Zygomatic fractures, pitfalls in management of. Symposium on maxillofacial trauma (Yanagisawa). Laryngoscope, *83:*527, 1973

Fracture of orbital floor: case report with serious delayed sequelae (Rogers, Nardi), PRS, *52:*205, 1973. M. J. Australia, *1:*175, 1973

Fractures of orbital floor repaired with premolded silicone prosthesis (Herrick), PRS, *54:*105, 1974. New Zealand M. J., *78:*159, 1973

Zygomatic arch, role of, in growth of skull in rabbits (Ritsila *et al*). Proc. Finn. Dent. Soc., *69:*164, 1973

Malar bone, osteotomy of (Gimenez). Rev. Asoc. Odontol. Argen., *61:*302, 1973 (Spanish)

Cheek fracture and karate (Serres *et al*). Rev. Stomatol. Chir. Maxillofac., *74:*177, 1973 (French)

Diplopia due to fracture of the roof of the orbit (Dupuis *et al*). Rev. Stomatol. Chir. Maxillofac., *74:*620, 1973 (French)

Use of Kirschner wires in facial fractures (Cadenat *et al*). Rev. Stomatol. Chir. Maxillofac., *74:*698, 1973 (French)

Fractures, blow-out, of orbital floor, non-surgical management (Putterman, Stevens, Urist), PRS, *55:*508, 1975. Am. J. Ophth., *77:*232, 1974

Orbital floor, exploration through conjunctival approach (David), PRS, *54:*500, 1974. Australian & New Zealand J. Surg., *44:*25, 1974

Use of the foley balloon catheter in zygomatic-arch fractures (Podoshin *et al*). Brit. J. Oral Surg., *12:*246, 1974

Fracture, orbital blowout (Fujino *et al*). PRS, *56:*352, 1975. Jap. J. Plast. Reconstr. Surg., *17:*427, 1974

Fractures, blowout, of medial orbital wall (Domarus), PRS, *54:*619, 1974. J. Maxillofacial Surg., *2:*55, 1974

Zygoma, malunited fracture with diplopia, treatment and comments on blowout fracture (Tajima *et al*), PRS, *55:*716, 1975. J. Maxillo-facial Surg., *2:*201, 1974

Zygomatic complex fracture with an avulsed tooth causing malocclusion: case report (Dunsworth). J. Oral Surg., *32:*131, 1974

Treatment of facial fractures (Calabretta *et al*). Pa. Med., *77:*62, 1974

Zygoma – Cont.

Cheekbones, building out as an addition to rhytidectomy (Gonzalez-Ulloa), PRS, *53:*293, 1974. Discussion by Stark, PRS, *53:*469, 1974

Zygomatic arch, experimental study of healing of fractures of membranous bone (Craft *et al*), PRS, *53:*321, 1974

Advantage of the endo-oral approach for the treatment of malar fractures (Hosxe *et al*). Rev. Stomatol. Chir. Maxillofac., *75:*867, 1974 (French)

Midfacial fractures from vehicular accidents (Schultz *et al*). Clin. Plast. Surg., *2:*173, 1975

Zygomatic fractures, pressure-plate osteosynthesis in (Harle *et al*). Dtsch. Zahnaerztl. Z., *30:*71, 1975 (German)

Fractures, orbital, prevention and treatment of complications of (Tenzel), PRS, *57:*670, 1976. Eye, Ear, Nose & Throat Month., *54:*305, 1975

Results of surgical management of zygomatic fractures (with special reference to fracture classification) (Schmoker *et al*). Fortschr. Kiefer. Gesichtschir., *19:*154, 1975 (German)

Indications for transcutaneous and surgical treatment of zygomatic fractures (Schroll). Fortschr. Kiefer. Gesichtschir., *19:*159, 1975 (German)

Reposition and retention of lateral mid-facial fractures by means of a balloon catheter (Worle *et al*). Fortschr. Kiefer. Gesichtschir., *19:*178, 1975 (German)

Treatment of lateral orbital fractures (Jacobs *et al*). Fortschr. Kiefer. Gesichtschir., *19:*180, 1975 (German)

Fracture, orbital, treated by internal indirect fixation with hooks (Mektubjian), PRS, *57:*394, 1976. J. Maxillo-facial Surg., *3:*132, 1975

Use of Scialom pins for fracture fixation (Bahn). J. Oral Surg., *33:*268, 1975

Middle-third facial osteotomies: their use in the correction of acquired and developmental dentofacial and craniofacial deformities (Epker *et al*). J. Oral Surg., *33:*491, 1975

Paget's disease of bone. Report of a case (Akin *et al*). Oral Surg., *39:*707, 1975

Le Fort III osteotomy to correct dish-face deformity resulting from facial trauma (Lewis *et al*). S. Afr. Med. J., *49:*1915, 1975

Fractures of the zygomatic-maxillary complex (Skokijev *et al*). Vojnosanit. Pregl., *32:*536, 1975 (Serbian)

Persistent sensory disturbances and diplopia following fractures of the zygoma (Nordgaard). Arch. Otolaryng., *102:*80, 1976

SUBJECT HEADINGS USED IN THIS INDEX